Medicine

The editors

John Axford is Director of The Sir Joseph Hotung Centre for Musculoskeletal Diseases. He is a Reader, and Consultant in Rheumatology and Clinical Immunology at St George's Hospital in London. In addition to this, he is the Coordinator of both the Undergraduate MBBS Rheumatology and Orthopaedics Programme and the Postgraduate Rheumatology CPD Programme at St George's. Since 1990 he has been the Rheumatology Representative on the University of London Examination MCQ Committee and since 1999 has been heavily involved with the Royal Society of Medicine as an Honorary Member.

Chris O'Callaghan is an MRC Senior Clinical Fellow and Senior Lecturer in the Nuffield Department of Medicine in the University of Oxford. He is an Honorary Consultant in General Internal Medicine and Renal Medicine in the Oxford Radcliffe Hospitals. After training and working in Oxford he has worked at Guy's, St Thomas', Hammersmith, Brompton and Lewisham hospitals in London and Stoke City General and North Staffordshire Royal Infirmary. He has worked and taught in the United States at the University of California, San Francisco and the California Institute of Technology. His other books include *The Kidney at a Glance*, *The MRCP Part I: a system based tutorial* and *The MRCP Medical Masterclass Nephrology* teaching module.

Medicine

SECOND EDITION

EDITED BY

John S. Axford

BSc MD FRCP
Director of the Hotung Centre
St George's Hospital Medical School
London

Chris A. O'Callaghan

BM BCh MA DPhil MRCP
MRC Senior Clinical Fellow, Senior Lecturer
Honorary Consultant Physician and Nephrologist
Nuffield Department of Clinical Medicine
John Radcliffe Hospital
University of Oxford
Oxford

Blackwell
Science

© 1996, 2004 by Blackwell Science Ltd
a Blackwell Publishing company
Blackwell Publishing, Inc., 350 Main Street, Malden, Massachusetts 02148-5020, USA
Blackwell Publishing Ltd, 9600 Garsington Road, Oxford OX4 2DQ, UK
Blackwell Publishing Asia Pty Ltd, 550 Swanston Street, Carlton, Victoria 3053, Australia

First published 1996
Second edition 2004

Library of Congress Cataloging-in-Publication Data
Medicine / edited by John S. Axford, Chris A. O'Callaghan.— 2nd ed.
    p.   cm.
   includes bibliographical references and index.
   ISBN 0–632–05162–0
  1. Internal medicine.
    [DNLM: 1. Clinical Medicine. WB 102 M489 2004]   I. Axford, John S.
II. O'Callaghan, C. A.
  RC46.M47582 2004
  616—dc22   2003028167

ISBN 0-632-05162-0

A catalogue record for this title is available from the British Library

Set in 9.5/11.5 Minion by Graphicraft Ltd, Hong Kong
Printed and bound in Spain by Mateu Cromo, S.A., Pinto (Madrid)

Commissioning Editor: Vicki Noyes
Managing Editor: Geraldine Jeffers
Production Editor: Lorna Hind
Production Controller: Mirjana Misina

For further information on Blackwell Publishing, visit our website:
http://www.blackwellpublishing.com

The publisher's policy is to use permanent paper from mills that operate a sustainable forestry policy, and which has been manufactured from pulp processed using acid-free and elementary chlorine-free practices. Furthermore, the publisher ensures that the text paper and cover board used have met acceptable environmental accreditation standards.

Contents

Contributors

R.L. Allen BSc (Hons) DPhil
Research Associate
Department of Pathology
University of Cambridge
Cambridge

J.S. Axford BSc MD FRCP
Director of the Hotung Centre
St George's Hospital Medical School
London

K. Baynes MRCP PhD
Clinical Lecturer
Department of Diabetes, Endocrinology and Internal Medicine
St Thomas' Hospital
London

G. Bell FRCPsych
Consultant Psychiatrist
Cancer Treatment Centre
Mount Vernon Hospital
Northwood
Middlesex

D.J. Betteridge BSc MB BS PhD MD FRCP FAHA
Professor of Endocrinology and Metabolism
Department of Medicine
Royal Free and University College London School of Medicine
The Middlesex Hospital
London

D.H. Bevan MB FRCP FRCPath
Senior Lecturer and Consultant in Haematology
St George's Hospital Medical School
Cranmer Terrace
London

J. Bolton MB BS BSc (Hons) MRCPsych
Consultant Psychiatrist and Honorary Senior Lecturer
Department of Liaison Psychiatry
St Helier Hospital, Carshalton
Surrey

C.B. Bunker MA MD FRCP
Consultant Dermatologist
Chelsea & Westminster and Royal Marsden Hospitals
Honorary Senior Lecturer, Imperial College School of Medicine
London

C. Carne MD FRCP
Consultant in Genitourinary Medicine
Addenbrooke's Hospital
Cambridge

E. Clark BSc MBBS MRCP
Clinical Research Fellow and Specialist Registrar in Rheumatology
University of Bristol
Bristol

G. Conway MD FRCP
Consultant Endocrinologist
Department of Endocrinology
The Middlesex Hospital
London

G.R. Davies MD FRCP
Consultant Physician and Gastroenterologist
Harrogate District Hospital
Harrogate

A.K. Fletcher BMedSci MB ChB MRCP FFAEM
Specialist Registrar in General Medicine and Emergency Medicine
Northern General Hospital
Sheffield

S.H. Gillespie MD FRCP (Edin) FRCPath
Professor of Medical Microbiology and Honorary Consultant
Royal Free and University College Medical School
University College London
London

C.R.K. Hind MD FRCP FRCP (Edin) FACP
Medical Director and Consultant Chest Physician
The Cardiothoracic Centre
Liverpool

F. Kaplan DCH FCP (SA)
Consultant in Diabetes and Endocrinology
Lister Hospital
Stevenage
Herfordshire

J.C. Kingswood MBBS FRCP
Consultant Physician
Renal Unit
Royal Sussex County Hospital
Brighton

A.C. Kurowska BSc BA FRCP
Consultant in Palliative Medicine
Whittington Hospital
Highgate Hill
London

M. Macleod MRCP PhD
Clinical Research Fellow
National Stroke Research Institute
Melbourne
Australia
and
Honorary Fellow and Specialist Registrar
Department of Clinical Neurosciences
School of Molecular and Clinical Medicine
University of Edinburgh
Edinburgh

A.J. Maycock MBBChir (Cantab) MA Leeds, MRCGP
General Practitioner and Tutor,
Guy's, Kings and St Thomas' Medical School
The Walworth Surgery
1 Manor Place
London

F.P. Morris FRCP FRCS
Consultant in Emergency Medicine
Emergency Department
Northern General Hospital
Sheffield

C.J. Mumford BMedSci DM FRCPE DIMCRCS
Consultant Neurologist
Department of Clinical Neurosciences
Western General Hospital
Edinburgh

J. Neuberger DM FRCP
Professor and Consultant Physician
The Liver and Hepatobiliary Unit,
Queen Elizabeth Hospital
Birmingham

C.A. O'Callaghan BM BCh MA MRCP
MRC Clinical Scientist and Clinical Lecturer
University of Oxford Institute of Molecular Biology
Nuffield Department of Clinical Medicine
Oxford

D.K. Packham MBBS FRCP FRACP MD
Consultant Nephrologist
Department of Nephrology
Royal Melbourne Hospital
Melbourne
Australia

C.W. Pumphrey DM FRCP
Consultant Cardiologist
St George's Hospital
London

D.S. Rampton DPhil FRCP
Professor of Clinical Gastroenterology
Department of Gastroenterology
Royal London Hospital
London
and
Barts and the London School of Medicine and Dentistry
Queen Mary College
London

C. Sonnex MA MB FRCP
Consultant Physician in Genitourinary Medicine
Department of Genitourinary Medicine
Addenbrooke's Hospital
Cambridge

J. Tobias MD PhD FRCP
Consultant Senior Lecturer
Rheumatology Unit
Bristol Royal Infirmary
Bristol

A. Tookman FRCP
Consultant in Palliative Medicine
Royal Free Hampstead NHS Trust
London
and
Medical Director
Marie Curie Hospice
Hampstead
London

M.J. Walshaw MB ChB (Hons) MD FRCP (London)
Consultant Physician in Respiratory Medicine
The Cardiothoracic Centre
Liverpool

Acknowledgements

We would like to thank the following for their help. Professor Philip Hawkins for writing the section on Amyloid in Chapter 11, Dr Jonathan Gleadle, Professor Oliver Fitzgerald and Dr David Kane for their help and contributions. At St George's Hospital: Dr Christine Heron, Dr Jo Sheldon, Dr Patrick Kiely, Dr Suzanne Donnelly, Dr Jade Chow, Lynda Carter, student, Simon Winn, student and especial thanks to Miss Caroline Cooper for keeping the text under control. At Blackwell Publishing: Fiona Goodgame, Geraldine Jeffers, Anita Lane, Vicki Noyes, Martin Sugden, Lorna Hind and Andrew Robinson.

Introduction

This book is designed for students who are learning medicine. It contains all the medicine that you need to know to qualify as a doctor and shows you how to develop the skills and attitudes that are essential for clinical practice. It is written by authors who are experts in their field as well as being experienced writers and teachers. In addition, this book has been strongly influenced by input from many students and other doctors. This input has formed part of an extensive writing and editorial process, each stage of which has involved repeated feedback from students from many medical schools. The result, we believe, is uniquely tailored to students' needs.

Each system is presented in an integrated style, with sections on the basic structure, function and biology of the system, on the clinical presentations and approach to the patient and on the diseases affecting the function of that system. Throughout the book, there is a clear focus on evidence-based medicine. In addition, there is significant attention given to discussion of the social, caring and communicative aspects of medicine and the impact of medicine and disease on the lives of patients.

Designed for learning

There are many textbooks of medicine on the market, but we believe that they are generally not well designed for learning from. Over recent years, the major student texts seem to have grown increasingly thicker with each edition and now incorporate much detail that is irrelevant to the student. This complicates learning, and makes it slower.

If you finish medical school without understanding the basics of medicine, then you will be in trouble. However, learning small print detail about a range of topics will seldom be of much use in your qualifying examinations or in clinical practice.

Both for the purposes of passing examinations and of learning medicine to practise it well, it is more important to understand the basics than to accumulate a series of unimportant details about a topic.

The body of medical knowledge increases every day, but the capacity of the human brain does not. Therefore, we believe that it is essential to present medicine in a way that is comprehensive, but also concise and free of irrelevant details. This allows the learner to focus on the key aspects of a topic.

In this book, we have aimed to present you, the student, with the necessary information to pass examinations and to learn medicine in order to practise it well.

To simplify learning, all the material in this book has been chosen and arranged to make it easy to learn. Important topics are readily identifiable. The amount of information on each topic has been carefully regulated and some topics are deliberately presented in detail because they are very important or very common. The number of illustrations has been increased and they have been used extensively to aid learning.

The book is written for students, but we hope that the focus on core information and the way the book is designed to aid learning will continue to be of use to doctors and other healthcare workers who are trying to understand or revise medicine. In this way we hope that the book will remain useful as you advance through your student years and into hospital or community medicine.

How to use this book

You should start with the first two introductory chapters, whatever your stage of learning. Chapter 1 provides an overview of the human dimension to the practice of clinical medicine, whereas Chapter 2 provides a review of the basic science, which will help you to understand much of modern medicine.

The chapters which follow provide a systematic and state of the art account of modern caring clinical practice. Although they have been carefully designed as separate units, which provide comprehensive coverage of the system or topics concerned, they have been closely integrated with each other and there is extensive cross-referencing to related material in other chapters. Within each chapter there are a number of features designed to make learning easy and logical.

The layout of the book is self-explanatory and there is a comprehensive index. Navigation is aided by the coloured page end-tabs that label each chapter. Drugs are referred to by their Recommended International Non-proprietary Name (rINN), but in a few cases older names are also provided if they are still in use.

Chapter layout

The main subject chapters have the following plan. A brief introduction puts the chapter into context and then there are three main sections:

- Structure and function
- Approach to the patient
- Diseases and their management

When you read each chapter you will develop a clear understanding of the disease processes that cause certain clinical presenting problems and will learn the skills and attitudes needed to make a diagnosis and put together a management plan.

Aids to learning

Within each chapter different boxes have been used to highlight important material

- **History & Examination boxes** summarize the relevant history to be taken and examination to be made for the system or topic being considered.
- **At a glance boxes** contain summaries of all the major information about core topics and are designed for rapid revision. The system chapters have an initial Clinical presentations at a glance, which summarizes the different problems caused by diseases of the relevant system. There is a list of all the At a glance boxes on the inside front cover.
- **Emergency boxes** provide a brief summary of essential information relating to emergency situations.
- **Keypoints boxes** are a crisp reminder of the key aspects of important topics.
- **Must know checklist boxes** are a brief reminder of the key elements of the chapter that you must know.
- **Further reading boxes** contain concise advice on useful sources of further information including websites, books and journals relevant to the evidence base for clinical practice.

The editors and authors have enjoyed editing the second edition of this book and applying new concepts to its design to make it useful and appropriate to the needs of today's medical students. We feel confident that we have fulfilled this aim and that students will find it a useful and enjoyable book as they learn medicine.

John Axford and Chris O'Callaghan
Editors

General references

Listed below are various useful sources of general information that are relevant to most of the chapters in the book. Sources of further specific information relevant to the subject matter in each chapter are contained within the **Further reading** boxes.

Books

Warrell DA, Cox TM, Firth JD, Benz EJ. *Oxford Textbook of Medicine*, 4th edn. Oxford: Oxford University Press, 2003 – a major authoritative textbook, but too detailed for most students' needs

British National Formulary – the standard UK reference for prescribing; it is full of useful information about drugs and their uses

Journals

The New England Journal of Medicine – http://content.nejm.org

The Lancet – www.thelancet.com

The British Medical Journal – www.BMJ.com

Journal of the American Medical Association – www.jama.amaassn.org

Annals of Internal Medicine – www.annals.org

Websites

Pubmed – www.ncbi.nlm.nih.gov/entrez/query.fcgi – a fantastic free resource providing abstracts of all the major world literature

National Electronic Library for Health www.nelh.nhs.uk – an excellent National Health Service website with many useful links and resources

National Institutes of Health – www.health.nih.gov – an extensive range of health resources including the excellent Medlineplus databases which include a useful illustrated online medical encyclopaedia

Bandolier http://www.jr2.ox.ac.uk/bandolier – a free evidence-based medicine journal from Oxford

Up To Date – www.uptodate.com – an excellent information service, which requires a subscription

Clinical evidence – www.nelh.nhs.uk/clinical_evidence.asp – a set of evidence-based medicine reviews

Cochrane Collaboration – www.cochraneconsumer.com/index.asp?SHOW=Topics – a database of evidence-based medicine

Abbreviations

Ab	antibody
ABC	adenosine triphosphate binding cassette
ACE	angiotensin-converting enzyme
ACTH	adrenocorticotrophic hormone
ADCC	antibody-dependent cell-mediated cytotoxicity
ADH	antidiuretic hormone
ADP	adenosine diphosphate
ADPKD	autosomal dominant polycystic kidney disease
AFP	α-fetoprotein
AGBM	antiglomerular basement membrane
AGE	advanced glycosylation end products
AGM	aorta-gonad-mesonephros
AIDS	acquired immune deficiency virus
AIHA	autoimmune haemolytic anaemia
AITP	autoimmune thrombocytopenic purpura
ALA	aminolaevulinic acid
ALG	antilymphocyte globulin
ALT	alanine aminotransferase
ANA	antinuclear antibody
ANCA	antineutrophil cytoplasmic antibody
APC	antigen-presenting cell
APECED	autoimmune polyendocrinology–candiasis–ectodermal dystrophy
APTT	activated partial thromboplastin time
APTTr	activated partial thromboplastin time ratio
ARDS	acute/adult respiratory distress syndrome
5-ASA	5-aminosalicylic acid
AS	ankylosing spondylitis
ASD	atrial septal defect
ASH	asymmetrical septal hypertrophy
ASO	antistreptolysin-O
ASOT	antistreptolysin-O titre
AST	aspartate aminotransferase
ATG	antithymocyte globulin
ATP	adenosine triphosphate
ATRA	all-$trans$-retinoic acid
AV	atrioventricular
AVM	atriovenous malformation
AVNRT	atrioventricular node re-entry tachycardia
AVRT	atrioventricular re-entry tachycardia
β_2m	β_2-microglobulin
BAER	brainstem auditory evoked response
BCE	basal cell carcinoma/epithelioma
BCG	bacille Calmette–Guérin
BCR	B-cell receptor
BMD	bone mineral density
BMI	body mass index
BMZ	basement membrane zone
BNF	British National Formulary
bp	basepair
BSE	bovine spongiform encephalitis
BV	bacterial vaginosis
CAM	cell adhesion molecule
cAMP	cyclic adenosine monophosphate
CD	Crohn's disease
CDK	cyclin-dependent kinase
CDKI	cyclin-dependent kinase specific inhibitor
cDNA	complementary deoxyribonucleic acid
CETP	cholesterol ester transfer protein
CFA	cryptogenic fibrosing alveolitis
CFTR	cystic fibrosis transmembrane regulator
cGMP	cyclic guanosine monophosphate
CHD	coronary heart disease
CIDP	chronic inflammatory demyelinating polyneuropathy
CIE	countercurrent immune electrophoresis
CJD	Creutzfeldt–Jakob disease
CMML	chronic myelomonocytic leukaemia
CMV	cytomegalovirus
CNS	central nervous system
CoA	coenzyme A
COMT	catechol-O-methyl transferase
COP	cryptogenic organizing pneumonia
COX	cyclo-oxygenase
CPPD	calcium pyrophosphate dihydrate
CPR	cardiopulmonary resuscitation
CRH	corticotrophin-releasing hormone
CRP	C-reactive protein
CSF	cerebrospinal fluid
CT	computerized tomography
CTL	cytotoxic T cell
DAT	direct antiglobulin test
DC	dendritic cell/direct current
DCCT	Diabetes Control and Complication Trial
DDAVP	desmopressin, 1-desamino-8-D-arginine vasopressin
DEFRA	Department for Environment, Food and Rural Affairs
DFA	direct fluorescence antibody

DIC	disseminated intravascular coagulation	FTA-abs	fluorescent treponemal antibody absorption
DIP	distal interphalangeal	FVC	forced vital capacity
DISH	diffuse idiopathic skeletal hyperostosis	G6PD	glucose-6-phosphate dehydrogenase
DKA	diabetic ketoacidosis	GABA	γ-aminobutyric acid
DLCO	diffusing capacity of lung for carbon monoxide	GAD	glutamic acid decarboxylase
		GALT	galactose 1-phosphate uridyl transferase
DLE	discoid lupus erythematosus	Gbp	giga-basepair
DM	dermatomyositis/diabetes mellitus	GBS	Guillain–Barré syndrome
DMSA	dimercapto succinic acid	GCS	Glasgow Coma Scale
DNA	deoxyribonucleic acid	GFR	glomerular filtration rate
DPG	diphosphoglycerate	GGT	gamma-glutamyl transferase
DSH	deliberate self-harm	GH	growth hormone
DTPA	diethylenetriaminepenta-acetic acid	GHRH	growth hormone-releasing hormone
DU	duodenal ulcer	GISA	glycopeptide-resistant *Staphylococcus aureus*
DXA	dual energy X-ray absorptiometry	GMC	General Medical Council
EAEC	enteroadherant *Escherichia coli*	GM-CSF	granulocyte macrophage colony-stimulating factor
EBM	evidence-based medicine		
EBV	Epstein–Barr virus	GnRH	gonadotrophin-releasing hormone
ECG	electrocardiography/electrocardiogram	GORD	gastro-oesophageal reflux disease
EDRF	endothelial-derived relaxing facor	GP	general practitioner
EDTA	ethylenediaminetetra-acetic acid	GPI	glycosylphosphatidylinositol
EEG	electroencephalography/electroencephalogram	GRE	glycopeptide-resistant enterococci
		G-CSF	granulocyte colony-stimulating factor
EFE	endocardial fibroelastosis	GTN	glyceryl trinitate
EHEC	enterohaemorrhagic *Escherichia coli*	GTP	guanine triphosphate
EHO	environmental health officer	GU	genitourinary/gastric ulcer
EIEC	enteroinvasive *Escherichia coli*	GVHD	graft-vs.-host disease
ELISA	enzyme-linked immunosorbent assay	HAART	highly active antiretroviral therapy
EMF	endomyocardial fibrosis	HAV	hepatitis A virus
EMG	electromyography/electromyogram	HBV	hepatitis B virus
EPEC	enteropathogenic *Escherichia coli*	hCG	human chorionic gonadotrophin
Epo	erythropoietin	HCV	hepatitis C virus
ER	endoplasmic reticulum	HD	Hodgkin's disease
ERCP	endoscopic retrograde cholangiopancreatography	HDL	high-density lipoprotein
		HDN	haemorrhagic disease of the newborn
ES	embryonic stem	5-HIAA	5-hydroxyindole acetic acid
ESR	erythrocyte sedimentation rate	HIG	human immunoglobulin
EST	expressed sequence tag	HIV	human immunodeficiency virus
ESWL	extracorporeal shock wave lithotripsy	HLA	human leucocyte antigen
ET	essential thrombocythaemia	HMB	hydroxymethylbilane
ETEC	enterotoxigenic *Escherichia coli*	HMSN	hereditary motor and sensory neuropathy
FACS	fluoresence activated cell sorter	HNPCC	hereditary non-polyposis colon cancer syndrome
FBC	full blood count		
FCH	familial combined hyperlipidaemia	HONK	hyperosmolar non-ketotic coma
FEO	familial expansile osteolysis	HPA	hypertrophic pulmonary arthropathy
FEV_1	forced expiratory volume in 1 second	HPLC	high-pressure liquid chromatography
FFP	fresh frozen plasma	HPV	human papilloma virus
FH	familial hypercholesterolaemia	H_2RA	H_2 receptor antagonist
FHF	fulminant hepatic failure	HRT	hormone replacement therapy
FISH	fluorescence *in situ* hybridization	HSC	haematopoietic stem cell
FRC	functional residual capacity	HSP	heat shock protein/Henoch–Schönlein purpura
FSGS	focal segmental glomerulosclerosis		
FSH	follicle-stimulating hormone	HSV	herpes simplex virus

5-HT	5-hydroxytrytamine	MEN	multiple endocrine neoplasia
5-HTP	5-hydroxytryptophan	MGUS	monoclonal gammopathy of undetermined significance
HU	hydroxyurea		
HUS	haemolytic–uraemic syndrome	MHC	major histocompatibility complex
IBD	inflammatory bowel disease	MIBG	metaiodo-benzylguanidine
IBS	irritable bowel syndrome	MIC	minimum inhibitory concentration
IEF	isoelectric focusing	MIF	microimmunofluorescence
ICA	islet cell antibody	MLF	medial longitudinal fasciculus
IDL	intermediate-density lipoprotein	MMP	matrix metalloproteinases
Ig	immunoglobulin	MMR	measles, mumps and rubella
IGF	insulin-like growth factor	MODY	maturity onset diabetes of the young
IGT	impaired glucose tolerance	MPO	myeloperoxidase
IL	interleukin	MRA	magnetic resonance angiography
^{131}I-MIBG	^{131}I-meta-iodobenzyl guanidine	MRFIT	Multiple Risk Factor Intervention Trial
IMA	inferior mesenteric artery	MRI	magnetic resonance imaging
INF-γ	γ-interferon	mRNA	messenger ribonucleic acid
INR	international normalized ratio	MRSA	methicillin-resistant *Staphylococcus aureus*
ITP	immune thrombocytopenic purpura	MS	multiple sclerosis
ITT	insulin tolerance test	MSH	melanocyte-stimulating hormone
IVIG	intravenous immunoglobulin	MTBE	methyl tert-butane ether
IVU	intravenous urogram	MTP	metatarsophalangeal
JIA	juvenile idiopathic arthritis	MUGA	multiple-gated acquisition scan
JNK	Jun-terminal kinase	NAD	nicotinamide adenine dinucleotide
JVP	jugular venous pressure/pulse	NADP	nicotinamide adenine dinucleotide phosphate
kb	kilobase	NAFLD	non-alcoholic fatty liver disease
KS	Kaposi's sarcoma	NGU	non-gonococcal urethritis
LBBB	left bundle branch block	NICE	National Institute for Clinical Excellence
LCAT	lecithin : cholesterol acyltransferase	NIPPV	nasal intermittent positive pressure ventilation
LCR	ligase chain reaction/locus control region		
LDH	lactic dehydrogenase	NK	natural killer
LDL	low-density lipoprotein	NNRTI	non-nucleoside reverse transcriptase inhibitors
LEC	leucocyte endothelial cell		
LGL	Lown–Ganong–Levine (syndrome)	NRTI	nucleoside reverse transcriptase inhibitor
LGV	lymphogranuloma venereum	NSAID	non-steroidal anti-inflammatory drug
LH	luteinizing hormone	NSF	National Service Framework
LINES	long interspersed repetitive elements	NSU	non-specific urethritis
LMWH	low-molecular-weight heparin	NYHA	New York Heart Association
LOD	logarithm of the odds	OA	osteoarthritis
LOS	lower oesophageal sphincter	OGD	oesophagogastroduodenoscopy
LPL	lipoprotein lipase	OMIM	Online Mendelian Inheritance in Man
LPS	lipopolysaccharide	ORT	oral rehydration therapy
LRC	leucocyte receptor complex	PA	pernicious ananemia
LT	heat-labile toxin	PABA	para-amino benzoic acid
MAC	membrane attack complex	PAN	polyarteritis nodosa
MAOI	monoamine oxidase inhibitor	PAS	periodic acid–Schiff
MAP	mitogen activated protein kinase	PBC	primary biliary cirrhosis
MBC	minimum bactericidal concentration	PBG	porphobilinogen
MBL	mannan-binding lectin	PBP	penicillin-binding protein
MCP	metacarpophalangeal	PBSC	peripheral blood stem cell
MCV	mean cell volume	PCI	percutaneous transluminal coronary intervention
MDR	multidrug resistance		
MDS	myelodysplastic syndromes	PCP	*Pneumocystis carinii* pneumonia
MEA	multiple endocrine adenomatosis	PCR	polymerase chain reaction

PD	Parkinson's disease	SAP	serum amyloid P component
PDA	patent ductus arteriosus	SARA	sexually acquired reactive arthritis
PDT	photodynamic therapy	SCA	sickle cell anaemia
PE	pulmonary embolism	SCD	sickle cell disease
PEFR	peak expiratory flow rate	SCF	stem cell factor
PEG	percutaneous endoscopic gastrostomy	SCID	severe combined immunodeficiency
PEP	postexposure prophylaxis	SDS-PAGE	sodium dodecyl sulphate-polyacrylamide
PET	positron emission tomography		gel electrophoresis
PEX	plasma exchange	SE	staphylococcal enterotoxin
PGI	prostacyclin	SERM	selective oestrogen receptor modulator
PI	phosphoinositide	SHBG	sex hormone-binding globulin
PID	pelvic inflammatory disease	SIADH	syndrome of inappropriate antidiuretic
PIP	proximal interphalangeal		hormone secretion
PLID	prolapsed intervertebral disc	SINES	short interspersed repetitive elements
PM	polymyositis	SLE	systemic lupus erythematosus
PML	progressive multifocal leucoencephalopathy	SMA	superior mesenteric artery
PMR	polymyalgia rheumatica	SPECT	single photon emission computed
PND	paroxysmal nocturnal dyspnoea		tomography
POMC	pro-opiomelanocortin	SSER	somatosensory evoked response
PPI	proton pump inhibitor	SSPE	subacute sclerosing panencephalitis
PR	proteinase	SSRI	selective serotonin reuptake inhibitor
PRR	pattern recognition receptor	SSSS	staphylococcal scalded skin syndrome
PRV	polycythaemia rubra vera	ST	heat-stable toxin
PSA	prostate-specific antigen	STI	sexually transmitted infection
PT	prothrombin time	SVT	supraventricular tachycardia
PTC	percutaneous transhepatic cholangiography	T_3	triiodothyronine
PTCA	percutaneous transluminal coronary	T_4	thyroxine
	angioplasty	TAP	antigen presentation transporter
PTH	parathyroid hormone	TCBS	thiosulphate citrate bile salt sucrose
PTHrP	parathyroid hormone-related peptide/	TCIA	transient cerebral ischaemic attack
	protein	TCR	T-cell antigen receptor
PTR	prothrombin time ratio	TEN	toxic epidermal necrolysis
PUO	pyrexia of unknown origin	TENS	transcutaneous electrical nerve stimulation
PUVA	psoralen and ultraviolet A	TF	tissue factor
PVNS	pigmented villonodular synovitis	TGF	transforming growth factor
QALY	quality adjusted life year	T_H	helper T cell
RA	refractory anaemia/rheumatoid arthritis	TIBC	total iron-binding capacity
RAEB	refratory anaemia with excess blasts	TIPS	transjugular intrahepatic portosystemic
RARS	refractory anaemia with ringed sideroblasts		shunt
RAST	radioallergosorbent test	TLC	total lung capacity
RBBB	right bundle branch block	TLR	toll-like receptor
REM	rapid eye movement	TNF	tumour necrosis factor
RF	rheumatoid factor	TPA	tissue plasminogen activator
RFLP	restriction fragment length polymorphism	TPHA	*Treponema pallidum* haemagglutination
RNA	ribonucleic acid		assay
RPR	rapid plasma reagin	Tpo	thrombopoietin
RSV	respiratory syncytial virus	TPPA	*Treponema pallidum* particle agglutination
RT-PCR	reverse transcription-polymerase chain	TRH	thyrotrophin-releasing hormone
	reaction	tRNA	transfer ribonucleic acid
RV	residual volume	TSH	thyroid-stimulating hormone
SA	sinoatrial	TSS	toxic shock syndrome
SACE	serum angiotensin-converting enzyme	TSS-1	toxic shock syndrome toxin-1
SAH	subarachnoid haemorrhage	TTP	thrombotic thrombocytopenic purpura

TURP	transurethral resection of the prostate		VSD	ventricular septal defect
UC	ulcerative colitis		VT	ventricular tachycardia
UDCA	ursodeoxycholic acid		VTEC	verotoxigenic *Escherichia coli*
UKPDS	UK Prospective Diabetes Study		VTED	venous thromboembolic disease
UMN	upper motor neurone		VWD	von Willebrand's disease
UV	ultraviolet		VWF	von Willebrand factor
VC	vital capacity		VZV	varicella zoster virus
VDRL	Venereal Disease Research Laboratory		WAGR	syndrome of Wilms' tumour, aniridia, genitourinary malformations and mental retardation
VER	visual evoked response			
VF	ventricular fibrillation			
VLDL	very low density lipoprotein		WBC	whole blood count
VMA	vanillylmandelic acid		WCC	white cell count
VNTR	variable number tandem repeat		WHO	World Health Organization
V/Q	ventilation–perfusion		WPW	Wolff–Parkinson–White (syndrome)

The Human Aspects of Medicine

Introduction

Learning to practise clinical medicine can seem daunting. On the one hand, there is a huge body of factual scientific information to assimilate and, on the other hand, there are many important human aspects, which need to be addressed. In this chapter we discuss some of the key human aspects of medical practice that have a role in the interactions between doctors and patients and doctors and their colleagues. An appreciation of such factors will help you to be an effective clinician. These factors include:

- Psychological and social factors in doctor–patient interactions
- Differences in how doctors and patients understand disease and illness
- Communication skills
- Organizational skills
- The value of reflecting on one's own practice in order to improve it

The chapter starts with a consideration of the patient–doctor consultation and the different factors affecting doctors and patients, especially in this context. This is followed by sections on the practical aspects of organizing clinical work, on learning and updating clinical skills and on approaching ethical dilemmas in clinical practice.

Science and compassion

Good medicine is based on good scientific evidence. You can help your patients more with science than without it. Science seeks to provide a rational basis for doctors' decision making. Health care should be delivered in the most appropriate and considerate way possible, given individual circumstances. When scientific evidence and a caring approach are combined, medicine has a human face and the best technical care is delivered with consideration for all the patient's needs, including their emotional, psychological and social well-being. Traditionally, the compassion of doctors towards their patients has been much valued and is often evident in representations of the doctor–patient relationship (Fig. 1.1).

Bedside manner

A doctor's 'bedside manner' is not a façade designed to put the patient at ease, but the authentic way in which the doctor practises medicine, trying to understand and address the patient's circumstances and needs. Being a caring doctor does not mean being soft or sentimental, it means dealing with patients honestly and with respect. This can take many forms, from the simple step of reassuring a patient that a trivial symptom has no sinister significance to more complex interactions with those who are seriously ill.

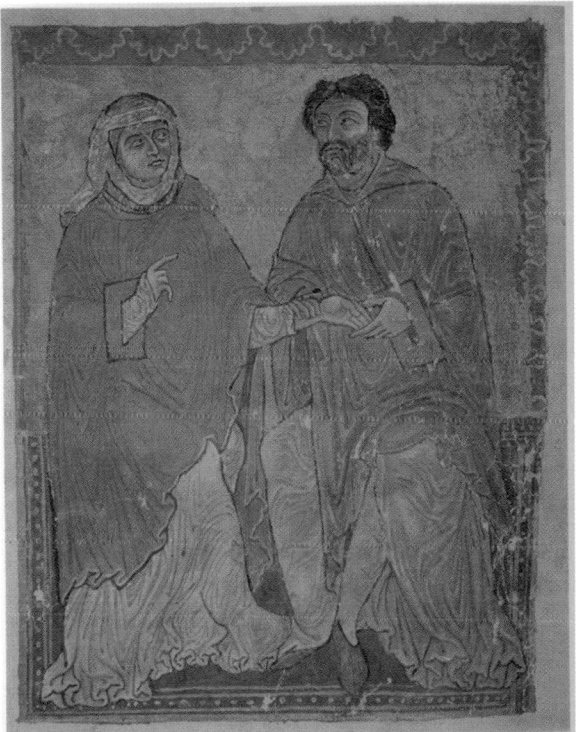

Figure 1.1 The doctor–patient interaction. This image shows a doctor taking the patient's pulse. The doctor appears to be handling the patient sensitively and paying attention to her.

Learning from doctors

The human aspects of clinical practice are increasingly incorporated into modern medical training. However, you can learn a great deal by observing your own behaviour and that of patients and colleagues in an open, analytical and reflective manner. In this way, you can learn much about how the actions of doctors can have positive or negative effects on patients' experiences. This chapter provides some pointers to help you to do this. The topics in this chapter will inevitably have a major role in your professional life and so merit serious informed consideration.

Learning from patients

Developing your own professional approach to the human aspects of medicine is a continuing process and can be worked on at any stage of your training. The most important aspect of this is simply spending time talking to patients, appreciating their circumstances and reflecting on your own responses. It can be tempting to shy away from contemplating the difficult lives of many patients. However, by contemplating what they face, you will understand how they might feel and what they might want or need from you. Such consideration will help you to empathize with worried patients or relatives. This means being able to demonstrate to patients that you can recognize both their problem and how they feel about it. This is one of the skills that patients value most in their doctors.

The consultation

To do their job well, clinicians need to communicate effectively with patients, their relatives or friends and with colleagues. Interactions between doctors and patients can take a variety of forms: clinic appointments, home visits, elective or emergency inpatient attendances, phone conversations and even letters or e-mails.

It is important for the patient, the clinician and health services in general that consultations are as effective as possible. Effectiveness in this context means not just reaching the right diagnosis, but also enabling patients to be fully informed and actively involved in their management plan. This type of consultation undoubtedly takes more time in the short term, but in the long term leads to greater patient responsibility and self-management, greater concordance (perhaps a better term than *compliance* with its implications of obedience to the doctor's orders) and more appropriate use (and less ignorance-based misuse) of health services. For example, patients are more likely to take their antihypertensive tablets if they understand why they need to keep their blood pressure at a certain level. Similarly, most asthmatics will increase their inhalers themselves when they experience a slight exacerba-

tion, if they understand how the inhaled medication works and how this can help their breathing. In addition to these benefits, good communication can relieve the anxiety and suffering that might otherwise arise in a one-sided or dogmatic consultation because of confusion or unaddressed fears. Time spent optimizing communication is usually well invested.

In broad terms, the aim of any consultation is to maximize the health and sense of well-being of the patient. This can be achieved via a number of more specific objectives as outlined in KEYPOINTS BOX 1.1.

Keypoints 1.1: Consultation objectives

- Make the correct diagnosis in physical, psychological and social terms that are meaningful to the patient
- Establish the impact of the problem on the patient
- Devise a management plan to which the patient is committed and can implement
- Develop the patient's health understanding and behaviour

These objectives can only be achieved if the doctor has good evidence-based clinical skills and knowledge, has good communication skills, respects the patient and aims for mutual cooperation. This latter point is sometimes called the partnership model of the consultation. The key attributes for an effective doctor in a consultation are summarized in KEYPOINTS BOX 1.2.

Keypoints 1.2: Characteristics of the effective doctor in a consultation

- Evidence-based clinical skills and knowledge
- Commitment to working in partnership with patients
- Communication skills

Evidence-based clinical skills are discussed throughout this book; here we discuss the other two features of the effective clinician.

Partnership model of the consultation

The traditional model of the doctor as an expert and the patient as a docile and grateful recipient of that expertise has been shown to be unsatisfying for both doctors and patients. It leads to burnout in the former, complaint making in the latter *and* is ineffective in terms of health outcome. A model of partnership has replaced it in which patients are empowered to take responsibility for, and be involved in, their own health decisions and management. Clearly, it would be naive to imagine that such a partnership could be one of complete equality in all aspects. The clinician has greater knowledge and familiarity with certain kinds of decision making and is usually less crucially affected by the outcome of a consultation. On the other hand, the views and desires of the patient are those that ultimately need to be addressed and met. The doctor should try to confine his or her opinions to the likely effectiveness of any proposed courses of action with regard to the particular situation in hand. Partnership implies a sense of moving through the discussion together with shared understanding and control so that the end point will be valued and meaningful to both parties. Partnership can only be achieved if communication is good.

Optimizing communication

Effective communication between doctor and patient depends on the environment in which the exchange takes place, on the doctor's (and the patient's) attitude, and on a number of techniques or skills employed by the doctor when talking to patients. These factors are outlined in Table 1.1 and some are illustrated in Fig. 1.2. Let us consider some of them in more detail.

Listening skills
- Not interrupting
- Use of silence
- Use of verbal cues: 'Go on . . .', 'and . . .', 'I see';

Table 1.1 Prerequisites for good communication

A quiet, private environment
A comfortable non-intimidating seating arrangement
Adequate time
The patient can hear, lip-read or read
Doctor and patient share the same language or have an appropriate translator (preferably not a relative of the patient)
Doctor's listening skills
Doctor's observing skills
Doctor's questioning skills
Doctor's empathizing skills
Doctor 's explaining skills
Doctor's manner is friendly, open, unhurried and responsive

echoing or reflecting back words or phrases: 'I feel frustrated', 'Frustrated . . . ?'
- Use of non-verbal cues: nodding, smiling, raising eyebrows, eye contact
- Summarizing your interpretation of the information (active listening)

Summarizing the patient's story is a powerful way of demonstrating that you have really heard and understood his or her problem. An example of this technique is, 'So this pain comes on two hours after you have eaten and lasts about half an hour, but nothing you do seems to make it better?'

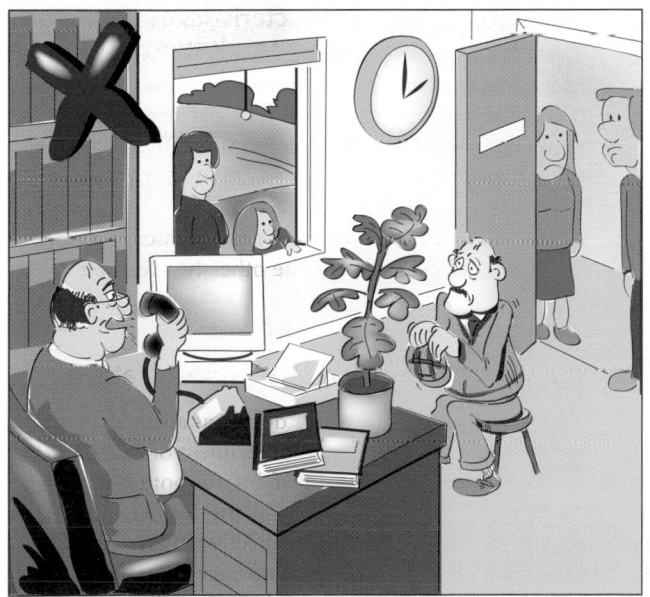 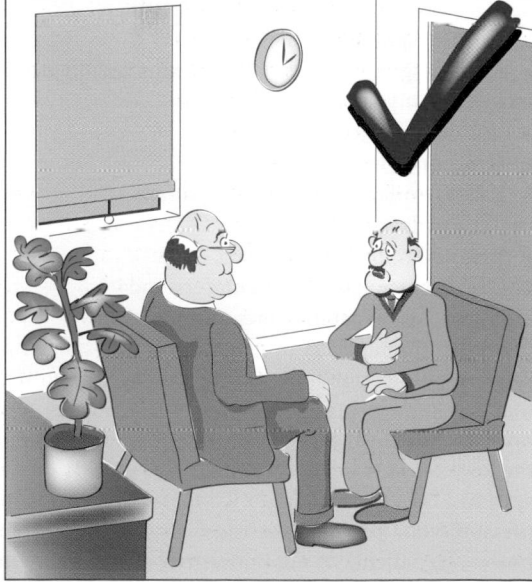

Figure 1.2 Optimizing communication. The first image shows a number of basic mistakes in establishing suitable conditions for a good consultation. The second illustrates how the situation can be improved.

Observing skills

Notice the patient's:

- appearance
- type and manner of movements
- body posture
- facial expression
- tone of voice
- direction of gaze

Do these observations reinforce or contradict what is being said?

Questioning skills

We must tailor our question to the type of information we are seeking. Open questions enable us to probe widely and deeply for hidden ideas and concerns. Precise closed questions are needed when we are after very specific, highly discriminatory details.

- *Open and wide questions:* e.g. What is the problem? How are you feeling? How does that make you feel?
- *Open and specific questions:* e.g. Does the pain ever go away?
- *Closed questions:* e.g. What time did you take your insulin last night? Does eating help the pain?

Beware of leading questions, which are often *mis*leading: 'This is the first time you have had a problem with your ears then?' 'You don't have a family history of breast cancer do you?'

Empathizing skills

To empathize means to identify a problem and demonstrate to the patient that you have understood its impact and significance for them.

Explaining skills

- Avoid jargon ('weakened heart muscle' might convey more than 'myocardial infarction')
- Use short words
- Use short sentences
- Tailor explanations to the patient's framework of health and illness
- Explain important items first
- Check that you have been understood
- Offer written material, including diagrams

It is easy for clinicians to forget how little others might know about human biology. The patient may not realize that the kidneys produce urine, or that nerves activate muscles. You must check what the patient understands of the key concepts being discussed. Ask specific questions such as, 'Do you know what we mean by arthritis/blood pressure/your pancreas/diabetes?' It is often surprising how many patients do not know their diagnosis or understand it and do not appreciate why they take certain treatments. This can lead to confusion, anxiety, suboptimal treatment and inappropriate behaviour.

Table 1.2 Factors inhibiting patient's questions

Concern about taking up the doctor's time
Discomfort with medical and bodily issues
Fear of being seriously ill
Custom in some cultures of not questioning authority figures
Fear of appearing ignorant

Interestingly, patients do not always ask for extra information, even when they are still unsure of the points being made. It is useful to consider and minimize the reasons for this. Potential factors are listed in Table 1.2.

Doctor's manner

- Adopt an open body posture and relaxed expression
- Look at the patient
- Allow them to show emotions
- Respond both verbally and non-verbally to what they are saying or doing
- Allow them to have a role in identifying, pursuing or changing topics for discussion
- Refrain from too rapid reassurances—hear their concerns out

Consultation tasks

Consultations can be very complex interactions. They deal with vastly varying medical, psychological, emotional and social problems, and involve individuals with very different concerns and expectations. To make the issues to be addressed more manageable, it is useful to break the doctor–patient encounter into discrete tasks or stages. These can be arranged with a sense of logical progression and are outlined in KEYPOINTS BOX 1.3. In practice, a consultation is very flexible, and the order and extent of the tasks may vary in whatever way is appropriate to the situation.

Let us consider what is involved in each stage.

Keypoints 1.3: Consultation tasks

- Prepare yourself and all the information you need before you meet the patient
- Achieve a rapport with the patient
- Invite the patient to express their problem
- Identify the patient's understanding, concerns and expectations
- Be aware of your own concerns and agenda
- Locate the problem in a medical framework
- Discuss your conclusions with the patient
- Agree on a management plan
- Close the consultation in a friendly and polite manner
- Record accurately salient features in the patient's notes

Prepare yourself
● Attend to thirst, hunger or other bodily requirements
● Recover from your previous task and focus on the next patient
● Collect necessary results, documents or equipment

Achieve a rapport with the patient
● Introduce yourself
● Check this is the correct patient
● Make eye contact
● Shake hands
● Smile

Invite the patient to express their problem
Use open questions such as:
● How can I help?
● What brings you here today?
● What's troubling you?
● How are you getting on?
Try hard not to interrupt. Studies show that 80% of patients speak for less than 2 min if left uninterrupted. You will gain much useful information and the patient will feel they are being taken seriously.

Identify the patient's understanding, concerns and expectations
Use questions that help establish the patient's key issues:
● What is it that particularly worries you?
● What is your main concern today?
● What would you like us to focus on today?
The patient may not immediately inform you of their underlying or 'hidden' concern; this may only emerge after you have addressed the problem they have presented with. Examples of hidden concerns are given in CLINICAL SCENARIO BOX 1.1.

Find out what the patient understands about their problem and tailor your line of inquiry and explanations to this. This makes the patient feel more engaged in the process, more confident that their problem is being addressed and more satisfied with the outcome of the consultation. Establishing the patient's views can also save time later, by guiding you to the key pieces of information they will need to be given to be satisfied with your assessment and the plan you suggest. The following questions are ways of exploring the patient's understanding:
● What do you think is going on? (open question)
● Do you know why we are treating your blood pressure? (closed question)

Clinicians and patients are likely to have different expectations or 'agendas'. Being aware of this helps communication. Examples of diverging agendas are given in CLINICAL SCENARIO BOX 1.2. It is vital that the doctor recognizes that there are different agendas afoot and makes this explicit, acknowledging that each is of value. For example, 'I can appreciate that this injury claim is important to you and I will prepare a report as soon as I can, but for today I am concerned about your kidneys and feel we need to look into that first.'

Clinical Scenario 1.2: Diverging agendas

The patient wants to complain about the side-effects of the tablets you gave her last time, whereas you want to talk to her about stopping smoking.

The patient wants an X-ray of his back because his wife, fed up with his chronic back pain, has told him to get this done. You want him to lose weight and advise him that this will help his back.

The patient wants you to write a report for an injury claim he is pursuing, you are alarmed at his rising creatinine level.

Patients' ideas can be based on past experience, experiences of friends or family or something the patient has read or seen on television or on the internet. Such ideas may not be clinically relevant to the situation from the doctor's perspective, but they are best brought out for discussion rather than remaining in the patient's mind as unresolved issues. Unresolved issues will be brought back in various guises again and again. Conversely, clinicians often assume patients want investigation and treatment for their problem, but sometimes they simply want explanations of their symptoms or reassurances that nothing is seriously wrong. They may simply want to have their complaint heard. Embarking on extensive investigations or elaborate treatments may be inappropriate and wasteful in these situations. Questions that help clarify these issues include:
● What is it you would like me to do?
● Do you have any specific ideas about what we should do?
● Which aspects of the problem do you want to address?
● What worries you about this problem?

Clinical Scenario 1.1: Examples of patients' hidden concerns

A 55-year-old-male patient presents with left-sided chest pain, which you think is muscular. He seems unconvinced by your reassurances and then reveals that his father died of a heart attack aged 54.

A 35-year-old woman presents with 1 month of pelvic pain, no other symptoms and no abnormalities on examination. She later informs you that she has been trying to conceive for 18 months.

A young man visits you with an innocuous sounding cough and on his way out mentions sexual problems.

Be aware of your own concerns and agenda

Clinicians are often unaware that they have agendas. Examples of such agendas include:

- I really must get Mr Smith's blood pressure down
- I want to try out this new drug
- I want my patients to like me
- I must reduce the number of follow-up patients in my clinic
- I don't know anything about gynaecology so I will ignore menstrual symptoms
- I must leave in 20 minutes

Self-reflection and the discovery of one's own agenda is a fascinating and crucial activity for the clinician.

Locate the problem in a medical framework

It is always best to let the patient describe problems in their own terms before we impose our medical terms on the situation. This gives us insight into the patient's conceptualizations of their problem. However, at some point the clinician needs to ask specific questions to characterize the complaint within the medical model. Within this model we have fairly specific and rigid ways of describing and conceiving of illnesses. These are very familiar to us, but may be unfamiliar to patients.

When we ask a patient, 'What kind of pain is it?' We want them to say 'burning' or 'stabbing' or 'dull' or 'colicky' but they may simply say 'a bad one' or 'it's just there' or 'a painful one'. In these situations we can offer our preferred descriptive terms as suggestions. Similarly, patients can find it difficult to estimate time. 'How long have you had this pain?' can be answered by 'a while' or 'a good while' or 'I don't know'. Questions like, 'When was the first time you felt the pain?' can help to focus the answer. Sample timescales such as, 'Have you had it for weeks or months or years?' can also help. Clinicians have to be both imaginative and flexible in order to extract the information they need to make sense of the patient's problem in medical terms.

If you are taking a detailed complete history for a major condition then this is the stage to explore the patient's past medical, family, social, drug and allergy history. You may

also conduct a full functional inquiry and perform an examination as appropriate.

Discuss your conclusions with the patient

Once you have made your clinical assessment you need to share a version of this with the patient in terms that they can clearly understand. If you have a differential diagnosis in mind, you may wish to discuss this with the patient as far as seems appropriate. If the diagnosis is equivocal, it is probably reasonable to mention the possible options. It may not be of benefit to mention a serious condition if it is very unlikely. However, if a serious condition, such as cancer, *is* likely, then you may wish to raise the possible diagnosis at this point. One must bear in mind the anxiety this will cause until a definitive diagnosis is made. In answering patients' questions, honesty is the best policy. Before finalizing your assessment, you may wish to consult with colleagues or carry out further research; if so, then be open in explaining this to patients. It is not necessary to make them think that you know everything. Clarity concerning what you know and about your limitations, and a willingness to take advice or refer on where necessary can inspire patients with greater confidence in your honesty and integrity—and rightly so.

Check the patient understands you by asking questions such as, 'Does that make sense?' 'Do you understand what happens during your menstrual cycle?'

Agree on a management plan

Discuss with the patient what you think the best course of action should be and your reasoning. The plan may include investigation, treatment and when they should be seen again for review and why they should be seen again. Ask the patient for suggestions and agree on a final version. KEYPOINTS BOX 1.4 outlines the ideal management plan.

You may be starting a young diabetic patient on insulin and teaching them the principles of self-management, which is a complicated business. To check on your message you would need to ask questions such as, 'So what would you do if your blood sugar reading was 18?' In other situations, more general questions are appropriate, such

---

Keypoints 1.4: The ideal management plan

A management plan should:

- Be clear and understood by both parties
- Make explicit the tasks and responsibilities of each party
- Take into account the concerns raised by the patient at the outset
- Be clinically appropriate given the differential diagnosis

- Maximize the patient's role in their management
- Develop the patient's understanding of the problem
- Develop the patient's health behaviour
- Be feasible for the patient to implement
- Anticipate future events and how to deal with them
- Use resources wisely

as, 'Do you have any questions?' 'Is everything clear?' 'Are you all right with that?' Sometimes a patient wishes to explore an issue in great detail and the internet, books and patient support groups can help them in this. It may still be necessary to help the patient weigh up the pros and cons of possible plans, or to give them time to do this.

Think ahead on the patient's behalf. Give specific advice about the likely occurrence of significant events and appropriate responses to them. For instance, as a community doctor treating a young patient with an exacerbation of their asthma late at night, you might say, 'Start these steroid tablets now and double your inhalers. I would like to review you tomorrow morning, but if your asthma gets significantly worse tonight, I think you should go straight to the accident and emergency department. There is no further treatment I can safely give you at home.' Or to a young woman with menstrual pain, 'Try these ibuprofen tablets. It is best to take then with food as they can irritate the stomach lining. If you get any indigestion stop them and use paracetamol instead.'

Doctors rarely have neutral views about management options and this may be reflected in the way we present the information. For instance, we might overemphasize the risks of high blood pressure and underemphasize the side-effects of antihypertensive medication because we want to control our patient's blood pressure. This may be for the patient's benefit, but it may also be to improve our audit results. It can be instructive to consider our own interests in the patient's management choices.

Close the consultation in a friendly and polite manner
- Smile
- Shake hands
- Open the door

Make accurate records
When you are rushed, it is tempting to skimp on record keeping. This is a mistake. Good records will help you and other colleagues involved with the care of your patients get up to speed quickly at each new encounter. This is an efficient way of working, avoids duplication and waste, benefits the patient and is helpful in the event of litigation. KEYPOINTS BOX 1.5 outlines the key features of good clinical records.

Clearly, the exact balance of the elements in a consultation varies according to the setting and the problem being presented. The overall shape of the discussion will be different for a young woman consulting her GP about contraception, compared to that if the same woman presented very ill in the accident and emergency department with an ectopic pregnancy. In the second scenario it is fairly obvious she has come to the accident and emergency department for immediate relief of severe pelvic pain and

---

> **Keypoints 1.5: Clinical records**
>
> Good clinical records should:
> - Be legible
> - State the significant positive and negative features of the case
> - Detail the impact of the problem on the patient's function, psychological and social states
> - List the working differential diagnoses
> - Outline the management plan
> - Be signed and dated

---

collapse. A long exploration of her ideas and expectations is not appropriate. There is relatively little time or scope for this patient to choose between different treatments. However, a clear brief explanation of your assessment and proposed treatment, with an opportunity for the patient to ask questions, should still be attempted. It would, for example, be extremely pertinent to discover that the patient is a Jehovah's Witness, who objects to blood transfusions. Continue to explain things to the patient as emergency events proceed. 'I am going to put a small plastic tube in your vein so that I can give you a drug to make your heart beat more regularly.' You will need also to spend some time explaining events to worried relatives, as far as patient confidentiality permits. Much of the consultation model also applies to these conversations.

Challenging scenarios—practical advice

Certain situations are particularly demanding in terms of the doctor's communication skills. Most clinicians find it challenging to convey uncertainty in diagnosis or prognosis, explain an error, break bad news or deal with angry patients. In addition, each of us may have subject areas or scenarios that we find difficult for personal reasons. Whatever the situation, we should apply the same rules of good communication and aim to cover the same tasks or stages in our consultations as outlined above.

How to approach breaking bad news
Bad news is difficult to deliver and difficult to receive. The clinician may feel that they or the medical profession are letting their patient down. Perhaps there is a diagnosis of cancer or infertility to convey or news that an unpleasant course of treatment has not been successful. The clinician may be apprehensive about the impact such news will have on the patient or their family.

In these situations it is especially important to be gentle in manner and give the information as clearly as possible. It is often useful to write down information or instructions

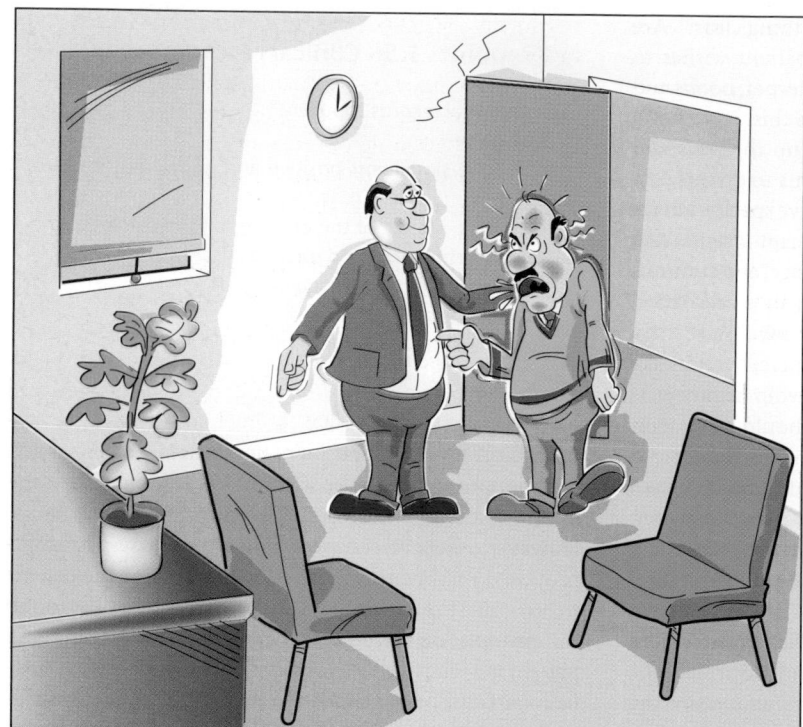

Figure 1.3 Dealing with angry patients. Try to stay calm with angry patients and give them an opportunity to air their concerns.

as patients may be too emotionally shocked to appreciate fully what is being said to them. It is difficult for patients to make decisions on the spot, so it can be useful to schedule a further meeting in the near future. Be honest and direct in answering any questions. Gauge how much information is desired. Questions such as, 'Do you want me to go into any more details?' may achieve this. In some circumstances, you may feel it necessary to gently offer information not explicitly requested.

How to approach angry patients

Being a patient is a role characterized by emotion. Sometimes patients are angry and frustrated with their health care; sometimes this is justified and sometimes not. It is inevitable that during our professional life we will have complaints made against us, either face-to-face or via other channels. It is never pleasant to face criticism but vital to so do calmly and openly. We have no interest in defensive confrontation, which will only make the situation worse. Indeed, sometimes, we may have something to learn. Even if there are no grounds for complaint, such a process is a form of feedback worth attending to, if only to avoid future similar episodes. When a complaint is made one must ascertain carefully what the grievance is. One must then offer the facts as clearly as possible. If an error has been made or a service delivered suboptimally then an apology is appropriate. A polite and sympathetic explana-

tion is often all the patient is seeking (Fig. 1.3). It is usually wise to sort out the complaint in person or verbally at an early rather than a late stage. However, in some instances patients may wish to proceed to litigation, and if you feel this may be a possibility then getting early advice from a medicolegal defence organization is sensible.

Violence

If a patient is really very angry, they may resort to violence. Consider this possibility and if you are worried about this and alone, then stay calm, leave the room and seek help at an early stage.

Acquiring consulting skills

Analysing and reflecting on your own interactions with patients is the best method for developing consultation skills. You can then use your observations to modify your future practice. You can do this informally in your head or in a notebook. Alternatively, you can do this more formally by case discussion or by recording your consultations on video and discussing them with a colleague or mentor (this last method requires explicit patient consent). Watching other people consult can also be extremely instructive. As a student you spend many hours on ward rounds and in clinics and you can use this time to observe how experienced clinicians interact with patients.

You are out of the 'hot seat' and so feel relaxed and can see more clearly and objectively the dynamics of the situation. You can identify just how messages are sent and received, what makes communication effective and what makes it fail.

The components of the consultation have been presented here in a linear, logical and coherent order. In real life, the consultation is often more free-flowing and organic. Different issues crop up at different times. A clinician skilled in the art of the consultation may cease to be consciously aware of going through the above stages, but will do so automatically. However, when starting out it is helpful to have a framework to follow consciously.

Medicine is now frequently regarded as a high-tech, objective and authoritative science. It is true that the application of science to health and illness has radically influenced what modern medicine can offer to society. However, that is not the whole picture; when we consider the point of delivery of medicine, which is our interaction with patients, we see, central to medical practice, the need for skills that are imaginative, creative and personal.

Patient factors

Why do patients consult doctors?

Patients usually visit their doctor for some combination of the following reasons:
- They have a health concern
- Their own coping mechanisms are failing
- They have tried other forms of therapy already, but these have not been completely successful
- They have a high regard for science and the scientific basis of medicine
- They have a high regard for the professional integrity of health care practitioners
- They feel entitled to health care because they have already paid for it by taxes or insurance schemes

Health concerns

What may count as a health concern is, to some extent, culturally determined, but is also highly personal. Identifying beliefs about health can help to explain the health behaviour of individuals in modern society. Such explanations can be framed in terms of an individual's general belief systems, values, personality and personal concerns and motivations. Working in multicultural societies can remind us how much some of these factors vary between individual patients or groups. Problems such as mental illness or infertility can be particularly stigmatized in certain cultures, and the social significance of such illnesses cannot be assumed but must be ascertained for each patient.

Patients may also consult doctors because they seek a medical diagnosis that validates some level of withdrawal from normal functioning. This aspect of health behaviour has been much studied. Similarly, we need to be aware that medical labelling can turn illness into a stigmatized deviation from normal when the reality is that illness is a part of normal human existence.

Failure of coping mechanisms

Studies have shown that patients consult their primary care physician for only 1 in 10 of their perceived problems. When they do consult, they have often been coping with their symptoms for some time. Often, an additional social or psychological stress is the 'final straw' that makes a patient seek professional help, rather than a deterioration in the symptom itself. It is useful to identify this social trigger as part of establishing the context for the current visit. These studies underline the fact that patients have substantial coping mechanisms and that they are active agents in their own health management. Doctors should aim to harness and maximize these factors in management plans.

Other forms of therapy

Orthodox western scientific medicine has never been and never will be the only form of therapy in the market place. There are some problems that orthodox medicine deals with poorly. Many types of pain persist, whether musculoskeletal or undiagnosed abdominal or pelvic pain, which we label as some form of 'chronic pain syndrome'. We might send such patients to a pain clinic but a significant number of them remain not only uncured but also unpalliated. Likewise, individuals with certain skin problems, functional bowel problems and psychological problems remain unsatisfied with what mainstream medicine has to offer and turn to other or complementary medicines. These include herbal medicine, massage therapy, aromatherapy, reflexology, acupuncture, chiropractic, osteopathy and spiritual healing.

Much of the appeal of complementary medicine is that its practice tends to focus on the person as a whole rather than on the abstracted symptom. The same individual usually delivers diagnosis and treatment over a variety of meetings and thus the interaction between therapist and patient feels more personal. We have little systematic evidence of the efficacy of many of the therapeutic interventions that fall outside our 'orthodox' medical model. This may be because of a genuine lack of efficacy, but may be brought about by the methodological difficulty in testing interventions that are so profoundly holistic and dependent on the quality of the relationship between healer and patient. The popularity of medical practices that are significantly more holistic than conventional medicine highlights how much this feature is valued by patients. This suggests that we should maximize this factor in our own dealings with patients.

High regard for the scientific basis of medicine

On the whole, society trusts the scientific basis of western medicine. The impression society has of medicine derives from a combination of the way in which science and medicine portray themselves and how they are portrayed by the media, in films, on television and in writing. For a particular individual, this general impression is modified by the beliefs of their immediate social group and their own previous experience of medicine or that of someone they know.

Usually, doctors are consulted by patients who regard them as highly trained specialists operating in an effective health care system. Indeed, individual patients may have unrealistic expectations of what current health care can offer them and it is important to outline clearly and honestly the current state of affairs with regard to any particular problem. Clinicians may be reluctant to face this head on for fear of sounding too pessimistic or taking away a patient's hope of cure or improvement. However, it is better to set a realistic stage and work with the patient to optimize the available outcomes.

High regard for the professional integrity of health care workers

There are, of course, bad doctors and suboptimal health care institutions. Such medical failures attract a great deal of media coverage, and can be disheartening for other members of the profession. However, despite high profile 'bad doctor' cases and a general increase in medical complaints and litigations in the UK, studies have shown that the general public still values doctors highly. The maintenance of professional integrity via professional self-monitoring and the setting of acceptable standards of professional conduct is discussed in more detail below in relation to medical ethics (see pp. 20–21)

Although there is generally a high regard for the scientific basis of medicine and the integrity of its practitioners, a particular individual may themselves have had or may know someone who has had a bad medical experience. If these can be unearthed and discussed, greater progress can often be made in the current situation. Patients may also hold certain views that oppose conventional medical practice. An example of this is the stand some homoeopathists take to immunizations. In these cases it is vital not to be defensive or irritated but to identify the areas of conflict or concern in order that useful common ground be established.

Sense of entitlement to medical attention

Some patients may feel that they are entitled to a certain amount of medical attention, especially from a public health maintenance organization such as the National Health Service. Regardless of their attitude, we should always aim to deliver the highest quality of care in our power. In any case, most patients really have, in some way, paid for their doctor's time and the services delivered. This can be either by taxes, insurance policies or direct payment.

Doctor factors

Clinical reasoning—making a diagnosis

Locating the patient's problem in a medical framework requires us to use the information that the patient supplies in a particular way. Clinicians reason backwards from a patient's complaint to the potential physical or psychological processes causing it. This is what we refer to as making a diagnosis. It is a form of inductive reasoning and is the same process that detectives use to solve a crime. The character of the fictional detective Sherlock Holmes was based on a famous clinician. To reason from symptom to disease, from effect to cause, we first need to know a certain amount about the symptom itself. Let us consider the example of a cough. We would ask questions such as:

- When did it start?
- What makes it better or worse?
- Does it interfere with activities?

However, a cough, like most common symptoms, is fairly non-specific. No matter how much we know about it, we cannot usually make a diagnosis on the basis of that information alone. To make a diagnosis, we need to know about any associated symptoms, such as discoloured sputum. We also need to know some demographic details about the patient. For example, we want to know:

- Is there any fever or difficulty in breathing or any sputum or chest pain or wheeze?
- Is our patient young or old or a cigarette smoker?

We then consider the patient's symptoms in the light of this additional information about associated features and demographic or other background details. A good clinician develops their history taking so that their questions elicit the most useful information in the most effective manner.

Recognizing patterns

Most diagnoses are based on the recognition of a pattern of typical features. We must learn to recognize these patterns and to identify those features that are the most useful discriminating factors. It would be unusual for a cough to be caused by severe asthma if there was no associated wheeze. However, the presence of wheeze does not guarantee that the diagnosis is asthma. Wheezing is highly suggestive of asthma in a child, but less so in an elderly smoker who is more likely to have chronic obstructive pulmonary disease.

Clinicians hone their diagnosis by a series of key questions that aim to clarify whether a pattern of symptoms and biographical features is present. This is done in such a way that it points to a shortlist of possible underlying disease processes and excludes as many others as possible. This is called formulating a differential diagnosis and is a vital aspect of clinical reasoning. We can only get so far with taking a history and examining our patient, we often need to use investigations and even trials of treatment to refine our differential diagnosis further. However, with an examination or investigation or even a trial of treatment, we are essentially using the same process of testing our hypotheses about the patient's underlying problem. We usually stop this process either when we have reached a final diagnosis or when to proceed further would not affect our management or add any other benefits.

Evidence-based medicine—how do doctors decide what to do?

Medical research attempts to provide a rational basis for determining whether a particular clinical intervention is likely to be helpful. Much emphasis has been placed on the practice of 'evidence-based medicine' (EBM) with its underlying scientific principle that doctors should have an explicit rational basis for their actions whenever possible. Moreover, if a doctor does not know the answer to a question posed by the patient's condition, then they should know how to find the answer or how to establish that there is no clear answer.

It is important to remember that evidence-based medicine is not simply the memorization of numerous clinical trial names and results. Clinical trials are very important, but they are only one type of clinical evidence. Other types include laboratory studies, studies of normal human physiology and epidemiological studies. Overall, evidence-based medicine is the application of scientific thought to a clinical problem, as illustrated in CLINICAL SCENARIO BOX 1.3.

The approach to the patient in Clinical Scenario Box 1.3 is all evidence-based medicine and at each stage the clinical thinking proceeded logically and rationally on the basis of well-conducted science. Only in the very last stage was a trial result useful. This highlights the benefits of learning basic clinical science as a student. Although the trial result may become out-of-date when a new clot-dissolving therapy is developed, the rest of the approach will still be relevant. It is worth remembering that even to evaluate clinical trials, you often need a good understanding of the basic science underlying the study.

> ### Clinical Scenario 1.3: A clinical example of evidence-based medicine: a cold painful foot
>
> Consider a patient with a cold painful bluish left foot. Your basic scientific knowledge suggests that the foot is blue because the haemoglobin in the blood of the foot is deoxygenated. The right foot is pink, so the heart and lungs are still oxygenating and pumping blood. The femoral artery pulse in the left groin is strong, but there is no pulse in the foot. From your anatomy knowledge, you know that the foot receives its blood supply from the femoral artery, so there must be an obstruction to blood flow below this. By injecting a radio-opaque dye into this artery and taking X-ray images, we see that there is a large clot in an artery below the knee. At this point, we know from clinical trials that a specific procedure to remove the clot is likely to save the foot from amputation.

Applying results from clinical trials

Clinical studies or trials are key sources of evidence-based medicine. Unfortunately, clinical situations are so diverse and some conditions are so rare that it is unlikely that we will ever have trial evidence addressing every possible question about every problem confronting every patient. However, for many well-defined clinical problems, good clinical trial evidence is now available. In using these sources, it is important to consider how well designed the trial was and how relevant the trial is to the patient you are dealing with.

The design of clinical trials is very important, because a poorly designed trial could give misleading results. Therefore, the strength of the conclusions that we draw from a trial depends on its design and methodology. The key types of clinical studies are summarized in Table 1.3.

Clinical decisions are made by considering the clinical situation of an actual patient in the light of the evidence that seems relevant to the patient (Fig. 1.4). A good clinician has to judge the extent to which an individual patient's situation is sufficiently similar to that of patients studied in a trial. This judgement determines whether a treatment recommendation can reliably be based upon the trial result. For example, consider a trial conducted in fit young women showing that there is no clear benefit from giving antibiotics for urinary tract infection. If you are presented with an 80-year-old man with a large prostate gland who is delirious and very unwell with a high fever caused by urinary tract infection, you would be wrong to apply these trial results to this patient. The trial did not address the treatment of people in his condition, even though both have 'urinary tract infection'. A trial of antibiotics for men in his position might show a clear benefit.

Table 1.3 Clinical trial design. The examples assume that the new treatment to be tested is a drug but, in principle, other types of intervention could be tested in an analogous fashion

Historically controlled trials
A new drug is given to patients and the outcome is compared to that documented previously with other treatments or no treatment. This is a poor trial design because there may be many differences other than just the treatment between the two groups

Placebo controlled trials
Patients are given either the new drug of interest or a placebo drug to test whether the new drug has more effect than placebo alone

Randomized trials
The decision to give a patient the new drug or another treatment (which could be a placebo) is made by a completely random process, such as tossing a coin. This ensures that the researchers do not bias the selection of the patients receiving the new drug

Single-blind trial
Patients receive either the new drug or another treatment (which could be a placebo). The patients do not know whether they have received the new drug or the other treatment, but the researchers do know

Double-blind trial
This is the same as a single-blind trial, except that the researchers who are analysing the trial results and conducting clinical assessments do not know which patients received the new drug and which received the other treatment

Randomized double-blind controlled trial
This is the best trial design and incorporates the best features of the simpler designs. It avoids bias in the allocation of patients to the new drug and avoids bias in the analysis of the outcome. The term 'controlled' refers to the attempts of the trial design to match closely the patients in both groups and ensure that the only major difference between them and their treatment is the drug therapy being tested

Crossover studies
This is a different type of design from those above. Each patient serves as their own control by spending some time taking the new drug and then some time taking the other treatment (which could be placebo). For example, an established drug for hypertension could be given to all the patients in the trial and the effect on their blood pressure noted. The patients could then be given the new drug and the effect of this noted and compared to that of the established treatment

The urinary tract infection example may seem straight-forward, but sometimes more subtle problems arise in interpreting trial results for individual patients. Consider a good double-blind randomized controlled trial showing

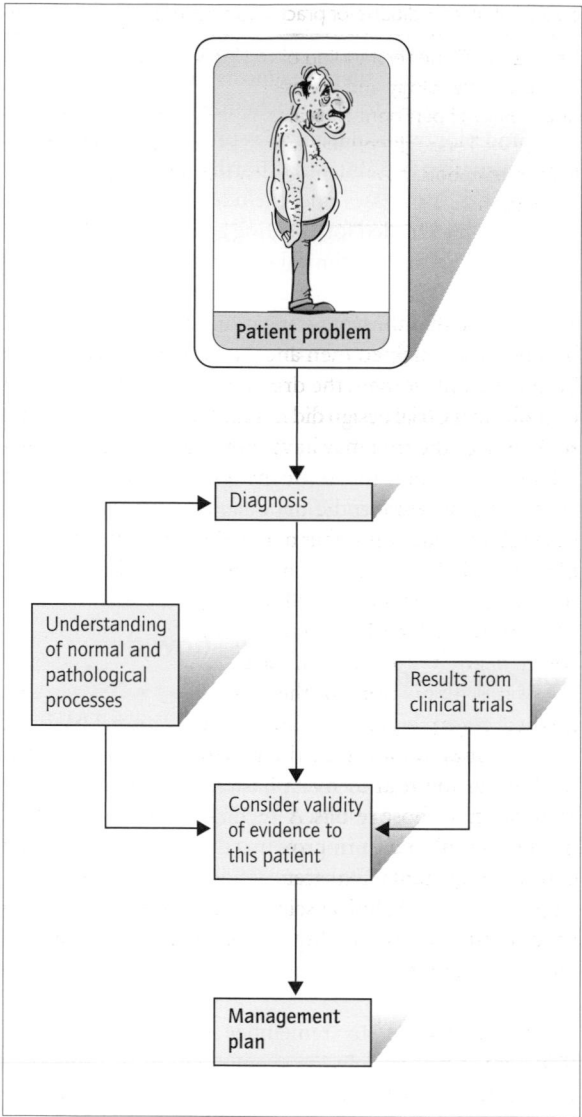

Figure 1.4 The use of evidence-based medicine in clinical decision making. Good clinical judgement is important in assessing the relevance of any evidence to the situation of an individual patient.

that a new drug reduces death from acute myocardial infarction, but only in patients under 65 years. If we encounter a woman aged 60 years, who we believe is having a myocardial infarction then, at face value, it would seem sensible to use the drug. However, there is no guarantee that this will benefit the individual patient.

● We may have made the wrong diagnosis and she is not having a myocardial infarction at all.

● Perhaps she has forgotten her age or is confused and is actually aged 70—an age group in which the drug is of no benefit.

Table 1.4 Preconditions for practising evidence-based medicine

Basic scientific understanding of the individual patient's altered physiology and disease

Knowledge of pertinent clinical trials and of whether they were well enough conducted to produce reliable results

Judgement about how relevant each trial is to the patient in question

---

● It may be that the drug is of no benefit to women at all but, because it helped men and the trial group contained both men and women, the drug appeared to be of benefit overall and the trial design did not explore gender difference.

● Although the trial may have shown overall benefit, that might mean that for some people with one type of myocardial infarction the drug made death more likely, but that for a larger number of people with a different type of myocardial infarction it made death less likely, so that the net result was that overall the drug reduced mortality. This individual patient may be one of the people for whom death is more likely if the drug is given.

We may know none of these variables, and if the trial showed a very significant increase in survival with the drug we may reason that the patient is similar enough to those in the trial to merit basing a treatment recommendation on those results. A key objective of your medical training should be to improve your ability to make such clinical judgements. Experience, reflection, a good knowledge of basic and clinical science and continued learning should improve your ability to make these clinical judgements (Table 1.4).

Evidence-based medicine and guidelines from expert bodies

Unfortunately, most doctors are too short of time and resources to investigate, in detail, the rational basis for everything they do, and much of the published literature is not easily available to them without significant financial cost. In addition, most clinicians are not expert in all the fields necessary to critically evaluate all studies relevant to their practice. For these reasons, expert panels often study evidence and produce practical guidelines for others to follow. Expert or consensus guidelines provide a basic framework for much of clinical practice. The UK government has established the National Institute for Clinical Excellence (NICE) to produce guidance on key issues. In addition, the UK National Health Service now produces National Service Frameworks (NSFs), which attempt to define the care that patients with specific conditions should receive. Similar guidelines are also produced in the USA and other countries. However, as with clinical trial evidence, guidelines need careful interpretation by the clinician to determine whether they apply to an individual patient under consideration. Factors that may differ between your patient and those referred to in the guidelines include:

● age
● gender
● diagnosis
● ethnicity
● comorbidity

Local audit-based guidelines

Local audit and the regular review of local clinical outcomes can provide evidence for a particular clinical practice in the local setting. For example, if all the patients in your practice with a particular sexually transmitted infection respond well to a particular antibiotic, then this suggests that the local organisms are sensitive to this antibiotic. The next patient you see with this infection from the local population is also likely to respond well to this therapy. Local guidelines based on such observations may sometimes be of more use and relevance than those of experts in a different part of the world, practising in a different environment.

Medicine and uncertainty

Uncertainty is an inevitable aspect of clinical practice. There are three major types of uncertainty in clinical practice (KEYPOINTS BOX 1.6). We cannot usually predict with certainty what the outcome of a particular disease will be for a given patient, nor can we always predict whether a patient will have an unexpected side-effect from a drug. Sometimes we cannot even make a certain diagnosis. Patients often seek absolute certainty and reassurance from doctors and uncertainty is something they may not have been expecting. Clinicians may feel that acknowledging uncertainty is an admission of failure or a threat to their expertise.

Keypoints 1.6: Major sources of uncertainty in clinical practice

■ Statistical basis of medical evidence on risk and prognosis —clinical trials are based on statistical probability
■ Limitations of medical definitions of disease
■ Human error

Uncertainty of prognosis and risk

Clinicians become familiar with the difficulty of predicting the future. It can be difficult to answer perfectly understandable questions about **prognosis** such as:

- Will this get better?
- What will happen to me?
- How long do I have?

Doctors often consider prognoses in statistical terms, using concepts that can be difficult for patients to apply to their own case, such as 'a 5-year survival rate' or a '15% risk of a cardiovascular event in 10 years'. These can be difficult for patients to understand in a meaningful way. Similarly, the communication skills of the doctor are critical in **communicating risk** to patients in terms they understand. It may be helpful to illustrate prognosis or risk with simple examples. 'If you carry on smoking then you have a 70% chance of amputation of your leg in a year. That means that if I see 10 patients like you today and they all carry on smoking, then 1 year from now 7 of them will have had a leg amputated.'

Furthermore, we each have our own approach to risk and while some people are concerned about the future and take out pensions and insurance, other people do not. There is a similar spectrum of attitudes to health. Weighing up present cost with future benefit (lowering cholesterol, adhering to a diabetic diet or stopping drinking or smoking) involves the patient's personal judgement and values. There are scales of risk that may help patients decide more logically about risks. One such scale attempts to give patients a comparison of different levels of risk with everyday risks that they take, such as crossing a road (http://www.johnpaling.com/perspectives3.html).

Statistical uncertainty

In most clinical situations, doctors are aware that they are dealing with probabilities and not certainties. Clinical trials usually show that a certain percentage of patients given a treatment derive benefit from the treatment. If a trial of a treatment shows that it benefits 80% of those who receive it, then we cannot be sure that an individual patient will benefit; we can only tell them that they have an 80% chance of benefiting. Statistical uncertainty is also well illustrated if we consider prescribing a drug for a patient. All drugs produce adverse reactions in some people, but usually we cannot predict who these will be. We are generally happy to prescribe the drug if we think that on balance the probability that the patient will benefit outweighs the small probability of an adverse reaction. However, we cannot tell the patient with certainty that they will not have an adverse reaction or that they will benefit from the drug.

Uncertainty of diagnosis

A different type of uncertainty can arise because not all ailments that patients complain of fit into a strictly medical model of disease. In some cases, we cannot identify a definite pathology or a clear disease process. Important examples of this are chronic pains for which no cause can be found. It can be frustrating for clinicians and patients alike when symptoms persist but no label can be attached. Labels are helpful to the clinician because they trigger an established set of management options and they are helpful for the patient because they can give their complaint greater validity. However, when we cannot label a patient's complaint as a well-defined illness, it is important to remember that this does not make it any less real for them. We must continue to consider the effects of the symptom on the patient seriously and to explore what palliative options there might be and how the patient can psychologically manage the ongoing problem. It may be helpful to explore the issue and the patient's expectations. Questions can be aimed at exploring the patient's own thoughts about what they think will help. This might include the following type of question: 'As you know, we haven't found any definite cause for your pelvic pain. How will you cope living with it? Are you keen to try stronger painkillers?'

Uncertainty in human judgement

A third type of uncertainty arises because there is a probability of human error in all human actions. A good doctor may weigh up all that he or she knows about a patient and then, in good faith, make a decision that is detrimental to the patient. However, this does not mean that the doctor is a bad or negligent doctor. The doctor tried to do the right thing, was well informed and conscientious, but the line of action that the doctor pursued led to a bad outcome. This may be especially true in emergency situations when decisions may have to be taken very rapidly. We cannot ever make a perfect doctor and, even with the best will in the world, unwanted outcomes will occur. The same applies in all human activities—even the best car driver can have an accident.

We should take all reasonable steps to reduce these risks, but must also realize that they can never be reduced to zero. A better-informed society will appreciate the limitations as well as the strengths of medicine. Medicine should improve over time as more knowledge is brought into the clinical arena, but it will never become perfect.

Management and organizational factors

Setting priorities

All patients deserve equal respect, but the extent to which they need medical input is not necessarily the same. For a given amount of time or resources, the benefits may be much greater for one patient or patient group than for another. The clinical skill lies in recognizing and judging the extent to which the patient will benefit from your attention and the extent to which devoting time to one patient will reduce the quality of care delivered to another.

Approaches to managing a busy workload

In some clinical situations, time is not pressing and it is reasonable to see patients in whatever order has been decided in advance. However, in other situations, such as a busy accident and emergency department, it is common for some patients to have conditions that need a more rapid response than others (CLINICAL SCENARIO BOX 1.4).

The principle of triage is applied during a major incident and even sometimes when an accident and emergency department or medical team is excessively busy. Historically, the triage principle was applied after a battle, when the injured were rapidly sorted to identify those most in need of and most likely to benefit from medical input. In the extreme case, there were three categories: those who would probably live without medical care, those who would probably only live if they received medical care and those who were so badly injured that they would probably die even with medical care. The second category received medical care first.

In normal clinical practice, such extreme judgements are not the rule, but with sick patients it is important, even with routine ward work, to be able to prioritize the work that needs to be done. Arranging a chest X-ray for an acutely breathless patient who may have a large pneumothorax takes priority over that for a stable patient with long-standing lung fibrosis who has been in hospital for weeks and just needs a follow-up radiograph.

In practice, flexibility and efficiency are important. In the example in CLINICAL SCENARIO BOX 1.4, it should be possible to start looking after the patient with the myocardial infarction first. Then, when the immediate potentially life-saving care has been administered, the care of the other patients, such as the prescribing of analgesia, can be started before returning to continue care of the patient with the myocardial infarction. Although such schemes of care sound somewhat chaotic and fragmented, much acute medicine is necessarily like this.

Setting priorities with an individual patient

Even an individual patient may have several problems that need to be prioritized. Often it is the patient's own prioritization that will decide what, if anything, they wish to do about their problems, but the doctor can inform the patient and give a professional opinion for the patient to consider. For example:

● The patient may be concerned about a grown-in toenail, but also mention that they have had mild chest pain while walking in to the clinic that day.
● The doctor, concerned that the chest pain is ischaemic heart disease may set a different priority to the patient and regard the chest pain as much more important.

Interacting with colleagues

Teamwork

Most clinicians work in teams and to do this effectively can be a challenge. Communication, respect and consideration for other team members are vital. In some situations, good leadership is also necessary. Try to learn about teamwork from:

● Observing colleagues
● Reflecting on your own experiences
● Discussing team issues with your colleagues

Medicine is a busy and stressful occupation, but a good team spirit will enhance your work experience and efficiency. It may be useful to work at building up this team spirit; at the most simple level, this could involve spending some time socializing or doing something together outside the busy atmosphere of work. You will undermine any team spirit by being unfair or difficult about holidays, shifts, rotas or clinic allocations. The social lives of all doctors are equally important and cannot be ranked on the basis of obvious domestic commitments. This can be difficult to remember, as a colleague may not wish to disclose their domestic circumstances. One person may have children to look after, but another may have a disabled partner with multiple sclerosis or an elderly dependant relative, or may themselves be under great stress and in need of their full quota of leisure time.

Continuity of patient care

In hospital, there are usually several levels of doctor, such

---

Clinical Scenario 1.4: Managing a busy workload

Consider three patients who attend hospital with chest pain:
■ One may have bruised a rib in a game of football
■ One may be in the early stages of a myocardial infarction with a dangerous heart rhythm
■ One may be known to be dying of advanced terminal lung cancer involving the ribs

All three patients need careful assessment and treatment for their pain. However, the immediate focus of attention is likely to be the second patient because rapid medical input could alter the outcome and there is an immediate potentially preventable risk of death from cardiac arrest. The man with the bruised rib is likely to be all right whatever the doctor does. The man with terminal cancer needs analgesia and palliative care, but it is evident that a delay of minutes in its delivery is not crucial.

as house officers, specialist registrars and consultants who are all looking after a patient. At each of these levels, there may even be several different doctors involved with a patient, for example if there are several house officers on a team. However, at each level of seniority, it should always be clear who has responsibility for each patient. In general practice, patients usually have a named doctor. Social and health care workers who operate in teams have 'keyworkers' for each patient, in recognition of both the importance of continuity of care and professional responsibility for each patient.

In most situations, one doctor should have continuing responsibility for each patient. The benefits of this are that:
● If anyone needs to communicate information about the patient, they can do so with a doctor who knows the patient and who can deal with any problems as they arise
● Patients get to know one doctor rather than seeing a different doctor each time they interact with the medical team
● Medicine is more satisfying if you establish relationships with your own patients rather than doing random jobs for many different patients

Allocating work

At any one time, it is desirable for all members of a team to know their individual responsibilities. If something needs to be done for a patient, this task must, at some point, be assigned to a specific individual. If it is not assigned, everyone may assume that somebody else is doing it and the task may be left undone.

If you are very busy and there are other members of your team, involve them at an early stage to maximize the number of people available to deal with the situation. When you are in charge, at whatever level, lead from the front and do not leave your juniors exposed to an unreasonable workload without your help. This will help morale, as well as helping to get the work done and reducing the time patients are kept waiting. Unnecessary work can often be prevented by early involvement of intermediate or senior colleagues. Acute medicine can be at its most rewarding when a team works well together in such circumstances. Clearly, if a rapid response is necessary because a patient is in a very dangerous situation, then it is usually wise for the most senior members of the team to take charge of this situation.

Professional standards within the medical team

Decisions should be made at an appropriate level and patient care should not be compromised by decisions taken at too junior a level. However, nor should patient care be made too slow by the unnecessary passing up of trivial decisions to more senior colleagues or specialists. In general, if a doctor is not competent to make a decision they should not be put in the position of having to do so. Senior doctors need to ensure that their junior colleagues are competent to bear any responsibility that is devolved to them. Senior doctors should provide the degree of supervision appropriate to the junior's experience and competence. Wherever you are in the hierarchy, always remember to respect your junior as well as your senior colleagues.

As a student or junior doctor, you may lack knowledge or experience, but you should be equally responsible in your professional capacity and have equally high standards of trustworthiness, honesty and reliability as your senior colleagues. If you are asked to do a task and agree to do it, your colleagues must be able to rely on you to keep your word or to inform them if you cannot complete the task.

Communicating with other doctors

If more than one doctor is involved with a patient's care, they must communicate to coordinate their actions. Similar principles apply to doctor–doctor communication as to doctor–patient communication. In particular:
● Be clear about what you want to communicate
● Do everything to maximize the chances of the other person understanding you
● Try to verify that they have understood you

There is a skill to communicating the essential aspects of a situation to a colleague without wasting too much of their time. The ability to present a patient's situation to a colleague succinctly is important if many hours are not to be wasted on ward rounds or referrals. It is usually helpful to start with a simple conventional phrase such as, 'Mr Smith is a 54-year-old man who was woken this morning with severe chest pain.' This gives everybody the key information and you can then elaborate as necessary. Do not assume that all medically qualified colleagues understand your practice or specialty—the last time they encountered your field may have been 30 years ago, when they were a medical student. Explaining or teaching medicine to colleagues or students is a professional obligation that will help them to make good critical decisions in the future when you are not there to help.

If you need advice from colleagues, seek it early rather than late. A formal referral may not be necessary and a simple conversation may establish whether anything needs to be done at a particular time. If you are the person whose advice is sought, make it easy for colleagues to communicate with you. This will encourage them to seek your advice at an earlier stage and, if you are available for simple conversations, this will save you the trouble of many inappropriate referrals. Colleagues, just like patients, deserve respect and may be very stressed about a problem that you can easily help them with.

The extended clinical team

Doctors work with a number of other skilled professionals in the delivery of modern health care. These include nurses, physiotherapists, occupational therapists, pharmacists, dietitians, radiographers, paramedics and social workers. An appreciation of the skills, needs and demands made on our coworkers helps the expanded clinical team to gel and work more efficiently. We should all strive to use each other as effectively as possible. It is good team practice to avoid making inappropriate requests or duplicating work and to be aware of others' workloads. Wherever possible, there should not be a conflict of interests between different members of the expanded team. For example, sending a patient home from the ward might reduce the workload of one team of doctors, but if the patient will be replaced by a more acutely ill patient under another team of doctors, then the nurses' workload will be increased. This might encourage the first team of doctors to send the first patient home, but encourage the nurses to keep that patient in hospital. Good communication, careful planning and mutual respect for our different types of contribution are at the heart of effective and enjoyable health work.

Communicating with non-clinical colleagues

Our working life also involves non-clinical colleagues such as cleaners, receptionists, secretaries and administrators. Some of these people may be paid little for their efforts, but can make a significant contribution to the smooth running of the health care system and our individual experience of work. They too deserve courtesy and respect.

Ethical factors

How does one recognize an ethical dilemma?

An ethical dilemma often becomes apparent as an obstacle to decision making. Suddenly, in the midst of a clinical problem, one feels unsure of what should be done for the best, even though the 'medical' problem itself is not difficult.

● Paediatricians resuscitate children as a routine part of their job. However, they might feel uneasy when called to resuscitate a child with advanced terminal cancer.

● A geriatrician may feel unsure whether it is a good thing

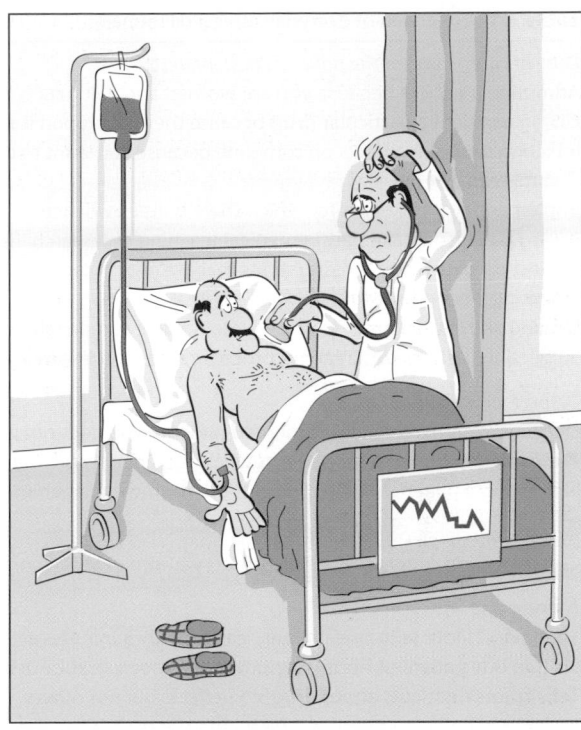

Figure 1.5 Recognizing an ethical dilemma. In clinical practice, ethical problems can arise in many forms, but sometimes they become apparent when the doctor feels unsure how to proceed, even though the medical issues are straightforward.

to continue artificially feeding an elderly patient who remains paralysed and unconscious some time after a major stroke.

Such pauses are the result of a 'moral alarm bell' ringing and making you ask 'is this the right thing to do?' (Fig. 1.5). When this happens, if you are the clinician with overall responsibility, you must analyse the situation with some care. You need to ask who benefits and who suffers in each of the different potential courses of action. Confronting each dilemma strengthens your moral analysing skills and increases your awareness of the moral dimensions in many more clinical situations.

Table 1.5 lists some ethical concerns that we have identified in our everyday clinical practice. Indeed, the list is seemingly endless once started and this emphasizes that moral dilemmas affect *all clinicians much of the time*, not just heart transplant surgeons or intensive care unit consultants. Each of us needs to be familiar with agreed ethical frameworks that enable us to address this dizzying variety of problems. A number of principles help us to organize the issues more clearly. These principles form the subheadings of the list in Table 1.5.

01

Table 1.5 A selection of everyday ethical dilemmas

Duty of care: acting in the patient's best interests
Admitting a patient because you are worried about litigation if they go home and something unexpected happens
Giving a patient a particular drug because they insist upon it and not because you think it is the best indicated
Inflicting drug side-effects on someone because you want to decrease their cholesterol for a small improvement in cardiovascular risk
Implementing treatments for which there is little evidence
Asking patients to take part in medical teaching or research
Subjecting patients to investigations that are not crucial to management
Practising a new skill while still learning it
Dealing with situations in which you do not feel completely competent
Subjecting patients to screening procedures for conditions for which they have low risk

Respect for patient autonomy
Deciding whether a mildly demented patient, who does not want to go into a nursing home, is fit to remain in their own home
Prescribing treatments for patients when you are not sure that they clearly understand what is at stake
Not asking a patient for their suggestions for the management plan

Respect for patient confidentiality
Giving out test results to patients' carers without explicit consent

Fairness and equity
Spending 1 hour with one patient, leaving only 5 minutes available for the next one
Visiting one patient at home inappropriately because they demand it and making the next one come to see you
Telling some patients about drug side-effects but not others
Giving one patient a range of treatment options, but not the next, because of time or language difficulties

Just use of resources
Deciding whether a patient who could possibly be managed at home should be admitted to your last bed
Deciding how much time you should spend with patients who have chronic deteriorating illnesses, but who persistently fail to follow advice or treatment
Signing relatively fit patients off sick for work
Referring patients for expensive investigations or treatments that they request but which are not obviously necessary

Maintaining professional competence
Not finding time to review your performance or level of knowledge or skill
Overlooking a colleague's suboptimal management
Not turning up to an important meeting with colleagues because you are too busy
Not discussing your management plan with other members of the team looking after a patient
Not taking a break when you are tired
Not identifying situations that you find difficult

Organizing principles

Duty of care

The whole of medical practice is underpinned by the assumption that clinicians have a duty of care to their patients. Patients approach health professionals on the basis that these professionals will act in the patient's best interests and will do so to a reasonable degree of professional competence. Trust in their doctor enables patients to divulge their problems and forms part of the therapeutic process. It is assumed that clinicians will not be swayed by motives such as financial gain, expediency, professional ambition or simply their own convenience.

Self-awareness on the part of the clinician is essential to ensure that partial but all too human interests are excluded from their clinical decision making.

To identify a patient's best interests we usually make a common sense cost–benefit analysis. In such an analysis we weigh up the pros and cons of different courses of action. For example, if we have a patient who has a very low risk of cervical cancer and who is terrified of having smears, we may advise them to have this procedure every 5 years rather than 3 years. The extra benefit of this particular patient having 3-yearly smears in terms of the likelihood of an abnormality being detected is small relative to the personal cost to her of having the smears done. These factors cannot be precisely measured; any solution is inevitably subjective to some degree. For this reason, it is important to include the patient's judgement in the weighing up process.

Respect for patient autonomy

Autonomy means self-government and in this context refers to the patients' ability to make their own decisions about their health. It is the role of clinicians to maximize this process by giving information, time and guidance in decision making rather than making decisions on behalf of the patient. Sharing the decision making between clinician and patient means that both the control of the situation and also the responsibility are shared. However, respecting patient autonomy does not mean simply passing the buck and the clinician must ensure that the patient is informed sufficiently for the decision in hand. This will probably involve careful communication about the weighing up of risks. It is advisable to document evidence of the level of information given to the patient and their competence in assessing it.

Consider the following scenarios:

● You discuss with a patient the pros and cons of being investigated in hospital or at home for melaena, but they decide to go home and later have a large bleed. You are unlikely to be deemed negligent if you can demonstrate that the patient fully understood what was at stake in the decision and opted not to go to hospital.

● One of your diabetic patients repeatedly fails to attend the diabetic clinic; you stop sending them appointments as you only have limited slots available. Your considered use of resources can be justified if you can prove that your patient fully understands the risks of poor blood pressure and glycaemic control.

Informed consent

The amount of information required to make consent adequately informed is context specific. This is reflected in the law, which requires a clinician to give the level of information a competent colleague would be likely to give in a comparable situation. It is best to think of this in terms of the need to establish, through discussion, the level of knowledge this particular patient requires to make a decision about this particular issue. A general rule is that common consequences should be mentioned, as should less common but serious possible outcomes. The clinician must provide the required information in an accessible way. Ideally, the clinician will have a good understanding of the treatment or procedure that the patient is consenting to and will be well informed about the relevant potential complications.

Strictly speaking, legal consent is required before touching a competent person to avoid a charge of a battery.

Conversely, in the same way, any competent individual can refuse any form of medical treatment, even if their life is thus endangered.

Competence

Competence is the ability to make judgements. It is a faculty that is context specific. To conclude that a patient is competent to make a particular decision, the clinician must assess that they have understood the information given and can deliberate upon it. Age is an arbitrary index of competence and adolescents under the age of 16 must be judged according to their merits. Different decisions require different levels of competence. A dementing patient may not be competent to judge how to invest their savings, but may be able to decide whether they want an influenza vaccine or their nails cut. With a patient who is no longer competent, it is the duty of the medical team to act in their best interests. This involves adhering as closely as possible to what is known about what the patient's wishes would have been if they were still competent. Relatives are often a good source of this type of information, as are advanced directives. However, the contributions of relatives are no substitute for a team assessment of the patient's best interests, as the relative's interest may be in conflict with that of the patient.

A special note should be made about discussing resuscitation of inpatients. Ideally, each competent patient should consent to the decision whether or not to resuscitate in the event of an arrest. They should be made aware of the pros and cons of such an intervention and their decision should be documented clearly in their notes. However, in practice this can be difficult and it may frighten a relatively well patient if they are asked about resuscitation. In the future, a better informed public may be better equipped to deal with such issues.

The euthanasia debate

Patient autonomy is at the heart of the euthanasia debate. If a perfectly competent individual with a distressing and terminal condition wants their life to end for palliative reasons, respecting their autonomy would seem to encourage us to comply. At the moment it is acceptable for doctors to withhold life-saving treatments from such patients but it is not acceptable in the UK to actively hasten death. Some people feel that any kind of killing is wrong, others that such a practice is open to unacceptable abuse, or that it would damage the trust that patients have in doctors. As with so many medical issues, this is something that society, rather than doctors alone, must address. Life-saving treatments can lawfully be withheld from an incompetent patient, who is severely and irreversibly brain damaged and deemed incapable of any future self-determination, or from an individual irretrievably

01

close to death on the basis that neither has an interest in their life being prolonged.

Respect for patient confidentiality

Patients divulge very personal information to health care workers on the—often tacit—assumption that the information will be treated with discretion. We should always make it clear to patients with whom we need to share their details and acquire consent to do so. Usually, this means other clinical team members involved in the patient's care. We should make every effort to avoid unnecessarily disclosing patient details. We do not need to identify patients we present in clinical meetings or for teaching purposes. In addition, we should be careful that we cannot be overheard when legitimately discussing patient details with our colleagues.

If a patient withholds consent to our sharing their medical details, then we must weigh up the cost–benefit of breaking or maintaining their confidence and inform them of our decision. In these situations, we are often weighing up the interests of our patient with those of particular or unknown other people. For example, a clinician might inform the authorities that a patient with uncontrolled epilepsy is continuing to drive, on the basis that the cost of the damage to the doctor–patient relationship is outweighed by the benefit of reducing the risk of possibly fatal accidents.

The law requires us to inform outside agencies in the case of certain infectious diseases, suspected terrorist activities or in response to certain court orders. The issue of patient competence is also a factor in issues of confidentiality—if a patient is not able to make decisions in their own interest because of an intellectual incapacity, perhaps because they are too young, or demented or psychotic, then one is justified in discussing their medical problems with their guardian, carer or legal custodian.

Fairness and equity

Most health systems have a notion that all patients should be treated with equal respect and priority should be given only according to clinical need. We certainly should not make judgements about people or offer privileged access to health care or our time on the basis of class, education, ethnic group, lifestyle habits or our personal reactions to the patients as individuals. We will all have patients we like and patients we dislike, but these feelings should not determine the kind of care we deliver.

Just use of resources

At all levels, our clinical practice has resource implications. At senior management levels we might deal with some very frank rationing issues. It is naive to think that in conditions of finite resources hard decisions can be

avoided. The principle of the 'maximization of utility' is a useful guide in these circumstances. This principle dictates that the course of action that produces the greatest good to the greatest number should be followed. This provides a means of ranking or prioritizing health care interventions so that precious resources are used to the greatest effect. Even at non-managerial level we all have a responsibility in this regard. Consider the following scenarios:

- 100 cataract operations restore 100 people to independent functioning and 10 hip replacements restore independence to 10 individuals but cost the same amount. If other factors are considered equal and pain and disability is controlled and costed then, according to the principle of the maximization of utility, the cataract operations should be chosen.
- A surgeon decides to perform coronary artery bypass surgery on a non-smoker rather than on a committed smoker with an otherwise similar profile, on the basis that the outcome for the former is likely to be better than for the latter.

Cost effectiveness is a duty incumbent on us all. A respect for resources underlies the imperative for a clinician to choose the cheapest efficacious drug or therapy for an individual patient. Our time is also a valuable resource and can be rationed along cost–benefit lines. For example, you may have a patient with a particularly complex psychological problem and thus justify spending an hour of hard-pressed clinic time with them in order to get a clear picture and embark on an effective management plan. This will save you time and the patient distress in the long run. By the same cost–benefit token, you might decide to limit how much time you continue to spend with your insoluble hypochondriac patients.

In some cases, the concept of the quality adjusted life year (QALY) has been useful. This is a way of assessing the usefulness of an intervention, by grading not only the quantity of extra years of life that an intervention provides, but also the quality of these extra years. It may seem an odd idea to do this, but consider a treatment for severe stroke that kept patients alive for an extra year but left them completely paralysed and comatose. The quality of this extra year would be very low and an analysis using QALYs would probably conclude that the treatment should not be introduced. However, in less extreme cases, it may be an insensitive way of assessing the benefit of a treatment.

The final arbiters of health priorities need not be clinicians. Society at large, if adequately informed, might be the most appropriate judge, as the resources expended are often from the common purse.

Maintaining professional competence

No individual clinician has perfect knowledge, perfect

skill or perfect judgement. However, we are required to have a certain standard of each of these features and, in the UK, the required standard is set by the medical profession itself. This is partly via the guidance published by the General Medical Council (GMC) and partly by the law's use of peer opinion in establishing acceptable medical practice when cases reach the courts. On the whole, we should be as good as our closest peers. For instance, if a patient has erythema nodosum it would be acceptable for a GP to decide that the patient has a rash of some significance and refer them to a dermatologist. It would not be acceptable for the dermatologist to fail to make a definitive diagnosis.

During our professional lives, all of us will have bad outcomes; some of these are inherent in the natural histories of the problems we deal with and the risk assessments we make and some result from our mistakes. The law allows us to make the mistakes a competent colleague would make. However, the onus is on us to maintain an acceptable level of competence. This requires ongoing active input and includes the following elements:
- Keeping up-to-date with developments in the field
- Making the most constructive use of continued professional development and appraisal processes
- Ensuring that we are trained in any new tasks we start performing
- Ensuring that we are physically and mentally fit to practise (doctors have an above average rate of alcohol and drug addiction)
- Responding to mistakes in a constructive manner
- Identifying and addressing weak areas
- Identifying significant substandard practice in colleagues and activating appropriate remedial measures

Improving skills in ethical decision making

Ethical issues affect a wide range of clinical decisions, but may be more obvious in some cases. The clinical decision maker needs to be aware of these moral dimensions to a problem and needs to be able to analyse them by identifying key principles, such as respect for patient autonomy, a duty to act in the patient's best interests and fairness in the use of resources. Most ethically challenging medical scenarios involve more than one of these issues. When these concerns are in conflict, they can be weighed against each other with a cost–benefit analysis or maximization of utility consideration. The weighting of each factor varies according to the particular situation and the decision maker.

Respect for confidentiality and autonomy is usually our patient's interest; fairness and the maximization of utility is often an interest of other groups of patients or society as a whole. As moral decision makers, we are often perform-

ing a cost–benefit analysis between these conflicting interests, loaded in favour of those to whom we feel we have the greatest duty. This is usually the patient before us. It is useful to discuss each case with as many of the relevant parties as confidentiality allows. This ensures that all viewpoints are considered and everyone feels that their position has been taken into account. It is also worth discussing matters in an anonymous way with colleagues and trusted lay people who may have useful and objective perspectives to offer. One may need to take time to establish the correct course of action, if the medical circumstances allow.

Regardless of the number of opinions we consider or perspectives, there remains an inevitable subjectivity to our judgement. We should be aware of any strong beliefs we hold that may bias our judgement. For example, a doctor may disagree with abortion on religious grounds. If this is relevant to the case, it might be appropriate to explain this to the patient and ask another colleague to take over their management.

The more we recognize the moral dimensions of our work, the more competent we will become in addressing them. This will give us a richer appreciation of the challenges inherent in clinical practice.

Life-long learning

After medical school, most doctors, whether in hospital or community practice, take further professional examinations during a training period that can range around 4–12 years. In the UK, each clinician must usually pass a set of examinations that admits them to a specialist college and enables them to practise as a specialist consultant or assistant specialist. After this training period, there is mandatory continuing medical education and revalidation to ensure that doctors remain up-to-date with scientific and clinical developments relevant to their field. Not only is the scientific and evidence basis of medicine always changing, but our roles may also change as we become more senior in the profession. We need to be alert to our changing educational requirements and resourceful in meeting them. They might include:
- Keeping up-to-date with scientific and clinical literature
- Keeping up-to date with the latest advice from the Chief Medical Officer, NICE or college guidelines
- Training in a new or modified procedure
- Acquiring new research or audit skills
- Acquiring people management or leadership skills
- Learning more about a particular patient group
- Learning teaching skills
- Improving communication skills

Portfolio learning can facilitate continuing education. In this system, an individual clinician keeps records of educational milestones met and identifies goals to be achieved in order to fulfil specified aims pertinent to their practice. The means proposed to achieve these goals are also documented. These might include:

- Reading journals in paper or electronic versions
- Attending courses
- Taking correspondence courses
- Videotaping consultations
- Auditing certain aspects of personal practice
- Seeking advice from colleagues
- Organizing meetings

Regular meetings with an educational mentor or a small group of colleagues can facilitate this process. The latter practice can be both a source of information and stimulation and also an effective support system. This is an important function, as senior clinicians are often in danger of being professionally isolated. Taking responsibility for our own continuing education is not only a professional requirement, it is also the means by which we continue to be interested in our work and develop both as clinical practitioners and as individuals.

Further reading

Books

Armstrong D. *Political Anatomy of the Body: Medical Knowledge in Britain in the Twentieth Century.* Cambridge: Cambridge University Press, 1983. [A consideration of the cultural context in which medicine is practised and understood.]

Atkinson P. *The Clinical Experience: The Construction and Reconstruction of Medical Reality.* Farnborough: Gower, 1981. [Similar to Armstrong.]

Berger J, Mohr J. *A Fortunate Man: The Story of a Country Doctor.* London: Allen Lane, 1967. [An extended illustrated essay about the role of a twentieth century doctor as healer in a remote impoverished rural community in England.]

Boyd KM, ed. *The New Dictionary of Medical Ethics.* London: BMJ Publishing, 1997. [A consideration of ethical aspects of medical practice.]

General Medical Council (GMC). *Good Medical Practice*, 3rd edn. London: GMC, 2001. [An exploration of the values and aims desirable in the modern doctor.]

Glover J. *Causing Deaths and Saving Lives.* Harmondsworth: Penguin, 1977.

Launer J. *Narrative-based Primary Care: A Practical Guide.* Abingdon: Radcliffe Medical Press, 2002. [A thought-provoking exploration of the ways in which doctors and patients construct stories about health and illness.]

Morgan M, Calnan M, Manning N. *Sociological Approaches to Health and Medicine.* London: Croom Helm, 1985.

Myerscough P. *Talking with Patients: A Basic Clinical Skill.* Oxford: Oxford University Press, 1989. [A slim volume concentrating on communication skills and the special considerations needed when talking with patients from particular groups, for example the elderly or adolescents.]

Neighbour R. *The Inner Consultation: How to Develop an Effective and Intuitive Consulting Style.* Netherlands: 1987. [This book emphasizes self-awareness and self-development of the clinician. It uses a lot of example dialogues and has an informal style. It breaks the consultation down into stages of a linear process.]

Ogden J. *Health Psychology.* Buckingham: Open University Press, 2000. [A psychological perspective on doctors' and patients' health beliefs and health behaviour.]

Pendleton D. *The Consultation: An Approach to Learning and Teaching.* Oxford: Oxford University Press, 1984. [This starts with a discussion of different models of the consultation: medical, psychological, sociological and anthropological. It defines the tasks, skills and strategies involved in the consultation and discusses the relevant evidence from research. Also explored are the means by which we learn and then teach consultation skills.]

Royal College of General Practitioners (RCCP). *What Sort of Doctor?* London: RCGP, 1985. [A discussion of the values and aims doctors should have.]

Sackett DL, Straus SE, Richardson WS, Rosenberg W, Haynes RB. *Evidence-Based Medicine: How to Practice and Teach EBM*, 2nd edn. London: Churchill Livingstone, 2000.

Stewart M *et al. Patient-Centred Medicine: Transforming the Clinical Method*, 2nd edn. Abingdon: Radcliffe Medical Press, 2002. [A full explanation of patient-centred medicine and how to practise it.]

Journals

British Medical Journal. What is a good doctor and how do you make one? (Theme Issue) *Br Med J* 2002; 325: Issue 7366.

British Medical Journal. Communicating risks: illusion or truth? (Theme Issue) *Br Med J* 2003; 327: Issue 7414.

British Medical Journal. From compliance to concordance. (Theme Issue) *Br Med J* 2003; 327: Issue 7419.

Websites

National Institute for Clinical Excellence: www.nice.org.uk
US National Institutes of Health medical site: www.ncbi.nlm.nih.gov/Entrez/
General Medical Council: www.gmc-uk.org

The Scientific Basis of Medicine

2

Introduction

Science provides a basis for rational clinical medicine. Improvements in modern medicine require the thorough scientific evaluation of potential therapies and have usually followed the careful application of science to clinical problems. The application of science in medicine must be conducted within a caring and compassionate framework as discussed in Chapter 1. The combination of the themes of good science and caring clinical practice recur throughout this book. In this chapter, we outline some of the scientific foundations upon which so much of modern medicine is based. These should serve as a quick précis of important concepts and provide a framework for understanding later chapters.

Organization

An ability to maintain an organism as large and complex as the human body requires many interactions between specialized features. Our bodies are composed of organs, tissues and cells, each fulfilling their own particular role. Vital functions (for example, nutrition, excretion and respiration) are implemented by **organ systems** whose functional units cooperate to provide for that need. **Organs** are formed from a combination of four **tissue** categories. Of these, **epithelial tissue**, arranged in one layer (**simple epithelium**) or multiple layers (**stratified epithelium**) forms the lining of all body surfaces. Consistent with their protective function, epithelial cells are packed tightly together and are polar in nature. **Connective tissue** has a supportive role and is found embedded within an extracellular matrix. **Muscle tissue** comprises specialized cells that are capable of contraction, allowing them to power movement and perform mechanical work. Muscle fibres are usually bound into groups by connective tissue. Highly excitable **nerve tissue** is specialized to transmit impulses. **Cells** are the basic structural unit of all living organisms. However, patterns of functional organization continue well beyond the boundary of the cell membrane.

Evolutionary pressures have selected a blueprint to provide all the functions necessary to maintain life at this basic level. Every cell contains a framework system of essential organelles, which are further partitioned into functional domains.

Biological macromolecules

Nucleic acids

Genetic information is stored and transferred in the form of the nucleic acids **deoxyribonucleic acid** (**DNA**) and **ribonucleic acid** (**RNA**). These molecules also provide the necessary information for protein production. Like many biological molecules, nucleic acids are multimers of smaller units; in this case known as nucleotides. Each **nucleotide** unit contains a 5-carbon sugar (pentose), a phosphate group and a nitrogenous base (Fig. 2.1a). A set of four nucleotide components is used to generate DNA or RNA. Two **purines**, **adenine** (**A**) and **guanine** (**G**) are common to both DNA and RNA. **Cytosine** (**C**) and **thymine** (**T**) are the **pyrimidine** bases found in DNA. Thymine is absent from RNA with **uracil** (**U**) present in its place.

The common unit of heredity for higher organisms is DNA, named for its deoxyribose sugar. DNA strands consist of nucleotides joined by **phosphodiester bonds** linking the sugar of one nucleotide to the phosphate group of the next. At one end of the molecule the terminal nucleotide carries a free 5′ pentose position and at the other end a free 3′ position. Nucleic acids are conventionally notated in the 5′-3′ direction. According to the structure determined by Watson and Crick in 1953, DNA coils into a **double helix** of two antiparallel strands (Fig. 2.1b). The **sugar–phosphate backbone** provides structural support, while the sequence of purine–pyrimidine bases encodes genetic information. To maintain stability, DNA strands are held together by **hydrogen bonding** between their constituent bases. **Complementary base pairing** of purine–pyrimidine dimers—adenine with thymine, and guanine with cytosine—also ensures the fidelity of DNA transcription and replication. When DNA is copied, each parental strand acts as a template for **semiconservative replication**: incoming nucleotides hydrogen bond to an appropriate base on the template strand. Base mispairing induced by damage or mutation introduces structural alterations to the molecule which can be detected and/or removed by a range of specific repair proteins. Defective excision repair is responsible for the ultraviolet-induced lesions seen in patients with xeroderma pigmentosum.

In addition to its sugar component, RNA differs from DNA in that it usually exists as a single strand. RNA is a versatile molecule that is fundamental to protein synthesis. During this process it appears in several functionally distinct forms. A number of viruses use RNA as their hereditary material; retroviruses such as human immunodeficiency virus (HIV) encode their genome on a single strand of RNA which is reverse transcribed into DNA in an infected cell.

Proteins

Proteins are long chains of **amino acids** held together by peptide bonds. Amino acids are composed of an amino group, a carboxyl group and the particular side-chain that defines their chemical nature (Fig. 2.2). Individual proteins are constructed from a library of 20 amino acids, which may be subgrouped according to the acidic, basic,

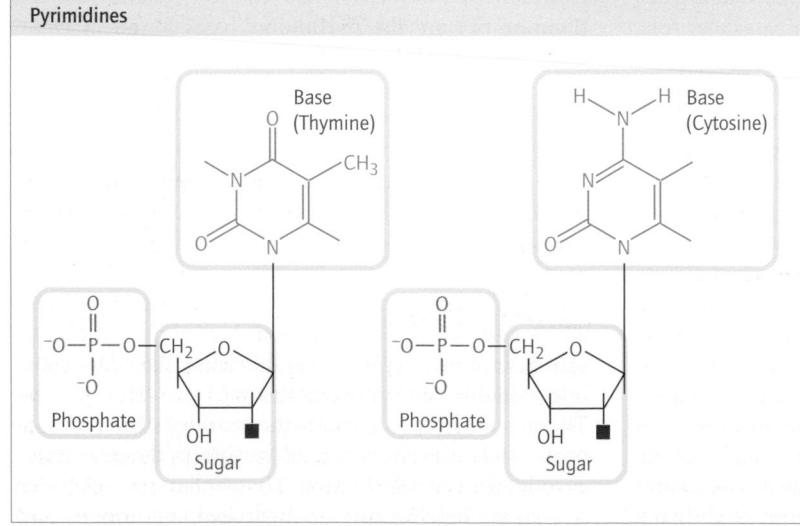

(a)

Figure 2.1 Nucleotides and nucleic acid structure. (a) Nucleotide subunits. Each nucleotide is composed of a base, a sugar and a phosphate group. For DNA, the position marked by the red square is taken by hydrogen and for RNA by a hydroxyl (OH) group.

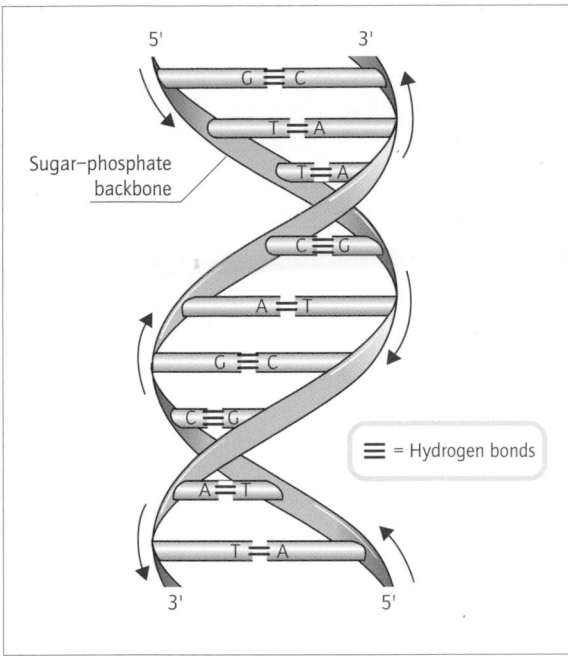

(b)

Figure 2.1 (*cont'd*) (b) The DNA double helix.

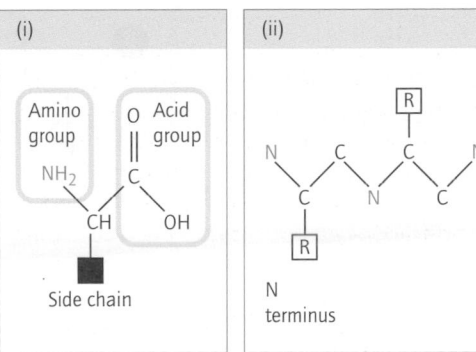

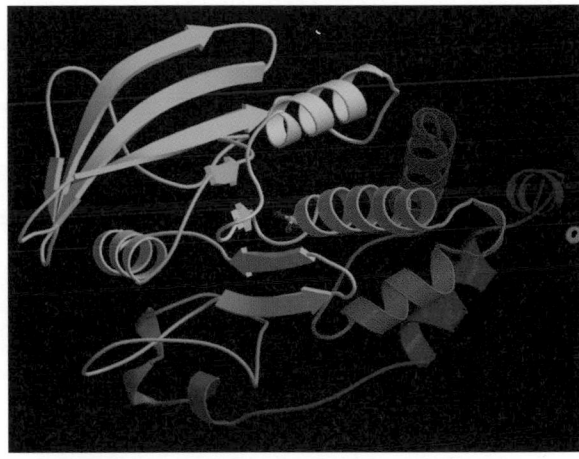

(iii)

Figure 2.2 (i) Amino acid side-chains (designated by a black box) may be acidic, basic or hydrophobic in nature. (ii) Amino acids join to form a polypeptide chain. (iii) Protein secondary structure is composed of α-helices and β-sheets, both of which can be seen in the structure of human tyrosine phosphatase 1B. An example of an α-helix is shown in red and an example of a β-sheet is shown in green.

uncharged polar or non-polar character of their side-chains. Four structural terms are used to describe proteins (Fig. 2.2). **Primary structure** refers to the number and sequence of amino acids, and the number of peptide chains. Like all large molecules, proteins adopt an energy-dependent conformation that confers the most stability. The spatial configuration of nearby amino acids is known as **secondary structure**. Two particularly stable conformations known as **α-helices** and **β-sheets** are a common feature of secondary structure. Within an α-helix, hydrogen bonds form between residues lying three positions apart in the chain. In a β-sheet, hydrogen bonds form between adjacent polypeptide chains. Beyond the level of secondary structure, α-helices and β-sheets can themselves assemble into complex shapes that determine the chemical nature of individual parts of a protein. Amino acids lying far apart in the linear sequence may be brought into close spatial contact; for example, to form active sites on enzymes. This, the **tertiary structure**, generates local areas of hydrophobic or charged polar residues. Two or more polypeptide chains can interact to form a multisubunit **quaternary structure**, as happens in haemoglobin molecules. Further modifications result from the addition of other substances to form **conjugated proteins**. Prosthetic groups include metal ions (for example,

iron in haemoglobin), carbohydrates (glycoproteins) or lipids (lipoproteins) and may be essential for protein function.

Carbohydrates

Members of this family of organic compounds are composed of carbon, hydrogen and oxygen with a general formula $C_x(H_2O)_y$. Carbohydrates range from simple **monosaccharides** of 3–6 carbons to large complex **polysaccharides** (Fig. 2.3). Monosaccharides are aldehydes or ketones bearing two or more hydroxyl groups and can be characterized according to their number of carbon

02

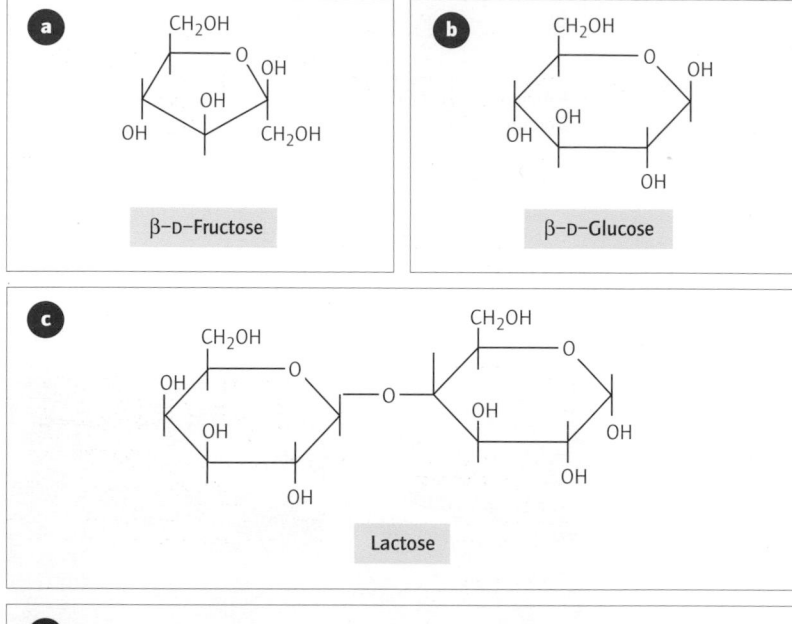

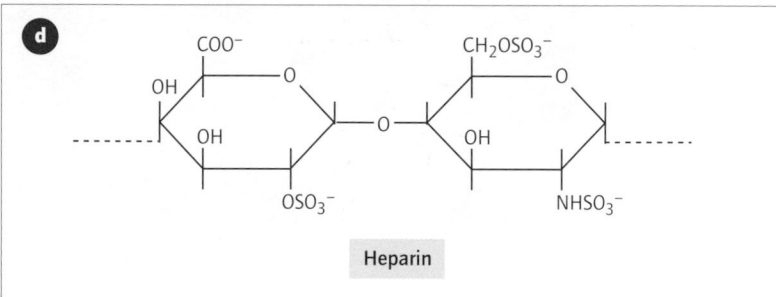

Figure 2.3 Carbohydrate structures. Most common monosaccharides adopt a ring conformation in aqueous solution. (a) Fructose and (b) glucose are examples of 5-carbon (pentose) and 6-carbon (hexose) monosaccharides, respectively. (c) Lactose is a disaccharide formed from galactose and glucose subunits. (d) Heparin is a polysaccharide formed from a series of acidic disaccharide units.

atoms. For example, glucose and fructose are 6-carbon sugar (hexose) isomers of one another. Derivative monosaccharides such as glucosamine and glucose-6-phosphate contain other elements in the form of phosphate or amino groups. As their name suggests, **disaccharides** and **trisaccharides** contain two or three monosaccharide units bound together. **Polysaccharides** can form complex structures. Unlike proteins, their primary structure need not be linear and, as a result, large branched structures can occur. Glycoproteins are usually generated by covalent attachment of carbohydrate groups to either the NH_2 group of the amino acid asparagine (*N*-linkage) or the OH group of threonine or serine (*O*-linkage).

The clinical relevance of glycosylation is the subject of much study. Some diseases, such as cancers and arthritis, may have characteristic patterns of glycosylation, which could be useful for their diagnosis and for predicting prognosis. In some cases, bacteria interact with their hosts using carbohydrate groups or carbohydrate recognizing proteins. Carbohydrate groups may also interact with inflammatory cytokines. The possibility of modulating the synthesis of carbohydrate molecules and glycosylation to treat disease is being actively explored.

Long-term complications associated with diabetes can result from hyperglycaemia. In a non-enzymatic process, glucose attaches to the amino group of proteins such as collagen; for example, in blood cell walls. Consequent chemical rearrangements generate irreversible advanced glycosylation end products (**AGE**). This process may be reflected in the levels of glycosylated haemoglobin circulating through the blood. AGE have a range of pathological effects including peptide cross-linking. Recognition of AGE by cell surface receptors can trigger various biological activities and may contribute to tissue damage.

Lipids

Lipids constitute the fourth major type of biological molecules. Their structural units are fatty acids, containing

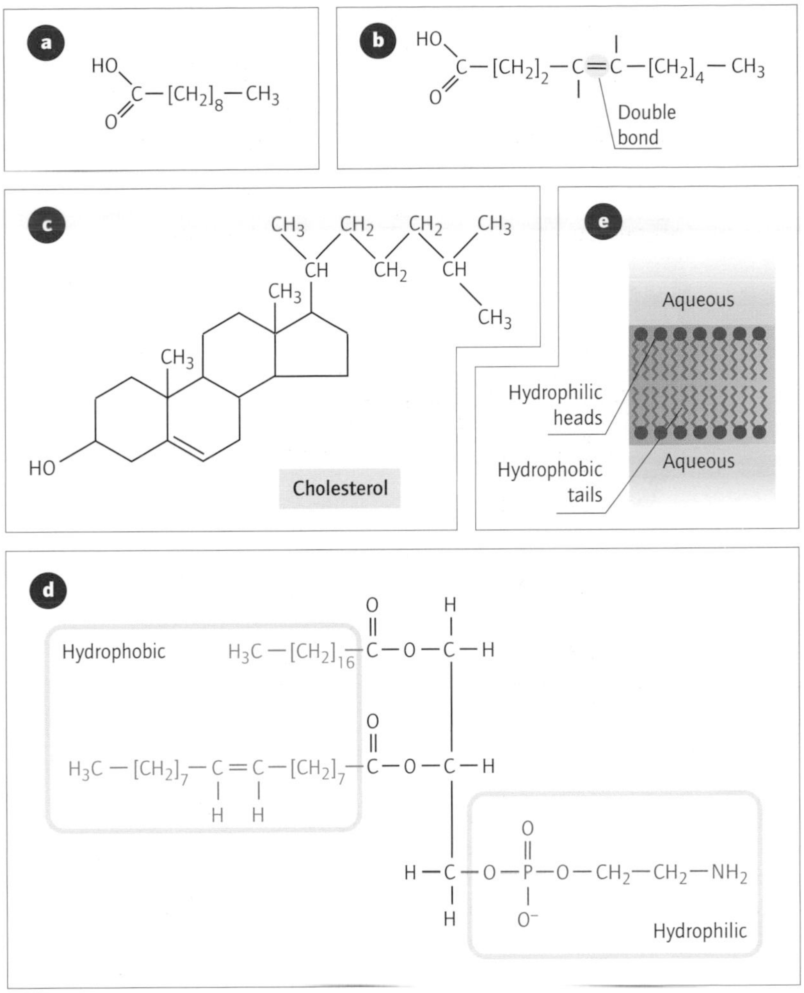

Figure 2.4 Lipids. (a) Saturated and (b) unsaturated fatty acids are termed according to the presence of double bonds within their hydrocarbon tail. (c) Steroid molecules such as cholesterol are based on a skeleton of four carbon rings. (d) Phospholipids are amphipathic molecules with two hydrophobic (green) hydrocarbon tails attached to a hydrophilic polar head group (blue). (e) In aqueous solution, phospholipids form a bilayer with a hydrophobic interior. This arrangement forms the basis for eukaryotic cellular membranes.

long chains of 4–24 carbon atoms joined to a carboxylic acid group (Fig. 2.4). Fatty acids may be **saturated** or **non-saturated** depending on the presence of double bonds within their hydrocarbon tail. **Polyunsaturated** fatty acids contain multiple double bonds. One of the most important *in vivo* functions performed by lipids is the formation of cellular membranes. **Phospholipids** contain a hydrophilic phosphate group, linked by glycerol to a hydrophobic fatty acid tail (Fig. 2.4). The amphipathic nature of phospholipids allows them to form a sealed membrane bilayer in aqueous solution. Another physiologically important group of lipids are the cholesterol derivatives (steroids). These molecules contain four hydrocarbon rings (Fig. 2.4), one of which carries a hydroxyl group to confer an amphipathic nature on the molecule.

Cell biology

Life and death of the cell

Cell structure

Cells are defined as the basic structural unit of all living organisms. Each is suitably equipped with the means to maintain itself within the organism and interact with other cells and body systems. Subcellular organelles compartmentalize various cellular process such as respiration or digestion (Fig. 2.5). Eukaryotic cells possess a standard set of organelles, although relative organelle sizes may vary according to cell specialization. For example, a large proportion of the B-lymphocyte-derived plasma cell is taken up with protein production machinery in order to fulfil its antibody secretory functions.

02

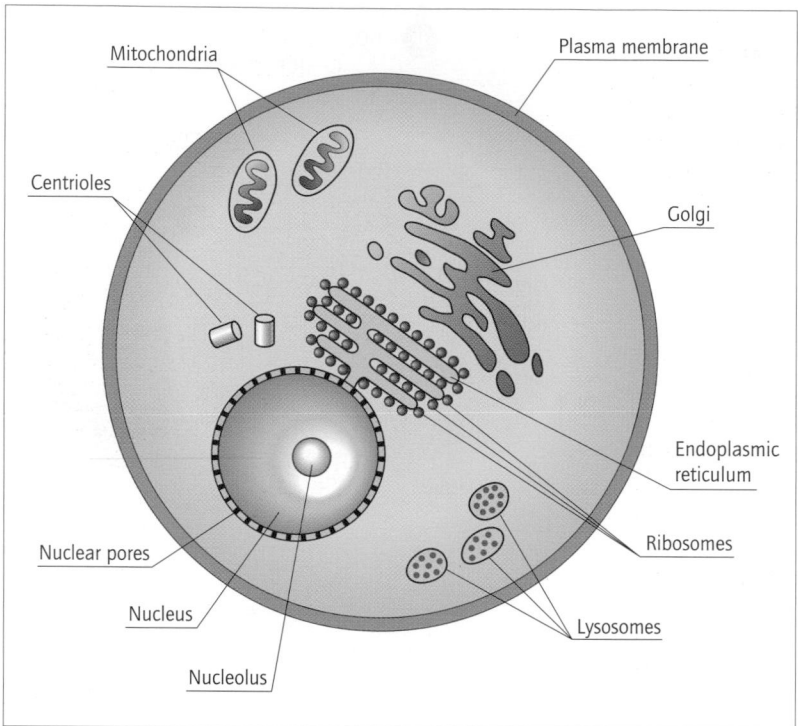

Mitochondria

Plasma membrane

Centrioles

Golgi

Endoplasmic
reticulum

Nuclear pores

Ribosomes

Nucleus

Lysosomes

Nucleolus

Figure 2.5 Cell structure.

An outer phospholipid **plasma membrane** separates a cell from the outside world. Membrane phosopholipids form a bilayer with a core of hydrocarbon side-chains. The amphipathic nature of this structure allows proteins to anchor themselves within the membrane using stretches of hydrophobic amino acids. **Transmembrane proteins** whose N terminus lies outside the cell are termed **Group 1** membrane proteins; **Group 2** proteins show a reversed orientation. Some proteins can span the membrane several times. In the absence of a hydrophobic anchor, proteins may still attach themselves to the cell membrane through a glycosylphosphatidylinositol (**GPI**) link. The fluid nature of membrane lipids allows proteins to move around the cell surface. GPI-linked proteins in particular can relocate themselves in structures known as **membrane rafts** to facilitate cellular signalling.

Containing all the necessary machinery for protein synthesis, the **cytosol** is the site of many cellular reactions. Components of the cytosol maintain the structure of the cell and provide transport, structure, motility and storage. A **cytoskeleton** of microfilaments, intermediate filaments and microtubules provides physical support for the various organelles and forms transport routes between them. Chemically heterogeneous **intermediate filaments** of keratin, desmin and vimentin extend from the nucleus to the cell surface. **Microtubules** of α and β tubulin exist in equilibrium with a pool of cytosolic monomers, allowing

rapid polymerization in response to various stimuli. These fibres have an important role in cell division and organelle movement. The major constituents of cellular contractile machinery are actin-based **microfilaments**, which are intimately involved in cell division, movement, muscle contraction and other processes.

The membrane-bound **nucleus** acts as a store for genetic information, determining the biochemical activity of a cell through gene transcription. Nuclear pores facilitate exchange of protein and RNA between the nucleus and the rest of the cell. A small dense **nucleolus**, rich in RNA and protein, is visible in non-dividing cell nuclei. This structure is responsible for the generation of ribosome components. **Centrioles** are located just outside the nucleus. During cell division, these structures form the poles of the mitotic spindle, separating two sets of DNA for daughter cells (see p. 30).

The **endoplasmic reticulum** (ER) is a system of folded membranes, continuous with the outer membrane of the nucleus. It is defined as **smooth** or **rough** depending on the presence or absence of ribosomes on its outer surface. The presence of ribosomes reflects the role of the ER in protein synthesis. Newly formed proteins destined for transport to lysosomes or the cell surface are inserted through the ER membrane as they are translated. Once inside, they may engage **chaperones** to facilitate protein folding. One of the best characterized chaperone families are the **heat shock proteins** (HSPs), which assist folding of newly synthesized proteins or those that have become denatured as a consequence of cellular stress. Initial **protein glycosylation** may also occur within the ER. From the ER, proteins progress through a related system of membrane compartments known as the **Golgi complex**, where further modifications such as carbohydrate trimming take place. The Golgi complex also sorts macromolecules for transport to other cellular compartments and, on leaving it, proteins progress through a system of vesicles until they reach their ultimate location.

Endocytosed proteins and other materials are degraded within membrane-bound **lysosomes**, which store the hydrolytic enzymes required for such degradation. To optimize the enzymatic activity of their hydrolytic enzymes, lysosomes maintain an acid pH. **Tay–Sachs disease** is a neurological disorder associated with the deficiency of a lysosomal hexosaminidase. The resulting accumulation of ganglioside in the brain triggers neural degeneration leading to early death.

Mitochondria are the powerhouses of the cell. These maternally inherited organelles carry their own small genome encoding various components of the respiratory process. Two membranes divide mitochondria into separate compartments. The inner membrane is heavily folded to form **cisternae**, thus generating a relatively large surface area. Enzymes of the **Krebs' cycle** are contained within the inner compartment while those of the **electron transport chain** are found on the inner membrane (Fig. 2.6). Pyruvic acid generated by glycolysis is transported into the inner compartment, where it is converted into acetyl coenzyme A (CoA) and enters the Krebs' cycle. Adenosine triphosphate (ATP) products of the Krebs' cycle are pumped from the mitochondria into the cytosol. Nicotinamide adenine dinucleotide (NAD) carries its electrons to the inner membrane where it enters the electron transport chain. The flow of H^+ ions from outer to the inner compartments is used to generate further ATP from adenosine diphosphate (ADP).

Cell division
Mitosis
In order to divide successfully, a cell must copy its DNA then organize this into chromosomes so that each daughter cell receives its full set of chromosomes. This is achieved by a tightly regulated mitosis following the cell cycle pathway (Fig. 2.7). Passage through the cell cycle is controlled by members of the **cyclin** protein family, in a cascade of phosphorylation events. **Cyclins** accumulate through the cell cycle and are destroyed after mitosis. Each cyclin acts as a catalytic subunit in partnership with a cyclin-dependent kinase (**CDK**). Upon cyclin binding, CDKs start to phosphorylate target proteins that are

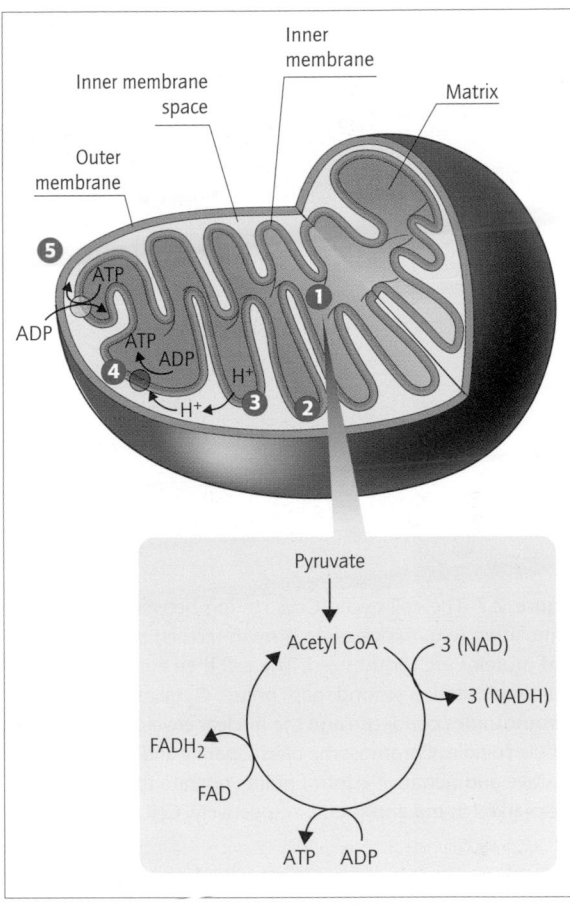

Figure 2.6 Mitochondria. (1) Pyruvic acid generated by glycolysis in the cytosol is converted to acetyl CoA which enters Krebs' (citric acid) cycle in the mitochondrial matrix. (2) Enzymes such as reduced nicotinamide adenine dinucleotide (NADH) reductase on the inner mitochondrial membrane transfer electrons from energy-rich products of Krebs' cycle to oxygen. (3) Energy released from this transfer is used to pump protons into the intermembrane space. (4) Protons return to the mitochondrial matrix through the adenosine triphosphate (ATP) synthase complex, which harnesses energy generated by their passage down the pH and electrochemical gradient to produce ATP. (5) The ATP–ADP translocase transfers ATP molecules from the mitochondria into the cytoplasm in exchange for adenosine diphosphate (ADP), thus coupling cytoplasmic ADP : ATP ratios with mitochondrial ADP : ATP ratios.

required for cell cycle progression. CDK-specific inhibitors (**CDKIs**) bind cyclin–CDK complexes to regulate their activity. CDKIs can themselves be regulated by other proteins. Various checkpoints ensure that every part of the mitotic process is completed correctly before the next stage begins. The cell does not commit to division until the end of the G_2 phase. During mitosis, one of each

02

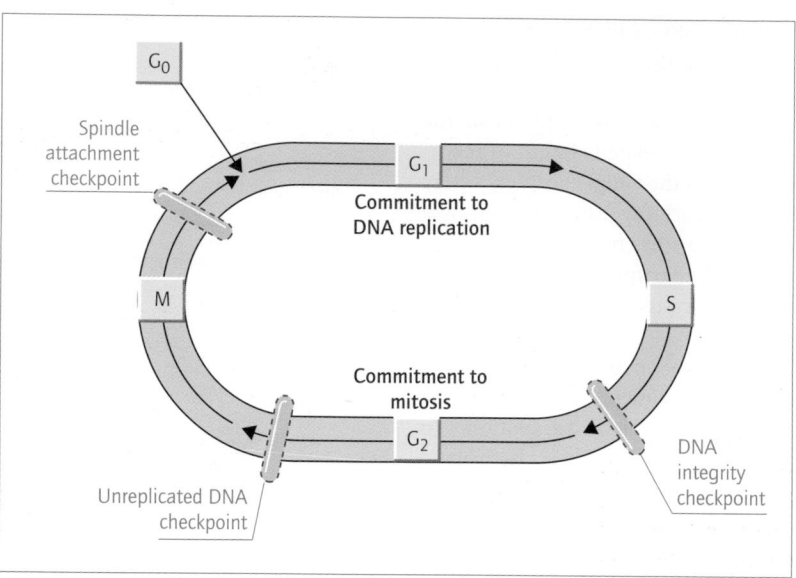

Figure 2.7 The cell cycle. Cells resting between divisions are held indefinitely in the quiescent (**G₀**) phase. Upon appropriate stimulation (e.g. exposure to growth factors) cells enter 'gap 1' (**G₁**), the first stage of the cell cycle, during which various RNAs and proteins are synthesized. The cell then enters a period of DNA synthesis termed the 'S phase'. Once each chromosome has been replicated, a second 'gap' phase, **G₂** takes place. When the cell is ready to divide, mitosis begins (**M** phase). During mitosis, chromosomes condense and the nuclear envelope breaks down, allowing paired chromosomes to attach to centrioles by a micro-tubule spindle. Chromosome pairs separate and are moved to opposite ends of the cell preceding cytoplasmic division (cytokinesis). Positive and negative control points operate throughout the cell cycle. Various commitment points and regulatory checkpoints are marked in red and green, respectively. Cell cycle control proteins include p21, p53 and Rb (the retinoblastoma protein).

chromosome pair becomes attached to a centriole by microtubules. Centrioles move to opposite ends of the cell, taking the chromosomes with them. Because uncontrolled proliferation is a hallmark of cancer, the cell cycle provides an obvious target for therapy. CDKIs often act as tumour suppressors and are potentially useful anticancer agents.

Meiosis

A more specialized form of cell division generates gametes bearing a single set of chromosomes for reproduction. **Meiosis** requires two rounds of cell division. DNA replication occurs during a complex prophase in the first round of division. As a means to increase genetic diversity, a physical exchange of genetic material takes place when equivalent or homologous DNA regions of the sister chromatids crossover during early meiosis. These crossover points or **chiasmata** become visible as the two chromatids begin to separate. Sister chromatids part during the second division, which proceeds without an interphase. Serious genetic diseases, such as Down's syndrome, can arise if a cell does not receive its correct quota of chromosomes or if there is inappropriate loss of part of a chromosome during meiosis. Mitochondria are carried within the cytoplasm of the female gamete (which, upon fertilization,

becomes the cytoplasm of the embryo) and are therefore maternally inherited. As mitochondria contain their own genetic material (see p. 29), there are a number of rare genetic disorders that result from maternal inheritance of mitochondrial DNA mutations. Some of these mutations cause muscle diseases or myopathies as the highly efficient energy generation required for muscle function is impaired.

Apoptosis

As a counterpoint to cell division, an effective mechanism is required to remove cells that are no longer necessary. Controlled cell death is generally known as **apoptosis** or programmed cell death (Fig. 2.8). Apoptosis is particularly relevant for clearing unwanted populations of cells, carving out tissues during development or removing damaged cells. Unlike necrotic cell death, cells undergoing apoptosis follow a carefully controlled programme of events allowing the cell to condense its cytoskeleton and fragment its DNA. Apoptosis is driven in a proteolytic cascade by members of the caspase protein family. Bcl proteins provide a control mechanism to regulate caspase activity. Programmed cell death can be triggered in response to cell surface signals or mitochondrial stress. Following ligand binding, cell-surface death receptors

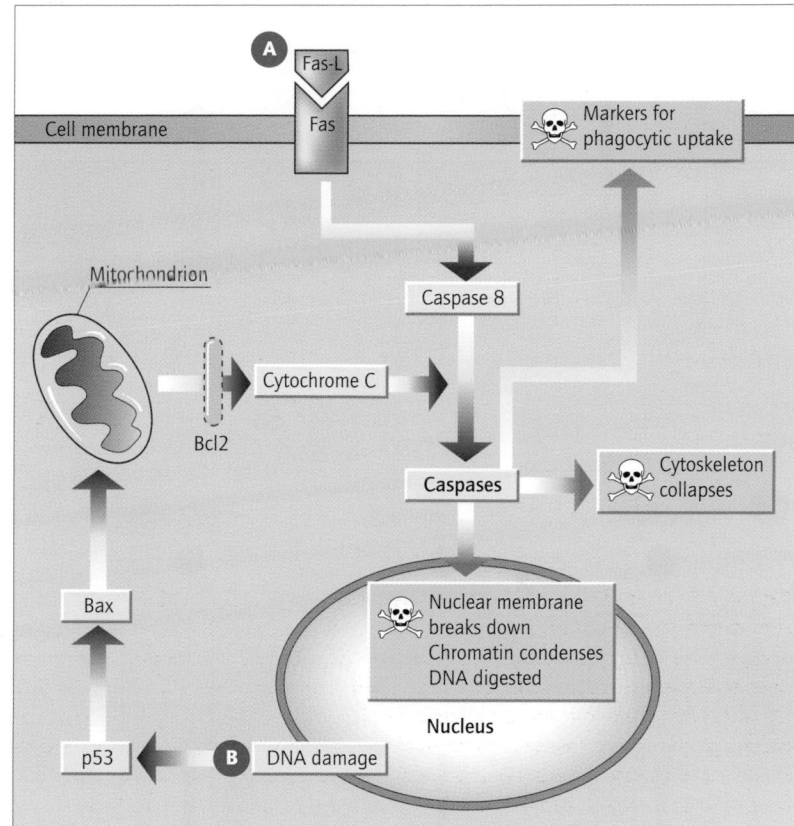

02

Figure 2.8 Apoptosis. There are two major pathways of apoptosis. (A) Death signals from cell surface receptors such as Fas (CD95) trigger activation of caspase 8 to initiate a signalling cascade through downstream enzymes. Mitochondria host a range of pro-apoptotic factors including cytochrome C, which is necessary for downstream caspase activation. A second apoptotic pathway (B) operates through these organelles. Triggers such as DNA damage (signalled through p53 and Bax) initiate the release of pro-apoptotic factors from mitochondria. Bcl2 acts as an anti-apoptotic regulator of this process.

such as Fas recruit adaptor proteins to trigger procaspase activation, and thus elicit apoptosis. Mitochondria are central targets for intracellular oxidative stress and can thus initiate an alternative apoptotic pathway. Correspondingly, mitochondria have been found to host a range of pro-apoptotic proteins. A dying cell will show membrane blebbing, cell shrinkage and protein fragmentation as it collapses in upon itself. Within the nucleus, chromatin condensation and DNA degradation occur. Finally, the cell is flagged for uptake by professional macrophages or by semiprofessional neighbouring cells acting as phagocytes. Professional uptake of apoptosed cells by phagocytes can trigger the release of anti-inflammatory molecules.

Cellular homoeostasis and communication

The human body maintains a stable environment for its cells and tissues through a combination of physiological and biochemical processes. Cell membranes form a barrier to large molecules, allowing the cell to maintain a constant internal environment. Specific transport mechanisms are therefore required to transfer material in and out of the cell. Small uncharged polar molecules such as water and urea can follow concentration gradients to cross the cell membrane unaided. However, membranes contain many different proteins that actively or passively facilitate the movement of ions or molecules across membranes. Three major classes of transport protein—membrane channels, pumps and transporters—are responsible for the import or export of specific substrates (Fig. 2.9).

Membrane channels

The movement of ions across a membrane is influenced by both electrical and concentration gradients. **Membrane channels** provide a simple mechanism for transfer of ions. Movement of multiple molecules down electrical or concentration gradients allows rapid import or export of ions from the cell. The physical and chemical nature of each channel ensures that only the correct substrate can pass through. **Gated channels** allow ions to enter the cell following specific membrane stimulation. Thus, opening and closing of Na^+, K^+ and Ca^{2+} channels allows control of ionic gradients across the membrane. The coordinated opening and closing of channels is responsible for the

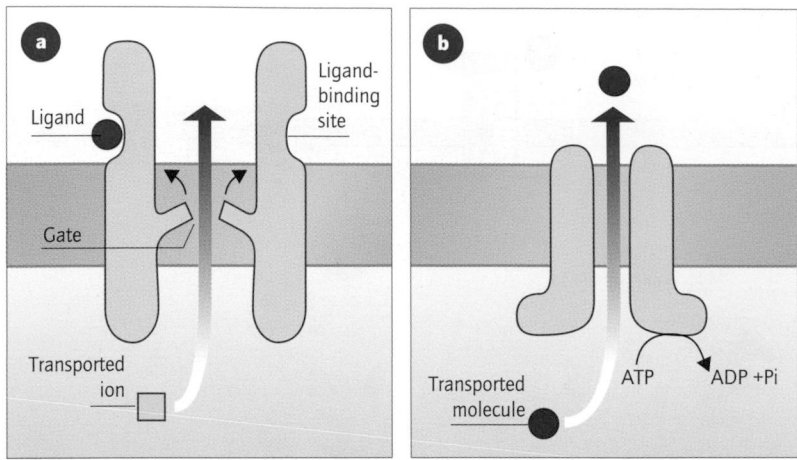

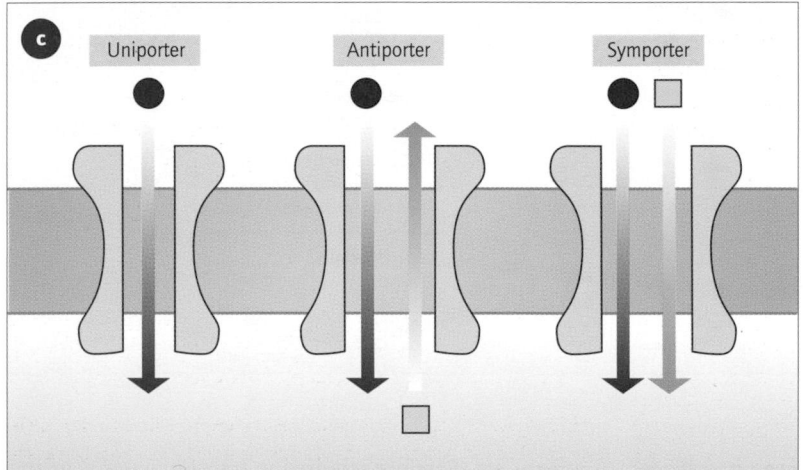

Figure 2.9 Membrane transport proteins. (a) Membrane channels allow passive transport of ions down their concentration or electrochemical gradient. For gated channels such as the acetylcholine receptor, an initial ligand-binding event is required to activate ion flow. (b) Pumps use energy generated by ATP hydrolysis to transfer solutes across the membrane. (c) Symporters such as the Na^+–glucose transporter couple transport solutes in the same direction across the membrane, for antiporters the ion and the transported molecule travel in opposite directions across the membrane.

electrical activity of nerve and muscle cells, including cardiac muscle.

Membrane pumps

Pumps use energy generated from ATP hydrolysis to move ions and small molecules, sometimes against concentration or electrical gradients. Such systems help maintain Ca^{2+} and Na^+ ion concentrations inside cells. There are four classes of ATP-driven membrane pumps. P-class ion pumps such as the Na^+/K^+ ATPase are composed of two subunits and become phosphorylated during substrate transport. Multisubunit **F- and V-class pumps** transport protons across the membrane. Finally, members of the **ATP-binding cassette (ABC) family** transport a variety of small molecules or ions. Each ABC transporter has four core domains, two of which mediate ATP binding while the other pair form a pathway through the membrane, thus determining substrate specificity. ATP hydrolysis is tightly coupled to substrate transport. Clinically

relevant members of the ATP family include multidrug resistance (MDR) proteins which expel hydrophobic drugs from the cytosol. Increased expression of MDR can provide tumours with resistance to various cytotoxic drugs. Mutations in CFTR, an ABC transporter responsible for regulation of transmembrane conductance, are associated with cystic fibrosis.

Transporters

Transporter proteins often work against their electric potential or concentration gradients to move substrates from one side of the membrane to another. Speed of transport is limited by a requirement for conformational change upon substrate binding. **Uniporters** such as the glucose transporter GLUT1 carry molecules in a single direction down their concentration gradient in a thermodynamically favourable reaction. More complex carrier proteins allow simultaneous transport of multiple substrates, combining the energetically favourable movement of one down its concentration gradient with the transport of the other against its gradient. Thus, energy stored in the electrochemical gradient of Na$^+$ or H$^+$ ions can be harnessed to drive the transport of another substrate. **Symporters** and **antiporters** carry their two solutes in the same or opposite directions, respectively.

Receptor-mediated endocytosis

Specific cell-surface receptors can directly bind to ligands, which may be large macromolecules such as low-density lipoprotein (LDL) and so transport them into the cell. This receptor-mediated endocytosis is triggered by the presence of a ligand-bound or activated receptor within a clathrin-coated pit. The clathrin pit detaches to form an intracellular vesicle which migrates to early endosomes where the acidic pH triggers release of the ligand. Receptors may then be recycled to the cell surface to compensate for the loss of cell membrane. One type of hypercholesterolaemia results from mutations within the LDL receptor causing the accumulation of excess LDL in plasma.

Surface receptors and signalling pathways

Cells use signalling pathways mediated by extracellular molecules or messengers to communicate with one another. Messengers can act on distant cells (**endocrine**), nearby cells (**paracrine**) or the secreting cells themselves (**autocrine**). Signal transduction pathways translate these stimuli into an appropriate cellular response through a series of phosphorylation reactions (Fig. 2.10). **Tyrosine kinase** enzymes transfer phosphate groups onto tyrosine residues, while **serine/threonine kinases** add phosphate groups onto serine or threonine residues of their substrates. Phosphatase enzymes perform the reverse process of dephosphorylation.

In addition to the gated ion-channels described above, common cell-surface receptors include G protein-coupled receptors, tyrosine kinase-linked receptors and receptors with their own intrinsic enzyme activity (Fig. 2.10). These proteins act as **first messengers** in a signalling pathway. Members of the **G protein-coupled receptor** family are serpentine receptors and span the membrane seven times. G protein-coupled receptors are found at the cell surface in association with a multimeric G protein that, upon receptor engagement, undergoes guanosine diphosphate–guanosine triphosphate (GDP–GTP) exchange to trigger the process of signal transduction. **Tyrosine kinase-linked receptors** often dimerize upon target recognition to activate cytosolic protein tyrosine kinases. Phosphorylation recruits second messengers, which are themselves phosphorylated in turn (**phosphorylation cascade**). Some receptors have intrinsic guanine cyclase activity and can autophosphorylate to trigger signalling cascades.

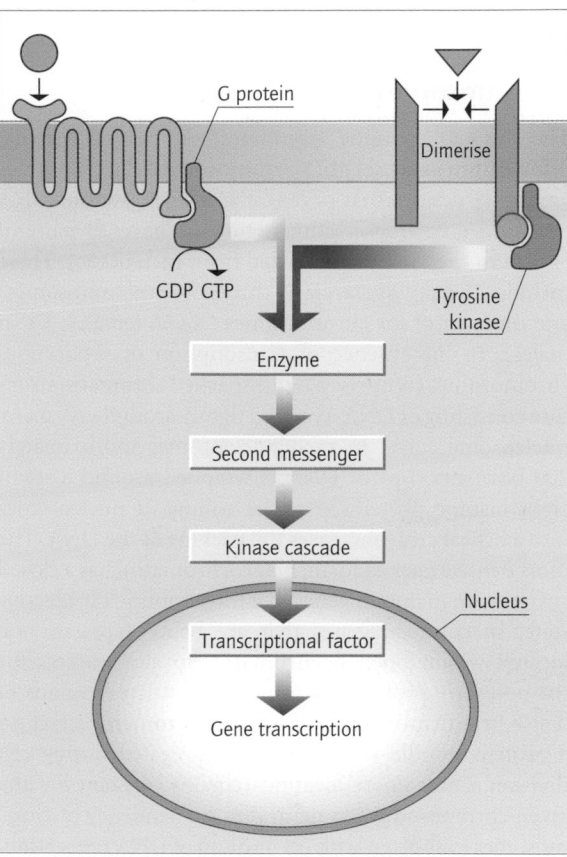

Figure 2.10 Signal transduction. Ligand binding by cell-surface receptors triggers a series of events leading to novel gene transcription in the nucleus. Second messengers and various proteins amplify the signal during this process.

Second messengers mediate the process of signal transduction from the cell surface to the nucleus. Accumulation of secondary messengers such as cyclic adenosine monophosphate (cAMP), cyclic guanosine monophosphate (cGMP) and phosphoinositide (PI) will have different effects in different cells. By acting on multiple substrates, a secondary messenger can amplify the original signal to provide an appropriate cellular response. Ras proteins act as molecular switches during signal transduction, dependent on their GTP (on) vs. GDP (off) binding. Activated Ras triggers a kinase cascade culminating in the activation of microtubule-associated protein (MAP) kinases, a serine–threonine kinase family which includes Jun-terminal kinases (JNKs). MAP kinases translocate to the nucleus in order to phosphorylate various nuclear substrates such as transcription factors. Members of these signalling pathways have a role in the development of many cancers.

Molecular biology

Chromosomes

The human **genome** combines our entire genetic information into a set of 26 **chromosomes**. Chromosomes are the structures that organize and segregate our DNA for storage or transcription. Humans have 23 pairs of chromosomes, one set inherited from each parent. These include 22 pairs of standard chromosomes (autosomes) and one pair of sex chromosomes (XX in females, XY in males). In the absence of transcription or replication, chromosomes comprise a tightly packed **chromatin** structure consisting of DNA wrapped tightly around very many **nucleosome** cores. In each nucleosome, approximately 200 basepairs (bp) of DNA is wrapped around a set of eight **histone** proteins. Further coiling of nucleosomes into a helical array increases the packing of the DNA. The most densely packed form, **heterochromatin**, has a closed structure to maintain genes in a transcriptionally inactive state. In contrast, genes that are being expressed are located within open **euchromatin**, to allow access for the necessary protein machinery. Constricted regions of dense heterochromatin known as **centromeres** attach to a protein spindle when DNA is segregated during cell division. Centromere location remains constant for any given chromosome. To neutralize the tendency of chromosomes to shorten with each round of DNA replication, telomerase enzyme elongates the end of each chromosome, adding C and G nucleotide repeats to form a blocked **telomere** structure. Telomerase is usually active in stem cells and germ cells or during oncogenesis, but is not found in healthy somatic tissues. Modulation of telomerase enzyme has therefore become a subject of interest for antiageing and anticancer research.

Gene structure

Every endogenous protein is encoded by a DNA sequence known as a **gene** found at a defined **locus** on a chromosome. **Codons** of three sequential nucleotides signify a single amino acid or a stop signal. There are 64 potential codons, and as most amino acids are encoded by more than one of these, the genetic code is referred to as **degenerate**. Regulatory regions containing target sites for various DNA-binding proteins flank the coding sequence and control gene expression. These regions form a vital part of the gene and their loss can have profound effects on protein expression. Mutations in control regions can cause disease as evidenced by some of the haemoglobin gene mutations that cause thalassaemia. An upstream **promoter** provides binding sites for RNA polymerase and transcription factors. Promoters usually contain a **TATA** box and a **CAAT** box sequence above the transcription start site. Functionally related **enhancer** sequences are located further afield, and recruit various DNA-binding proteins to increase the efficiency of gene transcription. The transcriptional unit contains **exons** of coding DNA separated by **introns**, which play no part in the finished protein. A large portion of our genome is composed of **repetitive DNA** with no known function. **Tandem repeats** range from short micro- and minisatellites of 1–30 kilobases (kb) to macrosatellites many megabases in length. These repeats are used for genetic studies and for forensic DNA studies in criminal investigations (see p. 56). **Single copy interspersed repeats** whether short (SINES) or long (LINES) are also common throughout the genome.

From gene to protein—transcription and translation

When a gene is active within a cell, DNA strands separate, allowing access for RNA polymerase to generate an anti-sense RNA molecule (Fig. 2.11). The messenger RNA (mRNA) precursor is then processed for translation into an amino acid sequence. Enzymatic nucleotide addition generates a 5′ protective cap on one end of the RNA strand. Similarly, the 3′ end of the molecule is tagged with a chain of adenylic acid nucleotides (the polyA tail) to aid mRNA transfer into the cytosol. Gene splicing removes introns from the coding sequences to leave a continuous series of exons for translation (Fig. 2.11). Once within the cytosol, mRNA attaches to large ribonucleoprotein particles known as ribosomes. Reading along mRNA, ribosomes generate proteins by polymerizing amino acids donated by transfer RNA (tRNA) molecules bearing an appropriate anticodon (Fig. 2.11).

Gene expression patterns

Undifferentiated **stem cells** divide without limit, acting as precursors for multiple cell types. Their division can be described as asymmetric because, after a single division, one daughter cell may be committed to a particular lineage while the other continues the stem cell line. Once committed to a particular lineage, cells will express an appropriate set of proteins. Developmental regulation of gene expression has clinical significance in a number of areas. For example, different haemoglobin genes are activated in the fetus compared to those expressed by adults. One therapeutic approach for thalassaemia is to attempt to reactivate fetal haemoglobin genes in order to compensate for abnormalities in their adult counterparts.

Every somatic cell carries an identical set of genes. **Housekeeping genes** are required for basic cellular functions and are constitutively expressed without any need

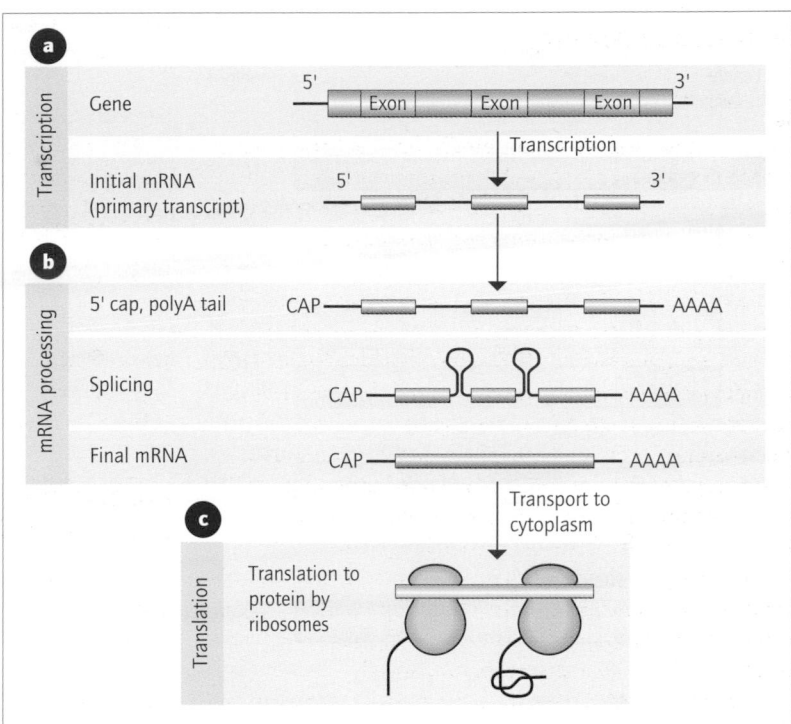

Figure 2.11 Gene transcription, messenger RNA (mRNA) processing and translation.

for further regulation. Additional subsets of expressed genes determine the phenotype and differentiation state of the cell. Gene control is generally imposed at the level of transcription initiation. Access of transcriptional proteins to the gene promoter will be restricted if it is tightly packed within heterochromatin. **CpG islands** are stretches of cytosine and guanine found at the 5′ end of genes. Methylation of cytosine (C) within CpG islands can prevent a gene from becoming expressed. An extreme form of methylation control is exercised on one of the X chromosome pair in every somatic female cell. This process, known as **lyonization**, results in hypermethylation of the inactive chromosome to prevent gene transcription.

Gene activation can occur in response to various internal or external stimuli through the action of receptor proteins and signalling pathways. The end point of these pathways is usually the expression or activation of a particular DNA-binding protein that, in turn, stimulates gene expression. Thus, transcriptional control can be imposed through a requirement for specific regulatory proteins to bind enhancer regions. DNA-binding proteins are classified according to the form of their DNA-binding domains. Of these, **zinc finger** proteins such as the steroid receptors and WT-1 (the Wilms' tumour suppressor protein) complex a zinc ion within a finger-shaped motif, **helix-turn-helix** proteins consist of two α-helices separated by a short β-turn and **leucine zipper** proteins contain leucine rich α-helices.

Beyond the level of transcription initiation, factors such as mRNA stability, transcriptional regulation and differential splicing may influence protein expression. Splicing patterns can create alternative protein forms from a single coding sequence. For example, different forms of CD45 are expressed on various lymphocyte subsets and at different stages of cell differentiation. CD45 isoforms are generated from the same initial mRNA by alternative selection of particular exons (Fig. 2.12).

Genetics

The Human Genome Project

The human genome has been estimated to contain 3.2 giga-basepairs (Gbp) of DNA encoding 25 000–35 000 genes. The first draft of the human genome sequence, covering 90% of the euchromatic sequence was published in 2001 after an international collaborative effort. Continuing efforts will extend the known sequence. Sequence data provide a first step to understanding genetic disease. The Human Genome Project has generated an important reference source for experimental studies and for the rapid identification of disease and cancer genes. Additionally, identification of single nucleotide polymorphisms has assisted genetic mapping studies and should prove particularly useful for dissecting the origins of multigene disorders.

02

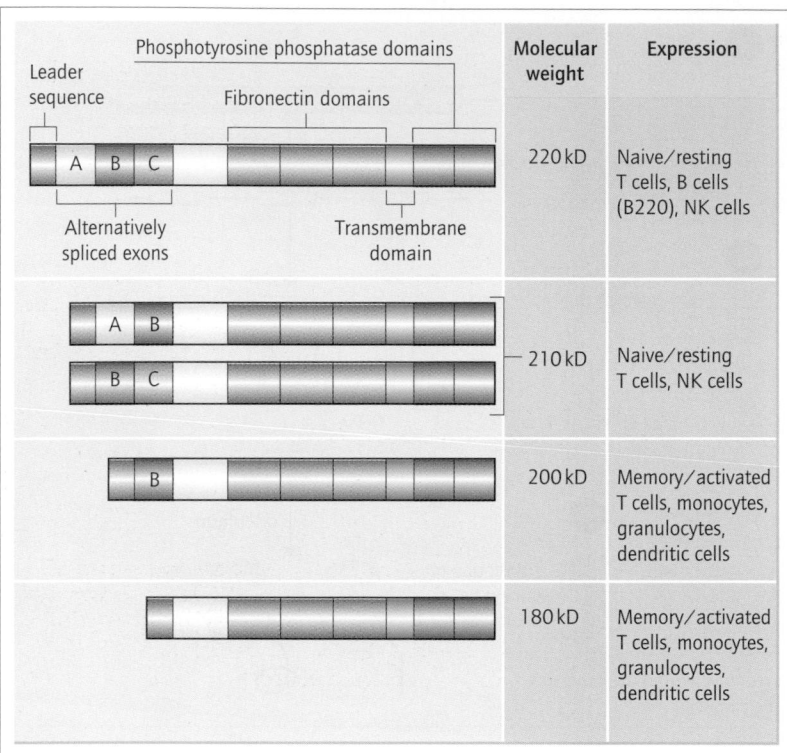

Figure 2.12 CD45 splicing patterns. CD45 (also known as LCA, T200 and B220) is expressed on the surface of haemato-poietic cells in a variety of isoforms generated by alternative splicing.

Data from the Human Genome Project are freely available (results are maintained at http://genome.ucsc. edu). Other genetic resources that are publicly available include the expressed sequence tag (**EST**) database (http://www.ncbi.nlm.nih.gov/dbEST/). On-line Mendelian Inheritance in Man or **OMIM**™ (http://www.ncbi.nlm.nih.gov/entrez/omim) is a search-able index that lists all inherited human diseases and the genes responsible. OMIM also links to Pubmed and sequence information.

Mutations

A certain degree of variation is required to maintain our genetic diversity. Polymorphic variants (alleles) of genes, differing slightly in their sequence are distributed throughout populations. One side-effect of genetic diversity is the potential for genetic disease. Genetic diseases and cancers result from the introduction and/or inheritance of pathogenic DNA mutations. Our genomes can acquire several kinds of mutation. Defects in a single gene may be responsible for a particular disease such as cystic fibrosis, but within that gene mutations may occur at multiple sites. These mutations vary in their penetration —the most common mutation seen for cystic fibrosis is a

3 nucleotide deletion (ΔF508) in the CFTR protein which causes protein misfolding, leading to its retention within the ER. A virtual absence of functional CFTR protein from the cell surface is reflected by a severe disease phenotype. Other mutations that allow CFTR protein to reach the cell surface but reduce its activity cause less severe forms of disease.

Point mutations are the simplest form of DNA alteration (Fig. 2.13). In this case, a single base of the DNA sequence is affected. Base **transitions** occur between purine (A,G) or pyrimidine (C-T) nucleotides. **Transversions** represent nucleotide substitution of purines for pyrimidines and vice versa. Resulting from degeneracy of the genetic code, some DNA substitutions may be **silent** at the amino acid level. A **missense** mutation occurs when DNA alterations introduce coding for a different amino acid. Sometimes the effects are more drastic; substitution for an early stop codon (**nonsense** mutation) will terminate protein translation and the full-length protein will be lost. Similarly, gain or loss of one or two nucleotides will alter the subsequent reading frame of the protein and the remainder of the correct sequence will be lost. Pathogenic mutations may also occur outside a protein coding sequence; alterations to promoter regions or splice sites can have profound effects on gene expression.

02

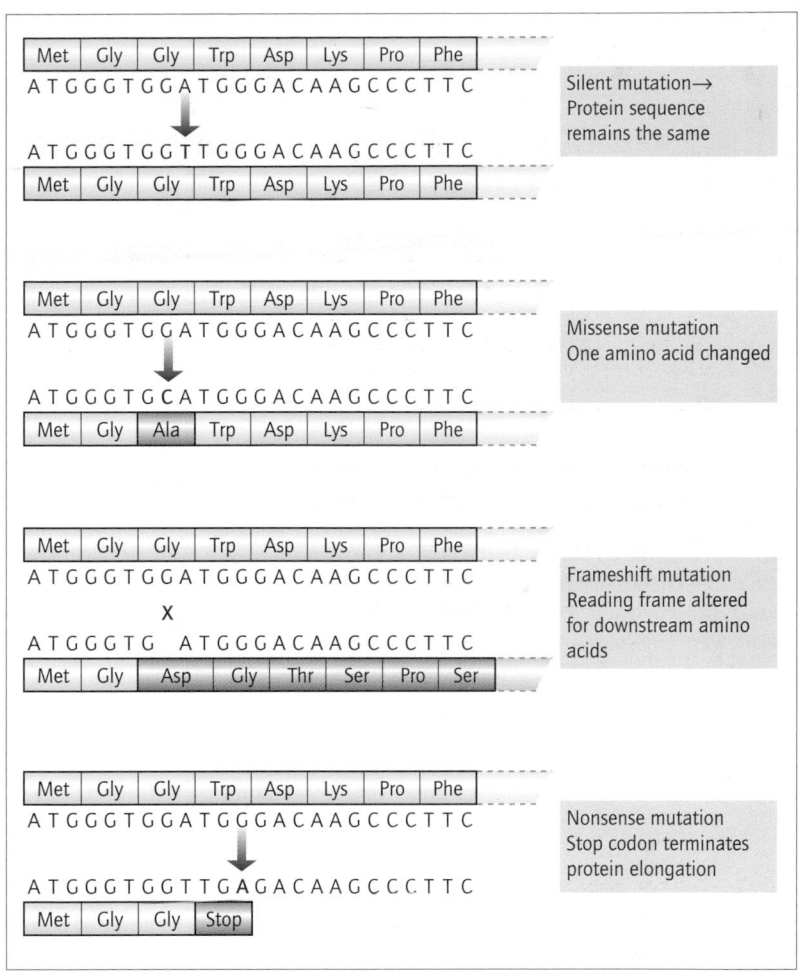

Figure 2.13 Point mutations.

Background levels of mutation arise from normal cellular and environmental interactions. Mutation rates also reflect the fidelity of DNA replication and its proofreading and/or correction potential. Trinucleotide repeats are known to be particularly unstable and are associated with a range of genetic diseases including Huntington's chorea, myotonic dystrophy and fragile X syndrome. Disease severity is usually proportional to the increase in repeat length.

Monogenic and polygenic disorders

Monogenic diseases are the simplest genetic disorders to study as they tend to follow Mendelian genetics. Dominant and recessive diseases have characteristic patterns of inheritance (Fig. 2.14). **Dominant** traits require only one defective copy to generate a disease phenotype. In contrast, **recessive** disorders are only visible when both copies of a gene are mutated. Recessive disorders often result from null mutations, leading to a loss in biological activity

for the relevant protein and a severe phenotype. Sex linkage alters Mendelian genetics, as males carry only one copy of the X chromosome; recessive mutations carried on this chromosome behave as if dominant in men, while heterozygous females act as asymptomatic 'carriers'. **Polygenic disorders** have a known genetic component, but involve many genes (Table 2.1). In such cases, disease results from a combination of multiple polymorphisms, acting in concert with external factors. Those who inherit susceptibility genes for polygenic disorders are at much lower risk of disease than those who inherit markers for a monogenic disease.

Chromosomal abnormalities

A range of clinical syndromes can be caused by chromosomal abnormalities such as inappropriate chromosome numbers or structural alterations (Table 2.2). Normal individuals carry two complete sets of chromosomes (**diploid**). Deviation from this rule (**aneuploidy**) can

02

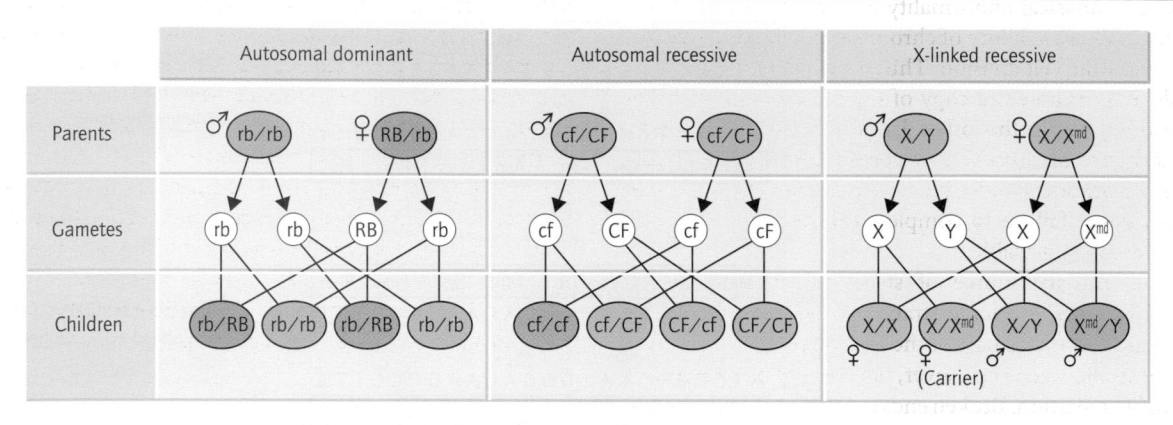

Figure 2.14 Inheritance patterns. Diseased phenotypes are indicated in pink, dominant alleles in capitals and recessive alleles in lower case. For autosomal dominant disorders such as retinoblastoma, children have a 50% chance of inheriting the disease allele (RB) from an affected parent. In the case of autosomal recessive disorders including cystic fibrosis, children of two carrier parents have a 25% chance of inheriting two copies of the disease allele (cf). Ratios are altered for X-linked recessive disorders such as muscular dystrophy where daughters have a 50% chance of inheriting the disease allele (X^{md}) from their mother to become carriers themselves. Sons have a 50% chance of inheriting the disease allele from their mother; as there is no compensatory allele on the Y chromosome these sons are affected with the disease.

Table 2.1 Common genetic diseases

Disease	Approximate frequency	Nature
Rheumatoid arthritis	1/100	Polygenic
Haemochromatosis	1/400	Monogenic; autosomal recessive, mutations in *HFE* gene
Type 1 diabetes mellitus	1/500	Polygenic
Familial hypercholesterolaemia	1/500	Monogenic; autosomal dominant, various mutations in LDL receptor gene
Von Willebrand's disease	1/1000	Monogenic; autosomal, usually dominant, mutations in *VWF* gene
Polycystic kidney disease	1/1000	Monogenic; autosomal dominant
Fragile X syndrome	1/1250 males	Monogenic; X-linked recessive, mutations in *FMR1* gene
Ulcerative colitis	1/1500	Polygenic
Cystic fibrosis	1/2000	Monogenic; autosomal recessive, mutations in *CFTR* gene
Huntington's disease	1/2000	Monogenic; autosomal dominant, repeat length mutation in Huntingtin (*HT*) gene
Haemophilia A	1/5000 males	Monogenic; X-linked recessive, mutations in factor VIII gene

Table 2.2 Chromosomal abnormalities

Disease	Approximate frequency	Genetic nature
Trisomy 21 (Down's syndrome, mongolism)	1/700 (at birth)	Usually three complete copies of chromosome 21 (4% of cases result from a balanced translocation involving chromosome 21)
Klinefelter's syndrome	1/1000 males	Trisomy of sex chromosomes: XXY
Hereditary motor and sensory neuropathy type 1 (Charcot–Marie–Tooth disease)	1/2600	Most cases are associated with a duplication of chromosome 17p11.2
Trisomy 18 (Edwards' syndrome)	1/3000	Three complete copies of chromosome 18
Turner's syndrome	1/5000 females	Monosomy of the X chromosome (XO)
Trisomy 13 (Patau's syndrome)	1/5000	Usually three complete copies of chromosome 13
Prader–Willi syndrome	1/10 000	75% of cases are associated with a deletion from chromosome 15

result in physical abnormality or prenatal death. Aneuploidy follows a failure of chromosomes to segregate correctly during cell division. Thus, one of the two daughter cells inherits an extra copy of the relevant chromosome (**trisomy**) while the other lacks a copy (**monosomy**). Inheritance of extra sets of chromosomes (**polyploidy**) arises from a diploid gamete, fertilization by two spermatozoa or failure to complete cell division. Polyploid zygotes are non-viable.

The primary source of structural abnormality for chromosomes is double stranded DNA breakage. DNA breakage occurs as part of the natural meiotic process in order to allow gene crossover, but can also be triggered by ionizing radiation. Broken ends of DNA are highly recombinogenic and are rapidly repaired by specific enzymes using pathways of homologous or non-homologous end-joining. Abnormal repair generates structural abnormalities including translocation, deletion, duplication and inversion. **Translocations** represent a transfer of DNA between two chromosomes. As this exchange does not result in any loss of DNA, an individual carrier may remain healthy. However, chromosome translocations can hinder normal meiotic division such that offspring may receive a partial trisomy or monosomy. **Deletions** result in a loss of genetic material, often spanning many genes. Their effects are usually severe, resulting in congenital malformation. Additional copies of a DNA stretch (**duplications**) originate from an abnormal meiosis, and are generally less harmful than deletions. Introduction of two separate double stranded breaks can generate an **inversion** if the chromosomal fragment is replaced back to front. Although no DNA is lost or gained in this process, inversions can obstruct chromosome pairing during meiosis.

Cancer genetics

Cancers result from an accumulation of genetic abnormalities within somatic cells. The majority of these defects arise spontaneously (often as a result of exposure to mutagens), although a subset may be inherited. An inherited predisposition to cancer is often characterized by early disease onset and other affected family members. The genetic component usually follows a recessive inheritance pattern. Cell proliferation is central to tumour formation, as cancers arise from a single cell. Thus, mutations in genes that promote or inhibit cell proliferation, control apoptosis or regulate DNA repair can have profound effects.

Oncogenes were first discovered by retroviral studies and subsequently termed c- or v- to denote their cellular or viral origins. Protein products of oncogenes promote cell division and differentiation (e.g. growth factors and

their receptors). In their non-activated healthy state they are referred to as **proto-oncogenes**. **Tumour suppressor genes** restrict cell proliferation and induce repair or apoptosis in response to DNA damage. *p53* is the classic example of a tumour suppressor gene, and is the most commonly mutated gene in tumours (Fig. 2.15). p53 is expressed in response to DNA damage, and localizes to the nucleus where it exerts transcriptional control on its target genes to trigger cell cycle arrest, DNA repair and, if necessary, apoptosis. Most common mutations in p53 affect its DNA-binding domain. **DNA repair genes** remove the damage induced by mutagenesis. Point mutations,

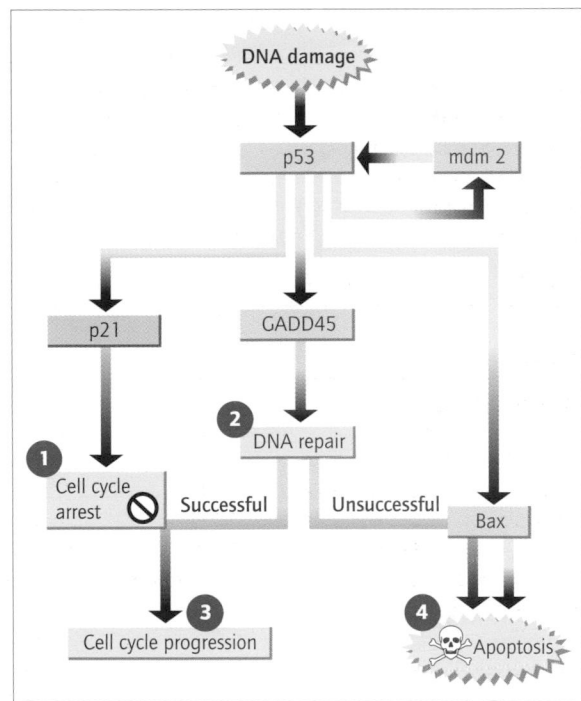

Figure 2.15 The tumour suppressor protein p53 acts to maintain genetic stability by controlling cell cycle and apoptosis pathways. The wide-ranging influence of p53 reflects its status as the most commonly mutated protein in cancer (p53 is implicated in 50% of colon cancers, 50% of lung cancers and over 50% of breast cancers). p53 is usually localized to the nucleus where it acts as a transcription factor, thus the majority of pathogenic p53 mutations affect its DNA-binding domain. In response to DNA damage, p53 triggers the expression of various proteins including p21, which arrests the cell cycle (1) by inhibiting cyclin-dependent kinases (CDKs), and GADD45, a DNA repair protein (2). Cell cycle block is lifted following successful DNA repair (3). If DNA repair is unsuccessful, however, pro-apoptotic factors such as bax (also induced by p53) trigger cell death (4). p53 also stimulates expression of its own negative regulator, mdm2.

translocations and gene amplification can all play a part in tumorigenesis. Chromosomal translocations can generate hybrid oncogenes. The Philadelphia chromosome is the result of a translocation that causes overexpression of an altered form of the protein kinase c-abl, which contributes to the pathogenesis of chronic myeloid leukaemia (Fig. 2.16).

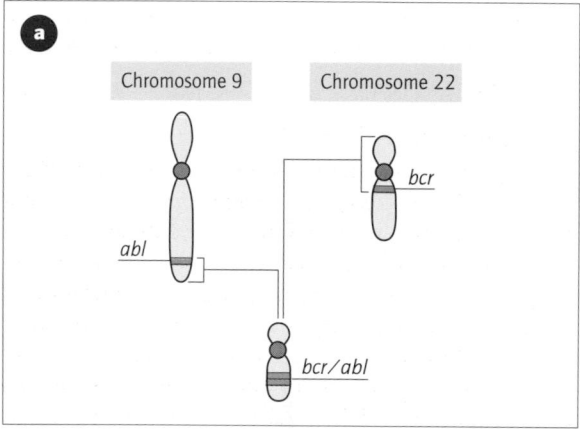

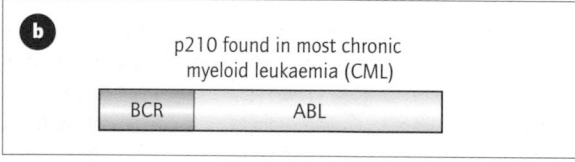

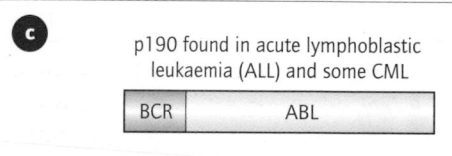

Figure 2.16 The Philadelphia chromosome. *Abl* is an oncogene located on chromosome 9. *Bcr* is an oncogene on chromosome 22. Ninety per cent of patients with chronic myeloid leukaemia (CML) possess a reciprocal translocation between chromosomes 9 and 22 to create a hybrid known as the Philadelphia chromosome (a). This balanced translocation fuses the *abl* and *bcr* oncogenes to encode a hybrid protein (BCR/ABL) with tyrosine kinase activity. Two major forms of BCR/ABL hybrid may be generated, depending on the location of the breakpoint in the *BCR* gene. A breakpoint in the major breakpoint cluster (Mbcr) region joins exons 2–3 of BCR to exon 2 of ABL to generate a hybrid protein of 210 kD (b) seen in the majority of CML cases. An alternative breakpoint, nearer the 5′ end of *abl* generates a hybrid protein of 190 kD (c) observed in both CML and acute lymphoblastic leukaemia (ALL).

Immunology and inflammation

Immunology is directly relevant to many clinical situations and is a key area of study in molecular medicine. In order to counter a daily attack from potentially infectious pathogens, the immune system has evolved complex strategies to detect and destroy anything it regards as foreign (or non-self). Following the development of tissue transplantation methods, transplanted organs can now be added to the list of 'foreign' matter that an immune system might encounter. The **innate** (non-specific) immune response involves the complement system, natural killer (NK) cells and phagocytes and is active against pathogens when they are first encountered, regardless of whether they have been seen before. The **adaptive** (specific) immune system, including T cells and antibodies secreted by B cells, becomes activated in response to foreign antigens. The term antigen refers to something, such as a molecule, that is recognized by the immune system. Individual **epitopes** are the actual sites on the antigen that act as direct immune targets.

Key immune cell types and functions

Phagocytes

Phagocytes are cells of the **myeloid** lineage which can destroy exogenous particles by phagocytosis (a specialized form of endocytosis). Pseudopodia engulf external particles into specialized vacuoles (**phagosomes**), which fuse with lysosomes where ingested material is broken down. Micro-organisms and whole cells can be destroyed in this way. The phagocyte cytoplasm is stocked with granules containing enzymes required for digestion of phagocytosed particles. Phagocytes also produce soluble immune mediators that can trigger inflammation and direct the responses of other immune cell types. Neutrophils, basophils and eosinophils (commonly known as granulocytes) possess segmented nuclei and are named for their acid, basic or neutral dye-staining tendencies. Mononuclear phagocytes (macrophages and monocytes) have simple-shaped unsegmented nuclei.

Although capable of phagocytosis, the primary functions of granulocytes are predominantly secretory in nature. **Eosinophils** are specialized to combat parasitic infection. Their peroxidase-rich granules stain readily with eosin. **Neutrophils** are recruited to sites of inflammation where they have a major role in the inflammatory process. **Basophils**, which form a small population of circulating leucocytes, are closely related to mast cells and their granules contain histamine, heparin and other vasoactive amines, which are released in response to antibody–antigen interactions. **Monocytes** are found in bone marrow and circulate through the blood. Upon leaving the blood, monocytes differentiate into **macrophages** with tissue-specific characteristics (e.g. alveolar macrophages, liver Kupffer cells). Macrophages play an important part in apoptosis by clearing away dead cells. Macrophage functions can be enhanced if they are activated during an inflammatory process.

Macrophages express a range of cell-surface molecules that enable them to recognize foreign particles. **Pattern recognition receptors** recognize certain microbe-specific molecules, alerting phagocytes to the presence of infection. Phagocytes also express receptors for immune system components. Thus, complement receptors bind complement-coated particles, while antibody–antigen complexes are primed for phagocytic uptake through their recognition by receptors for the Fc portion of the antibodies.

Megakaryocytes

Portions of cytoplasm bud off from megakaryocytes to form **platelets**. This is not a mitotic division, so platelets have no nucleus of their own. Platelets circulate through the blood providing soluble factors that are essential for blood clotting and inflammation and can aggregate to enhance haemostasis.

Natural killer cells

Natural killer cells are large granular lymphocytes with cytotoxic activity; they can destroy tumour or virally infected cells without any need for prior immunization or activation. Additionally, NK cells can lyse immunoglobulin G (IgG) coated targets by the process of antibody-dependent cell-mediated cytotoxicity (ADCC) or secrete cytokines to influence lymphocyte function. Natural killer cells appear to play a part in the early phase of host defence against intracellular pathogens including herpes viruses, *Leishmania* and *Listeria monocytogenes*. Cytokine stimulation can increase NK cell activity by up to 100-fold.

Dendritic cells

These cells are named for their long dendrite-like processes. An adaptive immune response may be initiated when an immature dendritic cell (DC) in peripheral tissue encounters a potential pathogen. Following antigen uptake, the DC differentiates into a professional **antigen-presenting cell (APC)**. Dendritic cells express very high levels of major histocompatibility complex (MHC) class 2 proteins on their cell surface in combination with peptide antigens. Dendritic cells returning through the lymphatic system carry potential antigens to lymph nodes where they deliver an activation signal to stimulate resting T-cell differentiation.

Lymphocytes and acquired immunity

B and T lymphocytes dominate the adaptive immune response, providing its specificity, diversity and memory. Lymphocytes are maintained in a resting state until activation, but when they encounter an appropriately presented antigen this triggers clonal expansion, generating a large population of cells with identical antigen specificity. Upon completion of an active immune response, the vast majority of these cells die by apoptosis, but some persist as memory cells. Maintenance of a memory cell population following an initial immune response enables lymphocytes to provide a stronger and more rapid response upon repeat exposure.

B lymphocytes (B cells)

B-cell specificity is conferred by the B-cell receptor (**BCR**), which can be expressed as a membrane-bound receptor or in a soluble form known as **antibody (Ab)** or **immunoglobulin (Ig)**. B-cell receptors recognize soluble antigens and extracellular micro-organisms encountered in body fluids. Following activation, and in response to cytokine stimulation, B cells differentiate into large **plasma cells** that secrete antibodies. Membrane-bound BCRs recognize and internalize antigen for processing and presentation to T cells. In contrast, secreted antibodies trigger various effector mechanisms to inactivate or remove foreign antigens from the body. When antibodies bind antigens on the surface of a pathogen, they can trigger ADCC by complement activation or by binding to Fc receptors on cells such as NK cells.

T lymphocytes (T cells)

T cells provide cellular immunity, and can be divided into cytotoxic and helper subsets. Instead of native antigen, T cells recognize short peptide fragments of approximately 8–25 amino acids in length when they are bound in the groove of the **MHC** (also known as **human leucocyte antigen (HLA)**) proteins. T-cell specificity is determined by the T-cell antigen receptor (**TCR**), an immunoglobulin-like heterodimer of either αβ or γδ chains. Resting T cells are activated by dendritic cells, but activated or memory T cells can respond rapidly to a wide variety of APCs. Cytotoxic T cells (**CTLs**) expressing the CD8 coreceptor are responsible for lysis of virally infected and possibly also tumour cells. Helper T cells (T$_H$ cells) expressing the CD4 coreceptor perform a range of functions mediated through the action of secreted cytokines. The T$_H$ cell population may be subdivided into T$_H$1, T$_H$2 or T$_H$0 subsets on the basis of cytokine secretion profiles. Secretion of soluble cytokine mediators enables T$_H$ cells to support cytotoxic T-cell responses, B-cell responses and monocyte activity.

B- and T-cell antigen receptors

The adaptive immune response depends upon antigen recognition by specific immune receptors. B and T cells express structurally related specific antigen receptors. Each receptor molecule can be divided into **variable** and **constant** regions. Antigen specificity is provided by the variable region, which forms an antigen-binding site, while the constant region forms a supporting structural scaffold. For antibodies, the antigen-binding site is often referred to as the **Fab** fragment, which can be separated from the constant **Fc** region by enzymatic digestion.

Four protein chains (two heavy and two light) held together by disulphide bonds form the basic structural unit of an antibody (Fig. 2.17a). Each unit has two antigen-

binding sites. Antibodies are subgrouped on the basis of their heavy chain determinants; humans have five classes of heavy chains, each designed for different effector mechanisms (Table 2.3). Unlike antibodies, the TCR exists only in a membrane-bound form with a single antigen-binding site. Approximately 95% of circulating T cells have a receptor consisting of a heterodimer of α and β chains (Fig. 2.17b), but a subpopulation of T cells uses an alternative receptor, composed of γ and δ chains. Each TCR chain has one variable and one constant domain, with the paired variable domains forming an antigen-binding site.

Specific immunity to a huge diversity of antigens requires a similarly huge diversity of specific receptors on lymphocytes. This level of protein variability is achieved

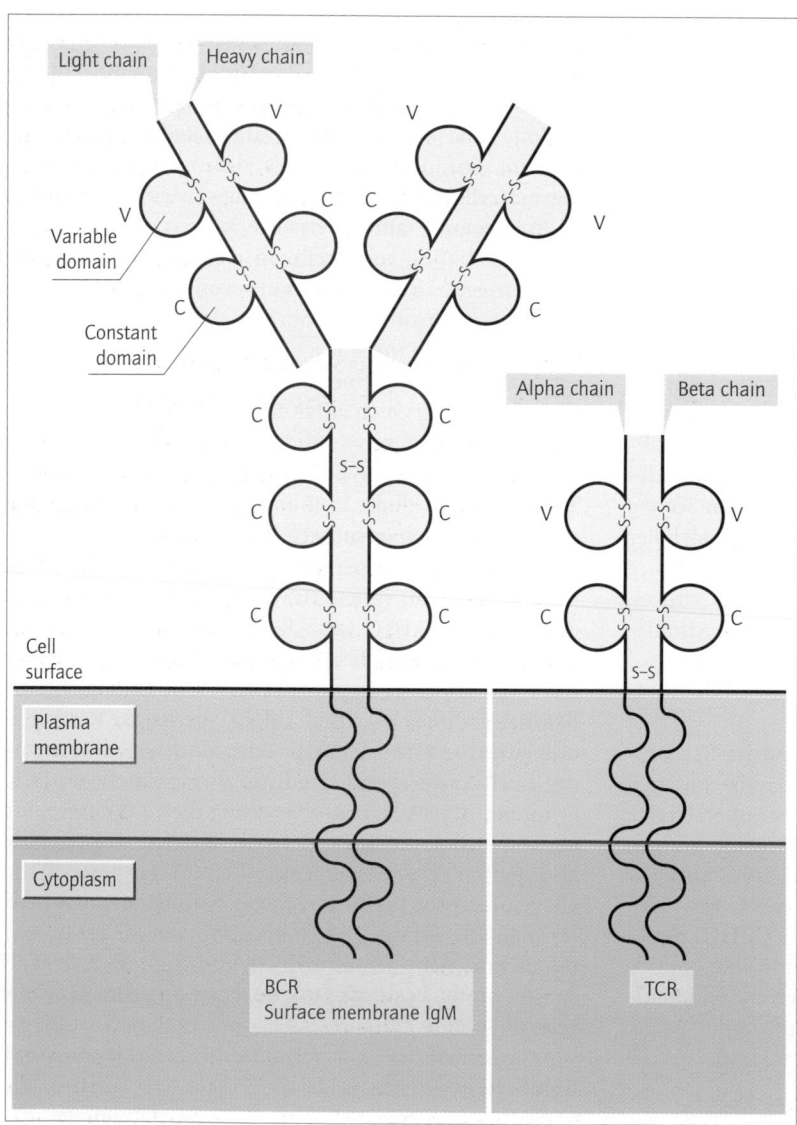

Figure 2.17 Schematic diagram of BCR and TCR. Both are comprised of variable (V) and constant (C) immunoglobulin-like domains. The structure of the BCR is a typical immunoglobulin molecule anchored within the membrane of the B cell. B cells produce immunoglobulins with the same specificity, but with different heavy chain constant regions which allow them to be secreted from the cell as soluble antibody molecules.

Table 2.3 Antibody isotypes

Isotype	Structure	Function
IgG	Monomer	Predominant form in plasma. Can cross placenta. Can activate complement and bind Fc receptors. Good opsonin
IgM	Monomer on B cell surface. Pentamer in serum	One of two predominant forms on B cells. First antibody produced during primary immune response, functions as receptor for antigen on B cells. Can activate complement. Good for complement fixation and agglutination. Binds some Fc receptors on some cell types
IgA	Monomer in serum. Dimer in secretions	Found in secretions such as milk, saliva, tears and in digestive tract. Provides local protection in these areas
IgE	Monomer	Binds Fc receptors on basophils and mast cells before interacting with antigen. Interacts with allergens to trigger Fc receptor degranulation of mast cells and histamine release
IgD	Monomer	Other predominant form on B cells, found at low levels in serum. Does not fix complement

Ig, immunoglobulin.

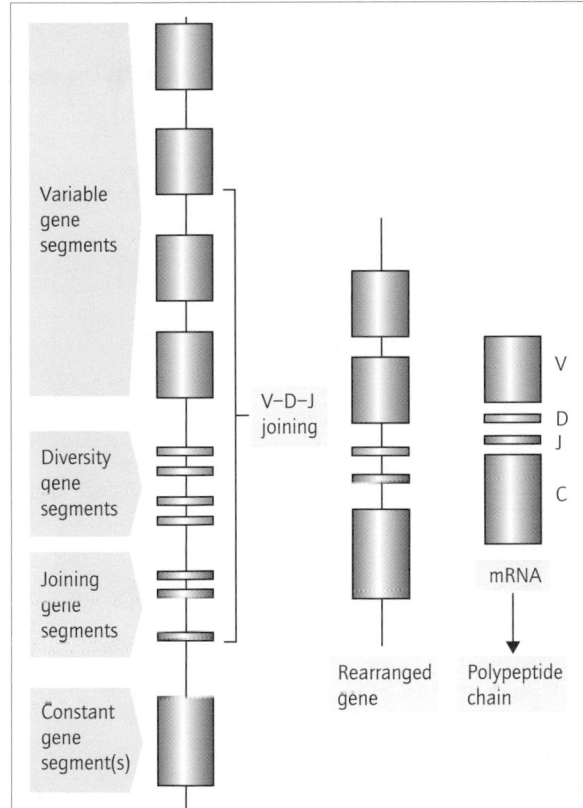

Figure 2.18 Generation of diversity within the immunological repertoire. Each of the polypeptides making up the BCRs and TCRs is encoded by a number of clusters of gene segments. Functional genes are produced by rearrangements that bring together a gene segment from each of the clusters, with a constant region gene segment. The larger the number of gene segments within each cluster the greater the number of gene combinations that can be produced by rearrangement.

by **combinatorial rearrangements** of multiple gene segments (Fig. 2.18). DNA rearrangement in developing B cells brings together a segment from each pool of V, D and J sequences to generate a functional immunoglobulin gene. **Somatic mutation** completes the mechanisms that add to antibody diversity. The residues most susceptible to change are those at the antigen-binding site. T-cell receptors display parallel gene organization and rearrangement but do not undergo somatic mutation.

Major histocompatibility complex proteins and antigen presentation

Major histocompatibility complex

The **MHC** is a gene cluster located on chromosome 6, first identified as the major genetic determinant of transplant compatibility. Antigen-presenting proteins encoded by the human MHC are generally referred to as **HLAs**. The MHC encodes two families of antigen-presenting proteins that play a fundamental part in the specific immune response. **MHC class 1** (HLA-A, HLA-B and HLA-C) proteins are expressed on the surface of virtually all nucleated cells where they present intracellular antigens for recognition by the TCRs of cytotoxic T cells. Expression of **MHC class 2** (HLA-DP, HLA-DQ and HLA-DR) is restricted to specialized APCs including B cells, macrophages and monocytes, but can be induced on other cell types such as endothelial cells during an active immune response. Antigens presented by MHC class 2 are recognized by the TCR of T_H cells. The MHC also encodes genes for cytokines, complement proteins and other antigen-processing factors.

MHC class 1 and class 2 proteins are members of the immunoglobulin superfamily (Fig. 2.19). Both form a peptide-binding groove, which presents antigenic peptides to the TCR. The MHC class 1 structure consists of a heavy chain, associated with β_2-microglobulin (β_2m).

02

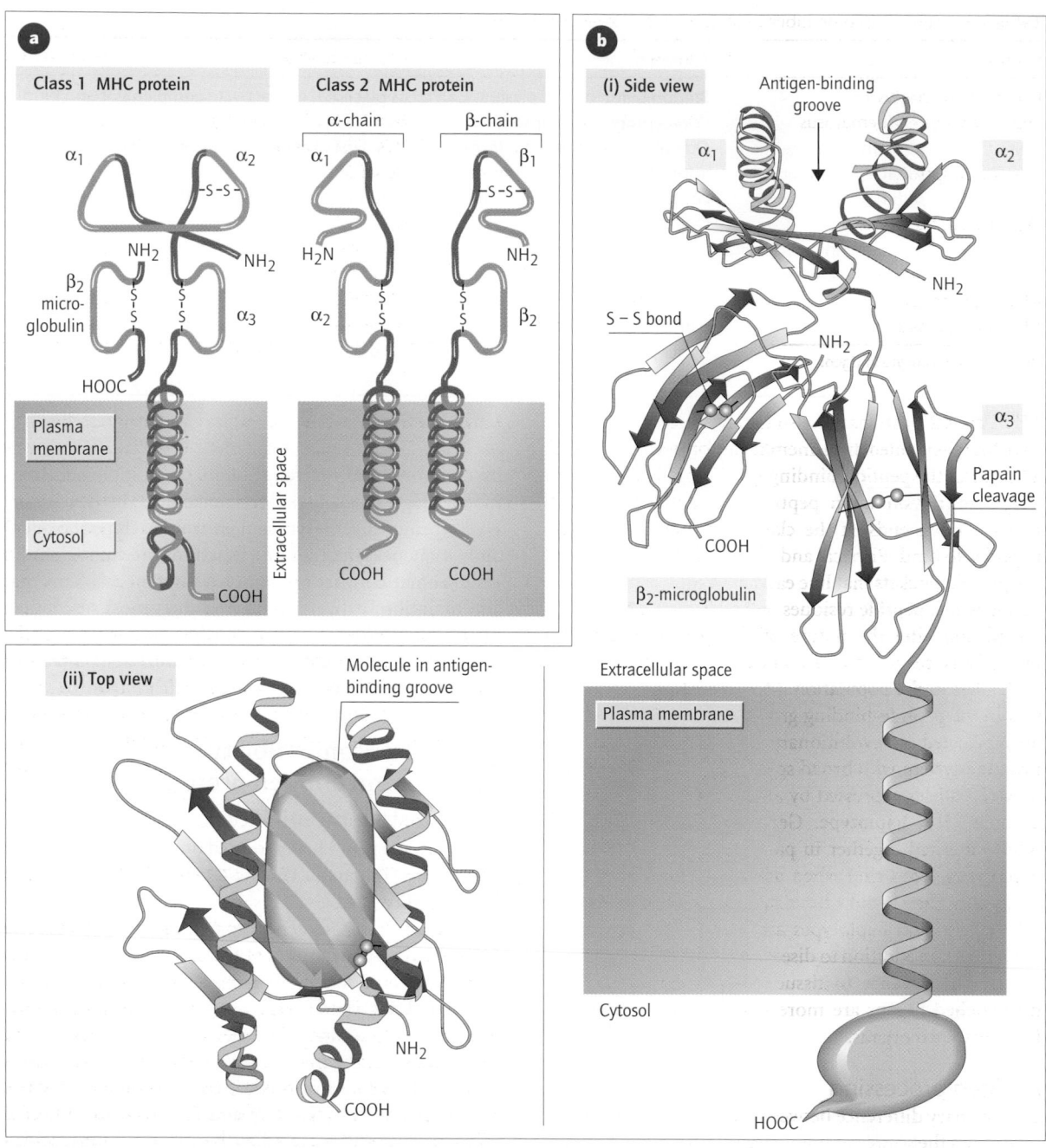

Figure 2.19 Structure of MHC class 1 and class 2 proteins. (a) Schematic diagrams of class 1 and 2 MHC proteins. The α-chain of the class 1 molecule has three extracellular domains. It is non-covalently associated with a smaller polypeptide chain, β_2-microglobulin, which is not encoded within the MHC. The β_2-microglobulin is invariable while the α-chains (especially α-1 and α-2) are extremely polymorphic. In class 2 MHC molecules, both α- and β-chains are polymorphic, mainly in the α-1 and β-1 domains. In both class 1 and 2 molecules, the two outermost domains interact to form a groove that binds foreign antigenic peptide and presents it to T cells. (b) (i) The three-dimensional structure of the class 1 MHC molecule as determined by X-ray crystallography. (ii) The antigen-binding groove containing a small peptide, as viewed from above. This is the part of the molecule that interacts with the T-cell receptor (TCR). Adapted from Bjorkman *et al.*, *Nature* 1987; **329**: 506–12 (Macmillan Magazines, London) with permission of the publishers and authors.

Table 2.4 Major histocompatibility complex (MHC) disease associations

Disease	Frequency	HLA association	Relative risk
Rheumatoid arthritis	1/100	HLA-DR4	2–6
Systemic lupus erythematosus	Varies between populations and sexes	HLA-DR3 (white people)	2–5
		HLA-DR2 (Japanese)	2
Ankylosing spondylitis	1/500 men	HLA-B27	90
	1/5000 women		
Type 1 diabetes mellitus	1/500	HLA-DR3	3–6
		HLA-DR4	2–7
		DR3/DR4 combined	14
Multiple sclerosis	1/1000 (approx.)	HLA-DR2	2–4
Myasthenia gravis	1/25 000	HLA-DR3	2–3

HLA, human leucocyte antigen.

02

MHC class 2 proteins are also heterodimers, comprising two MHC-encoded transmembrane proteins: α and β. The size of the peptide-binding groove imposes a general length restriction upon peptides presented by class 1, whereas open ends of the class 2 groove allow longer peptides to bind. Physical and chemical characteristics of the protein pockets that line each peptide-binding groove define which peptide residues will be bound. MHC polymorphisms alter the nature of the groove in different individuals, resulting in a unique binding specificity for each allele in the population. Most variations are located within the peptide-binding groove and are likely to have been selected by evolutionary pressure to generate an immune system with broad specificity. The combination of MHC alleles expressed by an individual is referred to as their HLA **haplotype**. Genes within the MHC are often inherited together in patterns known as extended haplotypes, occurring when alleles are associated more frequently than would be expected by chance. Certain HLA alleles and haplotypes are associated with disease (Table 2.4). In addition to disease association, HLA typing has direct relevance to tissue transplantation as HLA-mismatched organs are more likely to be rejected than HLA-matched organs.

Antigen processing

One primary difference between class 1 and class 2 MHC proteins is the source of their antigenic peptides. Peptides bound by class 1 are generally derived from intracellular proteins, which are degraded to short peptides by the action of specific processing factors, and in particular the multisubunit multicatalytic cytosolic complex known as the **proteasome**. These peptides are transported into the ER by the transporter associated with antigen presentation (**TAP**) in an ATP-dependent manner. In their early, empty forms, class 1 are stabilized by a series of chaperones including **calnexin**, **caltreticulin** and **tapasin**. Chaperones dissociate upon peptide binding, allowing newly assembled class 1 complexes to progress through the Golgi complex and on to the cell surface where they can interact with T cells.

Peptides presented by MHC class 2 are usually generated by degradation of endocytosed proteins. Initial class 2 assembly takes place within the ER. Early complexes are stabilized by interaction with **invariant chain** (Ii), which fills their peptide-binding groove to prevent premature peptide binding. As class 2 molecules progress towards the cell surface, the invariant chain is gradually degraded to a short peptide fragment known as **CLIP**. The endocytic pathway transports exogenous proteins to lysosomes, where they are degraded into short peptides. The transport pathways of MHC class 2 and endocytosed proteins intersect at or near the Golgi complex, where CLIP is replaced by antigenic peptide.

Immune receptor recognition of MHC proteins

Both αβ and γδ TCR are found in association with the CD3 signal transduction complex and are similar in shape to antibodies. The functional distinction between class 1 and class 2 restricted T cells is thought to result from the influence of CD4 and CD8, which act as coreceptors for MHC class 2 and class 1, respectively. CD8 binds class 1 MHC and thus favours binding by TCRs on the cytotoxic T cells upon which it is expressed. CD4 mediates a similar effect for class 2 recognition by helper T cells, which express this class 2 specific receptor. In the thymus, useful T cells are selected by positive and negative selection processes, which serve various purposes such as the elimination of autoreactive cells with the potential to cause autoimmune damage.

Superantigens are a unique class of proteins that trigger a large primary T-cell response. Various pathogens encode these proteins, which bind intact to the outer surface of MHC class 2. Each superantigen is specific for a subset of TCR variable regions, and will activate any T cell bearing these domains. Bacterial superantigens include the staphylococcal enterotoxins (SEs) involved in food poisoning and staphylococcal toxic shock syndrome toxin-1 (TSS-1).

Although specific recognition of individual MHC–peptide combinations is mediated by the TCR, MHC class 1 proteins are also ligands for a variety of other cell surface immune receptors whose functions are currently being elucidated. For example, NK cells express an alternative family of MHC class 1 specific receptors encoded within another immune receptor complex—the leucocyte receptor complex (**LRC**) on chromosome 19. MHC-specific LRC-encoded proteins are expressed on T and NK cells in addition to B lymphocytes and monocytic cells.

Key immune modulators

The complement system

Complement proteins are soluble acute phase proteins that have an important role in the innate immune response and are rapidly synthesized following injury or infection. The complement system is involved in inflammation, increased susceptibility of antibody-coated antigens to phagocytosis (a process known as **opsonization**), lysis of pathogens or infected cells and immune complex solubilization. Most complement proteins circulate within plasma as inactive proenzymes. Activation of the complement system triggers a cascade of proteolytic cleavage of these proenzymes into multiple fragments, some of which act as soluble immune mediators. Following activation, plasma levels of the various complement system proteins can be measured to track the pathway of activation.

Complement can become activated by multiple pathways (Fig. 2.20). Each generates an enzyme known as the **C3 convertase**, which binds pathogens, targeting them for destruction. The **classical complement pathway** plays a part in both innate and acquired immunity and is triggered by the binding of C1q to antibody–antigen complexes or to pathogen surfaces. Mannan-binding lectin (MBL) is a serum protein which is similar to C1q, and initiates the **mannan-binding lectin pathway** (MBL pathway) when it binds to microbial carbohydrate components. The **alternative pathway** allows complement to

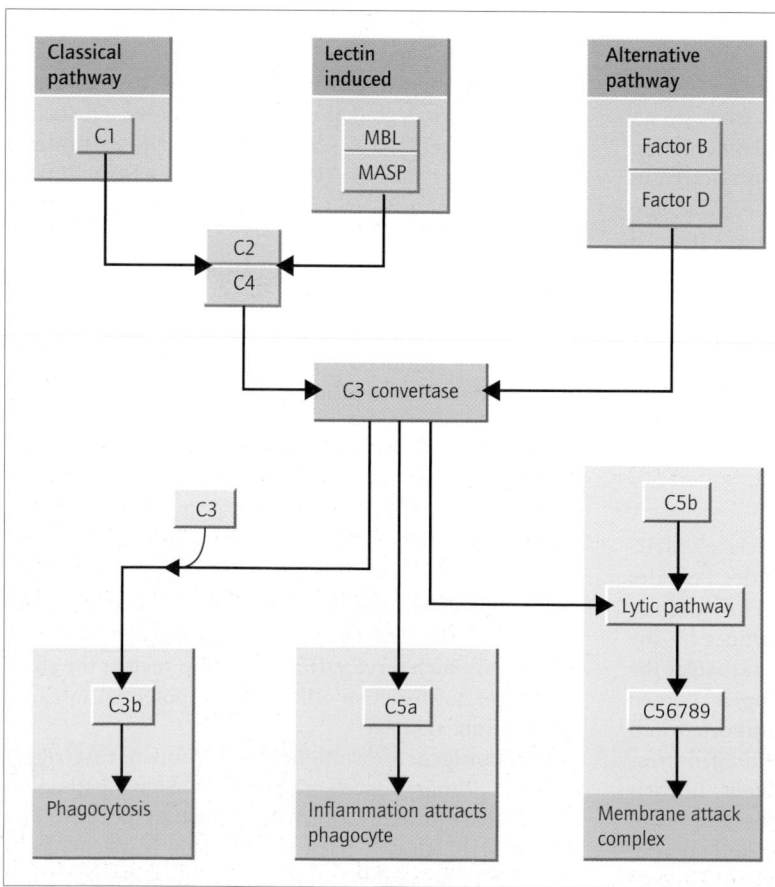

Figure 2.20 Complement activation pathways. Complement proteins are generally termed with a C prefix, followed by a number (corresponding to the order of their discovery); subsequent letters represent various cleavage products. The classical complement pathway is initiated by binding of C1 to antibody–antigen complexes or pathogen surfaces. The catalytic subunit of C1 in turn activates C2 and C4, the next two components of this pathway. Activated C4 and C2 together form the classical C3 convertase. The mannan-binding lectin (MBL) pathway is triggered by lectin to carbohydrate components on a pathogen surface. Mannan-binding lectin associates with the MBP-associated serum protease (MASP) to cleave C4 and C2. Both MBL and alternative complement pathway can proceed in the absence of specific antibodies.

02

Table 2.5 Cytokines

Cytokine	Structure	Major source(s)	Effects
GM-CSF	Bundle of 4 α-helices	T cells, macrophages	Survival and growth factor for cells of the haematopoietic lineage
Erythropoietin		Kidney or liver	Stimulates erythroid precursors to generate red blood cells
IL-2		T cells	Growth/differentiation for lymphocytes, NK cells, macrophages, etc.
IL-3		T cells	Colony formation for erythroid and myelomonocytic lineages
IL-4		T cells, mast cells	B- and T-cell growth/differentiation
IL-5		T cells, mast cells	Eosinophil colony formation and activation
IL-6		Lymphocytes, macrophages, etc.	Regulates lymphocyte function and haematopoiesis
IL-13		T cells, mast cells, NK cells	B-cell proliferation, suppresses inflammatory responses
IFN-α/IFN-β	(variant: altered topology)	Macrophages, lymphocytes	Inhibits cell proliferation, regulates MHC expression
IL-10	Homodimer	T cells	Proliferation of B cells, thymocytes and mast cells. Blocks activation of cytokine production by T cells, NK cells and monocytes
IFN-γ		T cells, NK cells	Activates lymphocytes, macrophages, NK cells, etc., enhances MHC expression
IL-1	β-trefoil	Myelomonocytic cells, lymphocytes, NK cells, etc.	Pyrogen, T-cell activation
TGF-β	Cysteine knot	T cell, macrophages, platelets	Inhibits cell growth, switch factor for IgA
TNF-α	Homotrimer ('Jelly roll' motif)	Macrophages, T cells	Inflammatory mediator, regulates growth/differentiation of various immune cells
IL-8	'Greek key' motif (3-stranded antiparallel β-sheet)	Monocytes, lymphocytes, etc.	Attracts and activates neutrophils

GM-CSF, granulocyte macrophage colony-stimulating factor; IL, interleukin; IFN, interferon; MHC, major histocompatibility complex; NK, natural killer; TGF, transforming growth factor; TNF, tumour necrosis factor.

be directly activated when one of its components binds the surface of certain infectious organisms. By proceeding in the absence of antibodies, the alternative pathway constitutes an important first line of innate defence. C3 convertase induces the formation of a membrane attack complex (**MAC**). MAC can disrupt plasma membranes, triggering lysis of the target cell. Soluble inhibitors control the complement cascade to prevent inappropriate binding and destruction of host tissue.

Cytokines

Cytokines are soluble immune mediators that behave in a similar manner to hormones: they can act locally on the cell that secreted them, on nearby cells or at a distance and their expression is tightly regulated. The many effects of cytokines, which often act in concert with one another, can make their precise functions difficult to dissect, although cytokine-deficient mice have provided some

clues to their individual roles. Cytokines have been systematically subgrouped in several ways, and may be categorized according to their structure, origin or effects (Table 2.5). **Haematopoietins**, such as granulocyte macrophage colony-stimulating factor (GM-CSF) are small single chain proteins that exert their influence on haemopoietic stem cells and their offspring. **Interferons** are named for their role in antiviral defence. **Tumour necrosis factors** (TNFs) exist as homotrimers and trigger a similar multimerization of their receptors upon engagement. **Interleukins** (ILs) are generally produced by T cells. Of these, IL-2 is produced by T cells and stimulates T-cell activation, proliferation and further cytokine production. Cytokines that favour a cellular and cytotoxic immune response are termed T_H1, and include γ-interferon (IFN-γ), IL-2, TNF and GM-CSF. T_H2 cytokines favour a humoral or antibody response and include IL-4 and IL-10, which influence B cells and macrophages, respectively.

02

Particular cytokine profiles are often observed in disease situations. This has therapeutic relevance as regulation of cytokine activity could be used to enhance or inhibit immune reactions. A number of novel immunotherapies are now in clinical use including basiliximab, a monoclonal antibody against the IL-2 receptor that has been used to prevent organ transplant rejection. Agents that target the interaction between TNF and its receptor can be used to treat rheumatoid arthritis. Such agents include infliximab, a TNF-α specific monoclonal antibody and etanercept, a soluble recombinant TNF receptor, which competes with the cell-surface receptor and so inhibits the normal TNF–TNF receptor interaction. An IL-1 receptor antagonist, anakinra, is also used to inhibit the inflammatory process in rheumatoid arthritis.

Chemokines

Chemokines (*chemo*tactic cyto*kines*) are involved in leucocyte activation and migration. Most members of this family exhibit a conserved motif of four cysteines (C) and are classified according to the pattern of these cysteines into **CXC chemokines**, **CC chemokines**, **CX3C chemokines** and **C chemokines**. Chemokines are recognized by G protein-coupled surface chemokine receptors (R), which are subgrouped according to their ligand (CR, CCR, CXCR and CX3CR). Two cytokine receptors (CCR5 and CXCR4) act as coreceptors for the entry of HIV into cells. Individuals who are homozygous for a CCR5 deletion have been observed to be resistant to acquired immune deficiency syndrome (AIDS) despite repeat exposure. The cells of these patients do not express normal CCR5 on their surface with the effect that viral entry is reduced.

Cell surface markers

Coreceptors and adhesion molecules

While B- and T-cell receptors mediate antigen specificity, additional leucocyte cell-surface molecules have other essential roles, as coreceptors, signal transduction molecules and adhesion molecules. Many of these molecules are members of the immunoglobulin superfamily and share structural similarities to immunoglobulins. Common cell-surface markers found on T cells include CD3, CD4 and CD8. CD3 is associated with the TCR and is required for TCR signal transduction. In contrast, CD4 and CD8 act as coreceptors to increase the avidity of T cell–APC interactions by engaging class 2 or class 1 MHC, respectively. Antibodies against these molecules have been used in transplantation to inhibit the immune system and prevent transplant rejection.

An important function of T cells is their ability to migrate into particular tissues. Circulating cells must first adhere to blood vessels at an appropriate site in order to pass into the tissue. Similarly, T cells must adhere to their targets in order to enable efficient antigen recognition. These functions are achieved by specific adhesion proteins (Table 2.6). Adhesion proteins include members of the immunoglobulin superfamily (**ICAM-1**, VCAM-1, **integrins**) and the **selectin** family of carbohydrate recognition receptors (also known at the leucocyte endothelial cell–cell adhesion molecules; LEC-CAMs).

Pattern recognition receptors

Pattern recognition receptors (PRRs) are receptors on innate immune effector cells that recognize particular molecular structures on foreign pathogens. These receptors typically recognize highly conserved microbial

Table 2.6 Cell adhesion molecules

Adhesion molecule	Properties and clinical relevance
E-selectin, P-selectin	Calcium dependent, mediate cell–cell adhesion interactions in the bloodstream. Characterized by their ability to bind carbohydrates. Increased expression on neutrophils during acute inflammation (e.g. septic arthritis)
VCAM-1	CAM adhesion proteins are members of the immunoglobulin superfamily and are calcium independent. VCAM-1 promotes the adhesion of lymphocytes, monocytes, eosinophils and basophils. Expression is elevated during chronic lymphocytic inflammation (e.g. sarcoidosis, graft rejection)
Integrin $\alpha_5\beta_1$	Integrins are heterodimeric transmembrane glycoproteins of α and β subunits and bind extracellular matrix proteins or ligands on other cells. Blocking the interaction between integrin $\alpha_5\beta_1$ and fibronectin can prevent melanoma cells from metastasizing
E-cadherin	Calcium-dependent glycoprotein expressed on epithelial cells. Upregulation of E-cadherin on breast carcinoma cells can inhibit their invasive properties
β_2 integrins	Deficiencies in β_2 integrins are associated with leucocyte adhesion deficiency caused by a lack of neutrophil migration

structures including bacterial or other microbial lipopolysaccharides (LPSs), lipids and DNA. Secreted PRRs can act in a manner analogous to antibodies by triggering the destruction of their targets by complement proteins or phagocytosis. Toll-like receptors (**TLRs**) are a family of PRRs that are activated in response to various microbial stimuli. Signalling through TLRs can trigger cytokine release and microbial killing mechanisms such as the production of reactive nitrogen species. Given that PRRs are expressed on cells that often act as APCs, these molecules may also influence responses of the adaptive immune system.

The immune system and disease

Immune evasion

While the immune system has been evolving to combat infection, pathogens have been evolving to evade recognition and destruction by the immune system. One simple approach used by intracellular bacteria such as *Chlamydia* and *Mycobacteria*, is to conceal themselves in privileged intracellular compartments in order to evade detection. Many viruses, such as the Epstein–Barr virus, can maintain themselves in a latent state. A classic example of host evasion is provided by trypanosomes, which, during the course of an infection, express a series of different antigenic coats to keep them one step ahead of antibody responses. As an immune response develops in response to one coat, the parasite switches to express another coat that the host has not yet developed a response to. In some cases, specific proteins are used to subvert the host immune system. For example, cytomegalovirus (CMV) and adenovirus encode proteins that block MHC class 1 antigen presentation. Other viruses express homologues of cytokines and their receptors. HIV provides an extreme example of host subversion, as it specifically infects immune cells, destroying their ability to function. The short lifespan of infectious pathogens allows a relatively rapid response to host selection pressures. An evolutionary process of immune evasion can also be seen in the development of cancers. Tumour-specific mechanisms of immune evasion are not fully defined, but loss of HLA molecules at the cell surface or expression of immunosuppressive cytokines such as TGF-β may have a role. Additionally, chemokine mechanisms may allow circulating tumour cells to home to particular tissues.

Immunodeficiency

Immunodeficiency can result from genetic or environmental factors. Inherited immunodeficiencies are usually recessive gene defects and, in the instance of minor deficiencies, other immune system components can usually compensate. When illness does occur, clinical features often reflect the nature of the defect. For example, increased susceptibility to certain bacterial infections could indicate a problem with antibody, complement or phagocytic responses. In contrast, problems with viral or fungal infections are more likely to indicate a problem with cellular immunity. Abnormalities in immunoglobulin production can cause immunodeficiency and are commonly associated with recurrent respiratory and sinus infections. These deficiencies are usually treated with regular infusions of normal human serum immunoglobulins. Deficiencies in MHC class 2 or T-cell function have profound effects, resulting in severe combined immunodeficiency (SCID). A similar effect is seen during AIDS following infection with HIV. HIV specifically infects immune cells by binding the CD4 coreceptor expressed on T_H cells, dendritic cells and macrophages. The subsequent loss of T-cell help affects the function of other immune populations including cytotoxic T cells, B cells and monocytes, leading to a generalized immunodeficiency. However, the genes responsible for immunodeficiency are not always obvious—patients with X-linked hyper IgM syndrome are actually deficient for a protein known as CD40 ligand, which is required for T-cell-dependant activation of B-cell proliferation, and its absence has an indirect effect on antibody production.

Hypersensitivity

Hypersensitivity results from an immune response that is inappropriate in terms of its target or its magnitude. Four main types of hypersensitivity have been defined, according to the immune mechanism involved and the nature of the target antigen (Table 2.7). **Type I hypersensitivity** (also known as atopic allergy) results from an inappropriate IgE response to soluble antigens. IgE antibodies prebound to the cell surface by FcεRI receptors will trigger mast cell degranulation to release histamine, vasoactive amines and inflammatory mediators when they complex with their cognate antigen. Immediate hypersensitivity involves vasodilatation and smooth muscle constriction. A late phase reaction occurs following recruitment of granulocytes, which release cytokines and chemokines. Severe anaphylaxis, as occasionally seen for nut allergies, can occur from disseminated mast cell activation following allergen absorption from the gut. **Type II hypersensitivity** is mediated through recognition of membrane-bound IgG immune complexes by complement, NK cells and macrophages. Fc receptor recognition of these membrane-bound immune complexes leads to ADCC or phagocytosis. Reactions to certain drugs can result in lysis of red blood cells (haemolytic anaemia) or platelets (thrombocytopenia) by this same mechanism. During **type III hypersensitivity**, small IgG–antigen complexes adhere to blood vessels or organs. This can arise during

Table 2.7 Hypersensitivity reactions

Type	Mediated by	Mechanism
Type I	IgE Soluble antigen	IgE immune complexes are recognized by high-affinity Fc receptors on mast cells. Fc receptor recognition triggers mast cell degranulation to release proinflammatory and vasoactive substances. Early phase response involves smooth muscle contraction and a drop in vascular permeability. Cellular infiltration occurs during late phase. Type I hypersensitivity requires previous sensitization to antigen. Clinical examples include anaphylaxis, hay fever and asthma
Type II	IgG/IgM Cell-associated antigen	Damage occurs via direct Fc-dependent mechanisms or through the classical pathway of complement activation. Cellular damage occurs as a result of antibody-dependent cellular cytotoxicity. Clinical examples include autoimmune haemolytic anaemia and Goodpasture's syndrome
Type III	IgG Soluble antigen	Mechanism is similar to type I hypersensitivity but involves a lower affinity Fc receptor. Clinical examples include Arthus' reaction, SLE, postinfective glomerulonephritis
Type IV	T cells Soluble antigen (T_H cells) Cell-associated antigen (CTL)	T-cell recognition triggers cytokine/chemokine production, resulting in cellular infiltration. Clinical examples include tuberculosis, contact dermatitis, thyroiditis, type 1 diabetes mellitus

CTL, cytotoxic T cell; Ig, immunoglobulin; SLE, systemic lupus erythematosus; T_H, helper T cell.

persistent infection or in some autoimmune conditions. A local inflammatory response is then triggered and tissue damage may occur through the action of activated complement proteins and recruited neutrophils. **Type IV (delayed) hypersensitivity** results from the action of cytokines produced by activated T cells, which recruit macrophages and other immune cells to the site of inflammation. Characteristic type IV hypersensitivity reactions include basophil infiltration into the skin, contact sensitivity and granulomatous responses as seen for tuberculosis.

Autoimmunity

Autoimmunity represents a breakdown of the control mechanisms that prevent the immune system from recognizing self-components. Under normal circumstances, **self-tolerance** ensures that B cells are unresponsive to self-components, and that self-peptides presented by MHC on the surface of healthy cells do not induce a T-cell response. **Central tolerance** is achieved by the clonal inactivation or deletion of autoreactive T lymphocytes in the thymus and of B cells in bone marrow. Because lymphocytes will not come into contact with all self-proteins within central lymphoid organs, **peripheral tolerance** mechanisms are also required. Tolerance in the periphery may be maintained by activation-induced cell death (deletion), a lack of costimulation (anergy), peripheral suppression (regulation) or by T-cell ignorance of antigens expressed in immunologically privileged sites. When these mechanisms break down, autoimmune disease can occur.

The nature of an autoimmune disease reflects the distribution of the target antigen(s). Type 1 diabetes mellitus and thyroiditis are organ-specific autoimmune diseases, where the main response is localized to particular tissues. Similarly, in antiglomerular basement membrane disease (Goodpasture's disease), the autoimmune antibodies are specific to collagen components in the basement membrane of the lungs and kidney, so disease is restricted to these sites. In contrast, systemic autoimmune diseases such as systemic lupus erythematosus (SLE) may feature a response directed against ubiquitously expressed proteins. These targets are often intracellular proteins that would not normally be exposed to immune surveillance. Susceptibility to autoimmune disease has a large genetic component, although environmental factors also have an important role. Autoimmune susceptibility often maps to the MHC where antigen-presentation molecules are encoded.

Transplantation

Organ transplantation is an important form of treatment in modern medicine, but a transplanted organ contains many foreign antigens that may constitute targets for the recipient's immune system. In this context, the foreign material is allogeneic rather than microbial in origin. Transplant rejection can occur as a result of disparities between MHC proteins (major histocompatibility differences) or between other molecules (minor histocompatibility (mHC) differences). HLA matching can improve transplant success by eliminating the major components of MHC-based rejection, but does not reduce the effect of mHC mismatches. A large number of circulating T cells in any individual can directly recognize foreign MHC molecules and this **direct allorecognition** is a major cause of transplant rejection. **Indirect allorecognition** occurs through presentation of donor MHC fragments or mHC antigens by the APCs of the recipient. Antibodies to alloantigens can also mediate transplant rejection. Therefore, some degree of ongoing immunosuppression is usually required to maintain graft survival. **Cyclosporin** inhibits T-cell activation, and is frequently used in human transplantation. Cyclosporin indirectly inhibits calcineurin, a kinase involved in T-cell activation. **Tacrolimus** and **rapamycin** have broadly similar effects and all three drugs are termed **calcineurin inhibitors**. Other immunosuppressive agents include steroids and drugs such as azathioprine inhibit cellular proliferation by interfering with purine synthesis. Antibodies against immune cells can also be used as immunosuppressive agents. The major problem with immunosuppression is that it increases the risk of opportunistic infection and, in the longer term, of cancers.

Bone marrow transplantation is a key treatment for various diseases, including leukaemias and immuno-deficiencies. This technique carries a greater risk of graft-vs.-host disease (GVHD) compared to solid organ transplants, because mature donor T cells are also trans-ferred with the bone marrow. When these donor T cells become activated within their new host, they can mount a vigorous response against the recipient's tissues, causing widespread damage, especially to the skin and gut.

Pharmacology

To prescribe drugs rationally, it is necessary to understand some basic pharmacological concepts. At their site of action, drugs interact with molecules termed 'drug recep-tors'. These are often actual biological receptors, such as hormone receptors, but may also be any other type of molecule, such as an enzyme or membrane channel. The **affinity** of a drug-receptor interaction is a measure of how tightly the two molecules bind. An **agonist** is a substance that has an effect on a specific drug receptor, causing activa-tion of the function of the receptor molecule. A **partial agonist** has the same type of effect on the function of the receptor molecule, but even at the maximal effect of the drug, the function of the receptor molecule is not activ-ated to its maximal level. An **antagonist** is a drug that binds to but opposes the natural activity of the receptor molecule. **Competitive antagonists** compete with agon-ists for the same receptor, but do not exert an agonist effect themselves and so reduce the effect of any agonist present. Under these circumstances, the overall effect

will depend on the relative concentrations of agonist and antagonist. A **non-competitive antagonist** does not compete for the same site, but opposes the effect of the agonist by another mechanism. Finally, an **irreversible antagonist** is an antagonist that inactivates the receptor molecule permanently once it has bound. This effect cannot be reversed, even at high concentration of agonist. Many drug receptors are bound by naturally occurring agonists and antagonists, including hormones and neurotransmitters.

Pharmacodynamics describe the distribution of a drug through various body compartments as a function of time. In contrast, **pharmacokinetic** studies follow the actions and effects of drugs on living tissue. **Dose–response curves** relate the biological effect of a drug to its administered dose. Sometimes this effect is directly proportional to the dose, so that doubling the dose will double the effect. However, this is often not the case and it may, for example, take a 10-fold increase in dose to achieve a doubling of effect. Drug dosage is affected by many factors including the absorption, distribution, metabolism and excretion of the drug. Although these effects are complex, clinically useful decisions about drug dosage can be made if the drug half-life is known. The **half-life** of a drug is the time taken for plasma levels of the drug to fall to half of their original value. Drugs are usually administered orally, intravenously, subcutaneously or intramuscularly. Before distribution to its site of action, a drug must first be absorbed from its administration site (e.g. gut, skin or muscle) unless it is injected intra-venously. The most rapid effects are obtained by intra-venous administration, which immediately delivers the drug into the blood for direct transport to the tissues. When a drug has been absorbed, it equilibrates through-out its **volume of distribution**, which may not include all tissues. Most orally administered drugs are absorbed in the small bowel and must pass through the liver before they can reach the systemic arterial circulation. This means that they may be altered by metabolism in the liver, a pro-cess known as 'first pass metabolism'. Once any drug has been administered, it may be inactivated by metabolism (especially in the lungs) or excreted by the kidney in urine or, less commonly, by the liver in bile. Metabolism fre-quently alters drug activity. **Phase 1 reactions** cause oxida-tion, reduction or hydrolysis of the drug and involve cytochrome p450 mixed-function oxidases. **Phase 2 reac-tions** add groups such as glucuronides or sulphates to the drugs, increasing their water solubility and making them suitable for excretion by the liver in bile or by the kidney in urine. Within the kidney, anion and cation transporters are capable of transporting drugs into tubules for excre-tion in the urine.

Many drugs are bound by **plasma proteins**; acidic drugs

bind albumin and basic drugs bind to $\alpha1$ acid glycoproteins. If a drug is strongly bound by a plasma protein, then it will tend to remain within the circulation. If a drug is poorly bound by plasma proteins, then its distribution will depend upon its **lipid-solubility**. Water-soluble drugs tend to remain within extracellular fluids, whereas lipid-soluble drugs cross cell membranes to enter cells and may even become concentrated in adipose tissue.

Statistics

The evaluation of both clinical and basic scientific studies can be complex if many individual observations have been made. Under these circumstances, it is useful to establish how likely or probable it is that measured similarities or differences between groups have occurred by chance rather than as a result of real differences between the groups.

Typically, the spread of characteristics for a group is communicated by providing some measure of the middle value and some measure of the overall range of values. For example, the weights of a group of patients could be communicated by providing the average weight in addition to the highest and lowest values. Other measures of the middle value are indicated in Table 2.8. Measures of the spread can include the range of values, which is simply the difference between the highest and the lowest value. The **standard deviation** measures the spread of values around the mean.

Clinical studies

Studies are usually performed on a sample of people drawn from a large population. A key use of statistics is to evaluate how well the information derived from studying this sample is likely to predict characteristics of the real population. The **standard error** of the data gives an indication of the reliability of the data by incorporating information about the number of observations. Standard error is calculated by dividing the standard deviation of the

data by the square root of the number of observations. The standard error of a study gets smaller as the size of the sample studied increases. **Confidence limits** can be calculated from the standard error of the mean to provide an indication of how reliably studies of the sample can predict the characteristics of the entire population. Thus, if the average weight of a sample from a population is 70 kg and the 95% confidence limits for this sample is 3 kg then that means that there is a 95% probability that the average weight of the population lies between 67 kg and 73 kg.

Risk factors for disease can also be evaluated statistically. In a retrospective study it is usual to calculate **odds ratios**, and in a prospective study to calculate **relative risk**. If, in a prospective study, smokers have twice the incidence of coronary artery disease than non-smokers, then the relative risk for coronary artery disease in smokers is 2. In a retrospective study, the odds ratio compares the ratio of non-smokers to smokers in the disease group to the same ratio observed for the disease-free group. The higher the ratio of smokers to non-smokers in the disease compared to the disease-free group, the higher the implied risk of smoking for developing disease.

Various tests have been devised to evaluate the strength of association for measured variables such as blood pressure with clinical outcomes. The **correlation** describes the strength of the association, while **regression** analysis can be used to evaluate the mathematical relationship between blood pressure and outcome. If multiple variables such as age, blood pressure and weight are studied, **multiple regression analysis** provides a method for determining the contribution of each variable to the outcome. Variables such as gender, which are **categorical** rather than **continuous**, can be studied as predictors of outcome using χ^2 analysis. For example, χ^2 analysis can be used to evaluate whether differences in observed numbers of men and women with stroke are likely to have occurred by chance or because of gender-related risk.

The **power** of a study determines whether it was appropriately designed to stand a good chance of detecting a difference between the groups analysed. For example, a study could have a 90% chance of detecting a 15% increase in survival from a new treatment for myocardial infarction. Usually, the main determining factor is the size of the study and the frequency of the event under study. A pilot study is often required to estimate the power of the main study. Different types of clinical studies can be identified. A **case–control study** is usually a retrospective examination to define risk factors for a disease. A **randomized control trial** is ideal for comparing the results of a therapy. Typically, patients should be allocated to either the treatment or a placebo, and the outcome of the two groups compared. If neither the study subjects, nor those evaluating the outcome know which subjects had

Table 2.8 Measures of middle value

Value	Definition
Arithmetic mean	The sum of the values of the data divided by the number of observations
Mode	The most frequent value
Median	The point that lies midway between the highest and the lowest values when the observations are put in order. If there are five observations, it is the value of the third highest observation

the new treatment or the placebo, then the trial is said to be '**double-blind**'.

Significance and *P* values

Many clinical studies are designed to establish whether there is a difference between two groups. In these circumstances, it is useful to have a statistical measure to determine the significance of any difference that is identified. For example, we might want to establish whether women have a different serum cholesterol level to men. We could measure the serum cholesterol levels in an equal number of men and women and find out what the average serum cholesterol level is for each group. Suppose that we find that the women have an average serum cholesterol of 4.2 and the men of 4.7. We then need to know how likely it is that this difference arises by chance and how likely it is that it arises because men really have higher cholesterol levels. If the number of people sampled is small, it might just be that by chance, the group of men we picked were all people with high cholesterol levels and if we chose another small set of men and women, we might find that they had similar cholesterol levels.

Statistical methods are available to assess this likelihood, or probability, by taking into account factors such as the number of measurements or observations in the study and the spread of the values. Usually, these methods produce a *P* **value**. A *P* value of 0.05 means that there is a probability of 5% that the difference occurs by chance and a probability of 95% that the difference is significant. Usually, it is considered that a *P* value of 0.05 is a useful cut-off for significance and a *P* value of greater than 0.05 is usually regarded as non-significant. However, it is important to remember that this cut-off is simply a convention and the *P* value may be poor because of the inadequate design of the study rather than because the difference is not real. *P* values can also be used to assess the significance of other statistics, such as those that define correlations or associations, such as those between high blood pressures and strokes. There are many different types of clinical studies that use *P* values and it is very important to be sure that the correct statistical test has been used to calculate the *P* value. Many clinical researchers take advice from statisticians for this reason.

Diagnostic tests

Diagnostic tests can be evaluated in a number of different ways. Consider a test for a viral infection (Table 2.9). The **sensitivity** and **specificity** define the probability of the diseased state being correctly identified. The sensitivity is the number of correctly identified infected individuals with a positive test result. Specificity describes the number of

Table 2.9 Test for viral infection

	Infected	Uninfected	Total
Test result positive (abnormal)	a	b	a + b
Test result negative (normal)	c	d	c + d
Total	a + c	b + d	n

Sensitivity = a/(a + c).
Specificity = d/(b + d).
Likelihood ratio = sensitivity/specificity.
Positive predictive value = a/(a + b).
Negative predictive value = d/(c + d).
Prevalence = (a + c)/n.

correctly identified uninfected individuals with a negative result. A **likelihood ratio** of sensitivity : specificity provides the probability of getting a positive test result if the patient is infected. As the sensitivity rises, so does the likelihood ratio.

Predictive values define the probability of the test result being correct for the population studied. The **positive predictive value** defines the number of people with a positive test result who are actually infected. The negative predictive value is the number of people with a negative test result who are uninfected. Predictive values are only correct for a population with the same prevalence as that in the studied sample group. Bayes' theorem can be used to calculate the predictive values for populations with different prevalences.

Diagnostic and research techniques in modern medicine

Nucleic acid techniques

Most nucleic acid techniques rely on the propensity of single DNA strands to anneal or **hybridize** to other strands of complementary sequence by complementary base pairing. Thus, single-stranded '**probes**' for DNA of a particular sequence can be labelled with a detectable marker then used to detect the appropriate sequence in a range of experimental situations. For sequencing and polymerase chain reactions (PCRs), short **primers** of complementary DNA hybridize with their templates and are extended by a polymerase enzyme.

DNA sequencing

Complementary primers to the sequence of interest are added to a DNA template along with a polymerase enzyme, the four normal nucleotide monomers and modified nucleotide monomers that can be incorporated instead of a particular base. Incorporation of modified

02

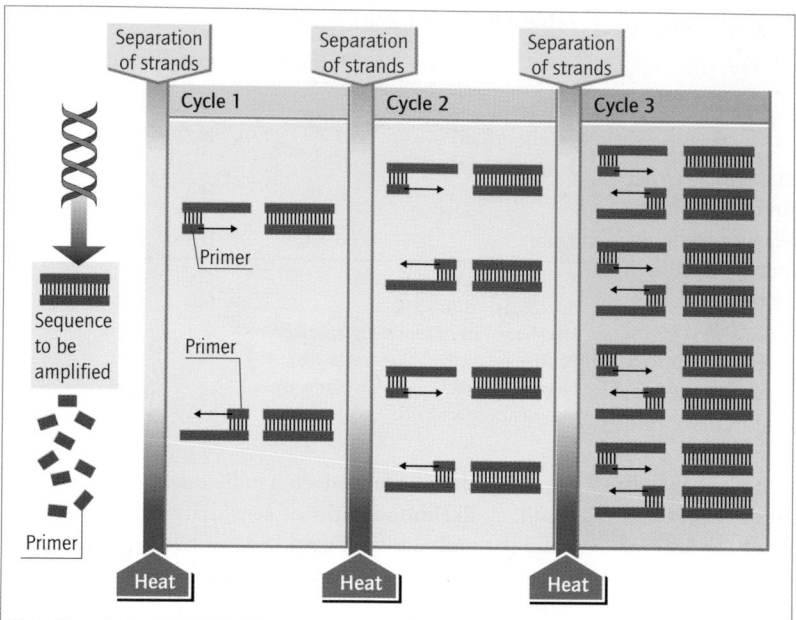

Figure 2.21 Polymerase chain reaction. The DNA sequence to be amplified is selected by short synthetic oligonucleotide primers that correspond to the sequences flanking the target DNA. Excess primers and a heat-stable polymerase is added and the mixture heated to separate the primers and the DNA. The mix is allowed to cool (annealing temperature), the primers bind and the polymerase elongates the primers on either strand, thus generating two new identical double stranded DNA molecules. Each cycle doubles the number of copies of the original DNA fragment.

nucleotides prevents further extension and the overall result is the production of many strands of different length, which can be separated according to their length. Ordering the strands according to their size gives the DNA sequence. Modern methods use a combination of fluorescent dyes (one for each modified base) read by an automatic sequencer.

Polymerase chain reaction

Polymerase chain reaction has revolutionized molecular research by allowing rapid cloning of genes and protein coding sequences. In each cycle of amplification, a double stranded DNA template is heated to separate the two strands, cooled to allow a primer to hybridize to the strands and then warmed slightly to allow a DNA polymerase enzyme to extend each primer, producing more double stranded template for the next cycle (Fig. 2.21). Repeating the amplification process over many cycles allows exponential generation of the DNA sequence between the two primers. This DNA can then be analysed by examining its length using gel electophoresis, or by determining its sequence.

DNA cloning

DNA cloning allows pieces of DNA to be isolated and incorporated into DNA vectors (Fig. 2.22). DNA vectors are often circular bacterial plasmids or modified viruses, which can be used to generate multiple copies of the cloned (recombinant) sequence or to express its encoded protein in a foreign situation. Specific enzymes, usually derived from bacteria, can be used to cut or join DNA, to

reverse-transcribe DNA from RNA and to polymerize complementary DNA (cDNA). Restriction enzymes bind to and cleave specific DNA sequences. Their targets are often palindromic; for example, the EcoR1 enzyme (purified from *Escherichia coli*) will cut DNA upon binding the sequence GAATTC. This means that if a piece of DNA is cut by a particular enzyme, then it must contain the relevant target sequence. Digested DNA fragments can be incorporated into an appropriately digested vector through the action of a ligase enzyme. Processes known as transfection or transformation are used to introduce recombinant DNA vectors into relevant host cells.

Microarrays

Microarray analysis uses precision technology to analyse the expression of numerous genes in a single experiment. DNA probes for thousands of individual genes are attached in microscopic spots to a glass slide. These probes can take the form of short primers or of longer amplified sequences. A bulk RNA preparation from the cell line or tissue of interest is fluorescently labelled then hybridized to the chip. Computer analysis is used to detect hybridization patterns and thus identify expressed genes.

Chromosomal techniques

Karyotyping/fluorescence *in situ* hybridization

As each human chromosome has its own characteristic shape, chromosome analysis can be used to detect structural abnormalities. Metaphase chromosomes (where

02

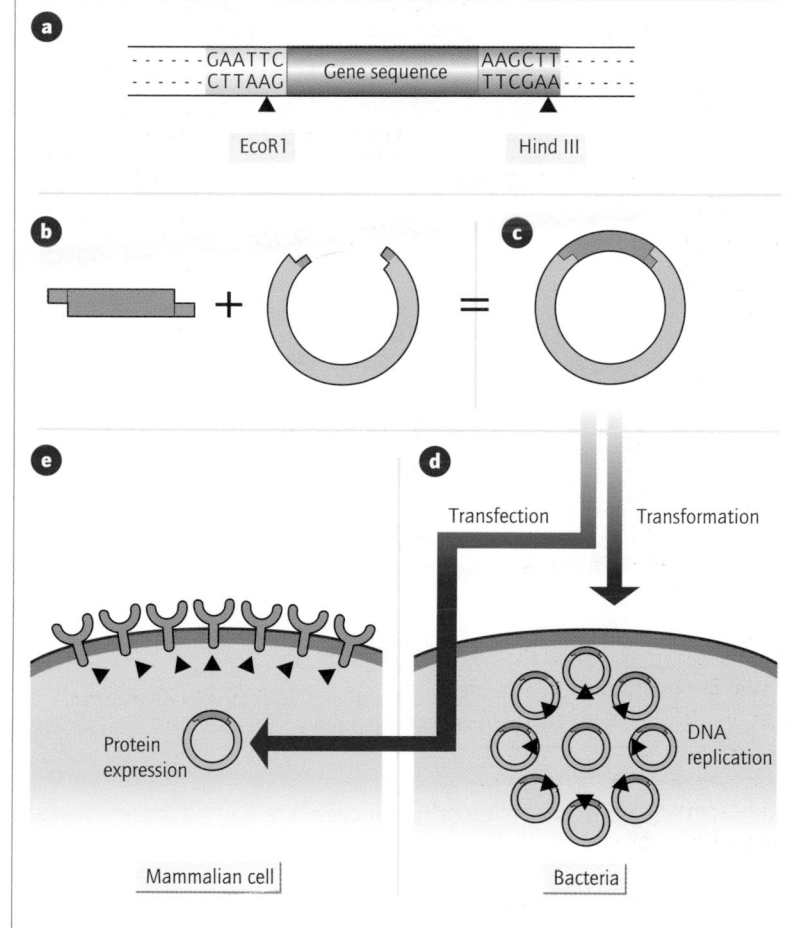

Figure 2.22 DNA cloning. (a) The DNA sequence of interest (e.g. a polymerase chain reaction product) is prepared by digestion with specific restriction enzymes (e.g. EcoR1 and Hind III). (b) The resulting DNA fragment is then ligated into a similarly digested DNA vector containing the sequences necessary to initiate DNA replication and/or protein expression. Recombinant DNA plasmid (c) can then be introduced into appropriate host cells as a means to generate further copies of the plasmid (d) or express the encoded protein (e) for experimental studies.

DNA is maximally contracted) were traditionally analysed by dye staining and normal microscopy. Characteristic banding patterns allowed sites of DNA loss or gain to be directly visualized. Modern developments in fluorescence technology allow complex chromosomal rearrangements to be observed in greater detail. Fluorescently labelled DNA probes are used to 'paint' each chromosome a different colour. DNA probes for each chromosome identify their complementary sequence in denatured metaphase chromosomes in a process known as fluorescence *in situ* hybridization (**FISH**). Multicolour analysis using different fluorescent dyes allows localization of individual genes to specific regions on chromosomes, in addition to identifying chromosomal translocations or aneuploidy (see p. 39).

Gene tracking

Genes located on the same chromosome are usually inherited together, a phenomenon known as **genetic linkage**. Genes located close to one another have an increased chance of being inherited together, but genes far apart may not be inherited together if there is a chromosomal recombination event between them during meiosis (see p. 30). **Linkage analysis** looks at the recombination frequencies between particular genes. Thus, known genes can be used to locate disease genes to which they show significant linkage. The logarithm of the odds (**LOD**) score measures the statistical significance of cosegregation between a marker and disease gene or, in other words, the likelihood that the disease gene is near the marker.

Genetic polymorphisms often affect the target sequences of restriction enzymes. Thus, genomic DNA taken from genetically disparate individuals can be digested using frequent-cutting enzymes such as EcoR1 to generate fragments of different length. These differences are termed **restriction fragment length polymorphisms** (**RFLPs**) (Fig. 2.23). If a particular restriction marker is associated with a phenotypic characteristic, the relevant gene is probably located nearby. Thus, RFLP analysis can also be used to track disease genes.

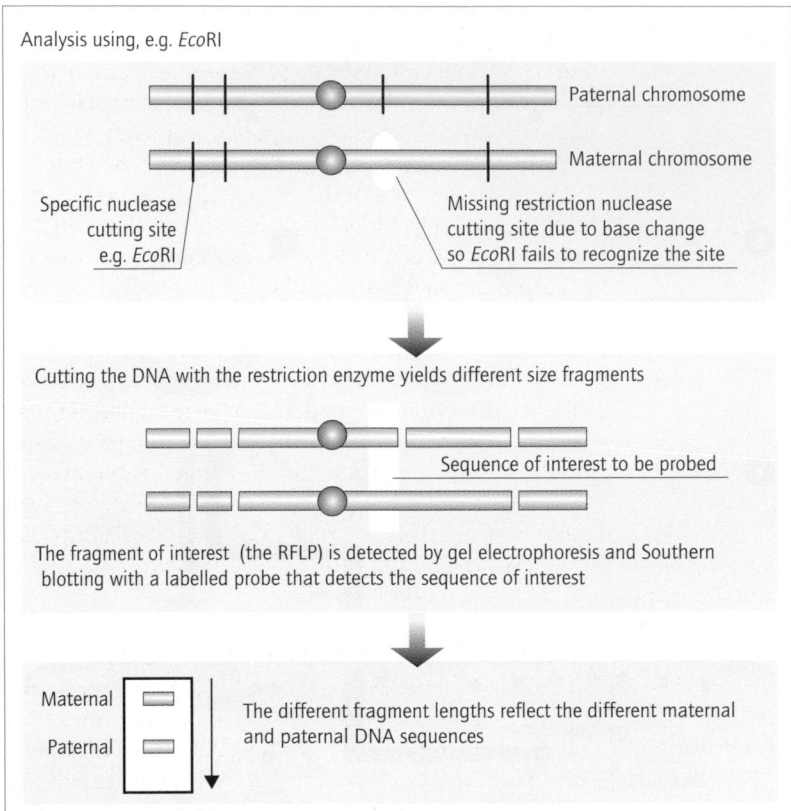

Analysis using, e.g. *Eco*RI

Paternal chromosome

Maternal chromosome

Specific nuclease cutting site e.g. *Eco*RI

Missing restriction nuclease cutting site due to base change so *Eco*RI fails to recognize the site

Cutting the DNA with the restriction enzyme yields different size fragments

Sequence of interest to be probed

The fragment of interest (the RFLP) is detected by gel electrophoresis and Southern blotting with a labelled probe that detects the sequence of interest

Maternal

Paternal

The different fragment lengths reflect the different maternal and paternal DNA sequences

Figure 2.23 Identifying genetic differences between individuals: restriction fragment length polymorphism (RFLP) analysis.

DNA fingerprinting

Non-coding regions of repetitive DNA such as minisatellites (see p. 34) are highly polymorphic. The hypervariable nature of variable number tandem repeats (**VNTRs**) (which differ in their length and number) allows them to be used as a source of genetic fingerprint. PCR amplification of a VNTR will produce a characteristic profile for an individual. Analysing two independent repeat variations increases the value of this technique. A child's amplification pattern is a combination of the patterns obtained for each parent. In addition to forensic analysis, DNA fingerprinting is used for paternity testing.

Biochemical techniques

Gel electrophoresis

Separation of nucleic acids or proteins by electrophoresis through a gel matrix is a fundamental laboratory technique. **Agarose** gels are commonly used to separate fragments of DNA, while **polyacrylamide** gels are used for protein analysis or high-resolution electrophoresis of DNA. Proteins can be separated on the basis of their size by polyacrylamide gel electrophoresis in the presence of sodium dodecyl sulphate (**SDS-PAGE**). Modifications of

the basic electrophoresis protocol include **isoelectric focusing** (IEF), a technique that separates proteins within a pH gradient, and **two-dimensional gel electrophoresis**, which separates complex mixtures of proteins, usually by IEF followed by SDS-PAGE.

Gel separated agents are usually visualized by incorporation of non-specific dyes and by comparison with molecular weight standards. To identify a specific molecule on a gel, a probe that binds only to the molecule of interest must be used. Molecular probes for nucleic acid sequences or proteins cannot be directly applied to the gel matrix. Once the gel has been run, the separated molecules must be transferred onto a solid support such as nylon or nitrocellulose membrane for further analysis. The process of **Southern blotting** (named after its inventor) transfers electrophoresed DNA onto a solid support, which can be hybridized with a labelled probe of single stranded DNA (Fig. 2.24). When this technique is applied to RNA rather than DNA, it is referred to as **northern blotting**. The equivalent technique for proteins (known as **western blotting**) transfers proteins onto a solid support where they are probed with antibodies. Many modern biochemical techniques employ antibodies to purify or detect proteins. Antibody bound to its target protein is identified by a directly conjugated marker or by use of a 'secondary'

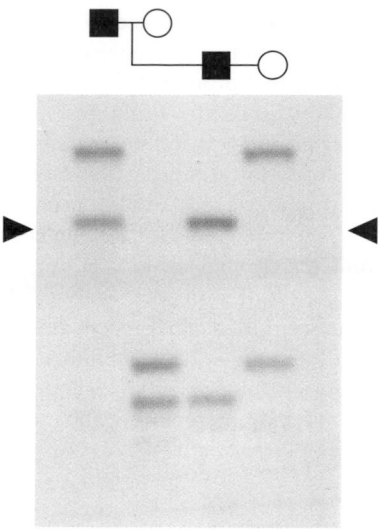

Figure 2.24 Nucleic acid blotting. Nucleic acid is run on an agarose gel to separate it into different sizes and then transferred to a membrane. Labelled DNA probes are added and bind to nucleic acid on the membrane with the complementary sequence. The position of the probes on the membrane can then be visualized as bands. This example shows a southern blot of DNA from four individuals which has been cut with a restriction enzyme and probed for a DNA sequence near the polycystic kidney disease gene. Two individuals carry the gene and, therefore, have a band of the size shown by the arrows.

immunoglobulin-specific antibody that has been prelabelled with a biochemical or fluorescent marker.

Monoclonal antibodies

Monoclonal antibodies are specific for a single epitope, and can therefore be used to study individual proteins in detail. Production of monoclonal antibodies has revolutionized biochemical research. According to this method, a rodent is immunized with the antigen of interest in order to trigger an antibody response. Antibody-secreting spleen cells from the immunized mouse are then fused to myeloma cells. Each of the resulting **hybridomas** secretes a single antibody. Clonal hybridoma populations can then be screened to identify those expressing antibody with the appropriate specificity. Slight differences exist between the framework regions of human and murine antibodies. Therefore, monoclonal antibodies used for therapy must be modified to prevent them from becoming a target for the recipient immune response. Protein engineering can be used to 'humanize' murine antibodies to prevent this type of antiglobulin reaction. **Polyclonal antibodies** are less specific as they recognize multiple epitopes. Although their precise targets are undefined, polyclonal antibodies are easier to produce as they are purified directly from the serum of an immunized animal.

Enzyme-linked immunosorbent assay

This antibody-based detection system harnesses the antigen-binding capacity of antibodies as a means of detecting their target antigen (Fig. 2.25). One example is the diagnostic detection of a viral antigen in serum. The sample is applied to a plate that has previously been coated with an antibody against the molecule of interest. A further antibody is then introduced and, if the target antigen has been captured, then this secondary antibody will also bind. The secondary antibody can be labelled with a chromogenic enzyme, allowing enzyme-linked immunosorbent assay (ELISA) results to be measured by spectrophotometry. ELISPOT is a modified form of ELISA that can be used to

Figure 2.25 The enzyme-linked immunosorbent assay (ELISA) can be used to detect antibodies to a given antigen. (a) In a traditional ELISA, for example, wells are coated with the target antigen, washed and then test serum applied. (b) If antibodies to the target antigen are present in the serum sample they will remain bound to the antigen-coated plate after washing. (c) Bound antibody can then be detected using 'secondary' antihuman antibodies to which a chromogenic enzyme (red circles) has been attached. (d) In the case of a 'sandwich' ELISA, antibody is bound first to the plate, and (e) used to capture soluble antigen. (f) Following a wash step, bound antigen is detected using a second antibody to which a chromogenic enzyme has been attached.

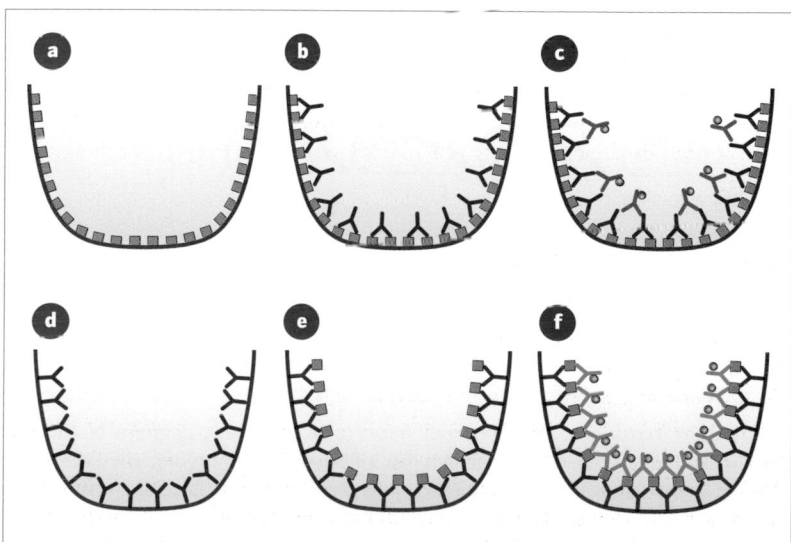

detect cells secreting particular cytokines. Cells are cultured in wells coated with cytokine-specific antibodies. If the cytokine is produced by cells in a particular well, it will be detected in the well by subsequent ELISA. T cells from a patient's blood can be incubated with a pathogen or pathogen component to test their cytokine secretion profile. A cytokine response would indicate a specific immune response, thus providing evidence of exposure to the pathogen.

Cell and tissue techniques

Flow cytometry

Flow cytometers (also known as fluorescence activated cell sorters; **FACSs**) analyse the size and fluorescence profiles of individual cells. Cellular expression of a protein can be studied by binding of fluorescence-tagged antibodies specific for that protein. A flow cytometer counts the number of cells stained with fluorescent antibody to determine the percentage of cells expressing the protein. For example, flow cytometry using fluorescent antibodies against the lymphocyte cell-surface protein CD4 can determine CD4 T-cell counts for HIV-infected patients. Multiple proteins on the same cell can be analysed together using a set of antibodies tagged with different coloured fluorescent markers. A recent development has been to substitute antibodies with fluorescently tagged protein ligands, generated *in vitro*. This approach has been applied to identify novel receptor–ligand interactions and to quantify peptide-specific T cells *ex vivo*.

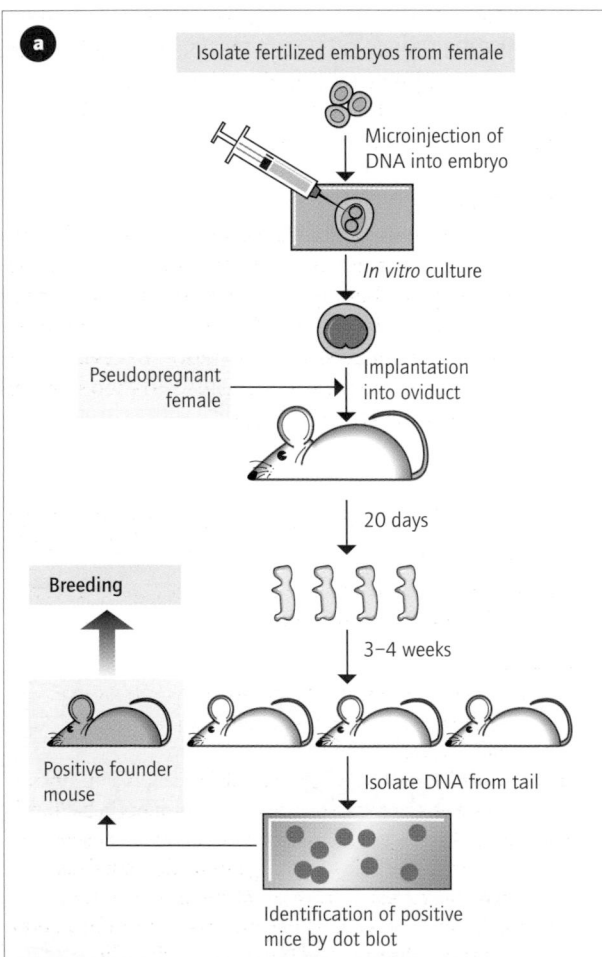

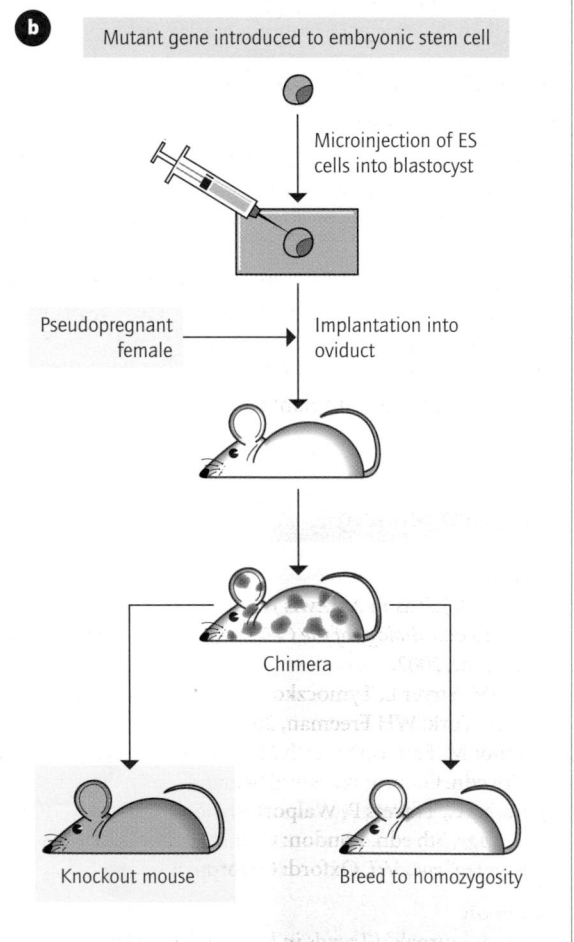

Figure 2.26 Transgenic and knockout mice. (a) A schematic diagram of the technology used to produce transgenic mice. (b) Knockout mice. The mutant gene is first introduced to embryonic stem (ES) cells in culture. The mutant ES cell is then micro-injected into a blastocyst for implantation into a female mouse. Resulting offspring are chimeric for the mutant gene, and are subsequently bred to homozygosity in order to obtain knockout mice.

Microscopy

Traditional light microscopy remains a commonly used technique to examine cells or tissue samples. **Immuno-histochemistry** using enzymatically tagged antibodies with a chromogenic substrate can be employed to identify proteins of interest in tissue sections. As an alternative, fluorescence microscopy visualizes proteins labelled by fluorescently tagged antibodies. **Confocal microscopy** provides high-resolution images using a focused laser to excite fluorescence in a single focal plane. The highest levels of resolution are provided by electron microscopy, as the wavelength of electrons is much smaller than that of light. Samples stained with gold-tagged antibodies are analysed by a **transmission electron microscope**. This apparatus focuses a beam of electrons through the specimen to visualize fine structural details and is often used on kidney biopsies. **Scanning electron microscopes** generate high-resolution surface images.

Gene modification *in vivo*

Transgenic animals

Advances in genetic manipulation allow us to study novel and disease-associated genes using *in vivo* animal systems. Human disease processes and novel treatments are increasingly analysed by comparison with transgenic models (usually rodents), which express a foreign gene. To create a novel transgenic, a DNA vector encoding the gene of interest is microinjected into an egg cell where it integrates at random within the host genome (Fig. 2.26a). Fertilized eggs are implanted into a female and the neonates are assessed for transgene expression. Several generations of backcrossing may be required to achieve transgene expression on a stable genetic background. Particular promoter elements can be used to regulate transgene expression; for example, to ensure that expression occurs only in certain tissues. Transgenic techniques have been used to generate pigs whose organs may be suitable for transplantation into humans. The long-term aim of this work is to allow xenotransplantation (transplantation across species) with organs expressing human markers to reduce the risk of rejection.

Gene knockout

The *in vivo* function of a gene can be investigated by removing it from an animal's genome using the 'knock-out' approach. Homologous recombination is used to remove functional gene copies from embryonic stem (ES) cells (Fig. 2.26b). Recombinant ES cells are injected into a blastocyst, which is then implanted into early mouse embryos to generate chimeric offspring. Mice that are homozygous for the mutant gene are derived from subsequent breedings from chimeric mice.

Human gene therapy

Although germ line modification of humans is unlikely to provide an acceptable option for treating human disease, somatic cell gene therapy may ultimately benefit patients with certain genetic disorders. For example, it may be possible to use homologous recombination to insert a non-mutated form of a haemoglobin gene into blood stem cells of patients with sickle cell disease.

Further reading

Books

Alberts B, Johnson A, Lewis J, Raff M, Roberts K, Walter P. *Molecular Biology of the Cell*, 4th edn. New York: Garland Science, 2002.

Berg JM, Stryer L, Tymoczko JL. *Biochemistry*, 5th edn. New York: WH Freeman, 2002.

Connor M, Ferguson Smith M. *Essential Medical Genetics*, 5th edn. Oxford: Blackwell Science, 1997.

Janeway C, Travers P, Walport M, Shlomchik M. *Immunobiology*, 5th edn. London: Churchill Livingstone, 2001.

Lewin B. *Genes VII*. Oxford: Oxford University Press, 2000.

Journals

'Trends journals' (*Trends in Immunology*, *Trends in Genetics*, etc.) give generalized reviews of current topics in each field (Elsevier Science).

'Insight' series of articles on a themed subject are regularly published in *Nature* magazine.

Websites

www.bmn.com [Biomednet contains a comprehensive source of web links, literature search and electronic journal listings.]

www.biomedcentral.com [This website contains a number of good reviews as well as a useful series of primers in biology.]

www.ncbi.nlm.nih.gov [This site contains an extensive range of resources for searching biomedical databases. It is possible to search most of the medical literature using the site. The OMIM database contains information about genetic diseases and the books section allows online searching of a number of standard basic science textbooks.]

Infectious Disease

3

Three hundred years ago most people in Britain died from infection and the average life expectancy is estimated to have been 30–40 years. In the middle of the last century, when comprehensive mortality figures were first compiled, the main causes of death included tuberculosis, smallpox, typhoid, cholera, dysentery, rheumatic heart disease, diphtheria and lobar pneumonia.

Clearly, a profound revolution has since occurred in the pattern of disease in developed countries. The traditional infective scourges are all but eradicated in the developed world and degenerative and neoplastic diseases now dominate the mortality statistics.

This dramatic reduction in the burden of infectious diseases in developed countries has occurred through a combination of factors:

● An enormous improvement in the nutrition and living conditions of most of the population has been at the root of the decline of most infectious diseases (Fig. 3.1).

● Public health measures, such as the provision of safe water and drainage, have limited epidemics of the faeco-oral infections.

● Specific measures, such as immunization (which has been most important for certain diseases) and effective chemotherapy, have become available for most of these conditions.

Meanwhile, developing countries continue to experience much the same pattern of infection-dominated pathology as developed countries in the last century, with the addition of some purely tropical parasitic infections. In some countries, many children die before their fifth birthday; acute respiratory infection, gastroenteritis, measles and malaria are among the biggest killers.

Infectious diseases remain important because:

● There are newly recognized diseases, such as acquired immune deficiency syndrome (AIDS), Lyme disease and Legionnaires' disease.

- There are new infective causes for old diseases, such as *Helicobacter pylori* in gastritis.
- There is a rising trend of antibiotic resistant organisms (e.g. multidrug-resistant tuberculosis).
- Infection is difficult to manage in patients receiving complex medical and surgical treatment.
- Widespread international travel means that many people from countries where infectious diseases have been eradicated put themselves at risk of tropical diseases.
- There is increasing recognition of the role of infectious agents in other areas of medicine—infections may be a trigger for arthritides, cardiomyopathy, dementing syndromes and tumour growth.

Infectious diseases affect all branches of medicine. The following is intended as a summary of the main infectious diseases. Diseases are discussed in groups according to their main presentation (e.g. fever with a rash), or by system (e.g. infections of the respiratory tract).

Pathogenicity and virulence

Introduction

Humans share the planet with a dizzying array of micro-organisms, most of which are completely harmless. Medicine is interested in the small minority of organisms that are capable of establishing themselves in the human host, paying particular attention to those that cause disease. Descriptions of this interaction depend on the definition of several terms used throughout this chapter and listed in Table 3.1.

There is often confusion about the terms communicable disease and infections. Not all infections are communicable; for example, endocarditis is an infection but it does not spread from one person to another. These non-communicable infections are usually derived from the body's normal flora that has been given an opportunity to invade a normally sterile site. The ability of micro-organisms to colonize the human host causing disease and then be transmitted on to another is the main factor that differentiates infectious from other diseases. Some infectious diseases are capable of rapid spread throughout the world; this is usually called a pandemic. Others may spread within a small area (a family or a ward) while others may spread within a locality, a town or province; both of these forms of spread are called epidemics. Other diseases are transmitted between hosts but at a low rate so

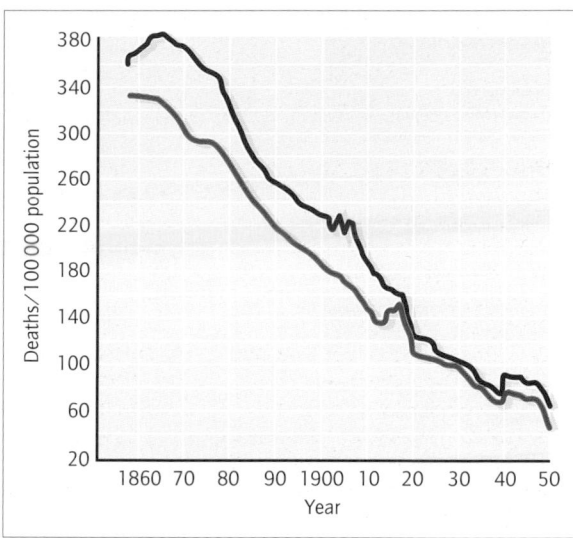

Figure 3.1 Historical decline in tuberculosis in England and Wales (blue), and Scotland (red).

Table 3.1 Definitions of terms

Pathogen	A micro-organism capable of establishing itself in the human body where it causes disease
Commensal	A micro-organism capable of establishing itself in the human body without causing disease
Pathogenicity	The ability of a micro-organism to invade the host
Virulence	The ability of an organism to cause serious disease

that there is a steady number of cases which only varies a little. This is known as endemic spread.

Sources of infection

There are four sources for micro-organisms that give rise to disease: the host's normal flora, other humans, animals and organisms in the environment.

Normal flora

The body is colonized by many micro-organisms, in fact bacterial cells outnumber the human cells. The bacteria colonize the pharynx, the lower small intestine and colon, the female genital tract and the skin (Fig. 3.2). The normal flora has a beneficial effect by competing with pathogens for colonization sites. Some bacteria produce antibiotic

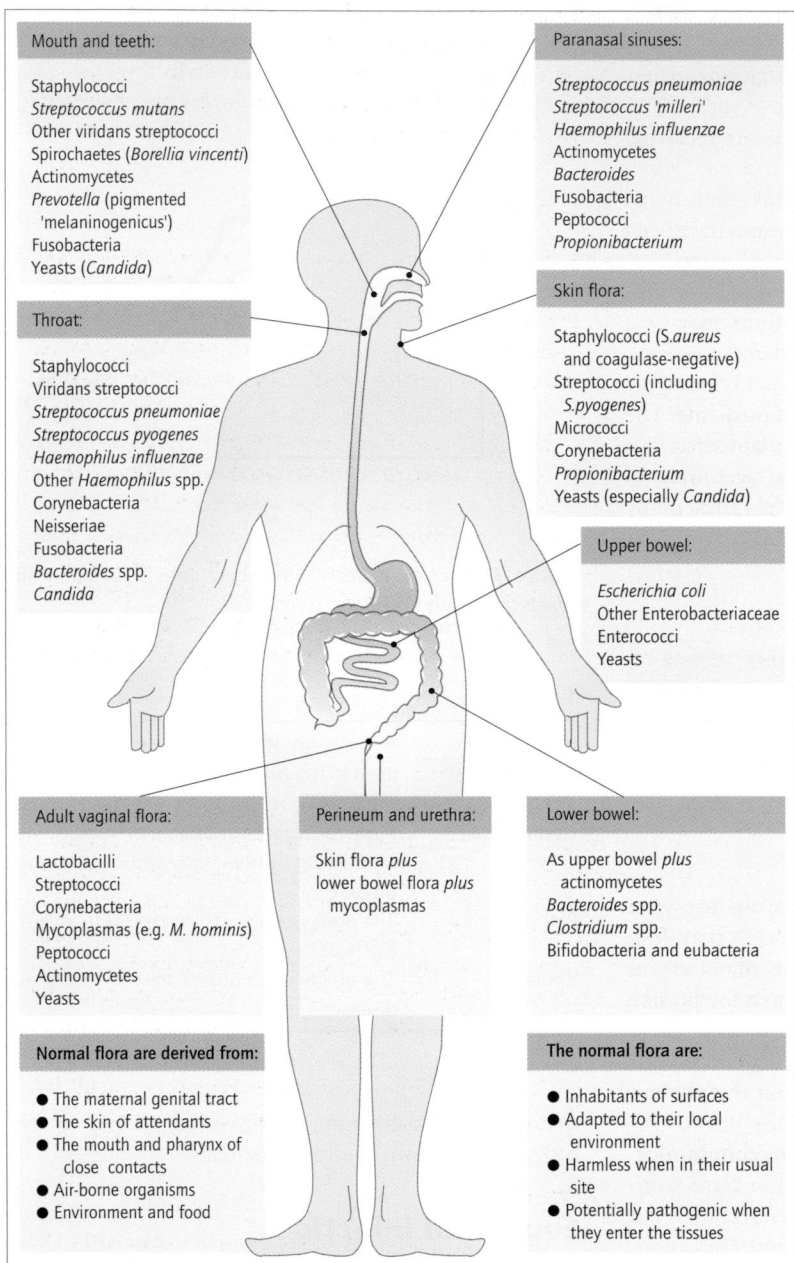

Mouth and teeth:

Staphylococci
Streptococcus mutans
Other viridans streptococci
Spirochaetes (*Borellia vincenti*)
Actinomycetes
Prevotella (pigmented
  'melaninogenicus')
Fusobacteria
Yeasts (*Candida*)

Throat:

Staphylococci
Viridans streptococci
Streptococcus pneumoniae
Streptococcus pyogenes
Haemophilus influenzae
Other *Haemophilus* spp.
Corynebacteria
Neisseriae
Fusobacteria
Bacteroides spp.
Candida

Paranasal sinuses:

Streptococcus pneumoniae
Streptococcus 'milleri'
Haemophilus influenzae
Actinomycetes
Bacteroides
Fusobacteria
Peptococci
Propionibacterium

Skin flora:

Staphylococci (*S.aureus*
  and coagulase-negative)
Streptococci (including
  S.pyogenes)
Micrococci
Corynebacteria
Propionibacterium
Yeasts (especially *Candida*)

Upper bowel:

Escherichia coli
Other Enterobacteriaceae
Enterococci
Yeasts

Adult vaginal flora:

Lactobacilli
Streptococci
Corynebacteria
Mycoplasmas (e.g. *M. hominis*)
Peptococci
Actinomycetes
Yeasts

Perineum and urethra:

Skin flora *plus*
lower bowel flora *plus*
  mycoplasmas

Lower bowel:

As upper bowel *plus*
  actinomycetes
Bacteroides spp.
Clostridium spp.
Bifidobacteria and eubacteria

Normal flora are derived from:

● The maternal genital tract
● The skin of attendants
● The mouth and pharynx of
  close contacts
● Air-borne organisms
● Environment and food

The normal flora are:

● Inhabitants of surfaces
● Adapted to their local
  environment
● Harmless when in their usual
  site
● Potentially pathogenic when
  they enter the tissues

Figure 3.2 Normal human flora. Reproduced from Bannister, Begg & Gillespie, *Infectious Disease*, 2000, 2nd edn (Blackwell Science Ltd) with permission.

substances (bactericines) that suppress competing organisms. Resident anaerobes produce toxic metabolic products and free fatty acids that inhibit the growth of other organisms. In the female genital tract, lactobacilli produce lactic acid in quantities that lower the pH, making colonization by pathogens more difficult.

Bacteria from the normal flora can get beyond their proper place in the intestinal tract or the skin, with severe consequences. During aspiration of stomach contents, bacteria from the oral cavity are transported to the lung, where a rapidly progressive lung infection may develop. When there is perforation of the stomach or large bowel, intestinal contents can escape into the peritoneum, resulting in peritonitis. Poor dental hygiene can result in oral bacteria such as *Streptococcus sanguis* being deposited on heart valves, leading to endocarditis.

Other humans

The most common source of pathogenic organisms is from other humans and infections can spread by a number of routes described below. Interrupting routes of transmission is important for everyone involved in the practice of medicine.

Animals

Infections derived from animals are known as zoonoses. This may be as a result of direct contact with animals either as pets or in the course of farming or other occupational exposure. Almost all of the human population is exposed to animals through the consumption of meat or other animal products such as milk. Even strict vegetarians can be at risk if meat products contaminate their food.

Environment

Most environmental organisms have little capacity to invade humans and cause disease. There are some notable exceptions that, in the right circumstances, can cause infection. *Legionella* is an environmental organism that lives in an aquatic environment, often invading amoebae. It is able to colonize air-conditioning systems and showers.

Routes of transmission

Micro-organisms have devised many different ways of spreading from one host to another, which is broadly related to their ability to survive outside a host. Organisms that are very hardy, like *Clostridium tetani*, which has a spore, survives in the environment and patients can become infected from the inoculation of infected soil or other material. In contrast, organisms like *Neisseria gonorrhoeae* are very delicate and highly susceptible to drying and are not able to survive outside the body so are transmitted by the sexual route.

Respiratory route (air-borne)

When an individual coughs or sneezes, a large number of particles are projected into the atmosphere. Some of these particles are of optimal size (5–/ μm) to be carried into the respiratory tract, some as far as the alveoli. These are known as droplet nuclei and may contain micro-organisms. Organisms that spread by the respiratory route include respiratory pathogens such as *Streptococcus pneumoniae* and influenza virus as well as organisms that colonize the upper respiratory tract then invade to cause disease at distant sites, such as *Neisseria meningitidis*. Infections that are spread by this route may be transmitted

very rapidly in a community; for example, the speed with which influenza spreads during the winter months. Some organisms that do not cause respiratory infections can be transmitted from person to person in the air, including *Staphylococcus* and *Streptococcus*.

Ingestion

Organisms that cause disease of the gastrointestinal tract are typically transmitted in food or water. Transmission by this route can give rise to an epidemic if a large number of individuals ingest food at the same time; for example, a turkey contaminated with *Salmonella* inadequately cooked and served at a communal Christmas lunch. Infection can also spread from person to person through poor hand hygiene: faeco-oral transmission. *Shigella* have a very low infectious dose, as few as 10 organisms, making it easy for the organism to spread from one patient with dysentery to another. Intestinal nematodes, such as *Ascaris lumbricoides*, have a tough egg that survives in the environment for many months. If an individual ingests food contaminated by these eggs, infection may follow.

Direct contact

Many organisms are spread by direct contact with other people or contaminated objects (fomites). Direct contact with people can permit organisms to be carried from one patient to another on the hands of medical staff attending the patient. Also, equipment such as stethoscopes can become contaminated, allowing organisms to spread. Equipment and materials used in operations must be scrupulously decontaminated to prevent inoculation of micro-organisms. Close contact also allows skin organisms to be transmitted between people, transmitting infections such as ringworm or scabies.

Parenteral

The parenteral route allows blood-borne organisms to be spread within populations. This route spreads hepatitis B and C and the human immunodeficiency virus (HIV). This may arise through inadequate decontamination of medical devices or the reuse of disposable syringes. Alternatively, non-medical procedures that pierce the skin can transmit infections, including scarification rituals, tattooing, acupuncture or intravenous drug misuse.

Sexual

Many organisms that are unable to survive in the environment and which colonize mucosal surfaces are transmitted

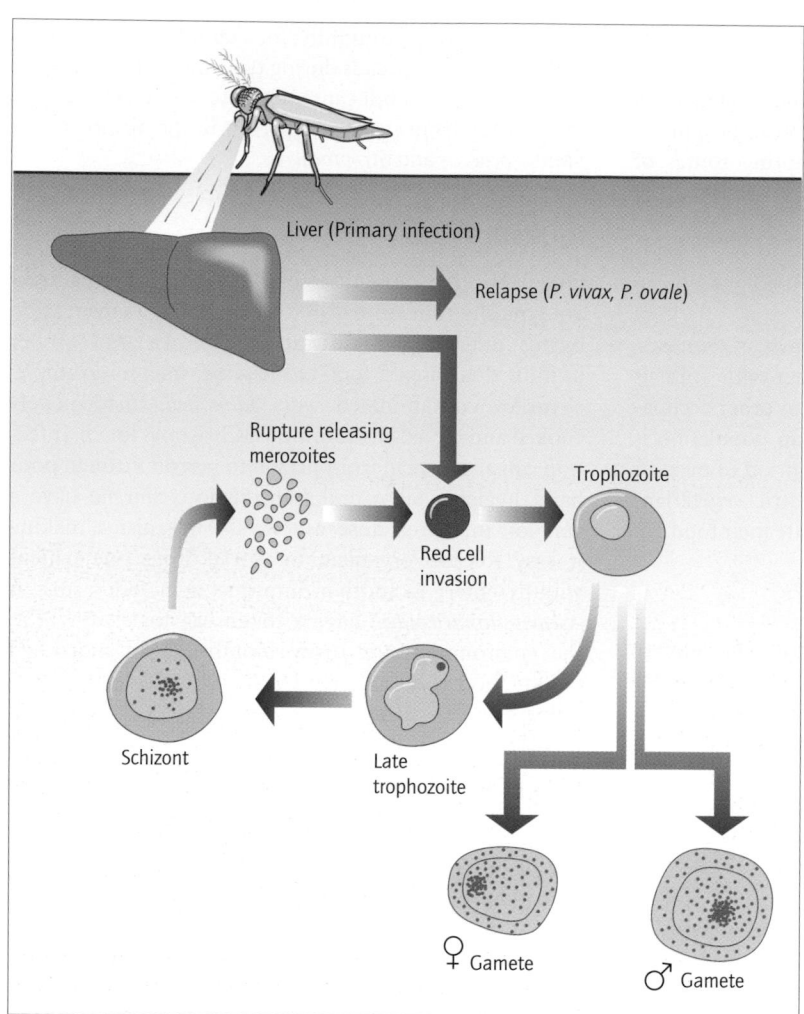

Figure 3.3 Malaria life cycle.

by the sexual route. Agents include *Neisseria gonorrhoeae*, *Treponema pallidum*, HIV and *Chlamydia trachomatis*.

Vectors

The physical barrier of the skin can also be breached by biting arthropods. All types of pathogen can be transmitted by this route. The most important example of this is malaria (Fig. 3.3) and some examples, together with their vector, are noted below (see p. 128).

Elements of pathogenicity

Survival in the environment

Some bacteria produce endospores that are resistant to environmental trauma and are almost metabolically inert so that nutrients are not required (Fig. 3.4a,b). Spores enable organisms to survive in severe adverse conditions where conditions for multiplication are unsuitable. Spores may remain dormant for many years in the soil only to become active and cause disease when inoculated into a wound.

Attachment to host surfaces

Invading micro-organisms must attach themselves to host tissues to colonize the body and the distribution of receptors will define the organs that are invaded. *Neisseria gonorrhoeae* adhere to the genital mucosa using specialized organelles of attachment known as fimbriae or pili. These are long protein structures that adhere to epithelial surfaces. Strains of *N. gonorrhoeae* that do not possess fimbriae are non-pathogenic. Influenza virus attaches to host cells via its haemagglutinin antigen and HIV has an antigen which binds CD4 receptors on host cells allowing the virus to invade T cells and macrophages. Staphylococci synthesize fibronectin binding protein to attach to this protein expressed on cell surfaces and intracellular matrix.

In the gut, organisms must bind to enterocytes to prevent being expelled by peristalsis. *Vibrio cholerae* excretes

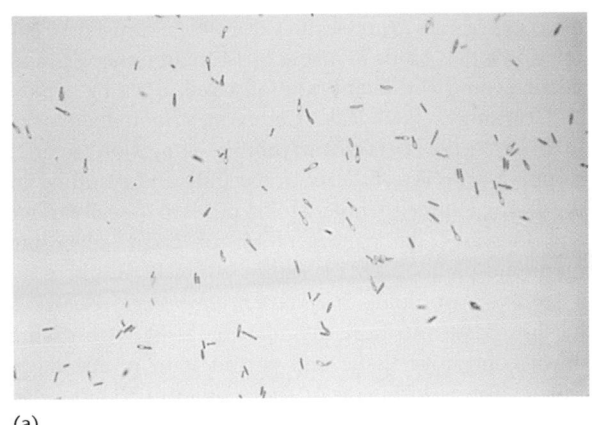

(a)   (b)

Figure 3.4 Examples of spore-forming bacteria: (a) sub-terminal spores, (b) terminal spores.

a mucinase to help it penetrate to the enterocyte, then attaches via a pilus and switches on fluid secretion. *Giardia lamblia* is attached to the jejunal mucosa by a specialized sucking disc and red cells infected by *Plasmodium falciparum* express a parasite encoded protein on knobs on the red cell surface which mediate adherence to host brain capillaries responsible for the often fatal complication of cerebral malaria.

Some bacteria form biofilms, which consist of a layer of cells attached directly to a surface and other layers attached to this basal layer by means of a polysaccharide matrix. Biofilms have an important part to play in colonization of indwelling prosthetic devices such as catheters. Organisms in the biofilm grow more slowly and antibiotics and immune components may not penetrate effectively. This has the effect of enabling the organism to survive in the face of antibiotic therapy and immune response.

Motility

The ability to move to locate new sources of food and in response to chemotactic signals should enhance pathogenicity; *V. cholerae* is motile by virtue of its flagellum but non-motile mutants are less virulent.

Immune evasion

To survive in the human host pathogens must overcome the host immune defence. *Neisseria meningitidis* and respiratory bacteria secrete an immunoglobulin A (IgA) protease which degrades host immunoglobulin. *Streptococcus pyogenes* expresses protein A which binds host immunoglobulin, preventing opsonization and complement activation.

Avoiding destruction by host phagocytes is an important evasive technique. *Streptococcus pneumoniae* has a polysaccharide capsule which inhibits uptake by poly-

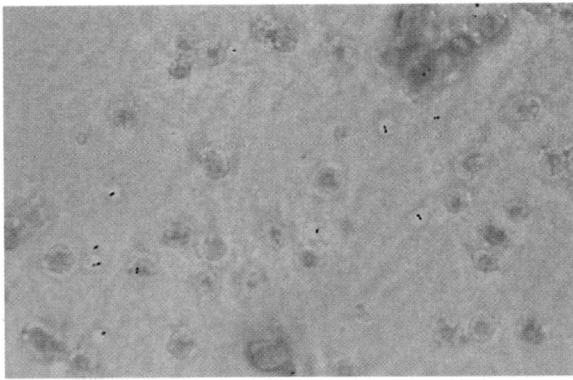

Figure 3.5 Capsulate *Strep. pneumoniae* in sputum. Reproduced from Gillespie, *Medical Microbiology Illustrated*, 1994 (Butterworth-Heineman, Oxford) with permission.

morphonuclear leucocytes; M protein performs a similar function in Streptococcus pyogenes (Fig. 3.5). Some organisms are specially adapted to survive inside host macrophages. *Toxoplasma gondii* and *Mycobacterium tuberculosis* prevent fusion of the phagosome with the digestive lysosome, *Leishmania donovani* excretes material that enables it to inhibit the effects of free radicals and enzymes inside the phagolysosome. The lipopolysaccharide of Gram-negative organisms prevents the formation of C3 convertase and the length of the polysaccharide chain prevents formation of an effective membrane attack complex. Organisms expressing a lipopolysaccharide are thus protected from the lethal effects of human serum.

The major surface antigen of *Trypanosoma rhodesiense* goes through a series of antigenic changes; thus, antibodies produced against the organism rapidly lose their effectiveness and a new wave of organisms continues the infection (Fig. 3.6). Other organisms that adopt this strategy are

03

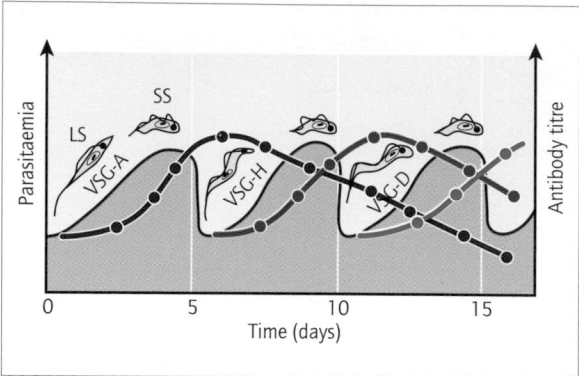

Figure 3.6 Trypanosome antigenic variation. Red, anti-VSG-A; blue, anti-VSG-H; green, anti-VSG-D; LS, long slender trypomastigotes; SS, short stumpy trypanomastigotes. VSG, variable surface glycoprotein.

Borrelia sp. Influenza virus survives as a pathogen by antigenic variation on a global scale, because of the nature of its genome to undergo antigenic 'drift and shift'. Drift is the process of minor changes in the genes coding for viral antigens that occur from year to year. This change means that many of the hosts infected in the previous influenza outbreak will also be susceptible in the next year. Shift is a major change in the antigenic structure of the virus which makes the whole population susceptible and worldwide pandemic develops.

Toxicity

Some organisms release substances that are directly damaging to the host. These are known as toxins (derived from the Greek word for poison). Toxins are classified into two broad categories: endotoxins and exotoxins.

Endotoxins

Endotoxins are part of the structure of bacteria that are released when bacteria cells die or during normal bacterial cell turnover. They are not directly toxic to the human host but require the activation of host immune cells. Gram-negative organisms express a lipopolysaccharide (LPS) on their outer membrane that causes disease by activating host macrophages to produce interleukin 1 (IL-1) and tumour necrosis factor (TNF). These proteins, called cytokines, stimulate changes in the body's metabolism that lead to fever, shock and metabolic disarray: the signs of severe sepsis (Fig. 3.7).

Exotoxins

Exotoxins work by a range of different mechanisms. *Strep-* *tococcus pyogenes* expresses an extracellular antigen, streptolysin O, that binds in a ring of 14 toxin molecules and dissolves into the membrane of a cell, opening a pore and causing a fatal leak. *Corynebacterium diphtheriae* toxin enters the host cell and inhibits elongation factor 2, stopping protein synthesis irreversibly and resulting in the death of the cell. Cholera toxin binds to the cell surface and increases the concentration of cyclic adenosine monophosphate (cAMP) within the cell, resulting in a secretion of fluid. *Streptococcus pyogenes* releases a hyaluronidase into the tissues that may assist it in breaking down connective tissue and permit it to invade more widely. The lechithinase of *Clostridium perfringens* also breaks down tissues, contributing to the rapid spread of gas gangrene in tissues once infection is established. Some organisms, including *Clostridium botulinum* and *Clostridium tetani*, release potent neurotoxins that are responsible for the symptoms and signs of disease.

Classification of infectious diseases

There are difficulties in classifying and presenting infectious diseases. Traditionally, they have been classified according to the organism that causes the condition. However, diseases do not present as organisms, but as clinical syndromes. A further problem arises from the 'many-to-many' relationship of organism and disease.

● One organism can cause many diseases: streptococci are the cause of sore throats, rheumatic fever, puerperal sepsis and bacterial endocarditis.

● Bacterial endocarditis can be caused by many organisms.

In this chapter, the organisms are first classified in a table form in a traditional microbiological manner. The tables also name some of the diseases the organism is associated with and refer to where a fuller description of the disease can be found.

The diseases that present with fever are the main focus of this chapter. They encompass:

● the main childhood infections such as measles and mumps

● tropical or other imported infections

● fever in special groups (the elderly and the immuno-compromised)

Tables 3.2–3.11 give a classification of infectious organisms with their associated diseases and a cross-reference to the appropriate page.

Structure and classification of micro-organisms

Classification of bacteria

The purpose of classification of micro-organisms is to define their pathogenic potential: for example, *Staphylo-*

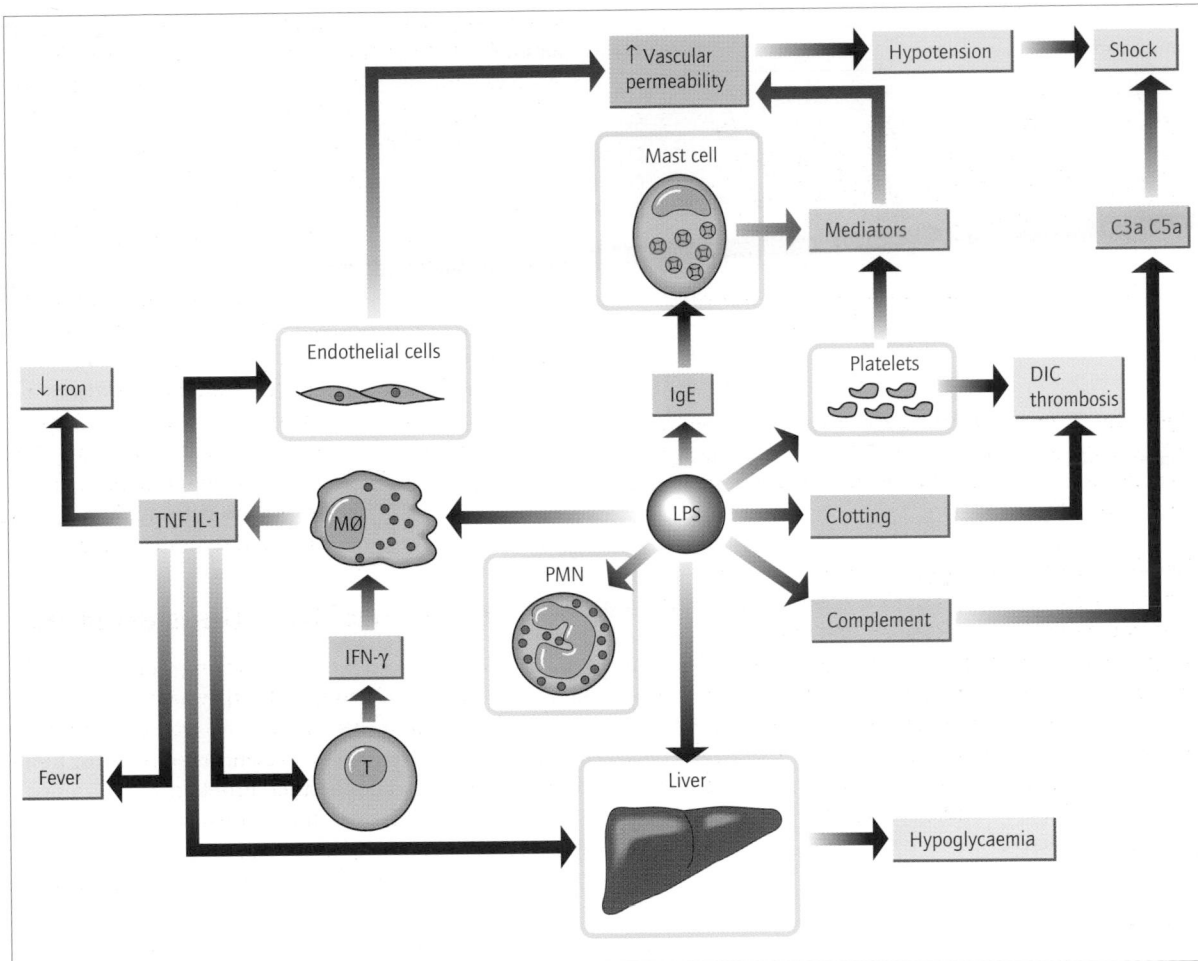

Figure 3.7 Action of bacterial lipopolysaccharide (LPS). Bacterial LPS (endotoxin) activates nearly all immune mechanisms and the clotting pathway, thus making LPS one of the most powerful immune stimuli recognized. DIC, disseminated intravascular coagulation.

coccus aureus isolated from blood is more likely to be acting as a pathogen than *Staphylococcus epidermidis* from the same site. Some bacteria have the capacity to spread widely in the community and cause serious disease; for example, *C. diphtheriae* and *V. cholerae*. Identification of these organisms has important public health implications. Bacteria are identified, or speciated by using a series of physical characteristics. Some of these are listed below.

- Gram reaction: Gram positive and Gram-negative bacteria respond differently to antibiotics.
- Cell shape: cocci, bacilli or spirals.
- Presence and shape of an endospore and its position in the bacterial cell: terminal, subterminal or central.
- Atmospheric preference: organisms are aerobic, requiring oxygen, or anaerobic, requiring an atmosphere with very little or no oxygen. Organisms that grow in either atmosphere are known as facultative anaerobes.

Microaerophiles prefer a reduced oxygen tension and capnophiles prefer increased carbon dioxide.

- Requirement for special media or intracellular growth. More detailed biochemical, antigenic and molecular tests are performed to identify organisms to species level.

Medically important groups of bacteria

Gram-positive cocci

Gram-positive cocci are divided into three main groups: the staphylococci, which include the major pathogen *S. aureus*; the streptococci, including *S. pyogenes*, an agent of sore throat and rheumatic fever, and *S. agalactiae*, which causes meningitis and pneumonia in neonates; and the enterococci (Table 3.2).

Table 3.2 Gram-positive cocci and associated diseases

Genus and species	Associated diseases	Page
Staphylococcus (aerobic, facultatively anaerobic, arranged in clusters)		
Staph. aureus (coagulase positive)	Skin infection (boils, impetigo, abscesses)	1135
	Osteomyelitis and postsurgical sepsis	261
	Pneumonia (especially postinfluenza)	319
	Acute endocarditis	478
Enterotoxin-producing	Food poisoning	751
Toxic shock syndrome toxin-producing	Toxic shock syndrome	125
Staph. epidermidis (coagulase negative)	Rarely pathogenic	
	Septicaemia in immunocompromised	123
	Infection of prostheses and cannulae	
	Peritoneal dialysis infection	560
Staph. saprophyticus (coagulase negative)	Urinary tract infection	568
Streptococcus (aerobic, facultatively anaerobic, arranged in pairs or chains, classified by α or β haemolysis, and by Lancefield grouping)		
Group A β haemolytic *Strep. pyogenes*	Scarlet fever	1136
	Erysipelas	1136
	Cellulitis	1136
	Pyoderma	
	Pneumonia	321
	Pharyngitis	318
	Septicaemia	123
	Rheumatic fever (postinfective complication)	477
	Acute glomerulonephritis (postinfective complication)	521
Group B *Strep. agalactiae*	Neonatal meningitis, pneumonia and septicaemia	
Group C *Strep. equi, Strep. dysgalactiae*	Pharyngitis, endocarditis	318, 478
Group D *Strep. bovis*	Endocarditis	478
	Bacteraemia associated with colonic carcinoma	
Viridans α haemolytic streptococci		
Strep. mitis	Endocarditis	478
Strep. sanguis	Endocarditis	478
Strep. anginosis, Strep. constellatus, Strep. intermedius	Deep-seated abscesses (e.g. liver abscess, empyema)	617, 552
Strep. pneumoniae	Pneumonia, bacteraemia	319
	Meningitis	111
	Otitis media	
	Osteomyelitis	261
Enterococcus		
E. faecalis	Urinary and abdominal infections	
E. faecium	Endocarditis	478
	Bacteraemia in intensive care	

Gram-positive bacilli

Pathogens include *Bacillus anthracis* and the pathogens of gas gangrene, tetanus, pseudomembranous colitis and botulism, all of which carry spores. Non-sporing pathogens include *Listeria*, and corynebacteria (Table 3.3).

Gram-negative cocci and coccobacilli

Gram-negative cocci include the pathogenic *N. meningitidis*, an important cause of meningitis and septicaemia, and *N. gonorrhoeae*, an agent of sexually transmitted urethritis and gonorrhoea. Among the coccobacilli are the

Table 3.3 Gram-positive rods and associated diseases

Genus and species	Associated disease	Page
Bacillus (spore-bearing aerobes)		
B. cereus	Food poisoning	751
B. anthracis	Anthrax	1138
Listeria		
L. monocytogenes	Neonatal meningitis	112
	Meningitis and septicaemia in pregnancy and immunocompromised	
Corynebacterium		
C. diphtheriae	Diphtheria	66, 319
C. pyogenes	Skin infection	1135
Clostridium (spore-forming anaerobes)		
Cl. tetani	Tetanus	114
Cl. botulinum	Botulism	115
Cl. perfringens	Food poisoning	751
	Wound infection	
	Gas gangrene	
Cl. difficile	Antibiotic-associated colitis	121, 754

Table 3.4 Gram-negative cocci, coccobacilli and associated diseases

Genus and species	Associated disease	Page
Neisseria		
N. gonorrhoeae	Gonorrhoea, pelvic inflammatory disease	155
N. meningitidis	Meningitis, septicaemia	110
Moraxella		
M. catarrhalis	Bronchitis (mucopurulent exacerbation)	
	Pneumonia	
	Sinusitis	
	Otitis media	
M. lacunata	Conjunctivitis	
Acinetobacter		
A. baumanii	Ventilator-associated pneumoniae, bacteraemia	
	Wound infection	
Haemophilus		
H. influenzae		
Capsulated	Meningitis	111
	Epiglottitis	
	Acute lower respiratory tract infection	319
	Sinusitis	319
	Otitis media	
	Bronchitis	319, 321
Unencapsulated	Sinusitis	319
	Mucopurulent exacerbations of chronic bronchitis	321, 343
H. aegyptius	Conjunctivitis	
	Brazilian purpuric fever	
H. ducreyi	Chancroid	169
Bordetella		
B. pertussis	Whooping cough	328
Brucella		
B. abortus	Brucellosis	133
B. melitensis		
B. suis		
Francisella		
F. tularensis	Tularaemia	80
Pasteurella		
P. multocida	Sepsis after an animal bite	

respiratory pathogens *Haemophilus* and *Bordetella* and zoonotic agents such as *Brucella* and *Pasteurella*. Acinetobacter are naturally resistant to many antibacterials and are important hospital pathogens (Table 3.4).

Gram-negative bacilli

The terms used to describe the Gram-negative rods are often confusing so it is better to use the species or genus name when describing these organisms. Some are grouped together in the family Enterobacteriaceae and form part of the normal flora of humans and animals but can also be found in the environment. This family includes many pathogenic genera: *Salmonella*, *Shigella*, *Escherichia*, *Proteus* and *Yersinia*. *Pseudomonas* is an environmental saprophyte naturally resistant to antibiotics that has come to be an important pathogen in the hospital environment and in patients with cystic fibrosis. *Legionella* is another environmental species that lives in water but can cause human infection if conditions allow. Anaerobic Gram-negative bacteria are an important part of the flora of the intestinal tract but may cause infection; for example, if the intestinal contents spill into the peritoneum (Table 3.5).

Spiral bacteria

Gastrointestinal pathogens include the small spiral *Helicobacter*, which colonizes the stomach leading to gastric

and duodenal ulcer and gastric cancer, and *Campylobacter* spp., which cause acute diarrhoea. *Borrelia*, spiral bacteria with a long wavelength, give rise to relapsing fever and Lyme disease, a chronic disease of the skin joints and central nervous system. *Leptospira* are zoonotic agents

Table 3.5 Gram-negative rods and associated diseases

Genus and species	Associated disease	Page
Enterobacteriaceae		
Serratia, Enterobacter	Urinary tract infection	568
Citrobacter, Proteus	Major hospital-acquired sepsis (e.g. peritonitis, pneumonia, septicaemia)	
Klebsiella	Urinary tract infection	568
	Hospital-acquired sepsis	
	Community-acquired pneumonia (uncommon)	321
Escherichia		
E. coli	Urinary tract infection	508
	Hospital-acquired sepsis	
	Traveller's diarrhoea	118
ETEC	Traveller's diarrhoea	118
EIEC	Dysentery	118
EHEC or VTEC (often serotype 0157)	Haemolytic–uraemic syndrome	531
Yersinia		
Y. enterocolitica	Enterocolitis	121
	Septicaemia	121
Y. pseudotuberculosis	Mesenteric adenitis	
Y. pestis	Plague	135
Salmonella		
S. typhi, S. paratyphi A, B	Enteric fever	131
Non-typhoid salmonellae	Enteritis	119
Shigella		
S. flexneri, S. boydii, S. dysenteriae, S. sonnei	Dysentery	119
Vibrio		
V. cholerae	Cholera	117
Pseudomonas		
P. aeruginosa	Urinary tract infection	568
	Hospital-acquired sepsis	
	Otitis externa	
Burkholderia		
B. pseudomallei	Melioidosis	
B. cepacia	Chronic destructive chest infection in cystic fibrosis	357
Legionella		
L. pneumophila	Legionnaires' disease	
	Pontiac fever	321
Bartonella		
B. bacilliformis	Oroya fever	
B. henselae		
Bacteroides		
B. fragilis	Surgical sepsis	
Prevotella		
P. ovatis		
Porphyromonas		
P. melaninogenicus		

EHEC, enterohaemorrhagic *E. coli*; EIEC, enteroinvasive *E. coli*; ETEC, enterotoxigenic *E. coli*; VTEC, verotoxin producing *E. coli*.

03

Table 3.6 Spiral organisms and associated diseases

Genus and species	Associated disease	Page
Treponema		
T. pallidum	Syphilis	166
T. endemicum	Endemic non-venereal syphilis	166
T. pertenue	Yaws	
T. carateum	Pinta	
Borrelia		
B. burgdorferi	Lyme disease	1137
B. hermsii (tick-borne)	Relapsing fever	
B. recurrentis (louse-borne)	Relapsing fever	
Leptospira		
L. interrogans	Aseptic meningitis	107
	Weil's disease	107
Spirillum		
S. minus	Rat-bite fever	
Campylobacter		
C. jejuni	Enteritis	120
Helicobacter		
H. pylori	Gastritis	711
	Peptic ulcer disease	703

Table 3.7 *Rickettsia, Chlamydia, Mycoplasma* and associated diseases

Genus and species	Associated disease	Page
Rickettsia		136
R. prowazekii (louse-borne)	Epidemic typhus	
R. typhi (flea-borne)	Murine typhus	
R. rickettsii (tick-borne)	Rocky Mountain spotted fever	
R. conorii (tick-borne)	Boutonneuse fever African tick fever	
R. akari (mite-borne)	Rickettsial pox	
R. tsutsugamushi (mite-borne)	Scrub typhus	
R. quintana (louse-borne)	Trench fever	
Coxiella		
C. burnetti	Q fever	136
Chlamydia		
C. trachomatis	Trachoma	
	Lymphogranuloma venereum	169
	Genital tract infection	156
C. psittaci	Psittacosis	321
C. pneumoniae	Pneumonia	321
Mycoplasma		
M. pneumoniae	Upper respiratory tract infection	318
	Pneumonia	321
	Otitis media	
M. hominis	Genital tract infection	159
Ureaplasma		
U. urealyticum	Genital tract infection	159

causing an acute meningitis syndrome that may be accompanied by renal failure and hepatitis. *Treponema* include the causative agent of syphilis (*Treponema pallidum*) (Table 3.6).

Rickettsia, Chlamydia and Mycoplasma

Only *Mycoplasma* can be isolated on artificial media, the others require isolation in cell culture or diagnosis by molecular or serological techniques. The chlamydiae and mycoplasmas are important pathogens of the respiratory and genital tract. Rickettsias are spread by insects to humans, causing serious systemic infection such as typhus (Table 3.7).

Mycobacteria

Mycobacteria are mainly environmental organisms that only cause disease in patients who are compromised (e.g. *Mycobacterium avium-intracellulare* in AIDS patients). It also includes two of the most important human pathogens: *M. tuberculosis* and *Mycobacterium leprae* (Table 3.8).

Table 3.8 Mycobacteria causing disease in humans. (Non-tuberculosis mycobacteria are often called 'atypical mycobacteria' or 'mycobacteria other than tuberculosis; MOTT'.)

Genus and species	Associated disease	Page
Mycobacterium		
M. tuberculosis	Tuberculosis	330
M. bovis	Tuberculosis	
M. avium-intracellulare	Bacteraemia and pulmonary infection	
	In AIDS patients	182
	Lymphadenopathy in children	
M. kansasii, M. xenopi	Tuberculosis-like syndrome in those with chronic chest disease	333
M. leprae	Leprosy	115

Structure and classification of viruses

DNA viruses

The DNA of viruses is either double or single stranded. Double stranded DNA viruses include a number of important species that cause human disease; for example, poxviruses (smallpox, molluscum contagiosum and vaccinia virus), herpes viruses (herpes simplex and zoster, cytomegalovirus, Epstein–Barr), adenoviruses, papova and polyoma viruses. Papova viruses are small viruses associated with benign tumours, such as warts and malignant tumours, such as cervical cancer. Hepatitis B virus is double stranded with single stranded portions.

Among the single stranded DNA viruses, parvoviruses are responsible for erythema infectiosum. DNA viruses usually replicate in the nucleus of host cells producing a polymerase, which reproduces viral DNA. Viral DNA is not usually incorporated into host chromosomal DNA (Fig. 3.8; Table 3.9).

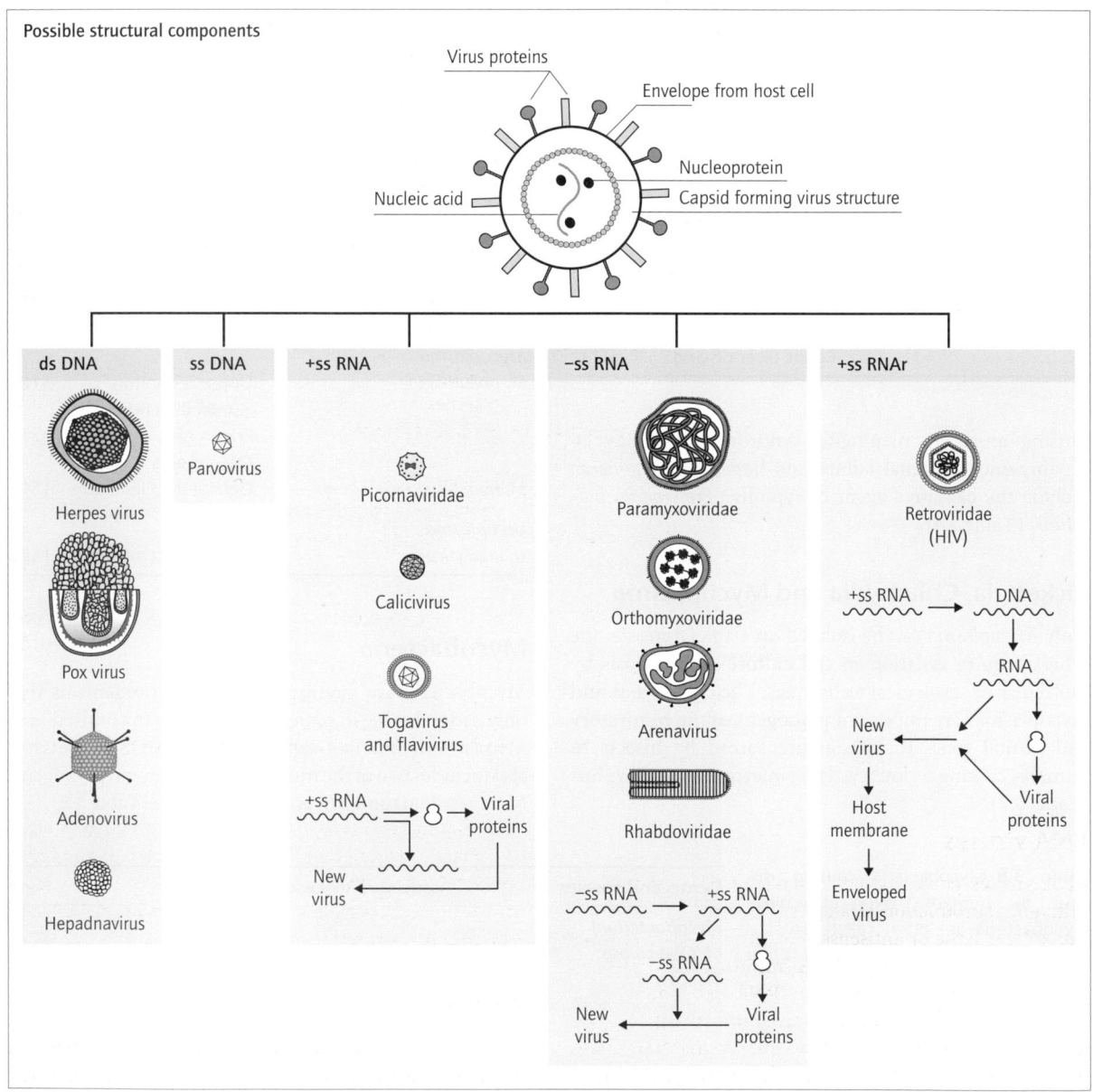

Figure 3.8 Viral classification. Reproduced from Gillespie & Bamford, *Medical Microbiology and Infection at a Glance*, 2000 (Blackwell Science Ltd, Oxford) with permission.

Table 3.9 DNA viruses

Family and virus	Associated disease	Page
Papovaviridae		
Human wart viruses	Warts	
Polyomaviridae		
JC virus	Progressive multifocal leucoencephalopathy	
BK virus	Haemorrhagic cystitis in the immunosuppressed	
Adenoviridae		
Influenza A–F	Upper respiratory tract infection	
	Conjunctivitis	
	Gastroenteritis (few types only)	
Herpesviridae		
Herpes simplex		
Type 1	Primary stomatitis	
	Orogenital herpes	113
	Encephalitis	113
	Keratitis	
Type 2	Herpes genitalis	163
	Neonatal infection	
Cytomegalovirus	Congenital infection	143
	Infection in the immunocompromised	180
Epstein–Barr virus	Infectious mononucleosis	142
	Burkitt's lymphoma	142
	Nasopharyngeal carcinoma	
Varicella-zoster virus		
Primary	Chickenpox	143
Recurrent	Shingles	145
Human herpesvirus 6	Roseola infantum	
Poxviridae		
Variola virus	Smallpox	
Molluscum contagiosum virus	Molluscum contagiosum (benign epidermal tumours)	1140
Orf	Orf	1139
Parvoviridae		
Parvovirus (B19)	Erythema infectiosum	150
	Aplastic crisis	150
Hepadnaviridae		
Hepatitis B	Acute, fulminant and chronic hepatitis	610
	Hepatocellular carcinoma	633

RNA viruses

RNA viruses possess a single stand of RNA and adopt different reproduction strategies depending on whether the RNA is sense or antisense. RNA sense (positive) may serve directly as messenger RNA (mRNA). It is translated into structural protein and an RNA-dependent RNA polymerase. A virus with RNA antisense (negative) contains an RNA-dependent RNA polymerase that transcribes the viral genome into mRNA. Alternatively, the transcribed RNA can act as a template for further viral (antisense) RNA.

Retroviruses possess single stranded positive (sense) RNA that cannot act as mRNA. It is transcribed into DNA by reverse transcriptase. The DNA is incorporated into host DNA. The subsequent transcription is under the control of host transcriptase enzymes to make mRNA and viral genomic RNA (Fig. 3.8; Table 3.10).

Protozoa

Protozoa are unicellular organisms, some of which are important pathogens of humans. They include the causative organism of malaria, which is responsible for many millions of deaths each year in children under the age of 5 in developing countries, and trypanosomiasis,

Table 3.10 RNA viruses

Family	Virus	Associated disease	Page
Picornoviridae			
Enteroviruses	Polioviruses 1–3	Polio	116
	Echoviruses	Aseptic meningitis	106
		Fever with rash	
	Coxsackie viruses	Aseptic meningitis	106
		Fever with rash	
		Pleurodynia	
		Hand, foot and mouth disease	150
		Myocarditis	482
		Pericarditis	488
	Hepatitis A virus	Acute hepatitis	609
Rhinoviruses		Coryza	318
Caliciviruses	Norwalk agent	Gastroenteritis	121
Astroviruses		Gastroenteritis	121
Togavirus			
Alphaviruses	Chikungunya	Fever with bone pain	135
(all arboviruses)	O'nyong-nyong	Fever with bone pain	135
	Ross River	Fever with rash	135
	Venezuelan equine encephalitis	Fever, encephalitis	135
Flaviviruses	Dengue 1–4	Fever with bone pain, haemorrhagic fever	114
(all arboviruses)	Yellow fever	Haemorrhagic fever and hepatitis	126
	Japanese encephalitis	Encephalitis	113
	St Louis encephalitis	Encephalitis	113
	Tick-borne encephalitis	Encephalitis	113
Rubiviruses	Rubella virus	Rubella	147
Orthomyxoviruses	Influenza viruses A, B, C	Influenza	321
Paramyxoviruses	Parainfluenza viruses 1–4	Acute respiratory infections	
	Mumps virus	Mumps	147
	Measles virus	Measles	146
	Respiratory syncytial virus	Bronchiolitis in infants	319
		Acute respiratory infections	319
Coronaviruses		Coryza	318
Arenaviruses	Lassa virus	Lassa fever	126
	Junin virus	Argentine haemorrhagic fever	126
	Machupo virus	Bolivian haemorrhagic fever	126
Bunyaviruses	Congo–Crimea haemorrhagic fever	Haemorrhagic fever	135
(all arboviruses)	Rift valley fever	Haemorrhagic fever	135
	La Crosse virus	Encephalitis	
	Colorado tick fever	Encephalitis	
Retroviruses	HTLV I	T-cell leukaemia and lymphoma	
		Tropical spastic paraparesis	
	HTLV II	Unknown	
	HIV	AIDS	170
Rhabdoviruses	Rabies virus	Rabies	115
Filoviruses	Marburg virus	Haemorrhagic fever	135
	Ebola virus	Haemorrhagic fever	135
Reoviruses	Rotavirus	Gastroenteritis	121
Unclassified RNA viruses	Norwalk-like viruses (SRSVs)	Gastroenteritis	121
	Hepatitis C virus	Transfusion-related hepatitis	613
		Chronic hepatitis	
		Hepatocellular carcinoma	633
	Hepatitis D virus	Acute and chronic hepatitis in the presence of coexistent (delta agent) hepatitis B virus infection	614
	Hepatitis E virus	Epidemic and sporadic faeco-oral acute and fulminant hepatitis	614

HTLV, human T-cell leukaemia/lymphoma virus; SRSV, small round-structured virus.

Table 3.11 Protozoa and associated diseases

Genus and protozoan	Associated disease	Page
Plasmodium		
P. vivax, P. ovale, P. malariae, P. falciparum	Malaria	128
Trypanosoma		
T. brucei gambiense, T. brucei rhodesiense	African trypanosomiasis	138
T. cruzi	South American trypanosomiasis	139
Leishmania		
L. donovani	Visceral leishmaniasis	136
L. infantum	Visceral leishmaniasis	136
L. aethiopica	Old World cutaneous leishmaniasis	136
L. tropica	Old World cutaneous leishmaniasis	136
L. major	Old World cutaneous leishmaniasis	136
L. braziliensis	New World cutaneous leishmaniasis	136
	Mucocutaneous leishmaniasis	136
L. mexicana	New World cutaneous leishmaniasis	136
	Mucocutaneous leishmaniasis	136
Giardia		
G. lamblia	Diarrhoea	122
Toxoplasma		
T. gondii	Congenital abnormalities	141
	Fever with lymphadenopathy	141
	Retinitis	141
	Encephalitis in AIDS	180
Acanthamoeba		
Various species	Amoebic meningitis	
	Keratitis	
Naegleria		
N. fowleri	Amoebic meningitis	
Entamoeba		
E. histolytica	Amoebic colitis	121
	Amoebic liver abscess	121
Cryptosporidium		
C. parvum	Acute diarrhoea	123
	Chronic diarrhoea in AIDS	
Isospora		
I. belli	Diarrhoea in AIDS	
Microsporidium		
Enterocytozoon bienusi	Diarrhoea in AIDS, also sinusitis, keratitis	
Trichomonas		
T. vaginalis	Vaginitis	162

03

which makes it impossible to raise cattle in some regions. Some may have a complex life cycle that includes a vector, whereas others spread from person to person by the faeco-oral route. Many protozoa such as *Leishmania* and *Trypanosoma* are adapted to an intracellular environment (Table 3.11).

Helminths

Parasitic worms are the most complex infectious agents (Table 3.12). They have evolved over millions of years in parallel with their hosts, acquiring ever more subtle adaptations:
- to help them evade the host's immune response
- to exploit idiosyncrasies of host behaviour

Unlike micro-organisms, such as protozoa and bacteria, most helminths do not complete their life cycle within one host individual. Typically, a host harbours one or more stages of the parasite but the complete life cycle includes a period outside the host, often involving another host species (Fig. 3.9). The species that harbours the adult reproductive stage of a parasite is the *definitive host*, while species parasitized by larval stages are *intermediate hosts*.

To ensure that its progeny are disseminated widely in the environment, the worm's definitive host should be long-lived. Illnesses caused by adult worms are therefore usually low grade and chronic. In contrast, because the intermediate host of some larval worms needs to be eaten by a suitable definitive host to complete the life cycle, a much more aggressive illness which disables the intermediate host may promote the propagation (see p. 140). Parasitic worms are classified into roundworms (nematodes), tapeworms (cestodes) and flukes (trematodes).

Table 3.12 Helminths and associated infections

Classification	Species	Associated disease
Filarial nematodes	*Wuchereria bancrofti*	Elephantiasis
	Onchocerca volvulus	River blindness
		Dermatitis
	Loa loa (African eye worm)	Calabar swelling
	Dracunculus medinensis (guinea worm)	Chronic leg ulcer
Gut nematodes	*Ascaris lumbricoides* (roundworm)	Minor abdominal symptoms
	Ancylostoma duodenale and	Anaemia
	Necator americanus (hookworm)	
	Trichuris trichiura (whipworm)	Minor abdominal symptoms
		Nutritional deficiency
	Enterobius vermicularis (threadworm)	Pruritus ani
Other nematodes	*Strongyloides stercoralis*	Larva currens
		Opportunistic hyperinfection
	Toxocara canis	Visceral larva migrans
		Retinitis
	Trichinella spiralis	Fever, muscle pain
Trematodes	*Schistosoma mansoni*	Colitis
		Portal hypertension
		Pulmonary hypertension
	Schistosoma haematobium	Haematuria
		Hydronephrosis
		Carcinoma of the bladder
	Clonorchis sinensis and *Opisthorchis* spp.	Cholangitis
		Cholangiocarcinoma
	Fasciola hepatica	Fever, painful hepatomegaly
	Paragonamus spp.	Chronic cavitating lung disease
Cestodes (tapeworm)	*Taenia saginata* (beef tapeworm)	Minor abdominal symptoms
	Taenia solium (pork tapeworm)	Cysticercosis, epilepsy
	Hymenolepis nana (dwarf tapeworm)	Minor abdominal symptoms
	Echinococcus granulosus	Hydatid cysts

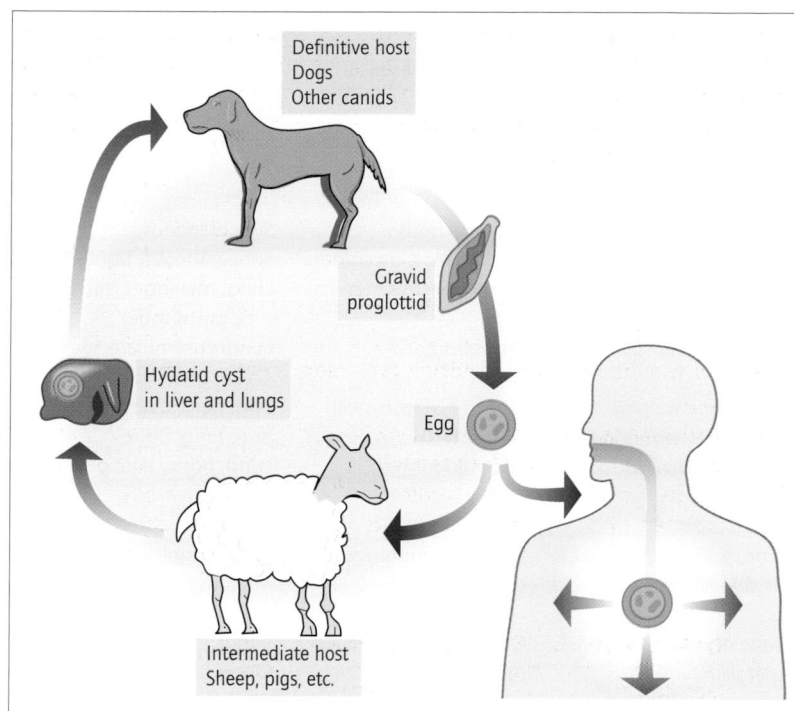

Figure 3.9 Hydatid life cycle.

03

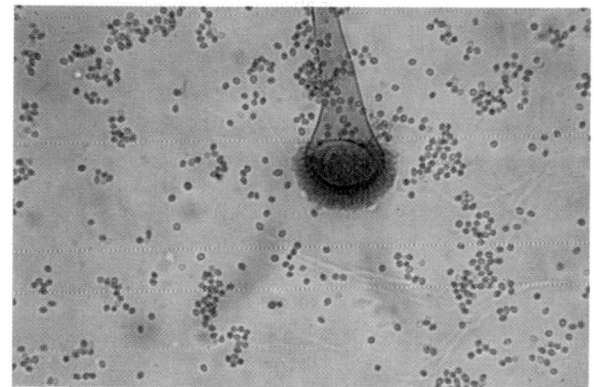

Figure 3.10 *Candida*.

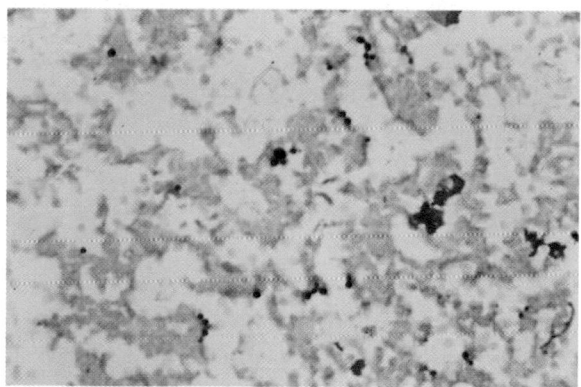

Figure 3.11 *Aspergillus*.

Fungi

Fungi are widely distributed in the environment and only rarely cause human disease. They may have a yeast-like morphology such as *Candida* and *Cryptococcus* (Fig. 3.10) or be filamentous (Fig. 3.11). A wide range of diseases can arise when invasion occurs, ranging from cutaneous dermatophyte infections to systemic *Candida* or *Aspergillus* infection in the severely immunocompromised patient (Table 3.13).

Table 3.13 Fungi and associated diseases

Organism	Associated disease	Principal target organs	Geographical distribution	Page
Microsporum sp.	Ringworm	Skin	Worldwide	1141
Trichophyton sp.	Ringworm, athlete's foot	Skin, nails	Worldwide	1141
Malassezia furfur	Tinea versicolor	Skin	More common in hot climates	
Sporothrix shenkii	Sporotrichosis	Subcutaneous	Tropics/subtropics	
Madurella sp. and others	Madura foot, mycetoma	Subcutaneous, bone	Tropics	
Cryptococcus neoformans	Cryptococcosis	Lung, meninges (often opportunistic)	Worldwide	179
Histoplasma capsulatum	Histoplasmosis	Lung/disseminated (opportunistic)	North America and many tropical areas	
Histoplasma duboisii	African histoplasmosis	Skin, bones, disseminated	Africa	
Blastomyces dermatitidis	Blastomycosis	Skin, lung, bone	North America and Africa	
Coccidiodes immitis	Coccidiodomycosis	Lung, bone, skin, disseminated	South-western USA, Mexico, Argentina, Paraguay	
Paracoccidiodes braziliensis	Paracoccidiodomycosis	Lung, lymph nodes, disseminated	South America	
Candida albicans	Candidiasis	Mucous membranes, commonly	Worldwide opportunistic, rarely disseminated	160
Pneumocystis carinii	Opportunistic infection	Lungs	Worldwide	177
Aspergillus fumigatus	Aspergillosis	Opportunistic (especially lungs)	Worldwide	367
A. flavus, A. niger		Also allergic bronchopulmonary aspergillosis		

Approach to the patient

History and examination

History

About the patient

Infection results from a complex interaction between an individual, an organism and the environment (HISTORY & EXAMINATION BOXES 3.1 and 3.2). Any feature of the individual, innate or acquired, may be relevant.
- Age, sex and race alter susceptibility.
- Occupation, lifestyle and level of education influence the range of organisms to which an individual is exposed.
- Intestinal conditions may increase the risk of infection because of immunodeficiency or organ damage.
- Skin conditions with a break in the protective surface surrounding the organism predispose to infection.
- Sickle cell anaemia results in a functional splenectomy.

History & Examination 3.1

Questions to be addressed by the history and examination of a patient with an infectious disease

What is the site of the infection?

What is the probable infecting organism?

Is there any associated tissue damage and/or organ failure?

Is there an underlying disease predisposing the patient to infection?

Are there other predisposing factors (e.g. lifestyle, travel)?

History of exposure to infection

Obtain a detailed history of factors that increase the risk of exposure to infectious agents including travel, occupational history and a history of exposure to animals or of insect bites. Any medical procedures, especially injections and transfusions, which may transmit a variety of agents (HISTORY & EXAMINATION BOX 3.2), should be noted. Contact with family members or others who have been unwell may be relevant. Always ask about sexual contacts.

History & Examination 3.2

Important questions to ask a patient with an infection

About the patient
Where have you been recently?
Have you been abroad? If so, where and for how long?
What is your occupation?
Have you been exposed to animals or insect bites?

Symptoms
When were you last well?
Do you have any localized features?
Does the fever have a pattern?
Do you have any symptoms other than fever (e.g. headache, joint aches, rash, diarrhoea, stomach upset, nausea)?
Have you lost any weight?
Do you have sweats during the night?

Drug history
Have you taken any antibiotics?
Have you taken any medicines to bring down your fever?
Are you taking any other medicines or tonics, either prescribed or obtained from other sources including health food shops?

Past medical history
What infections have you had in the past?
What immunizations have you had?
Have you had any transfusions?

Family history
Is anyone in your family immunosuppressed?
Has anyone in your family had an unusual infection?
Does anyone in your family have a skin condition?

Sexual history
(see History & Examination Box 3.4)

Table 3.14 Screening investigations performed on all patients presenting with pyrexia of unknown origin (PUO)

Full blood count
  Neutrophils
  Eosinophils
  Anaemia of chronic disease
  Low platelets
Blood culture (×3)
Sputum culture
Urine culture
Faeces
  Bacterial pathogens
  Ova, cysts and parasites
Chest X-ray
  Pneumoniae
  Tuberculosis or other chronic lung infection
Serum
  Save for investigation when a second sample collected after 10 days
C-reactive protein and erythrocyte sedimentation rate
  To set a baseline and monitor markers of inflammation

of travelling as well as people. The apparent lack of an appropriate travel history has not prevented people living near airports from acquiring malaria from mosquitoes transported in aircraft. Some parasitic infections may be very persistent too (e.g. amoebiasis, strongyloidiasis, schistosomiasis) and cause important clinical effects many years after the initial infection.

Animal contact

Animal contact can vary from simply entering the same environment as a wild animal (deer in the case of Lyme disease). Some patients have close contact by virtue of their occupation: veterinarians and farm workers (brucellosis, Q fever, leptospirosis). There are risks in keeping companion animals: birds (psittacosis, extrinsic allergic alveolitis), dogs (toxocariasis, rabies) and cats (toxoplasmosis, cat-scratch disease).

Occupational history

A person's occupation can bring them into contact with unusual infectious agents. The classic story associating leptospirosis and sewer workers is now an interesting historical example. It is now recognized that contact with sewage can result in infection with the leptospires, which can penetrate intact skin, but infection is rare because appropriate protective clothing is worn. Farmers, veterinarians and abattoir workers are exposed to a number of infectious hazards including leptospirosis, brucellosis, salmonellosis and Q fever.

Q fever is found in sheep and cattle and can be transmitted to individuals on farms or living in the countryside.

Travel history

Some infections occur within limited geographical areas to which they are restricted either by climate or by the range of a vector or an animal reservoir (e.g. malaria or leishmaniasis). Many others are associated with poor sanitation or poverty (e.g. amoebic dysentery). A detailed history of travel to the tropics is essential as many infections are found in this zone (HISTORY & EXAMINATION BOX 3.2), but there are some diseases limited by geography in developed countries (e.g. visceral leishmaniasis in the Mediterranean area and Rocky Mountain spotted fever in North America).

As with most aspects of clinical diagnosis, geographical ranges of disease are matters of probability rather than absolutes. Agents of disease and their vectors are capable

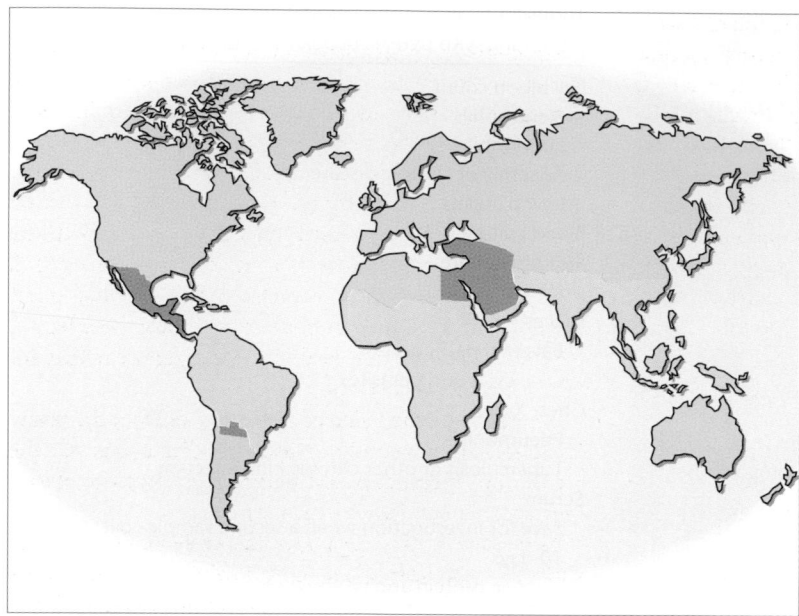

Figure 3.12 Geographical distribution of malaria. Blue, chloroquine-resistant *Plasmodium falciparum*; pink, chloroquine-sensitive malaria.

Brucella spp. infect herds of cattle, sheep and goats, causing abortion in cattle and reduced fertility and growth in goats. It is now rare because of control methods but may arise in people from countries without these measures, notably the Middle East.

Kennel maids and hydatid control officers are two occupations where close exposure to whelping bitches increases the risk of toxocariasis. People who work with birds have an increased risk of developing psittacosis and, more rarely, cryptococcosis. It is important to bear in mind that although a patient's occupation may be recorded as an apparently 'safe' occupation such as 'painter and decorator', their occupation may have exposed them to considerable hazard; for example, if recently painting a hen house, or repairing a roof that was heavily contaminated with bird droppings.

Many of the pneumoconioses such as silicosis or asbestosis predispose to pulmonary tuberculosis. Although many of the dust hazards are now well controlled in the work environment, the working population carries a continuing risk in those who have been exposed in the past.

Sport and recreation

This is an important subsection of the occupational history because a person's outdoor life may allow exposure to more unusual pathogens.
- People who walk in forests may be bitten by ticks infected with *Borrelia burgdorferi* or with the virus of louping-ill.
- Camping or hunting on the European mainland may allow exposure to *Francisella tularensis*.
- Cavers in more remote areas of Central or South America may be exposed to rabies in caves where infected bats roost.

Sexual history

A history of sexual exposure should be obtained from all patients. As many sexually transmitted diseases such as HIV and syphilis have a long incubation period, this should go back over a number of years (see p. 151).

Retaking the history

Infectious diseases are by nature dynamic processes, the symptoms and signs change quickly (in comparison to chronic diseases such as a cancer) and new symptoms may appear over a short time. It is valuable therefore to retake the history regularly, permitting patients to express the changes in the pattern of symptoms. Also, patients may remember new pieces of information or, on reflection, understand the aim of a question that may not first have been clear.

Presenting symptoms

Common presenting symptoms of infectious disease include fever, rash, arthritis, malaise, shortness of breath, headache, photophobia, lymphadenopathy, diarrhoea, vomiting and nausea.

Fever

Fever is a non-specific manifestation of many processes including malignancies and non-infectious inflammatory conditions, as well as infections. A constellation of related symptoms accompany a fever and include anorexia, aching limbs and mild headache. Patients feel cold and shiver as their temperature rises and sweat as it falls. An abrupt rise in temperature can cause *rigors* (uncontrollable shaking of the whole body). If a fever persists for more than a few days, there is rapid weight loss and increasing weakness and debility. These associated symptoms give some indication of the severity of a febrile illness, but are of little help in determining its cause (Fig. 3.13).

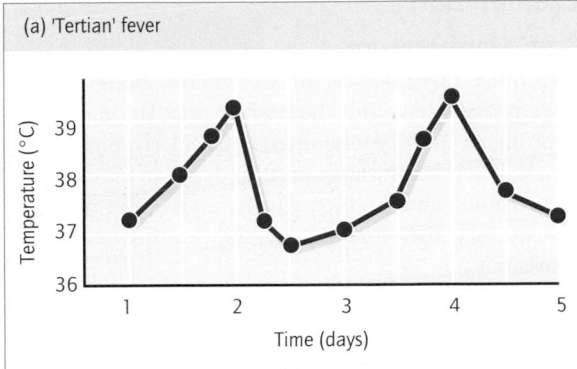

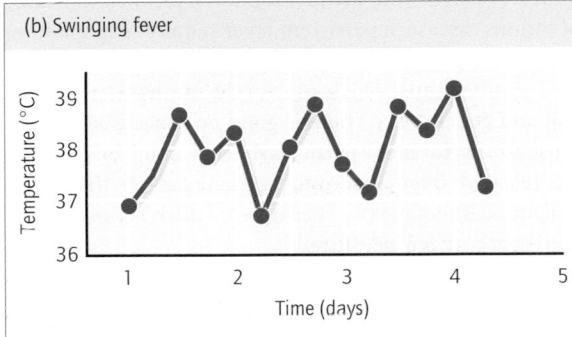

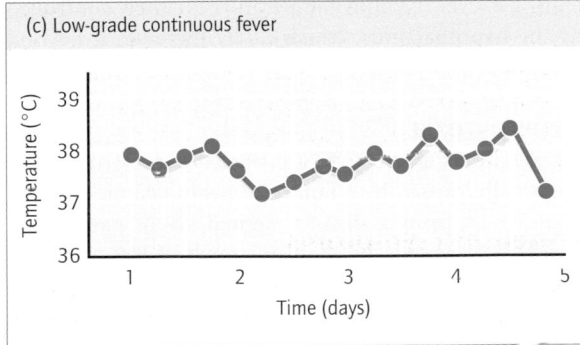

Figure 3.13 Examples of fevers. (a) Typical 'tertian' fever of *Plasmodium vivax* malaria with peaks on alternate days. (b) Swinging fever often found in occult abscess or tuberculosis. (c) Low-grade continuous pyrexia of endocarditis or line-related sepsis.

Rash

Characteristic rashes are common in childhood fevers and so rashes are often associated with infectious disease. The typical features of these rashes are discussed in more detail on p. 143. Naturally, infections of the skin such as impetigo or staphylococcal scalded skin syndrome present as a 'rash'. If a skin infection is suspected, the natural history of the process must be recorded, together with any predisposing injury such as a thorn puncture wound. Many skin infections are highly infectious and other members of the family or close contacts may be infected. The rash of scabies may be difficult to diagnose if the contact history is not available.

A rash may be the sign of systemic infection; the severity of the patient's condition usually indicates this (e.g. the purpura of meningococcal septicaemia), but not always (e.g. chronic meningococcaemia).

Skin rashes may also arise as embolic phenomena (infective endocarditis), or following acute urethritis (Reiter's syndrome), and the appropriate associated history should be sought. When a rash is a presenting symptom, a detailed drug history is essential. Many antibiotics used in the community cause a rash as an allergic response (e.g. beta-lactams).

Arthritis

Arthritis can result from direct infection of the joint or as a immune related postinfectious complication. The distribution of joints involved may indicate the diagnosis. A single swollen joint in a child may indicate an infective arthritis, but in older patients the diagnostic problem is greater. An acutely swollen joint in a patient with rheumatoid arthritis may result from either reactivation of the disease or infection in the damaged joint.

The history of the presenting symptoms must be recorded, making note of the temporal relationship of all symptoms. A viral infection such as rubella might be followed by arthritis in several joints a few days later.

Arthritis may also be an important symptom of infective and immunological conditions such as Reiter's syndrome (see p. 265) or rheumatic fever (see p. 477). Infections of the musculoskeletal system are discussed in Chapter 4.

Lymphadenopathy

Lymphadenopathy may be localized, regional or generalized. If lymphadenopathy is a symptom, a history of localized infection or trauma should be sought. In addition, the tissue drained by the node should be carefully examined.

- *Local lymphadenopathy:* may result from infection of the lymph node (e.g. by *Mycobacterium tuberculosis*)
- *Generalized lymphadenopathy:* a feature in many infections (e.g. infectious mononucleosis; see p. 142).

Headache

Headache is one of the most difficult symptoms to evaluate. It may be entirely trivial, indicating a tension headache, or it may be the harbinger of encephalitis or meningitis. Its natural history is a useful diagnostic indicator. Any associated symptoms should also be noted.

● People with acute meningitis may complain of sensitivity to light (photophobia).
● People with infective space-occupying lesions may have a lowered level of consciousness, or confusion.

Many other signs may be associated with infections of the nervous system and these are discussed in more detail below.

Diarrhoea

Diarrhoea is usually associated with infection, at least by the patient. Its nature will vary depending on the part of the bowel involved (see p. 117).

History suggesting localized infection

Any clues from the history suggesting a localized site of infection should be noted; for example:
● dysuria of urinary tract infection
● persistent low back pain of vertebral osteomyelitis

A vague localized symptom may be the only clue to the diagnosis of a troublesome infection (e.g. dental abscess).

Pattern of disease

Incubation and onset

If the time of exposure to infection is known, the interval until the appearance of symptoms (*incubation period*) is valuable diagnostically. This is especially valuable in travellers when the last date of possible exposure to an infectious agent (e.g. malaria) is known. Another useful parameter in the diagnosis of some infections is the period of onset or *prodrome*, which is the time from the first appearance of symptoms to the onset of some characteristic feature such as a rash. Many infections have a characteristic incubation period and prodrome (e.g. chickenpox).

Drug history

Self- or prescribed medication can affect the course of an infectious disease, modifying the symptoms and signs (e.g. antipyretics mask fever, antibiotics modify symptoms and reduce the likelihood of a positive culture). Self-medication of malaria may mask symptoms and produce a false-negative blood smear. A history of previous antibiotic therapy can suggest infection with a resistant organism (e.g. partially treated tuberculosis). Many of the features of a drug reaction (e.g. fever, rash, malaise) are similar to those of infection, and the presenting illness may be caused by medication. Abuse of drugs and alcohol predisposes to infectious disease. Intravenous drug abusers are at risk of endocarditis, osteomyelitis and AIDS, while alcoholics have an increased risk of pneumonia.

Past medical history and family history

The family history can reveal a possible infectious contact or a genetic susceptibility to infection (e.g. immunodeficiency syndrome or sickle cell disease). The past medical history may suggest that the patient is immunosuppressed and at risk of an opportunistic infection.

Examination

Body temperature

Like other physiological measurements, body temperature is variable within the healthy population. It tends to be higher in the young than in the elderly, higher after physical exercise or a large meal, and rises in the evenings, at ovulation and premenstrually. A few normal individuals may therefore have a temperature marginally above 37°C.

Fever

A temperature between 37.5 and 40.5°C almost always indicates a fever and, because it may be the only indicator of serious disease, a persistent fever requires explanation. Body heat is regulated by temperature-sensitive cells in the hypothalamus, which control the mechanisms of heat loss and generation. There is good evidence that fever is caused by cytokines (particularly IL-1 and TNF). These are released from macrophages and act on the hypothalamus, affecting the thermoregulatory set point and therefore core temperature.

Fever is probably beneficial during an infection; the immune system may be more effective and infecting organisms less well adapted to the higher temperature. During a fever the body temperature is closely controlled by the hypothalamus, which rarely increases it beyond about 40.5°C.

Hyperpyrexia

Temperatures above 41°C are termed *hyperpyrexias* and are usually caused by a failure of hypothalamic control. They result from a distinct limited set of pathologies in which either the mechanisms for heat loss are overwhelmed (e.g. heat stroke and thyrotoxic storm), or hypothalamic function is disrupted (e.g. intracranial haemorrhage and certain drug reactions).

Patterns of fever

It is traditional to ascribe certain patterns of fever to particular diagnoses. These patterns are useful as rules of thumb, but there is so much variation in the febrile response that they must be interpreted with caution.

• *Hectic fever* (Fig. 3.13): typical of the response to a deep-seated collection of pus; the temperature is at times very high, but falls back to normal between the 'spikes'.

• *Sustained fever* is typical of pneumococcal pneumonia and typhoid; the temperature remains high with little variation.

• *Remittent fever* is typical of most fevers; the temperature spikes, but seldom drops to normal.

• The classical *tertian fever* of malaria occurs on the afternoon of every second day, but is only common in relapses of *Plasmodium vivax* and *Plasmodium ovale* or in semi-immunes with *P. falciparum*. Malaria more often presents with a hectic or remittent fever.

• The typical *Pel–Ebstein fever* is characterized by episodes of fever lasting for a few days, interspersed by long periods of remission. It strongly suggests a lymphoma, but occurs in only a minority of cases.

• *Low constant fever*. A low-grade fever constant throughout 24 h with minor variation. This is typical of patients with endocarditis or with infected intravenous access catheters.

• *Low-grade fever* accentuates the normal diurnal change in temperature, which is highest in the evening and lowest in the small hours of the morning. The fall in body temperature at night is the most rapid change in this cycle and the accompanying sweats are likely to be the most prominent symptom.

• Night sweats are typical of tuberculosis, but can occur in many other conditions.

General examination

Any part of the physical examination can reveal signs relevant to an infection. It must therefore be as thorough as possible (HISTORY & EXAMINATION BOX 3.3). A full examination includes sigmoidoscopy and pelvic examination.

Look

Careful examination of the skin for inconspicuous lesions of which the patient is unaware can provide important information, for example:

• The eschar of a tick bite (Fig. 3.14)
• Signs of intravenous needle use
• The first few petechiae of meningococcaemia in an otherwise unremarkable febrile illness
• Finger clubbing associated with chronic diseases including infections such as tuberculosis, bronchiectasis and endocarditis
• Signs of rheumatic disease (e.g. nodules, capillary looping in the nail beds)

Inflammatory lesions may be seen in the fundus on examination of the eye (including ophthalmoscopy), the ears, buccal mucosa and throat. Fever blisters, brought about by a recurrence of a herpes simplex infection in response to a high fever, usually occur around the mouth

---

History & Examination 3.3

Examination of a patient with an infection

Look

Inspect the skin
Look for rashes, eschars and petechiae

Examine the eyes
Look for petechiae, keratitis and retinal lesions (e.g. tubercle)

Inspect the ears
Look for otitis media

Feel

Palpate the lymph nodes
Note any trochlear enlargement suggesting syphilis or HIV infection, or cervical enlargement suggesting rubella or trypanosomiasis

Palpate the liver and spleen
Hepatosplenomegaly may suggest a non-infective infiltrative cause of a fever (e.g. lymphoma)
Hepatomegaly may occur with a liver abscess
Splenomegaly is a feature of glandular fever and malaria

Feel for abdominal soft tissue, hot and cold abscesses

Feel the nerves
Note any thickening suggestive of leprosy

Palpate the sinuses
Note any tenderness suggesting sinusitis

Feel for nodules
Skin nodules can be felt in cysticercosis

Move

Move the joints
Look for septic arthritis

Move the neck
Look for meningeal irritation

Percuss

Percuss the chest
Look for evidence of an effusion (tuberculosis) or consolidation (pneumonia)

Listen

Note the whoop of pertussis (whooping cough)
Listen to the heart for the murmurs of subacute bacterial endocarditis
Listen to the lungs for signs of pneumonia

---

and must be noted (Fig. 3.15a,b). They may provide diagnostic clues; in pneumonia they are associated with pneumococcal infection and they are much more common in malaria than in typhoid.

Feel

An area of tenderness is often the clue to the site of a

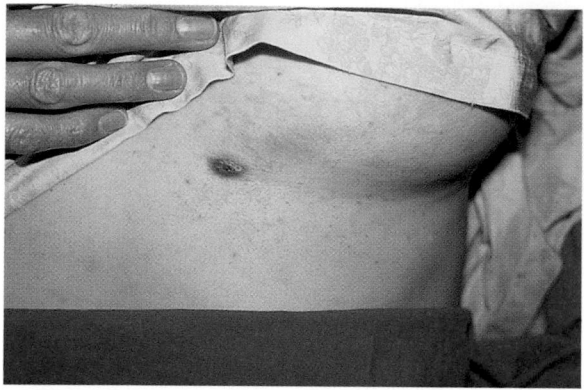

Figure 3.14 Tick typhus: a black eschar at the site of the infecting tick bite. Reproduced from Bannister *et al.*, *Infectious Disease*, 1996 (Blackwell Science, Oxford) with the permission of the authors.

localized infection (e.g. loin tenderness in pyelonephritis). A search for lymphadenopathy should include the trochlear nodes, situated anteromedially just above the elbow. Hepatomegaly and splenomegaly are also important signs of infection. Careful palpation of the superficial nerves is necessary in suspected leprosy to detect infiltration and enlargement.

Listen

Cardiac murmurs may be the only clinical sign of endocarditis.

A complete physical examination should be repeated regularly to detect changes such as a new soft systolic murmur or increasing abdominal tenderness. A spleen or liver that was impalpable on first examination, may have become so because of the development of the condition.

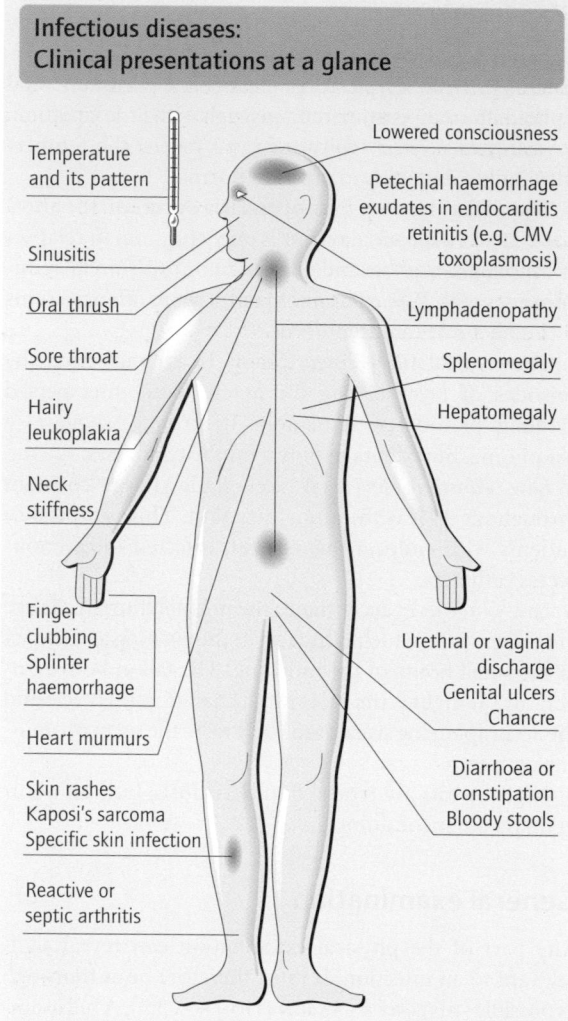

Infectious diseases: Clinical presentations at a glance

- Temperature and its pattern
- Sinusitis
- Oral thrush
- Sore throat
- Hairy leukoplakia
- Neck stiffness
- Finger clubbing
- Splinter haemorrhage
- Heart murmurs
- Skin rashes
- Kaposi's sarcoma
- Specific skin infection
- Reactive or septic arthritis
- Lowered consciousness
- Petechial haemorrhage exudates in endocarditis retinitis (e.g. CMV toxoplasmosis)
- Lymphadenopathy
- Splenomegaly
- Hepatomegaly
- Urethral or vaginal discharge
- Genital ulcers
- Chancre
- Diarrhoea or constipation
- Bloody stools

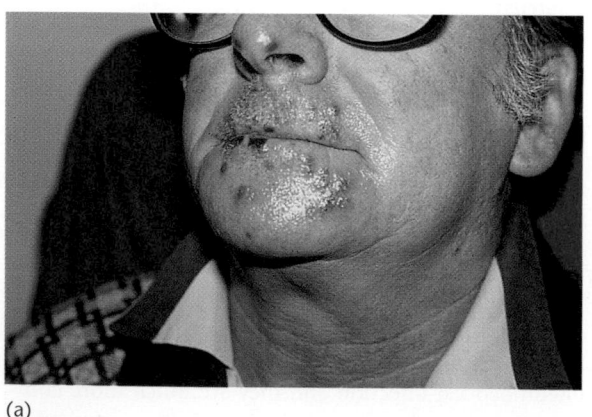

(a)

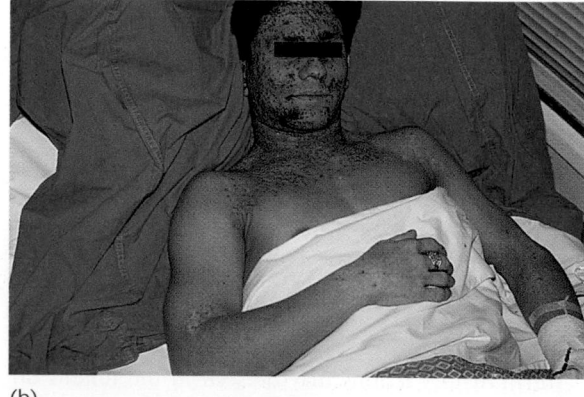

(b)

Figure 3.15 (a) Herpes simplex reactivation lesion (cold sore). (b) Eczema herpeticum originating from a cold sore. Both parts reproduced from Bannister *et al.*, *Infectious Disease*, 1996 (Blackwell Science, Oxford) with the permission of the authors.

Investigations

A careful history and examination of a febrile patient usually provides evidence implicating an organ or system as the site of disease, and therefore suggests appropriate investigations. The investigative process can be divided into three broad stages:

1 Screening investigations that are performed on all patients (Table 3.14).

2 Investigations that depend on the results of history and physical examination (e.g. fever and eosinophilia; Fig. 3.16).

3 Further screening tests and special imaging techniques: ultrasound, computerized tomography (CT), magnetic resonance imaging (MRI), echocardiography and dental X-ray (Fig. 3.16).

The results of the preliminary history and examination are taken together with the results of the primary investigations to plans the tests that are to be performed in the second round. These investigations are chosen based on syndrome groups (e.g. fever, eosinophila, tropical travel). If a diagnosis is not made, further imaging techniques are used to reveal an occult abdominal abscess or osteomyelitis. History and examinations are repeatedly made and the results synthesized to direct the diagnostic process. If a clear diagnosis is not made, a trial of chemotherapy may be considered (Fig. 3.16).

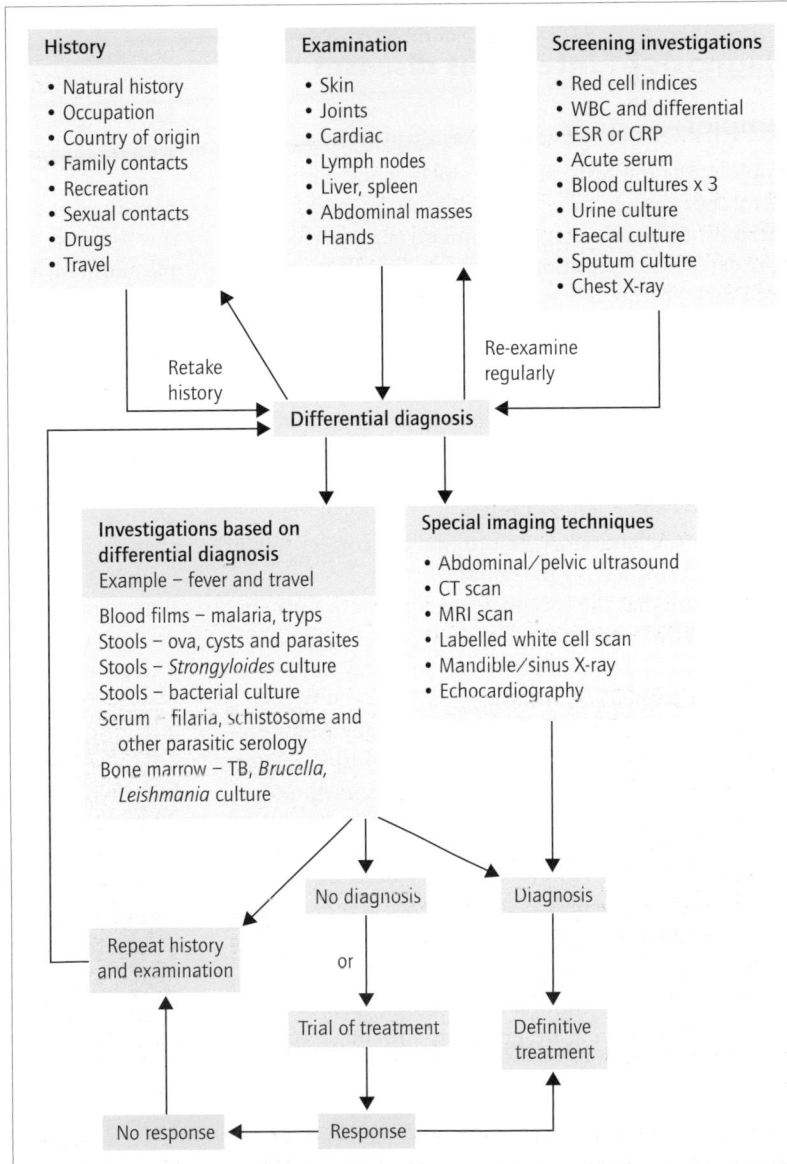

Figure 3.16 Pyrexia of unknown origin. Reproduced from Gillespie & Bamford, *Medical Microbiology and Infection at a Glance*, 2003 (Blackwell Science Ltd, Oxford) with permission.

Table 3.15 The infectious risk of therapeutic procedures

Procedure	Organism that may be introduced	Population at risk
Dental work	Streptococci from the mouth	Those with heart lesions are at risk of endocarditis
Oesophagoduodenogastroscopy		As for dental work
Injections	Staphylococci	Drug addicts
	Hepatitis B	
Blood transfusion	HIV	Transfusions where blood is inadequately screened
	Hepatitis B	
	Hepatitis C	
	Malaria	
Instrumentation of the genitourinary tract	Gram-negative or enterococcal septicaemia	The elderly
Colonoscopy	Gram-negative septicaemia	The elderly

Diagnosis of infectious diseases

Samples

Simple screening tests, such as a plain chest film, urine microscopy and culture, blood microscopy and culture, and routine biochemistry may similarly suggest a focus for more detailed investigation. Specimens for culture must be taken early, before any antibiotics are started and transported to the microbiology laboratory rapidly. Before precious (unrepeatable) samples are taken it may be useful to contact the laboratory first. Samples for serological studies should be stored at −20°C. Specialized radiological studies, ultrasound, CT scanning, MRI and isotope studies may be of value if a localized infection is suspected (see p. 85).

Advice about precious samples:
- Contact the laboratory first to find the correct way of taking and transporting the sample.
- Make sure that the specimen is *not* put into formalin. Many surgical specimens are put into formalin for histopathological examination and this may happen to infection specimens by mistake.
- Take the sample to the laboratory personally. Many precious samples are lost by entrusting it to a routine delivery method where specimens can be delayed and sometimes lost.

Haematological investigation

A full blood count (FBC) may reveal:
- normocytic normochromic anaemia of chronic disease (e.g. in tuberculosis or endocarditis)
- neutrophilia, indicating acute bacterial infection
- lymphocytosis, suggesting whooping cough or viral infection
- neutropenia, indicating underlying immunosuppression
- eosinophilia, suggesting a helminth infection

During acute infection, platelet counts may fall significantly; this may be a very sensitive sign of infection in neonates. The erythrocyte sedimentation rate (ESR) can be very high in chronic infections and tuberculosis.

Biochemical investigation

Measurement of renal function is vitally important in severe sepsis as acute renal failure is a common complication. Measurement of blood gases is useful in severe pneumonia and in monitoring the acidosis found in the sepsis syndrome. Liver function tests may be abnormal if there is localized disease in the liver (e.g. hepatitis or liver abscess) or generalized disease affecting the liver (e.g. miliary tuberculosis, septicaemia).

Markers of inflammation

During infection the body responds with non-specific changes in a range of serum proteins. C-reactive protein increases to high concentrations in inflammatory conditions. This can occur in bacterial infection but may also occur in malignancy, collagen vascular disease or trauma. There are changes in other serum proteins.

Microbiological investigation

Microbiological investigation has a crucial role in the diagnosis of infectious diseases. There are three main ways of making a microbiological diagnosis:
- microscopically
- by culture
- by serological methods

In addition, there are a number of new diagnostic techniques that do not fit easily into these categories, but which are discussed below.

Microscopy

The advantage of direct microscopic examination of patients' specimens is that a rapid presumptive diagnosis can be obtained. In addition, many of the techniques use simple equipment and inexpensive reagents and are therefore suitable for use as a side-room test or for laboratory diagnosis in less developed countries.

Wet preparations

Pathogens can be diagnosed by direct microscopic examination of unstained wet preparations. This technique can be used for the diagnosis of trichomoniasis (Fig. 3.17) and candidiasis in vaginal secretions or of intestinal parasites in a saline wet preparation of faeces (Fig. 3.18).

Fixed preparations

Dried fixed preparation of specimens can be examined using simple stains, such as Gram stain. This can provide a presumptive diagnosis in many clinical settings. This form of investigation is most valuable for fluids that are normally sterile, such as cerebrospinal fluid (CSF) and pleural fluid, because the presence of organisms is nearly always significant.

The sensitivity of Gram stain is relatively low and there must be more than 10 000 organisms/ml for a diagnosis to be made (Fig. 3.19a,b). Staining with acridine orange may increase sensitivity of such direct examination 10-fold. Special stains such as Ziehl–Neelsen are used to demonstrate acid-fast organisms such as mycobacteria and cryptosporidia (Fig. 3.20). A variation of this technique

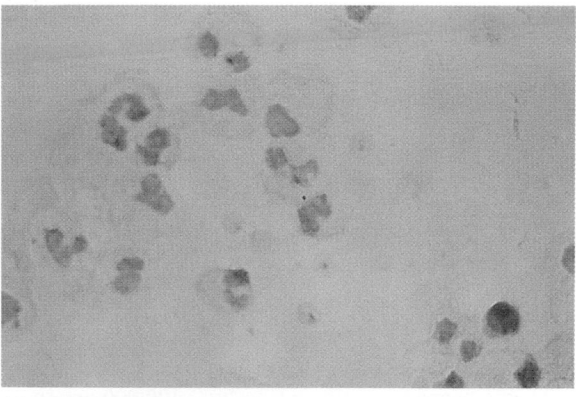

(a)

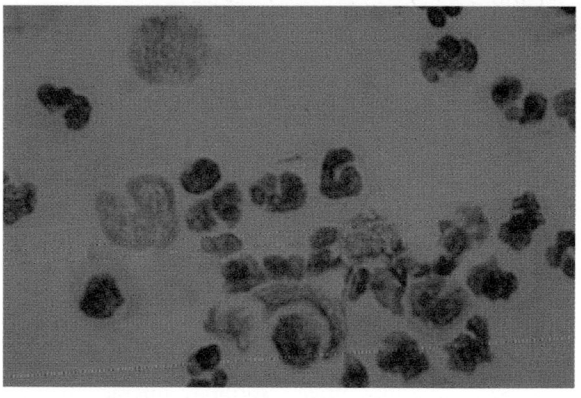

(b)

Figure 3.19 (a,b) Gram stain of bacteria.

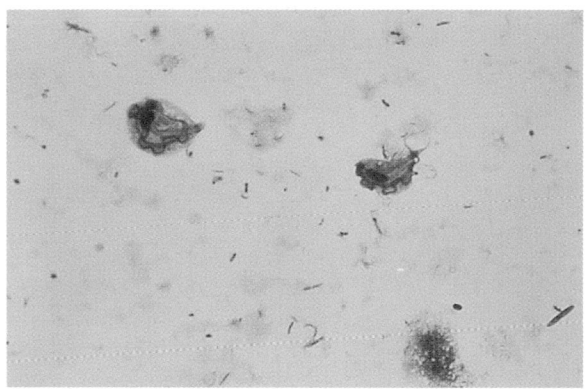

Figure 3.17 Trophozoites of *Trichomonas vaginalis* stained by Giemsa.

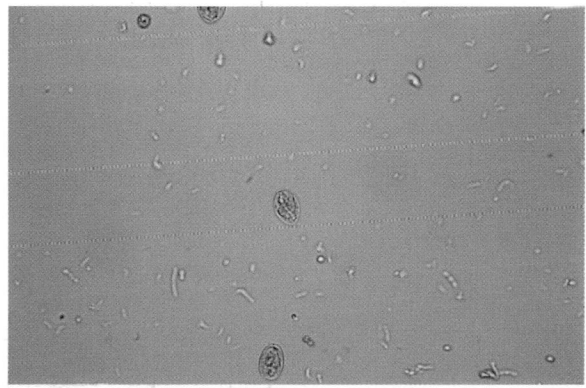

Figure 3.18 *Giardia* cysts in stool.

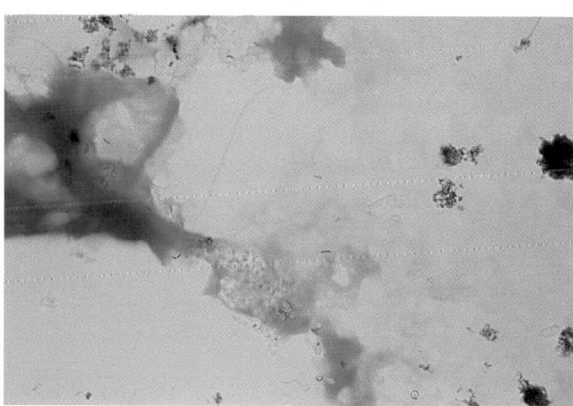

Figure 3.20 Ziehl–Neelsen-stained smear, showing acid-fast bacilli. Reproduced from Bannister *et al.*, *Infectious Disease*, 1996 (Blackwell Science, Oxford) with the permission of the authors.

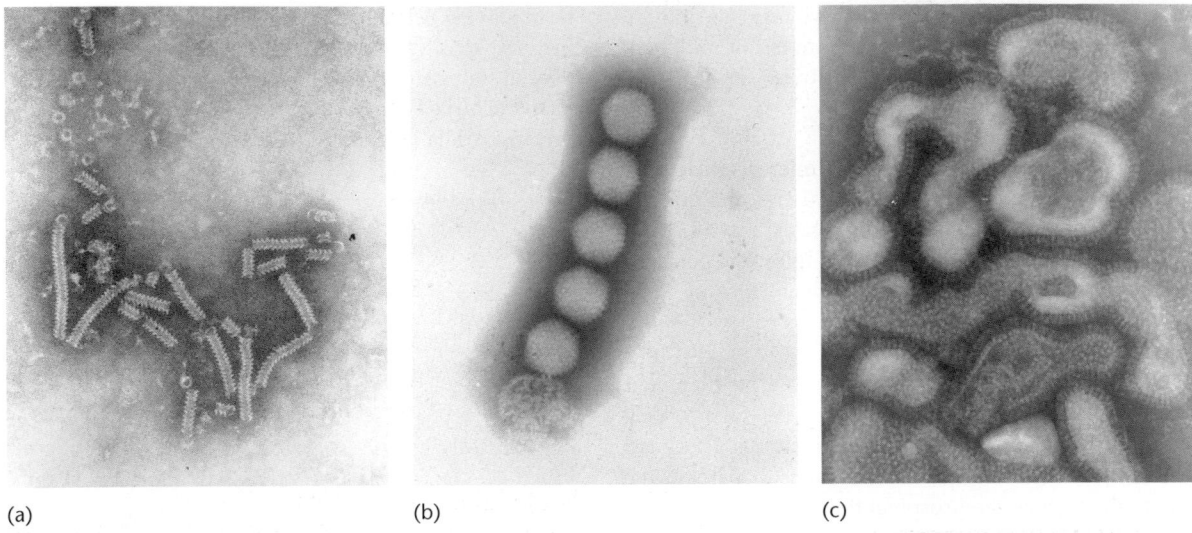

(a)   (b)   (c)

Figure 3.21 Viruses under electron microscopy. (a) A virus with helical symmetry, parainfluenza type 3 virus ×100 000. (b) A virus with icosahedral symmetry, adenovirus ×100 000. (c) An enveloped virus, influenza virus ×100 000. All parts reproduced from Bannister *et al.*, *Infectious Disease*, 1996 (Blackwell Science, Oxford) with the permission of the authors.

uses phenol-auramine, which makes acid-fast organisms fluoresce bright yellow under ultraviolet light.

Direct immunofluorescence

To examine a specimen using direct immunofluorescence it is first dried on a multiwell slide together with positive and negative controls. A specific antibody labelled with fluorescein is applied to the patient's specimen, which is then incubated at 37°C in a humidified chamber for approximately 1 h. The slides are then washed and examined under ultraviolet light.

Where a specific antigen–antibody interaction takes place, labelled antibody is bound to the pathogen and is evident as an apple-green fluorescence.

This technique is both sensitive and specific and provides a rapid presumptive diagnosis. Direct immunofluorescence is useful in the diagnosis of:

- *Chlamydia* urethritis
- influenza and parainfluenza virus infection
- respiratory syncytial virus (RSV) infection
- measles
- rhabdovirus infection

Electron microscopy

Electron microscopy is useful for the direct demonstration of (Fig. 3.21a–c):

- viruses
- pox virus in orf and molluscum contagiosum
- herpes simplex or varicella zoster virus in vesicle fluid
- gastrointestinal viruses (e.g. rotavirus)

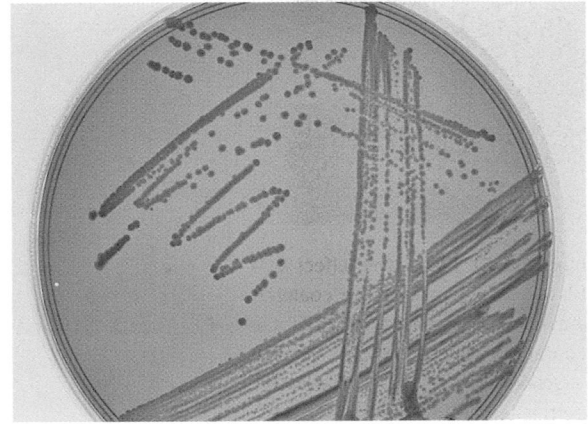

Figure 3.22 *E. coli* isolated on MacConkey's agar.

Bacterial culture

Microbiological culture can be attempted to provide a diagnosis in bacterial, parasitic and viral diseases. The main aim in bacteriological culture is to isolate bacteria on solid media so that they can be identified and appropriate sensitivity testing can be carried out. These methods are possible using agar, a gel-like substance derived from seaweed which melts at 90°C but solidifies at 50°C. It is a highly stable reagent to which nutrients such as blood, serum and protein digests can be added. Examples of bacteria growing on agar media are seen in Figs 3.22 and 3.23.

Viral culture

Viruses are obligatory intracellular pathogens. Viral

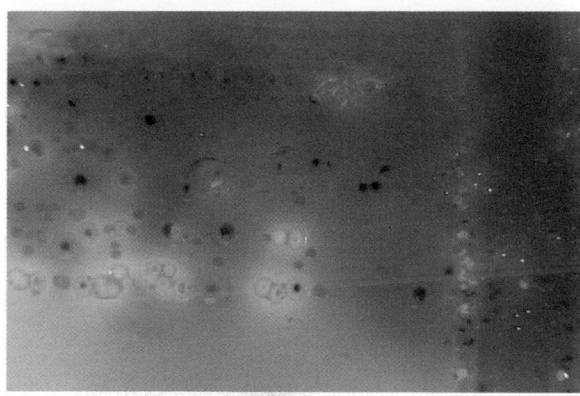

Figure 3.23 Xylose lactose desoxycholate (XLD) medium. Salmonellae are pale with black centres.

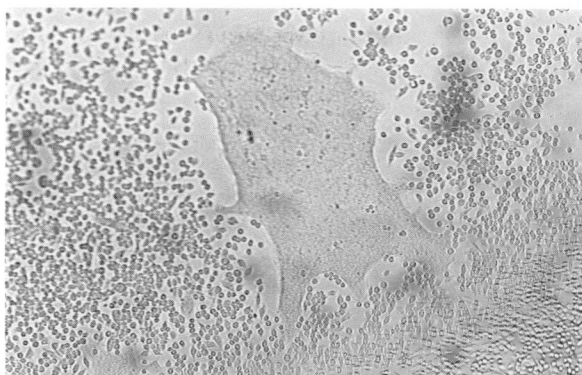

Figure 3.24 Cytopathic effect of measles virus on lympho-blastoid cells; progressive coalescence of infected cells into a syncytium has formed a giant cell. Such giant cells may contain up to 50 nuclei. Reproduced from Bannister *et al.*, *Infectious Disease*, 1996 (Blackwell Science, Oxford) with the permission of the authors.

culture must therefore be performed in primary tissue culture or a continuous cell line. Cell cultures use a cell monolayer onto which the specimen is inoculated. The monolayer is then inspected for the presence of viral damage to the cells—the 'cytopathic effect'. This pathological change takes place in tissue cells as a result of viral growth. Some viruses may be presumptively identified on the basis of a distinctive cytopathic effect (Fig. 3.24). Viral isolates can also be identified by electron microscopy and immunological and virus neutralization techniques.

Immunology

Serological techniques depend on an interaction between antigen and specific antibody. They are of particular value:

- when the pathogen is difficult or dangerous to isolate
- when the patient has been treated with antimicrobial agents
- when culture of the pathogen may be delayed

A secondary signal system detects the interaction between antibody and antigen. The natural secondary phenomena that follow antigen–antibody interaction can be used (agglutination, precipitation and complement fixation). Antibodies can also be manipulated in the laboratory by labelling with fluorescein, radioisotopes or enzymes to allow detection of the antibody–antigen interaction. These techniques include gel precipitation, agglutination, complement fixation, indirect fluorescence, enzyme-linked immunosorbent assay (ELISA) and radio immunoassay.

Molecular diagnostics

There are now a range of new diagnostic techniques that use molecular biology to identify the infectious organism. These include:

- Polymerase chain reaction (PCR) to amplify and detect small amounts of microbial nucleic acids (see p. 111)
- Southern blotting to detect specific DNA sequences from pathogens
- Western blotting to detect specific microbial proteins separated by sodium dodecyl sulphate-polyacrylamide gel electrophoresis (SDS-PAGE) and detected using enzyme-labelled antibodies

PCR is ideal for detecting very low concentrations of organisms and those that are difficult to culture. The sample is mixed with pathogen-specific nucleotide sequences, or primers, and a heat-stable DNA polymerase and subjected to a cycle of temperature changes that results in copying of the specific pathogen sequence. Successive repetition of these cycles results in an exponential amplification of the diagnostic pathogen sequence. Once sufficient pathogen nucleic acid has been generated, the sample is separated by electrophoresis on agarose gel and identified by molecular weight. PCR can be used to diagnose several viral diseases including HIV, cytomegalovirus (CMV), hepatitis (detecting RNA), and is also being used to diagnose bacterial pathogens including *M. tuberculosis* and *Chlamydia trachomatis*. Quantitative techniques can be applied and these have proved useful in monitoring antiviral therapy for HIV and hepatitis C.

Diagnostic imaging

Imaging should be tailored to the presenting syndrome; for example, patients with shortness of breath need a chest radiograph. Specific imaging techniques are discussed in association with specific infections.

Histopathology

Pathological examination of tissue is extremely important in the investigation of infectious disease. Biopsy material must be retained unfixed for culture whenever there is a possibility that underlying infection is a differential diagnosis. Pathological examination for fungi, acid–alcohol-fast bacilli (*M. tuberculosis*) and intracellular organisms should be performed whenever there is diagnostic difficulty. Molecular examination adds to the value of histopathological techniques through PCR-based methods that permit amplification of pathogen DNA/RNA from fixed tissue.

Principles of antimicrobial chemotherapy

Antimicrobial agents have their effect because of selective toxicity. They interfere with microbial metabolism or functions, but have minimal effect on the host. A number of different strategies have been used in their design.

DNA supercoiling and transcription

To conserve space within the confines of the cell, bacterial DNA is tightly coiled ('supercoiled'). When cell division occurs, the DNA is uncoiled, a process controlled by the tetrameric DNA gyrase enzyme system. 4-Fluoroquinolone antibiotics (e.g. ciprofloxacin) act to block this enzyme system, producing lethal double stranded DNA breaks. The transcription of mRNA is controlled by RNA polymerase: this is inhibited by rifampicin and rifabutin.

Bacterial protein synthesis

Bacterial protein synthesis is another important target and a number of different mechanisms are targeted (Fig. 3.25). These include:
- inhibition of transfer RNA (tRNA) binding to the 30S ribosome by tetracyclines
- inhibition of RNA-dependent protein synthesis at the 50S ribosome by macrolides
- binding to both subunits of the ribosome, interfering with protein synthesis and causing misreading of the genetic code by aminoglycosides
- prevention of binding of tRNA to the 50S subunit of the ribosome by chloramphenicol

Antimetabolites

Antimetabolites are compounds that mimic components essential to microbial survival. For example,

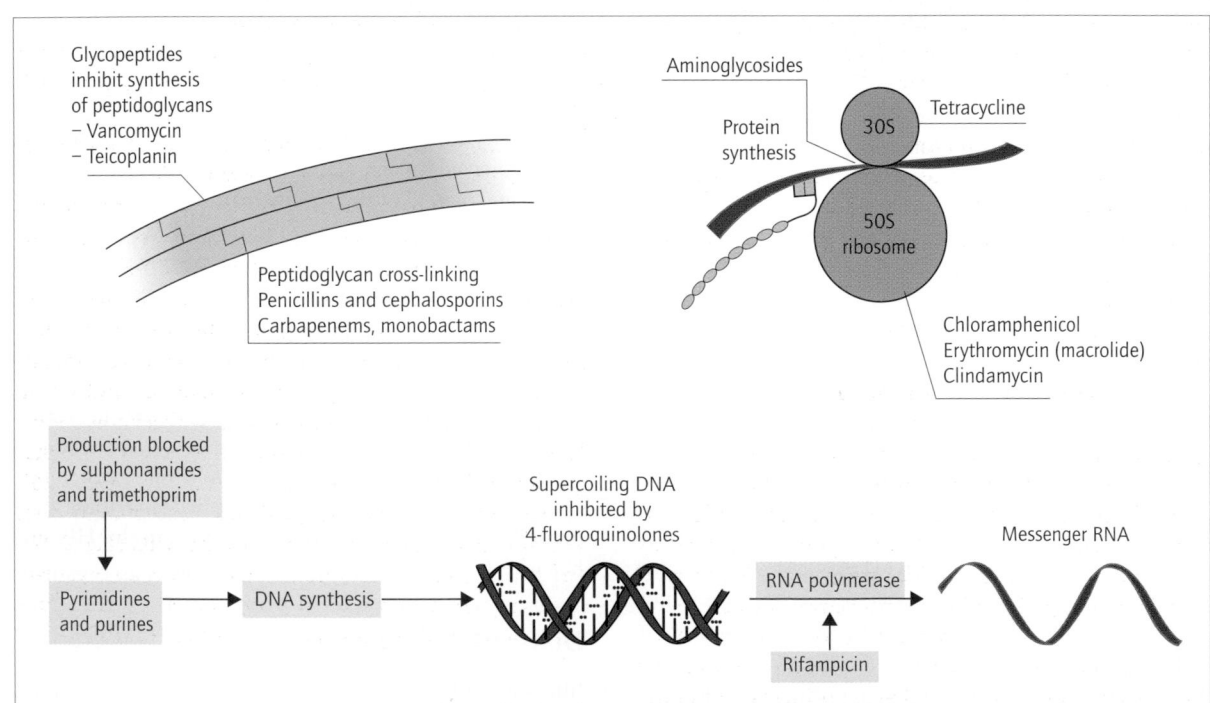

Figure 3.25 Mechanism of action of antibiotics. Reproduced from Gillespie & Bamford, *Medical Microbiology and Infection at a Glance*, 2000 (Blackwell Science Ltd, Oxford) with permission.

sulphonamides mimic *para*-amino benzoic acid (PABA) and competitively inhibit the conversion of PABA into dihydropteroic acid which is later converted in folate and is essential for bacteria in the nucleotide synthesis pathway. Bacteria must synthesize folate for survival but humans do not: it is one of the vitamins, so humans do not have this pathway.

Bacterial cell wall inhibitors

Beta-lactam antibiotics (penicillins, cephalosporins, monobactams and penems) inhibit transpeptidation. This action prevents cross-linking of the polysaccharide chains of peptidoglycans, which are essential for the structural integrity of the bacterial cell wall. Vancomycin also blocks transpeptidation but does so by a different mechanism (Fig. 3.25).

Pharmacology

Knowledge of the pharmacology of antimicrobial agents is required to ensure that adequate concentrations of free antibiotic are available at sites of infection. Infection is often localized to special sites such as the meninges or the peritoneum where penetration of antibiotics can be difficult.

The usual rules of pharmacology apply to the absorption and distribution of antimicrobials within the body:
- non-polar agents such as chloramphenicol are well absorbed and cross the blood–brain barrier
- more polar agents (e.g. penicillins and cephalosporins) are less well absorbed and are confined to extracellular compartments
- protein binding has an effect on the duration of action and bioavailability

In addition to conventional pharmacological considerations, remember that the conditions at the site of an infection can modify the effect of an antimicrobial agent. Concentrations of antimicrobial may be lower at the centre of an abscess than in the serum, and cellular and bacterial debris. At low pH some antibiotics such as aminoglycosides and macrolides are inactive; in contrast, pyrazinamide requires a low pH for activation. Low redox potential in abscesses may interfere with antimicrobial action of most antibiotics, whereas they are essential for the activation of metronidazole—the principal antibiotic used against anaerobes.

(This chapter presents brief information relating to some of the commonly used drugs in infectious diseases. However, the information, especially that relating to side-effects and contraindications, is not complete. Fuller information is given in a formulary, e.g. *British National Formulary* (*BNF*). Regimens should also be checked in the *BNF*.)

Drug excretion and metabolism

The route of excretion is an important factor when planning antimicrobial therapy. Agents excreted in the urine are likely to be effective in pyelonephritis and cystitis, antibiotics excreted in the bile are more likely to be effective in acute cholangitis; in each case the maximum concentration of antimicrobial agent will be available at the site of infection.

In renal failure, drugs may be retained causing toxicity, notably aminoglycosides, so the regimen of a drug excreted in the urine may need adjustment in renal failure. Hepatic disease may interfere with the metabolism of some drugs, resulting in an increased risk of side-effects or making it necessary to reduce the dosage.

Minimum inhibitory concentration and minimum bactericidal concentration

Two other important concepts in understanding antibacterial chemotherapy are as follows:
- *minimum inhibitory concentration* (MIC): the lowest concentration at which the growth of the organism is inhibited
- *minimum bactericidal concentration* (MBC): the lowest concentration at which the organism is killed

The concentration of antimicrobials at the site of the infection should exceed the MIC. In some specialized situations, such as infective endocarditis, it is usual to aim for a serum concentration of antibiotic more than eight times higher than the MBC throughout the treatment. Most sensitivity testing is performed using paper discs containing antimicrobials. This gives an estimate of sensitivity in comparison to that of a control strain with a known MIC. This is quicker and less expensive than MIC determination and suitable for most clinical situations (Fig. 3.26). Modern methods have adapted disc susceptibility tests so that they can give an estimate of the MIC (Fig. 3.27). The MIC may be determined by incubating an organism in varying concentrations of antibiotic. The lowest concentration at which growth is inhibited is the MIC.

Adverse effects

Most antimicrobial agents have a very favourable therapeutic index and are therefore effective without

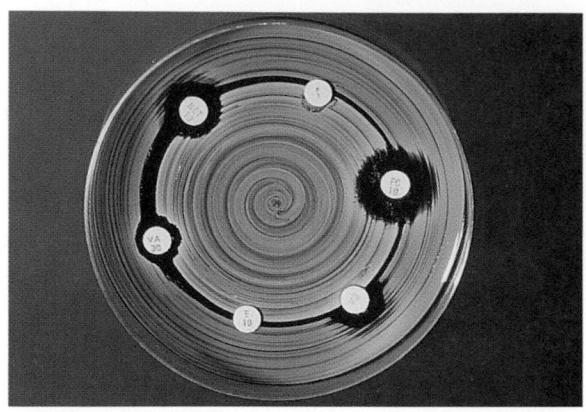

Figure 3.26 Disc sensitivity testing: antibiogram of an isolate of *Staphylococcus epidermidis* from the blood of a patient in intensive care. Reproduced from Bannister *et al.*, *Infectious Disease*, 1996 (Blackwell Science, Oxford) with the permission of the authors.

causing any major adverse effect. Adverse effects fall into two major groups:
● those that occur in a dose-dependent manner (e.g. aminoglycoside toxicity)
● idiosyncratic reactions (e.g. acute anaphylaxis with penicillin)

Renal toxicity

Renal toxicity resulting from the use of an antimicrobial agent can be:
● secondary to the systemic effects of the antimicrobial (e.g. acute tubular necrosis caused by hypotension in acute anaphylaxis; see p. 549)
● a direct effect of the antimicrobial agent
Direct effects include a toxic action on the renal cells (e.g. aminoglycosides), immunological effects (e.g. acute interstitial nephritis associated with cephalosporins, penicillins, rifampicin and sulphonamides) and obstructive uropathy (e.g. crystalluria with early sulphonamides). Other antibiotics with important renal side-effects include tetracyclines and amphotericin B.

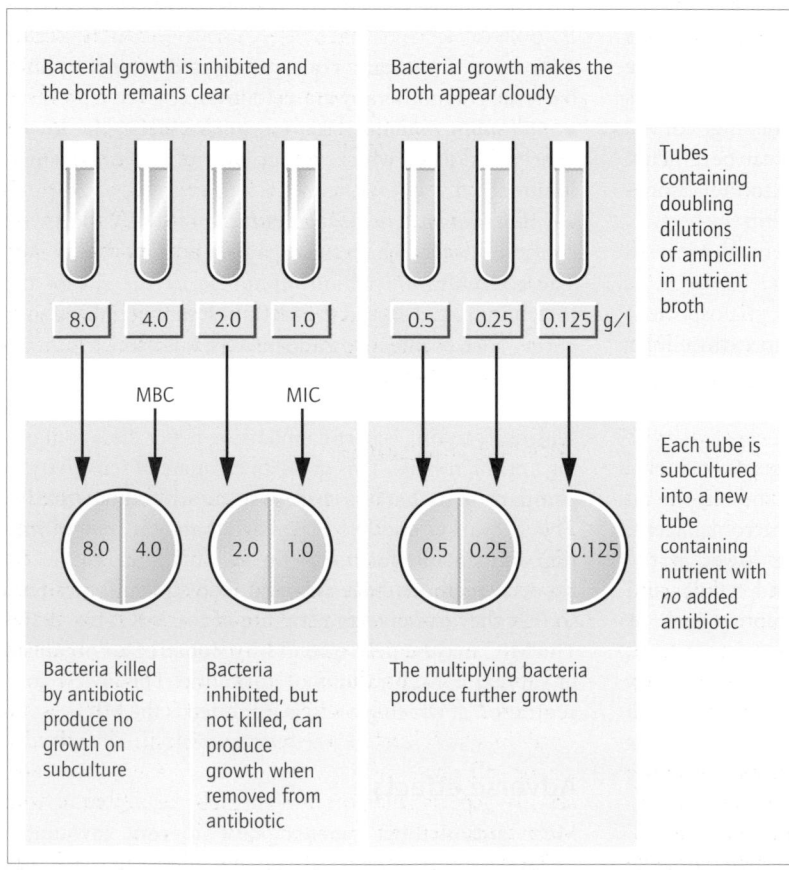

Figure 3.27 The principle of minimum inhibitory concentration (MIC) and minimum bactericidal concentration (MBC) determination. Reproduced from Bannister *et al.*, *Infectious Disease*, 1996 (Blackwell Science, Oxford) with the permission of the authors.

Liver toxicity

Damage to the liver may take the form of acute or chronic inflammatory hepatitis, cholestasis, fatty degeneration or a granulomatous hepatitis. Inflammatory hepatitis is the most common form of liver toxicity and is most often associated with the antituberculosis agents isoniazid and rifampicin. Acute hepatitis occurs in approximately 1% of patients given isoniazid for prophylaxis. The risk of liver damage is related to age, becoming more common in patients aged over 35 years. Hepatitis is most likely to develop in patients with previous liver disease, who have a history of alcohol abuse or who are elderly. Rifampicin may also induce hepatitis, of which there are two types: a transient transaminitis, in which jaundice is absent and transaminase concentrations are elevated but return to normal despite continued drug use; or a severe hepatitis associated with jaundice. Other antituberculous agents—pyrazinamide, ethionamide and cycloserine—can also cause hepatitis. The esteolate and proprionate salts of erythromycin can induce cholestasis associated with fever and eosinophilia. Subsequent challenge results in a rapid reappearance of symptoms, suggesting an immune mechanism. Fusidic acid can cause hepatotoxicity, which is more common if the drug is administered intravenously. Tetracyclines can induce fatty change in the liver if high doses are given intravenously or in patients predisposed by pregnancy or renal failure.

Bone marrow toxicity

A number of different agents including high-dose benzylpenicillin, zidovudine (AZT) or sulphonamides can induce bone marrow toxicity.

Aplastic anaemia may follow treatment with chloramphenicol, from 10 days to 6 months after the therapy. This idiosyncratic reaction must be distinguished from a dose-dependent bone marrow depression observed in patients on higher doses. Granulocytopenia can follow high-dose benzylpenicillin therapy (>12 MU/day), and thrombocytopenic purpura can result from treatment with sulphonamides. Antibiotics may act as haptens, inducing antibodies to red blood cells, resulting in an autoimmune haemolytic anaemia.

Cutaneous reactions vary from urticarial and maculopapular eruptions with penicillins and cephalosporins to life-threatening Stevens–Johnson syndrome (especially with sulphonamides). Of patients with infectious mononucleosis treated with ampicillin, 95% develop raised red urticarial-like lesions. This is not strictly an allergic reaction.

Acute anaphylaxis results when an antibiotic—usually a penicillin—generates a type I hypersensitivity reaction (see p. 49) as a result of hapten–drug sensitization. This complication is truly uncommon (approximately 1/100 000 people). Cephalosporins may also cross-react, but usually in fewer than 10% of penicillin-sensitive patients. New monobactam agents have even lower cross-sensitivity rates.

Sensitivity and resistance

Antimicrobial agents have a limited spectrum of activity: only some genera are susceptible to their action. This is usually because the metabolic process with which they interfere occurs in only a limited number of genera. For example, vancomycin interferes with peptidoglycan synthesis, but can only do this in Gram-positive organisms; all Gram-negative organisms are therefore naturally resistant (Fig. 3.28).

Naturally produced inactivating enzymes

Some organisms are resistant because they naturally produce inactivating enzymes. When penicillin was first introduced, more than 95% of *Staphylococcus aureus* were sensitive and 5% produced a beta-lactamase and were resistant. Since then an increasing number of strains have become beta-lactamase producers so that now it is almost the rule that hospital staphylococci produce this enzyme. It could be said that *Staph. aureus* has acquired resistance because of the selective pressure applied by antibiotics favouring survival of beta-lactamase-producing strains. Drugs such as methicillin (e.g. flucloxacillin) resists the effect of beta-lactamases and at one time bacteria resistant to this agent were rare. Now in many hospitals methicillin-resistant *Staphylococcus aureus* (MRSA) are commonplace and cause a significant morbidity and mortality.

Bacteria have also developed inactivating enzymes for other antimicrobial agents, including aminoglycosides and chloramphenicol.

Altered behaviour

The action of an antimicrobial agent can be inhibited as a result of altered binding to its target. An altered ribosome binding site may explain why organisms are resistant to macrolides and aminoglycosides. Resistance to sulphonamides and trimethoprim arises from alterations in the target enzymes dihydropteroate synthetase and dihydrofolate reductase, respectively (Fig. 3.28).

Altered permeability of bacterial outer membranes can result in a high level of resistance, which may be effective against all drugs of a particular class. Organisms may acquire a specialized pump that expels the antibiotic from the bacterial cell (e.g. pumping quinolones).

Bacteria can acquire DNA that alters the cell wall

03

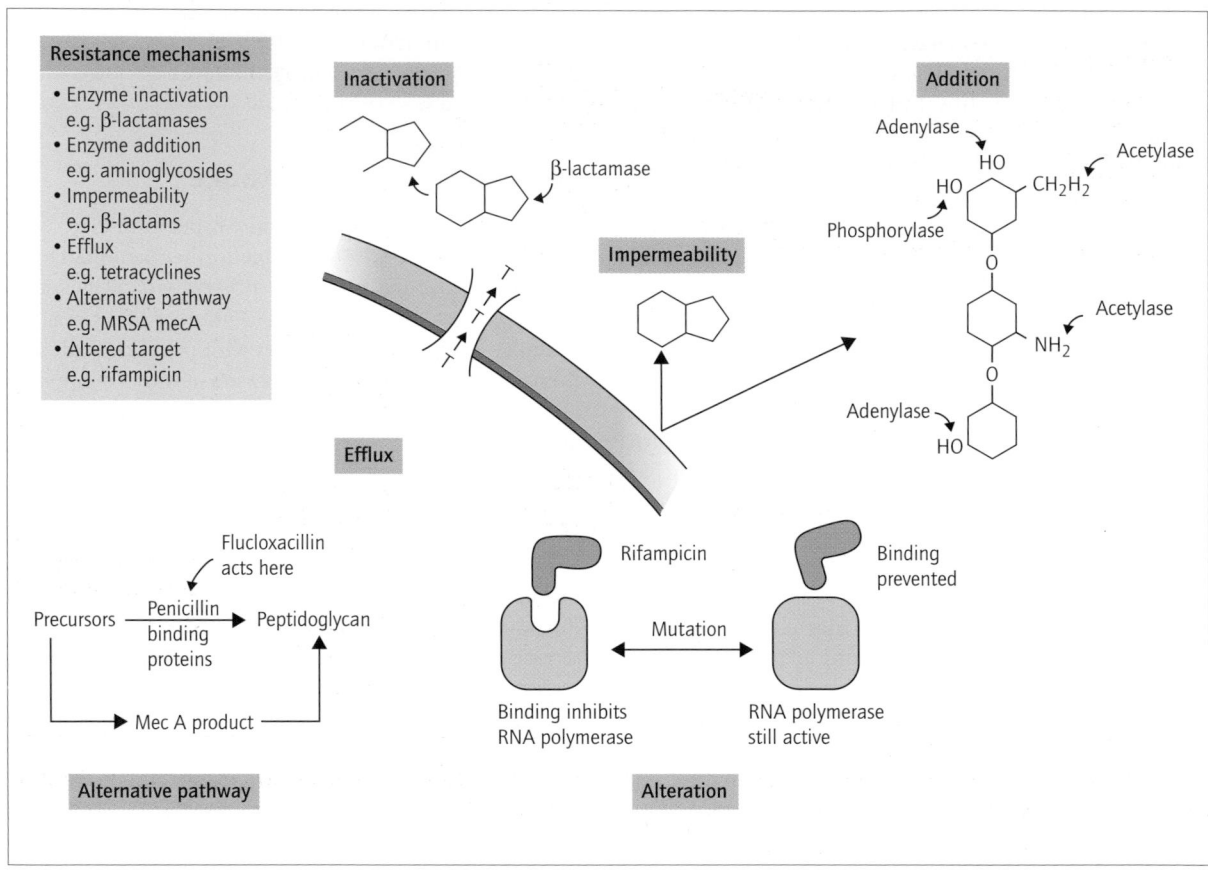

Figure 3.28 Mechanisms of resistance to antibacterials. Reproduced from Gillespie & Bamford, *Medical Microbiology and Infection at a Glance*, 2003 (Blackwell Science Ltd, Oxford) with permission.

synthesis enzymes, making them bind penicillin less efficiently, leading to resistance as in the case of *Streptococcus pneumoniae*. *Staphylococcus aureus* has acquired a new gene that encodes an altered penicillin-binding protein 2′ (PBP2′) which no longer binds methicillin, making the organism methicillin-resistant (MRSA).

Transfer of resistance

The bacterial genes coding for antimicrobial resistance can be transmitted not only between organisms of the same species, but also between different genera. Transfer of resistance means that organisms that are naturally resistant to an antimicrobial agent can transmit this ability to naturally sensitive organisms. This is achieved by:
- *Transduction:* small sequences of DNA are carried on bacteriophages
- *Transformation:* naked DNA from one bacterium is taken up by another
- *Conjugation:* DNA is transferred on a plasmid, which

induces the bacterium that carries it to mate with another and transfer a copy of the plasmid (Fig. 3.29)
- *Transposons:* small portions of DNA able to transfer resistance DNA from one strain to another, and between plasmids and the bacterial chromosome
- *Integrons:* small sections of DNA that can be transferred between bacteria and encode multiple resistance determinants

Beta-lactam antibiotics

Beta-lactam antibiotics include penicillins and cephalosporins, which have similar structures. They work by inhibiting cross-linking of bacterial peptidoglycan (Fig. 3.25).

Penicillins
Antibacterial activity
Natural penicillins have been modified to produce

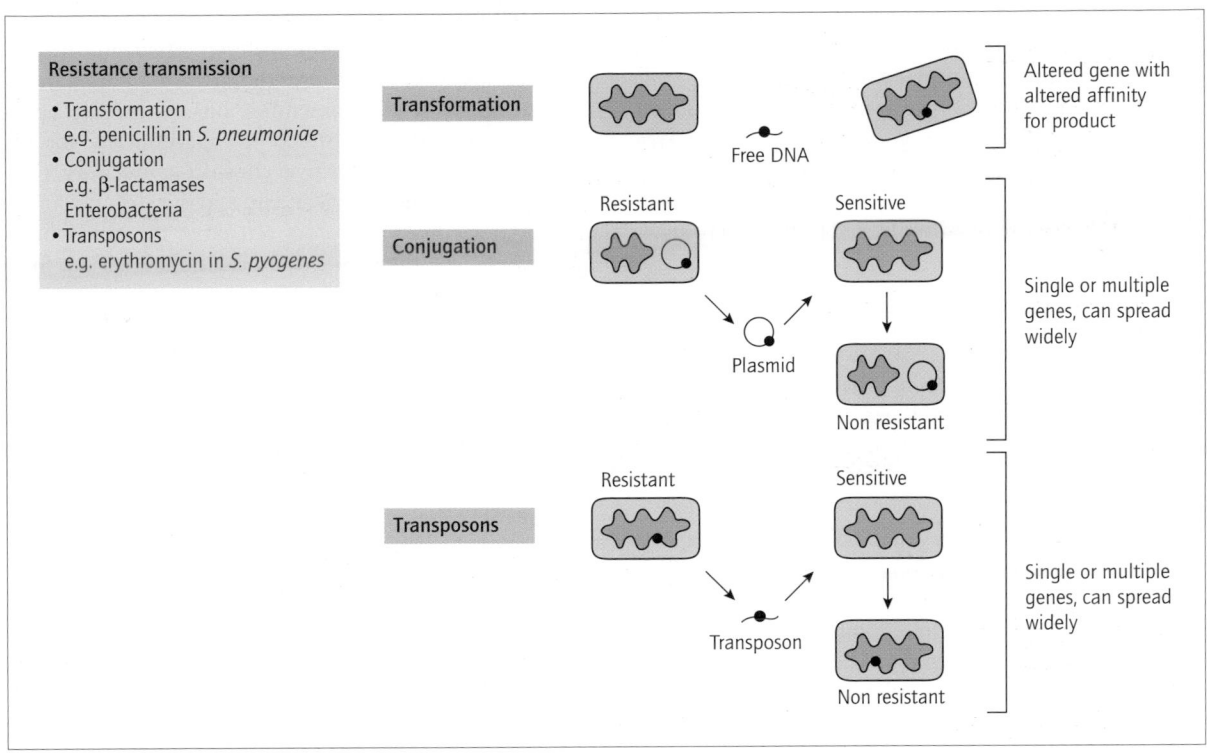

Resistance transmission

- Transformation
  e.g. penicillin in *S. pneumoniae*
- Conjugation
  e.g. β-lactamases
  Enterobacteria
- Transposons
  e.g. erythromycin in *S. pyogenes*

Transformation — Free DNA — Altered gene with altered affinity for product

Conjugation — Resistant — Sensitive — Plasmid — Non resistant — Single or multiple genes, can spread widely

Transposons — Resistant — Sensitive — Transposon — Non resistant — Single or multiple genes, can spread widely

Figure 3.29 Transfer of resistance to antibacterials. Reproduced from Gillespie & Bamford, *Medical Microbiology and Infection at a Glance*, 2003 (Blackwell Science Ltd, Oxford) with permission.

penicillinase resistance and an extended antibacterial spectrum. Penicillins can be conveniently divided into the following classes on the basis of their antibacterial activity:

- Natural penicillins (e.g. penicillin G, penicillin V)
- Penicillinase-resistant penicillin (e.g. flucloxacillin)
- Aminopenicillins (e.g. ampicillin-like agents)
- Expanded spectrum penicillins

Penicillins differ markedly in their oral absorption. Penicillin G is unstable in the presence of gastric acid and must therefore be given intravenously. In contrast, penicillin V is stable in the presence of gastric acid and can be used via the oral route. The aminopenicillins and flucloxacillin are also absorbed orally, while the remaining agents must be given intravenously. All the orally active penicillins yield peak levels in the serum 1–2 h after ingestion, this peak being delayed by food.

Penicillins are excreted and secreted by the kidney. Their excretion is rapid and so their half-life is very short, ranging from 30 to 72 min. Coadministration of probenecid, which competes with penicillin for the renal tubular secretory mechanism, increases the half-life. Protein binding is variable, ranging from 17% for aminopenicillins to 97% for dicloxacillin. Penicillins are distributed in extracellular fluid to most of the body tissues including the lungs, liver, kidneys, muscle, bones and placenta. They do not cross the blood–brain barrier unless the meninges are inflamed. High concentrations of penicillin are found in the urine, and penicillins are actively secreted into the bile.

Bacterial resistance to beta-lactam antibiotics is mediated by chromosomal or plasmid-encoded mechanisms. Organisms that become resistant may do so because they produce a beta-lactamase or by alterations in their penicillin-binding proteins.

Cephalosporins

Cephalosporins are closely related to penicillins, and are usually classified according to their route of administration and spectrum of activity.

- The first group comprises the orally active cephalosporins, which have a mainly Gram-positive spectrum. Some agents such as cefaclor also have activity against *Haemophilus influenzae*.
- The second group consists of the older injectable agents, such as cefamandole and cefuroxime. These all have a wide spectrum of activity against Gram-positive organisms and good activity against *Escherichia coli* and some species of *Proteus*.

- The third group comprises the newer injectable cephalosporin agents. These include cefotaxime, which is active against most Gram-negative organisms and *Streptococcus* spp. but is less active against *Staph. aureus*. Only some of these drugs have good activity against *Pseudomonas aeruginosa* such as ceftazidime and cefepime.
- The fourth group have the same wide spectrum as the third group, but can be administered by the oral route.

Aminoglycosides

The first aminoglycoside—streptomycin—was isolated from *Streptomyces griseus*. Since then a number of different agents have been developed including kanamycin, gentamicin, tobramycin, netilmicin and amikacin.

Pharmacokinetics

Aminoglycosides are given parenterally and have a narrow therapeutic index. They are polar, limited to the extracellular fluid, excreted in the urine and not metabolized by the liver. Aminoglycosides are toxic to cells of the proximal renal tubules, and renal toxicity will occur at doses close to those necessary for antimicrobial action. There is evidence of mild tubular effects in all patients and small reductions in the glomerular filtration rate occur in approximately 80%. Aminoglycosides can also damage hair cells of the organ of Corti, resulting in auditory or vestibular impairment. Toxicity is especially likely to arise in the elderly, in patients taking other drugs that are toxic to the kidney, or in circumstances where there are other conditions predisposing to renal failure (e.g. shock or endocarditis). The serum concentration of aminoglycosides must therefore be closely monitored.

Bacterial resistance

Some organisms have become resistant to aminoglycosides through the development of inactivating enzymes.

Glycopeptides (vancomycin, teicoplanin)

Antibacterial activity

Vancomycin is a glycopeptide antibiotic first isolated from *Streptomyces orientales*. It inhibits the formation of peptidoglycan polymers. Bacterial resistance was previously extremely uncommon, but has now often been found in enterococci isolated in hospitals (glycopeptide-resistant enterococci; GRE). Some *Staph. aureus* have developed intermediate resistance to glycopeptide antibiotics (glycopeptide-resistant *Staph. aureus*; GISA). Some species of staphylococci (e.g. *Staphylococcus haemolyticus*) are naturally resistant to teicoplanin and may cause line infections in patients in intensive therapy units.

Pharmacokinetics

Glycopeptides must be administered intravenously; they are not absorbed orally. Oral therapy is only used in the management of pseudomembranous colitis. Glycopeptides are often administered intraperitoneally for the treatment of Gram-positive chronic ambulatory peritoneal dialysis infection. Vancomycin is distributed in the extracellular fluid, and does not cross the blood–brain barrier unless there is meningeal inflammation. It is excreted by the kidney.

Quinolones

The quinolone agents have a similar structure; the first described was nalidixic acid, but it did not attain high tissue levels and was confined to the treatment of urinary tract infection.

Antibacterial activity

Development of the fluoroquinolones (e.g. ciprofloxacin) has resulted in antibacterial activity many times greater than that of nalidixic acid against Gram-negative pathogens including *Pseudomonas*. These agents are also active against *Chlamydia*, and they have been used for single dose treatment of genital infections (see p. 150). They have relatively poor activity against Gram-positive organisms. The excellent safety profile and favourable pharmacokinetics of ciprofloxacin and similar compounds means that they have a place in the management of Gram-negative sepsis. More recently synthesized quinolones such as gatifloxacin and moxifloxacin are very active against Gram-positive pathogens including *Streptococcus pneumoniae*.

Pharmacokinetics

Fluoroquinolones are absorbed orally and reach a peak concentration in serum about 90 min after oral administration. They are distributed widely in the tissues, and penetrate inside cells including macrophages and polymorphs.

Erythromycin

Erythromycin is derived from *Streptomyces erythreus* and is the prototype macrolide antibiotic. It acts by interfering with protein synthesis. Erythromycin is active against Gram-positive cocci, many anaerobes (but not *Bacteroides*), *Mycoplasma* and *Chlamydia*. It is absorbed orally, is distributed in the total body water, crosses the placenta, and is concentrated in alveolar macrophages and polymorphs, and in the liver. It is excreted in the bile. It is usually well tolerated, although some patients complain of nausea. Newer macrolide antibiotics are now available (clarithromycin and azithromycin) that have more favourable pharmacokinetics and toxicity profile but a similar spectrum of activity.

Streptogramins

Pristinomycin is a semisynthetic parenteral streptogramin consisting of two components, quinupristin and dalfopristin, that are designed to work synergistically. It acts by preventing peptide bond formation, resulting in release of incomplete polypeptide chains from the donor site. Although both quinupristin and dalfopristin are bacteriostatic, the combination is bactericidal.

Pristinomycin is active against a broad range of Grampositive pathogens, including staphylococci (irrespective of methicillin resistance), enterococci, streptococci (including penicillin-resistant strains), *Clostridium* and *Peptostreptococcus*. It has activity against some Gramnegative pathogens including *Moraxella*, *Legionella*, *Neisseria meningitidis* and *Mycoplasma*. It is used mainly for the treatment of resistant Gram-positive infections (e.g. GRE and GISA).

Pharmacokinetics
Pristinomycin should be administered through a central venous cannula. The metabolism of the drug is reduced in patients with cirrhosis or with reduced clearance (e.g. renal failure).

Oxazolidinones

The oxazolidinones represent a new class of antibiotic that has been developed to meet the challenge of resistant Gram-positive organisms. They inhibit protein synthesis by a unique mode of action competing for the same binding site on the 50S ribosomal subunit as chloramphenicol and clindamycin, but acts in a different way. The differing mechanism means there is no cross-resistance between oxazolidinones and other protein synthesis inhibitors.

Antibacterial activity
Oxazolidinones are most active against Gram-positive bacteria, including penicillin-resistant *S. pneumoniae* and MRSA. They are used mainly for the treatment of resistant Gram-positive infections.

Pharmacokinetics
Linezolid is rapidly and completely absorbed after oral administration, with near 100% bioavailability and peak serum concentrations 1–2 h after administration. The drug is cleared by both renal and non-renal routes, with an elimination half-life of 4.5 h following intravenous administration and 5.5 h after oral administration. However, in patients with renal failure, a reduction in dosage may not be required.

Metronidazole

Metronidazole is a nitroimidazole drug. It is active against all species of anaerobic bacteria and resistance is very rare. It is also active against some species of protozoa including *Giardia*, *Entamoeba histolytica* and *Trichomonas vaginalis*. It is absorbed orally and can be administered parenterally, and is not significantly protein bound. Metronidazole is widely distributed throughout the tissues, crossing the blood–brain barrier and penetrating into abscesses. It is metabolized in the liver and excreted in the urine, and is well tolerated. Metronidazole has mutagenic activity in prokaryotic systems, but no similar activity has been found in eukaryotic systems. There is no evidence of increased incidents of mutagenicity. Another nitromidazole derivative, tinidazole, may be better tolerated in some patients.

Tetracyclines

Tetracyclines were first isolated from *Streptomyces* spp. Many tetracycline compounds have been described, but they all have similar spectra of activity. They act by interfering with protein synthesis and are active against many Gram-positive and some Gram-negative pathogens (*Chlamydia*, *Mycoplasma*, *Rickettsia* and treponemes). Doxycycline has useful activity against some protozoa including *Plasmodium* and *E. histolytica*.

Pharmacokinetics
Tetracyclines are absorbed orally and their half-lives vary widely. Some, such as doxycycline, have a long half-life and adequate therapeutic levels may be obtained by a once daily regimen. They are distributed to many tissues including the lung, liver, kidney, brain and respiratory tract, and are concentrated in bile.

Chloramphenicol

Chloramphenicol was first isolated from *Streptomyces venezuelae*, but is now produced synthetically. It acts by inhibiting protein synthesis at the ribosome. It has a very wide spectrum of activity that includes Gram-positive, Gram-negative bacteria and anaerobes.

Pharmacokinetics
Chloramphenicol can be given parenterally, but is well absorbed orally. A special oily preparation of chloramphenicol is available for intramuscular use. This has proven valuable for use by primary health care workers in

03

developing countries for single dose treatment of bacterial sepsis.

Chloramphenicol is metabolized in the liver and is excreted in the kidney. In the neonatal period hepatic enzymes are unable to process chloramphenicol efficiently and the dose must be halved.

Chloramphenicol use is associated with a rare idiosyncratic aplastic anaemia and this now limits the use of this agent to life-threatening infections where its spectrum of activity, pharmacokinetics and safety in penicillin allergic patients make a useful alternative.

Sulphonamides and trimethoprim

Sulphonamides are the oldest antibacterial agents still in clinical use. They act by inhibiting the synthesis of tetrahydrofolate. They are rarely used in the treatment of bacterial infections but have an important role in the management of *Pneumocystis carinii* and protozoan infections including malaria. Many different types have been synthesized. Their antibacterial spectra are the same, but their half-lives vary remarkably.

Sulphonamides can be given intravenously and are well absorbed when given orally. They are distributed widely in the tissues and cross the blood–brain barrier. They are metabolized in the liver and excreted via the kidney.

Polyenes

There are two polyene cyclic macrolides in clinical use: nystatin and amphotericin B, the products of *Streptomyces* species. They have a wide spectrum of activity inhibiting the growth of almost all fungi implicated in human infection including *Candida*, *Aspergillus*, *Cryptococcus* and the agents responsible for systemic mycoses. More recently, amphotericin has been used successfully in the management of cutaneous and systemic leishmaniasis (see p. 136).

The polyenes are amphipathic molecules, which bind preferentially to ergosterol in the fungal membrane forming a pore, which leads to leakage of the intracellular contents and cell death. Primary and secondary resistance is rare but resistant variants of some *Candida* spp. including *C. krusei*, *C. lusitaniae*, *C. tropicalis* and *C. parapsilosis* have been described.

Nystatin is too toxic for systemic application and its use is confined to topical treatment of superficial *Candida* infections and the prevention of fungal infection in immunocompromised patients; it has no value for the treatment of dermatophyte infections. Amphotericin can be given parenterally. The older preparations are administered as a complex with sodium deoxycholate and are relatively toxic. Their use is associated with fever,

chills, thrombophlebitis and hypotension. The drug can also cause renal tubular damage that usually but not always recovers after treatment. Modern preparations with various lipid formulations, such as incorporation into liposomes, are much less toxic and higher doses can be safely given.

Azoles

The azole group of compounds (clotrimazole, miconazole, fluconazole and itraconazole) act by blocking the action of cytochrome p450 and sterol 14α-demethylase. This latter enzyme allows the incorporation of 14-methyl sterols in the fungal membrane, instead of ergosterol. In addition, the azoles also cause direct damage to the fungal membrane. Although some species of *Candida* are naturally resistant (e.g. *C. krusei*), resistance can develop during long-term treatment, as in the case of the immunocompromised patient.

Clotrimazole and miconazole are frequently used as topical preparations for minor infections.

Fluconazole

Fluconazole can be given orally, topically or parenterally. Fluconazole is widely distributed, crosses the blood–brain barrier and is active against *Candida* and *Cryptococcus* but not against filamentous fungi. It is used for the prophylaxis and treatment of cryptococcal infections, and treatment of superficial and systemic candidiasis. Although well tolerated, it may cause liver enzyme abnormalities. It has significant drug interactions, increasing the serum concentration of phenytoin, cyclosporin and oral hypoglycaemic agents and reducing the rate of warfarin metabolism.

Itraconazole

In addition to being effective against *Candida*, *Cryptococcus neoformans* and *Histoplasma*, itraconazole also displays activity against filamentous fungi including *Aspergillus* and the dermatophytes. It is indicated in treatment of invasive candidiasis, cryptococcosis, aspergillosis, superficial mycoses and pityriasis versicolor. Resistance is rare.

Highly lipid soluble, it is incompletely absorbed from the gastrointestinal tract; optimal absorption is achieved when taken with food. The drug achieves high tissue concentrations.

Adverse events are rare but there may be a transient increase in the transaminases and in the concentrations of cyclosporin, digoxin and phenytoin. Concomitant use of rifampicin or rifabutin lowers the serum concentration of itraconazole.

Other agents

Flucytosine

This synthetic fluorinated pyrimidine inhibits *Candida* sp., *Cryptococcus neoformans* and some moulds. Metabolized by the fungus to phosphorylated 5-fluorouracil, the drug disrupts protein synthesis by inhibiting thymidylate synthase and by being incorporated into RNA in place of uracil, distorting RNA structure. It is well absorbed orally and can be given intravenously. It may produce bone marrow suppression, thrombocytopenia and abnormal liver function tests. It is usually prescribed in combination with amphotericin or an azole agent as resistance readily develops on monotherapy.

Terbinafine

This drug acts by inhibition of squalene epoxidase resulting in accumulation of aberrant and toxic sterols in the cell wall. It is indicated for the oral treatment of superficial dermatophyte infections when infections are unlikely to or have failed to respond to local therapy. Stevens–Johnson syndrome, toxic epidermal necrolysis and hepatic toxicity are reported adverse effects. Treatment should be continued for up to 6 weeks for skin infections and 3 months or longer for nail infections.

Griseofulvin

This is the earliest antifungal compound derived from some species of *Penicillium*. It has activity only against dermatophytes and works by preventing the sliding of microtubules, thus inhibiting mitosis. Treatment is given orally and the drug is incorporated into the stratum corneum or nail where it inhibits fungal infection of new skin or nail. Thus, treatment must be continued until infected skin and nail is replace by uninfected tissue. This process may take many months in the case of toenails.

Adverse events are rare but include gastrointestinal upset. The drug is metabolized in the liver and is contraindicated in all patients. Griseofulvin reduces the anticoagulant effect of warfarin. Dermatophyte resistance to griseofulvin has been described but is rare.

Antiparasitic agents

Many of the agents used to treat bacterial infection have an application in protozoan infections; for example, metronidazole in the treatment of trichomoniasis and sulfadiazine in the treatment of toxoplasmosis. Malaria, which is usually treated with specific antimalarials, may sometimes be treated with agents usually associated with the treatment of bacterial infections, such as tetracyclines used in the accessory treatment of drug-resistant malaria.

The main antimalarials are discussed below.

Quinine

Quinine is the oldest specific anti-infective agent known. It was originally brought back to Spain from South America where it was used by Native Americans for the treatment of fever. It was known for some time as Jesuit bark.

The drug is extracted from the bark of the Cinchona tree, and although the active molecule has been synthesized this is so difficult to do that it is still extracted from bark to this day. The mode of action of the drug remains uncertain. It is indicated for the treatment of malaria from areas where chloroquine resistance is described (almost everywhere).

Pharmacokinetics
The drug can be administered orally or parenterally.

Toxicity
Most patients complain of tinnitus, known as cinchonism, at close to the therapeutic concentrations. It can give rise to hypoglycaemia and this complication is especially likely in malaria. It is dangerous in overdose where it may cause severe and permanent retinal toxicity.

Mefloquine

Mefloquine arose as a result of the research activity of the US army following their experience of drug-resistant malaria in Vietnam. It is a quinolone-carbinol possessing a quinine-like ring structure used in the treatment and prophylaxis of all species of human malaria. Mefloquine can be used for prophylaxis of *P. falciparum* that is resistant to chloroquine, but mefloquine resistance itself has now been reported in some areas. It is highly effective when used as prophylaxis.

Pharmacokinetics
It is administered orally and absorbed from the gut, reaching a peak between 2 and 12 h after administration. A weekly regimen is used for prophylaxis. The drug is mainly excreted in the bile and faeces.

Toxicity
Convulsions, dizziness, altered balance, vomiting, diarrhoea and psychological reactions have been reported, and mefloquine is teratogenic to rats and mice in early pregnancy, and relatively contraindicated for pregnant and lactating women. It may potentiate the convulsive properties of quinine.

03

03

Artemesin

Artemesin is derived from the plant *Artemisia annua* or qinghaosu, which has a long history of use in traditional Chinese medicine for the treatment of malaria. This drug is currently in evaluation but is likely to find a place in the therapy of multidrug resistance. It has a rapid action and is therefore particularly suitable for the treatment of serious complications of malaria, including cerebral malaria.

Atovaquone

This is a hydroxynamphthoquinone, which is a potent inhibitor of mitochondrial electron transport mechanisms. This is achieved by competing with ubiquinone in ubiquinone-linked dehydrogenases involved in adenosine triphosphate generation. It is used for prophylaxis of malaria in combination with proguanil and may be used in the treatment of *Pneumocystis carinii* and toxoplasmosis.

Pharmacokinetics

Atovaquone is absorbed orally. Plasma elimination half-life is 72 h. Bioavailability was variable especially in relation to food, with absorption being increased up to fivefold with food.

Major adverse events are not yet apparent, but many more patients will need to be treated to confirm this safety profile (i.e. a serious side-effect may develop rarely, which may be significant).

Ivermectin

Ivermectin is a semisynthetic macrocyclic lactone (macrolide), which is known to mimic the inhibitory neurotransmitter gamma-aminobutyric acid (GABA). This is thought to result in the paralysis of nematode muscle. It probably also has an immune modulatory effect. It is indicated for the individual and mass treatment of *Onchocerca volvulus* infection, treatment of lymphatic filariasis and *Strongyloides stercoralis* infection. One of the main attractions for the use of ivermectin is the relative lack of side-effects. There is minimal reaction after administration. Adverse reactions occurred at a rate of 3–13/1000 in a community-based *Onchocerca* study in Liberia. The main side-effects reported were oedema, pruritus and rash, painful lymph nodes and dizziness.

Albendazole

This is a benzimidazole compound which is indicated in the treatment of hydatid disease. In countries outside the UK it is used for the treatment of nematode infections including *Strongyloides*, hookworm, *Ascaris* and *Trichuris* infection. It may also have a role in the management of some microsporidial infections in AIDS patients. The drug is usually well tolerated but headache, dizziness, rashes and changes in liver enzymes, together with occasional reports of alopecia have been associated with the use of this drug.

Praziquantel

This is the drug of choice for the treatment of schistosomiasis. It is active against all of the species of schistosome that infect humans. It is also useful for the treatment of cestode infections including tapeworms, hydatid disease and cerebral cysticercosis. Treatment is given orally and few side-effects have been reported with its use.

Antivirals

The intracellular location of viruses and their use of host cell systems make it difficult to develop antiviral therapy. Despite this, there are a growing number available—some of the more important are listed below.

Amantadine and rimantadine

Amantadine prevents viral uncoating and release of viral RNA within the infected cell. It is active against influenza A, although resistance develops through mutation in the matrix protein gene. Short courses of oral therapy are indicated in the prevention and treatment of influenza during known outbreaks. Its use is usually restricted to individuals at high risk of severe illness.

Neuraminidase inhibitors

Until recently the only compounds with activity against influenza virus were amantadine and rimantadine. However, these need to be given prophylactically or very early in the course of infection if they are to modify the outcome.

Mechanism of action

Neuraminidase is essential in enabling the virus to penetrate the mucus layer. Neuraminidase permits viral release from infected cells as neuraminic acid is found on new progeny virus and agglutination would occur if these residues were not cleaved by neuraminidase. When neuraminidase is inactivated by therapy, the virus remains attached to infected cell membranes and to each other, thus preventing spread of the infection within the host.

Anti-influenza drugs are structural mimics of

neuraminidase: zanamivir is a guanidinyl derivative of neuraminic acid; oseltamivir uses a cyclohexene ring and more lipophilic side chains. Resistance occurs by two mechanisms: by mutations in, or close to, the genetic area coding for the haemagglutinin binding site or by alteration of the sequence in the active site of the gene encoding neuraminidase. Zanamivir must be given by nasal drops, spray, nebulized mist or dry powder aerosol. Oseltamivir, in contrast, is rapidly absorbed after oral administration and then metabolized to an active compound. Both drugs are well tolerated but zanamivir has been associated with increased bronchospasm in some asthmatic patients: one study of patients with chronic obstructive pulmonary disease showed that the FEV_1 was depressed. Zanamivir is well tolerated in patients with mild to moderate asthma.

Zanamivir and oseltamivir bring a modest reduction in the duration of influenza symptoms among patients treated within 48 h of the onset of symptoms. Neuraminidase inhibitors can prevent influenza in compromised patients when the drug is given for 14 days during an influenza epidemic.

Nucleoside analogues

Aciclovir

Herpes virus encoded thymidine kinase but not human enzymes phosphorylate aciclovir. This process must occur before incorporation into DNA and only occurs in virally infected cells. Aciclovir is active against herpes simplex virus (HSV) and varicella zoster virus (VZV), which code for their own thymidine kinases, and is used to treat herpes simplex infections including primary and secondary oral, genital infections and encephalitis. It is also used for prophylaxis against herpes infections in the immunocompromised. Resistance occurs through the development of deficient thymidine kinase production or alteration in the viral polymerase gene. The drug can be taken orally and crosses the blood–brain barrier. Most is excreted unchanged in the urine; toxicity is rare.

Ganciclovir

Virus-infected cells phosphorylate ganciclovir to a monophosphate form which is then metabolized further to a triphosphate form. The drug is active against HSV and CMV and is available as an intravenous or oral formulation. It is indicated in the treatment of life- or sight-threatening CMV infections in immunocompromised individuals. Ganciclovir causes bone marrow toxicity and this may limit therapy. Monitoring of haematological indices is required during therapy.

Ribavirin

Ribavirin is a guanosine analogue that has activity against RSV, influenza A and B, parainfluenza virus, Lassa fever and other arena viruses. It inhibits several steps in viral replication including capping and elongation of viral mRNA and its mechanism of action is probably by inhibition of cellular pathways. Usually, ribavirin is administered by aerosol for treatment of severe RSV infection in infants. It is used in the treatment of Lassa fever virus and Haantan virus infection.

Antiretroviral compounds

The introduction of highly active antiretroviral therapy (HAART) has transformed the clinical landscape of HIV care. For patients, this therapy has brought about improvement in the CD4 count and a fall in the HIV viral load.

Nucleoside reverse transcriptase inhibitors or nucleoside analogues

Nucleoside reverse transcriptase inhibitors (NRTIs) are nucleoside analogues that inhibit the action of reverse transcriptase, the enzyme responsible for the conversion of viral RNA into a DNA copy. These include the longest established antiretroviral drug zidovudine (AZT), and lamivudine (3TC), stavudine (d4T), didanosine (ddI) and zalcitabine (ddC). They are the mainstay of retroviral therapy and are used in combination in initial therapy (see p. 176). Lamivudine is highly active but selects for resistance and should only be used in completely suppressive regimens.

Protease inhibitors

These drugs inhibit HIV protease and are highly effective in reducing viral load. They are central to HAART (see p. 176). They include indinavir, ritonavir, saquinavir and nelfinavir. The activity of these drugs appears to be similar.

Non-nucleoside reverse transcriptase inhibitors (NNRTIs)

Non-nucleoside reverse transcriptase inhibitors (NNRTIs) inhibit reverse transcriptase by an alternative mechanism to NRTIs (e.g. nevirapine, delavirdine). They have been shown to be effective agents in combination regimens. Because of their potential to resistance after a single mutation event, they should only be used in regimens designed to be maximally suppressive.

03

Table 3.16 Some causes of fever and infection in a traveller

Area visited	Infection
Tropics and subtropics	Malaria, typhoid, tuberculosis, worldwide hepatitis A, hepatitis C
Africa (rural)	Filariasis (West Africa), typhus, viral haemorrhagic fever, yellow fever (West Africa)
Middle East	Brucellosis
Asia	Japanese encephalitis
South America	Viral haemorrhagic fever, Ororya fever
Oceania	Malaria, filariasis
North America	Rocky Mountain spotted fever, Lyme disease
Urban countries worldwide	Sexually transmitted diseases, HIV

Prevention of infection

Advice to the traveller

Many people travelling abroad become ill, often because of minor gastrointestinal infections or conditions caused by changes in environment such as sunburn, heat stroke and altitude sickness (Table 3.16). Occasionally, a traveller acquires a serious infection.

People travel increasingly to what were once considered exotic destinations and medical advice about possible health risks should be available.

Food and drink

In countries with a high risk of faeco-oral infections, water should be boiled or sterilized. Brief boiling or proprietary sterilizing tablets will destroy most pathogens, but it is necessary to boil for at least 10 min or sterilize with decolorized 2% iodine tincture to be certain of eliminating *Entamoeba histolytica* cysts.

All food, except fruit that can be peeled, should be eaten freshly cooked. Salads and ice in drinks should be avoided.

Malaria

All visitors to malarious areas and residents returning after prolonged absence should be advised to take prophylactic antimalarial drugs. The recommended regimen depends on the area to be visited and may alter as resistance patterns change. Up-to-date advice must therefore be obtained. No prophylactic regimen is completely effective and so it is important to reduce the risk of mosquito bites by sleeping under netting and using repellents, especially between dusk and dawn when *Anopheles* mosquitoes are active.

Immunization

- Travellers should be up-to-date with their domestic immunization programme including polio and tetanus (Table 3.17).
- Visitors to countries with poor hygiene should be immunized against typhoid and actively or passively immunized against hepatitis A.
- Killed whole-cell cholera vaccine has low efficacy and, because cholera is a rare infection for most types of traveller, is seldom recommended.
- Rabies vaccine should be offered to anyone visiting remote areas where medical care will be delayed and for long stays in tropical countries.
- Yellow fever vaccine is the only immunization required

Table 3.17 Example of a national vaccination schedule

Vaccine	Vaccine type	Age
DTP		
Diphtheria	Toxoid	
Tetanus	Toxoid	Three doses at 2, 3 and 4 months
Pertussis	Killed	
H. influenzae b/polio	Polysaccharide/attenuated	
MMR	Attenuated	Single dose 12–15 months
Booster DT and MMR	Toxoid/attenuated	3 years after completion primary course
Meningitis C	Polysaccharide conjugate	Young adults and adolescents
BCG	Attenuated	10–14 years or infancy
Booster tetanus, diphtheria, polio		
Rubella		Sero-negative women
Polio, tetanus, diphtheria		Previously unimmunized
Hepatitis A, B, influenza, *S. pneumoniae*		Individuals at increased risk

BCG, bacille Calmette–Guérin; DPT, diphtheria/pertussis/tetanus; DT, diphtheria/tetanus; MMR, measles/mumps/rubella.

at present as a condition of travel (to certain countries in tropical Africa and South America).

Many other vaccines are available and may be appropriate in certain circumstances. Detailed advice should be sought for unusual destinations or activities.

Control of infection in the hospital environment

Every hospital should have procedures to ensure that infection is not transmitted within the hospital environment. Together, these form the *infection control policy*, which, if it is to be successful, must have the support of the entire hospital staff. The control of infection team (consisting of a consultant microbiologist or infectious diseases specialist, and specialist nurses) promotes the policy by:
• Encouraging clinical practice that restricts the spread of infection
• Coordinating the response to outbreaks of infection
• Collecting infection statistics
• Identifying particular problems, e.g. waste storage and disposal
The team should arrange enhanced surveillance of particular organisms (e.g. MRSA) and the screening of suspected carriers, including members of staff. It also has an important role in hospital planning, both physical (e.g. alterations to buildings) and functional (e.g. new clinical services).

Good clinical practice

Infected individuals should be separated from non-infected people. Sources (infected or colonized [carriers] individuals) must be identified by appropriate screening measures (e.g. routine surveillance specimens from both patients and staff). Infected patients should be appropriately isolated (source isolation) and practical measures taken to interrupt possible transmission. Patients who are especially susceptible to infection require protective isolation. Isolation is often difficult to maintain when staff do not adhere to agreed practice. This can be compounded when simple measures (e.g. hand washing) are neglected because of work pressures. Large ward rounds where many staff can come in contact with a patient should be discouraged as they inevitably increase the risk of transmission of organisms.

Wound and enteric isolation

Wound and enteric isolation aims to prevent transmission of organisms spread by contact or ingestion, respectively. Patients are nursed in a side room that contains a wash-hand basin and a separate toilet facility. Disposable plastic aprons and gloves are used while handling the patient or performing a clinical procedure. The gloves and apron are disposed of, and hands are washed using liquid soap and disposable towels.

Respiratory isolation

In addition to the precautions listed above, hospital staff should also wear a face mask when in the room. If the patient is transferred to another department of the hospital, the patient should wear a face mask. Stricter respiratory isolation methods are necessary for the control of transmission of multidrug-resistant tuberculosis. This requires the use of negative pressure rooms and effective masks (dust/mist masks or personal respirators); such precautions are especially essential during procedures that are likely to generate aerosols (e.g. bronchoalveolar lavage). These measures are effective in controlling transmission, even among highly immunocompromised patients.

Strict respiratory isolation

This is required when a patient is known or suspected to be suffering from infection with multidrug-resistant *M. tuberculosis*. The side room should be under negative pressure, preventing the organisms from being transmitted to other patients. When entering the room staff members should wear high efficiency face masks.

Strict isolation

This form of isolation is designed to prevent the transmission of infections such as viral haemorrhagic fevers. Patients are nursed in an enclosed isolation unit that prevents aerosol transmission of the organism because of its enclosed air system and negative pressure (Fig. 3.30).

Protective isolation

Protective isolation is required for patients who are highly susceptible to infection (e.g. neutropenic patients). Protection includes single room isolation, provision of filtered air and measures to control the risk from organisms in food (e.g. resistant Gram-negative organisms in vegetables, or *Listeria* in soft cheeses).

03

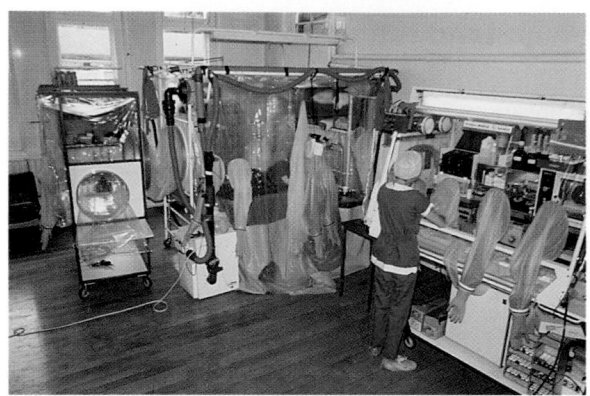

Figure 3.30 Trexlor isolator for management of patients with Category 4 pathogens.

Control of infection in the community

Control of infectious diseases in the community depends on national agencies, public health doctors, microbiologists, hospital clinicians and general practitioners (GPs).

Social and environmental factors

Factors in reducing the burden of infectious disease are improvements in social and environmental conditions. Improved sanitation reduces the risk of diarrhoeal diseases and better housing reduces the spread (e.g. tuberculosis). Better nutrition means that the population is less susceptible to disease.

Paradoxically, the incidence of some infectious diseases rises as living conditions improve. This occurs in conditions where the complication rate is greater in adults than in children (e.g. paralytic poliomyelitis).

Health education

There are many infection-related health education programmes covering safe sex, needle exchange, advice to pregnant women, guidance on food hygiene and advice to travellers.

Food safety

Food safety legislation has been harmonized across the European Community (the Food Safety Act in the UK).

The law is enforced by environmental health officers (EHOs) in food premises and officials of the Department for Environment, Food and Rural Affairs (DEFRA) on farms. Pasteurization of milk reduces the risk of infection with *M. bovis* and *Campylobacter* sp. In Scotland it is illegal to produce or sell unpasteurized milk, reducing milk-associated outbreaks of infection.

Vector control

This is particularly important in tropical countries where arthropods play an important part in many infections as vectors. Travellers to the tropics can reduce the risk of infection by taking measures to avoid insect bites (e.g. use of repellents, mosquito nets and protective clothing). Attempts to control insect populations by the use of pesticides have usually been unsuccessful because of the emergence of resistance.

Immunization

Many infectious diseases have been controlled by vaccination (e.g. polio and diphtheria). Smallpox has been completely eradicated by this means.

Immunization may be achieved **passively** by administration of an immunoglobulin preparation, or **actively** by use of a live or non-replicating vaccine.

Immunoglobulins are prepared from humans or, more rarely, plasma and provide short-term protection against certain infections and are used in the treatment of immune disorders. Human immunoglobulin (HIG) is prepared from pooled plasma and contains antibodies to viruses that are prevalent in the general population. It is used for postexposure prophylaxis of acute hepatitis A in normal individuals and measles in an immunosuppressed contact.

Specific immunoglobulins, prepared from hyperimmune donors, are available for postexposure management of specific infections (e.g. hepatitis B, varicella-zoster and tetanus). Tick-borne encephalitis immunoglobulin is available in countries where the disease is endemic for prophylaxis following tick bites.

The purpose of vaccination is to produce immunity in subjects without the complications of natural infection. Vaccines are derived from whole viruses and bacteria, or their antigenic components (acellular). Live vaccines consist of strains with severely reduced pathogenicity (attenuated). They induce protection but do not cause disease. Examples include mumps, measles, rubella, polio, yellow fever, bacille Calmette–Guérin (BCG). They usually produce durable immunity after a single dose. Live vaccines can cause disease in immunocompromised patients and are avoided in pregnancy because of the potential risk of fetal infection.

Non-replicating vaccines contain either inactivated whole organisms (e.g. pertussis) or antigenic components (e.g. capsular polysaccharide of *S. pneumoniae*). The toxins of tetanus and diphtheria are inactivated to produce toxoids that do not cause symptoms but are fully immunogenic. The immunogenicity of acellular vaccines can be increased by conjugation with proteins (e.g. *H. influenzae*). Genetic engineering is being harnessed for acellular vaccine production (e.g. hepatitis B). These vaccines are safe in immunocompromised patients because they are unable to replicate. Multiple doses may be required for optimum immunogenicity.

The aim of an immunization programme may be eradication, elimination or containment. **Eradication** is total absence of the organism in humans, animals and the environment. This can be attempted if the disease is easily recognizable, there is no long-term carriage or subclinical infection and no non-human hosts. **Elimination** is where the disease has disappeared but the organism remains in animal hosts, the environment, or is causing subclinical infection in humans.

Universal immunization is adopted for most childhood infections and selective programmes for those at risk from disease (e.g. hepatitis B in health care workers). Immunization schedules vary between countries; the UK uses the schedule in Table 3.17.

Chemoprophylaxis

This is used for control of more serious infections such as diphtheria and meningococcal disease. The aim of chemoprophylaxis may be to eliminate carriage of pathogenic organisms, thereby reducing the risk of infection in those not yet exposed. Single-dose regimens are the most effective.

Outbreak investigation

Outbreaks can be recognized if there is adequate surveillance. A case is defined and basic epidemiological information is collected, including date of onset of symptoms, age/sex and place of residence. Additional information will be required (e.g. a food poisoning outbreak requires detailed food history).

A hypothesis of causation is tested by a case–control or cohort study. In a case–control study, exposure histories are sought from cases and healthy controls. The relative risk of exposure to the postulated source is calculated for cases and controls. The controls are drawn from the same population as the cases. Case–control studies are suited to investigation of uncommon infections such as botulism. In a cohort study, the disease outcome is compared between those exposed and not exposed to the source and

are often used to investigate outbreaks with a high attack rate such as food poisoning incidents. In both cases, a structured questionnaire should be used.

The role of national agencies

Most countries have a national system to control communicable diseases and they have four main functions:
1 Surveillance of communicable diseases
2 Investigation of outbreaks
3 Surveillance of immunization programmes
4 Epidemiology research and training
Close collaboration between food and agriculture control agencies and the human infection control agency is required for zoonotic infections.

Infectious disease morbidity and mortality data are collected to identify trends or clusters of disease requiring preventative action, and to evaluate control measures. Data on common or less severe diseases, such as food poisoning, are collected by passive surveillance systems, and active surveillance is used for rare or serious conditions. Data can be obtained from statutory notification, microbiology laboratory reports, death certificates, GP surveillance schemes and infection reports from hospitals. Some conditions (e.g. sexually transmitted diseases) are reported by clinics to the Department of Health directly. Active reporting schemes include those for AIDS and HIV-related diseases, and some rare childhood infections are surveyed through a network of paediatric consultants.

The collected data must be interpreted and disseminated so that clinicians can use them in diagnosing infections and ensuring that vaccination levels are maintained (e.g. influenza epidemics). In the UK, infectious disease data are published by the Registrar General in the weekly *Communicable Disease Report* and other countries have similar systems (e.g. the *Morbidity and Mortality Weekly* published by the Centers for Disease Control in the USA).

03

Infections and their management

Infections of the nervous system
(Table 3.18)

Aseptic meningitis

This is inflammation of the meninges associated with

Table 3.18 Infections of the central nervous system

Syndrome	Organism	Page
Meningitis	*N. meningitidis*	107
Purulent (bacterial meningitis)	*H. influenzae*	108
	Strep. pneumoniae	108
	L. monocytogenes	112
Aseptic meningitis	Enterovirus	116
	Leptospirosis	107
	L. monocytogenes	112
	M. tuberculosis	330
	Fungal meningitis	179
Encephalitis	Herpes simplex	134
	Trypanosomiasis	138
Space-occupying lesions		
Brain abscess	Anaerobes	112
Toxoplasmosis	*T. gondii*	141
Neurosyphilis	*T. pallidum*	168
Tetanus	*Cl. tetani*	114
Botulism	*Cl. botulinum*	115
Poliomyelitis	Poliovirus	116
Rabies	Rabies virus	115
Slow virus infection		
Subacute sclerosing panencephalitis	Measles	146
Prion disease	Kuru	112
	Creutzfeldt–Jakob disease	
	Variant Creutzfeldt–Jakob disease	

Table 3.19 Causes of aseptic meningitis

Enteroviruses
Mumps virus
Other viruses
Leptospirosis
Tuberculosis
Cryptococcosis
Partially treated bacterial meningitis

produce a predominantly lymphocytic inflammatory response are therefore amongst the principal causes (Table 3.19). In developed countries, benign self-limited viral infections are the most common cause of aseptic meningitis. The most common viruses are the enteroviruses, Coxsackie, echo and polio viruses.

Clinical features
The patient complains of a prodromal sore throat in the preceding 5–7 days. Headache of 12–36 h develops associated with myalgia, nausea and vomiting. The level of consciousness is rarely disturbed. Neck stiffness is present and Kernig's sign is positive. Apart from cervical lymphadenopathy and pharyngitis other signs are rare.

Investigations
Diagnosis is by examination of CSF which is typically lymphocytic but neutrophils may be present in the first 24 h of the illness. Protein concentrations may be slightly raised and CSF sugars are usually normal (Table 3.20). It should be noted that in pyogenic infections lymphocytes tend to become more prominent as the inflammatory process becomes chronic. Lymphocytes may therefore come to predominate over neutrophils in the CSF in partially and inadequately treated bacterial meningitis. However, the accompanying high protein and low glucose levels should suggest the true bacterial nature of the problem.

A definitive diagnosis can be made by culture from throat or faecal swabs. Viral RNA can be amplified by reverse transcription-polymerase chain reaction (RT-PCR).

lymphocytes in the CSF. The term aseptic meningitis is used to distinguish it from bacterial meningitis in which the predominant cells are polymorphs.

Epidemiology
Infection is more common in the summer, in children aged 5–14 years and young adults. The causative viruses are usually spread by faeco-oral transmission and outbreaks may occur in closed institutions. Only a minority of the viral infections result in clinical signs of meningitis.

Disease mechanisms
Viruses and other intracellular organisms that tend to

Management
There is no specific treatment for the viruses responsible

Table 3.20 Important investigatory findings in meningitis

Investigation	Pyogenic meningitis	Viral or aseptic meningitis	Tuberculous meningitis
White cells	Predominantly polymorphs	Predominantly lymphocytes	Predominantly lymphocytes
White cell count	500–1000	<500	<500
CSF/blood glucose	<40%	60%	<40%
CSF protein	0.5–3.0 g/l	0.5–1.0 g/l	1.0–6.0 g/l
Other tests	Bacteria on Gram-stain antigen	Viral culture in CSF, throat swab or faeces	Acid-fast bacilli on Ziehl–Neelson or auramine stain

for aseptic meningitis so patients should be treated symptomatically.

Prognosis
Viral aseptic meningitis is usually a self-limiting condition with complete recovery within a few days.

Leptospirosis

A zoonotic infection that is now rare in developed countries.

Epidemiology
This infection is now rare in developed countries because of preventative measures. It is found throughout the world and is spread from animals to humans by direct spread or through contact with their excreta. It is excreted in the urine of infected animals and infection in humans is caused by contact with urine or urine-soaked soil. Many patients become infected while participating in country-side pursuits such as water sports. Agricultural and abattoir workers are also at increased risk of infection. The disease was once common in sewage workers until appropriate preventative measures were taken.

Disease mechanisms
Leptospirosis is a disease caused by the zoonotic genus *Leptospira*. The organism *Leptospira interrogans* consists of 130 serotypes in 16 serogroups.

Clinical features
The clinical spectrum of leptospirosis is wide and any one serotype can cause many different clinical presentations. Leptospirosis is characterized by a triad of meningitis, hepatitis and renal failure, of which meningitic symptoms may dominate the clinical picture in some cases. Following an incubation period of 7–13 days, the illness usually starts abruptly with headache, myalgia, conjunctival suffusion and fever. During this first phase, organisms are present in the blood and CSF. Following a week of illness the fever may settle, only to rise again after 3 days with further symptoms such as meningism. This later phase is associated with the development of the immune response and myocarditis, and can be accompanied by renal manifestations—proteinuria, pyuria and haematuria. Acute tubular necrosis and vasculitis can also occur.

The combination of leptospirosis with jaundice and uraemia is sometimes known as Weil's disease. Death is commonly associated with renal failure but is usually a result of myocarditis or massive blood loss. Leptospires occasionally persist in the aqueous humour, giving rise to anterior and posterior uveitis, retinitis and optic atrophy.

Investigation
● *FBC:* during the first phase of the illness there may be a leucopenia, although jaundice may be associated with neutrophilia.
● *Serum urea:* about one-quarter of patients have an elevated urea.
● *Microbiology:* a diagnosis can also be made by visualizing leptospires in the blood, CSF or urine under dark field illumination. Culture is possible in specialist centres, but rarely attempted.
● *Serology:* definitive diagnosis is usually made by the detection of serotype specific IgM in the patient's blood.

Management
Treatment with intravenous benzylpenicillin in the first 4 days probably reduces the severity of leptospirosis, but the response may not be dramatic.

Prevention
Infection can be prevented by doxycycline in people exposed to short-term high risk.

Prognosis
Prognosis is variable depending on the infecting species. The mortality is variable depending on the infecting species, but is 5–15% for icteric disease. Icteric disease, in turn, accounts for only 5–15% of leptospirosis.

Cryptococcal meningitis

See p. 179.

Pyogenic meningitis

An infective inflammation of the meninges usually caused by bacteria and typified by the presence of polymorphonuclear lymphocytes in the CSF.

Epidemiology
Patients of all ages are susceptible to pyogenic meningitis but the general incidence of the disease and that of each organism varies widely in different ages. Bacterial meningitis occurs throughout the world, but in the countries of the Sahel, *N. meningitidis* may produce intense epidemics every 10–12 years (Fig. 3.31). Infection with *H. influenzae* usually occurs in children under the age of 7 years, but is rarely seen in countries where a conjugate vaccine programme has been introduced.

Neisseria meningitidis (meningococcal) infections

Epidemics of meningococcal meningitis occur every

03

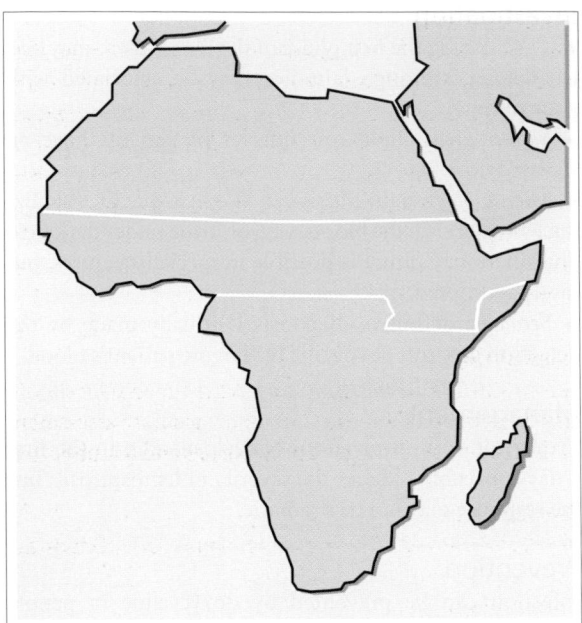

Figure 3.31 The meningitis belt of Africa.

10–12 years and peaks of incidence may reach 10–90 cases/100 000/year in a developed country. Between these peaks clinical infections continue at a lower rate, infection being most common in the second winter quarter (January–March) of each year. Similar patterns are found in the 'meningitis belt' of Africa (Fig. 3.31), but the background incidence is higher and during epidemics up to 1000 cases/1 000 000/year may occur. During epidemics the case : carrier ratio increases.

Cause

Common causes of pyogenic meningitis are:
- *E. coli*
- *Streptococcus agalactiae* (group B)
- *Listeria monocytogenes* in neonates caused by transmission of organisms from the female genital tract at birth and in immunocompromised individuals
- *Haemophilus influenzae* from 6 months of age until about 6 years when naturally acquired immunity gives protection. It is a rare cause in neonates because of maternal antibody
- *Neisseria meningitidis* in children and adolescents
- *Streptococcus pneumoniae* in young children and the elderly

Ventriculoperitoneal and ventriculoatrial shunts predispose to a subacute meningitis caused by organisms of low virulence such as *Staph. epidermidis*.

Otitis media, sinusitis, skull fracture, dural tear and splenectomy predispose to pneumococcal meningitis, as does severe lobar pneumonia, especially in those predisposed to invasive pneumococcal disease resulting from alcoholism, diabetes or sickle cell anaemia.

Disease mechanisms

Neisseria meningitidis circulates in the community and infection usually results in colonization without clinical disease. Carriage of the organism may continue for a few weeks or months. Specific antibody is produced by only about 50% of those infected. Colonization by other *Neisseria* spp. or other genera with cross-reacting antigens may assist in the development of immunity.

Clinical features

The incubation period of meningitis is not more than 2–3 days and there is rarely a history of contact with another case. The cardinal symptoms that point to the diagnosis of meningitis are fever, headache, photophobia and neck stiffness. In neonates and young children these symptoms are often absent, and listlessness and anorexia may be the only features.

The progression of symptoms is variable. Sometimes the first symptom may precede fulminant disease by only a few hours and usually symptoms have been present for not more than 48 h.

As the infection progresses, patients may lapse into coma. In adults, convulsions are uncommon, but occur in up to one-third of children. In young children the clinical picture is often more non-specific. The child may be unwell and unwilling to feed, and usually has a fever, which may be accompanied by diarrhoea. Neck stiffness may not be prominent. In babies the fontanelle may bulge but more commonly merely appears fuller and more resistant to depression.

Antibiotics given before admission to hospital diminish the intensity of clinical symptoms and signs. A diagnosis of meningitis should therefore be considered for any child with a persistent vague headache and fever.

Emergency: Meningococcal septicaemia

- Treatment depends on early diagnosis
- Recognizing the disease: fever, neck stiffness, associated with petechial rash, patient may be shocked
- Classical symptoms and signs may be absent early in the course of infection
- Progression can be rapid
- Emergency treatment: parenteral benzylpenicillin if diagnosis suspected
- Admission to hospital with intensive care facilities
- Treatment is with intravenous benzylpenicillin and intensive care support

Older children and adults complain of malaise and anorexia accompanied by a severe bursting headache. Patients are irritable and resist all movement, loud noises and, in particular, light (photophobia). The headache is often accompanied by anxiety. Fever is present and the patient may feel cold, but rigors are rare. Meningeal irritation causes spasm of the neck and spinal muscles and, in severe cases, opisthotonos. Vomiting is common and diarrhoea can occur, and so the illness may mimic a gastrointestinal infection. Meningitis can cause marked pain on stretching the lumbar plexus nerve roots. This may be demonstrated by Kernig's sign—extending the knee when the hip is flexed causes pain and muscle spasm.

Skin signs

Patients with pyogenic meningitis may have herpes 'cold sores', which often develop during the prodromal period. A rash can also occur in meningococcal meningitis (see p. 110), which may be macular, petechial or purpuric, and is associated with septicaemia. The skin may ulcerate as a result. The rash often starts as a few spots on the trunk, but once it appears may progress rapidly in association with a diminishing level of consciousness and symptoms and signs of endotoxic shock (Waterhouse–Friderichsen syndrome). Rashes are rarely reported in association with *H. influenzae* and *Strep. pneumoniae* meningitis.

Complications

Just as the prodromal period can vary in its speed of progression, so does the course of the disease. Complications of pyogenic meningitis are caused by inflammation and cerebral oedema and include the following:
- *Cranial nerve palsy:* especially after pneumococcal infection. This occurs late in the course and may resolve spontaneously.
- *Deafness:* a common complication of meningococcal disease.
- *Hydrocephalus:* resulting from a block in CSF flow or a blockage in the basal cisterns.
- *Mental retardation:* especially as a result of fulminant infection and delayed or ineffective treatment.
- *Epilepsy:* may occur as a late complication as a result of cortical scarring.
- *Subdural effusion:* occurs most commonly following *H. influenzae* infection in children in the first 2 years of life. It may manifest as deterioration in a patient previously responding well to therapy.
- *Reactive arthritis:* a late complication of meningococcal disease and thought to be mediated by immune complexes. Arthritis may occasionally be purulent.
- *Myocarditis:* occurs in severe meningococcal disease.

Investigation

Any suspicion of the diagnosis should prompt immediate preadmission antibiotic therapy and GPs should carry parenteral penicillin for this purpose. Investigation includes lumbar puncture in cases where this investigation is not contraindicated by the suspicion of raised intracranial pressure. Therapy should not be delayed while waiting to obtain a CSF sample or to discover the results. The results of these investigations may be interpreted using Table 3.20 (p. 106).

Haematology

Serum and CSF white cell counts. A Leishman stain should also be performed on the CSF for an accurate assessment of the relative percentage of polymorphs and lymphocytes.

Biochemistry

Blood glucose and CSF glucose, total protein and chloride.

Immunology

Bacterial antigens can be detected in serum, CSF and urine.

Microbiology

Blood and CSF culture and direct Gram stain, and Ziehl–Neelsen stain if indicated. Culture may yield the causative organism, but preadmission antibiotic therapy often renders CSF culture negative. PCR detection of the main pathogens may provide an aetiological diagnosis.

Diagnostic imaging

CT scanning may be used to exclude raised intracranial pressure before lumbar puncture.

Management

The treatment of meningitis depends on the administration of intravenous antibiotics to which the likely organisms are sensitive. For empirical treatment, ceftriaxone should be commenced pending the results of laboratory tests. Meningococcal disease can be successfully treated with benzylpenicillin intravenously. Most *S. pneumoniae* are also penicillin susceptible and can be treated like meningococci, but penicillin resistance is increasing throughout the world. Where there is a significant risk of reduced susceptibility to penicillin, ceftriaxone should be continued until susceptibility results are available. There are some reports of cephalosporin-resistant organisms and in those circumstances intravenous vancomycin can be added to the regimen. Increasing resistance to beta-lactam antibiotics in *H. influenzae* means that ceftriaxone must be continued until it is determined whether the organism expressed a beta-lactamase. Symptomatic treatment and intensive care may be needed.

03

Meningococcal infection at a glance

Epidemiology

Prevalence
One to 1000/100 000

Age
Children and young adults

Genetics
Congenital complement deficiency more susceptible

Geography
Sporadic disease worldwide. Epidemics in 'meningitis belt' of Africa

Clinical features
Septicaemia: fever with petechial rash
Neck stiffness and meningism
Fever
Photophobia
Reduced level of consciousness

Findings on investigation

Haematology
White blood cell count increased

Biochemistry
Blood : cerebrospinal fluid glucose ratio reduced

Microbiology
Culture of blood and cerebrospinal fluid
Specific meningococcal polymerase chain reaction

Treatment
Benzylpenicillin intravenously

Prevention
Prophylactic antibiotics to contacts
Meningitis C vaccine to adolescents

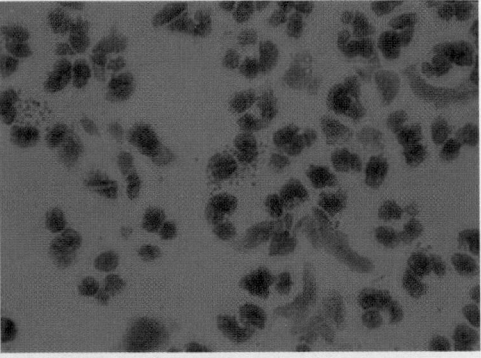

Fig. A Rapid diagnosis of meningococcal meningitis: cerebrospinal fluid shows neutrophils and intracellular and extracellular Gram-negative diplococci.

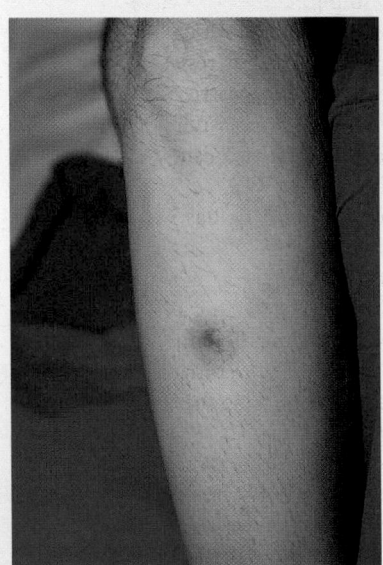

Fig. D Acute meningococcal meningitis: a vasculitic lesion on the shin; there were three others on the hand and arms.

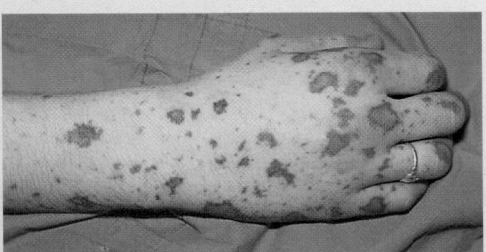

Fig. B Early meningococcal rash.

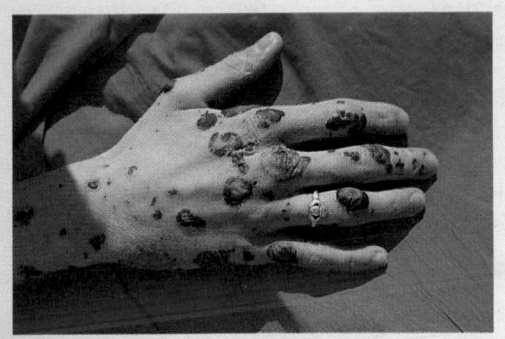

Fig. C The same rash as in Fig. B after 1 week's evolution.

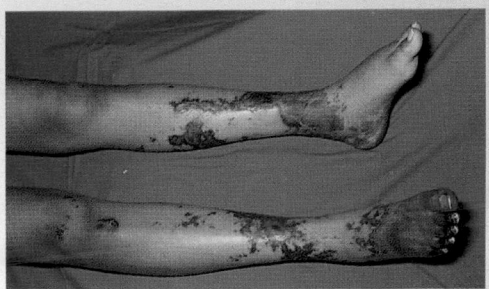

Fig. E Acute meningococcal meningitis: purpura fulminans. (All figures reproduced from Bannister *et al. Infectious Disease*, 1996 (Blackwell Science, Oxford) with the permission of the authors.)

Prevention and control

Meningococcal disease

Antimicrobial prophylaxis is beneficial in meningococcal disease and should be given to close contacts (those who share eating and sleeping accommodation and 'kissing partners', irrespective of age).

Rifampicin is the drug of choice and is more commonly used than sulphonamides, which have been used for this purpose but against which meningococci have now developed a high level of resistance. Ciprofloxacin and minocycline are also effective, but neither should be used in children. Successfully treated patients often continue to carry the organism and should also be given prophylaxis.

Meningococcal vaccine has similar problems to those for *H. influenzae*. A vaccine consisting of capsular carbohydrates of serotypes A, C and W135 is clinically available. Serotype B is poorly antigenic and so at present there is no vaccine against the most common organism in northern Europe. The conjugate meningitidis C vaccine has proved highly effective in reducing the incidence of infection with this serotype.

Meningococcal vaccine is valuable for travellers to areas of high endemicity or where epidemics are occurring. Its expense probably excludes its widespread use in developing countries. It is highly effective in arresting the spread of epidemic meningococcal meningitis when given to populations at risk.

Haemophilus influenzae infection

Carbohydrate–protein conjugates of capsular polysaccharide and protein stimulate strong antibody responses in young children and such a vaccine is now available and has brought about the almost complete eradication of this infection. The case for antimicrobial prophylaxis in *H. influenzae* infection is less clear. It should be given

to child contacts under the age of 4 years. Rifampicin is effective in eradicating carriage and should also be given to the index case who is still likely to carry the organism after effective therapy.

Pneumococcal disease

Recurrent pneumococcal meningitis may follow dural tear, splenectomy or hypogammaglobulinaemia. Dural reconstruction together with long-term penicillin should be used to control further recurrence.

The place of pneumococcal vaccine is less well-established. Full efficacy requires a functional spleen, and therefore this prophylaxis will have limited efficacy in patients with e.g. sickle cell disease. There is a new protein–polysaccharide conjugate vaccine with a limited number of serotypes. It is highly effective at producing antibodies in vulnerable patients.

Listeria monocytogenes infection

Epidemiology

This is an uncommon cause of meningitis, more likely to occur in patients who are immunocompromised. It occurs mainly in neonates and in older patients predisposed by other illness or immunosuppressive therapy. Human infection is probably acquired through food (unpasteurized soft cheeses and yoghurts). It is thought that listeriosis may have become more common with the rise of prepared refrigerated meals.

Disease mechanisms

Listeria are small motile microaerophilic Gram-positive bacilli that are widely distributed in the environment. They are notable for their ability to continue to multiply at temperatures as low as 4°C and so they survive and multiply in refrigerators.

03

Clinical features

In many instances *Listeria* gives rise to a mild influenza-like illness; however, in women infected during pregnancy, infection can spread to the neonate and result in severe meningitis. Infection can also spread to the newborn during delivery. In immunocompromised patients *Listeria* meningitis is an important differential diagnosis and must be considered, as the treatment differs from that for other causes of pyogenic meningitis.

Investigation

As for pyogenic meningitis above.

Management

Ampicillin is an effective treatment, and synergizes with aminoglycosides in severe infections.

Prognosis

Listeriosis is a severe illness with a high mortality.

Spongiform encephalopathies

The transmissible agent of spongiform encephalopathies is the prion protein: a conformationally abnormal, protease-resistant form of a protein that is a normal constituent of the brain. When ingested, the abnormal prion protein induces a conformational change in the native brain protein, leading to spongiform degeneration in the brain. There is an extended incubation period of more than 5 years.

Transmissible spongiform encephalopathies can affect humans. Scrapie, a disease of sheep is not considered transmittable to humans. 'Kuru' was described in cannibals from Papua New Guinea who ate human tissue, including brain. Recently, an epidemic of a spongiform encephalopathy in cattle (bovine spongiform encephalitis; BSE) has been recognized and is thought to have been caused by feeding animal brain protein to cattle. Transmission to humans, following ingestion of contaminated beef products, is thought to be responsible for variant Creutzfeldt–Jakob disease. The incidence of cattle BSE has diminished rapidly because of a selective slaughter policy and a ban on feeding animal protein to cattle. The size and scale of any human epidemic is not yet known.

Brain abscess

A brain abscess is a localized pyogenic infection in the cerebral substance.

Epidemiology

With a fall in chronic lung sepsis, brain abscess is relatively rare. It is more common in patients with chronic lung, sinus or dental infection.

Disease mechanisms

Brain abscess arises from metastatic spread of sepsis from other sites or local spread from parameningeal suppuration (Table 3.21). Spread may be from chronic bronchial sepsis, as in the case of bronchiectasis. Primary haematogenous brain abscesses may arise and these are usually polymicrobial infections in which one of the organisms isolated is often of the *Strep. anginosus–constellatus* group. Spread from contiguous structures —frontal, mastoid or maxillary sinuses— or chronic otitis media, is with organisms that infect these sites. Brain abscesses can arise after compound skull fracture or penetrating foreign body contaminated with bacteria. Brain abscesses are often polymicrobial, especially when the organisms have their origin in the gastrointestinal tract or arise as a result of bronchiectasis. Anaerobic organisms are frequently involved, including *Bacteroides* spp., *Porphyromonas* spp. and anaerobic cocci. *Streptococcus anginosus–constellatus–intermedius* is often a component (this group of organisms is often given the name *Strep. milleri*). Other aerobic and facultative anaerobes found include *Staph. aureus* and *Proteus* spp. Abscesses are found equally in the frontal, parietal and temporal regions.

Clinical features

Brain abscesses present clinically with the signs of infection (fever and malaise) together with lowered consciousness level and signs of an intracerebral space-occupying lesion. Patients may complain of headache and may vomit. Papilloedema is present in less than half of patients because of the rapid development of symptoms. Focal neurological signs may be present such as focal epileptic seizures or upper motor neurone lesions.

Diagnosis

The diagnosis of brain abscess is made on the basis of clinical suspicion of the condition and the use of imaging techniques such as CT and MRI. Surgical evacuation of the abscess pus is a part of the therapeutic process and brain abscess pus should be processed to provide a bact-

Table 3.21 Infective mass lesions in the brain

Pyogenic abscess
Tuberculoma
Cryptococcoma
Cysticercus
Hydatid cyst
Toxoplasmosis

eriological diagnosis. Fastidious anaerobes that are killed by oxygen often play an important part in the cause of brain abscess, so specimens should be transported to the laboratory quickly or inoculated onto bacteriological medium in theatre.

Differential diagnosis

Tuberculomas are small caseous foci found in the brains of patients with miliary tuberculosis and are often multiple. Fungal abscesses with *Aspergillus* spp. usually occur only in severely immunocompromised patients such as those undergoing liver or bone marrow transplantation. Cerebral toxoplasmosis is an important infectious complication of AIDS. Other rare parasitic causes of infective mass lesions include *Entamoeba histolytica* abscess and cysticercosis caused by the intermediate stage of *Taenia solium* developing in the human host instead of the pig (the natural intermediate host). Cerebral hydatid disease may also mimic brain abscess; this is most likely to arise in *Echinococcus multilocularis* infection.

Management

Surgery has an important role in the diagnosis and treatment of brain abscess. The antibiotic regimen should be prescribed on the basis of the possible origin of the infections and their penetration into the cerebral substance. It should be adjusted in the light of bacteriological results obtained from cultivation of brain abscess pus. In most cases, the regimen will include an agent active against anaerobes (e.g. metronidazole), against streptococci, staphylococci and Gram-negative facultative anaerobes (e.g. cefotaxime), with the possible addition of flucloxacillin or chloramphenicol.

Encephalitis

This is a generalized inflammation of the cerebral substance, often (but not always) caused by viral infection. It can sometimes develop days, weeks, months or years after an infection as with chickenpox (days) or measles (years).

Epidemiology

Encephalitis is uncommon. It is found throughout the world, although the spectrum of causative agents can vary significantly.

Disease mechanisms

Most cases of acute encephalitis are believed to be viral in origin, although commonly no specific agent can be identified. Among the recognized causes are enteroviruses (see p. 116), adenovirus and herpes simplex virus, which are most common in the northern hemisphere. Rarely, in Europe and North America arbovirus infections (transmitted by insects) can cause encephalitis (e.g. eastern equine encephalitis, West Nile fever). In the tropics, arboviral infections from a wide range of species can cause infection including dengue and Japanese B encephalitis (see p. 114).

Acute encephalitis is also a rare complication of many common viral infections, including measles, chickenpox, rubella and mumps, and may develop during the acute phase of illness or some weeks to years later (in the case of measles).

Clinical features

Patients can present with irritability, restlessness and personality change or, more seriously, seizures. Acute encephalitis is characterized by global changes in central nervous system (CNS) function such as drowsiness and irritability, together with signs of infection (such as fever and an elevated C-reactive protein), symptoms and signs of meningeal irritation. In some cases there may be focal neurological deficits. Tendon reflexes may be brisk and the plantars upgoing. Severe cases can progress to convulsions, coma and death.

Investigation

- *CSF examination:* usually reveals a lymphocytosis of 20–2000 cells/mm^3 and elevated protein. IgG may be increased in chronic infection. The CSF glucose is usually normal, whereas it is low in cases of tuberculosis, fungal and amoebic infection. The CSF should be stained for *M. tuberculosis* and fungi. If there is a relevant history of exposure, trypanosomes should be looked for.
- *Virology:* samples should be sent urgently to the laboratory for PCR to identify the presence of herpes simplex and other viral pathogens.
- *Serology:* may be helpful in the diagnosis of exotic viral infection and specialist advice should be sought.
- *Imaging with CT or MRI scanning:* excludes a space-occupying lesion or brain abscess.

Management

Where herpes simplex infection is suspected or proved, treatment with parenteral aciclovir should be instituted immediately. The response to treatment is slow and fever often does not subside for 48–72 h. Treatment is continued for 14 days. Physiotherapy and other treatment (e.g. speech therapy) may be necessary to manage continuing neurological deficits.

For other causes of encephalitis, treatment is supportive.

03

Prognosis

The prognosis is highly variable with some associated with a good outcome (e.g. herpes simplex) whereas others, such as Japanese B infection, are associated with high mortality up to 20%, with more than one-third of survivors having permanent neurological deficit.

Dengue

This mosquito-borne flavivirus is closely related to yellow fever virus. It has four serotypes. Infection is transmitted by *Aedes* mosquitoes and the incubation period is 2–15 days, with viraemia present at the onset of fever and persisting for several days. Dengue virus is found throughout the tropics: India, South East Asia, Pacific islands, Caribbean islands, South America, Africa and the Middle East.

Following the sudden onset of fever and chills, headache and malaise, patients complain of pains in the bones and joints. Fever may be biphasic and mild rash may also be present. Dengue haemorrhagic syndrome is a more severe form of disease with severe shock and bleeding. The mortality rate is 5–10%.

Dengue infection can be confirmed by serological means, culture and PCR-based amplification methods. Dengue can only be prevented by controlling mosquito populations. Treatment of acute cases is symptomatic.

Other infections of the nervous system

Tetanus

Tetanus is a cutaneous infection with *Clostridium tetani* that produces extensive tonic–clonic spasms which may compromise respiration through the secretion of a potent neurotoxin.

Epidemiology

There are more than 500 000 cases worldwide, but disease is rare in developed countries. Disease is common in neonates in developing countries and in older patients with soil-contaminated wounds who have not been vaccinated. Disease is more common in males through occupational exposure.

Causes

Tetanus results from infection with *Cl. tetani*. This is a common organism worldwide, occurring in the soil and in the gut of many species, including cattle and a small proportion of healthy humans (Fig. 3.32). *Cl. tetani* produces spores that are hardy and persist in the environment for many years. These may cause infection in wounds that

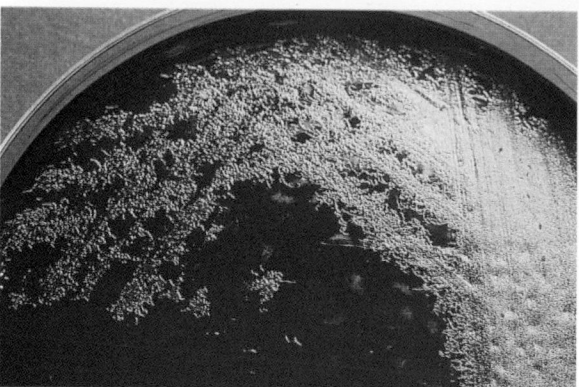

Figure 3.32 Spores of *Cl. tetani*. Reproduced from Gillespie, *Medical Microbiology Illustrated*, 1994 (Butterworth-Heinemann, Oxford) with the permission of the publisher and author.

they contaminate. Sometimes the wound is too trivial to be noticed (such as a rose thorn). Large and dirty wounds carry a higher risk of infection. Fortunately, tetanus has become rare in countries where there is a safe and effective immunization programme with tetanus toxoid.

Disease mechanisms

When *Cl. tetani* bacilli are introduced into a wound they multiply in any small focus of dead tissue that provides suitable anaerobic conditions. Here they produce an exotoxin called tetanospasmin. Tetanospasmin is carried up the axons of peripheral neurones and also via the blood to the anterior horns of the spinal cord and medulla where it blocks the normal inhibitory input to the motor neurones. There is a consequent increase in muscle tone and an exaggeration of any movement into uncontrollable, painful spasms.

Clinical features

The incubation period of tetanus is variable, ranging from a few days to several months; it is longer for wounds that are more distant from the CNS. The disease may present subtly and go unrecognized until more classical symptoms emerge. The features are of muscular rigidity and spasms with a normal level of consciousness. The rigidity leads to a tense abdomen, arched back (opisthotonos), clenched jaw (trismus) and a fixed smile (risus sardonicus). Respiration is often impaired as the direct result of frequent generalized spasms, because of laryngeal spasm or because of inhalation of secretions. Spasm of the respiratory muscles can compromise breathing.

Management

The organism must be eliminated by wound débridement and with penicillin or metronidazole. Unbound toxin

03

must be eliminated by passive immunization with human immunoglobulin. Muscular spasms must be controlled and respiration protected by sedation, paralysis and artificial ventilation until spontaneous recovery occurs—typically after 1 or 2 weeks (KEYPOINTS BOX 3.1).

Keypoints 3.1: Management of tetanus

Supportive treatment
Control spasms and protect respiration
Sedation, paralysis and artificial ventilation

Specific treatment
Drug treatment
Eliminate the organism: penicillin or metronidazole
Eliminate unbound toxin: human immunoglobulin

Surgery
Eliminate the organism
Wound débridement

Prognosis

With early recognition and intensive care management to provide ventilation and supportive therapy, the prognosis is good. Neonatal disease in developing countries is associated with a high mortality.

Botulism

Epidemiology and disease mechanisms

This is a rare form of food poisoning where multiplication of the anaerobic organism *Clostridium botulinum* in food produces an extremely potent neurotoxin that causes generalized paralysis. Botulism is rare in Europe where home preservation is usually with fruit where the low pH of the produce prevents multiplication of *C. botulinum*. In the USA, there are sporadic domestic outbreaks related to home preservation (e.g. of meat). Recent cases in Europe have been caused by process failures in the food industry allowing spores to survive, germinate and multiply to produce the toxin.

Clinical features

Botulism typically presents with signs of bulbar palsy, often double vision or palatal paralysis. Paralysis can be progressive until respiration is compromised. Botulism must be suspected by the unusual presentation. Suspect food can be tested for the presence of toxin by immunoassay. A detailed food history by a case–control study must be undertaken to identify the source of the outbreak and to prevent further cases.

Management and prognosis

Some cases may be mild and self-limiting, but severe cases require intensive care management to support respiration and protect the airway. Polyvalent antitoxin can be given to patients and to individuals who have ingested contaminated food but have not yet developed symptoms. Mortality may be more than 25%.

Leprosy

This is a chronic granulomatous disease caused by *Mycobacterium leprae* and spread by nasal secretions. It can affect many tissues, especially skin and nerves and develops slowly. Nerve damage causes motor and sensory loss which leads to traumatic damage to tissues.

- Lepromatous leprosy occurs with poor cellular immunity and high pathogen numbers cause tissue thickening and damage.
- Tuberculoid leprosy occurs with substantial cellular immunity and is usually localized within an area of hypopigmented anaesthetic skin supplied by a thickened nerve. Treatment is usually with a combination of rifampicin, dapsone and clofazimine.

Rabies

This is a viral encephalitis, universally fatal once symptoms have developed, that spreads to humans through the bite of an infected animal.

Epidemiology

This is a zoonotic infection sustained in the wild, often among foxes. Many thousand deaths are reported worldwide but the disease is rare in Europe and North America where imported cases are rarely seen. Seventy per cent of patients are male. The UK and New Zealand are rabies free.

Disease mechanisms

The causative organism of rabies is a bullet-shaped RNA virus (rhabdovirus) with no close relatives amongst human pathogens. Rabies infects a wide range of mammals, with reservoirs in such diverse species as skunks, mongooses and bats. In many areas, however, the most important hosts are wild or domestic canines. The virus is excreted in the saliva of infected animals. Spread by the inoculation of virus through the skin is encouraged by behavioural changes during the period of encephalitis, which make some animals more likely to bite. Domestic dogs are the most common source of human infection. Direct human–human transmission has never been recorded except, as a rarity, via corneal transplants.

03

Rhabdovirus has an affinity for the CNS where it produces characteristic Negri bodies, which are cytoplasmic inclusions seen in histological sections. A localized focus of infection is established in striated muscle at the site of inoculation. The virus is limited to this site during the often prolonged incubation period. It then spreads via the nerve axons to the CNS where it replicates rapidly, resulting in clinically apparent disease.

Clinical features

The incubation period of rabies varies from 3 weeks to several months. The onset of illness may be heralded by a brief febrile prodrome, and by pain or paraesthesia at the site of inoculation. There may be headache, irritability or insomnia. This is followed by a general deterioration of mental function with distressing outbursts of extreme agitation. Convulsions are common. At this stage the patient develops hydrophobia; swallowing, or even the sight of water, induces terrifying spasms of the pharyngeal muscles. If the patient survives this period he or she develops a progressive paralysis and lapses into coma.

Investigation

Immunology

Antibody tests may be used to diagnose the infection. Very high titres are associated with infection rather than previous vaccination. Rabies virus may be identified by PCR and the characteristic Negri bodies can be seen in brain and skin biopsy or corneal impression smears.

Management and prognosis

Treatment of the established disease depends on sedation and intensive supportive care. Established rabies is almost always fatal once symptoms have developed.

Prevention

This is based on two strategies:

1 The prevention of peridomestic spread, where it is most dangerous to humans, by the rigorous immunization of dogs and cats and the destruction of strays.
2 Control in the fox population, which is best achieved by immunization, by distributing as bait carrion that contains an oral vaccine. As a result of these measures, human rabies has remained very rare in western Europe.

A killed vaccine, cultured in human diploid cells, is effective and safe. It may be given before exposure to those at particular risk or as postexposure prophylaxis after a possibly infected bite, in which case immunoglobulin should also be given. Present regimens prevent the onset of rabies in the great majority of cases. However, it is essential that prophylaxis is started as soon as possible after any skin abrasion caused by any mammal in an endemic area.

Poliomyelitis (polio)

Polio is an enteroviral infection that destroys anterior horn cells, leading to severe paralysis. An international vaccination campaign is nearing completion to bring about its eradication.

Disease mechanisms

Polio is caused by one of three serotypes of poliovirus, which is an enterovirus.

The initial infection occurs in the throat and, like other enteroviruses, in the intestinal tract. After a few days there is a viraemic phase, which is usually asymptomatic, but may be associated with a minor febrile illness in about 10% of cases. Less than 2% of those infected will then go on to develop CNS involvement after a total incubation period of 10–17 days when a typical enteroviral aseptic meningitis is usually the only manifestation. However, in a proportion of those infected, the virus invades and kills spinal or bulbar lower motor neurones, leading to paralysis. Injections and trauma during the incubation period are believed to promote the onset of paralysis in the affected area.

Epidemiology

Only isolated cases are found in developed countries because of an international eradication campaign. Spread of polioviruses is either by the faeco-oral or respiratory routes.

Clinical features

Usually, the patient developing paralysis is febrile and looks ill. Pain or hyperaesthesia often herald the onset of paralysis, which characteristically manifests as an asymmetrical flaccid weakness evolving rapidly over a few hours or progressing more gradually over a week or more. Respiratory or bulbar paralysis may be dominant features. The asymmetry and complete absence of any sensory defect differentiates polio from Guillain–Barré syndrome (see p. 950) and peripheral neuropathies.

Investigation

Serology will confirm the diagnosis and poliovirus can usually be isolated from faeces, but not usually from the CSF. Alternatively, viral RNA can be amplified by RT-PCR.

Management

Bed rest and supportive care with mechanical ventilation

if necessary are all that can be offered. Intensive rehabilitation can reduce the eventual disability.

Prevention

An international vaccine programme has brought about the almost complete eradication of this disease using a combination of the killed and the live attenuated Sabin oral vaccine or the killed parenteral Salk vaccine.

Prognosis

A small proportion of patients have localized or more general permanent paralysis which may compromise respiration.

Infections of the gastrointestinal system

The common infections of the gastrointestinal system are listed in Table 3.22. Most of these are treated by gastroenterologists and hepatologists and cross-references to the appropriate pages are given.

Cholera

Cholera is a secretory diarrhoeal disease caused by *Vibrio cholerae*.

Epidemiology

The organism is spread rapidly in water or contaminated food. Disease is found in Asia, North Africa, the Middle East, South and Central America; particularly where socioeconomic conditions are poor, or during war, famine and other disasters. Cholera may remain endemic in a community. The disease is capable of spreading rapidly across the world: a phenomenon known as a pandemic.

Disease mechanisms

Cholera is caused by the comma-shaped Gram-negative bacillus *Vibrio cholerae* carrying O1 somatic 'O' antigen. The El Tor biotype has replaced the classical strain as the major cause of cholera. More recently, a cholera-like disease has been reported caused by a *V. cholerae* with a O139 serotype.

Pathogenesis

Cholera bacilli proliferate in the small intestine where they produce an enterotoxin with A and B subunits. The B subunit irreversibly binds to enterocytes by specific GM1 ganglioside receptors; the A subunit activates intracellular adenyl cyclase, leading to massive secretion of water and electrolytes into the gut lumen (see Fig. 8.31, p. 560).

Clinical features

The incubation period varies from a few hours to 6 days. There is profuse watery diarrhoea, up to 20 l/day, leading to death from fluid depletion, possibly within a few hours. Other complications include renal failure resulting from dehydration, muscle cramps from hypokalaemia, and fits from hypoglycaemia. Mild or subclinical attacks can occur.

Investigation

- Stool microbiology may reveal vibrios on direct microscopy. Inhibition of movement by specific antiserum makes a rapid diagnosis. Stool samples should be cultured on special selective medium (thiosulphate citrate bile salt sucrose; TCBS) agar.
- Plasma urea may be high and the potassium and glucose may be low.

Management

Treatment must not await confirmation of the diagnosis. Rehydration with oral rehydration therapy (ORT) or intravenous fluids is urgent, and tetracycline or doxycycline shorten the duration of the illness.

Prevention

The most effective preventive measures are good hygiene and sanitary living conditions.

Prognosis

Without treatment, mortality can vary widely depending on the virulence of the infecting strain, but treatment with intravenous fluids, ORT and antibiotics reduces it to 1%.

Escherichia coli infections

Escherichia coli is a normal commensal of the intestinal tract, but several strains may cause diarrhoea in humans.
- *Enterotoxigenic E. coli (ETEC):* probably the most common single cause of diarrhoea in travellers. It causes acute watery diarrhoea by activating small intestinal secretion by heat-labile (LT) and/or heat-stable (ST) toxins
- *Enteroinvasive E. coli (EIEC):* produces a dysenteric illness resembling shigellosis (see p. 119)
- *Enteropathogenic E. coli (EPEC):* attaches to and damages enterocytes, causing epidemics of diarrhoea in children under 2 years of age
- *Verotoxigenic E. coli (VTEC)* and enterohaemorrhagic *E. coli (EHEC):* may produce diarrhoea, which is sometimes severe and haemorrhagic, and complicated rarely by haemolytic–uraemic syndrome (see p. 531)

03

Table 3.22 Gastrointestinal infections

Location	Syndrome	Organism	Page
Mouth	Dental caries	*Streptococcus mutans*	
	Gingivitis	Anaerobes	
	'Cold sore' (herpes labialis)	Herpes simplex type 1	182
	Candidiasis (thrush)	*Candida*	160
	Vincent's angina	*Fusobacterium fusiformis*	
		Borrelia vincenti	
Stomach	Gastritis, ulcer	*Helicobacter pylori*	703
Small intestine	Malabsorption/chronic	Bacterial overgrowth	721
	diarrhoea	Traveller's diarrhoea	102
		Tuberculosis	330
		Yersinia enterocolitica	121
		(Tropical sprue)	752
	Enterotoxin	*Staphylococcus aureus*	751
		Bacillus cereus	751
		Vibrio parahaemolyticus	
		Vibrio cholerae	117
		Enterotoxigenic *E. coli*	117
	Renal dysfunction	*Giardia*	122
	Invasive	*Salmonella*	119
		Campylobacter	120
		Rotavirus	121
		Cryptosporidia	123
Large intestine	Dysentery	*Shigella*	119
		Amoebae	121
		Campylobacter	120
		Enteroinvasive *E. coli*	118
Liver	Acute hepatitis	Hepatitis A–E	609
		Epstein–Barr virus	142
		Cytomegalovirus	143
		Arboviruses (yellow fever)	135
		Leptospirosis	107
		Septicaemia	123
		Legionella	321
		Chlamydia	321
	Chronic hepatitis	Hepatitis B	610
		Hepatitis C	613
		Hepatitis D	614

● *Enteroadherent E. coli (EAEC):* occasionally causes chronic diarrhoea in young children

Management
Treatment involves ORT and, in severe cases, antibiotics (e.g. co-trimoxazole, ciprofloxacin).

Prognosis
Disease is often self-limiting, recovery occurring after a few days. Infection with VTEC may be more serious with patients suffering from the haemolytic–uraemic syndrome with which is associated a significant mortality.

Shigellosis

Shigellosis is an acute intestinal infection by *Shigella* spp., associated with superficial haemorrhagic disease in the colon, giving rise to frequent small volume stools.

Epidemiology
Shigella are spread by the faeco-oral route and the infective dose is very low. Shigellosis is common throughout the world and infection is most likely in children between the ages of 6 and 10 years, although all age-groups are at risk. Disease is more likely in insanitary

conditions and when services are disrupted by war or natural disaster.

Causes

Intestinal infection is caused by one of four species: *Shigella dysenteriae*, *S. flexneri*, *S. boydii* and *S. sonnei*. *Shigella flexneri* has a reservoir amongst monkeys and *S. sonnei* has been isolated from certain species of fruit-bat; otherwise, shigellosis is an exclusively human infection. *Shigella sonnei* is much the most prevalent species in Europe and causes the mildest disease. In the tropics, infection with *Shigella dysenteriae* is more important.

Disease mechanisms

Shigella spp. invade the colonic epithelium (see Fig. 8.32, p. 571) causing mucosal ulceration, which may be extensive but seldom invades deeply. Many strains of *Shigella* produce Shiga toxin, which is cytotoxic in nervous, gut and other tissue.

Clinical features

The incubation period is 2–3 days. Many *S. sonnei* infections result in only trivial symptoms. A brief dysenteric illness without conspicuous fever, abdominal pain or systemic upset is common. The untreated illness usually lasts less than 2 weeks, and resolves without sequelae. Occasionally, infection with *S. sonnei* follows a severe course more typical of the other *Shigella* spp., with the passage of profuse bloodstained mucus accompanied by fever, rigors, headache and abdominal pain. Death may result from dehydration, endotoxic shock, bowel necrosis and perforation, or haemolytic–uraemic syndrome.

Investigations

A neutrophil leucocytosis is usual. The diagnosis is made on the basis of the clinical features and isolation of the organism from stool. Sigmoidoscopy shows ulcerated and inflamed mucosa.

Management

Rehydration with intravenous fluids and ORT is the cornerstone of treatment. Antibiotic therapy may prolong diarrhoea and antibiotic resistance is widespread.

Prevention

Public health measures and good personal hygiene are essential.

Prognosis

Prompt diagnosis and treatment of serious cases leads to full recovery.

Salmonellosis

Salmonella are a common cause of intestinal infection that may spread beyond the gut to cause septicaemia.

Disease mechanisms

Salmonella is a Gram-negative bacillus. Different strains are identified by serological means in the laboratory. Important serotypes include *Salmonella typhi* and *S. paratyphi*, which usually give rise to a systemic infection known as enteric fever. The remainder of the serotypes cause intestinal disease of varying severity, with some more likely to spread beyond the gut to produce septicaemia.

After ingestion, salmonellae multiply in the small intestine. They then pass via lymphatics and the bloodstream to the reticuloendothelial system. In typhoid, there is a second bacteraemic phase and the organism reinvades the gut via the gallbladder. Infection localizes in Peyer's patches, resulting in ulceration, bowel perforation or haemorrhage.

Epidemiology

The organisms are found throughout the world and are spread from person to person through the faeco-oral route and in food and water. The risk of infection is increased particularly where poor hygiene and overcrowding are common. Transmission is through contaminated foods (e.g. eggs and poultry) or water, can be a problem in restaurants, hospitals or institutions.

Clinical features

Five main clinical syndromes can occur:
1 Enteric fever (typhoid and paratyphoid; see p. 131)
2 Enterocolitis
3 Gastroenteritis (food poisoning; see p. 751)
4 Carrier state
5 Localized infection (e.g. osteomyelitis, meningitis and arthritis)

Typhoid fever

The incubation period is 10–14 days. It starts gradually with a headache, cough, sore throat, initial constipation and gradually increasing remittent fever. Physical signs in the first week are a systemic upset, relative bradycardia, a transient erythematous maculopapular rash on the abdomen ('rose spots'), mild splenomegaly and abdominal tenderness. Diarrhoea occurs after the first week, and the third week may be complicated by intestinal perforation and haemorrhage osteomyelitis rarely, acute cholecystitis, lobar pneumonia, haemolytic anaemia, meningitis, peripheral neuropathy or urinary tract infection.

03

Enterocolitis

The illness consists of fever, malaise, abdominal pain, bloody diarrhoea and vomiting for 2–3 days.

Carrier state

This may complicate typhoid or enterocolitis, with the individual harbouring *Salmonella* in the gallbladder and excreting it in the stools for a year or more.

Investigation

Typhoid fever

- *FBC:* leucopenia is common
- *Blood cultures:* positive in the first and third weeks
- *Urine culture:* in the second week
- *Stool culture:* in the second to fourth week
- *Bone marrow culture:* may also be positive

Other *Salmonella* infections

Stool cultures usually give the diagnosis. It is important to instigate appropriate investigations of food sources where outbreaks are traced back to a single food source (e.g. hospital kitchen or restaurant).

Management

Full supportive treatment is necessary. Typhoid requires treatment with ciprofloxacin, ceftriaxone, ampicillin, co-trimoxazole or chloramphenicol. Ciprofloxacin is the drug of first choice but there are increasing reports of strains that are multidrug-resistant and which must be managed following susceptibility testing.

Antibiotics can increase the incidence and duration of asymptomatic carriage of salmonellae, and encourage drug resistance. They should be withheld in non-typhoidal salmonellosis unless the patient has a serious infection (i.e. high fever, rigors, hypotension, decreased renal function, localized extraintestinal infection). It may be difficult to eradicate the carrier state with antibiotics.

Prevention

Improved sewage disposal, clean water supplies and scrupulous personal hygiene, especially by food handlers, are crucial. Known carriers should not work in food-handling jobs until the organism has been shown to be eradicated.

Three vaccines are available for typhoid: killed whole-cell vaccine; subcellular vaccine containing the Vi antigen; and oral live attenuated salmonella Ty21A.

Prognosis

Prompt diagnosis and treatment leads to a full recovery from *Salmonella* infections. In developing countries, typhoid still has a substantial mortality. The elderly are especially prone to disseminated infection and there is a significant mortality.

Campylobacter jejuni

An intestinal infection caused by organisms of the *Campylobacter* spp., associated with fever and cramping abdominal pains.

Epidemiology

This is now the most common cause of infective diarrhoea in many developed countries. Infection is spread to humans in food. Food animals are the natural source of infection, which develops through contamination of uncooked food or by inadequate cooking.

Disease mechanisms

The most common cause of infection is *Campylobacter jejuni*, a Gram-negative spiral bacterium. The organism invades and colonizes the mucosa of the small intestine. It then translocates across the epithelial layer to the underlying tissues. The pathogenicity determinants of these organisms are uncertain. Guillain–Barré syndrome is associated with *Campylobacter* infection. It causes an acute enterocolitis, with the pathology in the colon resembling ulcerative colitis. The related species *C. fetus* and *C. coli* are more rarely implicated in diarrhoeal disease.

Clinical features

The incubation period is 2–5 days. Fever, headache and malaise are prominent symptoms which are followed by diarrhoea that is often bloody. Abdominal pain, and sometimes constitutional disturbances may be present.

Investigation

A peripheral leucocytosis is common. The organism should be cultivated from stools using specialist culture media. Blood culture is occasionally positive in severe disease.

Management and prognosis

Most patients recover within 7 days with supportive treatment. Erythromycin or ciprofloxacin can be used for individuals with a severe attack. Recovery is usually complete.

Pseudomembranous colitis

Pseudomembranous colitis is caused by a disturbance in the gut flora, usually caused by antibiotics, which allow *Clostridium difficile* to cause a toxin-mediated diarrhoeal disease. *Clostridium difficile* is normally found in the human intestine, especially in hospitalized patients. It produces enterotoxins, which cause fluid secretion and tissue damage.

Clinical features

Typically, the patient passes more than three loose or unformed stools per day and has a history of previous antibiotic exposure. Abdominal pain may develop and sigmoidoscopy reveals pseudomembranes: small white-yellow plaques situated on the mucosal surface of the rectum and sigmoid colon. The diagnosis is suspected by the history, suggested by the demonstration of pseudomembranes and confirmed by the laboratory demonstration of toxin in the stool by ELISA or tissue culture. Isolation is not diagnostic as many patients are asymptomatic carriers.

Treatment and prevention

The inciting agent should be stopped and the patient given oral vancomycin or metronidazole. Treatment with *Saccharomyces boulardii* may be beneficial. Patients with pseudomembranous colitis should be isolated from other patients with enteric precautions.

Yersiniosis

Yersiniosis is an intestinal infection with *Yersinia enterocolitica*.

Epidemiology

Rodents, pigs, sheep and cattle form a reservoir and infection is spread to humans by food and occasionally water. It is rare in Europe but infection can be acquired throughout the world.

Disease mechanisms and clinical features

Yersinia enterocolitica and *Y. pseudotuberculosis* can cause enterocolitis (with fever, abdominal pain and diarrhoea), mesenteric lymphadenitis (especially in children), terminal ileitis, or appendicitis after the ingestion of contaminated milk or pork. Complications include arthritis (Reiter's syndrome, particularly in HLA-B27 positive individuals) and erythema nodosum, both of which are thought to be immunologically mediated.

Investigation

● *Stool or blood cultures:* may detect the presence of *Yersinia* spp.
● *Serology:* may reveal *Yersinia* infection. Antibodies to *Yersinia* LPS (the somatic 'O' antigen) can be detected.

Management and prognosis

No treatment is usually necessary because the disease is usually self-limiting. Aminoglycosides and fluoroquinolones can be used for severe disease.

Viral diarrhoea

Rotavirus is a well-established cause of self-limiting, often severe diarrhoea in young children. Most people acquire immunity early in life, but because this wanes with increasing age the elderly are again vulnerable.

Winter vomiting disease occurs in epidemics of mild and short-lived gastroenteritis, often associated with upper respiratory tract symptoms and sometimes with a fever, and are extremely common in temperate climates. The aetiology of most of these illnesses is not established, but the Norwalk virus appears to be responsible in some instances.

Astroviruses, caliciviruses and fastidious **adenoviruses** have all been implicated as causes of transient diarrhoea. These organisms can cause outbreaks in the hospital environment.

Amoebiasis

Amoebiasis is an intestinal infection caused by the protozoan *Entamoeba histolytica*.

Epidemiology

Infection is found worldwide, mainly in the tropics and subtropics, but there are occasional outbreaks in temperate climates. It is a disease of poor sanitation. There are an estimated 50 million cases of invasive disease each year, causing 100 000 deaths worldwide. Cysts of *E. histolytica* are transmitted in contaminated food or water, or by direct person–person contact (Fig. 3.33).

Disease mechanisms

Entamoeba histolytica, the intestinal pathogen, is distinguished microscopically from other non-pathogenic enteric amoebae by its phagocytosis of red blood cells in the stool. It exists as both a motile trophozoite and a cyst that can survive outside the body.

Trophozoites excyst in the small intestine and multiply in the colon. Virulent strains attach to colonocytes using a surface lectin and release a proteolytic protein ('amoebapore') that damages the apical cell membrane and allows other cytotoxins to enter; the end result is frank mucosal ulceration. There is a morphologically indistinguishable organism that does not cause disease called *E. dispar*.

03

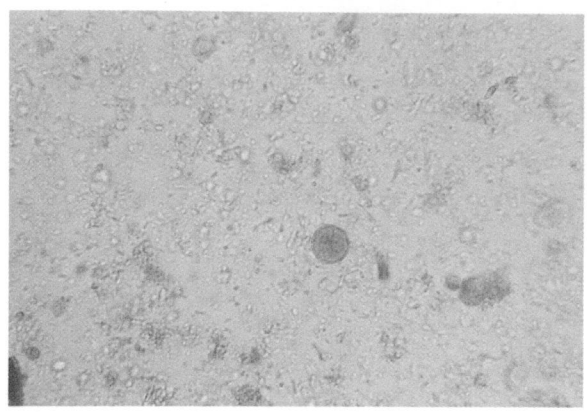

Figure 3.33 Cyst of *Entamoeba histolytica* in a stool.

Clinical features

The incubation period is variable, ranging from a few days to several months.

Amoebic colitis may start gradually, first with an intermittent diarrhoea, which later becomes bloody and mucopurulent. There may also be headache, nausea and anorexia. Occasionally, there is **fulminant amoebic dysentery** like that of shigellosis (see p. 119). Complications are unusual, but include amoebic liver abscess, toxic megacolon with perforation and peritonitis, colonic stricture, severe intestinal haemorrhage and a mass of fibrotic granulation tissue, usually in the caecum and occasionally causing bleeding or intussusception—an amaeboma.

Investigation

The diagnosis is made by identifying the presence of the organism in stool or jejunal fluid. Microscopy of repeated fresh liquid stool specimens or scrapings from ulcers collected at sigmoidoscopy shows motile amoebic trophozoites containing phagocytosed red cells. The presence of cysts alone in a patient with diarrhoea does not prove that amoebiasis is the cause. Detection of antibodies to *E. histolytica* may be helpful in the diagnosis of liver abscess. Ultrasound or CT can prove useful to identify liver abscess.

Management

It is essential to avoid mistaking amoebiasis for ulcerative colitis or Crohn's disease, as treatment with corticosteroids can cause a rapid deterioration and death in patients with invasive disease.

The combination of metronidazole, which is effective in the tissues, and diloxanide furoate, which is effective in the lumen of the gut, will eradicate the cyst stage and prevent relapse and late complications. Diloxanide alone is usually adequate for asymptomatic cyst passers.

Prevention

The main measures are personal hygiene and boiling drinking water for 10 min to destroy cysts.

Prognosis

Recovery is usually complete following treatment with appropriate antimicrobials.

Giardiasis

An intestinal infection caused by the protozoan *Giardia lamblia*.

Epidemiology

Giardia infections are very prevalent in tropical countries (affecting 10–20% of children under 10 years of age), and are not uncommon in developed countries (affecting 3–4% of children under 10 years of age). Water-borne epidemics, person–person faeco-oral spread and zoonotic infections all occur.

Disease mechanisms

Giardia lamblia is a flagellate protozoon that commonly infects the small bowel. The cysts are resistant to killing by standard methods of chlorination, and are excreted in the faeces.

Trophozoites of *G. lamblia* are found in the layer of mucus closely investing the enterocytes. There may be some mucosal inflammation, but enterocyte dysfunction is probably responsible for the diarrhoea. Mucosal immunity is important in controlling the infection—individuals with IgA deficiency are particularly prone to chronic or recurrent giardiasis.

Clinical features

Acute infections are characterized by watery small bowel diarrhoea, which may be profuse. The clinical features are not self-limiting and can be persistent. Symptoms in chronic infection are usually milder. Asymptomatic carriage is common, and some chronic infections are associated with partial villous atrophy and malabsorption.

Investigation

The diagnosis is made by identifying cysts and the trophozoites with their characteristic appearances by microscopy of stool or jejunal fluid (Fig. 3.18). At least three stools should be sent.

Management

Metronidazole and tinidazole are both effective. Short courses of high doses are now usually recommended.

Prognosis

Occasionally, there is a relapse requiring a second course of treatment. The organism can prove difficult to eradicate in immunocompromised individuals.

Cryptosporidiosis

This is an intestinal infection with the protozoan *Cryptosporidium parvum.*

Epidemiology

The incidence of infection varies greatly. The carriage rate is 0.6–20% in developed countries. Infection usually occurs in the young. Infection is particularly serious in patients with immunodeficiency, including AIDS.

Disease mechanisms

Cryptosporidia are coccidian protozoa and are gut pathogens of domestic animals, especially calves, undergoing part of their life cycle within enterocytes. Human infection occurs either as a sporadic zoonosis or in waterborne outbreaks.

Clinical features

The infection generally causes a mild and self-limiting watery diarrhoeal illness. Its main importance is in people with AIDS in whom it may be persistent or progressive and cause profound weight loss.

Investigation

The diagnosis is made by examining **stool or intestinal biopsies** for the presence of oocysts after Ziehl–Neelsen staining.

Management and prognosis

The disease is self-limiting in people who are immunocompetent and no specific treatment is needed.

In patients with AIDS, none of the many antimicrobials tried have proved effective. Some patients improve when their immune defence is boosted, for example with HAART (see p. 177), but most patients need prolonged treatment with antidiarrhoeal agents (e.g. loperamide).

Infections of the respiratory tract

The common infections of the respiratory tract are listed in Table 3.23. Many of these are treated by respiratory physicians and cross-references to the appropriate pages are given.

Infections of the cardiovascular system

The common infections of the cardiovascular system are listed in Table 3.24. Many of these are treated by cardiologists and cross-references to the appropriate pages are given.

Infections presenting mainly with fever

Septicaemia

Septicaemia is usually a condition of acute onset (the presence of organisms in the blood causes symptoms). It is often associated with hypotension and is then called 'septic shock'. The features of septic shock can occur in the absence of circulating organisms. Other causes of shock are listed in Table 3.25.

Epidemiology

Septicaemia is a common condition in hospitalized patients. There is an increased prevalence in the elderly and among individuals with underlying diseases. Septicaemia is found in all countries but reporting is more frequent where hospitalization and antibiotic use is common.

Causes

The organisms isolated in septicaemia depend on the age and underlying condition of the patient. Overall (in the absence of meningococcal and *Salmonella* epidemics), the most common organisms isolated in adults are:

- Gram-negative coliforms (40% of cases)
- *Staphylococcus aureus* (12% of cases)
- *Streptococcus pneumoniae* (10% of cases)

Disease mechanisms

Gram-negative organisms possess an LPS on their surface that, when injected in pure form into the circulation, reproduces most of the features of septic shock. LPS acts by causing the release of endogenous mediators such as TNF and IL-1 (see p. 66), which may mediate the shock and tissue damage by triggering the release of further vasoactive agents such as prostaglandins and nitrous oxide.

Clinical features

The patient may be too unwell to give a history, but useful clues include recent surgery or instrumentation (particularly of the bowel or urogenital tract), or symptoms of a recent infection (e.g. dysuria, diarrhoea or a cough). The clinical signs of septicaemia are legion. Early on, the patient may experience rigors, nausea and confusion. He or she usually has a tachycardia and is vasodilated with warm peripheries. The patient passes through a stage of **warm shock** with hypotension and vasodilatation

Table 3.23 Respiratory infections

Location	Syndrome	Organism	Page
Upper respiratory tract	Acute tonsillitis	Group A streptococci	
	Diphtheria	*Corynebacterium diphtheriae*	
	Pharyngitis	*Haemophilus influenzae*	318
		Mycoplasma	321
		Mycobacterium tuberculosis	330
	Coryza	Rhinovirus	318
	Whooping cough	*Bacillus pertussis*	328
Lower respiratory tract	Lobar pneumonia	*Streptococcus pneumoniae*	321
	Atypical pneumonia	*Mycoplasma*	321
		Legionella	321
		Chlamydia	321
		Staphylococcus aureus	321
		Viral	321
		Gram-negative bacteria	321
	Lung abscess	*Staph. aureus*	329
		Gram-negative bacteria	329
		Anaerobes	329
	Empyema	*Strep. pneumoniae*	321
		M. tuberculosis	330
	Tuberculosis	*M. tuberculosis*	330
	Mycotic infection	Bronchopulmonary aspergillosis	367
		Phycomycosis	
		Histoplasmosis	

Table 3.24 Infections of the cardiovascular system

Syndrome	Organism	Page
Infective endocarditis		478
Native valves	*Streptococcus viridans*	
	Other streptococci (*S. sanguis,* *S. mitior, S. milleri,* etc.)	
	Enterococci	
	Staphylococcus aureus	
	Coxiella burnetti (Q fever)	
Prosthetic valves	The above plus *Staphylococcus epidermidis*	
Myocarditis	Coxsackie and echovirus	482
	Influenza, mumps, EBV, CMV	Table 7.45
	Mycoplasma pneumoniae	
	Leptospira spp.	
	Pyogenic organisms	
	Trypanosomiasis (Chagas' disease)	
	Coxiella (Q fever)	
Acute pericarditis	Coxsackie and influenza viruses	488
	Mycoplasma pneumoniae	
	Streptococcus pneumoniae	
	Mycobacterium tuberculosis	

CMV, cytomegalovirus; EBV, Epstein–Barr virus.

Table 3.25 Causes of fever accompanied by shock

Disease	Causative agent
Septicaemia	Any organisms, but especially associated with Gram-negative infection
Leptospirosis	*Leptospira icterohaemorrhagiae* *Leptospira hebdomidis*
Meningococcaemia	Meningococcus (i.e. *Neisseria meningitidis*)
Toxic shock syndrome	Enterotoxin-producing *Staphylococcus aureus*
Malaria	*Plasmodium falciparum*
Typhoid	*Salmonella typhi*
Typhus	*Rickettsia*
Spotted fevers	*Rickettsia*
Viral haemorrhagic fevers	Lassa, Ebola, Marburg, arbovirus, Congo–Crimean haemorrhagic fever
Haemolytic–uraemic syndrome	Verotoxin-producing *Escherichia coli*

associated with confusion, to a state of cold shock. In **cold shock** the cardiac output falls as the heart can no longer maintain a high output, possibly because of circulating 'myocardial depressant factors'. Hypotension is then associated with cold clammy peripheries. During this period the patient can develop renal failure, progressive acidosis and adult respiratory distress syndrome. Signs may be absent in the elderly and the immunosuppressed. Some patients do not pass through a period of warm shock, and on presentation are cold and hypotensive.

Patients should be examined carefully for any sign of a localized or specific infection that may help to make an aetiological diagnosis. Female patients should be examined gynaecologically to ensure that there is no retained tampon. The skin should be inspected carefully. Ecthyma gangrenosum—a lesion with a necrotic centre 0.5–1 cm in diameter and an erythematous surround—is associated with Gram-negative infection. Meningococcaemia, gonococcaemia and rickettsial diseases can be suggested by their rash (see pp. 110 and 136).

Investigation

Blood culture is the most important investigation and up to three samples should be sent before antibiotics are administered.

Haematology
The white cell count is usually elevated but may be normal or depressed. The severity of infection cannot be determined from the white cell count because many patients with severe disease have a low white cell count.

Biochemistry
Biochemical examination is useful to determine the severity and course of infection. The blood gases, renal and liver function should be monitored.

Immunology
Serum should be stored for serological investigations. Some organisms that produce a septic shock-like picture may only be diagnosed on the basis of paired serological samples (e.g. *Chlamydia psittaci*).

Diagnostic imaging
Imaging should be directed towards uncovering an underlying cause. For example, ultrasound or CT imaging may reveal an intra-abdominal abscess or an underlying gastrointestinal malignancy. All patients with septicaemia will need a chest radiograph. This may reveal the underlying infection (e.g. pneumonia), a predisposing cause (e.g. carcinoma, lymphoma) or a complication (e.g. adult respiratory distress syndrome).

Management

Antibiotics should be given without delay. If the source of the infection is known because, for example, there has been a recent urinary tract infection or a concomitant pneumonia, antibiotic therapy can be directed at the likely organisms. Otherwise it is reasonable to use a combination of an extended spectrum penicillin and an aminoglycoside (e.g. tazobactam and gentamicin), or a third-generation cephalosporin. Many hospitals have an antibiotic policy with recommendations for treating septicaemia of unknown cause. The policy should be followed unless there are compelling reasons not to do so.

Patients with burns and those who are immunosuppressed have an increased risk of *Pseudomonas* infection and should receive tazobactam or ceftazidime. Treatment should be adjusted according to local sensitivity patterns. Organ failure is treated as necessary.

Prognosis

Mortality of septicaemia is related to the condition of the patient. It is four times higher in patients with an underlying serious disease than in those who are otherwise fit. Overall mortality ranges between 20 and 50%.

Staphylococcal toxic shock syndrome

This is a serious toxaemia that may be caused by a localized staphylococcal infection.

Disease	Causative agent	Page
Infections		
Gram-negative septicaemia accompanied by DIC	Enterobacteriaceae, *Pseudomonas* spp.	125
Leptospirosis	*Leptospira icterohaemorrhagiae*	107
Meningococcaemia	*Neisseria meningitidis*	110
Viral haemorrhagic fever	Lassa fever virus	126
Rickettsial disease	*Rickettsia* spp.	136
Non-infectious causes		
Leukaemia		1048
Any cause of DIC		1075

Table 3.26 Causes of fever accompanied by haemorrhage

DIC, disseminated intravascular coagulation.

Epidemiology

It is an uncommon condition but one that is easily over-looked if it is not considered. It is predominantly found in women and associated with contaminated tampons.

Disease mechanisms

Toxic shock syndrome (TSS) is caused by enterotoxin staphylococci. It was originally described in association with prolonged wearing of highly absorbent tampons, but has since been noted in association with staphylococcal colonization of other sites in both men and women.

Clinical features

Clinically, TSS presents as hypotension (resulting from vasodilatation and fluid extravasation) accompanied by a macular or petechial rash and multiorgan failure. There may have been severe diarrhoea. As the condition resolves there is often characteristic periungual desquamation.

Investigation

Staphylococci are not found in the blood, but may be found colonizing a site. The diagnosis is supported by isolating an enterotoxin-producing strain of *Staph. aureus*.

Management

As this condition is caused by a toxin, the treatment is primarily supportive with fluid replacement. The hypotension usually responds to this. A penicillinase-resistant antibiotic should be given to eradicate the *Staphylococcus*.

Prognosis

Case fatality rate is between 5 and 10%.

Fever with haemorrhage

Fever may present with haemorrhage into the skin (purpura), nose bleed or gastrointestinal bleeding. Some of the causes are shown in Table 3.26.

Viral haemorrhagic fever

The viral haemorrhagic fevers should be considered in travellers who have passed through an endemic area and who develop a fever with a bleeding tendency; other features include pharyngitis, hepatitis and shock (Table 3.27). Viruses from three groups are implicated in these illnesses: arboviruses, arenaviruses and the Marburg and Ebola viruses.

If viral haemorrhagic fever is suspected, the patient should be isolated in a specialist unit as several of the causative viruses can cause severe illness in secondary cases amongst clinical or laboratory personnel.

Infections presenting primarily as fever

Pyrexia of unknown origin

If a fever has lasted for more than 10 days (i.e. beyond the duration of common acute viral infections), it is unusual for there to be no strong presumptive diagnosis. In this situation the first step, before ordering numerous investigations, is to start again from scratch with a thorough repeat history and examination. The term pyrexia of unknown origin (PUO) artificially groups together patients with unrelated conditions. Its value is that it highlights certain conditions that might not be considered otherwise.

Disease mechanisms

Fevers of unknown origin commonly fall into several groups (Table 3.28):

- Infection, often low-grade intracellular or pyogenic

Table 3.27 Viral haemorrhagic fevers

Virus family	Virus	Disease	Endemic areas
Flavivirus	Yellow fever	Yellow fever	West Africa
	Dengue	Dengue	Worldwide
Arenavirus	Lassa	Lassa fever	West Africa
	Junin	Argentinian haemorrhagic fever	South America
	Machupo	Bolivian haemorrhagic fever	South America
Bunyavirus	Congo–Crimean	Congo–Crimean haemorrhagic fever	Africa, Asia
	Marburg	Monkey-related laboratory outbreak	
Ebolavirus	Ebola	Ebola	Zaire, Sudan

- Granulomatous inflammatory disease (e.g. sarcoidosis)
- Malignancy (e.g. lung, bone, renal tumours)
- Collagen vascular disease (e.g. rheumatoid arthritis or Still's disease)
- Factitious fever

Common infectious diagnoses of PUO include tuberculosis, abdominal or pelvic abscess. Dental abscess is a commonly missed diagnosis and can be present without dental pain. Some mysterious intermittent fevers will be found to be factitious (tinkering with the thermometer) or deliberately self-induced (e.g. by self-injection with infected material). Disease mechanisms depend on the underlying condition.

Clinical features

The clinical features depend on the underlying condition. Careful history taking and examination can reveal important clues. Ask about any history of exposure, especially through contacts at work, travel, hobbies and contact with animals.

A careful examination should include a thorough inspection of the skin for rashes, bites and needle marks. A rectal examination and a gynaecological examination are usually necessary.

The history and examination should be reviewed regularly in case symptoms are remembered or change, and to look for new signs that have developed as the disease progresses.

Investigation

After the initial history and examination is taken the investigative process can be divided into three phases:

1 Screening investigations that are performed on all patients (Fig. 3.16)

2 Investigations that depend on the results of history or physical examination

3 Further screening tests and special imaging techniques: ultrasound, CT, MRI, echocardiography, dental X-ray (Fig. 3.16).

Table 3.28 Causes of fever of unknown origin

Cause	Page
Infections	
Subacute bacterial endocarditis	478
Chronic pyelonephritis	571
Osteomyelitis	261
Chronic sinusitis	318
Liver abscess	617
Tuberculosis	330
Brucellosis	134
Q fever	136
HIV	170
Syphilis	166
Inflammatory	
Rheumatic fever	477
Inflammatory bowel disease	734
Polyarteritis nodosa	221
Chronic hepatitis	619
Systemic lupus erythematosus (SLE)	212
Rheumatoid arthritis	206
Temporal arteritis	220
Familial fevers	
Malignancy	
Haematogenous	
Lymphomas	1059
Leukaemias	1048
Polycythaemia rubra vera	1056
Solid	
Hepatocellular	567
Renal	
Ovarian	
Hepatoma	633
Lung	362
Other causes	
Recurrent pulmonary emboli	334
Atrial myxoma	500

03

The results of the preliminary history and examination are taken together with the results of the primary investigations to plan the tests to be performed in the second round. These investigations are chosen based on syndrome groups (e.g. fever, eosinophila and tropical travel). If a diagnosis is not made, further imaging techniques are used to reveal an occult abdominal abscess or osteomyelitis. History and examinations are repeatedly made and the results synthesized to direct the diagnostic process. If a clear diagnosis is not made, a trial of chemotherapy may be considered (see p. 85).

Appropriate plain films are required to reveal or exclude sinusitis or a dental abscess, both of which may present without the typical history of pain. A hidden infected or malignant mass, most often within the abdomen, may be demonstrated by modern imaging techniques.

Echocardiography
The heart should be investigated for clinically non-apparent lesions that could be the site of endocarditis.

A liver biopsy, especially in the presence of an elevated alkaline phosphatase, can be valuable in the diagnosis of granulomatous hepatitis and lymphomas. All biopsy material must be sent for culture as well as for histology. In addition to lymphomas and other reticuloendothelial neoplasms, microscopy of a bone marrow aspirate may reveal *Leishmania* or malaria parasites. The aspirate should also be cultured (see p. 137).

Management and prognosis
These depend on the underlying condition.

Fever in a traveller: imported and unusual infections

Ideally, anyone with an undiagnosed fever who has been in the tropics in the recent past should be seen by a clinician with infectious disease expertise. Fatal malaria can develop extremely rapidly in the non-immune and mimic influenza.

Disease mechanisms
A detailed travel history must be obtained from all patients with a fever. This should include details of where the patient has been, when, for how long and for what reason (HISTORY & EXAMINATION BOX 3.2). A banker visiting West Africa for 48 h who does not leave the capital city and an engineer who visits West Africa for 48 h but has been staying in a tented camp in the bush will be exposed to different infections (Table 3.16).

Investigation
Investigations should be guided by the clinical state of the patient and knowledge of the prevalent diseases in the places they have visited:

- *Three thick and thin blood films:* to exclude malaria for any patient who could have been exposed. It is not excluded by examination of a single blood film by an inexperienced observer, and many commonly prescribed antibiotics (e.g. tetracycline, co-trimoxazole) have an antimalarial action
- *Liver function tests:* results guide further investigations
- *Serology:* save serum for future study to diagnose, for example, brucellosis or arbovirus infection
- *Blood cultures:* should be taken early to exclude typhoid
- *Bone marrow culture:* should be considered
- *Chest radiography:* to exclude tuberculosis and lower respiratory tract infection
- *Abdominal ultrasound:* to exclude amoebic abscess if there is jaundice or right upper abdominal pain
- *Bone marrow biopsy:* should be considered

Malaria

Malaria is a systemic infection with one of the four species of *Plasmodium* protozoa.

Epidemiology
More than 1.5 billion people are exposed to the risk of malaria infection, and the number of cases occurring in endemic parts of the world is unknown. Malaria has been eradicated from Europe and North America but imported cases are common; for example, there are more than 2000 imported cases a year in the UK. All ages are susceptible. In areas of endemic transmission, the disease is less severe in those over 5 years of age. There is some evidence that females mount a stronger humoral response, but pregnant women are more likely to suffer severe disease. People with sickle cell trait have reduced susceptibility, but in sickle cell disease the risk is markedly increased. Malaria is endemic in more than 100 countries throughout Africa, Central and South America, Asia and Oceania.

Many people travel to infected areas, and the contribution of each species to imported malaria is related to the risk of infection and the number of visitors. There has been a major increase in the number of imported *P. falciparum* infections resulting from increased travel to and the failure of malaria eradication in Africa. It is therefore important that travellers are fully informed of the risks and take personal protection measures.

Disease mechanisms
Plasmodium falciparum and *P. vivax* are the most common species of *Plasmodium* to infect humans.
- *Plasmodium falciparum:* the main species in Africa

and Papua New Guinea, and the cause of an increasing proportion of malaria imported to Europe
- *Plasmodium vivax:* dominates in South America and Asia
- *Plasmodium malariae:* widely distributed, but much less common
- *Plasmodium ovale:* found mainly in West Africa

Disease mechanisms

Transmission of malaria depends on the interactions between the host, the vector, the environment and the parasite. All ages are susceptible, although variations in age and sex susceptibility may be explained by differences in vector exposure.

Host factors may enhance or decrease the severity of disease:
- Pregnancy and splenectomy increase the severity of the disease
- People who are negative for the red cell surface Duffy molecule are immune to *P. vivax*
- Sickle cell trait, α and β thalassaemia trait, glucose-6-phosphate dehydrogenase (G6PD) deficiency and malnutrition decrease the severity of the disease. Well-nourished children develop more severe disease

Clinical features

Malaria can present with almost any clinical pattern and must be considered when anyone has been exposed to the parasite as a result of travel or blood transfusion, or the rare 'airport' malaria (mosquitoes carried on an aircraft escape and bite people living near an airport in a non-endemic area). Delayed diagnosis of *P. falciparum* malaria is associated with an increased mortality.

Patients typically present with an elevated temperature, malaise and myalgia. This presentation can resemble the influenza-like symptoms that are commonly found in a general practice surgery but can pose a trap if a travel history is not taken and the risk not recognized. Travellers rarely have the classic tertian or quartan fevers (see p. 80) but have a sustained temperature.

The most classical symptom is the malarial rigor, which occurs when the schizonts rupture. The periodic nature of the attacks of fever may suggest the diagnosis. However, the classical 3- (tertian) or 4- (quartan) day cycle of fever occurs only in synchronized infections, when most of the parasitized red cells rupture together. This only occurs in patients from endemic countries who have a degree of immunity. Other clinical features of malaria are tiredness, lassitude and sometimes diarrhoea. Hepatosplenomegaly, which may be tender, and labial herpes are common.

Complications of *P. falciparum* malaria are related to high parasitaemia and are therefore more common in people with no immunity, children and travellers, and in areas of unstable transmission.
- Blackwater fever is characterized by haemoglobinuria causing 'Coca-Cola'-coloured urine. It results from severe haemolysis, which may be triggered by quinine or oxidant drugs in patients with G6PD deficiency or by severe parasitaemia. The free haemoglobin damages the glomeruli, leading to renal failure.
- Algid malaria is a syndrome of hypovolaemic shock associated with falciparum malaria.
- Cerebral malaria results from parasitized red cells obstructing the cerebral capillaries. It is associated with impaired consciousness ranging from mild clouding of consciousness to coma, fits and psychosis. Focal signs are uncommon. Concomitant meningitis should be excluded.
- Pulmonary oedema is a complication of malaria, and fluid balance needs attention to prevent fluid overload.

Investigations

The platelets are usually low but the white cell count (WCC) is normal. Low serum sodium and albumin and high bilirubin and urea are associated with a poorer prognosis. Serology has no part to play in diagnosis of acute malaria.

Malaria is diagnosed by demonstrating parasites in the peripheral blood. A minimum of three specimens should be taken at the height of fever and shortly afterwards. Antigen detection dipstick tests for blood are almost as sensitive as an experienced microscopist and should prove valuable in laboratories where this diagnosis is less common.

Management

Plasmodium falciparum infection. Because of the rise in chloroquine resistance there are few areas in the world where chloroquine can be relied on for the treatment of non-immune subjects. For clinically mild or moderate infections, oral quinine followed by Fansidar will be adequate.

Intravenous therapy is indicated if oral therapy is not tolerated, if there is a high parasite count, or if there is any sign of lowered consciousness or other complication. The volume of intravenous fluids given must be carefully monitored because there is a marked tendency for fluid retention and pulmonary oedema. Quinine should be given intravenously until the patient is fully conscious and the parasite count is falling. It can then be continued orally until thick blood smears are negative and the patient is apyrexial. Corticosteroid therapy worsens the outcome.

Quinine is nephrotoxic, and this is compounded when a severe infection predisposes to renal damage. Renal failure may need treatment. Quinine also stimulates insulin secretion, resulting in a potential hypoglycaemia, which is

03

Malaria at a glance

Epidemiology
More than 2 million deaths per year, 2 billion at risk
Transmitted by the bite of the female mosquito
Four species infect humans: *P. falciparum, P. vivax, P. ovale* and *P. malariae*
P. falciparum is the species that may cause rapidly progressive and fatal infection

Clinical features
Fever and muscle aches
Can resemble influenza
Temperature
Clinical signs are often absent but the spleen and liver may be enlarged in children

History
It is essential to take a history of travel to an endemic area

Diagnosis
Urgent blood smear (×3)
Dipstick antigen detection test

Treatment
P. falciparum infection must be treated with quinine
Infection with other species usually responds to chloroquine

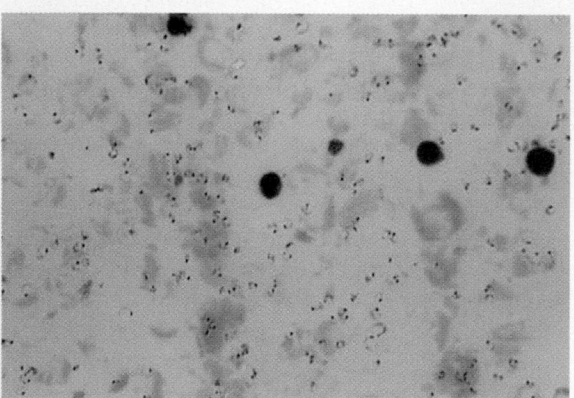

Fig. A Thick blood film showing *P. falciparum* trophozoites.

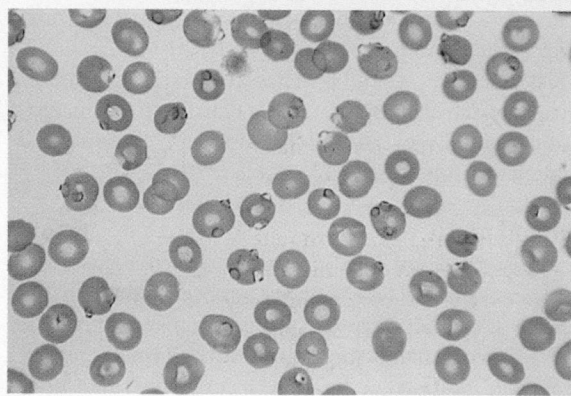

Fig. B Thin blood film showing *P. falciparum* trophozoites.

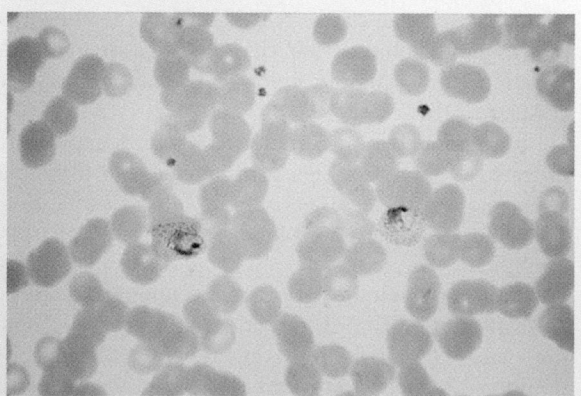

Fig. C Thin blood film showing *P. vivax* trophozoites

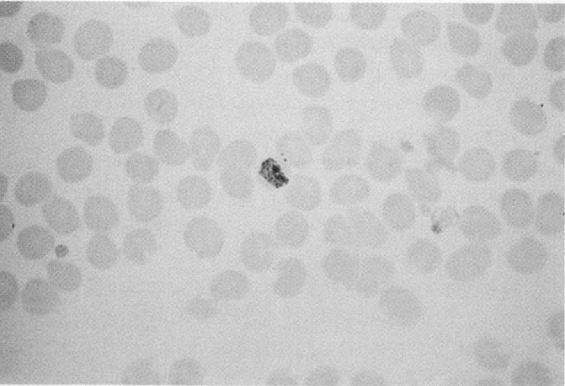

Fig. D Thin blood film showing *P. malariae* trophozoites. Figures C and D reproduced from Gillespie, *Medical Microbiology Illustrated*, 1994 (Butterworth Heinemann, Oxford) with the permission of the author and the publisher.

especially common in pregnant patients. Quinine levels must therefore be monitored where possible, together with blood glucose.

Patients should be reviewed 28 days after treatment to confirm parasitological and clinical cure. Those with splenic enlargement should avoid body contact sports and strenuous exercise because the enlarged spleen may rupture.

Plasmodium vivax, *P. ovale* and *P. malariae* infections are benign and fatal infections are rare in immunologically competent patients. Treatment with chloroquine is effective. *Plasmodium vivax* and *P. ovale* infections will relapse unless treatment is given to eradicate the liver hypnozoite stage (*P. falciparum* and *P. malariae* have no similar stage). Primaquine achieves radical cure in most cases. G6PD deficiency must be excluded as a haemolytic crisis may be provoked (see p. 1044). Radical cure is usually given only if there will be no further exposure to infective episodes (e.g. travellers returning from an endemic country).

Prevention

Personal protection against malaria depends on preventing mosquito bites, which occur mainly at night, and suppressing malaria parasites by chemoprophylaxis. Regular antimalarial prophylaxis should be taken for 1 week before travel to an endemic area and for 6 weeks after return, but the choice of regimen can be difficult because of changing patterns of resistance. Specialist advice should therefore be sought. The pattern of malaria drug resistance is changing all the time:
● In areas where there is no *P. falciparum* infection present, prophylaxis with chloroquine or proguanil alone is adequate.
● Where there is *P. falciparum*, and chloroquine and/or mefloquine resistance has also been reported, the situation is more complicated. In countries where chloroquine-resistant malaria is present, mefloquine or Malarone may be used. When mefloquine resistance is common, or as an alternative to mefloquine or Malarone, doxycycline can be prescribed.

In some places, multidrug resistance has been reported and the situation is changing rapidly, making prophylactic advice difficult. The public health services of most countries in Europe and North America publish recommendations for antimalarial prophylaxis, which are updated in the light of the changing situation and the availability of new antimalarial agents; these should be consulted before travelling.

Control of malaria in populations depends on reducing or eradicating the vector, the *Anopheles* mosquito. Methods include spraying houses with residual insecticide such as DDT, although mosquitoes have developed resistance to many of these agents, and destroying larval sites by removing standing water.

One of the major current research goals is the production of a malaria vaccine. Researchers are working on:
● Sporozoite vaccine directed against the stage injected by mosquitoes
● Merozoite vaccine, which attacks the blood stage
● Gametocyte vaccine, which will not prevent infection but is intended to reduce transmission, being directed against the parasite stage that infects mosquitoes
None of these vaccines has proved effective to date and a combined approach is probably necessary.

The cost of any future malaria vaccine is likely to be high and this may limit its value in the countries where it is most needed.

Prognosis

Plasmodium vivax, *P. ovale* and *P. malariae* infections are benign and fatal infections are rare in immunologically competent patients. *Plasmodium falciparum* infection can have a rapidly progressive course and high mortality in those with no immunity.

Typhoid and other enteric fevers
Epidemiology

Typhoid remains a common infection in many developing countries. It is rare in Europe, with many of these cases being imported; there are approximately 200 cases reported each year in the UK. In endemic countries, the peak incidence is in children under 5 years old. Imported cases are commonly adults. Infection is most common where sanitation is inadequate.

Causes

Typhoid fever is caused by *Salmonella typhi*. A closely similar, although usually less severe illness may be caused by *S. paratyphi* A or B or, less commonly, by other salmonellae. The collective name for these clinically indistinguishable conditions is enteric fever.

Disease mechanisms

Infection occurs following ingestion of water or food contaminated by human faeces, and is associated with poor sanitation. *Salmonella typhi* is extremely infectious: infection may occur with ingestion of as few as 10^3 organisms. Stomach acid, the resident gut flora, the spleen, and humoral and cell-mediated immunity all have a role in host defence. The natural history of infection is illustrated in Fig. 3.34.

Virulence (Vi) antigen is found almost universally on pathogenic strains. It is thought to prevent antibody binding to the somatic 'O' antigen. *Salmonella typhi* possesses

03

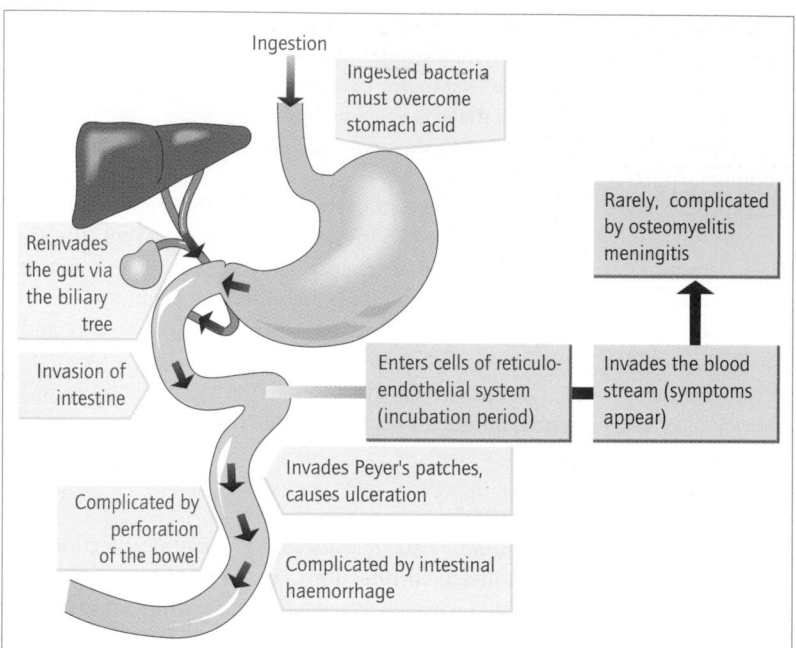

Figure 3.34 Typhoid pathogenesis.

LPS (see p. 66), which produces the characteristic symptoms of fever, chills, myalgia and anorexia by induction of cytokines such as TNF by macrophages.

Clinical features

The incubation period for typhoid fever is usually 1–3 weeks. The illness begins with a fever, increasing over 2 days to 38–40°C. Although fluctuating, the fever does not fall to normal and rigors may occur. Other symptoms include headache, cough, malaise and myalgia and, in the early stages, there may be constipation. Later, diarrhoea, abdominal tenderness, vomiting, delirium and confusion may occur.

Examination can reveal a relative bradycardia—the pulse rate is raised above normal, but less than would be expected for the height of the fever. A few inconspicuous pale red spots (rose spots) scattered over the trunk are seen in less than 20% of patients and are undetectable in pigmented skin. In paratyphoid, spots are more common and brighter red. The spleen may be enlarged and abdominal tenderness is common but not severe.

Complications typically arise in the third week. In the abdomen, ulcerated Peyer's patches may haemorrhage (1.7% of patients) or perforate (1–4% of patients). Osteomyelitis may develop, especially in those predisposed by sickle cell disease. Disseminated intravascular coagulation (DIC) and renal failure occur in severe infection. Other rare complications include cholecystitis, meningitis and typhoid pneumonia.

Investigation

The WBC is commonly suppressed and liver function tests may show a hepatic scenario.

Blood, urine and faecal cultures are indicated. A definitive diagnosis of typhoid is by culture of the organism from a normally sterile site such as the blood. In difficult cases when there is no growth, especially when some antibiotic treatment has already been given, culture of a bone marrow aspirate may be positive.

Management

Ciprofloxacin, which penetrates well into cells, is effective and is probably the first choice. Chloramphenicol remains standard therapy for typhoid in many developing countries. Co-trimoxazole is also effective and recent trials suggest good results with trimethoprim alone. Results with ampicillin are often disappointing. Alternative drugs in cases of multidrug resistance are ceftriaxone or azithromycin. Where facilities are adequate, surgery is the preferred treatment for complicating intestinal perforation.

Prevention

Control of typhoid, as with other enteric infections, depends on sanitation, clean water and personal hygiene. Vaccination is recommended for travellers to endemic countries. It has had a limited effect as a control measure, but provides useful protection in individuals. The first typhoid vaccine was a simple heat-killed vaccine provid-

Typhoid at a glance

Epidemiology

Prevalence
Up to 450/100 000 in some developing countries, rare in developed countries

Age
Most common in under-5-year-olds, imported cases often in adults

Geography
Worldwide, especially where there is poor sanitation

Findings on investigation

Haematology
Exclude malaria, WBC may be low

Biochemistry
Mild hepatitis may be present

Immunology
Standard agglutination ('Widal'), Vi and LPS test detect antigen

Microbiology
Culture blood, stool or bone marrow

Diagnostic imaging
Rarely required

Histopathology
Rarely required

Clinical features
Incubation 1–3 weeks
Fluctuating fever associated with diarrhoea, constipation, cough and generalized malaise
Spleen may be enlarged

Management

Drug treatment
Ciprofloxacin
Chloramphenicol
Co-trimoxazole
Trimethoprim

Surgery
Surgery for complicating intestinal perforation

Prevention
Sanitation
Clean water
Personal hygiene

Vaccination
Vaccination for travellers to endemic countries

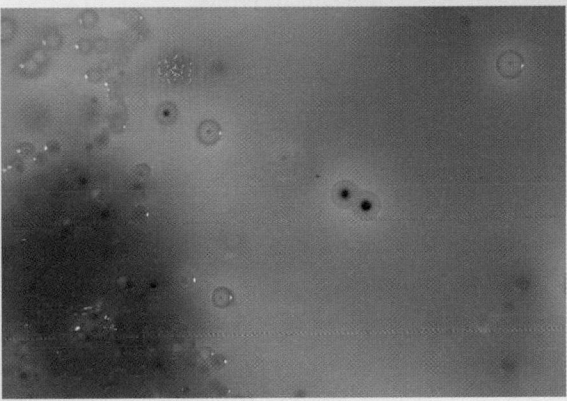

Fig. A Pink colonies of lactose-fermenting *Enterobacteriaceae* growing on MacConkey agar.

03

ing 65% protection, and a variant of this vaccine—the phenol-killed vaccine—is still in use. A live attenuated vaccine Ty21a has been produced, and extensive field trials have shown that it gives similar protection to phenol-killed vaccine but without the side-effects of local inflammatory response, fever and malaise that may accompany the phenol-killed vaccine. However, it is expensive and three doses on alternate days are required for adequate protection. An alternative approach is the use of purified Vi antigen vaccine administered parenterally.

Prognosis

The prognosis is good if treated early, but there is a significant mortality among patients who are shocked or who develop small bowel perforation.

Brucellosis

Other terms for brucellosis include undulant fever, Malta fever or Mediterranean fever. The causative organism was first isolated by Sir David Bruce from the spleens of soldiers dying of fever in Malta in 1886.

Epidemiology

This remains a common disease in developing countries but is a rare imported disease in Europe and North

America. Brucellosis is a zoonotic disease transmitted to humans from livestock, either directly or via food.

Disease mechanisms

The genus *Brucella* are small Gram-negative aerobic or carboxyphyllic coccobacilli. Three species are usually implicated in human disease: *B. melitensis*, which is usually found in goats; *B. abortus* in cattle; and *B. suis* in pigs.

Clinical features

The clinical manifestations of brucellosis are varied, and serological evidence in high-risk groups suggests that up to one-third of infections may be clinically non-apparent. About half the recognized cases present with an acute sys-temic febrile illness, which is often severe, and sometimes associated with cough, arthralgia or testicular pain. Others present with localized suppuration in a variety of sites but most often involving bones or joints, particularly the spine. Splenomegaly and lymphadenopathy occur in only about 15% of patients.

Very chronic disease can last for years and be characterized by non-specific features of fatigue and malaise but little or no fever. Neuropsychiatric features may predominate.

Investigation

The FBC may reveal anaemia of chronic disease, and the ESR is elevated. *Brucella* may be diagnosed by serological

Brucellosis at a glance

Epidemiology

Prevalence
Approximately 500 000 cases worldwide

Age
All ages, imported cases usually in adults

Geography
Eradicated in many developed countries, common in Middle East and South America

Findings on investigation

Haematology
Anaemia

Biochemistry
Not helpful

Immunology
Standard agglutination test, radio immunoassay or ELISA detect antibodies

Microbiology
Culture blood, bone marrow or other tissue

Diagnostic imaging
Radiograph of lumbosacral spine

Histopathology
Liver biopsy may reveal brucellosis as an unexpected diagnosis

Clinical features
3-week incubation period
Undulant fever
Myalgia
Sacroileitis
Splenomegaly

May be complicated by epidymitis, arthritis
Meningoencephalitis and neuropsychiatric symptoms have been associated

Management

Drug treatment
Tetracycline alone or with streptomycin for the first 14 days
Co-trimoxazole is an alternative
Rifampicin has been used in combination therapy

Surgery
Collections of pus may require surgical drainage

Prevention
Mass testing of cattle and slaughter of infected herds
Pasteurization of milk

Vaccination
A vaccine is available for cattle, but is unsuitable for human use

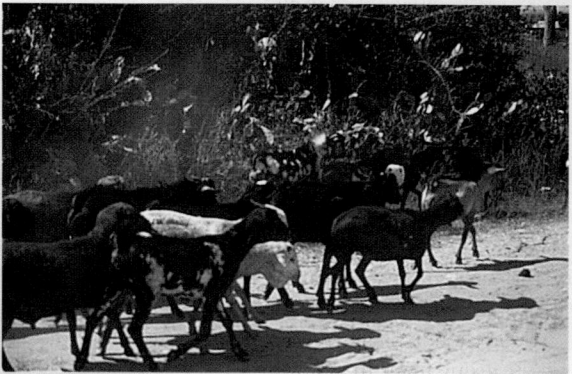

Fig. A Environment for transmission of brucellosis.

means. ELISA and radio immunoassay to detect IgG and IgM have been described and are available as a reference service.

Definitive diagnosis is made by culture of *Brucella* from blood, bone marrow or pus. This may take 10 days or longer so the microbiological laboratory should be alerted to the need for prolonged incubation. Bone marrow culture produces the highest diagnostic yield and will remain positive for some days after the commencement of antimicrobial chemotherapy.

Management

The intracellular location of *Brucella* makes treatment difficult and relapse is common. Tetracycline has been used alone, but the addition of streptomycin for the first 14 days is associated with a lower incidence of relapse. Co-trimoxazole is an alternative, and rifampicin has been used in combination therapy. Collections of pus may require surgical drainage.

Prevention

The prevention of human disease depends on controlling brucellosis in the animal population. Mass testing of cattle and slaughter of infected herds has virtually eliminated endemic brucellosis in northern Europe, USA, Israel and Japan. A vaccine is available for cattle, but is unsuitable for human use. Pasteurization of milk reduces the risk to urban populations in endemic countries.

Prognosis

With appropriate chemotherapy almost all patients make a full recovery but relapses are quite common. A small number may have chronic non-specific symptoms.

Arboviruses

The common characteristic of arboviruses is that they are arthropod-borne: they are transmitted by insect or arachnid vectors in which they can also replicate. This is a major adaptation for viruses, which tend to be very host specific.

Most arboviruses are concentrated into two specialized families of RNA viruses:
- Togaviruses: subdivided into alphaviruses and flaviviruses
- Bunyaviruses

Hundreds of arboviruses have been identified and most are purely animal pathogens. Forty or so are of medical importance, but cause a relatively restricted range of clinical syndromes including 'break bone fever', encephalitis and viral haemorrhagic fever. Most arboviruses are capable of causing more than one of these syndromes. Many also cause a non-specific febrile illness, often with a rash. Additional clinical features are associated with particular viruses; for example, polyarthritis with Ross River virus in Australia and the Pacific islands, and retinitis with Rift Valley fever in East Africa.

Plague (*Yersinia pestis*)

This is a vector-borne bacterial disease that has caused pandemics in the past, associated with high mortality.

Epidemiology

Plague is a zoonosis that is capable of spreading from person to person. Plague is a disease of rodents transmitted to humans by a flea bite. Contact with infected fleas results from disturbing the natural hosts (e.g. ground squirrels, gerbils) or if domestic rats acquire the disease. Pneumonic plague can be passed on by respiratory transmission. In past centuries there has been pandemic spread. Plague is now limited to a small number of endemic foci where the disease continues in North America, South America, Central Africa and the Far East. There are concerns that this organism could be used for bioterrorism purposes.

Disease mechanisms

Yersinia pestis is the bacterium responsible for disease. It possesses a capsule and potent toxins.

Clinical features

There are two major clinical presentations. Bubonic plague has an incubation period of 1–6 days and patients present with rapidly developing high fever, malaise and delirium. There is a regional adenopathy and tender buboes; drain the site of infection. Petechial or purpuric haemorrhages are common, and the disease progresses to septic shock.

Pneumonic plague is acquired from respiratory spread. A severe illness develops within 10–15 h of the onset of a high fever, and is characterized by tachypnoea, restlessness and shortness of breath. Respiratory signs are, however, often absent. Frothy blood-tinged sputum is usually produced as a preterminal event.

Mild plague (pestis minor) occurs occasionally. It is accompanied by few systemic signs, but organisms can be cultured from a bubo.

Investigations

In bubonic and pneumonic plague *Y. pestis* can be isolated from the blood, sputum and buboes. Organisms in smears can be Gram-stained. This work should only be performed in specialized laboratories.

Management

Streptomycin and tetracyclines or chloramphenicol are the drugs of choice, but treatment after 15 h probably does

03

not influence the course of pneumonic plague. Plague is highly infectious, and specimens must be handled with extreme care. Patients and their possessions must be disinfected of fleas and strictly isolated. Staff should be monitored carefully for fever and treated promptly, while household contacts should be offered tetracycline prophylaxis.

Prognosis

Untreated, the mortality of bubonic plague is 60–90% and of pneumonic plague 100%.

Typhus and other rickettsial infections

Rickettsia have a complex life cycle that includes a range of vectors. Different pathogens produce slightly different conditions in different parts of the world.

Disease mechanisms

Rickettsia are small bacteria that, like *Chlamydia* and viruses, are only capable of replication within another cell. They are transmitted between their mammalian hosts by an arthropod vector. Typically, the natural mammalian host is a rodent, with humans acquiring the infection as a zoonosis. Only epidemic typhus is primarily a disease of humans.

Clinical features

In many rickettsial infections the organism first replicates at the site of the infected arthropod bite. This may give rise to a characteristic skin lesion, called an eschar, which is a small painless ulcer with a black centre (Fig. 3.14). The infection then becomes generalized, with a predilection for skin and endothelial cells. There is an accompanying fever, which in the more severe infections is high and unremitting. If there is a rash it appears around the fourth or fifth day of the illness and may have either a dusky macular appearance or be petechial. In the most serious infections there are complications induced by multiorgan damage, which usually appear towards the end of the second week. A rickettsial infection should be suggested by the combination of fever with either the typical rash or an eschar and by an appropriate travel history.

Investigation

Confirmation of infection by specific serology is now available for many *Rickettsia* in reference laboratories.

Management

Tetracycline and chloramphenicol are both effective treatments if given early in the course of disease.

Q fever

Q (or query) fever is caused by *Coxiella* closely related to *Rickettsia* but not requiring a vector for transmission.

Epidemiology

Found throughout the world, the most common animal reservoirs are cattle, sheep and goats. It is principally an occupational condition of farm and abattoir workers who come into contact with grazing animals, which are the source of infection. Transmission is most often by aerosol, but infected milk may be another route.

Disease mechanisms

Q fever is caused by *Coxiella burnetti*, a small intracellular bacterium related to the *Rickettsia*.

Clinical features

The acute illness presents as a fever and atypical pneumonia, sometimes accompanied by granulomatous hepatitis. *Coxiella burnetti* is also an important cause of culture-negative endocarditis (see p. 478).

Investigation

The diagnosis is usually confirmed by serology.

Management

Chloramphenicol and tetracycline are effective if given early. Rifampicin may also be effective.

Prognosis

Usually good, although relapse may occur.

Leishmaniasis

Epidemiology

Leishmaniasis can be found in India, China, the Middle East, East Africa, the Mediterranean and South America.

Disease mechanisms

Leishmania are flagellate protozoan parasites that may be transmitted to humans by the bite of a sandfly. They have two stages in their life cycle: the motile promastigote in the salivary secretions of the sandfly; and the amastigote in the macrophages and cells of the reticuloendothelial system of the mammalian host. Infective blood meals may come from another human or from the animal reservoir host (Fig. 3.35), which may be a dog or rodent, depending on the species of *Leishmania*. Direct person–person spread can occur.

   Leishmania species are morphologically identical under the light microscope (Fig. 3.36). The major species are:
• *Leishmania donovani* and *L. infantum:* cause visceral leishmaniasis

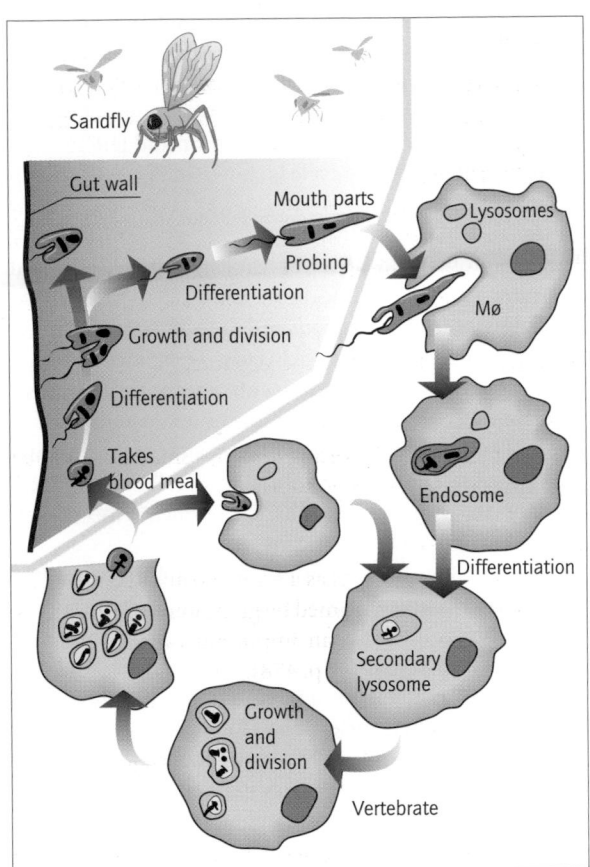

Figure 3.35 Life cycle of *Leishmania*.

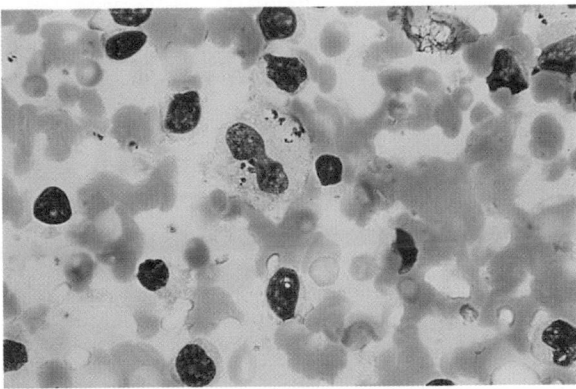

Figure 3.36 Amastigotes of *Leishmania donovani*. Reproduced from Gillespie, *Medical Microbiology Illustrated*, 1994 (Butterworth–Heinemann, Oxford) with the permission of the publisher and author.

extracellular excreted factor that interferes with the function of lytic enzymes, and scavenges toxic free radicals. Cells of the reticuloendothelial system are infected, resulting in hepatosplenomegaly. The cells of the macrophage lineage secrete cytokines such as TNF and IL-1, resulting in the characteristic features of fever and cachexia.

Clinical features
The incubation period of visceral leishmaniasis is usually 2–4 months, but may be as short as 10 days or longer than 1 year. The onset is usually insidious, but may be more acute in those from non-endemic countries. Patients present with anorexia, malaise and weight loss, and may complain of abdominal discomfort resulting from splenic enlargement.

Signs include anaemia and cachexia, and the liver and spleen are enlarged. There may be a primary cutaneous lesion resembling cutaneous leishmaniasis. Fever is intermittent and undulant and often spikes twice a day.

Investigations
There is a profound normocytic normochromic anaemia (haemoglobin <7 g/dl), thrombocytopenia and leucopenia. Immunoglobulin concentrations, especially IgM, are elevated, and specific antileishmania antibodies can be detected by a variety of techniques. *Leishmania donovani* amastigotes can be found by direct microscopy of the bone marrow or splenic aspirate. Occasionally, amastigotes can be demonstrated in the buffy coat cells. Culture can be performed.

Management
Liposomal amphotericin B has revolutionized the treatment of visceral leishmaniasis. Alternatives include pentamidine.

- *Leishmania tropica* and *L. major:* cause Old World cutaneous leishmaniasis
- *Leishmania braziliensis* and *L. mexicana:* agents of New World cutaneous (American) leishmaniasis. The former infection can be complicated by destructive mucocutaneous lesions known as espundia

Antigenic and DNA analysis has demonstrated a number of subspecies. The vectors fall into two genera: *Phlebotomus* (Old World) and *Lutzomyia* (New World).

Visceral leishmaniasis (kala-azar)
Causes and disease mechanisms
Two species are implicated: *L. donovani* and *L. infantum* (Mediterranean). Promastigotes are injected by the bite of an infected sandfly and are phagocytosed by macrophages using a mechanism that does not stimulate a respiratory burst which would have killed the parasite. The organism differentiates into the amastigote form, which is adapted for survival inside the phagolysosome by virtue of an

Prognosis

Untreated, patients slowly deteriorate and die, usually from secondary infections after about 2 years.

Cutaneous leishmaniasis

Disease mechanisms

Old World cutaneous leishmaniasis is caused by three species: *L. tropica*, *L. major* and *L. aethiopica*. *Leishmania mexicana* and *L. brasiliensis* occur in the New World. They are transmitted to humans by the bite of a sandfly or from a reservoir host.

Clinical features

The incubation period is variable—from a few days to more than 6 months. The lesion begins as a small itching papule, which increasingly infiltrates the dermis and crust. When scratched the lesion becomes a shallow discharging ulcer. After 3 months or more the lesion heals to form a depressed white or brown scar. The infection causes an associated regional lymphadenopathy. South American lesions can be very destructive of the nasal mucosa and relapse after a prolonged period.

Investigation

The diagnosis of cutaneous leishmaniasis is made as for visceral disease using serology and cutaneous biopsy.

Management

Pentavalent antimonials are the mainstay of therapy, although other drugs including amphotericin B have been used, especially for American (New World) leishmaniasis.

Trypanosomiasis

Three trypanosomes are pathogenic to humans. *Trypanosoma brucei gambiense* and *T. brucei rhodesiense* are transmitted to humans through the bite of a blood-sucking fly of the *Glossinia* genus (tsetse fly). *Trypanosoma cruzi* infects humans by inoculation of faeces from its blood-sucking insect vector, the triatomid bug.

African trypanosomiasis

Epidemiology

Up to 20 000 cases are reported each year in Africa. *Trypanosoma brucei gambiense* is an infection of river and lakeside areas of West and Central Africa; *T. brucei rhodesiense* is found in southern and eastern Africa.

Disease mechanisms

Humans are the main reservoir of infection of *T. brucei gambiense* and wild antelope, particularly the bush buck, is the main reservoir of infection for *T. brucei rhodesiense*.

The parasites spread through the lymphatics and circulation, first travelling from the inoculation site to the regional lymph nodes and then disseminating. Endarteritis, pericarditis and meningoencephalitis develop, and there may be polyclonal B-cell activation and DIC.

The trypanosome life cycle is shown in Fig. 3.37.

Clinical features

The symptoms and signs of *T. brucei gambiense* and *T. brucei rhodesiense* infections are similar except that the illness of *T. brucei gambiense* infection runs a more chronic course lasting up to 3 years. *Trypanosoma brucei rhodesiense* infection is more acute and untreated infection can cause death in a few months and usually within 1 year. The incubation period of African trypanosomiasis is 2–3 weeks. The original bite may be followed by local swelling (the trypanosomal chancre), which is more often seen in Europeans than Africans.

The next stage occurs with bloodstream invasion. It is characterized clinically by an intermittent fever (up to 41°C at regular intervals), which may be accompanied by erythema, and sometimes by a form of hyperaesthesia—the skin over the tibia is tender to touch, but the pain is only perceived after a brief delay (Kérandel's sign).

As the infection progresses, patients become increasingly debilitated and have a persistent tachycardia, generalized lymphadenopathy and splenomegaly. Prominent glands in the posterior cervical triangle in *T. brucei gambiense* infection are known as Winterbottom's sign. The skin, especially of the face, may be oedematous, and Europeans may have a flitting erythematous rash on the trunk. Death is brought about by encephalitis:

- In *T. brucei gambiense* infection, this is typically an insidious chronic process characterized by progressive mental deterioration. The patient is unable to exert him or herself, has a slow shuffling gait and a vacant expression, and does not readily take part in voluntary activity. He or she may lapse into sleep during the day and progressively lose weight. Tremor, convulsions, focal neurological signs and a persistent headache are features. The body wastes and the patient becomes comatose, finally succumbing to a secondary infection.

- An acute encephalitis accompanied by a rapid onset of coma and death within a few weeks is more typical of *T. brucei rhodesiense* infection.

Investigations

African trypanosomiasis should be suspected in a patient with fever and lymphadenopathy who has recently stayed in an endemic area. It must be differentiated from malaria, leishmaniasis, tuberculosis, brucellosis and lymphoma and, in the late encephalitic stage, from cerebral tumour, tuberculous meningitis, viral encephalitis and tertiary syphilis.

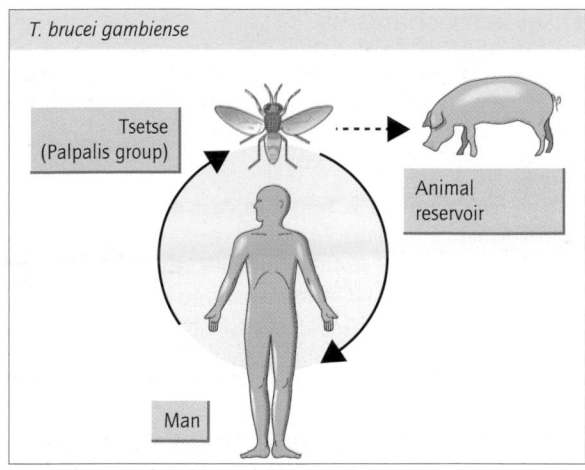

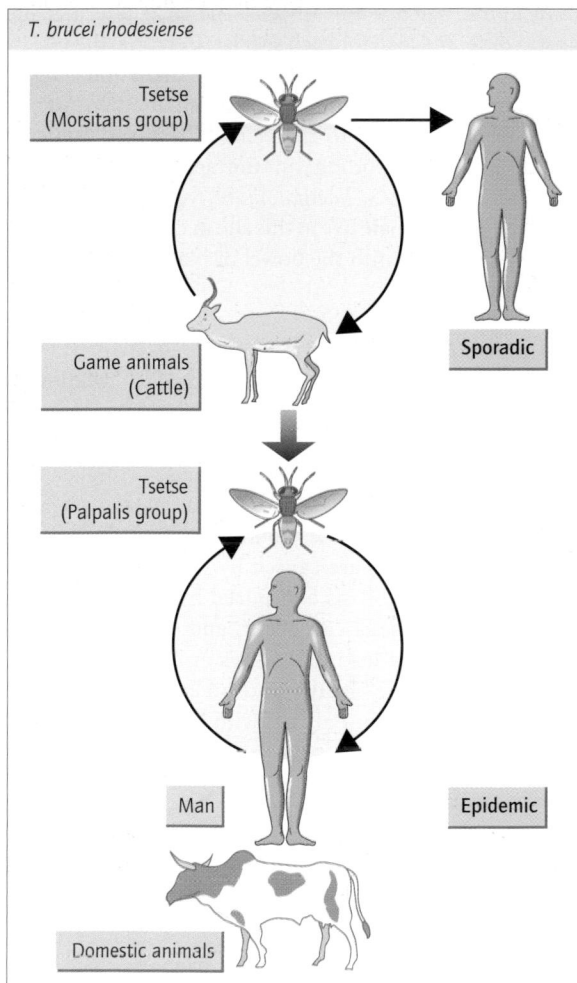

Figure 3.37 Life cycle of African trypanosomiasis differentiating the life cycle of West (*gambiense*) and East (*rhodesiense*) African trypanosomiasis. Reproduced from Bell, *Lecture Notes on Tropical Medicine*, 4th edn, 1995 (Blackwell Science, Oxford) with the permission of the author.

The ESR is typically very high and parasites can be identified by examining thick and thin blood films. A buffy coat preparation helps to concentrate the organisms (see Fig. 11.3, p. 768). Serum IgM is typically very high. An ELISA method is available for diagnosis, but is of more value for large-scale field surveys than for diagnosing individual patients.

On CSF examination, CSF cell count is increased if there is CNS involvement and protein is elevated.

Management

Suramin has been the treatment of choice for African trypanosomiasis before invasion of the CNS has occurred. Melarsoprol (MelB) is able to cross the blood–brain barrier and is therefore useful for the management of the later stages. Eflornithine is the treatment of choice for West African infection if available.

Prevention

Control strategies are based on eliminating tsetse flies, usually by widescale spraying of insecticides such as DDT from aircraft. This is often effective, but causes considerable ecological damage. More subtle tsetse traps, based on colour and odour attractants, have now been developed but have been used only in limited areas.

Prognosis

Untreated *T. brucei rhodesiense* infection can cause death in a few months and usually within 1 year. The prognosis is better when treatment is started in the early stages, but there is a 10% mortality if it is treated late.

South American trypanosomiasis

Epidemiology

Up to 10–12 million people are infected. Eighty five per cent of acute infections occur in children under 10 years of age. The mean age for chronic disease is 33–45 years of age.

Disease mechanisms

Trypanosoma cruzi is the aetiological agent of South American trypanosomiasis or Chagas' disease. *Trypanosoma cruzi* pass through three stages in their life cycle: amastigote, epimastigote and trypomastigote, and are transmitted to humans by triatomid or reduviid bugs. Triatomid bugs live in cracks and crevices in poorly constructed houses in South America. Infected bugs excrete infective epimastigotes in their faeces and the organism is inoculated into a bite when the victim scratches.

Trypanosomes can also be transmitted by transfusion of blood and blood products. This is an important public health concern in South America, and in countries where donors frequently travel to endemic countries.

03

Clinical features

Infection with *T. cruzi* falls into four stages:

1 Short incubation period.

2 *Acute stage:* often asymptomatic or unrecognized because the symptoms are non-specific, although there is a local inflammatory reaction at the site of the bite (the chagoma) accompanied by regional lymphadenopathy (Romaña's sign). There is an acute febrile illness associated with malaise, and oedema of the face and legs. Generalized lymphadenopathy and hepatomegaly may also be found. About 15% of people with acute infection develop myocarditis and most deaths are caused by this complication.

3 *Latent stage:* follows the acute stage and is an asymptomatic period lasting up to 25 years.

4 *Final stage:* Chagas' disease is characterized by cardiomyopathy and intractable congestive cardiac failure, cardiac arrhythmias and thromboembolism. In addition, there may be oesophageal dilatation resulting from achalasia or chagasic megacolon. These conditions were thought to result from parasympathetic nerve fibre degeneration, but more recent evidence indicates that they probably result from direct tissue damage.

Diagnosis

Diagnosis of acute South American trypanosomiasis can be made by examining Giemsa-stained preparations of peripheral blood for the presence of parasites. An ELISA is available to detect serum antibodies to *T. cruzi*. This is most useful for excluding Chagas' disease in patients who have lived in endemic countries, and in sero-epidemiological surveys.

Management

Nifurtimox and benznidazole are the only agents with activity against *T. cruzi*.

Prevention

South American trypanosomiasis may be controlled by improving housing construction to remove the vector breeding sites, and by spraying houses with residual insecticide.

Prognosis

The prognosis of Chagas' disease depends on the involvement of the heart, oesophagus and colon. Cardiac failure and arrhythmias may be alleviated by treatment. Oesophageal carcinoma, and chronic constipation and intestinal obstruction can develop.

Helminthic infections

Schistosomiasis

This is a chronic infection of the venous system with blood flukes of the *Schistosoma* genus.

Disease mechanisms

Schistosomiasis or bilharzia is caused by one of the three main species of blood fluke that infect humans: *Schistosoma mansoni*, *S. haematobium* and *S. japonicum*.

Epidemiology

Schistosoma mansoni is found in Africa, the Caribbean, South America and the Middle East; *S. haematobium* is found only in Africa and the Middle East; and *S. japonica* is found in the Far East. There are more than 200 million cases worldwide. The incidence of disease is highest in teenagers and there is a male predominance.

Life cycle

Eggs are shed in the urine or faeces and once in water a miracidium hatches and invades the snail intermediate host; a different snail for each species. Cercaria, the infective stage for humans, emerge from the snails and actively penetrate the human skin. The organism matures into an adult, which migrates to the veins of the mesenteric or vesical plexus depending on the species: *S. mansoni*, mesenteric plexus; *S. haematobium*, vesical plexus. The adult male and female live at this site in copula, producing eggs which escape into the bowel or bladder to complete the life cycle.

Clinical features

An intensely itchy, vesicular rash known as 'swimmer's itch' is found at the site of cercarial penetration. As the adult worms are maturing, patients may develop a syndrome characterized by fever, malaise arthralgia and splenomegaly (Katayama fever). When egg laying begins, patients may complain of bloody diarrhoea or haematuria. Complications are caused by the presence of eggs in the liver, liver fibrosis and portal hypertension. Lung fibrosis and dyspnoea can occur, and eggs in the brain or spinal canal can lead to seizures or transection of the cord. Fibrosis of the bladder leads to loss of capacity and may be premalignant. Patients with low egg counts may have few symptoms after the initial acute phase of the infection.

Investigations

The diagnosis is made by demonstrating the presence of eggs in the stool or urine (Fig. 3.38). Rectal biopsy may be used in patients likely to have a low egg burden. Serological diagnosis by ELISA supports the diagnosis.

Management and prognosis

Schistosomiasis is readily treatable with a single dose of praziquantel (see p. 100). When the egg count is low the prognosis is excellent but the long-term consequences of heavy infections, liver or lung fibrosis cannot be reversed by chemotherapy.

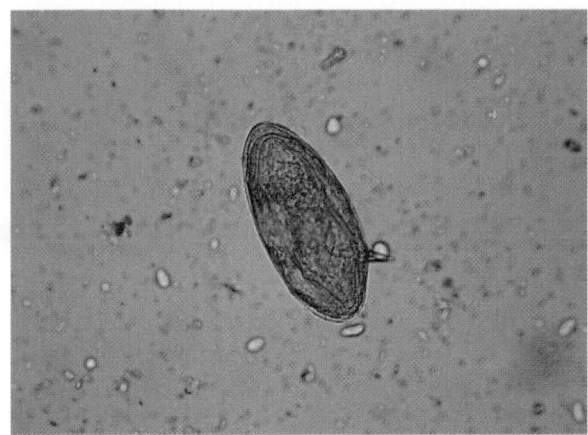

Figure 3.38 Egg of *S. mansoni* in the stool. The lateral spine is characteristic of this species. *S. haematobium* has a terminal spine and *S. japonicum* is more rounded with a small spine. Reproduced from Gillespie, *Medical Microbiology Illustrated*, 1994 (Butterworth–Heinemann, Oxford) with the permission of the publisher and author.

Hydatid disease

Causes
The two main species infecting humans are *Echinococcus granulosus* and *E. multilocularis.*

Epidemiology
Hydatid disease is endemic throughout the world. The life cycle is shown in Fig. 3.9.

Disease mechanisms and clinical features
Symptoms arise because of the presence of cysts, usually in the liver, sometimes in the lungs and brain and rarely in other tissues. The cysts may be asymptomatic or produce local pain. Release of cyst contents can result in multiple cysts in the peritoneum and the release of parasite antigens can produce acute anaphylaxis.

Investigation
Cysts are identified by ultrasound and CT scanning. ELISA methods to detect specific antibody and antigens support the diagnosis.

Management
Treatment depends on a combination of surgery and chemotherapy. Albendazole is active against the germinal epithelium of the cysts and praziquantel against the protoscolices. Prognosis depends on operability of the cysts, but some regress with chemotherapy.

Fever with generalized lymphadenopathy

The syndrome of fever with lymphadenopathy and atypical lymphocytes in the peripheral blood is usually known as infectious mononucleosis or glandular fever (see p. 142). Other infections can also cause similar syndromes of persistent fever with lymphadenopathy. A careful history of possible exposure to any of these organisms, such as a partner with a sore throat (infectious mononucleosis), should be taken (see HISTORY & EXAMINATION BOX 3.2). A sexual history may reveal behaviour that has put the patient at risk of HIV infection or syphilis.

The patient presents with acute or subacute sore throat and cervical gland enlargement. There is commonly malaise, which is usually worse in adult patients. The voice may have a nasal quality in infectious mononucleosis as a result of tonsillar swelling.

Toxoplasmosis

Epidemiology
Toxoplasma gondii is a protozoan parasite whose definitive host is the cat. Faecal shedding of the oocyst transmits the infection to other intermediate hosts. Humans are usually infected by eating undercooked meat, but contact with cats may be relevant. Seroprevalence varies from country to country depending on the culinary habits. In general, the rate of seropositivity rises with age. Toxoplasmosis can be spread from mother to infant *in utero.*

Cause
Toxoplasmosis is caused by the protozoan organism *Toxoplasma gondii.*

Disease mechanisms
Pathologically, acute infection is characterized by the rapid multiplication of tachyzoites (growing stages) in cells throughout the body. Increasing humoral and, more importantly, T-cell immunity force a change to a semidormant bradyzoite 'sleeping' stage confined to cysts in somatic tissue. If T-cell immunity fails later in life, the dormant bradyzoites may reactivate to tachyzoites to cause further pathology.

Clinical features
Toxoplasmosis causes three clinical syndromes: acute mononucleosis, neonatal infection and cerebral toxoplasmosis in the immunocompromised.

Acute mononucleosis
Acute mononucleosis represents the extreme of acute *Toxoplasma* infection, which is usually asymptomatic. It is

03

characterized by fevers, malaise, weakness and anorexia. Hepatosplenomegaly and generalized lymphadenopathy are common, and may be complicated by myocarditis. The duration of illness is variable, but usually self-limiting.

Congenital infection
Congenital infection—characterized by fetal hepatosplenomegaly, chorioretinitis and mental retardation—occurs when a mother suffers an acute infection during pregnancy. The risk of congenital toxoplasmosis when mothers are seropositive before the conception of the fetus are less than 5%.

Investigations
Evidence of acute infection during pregnancy is an indication for fetal blood sampling at 18 weeks and cord blood following delivery. The presence of IgM or amplification of *Toxoplasma*-specific DNA in neonatal blood indicates neonatal infection.

T-cell immunity is essential to control *Toxoplasma* infection. In patients with HIV infection, the risk of cerebral toxoplasmosis increases with the development of more severe immunosuppression. Other causes of severe T-cell deficiency (e.g. cytotoxic drug therapy) may also lead to reactivation of toxoplasmosis. Symptoms include headache, confusion and lethargy, progressing to a focal neurological deficit or seizures. Examination usually reveals a focal neurological deficit.

Diagnosis of cerebral toxoplasmosis is usually based on the clinical features, a history of immunosuppression, a positive agglutination test and characteristic CT scan appearance.

Management
Acute toxoplasmosis is usually asymptomatic, but some patients with severe or prolonged symptoms or with complicated infection require antimicrobial therapy. Acute infection in an immunocompromised person is an indication for treatment. Treatment consists of spiramycin or a combination of sulfadiazine and pyrimethamine.

Women who have a suspected acute infection in pregnancy should be prescribed spiramycin for the duration of pregnancy or until fetal blood sampling. If this reveals fetal infection, a termination of pregnancy may be considered. If the pregnancy is continued the chemotherapy should be changed to sulfadiazine and pyrimethamine.

Sulfadiazine and pyrimethamine, or dapsone and pyrimethamine are used for cerebral toxoplasmosis. Clindamycin and a spiramycin and pyrimethamine combination have also been used, but their comparative efficacy has not been assessed. In HIV infection, therapy should be continued indefinitely because relapse is common.

Prognosis
The prognosis is related to that of the underlying condition. Most patients respond to treatment.

Epstein–Barr virus infection
This is an acute systemic infection by the Epstein–Barr virus.

Epidemiology
Antibody studies show that about 50% of preteenage children have been exposed to Epstein–Barr virus (EBV), while more than 75% of over 25-year-olds have antibodies. In developing countries 75–90% of 5-year-olds have antibodies. Infection is often mild or asymptomatic in children. Symptomatic infection is most common in the teenager or young adult.

Disease mechanisms
Infectious mononucleosis results from EBV infection of B lymphocytes. The virus is present in saliva and is spread by close contact.

Clinical features
Infection is usually asymptomatic in children, but causes clinical disease in the 15–20-year age group. There are two major clinical presentations:

1 *Anginose type:* with exudative tonsillitis, palatal petechiae, facial and peritonsillar oedema, nasal intonation and cervical lymphadenopathy
2 *Juvenile type:* with generalized lymphadenopathy, mild sore throat and low-grade pyrexia

Complications include pharyngeal obstruction, hepatitis, pancreatitis, myocarditis, meningoencephalitis, malignant lymphoid proliferation (Duncan's syndrome) and chronic fatigue syndrome.

Investigations
The peripheral blood reveals a mononucleosis and 'atypical lymphocytes' in large numbers.

Paul–Bunnell test
Diagnosis is made by a rapid slide agglutination technique. Definitive diagnosis is by detection of specific IgM to EBV viral capsid antigen. Other causes of the glandular fever syndrome will need to be excluded (e.g. CMV, toxoplasmosis, HIV, lymphoma, syphilis). Specific EBV antibodies can be detected in acute infection.

Management
There is no specific treatment, but corticosteroids may be required if the airway is in danger of obstruction because of peritonsillar oedema. Sore throats should not be treated

with ampicillin because this drug causes a skin rash in patients with infectious mononucleosis.

Prognosis

This is good; most patients make an uncomplicated recovery.

Cytomegalovirus infection

Cytomegalovirus is an acute infection with the herpes virus cytomegalovirus.

Epidemiology

More than 50% of women of childbearing age living in developed countries have antibodies to CMV.

Disease mechanisms

Cytomegalovirus is a ubiquitous DNA virus of the herpes family. In developed countries, transmission occurs during infancy and most children have been exposed by the age of 5 years. CMV infection has become increasingly important because of infection in the immunosuppressed, especially following transplantation and in end-stage HIV infection.

Clinical features

In the immunocompetent, infection with CMV is usually asymptomatic. Occasionally, it causes a glandular fever-like illness without a sore throat, which is usually self-limiting. In the immunosuppressed, CMV infection may cause a progressive illness with severe organ involvement. Gastrointestinal infection can result in severe colitis with fever, diarrhoea and abdominal pain, and occasionally mucosal ulceration. Retinitis causes visual disturbance, eventually progressing to blindness. Fundoscopy reveals irregularity and luminal narrowing of the retinal vessels associated with granular white spots and, in more advanced infection, areas of haemorrhage and infarction. Other complications of CMV infection include interstitial pneumonitis, encephalitis, transverse myelitis, hepatitis cholangitis and adrenal necrosis.

Congenital infection occurs when there is a primary maternal infection. The incidence varies from 1/100 to 1/500, and 25–50 maternal infections/year result in congenital infection. About 50% of affected fetuses show signs of infection, which include hepatomegaly, splenomegaly, purpura and jaundice, all of which may resolve. Microcephaly is the most common neurological abnormality.

Investigations

Cytomegalovirus is frequently isolated from people with HIV in the absence of symptoms. Evidence of pathogenicity should therefore be obtained before attributing CMV to a particular disease complex. This usually requires identification of inclusion bodies in biopsy material or the growth of virus from tissue rather than body fluid.

Immunology

Monoclonal antibodies to early antigens can be used to detect virus in tissue samples. The virus can also be grown in tissue culture but this has now been superseded by PCR-based diagnosis.

Management

Treatment of CMV infection is only required if there is organ involvement. Ganciclovir is an analogue of deoxyguanosine (see p. 101), which can delay progression of CMV retinopathy. Pneumonitis and encephalitis respond less well. Phosphonoformate (foscarnet) is a pyrophosphate analogue that has proved successful in some patients.

Prognosis

The outcome of CMV disease in HIV infection in the long term is generally poor.

Common childhood fevers and exanthems

These diseases are usually thought of as diseases of children but, with increasing immunization against them, their incidence in children is falling (Table 3.29). They are then seen more commonly in adults, as some people missed immunization and did not meet the disease during childhood, while others have developed only poor immunity in response to immunization. In adults, the presentation of these diseases can be atypical and the course modified.

Varicella (chickenpox)

Varicella is caused by varicella zoster virus (VZV), also known as herpes zoster virus (HZV).

Epidemiology

This is predominantly a childhood infection but adult chickenpox is seen more frequently in populations amongst whom the disease is less common, especially if a person moves to an area of increased transmission. In non-immune populations chickenpox spreads readily, with an incubation period of 2–3 weeks.

Disease mechanisms

Chickenpox is caused by a DNA virus of the herpes group called VZV. The virus is highly infectious and is transmitted by droplets and fomites. A patient is infectious from the start of the illness until the last scab has cleared.

03

Table 3.29 Common childhood exanthema

Measles	Chickenpox	Rubella (German measles)	Erythema infectiosum	Mumps
Causative virus				
Paramyxovirus (RNA)	Herpesvirus (DNA)	Togavirus (RNA)	Parvovirus (DNA)	Paramyxovirus (RNA)
Spread				
Droplet	Droplet, fomite	Droplet	Droplet	Droplet
Incubation period				
8–14 days	14–21 days	14–21 days		4–18 days
Infectious period				
2–3 days before rash	Until crusts dry			15 days before to 4 days after parotitis
Prodrome				
Conjunctival suffusion, cough, fever, Koplik's spots on the palate	Fever, malaise of a few hours or no prodrome	Malaise or no prodrome	Malaise, arthralgia	Sore throat, fever, pain at angle of jaw
Rash				
Blotchy macular rash becoming confluent appears about day 4, beginning on the forehead, spreading onto trunk and limbs over 3–4 days. Clears after 4–5 days, often with fine desquamation and brown discoloration	Pink macules, mainly central (trunk, face)—rapidly evolve into papules and vesiculate, dry and crust over. Different stages present at the same time	Fine macular rash develops over face and upper arms and spreads down. Fades after 3 days	'Slapped cheek' appearance, and a lacy rash on thighs	None
Other clinical features				
	Mild conjunctivitis, sore throat and cervical adenopathy, especially postcervical, occipital, and postauricular Forscheimer's spots may be seen	Fever and generalized arthralgia		Meningitis
Complications				
Mainly respiratory—secondary viral pneumonia and rarely giant cell pneumonia, bronchitis and otitis media. Myocarditis, encephalitis, hepatitis and subacute sclerosing panencephalitis (SSPE) are rare complications	Secondary bacterial pneumonia, chickenpox pneumonitis, bacterial infection of spots, disseminated chickenpox (especially in the immunosuppressed), cerebellar ataxia (may precede or follow the rash), haemorrhagic chickenpox	Asymmetrical large joint arthropathy, teratogenicity	Persisting arthralgia, aplastic crisis in those with haemolytic disease	Swollen parotid, submandibular gland, pancreatitis, orchitis, mastitis, sterility (controversial—it has proved difficult to show that sterility following orchitis is a consequence of the orchitis and sterility is not inevitable), meningitis

03

Clinical features

The illness usually begins within 14–21 days with the appearance of a few non-specific small macules on the trunk. These become papular and then vesiculate over 24 h as new lesions appear. Lesions are mainly on the trunk although the hands and face can be involved. The rash may be itchy and the child miserable. The course is usually uncomplicated. A rare form of chickenpox where large bullae develop is occasionally seen.

The development of tachypnoea may herald the development of chickenpox pneumonia, which is more common in adult cases. Secondary bacterial pneumonia is another possible complication, and transverse myelitis and encephalitis have been reported. Zoster may develop many years later. Immunosuppressed individuals with shingles or chickenpox can develop severe disseminated disease.

Investigations

A laboratory diagnosis is rarely required as the clinical features are diagnostic. Fluid from herpetic vesicles has a characteristic appearance when stained by Tzanck stain (Fig. 3.39). Virus can be detected by immunofluorescence or electron microscopy examination of vesicle fluid. VZV DNA can be detected by PCR.

Management

There is no specific treatment for uncomplicated chickenpox. Adolescents, adults or children with complications or disseminated disease should be treated with aciclovir. Immunosuppressed individuals with chickenpox should receive intravenous therapy. Immunosuppressed individuals who come into contact with chickenpox should be given specific immunoglobulin prophylaxis and aciclovir.

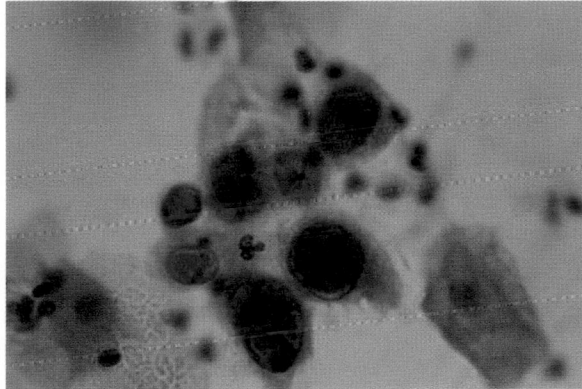

Figure 3.39 Microscopic appearance of a herpetic vesicle; Tzanck stain. Reproduced from Bannister *et al.*, *Infectious Disease*, 1996 (Blackwell Science, Oxford) with the permission of the authors.

Prognosis

Uneventful recovery is the rule following uncomplicated chickenpox, but pneumonia, encephalitis and disseminated disease in the immunocompromised are often fatal if not treated.

Zoster (shingles)

This is a recurrence of VZV that has lain dormant in sensory nerve ganglions.

Epidemiology

A common condition that occurs in up to 25% of patients over 50 years of age. Immunosuppressed individuals are more likely to develop zoster at an early age.

Disease mechanisms

Following primary VZV infection (chickenpox) the virus remains dormant in the sensory ganglia. Reactivation occurs as immunity wanes with age or following immunocompromise, and occasionally in fit young people.

Clinical features

The shingles rash is often preceded by a painful burning sensation in the affected dermatome. The skin may be slightly erythematous. The rash then develops as papules, which vesiculate and then crust. More widely disseminated zoster may be associated with a systemic upset. The lesions are largely confined to one dermatome, although careful inspection can reveal lesions in adjacent dermatomes. Any dermatome can be involved, but the thorax is the most commonly affected part of the body, and the ophthalmic division of the trigeminal nerve is the most commonly affected single dermatome.

Before the rash develops, the pain can be confused with many other possible diagnoses (e.g. myocardial infarction, abdominal perforation, migraine) depending on the dermatome involved.

Investigations

The diagnosis is usually made on clinical grounds but virus can be detected as noted above.

Management

Aciclovir given orally can reduce the severity and length of an attack if given early. It should be used in the immunocompromised. If the ophthalmic branch of the trigeminal nerve is involved and there is conjunctivitis, give aciclovir eyedrops and antibiotic eye ointment and seek an ophthalmic opinion. Adequate analgesia is essential.

Prognosis

Postherpetic neuralgia is most common in the elderly and

03

Varicella zoster at a glance

Epidemiology
Prevalence
Common, 90% infected by 15 years of age

Age
Childhood, but disease occurs in adults and may be severe with pneumonia

Clinical features
Fever with characteristic rash
Relapsing infection usually limited to one dermatome—'shingles'
Overwhelming infection in neonates and the immuno-compromised

Findings on investigation
Antibody detection by various techniques
Visualization of varicella zoster virus in lesion by electron microscopy

Microbiology
Culture rarely required, but indicated in diagnostic uncertainty and in some immunocompromised patients

Histopathology
Smear of lesion base (Tzanck smear) shows multinucleated giant cells

Prevention
A live attenuated vaccine is now available

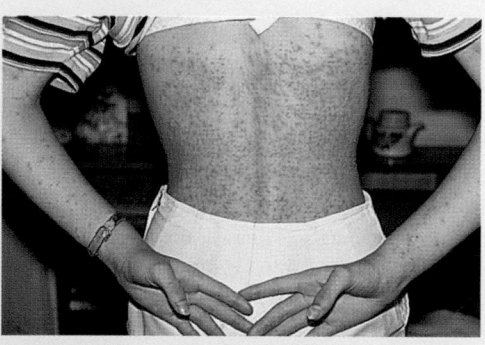

Fig. A Chickenpox: the very early rash. Many papules are seen, which will all become vesicles in the next few hours.

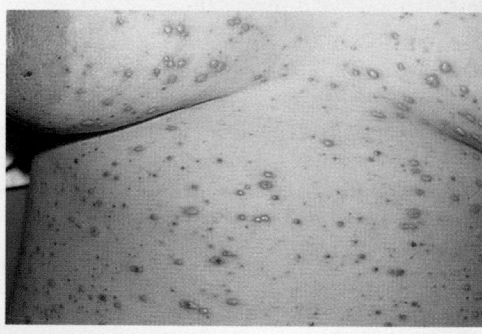

Fig. B Chickenpox: typical rash showing non-coalescing lesions at all stages of development. Both figures reproduced from Bannister *et al.*, *Infectious Disease*, 1996 (Blackwell Science, Oxford) with the permission of the authors.

may be difficult to control. There is no evidence that aciclovir reduces the incidence.

Prevention and control
A live attenuated vaccine is available and has been introduced into general use in USA, Japan and Korea.

Measles (rubeola)

Measles is a severe systemic infection with measles virus.

Epidemiology
Infection is found throughout the world wherever there is no effective vaccination programme. In the developing world, most attacks occur in children around 3 years of age, while in the developed world they occur later in life among individuals who have not developed natural immunity or have refused vaccination. It is endemic in all but isolated populations. Epidemics can occur as the proportion of non-immune people rises, about every 4 years.

Epidemics also occur when the disease is introduced into isolated communities.

There is concern that when vaccination rates fall, as a result of concerns about the vaccine, that epidemics will develop in Europe where measles has become a rare disease.

Measles virus is highly infectious, spreading rapidly in susceptible individuals. The incubation period is 8–14 days. Spread is by the respiratory route.

Disease mechanisms
Measles is caused by a highly infectious RNA paramyxovirus. There is a single antigenic type. Most outbreaks occur in the early spring. Infection confers life-long immunity. Characteristic round cell infiltration and giant cells are seen in mucosal lesions. Fatal cases of pneumonia show a mixture of interstitial giant cell infiltration and secondary bacterial infection.

Clinical features
After the incubation period, fever, malaise and headache

develop. There are usually pronounced catarrhal symptoms with cough and nasal discharge, and a conjunctivitis develops. During the prodrome, pathognomonic white spots 1–2 mm in diameter on an erythematous base appear on the buccal mucosa; these are called Koplik's spots. The measles rash appears on about the fourth day. Usually it starts behind the ears or on the cheeks as a blotchy reddish-brown erythema and spreads downwards. The lesions coalesce and then fade, leaving fine desquamation. During the febrile illness there may be tachypnoea and fine crackles in the chest.

Most of the complications of measles are a result of secondary bacterial infection, which is most common in the malnourished and accounts for the high mortality from measles in developing countries. The most serious common complication is secondary bacterial pneumonia, and *Strep. pneumoniae, Staph. aureus* and *H. influenzae* are the most common pathogens isolated. Giant cell pneumonia caused by the measles virus itself is less common and usually fatal.

Diarrhoea is common in the tropics and is often severe. Myocarditis and laryngitis are reported, and a rare complication is a demyelinating encephalopathy—the measles virus may remain latent within the CNS producing a rare encephalitis many years later called subacute sclerosing panencephalitis (SSPE).

Investigation
The diagnosis is usually made on the basis of the characteristic clinical features. Diagnosis can be confirmed by a significant serological response (specific IgM), by detecting the presence of the virus by immunofluorescence or (rarely) by isolating the virus.

Management
There is no specific treatment for measles, but suspected secondary infection must be treated vigorously.

Prevention and control
Attenuated live vaccine should be offered to all children without contraindications, as part of measles, mumps, rubella (MMR) vaccine (see p. 102).

Prognosis
The prognosis of uncomplicated measles is good. Morbidity is usually caused by secondary bacterial infection and is much higher in the developing world. The case fatality rate is highest in the youngest children.

Rubella (German measles)

This is an infection with a rubivirus that is usually mild but which can cause congenital infections.

Epidemiology
Eighty per cent of young adults have antibodies; many of them have had subclinical disease usually between the ages of 5 and 9 years.

Disease mechanisms
Rubella is caused by a small RNA togavirus, which is transmitted in droplets.

Clinical features
Fever, myalgia and posterior cervical node enlargement develop after an incubation period of 14–21 days. The rash becomes apparent on the first day of the illness, a faint macular erythema developing on the face and spreading down to the trunk. Occasionally, there is a diffuse erythema. The rash usually clears around the third day.

The infection is usually uncomplicated. Arthralgia, occasionally with joint swelling, is the most common complication. Rare complications include thrombocytopenic purpura, neuritis and heart block.

Rubella in pregnancy can cause persisting fetal infection with teratogenic effects—cardiac and ophthalmological lesions being the most common manifestations.

Investigation
The diagnosis is usually made on clinical grounds. A laboratory diagnosis is made by demonstrating the presence of IgM antibodies. Virus isolation is rarely attempted.

Management and prognosis
There is no specific treatment. All children should receive active immunization as part of the MMR vaccine. Prognosis of uncomplicated rubella is good. There are very rare deaths from meningoencephalitis.

Mumps

Mumps is an acute infection caused by a paramyxovirus, characterized by inflammation of the parotid and other glands.

Epidemiology
This disease is now uncommon because of vaccination. Infection in susceptible people occurs in children and teenagers up to 15 years of age but can also affect adults, when complications are more likely.

Disease mechanisms
Mumps is caused by an RNA myxovirus and is most common in the spring. Non-apparent infection with mumps is common.

03

Measles at a glance

Epidemiology

Prevalence
Uncommon in countries with effective vaccine programmes

Age
Most common in under-3-year-olds, but adult disease may occur and can be severe

Geography
Remains common in developing countries

Clinical features
Incubation 8–14 days
Fever, coryza and characteristic morbilliform rash associated with Koplik's spots in the mouth
May be complicated by primary or secondary pneumonia or encephalitis

Findings on investigation
Diagnosis is normally made clinically
Specific IgM tests in case of uncertainty or to confirm an outbreak

Microbiology
Culture of virus rarely required. RTPCR available

Diagnostic imaging
To detect primary or secondary bacterial pneumonia

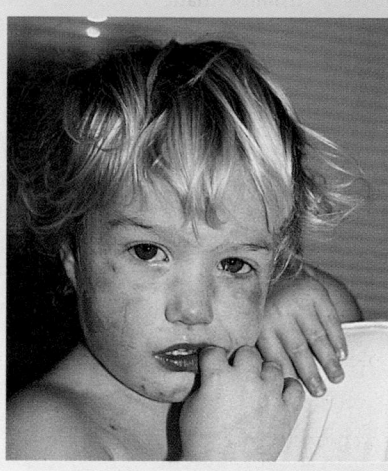

Fig. B Facies on the development of the rash.

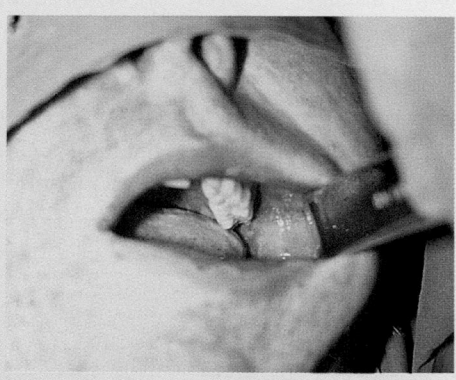

Fig. A Koplik's spots.

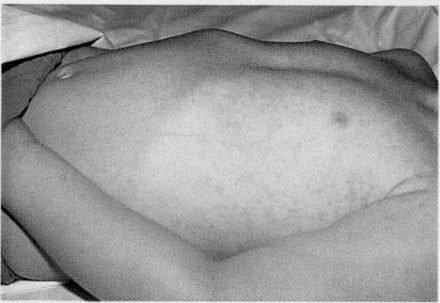

Fig. C Evolution of the maculopapular rash. Second day, the rash has reached the hips. All figures reproduced from Bannister *et al.*, *Infectious Disease*, 1996 (Blackwell Science, Oxford) with the permission of the authors.

Clinical features

Pain and swelling of the parotid develop after an incubation period of 17–21 days. The gland then increases in size over 2–3 days. The submandibular and submaxillary glands can also be affected. Constitutional symptoms are uncommon in children, with a high fever more commonly accompanying adult mumps. Complications of CSF lymphocytosis and severe headache are common in mumps, and clinical signs of meningism are not infrequent.

Aseptic meningitis occurs in up to approximately 25% of all cases of mumps. A low CSF glucose during mumps meningitis has been reported and occasionally leads to confusion with tuberculous meningitis. Preceding parotitis makes the diagnosis clear in many cases, but is absent in a substantial minority as mumps meningitis can precede parotid swelling or occur in its absence.

Rarely, deafness, labyrinthitis, facial neuritis and encephalitis have been reported. The condition is benign and self-limiting, unless there is a predominant encephalitis, which is fortunately rare. Orchitis occurs in adults and may present as gross painful swelling of the testis. It is usually unilateral, and resultant sterility is extremely rare. Oophoritis can present in women as high fever and back pain. Pancreatitis is indicated by fever, abdominal pain and vomiting.

Investigation

The diagnosis is usually made clinically and can be confirmed by demonstrating a significant rise in antibody titre. The virus can be isolated from saliva and CSF or viral RNA detected by RT-PCR.

Management and prognosis

There is no specific treatment for mumps. Pain relief should be offered and an ice bag applied to the parotid may help. Orchitis can be treated by scrotal support and analgesia. Corticosteroids do not alter the duration of

---

Rubella and mumps at a glance

RUBELLA
Epidemiology
Prevalence
80% of adults have antibodies

Age
5–9-year-olds

Sex
Disease in pregnancy can lead to congenital infection

Findings on investigation
Haematology
Lymphocytosis

Immunology
Rubella antibody detection by various techniques

Microbiology
Culture rarely required

Diagnostic imaging
Rarely required

Clinical features
Usually mild fever with erythematous rash
Infection in pregnancy can result in congenital infection resulting in deafness and mental retardation

MUMPS
Epidemiology
Prevalence
Rare in countries with a vaccination programme

Age
Under-15-year-olds

Findings on investigation
Haematology
Lymphocytosis

Biochemistry
Not usually helpful

Immunology
Specific antibody demonstrated by various techniques

Microbiology
Viral culture from CSF in cases of meningoencephalitis

Diagnostic imaging
Rarely required

Clinical features
Fever and painful swelling of parotid glands
May be complicated by orchitis and pancreatitis

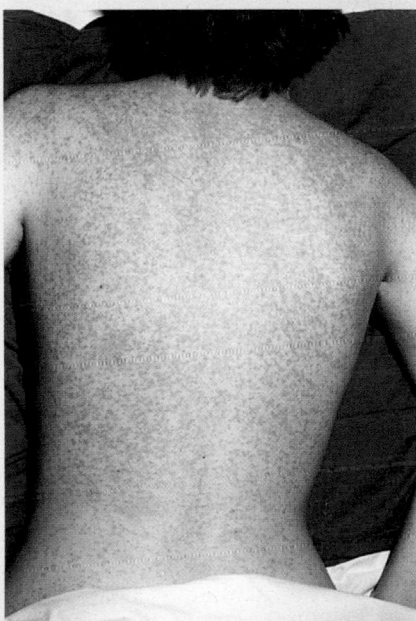

Fig. A The typical rash of rubella. Reproduced from Finch & Ball, *Infection*, 1991 (Blackwell Scientific Publications, Oxford) with the permission of the authors.

03

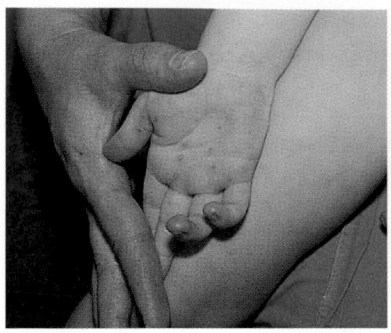 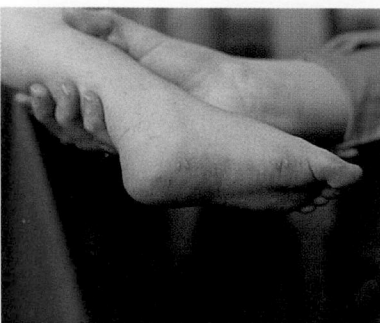

Figure 3.40 The typical blisters of hand, foot and mouth disease. Both parts reproduced from Bannister *et al.*, *Infectious Disease*, 1996 (Blackwell Science, Oxford) with the permission of the authors.

03

the illness, but may reduce very severe swelling and pain. Virtually all cases of mumps recover completely.

Prevention

Live attenuated mumps vaccine should be offered as part of MMR vaccination (see p. 101).

Erythema infectiosum (fifth disease)

This is an acute infection caused by parvovirus B19 associated with a characteristic red face rash (slapped cheek syndrome).

Epidemiology

Childhood infection is more common in spring and summer months, usually between 5 and 14 years of age. Infection occasionally occurs in adults.

Disease mechanisms

Erythema infectiosum or fifth disease is caused by parvovirus B19.

Clinical features

A fever associated with arthralgia, a 'slapped cheek' appearance and a lacy rash on the thighs develops after an incubation period of 8–14 days. The infection can lead to a severe anaemia because of marrow arrest in those who have high red blood cell turnover because of haemolysis.

Investigation

Serological tests show a rise in antiparvovirus antibody titres or detection of parvovirus DNA by PCR.

Management

There is no specific treatment but support may be required for patients with aplastic crisis.

Prognosis

The illness is usually self-limiting over 1 week, but there may be prolonged arthritis.

Hand, foot and mouth disease

Epidemiology and causes

This is an infection of toddlers, although family outbreaks are common. Adults are usually immune. It is caused by highly infectious Coxsackie A viruses.

Clinical features

Onset is heralded by fever followed by eruption of several blisters on the hands and feet and in the pharynx (Fig. 3.40). There is also a papular rash on the buttocks. There is mild discomfort as a result of the blisters, but the illness is short-lived and without complications.

Diagnosis and management

Diagnosis is most often on clinical grounds but if microbial diagnosis is required the virus can be identified by cell cultures of vesicle fluid, throat swab or faeces. No specific treatment is required as the disease is self-limiting.

Genital infections including sexually transmitted infections

Introduction

Sexually transmitted infections (STIs) are among the oldest and most common infectious diseases. The study and management of genital tract infection, including STIs, has become highly specialized, involving clinicians and health care professionals working from designated hospital clinics; in the UK these are called genitourinary (GU) medicine clinics or departments of GU medicine or sexual health.

In the UK, the highest rates of infection are amongst teenage women, and men aged 20–24 years. The highest male : female ratios for STIs are seen in developing countries, partly because STI detection in women in such countries is less efficient and partly because of promiscuous male behaviour, including frequent contact with prostitutes.

New cases of gonorrhoea, genital chlamydial infection and syphilis have increased appreciably in the UK over the past few years. Reports of increasing unsafe sexual practices (e.g. unprotected anal intercourse) amongst men who have sex with men, particularly between men of unknown HIV serostatus, is of concern. STIs are hyperendemic in many parts of the developing world because of changes in social structure, inadequate diagnostic facilities and increasing antimicrobial resistance. In addition, STIs are now recognized as important cofactors for the transmission and acquisition of HIV in the tropics.

Approach to the patient

People commonly present to a GU medicine clinic because they have genital symptoms or because they suspect that they may have contracted an infection. As patients are often embarrassed and anxious, it is essential to have a sensitive and non-judgemental approach. Confidence and trust should be gained early into the consultation.

History

All men and women attending a GU medicine clinic should be asked the questions listed in HISTORY & EXAMINATION BOX 3.4.

Genital tract symptoms

The most common presenting symptoms of patients attending GU medicine clinics are urethral discharge, vaginal discharge and genital ulceration. The causes of these symptoms are given in Tables 3.30–3.33.

Examination

Examination should be carried out in warm surroundings with good illumination.

General examination

Particular attention should be paid to the mouth, skin (including the soles of the feet), eyes and peripheral and sacroiliac joints.

History & Examination 3.4: Questions to ask a patient with a genital infection

About the patient

Sexual history
When did you last have sexual intercourse?
Was this with a regular partner, someone you know, or a casual acquaintance?
How many other sexual partners have you had in the last 3 months?
Were these all male or female?
Have you had sexual contact abroad or with partners from abroad?
Have any of your sexual partners had symptoms?

Contraception
What are you currently using for contraception?
How often do you use condoms?

Symptoms
For all symptoms ask:
When did you first notice it?
Is it improving or worsening?
Have you had anything like it before?

Men
Do you have any stinging pain passing water?
Do you have any penile discomfort or irritation?
Have you noticed any seepage or discharge from the penis or staining on your underwear?
Do you have any aching or discomfort within the scrotum?
Do you have any rashes, spots or sores?

Women
Do you have any vulval irritation or soreness?
Do you have any vaginal discharge? How heavy is it? What colour is it: white, offwhite, yellow, brown? Is there any smell or malodour?
Do you have any stinging or pain passing water?
Are you passing water more frequently than usual?
Do you have any intermenstrual bleeding?
Do you have any pelvic pain?

Non-genital tract symptoms
In particular, ask about joints, eyes and skin

Drug history
Current or recent antibiotic treatment can affect the clinical presentation. Various medications (e.g. tetracycline, sulphonamides) can cause genital fixed drug reactions

Past medical history
Have you had any genital infections before?
Do you have any allergies? (This is particularly relevant if there is a history of a genital rash or irritation)

Family history
Does anyone in your family have allergies or skin problems? (This is particularly relevant if there is a history of a genital rash or irritation)

03

Table 3.30 Vaginal infection

Causative organism(s)	Symptoms	Investigations			Treatment
		Microscopy	Culture	Other	
Candidiasis					
Candida albicans, occasionally *C. tropicalis*, *Torulopsis glabrata*	Variable, asymptomatic, vulval pruritis, oedema, ulceration, vaginal discharge, dyspareunia	Gram stain or wet mount, look for ovoid spores, pseudohyphae	e.g. Sabouraud's medium	Nil	Imidazoles: cream for vulva, pessaries or cream for vagina. Oral medication (e.g. fluconazole, itraconazole) may have a role in treating recurrent infection
Bacterial vaginosis					
Mixed infection with *Gardnerella vaginalis*, anaerobes (e.g. *Bacteroides* spp., *Mobiluncus* sp.), *Mycoplasma hominis*	Asymptomatic, discharge, malodour	Gram stain or wet mount, look for clue cells, curved rods (*Mobiluncus* sp.)	Not indicated	pH >4.5 Amine 'sniff' test	Oral metronidazole, intravaginal clindamycin cream
Trichomoniasis					
Trichomonas vaginalis vaginalis	Asymptomatic, vulval pruritis, vaginal discharge, dysuria, dyspareunia	Wet mount shows motile trichomonads	e.g. Feinberg–Whittington	Nil	Oral metronidazole (sexual partners should also receive treatment)

Table 3.31 Causes of urethral discharge

Physiological
Sexual arousal
Spermatorrhoea/prostatorrhoea

Pathological
Gonococcal urethritis

Non-gonococcal urethritis (non-specific urethritis)
Chlamydia trachomatis (30–50%) (serotypes D–K)
Ureaplasma urealyticum (10–15%)
Trichomonas vaginalis
Anaerobes
Escherichia coli
Candida albicans
Herpes simplex virus
Mycoplasma genitalium
Secondary to urethral lesion (e.g. warts, syphilitic chancre)
Secondary to cystitis
Foreign bodies (e.g. postcatheterization)
Reactive (e.g. postdysenteric Reiter's syndrome, Stevens–Johnson syndrome)
?Hypersensitivity reaction

Table 3.32 Causes of vaginal discharge

Physiological
1 Combination of cervical mucus, desquamated vaginal epithelial cells, water transudate through vaginal wall: may increase at time of ovulation and during sexual arousal
2 Cervical ectopy (excess mucus production)

Pathological
Non-infective
Cervical polyp(s)
Foreign bodies (e.g. retained tampon, condom)
Hypersensitivity reactions (e.g. to vaginal medications, spermicides, douches)
Trauma
Neoplasm

Infection
Candidiasis
Bacterial vaginosis
Trichomonas vaginalis
Chlamydia trachomatis
Neisseria gonorrhoeae
Herpes simplex virus
Non-specific cervicitis
Group B streptococci

Table 3.33 Causes of genital ulceration

Herpes
Syphilis
Chancroid
Lymphogranuloma venereum
Granuloma inguinale
Fixed drug eruption
Circinate balanitis
Behçets disease
Crohn's disease
Stevens–Johnson syndrome
Trauma

Genital examination

The essentials of the genital examination together with a summary of routine investigations are summarized in HISTORY & EXAMINATION BOX 3.5.

Investigation

Routine investigations performed on all patients, irrespective of symptoms, are listed in Table 3.34.

Men

Urethritis is present if more than four polymorphs per high power field are seen on the Gram stain of the urethral

---

History & Examination 3.5: Examination in genitourinary medicine

Men
Palpate the inguinal lymph nodes
Are they enlarged?
Are they tender?

Inspect the pubic area
Can you see evidence of lice?

Inspect the scrotal skin
Look for any rash, warts or ulceration
Palpate (gently) the scrotal contents
Check that the testes are present
Feel for testicular masses
Is there epididymal tenderness?

Inspect the penis with the foreskin fully retracted
Look for any rash, warts or ulceration
Is the glans inflamed (balanitis)?
Is the foreskin (prepuce) inflamed (posthitis)?
Inspect the meatus, coronal sulcus, frenulum and shaft

Gently milk the penis to check for urethral discharge
What is the appearance of the discharge?

Perform investigations (irrespective of symptoms and signs)
First urethral swab
Gram stain for number of polymorphs and to see if there are Gram-negative intracellular diplococci
Culture for *Neisseria gonorrhoeae*

Second urethral swab
Chlamydia trachomatis detection

Two glass urine test (see p. 154)

Syphilis serology (see p. 168)

Women
Palpate the inguinal lymph nodes
Are they enlarged?
Are they tender?

Inspect the pubic area
Can you see evidence of lice?

Inspect the vulva
Is the vulva inflamed (vulvitis)?
Inspect the labia for ulceration or warts
Inspect the fourchette and the introitus

Insert a warmed speculum to visualize the vagina and cervix
Is the vagina inflamed (vaginitis)?
Is there a vaginal discharge? If so, what is its appearance?

Perform investigations
Swab from the lateral vaginal wall
Gram stain for number of polymorphs, bacterial vaginosis type bacteria/'clue cells', hyphae, spores
Wet mount for *Trichomonas*
Culture for *Trichomonas* and *Candida*
Inspect the cervix, look for ectopy or cervicitis (they are often difficult to distinguish)
Gently wipe the vaginal secretions from the cervix

Swab from endocervix (just inside os)
Gram stain for number of polymorphs and to see if there are Gram-negative intracellular diplococci
Culture for *N. gonorrhoeae*

Second swab from endocervix
C. trachomatis detection

Cytology
Remove speculum

Urethral swab
Gram stain (assess number of polymorphs and look for Gram-negative intracellular diplococci)
Culture for *N. gonorrhoeae*

Perform bimanual examination
Is there any tenderness? Are there any masses?

Table 3.34 Routine investigations in genitourinary medicine

Specimen	Test	Results
Male		
Urethral smear	Gram stain and microscopy	■ >4 polymorphonuclear leucocytes per high-power field (×1000 magnification) confirms urethritis ■ Additional presence of Gram-negative intracellular diplococci suggests gonococcal urethritis
Urethral swabs ×2	Culture Culture or enzyme-linked immunoassay or MIF	■ For *Neisseria gonorrhoeae* (**definitive diagnosis**) ■ To detect *Chlamydia trachomatis*
Urine	Two-glass urine test	■ To detect urethritis and to differentiate anterior urethritis from a more proximal infection of the urinary tract
Female		
Vaginal smear	Gram stain and microscopy	■ Decreased or absent lactobacilli may suggest vaginal infection ■ Increased numbers of polymorphs indicate vaginitis ■ Hyphae or spores indicate candidiasis ■ Clue cells indicate bacterial vaginosis
Vaginal wet mount Vaginal secretions ×2	Phase contrast microscopy pH 'Amine sniff test' (drop 5% potassium hydroxide solution onto vaginal swab and sniff)	■ To identify *Trichomonas vaginalis* and clue cells ■ pH >4.5 suggests a pathological discharge ■ Sudden release of a fishy ammoniacal odour suggests a diagnosis of bacterial vaginosis
Vaginal swab	Culture	■ For *Candida* and *T. vaginalis*
Endocervical swabs ×3	Gram stain and microscopy	■ >30 polymorphs per high-power field suggests cervicitis ■ Gonorrhoea may be **presumptively** diagnosed by the presence of Gram-negative intracellular diplococci
	Culture Culture or enzyme-linked immunoassay or MIF	■ For *N. gonorrhoeae* (**definitive diagnosis**) ■ For *C. trachomatis*
Cervical smear	Cytology	■ Screen for subclinical human papillomavirus infection and dyskaryosis
Urethral swab	Culture	■ For *N. gonorrhoeae*
Men and women		
Genital ulcer swab	Culture	For herpes simplex virus
Genital ulcer serum	Dark ground microscopy	For treponemes (see p. 168)
Serum	Serology	For syphilis
	Serology	For HIV (with the patient's consent and after appropriate counselling) (see p. 175)

smear. The presence of 'threads' of pus in the first glass of the two-glass urine test is also suggestive of a urethritis. A presumptive diagnosis of gonococcal urethritis (gonorrhoea) can be made if Gram-negative diplococci are seen within the polymorphs. A definitive diagnosis of gonorrhoea requires the identification of *N. gonorrhoeae* on culture. Non-gonococcal urethritis (NGU) (non-specific urethritis; NSU) is diagnosed when the urethral Gram stain and two-glass urine test show the presence of urethritis and *N. gonorrhoeae* is not detected.

Mild urethritis may produce only minimal symptoms and the diagnosis can be missed on initial examination, particularly if the patient has urinated just a couple of hours before examination. In these circumstances, urethral swabs and a two-glass urine test should be repeated after the patient has held urine overnight. Examination of a centrifuged 'first-catch' urine may be more sensitive than urethral Gram stain for detecting mild urethritis.

Because both gonococcal and NGU can be carried asymptomatically, all male GU medicine clinic attenders should be routinely screened for these infections. Non-gonococcal urethritis (NSU) is the most common STI seen in men in the UK.

Women

Genital tract infection in women is often asymptomatic, yet gonorrhoea and chlamydial infection have potentially serious consequences (e.g. pelvic inflammatory disease with subsequent infertility, ectopic pregnancy, chronic pelvic pain).

Bacterial vaginosis and candidiasis are the most common female genital infections seen in the UK. Neither are sexually transmitted. The most common STIs affecting women are chlamydial infection, non-specific cervicitis and human papillomavirus (HPV) infection.

Principles of management

Supportive treatment

Once an STI has been diagnosed patients must be advised:
- To abstain from sexual contact until pronounced cured (a symptomatic improvement does not always signify cure)
- That sexual contacts should attend a GU medicine clinic for investigation
- That serological tests for syphilis should be repeated after 3 months (the maximum incubation period for the disease)
- How to avoid contracting infections in the future (e.g. use of condoms, avoiding casual sex)

Drugs

All patients attending a GU medicine clinic should receive treatment directly from the clinic doctor free of charge. This is to encourage patients with STIs to attend and comply with treatment.

Specific genital infections and sexually transmitted infections

A wide variety of organisms infect the genital tract, many of which are not sexually transmitted. Those organisms that can be sexually transmitted are listed in Table 3.35.

Gonorrhoea

Gonorrhoea is caused by the bacterium *N. gonorrhoeae*. All *Neisseria* spp. are Gram-negative diplococci and

Table 3.35 Organisms that can be sexually transmitted

Bacteria
Neisseria gonorrhoeae
Chlamydia trachomatis
Ureaplasma urealyticum
Mycoplasma hominis
Treponema pallidum
Group B haemolytic *Streptococcus*
Haemophilus ducreyi
Calymmatobacterium granulomatis
Shigella spp.

Viruses
Herpes simplex virus types 1 and 2
Human papillomavirus
Cytomegalovirus
Molluscum contagiosum virus
Hepatitis A, B and C viruses
Human immunodeficiency virus types 1 and 2

Protozoa
Trichomonas vaginalis
Entamoeba histolytica
Giardia lamblia

Fungi
Candida spp.

Ectoparasites
Phthirus pubis
Sarcoptes scabiei

differentiation between species relies on culture and confirmation by microimmunofluorescence (MIF) or sugar oxidation tests.

Epidemiology

Reported cases of gonorrhoea declined in most developed countries from mid-1980 to mid-1990. In the past few years, however, there has been a steady increase in the number of reported cases of gonorrhoea in developed countries, with younger age groups being particularly affected. Gonococcal infection tends to be concentrated in 'core groups', which in the UK includes men who have sex with men, and black ethnic minorities. In women, the highest rates are in those aged 16–19 years and in men, 20–24 years. The male : female ratio is 2 : 1.

Disease mechanisms

Gonorrhoea is caused by *N. gonorrhoeae* (the gonococcus), which has an affinity for mucous membranes lined by

03

non-squamous epithelium. The primary site of infection is:

- Anterior urethra in men
- Endocervical canal in women

Urethral infection can also occur in women, but is uncommon in the absence of cervical involvement. The gonococcus does *not* infect vaginal epithelium in the post-pubertal woman.

Other sites of infection in both men and women are the pharynx, rectal mucosa and conjunctiva.

Clinical features

Gonorrhoea usually has an incubation period of 2–8 days, but extremes varying from 1 day to more than 2 weeks have been reported.

Men

In men, the most common presenting symptoms are dysuria and urethral discharge. The discharge is usually profuse and purulent, but some men present with only a scant mucoid discharge that is indistinguishable from that of NGU. Local complications include preputial oedema (swollen foreskin), generalized penile oedema ('bull-headed clap'), infection of Cowper's and Tyson's glands, acute epididymitis, periurethral abscess and prostatitis.

Women

In women, presenting symptoms include an increased 'vaginal' discharge as a result of a cervical discharge secondary to cervicitis. An accompanying urethritis may produce dysuria. Spread to the upper genital tract produces an endometritis, which causes pelvic pain, intermenstrual bleeding or menorrhagia, or a salpingo-oophoritis (see p. 159). Other complications include Bartholin's abscess and infection of the periurethral (Skene's) glands.

Disseminated infection develops in approximately 1% of patients with gonorrhoea. In women this often occurs within 5 days of menstruation or during pregnancy. Certain subtypes of *N. gonorrhoeae* appear to have a propensity to disseminate, and are also associated with asymptomatic mucosal infection. Disseminated infection usually causes:

- Fever
- Characteristic sparse pustular rash affecting the extremities, particularly the skin near the small joints of the hands and feet, the lesions of which may be painful

Tenosynovitis and a migratory polyarthralgia are common in disseminated infection and may precede a septic oligoarthritis. Gonorrhoea is an important cause of an acute arthritis and can be difficult to differentiate from Reiter's syndrome. Endocarditis and meningitis are rare complications.

Investigation

Microbiology

- *Cervical or urethral Gram stain:* finding Gram-negative intracellular diplococci provides a presumptive diagnosis of gonorrhoea
- *Culture:* swabs taken from the urethra, cervix, pharynx and rectal mucosa provide a definitive diagnosis of gonorrhoea. Blood cultures should be taken if disseminated infection is suspected
- *DNA amplification techniques:* these are becoming available and increase the sensitivity of laboratory diagnosis

Management

Antibiotics that can be given as a single dose under supervision should be given as patients may not complete therapy or return to clinic once symptoms abate. Single dose treatments include ciprofloxacin, ofloxacin orally and ampicillin orally plus probenecid orally, or if the patient is allergic to penicillin or the infection is caused by ciprofloxacin- or penicillin-resistant strains (10% of cases in the UK), consider ceftriaxone or cefotaxime as a single dose given intramuscularly.

Patient review is necessary 3–7 days and 2 weeks after treatment. Microscopy and cultures must be repeated at each visit.

Treatment may fail as a result of reinfection by an untreated sexual partner. In women a rectal culture is necessary if initial treatment fails because infection may spread from the rectal mucosa to the genital tract.

All sexual partners *must* be assessed. This can be achieved by infected individuals contacting sexual partners directly (patient referral) or by health care workers (contact tracers) assisting in notifying at-risk partners (provider referral). 'Partner notification' is an essential part of STI control.

Chlamydia trachomatis genital infection

Chlamydia are obligatory intracellular parasites and show many of the features of bacteria: they multiply by binary fission, possess ribosomes and a discrete cell wall, contain both RNA and DNA, and are susceptible to certain antibiotics. Serovars A–C cause hyperendemic trachoma; serovars D–K cause genital tract infection. Serovars L_{1-3} cause lymphogranuloma venereum.

Epidemiology

Chlamydia trachomatis infection is the most common sexually transmitted bacterial infection in the developed

Gonorrhoea at a glance

Epidemiology

Age

Most commmonly affects those in their mid-teens to late twenties

Sex

Male : female ratio 2 : 1 in the UK

Findings on investigation

Microbiology

Neisseria gonorrhoeae grown on culture

Histopathology

Gram-negative diplococci can be seen within polymorphs on Gram stain

Clinical features

Men

Asymptomatic

Urethral discharge

Dysuria

Intrascrotal pain secondary to epididymitis

Women

Asymptomatic

'Vaginal' discharge secondary to cervicitis

Dysuria (secondary to urethritis)

Swollen and tender Bartholin's glands (bartholinitis)

Pelvic pain (if spread to endometrium or salpinges; i.e. pelvic inflammatory disease)

Men and women

Rectal pain ± discharge secondary to proctitis

Sore throat secondary to pharyngitis

Conjunctivitis

Arthritis and sparse rash (disseminated infection)

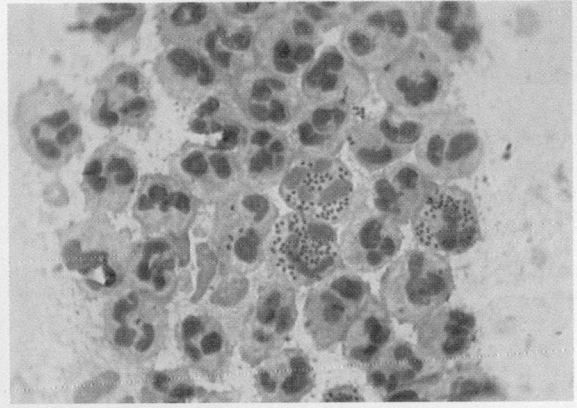

Fig. A Purulent urethral discharge.

Fig. B Gram stain appearance of urethral discharge showing Gram-negative intracellular diplococci.

03

world and is an important cause of morbidity in both adults and neonates.

Disease mechanisms

In men, the urethra is the most common site of infection by *C. trachomatis*. In women, the cervix and urethra are the common sites. Other sites of infection in both men and women are the rectal mucosa, the pharynx and the conjunctivae.

Chlamydia trachomatis causes about 30–50% of cases of NGU in men. It is also a major cause of cervicitis and pelvic inflammatory disease (PID) in women, and of epididymitis in young sexually active men. However, there is

no strong evidence to suggest that it is involved in the pathogenesis of prostatitis.

Clinical features

The clinical features of *C. trachomatis* genital infection are similar to those of *N. gonorrhoeae* infection.

Men

In men, symptoms occur after an incubation period of 1–3 weeks and are most commonly dysuria and/or urethral discharge. The discharge is usually mucoid or mucopurulent, but is occasionally frankly purulent and indistinguishable from that of gonorrhoea. These clinical features

Genital chlamydial infection at a glance

Epidemiology
Prevalence
Most common sexually transmitted bacterial infection in the developed world

Age
Most commonly affects those in their mid-teens to late twenties

Sex
Male : female ratio 2 : 1 in the UK

Findings on investigation
Immunology
Antigen detection (e.g. ELISA, microimmunofluorescence), DNA hybridization (polymerase or ligase chain reaction)

Microbiology
Microscopy. Not seen by Gram stain
Culture is less commonly performed than antigen detection tests

Clinical features
Men
Asymptomatic (common)
Urethral discharge (secondary to urethritis)
Dysuria
Epididymitis

Women
Vaginal discharge (secondary to cervicitis)

Dysuria (secondary to urethritis)
Pelvic inflammatory disease
Right hypochondrial pain (secondary to perihepatitis)

Men and women
Conjunctivitis
Pharyngitis
Proctitis
Reactive arthritis

Neonate
Conjunctivitis
Pneumonitis

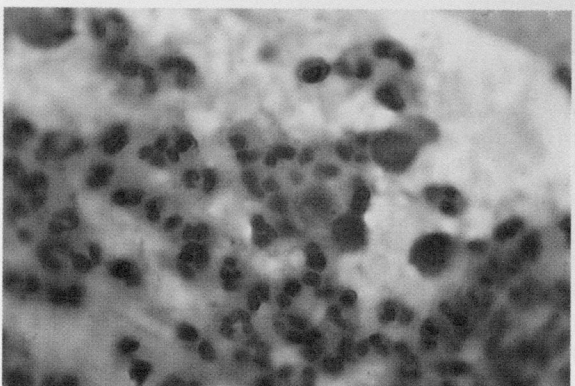

Fig. B Gram stain appearance of urethral discharge showing polymorphs. NB: *Chlamydia* cannot be seen on routine microscopy.

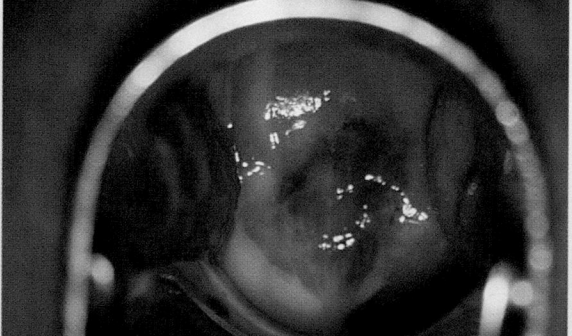

Fig. A Cervicitis: mucopurulent secretions.

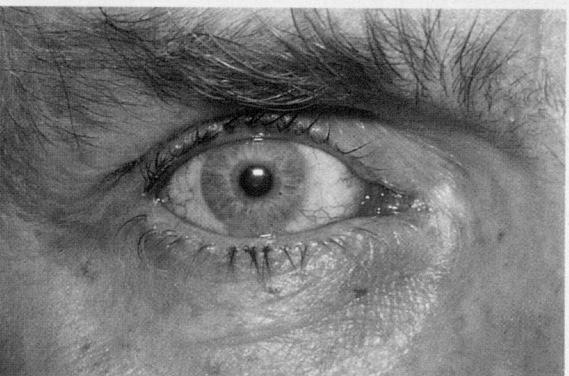

Fig. C Chlamydial conjunctivitis.

are the same as those of *C. trachomatis*-negative NGU. Asymptomatic infection is common.

Women

In women, *C. trachomatis* genital infection is frequently asymptomatic, but there may be an increased vaginal discharge resulting from cervicitis (not vaginitis) or dysuria from urethritis. Complications include bartholinitis, PID and perihepatitis (Fitz-Hugh–Curtis syndrome).

Investigation

Microbiology

● *Culture:* a costly and time-consuming method of diagnosis and less frequently used than ELISA, PCR and MIF
● *Urine smear and two-glass urine test:* usually evidence of a urethritis in men (more than four polymorphs per high powered field on a Gram-stained urethral smear and an abnormal two-glass urine test). This obviously does not distinguish chlamydial urethritis from non-chlamydial urethritis
● *ELISA, PCR and MIF:* the most commonly used methods for detecting urethral and cervical *C. trachomatis*
   DNA amplification techniques (PCR and ligase chain reaction; LCR) are potentially more sensitive. Swabs need to be taken from the appropriate site and positive tests are confirmed by a different testing method from the original screening test. Some laboratories are moving towards a PCR-based diagnostic service and have achieved good results using urine specimens in place of genital swabs.

Management

Tetracycline, azithromycin, ofloxacin and erythromycin are the drugs of choice for *C. trachomatis* infection.

Non-gonococcal urethritis (non-specific urethritis)

Non-gonococcal urethritis is the most common sexually transmitted condition affecting men in the UK. The clinical features are identical to those of *C. trachomatis* urethritis.

Non-gonococcal urethritis is diagnosed when investigations reveal a urethritis, but a causative agent is not identified (i.e. *Chlamydia*-negative and *N. gonorrhoeae*-negative). *Ureaplasma urealyticum* and *Mycoplasma genitulium* can cause up to 20% of cases but are difficult organisms to isolate.

Investigation

Microbiology

On urethral smear more than four polymorphs per high power field on a Gram-stained urethral smear indicates a urethritis.

Other

With the two-glass urine test there are threads or 'specks' of pus in the first glass of the two-glass urine test. *Mycoplasma* and *Ureaplasma* culture is not performed as a diagnostic test for NGU in the UK.

Management

Tetracycline or azithromycin are recommended treatments. Ofloxacin and erythromycin are alternative choices.

Reiter's syndrome (sexually acquired reactive arthritis)

For Reiter's syndrome or sexually acquired reactive arthritis (SARA) see Chapter 4.

Pelvic inflammatory disease

Pelvic inflammatory disease (PID) usually results from spread of infection from the lower genital tract. Spread of infection beyond the pelvis may result in perihepatitis, periappendicitis and perisplenitis. The term PID includes endometritis, parametritis, salpingitis, oophoritis, pelvic peritonitis and pelvic abscess formation.

Epidemiology

In developed countries, prevalence is approximately 1/100. It is most common between 15 and 24 years of age.

Disease mechanisms

Most PID is caused by sexually transmitted infection. In the UK, *C. trachomatis* is the most common cause, while *N. gonorrhoeae* is a less common cause. Other possible causative agents include anaerobic species, *Mycoplasma hominis* and *Ureaplasma urealyticum*. Infection with mixed facultative and obligate anaerobes (e.g. *Bacteroides* species, *Gardnerella vaginalis*, *Prevotella bivia*) may occur secondary to intrauterine contraceptive devices or obstetric complications and can complicate chlamydial and gonococcal upper genital tract infection.

Clinical features

Symptoms of PID include low abdominal or pelvic discomfort or pain, malaise, nausea, excessive vaginal discharge, intermenstrual bleeding and deep dyspareunia. Signs include a mildly increased temperature, pelvic

03

tenderness, pain on cervical movement during vaginal examination (cervical excitation) and a palpable adnexal mass.

Spread of infection to the liver capsule (perihepatitis or Fitz-Hugh–Curtis syndrome) may cause right upper quadrant pain and tenderness and is seen particularly with chlamydial infection.

Conditions that may be confused clinically with PID include ectopic pregnancy, acute appendicitis, corpus luteum bleeding, endometriosis, mesenteric lymphadenitis and ovarian tumour.

Investigation

A full genital infection screen should be performed (see p. 154). Chlamydial and gonococcal infection should be considered.

Haematology
- *FBC:* white blood count may be raised
- *ESR:* may be raised

Microbiology
- *Swabs:* specimens should be taken from the cervix and urethra for *Chlamydia* detection and *N. gonorrhoeae* microscopy and culture

Diagnostic imaging
- *Laparoscopy:* should be considered for all suspected PID as the diagnosis based on clinical findings alone often proves inaccurate

Management

Treatment must include an agent that is active against *Chlamydia*. Commonly used regimens include:
- Cefoxitin (intramuscular or intravenous) plus doxycycline plus metronidazole
- Ofloxacin plus metronidazole

All sexual partners must be advised to attend a GU medicine clinic for assessment. Asymptomatic urethritis is commonly found and can lead to reinfection if not treated.

Prognosis

Pelvic inflammatory disease carries a significant long-term morbidity so an accurate diagnosis is important.

Following a single episode of PID:
- 10–20% of women are infertile as a result of tubal damage
- 20% of women experience chronic pelvic pain
- 40% of women experience deep dyspareunia
- 80% of women have menstrual disturbances
- The risk of ectopic pregnancy is increased sevenfold

Candidiasis (thrush)

Approximately 15–20% of healthy adult women carry *Candida albicans* intravaginally without symptoms. In a proportion of cases, the yeast proliferates and causes a vulvitis and vaginitis. Various factors are known to encourage yeast proliferation (e.g. diabetes mellitus), but usually a precipitating factor cannot be identified.

Epidemiology

Candidiasis is a common cause of vulval irritation and vaginal discharge.

Disease mechanisms

Candida albicans causes more than 90% of cases of vulvovaginal candidiasis. Non-*albicans* strains, such as *C. glabrata*, account for about 5–10% of infections and may be resistant to antifungals.

Clinical features

Men may experience penile irritation immediately after coitus with an infected woman as a result of a hypersensitivity reaction to *Candida* antigen. Alternatively, a balanoposthitis may develop 1–3 weeks later. Women develop inflammation of the vulva and vagina associated with an increased vaginal discharge (Fig. 3.41).

Investigation
Microbiology
- *Microscopy:* diagnosis is based on the identification of Gram-positive yeast cells or pseudohyphae on microscopy (Fig. 3.42)
- *Culture:* because microscopy lacks sensitivity, vaginal secretions should also be cultured for *Candida*

Management

Topical antifungal agents (usually an imidazole) as pessaries (vaginal tablets) and cream are usually effective. Patients with frequent recurrences may benefit from an extended course of either pessaries or oral antifungals (e.g. fluconazole, itraconazole).

Bacterial vaginosis

Bacterial vaginosis (BV) is a condition characterized by an overgrowth of predominantly anaerobic organisms (*Gardnerella vaginalis*, *Prevotella* spp., *Mycoplasma hominis* and *Mobiluncus* spp.) in the vagina, leading to a replacement of lactobacilli and an increase in vaginal pH.

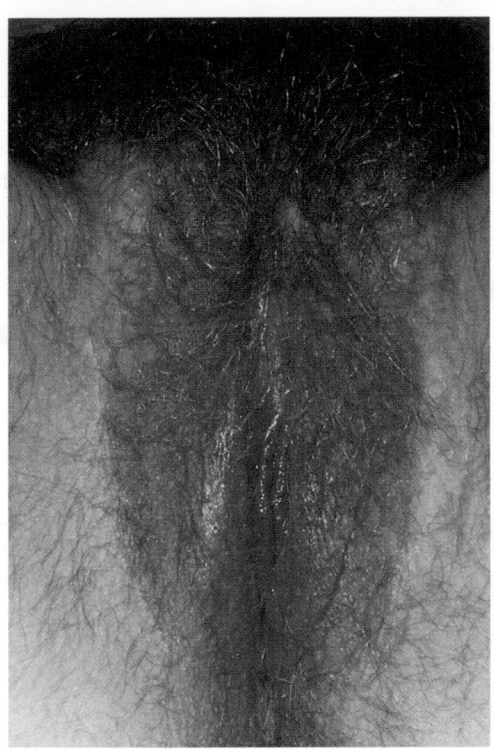

Figure 3.41 Vulvitis caused by *Candidiasis*.

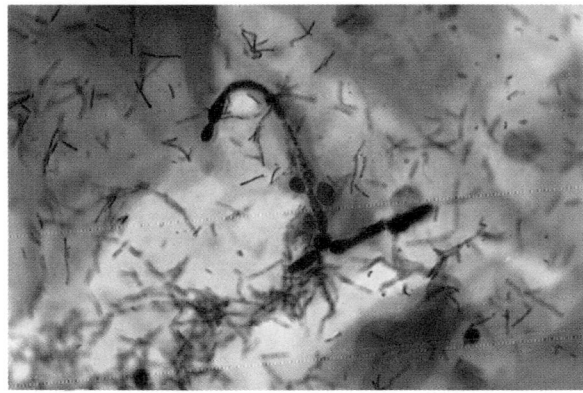

Figure 3.42 Gram stain appearance of candidal pseudohyphae and cells.

Epidemiology

Bacterial vaginosis is the most common cause of abnormal vaginal discharge in women of childbearing age (Fig. 3.43).

Disease mechanisms

Bacterial vaginosis can occur and remit spontaneously and is not regarded as a sexually transmitted infection.

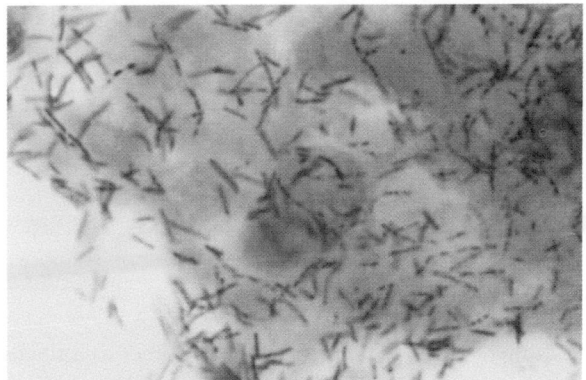

Figure 3.43 Bacterial vaginosis.

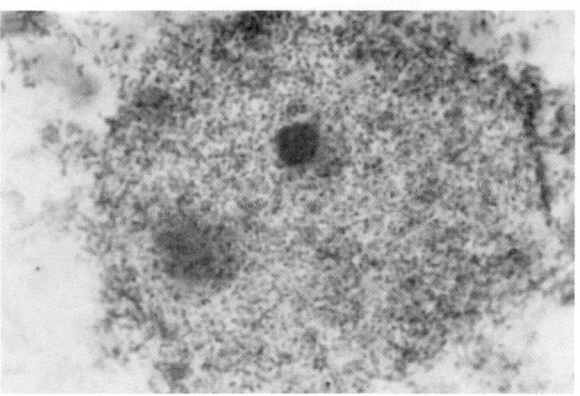

Figure 3.44 Gram strain appearance of a 'clue cell'—a vaginal epithelial cell covered with bacteria. No lactobacilli are present.

The reason for the change in vaginal microflora is unknown. Recurrent BV is sometimes associated with use of the intrauterine contraceptive device.

Clinical features

Malodour is an important clinical feature and is caused by the presence of amines (e.g. trimethylamine). These remain protonated at vaginal pH, but are volatilized by alkali, giving rise to a strong fishy odour. The malodour may be noticed only after coitus because of the sudden release of volatilized amines by alkaline semen. Clinically, there is no vaginal inflammation, which is why this condition is referred to as vaginosis rather than vaginitis.

Investigation

Microbiology

- *Culture:* of no help in the diagnosis unless quantitative microbiology is performed
- *Wet mount microscopy:* shows the presence of 'clue cells', which are epithelial cells covered with bacteria (Fig. 3.44)

03

- *Gram-stain microscopy:* reveals a loss of lactobacilli and an excess of secondary organisms (e.g. *Prevotella* sp., *Gardnerella vaginalis*), some of which will be covering epithelial cells
- *'Amine sniff test':* frequently positive (see p. 154). One per cent potassium hydroxide solution is dropped onto a vaginal swab and 'sniffed'. A distinct fishy odour is a positive result

Management

Treatment is with oral metronidazole, either as a single dose of suspension or as a 1-week course of tablets, topical intravaginal metronidazole gel or clindamycin cream.

Prognosis

Bacterial vaginosis is associated with late miscarriage, preterm labour, postpartum endometritis, posthysterectomy pelvic infection and post-termination of pregnancy pelvic infection.

Trichomoniasis

Trichomoniasis is primarily a sexually acquired protozoal infection.

Epidemiology

Although more than 200 million people worldwide are infected with this parasite annually, there has been a decline in reported cases in the developed world over the past 10 years.

Cause

Trichomonas vaginalis is a flagellated protozoan, which may be acquired concurrently with other sexually acquired infections, such as gonorrhoea.

Clinical features

Women with *T. vaginalis* infection may be asymptomatic, but more commonly present with profuse vaginal discharge. Associated symptoms include pruritus vulvae, dysuria and dyspareunia. The organism occasionally causes NGU in men, but is usually carried asymptomatically.

Investigation

- *Wet film microscopy:* diagnosis is made by finding motile *T. vaginalis* on wet film microscopy
- *Culture: T. vaginalis* may be missed on wet film

microscopy if present in low numbers, and so it is common practice to culture vaginal secretions as well

Management

Treatment is with oral metronidazole. A repeat test should be performed after treatment to ensure a cure. Sexual contacts should be advised to attend a GU medicine clinic for assessment, and a course of metronidazole is advised whether or not symptoms are present.

Genital warts

Genital warts represent one of the clinical manifestations of HPV infection. Most HPV infection is subclinical.

Epidemiology

Human papillomavirus infection is the most common viral STI in the developed world. It occurs mainly in the sexually active young person.

Cause

Human papillomaviruses are DNA viruses of the family Papovaviridae. More than 100 different types of HPV have been documented; 35 types have been isolated from lesions in the genital tract.
- HPV types 6 and 11 are associated with benign genital warts (condylomata acuminata)
- Types 16, 18 and, less commonly, 31, 33, 35 and 39 are found in malignant and premalignant ('intra-epithelial neoplasia') lesions

Disease mechanisms

Papillomaviruses replicate in differentiating squamous epithelium. They only undergo a full replicative cycle to produce infectious virus particles in the fully differentiated cells in the outermost cells of the epithelium. This close association between viral replication and cell differentiation has prevented the development of an effective *in vitro* culture system.

Genital warts may be solitary or multiple, and of variable morphology: jagged or pointed (acuminate), flat, polypoid or keratinized. They can occur in any genital site and commonly involve the anus and anal canal in both heterosexual and homosexual men and women.

Clinical features

Genital warts are usually asymptomatic, but occasionally cause mild skin irritation. Subclinical HPV infection is common and can be identified by applying 3–6% acetic acid solution, which whitens ('acetowhitening') an HPV-infected epithelium.

Complications of genital warts are uncommon. Secondary infection or bleeding can occur, and there have been reports of malignant transformation in long-standing warts, although this is rare. An unusual form of benign giant condyloma (Buschke–Lowenstein) may cause local tissue destruction.

Diagnosis is usually made by the clinical appearance of the lesions. The differential diagnosis of genital warts includes hirsuties papillaris penis or pearly penile papules (a normal finding in 10–40% of men), vulval micro-papillae, molluscum contagiosum, fibroepithelial polyps, condylomata lata (a feature of secondary syphilis) and neoplasms.

Investigation

The diagnosis is usually made clinically.

Microbiology
Human papillomavirus cannot be grown in culture. Human papillomavirus DNA can be detected by PCR and is commonly used in research and epidemiological studies of HPV infection.

Histopathology
Biopsy and histological examination is reserved for atypical or potentially premalignant lesions.

Management

Treatment of genital warts involves chemotherapy, cryotherapy, interferon or surgery.
- Podophyllin is a mixture of resins obtained from the dried rhizome and roots of the mandrake and mayapple plants. It acts by initiating mitotic activity and then arrests cell division in metaphase resulting in cell death. A 10% or 25% solution is applied topically 1–3 times/week under medical supervision, and may cause local inflammation and ulceration. The response is often variable and slow.
- Podophyllotoxin is one of the active ingredients of podophyllin. It produces less local side-effects and is therefore considered safer for self-treatment.
- Imiquimod is an immunomodulator that acts by stimulating a cell-mediated immune response against HPV. It is self-applied as a cream.
- Trichloracetic and monochloracetic acid act as caustic agents and remove warts by producing skin necrosis. They must be applied with extreme care.
- Cryotherapy (e.g. using liquid nitrogen) is a useful method for treating small numbers of warts or heavily keratinized lesions. The warts are sprayed with liquid nitrogen or touched by a frozen probe. This is generally well tolerated and does not require local anaesthesia.
- Interferon is a group of biologically active glycoproteins with antiproliferative, antiviral and immunomodulatory properties. It requires systemic or intralesional administration, and is very expensive.
- Surgery comprises electrocautery, scissor excision and laser ablation. It is useful for large warts or warts resistant to other forms of treatment.

All patients with genital warts must be screened for other STIs, which may be acquired at the same time as HPV and remain asymptomatic. Women with genital warts do not require more frequent cervical smears. Sexual contacts should be advised to attend the GU medicine clinic for assessment.

Prognosis

Recurrence is common after treatment. Subclinical infection may possibly persist for life.

Genital herpes

Genital herpes is caused by herpes simplex virus (HSV) types 1 and 2 and is acquired by sexual intercourse or orogenital contact.

Epidemiology

This is the second most common sexually transmitted viral infection in the developed world.

Causes

Approximately 60–90% of primary or first attacks of genital herpes are caused by HSV type 2. The remaining 10–40% are caused by HSV type 1 infection (the cause of oral cold sores). Herpes simplex virus is a DNA virus belonging to the herpesvirus family, which also includes CMV and EBV.

Studies documenting the prevalence of serum antibodies to HSV in various population groups have shown that most people acquiring HSV infection do not develop symptoms. All individuals infected with HSV may shed virus asymptomatically and transmit infection unknowingly to a sexual partner.

Disease mechanisms

Herpes simplex virus is neurotropic and remains as a latent infection in the sacral ganglia, resulting in relapsing infection.

03

Genital warts at a glance

Epidemiology
Prevalence
Most common sexually transmitted viral infection in the UK

Age
Predominantly young sexually active

Findings on investigation
Diagnosis made on clinical appearance

Microbiology
Virus cannot be grown in culture

Histopathology
Consider biopsy if there is diagnostic uncertainty

Clinical features
Any genital site can be involved
Anal warts are common in women and both homosexual and heterosexual men
Subclinical infection is very common
Can be detected by applying 5% acetic acid solution: 'acetowhitening' is suggestive of human papillomavirus infection

Management
Supportive treatment
Psychological support and counselling may be required if the warts are persistent or frequently recur

Specific treatment
Podophyllin

Podophyllotoxin
Trichloroacetic acid
Cryotherapy
Electrocautery
Scissor excision
Laser ablation

Screen for other sexually transmitted infections
Women should have regular cervical cytology

Sexual partners
Sexual partners should be assessed

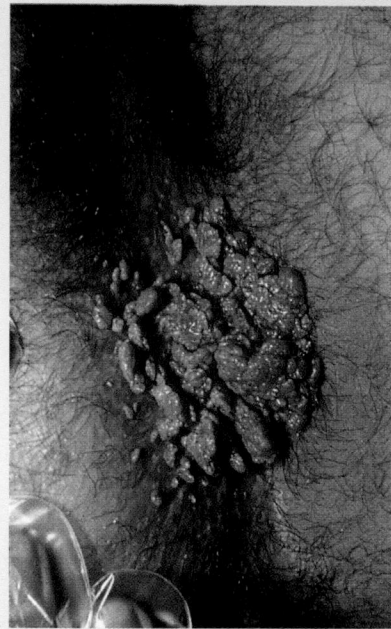

Fig. B Anal warts.

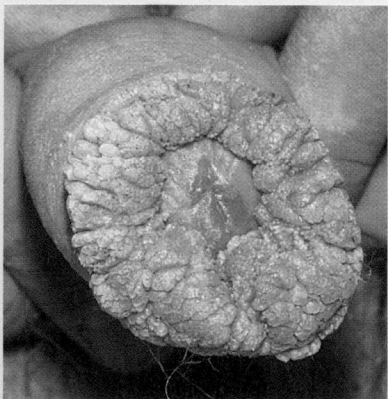

Fig. A Penile warts.

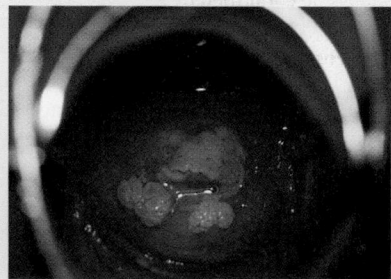

Fig. C Cervical warts.

Clinical features

Primary infection

After an incubation period of 2–6 days, small painful vesicles are noticed on the external genitalia. These are often accompanied, particularly in women, by systemic symptoms such as headache, fever, malaise and myalgia. The lesions ulcerate and are most painful at 8–10 days. They then slowly heal over the next 7–14 days. Virus may be shed for up to 12 days after the onset of the lesions. The inguinal lymph glands enlarge and become tender during the second and third week of the illness and are often the last manifestation to resolve.

Other features of primary genital HSV infection include urethritis in 80% of women and 40% of men, resulting in dysuria, and cervicitis in 80–90% of women, resulting in excessive vaginal discharge.

Complications of primary genital HSV infection are:
- *CNS manifestations:* meningism, photophobia, headache, aseptic meningitis
- *Autonomic nervous system dysfunction:* sacral radiculopathy, in which patients present with urinary retention or constipation
- *Transverse myelitis:* rare
- *Pharyngitis*
- *Extragenital lesions:* on the buttock, groin, fingers and/or lip
- *Disseminated infection*
- *Secondary infection:* with *Candida* spp.
- *Endometritis:* rare

Recurrent infection

This affects almost 90% of patients with primary genital HSV-2 infection, compared to 50% with HSV-1 infection. It is thought to result from reactivation of latent virus in the sacral ganglia. Some people report triggering factors such as sunlight, stress, febrile illnesses, menstruation or 'trauma' from sexual intercourse. The duration and severity of the clinical manifestations are less than in primary infection.

Diagnosis

A presumptive diagnosis of genital herpes may be made on the clinical appearance of the vesicles and ulcers.

Investigation

Immunology
- *MIF:* using monoclonal antibodies is being evaluated and may prove useful as a rapid diagnostic technique.

03

Genital herpes at a glance

Epidemiology

Prevalence
Second most common sexually transmitted viral infection in the UK

Findings on investigation
Usually a clinical diagnosis

Microbiology
Diagnosis should be confirmed by a positive viral culture

Clinical features

Lesion
Vesicle → ulcer → scab formation → healed

Associated features
Ulcers are usually painful
May be associated with painful inguinal lymphadenopathy
Primary infection often produces 'flu-like symptoms

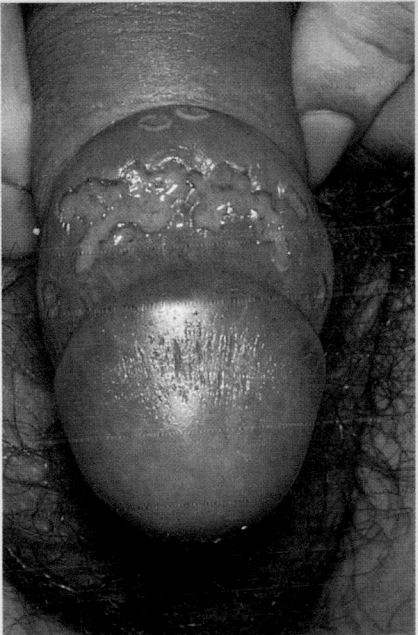

Fig. A Primary herpes affecting the penis.

Microbiology

- *Culture:* a swab should be taken from the genital lesion. A positive viral culture is required to make a definitive diagnosis of genital HSV infection. The sensitivity of the culture varies with the stage of the lesion. Virus is cultured from 95% of vesicular lesions, 90% of pustular lesions, 70% of ulcers but only 25% of crusted lesions. The detection of HSV DNA by PCR is currently generally unavailable for routine diagnostic purposes.

Management

There is no cure for genital herpes, and non-specific treatments are important. These include:
- Bathing the lesions with warm salt water
- Using ice packs (packets of frozen peas are effective)
- Simple analgesics (aspirin or paracetamol)

Aciclovir, famciclovir and valaciclovir are specific oral anti-herpes virus agents and are extremely effective in reducing the duration and severity of primary attacks. The small number of people who suffer frequent recurrences (e.g. more than 6/year) may benefit from long-term daily therapy (KEYPOINTS BOX 3.2).

Prognosis

Most patients with genital herpes suffer relapse (e.g. 2–3 episodes/year).

Syphilis

Venereal syphilis can be congenital or acquired and both are subdivided into early or late disease. The dividing line between early and late syphilis is arbitrarily placed at 2 years for both forms. This is about the length of time for which the body fluids (blood, semen, saliva) remain infectious. Although syphilis is relatively uncommon in the UK, there have been several outbreaks during the past few years associated with high rates of partner change and, in some cases, concurrent HIV infection.

Epidemiology

Prevalence is worldwide but uncommon in developed countries. It occurs with congenital infection and in the sexually active population.

Disease mechanisms

Syphilis is caused by a spirochaete belonging to the genus *Treponema. Treponema pallidum* causes venereal syphilis and endemic syphilis. It can be differentiated from other treponemes by its characteristic morphology and movement on dark ground microscopy. It is intolerant of heat and drying and can be effectively killed with soap and water.

Clinical features

Early acquired syphilis

Primary syphilis

A chancre appears at the site of inoculation after an incubation period of 2–4 weeks (range 9–90 days). This is macular at first, but soon progresses through a papular stage into a relatively painless and non-tender rounded ulcer with a well-defined margin and indurated base. The inguinal lymph nodes usually become moderately enlarged and are typically painless, non-tender and rubbery. Secondary infection of the chancre can cause pain and tenderness of both the ulcer and the inguinal lymph nodes. A chancre will heal in about 3–6 weeks and may pass unnoticed, particularly if it is sited at the anus, anal canal or cervix.

Secondary syphilis

Generalized signs of infection occur 4–8 weeks after the appearance of the primary lesion (Fig. 3.45). There may

---

Keypoints 3.2: Herpes in pregnancy

- Neonatal HSV infection is associated with high morbidity and mortality
- Transmission rate for vaginal delivery during a primary maternal infection is about 50%
- Transmission rate for vaginal delivery during a recurrent attack appears to be extremely uncommon (maternal antibody may contribute to this low rate)
- Sequential cultures for HSV in women with a past history of genital herpes appear to be of little value because most women shedding virus at delivery have no history of genital herpes and cervical HSV cultures taken in the weeks before delivery often fail to predict viral shedding during delivery
- Many obstetricians reserve caesarean section for women with clinical lesions at the onset of labour
- If an infant becomes ill in the first few weeks of life, neonatal herpes should be considered in the differential diagnosis, regardless of the maternal history

03

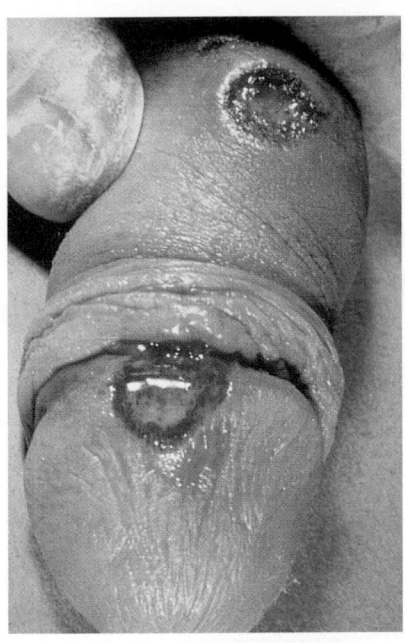

Figure 3.45 Penile chancres—primary syphilis.

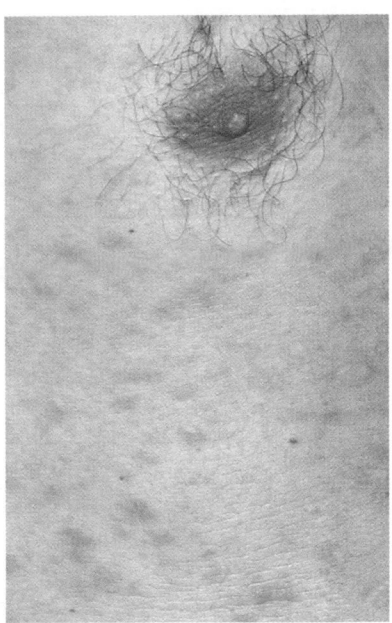

Figure 3.46 Macular rash of secondary syphilis affecting trunk.

be an initial prodromal phase with non-specific features such as headache, myalgia, malaise and low-grade fever, followed by a generalized skin rash, lymphadenopathy and mucosal ulceration.

The features of secondary syphilis include:
- Generalized macular, maculopapular, papular or pustulo-ulcerative skin rash involving the palms and soles (Figs 3.46 and 3.47)
- Pruritus, which is uncommon
- Condylomata lata, which are large fleshy skin lesions usually found in moist areas (e.g. anus) or at sites of skin irritation (e.g. axillae, vulva, submammary), which result from enlargement and fusion of skin papules
- 'Moth-eaten' or diffuse alopecia
- Onychia, paronychia
- Snail-track ulcers (mucous patches) in the mouth, under the prepuce, on the vulva, anus, larynx (causing hoarseness) and pharynx (causing a sore throat)
- Generalized rubbery non-tender lymphadenopathy
- Headache, optic neuritis, deafness, tinnitus
- Iritis, choroidoretinitis
- Fever, weight loss, anorexia, anaemia
- Periostitis, hepatitis, splenomegaly, nephrosis

Early latent syphilis refers to the latent period following secondary syphilis within 2 years of infection. It is usually diagnosed when syphilis serology is positive, but there are no overt symptoms or signs of disease and investigations do not show evidence of neurological or cardiovascular involvement.

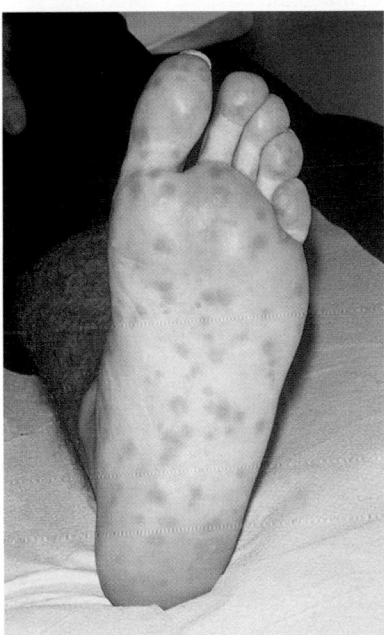

Figure 3.47 Macular rash of secondary syphilis affecting soles of the feet.

If infection is of more than 2 years' duration the diagnosis is late latent syphilis. Approximately 33% of people with untreated infection will develop the clinical sequelae of late syphilis. However, the frequent use of penicillin and other antitreponemal antibiotics for other conditions may modify the clinical picture of late syphilis.

03

Table 3.36 Classification of neurosyphilis

Asymptomatic	Early
	Late
Meningeal	Acute syphilitic meningitis
	Spinal syphilitic pachymeningitis (rare)
Parenchymatous	General paralysis of the insane
	Tabes dorsalis
	Taboparesis
	Optic atrophy
Meningovascular	Cerebral
	Spinal
	Cerebrospinal
Gummatous	Cerebral
	Spinal

Table 3.37 Causes of a false-positive Venereal Disease Research Laboratory (VDRL) result

Technical	Laboratory error
	Error in labelling specimen
Biological	
Acute	Pregnancy
(<6 months' duration)	Postimmunization
	Leptospirosis
	Relapsing fever
	Viral infection
Chronic	Old age
(>6 months' duration)	Malnutrition
	Malignancy
	Drug abuse
	Chronic infection (e.g. tuberculosis)
	Autoimmune disease
	Rheumatoid arthritis

Late acquired syphilis

Gummatous syphilis

Gummas are areas of tissue destruction surrounded by fibrosis and can vary in size from less than 1 mm to several centimetres in diameter. They usually appear within 10 years of infection and can affect the skin, mucous membranes, bones and, more rarely, the viscera.

Cardiovascular syphilis

Approximately 10% of people with untreated syphilis develop cardiovascular syphilis after a latent period of 10–20 years. *Treponema pallidum* induces a periarteritis and endarteritis within the wall of the thoracic aorta, resulting in a loss of elastic tissue and replacement fibrosis. Subclinical aortitis may persist for many years before the onset of symptoms. Complications include aneurysm formation, aortic regurgitation and coronary ostial stenosis.

Neurosyphilis

This develops in approximately 10% of people with untreated syphilis after 10–30 years. The classification and clinical features of neurosyphilis are summarized in Table 3.36.

Investigation

Immunology

● *Non-specific serological tests:* these detect antibody to cardiolipin-like substances carried by *T. pallidum*. The most widely used are the Venereal Disease Research Laboratory (VDRL) test and the rapid plasma reagin (RPR) test. Anticardiolipin antibodies can be produced excessively in other conditions (e.g. viral infections, postimmunization, autoimmune disease and pregnancy) so false-positive results may occur. The causes of a false-positive VDRL result are listed in Table 3.37. The VDRL test usually becomes positive 1–2 weeks after the appearance of the primary chancre and remains positive during the secondary stage. Approximately 33% of people with latent syphilis have a negative VDRL result and the test may become negative if treatment is started within 2 years of infection.

● *Specific tests:* the most commonly used tests for detecting antitreponemal antibody are the treponemal ELISA (may detect IgG and/or IgM), *T. pallidum* haemagglutination assay (TPHA), *Treponema pallidum* particle agglutination (TPPA) test and the fluorescent treponemal antibody absorption (FTA-abs) test.

The ELISA or VDRL/RPR and TPHA/TPPA are usually recommended for syphilis screening. The ELISA IgM test should be requested if primary syphilis is suspected. Specific tests often remain positive for life despite adequate treatment. In addition, they do not distinguish syphilis from other treponemal infections.

Histopathology

Dark ground microscopy is extremely important, allowing direct identification of treponemes in the serum exudate from a primary chancre or from the mucous membrane or skin lesions of secondary syphilis. *Treponema pallidum* may be distinguished from other treponemes by its characteristic movement involving rotation and central angulation while maintaining a regular spiral shape. In the early stages of primary syphilis, serological tests are frequently negative and a positive diagnosis can only be made by dark ground examination. The direct fluorescence antibody (DFA) test can be used for oral and other lesions where contamination with commensal treponemes is likely.

Management

Penicillin remains the drug of choice for all types of syphilis. Aqueous procaine penicillin intramuscularly daily is given for:
- 10 days for primary, secondary and early latent stages
- 15 days for late latent disease
- 20 days for cardiovascular syphilis and neurosyphilis

Doxycycline penetrates well into the CSF, and is gaining favour as a possible first-line treatment by some clinicians. Patients with primary or secondary syphilis should be warned that they may develop a 'flu-like illness on the first day of treatment. This is the Jarisch–Herxheimer reaction, thought to be caused by a reaction to killed treponemes and liberated toxins but the exact mechanism is not fully understood.

Follow-up

All patients with syphilis should be seen on a regular basis (e.g. 3–6 monthly) for 2 years after treatment. A physical examination and serological tests are necessary at each visit. Patients with late syphilis may require more prolonged follow-up.

Prognosis

Adequate treatment of primary, secondary and latent syphilis, and asymptomatic neurosyphilis will result in a cure and halt progression of the disease. The prognosis in cardiovascular syphilis and neurosyphilis is variable with aortic damage and paresis persisting or progressing despite adequate therapy.

Tropical causes of genital ulceration

Chancroid

Chancroid is a mostly tropical disease seen particularly in the developing countries of Africa and Asia. A few cases have recently been reported in Canada and the southern states of the USA.

Epidemiology

It is probably the most common cause of genital ulceration in the tropics and subtropics.

Disease mechanisms

Chancroid is caused by *Haemophilus ducreyi*, a small Gram-negative bacillus.

Clinical features

Multiple, very painful genital ulcers develop after an incubation period of less than 1 week. About 50% of patients also develop enlarged tender inguinal lymph nodes, which may become matted together and suppurate to form a bubo.

Investigation

Gram stain of serum exudate collected from the ulcer and culture confirm the diagnosis.

Management

Recommended treatments are ciprofloxacin, azithromycin, ceftriaxone (intramuscular) and erythromycin.

Lymphogranuloma venereum

Lymphogranuloma venereum (LGV) is a cause of genital ulceration, rare in industrialized countries.

Epidemiology

It is common in Africa, India, South East Asia, Papua New Guinea and some Caribbean islands.

Disease mechanisms

Lymphogranuloma venereum is caused by *Chlamydia trachomatis* serotypes L1, L2 and L3.

Clinical features

The primary lesion is a small painless papule or ulcer, which appears after an incubation period of about 1–3 weeks. It is frequently unnoticed and the patient often presents with constitutional symptoms (fever, sweats, malaise, nausea, myalgia, anorexia) together with enlarged tender suppurating inguinal lymph glands (buboes). Anorectal involvement results in abscesses, fistulae and proctitis, with the later development of rectal stricture.

Investigation

Culture and a rising or high antibody titre confirm the diagnosis.

Management

The treatments of choice are a tetracycline or erythromycin.

Granuloma inguinale

This is a cause of genital ulceration seen in small epidemic foci in all continents except Europe.

Epidemiology

It has been reported in India, Papua New Guinea, the Caribbean, South America, South Africa, some countries of the Far East and in Australian Aboriginals.

03

Disease mechanisms

Granuloma inguinale is a mildly contagious STI. The causative organism is *Calymmatobacterium granulomatis*, a Gram-negative bacillus, which is also known as *Donovania granulomatosis*.

Clinical features

The incubation period is variable. Lesions begin as papules that progress to form painless well-defined ulcers with rolled edges. Subcutaneous granulomas may form in the inguinal region and be mistaken for lymphadenopathy (pseudo-bubo).

Investigation

Diagnosis is made by finding the organisms on stained smears made from tissue scrapings or by histology of biopsy material.

Management

The treatments of choice are doxycycline, ciprofloxacin and azithromycin.

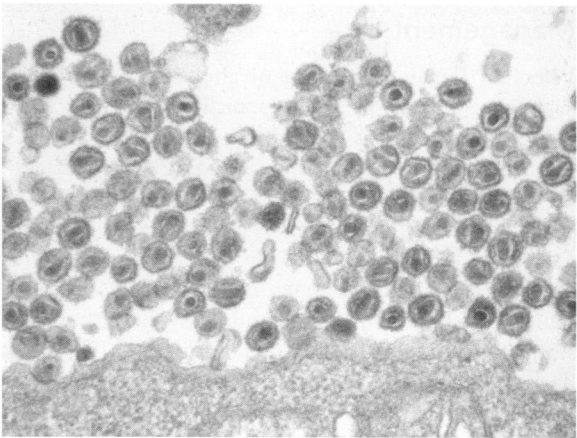

Figure 3.48 Electron micrograph of HIV particles. Courtesy of Professor D.J.P. Ferguson.

HIV and AIDS

HIV

Introduction

In 1981, in the USA, young homosexual men were noted to be dying from two previously rare conditions: *Pneumocystis carinii* pneumonia and a tumour that mainly affected the skin, Kaposi's sarcoma. These young men were found to be immunosuppressed. As this appeared not to be a congenital form of immunosuppression, it came to be known as the acquired immune deficiency syndrome (AIDS). Subsequently, it became clear that this new disease had originated in Africa where it was found predominantly in heterosexuals.

The causative agent was first identified in France in 1983, and was later named human immunodeficiency virus (HIV) (Fig. 3.48). AIDS can be defined as 'the life-threatening diseases caused by HIV'. These are categorized as opportunistic infections, tumours, AIDS dementia complex and HIV wasting syndrome.

Epidemiology

The common form of HIV is HIV-1. This appears to have originated in central Africa from a simian immunodeficiency virus found in chimpanzees. It is now widespread throughout the world. So far, 10 subtypes have been identified, each of which have different global distributions. HIV-2 is far less common and is found predominantly in West Africa. It appears to have originated from a simian immunodeficiency virus in sooty mangabey monkeys. Various risk factors for transmission have been identified (see p. 171). These risk factors vary between continents and between countries and so determine the epidemiology. In Africa, which has the majority of cases of HIV and AIDS in the world, the predominant means of transmission is sexual intercourse between heterosexuals. In North America, Australasia and most European countries, the predominant means of transmission is sexual intercourse between homosexual men, although injecting drug use is a particular problem in certain areas such as the Iberian peninsula and Italy. In South and South East Asia there is a rapidly growing epidemic where heterosexual transmission and injecting drug use are significant factors (Table 3.38).

Disease mechanisms

Both HIV-1 and HIV-2 commonly cause AIDS, but AIDS caused by HIV-2 has a longer latency period (KEYPOINTS BOX 3.3).

Sexual transmission

The sexual transmission of HIV takes place most easily through insertive anal intercourse (from the penis to the anal canal). It will also take place, although somewhat less easily, from the anal canal to the penis. The next most efficient means of transmission is through vaginal intercourse (from the penis to the vagina and, less easily, from the vagina to the penis). In addition, there is a significant although much lower risk of transmission through oro-

Table 3.38 UNAIDS Global HIV/AIDS Statistics (1 December 2001)

	Adults and children living with HIV/AIDS	HIV-positive adults (percentage women)
Sub-Saharan Africa	28.1 million	55
North Africa & Middle East	440 000	40
South & South East Asia	6.1 million	35
East Asia & Pacific	1 million	20
Latin America	1.4 million	30
Caribbean	420 000	50
Eastern Europe & Central Asia	1 million	20
Western Europe	560 000	25
North America	940 000	20
Australia & New Zealand	15 000	10
Total	*40 million*	*48*

Keypoints 3.3: Routes of transmission of HIV

Sexual
Anal intercourse
Vaginal intercourse
Orogenital sex

Blood and blood products

Injecting drug use—sharing 'works'

Vertical transmission
At delivery
Transplacental
Via breast milk

---

genital sex (from the penis to the mouth or vagina to the mouth). It does not appear biologically plausible for transmission to take place from the mouth to either penis or vagina. The higher the viral load (HIV RNA level) in the index case, the more likely that transmission will take place.

Rates of transmission also depend on other factors such as the amount of virus present in semen or cervicovaginal secretions. Cofactors such as coincident STIs, especially ulcerative diseases like chancroid, syphilis and genital herpes, increase the risk of transmission. Genetic factors, for instance those determining the structure of the cellular receptor for HIV, also affect susceptibility to infection. Men who are circumcised are between two and eight times less likely to acquire HIV than uncircumcised men when exposed to HIV. Condoms, when they remain on and intact, are an effective barrier against the transmission of HIV.

As a result of these factors and cofactors, there is a wide variation in the rates of transmission of HIV from HIV-positive people. At worst, when genital ulceration is present, transmission can take place at the rate of 30% per vaginal sexual intercourse. On the other hand, in the absence of cofactors, rates of transmission between regular partners in the absence of cofactors may be as low as 1/1000 per sexual intercourse.

Blood and blood products

Blood transfusion is an extremely efficient means of transmission of HIV. An estimated 90% of recipients of HIV-positive blood will acquire the virus. For this reason, in countries that can afford it, blood is screened for HIV antibodies. Nevertheless, there remains a risk of transmission if HIV-infected people donate in the period after infection before HIV antibodies become detectable (usually at some time in the first 3 months following infection). For this reason, people who perceive themselves to have been at risk of HIV are asked to refrain from donating blood. In developed countries with an efficient system for screening blood, it has been estimated that the risk of acquiring HIV from a blood transfusion is less than 1 in 1 million.

Early in the epidemic many haemophiliacs were infected by transfusions of factor VIII. Now screening and heat treatment renders this and other blood products safe.

In much of the developing world it is not feasible to screen donated blood for HIV and the risk of transmission by this route remains.

Injecting drug use

Injecting drug users who share needles and/or syringes run the risk of acquiring HIV infection. According to a World Health Organization estimate, the risk of acquisition of HIV by this means is between 0.5 and 1% each time an HIV-positive drug user shares needles.

Vertical transmission

Transmission from mother to baby mainly takes place at the time of delivery, but can also take place earlier in pregnancy across the placenta or, in a smaller number of cases, through breastfeeding. Rates of transmission vary from country to country. At worst, some areas of the developing world have transmission rates of approximately 50%. In industrialized countries, transmission occurred in between 10 and 15% of pregnancies before modern interventions were introduced. Nowadays, antiretroviral drugs are given to the mother and infant where possible to cut down the risk of transmission. Another useful intervention can be the use of caesarean section. By the use of these means, the rate of transmission can be cut to less than 1%.

Health care workers

Carers, mainly health care workers, run the risk of acquiring HIV mainly as a result of needlestick injuries. Someone who acquires a needlestick injury with HIV-positive blood runs a 1 in 300 risk of acquiring HIV, unless antiretroviral drugs are started quickly. After encouraging the wound to bleed freely under flowing warm water, the carer should access one of the relevant hospital departments (occupational health, accident and emergency or infectious diseases). Ideally, triple antiretroviral therapy should be started within 1 h and continued for 1 month. This will greatly diminish the risk of the carer acquiring HIV infection. When a needlestick injury has occurred from a patient of unknown HIV status, any approach to the patient seeking consent to perform an HIV test should be made by another health care professional rather than the recipient of the needlestick injury.

Emergency: HIV-positive needlestick injuries

- Encourage bleeding under warm running water
- Seek immediate advice (e.g. occupational health, accident and emergency, infectious diseases)
- 1 in 300 risk of acquiring HIV if no drugs given
- Postexposure prophylaxis (PEP) with AZT alone cuts risk fivefold
- PEP now recommended with three antiretrovirals for 1 month
- Start PEP as soon as possible (ideally within 1 h)

Disease mechanisms

The HIV life cycle is shown in Fig. 3.49. The envelope of HIV attaches to the CD4 epitope on various cells. Langerhans' cells are infected early on. Subsequently, cells in the monocyte–macrophage series are infected. Activated macrophages cross the blood–brain barrier and set up infection in the CNS, predominantly in microglial cells (KEYPOINTS BOX 3.4).

Keypoints 3.4: Cells infected by HIV

T-helper lymphocytes
Langerhans' cells
Macrophages
Microglial cells

The presence of HIV in the CNS can uncommonly cause symptoms at the time of seroconversion (see below). More commonly, HIV can have direct effects on the CNS late on in the disease. HIV also infects the T-helper lymphocyte, which also bears the CD4 epitope. Ultimately, the consequence of this infection is depletion in the number of T-helper lymphocytes giving rise to severe immunosuppression and the manifestations of AIDS. Another feature of the immune perturbation is B-cell activation resulting in hypergammaglobulinaemia. A further consequence is immune thrombocytopenia. When the T-helper cell count (CD4 count) drops below approximately 200/µl, HIV-positive people become vulnerable to the various life-threatening conditions that characterize AIDS.

Clinical features

Seroconversion

Seroconversion is symptomatic in an estimated 50% of people who acquire HIV. The symptoms are enormously variable and may mimic any acute viral infections. 'Flu-like symptoms accompanied by a maculopapular rash, symptoms suggestive of glandular fever, respiratory infection, gastrointestinal infection and even infection of the CNS also occur. Therefore cough, nausea, vomiting, diarrhoea and headache are possible symptoms as well as rash. Nervous system manifestations are unusual, but include meningitis, encephalitis, cranial nerve palsy, acute myelopathy and Guillain–Barré syndrome. A seroconversion illness can last days, weeks or months. Symptomatic seroconversion is associated with a worse prognosis for the development of AIDS.

Asymptomatic disease

All patients with HIV, whether or not they experience a symptomatic seroconversion, will shortly enter an asymptomatic phase, which may be prolonged for many years. During this period, HIV antibodies are detectable and the CD4 count almost always gradually declines. Thrombocytopenia is present in a small minority of patients. If untreated, this may lead to abnormal bleeding.

Persistent generalized lymphadenopathy

Approximately 50% of patients with HIV develop persistent lymphadenopathy. This is characteristically bilateral and

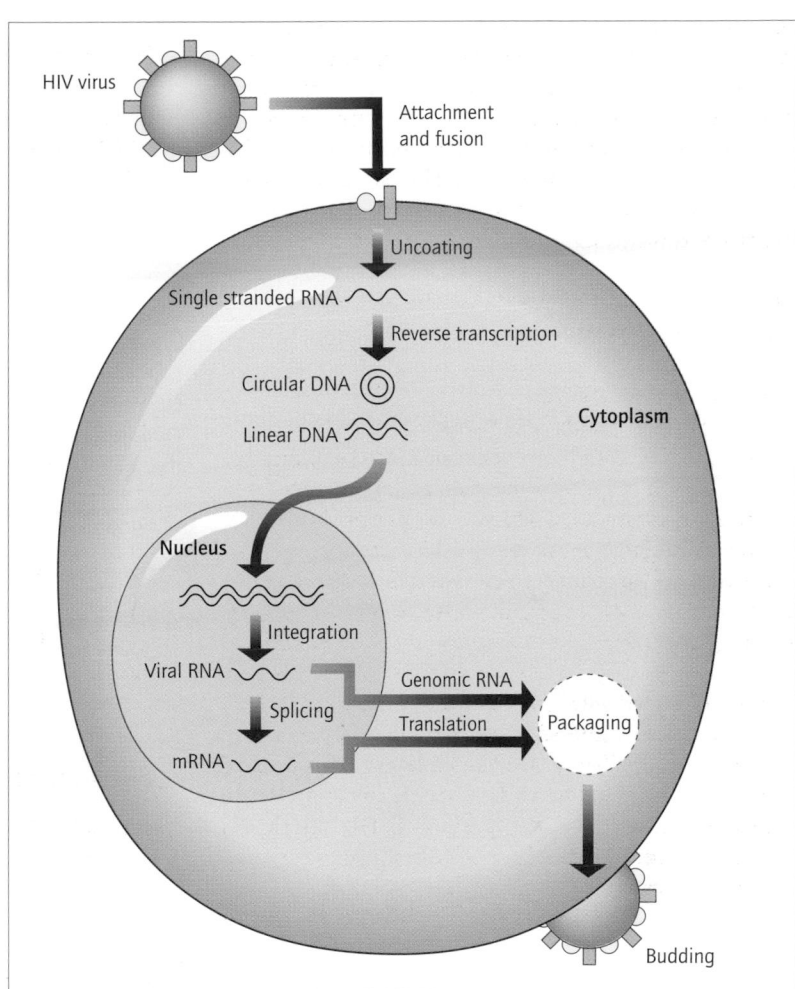

Figure 3.49 HIV life cycle.

symmetrical and most commonly found in the axillary, posterior cervical and inguinal lymph nodes. Strictly speaking, to meet the definition of persistent generalized lymphadenopathy, the lymph nodes should measure at least 1 cm in diameter. However, lymphadenopathy in this distribution should alert the clinician to the possibility of HIV infection whatever the size of the lymph nodes. When significant immunosuppression develops the lymphadenopathy subsides, so patients presenting with a manifestation of AIDS are unlikely to show this distribution of lymphadenopathy.

Constitutional symptoms

It is reasonably common for people with HIV to suffer occasional night sweats. This of itself does not indicate a poor prognosis. Herpes zoster (shingles) can arise when there is a relatively small degree of immunosuppression. When it is multidermatomal, this carries a worse prognosis and is classed within the definition of AIDS. Two oral conditions carry a poor prognosis and antiretroviral treatment should be started to diminish the risk of imminent

progression to AIDS. The first and more common of these is oral candidiasis. This causes soreness of the mouth and commonly white flecks of *Candida* are seen on the palate and the inner surface of the cheeks. Less commonly, oral hairy leucoplakia is seen as furring on the lateral borders of the tongue. This is usually asymptomatic and is caused by a reactivation of Epstein–Barr virus infection. Unexplained weight loss or unexplained diarrhoea (caused by an HIV enteropathy) are other symptoms that may herald rapid progression to AIDS (KEYPOINTS BOX 3.5).

Keypoints 3.5: Stages of HIV infection

Seroconversion (symptomatic in approximately 50%)
Asymptomatic
Persistent generalized lymphadenopathy (in approximately 50%)
Symptomatic
■ Non-AIDS-defining
■ AIDS defining

HIV infection at a glance

Epidemiology
Prevalence
Global pandemic

Age
Predominantly young adults and children born to mothers with HIV

Findings on investigation
Haematology
Platelets decrease in some patients
Haemoglobin decreases in some people with end-stage disease

Serology
HIV antibody positive

Immunology
CD4 lymphocyte count decreases with time

Clinical features
Seroconversion illness
'Flu-like symptoms 2–3 months after infection

Asymptomatic phase
Lymphadenopathy
Symptomatic disease
Fever
Weight loss
Lethargy
Diarrhoea
Opportunistic infection
Neoplasia
Dementia
Wasting

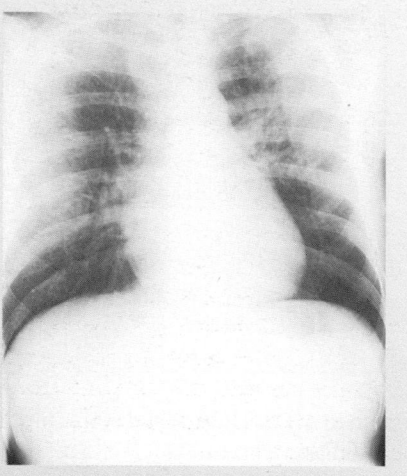

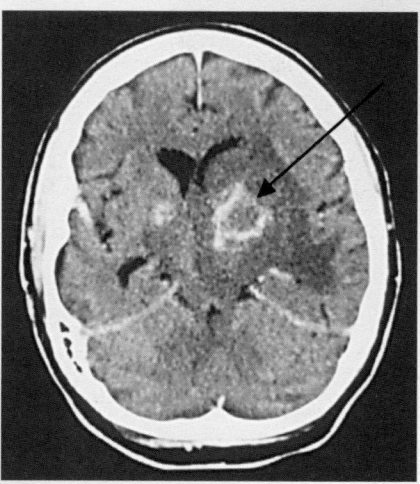

Fig. A Chest X-ray showing lung shadowing consistent with *Pneumocystis carinii* pneumonia.

Fig. B Ring enhancement in Toxoplasmosis. Reproduced from Leach, *Critical Care at a Glance* (Blackwell Publishing, Oxford) with permission.

AIDS

There are four broad categories of life-threatening disease that characterize AIDS:
● Opportunistic infections
● Tumours
● HIV-1 associated encephalopathy (AIDS dementia complex)
● HIV wasting syndrome (weight loss of greater than 10% of body weight with at least 1 month of unexplained fever)

Investigations

Keypoints 3.6: Special investigations in HIV infection

HIV antibody test (plus confirmatory tests)
Lymphocyte subsets
HIV RNA level
Resistance assays
Antiretroviral drug levels

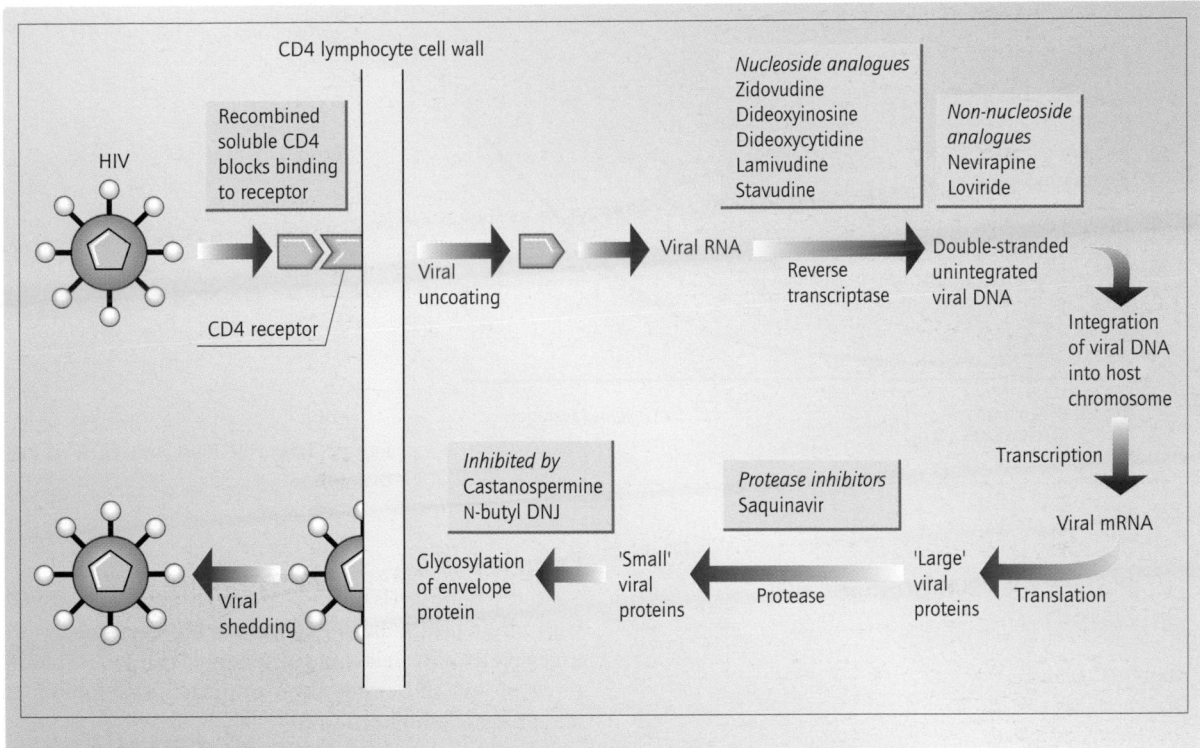

Fig. C The HIV replicative cycle.

HIV antibody tests

A diagnosis of HIV infection is made by demonstrating reliably the presence of HIV antibodies. Informed consent must be obtained, except in the rarest of circumstances. In order to obtain informed consent, a pretest discussion should take place to try to ensure that the patient is as well prepared as possible to receive the result, should it be positive (KEYPOINTS BOX 3.7)

Keypoints 3.7: Pretest discussion

Explore level of risk
Check symptoms
Feedback on assessment of risk
Explain implications of positive or negative result
Explain 'window period' to development of antibodies
Agree need to inform partner and expartner(s) if positive
Ensure adequate support if positive
Explain problems with life insurance
Invite further questions and discussion
Arrange to give result face to face

Confirmatory HIV antibody tests must be performed on the specimen using a variety of different methods, preferably prior to giving a result to the patient. If the result of these tests is positive, the patient should be informed, but at the same time a second blood sample should be taken for confirmation to rule out the possibility of a muddle in specimens or false-positive result.

Lymphocyte subsets

Lymphocyte subsets should be monitored every 2–3 months in order to establish the degree of immunosuppression. Early on in the course of HIV infection, patients are likely to have a CD4 count above 500/µl (within the normal range for the general population). This tends to fall at a variable rate until it is below 200/µl, when the patient becomes susceptible to the life-threatening diseases that characterize AIDS (Fig. 3.50; KEYPOINTS BOX 3.8).

HIV RNA level

This is measured in copies per millilitre. High levels of HIV RNA (viral load), e.g. over 100 000 copies/ml, are associated with a more rapid decline in the immune system (see Fig. 3.54). HIV RNA levels are especially

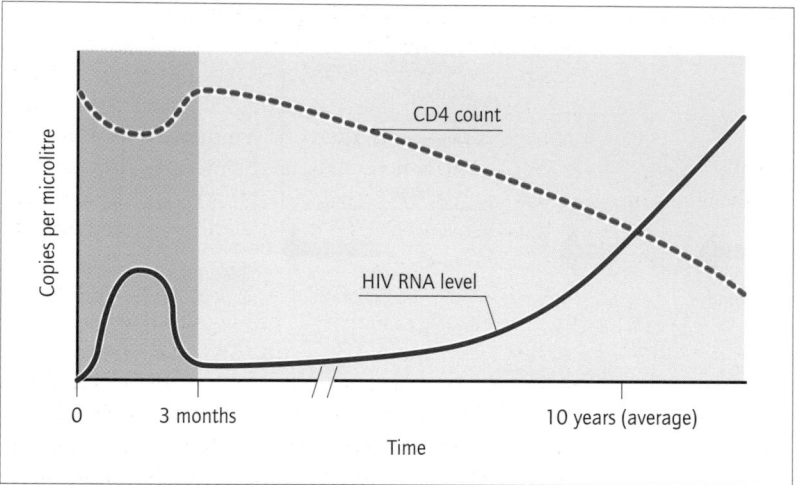

Figure 3.50 HIV RNA and CD4 counts over time.

> ### Keypoints 3.8: Symptomatic HIV infection
>
> *Non-AIDS-defining*
> Oral candidiasis
> Oral hairy leucoplakia
> Unexplained weight loss
> Unexplained diarrhoea
> Herpes zoster
> Night sweats
>
> *AIDS-defining illnesses*
> Opportunistic infections
> Tumours
> HIV-1 associated encephalopathy
> HIV wasting syndrome

important in monitoring antiretroviral treatment. Ideally, treatment produces sustained undetectability of HIV RNA at less than 50 copies/ml.

Resistance assays

Two main types of resistance assay are available: genotyping and phenotyping. The former is more often used. This involves sequencing the reverse transcriptase and protease genes. Point mutation assays can also be employed for the reverse transcriptase gene. These assays provide an indication of which resistance mutations exist in HIV. A knowledge of which mutations are associated with resistance to which drugs allows the clinician to select a regimen that should suppress the virus effectively. Ideally, genotyping is performed prior to starting the first regimen and at every change of regimen.

Drug levels

Subtherapeutic levels of antiretroviral drugs are associated with virological failure. High levels are associated with excessive toxicity. It is currently possible to measure blood levels of non-nucleoside reverse transcriptase inhibitors and protease inhibitors.

It is particularly important to monitor these levels in situations where drug interactions may interfere with drug levels.

Haematology

A full blood count is performed at baseline and at least 3 monthly thereafter. Anaemia can be seen in HIV and AIDS for a variety of reasons, including deficiencies of iron, vitamin B_{12} or folic acid. Zidovudine may suppress the bone marrow, causing anaemia and neutropenia. Thrombocytopenia and commonly neutropenia can result from the immune perturbation.

Biochemistry

Urea and electrolytes and liver function tests require regular monitoring as these can be affected either by HIV-related disease or by its treatment. Patients on treatment with protease inhibitors or efavirenz or stavudine require 6-monthly monitoring of fasting lipids, which may be raised as an adverse drug reaction.

Coexistent infections

Patients should be tested at baseline for other infections, which may have been acquired by the same route as the HIV, e.g. hepatitis B, C and syphilis. Repeat monitoring for STIs must be performed if the patient remains at risk. Antibodies to CMV and *Toxoplasma* must be performed to alert the clinician to the possibility of reactivation of these infections when the patient becomes immunosuppressed.

Chest X-ray

A baseline chest X-ray is advised. Patients from the developing world and injecting drug users are at increased risk of tuberculosis.

Management

The management of HIV infection is a rapidly advancing field. At the time of writing, the British HIV Association advises starting antiretroviral drugs when the CD4 count is between 200 and 350/µl (Table 3.39). People with a rapidly falling CD4 count or a high viral load may be considered for an earlier intervention. There may also be a case for starting treatment during or soon after seroconversion when this is recognized. However, proof of clinical benefit is still awaited. It is likely that treatment in this situation should be of limited duration. When antiretrovirals are started later in the course of HIV infection, the current intention is to continue treatment for life.

Three or more antiretroviral drugs are usually prescribed as a combination. Commonly, two nucleoside analogue reverse transcriptase inhibitors will be combined with one non-nucleoside transcriptase inhibitor or with one or two protease inhibitors. The initial aim of treatment is to lower the HIV RNA level as much as possible, preferably to undetectable levels, which correlate with prolonged survival. Adherence to the regimen is critical to long-term success. Unless 95% or more of doses are taken at the correct time, resistance mutations occur leading to failure of the regimen.

Unfortunately, antiretroviral drugs cause a wide variety of side-effects, some serious. Among the most important is a painful peripheral neuropathy caused especially by stavudine and didanosine and the little used zalcitabine. Any of the currently licensed protease inhibitors can cause hyperlipidaemia (raised cholesterol and/or triglyceride levels) and/or lipodystrophy. Lipodystrophy is an abnormal accumulation of fat in the abdominal organs and between the shoulder blades ('buffalo hump'). Protease inhibitors and nucleoside analogue reverse transcriptase inhibitors combine to cause lipoatrophy (wasting of fat in the face and limbs).

Prevention of secondary infections

Primary prophylaxis against *Pneumocystis carinii* pneumonia should be started prior to the CD4 count falling below 200/µl.

Immune modulation

This form of treatment is in its infancy. The drug that has been evaluated most is IL-2, which is given subcutaneously to boost the CD4 count in patients who are obtaining a disappointing immune response while on antiretroviral treatment.

Prognosis

In the developed world, the median interval between acquisition of HIV and the development of AIDS is just over 10 years. In the developing world it is 3–4 years. In the developed world, for all patients except those presenting in extremis, the outlook is good, although uncertain. With good adherence to therapy and intelligent prescribing and a steady development of new drugs by the pharmaceutical industry, a patient with HIV or AIDS can often look forward to an extended healthy life. The exact duration is difficult to predict.

Opportunistic infections

Pneumocystis carinii pneumonia

Pneumocystis carinii (some now call this organism *Pneumocystis jiroveci*) pneumonia is common among

Table 3.39 Antiretroviral drugs

Nucleoside-analogue reverse transcriptase inhibitors
Zidovudine (AZT or ZDV)
Didanosine (ddl)
Zalcitabine (ddC)
Stavudine (d4T)
Lamivudine (3TC)
Abacavir (ABC)

Nucleotide-analogue reverse transcriptase inhibitors
Tenofovir

Non-nucleoside reverse transcriptase inhibitors
Nevirapine (NVP)
Delavirdine* (DLV)
Efavirenz (EFV)

Protease (proteinase) inhibitors
Saquinavir (SQV) hard or soft gel capsules
Ritonavir (RTV)
Indinavir (IDV)
Nelfinavir (NFV)
Amprenavir (APV)
Lopinavir/ritonavir (Kaletra)

Ribonucleotide reductase inhibitor
Hydroxyurea

---

*Not licensed but available in expanded access programme.

HIV-positive adults in the developed world and among HIV-positive children throughout the world.

Epidemiology

In the absence of primary prophylaxis, approximately 80% of all HIV-positive adults in the developed world progressing to AIDS will at some stage develop *P. carinii* pneumonia.

Disease mechanisms

Most humans are infected with this organism as young children and *P. carinii* pneumonia among adults usually represents reactivation of latent infection rather than reinfection. However, person–person transmission can take place, particularly among children. *Pneumocystis carinii* pneumonia almost always occurs when the CD4 count is lower than 200/μl.

Clinical features

Patients with *P. carinii* pneumonia tend to present with dry cough, increasing breathlessness and fever; the breathlessness is exacerbated by exercise. Sometimes patients present with pyrexia of unknown origin. On examination the patient is usually pyrexial, may have an increased respiratory rate and may be cyanosed. Auscultation of the lungs is usually normal.

Investigation

A chest X-ray is often normal in the early stages but later shows a typical diffuse interstitial infiltration through both lung fields (Fig. 3.51). Arterial blood gas analysis may show hypoxaemia, which is exacerbated on exercise. Because there is no sputum, definitive diagnosis is usually made by bronchoalveolar lavage followed by microscopy of the lavage fluid looking for pneumocysts. It is not possible to culture *Pneumocystis*. Alternatively, a less invasive method employed in some centres is to induce sputum by inhalation of hypertonic sputum. The sputum is then stained and examined for pneumocysts, or demonstrated by immunofluorescence (Fig. 3.52).

Management

Co-trimoxazole is first-line treatment for *P. carinii* pneumonia, but HIV patients may experience a hypersensitivity reaction. Second-line treatments include pentamidine by infusion, dapsone–trimethoprim, or clindamycin–primaquine. Treatment is continued for 14–21 days. A 5-day course of corticosteroids is recommended for patients where the Po_2 levels are below 8 kPa.

Prevention

Primary prophylaxis is given when the CD4 count falls below 200/μl. Secondary prophylaxis is given after a

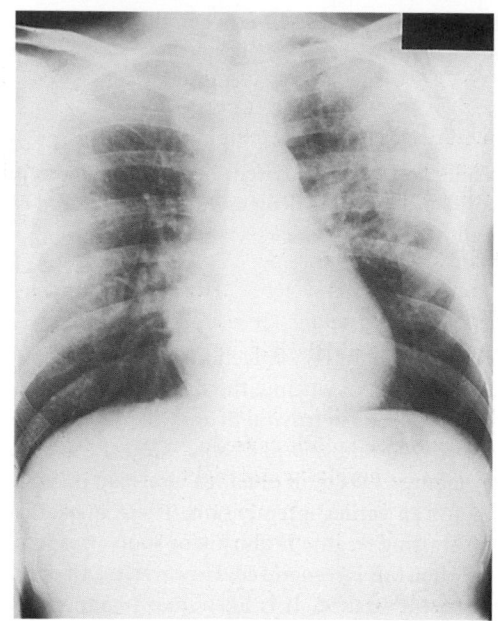

Figure 3.51 Chest X-ray showing lung shadowing consistent with *Pneumocystis carinii* pneumonia.

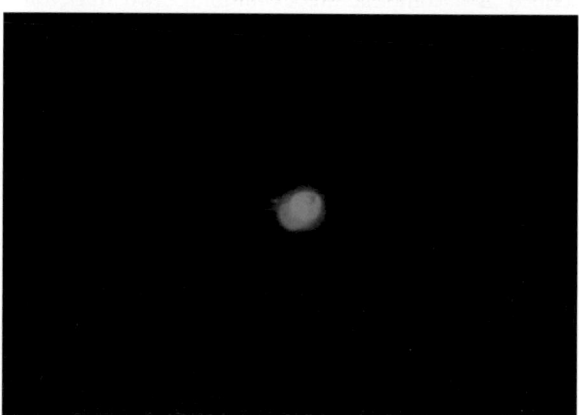

Figure 3.52 *Pneumocystis carinii* pneumonia: IFAT staining.

patient contracts *P. carinii* pneumonia. In each case the preferred agent is co-trimoxazole given either daily or three times a week. Alternatives include daily dapsone or monthly pentamidine via a nebulizer.

Prognosis

The prognosis of most patients with *P. carinii* pneumonia is good, provided that adherence to secondary prophylaxis and to antiretroviral drugs is satisfactory. However, patients who present in extremis may still die from the pneumonia.

Tuberculosis in HIV

Tuberculosis is widespread in the developing world and is seen in industrialized countries, particularly among immigrants from the developing world, people whose ancestors came from areas in the developing world and injecting drug users with HIV.

Disease mechanisms

Tuberculosis is caused by *Mycobacterium tuberculosis* bacillus. This can either cause a primary infection or can subsequently be reactivated.

Clinical features

Pulmonary tuberculosis causes a productive cough, with or without haemoptysis, and night sweats. Extrapulmonary tuberculosis can cause meningitis, lymphadenopathy, gut, urinary tract or bone involvement.

Investigation

Chest X-ray shows infiltration, which may or may not be in the upper lobes, with or without cavitation and with or without fibrosis. Sputum should be sent for acid-fast bacilli and/or PCR. Blood can be cultured for *M. tuberculosis* in HIV infected individuals. In the case of extrapulmonary involvement, blood culture, bone marrow culture, liver biopsy or lumbar puncture can yield a positive diagnosis.

Management

Patients with pulmonary tuberculosis require isolation in negative pressure ventilation rooms. Those with extrapulmonary tuberculosis require isolation until pulmonary involvement has been excluded on chest X-ray and there have been three negative sputum samples. Antibiotics are prescribed in the same way as for immunocompetent patients.

Pneumococcal pneumonia

Disease mechanisms

This is a pneumonia caused by *Streptococcus pneumoniae*. Although not strictly an opportunistic infection, this occurs more frequently in people with HIV infection, and patients with recurrent infection fall within the definition of AIDS.

Clinical features

Patients suffer with fever, productive cough, breathlessness and, occasionally, haemoptysis.

Investigation

Chest X-ray may show changes of lobar pneumonia or bronchopneumonia or be normal. Sputum and blood cultures should be performed.

Management

Treatment with penicillin is usually successful. However, sensitivity testing may reveal penicillin resistance in which case treatment with another agent is indicated (e.g. cefuroxime).

Prevention

It is usually advised that all HIV-positive people should be vaccinated against *Strep. pneumoniae*. Response to the vaccine in patients with HIV, however, is variably effective.

Nervous system

Cryptococcal meningitis

Epidemiology

Approximately 5–10% of patients with AIDS in the UK develop cryptococcal meningitis. Rates are much higher in Africa.

Disease mechanisms

Cryptococcus neoformans is a ubiquitous fungus, present in soil and found in pigeon faeces.

Clinical features

Cryptococcus most commonly causes meningitis with headache and fever. Photophobia and neck stiffness are seen in a minority of patients. Sometimes *Cryptococcus* involves the lungs and causes umbilicated papules on the skin.

Investigation

Lumbar puncture should be performed in cases of suspected meningitis. CSF can then be subjected to India ink staining, which shows spherical yeast cells without mycelia. Cryptococcal antigen should be sought in CSF and blood, and blood cultures performed.

Management

Intravenous amphotericin B is the most effective agent for seriously ill patients. Toxicity is reduced when the liposomal form is used. After at least 2 weeks, therapy can be switched to high-dose fluconazole. In less ill patients, the far less toxic oral fluconazole is used from the outset and continued for up to 6 weeks.

Prevention

Secondary prophylaxis using daily high-dose fluconazole is used.

Prognosis

Up to one-third of patients die during their first episode of cryptococcal meningitis. In those who do recover, relapse is common and carries a high mortality. Patients presenting with reduced consciousness have a worse prognosis.

Cerebral toxoplasmosis in HIV

The protozoan *Toxoplasma gondii* can cause brain abscesses in patients with AIDS. *Toxoplasma* cysts can be ingested through contact with cat faeces or ingestion of undercooked meat (see p. 142).

Clinical features

The cerebral abscesses of toxoplasmosis cause significant headache plus pyrexia. In addition, the level of consciousness may be reduced and signs such as hemiparesis, ataxia and cranial nerve palsies may be present. Fitting occurs in a minority of cases.

Investigation

Computerized tomography demonstrates focal brain lesions. Following the injection of contrast medium, these show ring enhancement. Magnetic resonance imaging is a more sensitive technique for demonstrating these lesions. Serology is used to detect antibodies to *Toxoplasma* but is not diagnostic.

Management

First-line treatment is usually with sulfadiazine and pyrimethamine and folinic acid for 6–8 weeks. In cases of sulphonamide allergy, clindamycin is used instead of sulfadiazine.

Prevention

Co-trimoxazole used either three times a week or daily (the first choice for *Pneumocystis* prophylaxis) is effective as primary prophylaxis against cerebral toxoplasmosis. Patients at risk of reactivation of a latent *Toxoplasma* infection can be identified by demonstrating anti-*Toxoplasma* titres above 1 : 16. When the CD4 count drops below 200/µl, such patients should, if at all possible, take co-trimoxazole as prophylaxis. However, an alternative would be dapsone and pyrimethamine, which is also a good prophylactic against *P. carinii* pneumonia. For secondary prophylaxis, a lower dose of sulfadiazine, pyrimethamine and folinic acid should be continued until the CD4 count has increased to above 200/µl for 3 months in response to antiretroviral treatment.

Progressive multifocal leucoencephalopathy

Progressive multifocal leucoencephalopathy (PML) is a demyelinating disease most often seen in association with HIV infection. It usually occurs when the CD4 count is less than 100/µl.

Disease mechanisms

It is caused by the JC papovavirus. This common virus is probably spread by droplets, usually causing few if any symptoms unless the person becomes immunocompromised, in which case reactivation can cause disease.

Clinical features

Patients usually undergo a rapid neurological deterioration with visual field defects, weakness of the limbs and cerebral ataxia being common. Cognitive impairment is present in a significant minority of cases.

Investigation

Magnetic resonance imaging shows characteristic appearances. Confirmation of the diagnosis is obtained by using PCR to demonstrate JC virus DNA in CSF.

Management

The antiviral agent cidofovir is used intravenously. This nucleoside analogue inhibits the DNA polymerase of JC papovavirus. The immune reconstitution that accompanies antiretroviral treatment is useful in combating the disease. In addition, the nucleoside analogue cidofovir is being evaluated.

Prevention

There are no strategies for prevention.

Prognosis

Most patients survive only a few weeks or a few months, although a few enjoy a prolonged survival.

Cytomegalovirus retinitis

This is an inflammation of the retina caused by cytomegalovirus (CMV).

Epidemiology

In the developed world, over 50% of adult heterosexuals and over 90% of adult homosexuals have antibodies to CMV. Retinitis can occur in anyone with CMV antibodies when the CD4 count drops below 100/µl.

Cause, clinical features, investigations and prognosis
(See p. 143.)

Management

Ganciclovir, given by intravenous infusion, is the first-line

Toxoplasmosis at a glance

Epidemiology
Prevalence
Up to 70% infected

Age
Infection more common with increasing age

Findings on investigation
Immunology
ELISA, dye test and agglutination techniques to demonstrate antibodies

Microbiology
Culture rarely indicated

Diagnostic imaging
Cerebral CT scan to detect cerebral toxoplasmosis

Histopathology
Biopsy of lymph nodes may reveal toxoplasmosis
Brain biopsy may be required to confirm diagnosis of cerebral disease

Clinical features
Majority of infections are asymptomatic
Self-limiting febrile illness may develop
Congenital infection can result in retinitis and mental retardation
Immunocompromised patients may reactivate cerebral lesions
Overwhelming infection in transplant patients

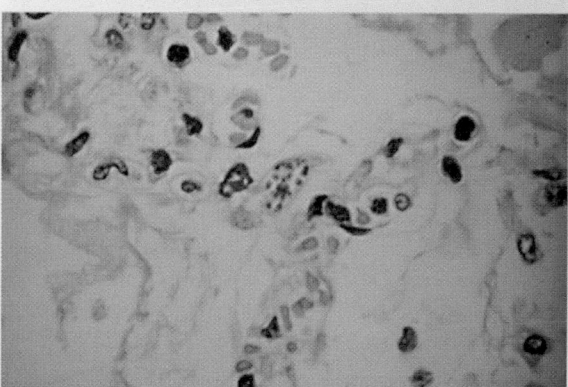

Fig. A Toxoplasma. Tachyzoites in lung tissue.

treatment for retinitis. Less well-tolerated alternatives are phosphonoformate (foscarnet) or cidofovir. Sometimes, in relapsing disease, intravitreal injections of ganciclovir are used.

The preferred agent for secondary prophylaxis is valganciclovir, a prodrug of ganciclovir, which is well-absorbed orally.

Gastrointestinal infections

Candidiasis

Candidiasis is an infection with the yeast *Candida albicans*.

Epidemiology
Candida is often present in the gastrointestinal tract and will multiply to cause problems in immunosuppressed patients. Oral candidiasis is experienced by almost all patients who develop AIDS and it is very often one of the first signs of immunosuppression prior to the development of AIDS.

Disease mechanisms
Most candidiasis is caused by *Candida albicans*, although other strains such as *Candida glabrata* may cause problems.

Clinical features
Oral candidiasis has been alluded to on p. 160. Oesophageal candidiasis is an AIDS-defining illness and causes dysphagia and/or odynophagia plus nausea.

Investigation
The definitive investigation is endoscopic biopsy. However, the diagnosis is often made clinically by the finding of oral candidiasis in association with typical symptoms of oesophageal candidiasis.

Management
Oral candidiasis often responds to topical treatment with nystatin suspension or pastilles, or amphotericin lozenges. In the large majority of cases, patients with oesophageal candidiasis can easily use an oral anti-*Candida* agent such as fluconazole for 2 weeks. In patients who either fail to respond or have abnormal liver function, itraconazole is a useful oral alternative. Patients whose symptoms fail to respond require a definitive diagnosis by endoscopy and may require admission for intravenous amphotericin B.

Prevention

Primary and secondary prophylaxis against oesophageal candidiasis is avoided if at all possible because they predispose to the development of resistant *Candida*.

Prognosis

The prognosis of both oral and oesophageal candidiasis is excellent. When antiretroviral treatment stimulates immune reconstitution, these no longer tend to recur.

Diarrhoeal diseases

The causes of the prevalent diarrhoeal diseases vary according to geography.

Disease mechanisms

Any of the common causes of diarrhoea in immunocompetent people (e.g. enteric viruses, *Salmonella* and *Shigella*) may cause diarrhoea in immunocompromised patients. In addition, the following opportunistic infections are found: *Cryptosporidium*, *Isospora*, microsporidia and CMV.

Clinical features

Cryptosporidium in particular may, on occasion, cause a very high volume, watery diarrhoea. Cytomegalovirus may cause bloody diarrhoea.

Investigation of intestinal infection

Between three and six stool samples should be examined for ova, cysts, parasites and culture. Special stains are required for *Cryptosporidium* and microsporidium. Ideally, electron microscopy is also performed to look for enteric viruses. If stool samples fail to yield the diagnosis, gut biopsy is required. Rectal biopsy is usually performed first, progressing to duodenal biopsy if necessary. Diarrhoea may also occur as a result of malignancy. The possibility of small bowel lymphoma or Kaposi's sarcoma may be investigated by either barium meal and follow-through, or enteroscopy. If still no cause is found, colonoscopy plus biopsy may yield a diagnosis.

Herpes simplex

Clinical features

Ulceration tends to be prolonged in immunosuppressed patients. Homosexuals, in particular, are at risk of severe perianal ulceration. When ulceration persists for more than a month, this is classed as an AIDS-defining illness.

Management

Oral treatment with aciclovir, valaciclovir or famciclovir usually heals the lesions within several days.

Prevention

Primary prevention is not necessary, but in the case of frequently recurring herpes, secondary prophylaxis with either aciclovir, valacivlovir or famciclovir is usually extremely effective.

Prognosis

The prognosis of patients with ulceration from herpes is excellent. Even in those cases where secondary prophylaxis is necessary, this can usually be stopped when immune restoration is obtained by the use of antiretroviral drugs.

Atypical mycobacterial infection

Atypical mycobacteria cause disseminated disease in approximately one-quarter of people with late stage HIV infection, usually when the CD4 count is below 50/μl.

Disease mechanisms

The major causative organism is *Mycobacterium avium-intracellulare*. Less commonly, *M. kansasii* and other non-tuberculous mycobacteria cause disease. These organisms enter the body through the respiratory or gastrointestinal tracts.

Clinical features

Typical features of disseminated disease are malaise, fever, night sweats, anorexia and wasting. Sometimes diarrhoea and abdominal pain may also feature. On examination hepatosplenomegaly may be present.

Investigation

The patient is commonly anaemic and there is commonly a raised alkaline phosphatase. Atypical mycobacteria may be cultured from blood, bone marrow, lymph nodes or liver. CT scanning may reveal enlarged lymph nodes in the abdomen. Treatment is with a combination of three or four drugs. Commonly, clarithromycin and ethambutol are combined with either rifabutin or rifampicin. Other options are ciprofloxacin, clofazimine, azithromycin or amikacin.

Prevention

Primary prophylaxis, usually with clarithromycin or azithromycin, should be used in patients with a CD4 count of less than 50/μl. Prophylaxis should be continued until the CD4 count has risen above 100 for at least 3 months (primary) and 6 months (secondary.)

Tumours

Kaposi's sarcoma

Epidemiology
Kaposi's sarcoma is sometimes seen in patients without HIV infection, e.g. Africans, elderly men of Mediterranean or eastern European origin, and in people who are immunosuppressed for other reasons, such as renal transplant recipients. Among HIV-positive people, Kaposi's sarcoma is mainly seen among homosexual men and Africans.

Disease mechanisms
Kaposi's sarcoma is caused by infection with the human herpes virus type 8.

Clinical features
Any organ can be involved, especially the lymph nodes (Fig. 3.53). New lesions arise until the lesions are widespread. Other organs that may be involved are lymph nodes, giving rise to lymphadenopathy, the gastrointestinal tract (a lesion is visible on the palate in approximately one-third of patients at presentation) and the lungs. Lesions in the gastrointestinal tract may bleed. Pulmonary Kaposi's sarcoma causes breathlessness and sometimes haemoptysis and is a life-threatening condition.

Investigation
Depending on the site of the symptoms, chest X-ray, lymph node biopsy and endoscopy may be warranted.

Management
Lesions on the skin can either be left alone or disguised with cosmetics, or treated with local radiotherapy, or with intralesional injections of low-dose interferon. In the case of visceral Kaposi's sarcoma or very advanced skin disease, systemic chemotherapy with liposomal doxorubicin or daunorubicin may be used.

Prevention
Human herpes virus type 8 appears to be sexually transmitted. This is one of various reasons why people with HIV should avoid penetrative sex.

Prognosis
Immune restoration by the use of antiretroviral treatment is helpful in causing lesions of Kaposi's sarcoma to regress.

Non-Hodgkin's lymphoma

Epidemiology
B-cell non-Hodgkin's lymphomas (high-grade B-cell lymphoma, diffuse large B-cell lymphoma and Burkitt's lymphoma) are seen many times more commonly among HIV-positive people than in the general population. Overall, 5–10% of patients with AIDS develop non-Hodgkin's lymphoma.

Clinical features
Most patients present with the symptoms of weight loss of greater than 10%, unexplained fever and night sweats. Although the disease may only be found in lymph nodes, it is commonly extranodal and can involve the gastrointestinal tract or respiratory tract and in some patients there is primary cerebral lymphoma. Symptoms are dictated by the site of the lymphoma.

Investigation
CT scanning is useful to localize the tumours and biopsy is necessary for histological diagnosis.

Management
Chemotherapy is used, taking care not to use overly toxic regimens.

Prognosis
Treatment of systemic or non-Hodgkin's lymphoma in HIV infection can be extremely rewarding and patients can survive for several years or more. However, the prognosis of primary cerebral lymphoma is usually measured in months.

Primary central nervous system lymphoma

Epidemiology
These lymphomas tend to occur in patients with very low CD4 counts who have often been immunosuppressed for a long period.

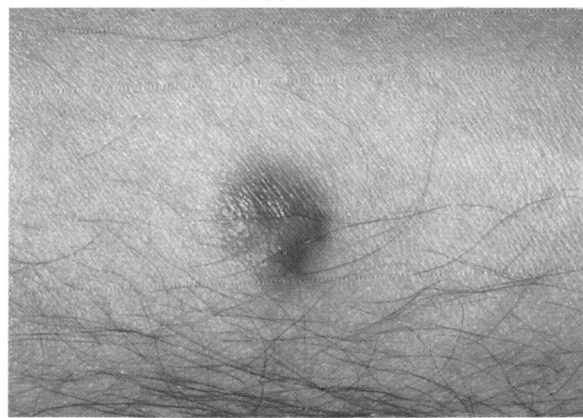

Figure 3.53 Lesion of Kaposi's sarcoma.

Disease mechanisms

Epstein–Barr virus causes CNS lymphoma, usually a high-grade diffuse large-cell immunoblastic B-cell lymphoma.

Clinical features

Clinical features vary according to the site of the lymphoma.

Investigation

Single or multiple lesions can be demonstrated by either CT or MRI. Biopsy is occasionally performed when the diagnosis is unclear.

Management

Dexamethasone is used initially to reduce cerebral oedema. Whole brain irradiation can then be administered.

Prognosis

Without treatment patients survive for about 1 month. Those who respond well to radiotherapy nevertheless die within the year.

Hodgkin's disease

Hodgkin's disease appears to be somewhat more common in patients with HIV infection compared to the general population. Patients generally present with 'B' symptoms and are treated with standard chemotherapeutic regimens.

Carcinoma of the cervix

Epidemiology

Carcinoma of the cervix occurs more frequently in patients with HIV who are immunosuppressed.

Disease mechanisms

The major types of HPV linked to carcinoma of the cervix are 16 and, to a lesser extent, 18.

Clinical features

Carcinoma of the cervix can cause bleeding per vaginam and pain through local invasion.

Management

Surgery is the treatment of choice.

Prevention

Women with HIV infection should undergo regular cytology and colposcopy to pick up precancerous changes so that loop diathermy or cone biopsy can be performed before the disease progresses to invasive carcinoma.

Prognosis

Provided that the disease is picked up early, the prognosis is good.

HIV-1 associated encephalopathy

Epidemiology

HIV-1 associated encephalopathy or AIDS dementia complex tends to be a late feature of AIDS. It is seen less frequently nowadays in countries where highly active antiretroviral treatment is used.

Disease mechanisms

HIV is neurotropic and crosses the blood–brain barrier to set up infection in the CNS very early on in the course of HIV infection.

Clinical features

In the early stages, AIDS dementia complex can be mistaken for depression. There is a gradually increasing level of cognitive impairment. In addition, there may be involvement of the nervous system elsewhere, for instance, HIV myelopathy causing gait problems and a symmetrical peripheral neuropathy, which is commonly painful.

Investigation

It is necessary first to verify a decline in recent memory and intellectual abilities. CT scan (or MRI) almost always demonstrate cerebral atrophy. Lumbar puncture is performed to exclude other diagnoses.

Management

Zidovudine is the first choice treatment in that it has been shown to improve neuropsychological performance in patients with HIV-1 associated encephalopathy. In the case of resistance to zidovudine, other drugs that penetrate well into the central nervous system, such as stavudine, abacavir and nevirapine, can be of use.

Prevention

The incidence of HIV-1 associated encephalopathy has reduced coincident with the widespread use of antiretrovirals, including zidovudine.

Prognosis

Without treatment, the patient commonly declines over the course of several months into an almost vegetative state, accompanied by paraparesis and double incontinence. With appropriate antiretroviral treatment, neuropsychological functioning can improve so that patients may live a satisfactory life for a period of years.

HIV wasting syndrome

Epidemiology
HIV wasting syndrome is seen only in advanced HIV infection.

Disease mechanisms
HIV can cause villous atrophy in the small bowel resulting in malabsorption. Together with the increased resting energy expenditure in HIV-positive people and disturbed protein metabolism, wasting can result.

Clinical features
HIV wasting syndrome can be defined as unexplained weight loss of greater than 10% of body weight or unexplained fever for more than 1 month.

Investigation
Opportunistic infections and tumours need to be excluded.

Management
Combination antiretroviral treatment is usually successful in restoring body weight and abolishing fevers.

Prevention
Antiretroviral therapy that suppresses viral load effectively will prevent the development of HIV wasting syndrome.

Prognosis
Provided there is not widespread resistance to antiretrovirals, the prognosis is good.

! Must know checklist

- Know how to take a history and examine patients with infections

- Understand the routes of transmission of infective agents and how to prevent their spread in the hospital and the community

- List the main organisms infecting humans

- Know the spectrum of the main anti-infective agents

- Understand the ways in which the laboratory can be used to make a diagnosis of infectious diseases

- Understand the process of immunization and outline the main components of an effective vaccination programme

- Sexual history taking requires an understanding non-judgemental approach

- Always warm a vaginal speculum

- Dysuria in sexually active young men is usually caused by urethritis not cystitis and is sexually acquired

- The most common cause of genital ulceration in the UK is genital herpes but syphilis is beginning to reappear

- The most common causes of genital 'lumps' are genital warts, molluscum contagiosum and normal anatomical structures (e.g. hirsuties papillaris penis, vulval micropapillae)

- Bacterial vaginosis and candidiasis are the most common causes of pathological vaginal discharge and neither are sexually transmitted

- *Chlamydia trachomatis* is the most common sexually transmitted bacterial infection in the developed world and the most common cause of tubal infertility

- Human papillomavirus (HPV) is the most common sexually transmitted viral infection

- Subclinical infection is more common than clinically overt disease. HPV types 6 and 11 cause genital warts. HPV types 16 and 18 cause dysplastic disease ('intra-epithelial neoplasia') and anogenital carcinoma

- Acquired immune deficiency syndrome (AIDS) can be defined as the life-threatening diseases caused by human immunodeficiency virus (HIV)

- Common routes of transmission of HIV are sexual, via blood, via sharing of equipment by injecting drug users and by vertical transmission

03

Further reading

Books

Adler MW, ed. *ABC of AIDS*. London: BMJ Books, 2001.

Bannister B, Begg N, Gillespie S. *Infectious Disease*, 2nd edn. Oxford: Blackwell Publishing, 2000.

Crowe S, Hoy J, Mills J, eds. *Management of the HIV-Infected Patient*, 2nd edn. London: Martin Dunitz, 2002.

Dolin R, Masur H, Saag MS, eds. *AIDS Therapy*. London: Churchill Livingstone, 2002.

Gazzard B, ed. *AIDS Care Handbook*, 2nd edn. Mediscript Ltd, 1 Mountview Court, 310 Friern Barnet Lane, London N20 0LD, 2002.

Gillespie S, Bamford K. *Medical Microbiology and Infection at a Glance*, 2nd edn. Oxford: Blackwell Publishing, 2003.

Greenwood D, Slack R, Peutherer J. *Medical Microbiology*. London: Churchill Livingstone, 1998.

Mims C. *The Pathogenesis of Infectious Diseases*. London: Academic Press, 2001.

Mims C *et al. Medical Microbiology*. London: Mosby, 1998.

Journals

Reviews in Medical Microbiology http://www.revmedmicrobiol.com/ (Lippincott Williams and Wilkins)

Clinical Infectious Diseases (Infectious Disease Society of America) http://www.journals.uchicago.edu/CID/home.html (Chicago University Press)

Lancet Infectious Diseases http://www.sciencedirect.com/science/journal/14733099 (Elsevier)

AIDS http://www.aidsonline.com (Lippincott Williams & Wilkins)

Websites

http://www.microbelibrary.org/
http://www.microbe.org/
http://www.sgm.ac.uk/
http://www.microbiologyonline.org.uk/
www.sextransinf.com
www.aidsmap.com
www.medscape.com
www.unaids.org/
www.mssvd.org.uk

Rheumatic Disease

Introduction

Rheumatic diseases are common, and osteoarthritis (OA) is one of the most frequent causes of disease. They form a significant part of a doctor's workload and lead to large annual health bills for doctors, drugs and hospital care. Approximately 15% of patients on an average GP's list have an arthritis-related condition and take up approximately 27% of consulting time. Many working days are lost each year because of arthritis and related conditions.

Rheumatic diseases affect people of all ages and both sexes, but some are more common in certain age groups and races, and in males or females.

Joint pain is a feature of most rheumatic diseases, but these disorders may present in different guises with other symptoms to a variety of specialist clinics ranging from dermatology to genitourinary medicine.

Structure and function

Arthritis is the most common factor linking the rheumatic diseases, and a knowledge of joint structure is required to understand the disease processes. Extra-articular manifestations involve skin, lung and kidney for example, and an understanding of the structure of such organs is also necessary (see pp. 503 and 299).

Connective tissue

The interstitial tissue of the musculoskeletal system is called **connective tissue** and its structural and functional properties depend on the relative proportions of the tissues of which it is composed. Connective tissues may be involved in rheumatic disease as a result of:

- Inflammatory cell infiltration
- Crystal deposition
- Enzyme degradation
- Structural abnormalities

Composition

The main components of connective tissue are **transitory and resident cells**, and the **macromolecules** they synthesize.

Connective tissue cells

Connective tissue cells include **transitory lymphocytes, monocytes and neutrophils**. Their numbers depend on several factors such as cell adhesion molecules (CAMs) directing the traffic of lymphocytes (see pp. 41 and 48), and cytokines attracting monocytes into the tissues (see p. 47).

Fibroblasts are the **resident** cells that synthesize and maintain the extracellular matrix. They may differentiate into more specialized cells, such as **chondrocytes, osteoblasts and endothelial cells**.

Macromolecules

The macromolecular components are:
- *Collagens:* a large family of related proteins that contain triple-helical protease-resistant domains and a high content of hydroxyproline residues, which have a supportive function (Fig. 4.1)
- *Fibronectin and laminin:* involved in the adhesion of cells to each other or to macromolecular components
- *Elastin:* a cross-linked polymer with elastic properties that are valuable in distensible tissue such as lung parenchyma and arterial wall

04

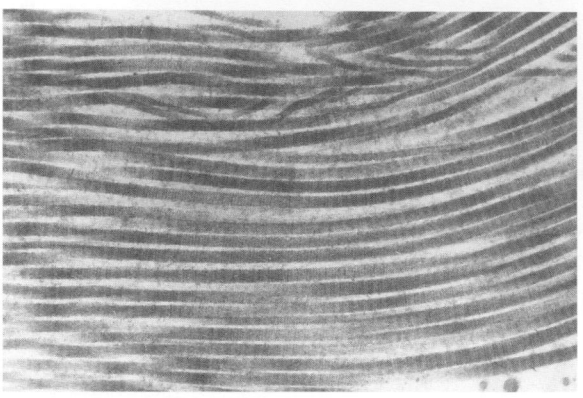

Figure 4.1 Structure of rabbit periosteal collagen. Magnification ×20 000.

● *Complex polysaccharides:* predominantly proteoglycan molecules containing long chains of repeating disaccharide units (glycosaminoglycans and hyaluronic acid) and which confer compressibility

Joints

In the context of musculoskeletal disease, joints may be either **fibrocartilaginous** (allowing moderate movement) or **synovial** (allowing considerable mobility).

Fibrocartilaginous joints

Fibrocartilaginous joints include the pubic symphysis, the sacroiliac joint and the intervertebral discs.

Synovial joints

In the normal human body there are 187 synovial joints divided into four general types:

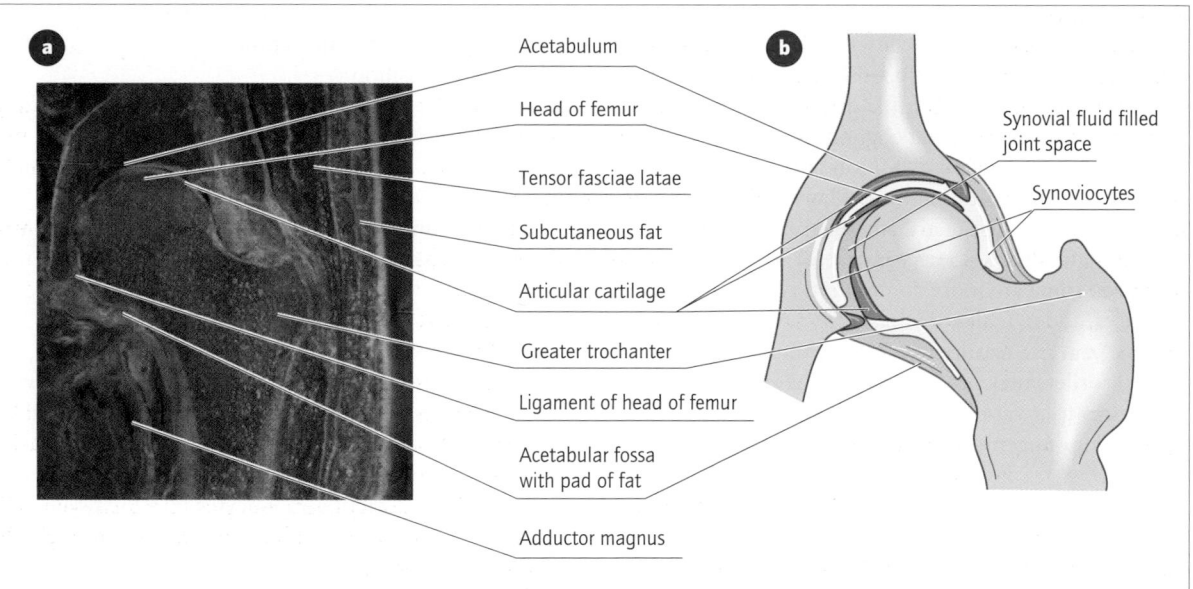

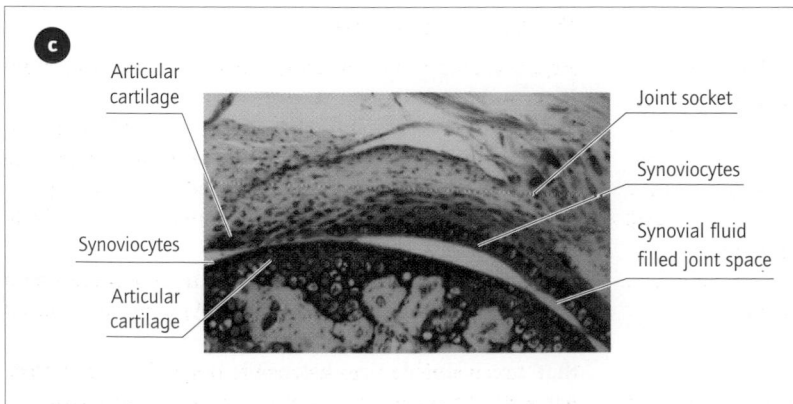

Figure 4.2 The hip joint is a synovial joint. (a) Cross-section. (b) Diagram of a cross-section. (c) Photomicrograph of section through joint (stained with toluidine blue). Synoviocytes are located on the periarticular surfaces of the joint.

1 Ball and socket (e.g. hip joint)
2 Hinge (e.g. interphalangeal joint)
3 Saddle (e.g. first carpometacarpal joint)
4 Plain (e.g. patellofemoral joint).

Design variations have evolved to allow movement in combinations of flexion, extension, abduction, adduction and rotation. Joints can act in one, two or three axes of movement; examples of such joints are the humero-ulnar, wrist and shoulder joints, respectively.

A typical synovial joint consists of articulating bone surfaces, **articular cartilage, synovium, synovial fluid, capsule and tendons** inserting into the capsule (see below) together with nerve and blood supply. It may contain fibrocartilage (e.g. knee menisci), and be surrounded by tendons, ligaments and bursae (Fig. 4.2).

Joint stability depends on the shape of the joint, its associated tendons, ligaments and muscles, and the presence of synovial fluid, which seals the joint surfaces together.

Articular cartilage

Articular cartilage provides a low-friction surface between opposing joint surfaces. It lines the bone and consists of:
● *Collagen fibres:* maintain the integrity of the cartilage and are densely packed and aligned parallel to the axis of movement at the surface
● *Matrix of proteoglycans:* linked to hyaluronate contained within the collagen framework, making it springy and resilient—the water it binds making it resistant to deformation
● *Chondrocytes:* specialized fibroblasts synthesizing proteoglycans and collagen

Synovium

Synovium is the main intracapsular tissue and consists of one to three layers of macrophage- and fibroblast-like cells. It covers all intracapsular structures other than articulating areas of cartilage, and produces synovial fluid. Fenestrated microvessels lie among the cells, along with lymphatic vessels and nerve fibres.

Synovial fluid

Synovial fluid has a similar composition to blood plasma, but also contains hyaluronic acid, which is secreted by synoviocytes and increases its viscosity. Albumin is its main protein constituent.

A thin film of synovial fluid covers the surfaces of the synovium and cartilage within the joint space in normal human joints and serves as a joint lubricant and nutrient supply to the articular cartilage. In disease, the volume of synovial fluid may increase, resulting in an effusion.

Joint capsule

The capsule of a synovial joint is continuous with the periosteum covering the bone and is composed of an irregular spiral of collagenous fibres. As in ligaments and tendons, these fibres are aligned with the axis of stress.

Joint sensation and blood supply

Joint sensation is derived from the joint capsule and its ligaments, the periosteum and the bone itself. Pain is transmitted by nerve fibres, while proprioceptive information is obtained from the nerve root supplying the associated muscles. An arterial plexus of blood supplies the synovial tissue, the capsule and the juxta-articular bone.

Approach to the patient

History

Most rheumatological diagnoses can be made clinically, although some diseases may resemble each other at first and evolve over time, for example autoimmune rheumatic diseases.

It is important to obtain a good history and to examine a patient thoroughly. Your aims should be to define:
● Symptoms and their location and effect
● Differential diagnosis
● Useful investigations
● Appropriate treatment
If the patient is managed over many years, a well-recorded presenting history and examination will prove valuable for charting disease progression.

A description of a patient as a 'poor historian' generally indicates a failure in guiding the patient through the history taking process.

About the patient

Age, sex, race and occupation are associated with certain rheumatic diseases:
● Sexually acquired reactive arthritis (SARA) and systemic lupus erythematosus (SLE) are more common in a younger age group (25–35 years) than OA and polymyalgia rheumatica (PMR), which are more common in those over 50 years of age
● Gout and ankylosing spondylitis (AS) are more common in men, but rheumatoid arthritis (RA) is more common in women
● White people are more prone to polymyalgia rheumatica, while Afro-Caribbeans are more susceptible to SLE

04

● Musicians, dancers, keyboard operators and labourers may repetitively traumatize certain joints or surrounding structures, and exposure to toxic agents (e.g. polyvinyl chloride) is associated with a scleroderma-like disease

Rheumatic symptoms

Some symptoms are common in rheumatic diseases so pain, stiffness and joint swelling should be explored in depth. The important questions to ask a patient are listed in HISTORY & EXAMINATION BOX 4.1.

Joint pain may arise from the joint itself, or from adjacent bone or surrounding soft tissue, or be referred from other systems (e.g. cardiac pain may be referred to the arm). Joint swelling always indicates disease.

First symptoms

First symptoms may provide clues to the diagnosis:

History & Examination 4.1: Important questions to ask a patient with rheumatic disease

About the patient
How old are you?
What is your occupation?

Joint symptoms
Joint pain
Where is it?
How long does it last?
Is it persistent, intermittent or flitting?
What is its character (e.g. ache, sharp pain)?
Where does it radiate?
What relieves or exacerbates it?
How does it affect your mobility?

Stiffness
When does it occur (e.g. morning or evening)?
How long does it last?
How severe is it?

Joint swelling
Is it persistent, intermittent or progressive?

Pattern of disease
Onset and progression
What were your first symptoms?
Over what period of time did they develop?
How many joints were affected (is it a mono-, oligo- or polyarthritis)?
Which joints were affected (symmetrical or asymmetrical)?
How many joints are affected now?
Which joints are affected now?
When are your symptoms most severe?
Does the overall severity of your symptoms change?
How have your symptoms responded to different treatments?

Associated features
Have you lost weight?
Do you have a fever?
Have you noticed any changes in your skin (indicating vasculitis, psoriasis or inflammation)?
Have you lost any hair and/or noticed any changes in your nails (suggesting SLE or psoriasis)?

Do you get eye pain and/or irritation (features of kerato-conjunctivitis sicca and AS)?
Has your bowel habit changed (suggesting systemic sclerosis or inflammatory bowel disease)?
(Men only) Do you have a urethral discharge (indicating SARA)?
Do you have any unusual sensations or loss of sensation in your arms and/or your legs (a feature of vasculitis and some compression syndromes)?

Disease impact
Work
Has there been any change in ability to perform certain types of work?
Has early retirement been necessary?
Has hospitalization affected career plans?

Home
Can household jobs be carried out?
Is assistance needed for personal care?
Are household aids necessary?

Social
Have social and sporting activities changed?
Is transport now necessary?

Drug history
What medication are you taking?
For how long has any treatment been prescribed?
Have there been any favourable or adverse reactions?
Have any drugs been discontinued and if so why?
Do you take your medication as prescribed?

Past medical history
(Women only) Have you ever had a miscarriage?
Have you ever had a peptic ulcer?

Family history
Does anyone in your family have:
A rheumatic condition?
An autoimmune condition?
A skin condition?
Inflammatory bowel disease?

- Patients with AS often have peripheral arthritis early in the disease
- Infection and gout are typified by an acute onset
- OA has chronic characteristics

Joint involvement

- *Monoarthritis* (involvement of one joint) may indicate infection; *oligoarthritis* (two to four joints) occurs in psoriatic arthritis; and *polyarthritis* (at least five joints) is common in RA
- Any joint may be involved in any disease but some joints are commonly associated with certain diseases
- Osteoarthritis—interphalangeal hand joints, cervical and lumbar spine, hips and knees
- Rheumatoid arthritis—metacarpophalangeal (MCP) joints, wrists, cervical spine, knees, ankles and metatarsophalangeal joints
- RA can usually be distinguished from spondyloarthropathies because of its symmetrical joint involvement
- RA and seronegative spondyloarthritis are characterized by exacerbations and remissions
- Gout is episodic
- RA is associated with early morning joint stiffness
- OA is characterized by an increase in symptoms during the day

Other symptoms

Do not disregard associated features that do not seem to be relevant. Many rheumatic diseases are accompanied by non-rheumatic manifestations (see p. 192)

Pattern of disease

The pathophysiological processes of some rheumatic diseases give rise to recognizable disease patterns in terms of first symptoms, progression and associated features. Certain events (e.g. trauma, drugs, illness) may trigger the disease. Important questions to ask in order to find out the pattern of a rheumatic disease are given in HISTORY & EXAMINATION BOX 4.1.

Disease progression

The number, location and pattern (symmetrical or asymmetrical) of the joints affected, the severity of the joint symptoms and the presence of associated symptoms may reveal milestones or stages of disease progression.

Disease impact

Chronic rheumatic diseases may not only alter a patient's way of life at home and work and socially, but can also test personal relationships and strain financial resources. It is important therefore to find out whether there has been any functional change in the patient in these settings. Particularly important questions to ask are listed in HISTORY & EXAMINATION BOX 4.1. To answer them it may be necessary to observe the patient at home or at work to assess his or her functional abilities and use of community resources.

Try to understand the patient's views of his or her disease and expectations of treatment. Expert counselling may be required.

Drug history

A detailed summary of past and present medication and physical therapy is essential. Important questions to ask about drug treatment are given in HISTORY & EXAMINATION BOX 4.1. Some drugs can trigger rheumatic disease: thiazide diuretics can induce gout; hydralazine and minocycline can cause lupus syndrome; and corticosteroids can cause avascular necrosis of bone.

Past medical history

Consider whether previous illnesses are:
- Related to the presenting complaint (e.g. spontaneous miscarriage and SLE)
- Affected by the current condition (e.g. subacute bacterial endocarditis and septic arthritis)
- Relevant to drug management (e.g. peptic ulcer and non-steroidal anti-inflammatory drug [NSAID] therapy)

Family history

Ask whether there is any family history of rheumatic disease or diseases that may have an arthritic component, such as psoriasis, Crohn's disease or haemochromatosis.

Examination

Examination of a rheumatological patient should not differ from that for other patients, except in its increased emphasis on the musculoskeletal system. All other systems should be examined in detail, especially those commonly involved in rheumatic disease, such as the skin, respiratory system and neurological system. In particular, look for the extra-articular manifestations listed in CLINICAL PRESENTATIONS AT A GLANCE BOX.

To avoid missing the unexpected, a methodical approach to rheumatological examination is advised. Examination is best conducted with the patient standing, then sitting, supine and prone (in that order). First look, then feel and then move the area under examination as appropriate (Fig. 4.3).

Specific details for a regional examination are given in

04

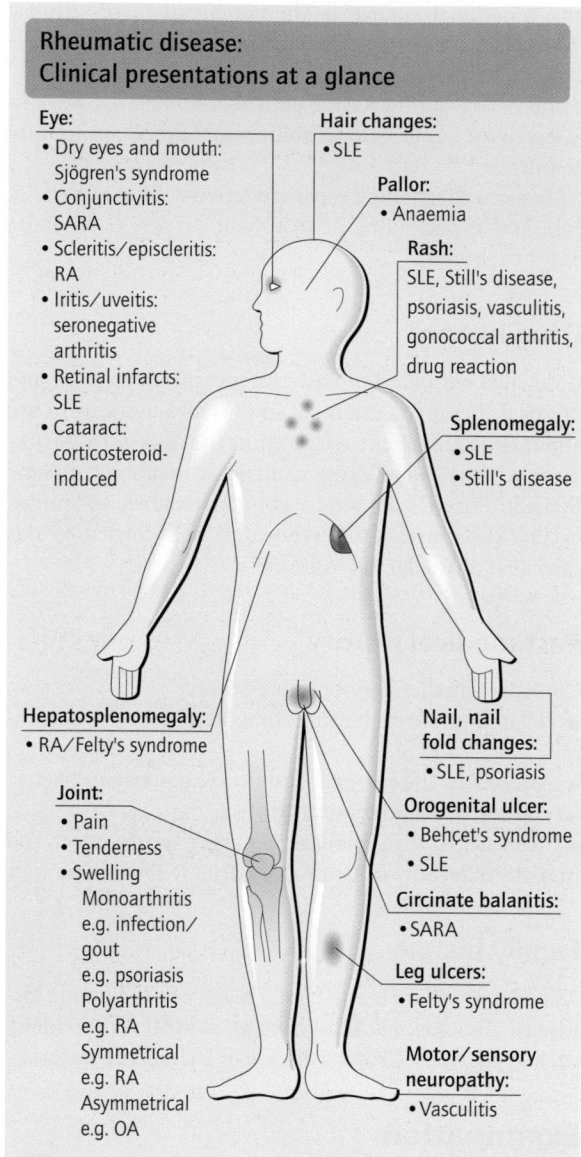

Rheumatic disease:
Clinical presentations at a glance

Eye:
- Dry eyes and mouth: Sjögren's syndrome
- Conjunctivitis: SARA
- Scleritis/episcleritis: RA
- Iritis/uveitis: seronegative arthritis
- Retinal infarcts: SLE
- Cataract: corticosteroid-induced

Hair changes:
- SLE

Pallor:
- Anaemia

Rash:
SLE, Still's disease, psoriasis, vasculitis, gonococcal arthritis, drug reaction

Splenomegaly:
- SLE
- Still's disease

Hepatosplenomegaly:
- RA/Felty's syndrome

Joint:
- Pain
- Tenderness
- Swelling
  Monoarthritis e.g. infection/gout e.g. psoriasis
  Polyarthritis e.g. RA
  Symmetrical e.g. RA
  Asymmetrical e.g. OA

Nail, nail fold changes:
- SLE, psoriasis

Orogenital ulcer:
- Behçet's syndrome
- SLE

Circinate balanitis:
- SARA

Leg ulcers:
- Felty's syndrome

Motor/sensory neuropathy:
- Vasculitis

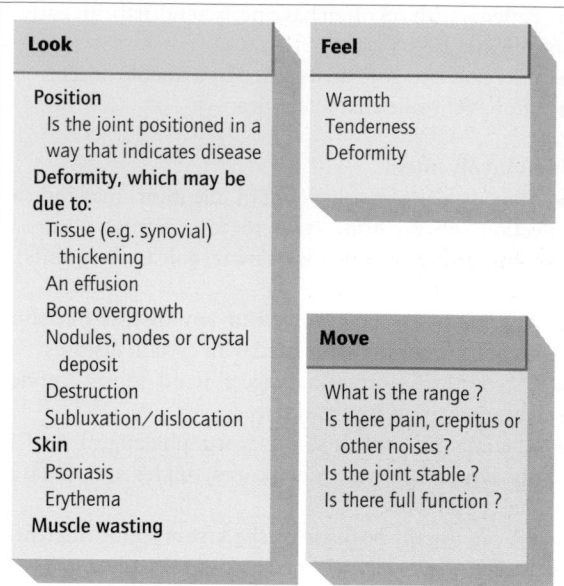

Look	Feel
Position Is the joint positioned in a way that indicates disease **Deformity, which may be due to:** Tissue (e.g. synovial) thickening An effusion Bone overgrowth Nodules, nodes or crystal deposit Destruction Subluxation/dislocation **Skin** Psoriasis Erythema **Muscle wasting**	Warmth Tenderness Deformity

Move

What is the range ?
Is there pain, crepitus or other noises ?
Is the joint stable ?
Is there full function ?

Figure 4.3 How to examine a joint.

be investigated. Tell the patient what is happening, particularly if it may hurt.

Neurological features of rheumatological disease include:
- Spastic paraparesis caused by cervical cord compression resulting from OA or RA involvement of the cervical spine
- Signs of root and nerve entrapment in disease of the lumbosacral spine and carpal tunnel syndrome
- Sensory motor neuropathy in vasculitis

Investigation

Investigations should be interpreted in the context of a careful history and physical examination.

Haematology

Full blood count
Haemoglobin
Anaemia. This is common in rheumatic disease. It may be:
- *Microcytic* (e.g. blood loss resulting from treatment with analgesics or NSAIDs)
- *Normocytic* (e.g. a manifestation of chronic disease)
- *Macrocytic* (e.g. folate deficiency, as may occur in RA)

White cell count. This may be increased or decreased:
- *Neutrophilia:* may accompany septic arthritis
- *Eosinophilia:* may occur in polyarteritis nodosa (PAN)

HISTORY & EXAMINATION BOX 4.2. It can be useful to sequentially measure the range of movement of specific joints to find out how a disease is progressing. An indication of the ranges found normally are included in HISTORY & EXAMINATION BOX 4.2 as a guide. It may be that your patient is not presenting primarily with a rheumatic disorder. In which case, screening history and examination would usually be appropriate (KEYPOINTS BOX 4.1).

Compare affected joints or muscles with their counterparts. Passive movement (measured with a goniometer) is a reliable measure of range of movement. Muscle tenderness may indicate an inflammatory disorder and should

04

History & Examination 4.2: Rheumatological examination

Standing

General inspection

Inspect front, back and sides for muscle bulk and symmetry, and for rashes

Gait

Look for any abnormality while walking and turning, and note whether walking aids are required. Normal gait involves stance (60%) and swing phases (40%)

Back

Look for any abnormality including scoliosis, cervical lordosis, thoracic kyphosis and lumbar lordosis

Check for localized tenderness (e.g. caused by infection)

Progression of thoracic kyphosis—a useful measure is the distance from the wall to the tragus (ear lobe) when the patient stands with his or her back to the wall

Forward bending—measure the increase in length between L5/S1 and points 10 cm above and 5 cm below on flexion (Schober's test). It should be greater than 4 cm (finger to floor distance is not a good measure of spinal stiffness as it may vary with hip mobility)

Lateral flexion—ask the patient to reach down laterally to the knee joint. This can normally be achieved, but may be restricted in ankylosing spondylitis

Hyperextension—usually 10° from the vertical can be achieved

Pelvis

Look for asymmetry, which may suggest unequal leg length

Trendelenberg's test—ask the patient to stand on one leg. A dropped pelvis on the side of the raised leg (positive Trendelenberg's test) suggests muscle weakness or hip pathology

Legs

Look for bow legs (genu varum—knees pointing out) or knock knees (genu valgum—knees pointing in), and popliteal swelling

Feet

Look for Achilles tendon swelling and hindfoot deformity (valgus/varus)

Sitting

Hand

Examine for tenderness, swelling bony enlargement and movement

Grip strength—squeezing a rubber air-filled bag inflated to 30 mmHg and recording the pressure increase is a useful measurement

Wrist

Extension and flexion—extension is normally 70° and flexion is normally 90°

Elbow

Look for tophi or subcutaneous rheumatoid nodules on the extensor surface of the elbow and forearm, and for olecranon bursae

Feel the elbow—this will cause pain if there is medial or lateral epicondylitis (golfer's or tennis elbow, respectively)

Flexion and extension—normal range is 0–150°. The amount of flexion deformity is a measure of any inability to extend the elbow fully

Pronation and supination—range of forearm pronation and supination (a combination of elbow and wrist movement) is normally to 80° from the neutral position to forearm horizontal and thumb pointing up

Shoulder

Look for squaring resulting from deltoid atrophy

Feel anteriorly for swelling and tenderness of the long head of biceps tendon, and laterally, under the acromion, for supraspinatous tendon insertion tenderness

Abduction—abduct arms through 180° from the sides of the body. In supraspinatous tendonitis pain is between 60° and 120°; in OA of the acromioclavicular joint pain is worse between 160° and 180°

Flexion (normal range 160°) and extension (normal range 60°)

Internal rotation—ask the patient to reach behind his or her head and neck, and record the lowest spinal level reached

Cervical spine

Flexion, extension, lateral flexion and rotation—measure from the face forward position. Normal ranges are: flexion and extension, 40°; lateral flexion, 40°; rotation, 45°

Costovertebral joint movement

Chest expansion—measure chest expansion along nipple line during deep inspiration. It should be more than 6 cm

Temporomandibular joint

Watch and feel the temporomandibular joint as the patient opens his or her mouth

Supine

Pelvis

Sacroiliac tenderness—press the anterior superior iliac spines gently apart. This will cause sacroiliac pain if they are inflamed

True and apparent leg lengths—measure from the anterior superior iliac spine and umbilicus, respectively, to the medical malleolus. An apparent difference may indicate lateral tilting of the pelvis

Hip flexion—bring the leg in towards the chest with the knee flexed. The normal limit is 110°

Continued on p. 194

04

Hip extension (see Rheumatological examination: prone below)

Internal and external rotation, abduction and adduction of the hip. Rotate each hip internally (normal range 25°) and externally (normal range 35°) with the hip flexed, then measure the range of abduction (normal 50°) and adduction (normal 30°)

Traction manoeuvres—assess the sciatic nerve by straight leg raising (and record the angle of elevation). Dorsiflex the foot while raised (Lasègue's test). This will exacerbate symptoms of lumbosacral root compression

Knee

Look—inspect the position and note any movement of the patella. Quadriceps wasting is a useful sign of knee pathology

Effusion—detect an effusion bimanually by compressing the patella onto the underlying femoral condyle (patella tap) and shifting fluid between medial and lateral sides (bulge sign)

Popliteal cyst—examine the popliteal area for a fluctuant swelling

Knee flexion and stability—assess knee flexion (0–110°) and

stability in both the mediolateral and anteroposterior planes

Ankle and subtalar joints

Feel for tenderness and swelling

Ankle—note flexion (normal 15°) and extension (normal 35°)

Subtalar joint—examine for eversion (normal range 0–20°) and inversion (normal range 0–30°)

Toes

Look—toes are numbered 1–5 from the big toe; note alignment, deformity (hammertoe, claw toe, hallux valgus), movement

Feel—gently squeeze the metatarsophalangeal joint. This causes pain if it is inflamed

Prone

Pelvis

Feel—press on the sacrum. This will cause pain if there is sacroiliac joint irritation

Hip extension—normal range 0–30°. Also the femoral nerve will be stretched causing pain if there is nerve root irritation

---

Keypoints 4.1: Musculoskeletal examination

Useful screening questions

To detect significant musculoskeletal abnormalities

Do you suffer from any pain or stiffness in your arms or legs, neck or back?

Do you have any difficulty with washing and dressing or with stairs and steps?

Useful screening examination

To detect significant musculoskeletal abnormalities

Check for joint swelling and deformity, plus pain and difficulty with movements (Fig. 4.3)

Four components of the musculoskeletal system need to be assessed (in any order)

Gait

Observe patient walking

Arms (sitting)

- Hold out hands
- Turn the hands over
- Make a fist
- Pinch the tip of the index and middle finger to the thumb
- Flex and extend the elbows
- Put hands behind head

Legs (lying)

- Inspect the feet
- Flex each knee
- Internally rotate the hip
- Extend each knee
- Palpate the knee

Spine (sitting and standing)

- Bend the neck from side to side
- Inspect the whole spine
- Bend forward and touch the toes
- Palpate lumbar vertebrae

Record the outcome of the examination in the notes (e.g. GALS) as simply as possible

---

- *Neutropenia:* a feature of Felty's syndrome and drug sensitivity
- *Leucopenia:* a manifestation of SLE and treatment with cytotoxic drugs (e.g. azathioprine)

Platelet numbers. These may be increased (e.g. in RA), or

reduced, as in SLE and as a side-effect of treatment with D-penicillamine, gold or cytotoxic agents.

Erythrocyte sedimentation rate and acute phase proteins

Erythrocyte sedimentation rate (ESR) is an indirect

Table 4.1 Antigen binding and disease associations of commonly measured autoantibodies

Bound antigen	Disease
IgG-Fc (rheumatoid factor)	RA (associated with severity)
Cyclic citrallinated peptide	RA
DNA (double stranded)	SLE (correlates with disease activity)
DNA (single stranded)	Infections and inflammation (non-specific)
Extractable nuclear antigens	
SSA/Ro	Sjögren's syndrome
	SLE; fetal heart block
SSB/La	Sjögren's syndrome
	SLE
SM/RNP	SLE (highly specific)
U1 RNP	Overlap syndromes
Jo-1 (t-RNA synthetase)	Myositis
SCL70 (topoisomerase)	Systemic sclerosis
Centromere	Systemic sclerosis
Phospholipids (anticardiolipin, lupus anticoagulant)	SLE; associated with thrombotic events, thrombocytopenia, fetal loss
Neutrophil cytoplasmic antigen classified as c- and p- (Fig. 4.4e & f)	Vasculitis
Proteinase III (c-ANCA)	Wegener's granulomatosis, microscopic polyangiitis
Myeloperoxidase (p-ANCA)	Rapidly progressive crescentic GN
	Microscopic arteritis (with GN)
	Polyarteritis nodosa
	Churg–Strauss syndrome
Histone	

ANCA, antineutrophil cytoplasmic antibody; c-, cytoplasmic; GN; glomerulonephritis; p-, peripheral; RNA, ribonucleic acid; RNP, ribonuclear protein; SLE, systemic lupus erythematosus.

04

measure of acute phase protein concentration; when increased it causes red cell rouleaux formation and results in a faster ESR. ESR and C-reactive protein (CRP), an acute phase protein, are both non-specific guides to inflammatory activity, as seen for example in RA and SLE. Normally, ESR is less than 20 mm/h and CRP is less than 10 mg/l.

A normal ESR generally excludes active inflammation. A falsely low ESR can occur in sickle cell disease, anisocytosis, spherocytosis, polycythaemia and heart failure. A falsely raised ESR can result from prolonged blood storage or a measurement error. ESR and CRP levels may be inappropriately low in some patients (e.g. seronegative arthritis and SLE, respectively) and are not infallible markers of inflammation.

Biochemistry

Diagnostically useful plasma biochemistry includes:
• *Uric acid:* may be raised in gout
• *Urea and creatinine levels:* may increase when there is renal involvement

• *Alkaline phosphatase and other tests of liver function:* may be altered as a result of drug therapy with, for example, methotrexate

Immunology

A number of markers of immune system function (e.g. antibodies, complement) that may be associated with specific diseases or disease groups can be measured. Autoantibodies and complement tests are discussed here because they are reliable and are commonly carried out.

Autoantibodies

Autoantibodies bind to a wide spectrum of antigens (Table 4.1), but their pathogenic relationship to disease has not been determined in most cases. The presence of autoantibodies may, however, be used clinically to:
• *Confirm a diagnosis:* rheumatoid factor (RF) may confirm a diagnosis of RA
• *Point to a diagnosis:* antinuclear antibody (ANA) may indicate a diagnosis of SLE

Disease	Incidence of RF (%)	Incidence of ANA (%)
RA	75	30
Primary Sjögren's syndrome	50	70
SLE	40	> 90
Systemic sclerosis	30	> 70

Table 4.2 Incidence of rheumatoid factor (RF) and antinuclear antibody (ANA) in autoimmune rheumatic disease

- *Forecast disease:* anticentromere antibodies are associated with the development of systemic sclerosis
- *Indicate an exacerbation of disease:* anti-DNA is associated with a relapse of SLE
- *Suggest early treatment:* coexistence of RF and reduced immunoglobulin G (IgG) galactosylation in RA is associated with severe disease later

Low concentrations of autoantibodies are present in the plasma of normal individuals, especially in the elderly.

Rheumatoid factors are autoantibodies against antigenic determinants on the Fc fragment of IgG. They may be IgM, IgG or IgA. At least 70% of RA patients have a positive RF test.

RF tests are also positive in:
- Other rheumatic diseases (Table 4.2).
- Viral infections (e.g. infectious mononucleosis).
- Chronic inflammatory diseases (e.g. tuberculosis).
- Neoplasms or chemotherapy.
- Four per cent of healthy individuals. RFs may have a physiological role in immune regulation.

Antinuclear antibodies bind to cell nuclear components (DNA and RNA). Immunofluorescent cell staining is a useful screening test for them, and their specificity can be further defined by testing for the antibodies referred to in Table 4.1. The pattern of ANA immunofluorescence is valuable diagnostically, but is not as specific as the identification of a specific antigen–antibody reaction.

Four patterns of immunofluorescence (Fig. 4.4a–d) are commonly recognized: homogeneous, peripheral, speckled nucleolar and centromere:
- *Homogeneous pattern* (antibody to nuclear protein) and a *peripheral pattern* (antibody to DNA) are features of SLE
- *Speckled pattern* (antibody to extractable nuclear antigens; e.g. ribonuclear protein) is seen in SLE, RA, systemic sclerosis and Sjögren's syndrome

- *Nucleolar pattern* (antibody to nuclear RNA) is most common in systemic sclerosis
- *Centromere pattern* is seen in limited cutaneous systemic sclerosis

ANA testing may also be positive, usually of low titre, in fewer than 20% of patients with chronic active hepatitis, infectious mononucleosis or lepromatous leprosy.

Complement

Total haemolytic complement, C3 and C4, are the factors usually measured to assess complement levels.

The main indication for these measurements is to diagnose SLE where immune complex activation of the classical pathway is thought to cause a reduction in these components. A genetic deficiency of the protein C2 is associated with SLE.

Complement proteins may show a rise in inflammatory rheumatic diseases (e.g. rheumatoid arthritis).

HLA typing

Class I and II typing may be useful in diagnosis and prognosis, for example HLA B27 (class I) in ankylosing spondylitis and HLA DR4 (class II); subtype specificity can also be useful (see Table 4.8).

Synovial fluid

Arthrocentesis

Arthrocentesis or joint puncture is safe and easy to perform.

Synovial fluid examination

Synovial fluid obtained by joint aspiration is described in terms of its:
- *Colour:* normally yellow, may become green in RA and purulent in bacterial arthritis

Figure 4.4 (*opposite*) (a–d) Antinuclear antibodies (ANA) detected by indirect immunofluorescence cultured human epithelial cells (HEp-2 cells). The HEp-2 cells are grown in culture and coated onto the microscope slides. Any antibodies in the patient's serum bind to antigens in the HEp-2 cells and are finally detected using rabbit antihuman immunoglobulin G (IgG) that is conjugated to fluorescein isothiocyanate (FITC). (a) Homogeneous pattern: note the chromosomal staining in the dividing cells. (b) Speckled pattern: note no chromosomal staining. (c) Centromere pattern: note the staining at the poles of the chromosomes. (d) Nucleolar staining: note the multiple nucleoli in each cell. (e-f) Antineutrophil cytoplasmic antibodies (ANCA) detected on normal human neutrophils coated onto microscope slides and then treated with ethanol. Any antibodies in the patient's serum bind to antigens

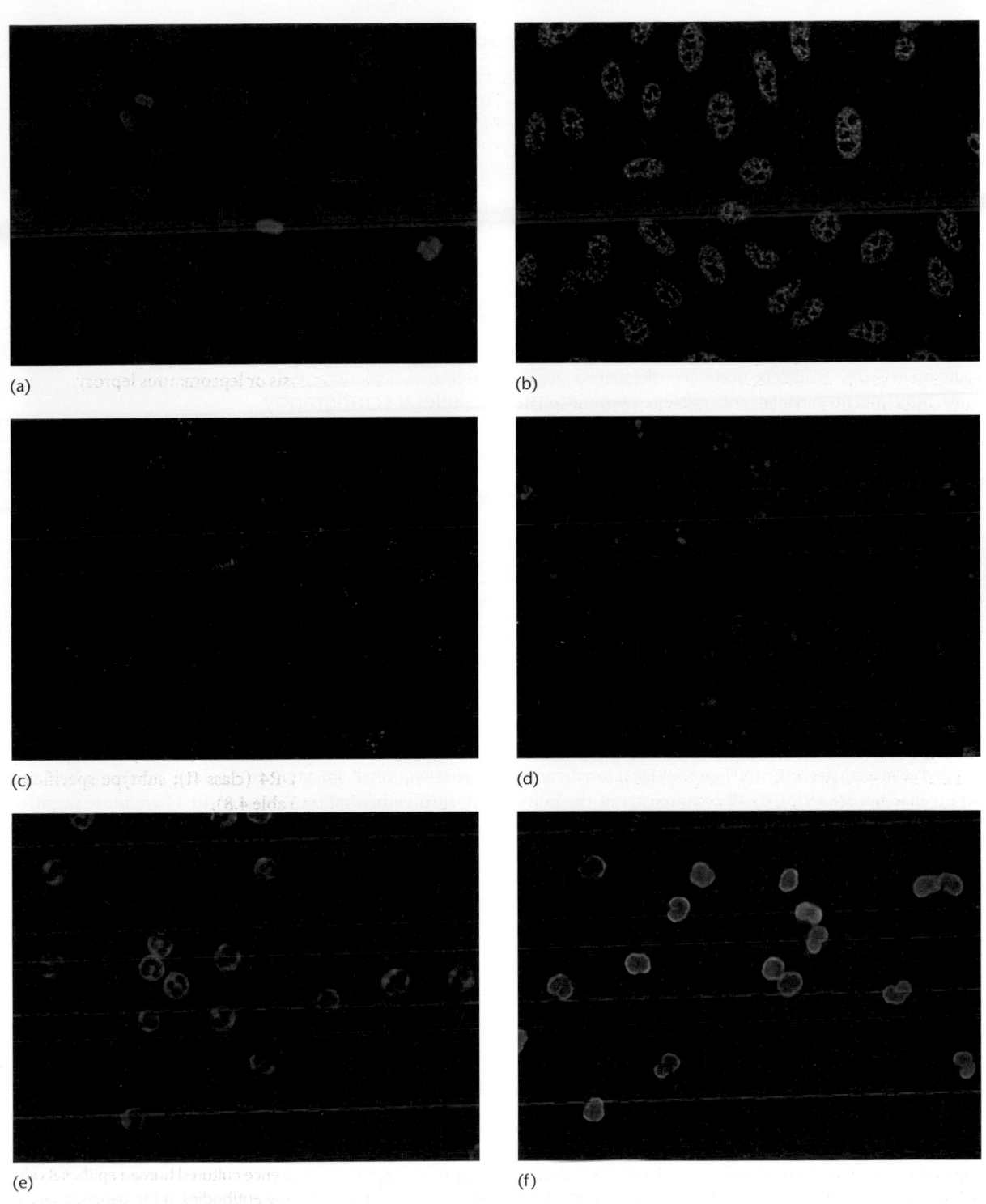

(a)

(b)

(c)

(d)

(e)

(f)

04

in the neutrophils detected using FITC conjugated rabbit antihuman immunoglobulin G (IgG). (e) Cytoplasmic ANCA (c-ANCA): note the staining in the cytoplasm and some accentuation in the clefts between the nuclear lobes (associated with antibodies to proteinase 3; typical disease Wegener's granulomatosis). (f) Perinuclear ANCA (p-ANCA): note the fluorescence localized around the nuclear lobes (associated with antibodies to myeloperoxidase but also seen non-specifically with antinuclear antibodies; typical disease, PAN, vasculitis of autoimmune rheumatic disease).

- *Clarity:* may become turbid in RA and bacterial arthritis
- *Viscosity:* usually high but will reduce because of inflammation. White cell count usually less than 200×10^6/l but will be significantly increased in bacterial arthritis to more than $50\,000 \times 10^6$/l.

Investigations when appropriate include:
- White cell count.
- Gram stain, acid-fast methods and culture for bacteria (including *Mycobacterium tuberculosis*) and fungi. **Synovial fluid culture** in suspected infectious arthritis should be accompanied by **sputum, blood, urine** (early morning if *M. tuberculosis* suspected) and **faecal cultures** to detect a further source of infection.
- Crystal identification (using compensated polarized light microscopy to detect urate (needle-shaped negatively birefringent crystals) and calcium pyrophosphate (rectangular-shaped positively birefringent crystals) (see p. 240).

Synovial biopsy may be necessary, for example to detect the presence of a reactive arthritis or *M. tuberculosis* infection.

Diagnostic imaging

Diagnostic imaging is often necessary to allow an accurate diagnosis in rheumatology, and some techniques are more appropriate than others for certain disorders.

Plain radiography
Radiography is the first and usually only imaging test needed to investigate arthritis (Fig. 4.5a–h). It can demonstrate changes occurring in all components of the joint, and characteristic changes are seen for example in OA, RA and AS. Serial radiography can be useful as it will document disease progression.

Ultrasonography
Ultrasound is a useful non-invasive technique, especially for distinguishing synovial cysts (e.g. popliteal cyst) from solid tissue and in the examination of tendons (e.g. rotator cuff and biceps).

Computed tomography
Computed tomography (CT) is useful for visualizing cross-sectional anatomy of calcified tissue (e.g. cortical and trabecular bone; Figs 4.5b,h) and may be used to create a three-dimensional image.

Magnetic resonance imaging
Magnetic resonance imaging (MRI) is a valuable imaging tool (Fig. 4.5c). It works by detecting hydrogen ion mobility when tissues are subjected to pulsed radiowaves and a strong magnetic field causes them to emit a transient signal. The magnetic fields are known by their relaxation times, T1 and T2, which are characteristics of the tissues being measured.

MRI imaging is especially useful for visualizing organs in which there are contrasts of soft tissues (e.g. the spinal cord). Cortical bone contains virtually no mobile hydrogen ions and is therefore better evaluated by radiography or CT.

MRI of the musculoskeletal system has been most useful for viewing the spinal cord, intervertebral discs, hip joints and knee joints, and offers significant potential as it allows three-dimensional imaging and multiple plane examination.

Skeletal scintigraphy
The typical radionuclide scan uses technetium-99m methylene diphosphonate complexes to detect physiological changes in the bone in contrast to the anatomical changes depicted by plain radiography and MRI.

An increased uptake of the isotope into the bone can result from many causes including infection, tumour, fractures and synovitis. This type of scanning is therefore non-specific and needs to be correlated with radiography and clinical findings. It is useful when clinical symptoms and radiography have proved inconclusive.

Gallium-67 citrate and indium-111 scans can be used to define sites of infection in bones and soft tissues, which appear as areas of increased uptake.

Single proton emission CT (SPECT), which provides cross-sectional imaging in skeletal scintigraphy, and positron emission tomography (PET) are more sensitive techniques, but have limited availability.

Arthroscopy

Arthroscopy is useful both diagnostically and therapeutically. Unlike needle biopsy, it allows a direct view of the joint and synovial fluid, and biopsy samples can be taken from multiple sites within the joint.

The joint most commonly examined by arthroscopy is the knee. The technique is often used to investigate trauma (e.g. sport injury). Most arthroscopies are carried out as day cases; the anaesthetic depending on the extent of the procedure.

Histopathology

It may sometimes be necessary to take an organ biopsy to help make a diagnosis, for example:
- *Synovial membrane and bone biopsy:* in suspected infection

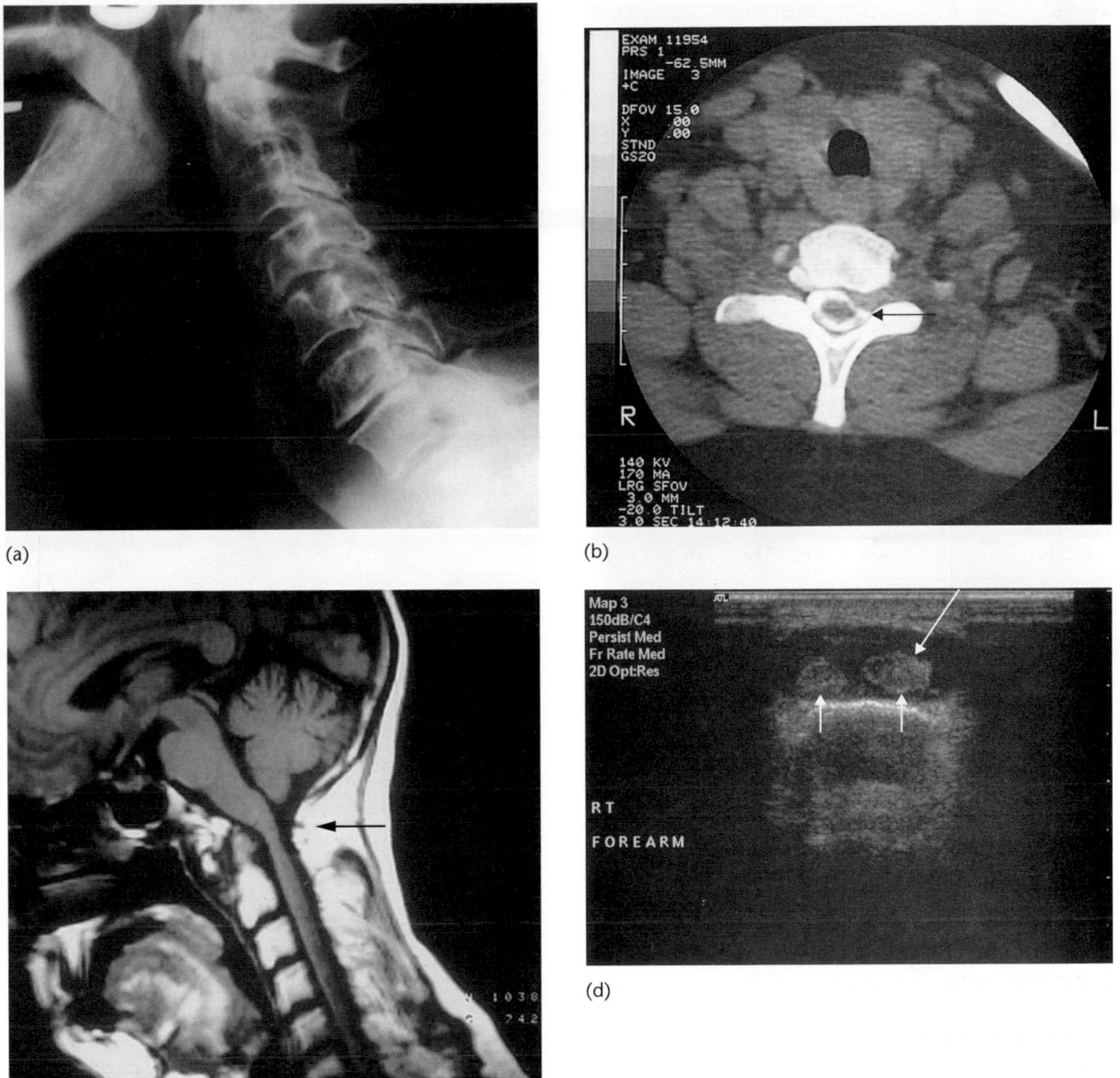

(a)

(b)

(c)

(d)

04

Figure 4.5 (a) Cervical spine radiograph showing typical changes resulting from osteoarthritis (OA): joint space narrowing, sclerosis and osteophyte formation. (b) Computed tomogram (CT) of the cervical spine (axial view after intrathecal contrast injection) of the same patient as in (a) demonstrating a prolapsed intervertebral disc causing extradural impingement on the theca (arrow). (c) Magnetic resonance image of cervical spine in a patient with rheumatoid arthritis (RA) (T_1-weighted image). Atlanto-axial subluxation is shown and in this patient the distance between the anterior arch of the atlas and the odontoid is approximately 1 cm; the upper limit of normal is 3 mm. There is erosion of the odontoid peg and narrowing of the spinal canal at this level (arrow). (d) Ultrasound image showing hypoechogenic fluid (long arrow) is seen in the tendon sheaths of the extensor tendons (short arrows) of the forearm. These ultrasound appearances are in keeping with severe tenosynovitis. *Continued on p. 200.*

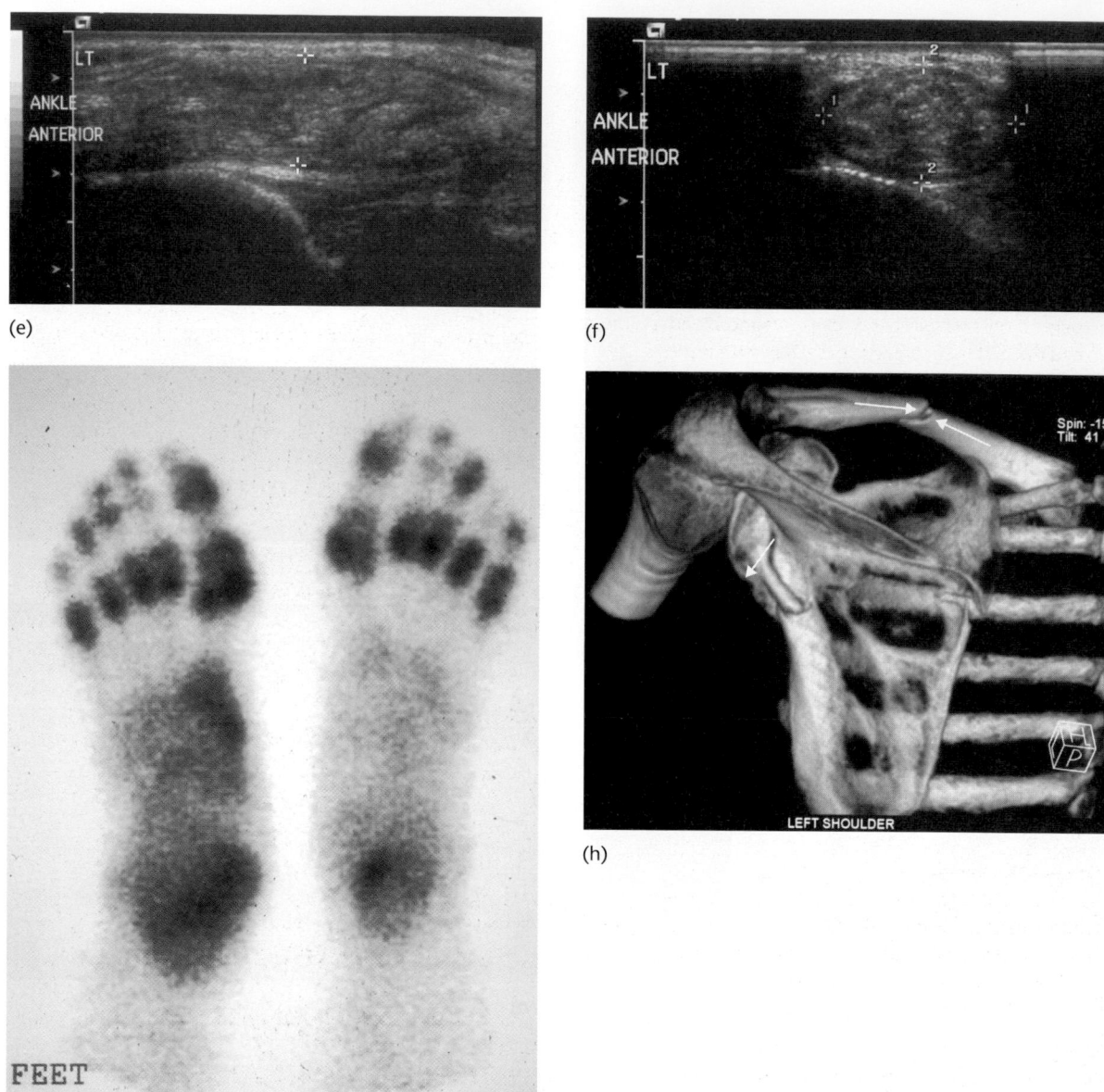

(e)

(f)

(g)

(h)

Figure 4.5 (*cont'd*) (e) Ultrasound image (longitudinal) of the tibialis anterior tendon at the level of the ankle joint. The markers indicate the boundary of the tendon, which is markedly enlarged. The tendon is inhomogeneous in appearance, with areas of decreased echogenicity within the tendon. The ultrasonic appearances are in keeping with severe tendonopathy. (f) Ultrasound image (transverse) of the tibialis anterior tendon at the level of the ankle joint as seen in part (e). (g) Radionuclide scan showing hot spots resulting from arthritis affecting joints of the feet. (h) Three-dimensional CT scan of the left shoulder viewed posteriorly. There is an oblique fracture of the upper scapular (arrows), in addition to a fracture of the mid-shaft of the clavicle (arrows).

- *Kidney biopsy:* in suspected SLE
- *Liver biopsy:* in suspected iatrogenic and autoimmune liver disease
- *Lung biopsy:* in suspected Wegener's granulomatosis

Differential diagnosis

The differential diagnoses of arthritis are shown in Table 4.3.

General principles of management

Keypoints 4.2: Managing rheumatic diseases

An integrated approach to treatment between hospital and community is essential. Regular patient follow-up is useful to reinforce treatment

Support
Education
Patients should be fully aware of the diagnosis and treatment and the part they should play to maximize therapy
Encourage walking, swimming and jogging if joint inflammation is controlled. Joining support groups can be useful in chronic disease. Dress warmly, no smoking, avoid drugs causing vasoconstriction in Raynaud's disease
Dietary advice is useful in most rheumatic disorders

Physiotherapy
To maintain joint function and increase mobility

Occupational therapy
To maintain activities in daily life
Splinting may be required to prevent contractions and regain muscle strength
Advice on work environment may be useful

Podiatry
Improves foot and toe posture and function
Foot care advice may be useful (e.g. to prevent local infection)

General treatment
Sunscreens to help prevent lupus skin involvement
Ointments and creams and attention to ulcers may be useful for cutaneous manifestations in systemic sclerosis
Artificial tears, saline nasal sprays and mouthwashes in Sjögren's syndrome

Drugs
Analgesics (e.g. paracetamol, codeine phosphate)
Tricyclic antidepressants for pain control
NSAIDs: meloxicam, rofecoxib, celecoxib, etoricoxib
Corticosteroids: prednisolone, Depo-Medrone injection may be useful for painful trigger spots, inflamed tendon sheaths, bursitis and synovitis

Immunization
Immunization should be considered for children and adults
Immunization status, particularly with regard to chickenpox, should be checked before starting corticosteroids and immunosuppressant drugs
Immunization with live vaccines (e.g. rubella in children) are contraindicated if immunosuppressant drugs are being taken

Disease-modifying drugs
Methotrexate, sulfasalazine, gold salts, leflunomide, penicillamine

Immunosuppressive drugs
Azathioprine, cyclophosphamide, anticytokine therapy (e.g. etanercept, infliximab, Anakinra and adalimumab)

Complementary therapies
Complementary therapies are popular. You should be aware of what is available and what your patient may be receiving

Surgery
Joint aspiration and washout: this may be carried out arthroscopically
Joint replacement—hip, knee, elbow, shoulder
Joint removal—metatarsal head
Joint reconstruction—hands

Orthodontic assessment
May be necessary if there is temperomandibular joint involvement (e.g. juvenile idiopathic arthritis)

Ophthalmology
Eye examination may be necessary as the following can occur:
Scleritis—rheumatoid arthritis
Uveitis—ankylosing spondylitis, juvenile idiopathic arthritis, especially antinuclear antibody-positive pauciarticular disease
Retinitis—lupus

04

Supportive treatment

The multidisciplinary team
Patients with rheumatic disease may require medical supervision for many years, perhaps a lifetime. Care on this scale can only be provided by a multidisciplinary team of specialists who educate, treat and support the patient. Such a team will include:
- Specialist nurses
- Physiotherapists
- Occupational therapists
- Physicians

Type of arthritis	Causes
Monoarthritis/oligoarthritis	Infectious arthritis (bacterial, viral, fungal)
	Crystal arthritis
	Trauma
	Haemarthrosis
	Juvenile idiopathic arthritis (pauciarticular)
	Lyme disease
	Neuropathic joint (e.g. diabetes mellitus)
	Sarcoidosis
	Malignancy (osteogenic sarcoma, lymphoma, leukaemia)
	Seronegative spondylarthritis (e.g. psoriatic, reactive)
Polyarthritis	OA
	RA
	Other autoimmune rheumatic diseases
	Juvenile idiopathic arthritis
	Haemochromatosis

Table 4.3 Differential diagnosis of arthritis

- Social workers
- Orthopaedic surgeons

Rheumatic disorders such as RA bring social, financial, emotional and physical disadvantage, and as the disease fluctuates so does the patient's ability to cope with it. Psychological support is very important.

Patient education

The patient and his or her family need to understand how the disease will affect them and what the probable outcome will be. He or she should also understand his or her role in the treatment programme. Reassure the patient that disease progression can usually be slowed, and that sometimes it can be halted with few sequelae.

This information can be built up and reinforced over successive visits to the rheumatology team. Free literature describing the disease and its treatment is helpful.

Physiotherapy

Movement can be severely limited by a single attack of an inflammatory arthritis. To retain maximum use for the maximum time, it is essential to maintain joint integrity and adjacent muscle function. A number of modalities are used and patients are generally instructed when to rest and exercise their joints. Treatment may include splints during the day (wrist) or at night (cervical spine and knees), heat treatment with sand, wax, or a hot shower or bath, and hydrotherapy.

Occupational therapy

Where necessary, activities of daily living should be reviewed by the occupational therapist. Advice can then be given about work and household aids that may help with standing, sitting and transferring.

Expert provision of joint splints, home appliances and orthotics is an essential and important resource.

Table 4.4 Corticosteroids and rheumatic disease

Potent anti-inflammatory action

Indications. Oral therapy generally reserved for complications with high morbidity or mortality (for local corticosteroid injection)

Prednisolone

Used for most purposes; high initial doses (60 mg/day) are required to induce remissions; maintenance regimen may be required and should be as low as possible (usually 7.5 mg/day)

Side-effects. Hypertension, sodium and water retention, potassium loss, diabetes mellitus, osteoporosis, avascular necrosis of the femoral head, mental disturbances, peptic ulceration (weak association), Cushing's syndrome, spread of infection, adrenal suppression

Specific treatment

Drug treatment

In rheumatic disease drug treatment is aimed at:

- *Alleviating pain:* analgesics (Table 4.5)
- *Modifying the inflammatory events themselves once they have been triggered:* drugs (Table 4.6)
- *Modifying the immunological events leading to inflammation:* drugs that suppress the disease process (Table 4.7)

Table 4.5 Analgesics commonly used in rheumatic disease

Aspirin

Aspirin has both analgesic and anti-inflammatory actions

Indications. Pain relief and as an anti-inflammatory and antipyretic

Side-effects (mild and infrequent). Gastrointestinal irritation, increased bleeding time, bronchospasm, skin reactions, rash, blood dyscrasis, acute pancreatitis, hepatic and renal damage after overdose

Contraindications. Children under 12 years of age, breastfeeding women, gastrointestinal ulceration, haemophilia, gout, asthma, hepatic and renal impairment, alcohol dependence

Paracetamol

Indications. Non-narcotic analgesia

Side-effects (rare). Rash, blood dyscrasias, acute pancreatitis, hepatic and renal damage after overdose

Contraindications. Hepatic and renal impairment, alcohol dependence

Aspirin and paracetamol may be usefully combined with certain opiate analgesics (e.g. codeine phosphate and dihydrocodeine)

Opiate analgesics

Indications. For moderate to severe pain, but rarely necessary in rheumatic disease

Common examples

Codeine phosphate

Co-codaprin

Tramadol

Meptazinol

Dihydrocodeine

Co-dydramol

Pentazocine

Buprenorphine (sublingual)

Dextromoramide

Side-effects. Nausea, vomiting, constipation, drowsiness. Large doses may cause respiratory depression and hypotension

Table 4.6 Non-steroidal anti-inflammatory drugs (NSAIDs)

Analgesic and anti-inflammatory activities to varying degrees as a result of decreasing the synthesis of prostaglandins, prostacyclin and thromboxane

Indications

Continuous or regular pain associated with inflammation. Generally not indicated for pain secondary to joint destruction (e.g. OA), where simple analgesics are more appropriate. It may be necessary to try several before finding one that suits an individual patient

Common examples

Selective COX-2 inhibitors: rofecoxib, etoricoxib, celecoxib

Ibuprofen

Diclofenac sodium

Naproxen

Piroxicam

Indomethacin

Side-effects (vary in severity and frequency and from one drug to another)

Dyspepsia (minimized by administration with food or milk), nausea, diarrhoea, intestinal bleeding and ulceration, hypersensitivity reactions (rash), headache, dizziness, vertigo, tinnitus, blood dyscrasias, fluid retention, acute renal failure

Use NSAIDs with care in the elderly, people with allergic disorders and asthma, pregnant women and people with renal impairment. NSAIDs vary in their selectivity for inhibiting cyclo-oxygenase. Selective inhibition of cyclo-oxygenase 2 may improve gastrointestinal tolerance and short-term studies support this

Important interactions between NSAIDs and other drugs

Altered activity of other drugs. NSAIDs enhance the anticoagulant effect of warfarin and decrease methotrexate and lithium excretion

Altered NSAID activity. Diuretics increase the risk of NSAID nephrotoxicity. Probenecid and other uricosurics may delay NSAID excretion

04

Further information, especially that relating to side-effects and contraindications, is given in a formulary, for example the *British National Formulary (BNF)*. Patients should be provided with written information detailing the drug treatment they should be taking, especially if they are taking corticosteroids.

Non-steroidal anti-inflammatory drugs

The use of NSAIDs has been limited by their adverse effects (e.g. upper gastrointestinal toxicity, nephrotoxi-

city). With the description of two classes of cyclo-oxygenase enzymes—COX-1 and COX-2—advances have been made in the development of NSAIDs with fewer adverse effects. COX-1 enzymes are expressed constitutively in gastric mucosa, kidneys and other organs and are not thought to be inducible. COX-2 enzymes are not constitutively expressed in tissues but can be induced by certain molecules (e.g. cytokines at sites of inflammation). Selective COX-2 inhibitors have now been developed that have minimal effects on the COX-1 enzyme. These

Table 4.7 Drugs that suppress the rheumatic disease process. These drugs are usually used in the treatment of autoimmune rheumatic diseases and spondyloarthritis

Pharmacological action

Disease-modifying antirheumatic drugs are thought to affect the disease process

They do not produce an immediate therapeutic effect—it may take up to 4–6 months of treatment to obtain a full response

The treatment should be discontinued at 6 months if no objective benefit has been achieved

Indications

Start early in rheumatic disease before joints start to become destroyed because joint components, principally articular cartilage, have little regenerative potential

Use in children requires early referral to a specialist and expert advice

Methotrexate

A folic acid analogue interfering with thymidylate synthesis, which explains its antiproliferative effects

Inhibits purine nucleotide synthesis and causes errors in DNA transcription

Sulfasalazine

An acid azo compound of 5-aminosalicylic acid and sulfapyridine

Leflunomide

Similar in efficacy to sulfasalazine and methotrexate

Gold

Sulphydryl-containing organic gold compounds were first used to treat arthritis in the 1920s. Sodium aurothio malate (IM injection) or Auranofin (oral) may be given

Hydroxychloroquine

An antimalarial drug. Better tolerated than gold or penicillamine

Penicillamine

Similar action to gold

Ciclosporin

For severe active RA

Etanercept, infliximab and adalimumab

Selective immunosuppressants that inhibit the activity of tumour necrosis factor-α

Anakinra

Selective immunosuppression by IL-1 receptor antagonism

Azathioprine

Inhibits purine nucleotide synthesis and causes errors in DNA transcription

Cyclophosphamide

Alkylating agents substitute alkyl radicals into other molecules and interfere with their function

NSAIDs are effective with less upper gastrointestinal toxicity (Table 4.6).

Corticosteroids

Corticosteroid has been demonstrated to retard the development of radiological bony erosions. Corticosteroids:

- Inhibit leucocyte chemotaxis
- Prevent circulating polymorphs, monocytes and lymphocytes from reaching sites of inflammation
- Reduce vascular permeability
- Inhibit the production of cytokines and arachadonic acid metabolites such as prostaglandins and leukotrienes

However, corticosteroids may:

- Affect bone metabolism resulting in osteoporosis
- Interfere with glucose metabolism and be diabetogenic
- Cause salt and water retention and precipitate or exacerbate hypertension
- Interfere with ocular lens metabolism resulting in cataract formation
- Be immunosuppressive because of increased susceptibility to bacterial and opportunistic infections (e.g. herpes zoster virus and fungal infections)

Corticosteroid side-effects are dose- and time-related and should therefore be used in as low a dose and for as short a time as possible. It may be more appropriate to deliver corticosteroids directly into the joint (Table 4.8).

In patients receiving prolonged periods of treatment it is important to protect against the development of osteoporosis. Dietary advice should therefore be provided and drugs such as vitamin D and calcium and bisphosphonates should be used (see Chapter 5).

Biological therapies

As the fundamental mechanisms of the immune response are becoming clearer (see p. 40), novel approaches to therapy are being developed; such therapies may be directed against B and T cells, cytokines (e.g. tumour necrosis factor-α; TNF-α), and cytokine receptors (e.g. interleukin-1 [IL-1] receptor antagonist) or involve the cytokine receptors themselves (e.g. TNF receptor).

Complementary therapy

Complementary therapy is defined as the practice of health care not considered part of conventional management. A significant proportion of patients with musculoskeletal disorders will be taking some form of complementary therapy. Ideally, clinical trials should be carried out on all complementary therapies available; however, in practice this is not the case

Table 4.8 Arthrocentesis and intra-articular corticosteroid injection: when, what, where, how?

Indications for arthrocentesis
To diagnose the cause of a joint effusion, particularly if there is a monoarthritis that could be caused by infection
To relieve pain by draining an effusion and injecting corticosteroids and/or local anaesthetic
Contraindicated if there is infection in the overlying skin or soft tissue, or if the patient has a coagulation disorder

Corticosteroid preparations
Range from shorter acting hydrocortisone acetate, to drugs with more prolonged action (e.g. triamcinolone hexacetonide)
1% lidocaine may be added to provide immediate anaesthetic benefit from the injection

Technique
The techniques for injecting into painful soft tissue or into a synovial space (e.g. joint, tendon sheath, bursa) are similar and can
    be easily learned with expert tuition

Procedure
Anaesthetize the skin. Local skin anaesthesia is usually necessary, using a refrigerant spray (e.g. ethyl chloride) or injecting 1%
    lidocaine intradermally and down to the joint capsule

Complications
Infection introduced by the procedure
Spread of infection from a septic joint
Trauma from the injection procedure
Aseptic necrosis of the joint surface resulting from repeated injections into a joint
Atrophy and hypopigmentation of skin following injection near the skin surface
A transient increase in inflammation resulting from a reaction to the presence of corticosteroid crystals

Advice for the patient
Minimize joint use for 24 h to reduce the amount of corticosteroid leaving the joint via lymphatics
Pain and inflammation may increase transiently because of the presence of corticosteroid crystals
The anaesthetic effect of the lidocaine will wear off within 2–4 h
The corticosteroid effect will not become apparent until 24–48 h after the injection
Infection is a complication—if inflammation is increased for more than 24 h the patient should report back to the clinic

04

and treatment with these therapies should therefore be recommended with caution. Complementary therapies for which some clinical trials have been carried out are as follows:

- Diet manipulation (e.g. avoidance of foods such as dairy products, cereals and eggs)
- Dietary supplementation with unsaturated fatty acids and glucosamine sulphate
- Acupuncture, osteopathy and chiropractic treatment

Surgery

Surgery is carried out mainly for pain relief, but large joint replacement—hip, knee or shoulder—can also increase functional ability in a selected population. Operations that are now commonly available are:

- *Joint replacement:* hip, knee, elbow, shoulder
- *Joint removal:* metatarsal heads
- *Joint reconstruction:* hand joints

Diseases and their management

Autoimmune rheumatic disease

The term 'connective tissue disease' has been used to describe rheumatic diseases associated with autoimmunity. 'Autoimmune rheumatic disease' is, however, a more precise description as the pathogenesis is a primary dysfunction of the immune system (see Chapter 2) in contrast to specific disorders of bone and connective tissue (e.g. Paget's disease and osteogenesis imperfecta). Autoimmune rheumatic diseases include:

- Rheumatoid arthritis (see below)
- Sjögren's syndrome (see p. 211)
- Systemic lupus erythematosus (see p. 212)

- Vasculitis syndromes (see p. 216)
- Myositis (see p. 222)
- Systemic sclerosis (see p. 225)

Rheumatoid arthritis

Rheumatoid arthritis is a multisystem disorder in which immunological abnormalities characteristically result in symmetrical joint inflammation, articular erosions and extra-articular complications. It is the most common and disabling autoimmune arthritis, and genetic susceptibility is well defined.

Epidemiology

Prevalence. Affects approximately 1–3% of the UK population.

Age. Prevalence increases with age, but peaks between 30 and 55 years.

Sex. Premenopausal women are two to three times more susceptible than men. There is no apparent sex difference in the elderly.

Race. There is increased incidence in certain racial groups (e.g. Pima Indians, Afro-Caribbeans and Asians).

Genetics. There are associations with the major histocompatibility complex (MHC; see p. 43), as well as an increased prevalence in first-degree relatives and monozygotic twins.

Geography. There is an increased incidence in urban black Africans compared to those living in rural communities.

Disease mechanisms

Rheumatoid arthritis is thought to be caused by genetic, microbiological and immunological factors.

Genetic factors

Genetic susceptibility is associated with the genes of the MHC.
- Certain class II human leucocyte antigen (HLA) types are disease-associated and HLA-DR4 is present in 70% of white people with rheumatoid factor (RF)-positive RA, compared to 15% of the healthy population.
- Of the subtypes of HLA-DR4, DRB1*0401 and DRB1*0404 are associated with disease in white people. It is thought that there are shared amino acid sequences that are critical for the predisposition of RA.

    In monozygotic twins, up to 30% twin concordance has been reported.

Microbiological factors

Infectious agents such as *Mycoplasma*, *Mycobacteria*, Epstein–Barr virus (EBV) and retroviruses have been associated, but there is no convincing evidence as to causation.

Immunological factors

Whatever the initiating event, autoreactive CD4$^+$ T-helper cells are triggered. This results in the generation of inflammation. Cells such as macrophages, neutrophils, fibroblasts and dendritic cells are predominantly involved. Macrophages are the most active and secrete pro-inflammatory cytokines (e.g. TNF-α) that are involved in perpetuating and amplifying the inflammatory response. Enzymes released from these cells such as the matrix metalloproteinases (MMP) collagenase, gelatenase, stromolysin mediate the degradation of joint tissues.

Rheumatoid factors are also present in 75% of patients with RA. RFs are antibodies directed against the Fc fragment of IgG (see pp. 42–43). Naturally occurring RFs are thought to have a role in the clearance of foreign antigen from the body. In RA, RFs are produced in synovial plasma cells and have the ability to form immune complexes, activate complement and participate in the inflammatory response. In RA, immunoglobulins have reduced galactose in their sugar component and it is thought that this is also associated with inflammatory mechanisms.

Pathology

Histologically, the RA inflammatory response is referred to as being granulomatous. Features include:
- Damage to synovial joints and tendons, leading to secondary osteoarthritis, bony ankylosis, loss of joint mobility, joint instability and subluxation
- Periarticular osteoporosis
- Vasculitis causing infarcts of the fingertips or nailfolds
  RA disease pathology may result in different patterns of clinical manifestation:
- Prolonged periods of remission
- Fluctuation of disease activity
- Progressive deforming joint damage

Clinical features
Systemic

Systemic manifestations can arise weeks or months before the arthritis and affect approximately 70% of patients. There may be significant weight loss.

Musculoskeletal

Joint involvement in RA is characteristically symmetrical,

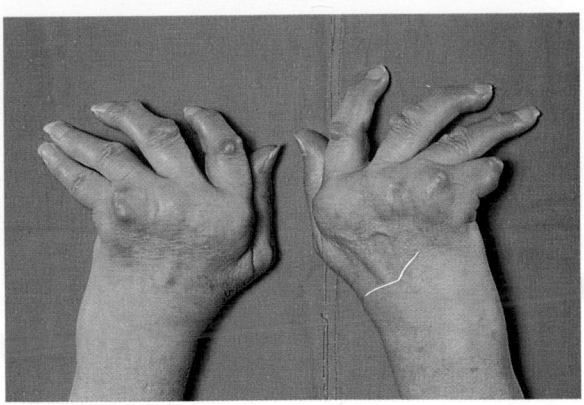

Figure 4.6 Metacarpophalangeal (MCP) destruction causing ulnar deviation of the digits. There is relative sparing of the distal and proximal interphalangeal (PIP) joints and multiple rheumatoid nodules are present.

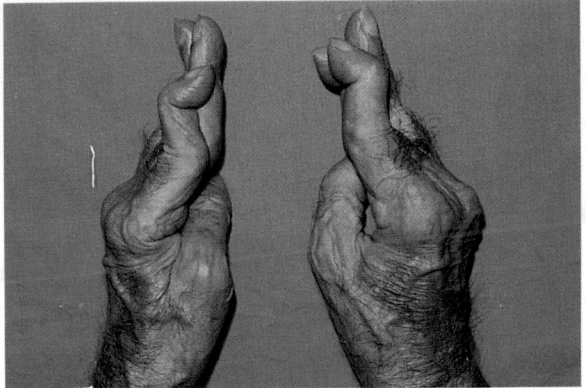

Figure 4.7 Swan-neck deformity of the forefingers caused by hyperextension at the PIP joint with flexion at the distal interphalangeal (DIP) joint.

affecting any synovial joint. Symptoms and signs include:
- *Stiffness:* common and most severe on waking, the joints becoming more mobile as the day progresses
- *Pain*
- *Warmth:* resulting from joint inflammation
- *Joint swelling:* usually results from an effusion or synovial hypertrophy (rings feel tight)
- *Deformity:* may develop insidiously

Specific joint and tendon involvement
Hand and foot changes. In RA, there are characteristic changes in the hands and feet. Distal interphalangeal (DIP) joints are not usually involved, in contrast to their frequent involvement in OA and psoriatic arthritis.

Hand changes
- Spindle-shaped deformity of the fingers
- Muscle atrophy
- Ulnar deviation of the fingers (Fig. 4.6)
- Extensor tendon subluxation or rupture

Finger deformities
- *Swan-neck deformity* (Fig. 4.7)
- *Boutonnière deformity:* flexion at the proximal interphalangeal (PIP) joint and hyperextension at the DIP joint
- *Z-shaped deformity:* palmar subluxation of the proximal phalanges and flexion at the MCP joint, making it difficult to pinch the thumb

Foot changes
- Eversion of the foot (subtalar joint)
- Forefoot widening

- Lateral deviation and dorsal subluxation of the toes
- Metatarsophalangeal (MTP) joint subluxation

Other changes
- The upper cervical spine is often involved, and subluxation of the vertebrae is a serious complication

The earliest and most common symptom of cervical subluxation is pain radiating up into the occiput (Fig. 4.5c). Other symptoms include:
- Paraesthesia
- Sudden deterioration of hand function
- Sensory loss
- Abnormal gait
- Urinary retention or incontinence
- Subluxation of the ulnar head
- Hip involvement is usually late and may be associated with marked restriction in movement
- Fixed flexion deformity at the elbow can be an early manifestation
- Popliteal (Baker's) cysts may accompany knee involvement, and rupture into the popliteal fossa, which may clinically resemble deep-vein thrombosis
- Inflammation of the olecranon bursa and other bursae such as the prepatellar bursa (housemaid's knee), the subacromial bursa (shoulder pain) and the greater trochanteric bursa (anterolateral thigh pain)
- Tendon sheaths of the fingers and wrists may be involved, resulting in rupture of finger extensor tendons and synovitis of wrist flexor tendons, which may result in carpal tunnel syndrome

Muscle and bone involvement
- Muscle weakness may result from the disease process itself or from disuse muscular atrophy.

04

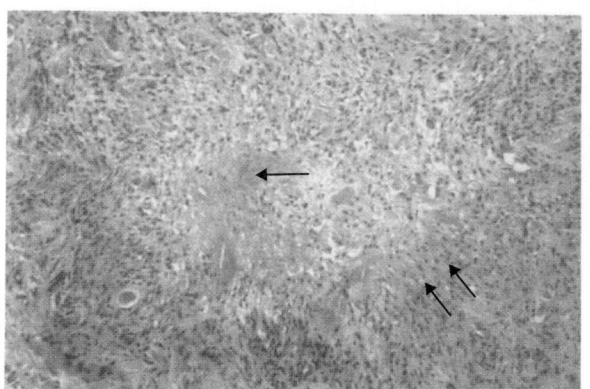

Figure 4.8 A rheumatoid nodule comprises a central area of degenerate collagen (arrow) surrounded by palisaded histiocytes (arrows) (haematoxylin and eosin stain; high power).

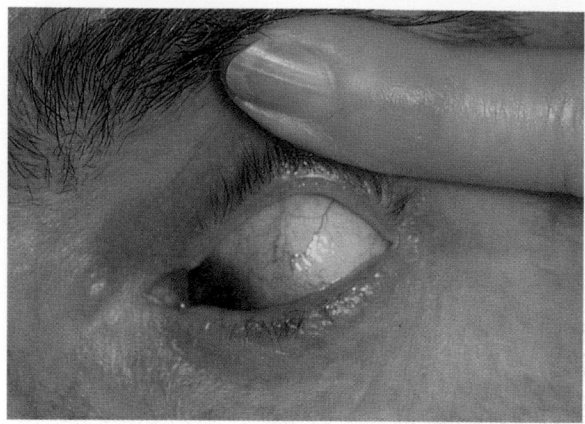

Figure 4.9 Scleritis is common in RA and causes painful red eyes.

● Osteoporosis may be associated with active disease or complicate corticosteroid treatment. It may cause spontaneous fractures.

Dermatological involvement

Rheumatoid nodules. These are firm, round, non-tender and often multiple cutaneous lesions (Fig. 4.8). They are:
● Found in approximately 20% of patients, commonly at pressure points in association with friction (particularly extensor surfaces of forearms, occiput, sacrum and back of heels)
● Associated with more severe disease and the presence of IgM RF

Rheumatoid vasculitis. This affects up to 20% of patients and may present with palmar erythema, dermal (especially nailfold) infarcts, peripheral sensory neuropathy, mononeuritis multiplex (may cause foot-drop), bowel infarcts and cerebral or coronary artery occlusion. Active treatment is necessary because it is life-threatening.

Ocular involvement

Painful eyes are:
● Usually caused by Sjögren's syndrome, which occurs in 15–20% of people with RA
● Characterized by dryness and grittiness (together with a dry mouth), or episcleritis and scleritis, which cause red inflamed eyes
   Repeated attacks of scleritis (Fig. 4.9) may lead to secondary infection and perforation (scleromalacia perforans). Visual loss is rare, and may be caused by scleritis and scleromalacia perforans, or by corticosteroid-induced cataract.

Nervous system involvement

Peripheral and central nervous system involvement is uncommon. Consequences include numbness, paraesthesiae and weakness resulting from:
● Peripheral nerve and root compression (e.g. carpal tunnel syndrome)
● Rheumatoid vasculitis affecting peripheral nerves (see above)
● Atlanto-axial or mid-cervical subluxation causing cord compression (cervical myelopathy)
   The most common symptom of cervical subluxation is pain radiating up into the occiput. Other symptoms include paraesthesiae, sudden deterioration in hand function, sensory loss, abnormal gait and urinary retention or incontinence.

Cardiac and lung involvement

Pericarditis with effusion and, rarely, mitral valve disease and conduction defects may occur.
   Pleuritis with effusion, fibrosing alveolitis and the occurrence of rheumatoid nodules occur but may be asymptomatic (Fig. 4.10).

Renal involvement

Kidney involvement is uncommon and may result from:
● Amyloidosis, causing proteinuria
● Drug toxicity (e.g. NSAIDs)

Gastrointestinal involvement

Splenomegaly may occur in Felty's syndrome (see below), hepatosplenomegaly may result from amyloidosis and hepatomegaly caused by disease-associated fatty changes.

04

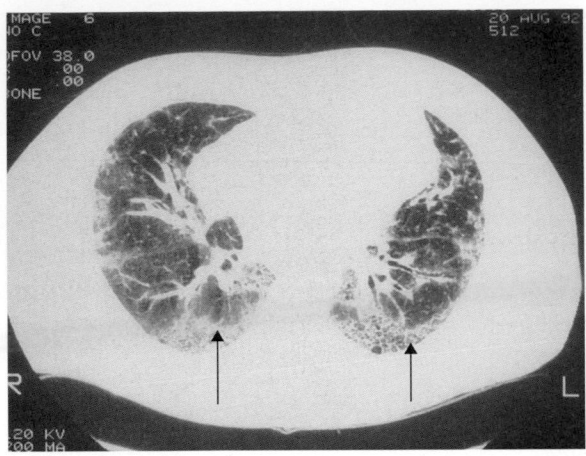

Figure 4.10 High resolution CT. Lung fibrosis in RA. Interstitial changes are present predominantly in the periphery (arrows).

Felty's syndrome

Felty's syndrome affects 1% of patients and consists of the triad of RF-positive RA, splenomegaly and neutropenia. Synovitis is usually severe, and is accompanied by an increased incidence of extra-articular features, including weight loss, leg ulcers and infections.

Iatrogenic factors

Drugs used to treat RA may cause peptic ulceration (NSAIDs), kidney damage (NSAIDs) and suppression of the bone marrow (methotrexate).

Disease pattern in rheumatoid arthritis

Clinical progression in RA is variable. The onset may be rapid or insidious, and there may be single or multiple but usually symmetrical joint involvement, with exacerbations and remissions. Season and climate change affect some patients (e.g. reduced symptoms in warm weather).

The following patterns of disease can be observed:
● Self-limiting disease with recovery and limited sequelae over 2 years.
● Distinct episodes of relapse and remission with residual joint damage and retention of reasonable function.
● Severe unresponsive disease. The patient may become largely wheelchair-bound 5–7 years from onset.
● Palindromic RA characterized by repeated brief attacks usually affecting one joint and rapidly resolving. It may progress into one of the other disease patterns.
● Unusual patterns (e.g. asymmetrical monoarthritis or oligoarthritis).

Investigation

Investigations are carried out to:

● Support the diagnosis
● Assess disease activity and response to treatment
● Assess internal organ involvement
● Identify drug toxicity

Haematology

● *Full blood count (FBC):* anaemia is common in RA, resulting from many factors, and is normally normochromic and normocytic but may be hypochromic and microcytic, reflecting a failure of iron utilization (see pp. 1026 and 1029). Thrombocytosis is common in active RA. The white cell count may be low in Felty's syndrome.
● *ESR:* often raised in active RA.

Biochemistry

Liver function tests (LFTs). Active disease is associated with a slight increase in alkaline phosphatase and transaminase. CRP (an acute phase reactant) can be used to monitor disease activity.

Immunology

Autoantibodies. Seventy-five per cent of adults with RA are IgM RF-positive. This may be absent early in the disease, and should be sought on repeated occasions. The level of RF may be used prognostically at diagnosis, but fluctuations are unhelpful in monitoring the disease. ANAs are present in 30% of patients.

Microbiology

Synovial fluid culture is always necessary when arthrocentesis is carried out because there may be a coexistent infection.

Diagnostic imaging (Fig. 4.10; Fig. B, p. 210)

● *Joint radiography:* reveals the extent of joint destruction. Characteristic radiological findings are soft-tissue swelling, joint space narrowing, periarticular osteoporosis, bony erosions, deformities and, rarely, atlanto-axial subluxation. Serial radiographs will document progress, particularly in relation to drug treatment. Usually radiography shows little in early disease, but changes in the hands and feet may be seen in the absence of symptoms.
● *Chest radiography:* may show heart and/or lung involvement.
● *MRI:* should be performed if atlanto-axial subluxation is suspected.

Histopathology

● *Liver biopsy:* rarely indicated in RA and usually carried out to find out whether drug-induced liver damage (e.g. resulting from methotrexate) has occurred
● *Lip biopsy:* useful in the diagnosis of secondary Sjögren's syndrome

04

Rheumatoid arthritis at a glance

Clinical features

Constitutional
Lethargy
Anorexia
Weight loss
Mild pyrexia

Joints
Symmetrical joint involvement causing:
- Pain
- Swelling
- Stiffness
- Deformity

Rheumatoid arthritis (RA) has a predilection for the metacarpophalangeal (MCP) and proximal interphalangeal (PIP) joints of the hands, wrists, shoulders, cervical spine, knees and feet, although any synovial joint may be affected.

Immunological
Lymphadenopathy
Amyloidosis

Haematological
Anaemia

Skin
Rheumatoid nodules
Vasculitis

Bones and muscles
Muscle weakness
Osteoporosis

Eyes
Sjögren's syndrome: keratoconjunctivitis
Scleritis

Nervous system
Peripheral nerve and cord compression

Heart
Pericarditis and effusion

Lungs
Pleuritis and effusion
Fibrosing alveolitis

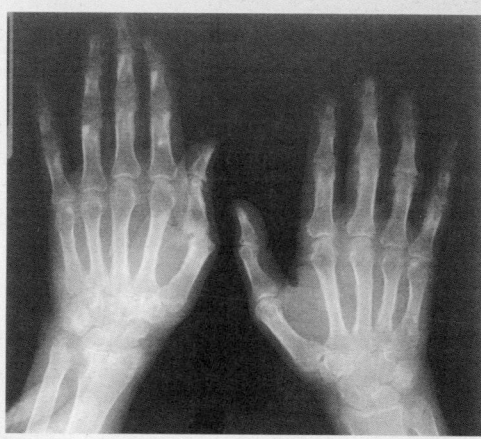

Fig. B Rheumatoid arthritis: radiography of hand demonstrate erosive changes in the proximal interphalangeal joints of the right hand, the interphalangeal joints (IPJ) of the thumbs, the metacarpophalangeal joint (MCPJ) of the left thumb, several of the carpal bones and the wrist and distal radio-ulnar joint of the left hand. In addition, there is characteristic juxta-articular osteopenia.

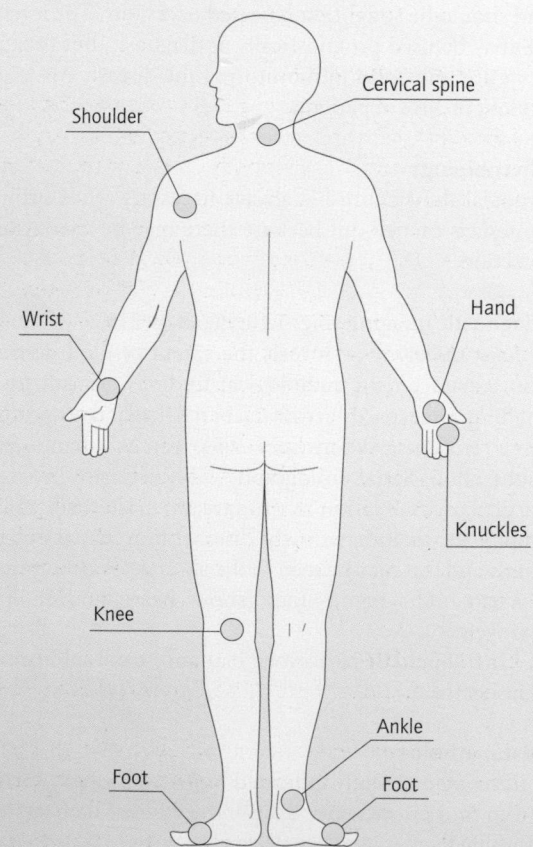

Fig. A Pattern of joint involvement in rheumatoid arthritis.

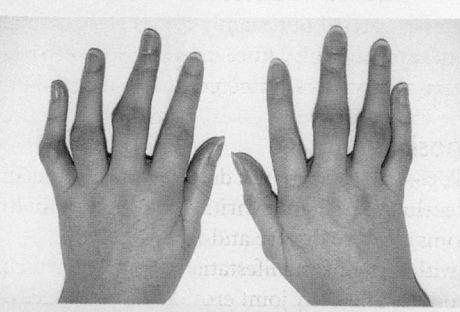

Fig. C MCPJ and IPJ synovitis and deformity in a patient with 5-year history of rheumatoid arthritis.

Other investigations
- *Synovial fluid investigation:* may be a useful confirmatory investigation as it is commonly turbid, with increased protein and white cells
- *Schirmer's tear test* (see p. 212): demonstrates reduced tear production
- *Rose bengal staining of the surface of the eye and slit-lamp examination:* used to determine the extent of the eye disease
- *Neurophysiological testing:* useful in suspected carpal tunnel syndrome
- *Urinalysis:* proteinuria may occur with drug toxicity (gold) or renal amyloidosis

Diagnosis
A disease pattern may not be evident in early disease; clinical suspicion may be all there is.

There is no diagnostic test for RA and a diagnosis is based upon symptoms (e.g. significant early morning joint stiffness) and clinical signs (e.g. symmetrical arthritis and rheumatoid nodules), together with investigations, such as the presence of serum RFs and characteristic radiographical changes. To assist with clinical trials the American College of Rheumatology have defined criteria for the classification of RA.

Management
The multidisciplinary team is central to efficient and effective treatment of the patient with RA.

Drug treatment in RA is outlined on pp. 202–204 and a summary is provided in KEYPOINTS BOX 4.2. Most patients will require a combination of drug therapies at some stage in the disease process. Immunomodulatory drugs have been shown to be of significant benefit to those patients unresponsive to other drug therapies. As trial data become available, so the appropriate use of these therapies will be better understood.

Gene therapy, where genes expressing anti-inflammatory cytokines are selectively delivered to arthritic joints, have significant potential for future treatments.

Surgery is carried out mainly for pain relief, but large joint replacement (hip, knee or shoulder) can increase functional ability in a selected population.

Prognosis
Overall, 5–10% of patients develop severe disease, and 70% develop persistent arthritis (30% with palindromic symptoms). Severe disease and a poor outcome are associated with systemic manifestations, raised RF, subcutaneous nodules and early joint erosions. In severe cases, RA can reduce life expectancy by 4 years in men and 10 years in women.

Sjögren's syndrome
Sjögren's syndrome is a chronic autoimmune disorder characterized by the progressive destruction of exocrine glands, which leads to mucosal and conjunctival dryness (xerostomia and keratoconjunctivitis sicca, respectively), and polyarthritis.

The syndrome may occur in isolation (primary Sjögren's syndrome) or be accompanied by a variety of other autoimmune rheumatic diseases (secondary Sjögren's syndrome). Secondary Sjögren's syndrome is evident in 15–20% of patients with SLE, 10–15% of patients with RA and 1–5% of patients with systemic sclerosis.

Epidemiology
Age. Primary Sjögren's syndrome commonly presents between 30 and 50 years of age.

Sex. Ninety per cent of patients are female.

Race. No known associations.

Genetics. Primary Sjögren's syndrome is associated with HLA B8 and DR3 in white people.

Disease mechanisms
A viral aetiology is suspected and EBV is a possible cause.

Sjögren's syndrome is characterized by salivary gland involvement and autoantibody production, although other organs may also be affected.

Environmental, genetic and immune factors are thought to be involved. Associated autoantibodies are IgM RF, SS-A (anti-Ro) and SS-B (anti-La), which are present in at least 90%, 70% and 48%, respectively, of patients with primary Sjögren's syndrome (Table 4.1).

Histologically, the salivary glands are infiltrated predominantly by CD4$^+$ T cells. The lobular architecture is preserved, but myoepithelial cell proliferation may produce myoepithelial 'islands' and duct occlusion.

The lymphocyte infiltration may become progressive and is termed pseudolymphoma when gland enlargement occurs; rarely, a malignant B-cell lymphoma may develop.

Clinical features
The clinical features of primary Sjögren's syndrome result from:
- *Exocrine gland involvement:* affects the eyes, mouth, respiratory system, gastrointestinal system, kidneys and skin
- *Extraglandular involvement:* affects the musculoskeletal system, thyroid, nervous system and blood vessels

04

Salivary glands

Salivary gland involvement is usually unilateral and episodic. It results in reduced pooling of saliva in the floor of the mouth. When severe, there may be lip cracking or ulceration, angular stomatitis, oral soreness, fissuring and ulceration of the tongue, atrophy of the oral mucosa, secondary candidiasis and dental caries.

Eyes

Keratoconjunctivitis sicca causes various ocular symptoms, including the sensation of a foreign body, burning, tiredness, dryness, redness, blurred vision, itchiness, soreness, pain, photosensitivity and excessive secretion. On examination the conjunctival vessels may be dilated, and there may be photophobia and irregularity of the corneal edge.

Skin

Common symptoms are skin dryness (xeroderma)—vaginal dryness causes a burning sensation and dyspareunia.

Musculoskeletal

Myalgia and arthralgia. Some patients develop a mild relapsing non-erosive polyarthritis that usually affects the large joints.

Lung

Recurrent bronchitis and pneumonitis are common.

Gastrointestinal

- Mild dysphagia or chronic gastritis resulting from gastrointestinal involvement
- Acute or chronic pancreatitis, enlargement of the liver and spleen (Sjögren's syndrome is associated with primary biliary cirrhosis and other autoimmune liver diseases)

Renal

Nephrogenic diabetes insipidus, renal tubular acidosis, interstitial nephritis or glomerulonephritis caused by renal involvement in approximately 10% of patients.

Neurology

Peripheral sensory, sensorimotor and cranial (especially trigeminal) neuropathy, and other manifestations of CNS involvement (e.g. seizures, movement disorders).

Vessels

Vasculitis of small- and medium-sized vessels in approximately 20% of patients, which may lead to skin and neurological features.

Pregnancy

The presence of anti-Ro/La antibodies is associated with the development of complete heart block and heart failure in neonates.

Diagnosis

Diagnosis of Sjögren's syndrome can generally be made from the combination of eye and mouth symptoms, abnormal Schirmer's test and a positive lip biopsy and the presence of serum autoantibodies (see below).

Investigation

Haematology

ESR is increased.

Immunology

Autoantibodies are common in both primary and secondary Sjögren's syndrome and include RF, ANA, SS-A (anti-Ro), SS-B (anti-La).

Diagnostic imaging

Diagnostic imaging of lungs, liver and kidneys may be useful.

Histopathology

- *Lip biopsy:* provides histological evidence of Sjögren's syndrome
- *Liver and kidney biopsy:* may be useful

Other investigations

- *Schirmer's tear test:* a useful test of lacrimal gland involvement. Unstimulated wetting of filter paper hooked over the lower eyelid normally exceeds 35 mm in 5 min. In Sjögren's syndrome it is often less than 5 mm.
- *Rose bengal dye test:* a 1% solution of rose bengal dye is instilled into the conjunctival sac and slit-lamp examination is performed to look for punctate filamentous keratitis resulting from eye involvement.
- *Salivary flow rate:* can be measured and, when unstimulated, will be 1.5 ml/15 min or less.

Management

Sjögren's syndrome is initially treated symptomatically. Additional management is similar to that for other rheumatic disorders (see KEYPOINTS BOX 4.2, p. 201). The management of autoimmune liver disease is discussed on p. 619.

Prognosis

Primary Sjögren's syndrome is rarely life-shortening. The prognosis of secondary Sjögren's syndrome relates to the severity of the underlying disease.

Systemic lupus erythematosus

Systemic lupus erythematosus is a multisystem disease

in which autoantibodies and immune complexes may cause cellular and tissue damage. This results in a wide spectrum of clinical manifestations, which have a tendency towards exacerbation and remission. There may be significant overlap with other autoimmune rheumatic disorders such as rheumatoid arthritis and systemic sclerosis.

Epidemiology

Prevalence. Estimates range between 1 in 1000 and 1 in 6000 worldwide.

Age. Usually 25–35 years old.

Sex. Ninety per cent of patients are women (99% in childbearing years).

Race. Some studies have found that Afro-Caribbean females are affected more commonly than white females.

Genetics. Genetic susceptibility is present (see below).

Geography. SLE is more common in urban than in rural areas and prevalence may vary according to country (e.g. it is as common as RA in Jamaica, but much less common in Scandinavia).

Disease mechanisms

The aetiology of SLE is probably multifactorial and, as with other autoimmune rheumatic disease, involves environmental factors and genetic susceptibility.

Environment

Potential disease triggers are:
- Stress
- Ultraviolet sunlight
- Drugs (e.g. captopril procainamide, hydralazine, phenytoin, minocycline and nitrofurantoin)
- Chemicals (e.g. pollutants, toxins and hairspray)
- Diet
- Infections (e.g. viruses, cytomegalovirus, EBV and retroviruses)

In addition, it is thought that antigens from bacteria may result in T-cell activation, pro-inflammatory cytokine release and polyclonal B-cell activation with antibody secretion.

Genetics

The monozygotic twin concordances are between 24 and 60% and dizygotic 5%. A number of MHC gene associations have been made (e.g. the B8DR3 haplotype in white individuals). Complement deficiencies C1q-r-s and C4 are strongly associated with lupus. C2 deficiency is associated with a lupus-like disease with cutaneous manifestations. Lupus is more common in women.

The basic abnormalities in SLE are thought to be the production of autoantibodies and immune complexes, and the inability of the immune system to suppress them. In SLE, antibodies are directed mainly against the cell nucleus (antinuclear and cytoplasmic proteins). These nuclear and cytoplasmic molecules may have important cellular functions that include storage of genetic materials (e.g. histone) and gene transcription (e.g. smRNA). A detailed list of SLE-associated antibodies is given in Table 4.1.

Autoantibodies are thought to result in:
- Cell death (e.g. anti-erythrocyte antibodies, lymphocytotoxic antibodies)
- Deposition of antigen–antibody complexes, resulting in complement activation (e.g. skin and kidney)
- Platelet aggregation and clot formation, resulting in microthrombus formation and tissue ischaemia

Pathology

Specific histological changes in the skin include depigmentation and degeneration of the basal layer of the epidermis with disruption of the dermal–epidermal junction—where immunoglobulin (Ig) and complement are deposited—and mononuclear cell infiltration.

The initial lesion of acute cutaneous lupus is typified by raised erythematosus, hyperkeratotic lesions, but in subacute cutaneous lupus there may be small raised erythematous plaques that can coalesce. Discoid lupus erythematosus describes severe skin involvement consisting of circular lesions with raised, scaly and erythematous rims, follicular plugging and telangiectasia.

Glomerulonephritis may develop and histologically may be focally proliferative, membranous, diffusely proliferative or mesangial (see Chapter 8).

Synovial effusions are unusual and of small volume. The fluid is clear or cloudy, has a low protein level (transudate) and the white cell count is not usually elevated.

In the blood, neutropenia and lymphocytopenia are common and there may be a mild thrombocytopenia. Avascular necrosis of bone is associated with the presence of anticardiolipin antibodies.

Clinical features

The multisystem involvement of SLE gives rise to a spectrum of clinical features that vary in severity. Systemic manifestations are common. Fatigue or general malaise are a common feature and may reflect a flare of the disease,

04

other causes may be associated with depression and cardiovascular disease.

Skin

A malar 'butterfly' rash over the cheeks and the bridge of the nose, exacerbated by ultraviolet light, is characteristic of SLE. Livedo reticularis may be present. Raynaud's phenomenon will occur in approximately 50% of patients at presentation. This describes the colour changes of the hands that occur as a result of digital vasospasm usually associated with cold weather. Typically, the fingers turn white (ischaemia), blue–purple (deoxygenation of the blood) and then red (reperfusion hyperaemia).

Discoid lupus may occur in isolation. Patchy alopecia can be permanent but usually rapid hair loss is associated with active disease and regrowth will occur when the disease remits. Other cutaneous manifestations are oral and vaginal mucosal ulceration, periungual erythema, angio-oedema and cutaneous vasculitis.

Musculoskeletal

Musculoskeletal involvement is manifest as arthralgia and a symmetrical non-erosive arthritis (Jaccoud's) affecting mainly the PIP and MCP joints, wrists and knees. Deformity is unusual. Myalgia caused by muscle involvement is common, but myositis is uncommon.

Kidneys

Renal disease (lupus nephritis) develops in 50% of patients with SLE at some time. There is a broad spectrum of severity; it is often asymptomatic, but may result in hypertension or renal failure.

Central nervous system

CNS involvement is an important cause of morbidity. Brain, meninges, spinal cord and peripheral nerves can all be affected, giving rise to many different features, which may fluctuate with disease activity (Fig. 4.11). Neuropsychiatric symptoms may range from cognitive impairment through seizures to strokes. Migraine is more common in patients with lupus than in the general population, particularly those with antiphospholipid antibodies. Neuropsychiatric features may also be a result of drug treatment (e.g. corticosteroids), infection, hypertension, renal failure (e.g. uraemia) or increased coagulation (e.g. antiphospholipid syndrome). Depression may also be a feature associated with any chronic disorder.

Blood

Haematological abnormalities include haemolytic anaemia and lymphopenia and occur in 10% of patients. Pancytopenia may occur as a result of drug-induced immunosuppression (e.g. azathioprine treatment).

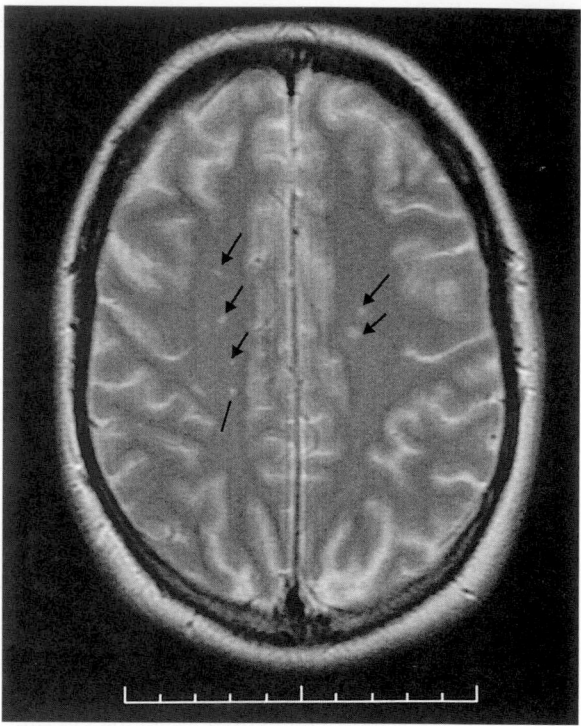

Figure 4.11 T_2-weighted axial image through the brain, demonstrating small foci of high signal intensity within the deep white matter (arrowed). These magnetic resonance appearances are non-specific, but in the correct clinical context are in keeping with small vessel ischaemia.

Heart and lungs

Heart and lung involvement can result in:

- *Pericarditis:* may be associated with a pericardial effusion
- *Myocarditis:* can cause arrhythmia and cardiac failure
- *Libman–Sacks endocarditis:* rarely, gives rise to emboli and aortic and mitral regurgitation
- *Peripheral vasoconstriction:* causing Raynaud's phenomenon in 50% of patients
- *Pleural effusion*
- *Pneumonitis:* may cause fever, dyspnoea and cough, and, rarely, leads to fibrosis
- *Loss of lung volume:* resulting in elevation of both hemidiaphragms and restricted lung fields (Fig. 4.12)
- *Adult respiratory distress syndrome and intra-alveolar haemorrhage:* rare
- *Pulmonary embolism:* as a result of increased coagulation in antiphospholipid syndrome

Eyes

Conjunctivitis, episcleritis and optic neuritis are features of SLE, and retinal vasculitis can cause infarcts

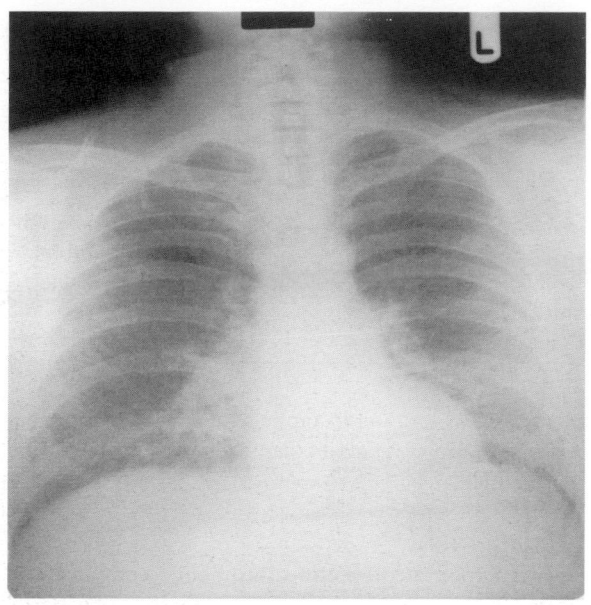

Figure 4.12 Volume loss and small reticulonodular densities are seen in both lung bases in a patient with systemic lupus erythematosus.

(cytoid bodies). Approximately 15–20% of patients have Sjögren's syndrome.

Abdomen

Abdominal pain and epigastric tenderness may be a result of:

- Drugs (e.g. NSAIDs)
- Abdominal serositis
- Vasculitis of mesenteric blood vessels
- Pancreatitis
- Non-specific hepatitis
- Hepatosplenomegaly

Investigation

Haematology

- *FBC:* anaemia may result from the chronic disease process and the use of NSAIDs
- *Coagulation tests:* abnormalities may be detected predisposing to thrombosis (see p. 1076)
- *ESR:* may correlate with disease activity

Biochemistry

- *Renal function:* can be assessed initially by serum creatinine estimation. Urinalysis by dipstick testing and microscopy of the urine will indicate renal abnormality (see p. 508)
- *CRP:* usually normal and when increased may be an indication of infection.

Immunology

- *Autoantibodies:* autoantibodies to nuclear and cytoplasmic antigens may be present (see Table 4.1). The ANA test is the best screening test for SLE as it is usually positive. Anti-dsDNA antibodies are specific for SLE and may reflect disease activity, while RF is found in 30–50% of patients. Anti-smRNA antibodies are also virtually confined to individuals with SLE, but are present in less than 20% of such patients.
- *Antiphospholipid antibodies:* may be associated with a thrombotic tendency (see below).
- *Complement:* low levels of total C3 and total C4 may reflect disease activity.

Microbiology

Synovial fluid culture is always necessary as infection may coexist.

Diagnostic imaging

Magnetic resonance imaging and spectroscopy, and CT scanning of the brain is useful in the diagnosis of neuropsychiatric lupus and may reflect electroencephalogram (EEG) abnormalities (Fig. 4.11).

Histopathology

- *Renal biopsy:* may be indicated to diagnose glomerulonephritis
- *Skin biopsy:* may be useful

Diagnosis

Diagnosis of SLE rests on recognizing a constellation of clinical and laboratory findings. Because it may be drug-induced, a detailed drug history is essential.

Differential diagnosis of SLE includes RA, epilepsy, psychiatric disorders, multiple sclerosis, idiopathic thrombocytopenic purpura, urticaria, erythema multiforme, rosacea and lichen planus.

Management

Patients with SLE need assiduous care so that any increase in disease activity can be treated immediately and appropriately (for a general summary of management see KEYPOINTS BOX 4.2, p. 201). Systemic corticosteroids and cytotoxic agents are required for severe life-threatening events (e.g. lupus nephritis).

There is no evidence that treatment during remission alters progression of the disease. It is safe and useful to immunize patients with influenza, tetanus and pneumococcal vaccine to prevent infection and the likelihood of a possible disease flare. A low-oestrogen oral contraceptive is safe but contraindicated in patients with migraine, hypertension, high titres of anticardiolipin antibodies and previous history of thrombosis. Progesterone-only

04

contraceptives can be used. Low-dose oestrogen hormone replacement therapy is safe as long as the patient is regularly monitored. Avoid sulphonamides as they may cause rash or neutropenia.

Prognosis

Complete remission is rare but, with optimal diagnostic awareness and management, the overall 10-year survival of SLE is 90% and most patients live a normal lifespan and die from non-SLE causes. Infection is the main cause of death now that renal support and transplantation are so successful. The complications of corticosteroid therapy can cause considerable morbidity (see Table 4.5).

Antiphospholipid syndrome

Antiphospholipid syndrome (APS) can occur as a primary condition or in association with SLE and other autoimmune rheumatic diseases.

Clinical features

Antiphospholipid syndrome is characterized by vascular thrombosis, thrombocytopenia and recurrent spontaneous miscarriage, and there are associated antibodies reactive with phospholipid.

Investigation

Phospholipid antibodies are specific markers for APS. There are a wide range; for example, cardiolipin, phosphatidylserine, phosphatidylethanolamine and phosphatidylinositol. Antibodies in APS are directed mainly to phospholipid binding plasma proteins and in particular β_2-glycoprotein-1. The functional activity of phospholipid antibodies (lupus anticoagulants) are detected using coagulation assays (e.g. activated partial thromboplastin time and dilute Russell's viper venom time). Both types of assay should be used in evaluating a patient for APS.

Systemic lupus erythematosus and pregnancy

Pregnancy is not contraindicated in a patient in remission with good renal function.

Fertility rate is normal, but there is a high spontaneous miscarriage rate (30–50%), especially if antiphospholipid antibodies are present.

Adverse fetal outcomes include miscarriage, prematurity and stillbirth, and a disease flare may occur, usually in the first trimester or postpartum.

Treatment with prednisolone is safe during pregnancy.

Neonatal SLE is rare. Clinically, there may be a transient rash or permanent congenital heart block, which is related to SS-A (Ro), SS-B (La) antibody in maternal serum and causes a high morbidity. The neonate may have a transient

Table 4.9 Classification of primary vasculitis

Vessel	Disease
Large and medium arteries	Giant cell arteritis
	Takayasu's arteritis
Medium arteries or small vessels	Polyarteritis nodosa
	Kawasaki's disease
	Wegener's granulomatosis
	Churg–Strauss syndrome
	Microscopic polyangiitis
Small vessels	Henoch–Schönlein purpura
	Leukocytoclastic vasculitis

positive ANA test and thrombocytopenia resulting from maternal antiplatelet antibodies, haemolytic anaemia and leucopenia.

Management

This is aimed at preventing thrombolic complications using aspirin, intravenous immunoglobulin and heparin. Pregnancy outcome in APS-positive mothers with recurrent fetal loss is also improved with regular fetal and maternal monitoring.

Vasculitis syndromes

The primary vasculitis syndromes are a heterogeneous group of autoimmune diseases characterized by inflammation and damage to blood vessels. The resulting disease depends on the type, size and location of involved blood vessels (Table 4.9). Secondary vasculitis may be associated with other autoimmune diseases such as rheumatoid arthritis and lupus, infection such as hepatitis B and HIV and drugs such as sulphonomides, penicillins and thiazide diuretics (for a summary see VASCULITIS AT A GLANCE, p. 219).

Vasculitis may be the main component of a disease or a secondary component, as in RA, and may involve single or multiple organs.

Epidemiology

Prevalence. Estimates range from 2 to 6 in 100 000 population, but the syndromes are more common in association with autoimmune rheumatic disease and malignancy.

Disease mechanisms

Disease is thought to be triggered by an antigen and can be categorized according to whether the antigen is thought to be:

- *Exogenous:* for example, resulting from drugs, microbe (e.g. streptococci) or foreign protein (e.g. immunization)
- *Endogenous:* for example, resulting from immunoglobulin in RA, DNA in SLE, and tumour antigens

Systemic lupus erythematosus at a glance

Clinical features

Constitutional
Malaise
Fever

Skin
Mucocutaneous
Alopecia
Malar 'butterfly' rash
Discoid lupus
Mucosal ulcers
Vasculitic rash
Raynaud's phenomenon
Nailfold/pulp infarcts

Joints
Arthralgia
Symmetrical arthritis (Jaccoud's)

Muscles
Myalgia
Myositis

Kidneys
Hypertension
Lupus nephritis

Neuropsychiatric
Psychomotor changes
Epilepsy
Stroke

Blood
Lymphopenia
Haemolytic anaemia
Coagulation abnormalities

Heart and circulation
Raynaud's phenomenon
Accelerated atherosclerosis
Pericarditis
Myocarditis (Libman–Sacks)

Lungs
Pleural effusion
Loss of lung volume
Pulmonary embolism

Eyes
Sjögren's syndrome: episcleritis
Retinal infarcts
Optic neuritis

Abdomen
Hepatosplenomegaly

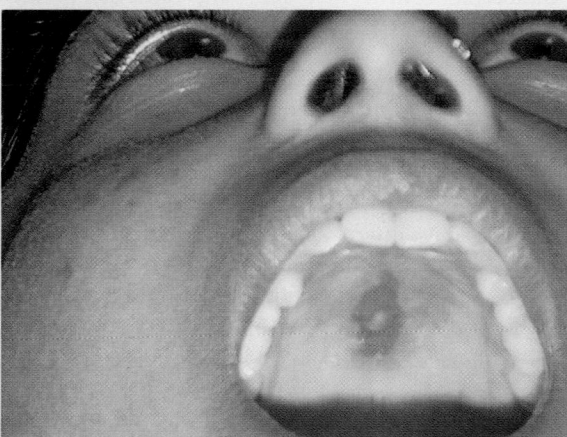

Fig. A Mucosal ulceration of the roof of the mouth.

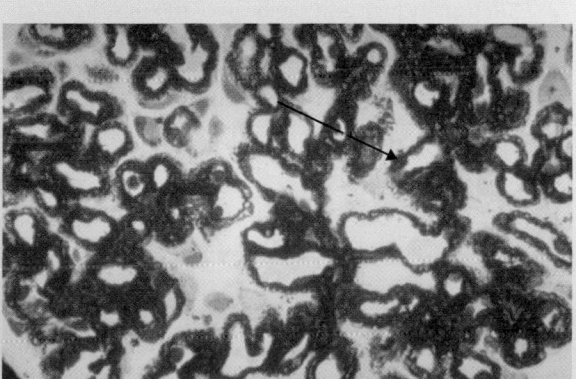

Fig. B Membranous glomerulonephritis. The peripheral capillary loops of the glomerulus exhibit spikes (arrow), some of which show cross-linking (arrows) (Jones silver stain: high power).

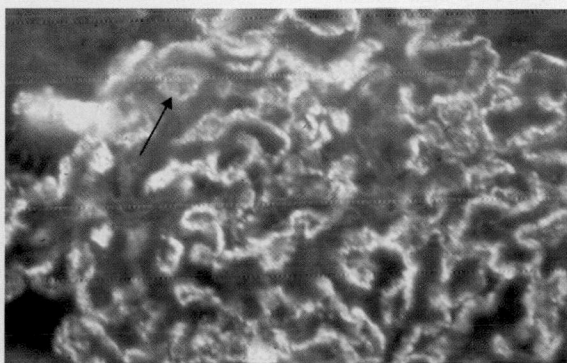

Fig. C Membranous glomerulonephritis–IgG. The peripheral capillary loops exhibit granular ('lumpy-bumpy') deposition of IgG (arrow).

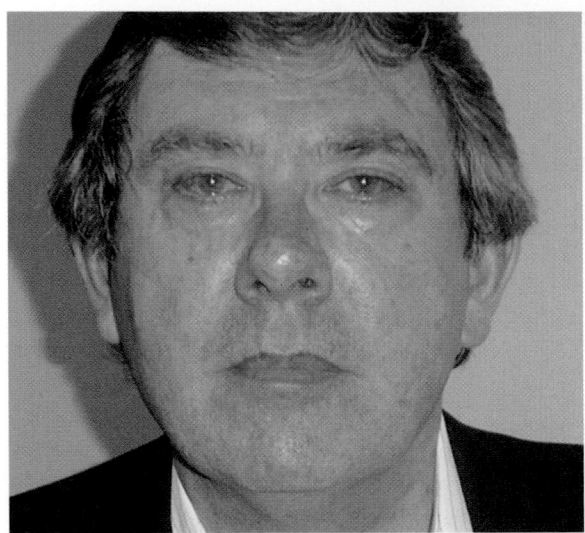

Figure 4.13 Episcleritis in Wegener's granulomatosis.

Pathology

The predominant pathological processes involved in these syndromes are thought to be:

- Immune complex deposition
- Cell-mediated and direct cellular cytotoxicity

There is also thought to be a genetic predisposition.

Common clinical features

Systemic symptoms

Fever, malaise, weakness, arthralgia, anorexia and weight loss. There may be features specific to the disease associated with vasculitis (e.g. SLE, malignancy).

Heart and lungs

Cough, sinusitis, haemoptysis, dyspnoea, wheeze, chest pain resulting from pericarditis and coronary vasculitis.

Joints

Arthralgia and arthritis.

Eyes

Conjunctivitis, episcleritis, scleritis and uveitis (Fig. 4.13).

Skin

Cutaneous vasculitis, palpable purpura, macules, papules, vesicles, bullae, subcutaneous nodules, ulcers (Fig. 4.14) and recurrent or chronic urticaria.

Neurology

Cranial neuritis, mononeuritis multiplex, cerebral vasculitis, sensory motor impairment and deafness.

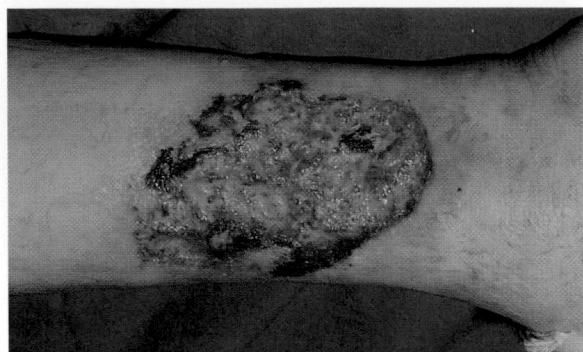

Figure 4.14 Vasculitis can cause skin infarction and ulcer formation. These ulcers may take many weeks to heal, and are a significant cause of morbidity.

Kidneys (see p. 514)

Glomerulonephritis may occur and cause symptoms of renal failure. Haematuria may be present.

Gastrointestinal

Mouth ulcers, abdominal pain and diarrhoea (for a summary see VASCULITIS AT A GLANCE).

Investigation

Investigations utilize blood and tissues (e.g. skin and kidney) to define inflammation, immunopathology and organ involvement. Imaging further aids the diagnosis of specific organ involvement (e.g. vessels, lung, brain and kidney).

Haematology

- *FBC:* reveals a normochromic anaemia, leucocytosis, thrombocytosis and chronic eosinophilia (Churg–Strauss syndrome)
- *ESR:* usually high and can be over 100 mm/h.

Biochemistry

- *Alkaline phosphatase:* may be raised
- *Muscle enzymes:* normal

Immunology

- *Serum antibodies:* increased (Fig. 4.4e,f). In Henoch–Schönlein purpura (HSP), IgA is the antibody class commonly involved in the immune complexes. Antibodies to both cytoplasmic (c-) serine proteinase 3 (PR3) and peripheral (p-) myeloperoxidase (MPO) associated neutrophil cytoplasmic antigens (ANCA) may be detected (see p. 522). Disease association with these antibodies may overlap, although 90% of Wegener's granulomatosis patients are c-ANCA/PR3 positive.
- *Other investigations* (e.g. ANA, RF, complement): may be useful for excluding other causes.

Diagnostic imaging
● *Echocardiography:* to detect heart involvement
● *Arteriography* (MRI can be used): may show characteristic aneurysms in the small and medium-sized renal and visceral arteries (Fig. 4.15)

Histopathology (biopsy)
● *Vessel:* temporal artery biopsy should be carried out if temporal arteritis is suspected and may show a panarteritis. This should be performed before corticosteroids are commenced if possible. The biopsy may be normal if there is segmental involvement.
● *Skin:* showing vasculitis, IgA deposits in HSP
● *Organ*
● *Nasal:* to show granulomas in Wegener's granulomatosis
● *Renal:* provides a histological diagnosis of glomerulonephritis

Urinalysis
Haematuria may be present.

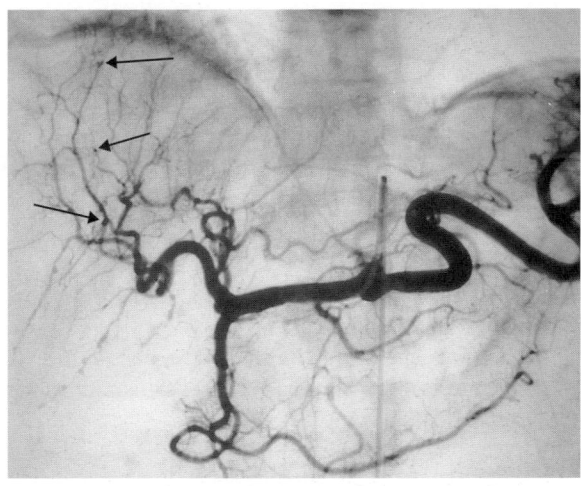

Figure 4.15 Digital subtraction angiography of the coeliac axis in polyarteritis nodosa (PAN). Microaneurysm formation can be seen affecting branches of the hepatic artery (arrows).

Vasculitis at a glance

A heterogeneous group of autoimmune diseases characterized by inflammation and damage to blood vessels

Aetiology
Antigen trigger
• *Exogenous:* drug, microbe, immunization
• *Endogenous:* immunoglobulin, DNA, tumour antigen

Clinical features
Constitutional: fever, weight loss

Heart and lungs
Cough
Chest pain

Joints
Arthralgia
Arthritis

Eyes
Conjunctivitis
Scleritis

Skin
Purpura
Macules
Ulcers

Neurology
Cerebral vasculitis
Sensory motor impairment

Kidneys
Renal failure

Gastrointestinal
Mouth ulcers
Abdominal pain
Other diseases associated (e.g. lupus, malignancy)

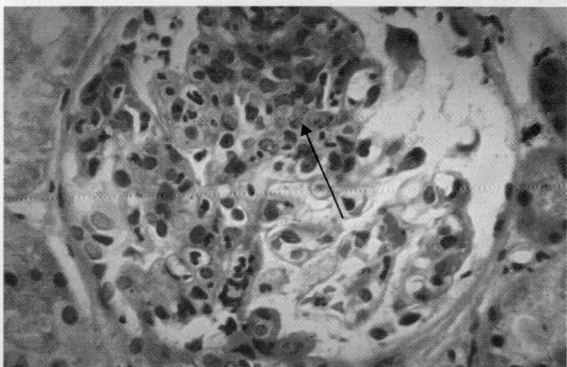

Fig. A The kidney shows a focal and segmented necrotizing glomerulonephritis. Part of the glomerulus shows an increase in cellularity, necrosis and infiltration by neutrophils (arrow).

04

Management

Treatment depends on the size of vessel and organ involvement, and small vessel vasculitis such as HSP may require no therapy. However, there is a wide spectrum of treatments available:

- High doses of corticosteroids (e.g. 40–60 mg prednisolone) may be required in systemic necrotizing vasculitis
- Cytotoxic drugs (cyclophosphamide, azathioprine, methotrexate)
- Plasmapheresis in patients with pulmonary haemorrhage and severe renal disease
- Intravenous immunoglobulin in Kawasaki's disease
- Co-trimoxazole for limited Wegener's granulomatosis (without renal involvement)

Primary vasculitic diseases

Temporal arteritis and polymyalgia rheumatica

Epidemiology

Prevalence. Temporal arteritis is relatively common in Europe and USA with a prevalence of 2 in 1000. PMR has a prevalence of approximately 5 in 1000 population.

Age. Usually over 55 years of age.

Sex. Most common in women.

Race. Rare in Afro-Caribbeans.

Genetics. Familial aggregation and association with the MHC have been reported.

Pathology

Temporal arteritis is a systemic disease involving medium- and large-sized arteries. Characteristically, one or more branches of the carotid artery are involved. PMR is a syndrome closely associated with temporal arteritis, and is usually benign in the absence of arteritis.

Temporal arteritis is characterized histologically by a panarteritis with inflammatory mononuclear cell infiltrates and giant cell formation. The mononuclear cell infiltrates and giant cell formation are associated with the media and internal elastic lamina. The intima may be thickened and oedematous and the vessel lumen restricted. Inflammatory changes may not affect the entire length of the artery and 'skip' lesions are common.

Clinical features

Temporal arteritis

Non-specific systemic symptoms include malaise and weight loss, and 50% of patients will have symptoms of

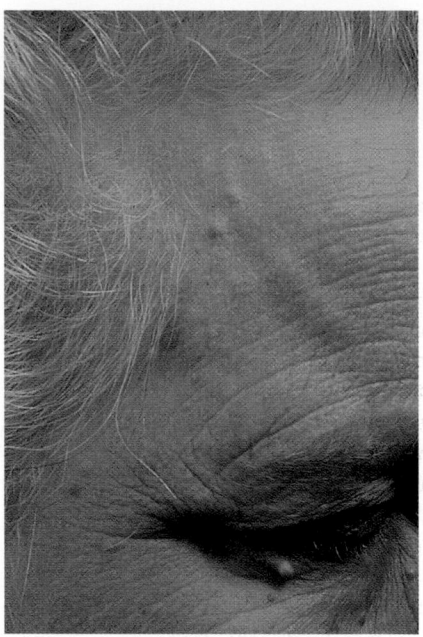

Figure 4.16 Temporal arteritis. The temporal artery may be visible and tender to the touch.

PMR. If the temporal artery is involved it may be nodular and tender to touch (Fig. 4.16). Pulsation may be absent or reduced. There may be associated scalp pain and pain on chewing, resulting from jaw claudication. Ischaemic optic neuritis may lead to severe visual impairment (amaurosis fugax) and sudden blindness, and may occur within weeks or months of the systemic symptoms. Large vessel vasculitis is uncommon, but may cause intermittent claudication and paraesthesiae.

Polymyalgia rheumatica

Bilateral muscle stiffness and ache, and pain in the neck, shoulders, lower back, hip and thigh are characteristic. These symptoms may also be associated with early RA. Approximately 15% of patients will have giant cell arteritis.

Diagnosis

The diagnosis may be difficult and is often delayed. It is based on clinical and laboratory findings, and is aided by a positive temporal artery biopsy.

Management

Temporal arteritis

Drug treatment. High-dose prednisolone (60 mg/day) at first; gradually decrease to maintenance regimen (7.5–10 mg/day) for 3–4 years.

Azathioprine or methotrexate may additionally be required in more severe cases.

04

Polymyalgia rheumatica
Drug treatment. Low-dose corticosteroid (prednisolone starting at 10 mg/day) and then gradually reducing each month for 6 months to 2 years.

Follow-up. Close follow-up to detect symptoms of temporal arteritis. The ESR is used to monitor disease activity and to titrate the dosage of corticosteroid.

Prognosis
Temporal arteritis and PMR both have a good prognosis if treatment is started promptly because corticosteroids prevent blindness and other vascular complications. PMR usually remits after 6 months to 2 years. Relapses may occur upon lowering prednisolone to below 5 mg/day.

Takayasu's arteritis
Takayasu's arteritis (aortic arch syndrome) has a predilection for the aortic arch and its branches. It may result in loss of pulses, claudication—especially effecting the upper limbs—as well as arterial bruits.

Polyarteritis nodosa
Epidemiology
Prevalence. Uncommon.

Sex. Approximately 67% of patients are male.

Pathology
Polyarteritis nodosa (PAN) is caused by necrotizing vasculitis. It characteristically affects bifurcations and branches of the renal and visceral arteries. There is an acute neutrophil infiltration of all layers of the vessel wall and perivascular areas, resulting in intimal proliferation, degeneration, fibrinoid necrosis, immune vessel narrowing, infarction of the tissues supplied by the vessel and, sometimes, haemorrhage.

Aneurysmal dilatation (up to 1 cm) is characteristic along involved arteries (Fig. 4.15). Glomerulonephritis occurs in 30% of patients (see SYSTEMIC LUPUS ERYTHEMATOSUS AT A GLANCE, p. 217).

Clinical features
The disease may have an abrupt onset, and 50% of patients experience fever, weight loss and malaise. Specific features reflect the location and degree of involvement of affected vessels. For example, a patient with PAN may present with nephritis and hypertension, an acute abdomen, mononeuritis multiplex or polyarthritis.

Cutaneous lesions are often present and include palpable purpura, digital infarcts, livedo reticularis and mucocutaneous ulceration. Approximately 70% of patients have renal involvement, and proteinuria is common.

Management
Long-term remission can be obtained using corticosteroids and cytotoxic drugs (e.g. cyclophosphamide).

Prognosis
The 5-year survival rate for untreated PAN is 13%. Death is usually brought about by renal failure and intestinal and cardiovascular complications, which may be compounded by hypertension.

Kawasaki's disease (mucocutaneous lymph node syndrome)
This is one of the most common vasculitides of childhood. The majority are children under 5 years of age, with greater prevalence in Japanese children. It is a self-limiting condition with an average duration of 12 days without therapy. Rash occurs involving lips, oral cavity, limbs, trunk, palms and soles of feet. There may be skin desquamation. In addition, conjunctivitis and other manifestations of inflammation including fever and lymphadenopathy are common. There is significant mortality associated with coronary artery vasculitis, reported in up to 25% of children. Treatment with anti-inflammatory and immunomodulation, principally with intravenous immunoglobulin, may be necessary.

Wegener's granulomatosis
Wegener's granulomatosis is a vasculitis affecting the upper (bloody nasal discharge and saddle nose deformity) and lower respiratory tracts (Fig. 4.13). An association with renal impairment resulting from glomerulonephritis is seen is some patients.

Churg–Strauss syndrome
Patients may specifically present with atopy (late-onset asthma), lung infiltrates, rash and arthritis. This may occur several years before the start of systemic disease. There may be associated cardiac and neurological involvement.

Microscopic polyangiitis
Patients may present with clinical symptoms and signs reflecting renal and lung involvement.

Henoch–Schönlein purpura
Epidemiology
Prevalence. Described as common, but exact data are not available.

Age. Peak incidence in children aged 4–11 years.

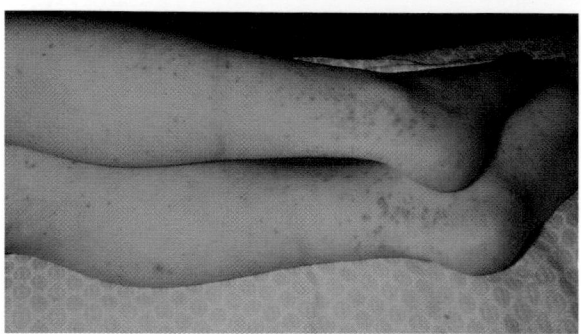

Figure 4.17 Henoch–Schönlein purpura. Palpable purpuric plaques occur on the lower legs. There may also be multifocal areas of haemorrhage or necrosis.

Disease mechanisms

Usually HSP occurs without a known antecedent event, but antigens implicated as triggers include viruses and bacteria (especially *Streptococcus*), drugs, foods, insect bites and immunizations.

Clinical features

Clinically, the disorder is characterized by an abrupt onset with malaise. 'Flu-like symptoms are common. Other features include:

● *Palpable purpura:* usually distributed over the buttocks and lower limbs (Fig. 4.17)
● *Transient non-migratory polyarthritis:* a common symptom
● *Intestinal symptoms:* including colicky pain, nausea and vomiting, diarrhoea, constipation and the passage of blood and mucus rectally
● *Haematuria, moderate proteinuria and casts:* indicating glomerulonephritis, occurs in 50% of patients
   The diagnosis is made on clinical grounds.

Management

The condition is generally self-limiting and treated symptomatically, although corticosteroids may be required for severe renal disease, but benefit is unproven.

Prognosis

The symptoms may recur over weeks or months, and there is a 40% recurrence rate in adults. It rarely becomes chronic.

Leukocytoclastic vasculitis

This disease is usually confined to the skin where there may be purpura, which may become bullous and ulcerate. Nailfold infarcts may be evident.

Myositis

Polymyositis (PM) is an inflammatory disease of striated skeletal muscle. It may be a primary disorder or a secondary manifestation of autoimmune rheumatic diseases such as RA and SLE. Dermatomyositis (DM) describes PM with skin involvement.

Epidemiology

Prevalence. Approximately 8 in 100 000 for primary PM/DM, 2–3/million for childhood-onset DM.

Incidence. 5 in 10 million/year

Age. Commonly 40–60 years of age.

Sex. More common in women.

Race. No association.

Genetics. An increased frequency of certain HLA genes in PM/DM (e.g. HLA-B8) suggests a genetic predisposition.

Geography. Worldwide.

Disease mechanisms

The aetiology is unknown. There are probably many different causes of PM/DM. The two main theories, which are not mutually exclusive, suggest viral and autoimmune aetiologies.

● *A viral role:* has been suggested, but no evidence has been revealed by investigations using serological methods, electron microscopy, culture, immunostaining or polymerase chain reaction (PCR).
● *An autoimmune mechanism:* suggested by lymphocyte infiltration and Ig deposition in the affected muscle, and by autoantibody production (anti-Jo1 antibody).

Pathology

The main feature is an inflammatory cell infiltration of muscle, predominantly lymphocytes, with associated degeneration and destruction of muscle fibres. Interstitial fibrosis may also be a feature. Calcinosis is present more frequently in the childhood form. In DM, there is a dermal infiltrate of inflammatory cells (Fig. 4.18).

Clinical features

Myositis can be classified into five categories:

1 *Primary PM:* 40% of patients
2 *Primary DM:* 25% of patients
3 *PM/DM associated with autoimmune rheumatic disease:* 15% of patients

04

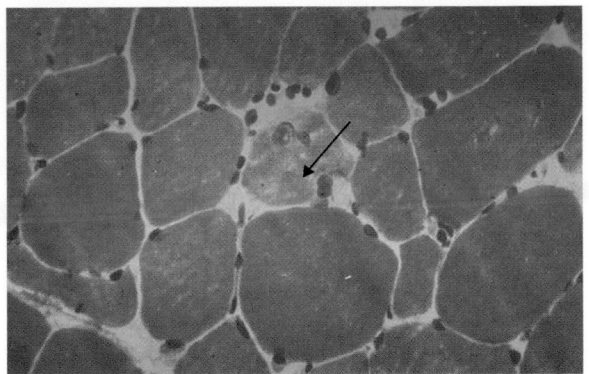

Figure 4.18 Dermatomyositis. The muscle fibres are seen in transverse sections. Centrally, there is a necrotic fibre showing flocculation of the cytoplasm (arrow).

4 *PM/DM associated with cancer:* 10% of patients
5 *Childhood-onset DM:* 10% of patients
   Progressive proximal muscle weakness is the dominant clinical feature.

Primary polymyositis

The onset of primary PM is insidious and progressive, usually over weeks or months; it is rarely acute. It may occur at any age and the female : male ratio is 2 : 1. Symptoms include:

- *Systemic features:* such as fever, weight loss, fatigue and malaise
- *Raynaud's phenomenon:* may occur in approximately 20–30% of patients
- *Symmetrical muscle weakness:* of the proximal limb muscles (especially hips and thighs), pharyngeal and upper oesophageal muscle (causing dysphagia) and the diaphragm (causing respiratory impairment)
- *Muscle pain and tenderness:* causing aching in the buttocks, thighs and calves
- *Cardiac abnormalities:* causing ECG changes, arrhythmias, myocarditis and heart failure
- *Lung involvement:* as a result of interstitial lung disease (30–40%), muscle weakness and, in severe disease, as a consequence of aspiration pneumonia

Primary dermatomyositis

Skin changes may precede or follow muscle involvement and include:

- Classic lilac-coloured (heliotrope) rash and oedema on the upper eyelids (Fig. 4.19a)
- Scaly violaceous eruption over the extensor surfaces of joints, commonly the knuckles, elbows and knees (Gottron's papules or collodian patches) (Fig. 4.19b)
- Subcutaneous calcification and ulceration

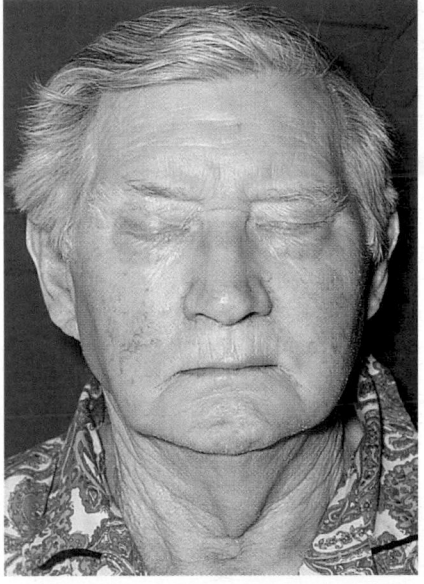

(a)

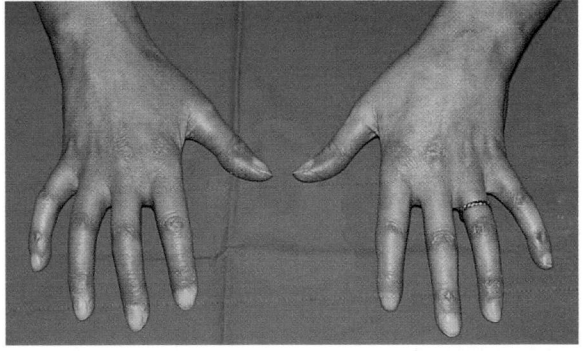

(b)

Figure 4.19 PM. (a) Primary dermatomyositis (DM). This patient has the classic lilac-coloured (heliotrope) rash on the eyelids, together with periorbital oedema. (b) Primary DM causes a characteristic rash over the knuckles, sometimes referred to as Gottron's papules or collodian patches.

PM/DM associated with autoimmune rheumatic disease
Autoimmune rheumatic diseases commonly associated with PM/DM are RA, systemic sclerosis and SLE. In these cases, Raynaud's phenomenon, sclerodactyly, arthralgia and myalgia are common presentations.

PM/DM associated with cancer
Malignancy may predate or postdate the myositis by up to 2 years, and the incidence is higher in patients aged over 55 years. The most commonly associated malignancies are those of the lung, ovary, breast and gastrointestinal tract, as well as myeloproliferative disorders.

04

Childhood-onset DM

Childhood-onset DM is not associated with malignancy, and its characteristic manifestations are:
- Inflammatory myopathy, with atrophy and contractures
- Subcutaneous calcification
- Vasculitis affecting the skin, muscle and gut
  Peak incidence is between 5 and 10 years.

Diagnosis

Diagnosis of PM is based on a typical clinical picture accompanied by characteristic electromyograph (EMG) changes, an elevated serum creatinine kinase and a characteristic muscle biopsy. The muscle biopsy may be normal in 10% of patients with myositis because of the patchy nature of the disease.

Differential diagnosis of primary PM include:
- *Neuromuscular disorders:* myasthenia gravis, muscular dystrophy, myopathies (e.g. metabolic) and myotonic disorders (see pp. 953 and 954)
- *Other forms of myositis* (e.g. inclusion body myositis)
- *Endocrine and metabolic disorders* (e.g. hypokalaemia, hypocalcaemia, hypomagnesaemia, hypothyroidism, Cushing's syndrome, alcohol abuse, corticosteroids)
- *Vitamin D deficiency*
- *Glycogen and lipid storage diseases*
- *Drugs:* alcohol, vincristine, lithium, cimetidine and ciclosporin
- *Infection:* viral (e.g. EBV, coxsackie), bacterial (e.g. *Staphylococcus* spp., *Mycobacterium leprae*) or parasitic (e.g. *Toxoplasma* spp., *Trichinella* spp.)
- *Other autoimmune disease* (e.g. PMR, RA, SLE)

Investigation

Haematology

ESR is raised in active disease.

Biochemistry

- *Muscle enzymes:* serum skeletal muscle enzymes creatine kinase, aldolase, asparate-amino transferase, lactate dehydrogenase and alanine-amino transferase are elevated
- *Urine myoglobin:* myoglobinuria may be detected if there is acute muscle destruction

Immunology

Autoantibodies that are commonly tested and may be present are RF and ANA (in less than 50% of patients) and anti-Jo1 (see Table 4.1). Anti-Jo1 is found in approximately 5% of those with polymyositis without lung disease and 6–7% of those with lung involvement; it binds to histididyl tRNA synthetase and blocks its aminoacylation.

Microbiology

A viral, bacterial or parasitic aetiology should always be excluded.

Diagnostic imaging

Chest radiography to look for diaphragmatic involvement and suspected malignancy. MRI of muscles involved (e.g. thigh) may aid diagnosis and assist biopsy.

Histopathology

Muscle biopsy serial sections should be examined, and changes include necrosis, muscle fibre regeneration and lymphocyte infiltration.

Other investigations

- *EMG abnormalities:* present in 90% of patients. Characteristic changes are low-amplitude polyphasic action potentials, pseudomyotonic high-frequency pattern and spontaneous fibrillation with positive sharp waves in resting muscle.
- *ECG abnormalities:* present in 5–10% of patients.
- *Respiratory function tests:* should be carried out if lung involvement is suspected.

Management

Treatment with high-dose corticosteroids may be necessary for several months and long-term maintenance therapy may be required.

Regular muscle strength and serum creatine kinase level tests are necessary to detect any relapse, together with tests of respiratory function, as diaphragmatic involvement is common.

Immunosuppressive and cytotoxic drugs may be required if the disease is severe, fails to respond to corticosteroids or relapses (Table 4.7).

Physiotherapy is required at all stages of the disease to prevent contractures, and occupational therapy may be necessary for those patients left with residual deformity.

Prognosis

The overall mortality rate of myositis patients is approximately four times higher than that of the normal population. Women, Afro-Caribbeans, patients over 45 years of age and patients with malignancy have a worse prognosis. The prognosis of childhood-onset DM is better than that for adult disease.

Death is usually brought about by malignancy, infection and pulmonary complications. Early treatment improves the prognosis. The 5-year survival rate is 68–80%. Within 5 years, 25% make a full recovery and discontinue therapy, 50% have inactive disease but residual weakness and 25% have active disease.

Fibromyalgia

This is a condition characterized by muscle pain with tender points, fatigue and sleep disturbance. It occurs most frequently in the 30–60-year age group and women predominate. Synonyms include:
- Chronic fatigue syndrome
- Postviral syndrome
- Myalgic encephalopathy
  Other features include:
- Irritable bowel syndrome
- Headaches
- Urinary urgency
- Anxiety

All investigations, including those of inflammation and immunopathology, are normal. If any tests are abnormal, then other causes of fatigue and muscle pain must be sought.

The aetiology of the disorder is multifactorial and poorly understood. In some cases there is a significant psychological component. Treatment is therefore patient-specific and usually responds to a graded exercise programme in association with tricyclic antidepressants. Patients require significant support. It is estimated that 60% of patients still have moderate symptoms 3 years after diagnosis.

Systemic sclerosis syndromes

Systemic sclerosis is a multisystem syndrome causing inflammation, fibrosis and vascular damage to the skin and internal organs; the gastrointestinal tract, lungs, heart and kidneys are predominantly involved. A wide spectrum of disease (Table 4.10) may result and need not be progressive. Scleroderma is a descriptive word for the skin involvement and means 'hard skin'.

Epidemiology

Prevalence. Uncommon. Annual incidence is 12 in 1 million.

Age. Any age, but most common in 30–50-year-olds.

Sex. Approximately 80% of patients are female.

Race. All races.

Genetics. A familial tendency and associated with the MHC.

Geography. Worldwide.

Disease mechanisms

Systemic sclerosis may be familial and there are certain associations with HLA class II genes (DR3). The risk of patients with Raynaud's phenomenon developing systemic

Table 4.10 Systemic sclerosis syndromes

Raynaud's phenomenon
Digital vasoconstriction producing pallor or cyanosis

Localized scleroderma
Morphoea (patch or linear area of skin thickening)

Limited cutaneous systemic sclerosis
Anticentromere antibody (ACA) association
Raynaud's phenomenon for many years (occasionally decades)
Skin involvement limited to hands, face, feet, or absent
Significant late incidence of pulmonary hypertension, with or without interstitial lung disease, gastrointestinal symptoms, skin calcification and telangiectasia
Nailfold capillary dilatation without capillary destruction

Diffuse cutaneous systemic sclerosis
Scl-70 and RNA polymerase antibody association
Raynaud's syndrome within 1 year of skin changes
Skin involvement of face, trunk and extremities
Early significant interstitial lung disease, oliguric renal failure, diffuse gastrointestinal disease and myocardial involvement
Nailfold capillary dilatation and capillary destruction

sclerosis is approximately 2% for females and 6% for males.

Similar fibrotic changes to those of systemic sclerosis can occur after exposure to drugs or chemicals, such as:
- *Silica* (e.g. stonemasons and coalminers);
- *Organic chemicals:* including chlorinated aliphatic hydrocarbons (e.g. vinyl chloride)
- *Toxic oil:* aniline-treated rapeseed oil
- *Drugs* (e.g. L-5-hydroxytryptophan)

A variety of local factors such as transforming growth factor β (TGF-β), epidermal growth factor, platelet-derived growth factor and tumour necrosis factor may stimulate fibroblast activity and growth. Autoantibodies may be present although their role in the pathogenesis is uncertain.

Pathology

Systemic sclerosis is characterized by fibrosis or scleroderma. Increased amounts of collagen in the skin and gastrointestinal tract are covered by a thin epidermis or mucosa, respectively. The muscles may atrophy in association with an infiltration in the muscle of lymphocytes and plasma cells.

Immunopathologically there may be complement activation and increased CD8 T cells, IL-2 levels, IL-2 receptor levels and γ/δ T-cell receptor expression.

Clinical features

Systemic sclerosis may develop rapidly or insidiously. Systems affected are mainly skin, kidneys, gastrointestinal

04

tract, musculoskeletal system, lungs and heart. Some features of the different systemic sclerosis syndromes are (Table 4.10):

● *Raynaud's phenomenon:* characteristically affects the fingers, but may involve the toes, nose and ears (SYSTEMIC SCLEROSIS SYNDROMES AT A GLANCE, Fig. E) and in 90% of patients is the first sign of systemic sclerosis. It is episodic and there are clearly demarcated colour changes from white (ischaemia) then blue (stasis) then red (reactive hyperaemia). Usually these changes are in response to cold, but may occur in response to stress.

● *Skin:* firm, thick (morphea), dry and leathery, tightly bound to subcutaneous tissue with associated hair loss; this is called sclerodactyly when involving fingers (Fig. 4.20). Ulceration of the skin may occur and the fingertip is the most common site. If digital ulceration and ischaemia is severe, irreversible tissue damage may occur and may be associated with gangrene (Fig. 4.20). There may be hypo- and/or hyperpigmentation. Calcitosis cutis describes calcium hydroxyapatite-containing nodules that appear on the digits, extensor surface of the forearms, elbows and knees. These may ulcerate and result in inflammation and considerable pain. Telangiectasia typically occurs in association with the limited form on the fingers initially. There may be a decreased number of nailfold capillary loops, the presence of giant loops and overall vascular derangement.

● *Lung involvement:* responsible for significant morbidity and mortality resulting from pulmonary hypertension, interstitial fibrosis and effusion.

● *Renal involvement:* associated with severe hypertension, renal insufficiency and microangiopathic haemolytic anaemia.

● *Heart:* any structure in the heart may be involved and heart failure may develop as a result of pulmonary hypertension.

● *Gastrointestinal involvement:* may cause regurgitation and aspiration, malabsorption and pseudo-obstruction.

● *Arthralgia, asymmetrical arthritis and a mild myopathy:* can occur but are relatively uncommon.

Diagnosis

Systemic sclerosis is diagnosed when Raynaud's phenomenon is associated with skin and visceral involvement and serological abnormalities. Raynaud's phenomenon may additionally be associated with:

● Other autoimmune rheumatic diseases, such as lupus
● Vascular obstruction (e.g. cervical rib), vibratory tools (e.g. vibration white finger)
● Drug treatment (e.g. β-blockers)
● Increased blood viscosity (e.g. paraproteinaemia, cryoglobulinaemia)

Approximately 90% of patients with Raynaud's phenomenon are female and 5% will eventually develop

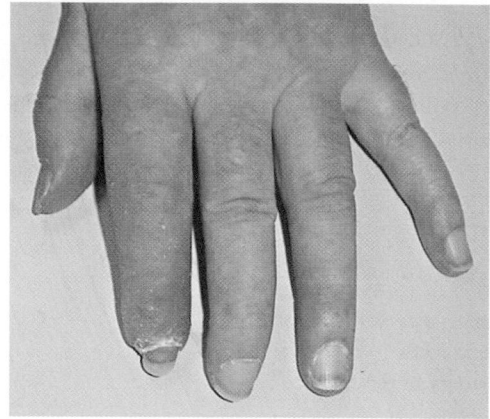

(a)

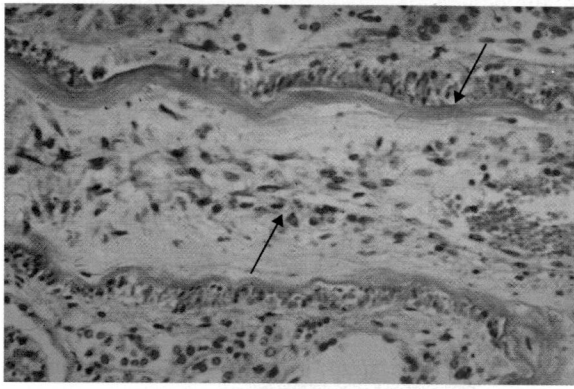

(b)

Figure 4.20 (a) Scleroderma of the fingers and irreversible ischaemia. (b) A medium-sized artery shows near-obliteration of the lumen. There is a myxoid thickening of the intima typical of scleroderma arrows.

an autoimmune rheumatic disease. A negative ANA test in a healthy patient usually excludes the subsequent development of an autoimmune rheumatic disease (for differential diagnosis of Raynaud's phenomenon see Table 4.11).

Investigation

Haematology

● *FBC:* anaemia is chronic and macrocytic because of malabsorption, or haemolytic resulting from renal involvement
● *ESR:* raised ESR is rare

Biochemistry

Muscle enzymes are not usually elevated.

Immunology

Serum immunoglobulins are increased.

Autoantibodies are present. Those commonly found are:

Systemic sclerosis syndromes at a glance

Clinical features

Skin
Raynaud's phenomenon
Sclerodactyly
Fixed flexion contractures
Ulceration
Increased pigmentation
Vitiligo
Telangiectasia
Disorganization of the nailfold capillary bed
Subcutaneous and periarticular calcium deposits

Kidney
Hypertension
Progressive renal failure

Gastrointestinal
Gastro-oesophageal regurgitation
Malabsorption
Constipation
Diarrhoea

Musculoskeletal
Arthralgia
Asymmetrical polyarthritis (25%)
Carpal tunnel syndrome
Acute myositis (15%)

Lung
Pulmonary fibrosis
Pulmonary hypertension

Heart
Cardiac failure
Arrhythmias
Cardiomyopathy
Pericarditis

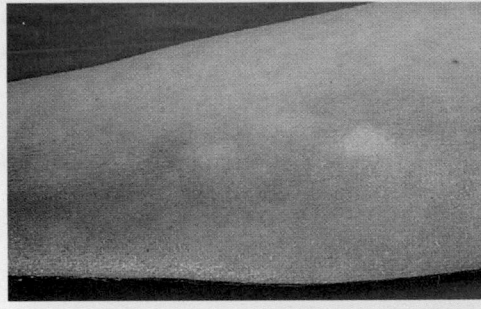

Fig. C Morphoea. This is a localized patch of skin thickening.

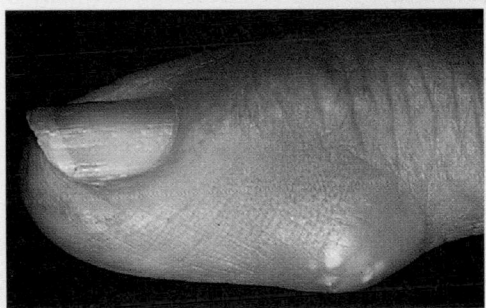

Fig. D Subcutaneous and periarticular calcium deposits may occur and can be extemely painful.

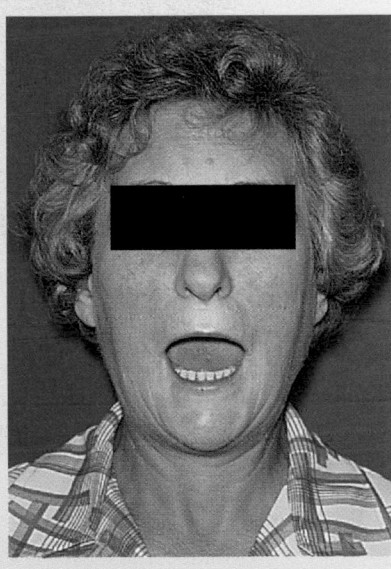

Fig. A Scleroderma may cause thickening of the skin around the mouth and an inability to open the jaw fully.

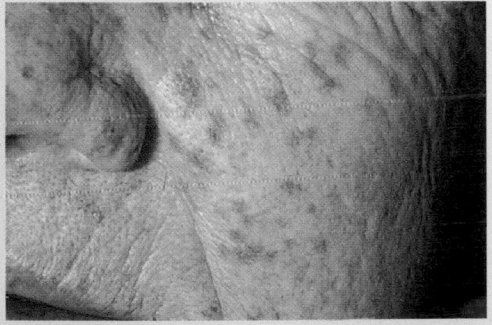

Fig. B Telangiectasia in a patient with systemic sclerosis.

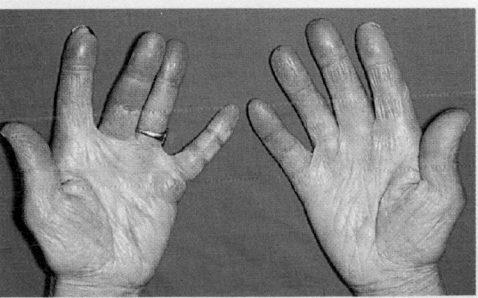

Fig. E Raynaud's disease. Cyanosis of the fingers occurs because of arterial vasoconstriction, which in the patient has resulted in an area of infarction of the left forefinger.

04

Table 4.11 Differential diagnosis of Raynaud's phenomenon

Primary Raynaud's phenomenon
Secondary Raynaud's phenomenon
   Autoimmune rheumatic disease (e.g. systemic sclerosis)
   Inflammatory muscle disease
   Systemic lupus erythematosus
   Overlap syndromes
Mechanical vascular obstruction (e.g. cervical rib)
Use of vibratory tools
   Vibration white finger
Drugs (e.g. β-blockers)
Increased blood viscosity
   Paraproteinaemia
   Cryoglobulinaemia

- *ANA:* 33–96%
- *Rheumatoid factor:* low level (30%)
- *Anticentromere antibody:* associated with limited cutaneous scleroedema
- *Anti-Scl 70* (topoisomerase-1): associated with diffuse cutaneous scleroedema
- *Anti-RNA polymerase:* associated with renal disease

Diagnostic imaging
- *Radiography of the hand:* may show resorption of the tuft of the distal phalanx
- *Chest radiography:* may show linear or nodular interstitial fibrosis if the lungs are involved
- *Barium meal:* typically shows dilatation, atony and delayed gastric emptying

Histopathology
Renal biopsy may show changes of arterial intimal proliferation as well as fibrinoid necrosis caused by hypertension.

Other investigations
- *EMG:* abnormalities are common
- *Pulmonary function tests:* reveal low diffusion capacity and Po_2 on exercise

Management

No drug has been shown to stop progression of diffuse systemic sclerosis, but palliative therapy directed at specific organs can help to maintain a good quality of life (for a general summary of management see KEYPOINTS BOX 4.2, p. 201). Digital sympathectomy may be of value in some patients. The patient should be watched closely to ensure that the following are recognized:
- *Hypertensive renal crisis:* renin–angiotensin blocking drugs (e.g. captopril, enalapril) are useful
- *Cardiac arrhythmias:* antiarrhythmics should be used as necessary

- *Pulmonary vascular disease*
- *Bacterial overgrowth of the bowel*
- *Oesophageal reflux*

Prognosis

The prognosis of systemic sclerosis depends on the extent of heart, lung and kidney involvement. If systemic, the disease often follows a prolonged relentless course. Mean 5- and 10-year survival rates are 60–70% and 40–50%, respectively. Pulmonary hypertension is a major cause of morbidity and mortality, and renal involvement must be promptly recognized and treated.

Spondyloarthritis

Spondyloarthritis is characterized by the involvement of the axial skeleton and the absence of serum RFs. Spondyloarthritic diseases include:
- Ankylosing spondylitis (AS) (see below)
- Psoriatic arthritis (see p. 232)
- Sexually acquired reactive arthritis (SARA) (see p. 232)
- Arthritis associated with gastrointestinal disease (see p. 234)

Ankylosing spondylitis

Ankylosing spondylitis is a chronic disease of unknown aetiology. It has a progressive course and involves mainly the axial skeleton, large proximal joints and adjacent soft tissue. Extra-articular manifestations may also occur.

Epidemiology

Prevalence. Affects 0.1–0.5% of the population.

Age. Commonly 15–40 years old.

Sex. Seems to be more common in men, but this is probably because it is more severe in men than women.

Race. Rare in Japanese people and black Africans.

Genetics. Associated with the HLA-B27 gene, which is equally distributed between males and females.

Geography. Worldwide.

Disease mechanisms

A wide variety of organisms may trigger the disease and *Klebsiella* has been suggested as a likely candidate. HLA-B27 seems to be a major susceptibility gene. This may be related to the unique amino-acid sequence motif: cysteine at residue 67, lysine at residue 70 and asparagine at residue 97. More than 95% of white people with AS have the

HLA-B27 gene compared to 8% of white people without AS. The prevalence of HLA-B27 is less than 1% in Japanese people and black Africans, and the disease is rare in these two groups.

Children of an HLA-B27 individual have a 50% chance of carrying the gene, and the risk of a child of an HLA-B27 AS patient developing AS is approximately 17%. Randomly selected HLA-B27 individuals have a 2–10% risk of developing AS.

Twin concordance is reported as 75% for monozygotes and 12.5% for dizygotes.

Several hypotheses relate the HLA-B27 gene to AS. HLA-B27 may:
● Predispose to an increased susceptibility to infectious and/or environmental agents
● Mimic foreign antigen and stimulate an immune response
● Be linked to an immune response gene
● Act as a receptor for exogenous antigen (e.g. bacteria) resulting in an autoimmune response

Pathology
Pathological changes are seen at skeletal and extraskeletal sites. In affected joints, hyperplasia and focal accumulation of lymphoid and plasma cells, similar to that seen in RA, lead to erosion of bone and destruction of cartilage and, later, fibrosis and bony ankylosis.

Involvement is common in:
● *Synovial joints:* apophyseal, costovertebral, sacroiliac, hip, shoulder and peripheral joints
● *Cartilaginous joints:* intervertebral discs, the manubriosternal joint and symphysis pubis
● *Entheses:* where ligaments, tendons and the joint capsule attach to bone

Sites commonly involved are the annulus fibrosus (leading to syndesmophyte formation and the radiographical appearance of bamboo spine), iliac crests, ischial tuberosities, greater trochanters, calcaneae and patellae.

Clinical features
Bones and joints
● *Low back pain and stiffness:* a common presentation, most severe in the early morning and after prolonged rest, and may be relieved by activity. Pain in the hips, buttocks and shoulders may be a feature, but neurological abnormalities are unusual. Advanced disease results in the classic bamboo spine and marked thoracic kyphosis ('question mark' posture(see ANKYLOSING SPONDYLITIS AT A GLANCE)). Cauda equina syndrome (see pp. 940 and 253) is a rare late complication. Symptoms may be persistent or intermittent, with deformities evolving over 10 or more years. Pain is usually lessened once ankylosis develops.
● *Asymmetrical peripheral arthritis:* approximately 20% of patients have asymmetrical peripheral arthritis at the same time as the back symptoms, although it may precede back symptoms in 10–20% of patients, particularly teenagers. Thirty per cent of those under 20 years of age have hip disease.
● *Enthesitis:* inflammation at a ligamentous bone junction (e.g. Achilles tendon or plantar fascia), pleuritic chest pain can occur on deep breathing as a result of inflammation at the costosternal and vertebral muscle insertions.

Extra-articular manifestations
Systemic manifestations are common:
● *Eye involvement:* causes acute anterior uveitis in 4–5% of patients at some time and patients may present with red painful gritty eyes and blurred vision
● *Lung involvement:* may result in fibrobullous apical disease
● *Carditis:* may lead to aortic insufficiency and conduction defects and a varying degree of heart block can occur

Diagnosis
AS is diagnosed on clinical grounds supported by characteristic findings on investigation. There may be:
● Peripheral joint involvement
● Decreased anterior flexion of the spine. Schober's test is the increase between 2 marks 10 cm apart centred upon L4/5 on lumbar flexion. Normal is more than 5 cm
● Increased wall to tragus (ear lobe) measurement indicative of thoracic kyphosis. Normal is usually approximately 12 cm
● Decreased chest expansion (less than 5 cm) if there is costovertebral involvement

Features of AS may resemble other diseases. For example:
● Low back pain may occur in AS and lumbar disc disease
● Peripheral arthritis in early AS may resemble RA
● Spondylarthropathy associated with ulcerative colitis and Crohn's disease may be indistinguishable from AS, whereas SARA and psoriatic arthritis are usually associated with less severe spinal involvement
● Diffuse idiopathic skeletal hyperosteosis (DISH) may be similar to AS radiographically, but the apophyseal and sacroiliac joints are not involved and DISH is more common in men over 50 years of age

Investigation
Haematology
● *FBC:* chronic anaemia is a feature
● *ESR:* may be raised, but does not reflect disease activity

Immunology
● *Autoantibodies:* RF is absent even if there is peripheral joint involvement
● *Serum IgA:* may be raised

04

Table 4.12 Radiographical changes in ankylosing spondylitis (AS)

Location	Radiographical change
Vertebral bodies	Early squaring; later bony bridging and fusion of adjacent vertebrae (syndesmophytes) leads to a bamboo spine appearance; erosion and sclerosis at vertebral body margins (Romanus sign)
Sacroiliac joint (anteroposterior view) (may involve lower third on one side early in disease)	Blurring of the joint margins, irregular subchondral erosions and patchy sclerosis, at first. Later, sclerosis becomes marked, joint space is lost and osteoporosis becomes evident
Ligamentous bony junctions (most commonly the pelvis, greater trochanters, plantar fascia and Achilles tendons)	Inflammation (enthesitis) and secondary ossification lead to proliferative bone margins, spicules and spurs
Atlanto-axial joint	Subluxation

- *Tissue typing:* HLA-B27 may be recognized but is not a reliable guide to prognosis

Microbiology

The possibility of genitourinary or gastrointestinal infection should be investigated in suspected reactive arthritis (see pp. 119, 232 and 749).

Diagnostic imaging

- *Radiography:* there may be no radiographical changes early in the disease, but changes that may be seen as the disease progresses are described in Table 4.12. Chest X-ray is necessary if interstitial lung disease is suspected.

- *Radionuclide imaging, CT and MR scanning:* can detect areas of active inflammation before there are radiographical changes.

Other investigations

- *Synovial fluid examination:* usually reveals a moderate neutrophil leucocytosis
- *Respiratory function tests:* may show reduced vital lung capacity and total lung capacity, with an increased residual volume and functional residual volume, indicating a restrictive abnormality
- *Cardiac imaging* (e.g. echo and MRI): useful if heart involvement is suspected

04

Ankylosing spondylitis at a glance

Clinical features

Joints
Low back pain and stiffness
Pain in hips, buttocks and shoulders
Asymmetrical peripheral arthritis

Muscles
Costosternal and vertebral muscle enthesitis

Constitutional
Fatigue
Fever
Weight loss

Haematological
Anaemia

Eyes
Acute anterior uveitis

Heart
Aortic valve incompetence
Cardiac conduction defects

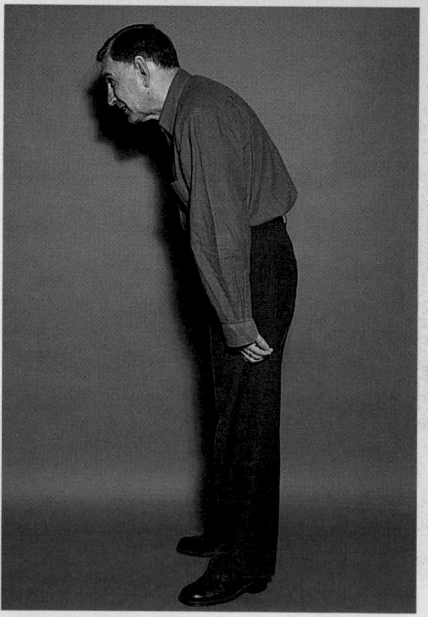

Fig. A Spine. Ankylosing spondylitis can cause a marked thoracic kyphosis with increased wall–tragus measurement.

Lungs
Bilateral upper lobe fibrosis

Metabolic
Secondary amyloidosis

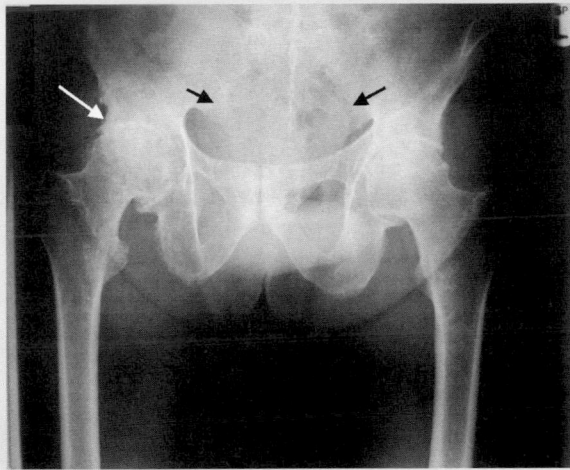

Fig. B The sacroiliac joints are fused (black arrows). Both hips show concentric reduction in joint space, in keeping with an inflammatory arthropathy. In the right hip there is also mild subarticular sclerosis in the superolateral aspect of the joint and marginal osteophyte formation in keeping with super-imposed degenerative change (white arrow).

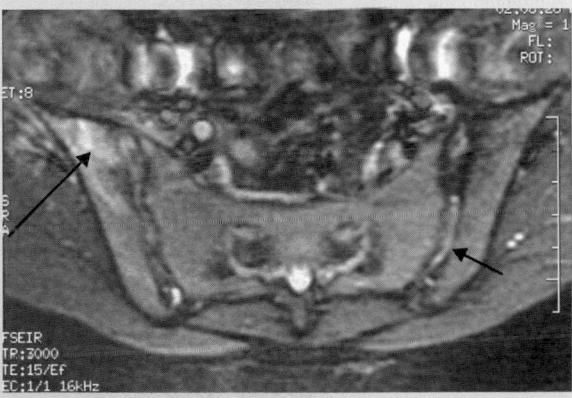

Fig. D Arial STIR MRI image of the sacroiliac joints. There is high signal intensity (fluid and/or oedema; short arrow) in both sacroiliac joints and in the subarticular region anterior (marked on the right) indicating sacroiliitis (long arrow).

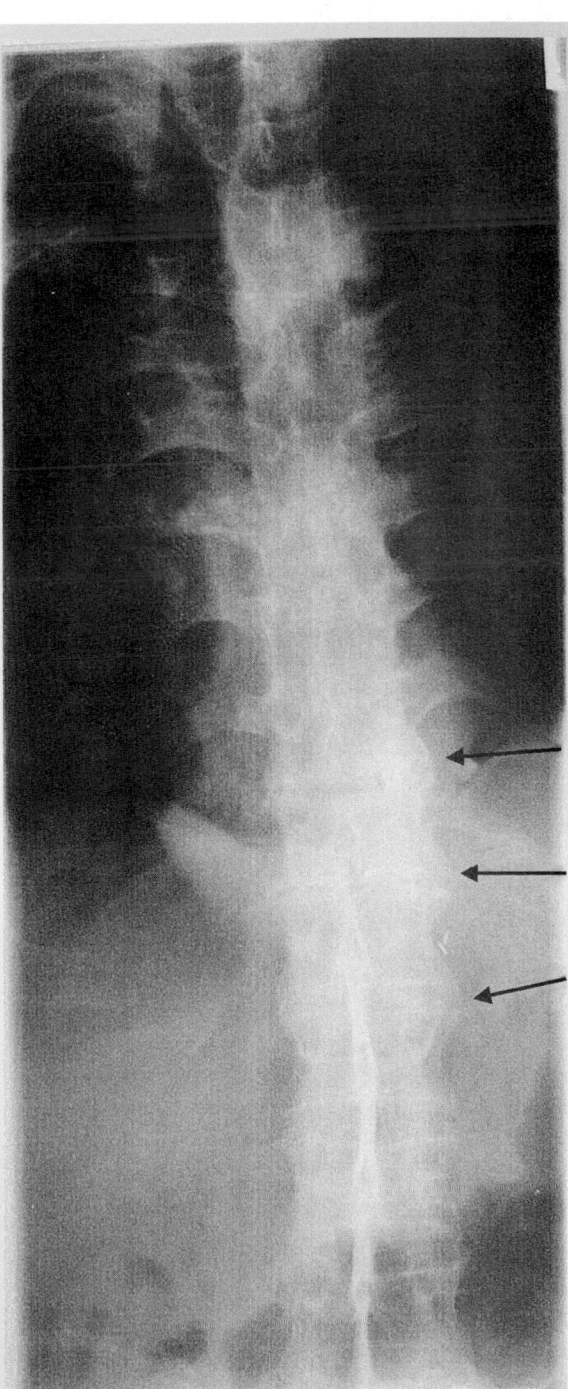

Fig. C Thoracic and lumbar spine radiograph. There is fusion of the vertical bodies in the thoracic and lumbar spine. Widespread syndesmophyte formation has resulted in the typical bamboo spine appearance (arrowed).

04

Management

The aims of management are to prevent or minimize spinal deformities and to maximize skeletal mobility (for a general summary of management see KEYPOINTS BOX 4.2, p. 201).

Prognosis

Approximately 10% of patients with AS develop progressive crippling disease. With physiotherapy and anti-inflammatory drugs and disease-modifying drugs, however, most patients should lead a normal life and have a normal life expectancy.

Psoriatic arthritis

Epidemiology

Prevalence. Affects approximately 10% of patients with psoriasis (0.1–0.2% of the population).

Age. Usually 30–40 years old.

Sex. No association.

Race. No association.

Genetics. Approximately 50% of those with psoriatic spondylitis, but not peripheral arthritis, have the HLA-B27 gene.

Geography. Worldwide.

Disease mechanisms

Aetiology and pathogenesis of psoriatic arthritis are unknown, but the pathological changes are similar to those of AS (Fig. 4.21). Synovial histology may resemble that of RA and the pattern of pro-inflammatory cytokines in synovial fluid is similar to that in RA.

Clinical features

Generally, psoriatic arthritis is mild and intermittent and affects few joints. Spontaneous remission may occur.

For 15% of patients, arthritis precedes the rash (Fig. 4.21), but these manifestations often begin together. A search for psoriasis should include scalp, natal, cleft and feet, and lesions may also affect genitalia and tongue. Severe skin lesions may occur in patients affected with HIV. There is no correlation between the extent of skin involvement or nail onychodystrophy and severity of the arthritis. Peripheral joints may be warm, swollen and tender, and flexion contractures and ankylosis may occur (Fig. 4.21). The characteristic patterns of joint involvement are detailed in Table 4.13. Ocular disease (conjunctivitis, iridocyclitis, episcleritis) is rare.

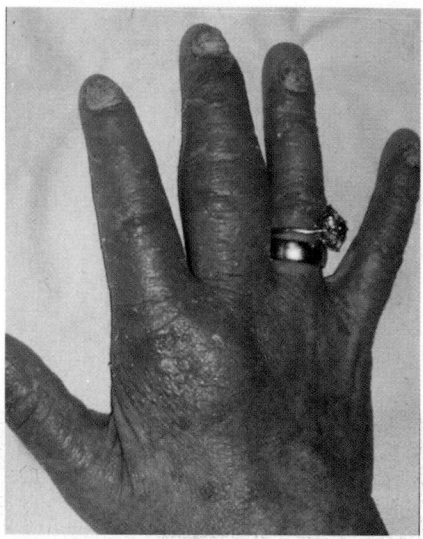

Figure 4.21 Right hand showing middle finger dactylitis, rash and nail dystrophy.

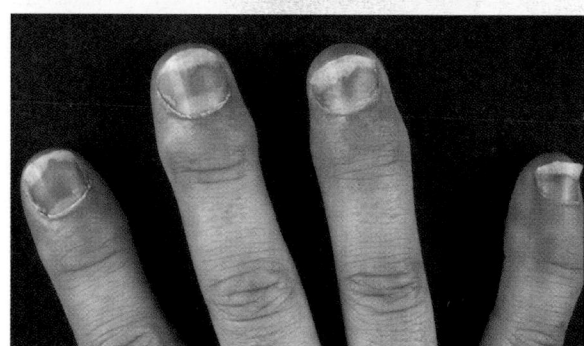

Figure 4.22 Nail dystrophy with adjacent distal interphalangeal joint arthritis.

Investigation

As for AS; 10–20% of patients have hyperuricaemia proportional to the degree of skin involvement. Diagnostic imaging can reveal joint destruction (Fig. 4.23).

Management

(See KEYPOINTS BOX 4.1, p. 194.)

Prognosis

Approximately 5% of patients develop a severe disabling and deforming arthritis. Axial spondyloarthropathy is associated with the same extra-articular manifestations as AS.

Sexually acquired reactive arthritis

Sexually acquired reactive arthritis (SARA) is characterized by seronegative oligoarticular asymmetrical arthritis,

Table 4.13 Characteristic patterns of joint involvement in psoriatic arthritis

Pattern	Percentage of patients	Features
Asymmetrical oligoarthritis	70	Commonly involves proximal joints of hands and feet. Finger dactylitis, similar to those in SARA (Fig. 4.21)
Axial spondylitis	25	May occur alone or with the other forms of arthritis
Symmetrical polyarthritis	10	Similar to RA with systemic symptoms
DIP joint involvement	10	Nail changes are usual, and associated with dactylitis (Fig. 4.21)
Arthritis mutilans	5	Destructive and deforming polyarthritis, ankylosis, dissolution of bone and telescoping of fingers, and spinal ankylosis may occur (Figs 4.23 and 4.24)

DIP, distal interphalangeal; SARA, sexually acquired reactive arthritis.

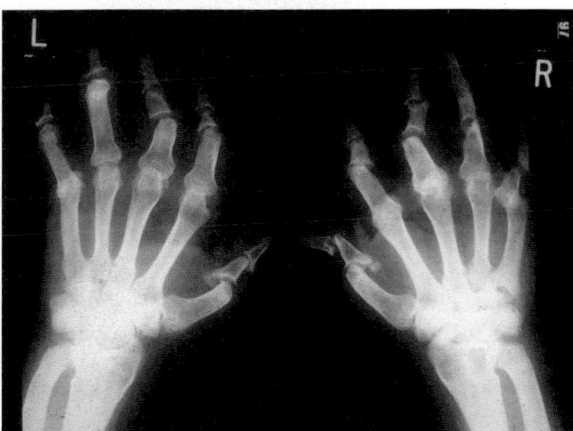

Figure 4.23 Radiograph of hands showing joint destruction resulting from arthritis mutilans.

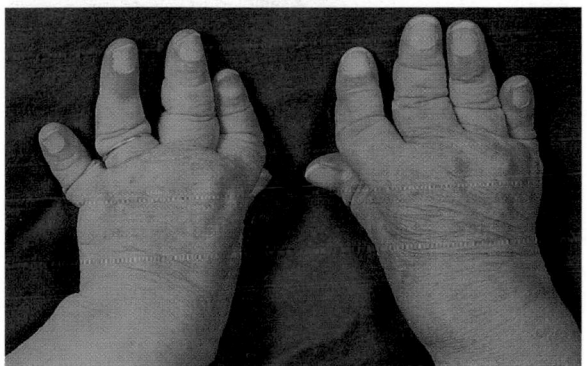

Figure 4.24 Arthritis mutilans. Joint destruction has caused dissolution of bone and telescoping of fingers. Remarkably, some function may be preserved.

urethritis and/or cervicitis and conjunctivitis. This may also be referred to as Reiter's syndrome.

Epidemiology

Incidence. Uncommon. Approximately 1% of people with urethritis develop SARA.

Age. Usually 16–35 years of age.

Sex. Approximately 95% of patients are male.

Race. No association.

Genetics. HLA-B27 gene is present in 60–90% of patients.

Geography. Worldwide.

Disease mechanisms

SARA is probably triggered by an infectious agent in the urogenital system interacting with a predisposing genetic background. Organisms thought to be responsible are *Chlamydia trachomatis* and *Ureaplasma urealyticum*. The arthritis is 'reactive' because it is not caused by a direct infection of the joint.

Pathology

There is no specific histological lesion. Acute SARA is associated with hyperaemia and leucocyte infiltrates. Findings in chronic SARA may resemble those in RA, and skin biopsy is indistinguishable from that of psoriasis.

Clinical features

There may be mild systemic symptoms, malaise and fever at first in both sexes and an associated intermittent mucopurulent penile discharge in men. It may be difficult to diagnose in women at this stage, but urethral ulcers may be present.

Musculoskeletal involvement

Rheumatic features arise later and include arthritis, Achilles tenosynovitis, enthesitis and plantar fasciitis (Fig. 4.25). The characteristic sausage-shaped digits (dactylitis) are caused by enthesitis and arthritis. The arthritis is usually acute, asymmetrical and oligoarticular, and affects mainly the knees, ankles, metatarsophalangeal joints and interphalangeal joints of the feet. Sacroiliitis is common and the presenting feature for 20% of patients. The spine may also be involved.

04

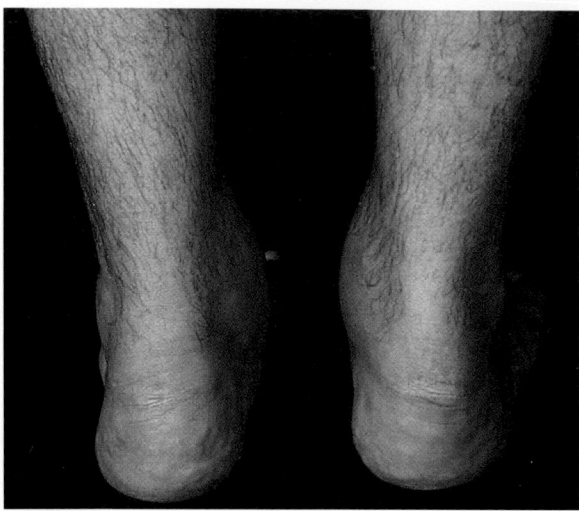

Figure 4.25 Sexually acquired reactive arthritis (SARA). Achilles tendinitis (on the left side in this patient) is sometimes a feature of SARA.

Skin involvement

Keratoderma blenorrhagica is common and indistinguishable from pustular psoriasis; the papules are commonly on the palms, soles and glans penis. Painless mucocutaneous lesions in the mouth and on the glans penis (circinate balanitis) are also common. Subungual cornification can accumulate and lift the nail plate, but there is no pitting.

Eye involvement

Conjunctivitis, uveitis, keratitis and optic neuritis are rare.

Diagnosis

No specific tests confirm SARA. It is diagnosed when asymmetrical seronegative oligoarthritis has been present for 1 month and is accompanied by non-specific urethritis and/or cervicitis.

The main differential diagnosis is gonococcal arthritis, for which there is a greater female incidence, no family history and usually a response to penicillin. There is no association with HLA-B27, and the arthritis is usually acute and non-recurrent.

Investigation

The investigations and their results are the same as those for AS.

Management

Ensure that the predisposing infection has been adequately treated in the patient and his or her partner (for a general summary of management see KEYPOINTS BOX 4.2, p. 201).

Prognosis

Most patients recover from the initial symptoms within several months, but 33% have recurrent or sustained disease and 15–25% of these develop permanent disability.

Arthritis associated with gastrointestinal disease

Gastrointestinal diseases associated with arthritis (enteric reactive arthritis) include:
- Dysentery, causing postdysenteric reactive arthritis
- Inflammatory bowel disease (IBD), Crohn's disease (CD) and ulcerative colitis (UC)

Epidemiology

Prevalence. Prevalence of postdysenteric reactive arthritis is up to 27 in 100 000. The two patterns of IBD-associated arthritis are peripheral arthritis, which affects 12% of patients with UC and 20% of patients with CD, and axial arthritis, which affects 6% of patients in each group.

Age. IBD-associated peripheral arthritis most commonly presents at 25–45 years of age.

Sex. No association.

Race. No association.

Genetics. IBD-associated axial arthritis is associated with the presence of HLA-B27 in approximately 50% of patients.

Geography. Postdysenteric reactive arthritis is more common in mainland Europe than in the UK.

Disease mechanisms

The organisms thought to be responsible for postdysenteric reactive arthritis are *Shigella dysenteriae, Shigella flexneri, Salmonella typhimurium, Yersinia enterocolitica* and *Campylobacter jejuni*. It is thought that bacterial antigens escape from the bowel across damaged intestinal mucosa and form immune complexes in the circulation. These complexes could then enter the joints and trigger an inflammatory reaction, resulting in synovitis.

Clinical features

The peripheral arthritis usually follows IBD by 6 months to several years and there is a close temporal relationship between exacerbations of IBD and the arthritis. Arthritis is more common when:
- Clinical features of UC include extensive colitis, pseudopolyps and perianal disease

- Clinical features of CD include colonic involvement or extra-intestinal manifestations, such as aphthous stomatitis, erythema nodosum or uveitis

A typical IBD-associated arthritic attack is acute and peaks in 24 h. A single joint may be involved at first, but the arthritis spreads asymmetrically to involve other joints (usually less than four). The knee and ankle are most often involved and usually appear red, swollen and painful. The spondylitis is indistinguishable from AS. Sacroiliac joint involvement is evident in 5–15% of patients, but will not usually become symptomatic or progress.

The clinical features of postdysenteric reactive arthritis are similar to those of SARA.

Investigation

Investigations and their results are as for AS. If IBD is suspected, specific investigations are required (see Chapter 10).

Management

IBD-associated arthritis is managed by controlling the IBD; topical corticosteroids may help. Bowel resection may prevent acute attacks of peripheral disease associated with UC, but not those associated with CD. Otherwise the treatment for enteric reactive arthritis is similar to that for AS (see p. 228).

Prognosis

Peripheral joint destruction in IBD-associated arthritis is rare. An attack of peripheral arthritis subsides within weeks and resolves without damage. The axial type of arthritis usually progresses despite any remission of IBD or colectomy.

The prognosis for postdysenteric reactive arthritis is similar to that for SARA (see p. 232).

Rheumatic disease in children

Children may present with a wide variety of musculoskeletal complaints, most of which are benign. Most conditions are unique to childhood, but may overlap with adult disease, even though their presentation may be similar to those in adults (e.g. gait disturbance or joint pain stiffness and swelling). This uniqueness may be as a result of congenital anomalies (e.g. scoliosis) or developmental anomalies (e.g. slipped femoral capital epithesis). This section highlights the variety of conditions that may occur.

Juvenile idiopathic arthritis

There are a variety of different causes of childhood arthritis

Table 4.14 Causes of childhood arthritis

Trauma
Sports injury
Non-accidental injury

Mechanical
Slipped capital femoral epiphysis

Viral infection
Rubella
Mumps
Chickenpox
Parvovirus

Bacterial (infective)
Haemophilus influenzae (especially neonates)
Staphylococcus aureus
Mycobacterium tuberculosis

Bacterial (reactive)
β-Haemolytic *Streptococcus* (rheumatic fever)
Borrelia burgdorferi (Lyme arthritis)
Sexually acquired reactive arthritis (see p. 232)
Enteropathic (see p. 749)

Idiopathic
Juvenile idiopathic arthritis
Autoimmune rheumatic disease
Henoch–Schönlein purpura
Dermatomyositis
SLE

Malignancy
Leukaemia
Lymphoma
Haemophilia
Haemarthoses

as listed in Table 4.14. Juvenile idiopathic arthritis (JIA) is the principal form of chronic idiopathic synovitis.

There are different patterns of JIA (Table 4.15), which have different characteristics and prognoses and are probably distinct diseases. Remember children will not describe their symptoms as adults may; for example, a parent may describe inability to walk or participate in games, but children with arthritis may avoid sporting activity. The criteria for diagnosis are arthritis for at least 6 weeks in a patient of 16 years of age or less.

Epidemiology

Prevalence. Incidence 1 in 10 000 in the UK.

Age. All age groups of children.

Sex. Depends on the type.

04

Table 4.15 Subtypes of juvenile idiopathic arthritis (JIA)

Pauciarticular onset (four joints or fewer, or oligoarthritis; 50% of patients)
70% are female, who are usually ANA-positive
Extended oligoarthritis may develop (more than four joint involvement) after the first 6 months of disease

Pauciarticular subtypes
- *Type I:* 25% of patients. Early childhood, large joints
- *Type II:* 15% of patients. Late childhood, subsequent spondyloarthropathy
- *Type III:* 15% of patients. Throughout childhood, subsequent psoriasis

Polyarticular onset (five joints or more; 40% of patients)
25% are rheumatoid factor (RF)-positive
75% are RF-negative

Systemic onset or Still's disease (10% of patients)

Race. No association.

Genetics. There are HLA associations according to the disease subtype (e.g. HLA-DR4 in systemic and polyarticular, RF-positive disease; HLA-B27 and male pauciarticular disease).

Geography. Worldwide.

Disease mechanisms
The aetiology of JIA is unknown and some of its causal hypotheses are similar to those for adult disease (RA and AS; see pp. 206 and 228).

Clinical features
Pauciarticular-onset juvenile idiopathic arthritis
For 50% of those with JIA the onset is pauciarticular (JUVENILE IDIOPATHIC ARTHRITIS AT A GLANCE, Fig. A(i)):
- *Type I:* the majority of these patients are girls under 5 years of age who are likely to be ANA-positive and have an asymmetrical mild arthritis that most commonly affects the knee, followed by the ankle, wrist and hip. ANA-positive JIA is associated with chronic uveitis. A small proportion of these children develop extended oligoarthritis affecting more than four joints.
- *Type II:* this group usually comprises adolescent boys, commonly with a family history of arthritis and who develop arthritis of the hips, knees and sacroiliac joints, enthesopathy and acute iritis. They are often ANA-negative and 70% are HLA-B27-positive. This pattern of disease may be considered as the juvenile form of AS.
- *Type III:* these children develop arthritis associated with psoriasis and have a similar pattern of disease as is found in adults (see p. 232).

Polyarticular-onset juvenile idiopathic arthritis
A polyarticular onset affects 40% of those with JIA (Fig. A(ii) opposite).
- Seventy-five per cent of these patients (usually children 1–3 years old) are RF-negative. This type is more common in girls and can be as destructive as RF-positive JIA (see below), but systemic symptoms are rarely severe. Micronathia may result from temperomandibular joint involvement and these children require an orthodontic assessment.
- The remaining 25% of children in this group (commonly adolescent girls with severe symmetrical arthritis) are RF-positive, and often ANA-positive too. The cervical spine is often involved. Joint stiffness is prominent but systemic symptoms are not.

Systemic-onset juvenile idiopathic arthritis (Still's disease)
Of those with JIA, 10% have Still's disease (Fig. A(iii) opposite). This can occur at any age, has no sex predisposition and is characterized by systemic symptoms, a rash and arthritis. Systemic symptoms include general malaise and a daily spiking fever that often develops in the evening and returns to baseline at least once a day.

The rash of pale pink macules of variable size that appear on the trunk, proximal extremities and face is evanescent and associated with fever and mild trauma (Köbner's phenomenon). There may also be lymphadenopathy, hepatosplenomegaly and polyserositis (e.g. pericarditis).

Arthritis may appear after weeks or months, and there may be only one episode, or it may progress to severe chronic polyarthritis.

A similar presentation may occur in adults. It is rare, with similar laboratory features and may become intermittent or chronic. Treatment is similar.

Diagnosis
The criteria for the diagnosis of JIA are:
- Persistent arthritis of one or more joints for at least 6 weeks
- Exclusion of other causes of arthritis (Table 4.14)

Investigation
Haematology
- *FBC:* usually reveals anaemia, a raised white cell count and thrombocytosis
- *ESR:* usually raised

Immunology
- *Autoantibodies:* ANA and RFs may be present
- *Viral antibodies:* rarely useful, but should be requested if a specific infection is suspected (e.g. parvovirus B19)

Juvenile idiopathic arthritis at a glance

Juvenile idiopathic arthritis (JIA) is arthritis for at least 6 weeks in a patient of 16 years of age or less
There are three different patterns of JIA
1 Pauciarticular (50%)
2 Polyarticular (40%)
3 Systemic (10%)

Clinical features
Arthritis

Skin
Köbner's phenomenon
Pale pink macular (Still's) rash

Systemic
Temperature chart spiking temperature (Fig. B)
Malaise and lymphadenopathy

Eyes
Chronic uveitis
ANA is strongly associated with occurrence of uveitis. This is a common cause of childhood blindness

Heart and lungs
Pericarditis
Pleural effusion

Patients may be of small stature and have limb growth discrepancy because of inflammation and corticosteroid treatment

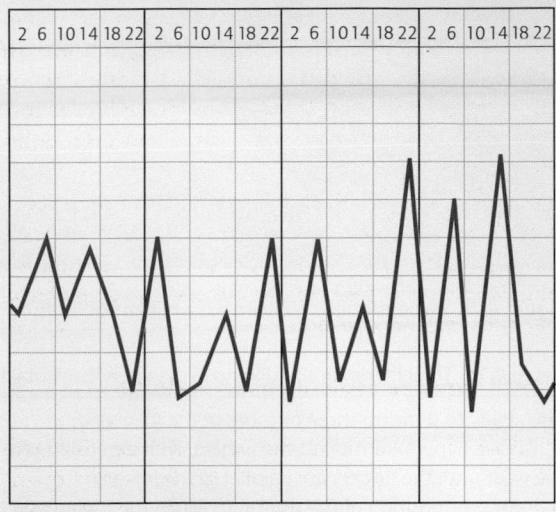

Fig. B Temperature chart for a patient presenting with systemic-onset JIA.

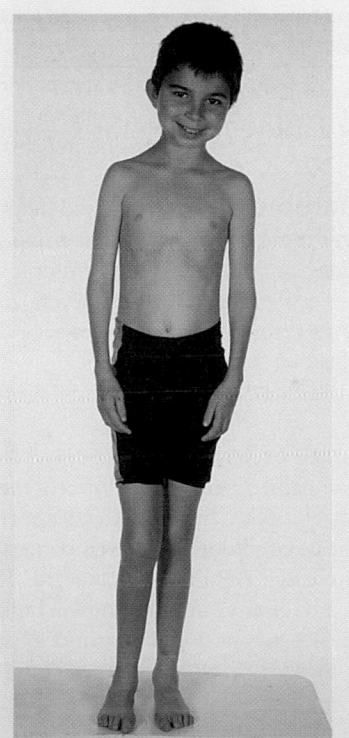
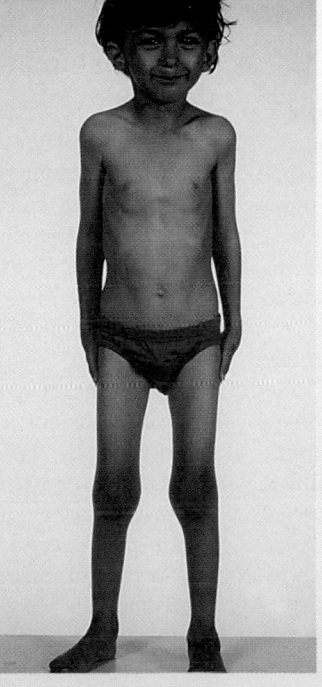
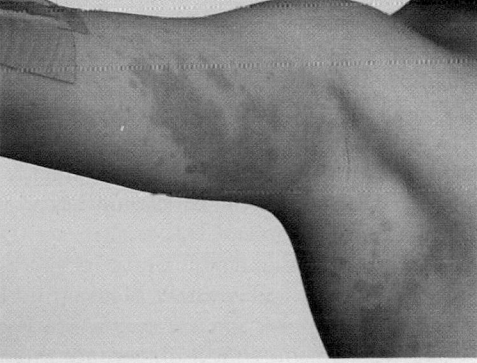

(i)   (ii)   (iii)

Fig. A JIA. (i) Pauciarticular JIA: this child has a monoarthritis affecting the right knee. (ii) Polyarticular JIA: this child has arthritis principally affecting the knees, hips, wrists, elbows, cervical spine and temporomandibular joints. (iii) Systemic JIA: the pale pink evanescent macular rash is found in the child's axilla.

• *Antistreptolysin O titre:* raised in β-haemolytic strepto-coccal infection

Microbiology
Appropriate culture (e.g. throat swabs, stool, synovial fluid) should be carried out if infection is suspected.

Diagnostic imaging
• *Radiography:* there may be changes similar to those of RA and AS
• *Ultrasound and echocardiography:* may be necessary to detect hepatosplenomegaly and pericarditis

Management
Treatment is most successful when there is prompt and long-term attention to maintaining joint mobility and avoiding or controlling complications.

Drug treatment includes symptomatic anti-inflammatory therapy (Tables 4.4 and 4.6): NSAIDs (e.g. naproxen) and intra-articular corticosteroids. Gold, sulfasalazine or methotrexate, for example (see Table 4.7), are required for progressive polyarticular disease. Severe systemic disease and chronic uveitis are indications for systemic corticosteroids, which should otherwise be avoided. For severe unremitting disease, immunomodulation therapy with etanercept (TNF-α receptor) is indicated. Great emphasis is placed on support for the child's family. Liaison between GP, hospital social worker and educational services is paramount.

Physiotherapy is of prime importance and is aimed at preventing joint deformity and maintaining function.

Regular slit-lamp examinations are necessary, especially for those with ANA-positive pauciarticular-onset JIA, who should be screened every 3 months for at least 7 years after diagnosis. Up to 50% of children with uveitis are asymptomatic and, if untreated, disease may lead to blindness.

Prognosis
The overall prognosis of JIA is variable. Of those affected, 40–50% (usually those with systemic or polyarticular RF-positive JIA) may have significant disability. Mortality is usually caused by infection, pericarditis or chronic renal disease secondary to amyloidosis.

Morbidity is substantial and may be psychological, educational, social and medical. Medical morbidity is associated with chronic anterior uveitis, which may lead to visual impairment, growth disturbance as a result of localized inflammation or corticosteroid treatment and joint failure. Poor prognostic indicators are polyarticular RF-positive disease associated with joint erosion. Poor drug compliance is also a significant prognostic factor. Five per cent of children require joint replacement.

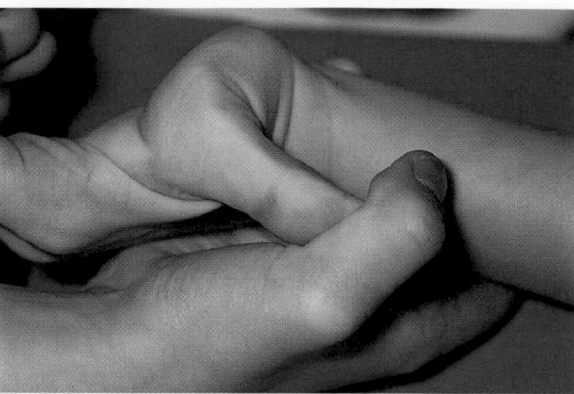

Figure 4.26 Hypermobility. William has a hypermobile thumb!

Table 4.16 The criteria for the diagnosis of joint hypermobility

The ability to perform three or more of the following:
• Passive hyperextension of the fingers, with extension of the wrist until the fingers are parallel to the forearm
• Passive opposition of the thumb to touch the forearm with the wrist flexed
• Hyperextension of the elbow greater than 10°
• Hyperextension of the knees greater than 10°
• Flexion of the trunk and hips with the knees extended until the palms of the hands touch the floor

Non-inflammatory musculoskeletal disorders

Hypermobility syndrome
Joint hypermobility syndrome in children is a common clinical finding and does not usually cause symptoms (Fig. 4.26). The criteria for diagnosis are given in Table 4.16.

Prevalence. Estimated to affect 7–12% of school children.

It is probable that up to 40% of children with hypermobility have recurrent joint pain. This typically affects the knees, but may also affect ankles, hips, back and upper limbs to a lesser extent. The condition is relatively benign, but there may be an increased risk of OA in later life. If treatment is necessary, exercises to increase muscle bulk may be helpful and orthoses may be useful to correct joint deformity.

Pain syndromes
Approximately 15–20% of children experience idiopathic musculoskeletal pain, which may become chronic. Specific causes need to be considered (e.g. infection, tumour, metabolic, endocrine) before a diagnosis of idiopathic pain is made. Awareness of the nature of this syndrome

will prevent unnecessary laboratory investigations, multiple referrals and perhaps the disease becoming chronic.

The syndrome may either be localized, when lightly touching the affected area may cause significant pain (allodynia), or alternatively may manifest as generalized musculoskeletal aches and pain, fatiguability and lethargy.

Nocturnal musculoskeletal pain

This has a number of common characteristics and is sometimes referred to as 'growing pains'. The pain occurs at night, commonly affects the knees and may wake the child from sleep. Episodes last 15–30 min, the pain usually settling with local massage or heat and simple analgesia. The frequency of attacks may vary, ranging from once every few months to virtually every night, and may be precipitated by physical activity.

Management

Treatment usually involves the resources of the rheumatology team and is aimed at educating both patients and their parents about the benign nature of these disorders. Physiotherapy and a graded exercise programme have been shown to be beneficial. Psychological support and coping strategies, and drug treatment with analgesia and NSAIDs may be helpful. Patients and parents need reassurance that the condition will improve spontaneously.

Congenital dislocation of the hip

Congenital dislocation of the hip is one of the most common causes of hip disability in children and of OA in later life.

Epidemiology

Sex. Most common in girls.

Incidence: 1 in 15 000 births.

Race. More common in white people from northern Italy and Scandinavia than in Orientals in whom there may be familial tendency.

Clinical features

The left hip is more often involved. Congenital dislocation of the hip should be recognized at birth by detection of an abnormal click as the infant's hip is abducted and adducted. Later, abnormalities of hip movement, femoral shortening and pain may become evident.

Investigation

Radiography shows that the acetabulum is oblique (increased angle from the horizontal), shallow and directed anterolaterally (Fig. 4.27). It is insufficient to cover the femoral head, which is usually anteverted

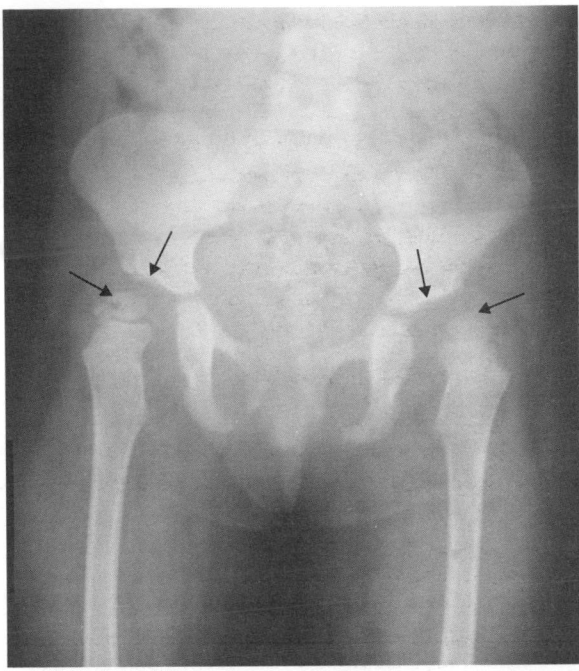

Figure 4.27 Congenital dislocation of the hip. In this patient the acetabula are shallow and the femoral heads are dislocated (arrows).

relative to the femoral shaft and is small and often deformed.

Management

Treatment is splinting in abduction.

Prognosis

Prognosis for full restoration to normal anatomy is excellent. Late diagnosis requires more complex treatment and is accompanied by an increased risk of OA in later life.

Slipped femoral capital epiphysis

Epidemiology

Prevalence. Common in 10–17-year-old boys.

Disease mechanisms

Slipped femoral capital epiphysis may result from acute trauma to the hip. However, before closure of the proximal femoral epiphysis, the femoral head can slip, displacing medially and posteriorly in relation to the shaft of the femur. There may be associated endocrine abnormalities.

Clinical features

The disorder produces an abduction, lateral rotation and extension deformity and there may be shortening of the leg and associated pain. The child is frequently

04

hypogonadal and obese. Avascular necrosis of the femoral head may occur.

Investigation
Lateral hip radiography is usually diagnostic.

Management
Surgical correction is often necessary.

Prognosis
Usually good.

Ischaemic bone disease

Ischaemic bone disease in childhood or osteochondrosis are conditions that refer to non-traumatic ischaemic necrosis, which typically affects a growth or ossification centre.

Osgood–Schlatter disease
Disease mechanisms
Osgood–Schlatter disease is idiopathic osteochondrosis of the tibial tubercle and may represent a partial avulsion of the tibial tubercle.

Clinical features
This disorder is most common in boys aged 10–16 years, who may present with pain, prominence and tenderness over the patellar tendon insertion into the distal extension of the proximal tibial epiphysis.

Investigation
Radiography may show soft tissue swelling, as well as irregular ossification of the anterior portion of the epiphysis. Small fragments of bone may also be noted in the tendon.

Management
Pain usually disappears when the ossicle fuses to the underlying tibia. Athletic activity should be discontinued or reduced until pain resolves. Analgesics and NSAIDs may be useful (see Tables 4.6 and 4.7).

Prognosis
Osgood–Schlatter disease is self-limiting and resolution usually occurs 1–2 years after epiphyseal closure.

Perthes' disease (Fig. 4.28)
Disease mechanisms
Perthes' disease is idiopathic osteonecrosis of the proximal femoral capital epiphysis. Its aetiology is unknown.

Clinical features
Clinically the patient (most commonly a boy 3–12 years

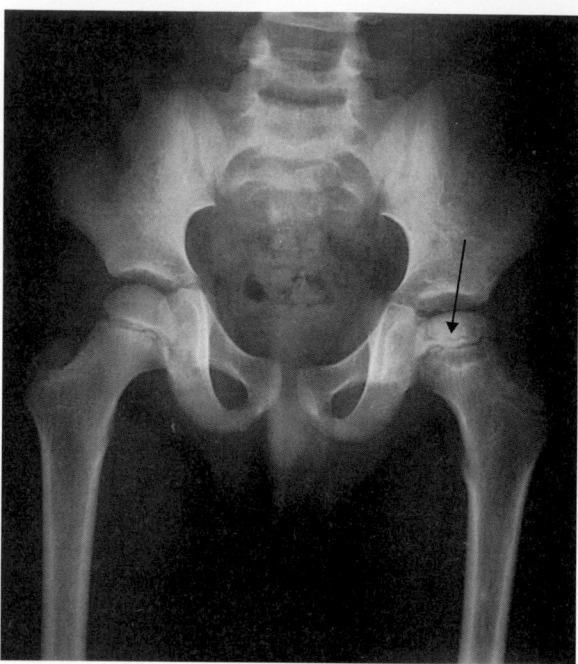

Figure 4.28 Perthes' disease (avascular necrosis) of the left hip. There is patchy sclerosis and structural collapse of the femoral head (arrow).

of age) presents with a limp, which may be painful and associated with limited abduction and internal rotation, and a fixed flexion deformity. It is bilateral in 15% of patients and may be associated with a modest degree of delayed skeletal maturation.

Investigation
Radiography shows disease progression through four phases: death of the bone, fragmentation, gradual revascularization and restoration of structure.

Management
Restoration of normal bone structure may result in a large flat femoral head with a wide short neck (coxa magna et plana). Treatment is based on the extent of the lesion. Surgical realignment may be necessary.

Prognosis
Therapy is most beneficial if started early in young children. Otherwise, the prognosis is relatively poor and many patients will develop painful hips in adult life.

Crystal arthritis

Three types of crystals may be deposited in joints and cause arthritis:

1 *Monosodium urate deposition:* causes gout and commonly affects the first toe

2 *Calcium pyrophosphate dihydrate (CPPD) deposition:* causes pseudogout and commonly affects the knee

3 *Basic calcium phosphate (apatite) deposition:* commonly affects the knee and shoulder

Gout

Gout is a heterogeneous group of diseases, which are manifest by increased serum urate concentration, recurrent arthritis, aggregated urate deposits (tophi), renal disease and nephrolithiasis.

Gout is associated with hypercholesterolaemia and hypertension, and hence with cardiovascular disease.

Epidemiology

Prevalence. Prevalence of hyperuricaemia and gout is approximately 2 in 1000 population.

Age. Prevalence increases with increasing age.

Sex. Ninety per cent of people with primary gout are male. Normal urate levels increase at puberty and the menopause, and are higher in men. Gout is extremely unusual in premenopausal women who are not taking diuretics.

Race. All races.

Genetics. Studies suggest a multifactorial inheritance, and a family history may be obtained from 6–18% of patients with gout. There is an association with high social status, alcohol intake, achievement and increased intelligence.

Geography. High serum urate levels correlate with a warm ambient temperature.

Climate

There is a significant seasonal variation in the incidence of acute gouty attacks with studies in North America and Europe both demonstrating more acute gouty episodes during the spring.

Disease mechanisms

Hyperuricaemia may be a primary or secondary manifestation, occurring as part of another disease or as an effect of drug treatment.

Hyperuricaemia may be caused by (Table 4.17) renal disturbances, resulting in reduced uric acid excretion, accounting for 90% of cases.

Reduced uric acid excretion may result from reduced glomerular filtration, enhanced tubular reabsorption or

Table 4.17 Causes of hyperuricaemia and gout

Primary
Reduced uric acid clearance
Undefined abnormality in otherwise normal kidneys

Overproduction of uric acid
Specific X-linked enzyme defects (increased PRPP synthetase activity, partial deficiency of HGPR transferase)

Secondary
Reduced uric acid clearance
Renal failure (permanent or reversible)
Lead poisoning
Drugs (e.g. diuretics, which enhance reabsorption and decrease filtration of uric acid, low-dose aspirin, pyrazinamide, nicotinic acid, ethambutol, alcohol, ciclosporin)

Competitive inhibition of uric acid excretion
Starvation, alcoholic ketosis, diabetic ketoacidosis, lactic acidosis
Overproduction of uric acid
Increased purine biosynthesis
Deficiency or absence of glucose-6-phosphatase (e.g. autosomal recessive glycogen storage disease type I or Von Gierke's disease)
X-linked HGPR transferase deficiency (Lesch–Nyhan syndrome in which the major clinical manifestations are unrelated to hyperuricaemia)
Increased nucleic acid turnover
Myeloproliferative and lymphoproliferative disorders, carcinoma
Severe psoriasis
High alcohol consumption
Obesity

HGPR, hypoxanthine guanine phosphoryl; PRPP, phosphoryl pyrophosphate.

decreased tubular excretion. Most hyperuricaemia is related to decreased renal excretion of urate by otherwise normal kidneys. Defects in renal function may be primary, resulting from renal disease (e.g. glomerulonephritis) or secondary, resulting from a disease affecting renal function (Table 4.17).

It is not clear why some people develop gouty arthritis, but factors that can cause an attack of gouty arthritis include:

(a) Trauma

(b) Lowered joint-space temperature

(c) Unequal reabsorption of water and urate from the synovial fluid

(d) Rapid reduction of serum uric acid level

● *Metabolic disturbances:* resulting in an overproduction of uric acid, accounting for 10% of cases. In these patients,

04

the rate of purine biosynthesis or turnover is increased. By definition, they excrete more than 3.6 mmol/day (600 mg/day) after a 5-day diet of purine restriction. This may be primary, as a manifestation of a molecular or enzyme defect, or secondary to increased turnover of nucleic acids or increased rate of purine biosynthesis (Table 4.17).

Uric acid is formed from the oxidation of purine bases and approximately 70% is excreted in the urine; the rest is excreted into the gastrointestinal tract.

The mean serum urate level in healthy individuals is approximately 0.30 mmol/l in males and 0.24 mmol/l in females, while the saturation value of serum urate is approximately 0.42 mmol/l. The risk of gouty arthritis and/or renal stones increases with increasing serum urate level and with duration of hyperuricaemia.

Microtophi of urate develop in the synovial lining cells and cartilage, and urate crystals may be released episodically into the synovial fluid where they act as a foreign substance in the joint space. This triggers an acute inflammatory attack, stimulating macrophages and resulting in neutrophil migration into the joint (see p. 40). The self-limiting nature of this process is not understood.

The systemic features of gout are probably explained by the release of cytokines such as IL-1, TNF-α, IL-6 and IL-8 (see p. 47).

Clinical features

The natural history of gout can be considered in four stages: asymptomatic hyperuricaemia; acute gouty arthritis; intercritical gout; and chronic tophaceous gout (GOUT AND PSEUDOGOUT AT A GLANCE).

Asymptomatic hyperuricaemia

The tendency to develop acute gouty arthritis increases with the level and duration of hyperuricaemia. Nearly all patients with gout have hyperuricaemia, but only approximately 5% of those with hyperuricaemia develop gout. The first attack of gouty arthritis (or nephrolithiasis) comes after many years of sustained hyperuricaemia.

Acute gouty arthritis

This usually manifests as exquisitely painful monoarthritis—first affecting the big toe in 50% of patients (Fig. 4.29a). Adjacent skin may become red and peel. As there may be a fever and polyarticular symptoms, it needs to be differentiated from infective arthritis (see p. 259). There may be asymptomatic periods between attacks, which commonly occur spontaneously at night, but they may be triggered by a specific event (e.g. trauma). The duration of an attack varies, but if treated is rarely longer than 2 weeks. Although acute gout most commonly affects the lower, more distal areas, it should always be considered in the diagnosis of an arthritis affecting any joint.

Intercritical gout

After the first attack there is an asymptomatic intercritical period, which may last up to 10 years, although approximately 60% of patients have a further attack within the first year. Each successive attack may last longer and resolve less completely, and is often associated with fever. Differentiation from other polyarticular arthritides (e.g. RA) may be difficult.

Chronic tophaceous gout

If gout is not treated, crystals of monosodium urate (tophi) will deposit in cartilage (e.g. in the helix of the ear) (Fig. 4.29b,c), in synovial membranes (e.g. in the olecranon bursa), in tendons (e.g. in the Achilles tendon) and in soft tissues (e.g. of the ulnar surface of the forearm). Tophi may resemble rheumatoid nodules, and may ulcerate and exude urate crystals.

Renal manifestations

Approximately 90% of patients with gouty arthritis have reduced renal uric acid clearance. The prevalence of uric acid stones in gouty patients ranges from 10 to 25%, compared with 0.01% in the general population. Parenchymal renal damage may be caused by deposition of urate crystals within renal interstitial tissue (urate nephropathy), or by formation of uric acid crystals within the collecting tubules, renal pelvis or ureter (obstructive uropathy). Gouty patients also have an increased incidence of calcium-containing renal stones.

Differential diagnosis

The most important differential diagnosis of gout is infective arthritis. Others include soft-tissue infection, inflamed bunions, local trauma, RA, OA with acute inflammation, acute sarcoidosis, psoriatic arthritis, pseudogout, acute calcific tendonitis, SARA and xanthomatosis.

Investigation

Haematology
- *ESR:* may be raised
- *Synovial fluid leucocyte count:* increased and composed mainly of neutrophils

Biochemistry
- *Serum uric acid:* elevated in 90% of patients with gout, but may be normal during an acute attack.
- *Serum creatinine and urea:* elevated in renal failure.
- *Urine uric acid:* healthy individuals on a normal diet excrete 300–800 mg/day of uric acid in urine. Excretion

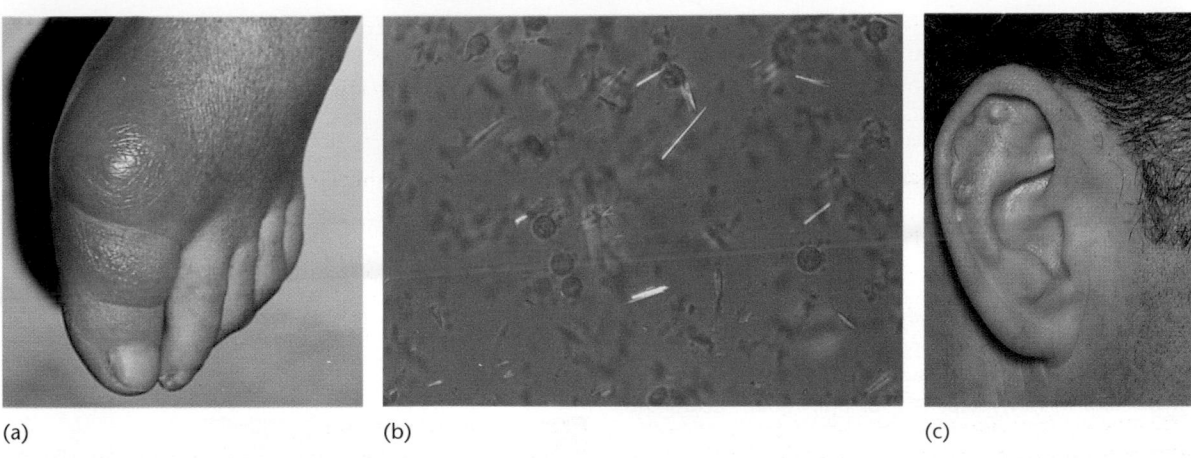

(a)   (b)   (c)

Figure 4.29 Gout. (a) Acute gouty arthritis affecting the big toe. This is exquisitely painful. (b) Synovial fluid microscopy under compensated polarized light showing the slender needle-shaped and negatively birefringent urate crystals. The axis of slow vibration is from bottom left to top right. (c) Urate crystal deposition in the cartilage of the ear.

greater than this suggests the presence of one of the diseases causing overproduction of uric acid.

Immunology
Autoantibodies. Test for ANA and RF if autoimmune rheumatic disease is suspected.

Microbiology
Gram stain and culture of synovial fluid should be performed to exclude infection.

Diagnostic imaging
● *Joint radiography:* shows soft-tissue swelling at first, but later tophi and periarticular erosions are seen. (Rheumatoid erosions are articular.)
● *Pyelography:* required to identify pure urate stones, which are radiolucent, in the kidneys or urinary tract.

Other investigations
Synovial fluid monosodium urate crystals are slender needle-shaped and negatively birefringent (bright yellow when parallel to the axis of slow vibration) under compensated polarized light microscopy. Crystals remain detectable after weeks or months of storage.

Management
Treatment of gout is aimed at relieving the acute synovitis with anti-inflammatory medication and preventing further crystal formation. Dietary advice for patients with hyperuricaemia is listed in Table 4.18.

Asymptomatic hyperuricaemia
There is no evidence that chronic renal disease or joint

Table 4.18 Advice for patients with hyperuricaemia to prevent gout and nephrolithiasis

Dietary
  Lose weight (if indicated)
  Avoid foods containing large amounts of purine (e.g.
    sardines, bacon, liver, kidneys)
  Supplement diet with foods containing small amounts of
    purines (e.g. cereals, cheese, vegetables)
  Avoid excess alcohol
  Drink plenty of fluid
Avoid aspirin and diuretics
Make sure that shoes fit and are comfortable

04

deformity will develop if it is not treated. Diuretic substitution and dietary change are advisable, but the only indications for hypouricaemic drug treatment are:
● Family history of renal stones with a similar degree of hyperuricaemia
● Clear-cut uric acid overproduction (over 1100 mg/day urinary excretion on a controlled diet or resulting from chemotherapy for haematological malignancies)
● Repeated uric acid levels above 775 mmol/l in males and 550 mmol/l in females

Acute gout
Acute gout is treated with indometacin or a similar NSAID. If an NSAID is contraindicated (e.g. because of asthma, congestive cardiac failure or duodenal ulceration) or if it is ineffective, colchicine can be used instead, until the attack subsides. If oral therapy is not effective, the attack can usually be terminated by an intramuscular corticosteroid injection or if possible (knee involvement)

Gout and pseudogout at a glance

Gout
Increased serum urate concentration (Fig. 4.29b), recurrent arthritis, aggregated urate deposits: tophi, renal disease and nephrolithiasis. Associated with hypercholesterolaemia, hypertension and cardiovascular disease.

Pseudogout
Calcium pyrophosphate dihydrate (Fig. 4.29a) (CPPD) deposition disease. May be secondary to another disease, e.g. haemochromatosis, hypomagnesaemia, hypophosphatasia, hypercalcaemia, hyperparathyroidism, gout, ochronosis, Wilson's disease.

Clinical features
Gout
• *Asymptomatic hyperuricaemia:* 5% of hyperuricaemics develop gout. The first attack of gouty arthritis comes after many years of hyperuricaemia
• *Acute gouty arthritis:* first affecting the big toe in 50% of patients (Fig. 4.29a)
• *Intercritical gout:* an asymptomatic period after the first attack. May last up to 10 years. Sixty per cent of patients have a further attack within the first year
• *Chronic tophaceous gout:* urate crystals (tophi) about the body (e.g. helix of ear) (Figs B and 4.29c)
• *Renal manifestations:* 10–25% of patients will develop renal stones, causing urate nephropathy and obstructive neuropathy

Pseudogout
• *Acute* (pseudogout): symptoms peak within 36 h and may last for 1–4 weeks
• *Subacute* (pseudorheumatoid): may develop over weeks to months in 5% of patients
• *Chronic* (pseudo-osteoarthritis): progressive symmetrical polyarthritis with acute attacks
• *Asymptomatic:* a coincidental finding of chondrocalcinosis

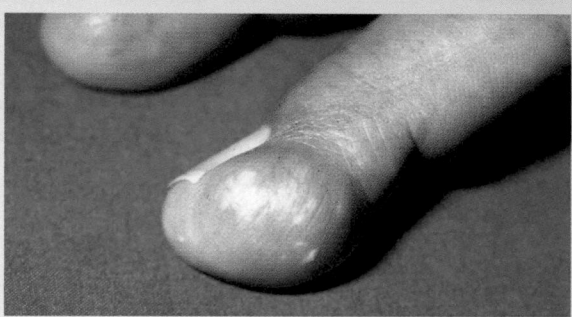

Fig. B Gouty tophus with uric acid crystals exuding from the fingertip.

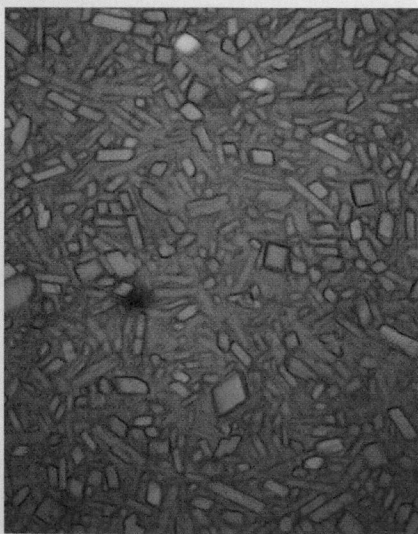

Fig. A Calcium pyrophosphate dihydrate (CPPD) crystals (extracted from synovial fluid). These are pleomorphic, rectangular and weakly positively birefringent. The axis of slow vibration is from bottom left to top right.

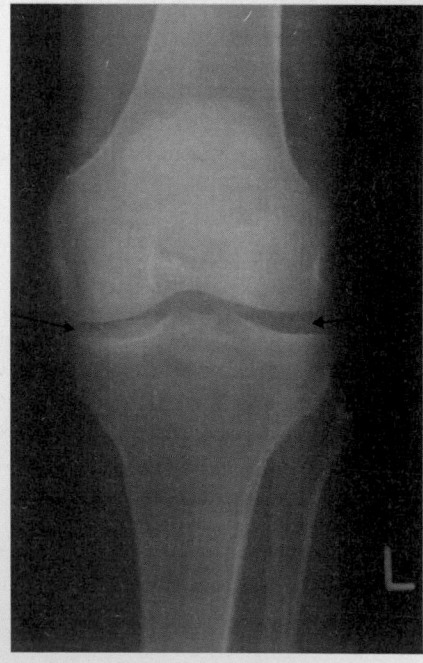

Fig. C AP radiograph of the knee: there is increased density between the femoral and tibial condyles in keeping with the calcification in the menisci (arrows) (chondrocalcinosis).

joint aspiration and an intra-articular corticosteroid injection (see Table 4.8).

Treatment is not indicated for intercritical gout unless there is a history of renal calculi or uric acid excretion and/or uric acid levels are raised (see above).

If there are repeated attacks of gout and the disease is likely to become chronic, allopurinol or sulfinpyrazone are used to reduce serum uric acid levels and prevent further attacks. The aim is to keep serum uric acid levels below 0.45 mmol/l. Neither allopurinol nor sulfinpyrazone should be started during an acute attack because their use will lead to a worsening of the inflammation. Both drugs should be given with indometacin or another NSAID for 1 month after the hyperuricaemia has been corrected. Neither allopurinol nor sulfinpyrazone need be stopped if an acute attack occurs during treatment (Table 4.19).

Dietary advice aimed mainly at decreasing purine intake together with measures to prevent gout and nephrolithiasis are listed in Table 4.18.

Prognosis
Unless chronic renal failure develops, which is uncommon, a normal lifespan is expected.

Calcium pyrophosphate dihydrate deposition disease or pseudogout

CPPD deposition disease is the most common cause of acute monoarthritis in middle-aged and elderly adults.

Epidemiology
Prevalence. Estimated 1 in 1000 population.

Age. Increasing prevalence with increasing age.

Geography. Worldwide.

Disease mechanisms
CPPD deposition disease may be primary. If present in a person under 55 years of age, CPP deposition disease may arise secondary to other diseases such as haemochromatosis, hypomagnesaemia, hypophosphatasia, hypercalcaemia (caused by primary hyperparathyroidism), hypothyroidism, gout, ochronosis and Wilson's disease.

The pathogenesis of pseudogout is unknown.

Clinical features
Acute attacks (pseudogout)
Acute attacks (pseudogout) are characterized by rapidly developing arthritis, which peaks within 36 h and lasts for 1–4 weeks. An attack may be provoked by trauma, surgery or illness. A single joint (commonly the knee) is usually affected, and becomes erythematous, warm and painful. There may be associated fever. Other joints may be

Table 4.19 Drugs used for hyperuricaemia and gout

Indometacin
Pharmacological action. An NSAID (see Table 4.6)
Indications. Acute gout
Side-effects. Gastrointestinal disturbances, headache, dizziness
Contraindications. Breastfeeding, epilepsy

Colchicine
Pharmacological action. Not known
Indication. Acute arthritis
Side-effects. Most common are nausea, vomiting, intestinal colic, diarrhoea
Contraindications. Gastrointestinal disease, renal impairment, pregnancy, breastfeeding

Allopurinol
Pharmacological action. A xanthine oxidase inhibitor. Decreases production of uric acid from purines
Indication. To prevent arthritis and nephrolithiasis
Side-effects. Fever, rash
Contraindications. Hepatic impairment, renal impairment

Sulfinpyrazone
Pharmacological action. A uricosuric. Increases urinary uric acid excretion
Indication. To prevent arthritis and nephrolithiasis
Side-effects. Infrequent
Contraindications. Blood disorders, nephrolithiasis, porphyria

Potassium citrate
Pharmacological action. Alkalinizes urine
Indication. To prevent nephrolithiasis
Side-effects. Hyperkalaemia in association with angiotensin-converting enzyme inhibitors, potassium-sparing diuretics and ciclosporin
Contraindications. Renal impairment, cardiac disease, the elderly

Acetazolamide
Pharmacological action. Inhibits carbonic anhydrase. Increases bicarbonate excretion
Indication. To prevent nephrolithiasis
Side-effects. Hypokalaemia
Contraindications. Renal failure

04

affected, including the MTP joint of the great toe. Radiography may show chondrocalcinosis.

Subacute attacks (pseudorheumatoid)
Five per cent of patients present with subacute attacks. Many joints (commonly knees, wrists and elbows) become involved over weeks to months, and there may be morning stiffness, pain, deformity and fatigue.

Chronic calcium pyrophosphate dihydrate deposition disease (pseudo-osteoarthritis)
Chronic deposition disease affects mainly middle-aged

women and causes progressive symmetrical multiple joint (knees, wrists, MCP joints, hips, shoulders, elbows and ankles) degeneration associated with acute attacks.

Asymptomatic calcium pyrophosphate dihydrate deposition disease

Asymptomatic CPPD deposition disease is detected by coincidental finding of chondrocalcinosis.

Diagnosis

Diagnosis of CPPD deposition disease is based on the pattern of clinical features, the presence of chondrocalcinosis and CPPD crystal identification. The differential diagnosis is mainly between gout and infective arthritis—but pseudogout, gout, OA and sepsis may occur together.

Investigation

Haematology

Synovial fluid leucocyte count is 50–75 000 10^6/l, and the cells are mainly eosinophils.

Biochemistry, immunology and microbiology

As for gout (see p. 241).

Diagnostic imaging

Joint radiography shows chondrocalcinosis in the articular hyaline cartilage, fibrocartilage and tendons in 75% of patients. In the articular cartilage, fine linear densities are seen parallel to and separated from the underlying bone, while fibrocartilage contains thick irregular densities within the central portion of the joint cavity. Commonly involved fibrocartilage includes the menisci of the knee, the triangular cartilage of the wrist, the symphysis pubis and the annulus fibrosus of the intervertebral discs. Additional radiographical findings are similar to those seen in OA (sclerosis of the subchondral bone, joint narrowing and subchondral cysts).

Other investigations

• *Synovial fluid:* CPPD crystals are pleomorphic, rectangular and weakly positively birefringent (yellow when at right angles to the axis of slow vibration). There is a marked decline in CPPD crystals if the fluid is stored for more than 1 day.
• *Look for an underlying cause* (e.g. haemochromatosis): in patients with early-onset disease (those who are under 55 years of age).

Management

Specific treatment may be required for protracted recurrent cases (KEYPOINTS BOX 4.2, p. 201).

Prognosis

CPPD disease is usually self-limiting and resolves within 1–3 weeks.

Basic calcium phosphate (apatite) disease

Basic calcium phosphate crystals are deposited mainly in the knee and shoulder (Milwaukee shoulder), and may also cause calcific periarthritis, tendonitis and bursitis.

The crystals are too small to be seen with light microscopy, but are visible with electron micrography, and joint radiographs are similar to those of CPPD deposition disease. Alizarin-positive red staining of synovial fluid has been suggested as a diagnostic test, but it is non-specific.

NSAIDs and intra-articular corticosteroids are the treatment of choice.

Regional musculoskeletal disorders

Regional musculoskeletal disease refers to localized rheumatic disorders that cause pain. They may be associated with systemic disease (e.g. diabetes mellitus, malignancy, other rheumatic disorders such as RA and SARA) but for most the cause is non-specific and multifactorial. These disorders are sometimes referred to as 'soft-tissue' disorders because they describe the extra-articular structures that are often involved.

Epidemiology

Regional musculoskeletal disorders are common and affect a broad spectrum of the population. General epidemiological data are not available.

Investigation

Investigations are required only if there is a suspected underlying disease (e.g. SARA or diabetes mellitus).

Management

Treatment is with analgesics, NSAIDs, ultrasound and local ice application. Local injections of corticosteroid and lignocaine (lidocaine) can be useful when the pain is acute and well localized. Hydrocortisone is the corticosteroid of choice for injection (see Table 4.4) because it is less commonly associated with complications such as subcutaneous fat necrosis and scarring than the long-acting corticosteroids. Specific treatment is discussed for specific conditions.

Hand and wrist disorders

Common disorders in the hand and wrist are trigger finger, ganglions, Dupuytren's contracture, de Quervain's tenosynovitis and carpal tunnel syndrome.

Patients may express considerable anxiety with regard to hand pain, especially if there is occupation involvement (e.g. musicians and keyboard operators).

Trigger finger
Disease mechanisms
Trigger finger is caused by stenosing tenosynovitis and most commonly affects the flexor tendons of the third and fourth fingers. It is often associated with repeated manual trauma and results from a nodular enlargement of the tendons.

Clinical features
Characteristically, when the nodule impacts on one of the fibrous tethers that anchor the tendon in its sheath, the movement stops until the nodule pops through the constraint.

Management
For a general summary of management see KEYPOINTS BOX 4.2, p. 201.

Ganglions
Clinical features
Ganglions may be painful and are firm dorsal swellings that contain synovial and mucinous material and are connected to joints or tendon sheaths, usually around the wrist and in the hand.

Management
They are treated by aspiration and/or corticosteroid injection. Recurrence is common, and surgical removal may be necessary.

Dupuytren's contracture
Epidemiology
Sex. Most common in males and there may be a family history.

Disease mechanisms
Associated with diabetes mellitus, alcoholism, trauma and HIV infection.

Clinical features
The contracture is a painless thickening of the palmar aponeurosis that produces gradual flexion initially of the little and ring fingers.

Management
Surgery to release the contracture may be required if it is severe.

De Quervain's tenosynovitis
De Quervain's tenosynovitis is a form of wrist tenosynovitis

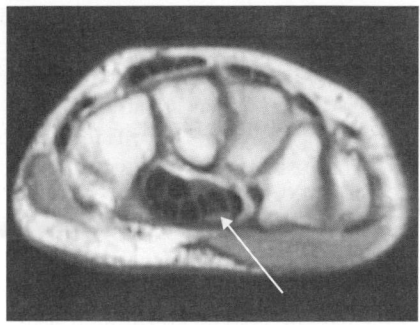

Figure 4.30 MRI of the wrist demonstrating the carpal tunnel. The median nerve and flexor tendons pass through the carpal tunnel, which is bound dorsally and laterally by the carpal bones, and on the anterior aspect by the transverse carpal ligament.

involving the tendons of extensor pollicis brevis and abductor pollicis longus in the most lateral compartment of the wrist adjacent to the radial styloid.

Clinical features
Pain is located in the anatomical snuff box, and can be elicited by forced ulnar deviation, placing the patient's thumb in the palm (Finkelstein's test). In more elderly patients, differentiation with osteoarthritis of the first carpal metacarpal joint (base of thumb) may be necessary.

Management
For a general summary of management see KEYPOINTS BOX 4.2, p. 201.

Carpal tunnel syndrome
Epidemiology
Sex. Most common in females.

Disease mechanisms
Carpal tunnel syndrome is the most common entrapment neuropathy and results from compression of the median nerve in the carpal tunnel of the wrist (Fig. 4.30). The median nerve supplies the sensory branches to the thumb, index and middle fingers, and half of the ring finger, together with motor branches to all anterior forearm muscles except flexor carpi ulnaris and flexor digitorum profundus to the ring and little fingers. It may be occupational because of repeated deviation of the wrist from neutral position, force, vibration and mechanical stress or be associated with RA, gout, myxoedema, acromegaly, diabetes mellitus, pregnancy, the contraceptive pill and neoplasia.

Clinical features
Early symptoms are painful tingling in the wrist and hands

04

at night that mainly affects the thumb and index and middle fingers, which may extend up the arm. The patient may also complain of numbness in the median nerve supply, as well as thenar weakness and atrophy.

Examination may reveal a positive Tinel's sign (percussion of the wrist causing finger paraesthesiae) and reproduction of the pain and paraesthesiae with the Phalen manoeuvre (flexing the patient's hand at the wrist). To determine motor loss, test the thenar muscles: abductor pollicis brevis (with the thumb adducted towards the fifth finger, ask the patient to abduct the thumb against resistance); opponens pollicis (ask the patient to oppose the tip of the thumb with the tip of the fifth finger and try to break the pinch). Inspection of the hand may reveal atrophy of the thenar muscles.

Investigation

Electrophysiology. Nerve conduction testing will show a prolonged distal median nerve motor latency, as well as delayed sensory latency across the wrist.

Management

Initial treatment includes wrist splinting, analgesia and local corticosteroid injection. If the symptoms are not relieved, especially if weakness is present, hand surgery is recommended.

Prognosis

Rarely incapacitating.

Elbow disorders

Common disorders at the elbow are humeral epicondylitis and olecranon bursitis (Fig. 4.31).

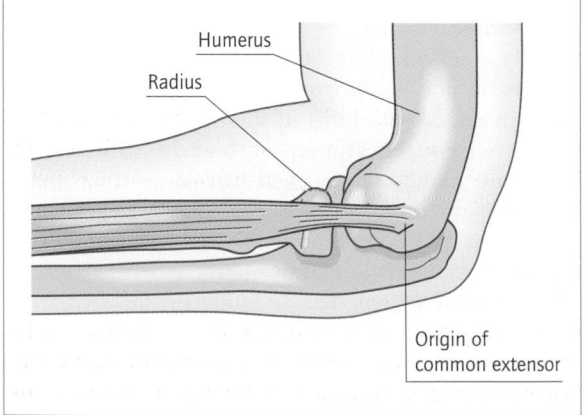

Figure 4.31 The elbow joint. Tennis elbow is caused by inflammation at the common extensor tendon origin at the lateral humeral epicondyle.

Humeral epicondylitis

Disease mechanisms

Lateral or medial humeral epicondylitis is usually caused by mechanical overload on the tendons.

Clinical features

Lateral involvement (tennis elbow) causes localized tenderness that is exacerbated by resisted wrist extension and supination. Grip strength may be reduced. Medial involvement (golfer's elbow) causes localized tenderness induced by resisted flexion of the wrist and pronation. A neurological examination should be carried out to look for medial or ulnar nerve entrapment.

Investigation

Radiographs are usually normal.

Management

Treatment is conservative at first with rest, but local corticosteroid injection is often required. Muscle strengthening exercises are necessary when the pain subsides. If the cause is sport- or occupation-related, preventive advice should be given. Elbow splints may be useful.

Chronic epicondylitis is rarely incapacitating, but surgery may be indicated to divide the extensor aponeurosis.

Olecranon bursitis

Disease mechanisms

Olecranon bursitis is commonly caused by acute trauma, gout, RA or infection.

Clinical features

These are pain, swelling and inflammation.

Management

Treatment is by aspiration and subsequent compression with an elastic bandage. Surgical excision may be necessary if bursae are fibrotic and chronically inflamed.

Shoulder disorders

The shoulder consists of three joints (the acromioclavicular, sternoclavicular and glenohumeral joints) all of which can be involved by inflammation.

Arm elevation is facilitated by the rotator cuff of muscles consisting of supraspinatus, infraspinatus, terres minor and subscapularis. These muscles act together to depress the humoral head to allow the deltoid muscle to elevate the arm. They are also involved in assisting internal and external rotation of the shoulder.

Causes of shoulder pain are listed in Table 4.20.

Table 4.20 Causes of shoulder pain

Referred pain from the cervical spine
Cervical spondylosis (see p. 255)
Tendinitis
Rotator cuff tendinitis (commonly affects the supraspinatus
 insertion into the humeral head), biceps tendinitis
Bursitis
The subacromial bursa may become inflamed with a
 coexistent rotator cuff tendinitis
Joint disease
Adhesive capsulitis
Sympathetic reflex dystrophy
Associated with minor trauma or myocardial infarction (see
 below)

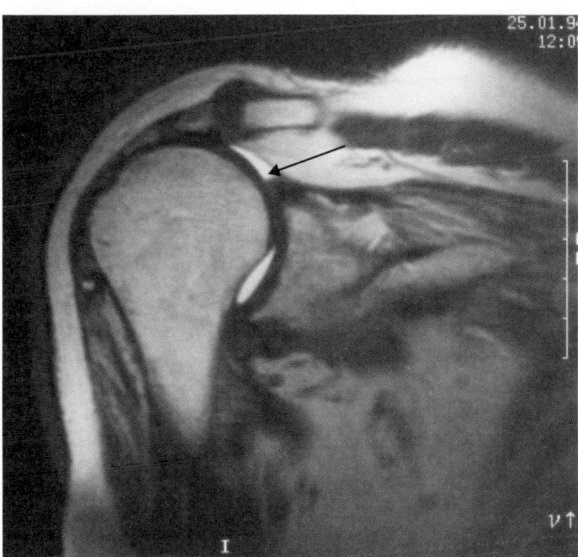

Figure 4.32 MRI of the shoulder. This shows a supraspinatus tendon tear and muscle retraction (arrow).

Rotator cuff tendinitis

Tendinitis may be associated with mild trauma (e.g. a sports injury) or in older patients may be caused by repeated impingement of the rotator cuff under the acromion. Partial or complete tears may result and this can be associated with severe pain (Fig. 4.32).

Clinical features

Inflammation of the rotator cuff causes a painful arc on abducting the arm (especially between 60° and 120° of abduction) and by palpating the rotator cuff at the anterior superior humoral head and proximal biceps tendon. Acromioclavicular joint pain is greatest on shoulder abduction between 160° and 180°.

Management

For a general summary of management see KEYPOINTS BOX 4.2, p. 201.

Calcific tendinitis

Disease mechanisms

Calcific tendinitis is a painful disorder of the rotator cuff, resulting from crystal deposition, primarily basic calcium phosphate.

Clinical features

The condition may present acutely or chronically and pain is elicited by palpation. There may be visible swelling over the humoral head.

Investigation

Radiographs may show calcium within the supraspinatus tendon.

Management

For a general summary of management see KEYPOINTS BOX 4.2, p. 201.

Adhesive capsulitis (frozen shoulder)

Disease mechanisms

Adhesive capsulitis can result from a variety of shoulder joint disorders such as tendinitis, and glenohumeral arthritis or may be associated with lung disease, myocardial infarction or stroke. Polymyalgia rheumatica may also be associated with bilateral shoulder pain and stiffness.

Clinical features

Pain is present on movement, is associated with a decreased range of movement and may be elicited on palpation. Patients are often unable to lie on the affected side at night.

Management

If arthritis is suspected, the joint should be aspirated to detect infection or other inflammatory conditions. In the absence of infection, intra-articular corticosteroid injection may be useful.

Sympathetic reflex dystrophy

Disease mechanisms

Sympathetic reflex dystrophy is usually associated with minor trauma or myocardial infarction, but may complicate adhesive capsulitis. It is thought to result from abnormalities of the sympathetic nervous system. Other names are shoulder–hand syndrome, Sudeck's atrophy and algodystrophy.

04

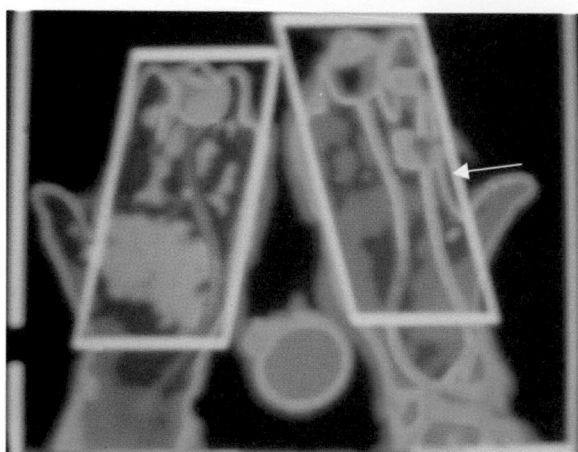

Figure 4.33 Thermography of sympathetic reflex dystrophy of the right hand (arrow). This demonstrates the hypervascular phase, which is coloured blue–purple because of increased temperature.

04

Clinical features

There are three phases:

1 Sympathetic overflow with diffuse swelling, pain, increased vascularity (Fig. 4.33) and radiographical demineralization

2 Progression to atrophy of the skin (which appears cold and shiny) and muscles after 3–6 months

3 Irreversible flexion contractures and a pale cold painful arm

Investigation

There are no specific laboratory findings.

● *Radiographical imaging:* of the affected limb may show patchy osteoporosis in a diffuse or juxta-articular distribution. Erosions may be seen 6–12 weeks after the onset of symptoms, particularly in MCP, MTP and DIP joints.

● *Radioisotope scan* (technetium-99): may show uptake in the affected extremity in a periarticular distribution.

Management

Treatment mainly involves physiotherapy to maintain function and is more effective if started within 6 months of the onset of symptoms.

Hip and knee disorders

Hip and knee disorders include trochanteric bursitis, chondromalacia patellae, patella tendinitis, prepatellar tendinitis, popliteal cyst, meniscal tears and ligament injuries.

Trochanteric bursitis

Clinical features

The trochanteric bursa lies over the lateral aspect of the greater trochanter and under the fascia lata.

Bursitis causes acute pain over the lateral side of the hip and proximal thigh that usually radiates distally and may cause swelling. The pain is often worsened by sitting.

Investigation

Hip joint disease, especially infection, should be ruled out, and a biomechanical cause (e.g. unequal leg length) should be looked for on examination.

Differentiation from polymyalgia rheumatica and radiating pain as a result of sacroiliitis may be necessary.

Chondromalacia patellae

Clinical features

Chondromalacia patellae results from fibrillation of the patellar articular surface.

At first there may be a localized dull ache that is aggravated by sitting and walking up and down stairs, and may be relieved by extending the knees. This may be accompanied by clicking and crepitus and a sensation of the knees giving way or locking. Destruction of the patella cartilage may cause swelling and stiffness.

Pain may be elicited by compressing the patella in knee extension, and crepitus may be detected on knee movement.

Investigation

Radiographs may show patellofemoral OA, but the changes are usually minimal.

Management

Treatment involves rest and avoidance of activities that precipitate the pain. NSAIDs are used if necessary. Rehabilitation is aimed at strengthening the quadriceps. Surgery may be indicated for specific mechanical problems.

Prognosis

This depends on the cause, but usually the disorder resolves.

Patella tendinitis (jumper's knee)

Patella tendinitis is commonly caused by jumping, hurdling and running. The ligamentum patellae may be painful and tender at its attachment to the upper or lower pole of the patella or at its distal attachment to the tibia. The differential diagnosis in young patients is tibial osteochondrosis (Osgood–Schlatter disease; see Table 4.33).

Prepatellar bursitis (housemaid's knee)

Prepatella bursitis can result from repetitive local trauma.

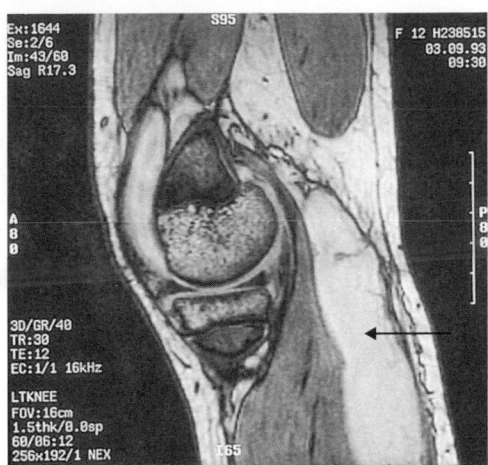

Figure 4.34 MRI of the knee showing a popliteal cyst (arrow).

Clinical features

Stiffness and limited movement. Pain on kneeling. Synovial fluid should be removed if infection is suspected. Knee protection with a foam cushion may be necessary if recurrence is likely.

Popliteal cyst (Baker's cyst)

A popliteal cyst usually arises from a posterior rupture of the knee joint. Popliteal cyst arises from the posterior surfaces of the knee joint capsule. It may be an incidental finding or may cause pain because of its size. When large, it may rupture into the calf causing severe pain and may mimic an acute deep-vein thrombosis (Fig. 4.34). Treatment is aimed at the knee abnormality.

Meniscal tears

Menisci are torn by compressive, rotational and shearing forces in the knee. Pain from medial and lateral tears is common, particularly after twisting injuries. Examination will reveal specific joint line tenderness. There may be swelling and a reduced range of movement.

- *Plain radiography and MRI:* may help with the diagnosis (Fig. 4.35)
- *Arthroscopy:* allows direct visualization

Treatment is conservative, with rest and pain relief. If a full range of movement is not possible and pain does not subside, partial or total meniscectomy or repair may be necessary.

Ligament injuries

Four major ligaments provide knee stability: the anterior and posterior cruciate, and the lateral and medial collateral ligaments. Injury to the knee may involve these ligaments, the joint capsule and other joint structures. Pain, swelling and a reduced range of movement can result.

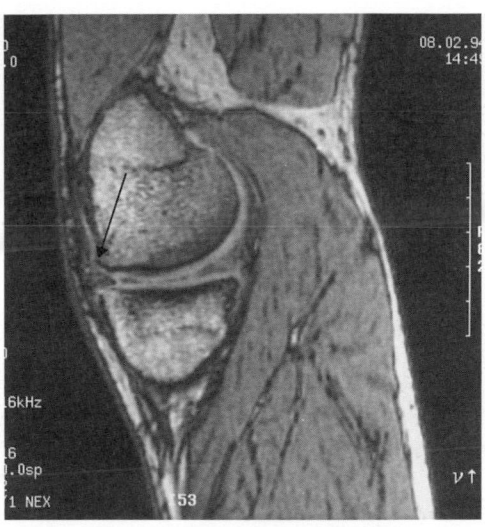

Figure 4.35 MRI of the knee demonstrating a meniscal tear (arrow).

Lower leg disorders

Common problems of the soft tissues of the lower leg, ankle and foot include compartment syndromes, ligament injuries, Achilles tendinitis, plantar fasciitis and hallux valgus.

Compartment syndromes
Clinical features

There are anterior, lateral and posterior, superficial and deep compartments in the lower leg. A tight fascial sheath surrounds the muscles and ischaemic pain may result from muscle hypertrophy as a result of training.

The differential diagnosis includes stress fractures, which are most common in the proximal tibia, distal fibula and metatarsals, and typically result from excessive exercise by an insufficiently trained athlete. There is tenderness directly over the fracture site, but plain radiographs may not show the fracture for at least 4–6 weeks.

Ligament injuries

The common mechanisms of injury to the major ankle ligaments are plantar flexion and inversion, dorsiflexion and eversion. The lateral ankle ligaments are most commonly injured. There may be swelling because of haemarthrosis and local swelling over the site of the ligament damage. The area of maximal tenderness is defined by palpation, and the entire length of the fibula should be palpated as there may be associated proximal fibular fractures.

Achilles tendinitis

Achilles tendinitis is associated with gout and spondyloarthritis. The peroneus longus and posterior tibial

04

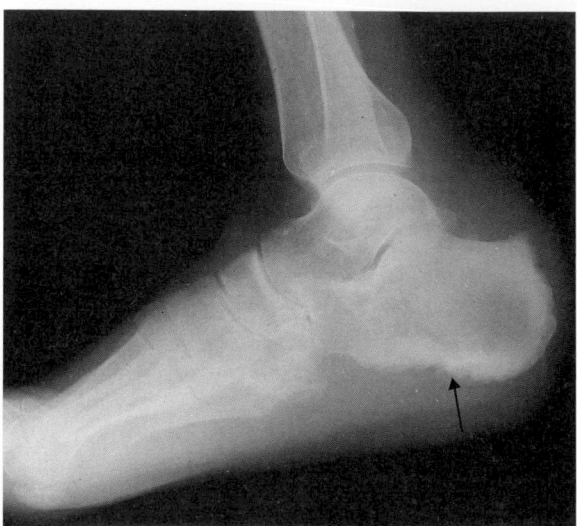

Figure 4.36 Radiograph of the foot demonstrating a plantar spur as a result of plantar fasciitis (arrow).

tendons commonly become inflamed. The pain of Achilles tendinitis is usually in the region of the tendon insertion into the calcaneal tuberosity.

Plantar fasciitis

Usually idiopathic, but may be associated with a spondyloarthritis. Plantar fasciitis causes tenderness on weight-bearing along the plantar surface of the metatarsal heads at the inferomedial surface of the calcaneus at the site of attachment of the plantar fascia.

Radiographs may show a plantar spur caused by calcification at the fascial attachment (Fig. 4.36).

A metatarsal head support and a foam doughnut over the painful area may provide relief. If not, a local corticosteroid injection around the attachment of the plantar fascia to the calcaneus is usually beneficial.

Hallux valgus (bunion)

Hallux valgus causes bursal inflammation because of prolonged pressure over the bony prominence. It commonly results in valgus deformity that may require surgical correction of the hallux.

Low back pain

Low back is defined as the area of the back and spine below the thoracolumbar junction (T12/L1) and the costophrenic angles. Movement in the spine occurs at the synovial apophyseal joints, and at the intervertebral discs. In the lumbar region there is little rotation and maximum flexion is approximately 45°.

Table 4.21 Causes of low back pain

Mechanical
Prolapsed intervertebral disc
Vertebral body and apophyseal OA
Spinal stenosis
Spondylolisthesis
Fracture
Non-specific abnormal posture

Neoplastic
Bone primary or secondary (bone metastases commonly originate from carcinoma of the breast, bronchus, kidney, thyroid and prostate)
Myeloma
Spinal cord and coverings

Inflammation
AS and other spondyloarthritis

Infection
Mycobacterium tuberculosis
Salmonella
Brucella

Metabolic
Osteoporosis
Osteomalacia
Haemochromatosis
Ochronosis
Wilson's disease
Paget's disease

Referred pain
Pelvic pathology
Gastrointestinal tract (e.g. pancreatitis)
Vasculature (e.g. aortic aneurysm)

Epidemiology

Low back pain is a serious cause of morbidity in the population and results in considerable time off work. It is also an expensive occupational health problem, accounting for many work-related injuries and subsequent litigation.

Prevalence. Common. It accounts for approximately 4% of GP consultations and 33% of all rheumatological symptoms.

Age. Prevalence increases with age.

Disease mechanisms

Low back pain can be caused by:
• *Any component of the thoracolumbosacral area:* vertebrae, intervertebral discs, apophyseal joints, ligaments and paraspinal and abdominal muscles
• *Associated structures:* may be retroperitoneal (kidneys,

Table 4.22 Clinical features of inflammatory and mechanical back pain

Clinical feature	Inflammatory back pain	Mechanical back pain
Nature	Constant	Precipitated by movement, etc.
Onset	Gradual	Sudden
Worst pain	On rest or in the morning	Evening
Location	Bilateral	Unilateral leg and buttock
Morning stiffness	Present	Absent
Effect of exercise	Relieves pain	Aggravates pain
Relieving factors	Exercise	Rest

uterus and associated structures), genitourinary (bladder, prostate) or vascular (aortic aneurysm)

- *Systemic disease:* sickle cell disease, infection

Specific causes are listed in Table 4.21. Common causes of low back pain in children are osteochondrosis (Scheuermann's disease) and scoliosis. Abnormal posture is a common cause of back pain. This may be associated with seating that may not offer sufficient back support or wearing high-heeled shoes, which may cause an exaggeration of lumbar lordosis. Additionally, unequal leg length may be present.

Associated risk factors include occupation (e.g. heavy manual work), anxiety, depression and pregnancy.

In the healthy disc, the nucleus pulposus behaves like a gel and distributes pressure equally in all directions, but with ageing localized points of high pressure develop. The pressure within a disc is increased by lifting while bending forward or sitting.

Lumbar disc disease usually causes root syndromes, because the spinal cord ends at L2. The lumbar nerve root exits high in its foramen and is usually above a prolapsing disc, which compresses the nerve root passing to the interspace immediately below.

Clinical features

Clinical features that may help in the diagnosis of back pain are:

- *History of previous trauma*
- *Characteristics of the pain:* acute pain suggests bone or soft-tissue injury; radiating pain, nerve root compression; early morning stiffness, inflammatory arthritis; and neurogenic claudication, characterized by pain on exertion—especially walking—and relieved by rest and stooping forward, suggests spinal stenosis

- *Symptoms of malignancy or systemic infection*
- *Peripheral arthritis:* the spondyloarthropathies
- *Metabolic bone disorders* (e.g. Paget's disease; see Chapter 5)
- *Aggravating and relieving factors:* coughing and sneezing aggravates compression on nerve roots, whereas bed rest may be beneficial, and anti-inflammatory drugs may relieve inflammatory arthritis
- *Other neurological symptoms:* paraesthesiae indicate nerve route compression and may indicate the level of involvement, while weakness, numbness and bowel or bladder dysfunction suggest significant nerve root or corda equina compression

The contrasting nature, onset, location and characteristics of inflammatory and mechanical back pain are shown in Table 4.22.

On examination, spinal alignment, tenderness and movement should be noted. Straight leg raising is useful for eliciting sciatic nerve irritation (L4, L5 and S1 roots). Restriction to 45° or less indicates significant root irritation. The level of the lesion will be revealed by the sensory motor and reflex findings of a neurological examination (Table 4.23; see Chapter 13).

A prolapsed intervertebral disc is unlikely if:

- There is no evidence of nerve root compression
- More than one root is involved
- There is bilateral nerve involvement
- There is diffuse pain and tenderness
- Pain is worse on resting

Corda equina compression may result from a central protrusion and causes saddle-shaped sacral anaesthesia, flaccid paralysis of the legs and sphincter involvement. **This is a surgical emergency.**

Table 4.23 Neurological features of lumbar disc prolapse

Disc (nerve root)	Sensory features (pain and dysthaesia)	Motor signs (weakness and wasting)	Decreased reflexes
L3–4 (L4 root)	Anterior leg, medial foot	Ankle dorsiflexion (tibialis anterior)	Knee
L4–5 (L5 root)	Lateral leg and thigh, central foot	Extension of great toe, extensor hallucis longus	Non-specific
L5–S1 (S1 root)	Posterior leg, lateral foot	Eversion of foot (peroneals)	Ankle

Low back pain at a glance

Mechanical
Osteoarthritis
Spondylolisthesis
Malignancy
Infection
Osteoporosis
Inflammatory
Ankylosing spondylitis

Referred
Prolapse intervertebral disc

Red flags for possible serious spinal pathology:
Age of presentation
Violent trauma
Constant progressive non-mechanical pain
Thoracic pain
Previous history of carcinoma
Systemic steroids
Drug abuse/HIV infection
Systemically unwell
Weight loss
Persisting severe restriction of lumbar flexion
Widespread neurological signs and symptoms
Structural deformity

Investigation

Haematology
- *FBC:* may reveal malignancy (e.g. lymphoproliferative disorder such as myeloma) or chronic anaemia (e.g. spondylitis)
- *ESR:* may be increased in infection, an inflammatory arthritis or malignancy

Biochemistry
Calcium, phosphate, alkaline phosphatase may reveal evidence of metabolic disease (e.g. osteomalacia, Paget's disease).

Microbiology and histopathology
Needle aspiration is usually necessary for culture or cytology to identify a source of infection (see Table 4.8).

Diagnostic imaging
- *Radiography:* plain radiographs may show the degenerative and regenerative changes of OA; osteoporosis, spondylitis, scoliosis or kyphosis; vertebral anomalies (hemivertebrae, spina bifida occulta); vertebral body or pedicle destruction (caused by neoplasia or infection); pathological fracture; or spondylolisthesis (forward subluxation of the body of one vertebra onto the one below, usually at L5/S1). Plain radiographs are rarely helpful, particularly if taken early in the course of an episode of back pain.
- *Bone scan:* useful for detecting infection, but will also appear abnormal in degenerative disease.
- *CT scan:* may be used to visualize the spinal canal.
- *MRI:* may be used for detecting disc lesions (Fig. 4.37).

Management
When there is no evidence of serious underlying disease,

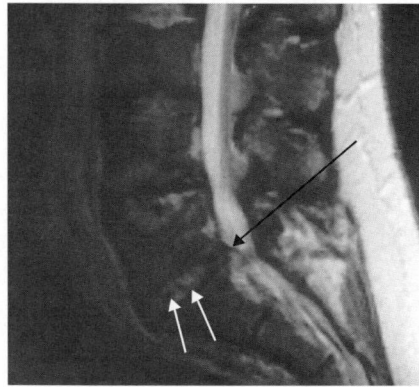

Figure 4.37 MRI of the lumbar spine. The L5/S1 disc is abnormal. There is decreased signal intensity indicating a reduced water content and hence disc degeneration (arrow). The disc is also prolapsed and disc material is protruding into the spinal canal (arrows).

a reduction in daily activities may be advised, but total bed rest should be avoided if at all possible (KEYPOINTS BOX 4.2, p. 201). Pelvic traction is of little use apart from causing immobilization. Physiotherapy, particularly to correct posture, and a progressive exercise programme with weight reduction may be useful when acute symptoms have resolved. This may be carried out in a back school where support may be obtained from other patients.

Drug treatment includes diazepam for muscle relaxation, and simple analgesics for pain relief (Table 4.5). NSAIDs and low-dose antidepressants (e.g. amitriptyline) may be useful. Transcutaneous nerve stimulation may be used to inhibit the sensation of pain. Further medical or surgical treatment may be indicated according to the diagnosis. Surgery is required if there is severe unremitting pain and/or significant neurological impairment.

Table 4.24 Neurological features of cervical disc prolapse

Disc	Nerve root	Sensory features	Motor loss	Decreased reflexes
C4–5	5	Neck to outer shoulder and arm	Deltoid	Biceps/supinator
C5–6	6	Outer arm to thumb and index finger	Biceps and brachioradialis	Biceps/supinator
C6–7	7	Posterior forearm to dorsum middle finger	Triceps and forearm extensors	Triceps
C7–T1	8	Inner arm to fourth and fifth fingers	Thumb and finger extensors	None

Prognosis

The symptoms of mechanical back pain usually resolve with treatment and at least 92% of acute back pain symptoms will settle within 6 weeks. A few patients develop chronic pain, which is associated with considerable morbidity.

Neck pain

Neck pain is common and probably has a similar prevalence to low back pain.

Disease mechanisms

The causes of neck pain are similar to those of low back pain and may be summarized as in Table 4.21, except that mechanical pain is limited to OA or prolapsed cervical disc or is non-specific in nature (e.g. posture) and referred pain commonly relates to visceral or cardiovascular disease (e.g. cardiac ischaemia). Whiplash injury is a specific trauma-related neck pain syndrome that may be associated with significant morbidity.

Clinical features

These may be similar to those described for low back pain (see Table 4.22) apart from those features specific to the lumbar spine and pelvis. The cervical spine is specifically involved in RA and AS, and in these conditions there is a consequent increase in the incidence of atlanto-axial subluxation (Fig. 4.5c). The features of cervical disc prolapse may be difficult to diagnose because of the referred nature of pain away from the neck, which is summarized in Table 4.24.

Investigation

Investigations and their results are as for low back pain.

Management

This is similar to that of low back pain. Cervical spine rest may be achieved using a soft collar and this may be particularly useful at night. However, neck collars should only be worn for short periods of time and not used for more than 2 or 3 weeks. Simple analgesics, NSAIDs, physiotherapy and surgery are all useful.

Disorders of bone, cartilage and connective tissue

Bone, cartilage and connective tissue can be involved in a wide variety of pathological conditions, from infection to genetic abnormalities (Table 4.25). Examples of the more common conditions are covered in this section, while bone metabolism and metabolic bone disease are discussed in Chapter 5.

Osteoarthritis

This is a multifactorial disease and can affect all joints, particularly those that are weight-bearing and frequently used.

Epidemiology

Prevalence. Approximately 50% of the population will have clinical symptoms by 60 years of age.

Age. Prevalence increases with age.

Sex. Under 45 years of age the prevalence is higher in men than in women, between 55 and 75 years it is higher in women, and over 75 years the sex distribution is equal. Women experience more severe hand and knee involvement and greater symptoms.

Race. Hip OA is uncommon in black and Asian populations. Polyarticular hand OA is uncommon in black Africans and Malaysians.

Genetics. OA of the hand may be associated with an inherited predisposition.

Geography. Worldwide.

Disease mechanisms

OA is not a result of ageing joint tissues. It has a multifactorial aetiology and may result from a primary abnormality, or be secondary to a predisposing factor. Aetiological factors include biochemical abnormalities of cartilage (probably as a result of gene defects), genetic predisposition, obesity and mechanical abnormalities. Causes of secondary OA are listed in Table 4.26.

04

Table 4.25 Disorders of bone, cartilage and connective tissue (page numbers are given for those not covered in the next few pages)

Osteoarthritis
Metabolic bone diseases (see Chapter 5)
Osteomalacia (see p. 280)
Osteoporosis (see p. 283)
Hyperparathyroidism (see p. 290)
Hypocalcaemia disorders (see p. 293)
Renal bone disease (see p. 561)
Bone and joint infection
Paget's disease of bone
Primary tumours of bone and synovium
Benign bone-forming tumours
Malignant bone-forming tumours
Benign cartilage-forming tumours
Malignant cartilage-forming tumours
Marrow tumours
Benign synovial-forming tumours
Malignant synovial-forming tumours
Ischaemic bone disease
Osteonecrosis
Dysplastic bone disease
Fibrous dysplasia
Osteopetrosis
Achondroplasia
Hypertrophic osteoarthropathy

Inheritable disorders of connective tissue
Disorders of fibrous elements
    Osteogenesis imperfecta
    Ehlers–Danlos syndrome
    Marfan's syndrome
    Pseudoxanthoma elasticum
Disorders of proteoglycan metabolism
    Mucopolysaccharidoses
Inborn errors of metabolism
    Ochronosis
    Homocystinuria

Table 4.26 Causes of secondary osteoarthritis

Mechanical causes
Congenital and developmental disorders
Hip dysplasia, slipped femoral capital epiphysis, hypermobility disorders
Trauma
Major trauma, repetitive occupational trauma, surgery
Bone disease
Paget's disease, osteonecrosis (Perthes' disease)
Neuropathic joints
Diabetes mellitus, syphilis, syringomyelia
Endocrinopathies
Acromegaly, Cushing's syndrome
Metabolic
CPPD disease, gout, ochronosis, Wilson's disease, haemochromatosis
Inflammatory arthritis
RA, infection

Drugs
Intra-articular corticosteroid

Haematological
Haemophilia, sickle cell disease

CPPD, calcium pyrophosphate dihydrate; RA, rheumatoid arthritis.

OA involves all joint structures, but characteristic changes affect the cartilage, subchondral bone and synovium:

- *Loss of cartilage:* this is thought to result from excessive secretion of cartilage matrix-degrading enzymes by chondrocytes, and there are changes in its proteoglycan, collagen and water content.
- *Increased bone and cartilage remodelling:* there is **subchondral bone sclerosis**, and a thick dense bony plate forms (eburnation) with cyst formation and new bone proliferation (osteophytes), changing the contour of the joint. There may be small areas of bone necrosis.
- *Patchy synovial inflammation:* this is probably a result of apatite and CPPD crystal deposition, accompanied by fibrotic thickening of the joint capsule and ligaments.

Synovial fluid may be increased in quantity and contains few, predominantly mononuclear, cells.

In view of the proliferative changes described above, OA can be best described as a metabolically active regenerative disease.

Specific changes may occur in the spine where OA affects the two principal joints (the synovial posterior apophyseal joints and the cartilaginous intervertebral discs). C5–C7 and L3–L5 involvement is common.

Secondary OA may result from mechanical or biochemical abnormalities (Table 4.26). It may involve joints not usually affected in primary disease.

Clinical features

OA results in painful stiff joints with limited movement but, unlike RA, there is no systemic involvement. The pain develops gradually on use and weight-bearing, and is usually limited to only one or a few joints. Stiffness increases with inactivity (gelling), may occur at night, be aggravated by cold or damp and lasts no longer than 30 min. Deformity can result from swelling, osteophytes, subluxation and node formation around the interphalangeal joints, and is not usually associated with pain. An effusion may also develop.

Primary OA may be:
- *Localized:* consisting only of Heberden's nodes with no other joint involvement

Table 4.27 Useful radiographs in osteo-arthritis

View	Use
Knee	
AP and lateral, weight-bearing	To assess cartilage loss
Tangential 'sky line'	To evaluate patellofemoral articulation
Spine	
AP	To evaluate disc degeneration
Lateral	To visualize anterior and anterolateral osteophytes
Oblique	To inspect neural foramina
Ankle and foot	
AP and lateral	First MTP joint is one of the most common sites of OA, but OA of the ankle and tarsal joints is rare

AP, anteroposterior; MTP, metatarsophalangeal; OA, osteoarthritis.

● *Generalized:* involving three or more joints
● *Erosive:* involving the DIP and PIP joints of the hands, with osteophyte and erosive changes on radiography

OA has a characteristic pattern of hand, hip, knee and spine involvement, and this is discussed below and illustrated in OSTEOARTHRITIS AT A GLANCE.

Hand involvement causes flexion and lateral deviation of the DIP joints, and enlargement of the first carpometacarpal (thumb) joint with radial subluxation, giving the hand a square appearance. Bony swellings over the DIP and PIP joints are called Heberden's and Bouchard's nodes, respectively. Involvement of the trapezeoscaphoid joint causes pain and swelling over the base of the thumb.

Hip involvement is equally common in men and women and is often unilateral. It causes pain in the groin over the greater trochanter, in the buttock or down the inner or anterior thigh. Standing may be difficult, and the patient may limp. All movements can be affected but at first only internal rotation may be limited. Contralateral disease often develops later.

Knee involvement is more common in women and is associated with obesity. It causes pain on kneeling, climbing stairs and getting in and out of cars. The knee may lock because of the presence of loose joint bodies, and the quadriceps atrophies.

Medial compartment disease results in a genu varus deformity and instability, while patellofemoral disease causes loss of side to side patellar mobility and anterior knee pain. An effusion with inflammation may be associated with a popliteal (Baker's) cyst if intra-articular pressure is raised.

Spine involvement may cause localized pain or neurological symptoms, for example sciatica (see p. 252).

Acute inflammation may result from trauma or from crystal-induced (CPPD or hydroxyapatite) deposition. Bursal inflammation on the medial side of the metatarsal head may cause pain and swelling (a bunion).

Diagnosis

OA is a clinical diagnosis aided by joint imaging. The main clinical features to note are:
● Characteristic pattern of joint involvement
● Early morning stiffness of 30 min or less
● Inactivity-associated joint stiffness (gelling)
● Use-related pain
● Absence of extra-articular manifestations
● Absence of wrist and MCP joint disease, which may distinguish it from RA
● Heberden's and Bouchard's nodes with swelling and erythema

Investigation

Routine investigations are usually normal in primary OA, but are helpful for evaluating associated conditions (e.g. haemochromatosis and Paget's disease) and the causes of secondary OA.

Diagnostic imaging
● *Joint radiography:* may reveal specific changes in OA. These are loss of joint space, sclerosis, cysts, osteophytes, soft-tissue swelling, mineral deposits (e.g. CPPD deposition) and calcification within soft tissue deriving from ossicles or loose bodies. Useful joint radiographs in the investigation of OA are listed in Table 4.27. There may be complete discordance between radiography and clinical features.
● *MRI and CT:* useful for visualizing disc prolapse and the neural canal.

Management

It is important to determine whether osteoarthritis is the cause of the patient's complaint. Once this has been done, education and reassurance that the disease has a good prognosis are important. This may help alleviate anxiety and depression.

The treatment of OA is aimed at relieving pain and

04

Osteoarthritis at a glance

Osteoarthritis is the most common condition to affect synovial joints and is a major cause of disability.

It is characterized by focal cartilage loss and bone regeneration. Osteoarthritis has a characteristic pattern of hand, hip, knee and spine involvement

Clinical features

Joint
Pain
Gelling
Crepitus
Instability
Limited movement
Deformity
Effusion

Imaging

Radiology
Loss of joint space, sclerosis, cysts, osteophytes, soft-tissue swelling, chondrocalcinosis

MRI, CT
Useful for visualizing disc prolapse and the neural canal

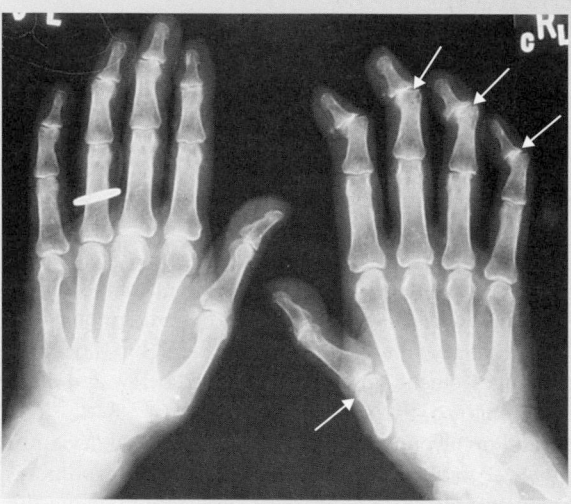

Fig. B Radiograph of the same hands showing typical osteoarthritic changes. There is significant DIP joint space narrowing, with subluxation and osteophyte formation (arrow). On the right, surgery has been carried out to remove part of the first metacarpal because of severe degenerative changes (arrows).

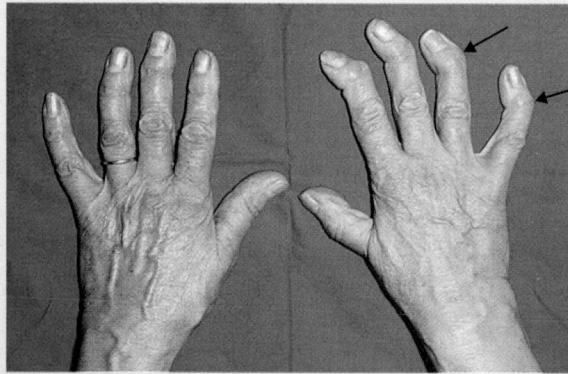

Fig. A Osteoarthritis primarily affecting the distal interphalangeal (DIP) joints with Heberden's nodes (arrows).

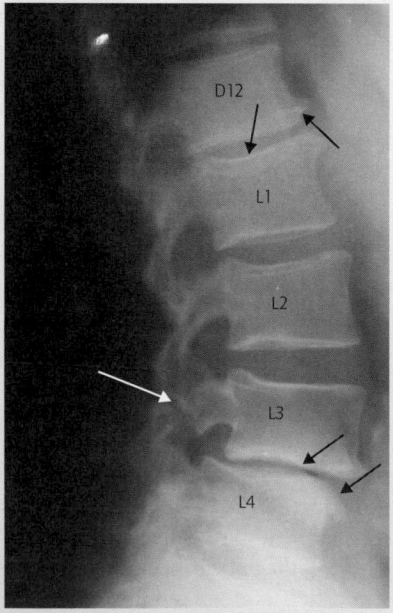

(i)

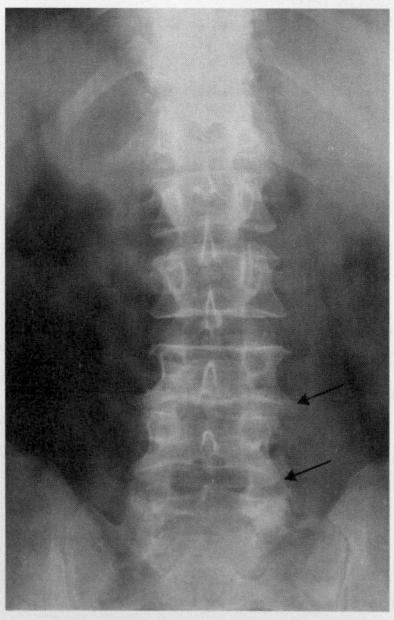

(ii)

Fig. C Lumbar spondylitis. (i) Anteroposterior and (ii) lateral radiographs of the lumbar spine. At L3/4 there is a spondylolisthesis with approximately 1 cm anterior displacement of L3 or L4. There is also a spondylolysis (long arrow). Degenerative changes are noted in addition (reduction and height of the disc space and marginal osteophyte formation; arrows).

Table 4.28 Micro-organisms and arthritis

Class	Infection known	Live micro-organism	Microbial structures	Examples in joint tissue
Infective	Yes	Yes	Yes	Septic arthritides, viral arthritides
Reactive	Yes	No	Yes	Arthritides following infection with *Chlamydia, Salmonella, Yersinia* spp.
Inflammatory	No	No	Yes	Rheumatoid arthritis, ankylosing spondylitis

stiffness, increasing joint mobility, strengthening supporting muscles and helping the patient adapt to any disability. A summary is presented in KEYPOINTS BOX 4.2, p. 201. The following measures need to be considered:

- *Joint rest:* achieved by use of a stick, crutches, walker, lumbar corset or cervical collar. Weight loss and an occupational change may help too.
- *Physiotherapy:* to relieve pain and stiffness, increase joint mobility and strengthen supporting muscles.
- *Occupational therapy:* to help the patient adapt to disability, and to provide advice on minimizing joint stress in activities of daily living. Wearing shoes with shock-absorbent soles may be of appreciable benefit.
- *Drug treatment:* analgesics for pain (Table 4.5), salicylates and NSAIDs (Table 4.6) for inflammation, and intra-articular corticosteroids (Table 4.4) for acute inflammation. Intra-articular hyaluronic acid may be useful to relieve joint pain. Systemic corticosteroids have no role.
- *Surgery:* to relieve pain, increase range of movement in severe disability or correct any mechanical derangement leading to OA. Total hip and knee replacement can successfully relieve pain, but may not increase the range of movement.

Prognosis

OA progresses slowly, and may stop altogether and remain static. Joint failure is rare.

Bone and joint infection

Micro-organisms causing joint and bone disease include bacteria, viruses, fungi and parasites. There are three mechanisms by which they can cause disease:

1 Active infection with live organisms
2 A reaction induced by inactive or degraded organisms (e.g. *Chlamydia*)
3 Inflammation induced by auto-activation of the cellular and/or humoral immune system (e.g. possibly rheumatoid arthritis and Lyme disease).

For a summary of micro-organisms and arthritis see Table 4.28. Bone and joint infection requires prompt recognition and treatment (KEYPOINTS BOX 4.3).

> ### Keypoints 4.3: Joint and bone infection
>
> Most patients with septic arthritis present acutely with a red, hot, painful joint
> Gram-positive cocci are the likeliest cause (e.g. *Staphylococcus aureus*), except in very young or immunosuppressed patients
> Aspiration of synovial fluid, biopsy of resected tissue (e.g. bone) and blood cultures should be performed immediately
> Intravenous antibiotics should be given for 2 weeks and oral treatment for a further month if the diagnosis is confirmed

Acute bacterial arthritis

Specific bacteria may be associated with septic arthritis, osteomyelitis and the triggering of reactive arthritis (Table 4.30). Factors such as source of infection, age of the patient and underlying disease can determine the organism causing infection. Patients with rheumatoid arthritis are of greater risk of septic arthritis.

Epidemiology

Incidence. Approximately 10 in 1 000 000, higher in warm and humid geographical areas and may relate to socioeconomic conditions.

Age. All ages, but most common at the extremes of life.

Disease mechanisms

The common causes of infection are listed in Table 4.29.

Infective arthritis is most common at the extremes of life and in immunosuppressed patients (especially those with HIV infection). Increased susceptibility is associated with diabetes mellitus, cancer, hypogammaglobulinaemia, chronic liver disease, damaged joints (e.g. resulting from RA, trauma or surgery) and treatment with corticosteroids or immunosuppressive drugs.

The organism may reach the synovial membrane by:
- Dissemination via the bloodstream from abscesses or infected wounds (most common)

04

Bacteria	Comment
Staphylococcus aureus	In adults
Haemophilus influenzae	In children under 6 years of age
Neisseria gonorrhoea	In young adults
Escherichia coli	In elderly, seriously ill and intravenous drug abusers
M. tuberculosis, *Salmonella* spp., *Brucella* spp.	Preferentially involve the spine
Salmonella spp.	Sickle cell anaemia

Table 4.29 Common bacterial causes of joint and bone infection

● Dissemination from an acute osteomyelitic focus (common in children because vessels through the metaphysis and epiphysis are not occluded)
● Spread from an adjacent soft-tissue infection
● Iatrogenic means (e.g. joint puncture by needle or arthroscope)
● Penetrating trauma (e.g. puncture, plant thorns have been implicated)

It is likely that bacterial cell wall components elicit the intra-articular production of the pro-inflammatory cytokines TNF-α and IL-1 (see p. 47).

Enzymes within the synovial fluid (e.g. elastase, collagenase) increase and the total effect is to degrade cartilage. Tissue changes may become irreversible even after a few days. Necrotic debris can collect in the joint space. Joint ankylosis during healing is caused by fibroblast proliferation.

Staphylococci are the most common organisms in adult septic arthritis and osteomyelitis; for example, *Staphylococcus aureus* (usually the causative agent in primary septic arthritis), *Staph. epidermidis* (usually in association with articular prostheses) and *Staph. saprophyticus* (Fig. 4.38). Surface factors may be important in pathogenesis; for example the cell wall activates complement and stimulates

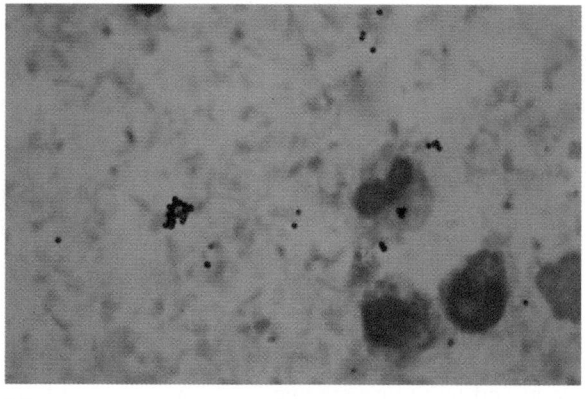

(a)

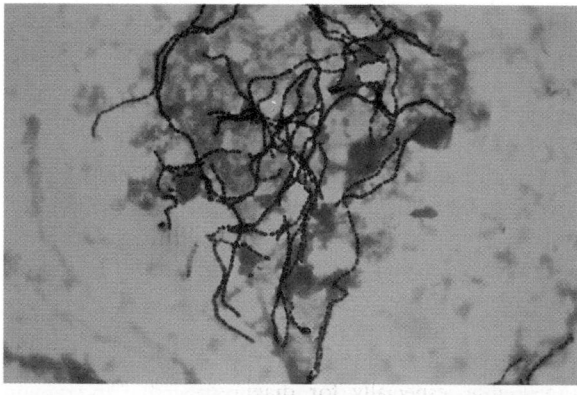

(b)

Figure 4.38 *Staphylococcus*. Gram-positive cocci (dark violet): (a) in clusters; and (b) in long and short chains, with pus cells (red) (Gram stain). (c) This patient had a 10-day history of acute pain and inflammation of the right shoulder. Joint aspiration and microscopy revealed staphylococci and the patient responded well to a joint drainage and antibiotic therapy. She regained almost a full range of movement at the shoulder. Reproduced from Axford JS. Joint and bone infections. *Medicine* 2002; **30**: 9 by kind permission of the Medicine Publishing Company.

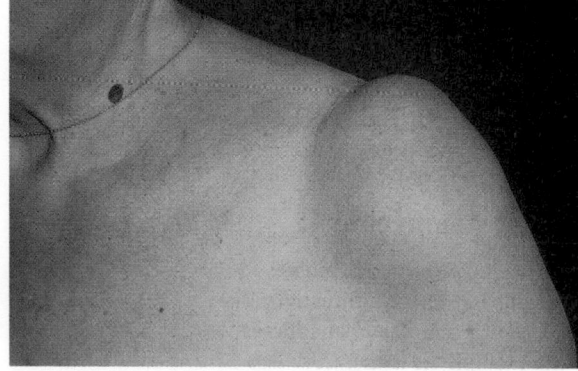

(c)

cytokine release. *Staph. aureus*, associated with staphylococcal toxic shock syndrome, may cause more severe joint infection.

Haemophilus influenzae is a common cause of haematogenous arthritis in children aged between 1 month and 5 years.

Clinical features

Septic arthritis is most common in children, the elderly and individuals who are immunosuppressed (e.g. AIDS patients, stem cell transplant recipients or those taking immunosuppressive agents or have damaged and artificial joints).

Signs of acute bacterial arthritis may develop over several days, and be accompanied by a fever, but may be minimal in those treated with corticosteroids and in infants.

Diagnosis

Diagnosis is clinical and is usually confirmed by detecting the organism in a culture of synovial fluid and blood. The following clinical features should be considered:
- Malaise, high fever and leucocytosis may be the only apparent abnormalities.
- The hip and knee joints are most commonly involved.
- Joints may be held in flexion and adults may complain of pain, and be reluctant to move joints or bear weight on them.
- Approximately 1% of all septic skeletal infections are spinal, and cervical involvement occurs in 3–6% of these.
- Recognition of hip disease is often delayed as pain may be felt in the groin, buttock and lateral upper thigh, or be referred to the knee. The thigh may be held in adduction, flexed and internally rotated.
- There may be an erythematous rash, which may be macular, vesicular or pustular.

Histology and microbiology of a synovial biopsy may be valuable, especially for diagnosing *M. tuberculosis* infection, as these organisms are difficult to grow from synovial fluid. Needle biopsy of the spine or sacroiliac joint may be necessary if infection is suspected at these sites.

Osteomyelitis should be suspected if the area of maximal tenderness extends beyond the joint. It is important to begin treatment early to prevent joint destruction.

Acute osteomyelitis

The metaphysis has a rich blood supply and a slow circulation time and phagocytic activity at sinusoid endothelial levels is reduced. Bacterial adherence and multiplication in the metaphysis is therefore favoured. Osteomyelitis is more common in children and young adults. The bone

may be locally tender to touch and there may be swelling and warmth. If treatment is established within 2–3 days the prognosis is good and chronic complications are uncommon.

Epidemiology

Incidence. In Europe, 10 in 100 000 children/year (the same as bacterial arthritis). Improved surgical technique and antibiotic prophylaxis has led to a significant reduction of infection rate in hip and knee prosthetic surgery.

Age. Usually affects children and young adults. An affected child will not move or put weight on the affected limb. The bone will be tender to touch and there can be swelling and warmth.

If treatment is prompt the prognosis is good and complications are rare.

Chronic osteomyelitis

Epidemiology

Incidence. 15–30 in 100 000/year.

Clinical features

Chronic osteomyelitis is usually post-traumatic or post-operative and the long tubular bones in the lower extremities are most often affected. In adults, chronic osteomyelitis usually occurs following trauma or surgery. The postoperative infection rate for prosthetic surgery is less than 2%. There is usually pain, swelling and increased temperature associated with the affected area, and there may be pyrexia. Skeletal malformation is common. Subacute osteomyelitis is referred to as a Brodie's abscess (Fig. 4.39). There may be pain without inflammatory signs or a sinus.

The recurrence rate is high (10–20%) and definitive healing is uncommon, even after adequate treatment.

Investigation

Haematology

FBC may show increased peripheral blood leucocytes.

Biochemistry
- *Serum uric acid:* to exclude gout
- *Synovial fluid:* contains less than 50% of blood glucose level 6 h after a meal
- *Acute phase response:* ESR and CRP are raised

Immunology
- *Autoantibodies:* RF may be present in chronic infection (e.g. *M. tuberculosis*)
- *Immune tests* (e.g. IgM and IgG antibodies to parvovirus B19)

04

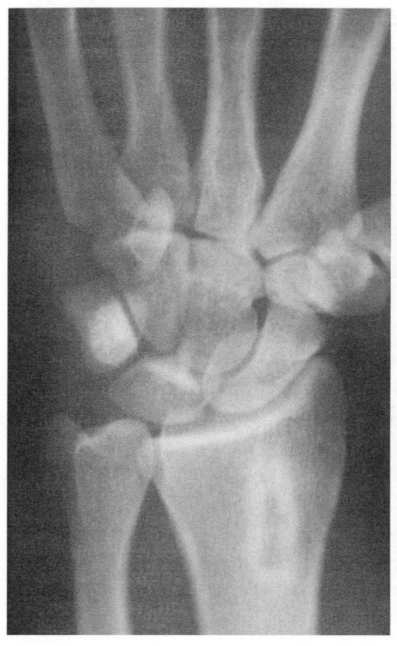

(a)

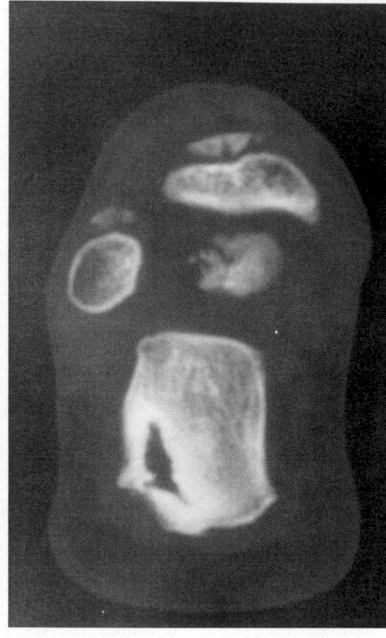

(b)

Figure 4.39 (a) Radiograph of the wrist showing a lytic lesion in the distal ulna. The lesion has sclerotic margins and the appearances are typical of a Brodie's abscess. (b) CT scan of the calcineum showing a lytic lesion with sclerotic margins and a defect in the bony cortex. The appearances are typical of a Brodie's abscess. Reproduced from Axford JS. Joint and bone infections. *Medicine* 2002; **30**: 9 by kind permission of the Medicine Publishing Company.

Table 4.30 Bacteriological findings in joint and bone infections. Reproduced from Axford JS. Joint and bone infections. *Medicine* 2002; **30**: 9 by kind permission of the Medicine Publishing Company.

	Acute septic arthritis	Acute haematogenous osteomyelitis	Chronic osteomyelitis
Staphylococcus aureus	+++	+++	+++
β-haemolytic streptococci	++	++	
Other streptococci	+	+	
Skin anaerobes	+	+	+
Gram-negative cocci	+		
Haemophilus influenzae	+	+	
Gram-negative aerobes	+	+	+
Salmonella	+	+	+
Intestinal anaerobes			+
Mycobacteria	+		+

Microbiology

Bacteriological findings in joint and bone infections are shown in Table 4.30.

- Synovial fluid culture, microscopic smears and arthroscopic or open synovial biopsy may be negative in 30% of *M. tuberculosis* infections.
- Blood and urine cultures and samples from suspected infectious foci are examined. In chronic osteomyelitis, tissue biopsy is necessary because cultures from the superficial orifice may be irrelevant.
- Urethral, cervical and anorectal swabs for culture, especially if gonococcal infection is possible.
- Mantoux test (purified protein derivative) is positive in *M. tuberculosis* infection.

Diagnostic imaging

- *Joint radiography:* commonly shows soft-tissue swelling and joint distension, and later juxta-articular osteoporosis, periosteal elevation, joint space narrowing, bony erosions and possibly osteomyelitis (Fig. 4.40). Spine changes may not be seen for a few months, but typically the disc space or vertebra is narrowed and there is bone proliferation at the vertebral margins. Lytic lesions in the vertebra may extend to the disc. Adjacent vertebrae may fuse during healing.
- *Chest radiography:* required to detect pneumonia.

Scintigraphy

- *CT and MRI:* may be helpful when cord compression

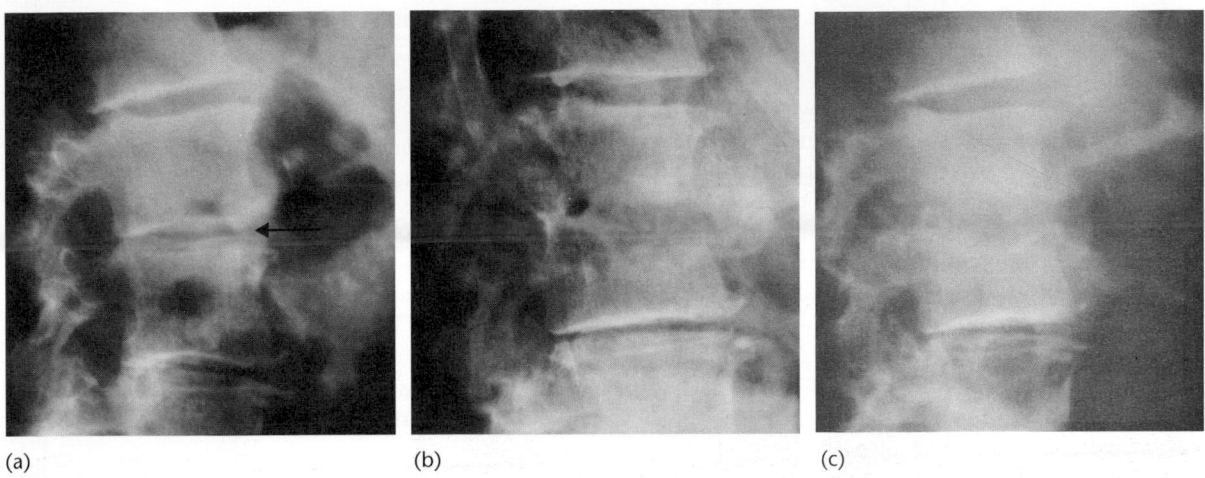

(a) (b) (c)

Figure 4.40 Radiographs showing the development of infective discitis. The initial radiograph (a) shows early bony destruction of the anteroinferior aspect of L2 (arrow). Subsequent radiographs (b,c) show destruction of the end-plates and adjacent vertebral bodies of L2 and L3. Reproduced from Axford JS. Joint and bone infections. *Medicine* 2002; **30**: 9 by kind permission of the Medicine Publishing Company.

is suspected. MRI can provide multiplanar images of the spine and surrounding soft tissues. T_1-weighted, T_2-weighted and gadolinium-enhanced MRI improves the accuracy when diagnosing spine infections.

- *Technetium, gallium or indium radioisotope scanning:* has little role in initial evaluation as it may be positive in other inflammatory conditions, such as cellulitis and OA.
- *^{111}In-labelled leucocytes and scintigraphy* (^{99m}Tc phosphate): may be helpful.

Management

If infection is suspected, the principles of management are:

- Prompt diagnosis
- Early therapy with appropriate antibiotics to prevent joint destruction and reduce mortality

Abscesses should be drained because decompression prevents further obstruction of blood vessels and resulting bone necrosis. Early rehabilitation is advisable; in joint infections patients can be mobilized once the pain has subsided. Full weight-bearing should be avoided for approximately 6 weeks. In osteomyelitis, weight-bearing should be avoided until radiographical signs of bone restoration are present.

If the joint is distended it may need aspiration daily. Irrigation with saline to remove inflammatory substances may be useful. Open surgical drainage may be necessary for hip infections, for failure of needle aspiration because of loculation or where there is lack of response to treatment.

Splinting may make the joint more comfortable and

will reduce flexion deformity. Passive movement is necessary once the pain lessens and an exercise programme is required later to restore strength and mobility.

Before dental procedures associated with bleeding and bacteraemia, antibiotic prophylaxis against bacterial endocarditis is recommended in high-risk patients.

Antibiotic treatment is usually necessary for up to 6 weeks in septic arthritis and 2–3 months in osteomyelitis. *Streptococcus aureus* is showing increasing resistance to beta-lactam antibiotics.

When acute bacterial arthritis is diagnosed and microscopy fails to identify a particular organism, start an antibiotic combination. The antibiotics of choice should be able to treat *Staph. aureus* and other Gram-positive cocci in adults (e.g. flucloxacillin and fusidic acid or clindamycin), *H. influenzae* in children under 3 years of age (e.g. ampicillin or a cephalosporin such as cefotaxime or ceftriaxone) and Gram-negative organisms in the elderly and in those with predisposing diseases such as RA (e.g. a cephalosporin such as cefotaxime or ceftriaxone). Switch to specific treatment when the culture results are known. Do not start an antibiotic until bacterial culture samples have been taken. Do not give the antibiotic by injection into the joint.

For a summary of management of infective diseases see KEYPOINTS BOX 4.3, p. 260.

Prognosis

Full recovery without joint damage is usual if treated promptly.

04

Mycotic (fungal) arthritis

Fungal infections

Fungal infections may be associated with immunosuppression, and joint and bone lesions may be associated with infection elsewhere. Such fungi include *Actinomyces*, *Aspergillus* and *Candida*. Fungal arthritis is uncommon. Patients usually have underlying debilitating conditions or are immunocompromised. Osteomyelitis, bursitis and tenosynovitis may also develop.

Viral arthritis

Viral infections

Few viruses have been unequivocally identified as the direct cause of human joint inflammation. The reason for this may be that the method for detecting viral infection is not sufficiently sensitive. Alternatively, the virus may be cleared early in the course of the disease or inflammatory joint diseases may co-occur with viral infections. Some viral infections are accompanied by arthritis more often than others (e.g. rubella, parvovirus, hepatitis, arboviruses, mumps, chickenpox, HIV).

Disease mechanisms

There are several possible mechanisms by which viruses can induce arthritis:
- *Direct toxic effect on target cells*
- *Immune complex formation:* inducing vasculitis and/or synovitis
- *Virus or viral antigen persistence:* causing perpetuation of chronic inflammatory mechanisms
- *Molecular mimicry:* causing tissue destruction by cross-reactivity of antibodies and cellular immune reactivity with homologous tissue structures
- *Superantigen function:* initiating production of lymphokines, which can stimulate B cells to produce immunoglobulins including antibodies
- *Modification of the immune response:* resulting in immunosuppression or infection of lymphohaemopoietic cells.

Rubella arthritis and arthralgias

These may occur in up to 50% of infected women, compared with up to 6% of men; it is uncommon in children. Live virus and viral antigens have been detected in synovial fluid. However, rubella vaccine is not associated with clinically important acute or chronic joint disease. There is still controversy as to whether rubella causes chronic arthropathy, but studies to date have been negative. The symptoms of arthritis occur within 1 week of the rash. The fingers, wrists, elbows, knees, and hip and toe joints are most commonly affected, usually asym-

Table 4.31 Rheumatic syndromes associated with HIV infection

Infective arthritis and osteomyelitis
Arthralgia syndrome, which is similar to that of other viraemic diseases
Reactive arthritis similar to SARA and psoriatic arthritis and characterized by peripheral arthritis, enthesopathy and spondyloarthritis
Sjögren's syndrome characterized by xerostomia and parotid enlargement
Vasculitis: with skin and nerve involvement

metrically. Tenosynovitis and carpal tunnel syndrome may occur. The arthritis usually resolves in approximately 30 days.

Parvovirus B19

This usually causes acute benign self-limiting disease, but it may be associated with rheumatoid-like polyarthritis. There may be symmetrical polyarthritis in association with erythema infectiosum (fifth disease), which gives a 'slapped-cheek' appearance. Rheumatic symptoms occur in 95% of infected children and may also affect adults; they are more common in women. Acute costochondritis and acute bilateral carpal tunnel syndrome have been reported.

Hepatitis viruses

During the prodromal stage of acute hepatitis B virus infection, transient polyarthritis occurs in 30% of patients; it usually resolves with the onset of jaundice. Small joints are usually symmetrically affected. The incidence is similar in men and women.

There is a well-recognized association of hepatitis C virus with type II mixed cryoglobulinaemia. Immunosuppressive agents should be avoided in these patients.

Human immunodeficiency virus (see Chapter 3)

HIV affects approximately 8–10 million individuals worldwide. It has been reported in more than 150 countries, but is most prevalent in Africa and the Americas.

HIV is associated with the following musculoskeletal presentations (Table 4.31).

Arthralgia

Arthralgia is the most commonly observed problem. It is intermittent, mild and polyarticular and more common in the later stages of HIV infection.

Arthritis

It commonly affects the knees and ankles and lasts from hours to a few days.

Acute symmetrical polyarthritis has also been reported.

Table 4.32 Common tumours of bone and synovium

Type	Benign/malignant	Tumour
Bone forming	Benign	Osteoma
		Osteoid osteoma
	Malignant	Osteosarcoma
Cartilage forming	Benign	Chondroma
	Malignant	Chondrosarcoma
Marrow tumour	Malignant	Ewing's sarcoma
		Lymphoma (see p. 1059)
		Myeloma (see p. 1064)
Synovial tumour	Benign	Pigmented villonodular synovitis
	Malignant	Synovial sarcoma

Reiter's syndrome

In which peripheral arthritis occurs with extra-articular features including urethritis, ocular inflammation and skin lesions. The rash ranges from seborrhoea to frank kerotoderma blenorrhagicum. There is a strong association with HLA-B27 antigen.

Psoriatic arthritis

Arthritis and enthesopathy occur in association with psoriasis.

Avascular necrosis of bone

This may be associated with anticardiolipin antibodies.

Septic arthritis

Opportunistic infections can occur (e.g. *Candida, M. avium*).

Autoimmune rheumatic disease-like syndromes

Patients may present with a Sjögren's syndrome-like disease, inflammatory or non-inflammatory myopathy, systemic vasculitis or a lupus-like syndrome.

Management

Virus-associated arthritis is usually self-limiting and most patients can be managed symptomatically and with NSAIDs.

In a few patients, the disease is severe and unresponsive, and joint disease must be controlled with corticosteroids and disease-modifying drugs, ideally without exacerbating the underlying retroviral infection.

In established RA, HIV causes a reduction in the inflammatory component, but the disease process causing joint erosion and destruction continues. HIV patients can develop RA.

Chronic fatigue syndrome

Chronic fatigue syndrome occurs in epidemics or sporadically. The incidence is biomodal and similar in males and females, and peaks at 25–30 years and 40–45 years. Clinical features include debilitating fatigue, muscle aches, pains, lymph node tenderness and pain, pyrexia, exhaustion and invariable psychiatric symptoms (e.g. depression, poor memory, loss of concentration).

Some patients may relate chronic fatigue syndrome to an infectious episode (e.g. EBV, *Borrelia burgdorferi*).

Primary tumours of bone and synovium

Primary tumours of bone and synovium are rare (Table 4.32). Most are benign.

Secondary malignant tumours may be complications of primary bone sarcomas or metastatic tumours, or result from invasion by leukaemia, lymphoma or myeloma. Primary tumours of the lung, breast and colon are the most common sources.

Investigation
Diagnostic imaging
- *Radiography:* bone may be sclerotic or osteolitic. Chest radiography to help determine whether primary or secondary tumour.
- *CT scanning, bone scintigrams, MRI.*

Other investigations
- Biopsy
- Joint aspiration
- Arthroscopy

Management
- Surgical local resection/limb amputation
- Chemotherapy
- Local radiation

Prognosis
If malignant the 5-year survival is between 25 and 60%, depending upon the tumour.

04

Benign bone-forming tumours

Osteoma

An osteoma is a slow-growing benign tumour consisting of well-differentiated mature bone.

Epidemiology

It may occur at any age, but is most common in 20–50-year-olds.

Clinical features

Osteomas may be asymptomatic or present as a hard swelling that slowly increases in size. Radiologically they are radio-opaque and usually less than 3 cm in diameter.

Treatment is only necessary for symptoms or cosmetic reasons.

Osteoid osteoma

An osteoid osteoma is a small (less than 1 cm) benign osteoblastic lesion that may be surrounded by reactive bone formation. The femur and tibia are most commonly affected.

Epidemiology

Prevalence. Relatively common.

Age and sex. Approximately 70% of patients are males aged 5–30 years.

Clinical features

Patients usually present with a constant pain, which may be worse at night and worsened by alcohol. There may be associated muscle atrophy and, if the lesion is superficial, there is localized swelling or tenderness.

Malignant bone-forming tumours

Osteosarcoma

An osteosarcoma is a malignant tumour characterized by the direct formation of bone tissue by the tumour cells (Fig. 4.41). Overall it is an uncommon malignant tumour. Any bone may be affected, but usually long bones. They grow rapidly and metastasize through the bloodstream, most commonly to the lungs.

Epidemiology

Prevalence. Incidence is approximately 2–3/million population/year.

Age and sex. Usually occurs in males 10–30 years of age.

Clinical features

Pain is the most common symptom and this may be well-localized or radiate to an adjacent joint. As the tumour

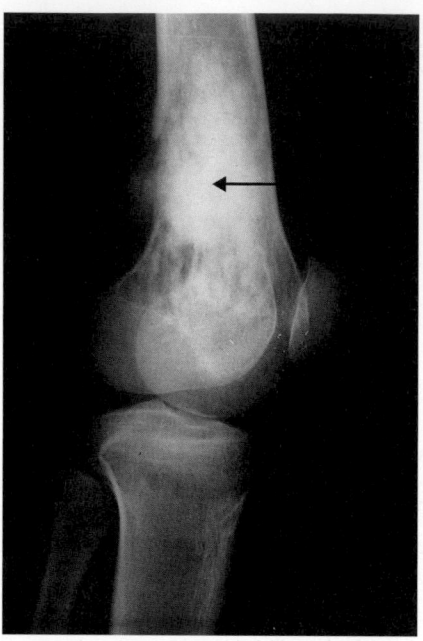

Figure 4.41 Radiograph demonstrating osteosarcoma of the knee. There is a destructive lesion in the distal femur and marked associated new bone formation (arrow).

increases in size it may be palpable, and the superficial skin may feel warm because of tumour vascularity.

Benign cartilage-forming tumours

Chondroma

A chondroma is a benign tumour characterized by the formation of mature cartilage.

Epidemiology

Age. Rare under 20 years of age.

Disease mechanisms

Most chondromas are isolated lesions within the medullary cavity. The hands, femur, humerus, fibula and ribs are common sites of involvement.

Clinical features

Chondromas may be asymptomatic or cause swelling and pain if there is a pathological fracture. Approximately 15–30% of multiple chondromas undergo malignant transformation.

Malignant cartilage-forming tumours

Chondrosarcoma

Chondrosarcoma is a malignant tumour characterized by the formation of cartilage.

Epidemiology
Prevalence. Chondrosarcomas comprise 10–13% of malignant bone tumours.

Age. Peak incidence 30–60 years of age.

Sex. More common in males.
   Secondary chondrosarcomas are a complication of multiple chondromas.

Clinical features
Pain is usually the first symptom. Swelling may also be noticed. The most common site of metastasis is the lung.

Marrow tumours

Ewing's sarcoma
Ewing's sarcoma is a malignant tumour characterized by the presence of densely packed small cells with round nuclei, without distinct cytoplasmic outlines or prominent nucleoli.

Epidemiology
Prevalence. Accounts for approximately 6–9% of malignant bone tumours.

Age. Usually under 25 years of age.

Sex. Males are more often affected than females.

Clinical features
Pain, tenderness and swelling are the most common presenting symptoms, but additionally there may be fever, anaemia and a raised white cell count. The most common site is in long bones.

Benign synovial tumours

Pigmented villonodular synovitis
Epidemiology
Prevalence. Uncommon.

Age. Most common in young adults.

Geography. Worldwide.

Disease mechanisms
Pigmented villonodular synovitis (PVNS) is characterized by a thickened synovial lining of joints, tendons, sheaths and bursae. The synovium forms reddish brown villous projections that invade the articular cartilage and subchondral bone causing erosions and thin-walled cysts

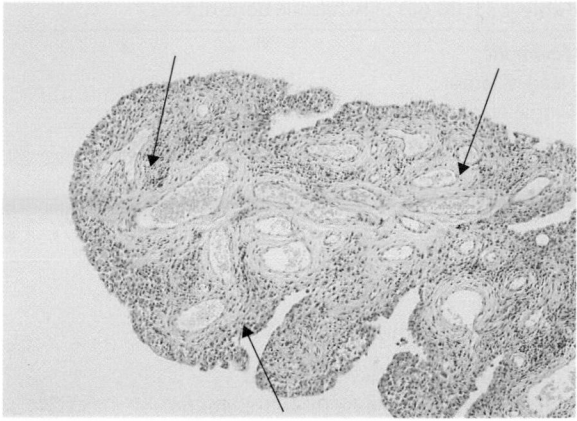

Figure 4.42 Photomicrograph of pigmented villonodular synovitis (PVNS) showing the villous architecture. Inflamed synovium covers the fibrovascular core which contains haemosiderin-laden macrophages to give it a pigmented appearance (arrows).

(Fig. 4.42). The discoloration is produced by areas of haemorrhage associated with deposits of brown haemosiderin and haemosiderin-laden macrophages. There may be a spectrum of disease.

Clinical features
Diffuse PVNS involves the knee, hip or ankle. The joint may be swollen and tender with a limited range of movement, synovial thickening and recurrent effusions.

Malignant synovial tumours

Malignant joint tumours are rare; synovial sarcoma is the most common.

Synovial sarcoma
Epidemiology
Prevalence. Rare: 2.75 in 100 000 population.

Age. Most common in 15–40-year-olds.

Geography. Worldwide.

Disease mechanisms
Synovial sarcoma may arise from a fascial aponeurosis, tendon, tendon sheath or synovial bursa, and is highly malignant. It commonly originates within the fascial planes of the thigh or leg adjacent to the knee.

Clinical features
Clinically synovial sarcoma often presents as a palpable swelling, which may be painful.

04

Table 4.33 Causes of ischaemic bone disease

Traumatic
Head of femur
Carpal scaphoid (wrist)
Knee joint (osteochondritis dissecans)

Non-traumatic (associated with specific diseases)
Endocrine (Cushing's disease and corticosteroid therapy)
Storage disease (e.g. Gaucher's disease)
Decompression sickness (e.g. Caisson's disease)
Pancreatitis
Haemoglobinopathies (e.g. sickle cell disease)

Conditions associated with childhood
Osgood–Schlatter disease (tibial tuberosity)
Perthes' disease (hip)
Sever's disease (os calcis)
Slipped femoral epiphysis

Table 4.34 Dysplastic bone disease

Osteopetrosis
Increased bone density on radiography
Aplastic anaemia
Renal tubular acidosis

Fibrous dysplasia
McCune–Albright syndrome—associated in females with *café au lait* spots and sexual precocity

Achondroplasia
Dwarfism
Reduction in endochondral bone formation

Hypertrophic osteoarthropathy
Chronic periosteal hyperplasia of long bones
Finger and toe clubbing
Arthritis associated with neoplasia, infection or hyperthyroidism

Ischaemic bone disease

Osteonecrosis

Osteonecrosis is a term given to cell death within bone and may be caused by a number of conditions, most of which lead to an impaired blood supply. The femoral head is commonly involved, although other bones may be affected (e.g. carpal scaphoid).

Osteonecrosis may be caused by trauma, but may also be associated with certain diseases (Table 4.33). There is an idiopathic group of conditions associated with osteonecrosis that occur predominantly in childhood.

Clinical features
Pain, swelling, crepitus and mechanical locking, depending upon location.

Investigation
MRI and radiography may be diagnostic.

Management
Physiotherapy and surgery.

Dysplastic bone disease

Dysplastic bone diseases (Table 4.34) are a group of heterogeneous diseases caused by a disturbance of the formation or modelling of bone and/or joints. There is a wide spectrum of clinical features from OA to pathological fracture and, in addition, there may be extraskeletal manifestations such as malabsorption and nerve palsy. Some more common diseases are described here. A group of inheritable disorders of connective tissue that cause osteoarticular dysplasia are described in the next section.

Inheritable disorders of connective tissue

Molecular biology has led to significant advances in our understanding of the aetiology of these primary connective tissue disorders. Gene mutations for connective tissue proteins have been associated with a variety of disorders, which are classified according to their phenotype as shown in Table 4.35.

Epidemiology
Prevalence. The most common heritable disorders of connective tissue affect from 1 in 10 000 to 1 in 50 000 of the UK population.

Management
Diagnosis is usually made by phenotypic appearance, and molecular techniques may be available to confirm it. Unless stated, management is usually symptomatic and supportive.

Disorders of fibrous elements

Osteogenesis imperfecta
Osteogenesis imperfecta can be classified into four types using clinical and inheritance pattern criteria. All are characterized by bone, ocular, dental, aural and cardiovascular involvement, and brittle bones, to a varying degree. Limbs may be short and bent at birth. Blue sclera and deafness may also be features. The diagnosis can usually be made clinically (Fig. 4.43).

Table 4.35 Classification of inheritable disorders of connective tissue according to phenotype

Phenotype	Inheritable connective tissue disorder
Disorders of fibrous elements	Osteogenesis imperfecta Ehlers–Danlos syndrome Marfan's syndrome Pseudoxanthoma elasticum
Disorders of proteoglycan metabolism	Mucopolysaccharidoses
Osteochondrodysplasias	Achondroplasia Spondyloepiphyseal and metaphyseal dysplasias
Inborn errors of metabolism	Homocystinuria Ochronosis

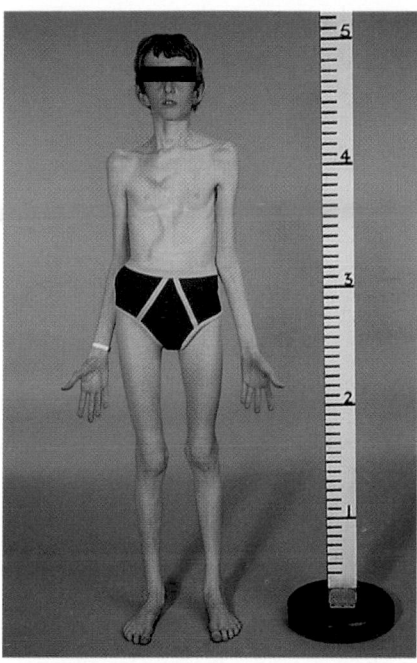

Figure 4.44 Marfan's syndrome. This man has characteristic musculoskeletal abnormalities.

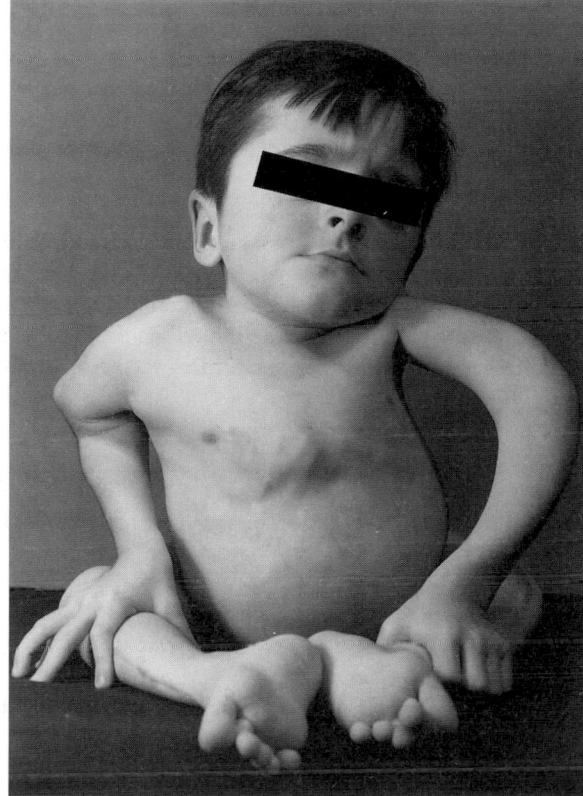

Figure 4.43 A child with the skeletal features of osteogenesis imperfecta.

Ehlers–Danlos syndrome
Clinical features
These involve joints, skin, vessels and internal organs:
- *Joints:* there may be hyperextensibility of large or small joints, which can dislocate.
- *Skin:* this may be soft with a velvet-like texture and hyperextensible. 'Cigarette paper scars' may occur because of its fragility.
- *Vessels and organs:* there may be easy bruising, but also life-threatening arterial rupture and rupture of the colon or uterus.

Marfan's syndrome
Marfan's syndrome was the first inheritable connective tissue disorder to be described.

Clinical features
Marfan's syndrome is characterized by musculoskeletal, cardiovascular and ocular features:
- *Musculoskeletal:* Marfan's syndrome is characterized by tall stature and abnormal body proportions—a long arm span and an abnormally low ratio of upper segment to lower segment—and elongated digits (Fig. 4.44). Other musculoskeletal features include anterior thoracic deformity (pectus excavatum and carinatum); abnormal vertebral column curvature (loss of thoracic kyphosis and scoliosis); hyperextensibility or contracture of peripheral joints; and pes planus, with long narrow feet.
- *Cardiovascular:* ascending aortic dilatation, which may result in aortic regurgitation and dissection; mitral valve prolapse resulting in mitral regurgitation.
- *Ocular:* myopia, subluxation of the lens.

04

Pseudoxanthoma elasticum

Clinical features

The main features of pseudoxanthoma elasticum are:

- *Ocular angioid streak:* resulting in progressive visual loss because of retinal haemorrhage
- *Intermittent claudication:* resulting from degeneration of elastic fibres in muscular arteries—stroke, myocardial infarction and gastrointestinal haemorrhage can occur
- *Wrinkled inelastic skin:* particularly in regions of flexural stress—resembles plucked chicken skin

Disorders of proteoglycan metabolism

Mucopolysaccharidoses

Mucopolysaccharidoses are lysosomal storage diseases that arise from errors of mucopolysaccharide metabolism, leading to mucopolysacchariduria and mucopolysaccharide deposition in tissues. The most frequent forms are Hurler's disease and Morquio's disease.

Clinical features

Relatively short stature is the rule for all types. Patients with certain types survive to adulthood without severe mental retardation.

Inborn errors of metabolism

Ochronosis

Ochronosis is rare and is a feature of alkaptonuria, which results from a lack of homogentisic acid oxidase. There is autosomal recessive inheritance (see p. 37).

Clinical features

- *Pigmentation of the sclera or the ear:* rarely seen before 20–30 years of age. The pigment gives a slate-blue–grey coloration.
- *Ochronotic arthritis:* hips, knees and shoulders are generally involved. There may be a reduced range of movement and episodes of acute inflammation.
- *Urinary changes:* in some patients the urine turns dark on standing because of oxidation of the large amounts of excreted homogentisic acid.

Homocystinuria

Homocystinuria results from an inborn error in the metabolism of methionine because of deficient activity of the enzyme cystathion β synthase.

Clinical features

Some of the clinical features are similar to those of Marfan's syndrome—lens subluxation, tall stature, abnormal body proportions, elongated digits, and anterior chest and spinal deformities—but aortic aneurysm and mitral valve prolapse do not occur.

Other clinical features are specific, including generalized osteoporosis, arthropathy, arterial and venous thrombosis, a malar flush and mental retardation.

04

! Must know checklist

- That there are genetic and environmental influences predisposing to arthritis
- The common major presenting clinical features
- Blood tests used in diagnosis
- Imaging techniques used in diagnosis
- What analgesics and NSAIDs to use and their side-effects
- When to use drugs that suppress rheumatic disease and their side-effects

- How to diagnose and treat bone and joint infection
- Supportive treatment available for patients (e.g. physiotherapy and occupational therapy)
- The importance of eye examination in juvenile idiopathic arthritis
- Important factors (red flags) in the diagnosis of back disease

Further reading

Books

Isenberg D, Maddison P. *Oxford Textbook of Rheumatology*. Oxford: Oxford University Press, 1998.

Klippel JH, Dieppe PA. *Rheumatology*. London: Mosby, 1998.

Provan D, Krentz A. *Oxford Handbook of Investigation*. Oxford: Oxford University Press, 2002.

Journals

Rheumatology, British Society for Rheumatology. https://www.msecportal.org/

Annals of Rheumatic Diseases, BMJ Publishing Group. http://ard.bmjjournals.com/

Journal of Rheumatology, Journal of Rheumatology Publishing. http://www.jrheum.com/

Arthritis and Rheumatism, American College of Rheumatology. http://www.rheumatology.org/ar/ar.html

Lupus. http://www.lupusuk.com/

Current Opinions in Rheumatology, Lippincott Williams & Wilkins. http://www.lww.com/product/0,1255,1040%252D8711,00.html

Baillière's Best Practice & Research: Clinical Rheumatology, Elsevier. http://www.us.elsevierhealth.com

Clinical Rheumatology, Elsevier. http://www.hbuk.co.uk/journals/berh/

Websites

Arthritis Research Campaign (ARC). www.arc.org.uk

American College of Rheumatology (ACR). www.rheumatology.org

British Society of Rheumatology (BSR). www.rheumatology.org.uk

British Society of Immunology (BSI). www.immunology.org/

Hotung Centre for Musculoskeletal disorders. www.hotungcentre.sghms.ac.uk/index.htm

LUPUS UK. www.hamline.edu/lupus/strathclyde.html

Arthritis Care. www.arthritiscare.org.uk

National Rheumatoid Arthritis Society (NRAS). www.rheumatoid.org.uk

National Ankylosing Spondylitis Society (NASS). www.nass.co.uk

European League Against Rheumatism. www.eular.org

Hospital for Special Surgery. www.rheumatology.HSS.edu.

International League Against Rheumatism. www.ilar.org

Johns Hopkins Arthritis Website. www.hopkins-arthritis.org

Primary Care Rheumatology Society. www.pcrsociety.com

04

Metabolic Bone Disease

5

Introduction

Metabolic bone diseases are a heterogeneous group of disorders characterized by abnormalities in calcium metabolism and/or bone cell physiology. They lead to an altered serum calcium concentration and/or skeletal failure. The most common type of metabolic bone disease in developed countries is osteoporosis. Because osteoporosis is essentially a disease of the elderly, the prevalence of this condition is increasing as the average age of people in developed countries rises. Osteoporotic fractures may lead to loss of independence in the elderly and is imposing an ever-increasing social and economic burden on society. Other pathological processes that affect the skeleton, some of which are also relatively common, are summarized in Table 3.20 (see Chapter 4).

Structure and function

Structure of bone

Bone consists of an extracellular matrix and cellular constituents. The structure of the extracellular matrix is maintained throughout life by constant remodelling by its cellular constituents.

Extracellular matrix

● *Type 1 collagen:* forms a fibrillar structure by cross-linkage of the precursor peptide procollagen, and provides tensile strength. The fibrils are generally arranged in parallel or concentric sheets to form lamellar bone, but in newly laid 'woven bone' this arrangement appears more random.

● *Calcium- and phosphate-containing crystals:* set in a structure similar to hydroxyapatite and deposited in holes between adjacent collagen fibrils, which provide rigidity.

● *At least 11 non-collagenous matrix proteins* (e.g. osteo-calcin, osteonectin): these form the ground substance and include glycoproteins and proteoglycans. Their exact function is not yet defined, but they are thought to be involved in calcification.

Cellular constituents

● *Mesenchymal-derived osteoblast lineage:* consist of osteoblasts, osteocytes and bone-lining cells. Osteoblasts synthesize organic matrix in the production of new bone.

● *Osteoclasts:* derived from haemopoietic precursors, and resorb bone tissue by the local release of hydrolase enzymes.

Anatomy of bone

● *Cortical bone:* the external part of each bone consists of dense skeletal tissue known as cortical (compact) bone, which contributes to most of the skeleton's mechanical strength.

● *Trabecular bone:* within the vertebrae and the ends of long bones, the internal space is filled with a fine network of bone tissue called trabecular (cancellous) bone. This is in intimate contact with the bone marrow and is largely responsible for the skeleton's metabolic role as a reservoir for body calcium. In addition, trabecular elements are thought to contribute to the ability of vertebrae to withstand compressive forces, with loss of these contributing to the vertebral collapse seen in osteoporosis.

Function of bone

Bone has two main functions: to provide an endoskeleton and to act as a reservoir for body calcium (bone contains

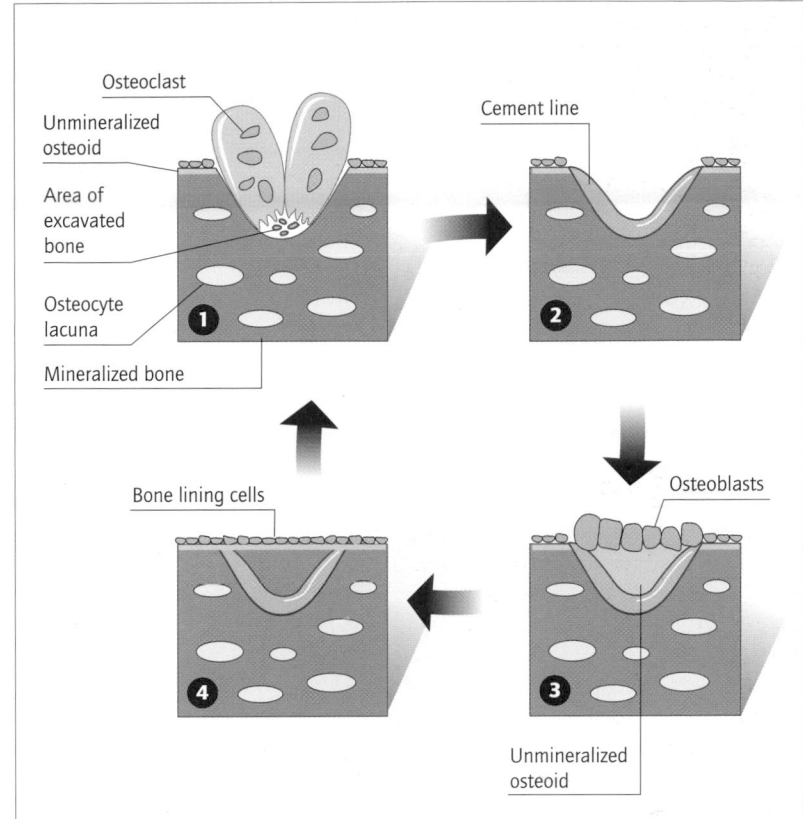

Figure 5.1 The remodelling cycle. (1) On activation of bone resorption the surface layer of unmineralized osteoid is removed and bone resorption by osteoclasts starts, the membrane of the osteoclasts taking on a ruffled appearance at the site of active bone resorption. (2) When bone resorption is complete the cement line is laid down during the reversal phase. (3) The unmineralized osteoid synthesized by osteoblasts fills the resorption cavity. (4) The osteoid is then mineralized, the bone surface finally being covered by lining cells and a thin layer of unmineralized osteoid.

1–2 kg of calcium compared with 1–2 g of calcium in the extracellular fluid). These two functions are normally independent. However, as 25% of extracellular calcium is replaced daily, prolonged calcium stress can ultimately affect skeletal integrity.

Skeletal maintenance

During growth, bone formation and resorption are regulated as part of the modelling process that results in the micro- and macroarchitecture of the adult skeleton.
- *Modelling:* involves resorption secondary to bone formation
- *Remodelling:* consists of repeated cycles of bone resorption followed by formation, at discrete sites throughout the skeleton (Fig. 5.1)

The mechanisms regulating modelling and remodelling are not clear, but local responses to mechanical stimuli are thought to have a major role.

Calcium balance

Many essential intracellular processes are critically dependent on the concentration of ionized extracellular calcium. The average western diet provides 0.5–1.0 g calcium/day; 20–40% of this is absorbed, which is usually sufficient to match minimal renal and intestinal losses (Fig. 5.2). However, if calcium intake or absorption is reduced, or requirements increase, a negative calcium balance may ensue. As powerful homoeostatic mechanisms preserve the concentration of extracellular calcium by using skeletal calcium stores, this can ultimately lead to a significant loss of calcium from bone. The homoeostatic mechanisms affecting bone include parathyroid hormone, vitamin D and other factors.

Parathyroid hormone

Parathyroid hormone (PTH) is an 84 amino acid polypeptide that is secreted by the chief cells of the parathyroid gland in response to hypocalcaemia. It is the principal regulator of extracellular calcium concentration (Fig. 5.3) and increases it by:
- Stimulating calcium release from bone by increasing osteoclast bone resorption
- Promoting renal tubular calcium reabsorption
- Increasing renal tubular phosphate excretion
- Enhancing renal conversion of 25-hydroxyvitamin D (25-OH-D) to 1,25-dihydroxyvitamin D (1,25-$(OH)_2$-D).

05

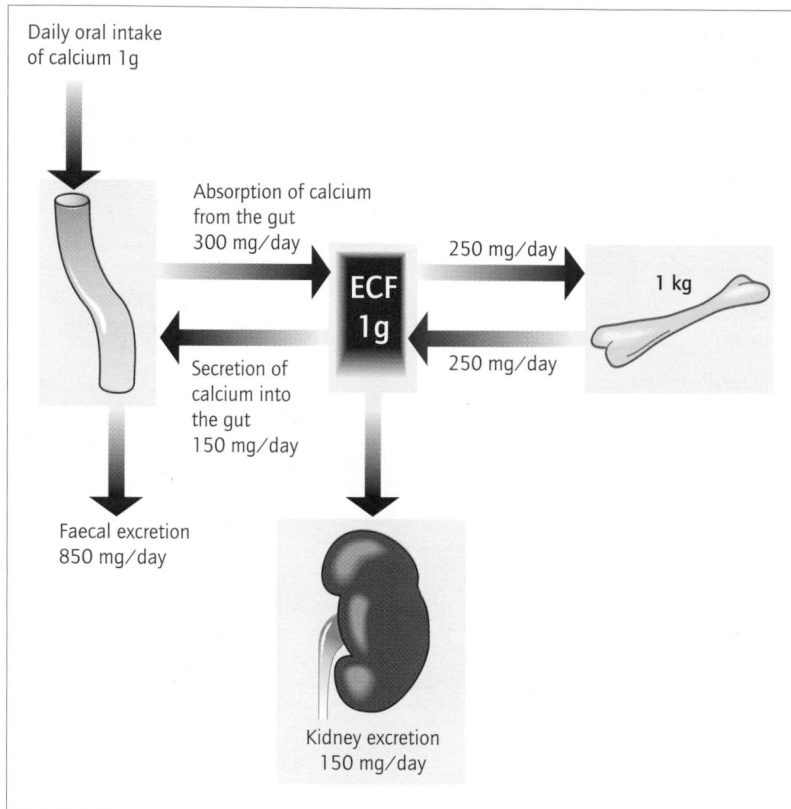

Figure 5.2 Pathways in calcium balance. The size of the extracellular fluid (ECF) and skeletal calcium compartments (1 g and 1 kg, respectively), the degree of exchange between them, the daily oral intake of calcium and the daily faecal and urinary excretion of calcium refer to a typical subject in zero calcium balance. A negative calcium balance may occur if calcium intake falls, the efficiency of calcium absorption from the gut is reduced and/or urinary calcium excretion is increased.

Vitamin D

Vitamin D is a steroid hormone, which is either ingested in the diet or produced in the skin from 7-dehydrocholesterol after exposure to sunlight.

Vitamin D is a pro-hormone; the active form (1,25-$(OH)_2$-D) is produced by successive hydroxylations in the liver and kidney by the enzymes 25-hydroxylase and 1-α-hydroxylase, respectively (Fig. 5.3). 1-α-Hydroxylase is stimulated not only by PTH, but also by low ambient inorganic phosphate, growth hormone, prolactin and oestrogen. This enables vitamin D levels to become adapted to the higher calcium requirements of growth and reproduction.

In conjunction with PTH, 1,25-$(OH)_2$-D acts to maintain serum calcium levels by:
- Increasing the efficiency of calcium absorption from the proximal small intestine
- Stimulating calcium release from bone

1,25-$(OH)_2$-D also acts to maintain phosphate levels by promoting phosphate absorption from the gut. In vitamin D deficiency, renal phosphate excretion is increased as a consequence of raised levels of PTH.

Other factors

- *Other hormones*: steroid hormones such as glucocorticoids, oestrogen and androgens are thought to influence bone metabolism
- *Local factors*: regulate bone cell activity in response to systemic hormones and mechanical strain such as members of the transforming growth factor-β (TGF-β) superfamily and osteoclast stimulatory factor
- *Local mechanical strain*: also an important controlling influence on osteoblast and osteoclast activity, with its loss in disuse states leading to rapid bone loss

Calcium measurement

Most calcium in the blood is bound or complexed to plasma proteins. However, only ionized calcium is biologically active.

Ionized serum calcium can be measured directly, but conventional analysers measure only total levels (normal range 2.2–2.6 mmol). Such total levels require correction for albumin concentration because albumin is the predominant calcium binder. The most convenient correction is to:

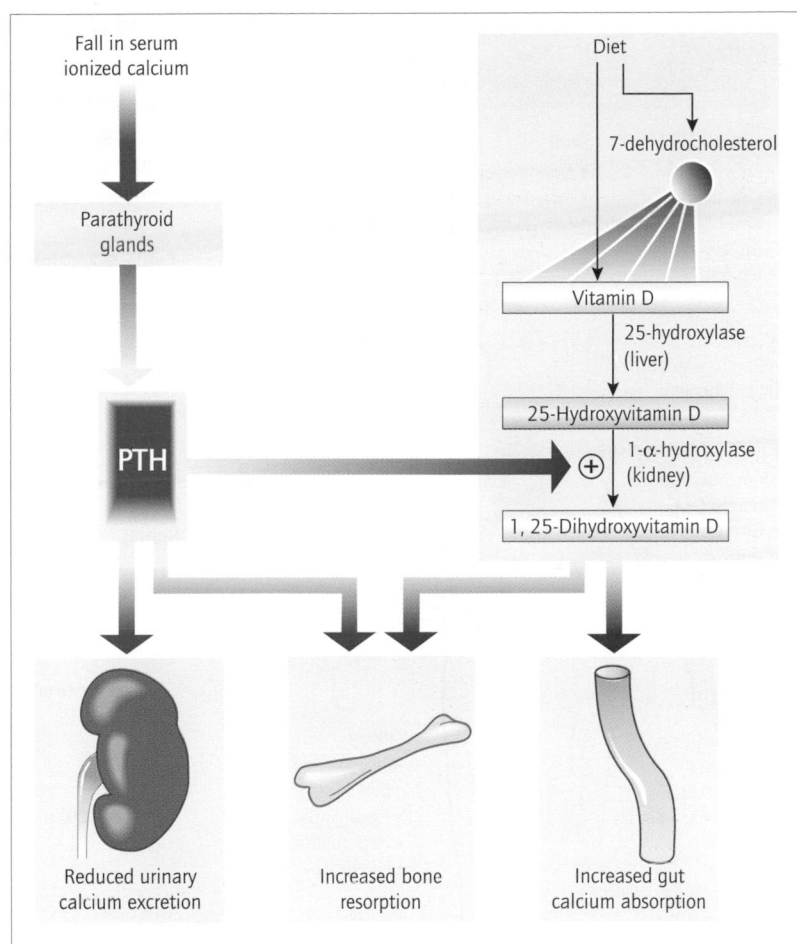

Figure 5.3 Regulation of calcium metabolism by parathyroid hormone (PTH) and vitamin D. PTH and vitamin D are the principal hormones responsible for calcium homoeostasis. Note that these two regulatory mechanisms are interdependent because of the stimulatory action of PTH on renal 1-α-hydroxylase.

● Add 0.02 mmol to the total calcium level for every g/l that the albumin is below 40 g/l
● Subtract 0.02 mmol from the total calcium level for every g/l that the albumin is above 40 g/l

Approach to the patient

History and examination

Findings from the history and examination vary according to the metabolic bone disease in question (see under separate disease headings). In general, people with chronic diseases such as rickets, osteomalacia and osteoporosis present with features specific to the musculoskeletal system such as bone pain, proximal weakness and deformity (Table 5.1). In contrast, people with disorders of short duration associated with an acute disturbance in calcium metabolism, such as hypercalcaemia of malignancy or postparathyroidectomy hypocalcaemia, present with features of hyper- or hypocalcaemia (Tables 5.2 and 5.3). Musculoskeletal features may occur in combination with long-standing symptoms of altered serum calcium concentration as in rickets and primary hyperparathyroidism. There are rare familial forms of metabolic bone disease such as X-linked hypophosphataemic rickets, so a family history should always be sought (see HISTORY & EXAMINATION BOXES 5.1 and 5.2).

05

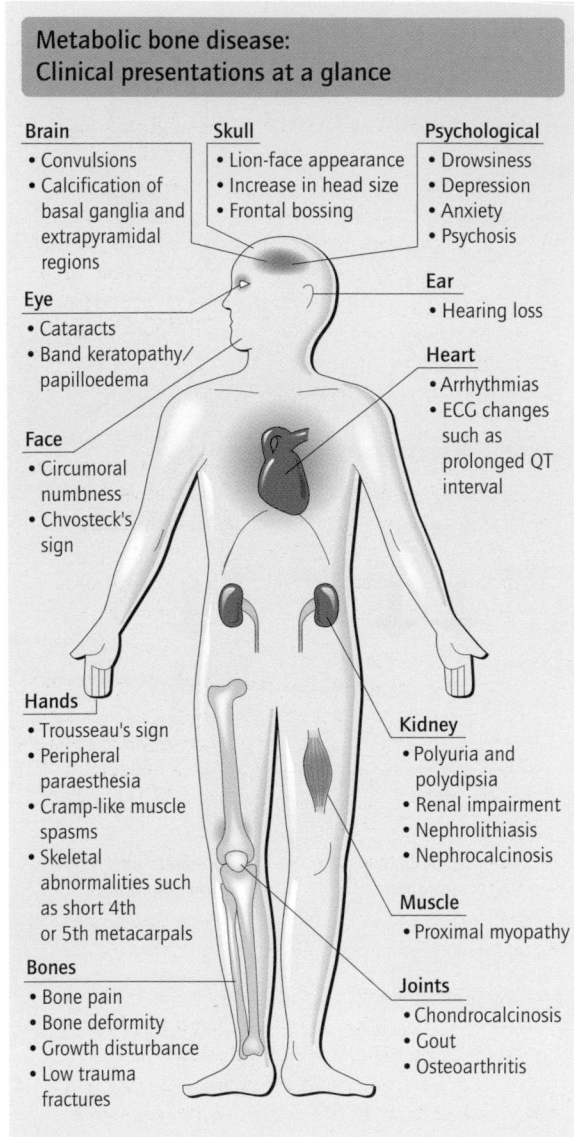

Metabolic bone disease:
Clinical presentations at a glance

Brain
- Convulsions
- Calcification of basal ganglia and extrapyramidal regions

Skull
- Lion-face appearance
- Increase in head size
- Frontal bossing

Psychological
- Drowsiness
- Depression
- Anxiety
- Psychosis

Eye
- Cataracts
- Band keratopathy/papilloedema

Ear
- Hearing loss

Face
- Circumoral numbness
- Chvosteck's sign

Heart
- Arrhythmias
- ECG changes such as prolonged QT interval

Hands
- Trousseau's sign
- Peripheral paraesthesia
- Cramp-like muscle spasms
- Skeletal abnormalities such as short 4th or 5th metacarpals

Kidney
- Polyuria and polydipsia
- Renal impairment
- Nephrolithiasis
- Nephrocalcinosis

Muscle
- Proximal myopathy

Bones
- Bone pain
- Bone deformity
- Growth disturbance
- Low trauma fractures

Joints
- Chondrocalcinosis
- Gout
- Osteoarthritis

Table 5.1 Musculoskeletal abnormalities in rickets and osteomalacia

Hypotonia, proximal muscle weakness and waddling gait
Impaired skeletal growth
Bowing deformity of long bones
Rib deformities
    Prominence of costochondral junction (rachitic rosary)
    Indentation of the lower ribs (Harrison's groove)
Kyphosis and lordosis of the thoracolumbar spine
Skull abnormalities
    Softened calvarium (craniotabes)
    Parietal flattening and frontal bossing
Delayed eruption of permanent dentition and enamel defects

Investigation

In metabolic bone disease, the findings of the history and examination are usually relatively non-specific. Further investigations are therefore needed to diagnose the nature of any underlying metabolic bone disease before starting treatment.

Table 5.2 Clinical features of hypercalcaemia

System	Feature
Neurological and psychiatric	Drowsiness and altered conscious level Headache Sleep disturbance Depression Muscle weakness Hyporeflexia
Renal	Polyuria Polydipsia Nephrolithiasis Nephrocalcinosis Renal impairment
Gastrointestinal	Constipation Nausea and anorexia Peptic ulceration Pancreatitis
Cardiovascular	Hypertension ECG abnormalities (shortened QT interval, first-degree heart block)
Articular	Chondrocalcinosis Gout
Miscellaneous	Pruritus and skin necrosis Band keratopathy

Table 5.3 Clinical features of hypocalcaemia

System	Feature

Neurological and psychiatric	Peripheral paraesthesia
	Circumoral numbness
	Tetany
	    cramp-like spasms
	    laryngeal stridor
	    Chvostek's and Trousseau's signs
	Convulsions
	Anxiety
	Psychosis
	Basal ganglia and/or extrapyramidal calcification (if long-standing)

Cardiovascular	Arrhythmias ECG abnormalities (prolonged QT interval)
Ocular	Papilloedema Cataracts (if long-standing)

History & Examination 5.1: Important questions to ask a patient with a metabolic bone disease

About symptoms

Do you have any bone, joint or muscle symptoms such as pain, tenderness or weakness? (People with metabolic bone diseases may have a history of musculoskeletal symptoms)

Have you ever broken a bone with only minimal trauma? (Low impact fractures, e.g. fall from a standing height or less, are a feature of many metabolic bone diseases)

Is your sleep disturbed? Do you have headaches? Nausea? Constipation? Do you pass much water? Are you particularly thirsty? (Ask about symptoms of hypercalcaemia that can occur with primary hyperparathyroidism or disseminated malignancy)

Do you have any pins and needles or tingling in your hands and/or feet? Do you have any numbness around your mouth? Do you have any muscle twitching or cramps? (Ask about symptoms of hypocalcaemia that can occur with severe osteomalacia, chronic renal failure or after a parathyroidectomy)

About the onset and progression of disease

When did your symptoms start? How old were you? (Onset in childhood is a feature of rickets and hereditary hypocalcaemic disorders)

Over how long have your symptoms been getting worse? (Metabolic bone diseases usually progress slowly over months or years but hypercalcaemia of malignancy can progress rapidly)

About past medical history

Do you have or have you had any intestinal or liver disorder? (Osteomalacia and osteoporosis are relatively common complications of gastrointestinal diseases associated with malabsorption and/or liver dysfunction)

Do you have or have you had any kidney disorders? (Chronic renal failure can cause osteomalacia and/or hypocalcaemia)

Have you had cancer, and if so what sort? (Patients with hypercalcaemia should be asked about a history of malignancy, particularly breast or lung cancer)

What age were you at your menopause and were your periods previously regular? Have you ever had a disorder of the thyroid or adrenal gland? (Osteoporosis can occur at a relatively young age following hysterectomy and in association with ovarian dysfunction. It may also occur in association with endocrine disorders such as hyperthyroidism and Cushing's disease)

About drug history

Have you received treatment for epilepsy? Have you received prolonged treatment with steroids? What medicines and tonics are you currently taking? (Glucocorticoids can cause osteoporosis; use of phenytoin can lead to osteomalacia; hypercalcaemia can result from vitamin A or D intoxication, antacids and thiazide diuretics)

About social history

Do you have a balanced diet? (A poor diet lacking in vitamin D-enriched foods such as milk products and cereals can cause osteomalacia. Osteomalacia is also associated with a strict vegetarian diet and increased intake of phytic acid, which are common in certain Asian populations. Calcium insufficiency in the elderly is common)

Do you smoke and if so how much? Do you drink alcohol and if so how much? Do you take regular exercise? (Osteoporosis is associated with cigarette smoking, increased alcohol intake and lack of exercise)

About family history

Has anyone in your family had similar symptoms? (Rare metabolic bone diseases can be inherited, e.g. X-linked hypophosphataemic rickets and primary hyperparathyroidism may be part of multiple endocrine neoplasia (MEN) which is autosomal dominant)

Has your mother broken her hip? (There is an increased risk of osteoporosis associated with maternal hip fracture)

05

Haematology

Full blood count. Anaemia can be caused by conditions that underlie metabolic bone disease such as gastrointestinal malabsorption and chronic renal failure. It is not a direct result of the metabolic bone disease itself.

Biochemistry

Serum biochemistry results are frequently diagnostic of the underlying metabolic bone disease (Table 5.4):

- *Serum creatinine:* may be elevated in associated chronic renal failure or multiple myeloma, or caused by dehydration resulting from polyuria resulting from hypercalcaemia.
- *Serum calcium:* may be increased (Table 5.5), normal in osteoporosis or decreased (Table 5.6).
- *Serum phosphate:* increased in chronic renal failure and hypoparathyroidism, and decreased in primary hyperparathyroidism and hyperparathyroidism secondary to deficiency, malabsorption or abnormal metabolism of vitamin D.
- *Serum alkaline phosphatase:* increased when there is

History & Examination 5.2: Examination of a patient with a metabolic bone disease

General examination

Is there evidence of underlying gastrointestinal disease? [Look for cholestasis (see EXAMINATION BOX 9.1) or signs of malnutrition]

Is there evidence of endocrine disorders? [Such as Cushing's disease (see p. 852) and hyperthyroidism (see p. 843)]

Is there evidence of malignancy? [Such as lung or breast the patient has hypercalcaemia]

Is there evidence of renal disease? [If the patient has osteomalacia and/or hypocalcaemia]

Neurological examination

Look for signs of hypercalcaemia such as hyporeflexia and band keratopathy (in long-standing cases)

Look for signs of hypocalcaemia such as papilloedema and tetany

Look for hypotonia and proximal myopathy, which are features of rickets and osteomalacia

Examination of the locomotor system

General

Stunted growth, rib deformities and long bone deformities occur in rickets. Abnormal skeletal development is a feature of congenital disorders such as pseudohypo-parathyroidism

Record the patient's height

Height records are of vital importance in the diagnosis and monitoring of metabolic bone disease in both children and adults. Normally, height is equal to span

Observe the gait

A waddling gait is a feature of rickets and osteomalacia, and occurs secondary to skeletal deformity and/or proximal myopathy

Look at the spine

A kyphotic deformity is a common feature of osteoporosis

	Calcium	Phosphate	ALP	PTH
Osteomalacia	N or ↓	↓	↑	↑
Osteoporosis	N	N	N	N
Hyperparathyroidism	↑	↓	↑	↑
Hypercalcaemia of malignancy	↑	N or ↓	N or ↑	↓
Hypoparathyroidism	↓	↑	N	↓

Table 5.4 Serum biochemistry in metabolic bone disease

↑ Increased; ↓ decreased; ALP, alkaline phosphatase; N, normal; PTH, parathyroid hormone.

osteoblastic hyperactivity (e.g. in osteomalacia/rickets, hyperparathyroidism, osteoblastic skeletal malignant deposits).

• *Serum PTH:* increased in deficiency, malabsorption or abnormal metabolism of vitamin D, and in primary, secondary and tertiary hyperparathyroidism; it is reduced in hypocalcaemia resulting from hypoparathyroidism. Relatively rapid degradation of PTH can result in falsely low levels of PTH where the assay uses an antibody against intact PTH.

• *Serum 25-OH-D levels:* may be increased or reduced in abnormal vitamin D metabolism, according to the site of the metabolic defect. 25-OH-D levels are measured in preference to other vitamin D metabolites because they give a better reflection of current vitamin D nutritional status.

• *Bone markers:* urinary and serum markers such as telopeptides (e.g. N-telopeptide) measure breakdown products of type I collagen and indicate the level of bone resorption. They can be used to measure the effectiveness of therapy with antiresorptive agents such as bisphosphonates.

Diagnostic imaging

Plain radiography

Metabolic bone disease can be associated with adverse effects on the skeleton that can be readily recognized on plain radiographs. Although changes such as low bone density are non-specific, specific changes pointing to a particular diagnosis such as Looser's zones in osteomalacia may be evident.

Isotope bone scan

Metabolic bone diseases can be associated with local areas of increased technetium uptake, especially if there are associated fractures. Widespread changes are most commonly a result of skeletal secondary malignant deposits but also occur in osteomalacia and Paget's disease of bone.

Bone densitometry

A number of techniques have been developed to quantify the amount of bone mineral present at a given skeletal site, from which other values such as bone mineral density can be derived. They largely consist of dual energy X-ray

Table 5.5 Causes of hypercalcaemia

Endocrine disorders
Primary hyperparathyroidism
Tertiary hyperparathyroidism
Hyperthyroidism
Addison's disease
Phaeochromocytoma

Malignancy
Solid tumours, especially breast and lung
Haematological tumours

Drugs
Thiazides
Lithium
Theophylline toxicity
Vitamin A intoxication
Vitamin D intoxication

Renal disorders
Acute and chronic renal failure

Granulomatous disorders
Sarcoidosis
Tuberculosis
Histoplasmosis

Familial
Multiple endocrine neoplasia (MEN) I and II
Familial hypocalciuric hypercalcaemia

Prolonged immobilization
Paget's disease of bone
Young patients

Table 5.6 Causes of hypocalcaemia

Vitamin D-dependent
Vitamin D deficiency or malabsorption
Impaired vitamin D metabolism
    Chronic renal failure
    Chronic liver failure
    Phenytoin
    Congenital renal 1-α-hydroxylase deficiency

Hypoparathyroidism/PTH resistance
Hypoparathyroidism
    Postoperative
    Idiopathic
DiGeorge's syndrome
Infiltrative (e.g. haemochromatosis)
Hypomagnesaemia
Pseudohypoparathyroidism

Miscellaneous
Phosphate therapy
Acute rhabdomyolysis
Pancreatitis
Massive citrated blood transfusion

it is invasive and so its use is generally confined to patients in whom there is diagnostic difficulty.

Management

Lifestyle modification

Lifestyle modification is an important aspect of management of all diseases. In metabolic bone diseases it can be very useful but should not be used in isolation; correction of dietary deficiency of calcium and vitamin D, stopping smoking, reducing alcohol consumption and increasing exercise is beneficial in patients with osteoporosis.

Physiotherapy

Increasing exercise capacity is important for all patients with skeletal diseases. Improving strength and balance can help prevent fractures by decreasing the likelihood of falls. Transcutaneous electrical nerve stimulation (TENS) and acupuncture, for example, can all help in the management of skeletal pain.

Occupational therapy

A thorough assessment of impairment and disability can be provided by occupational therapists so that intervention is appropriate to the social context.

Drug treatments

Drug treatment in metabolic bone disease is aimed

absorptiometry (DXA) and ultrasound-based approaches to assess fracture risk when preventative therapy is being considered.

DXA measures bone mineral density (BMD), which is bone mineral content partially corrected for size, either centrally (spinal BMD) or peripherally (forearm or heel BMD). Quantitative ultrasound analyses transmission of high-frequency sound through bone at the calcaneus, phalanges and other skeletal sites.

Histopathology

Bone biopsy

Because metabolic bone diseases generally affect the whole skeleton, the underlying diagnosis can usually be confirmed by performing a bone biopsy at a convenient site such as the iliac crest. In this way, abnormalities such as defective osteoid mineralization, loss of trabecular bone and excessive osteoclastic activity can be detected. However, although bone biopsy may be the most accurate means of defining an underlying metabolic bone disease,

05

at correcting the underlying metabolic disturbance, which may be calcium deficiency, vitamin D deficiency, malabsorption or abnormal metabolism, or a result of excessive bone breakdown. Brief information is presented below; however the information—especially that relating to adverse effects and contraindications—is not complete. Fuller information is given in a formulary; for example, the *British National Formulary* (*BNF*). Drug regimens should also be checked in the *BNF*.

Bisphosphonates

The bisphosphonates disodium etidronate, risedronate sodium, alendronic acid and intravenous disodium pamidronate are used for the prevention and treatment of postmenopausal osteoporosis including corticosteroid-induced osteoporosis. Alendronic acid is also licensed for the prevention and treatment of osteoporosis in men. In addition, bisphosphonates can be used in Paget's disease of bone (e.g. risedronate sodium or tiludronic acid) or hypercalcaemia of malignancy (e.g. intravenous disodium pamidronate).

The main adverse effects are on the gastrointestinal system, ranging from nausea to oesophageal ulceration and stricture formation. They are contraindicated in pregnancy and breastfeeding, and should be used with caution in renal impairment or hypocalcaemic states.

Hormone replacement therapy and selective oestrogen receptor modulators

Hormone replacement therapy (HRT) may be useful in postmenopausal women at risk of osteoporosis. Selective oestrogen receptor modulators (SERMs) such as raloxifene are indicated for the prevention of postmenopausal osteoporosis and the treatment of osteoporotic fractures in postmenopausal women. Adverse effects include thromboembolism, leg cramps and mastalgia. HRT is contraindicated in women with oestrogen-dependent cancers (e.g. breast) and both HRT and SERMs should not be used in women with active thromboembolic disorders.

Calcium

Calcium salts are used where there is dietary deficiency of calcium, and also in the treatment of osteoporosis and chronic hypocalcaemia. Adverse effects are mild and usually related to gastrointestinal upset.

Vitamin D and its metabolites

Vitamin D (cholecalciferol) and its metabolites (ergocalciferol, alfacalcidol, calcitriol, dihydrotachysterol) are used in dietary deficiency of vitamin D, chronic renal failure, vitamin D malabsorption or abnormal metabolism, and in hypoparathyroidism. It can be given orally or via the intramuscular approach. Adverse effects include symptoms of hypercalcaemia from overdosage, and so it is contraindicated in hypercalcaemia or hypercalciuria.

Calcitonin

Calcitonin is given via subcutaneous injection, or intranasally for the treatment of hypercalcaemia, postmenopausal osteoporosis or Paget's disease of bone. Adverse effects include inflammatory reactions at injection sites and nausea or diarrhoea.

Surgery

(See primary hyperparathyroidism, p. 293.)

Diseases and their management

Rickets and osteomalacia

Rickets and osteomalacia consist of a number of heterogeneous disorders characterized by defective mineralization of newly synthesized organic bone matrix. Rickets results when defective mineralization during skeletal growth leads to impaired epiphyseal growth plate calcification and bony deformity. Osteomalacia refers to defective mineralization of the adult skeleton.

Epidemiology

Prevalence. Osteomalacia and rickets brought about by dietary deficiency are relatively common. Non-nutritional causes are rare.

Age. In childhood and the elderly.

Sex. X-linked hypophosphataemic rickets most commonly affects males.

Race. Osteomalacia is relatively common amongst Asian immigrants in the UK.

Genetics. Rare causes may be familial (e.g. congenital renal 1-α-hydroxylase deficiency, hypophosphatasia, hereditary renal tubular disorders).

Geography. Vitamin D deficiency is most frequently seen in those developing countries where food is not fortified with vitamin D and reduced sunlight exposure is common.

Disease mechanisms

The cause of osteomalacia and rickets is usually a reduced serum level of $1,25\text{-}(OH)_2\text{-}D$. This results in lowering of the calcium-phosphate product to below normal, leading to impaired matrix mineralization. A direct effect of $1,25\text{-}(OH)_2\text{-}D$ on osteoblast activity and the mineralization process has also been suggested.

There are many causes of reduced $1,25\text{-}(OH)_2\text{-}D$ levels (Table 5.7). Insufficient dietary intake of vitamin D associated with reduced skin synthesis because of low levels of sunlight is the most common. Rarely, rickets and osteomalacia are unrelated to deficiency or abnormal metabolism of vitamin D (e.g. excessive use of phosphate-binding antacids).

Skeletal deformities caused by childhood rickets are now rare since the widespread supplementation of food and milk with vitamin D. However, osteomalacia is relat-ively common amongst the elderly and in immigrant Asian populations, especially those who adhere to a strict vegetarian diet.

Rickets and osteomalacia are characterized by defective mineralization of newly synthesized organic bone matrix. This leads to impaired epiphyseal growth in children, resulting in the characteristic skeletal deformities of rickets. In adults, unmineralized osteoid accumulates on bone surfaces, leading to a deficit in skeletal bone mineral. Ultimately, this compromises the mechanical strength of the skeleton, resulting in an increased susceptibility to fractures.

Clinical features

The clinical features of rickets are impaired skeletal growth, bony deformities such as bowing of long bones and rib deformities (rachitic rosary, Harrison's groove) (Table 5.1), weakness and symptoms of hypocalcaemia (see Table 5.3).

Osteomalacia is characterized by widespread bone pain and tenderness, muscle weakness, proximal myopathy (causing a waddling gait) and an increased risk of fracture.

Diagnosis

Childhood rickets is readily diagnosed from its characteristic skeletal deformities. However, the clinical manifestations of osteomalacia in the adult are relatively non-specific. Although typical radiographical changes such as Looser's zones may be seen, osteomalacia is most commonly diagnosed from serum biochemistry on the basis of a decreased phosphate concentration and an elevated alkaline phosphatase. Measurement of 25-OH-D provides useful confirmatory evidence of vitamin D deficiency, but this may be normal (e.g. in chronic renal failure). Iliac crest bone biopsy should be carried out if there is diagnostic difficulty.

Differential diagnosis

The differential diagnosis of osteomalacia includes:
- Other causes of proximal myopathy (see p. 954)
- Other causes of increased skeletal fragility (Table 5.8)

Investigation

If vitamin D deficiency is confirmed, further investigation to detect malabsorption is indicated if dietary deficiency seems unlikely, or if there are other features to suggest malabsorption (e.g. a history of gastric surgery, associated iron or folic acid deficiency).

If vitamin D levels are normal in a child with rickets, primary urinary phosphate wasting is the probable cause. Further studies of renal tubular function should then be

---

Table 5.7 Causes of rickets and osteomalacia

Vitamin D deficiency
Increased vitamin D requirements in childhood because of skeletal growth
Poor diet combined with reduced sunlight exposure

Vitamin D malabsorption
Gastric surgery
Small bowel malabsorption syndrome (e.g. coeliac disease, Crohn's disease)
Chronic cholestasis
Chronic pancreatic insufficiency

Impaired vitamin D metabolism
Chronic renal failure
Chronic liver failure
Drugs (e.g. phenytoin, barbiturates)
Congenital renal 1-α-hydroxylase deficiency (vitamin D-dependent rickets)

Drugs, toxins
Fluoride therapy
Bisphosphonates
Aluminium poisoning

Hypophosphataemia
Isolated renal tubular defects in phosphate handling (e.g. X-linked hypophosphataemic vitamin D-dependent rickets)
Urinary phosphate wasting resulting from a generalized renal tubular defect (Fanconi's syndrome)

Miscellaneous
Distal renal tubular acidosis
Hypophosphatasia (inherited alkaline phosphatase deficiency)
Malignancy

Rickets and osteomalacia at a glance

A heterogeneous group of disorders characterized by defective bone matrix mineralization. Rickets occurs in childhood and consequent bone softening leads to characteristic skeletal deformities. Osteomalacia is defective mineralization of the adult skeleton.

Epidemiology

Prevalence
Nutritional vitamin D deficiency is common

Age
In childhood and the elderly

Race
Asian immigrants in the UK are particularly at risk

Genetics
Rare causes may be familial

Geography
Nutritional vitamin D deficiency in childhood is largely confined to developing countries

Aetiology

Dietary
Dietary deficiency of vitamin D combined with reduced vitamin D skin synthesis because of poor sunlight exposure

Malabsorption
Of vitamin D

Impaired vitamin D metabolism

Hypophosphataemia

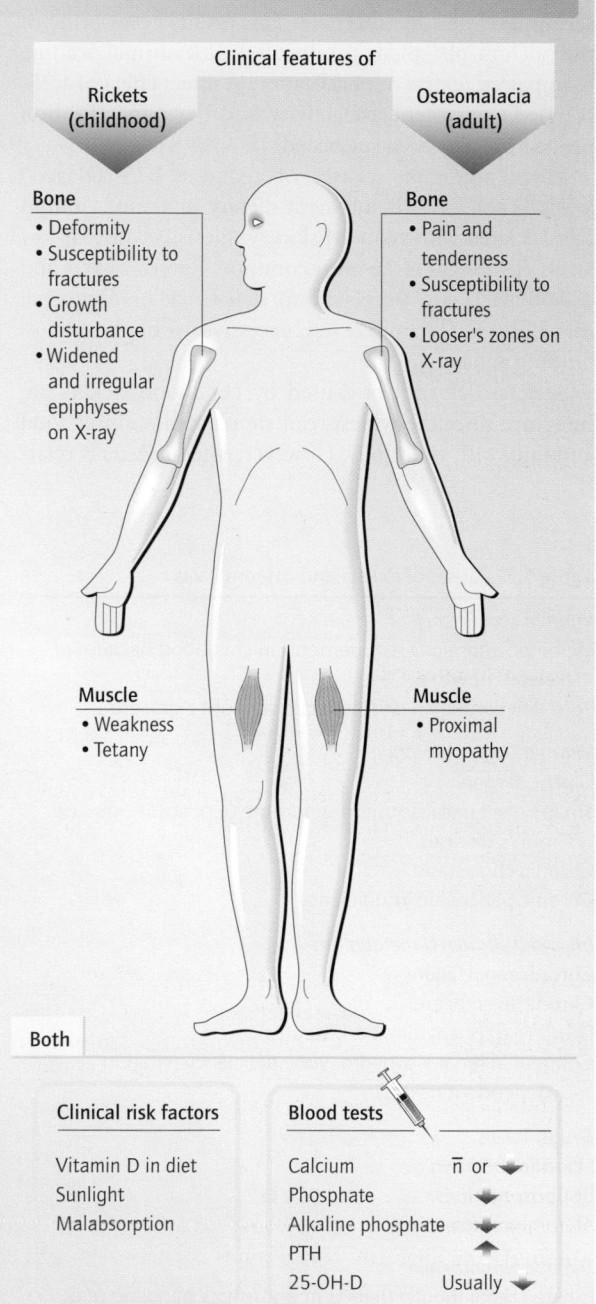

Clinical features of

Rickets (childhood)

Bone
- Deformity
- Susceptibility to fractures
- Growth disturbance
- Widened and irregular epiphyses on X-ray

Muscle
- Weakness
- Tetany

Osteomalacia (adult)

Bone
- Pain and tenderness
- Susceptibility to fractures
- Looser's zones on X-ray

Muscle
- Proximal myopathy

Both

Clinical risk factors	Blood tests	
Vitamin D in diet	Calcium	n̄ or ⬇
Sunlight	Phosphate	⬇
Malabsorption	Alkaline phosphate	⬇
	PTH	⬆
	25-OH-D	Usually ⬇

carried out to investigate whether this is part of a generalized tubular disorder (e.g. Fanconi's syndrome).

Haematology

There may be evidence of associated iron or folic acid deficiency if malabsorption is responsible.

Biochemistry

- *Serum calcium:* usually at the lower end of the normal range, but in children there can be a severe hypocalcaemia
- *Serum phosphate:* reduced in the absence of renal failure
- *Serum alkaline phosphatase:* may be elevated
- *Serum PTH:* elevated

05

Table 5.8 Common causes for an increased fracture tendency

Increased skeletal fragility
Osteoporosis
Osteomalacia
Malignant deposits
Paget's disease of bone

Increased risk of falling
Neurological disorders
   Stroke
   Cognitive impairment
   Parkinson's disease
Poor visual acuity
Locomotor disorders and other causes of postural instability
Cardiovascular disease
Drugs
   Diuretics
   Antihypertensives
   Sedatives

- *Serum 25-OH-D:* usually reduced in vitamin D deficiency or malabsorption

Diagnostic imaging
Plain radiography may show:
- Appearance of low density because of impaired mineralization and may resemble that of osteoporosis
- Bone deformity and widened irregular epiphyses in rickets
- Pseudofractures (Looser's zones) in osteomalacia most commonly seen in the scapulae, ribs, pubic rami and proximal femur.

Histopathology
Iliac crest bone biopsy can be useful if there is diagnostic difficulty. Impaired mineralization of collagenous bone matrix leads to its accumulation on actively forming bone surfaces. This is recognized as a widening of the layer of unmineralized osteoid on undecalcified sections.

Management
Dietary deficiency of vitamin D
Dietary vitamin D deficiency is readily corrected by giving vitamin D supplements. Body stores of vitamin D can be replenished by administering a single oral dose of ergocalciferol (vitamin D_2) 150 000–300 000 IU (1.25 mg). Low-dose ergocalciferol 200–400 IU (5–10 µg/day), which is available in combination with calcium supplements, should be taken if a continued dietary deficiency is anticipated. Regular administration of high-dose vitamin D should be avoided as it can cause hypercalciuria and/or hypercalcaemia.

Vitamin D malabsorption
Vitamin D malabsorption can usually be overcome with daily high-dose vitamin D and calcium supplements taken orally, although parenteral administration may be necessary. Alternatively, small doses of more potent metabolites such as calcitriol (1,25-$(OH)_2$-D) and alfacalcidol (1-α-OH-vitamin D) may be used. In either case, serum calcium should be regularly monitored.

Osteomalacia associated with renal disease
Although many forms of renal disease respond to high-dose vitamin D supplementation, there is often significant 1-α-hydroxylase deficiency and so α-hydroxylated vitamin derivatives (e.g. calcitriol or alfacalcidol) should be prescribed.

Prognosis
Vitamin D deficiency resulting from dietary deficiency or malabsorption usually responds well to vitamin D replacement. Osteomalacia associated with chronic renal failure can be difficult to manage in the long term, particularly if there is associated hypocalcaemia, which may be hard to correct.

Osteoporosis

Osteoporosis can be defined as a decrease in the quantity of bone per unit volume that is sufficient to compromise its mechanical function. The bone tissue is mineralized normally, but there is not enough of it to preserve the normal skeletal architecture.

Epidemiology
Prevalence. Thirty per cent of women living in developed countries are likely to sustain an osteoporotic fracture at some time in their life.

Age. Osteoporotic fractures are more common with increasing age. The annual UK incidence of hip fractures is 4.3/100 000 women aged 45–64 years, rising to 90.1/100 000 women aged 75–85 years. UK prevalence of vertebral fractures rises from 1–2% in women aged 44–54 years, to more than 10% in women over 65 years of age.

Sex. Osteoporotic fractures at all sites are more common in women than men (about 70% occur in women).

Race. The incidence of osteoporotic fractures is similar in different ethnic groups living in the same country, except in Afro-Caribbeans in whom it is relatively low.

Genetics. There may be a family history, and twin studies suggest a significant genetic component.

Geography. Osteoporosis is most common in developed countries.

Table 5.9 Causes of secondary osteoporosis

Endocrine causes
Cushing's disease
Thyrotoxicosis
Hypogonadism
Hyperparathyroidism

Drugs
Glucocorticoids
Heparin
Antiepileptics

Inflammatory
Rheumatoid arthritis
Ankylosing spondylitis
Ulcerative colitis

Gastrointestinal
Malabsorption
Primary biliary cirrhosis

Hereditary causes
Osteogenesis imperfecta
Homocystinuria
Ehlers–Danlos syndrome

Miscellaneous
Chronic renal failure
Immobilization (e.g. long-term bed rest)
Weightlessness (e.g. astronauts)
Alcohol

Table 5.10 Predisposing factors for postmenopausal osteoporosis

Age
Family history of osteoporosis (particularly history of maternal hip fracture)
Episodes of unexplained amenorrhoea for more than 6 months
Early menopause
Low calcium and vitamin D dietary intake
Smoking
Prolonged immobilization

Classification
Idiopathic osteoporosis
Osteoporosis usually occurs in the absence of any disorder known to cause osteoporosis (Table 5.9), when it is termed idiopathic osteoporosis. A combination of low adult peak bone mass and excessive age-related bone mass is thought to be responsible. Because bone loss is relatively rapid for 5–10 years following the menopause, idiopathic osteoporosis is most common in postmenopausal women (postmenopausal osteoporosis). A number of factors that predispose to postmenopausal osteoporosis by adversely affecting peak bone mass or subsequent bone loss have been identified (Table 5.10). Occasionally, idiopathic osteoporosis occurs in childhood before puberty (juvenile osteoporosis), and in younger adults of either sex when the cause is unknown.

Secondary osteoporosis
Secondary osteoporosis develops as a result of a disorder known to cause osteoporosis. Of these disorders ovarian hormone deficiency (premature ovarian failure) and glucocorticoid treatment are relatively common (Table 5.9).

Localized osteoporosis
Localized osteoporosis frequently develops where a limb is immobilized, such as after wearing a plaster cast, and in association with paraplegia and poliomyelitis. Localized osteoporosis can also be caused by algodystrophy (reflex sympathetic dystrophy, Sudeck's atrophy), whereby pain, swelling and autonomic dysfunction of a limb extremity develops after a precipitating event such as trauma.

Transient regional osteoporosis can occur in association with pregnancy. The spine and hip are the most commonly involved sites, and bone loss may largely recover.

Disease mechanisms
Osteoporosis arises as a result of a low peak bone mass and/or excessive bone loss.
- *Low peak bone mass:* insufficient bone tissue is formed during skeletal development. This may be because of genetic or environmental factors such as poor dietary calcium intake.
- *Excessive bone loss:* bone loss normally occurs as an age-related process following the attainment of peak bone mass. It may be excessive resulting from elevated bone resorption and/or reduced bone formation.

A significant reduction in bone mass (osteopaenia) does not necessarily cause any adverse effects. However, it is usually associated with an increase in skeletal fragility. This leads to a high risk of skeletal fractures, resulting in low trauma fractures and established osteoporosis. Any bone can be involved, but fractures of the hip, wrist and vertebral bodies are the most common.

Clinical features
Osteoporosis may predispose to fractures of any part of the skeleton. The most common sites are vertebral bodies, wrist and hip:

Vertebral body osteoporosis. This leads to wedge fractures of the vertebral body that may progress to near-complete vertebral body collapse. It is particularly associated with osteoporosis secondary to sex-hormone deficiency or glucocorticoid excess, and patients present either with sudden pain during an episode of vertebral collapse, or with a

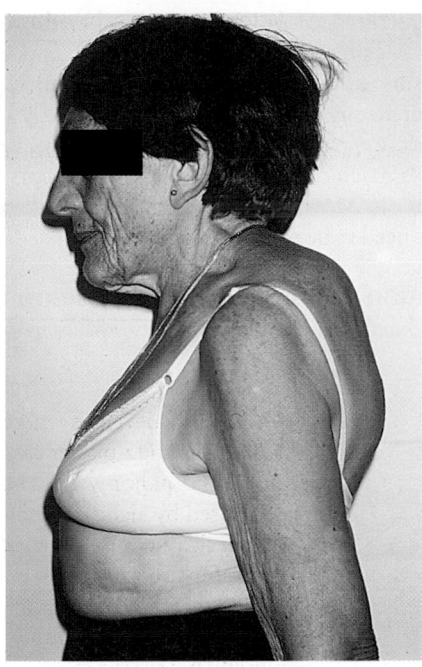

Figure 5.4 Dowager's hump. Kyphotic deformity of the thoracic spine in a patient with osteoporosis.

progressive kyphotic deformity (dowager's hump) associated with a loss of height (Fig. 5.4). The cumulative effect of vertebral collapse and associated deformity may reduce mobility. Although spinal cord compression is extremely rare, aggravation of nerve root irritation resulting from coexisting lumbar spondylosis is relatively common.

Wrist osteoporosis. A Colles' fracture in a middle-aged woman should be assumed to be secondary to osteoporosis until proven otherwise.

Hip osteoporosis. Osteoporotic hip fractures usually occur in people over 65 years of age. The risk of such fractures is considerably influenced by the presence of factors that increase the risk of falling (Table 5.8).

Diagnosis

Osteoporosis should be considered when a person in a high-risk group for osteoporosis (e.g. postmenopausal women) presents with a fracture at a typical site such as the hip, wrist or spine associated with relatively low levels of trauma (e.g. falling from a standing height).

Differential diagnosis

Secondary causes of osteoporosis should be excluded by clinical assessment and serum biochemistry.

Other causes of increased skeletal fragility should be considered for minimal-trauma fractures, particularly

those of the vertebrae (Table 5.8). In general, symptoms from a single episode of osteoporotic vertebral body collapse tend to improve over a few days, whereas malignant spinal deposits cause continuous pain that fails to resolve. In addition, laboratory investigations may be helpful (e.g. to exclude osteomalacia and multiple myeloma).

Investigation
Haematology
Full blood count is normal.

Biochemistry
- *Serum biochemistry:* characteristically normal
- *Serum alkaline phosphatase:* may be marginally elevated if there has been a recent fracture

Diagnostic imaging
Plain radiography. This is essential for the diagnosis of a fracture. In patients with established osteoporosis, early changes consist of wedge fractures and/or vertebral body height loss. In patients with more advanced osteoporosis, marked vertebral body compression or biconcave vertebral body fractures may occur. Plain radiographs may also be suggestive of osteopaenia, pointing to an underlying diagnosis of osteoporosis.

Isotope bone scan. This may differentiate between vertebral body collapse resulting from osteoporosis and that from malignant deposits. Multiple areas of uptake throughout the skeleton suggest malignancy.

Bone densitometry. This may reveal that the bone mineral density is below the threshold for diagnosis of osteoporosis according to the World Health Organization (WHO) criteria defining those who need further treatment (Fig. 5.5). Bone densitometry has also been used as a means of

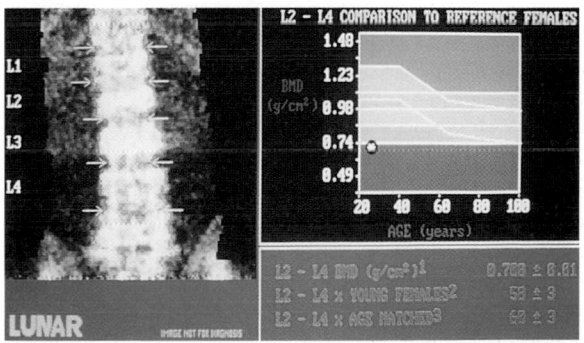

Figure 5.5 Bone densitometry. Bone densitometer reading of a female patient with spinal osteoporosis. Note the normal range for bone mineral density (BMD) at different ages (blue band) and the patient's result plotted according to age.

assessing future risk of osteoporosis in those with other risk factors, thereby targeting possible patients for preventive therapy (Table 5.10).

Histopathology

Iliac crest bone biopsy. This is useful for distinguishing between osteoporosis, osteomalacia, malignant deposits and Paget's disease of bone. Osteoporosis is seen as a generalized loss of trabecular bone and thinning of the cortex. However, a bone biopsy is only indicated if there is diagnostic difficulty.

Management of acute vertebral collapse

Initially, this should be treated with bed rest and analgesia followed by early mobilization. In addition, calcitonin by subcutaneous injection or intranasally may be given during acute episodes to relieve bone pain. Physiotherapy and TENs machines can play an important part in early mobilization. Measures to prevent further osteoporotic fractures need to be remembered.

Prevention of postmenopausal osteoporosis

Lifestyle modification. This is an important part of the

Osteoporosis at a glance

A decrease in the amount of bone tissue, resulting in a reduction of skeletal strength and an increased tendency to sustain fragility fractures.

Epidemiology

Prevalence
Occurs in up to 30% of menopausal women

Age
Predominantly a disease of the elderly

Race
Low prevalence in Afro-Caribbeans

Genetics
Significant genetic component

Geography
Most common in developed countries

Aetiology

Idiopathic osteoporosis
Most commonly affects postmenopausal women

Secondary osteoporosis
Endocrine disorders: sex hormone deficiency, Cushing's syndrome and thyrotoxicosis
Prolonged treatment with glucocorticoids
Metabolic disorders: chronic renal failure, malabsorption states
Hereditary causes: osteogenesis imperfecta, homocystinuria, Ehlers–Danlos syndrome
Miscellaneous: multiple myeloma, arthritides, alcoholism, chronic heparin therapy, systemic mastocytosis, anorexia nervosa

Localized osteoporosis
Limb immobilization
Algodystrophy (reflex sympathetic dystrophy, Sudeck's atrophy)
Transient regional osteoporosis

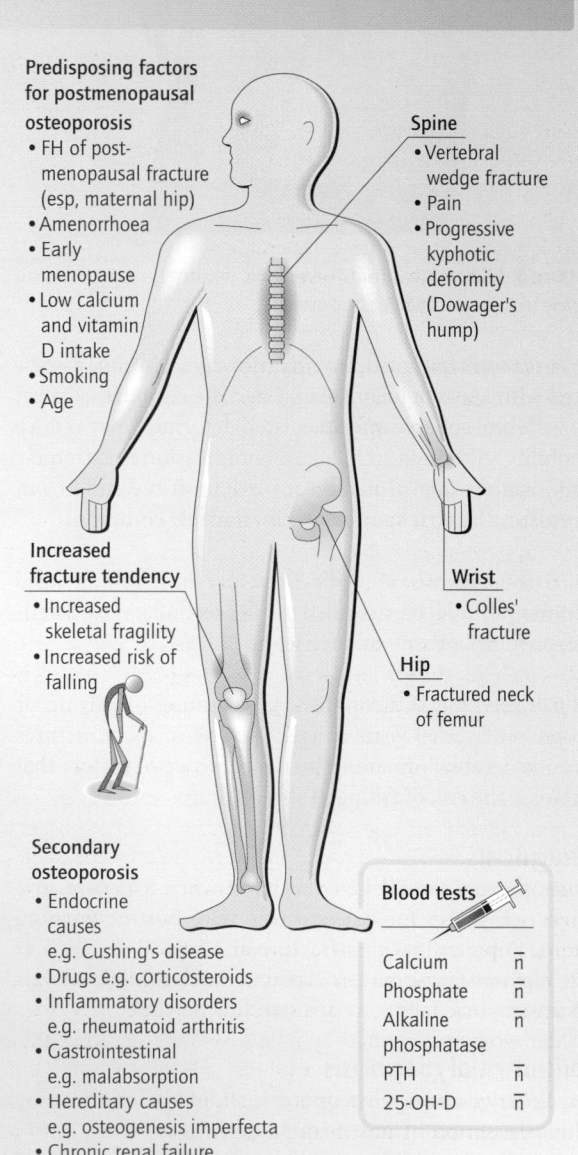

Predisposing factors for postmenopausal osteoporosis
- FH of post-menopausal fracture (esp, maternal hip)
- Amenorrhoea
- Early menopause
- Low calcium and vitamin D intake
- Smoking
- Age

Spine
- Vertebral wedge fracture
- Pain
- Progressive kyphotic deformity (Dowager's hump)

Increased fracture tendency
- Increased skeletal fragility
- Increased risk of falling

Wrist
- Colles' fracture

Hip
- Fractured neck of femur

Secondary osteoporosis
- Endocrine causes e.g. Cushing's disease
- Drugs e.g. corticosteroids
- Inflammatory disorders e.g. rheumatoid arthritis
- Gastrointestinal e.g. malabsorption
- Hereditary causes e.g. osteogenesis imperfecta
- Chronic renal failure

Blood tests

Calcium	n̄
Phosphate	n̄
Alkaline phosphatase	n̄
PTH	n̄
25-OH-D	n̄

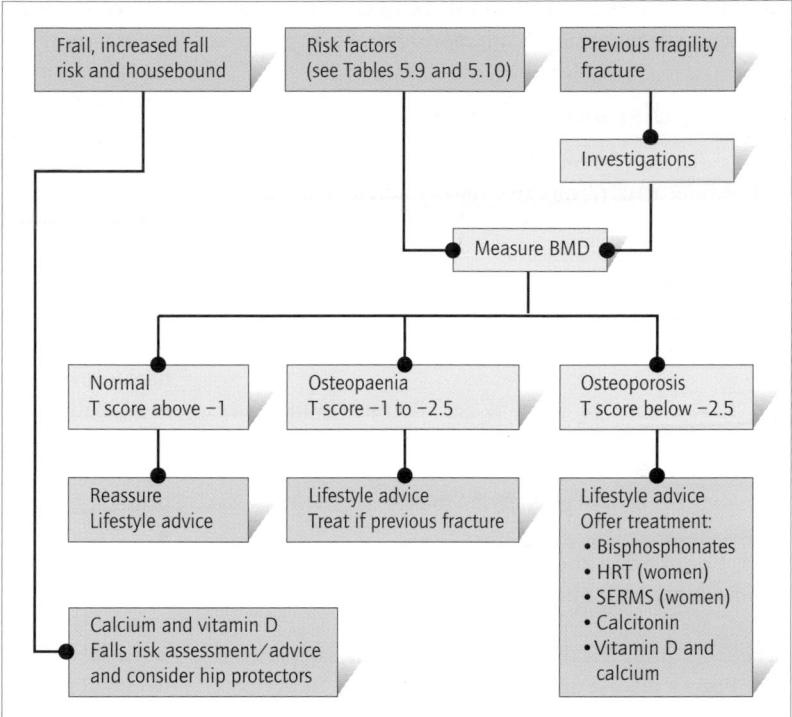

Figure 5.6 Management of women aged over 45 years who have or are at risk of osteoporosis. (Adapted from the Royal College of Physicians and Bone and Tooth Society of Great Britain Osteoporosis Clinical Guidelines for Prevention and Treatment, July 2000.)

management of osteoporosis. Encouraging people to stop smoking, take regular exercise and improve their dietary intake of calcium can help.

Medical therapy. Several drugs are available for the prevention and treatment of postmenopausal osteoporosis:
1 *Bisphosphonates:* the most widely used drugs to treat osteoporosis. They have been shown to reduce the risk of further fractures at both the spine and hip. Examples include disodium etidronate, risedronate sodium, alendronic acid, disodium pamidronate and tiludronic acid. They are indicated for the prevention and treatment of postmenopausal osteoporosis including corticosteroid-induced osteoporosis. Alendronic acid is also licensed for the prevention and treatment of osteoporosis in men. The main adverse effects are on the gastrointestinal system ranging from nausea to oesophageal ulceration and stricture formation. They are contraindicated in pregnancy and breastfeeding, and should be used with caution in renal impairment or hypocalcaemic states.
2 *Hormone replacement therapy:* reduces bone loss and fracture incidence in postmenopausal women. Its use in older women is limited by patient tolerance rather than lack of efficacy (e.g. withdrawal bleed; Fig. 5.6).
3 *Selective oestrogen receptor modulators:* can be used for prevention of postmenopausal osteoporosis and for the treatment of osteoporotic vertebral fractures in postmenopausal women.

4 *Anabolic agents:* these are currently under investigation for their role in stimulating osteoblastic activity; e.g. PTH, which has powerful effects on bone density.

Prevention of osteoporotic fractures in frail housebound people
- *Calcium and vitamin D supplementation:* many people who are frail or institutionalized are vitamin D-deficient and have a poor calcium intake. Use of these supplements in this population has been shown to decrease the risk of fracture.
- *Falls risk assessment and advice:* in this population it is especially important to look not only for increased skeletal fragility but also an increased risk of falling (Table 5.8).
- *Hip protectors:* foam or rubber shields that are worn over the greater trochanter and reduce the likelihood of hip fractures if the patient falls. However, they can be uncomfortable, conspicuous and difficult to put on, and this probably limits their usefulness.

Prognosis
Hip fracture is the most serious complication of osteoporosis, being associated with a 20% mortality within the first 3 months. In addition, many patients fail to regain their premorbid level of mobility and independence, with approximately 30% of patients requiring some form of institutional care.

Recurrent vertebral fractures in spinal osteoporosis

05

can cause pain and progressive deformity, and in some patients this leads to significant morbidity.

Paget's disease of bone

Paget's disease of bone is a localized disorder of bone remodelling that results in a disorganized structure of woven and lamellar bone.

Epidemiology

Prevalence. Approximately 3.6% of the population over 40 years of age in the UK.

Age. Rare before 40 years of age. Prevalence increases with age.

Sex. Sixty per cent of patients are male.

Race. Common in the UK. Rare in Scandinavia, India, Japan, China, Arab Middle East and black Africans.

Genetics. Family clustering occurs and siblings of patients with Paget's disease are 10 times more likely to develop the condition. In some families, Paget's disease is linked to a susceptibility locus on chromosome 18q21-22, which also contains the gene responsible for familial expansile osteolysis (FEO). FEO is a rare bone dysplasia with many similarities to Paget's disease of bone.

Disease mechanisms

Measles virus, respiratory syncytial virus and canine distemper virus have been suggested as causative agents.

There are three pathological stages:

1 Initially the bone is invaded by huge multinucleated osteoclasts, resulting in intense bone resorption and accompanied by vascular hypertrophy.

2 The bone resorption is then accompanied by disorganized woven bone formation.

3 The amount of bone resorption then decreases, resulting in irregularly shaped trabecular bone and bone enlargement.

Clinical features

About 30% of pagetic lesions are associated with pain, which is the presenting symptom in 80% of cases. Any bone may be involved, but most commonly affected sites are the pelvis, lumbar spine and femur. The skeletal distribution of these lesions in any one individual tends to be multifocal and asymmetrical. Whereas lesions at any one anatomical site may progress relentlessly within the same bone, contiguous spread to adjacent bones is not seen.

● *Limb involvement:* causes pain at the affected site. Deformity may be present such as the 'sabre tibia', which

is caused by a combination of bony enlargement and bowing as a result of skeletal softening. Long bone deformities can also cause osteoarthritis of adjacent joints. Paget's disease may result in transverse fractures because of localized skeletal fragility, particularly where aggressive lytic lesions are present in weight-bearing bones. In addition, small fissure fractures can occur along the convex surface of bowed lower limb bones.

● *Skull involvement:* leads to an increase in head size with or without frontal bossing. Hearing loss may also occur (conductive and/or sensorineural), while other cranial nerves may be affected less commonly. When the skull base is involved, the resulting softening can lead to basilar invagination. Increased vascularization of skull lesions may also result in the so-called vascular steal syndrome, which causes blood to be diverted away from the cerebrum, leading to somnolence and apathy.

● *Vertebral involvement:* may lead to vertebral compression fractures and secondary degenerative changes. Rarely, spinal cord compression and caudal ischaemia secondary to vascular steal syndrome may occur.

● *Facial involvement:* may cause facial deformity, leading to dental problems and a characteristic 'lion face' appearance (leontiasis ossea).

● *Osteosarcoma:* the most devastating complication of Paget's disease, occurring in approximately 0.2% of patients. Patients present with new pain in an existing affected site, the pelvis, femur and humerus being affected most commonly.

● *High output cardiac failure:* a rare complication of Paget's disease, which results from excess skeletal blood flow.

● *Hypercalcaemia:* may occur during periods of prolonged immobilization.

Diagnosis

Paget's disease of bone is readily diagnosed in patients presenting with localized bone pain by performing X-rays of the affected site. Alternatively, Paget's disease may be diagnosed in asymptomatic individuals with an isolated elevation in serum alkaline phosphatase.

Differential diagnosis

Other causes of localized bone pain need to be considered such as malignant deposits.

Investigation
Biochemistry

Serum alkaline phosphatase. This is nearly always elevated, and may reach beyond 10 times the upper normal limit, highest levels being found in association with skull involvement. This measure is particularly useful in monitoring the response of patients to therapy.

Paget's disease at a glance

A localized disorder of bone remodelling that results in a disorganized structure of woven and lamellar bone.

Epidemiology

Prevalence
Occurs in approximately 3.6% of people over 40 years old in the UK

Age
Rare before 40 years old. Increases with age

Sex
60% are male

Race
Common in the UK

Genetics
Familial clustering occurs

Aetiology

Unknown

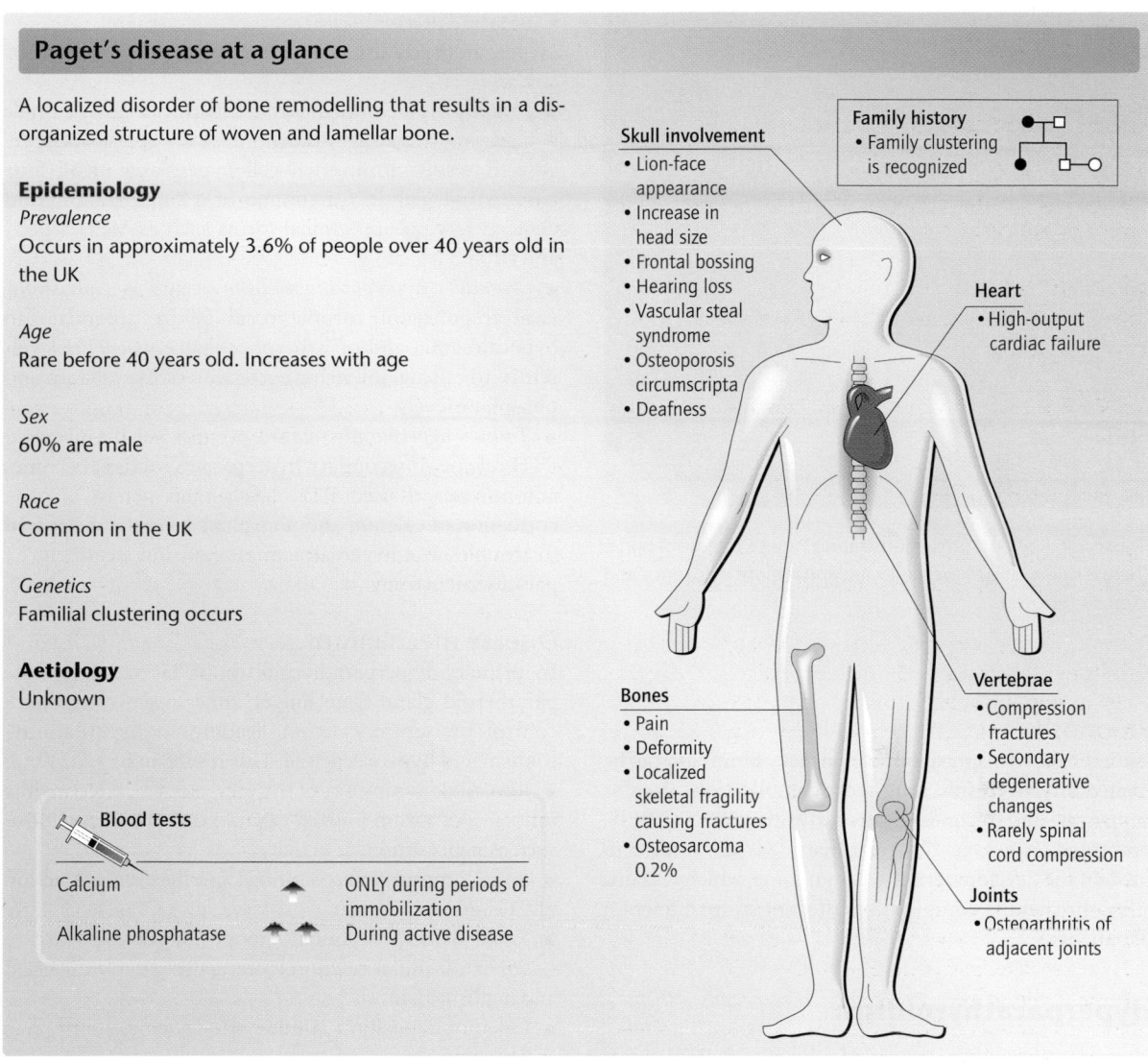

Skull involvement
- Lion-face appearance
- Increase in head size
- Frontal bossing
- Hearing loss
- Vascular steal syndrome
- Osteoporosis circumscripta
- Deafness

Family history
- Family clustering is recognized

Heart
- High-output cardiac failure

Bones
- Pain
- Deformity
- Localized skeletal fragility causing fractures
- Osteosarcoma 0.2%

Vertebrae
- Compression fractures
- Secondary degenerative changes
- Rarely spinal cord compression

Joints
- Osteoarthritis of adjacent joints

Blood tests

Calcium	▲	ONLY during periods of immobilization
Alkaline phosphatase	▲ ▲	During active disease

Diagnostic imaging

Plain radiography. This reveals generalized expansion and deformity of affected long bones, with a characteristic lytic leading edge ('blade of grass' appearance). There may also be areas of sclerotic bone at sites of osteoblastic reaction. When Paget's disease affects the skull, characteristic widening of the skull vault may be seen (Fig. 5.7), or broad scalloped areas of lysis (osteoporosis circumscripta).

Isotope bone scan. This is useful for showing the extent of pagetic involvement. Characteristically, affected bones show intense and uniform uptake over a considerable length.

Management

Bisphosphonates. These are the mainstay of treatment for Paget's disease of bone. Treatment should be offered to all symptomatic individuals, and should be considered in younger asymptomatic patients particularly where a weight-bearing bone is affected.

Bisphosphonates act to suppress osteoclast activity following their uptake within the skeleton. Higher doses for a shorter duration are used, compared to the treatment regimen for osteoporosis (e.g. risedronate sodium 30 mg/day for 8 weeks for Paget's disease of bone but 5 mg/day continuously for postmenopausal osteoporosis). In the great majority of cases, bisphosphonates cause significant symptomatic relief and lowering—if not normalization—of the serum alkaline phosphatase. Although patients frequently relapse within a few years, they generally respond to further courses of treatment.

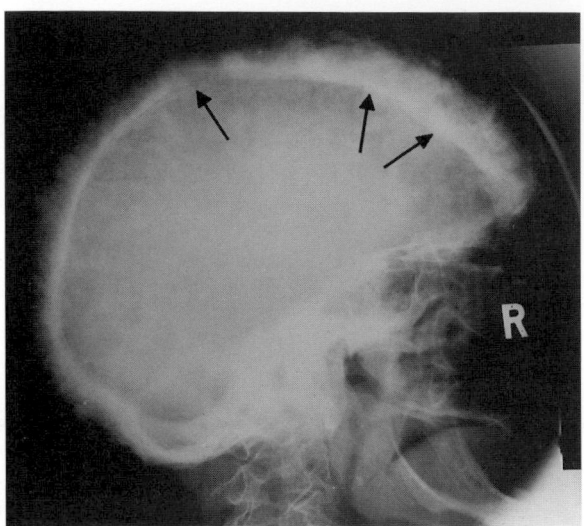

Figure 5.7 Radiograph demonstrating Paget's disease of bone. There is thickening of the skull vault and regions of lucency and sclerosis (arrows).

Prognosis

With the use of bisphosphonates, pagetic bone pain can be treated effectively and long-term complications such as deformity and secondary osteoarthritis can largely be prevented. However, this treatment does not appear to prevent the development of osteosarcoma, which remains a life-threatening complication affecting a small fraction of patients.

Hyperparathyroidism

Hyperparathyroidism is defined as increased PTH secretion from the parathyroid glands. The most common form, primary hyperparathyroidism, is a common endocrine disorder characterized by chronic hypercalcaemia (Table 5.2).

Epidemiology

Prevalence. Approximately 1/1000 men and 2/1000 women at 60 years of age.

Age. Incidence of primary hyperparathyroidism increases with age.

Sex. Approximately 70% of patients are female.

Genetics. A small proportion of cases are familial, when primary hyperparathyroidism is usually a component of multiple endocrine neoplasia (MEN) type I or II.

Classification

Hyperparathyroidism may be primary, secondary or tertiary:
- *Primary hyperparathyroidism:* usually caused by a single benign parathyroid gland adenoma (85% of cases). Otherwise, it results from chief cell hyperplasia of all four parathyroid glands. Carcinoma of a single parathyroid gland is rare, as are familial forms such as MEN types I and II.
- *Secondary hyperparathyroidism:* occurs as a physiological response in chronic renal failure secondary to hypocalcaemia and/or hyperphosphataemia. PTH levels return to normal following correction of the calcium and phosphate levels.
- *Tertiary hyperparathyroidism:* occurs when the increased PTH release of secondary hyperparathyroidism becomes autonomous. Raised PTH levels then persist, despite correction of calcium and phosphate levels, and can lead to troublesome hypercalcaemia, requiring treatment by parathyroidectomy.

Disease mechanisms

In primary hyperparathyroidism, PTH release by the parathyroid gland is no longer under negative feedback control by serum calcium, leading to hyperparathyroidism and hypercalcaemia. This results in:
- Reversible symptoms of hypercalcaemia, reflecting the influence of serum ionized calcium on cellular functions such as neuromuscular activity
- Bone complications resulting from the excessive action of PTH on the skeleton
- Renal damage secondary to prolonged exposure to raised extracellular calcium levels causing nephrolithiasis and nephrocalcinosis
- Calcium deposition at other sites, such as joints, eyes and the skin

Clinical features of primary hyperparathyroidism

Primary hyperparathyroidism most commonly presents as incidental hypercalcaemia on routine serum biochemistry. Symptoms of hypercalcaemia are likely if the serum calcium concentration is higher than 3.0 mmol and consist of:
- Polyuria and polydipsia
- Nausea, anorexia and constipation
- Depression and sleep disturbance

Such symptoms may have existed for some time before diagnosis, but older patients can present acutely with dehydration, drowsiness and confusion. Alternatively, hyperparathyroidism may manifest with complications as a result of organ damage, most commonly involving the kidney or skeleton.

Renal involvement. This is the most common complication of primary hyperparathyroidism, affecting 20–40% of patients. It manifests as either nephrolithiasis or nephrocalcinosis, which do not usually coexist in the same patient; nephrolithiasis is the more common. Primary hyperparathyroidism is detected in 5–10% of people with recurrent calcium-containing renal stones. In nephrocalcinosis, calcium and phosphate precipitate in the renal tubules and interstitium, leading to renal impairment.

Skeletal involvement. In primary hyperparathyroidism this comprises the characteristic histological and clinical entity of osteitis fibrosa cystica. Early histological changes are present in most people with primary hyperparathyroidism, but less than 15% have symptoms such as bone pain at the time of diagnosis. The full clinical picture of osteitis fibrosa cystica is now rare. It consists of bone cysts, fractures and deformity. Osteopenia on bone densitometry is a fairly common finding.

Hypertension. This frequently coexists with primary hyperparathyroidism, but hyperparathyroidism has not been found to have a causal role and the hypertension does not usually resolve following parathyroidectomy.

Gastrointestinal complications. In MEN type I there is an association between primary hyperparathyroidism and peptic ulceration resulting from Zollinger–Ellison syndrome. There is also an association between primary hyperparathyroidism and peptic ulceration in the absence of MEN type I, with peptic ulceration reported by up to 20% of patients with primary hyperparathyroidism. There is an infrequent association with pancreatitis, but the pathophysiological basis for this is unknown.

Neurological complications. A syndrome of reversible proximal muscle weakness and wasting resulting from denervation and atrophy of type II muscle fibres can occur.

Articular manifestations. Chondrocalcinosis.

Pruritus and skin necrosis. Resulting from skin involvement.

Band keratopathy. Occurs following the deposition of calcium salts below the corneal epithelium.

Diagnosis

Increased PTH in the presence of raised serum calcium is considered diagnostic of primary and tertiary hyperparathyroidism.

Differential diagnosis

Other causes of hypercalcaemia should be considered (Table 5.5). It is particularly important to exclude malignancy which, together with primary hyperparathyroidism, accounts for more than 90% of patients with hypercalcaemia. In general, mild hypercalcaemia that remains asymptomatic suggests primary hyperparathyroidism.

Investigation
Haematology
Full blood count. Anaemia is common in secondary and tertiary hyperparathyroidism resulting from the associated chronic renal failure.

Biochemistry
- *Serum creatinine:* increased, and creatinine clearance decreased if there is renal impairment.
- *Serum calcium:* elevated in primary and tertiary hyperparathyroidism. Repeated measurements are required to confirm the elevation.
- *Serum phosphate:* usually reduced in primary hyperparathyroidism (urinary phosphate wasting) and elevated in secondary hyperparathyroidism resulting from renal failure.
- *Serum alkaline phosphatase:* increased if there is any associated bone disease.
- *Serum PTH:* usually elevated. It is usually suppressed in hypercalcaemia from other causes.
- *Serum 25-OH-D:* usually elevated. It is also elevated in hypercalcaemia caused by granulomatous diseases and lymphoma.
- *24-h Urinary calcium excretion:* normal or increased, and should be measured to exclude familial hypocalciuric hypercalcaemia in which it is less than 100 mg/g creatinine. Familial hypocalciuric hypercalcaemia can mimic asymptomatic primary hyperparathyroidism.

Diagnostic imaging
Plain radiography. This commonly shows a diffuse reduction in bone density. Radiological evidence of osteitis fibrosa cystica is present in less than 5% of patients at diagnosis. It consists of subperiosteal bone resorption (best seen along the radial aspect of middle phalanges), erosions of the tufts of the terminal phalanges, mottling of the skull vault ('salt-and-pepper appearance'), cystic lesions and loss of the lamina dura. There may also be radiological evidence of nephrocalcinosis.

Bone densitometry. Measurement of skeletal calcium at both cortical and trabecular sites may reveal osteopaenia, which may be monitored by serial measurements.

Other techniques. High-resolution ultrasonography, high-resolution computed tomography, subtraction scan with technetium and thallium radioisotopes and parathyroid arteriography with selective venous sampling may

Hyperparathyroidism at a glance

Increased parathyroid hormone (PTH) secretion from the parathyroid glands.

Epidemiology
Prevalence
1/1000 men and 2/1000 women of 60 years of age

Age
Increased incidence with increasing age

Sex
Approximately 70% of patients are female

Genetics
Familial hyperparathyroidism with multiple endocrine neoplasia (MEN) types I and II

Aetiology
Primary hyperparathyroidism
Most commonly caused by a benign adenoma of a single parathyroid gland (85% of all cases), or hyperplasia of all four glands

Secondary hyperparathyroidism
Increased PTH secretion in response to hypercalcaemia and/or hyperphosphataemia of chronic renal failure

Tertiary hyperparathyroidism
Autonomous increase in PTH secretion in patients with secondary hyperparathyroidism

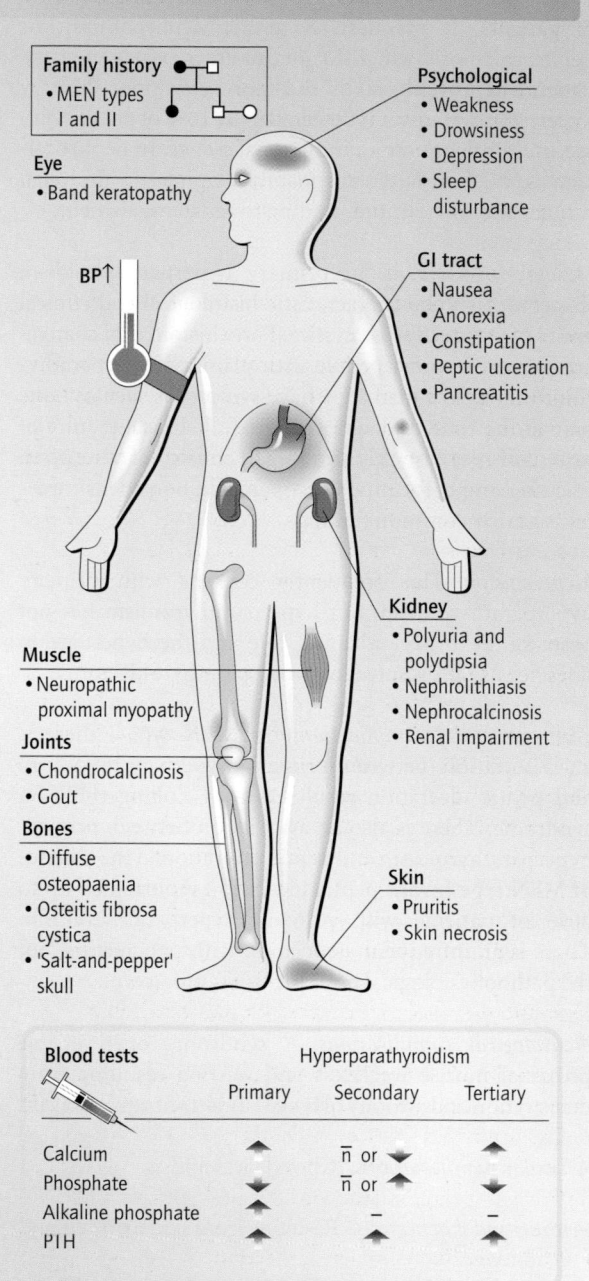

Blood tests	Hyperparathyroidism		
	Primary	Secondary	Tertiary
Calcium	↑	n or ↓	↑
Phosphate	↓	n or ↑	↓
Alkaline phosphate	↑	–	–
PTH	↑	↑	↑

localize parathyroid adenomas prior to surgical removal.

Histopathology
Biopsy of cystic lesions seen on plain radiography reveals either a true bone cyst filled with fibrous tissue, or an appearance similar to an osteoclastoma ('brown tumour').

Management
Life-threatening hypercalcaemia
Life-threatening hypercalcaemia needs prompt treatment with:

● Intravenous fluids such as 0.9% saline, 4–6 l in 24 h as needed

● Intravenous disodium pamidronate

- Glucocorticoids (intravenous hydrocortisone, oral prednisolone)
- Calcitonin

Symptomatic hypercalcaemia in people unfit for surgery

People with symptomatic hypercalcaemia who are unfit for surgery may benefit from long-term oral treatment with phosphate or a bisphosphonate drug; postmenopausal women may benefit from oestrogen replacement.

Asymptomatic primary hyperparathyroidism with no evidence of renal or skeletal impairment

Asymptomatic primary hyperparathyroidism in people with no evidence of renal or skeletal impairment at the time of diagnosis may follow a benign course, with little organ damage developing. It may therefore be reasonable to treat these people, particularly older patients with mild hypercalcaemia (serum calcium less than 2.9 mmol/l), conservatively if there are facilities for regular monitoring of renal function and bone density.

Surgery

Surgery is the only curative treatment for primary hyperparathyroidism. It should be offered to patients with symptomatic hypercalcaemia or evidence of skeletal or renal complications. Unfortunately, there are no definitive means of predicting the development of complications in asymptomatic people. Surgery is usually considered for younger patients, who have longer to develop complications, and those with a higher serum calcium (e.g. more than 2.9 mmol/l), who are presumed more likely to sustain significant organ damage.

Parathyroid surgery should only be undertaken by experienced surgeons as there may be associated complications which include:
- Difficulty in identifying parathyroid tissue at surgery (an ectopic site occurs elsewhere within the neck or upper mediastinum in 5–10% of patients)
- Transient postoperative hypocalcaemia, which is maximal 4–7 days postoperatively and persists for up to 2–3 weeks
- Prolonged hypocalcaemia secondary to significant parathyroid gland damage (hypocalcaemia persisting for longer than 6 months suggests permanent hypoparathyroidism)

Prognosis

Surgery cures 90% of patients with uncomplicated primary hyperparathyroidism. For the remaining 10%, re-exploration of the neck following preoperative localization of parathyroid tissue may be successful.

Untreated hyperparathyroidism can lead to irreversible renal failure and skeletal deformity, but this is now rare. In secondary and tertiary hyperparathyroidism, the prognosis largely depends on that of the underlying renal failure.

Hypercalcaemia of malignancy

Hypercalcaemia of malignancy is usually an indicator of advanced disease with secondary skeletal deposits and is rarely the first manifestation.

Epidemiology

Prevalence. Five per cent of hospital inpatients with malignancy.

Disease mechanisms

Nearly 50% of people with hypercalcaemia of malignancy have squamous cell carcinoma of the lung or adenocarcinoma of the breast. Hypercalcaemia is also a common feature of squamous cell tumours of the head and neck, renal and ovarian tumours, and haematological tumours such as multiple myeloma.

Hypercalcaemia of malignancy is most commonly associated with secondary malignant deposits in the skeleton. Such deposits stimulate osteoclast activity. This results in hypercalcaemia when calcium release from the bone exceeds renal calcium excretion.

Two mechanisms have been implicated in this increased osteolysis and involve the release of local factors or PTH-related peptide (PTHrP):

1 *Release of local factors:* skeletal secondary deposits are thought to stimulate resorption of surrounding bone by locally releasing bone-resorbing cytokines such as interleukin-1, tumour necrosis factor and prostaglandins.
2 *PTHrP:* hypercalcaemia of malignancy sometimes resembles hyperparathyroidism biochemically (reduced renal calcium excretion, increased phosphate excretion) despite reduced serum PTH levels. This is now attributed to the release of PTHrP by tumour cells. PTHrP is a calcium-regulating peptide with PTH-like activity and has been isolated from a number of solid tumours causing hypercalcaemia. As well as contributing to the hypercalcaemia complicating skeletal deposits, PTHrP is probably responsible for the hypercalcaemia that occasionally occurs as a non-metastatic paraneoplastic manifestation of malignancy.

Clinical features

The elevated serum calcium that occurs in malignancy is frequently high enough to cause symptoms of hypercalcaemia (Table 5.2). These may be relatively non-specific, and hypercalcaemia should therefore be sought in all patients with malignancy who feel unwell.

05

Bone pain from skeletal secondary deposits is common. There is often mild renal impairment because of dehydration, but significant renal failure is suggestive of multiple myeloma.

Diagnosis

Hypercalcaemia of malignancy usually presents in patients with malignancy associated with metastatic bone disease, in which case the diagnosis is clear and further investigation of the cause of hypercalcaemia is not usually helpful. Although occult malignancy is an infrequent cause of hypercalcaemia, it should be sought if primary hyperparathyroidism and rarer causes such as sarcoidosis and familial hypocalciuric hypercalcaemia have been excluded.

Differential diagnosis

Other causes of hypercalcaemia should be considered if hypercalcaemia is found in patients with malignancy rarely associated with hypercalcaemia such as cancer of the colon or cervix, or in those without skeletal metastases (Table 5.5).

Investigation

If hypercalcaemia is discovered when there is no history of malignancy, and the PTH level is suppressed, investigations should be carried out to look for an underlying malignancy. If no malignancy is discovered, and the patient remains asymptomatic during follow-up, a rarer cause of hypercalcaemia such as sarcoidosis should be considered.

Haematology
- *Full blood count:* There may be anaemia
- *ESR:* May be elevated, particularly in multiple myeloma

Biochemistry
- *Serum creatinine:* frequently elevated because of dehydration
- *Serum calcium:* elevated
- *Serum phosphate:* may be reduced (urinary phosphate wasting)
- *Serum alkaline phosphatase:* may be increased if there are solid tumour metastases to bone causing an osteoblastic response, but normal in the presence of osteolytic metastases (e.g. in association with multiple myeloma)
- *Serum PTH:* usually suppressed
- *Serum 25-OH-D:* usually suppressed, but may be elevated if hypercalcaemia is associated with lymphoma

Diagnostic imaging
- *Plain radiography:* may reveal an osteolytic bone lesion or evidence of a primary malignancy such as lung neoplasm
- *Isotope bone scan:* may reveal previously unsuspected secondary malignant deposits of the skeleton

Management

Hypercalcaemia should generally be treated aggressively if there are associated symptoms. However, if there is severe life-threatening hypercalcaemia, the overall prognosis and quality of life may be such that aggressive treatment is not indicated.

Intravenous saline

People with hypercalcaemia are frequently dehydrated as a result of polyuria from renal tubular impairment. This reduces renal calcium excretion further and aggravates the hypercalcaemia. Mild hypercalcaemia may respond to an increase in oral fluid intake, but volume replacement with intravenous normal saline is mandatory for severe hypercalcaemia. This treatment usually lowers calcium levels significantly but only transiently in the absence of additional therapy to inhibit bone resorption.

Bisphosphonates

Intravenous administration of bisphosphonates (e.g. disodium pamidronate) combined with intravenous saline is an effective treatment for acute hypercalcaemia.

Glucocorticoids

Glucocorticoids (e.g. prednisolone 30–60 mg/day) are usually a helpful treatment for hypercalcaemia caused by haematological tumours such as multiple myeloma. They may be conveniently administered orally if the hypercalcaemia is long-standing. They are less effective for hypercalcaemia resulting from solid tumours. Glucocorticoids are also useful in the treatment of hypercalcaemia associated with non-malignant causes such as sarcoidosis and vitamin D intoxication.

Calcitonin

Calcitonin is a non-toxic agent that usually causes a rapid lowering of calcium levels in acute hypercalcaemia. Its action is relatively transitory, but may be prolonged if used in combination with glucocorticoids.

Specific treatment

Hypercalcaemia of malignancy is usually caused by disseminated malignancy, in which case specific therapy aimed at eradicating the underlying tumour is not usually helpful. The exception to this is hypercalcaemia occurring as a non-metastatic paraneoplastic manifestation of malignancy, in which case the hypercalcaemia may resolve following successful ablation of the primary tumour.

Prognosis

Hypercalcaemia of malignancy can generally be satisfactorily treated with the measures outlined above. The overall prognosis is dictated by that of the underlying malignancy.

Hypocalcaemia

Hypocalcaemia is a less common clinical problem than hypercalcaemia and has fewer causes. Like hypercalcaemia, its presentation varies from an asymptomatic biochemical abnormality to a life-threatening condition.

Disease mechanisms

Hypocalcaemia usually results from chronic renal failure or other vitamin D-dependent causes (Table 5.6). Alternatively, it may be caused by hypoparathyroidism, which is most frequently seen as a postoperative complication of parathyroidectomy. There are a number of rare hypocalcaemic disorders characterized by hypoparathyroidism or PTH resistance (Table 5.11).

A decrease in ionized calcium concentration increases neuromuscular irritability. In addition, chronic hypocalcaemia can lead to mineralization of soft tissues, causing basal ganglia calcification and cataracts.

Hypocalcaemia caused by chronic renal failure results from a combination of phosphate retention and impaired vitamin D metabolism.

Clinical features

Clinical features of hypocalcaemia include (Table 5.3):
- *Paraesthesia:* peripherally and/or circumoral numbness.
- *Tetany:* cramp-like muscle spasms, which in milder forms are predominantly distal (carpopedal spasm) but may become generalized, causing, for example, laryngeal stridor.
- *Convulsions.*
- *Mental changes:* anxiety, psychosis.
- *Chvostek's sign:* gentle tapping over the facial nerve causes twitching of the muscles within its distribution. This is positive in 10% of people who do not have hypocalcaemia.
- *Trousseau's sign:* inflation of a sphygmomanometer cuff above diastolic pressure for 3 min to obliterate the radial pulse causes distal tetanic spasm.
- *Papilloedema:* if hypocalcaemia is long-standing.
- *Arrhythmias and/or ECG changes* (e.g. prolonged QT interval).

Differential diagnosis

The differential diagnosis of hypocalcaemia is shown in Table 5.6. If it is not caused by chronic renal failure, severe osteomalacia (associated with a raised PTH and reduced serum phosphate) can be readily distinguished from hypoparathyroidism (associated with a

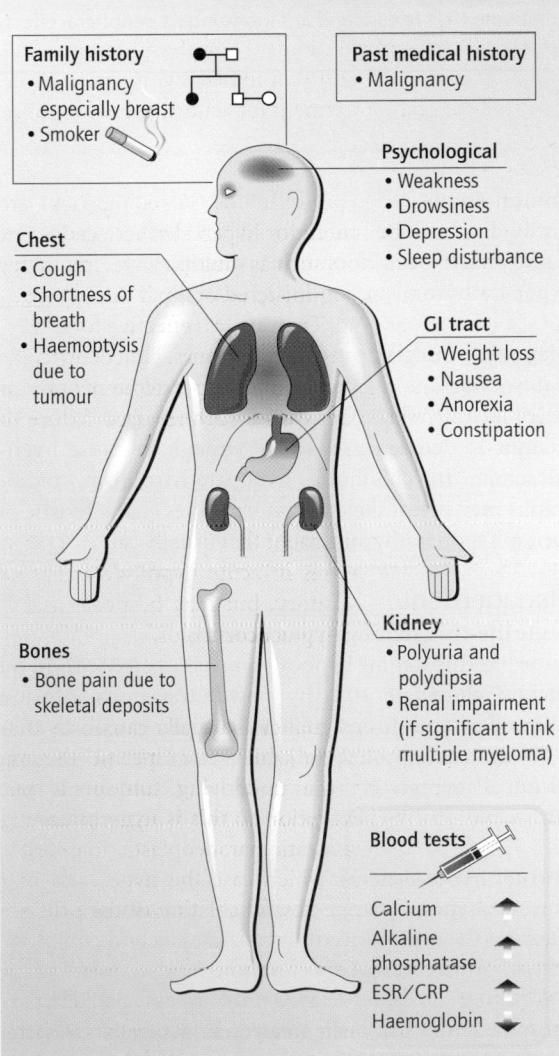

Hypercalcaemia of malignancy at a glance

A high serum calcium occurring with malignancy usually indicating advanced disease with secondary skeletal deposits.

Epidemiology
Prevalence
5% of hospital inpatients with malignancy

Aetiology
Squamous cell carcinoma of the lung
Adenocarcinoma of the breast
Squamous cell tumours of the head and neck
Renal carcinoma
Ovarian carcinoma
Haematogenous tumours, especially multiple myeloma

Family history
- Malignancy especially breast
- Smoker

Past medical history
- Malignancy

Psychological
- Weakness
- Drowsiness
- Depression
- Sleep disturbance

Chest
- Cough
- Shortness of breath
- Haemoptysis due to tumour

GI tract
- Weight loss
- Nausea
- Anorexia
- Constipation

Bones
- Bone pain due to skeletal deposits

Kidney
- Polyuria and polydipsia
- Renal impairment (if significant think multiple myeloma)

Blood tests

Calcium ↑
Alkaline phosphatase ↑
ESR/CRP ↑
Haemoglobin ↓

05

Table 5.11 Hypocalcaemic disorders caused by hypoparathyroidism or parathyroid hormone (PTH) resistance

Cause	Features
Idiopathic hypoparathyroidism A rare autoimmune disorder	Often associated with cutaneous candidiasis and other autoimmune disorders such as Addison's disease. It usually presents in childhood. There is also an adult-onset form
DiGeorge's syndrome Congenital absence of the parathyroid and thymus glands	Severe hypocalcaemia and T-cell immunodeficiency
Pseudohypoparathyroidism Hereditary disorder characterized by end-organ resistance to PTH	Hypocalcaemia. It is associated with intellectual impairment, short stature and skeletal abnormalities such as short 4th and 5th metacarpals and metatarsals (Albright's hereditary osteodystrophy)
Pseudopseudohypoparathyroidism Hereditary disorder	Skeletal and developmental abnormalities of pseudohypoparathyroidism, but calcium metabolism is normal
Hypomagnesaemia Most commonly caused by malabsorption	Causes hypocalcaemia by inhibiting PTH release and antagonizing its peripheral effects

reduced PTH and elevated phosphate). Hypomagnesaemia should be excluded by measuring serum magnesium concentration.

If hypoparathyroidism is suspected, skeletal abnormalities such as short stature and short fourth and fifth metacarpals and metatarsals may suggest pseudohypoparathyroidism.

Investigation
Haematology
Full blood count. There may be anaemia if there is underlying chronic renal failure.

Biochemistry
- *Serum calcium:* reduced
- *Serum phosphate:* increased in chronic renal failure and hypoparathyroidism; decreased in vitamin D-dependent causes other than chronic renal failure
- *Serum PTH:* increased in chronic renal failure and other vitamin D-dependent causes; decreased in hypoparathyroidism
- *Serum magnesium:* reveals or excludes hypomagnesaemia
- *Urinary cyclic adenosine monophosphate (cAMP) response to PTH:* absent in pseudohypoparathyroidism, confirming the end-organ resistance to PTH
- *Assay of the GS protein on red cells:* this protein binds guanine triphosphate (GTP) and is deficient in most patients with pseudohypoparathyroidism

Immunology
Antibodies to the parathyroid and other endocrine glands have been found in patients with idiopathic hypoparathyroidism.

Diagnostic imaging
Plain radiography. Changes of renal osteodystrophy or osteomalacia/rickets are likely if chronic renal failure or vitamin D deficiency is severe enough to cause hypocalcaemia. In childhood hypoparathyroidism, radiographs may reveal skeletal abnormalities characteristic of pseudohypoparathyroidism.

Management
Acute life-threatening hypocalcaemia
Acute life-threatening hypocalcaemia is treated with 10 ml calcium gluconate 10% by slow intravenous infusion followed by an infusion of 20 ml calcium gluconate 10% in 5% dextrose 6-hourly, adjusted according to the serum calcium. Patients receiving intravenous calcium should have cardiac monitoring because of the risk of arrhythmias.

Chronic hypocalcaemia
Chronic hypocalcaemia is difficult to manage. Recurrences of the symptoms of hypocalcaemia and complications of overtreatment are common.
- *Calcium:* should be delayed until any associated hyperphosphataemia has been treated, to avoid extraskeletal calcification.

Hypocalcaemia at a glance

Low serum calcium ranging from an asymptomatic biochemical abnormality to a life-threatening condition.

Aetiology
Hypoparathyroidism
Chronic renal failure
Severe vitamin D deficiency
Pseudohypoparathyroidism

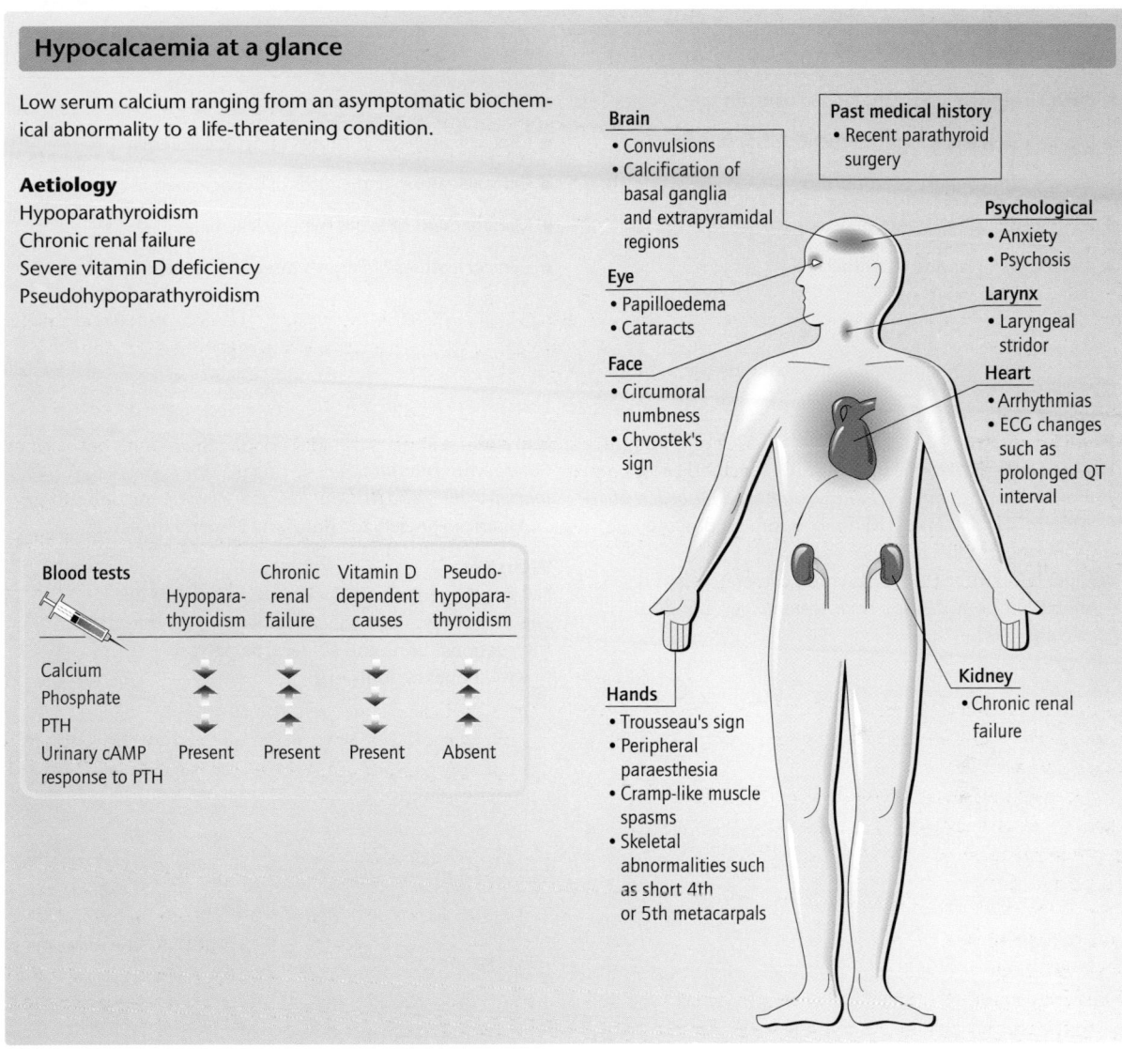

Brain
- Convulsions
- Calcification of basal ganglia and extrapyramidal regions

Eye
- Papilloedema
- Cataracts

Face
- Circumoral numbness
- Chvostek's sign

Past medical history
- Recent parathyroid surgery

Psychological
- Anxiety
- Psychosis

Larynx
- Laryngeal stridor

Heart
- Arrhythmias
- ECG changes such as prolonged QT interval

Hands
- Trousseau's sign
- Peripheral paraesthesia
- Cramp-like muscle spasms
- Skeletal abnormalities such as short 4th or 5th metacarpals

Kidney
- Chronic renal failure

Blood tests	Hypoparathyroidism	Chronic renal failure	Vitamin D dependent causes	Pseudohypoparathyroidism
Calcium	↓	↓	↓	↓
Phosphate	↑	↑	↓	↑
PTH	↓	↑	↓	↑
Urinary cAMP response to PTH	Present	Present	Present	Absent

- *Vitamin D formulations:* usually given in combination with calcium supplements and include ergocalciferol, dihydrotachysterol, alfacalcidol and calcitriol. In general, the more potent metabolites of vitamin D are preferred because their shorter half-life allows more rapid restoration of normocalcaemia and faster recovery in the event of vitamin D intoxication. Vitamin D intoxication causes hypercalcaemia or hypercalciuria, leading to nephrolithiasis and/or nephrocalcinosis. It should be prevented by regular monitoring of serum and urinary calcium during treatment with vitamin D.

Prognosis
Complications of hypocalcaemia depend largely on its severity and duration, which in turn reflect the underlying cause:
- *Hypocalcaemia of chronic renal failure:* may be associated with osteomalacia and/or secondary hypoparathyroidism, leading to renal osteodystrophy
- *Hypocalcaemia resulting from hypoparathyroidism and pseudohypoparathyroidism:* usually long-standing, and basal ganglia or extrapyramidal calcification may result, causing significant mental impairment

05

❗ Must know checklist

- Useful investigations in metabolic bone disease
- Predisposing factors for postmenopausal osteoporosis
- Causes of secondary osteoporosis
- Diagnosis and treatment of osteoporosis
- Causes of rickets and osteomalacia

- Clinical features of osteomalacia
- Clinical features and causes of hypercalcaemia
- Clinical features and causes of hypocalcaemia
- Management of acute hypercalcaemia
- Clinical features of Paget's disease of bone

Further reading

Books

Favus MJ, Christakos S, Goldring SR, Holick MF, eds. *Primer on the Metabolic Bone Diseases and Disorders of Mineral Metabolism*, 4th edn. London: Lippincott Williams & Wilkins, 1999.

Klippel JH, Dieppe PA. Chapters on osteoporosis and metabolic bone disease. In: *Rheumatology*. London: Mosby, 1997.

Journals

Osteoporosis International, Springer Verlag.
Journal of Bone and Mineral Research (www.jbmr-online.org), American Society for Bone and Mineral Research.

Websites

National Osteoporosis Society: www.nos.org.uk
Paget's Society: www.paget.org.uk
International Bone and Mineral Society: www.bonekey-ibms.org

Introduction

Diseases of the respiratory system are a major cause of illness worldwide. In the UK they are the most common reason for consulting a general practitioner (GP), and result in more days lost from work than any other type of illness.

There are many presentations of respiratory disease (see CLINICAL PRESENTATION AT A GLANCE BOX, p. 306). More than 20% of all deaths in the UK are caused by respiratory disease, which ranks second to heart disease as the most common cause of death. Bronchial carcinoma is the most common cancer to cause death, and other lung disorders related to cigarette smoking (e.g. chronic bronchitis and emphysema) are associated with significant mortality and morbidity and have a high economic cost (e.g. lost working days).

Changing pattern of respiratory disease

The pattern of some respiratory diseases is changing.
● Although uncommon in the western world, **pulmonary tuberculosis** remains endemic in developing countries.
● New respiratory infections such as Legionnaires' disease and *Chlamydia pneumoniae* have emerged.
● **Opportunistic pneumonias** such as *Pneumocystis carinii* pneumonia remain a common presentation of acquired immune deficiency syndrome (AIDS). These pneumonias are also common in patients receiving immunosuppressive therapy; for example, following an organ or bone marrow transplant.

In addition, therapies have emerged to prolong life in previously terminal respiratory conditions.
● More children with cystic fibrosis survive to adult life, and heart–lung or lung transplants are now possible not only for these individuals but also for those with end-stage respiratory failure resulting from pulmonary fibrosis or α_1-antitrypsin deficiency.

● Long-term oxygen therapy at home can prolong life for patients with respiratory failure resulting from chronic bronchitis and/or emphysema; some centres in the USA even perform heart–lung transplants in these patients.

Structure and function

Structure of the respiratory tract

The upper respiratory tract comprises the nose, pharynx and larynx. The nose is the organ of smell; it also heats, moistens and removes particulate matter from inhaled air. The lower respiratory tract is composed of a series of branching tubes that eventually connect to the alveolar air spaces (Fig. 6.1).

The sites of gas exchange receive a blood supply from the pulmonary arteries, which receive the total output of the right side of the heart. There is also a much smaller supply from the left side of the heart, via the bronchial arteries, which arise from the descending aorta or internal mammary or intercostal arteries. The bronchial arteries supply the bronchi as far down as the terminal bronchioles. Most of the blood is carried away from the lung via the pulmonary veins. Lymph drains from the lungs into nodes in the hilar (i.e. tracheobronchial and subcarinal nodes) and paratracheal regions.

The lung is innervated by the autonomic nervous system and has sympathetic and parasympathetic peptidergic supplies, but the inter-relationship between them is not clear. The parasympathetic and peptidergic supplies appear to have a bronchoconstrictor effect. Both lungs are enclosed by invaginated sacs of thin mesothelial tissue

06

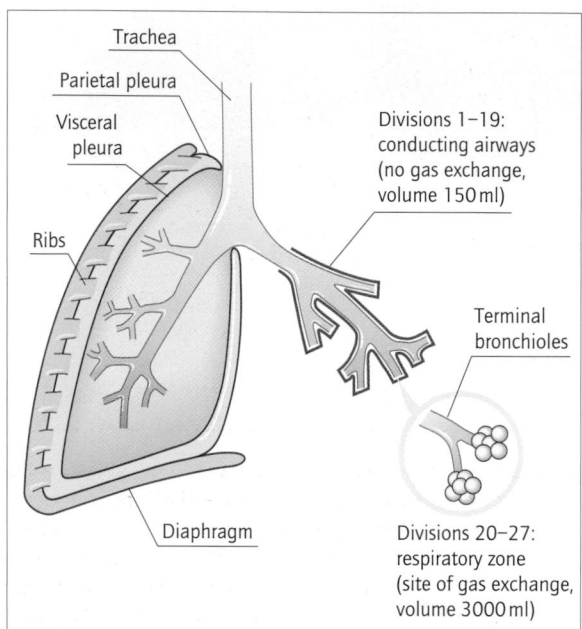

Figure 6.1 Diagram of the respiratory tract. The first 19 divisions of the airway (from the trachea to the terminal bronchioles) are conducting airways and transmit inspired air into the last seven divisions (the terminal respiratory zone), where gas exchange occurs. The distance from the terminal bronchiole to the most distal alveolus is about 5 mm.

(the pleura), which allow movement between the lung and the chest wall. The pleural surfaces are lubricated by a few millilitres of serous fluid, which is secreted by the parietal pleura and absorbed by the visceral pleura at the rate of about 700 ml/day. The parietal pleura is well equipped with somatic sensory fibres, but the visceral pleura has only an autonomic nerve supply and is relatively insensitive.

Function

The main function of the lung is to facilitate gas exchange between air and blood, by allowing oxygen (O_2) to move from the air into the venous blood and carbon dioxide (CO_2) to move from the venous blood into the air. This is achieved by four interdependent functional components:
1 *Adequate ventilation* of the airways to bring air into the lungs
2 *Ventilatory control mechanisms* to regulate ventilation according to the metabolic needs of the body
3 *A large air–blood interface* to allow the exchange of O_2 and CO_2
4 *A suitable pulmonary blood flow* to transport O_2 and CO_2 between the lungs and the rest of the body

The lung is elegantly designed to perform its functions, and disorders of these four functional components form the basis for understanding the pathophysiology of many respiratory disorders.

Ventilation

Ventilation is the bulk movement of air (10 000 l/day) from outside the body through the upper air passages and down the subdivisions of the conducting airways into the terminal respiratory units. The conducting airways do not contain alveoli and therefore do not take part in gas exchange. This anatomical dead space of 150 ml is small compared to the 3000 ml volume of the terminal respiratory units where gas exchange occurs.

The amount of inspired air reaching the sites of gas exchange is determined by:
● *Mechanical factors:* which include the elasticity of the lung and chest wall, and factors that govern the resistance of the airways to gas flow (e.g. airway diameter)
● *Nervous control mechanisms:* which regulate the ventilatory rate according to the body's need

Mechanical factors

Inspiration is an active process requiring muscular effort. The most important inspiratory muscle is the diaphragm, which is supplied by the phrenic nerve (C3–5). The diaphragm descends as it contracts and thereby increases the vertical dimension of the chest. In addition, the cross-sectional area of the chest is increased by contraction of the intercostal muscles, causing the ribs to move upwards and outwards (the 'bucket handle' effect). These two processes increase the intrathoracic volume; pleural and airway pressures become more negative, resulting in inspiratory flow down to the terminal bronchioles (Fig. 6.2). Ventilation of the terminal respiratory units takes place by rapid diffusion of gas, equalizing any difference in gas concentrations within 1 s.

The change in lung volume per unit of pleural pressure change is the compliance or distensibility of the lung, and is determined by many factors; for example, the elasticity of the lung tissue and the surface tension of the liquid film lining the alveoli (Fig. 6.3). Over 80% of the resistance to airflow is in the nose, oropharynx and large airways (trachea and all branches down to 2 mm in diameter). There has to be considerable disease of the smaller airways (those less than 2 mm in diameter) before the usual measurements of pulmonary function (e.g. spirometry) can pick up an abnormality; this part of the lung is therefore called the 'silent zone'. Lung volume has an important effect on airway resistance because of the support the bronchi receive from the radial traction of the surrounding lung tissue (Fig. 6.4).

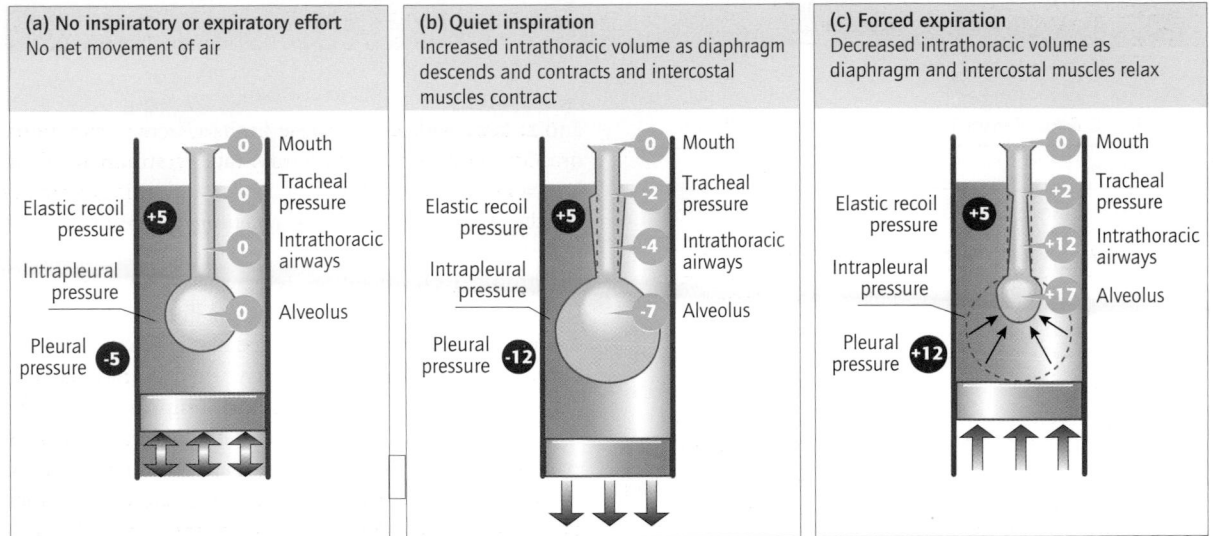

Figure 6.2 Pressure changes in the pleural cavity, alveoli and airway during breathing. (a) When there is no inspiratory or expiratory effort the alveoli are kept open by a distending, negative pleural pressure, which exactly balances the elastic recoil pressure of the lung. (b) During quiet inspiration a pressure gradient is set up and gas flows into the lung. The pressure difference needed to move gas through the airways is very small; a flow rate of 1 l/s requires a drop of less than 2 cm H_2O along the airway. (c) Forced expiration produces a pressure gradient not only down the airway, but also across the wall of the intrathoracic airway, which must narrow if it is at all compliant. Once this dynamic compression of the airways has occurred, the flow rate of air from the alveoli cannot be increased by greater expiratory effort. The higher the pleural pressure becomes because of increased muscular effort, the greater the extent of this dynamic compression of the airways themselves, and so there can be no further increase in flow rate. In practice, flow limitation occurs when one-third of the vital capacity has been expired. Thereafter expiratory flow depends solely on the elastic recoil of the lung and the resistance of the small airways (see Fig. 6.4).

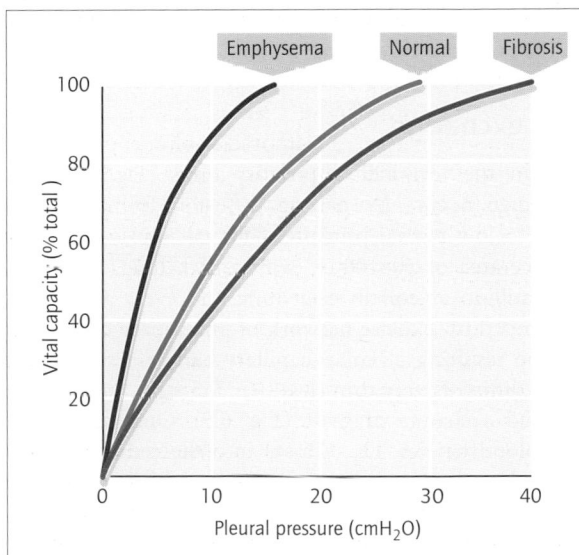

Figure 6.3 Lung volume–pressure curves. Green: normally the lung is easier to inflate at low volumes than at high volumes, so the curve is steeper at the beginning. Red: in emphysema the lungs are less elastic and the curve is shifted to the left. Blue: in pulmonary fibrosis elastic recoil is increased and the curve is shifted to the right (the lungs are stiffer).

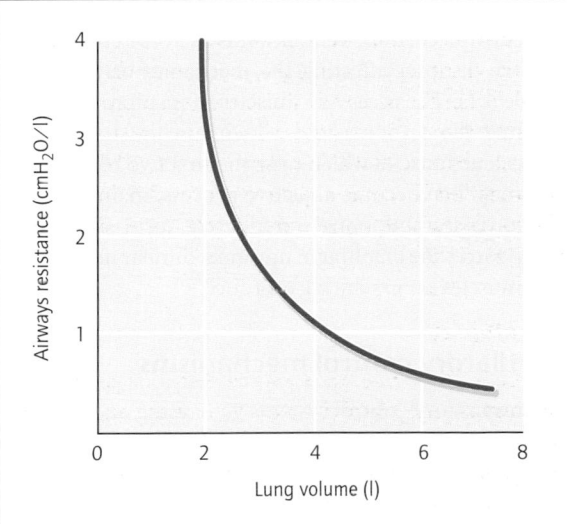

Figure 6.4 Airways resistance and lung volume. Airways resistance varies inversely with lung volume because the expanding lung parenchyma pulls on the walls of the airways. People with increased airways resistance (e.g. chronic obstructive airway disease) often breathe at a higher lung volume (and therefore appear barrel-chested; see p. 344) because this reduces the resistance to airflow.

Table 6.1 Causes of disordered mechanics of ventilation

Mechanism	Disorder
Increased resistance to airflow	Chronic airflow limitation
	Asthma
Decreased lung compliance	Pulmonary fibrosis
	Pulmonary oedema
Interference with thoracic cage movement	Spinal scoliosis
	Myasthenia gravis
	Respiratory muscle weakness
	Diaphragm weakness

Expiration

In contrast to inspiration, expiration is a passive process during quiet breathing. As the inspiratory muscles relax, the chest wall falls and the intrathoracic volume diminishes. Pleural and airway pressures therefore become less negative and, encouraged by the natural elastic recoil of the lungs, air is expelled from the chest. Unlike inspiration, there is a maximum flow rate that can be obtained during expiration and this cannot be increased by greater muscular effort because of the dynamic compression of the airways that occurs during expiration (Fig. 6.2c).

At the end of expiration the retractive elastic forces within the lungs are balanced by the natural tendency of the chest wall to move outwards. The respiratory muscles are relaxed and the lungs are at their functional residual capacity (FRC).

Disordered mechanics

The effort needed for ventilation is increased by any pulmonary disorder affecting the mechanics of ventilation (Table 6.1). The accessory muscles of inspiration may be required: the sternomastoids which raise the sternum, and the scalene muscles which raise the first two ribs. Expiration may then become an active process, mainly by contraction of the abdominal muscles (e.g. rectus abdomini), which forces the diaphragm upwards. Similar use of accessory muscles occurs during exercise.

Ventilatory control mechanisms

The respiratory control systems generating and coordinating the complex movements required for ventilation lie in the floor of the fourth ventricle in the brainstem medulla. From here efferent impulses travel to the respiratory musculature via the phrenic and intercostal nerves. These systems are influenced by chemical and peripheral stimuli, and are modified by complex interactions throughout the central nervous system (CNS).

Arterial blood P_{CO_2}

Under normal circumstances, the arterial blood P_{CO_2} (Pa_{CO_2}) is the most important factor controlling ventilation and is kept within very close limits (Pa_{CO_2} 4.8–6.0 kPa or 35–45 mmHg). Ventilatory rate is stimulated and increased by a rise in H^+ ion concentration in the extracellular fluid near the central receptors resulting from an increased P_{CO_2}.

Chronic CO_2 retention (e.g. caused by respiratory failure secondary to chronic airflow limitation) reduces the sensitivity of the respiratory centre. Hypoxaemia then becomes a more important drive to respiration. This drive is abolished by administration of supplementary O_2, which can, therefore, further elevate the P_{CO_2}, and lead eventually to CO_2 narcosis. Ventilation is also increased by rises in H^+ concentrations from non-respiratory causes; for example, diabetic ketoacidosis causes the deep sighing 'Kussmaul' respiration.

Some drugs (e.g. aspirin and doxapram) can stimulate the respiratory control centres directly. Other drugs (e.g. sedatives) may depress it.

Disordered ventilatory control mechanisms

Many cerebral disorders can interfere with the respiratory centres or their connecting pathways, and the resultant ventilatory pattern may help in localizing the problem (Table 6.2).

Cheyne–Stokes respiration, which is the most common form of this type of respiration, is a regular waxing and waning of total tidal volume with brief apnoea in between. It can result from bilateral interruption of the descending inhibitory cortical pathways (e.g. following a severe stroke) or from chronic hypercapnia.

Gas exchange

Within the terminal respiratory units (Fig. 6.1), gas exchange occurs by passive diffusion from areas of high to low partial pressure. This takes place across a surface area of 50–100 m^2 within each lung. There are 300 million alveoli in each lung and every alveolus is enveloped by a dense network of pulmonary capillaries. As the resulting alveolar–capillary barrier across which gases diffuse is very thin (less than 0.5 μm), there can be a rapid exchange of gases (Fig. 6.5). Once across the gas–blood barrier, O_2 diffuses into the red blood cells where it undergoes a chemical reaction with haemoglobin (Fig. 6.6).

In some diseases (e.g. pulmonary fibrosis) the blood–gas barrier is thickened. Gaseous diffusion can be so slow that O_2 equilibration may not be completed within the 1-s contact time the blood has with the alveolus. This may result in hypoxaemia but, because CO_2 is 20 times more soluble than O_2, CO_2 retention does not occur. In fact, in pulmonary fibrosis Pa_{CO_2} is often low as a result of overbreathing.

Table 6.2 Disorders of central ventilatory control

Breathing pattern	Level of disorder	Clinical features	Causes
Cheyne–Stokes respiration	Cerebral cortex	Regular waxing and waning of total tidal volume with brief apnoea in between	Vascular event, chronic hypercapnia, imminent death
Central neurogenic hyperventilation	Midbrain tegmentum	Hyperventilation	Vascular event
Apneustic breathing	Rostral pons	Pause at full inspiration	Vascular event, hypoglycaemia, meningitis
Ataxic breathing	Dorsal medulla	Irregularly irregular breathing	Vascular event, demyelination, encephalitis
Primary alveolar hypoventilation	Bilateral lateral medulla Anterolateral cervical cord	Apnoeic episodes (especially in non-REM sleep)	Vascular event, cervical cordotomy, congenital

REM, rapid eye movement.

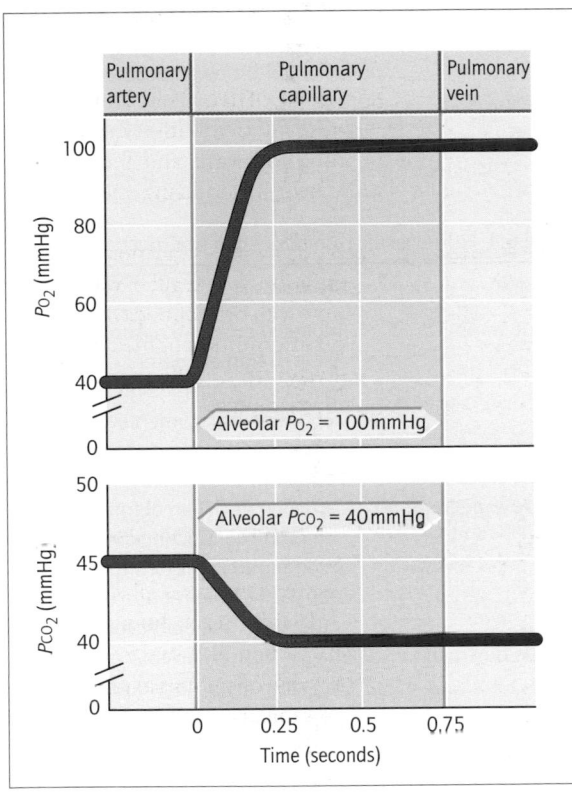

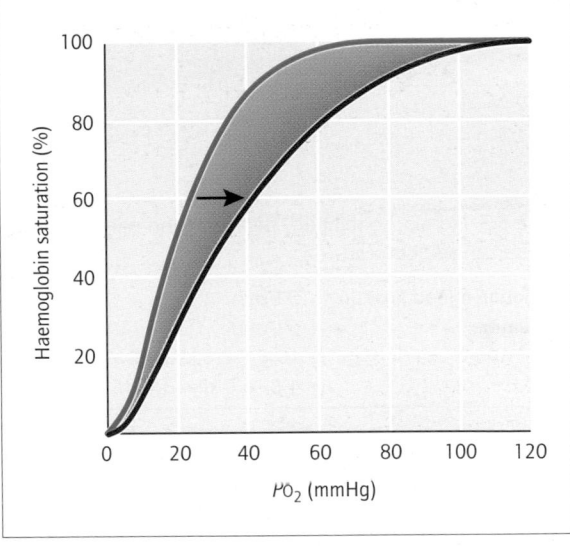

Figure 6.6 O_2 dissociation curves for haemoglobin. The sigmoid curve allows greater O_2 uptake at low O_2 tensions. Green: as 1 g of haemoglobin can combine with 1.39 ml of O_2, the O_2 capacity of blood with a normal haemoglobin concentration of 15 g/100 ml is 20.8 ml O_2/100 ml of blood. Purple: the normal dissociation curve is shifted to the right by a fall in pH, a rise in P_{CO_2} and a rise in temperature (e.g. as in exercising muscle), which increase O_2 release to the tissues.

Figure 6.5 P_{O_2} and P_{CO_2} changes in red blood cells. The normal changes in P_{O_2} and P_{CO_2} in red blood cells as they travel through the pulmonary capillaries and are exposed to an alveolar P_{O_2} of 100 mmHg and an alveolar P_{CO_2} of 40 mmHg are shown. At rest these changes are completed within 0.25 s. During exercise the time available for gas exchange falls as cardiac output increases (1 kPa = 7.5 mmHg).

Perfusion

For efficient gas exchange the ventilation of the terminal respiratory units (V_A) must be matched by an appropriate pulmonary capillary blood flow (Q) (Table 6.3). In the normal lung there is a wide range between the V_A/Q ratios, with a tendency for higher ratios towards the apex. Disruption of this relationship is the most common cause of

06

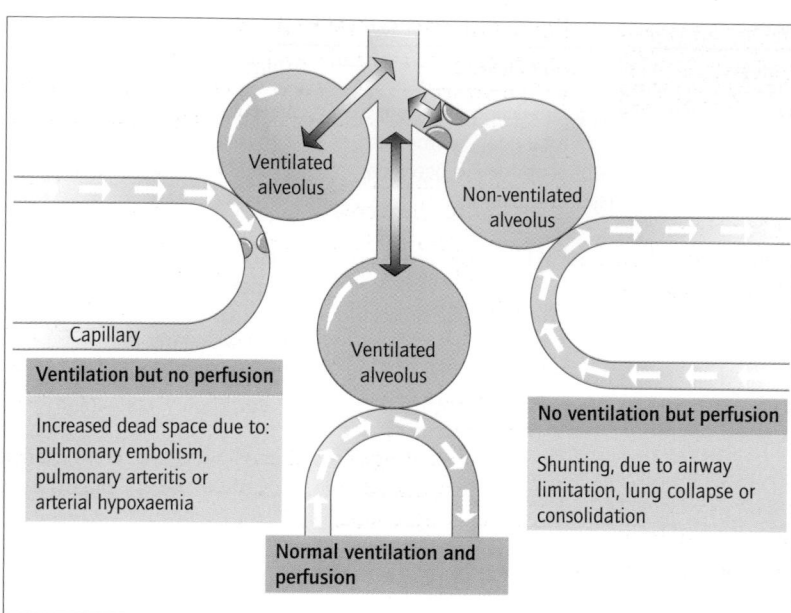

Figure 6.7 Ventilation and perfusion in health and disease. Diagram showing the relationship between ventilation and perfusion, and how various diseases can disrupt this.

Table 6.3 Normal ventilation, perfusion and partial pressure values in an adult at rest

Pulmonary blood flow	5 l/min
Ventilation	6 l/min
P_{O_2}	10.6–13.3 kPa (80–100 mmHg)
P_{CO_2}	4.8–6.0 kPa (35–45 mmHg)

Table 6.4 Non-specific respiratory defence mechanisms

Defence	Mechanism
Particle trapping	Impact in nose and nasopharynx if > 10 mm diameter
	Impact in carina if > 5 mm diameter
	Deposition by sedimentation in distal lung if 0.2–5 mm diameter
Particle expulsion	Coughing, sneezing
Particle expectoration	Carried in thick film of mucus, which lines the conducting airways and is continuously propelled proximally by the beating motion of the cilia that cover the epithelium
Particle destruction	Phagocytosis by alveolar macrophages, immune destruction

arterial hypoxaemia (Fig. 6.7). The conducting airways are supplied by an additional blood system, the bronchial arteries, but can function without it (e.g. following lung transplantation).

Pulmonary defence

The lungs are exposed daily to more than 10 000 l of ambient air containing infectious micro-organisms and hazardous dusts or chemicals. They are therefore equipped with:

● *Non-specific innate defences:* which normally protect them (Table 6.4)
● *Specific (immunological) defence mechanisms* (e.g. B lymphocytes and T-lymphocyte dependent) within lymphoid aggregates amongst the bronchi and bronchoalveolar cells

Defects in any pulmonary defence may result in lung disease:

● Smoking decreases mucociliary clearance and contributes to recurrent chest infections
● Congenital dyskinesia of tracheobronchial cilia (Kartagener's syndrome) leads to recurrent chest infections, and eventually to bronchiectasis (other features are situs inversus and absent frontal sinuses)
● T-cell deficiency (e.g. caused by human immunodeficiency virus infection; HIV), predisposes to infection with *Pneumocystis carinii* or *Mycobacterium tuberculosis.*

Approach to the patient

History

The history commonly provides the most important clue to the cause of a respiratory disorder, and a systematic inquiry should be made as outlined below (HISTORY & EXAMINATION BOX 6.1).

About the patient

Ethnicity

Some respiratory disorders are associated with ethnicity. For example, more than 30% of people with pulmonary tuberculosis in the UK are Asians. Pulmonary sarcoidosis, on the other hand, is rare in Asians but common in West Indians and young Irish women.

Personal and social history

Important personal and social factors are:
- *Contact with feathered pets:* can cause extrinsic allergic alveolitis (e.g. budgerigar-fancier's lung, pigeon-fancier's lung)
- *Contact with asbestos:* associated with the development of asbestosis, bronchial carcinoma or pleural mesothelioma decades later (see pp. 366 and 378)
- *Foreign travel:* tuberculosis is still common in developing countries
- *Sexuality:* homosexuals are an at-risk group for HIV infection and therefore pneumonia, most commonly from infection with *P. carinii*. This may be the first indication of AIDS (see p. 327)
- *Intravenous drug abuse:* if using dirty needles or sharing needles (associated with staphylococcal pneumonia, tuberculosis, HIV infection)

History & Examination 6.1

History
Respiratory symptoms
Cough
When do you cough?
How long does it last?
Do you produce any sputum?
Do you ever cough up blood?
Is there a wheeze associated with the cough?

Breathlessness
How far can you walk on the flat?
How many stairs can you climb?
Has the breathlessness developed suddenly over
    seconds or hours, or more slowly over weeks, months
    or years?
Does the breathlessness come and go?
Are you breathless on lying flat?
Do you get breathless at night?
Do you wheeze or pant?

Pain
Where is the pain?
How long have you had it?
What kind of pain is it: sharp, dull, aching?
What causes the pain?
What relieves the pain?

Disease impact
Do your symptoms interfere with your work? How?
Do they interfere with your social activities? How?
Do they interfere with your daily life? How?

About the pattern of disease
Onset and progression
Are your symptoms seasonal?
Have they developed slowly or rapidly?
Do they start suddenly?
Are your symptoms intermittent?

Associated features
Have you lost weight recently?
Do you have night sweats?
Have you noticed any swelling of your ankles or wrists?

Social history
Do you smoke?
Do you keep any pets?
What is your occupation? Is it industrial?

Drug history
Are you taking any medication (aspirin,
    beta-blockers, angiotensin-converting enzyme (ACE)
    inhibitors)?

Past medical history
As a child did you have asthma/eczema/hay fever or
    pneumonia?
Have you had tuberculosis?
Have you ever had general anaesthesia?
Have you ever had a tracheostomy?

Family history
Has anyone in your family had an allergy, cystic fibrosis or
    tuberculosis?

06

Respiratory symptoms

Cough

Cough is the most common symptom of lower respiratory tract disease, and can occur in a variety of situations:

- Cigarette smokers often complain of an **early morning cough**, which usually produces a small amount of sputum ('smoker's cough'). The presence of a continuous cough with daily sputum production for at least 3 months of the year for more than 1 year is the definition of chronic bronchitis (see p. 343).
- A more **persistent cough** or a change in character of a smoker's cough may indicate bronchial carcinoma.
- A **'bovine' cough** suggests left recurrent laryngeal nerve palsy, the most common cause being bronchial carcinoma.
- A cough may **persist for several weeks** after successful treatment of a lower respiratory tract infection due to bronchial hyper-responsiveness (see p. 338). It usually settles spontaneously, but a minority of patients go on to develop asthma (see p. 338).
- **Cough at night** may be the only symptom of asthma in a child or young adult.

Sputum

Causes of sputum production are as follows:

- *Cigarette smoking:* the most common cause of clear mucoid sputum
- *Lower respiratory tract infection:* associated with yellow or green mucopurulent sputum, although non-infected asthmatics often cough up yellow sputum (because of the presence of eosinophils)
- *Bronchopulmonary aspergillosis:* suggested by the production of firm plugs of sputum ('headless prawns') by an asthmatic (see p. 367)
- *Bronchiectasis:* characteristically results in copious quantities of yellow or green sputum

Haemoptysis

Common and rare causes of blood-stained sputum (haemoptysis) are listed in Table 6.5. Haemoptysis in a smoker must never be attributed to chronic bronchitis

Table 6.5 Causes of haemoptysis

Common causes	Rare causes
Bronchial carcinoma	Pulmonary aspergilloma
Bronchiectasis	Benign bronchial tumour
Pulmonary infarction	Inhaled foreign body
Pneumonia	Pulmonary–renal syndrome
Tuberculosis	(e.g. Goodpasture's disease)
	Blood dyscrasias
	Chest trauma

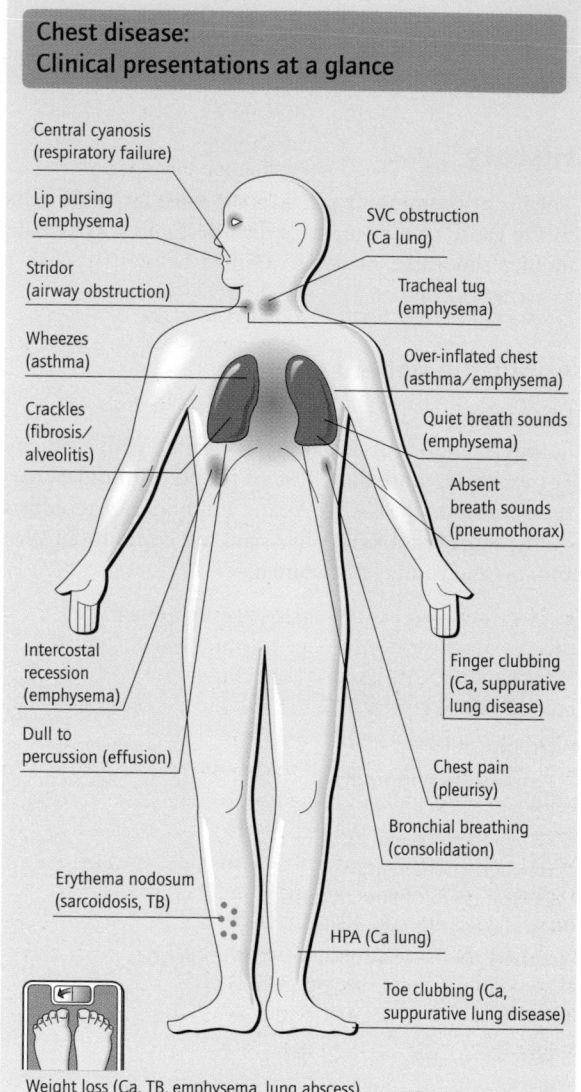

Chest disease: Clinical presentations at a glance

Central cyanosis (respiratory failure)

Lip pursing (emphysema)

Stridor (airway obstruction)

Wheezes (asthma)

Crackles (fibrosis/alveolitis)

SVC obstruction (Ca lung)

Tracheal tug (emphysema)

Over-inflated chest (asthma/emphysema)

Quiet breath sounds (emphysema)

Absent breath sounds (pneumothorax)

Finger clubbing (Ca, suppurative lung disease)

Intercostal recession (emphysema)

Dull to percussion (effusion)

Chest pain (pleurisy)

Bronchial breathing (consolidation)

Erythema nodosum (sarcoidosis, TB)

HPA (Ca lung)

Toe clubbing (Ca, suppurative lung disease)

Weight loss (Ca, TB, emphysema, lung abscess)

until it has been fully investigated to exclude bronchial carcinoma. Massive life-threatening haemoptysis can be a manifestation of bronchial carcinoma, bronchiectasis, pulmonary aspergilloma (see p. 367), Goodpasture's syndrome and the systemic vasculitides (see p. 372), blood dyscrasias (see pp. 1048, 1068) and idiopathic pulmonary haemosiderosis (see p. 372).

Breathlessness

Breathlessness or dyspnoea is an awareness of increased respiratory effort, which is uncomfortable and inappropriate. It must be distinguished from:

- *Tachypnoea:* rapid breathing
- *Hyperpnoea:* increased ventilation in proportion to an increased metabolism (e.g. during exercise)

06

Table 6.6 Causes of breathlessness according to rate of onset

Rate of onset	Disorder
Acute (seconds–hours)	Pneumothorax
	Pulmonary embolus
	Asthma
	Pulmonary oedema
	Respiratory infection
	Cardiac tamponade
Paroxysmal	Pulmonary oedema
	Asthma
Weeks/months	Cardiac failure
	Recurrent pulmonary emboli
	Pleural effusion
	Pulmonary fibrosis
	Pulmonary infiltration
	Lung cancer
Years	Emphysema
	Pneumoconioses

Table 6.7 Causes of breathlessness according to mechanism

Mechanism	Disorder
Obstruction to airflow	Asthma
	Chronic bronchitis
	Emphysema
	Collapse of a lobe or lung (e.g. lung cancer)
Impaired gas exchange	Pneumonia
	Pulmonary oedema
	Pulmonary fibrosis
	Lung infiltration
Pleural disease	Pneumothorax
	Pleural effusion
Vascular disease	Pulmonary embolism
Neuromuscular disease	Polio
	Myasthenia gravis
	Guillain–Barré syndrome
	Polymyositis
Extrapulmonary	Obesity
	Pregnancy
	Anaemia

● *Hyperventilation:* increased ventilation in excess of metabolic requirements (e.g. in panic attacks)

Causes of breathlessness according to rate of onset and mechanism are given in Tables 6.6 and 6.7. Breathlessness on lying flat (orthopnoea) with episodes of breathlessness at night (paroxysmal nocturnal dyspnoea) is a feature of pulmonary oedema, usually resulting from left ventricular failure (see p. 390). Asthmatics may also wake at night with breathlessness, which is usually associated with chest tightness and wheeze. Allergic and non-allergic stimuli may trigger an episode of breathlessness in asthmatics and such patients should be questioned carefully about all possible triggers (see pp. 338–339). Haemoptysis and breathlessness associated with weight loss in a smoker suggests bronchial carcinoma.

Chest pain

Pleuritic pain is the most common type of chest pain in respiratory disease, and is described as a localized, sharp ('stabbing') pain aggravated by coughing and inspiration. Pleuritic pain indicates pleural inflammation (e.g. caused by dry pleurisy, pneumonia or pulmonary infarction), and is also a feature of spontaneous pneumothorax or a rib fracture (e.g. following trauma or a bout of coughing).

Other causes of chest pain are given in Table 6.8.

Table 6.8 Causes of chest pain

	Disorder
Local pain and tenderness	Fractures (simple or pathological)
Pain and swelling of costochondral junction, particularly of second ribs bilaterally (Tietze's disease)	Perichondritis
Pain within the distribution of one dermatome	Herpes zoster of the thoracic nerves (often precedes vesicular rash)
Nerve root pain often described as burning	Intervertebral disc or malignant and inflammatory disease of the spine
Local pain and tenderness of chest wall muscles (may involve the diaphragm)	Coxsackie B virus (Bornholm disease)
Localized muscle pain	Breathlessness and coughing
Retrosternal 'raw' pain aggravated by deep inspiration	Inflamed trachea
Poorly localized, often dull, central chest pain	Large central tumours
Pleuritic pain	Pleuritic disease, pleurisy, pulmonary emboli, pneumonia, pneumothorax
Chest pain worsened by exercise	Ischaemic heart disease
Burning retrosternal discomfort	Gastro-oesophageal reflux

06

Wheeze, stridor

'All that wheezes is not asthma': the emission of high-pitched noises (wheezes) when the patient exhales simply implies intrathoracic airway obstruction. For example, generalized wheezing may be noted in a chronic bronchitis, and localized wheezing occurs when the airway is obstructed by bronchial carcinoma or a foreign body.

The presence of a lower-pitched noise on inspiration (stridor) implies extrathoracic airway obstruction (e.g. obstruction to the trachea or a major bronchus by carcinoma or a foreign body).

Associated symptoms

Weight loss and night sweats may be features of bronchial carcinoma or pulmonary tuberculosis, while painful wrists or ankles suggest hypertrophic pulmonary arthropathy (HPA). Ankle swelling in a patient with chronic bronchitis and emphysema is characteristic of cor pulmonale (see p. 343).

Drug history

Important drugs to ask about are:
- *Beta-blockers:* may worsen the symptoms of asthma
- *Cytotoxics* (e.g. bleomycin, busulfan): may cause pulmonary fibrosis
- *Diuretics* (e.g. frusemide): may cause pulmonary eosinophilia (see p. 373)
- *Contraceptive pill:* a risk factor for pulmonary emboli

Social history

Enquire about:
- *Cigarette smoking:* note duration (years) and extent (number of pack years: 1 pack/day for 1 year is 1 pack year)
- *Alcohol abuse:* such individuals are an at-risk group for pulmonary tuberculosis

Past medical history

Enquire about any history of whooping cough or tuberculosis in childhood, because either may be complicated by bronchiectasis in adult life. In addition, tuberculosis may reactivate decades later, particularly if the infection occurred prior to the anti-tuberculosis chemotherapy era (before 1950). Previous general anaesthesia can be associated with aspiration pneumonia and, later, bronchiectasis. Also ask about atopy, as many patients with asthma have a previous history of eczema and/or hay fever.

Family history

A family history of atopy, tuberculosis or cystic fibrosis may give clues to the diagnosis.

Examination

General examination

The patient should be undressed to the waist and either sitting or standing. Note general features of the patient's well-being (e.g. mental alertness), as well as the presence of obesity, cachexia or jaundice (HISTORY & EXAMINATION BOX 6.2).

History & Examination 6.2

Examination
General
Examine the hands
Note any tar staining, finger clubbing, peripheral cyanosis or flap/tremor

Examine the face and neck
Look at the conjunctivae for evidence of anaemia, and tongue and lips for central cyanosis
Note the height of the jugular venous pressure (JVP) and observe the effect of respiration
Look for any facial features of systemic disease

Chest
Inspection
Sputum pot
Look inside any sputum pot by the bedside
Chest wall
Note the shape of the chest
Look for evidence of previous surgery or radiotherapy
Look for engorged veins, subcutaneous nodules or use of accessory muscles
Measure the respiratory rate

Palpation
Determine the position of the trachea and apex beat
Check the symmetry of movement of the two sides, and measure the amount of movement
Palpate for cervical and axillary lymphadenopathy
Test for vocal fremitus

Percussion
Compare the percussion note in comparable areas on both sides of the chest and do not forget the lung apices

Auscultation
Note the nature and intensity of the breath sounds
Listen for added sounds (wheezes, crackles, pleural rub)
Note the character and intensity of vocal resonance

Table 6.9 Causes of finger clubbing

Common
Bronchial carcinoma
Suppurative lung infection (e.g. empyema, lung abscess,
    bronchiectasis, extensive pulmonary tuberculosis)
Fibrosing alveolitis

Rare
Bacterial endocarditis
Inflammatory bowel disease
Liver cirrhosis
Cyanotic congenital heart disease
Atrial myxoma
Pleural mesothelioma or fibroma
Familial
Idiopathic

Hands

Examine the hands for:
• *Tar staining:* from smoking
• *Finger clubbing* (see pp. 358 and 363; Table 6.9)
• *Peripheral cyanosis:* compare the patient's nail beds and
palms with your own
• *Coarse tremor or flap:* of the outstretched hands (a feature of CO_2 retention)
• *Fine tremor:* seen in some patients receiving nebulized
β_2-agonist therapy)
    Feel the pulse, which is 'bounding' in CO_2 retention.

Face and neck

Look at the conjunctivae for evidence of anaemia and look
at the tongue and lips for central cyanosis, the causes
of which are given in Table 6.10. Note the height of the
jugular venous pulse (JVP) and observe the effect of
respiration (e.g. JVP is raised in right heart failure; fixed
and raised in superior vena cava obstruction). Look for
facial features of systemic diseases that may have respiratory complications.

Examination of the chest

Examination of the respiratory system can be divided into
four parts: inspection, palpation, percussion and auscultation. The findings contribute to a pattern of physical
signs, which can then be compared with the typical signs
found in particular chest diseases (Table 6.11).

Inspection
Sputum pot
If there is a sputum pot by the bedside, look in it. This may
give an immediate clue to the diagnosis (see p. 356).

Chest wall
Note:
• Shape of the chest
• Any evidence of previous surgery (e.g. thoracotomy,
thoracoplasty) or radiotherapy (such as telangiectasia)
• Engorged veins
• Subcutaneous nodules (e.g. metastases)
• Rate of respiration (usually 14–18 breaths/min)
• Use of accessory muscles of respiration
• Whether chest expansion is symmetrical and adequate
(normal expansion is at least 3 cm)

Palpation
Determine the position of the trachea (upper mediastinum)
and apex beat (lower mediastinum). Check the symmetry

Table 6.10 Causes of cyanosis

Mechanism	Disorder
Peripheral cyanosis (hands will be cold, blood leaving the lungs is oxygenated adequately, but is not circulating adequately to peripheral tissues)	
Physiological	Cold temperature
Reduced cardiac output	Shock, heart disease
Large vessel obstruction	Peripheral vascular disease
Peripheral vasospasm	Raynaud's phenomenon
Central cyanosis (hands will be warm and there is arterial hypoxia)	
Common causes	
Respiratory disease	Many conditions including chronic obstructive airways disease, lung fibrosis, etc.
Congenital heart disease	Ventricular septal defect, Fallot's tetralogy
Polycythaemia	Polycythaemia rubra vera
Rare causes	
V/Q mismatch	Massive pulmonary embolism
Haemoglobin desaturation	Met- or sulph-haemoglobinaemia

06

Table 6.11 Typical physical signs found with particular chest disorders

Chest wall movement	Mediastinal shift	Tactile vocal fremitus and vocal resonance	Percussion note	Breath sounds	Added sounds
Consolidation (e.g. lobar pneumonia)					
None	None	↑ Increased (whispering pectoriloquy)	Dull	Bronchial	Fine inspiratory crackles during early stages and during recovery
Collapse or removal					
↓ Reduced on affected side	Towards affected side	↓ Reduced	Dull	↓ Absent (or bronchial)	None
Localized fibrosis (e.g. previous tuberculosis)					
↓ Reduced on affected side	Towards affected side	↑ Increased	Dull	↑ Bronchial	Coarse crackles
Generalized fibrosis (e.g. cryptogenic fibrosing alveolitis)					
↓ Reduced on both sides	None	↓ Reduced or bronchophony	Dull	Vesicular (or bronchial)	Fine inspiratory crackles
Large pleural effusion					
↓ Reduced on affected side	Away from affected side	↓ Reduced (aegophony)	'Stony' dull	↓ Reduced*	None
Large pneumothorax					
↓ Reduced on affected side	Away from affected side	↓ Reduced	Normal or hyper-resonant	↓ Absent†	None
Asthma					
↓ Reduced on both sides	None	Normal	Normal	Vesicular with prolonged expiration	Expiratory polyphonic wheezes
Chronic airflow limitation					
↓ Reduced on both sides	None	Normal	Normal	Vesicular with prolonged expiration	Expiratory polyphonic wheezes, coarse inspiratory crackles

* Bronchial breathing may be heard at the upper level of the dull percussion note.
† A click synchronous with cardiac systole may sometimes be heard with a left-sided pneumothorax.

Table 6.12 Causes of reduced chest wall movement

Unilateral
Pleural effusion
Pneumothorax
Consolidation
Collapse
Previous lobectomy/pneumonectomy
Fibrosis (e.g. apical tuberculosis)

Generalized
Emphysema
Bilateral pleural effusions
Ankylosing spondylitis
Respiratory muscle weakness

of movement of the two sides of the chest wall, and test for tactile vocal fremitus. Causes of reduced chest wall movement are given in Table 6.12. Palpate for cervical and axillary lymphadenopathy.

Percussion
Compare the percussion note in comparable areas on both sides of the chest (Table 6.11). Map out the limits of lung resonance, bearing in mind the anatomy of the lung and pleura.

Auscultation
Note:
• *Nature of the breath sounds:* bronchial or vesicular
• *Intensity of the breath sounds:* normal, diminished or increased

Table 6.13 Clinical features and causes of different types of breath sounds

Mechanism	Clinical features	Clinical causes
Vesicular breath sounds (normal breath sounds)		
Passage of air into the alveoli and terminal airways	Expiratory sound follows inspiratory sound without a distinct pause and is audible only during the earlier part of the expiratory phase	Normal breath sounds are vesicular There may be a prolonged expiratory sound in asthma and emphysema
Bronchial breath sounds		
Turbulent air flow through the trachea and major bronchi	Inspiratory sounds become inaudible before end of inspiration producing a gap between inspiration and expiration. Expiratory sound is usually more intense, higher pitched and more prolonged than the inspiratory sound	Consolidation, collapse (especially of the upper lobe), top of a pleural effusion, pneumothorax (occasionally), large air-filled cavity near lung surface (e.g. lung abscess), over the right apex in normal people
Wheezes or rhonchi		
Produced by vibration of airway walls	May be heard during expiration and inspiration	*Generalized wheeze:* smooth muscle contraction (e.g. asthma), mucus plugging (e.g. asthma, chronic bronchitis), pulmonary oedema (occasionally) *Localized wheeze:* local bronchial obstruction (e.g. carcinoma, foreign body)
Crackles or crepitations		
Produced by the explosive reopening of collapsed airways ('opening snaps') or air bubbling through bronchial secretions	May be heard during inspiration and expiration	*Fine crackles:* lung fibrosis, pulmonary oedema, early or resolving stages of pneumonia, lung collapse (occasionally) *Coarser crackles:* chronic bronchitis, bronchiectasis

● *Any added sounds* (wheezes or crackles) and their distribution (scratchy sound in time with the respiratory cycle suggests a pleural rub, e.g. caused by dry pleurisy)
● *Character and intensity of vocal resonance*
The clinical features and causes of different types of breath sounds are given in Table 6.13.

Investigation

Lung function tests

The aims of pulmonary function tests are to detect and define abnormal lung function and to allow serial assessment of lung function to monitor the progression of a disease or the effect of treatment.

Normal values are required because the results of these tests vary with age, height and sex. Ideally, the best result obtained from three tests is recorded. Pulmonary function tests are not diagnostic of particular diseases.

Measurement of ventilatory function during forced expiration

Measurements of ventilatory function during forced expiration are simple to perform and do not require complex expensive equipment. Peak expiratory flow rate (PEFR) records the greatest flow that can be sustained for 10 ms on forced expiration starting from full inflation of the lung, and is measured using a Wright peak flow meter or equivalent device. Its main use is in monitoring patients with reversible airflow limitation (Fig. 6.8).

A vitalograph spirometer (Fig. 6.9) measures both the volume of air expelled in the first second by a forced expiration (forced expiratory volume in 1 second; FEV_1) starting at full inspiration, and the total volume of air that can be expired (forced vital capacity; FVC). Normally FEV_1 is more than 70% of FVC (FEV_1/FVC = FEV%). With increasing airflow limitation, however, there is a proportionately greater fall in the FEV_1 than the FVC, and so the FEV% falls. In contrast, in restrictive lung diseases the FEV% remains normal (Table 6.14).

The physiological principle of dynamic compression can be measured by plotting maximum expiratory flow against change in lung volume during a FVC manoeuvre [i.e. breathing from total lung capacity (TLC) to residual volume (RV); Fig. 6.10]. Measurements of flow rates at 50% and 25% of vital capacity (VC) are a more sensitive

06

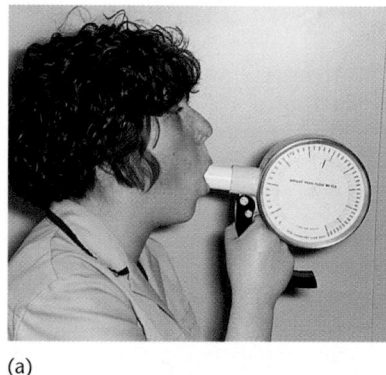

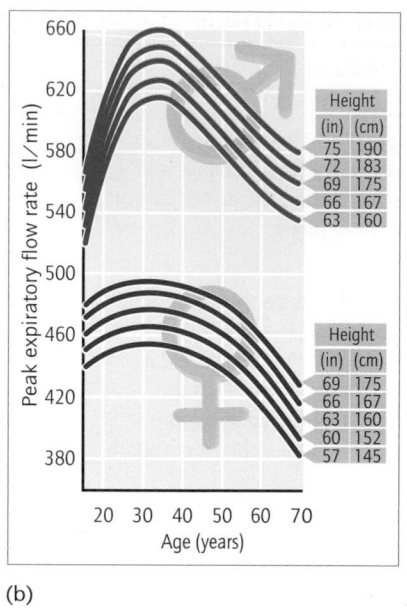

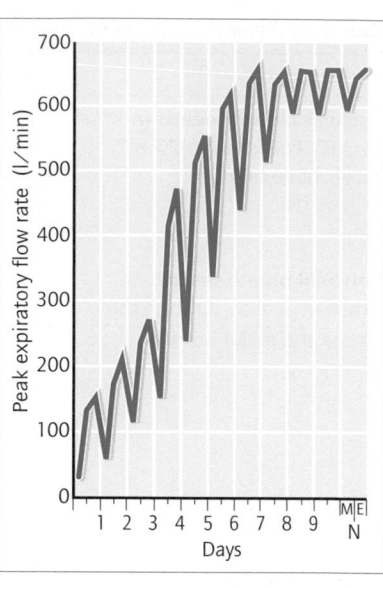

(a)

(b)

(c)

Figure 6.8 Peak flow measurement. (a) Blowing into a peak flow meter. (b) Normal peak expiratory flow rate (PEFR) readings (males, blue; females, red). (c) Changes in PEFR during recovery from acute severe asthma. Note the diurnal variation in PEFR with marked 'morning dips' (M, N, E, morning, noon and evening).

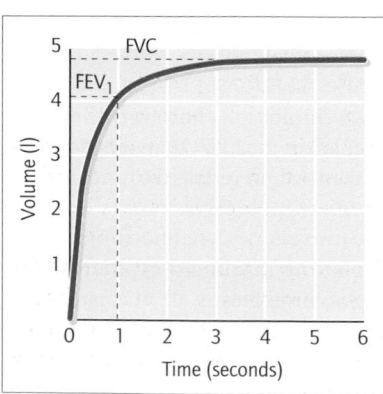

(a)

Figure 6.9 Lung spirometry. (a) Blowing into a dry vitalograph. (b) Spirogram trace of a normal adult male: FEV_1 4.1 l; FVC 4.9 l; FEV_1/FVC 84%. (c) Spirogram tracing of a person with airways obstruction (e.g. emphysema, chronic bronchitis): FEV_1 1.2 l; FVC 3.5 l; FEV_1/FVC 32%. (d) Spirogram tracing of a person with a restrictive defect (e.g. fibrosing alveolitis): FEV_1 1.9 l; FVC 2.1 l; FEV_1/FVC 90%.

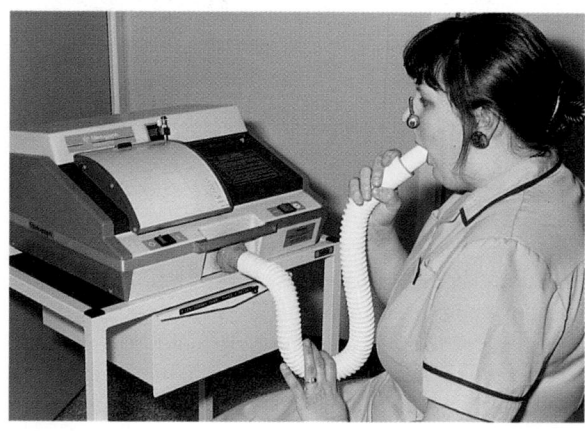

(b)

(c)

(d)

06

Table 6.14 Changes in ventilatory function during forced expiration in different diseases

Disease	FEV$_1$	FVC	FEV$_1$/FVC%	PEFR	Increased after inhaling bronchodilator (%)
Obstructive lung disease					
Chronic bronchitis	↓↓	↓	↓	↓	< 15
Emphysema	↓↓	↓	↓	↓	< 15
Asthma	↓↓	↓	↓	↓	> 20
Restrictive lung disease					
Pulmonary fibrosis	↓	↓	Normal or ↑	Normal	0

FEV$_1$, forced expiratory volume in 1 second; FVC, forced vital capacity; PEFR, peak expiratory flow rate.

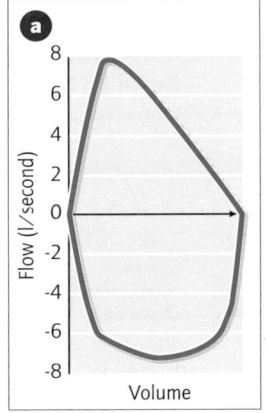
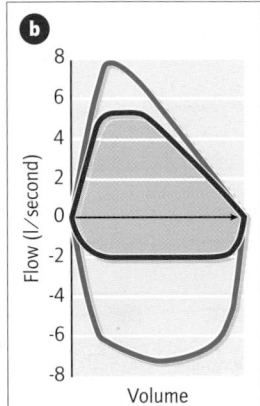
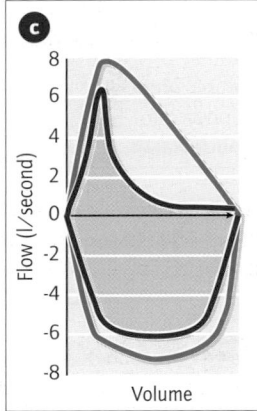

Figure 6.10 Maximum expiratory flow–volume curves. In each curve, the area above the zero line represents flow outwards during expiration and the area below zero represents flow inwards during inspiration. (a) Normal curve. (b) Extrathoracic large airway narrowing (e.g. resulting from a tracheal tumour) is shown in red. (c) Intrathoracic airway narrowing (e.g. asthma) is shown in red.

index of disease of the smaller airways than the FEV$_1$. Causes of a reduced VC are given in Table 6.15.

Measurement of subdivisions of lung volumes

This requires more complex equipment (e.g. helium dilution, body plethysmography) and a pulmonary function technician. Of the various divisions within the TLC (Fig. 6.11), only four need to be remembered: total lung capacity (TLC); residual volume (RV); functional residual capacity (FRC); and vital capacity (VC). Patients with airflow limitation tend to have evidence of lung hyperinflation, whereas those with pulmonary fibrosis have a reduction in all lung volumes (Table 6.16).

Measurement of gas exchange

Transfer factor (diffusing capacity of lung for carbon monoxide; DLCO) is a measure of the ability of the lungs to transfer gas from alveolar air into capillary blood (Table 6.17). The KCO is the gas transfer adjusted for the lung volumes. A low concentration of carbon monoxide (0.03% CO) is inhaled, and its uptake is measured while the breath is held for 10 s at full lung inflation. Its value depends on:

- Surface area of the alveoli available for gas exchange
- Thickness of the alveolar–capillary membrane
- Pulmonary capillary blood volume
- Capillary blood haemoglobin concentration

Haematology

There may be secondary polycythaemia in response to chronic hypoxaemia.

Biochemistry

Measurement of arterial blood gases

Direct measurement of the partial pressure of both O$_2$ (Pao$_2$) and CO$_2$ (Paco$_2$) within arterial blood is an essential part of the management of many respiratory disorders (e.g. in monitoring O$_2$ therapy in respiratory failure; see p. 347). Causes of hypoxaemia are given in Table 6.18.

Samples of arterial blood are usually obtained from the radial artery by withdrawing blood into a heparinized syringe. Alternatively, cutaneous O$_2$ saturation (Sao$_2$) may be measured by pulse oximetry, which is particularly useful in intensive care units.

Normal Pao$_2$ is 10.6–13.3 kPa (80–100 mmHg), and

06

Table 6.15 Reduced vital capacity

Skeletal abnormality
Kyphoscoliosis

Weak respiratory muscles
Myopathies
Poliomyelitis
Myasthenia gravis

Reduced lung volume
Diffuse pulmonary infiltration
Pulmonary fibrosis
Large pleural effusion
Collapsed lobes/lung
Pulmonary oedema

Severe airways obstruction
Asthma
Chronic bronchitis
Emphysema
Bronchiectasis

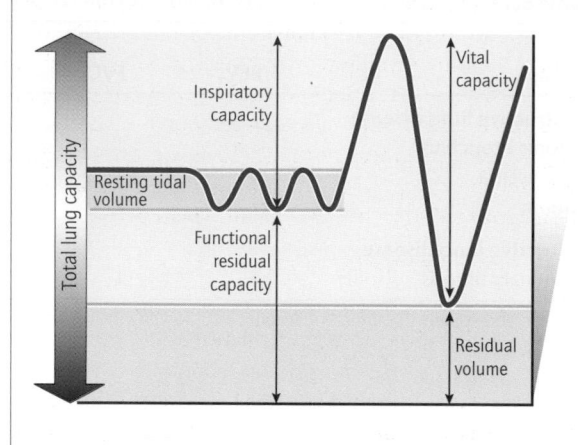

Figure 6.11 Lung volumes. Spirogram tracing showing static lung volumes.

Table 6.16 Changes in lung volumes in different respiratory diseases

Disease	TLC	RV	RV/TLC%
Obstructive lung disease (e.g. emphysema)	↑	↑↑	↑
Restrictive lung disease (e.g. pulmonary fibrosis)	↓	↓	Normal

TLC, total lung capacity; RV, residual volume.

Table 6.17 Changes in transfer factor (DLCO) in different diseases

Disorder	Gas transfer (DLCO)
Respiratory	
Asthma	Normal or ↑
Chronic bronchitis	Normal or ↓
Pulmonary fibrosis	↓
Alveolar haemorrhage	↑
Cardiovascular	
Low cardiac output	↓
Anaemia	↓
Polycythaemia	↑

DLCO, diffusing capacity of lung for carbon monoxide.

Table 6.18 Causes of hypoxia

Mechanism	Disorder	Cardinal features
Mismatching of pulmonary blood flow (Q) and alveolar ventilation (V)	Acute severe asthma or exacerbation of obstructive airways disease (most common cause of hypoxia)	Variable Pa_{CO_2}; increased alveolar–arterial O_2 gradient
Alveolar hypoventilation	Respiratory depression (e.g. sedatives), respiratory muscle weakness (e.g. myasthenia), thoracic cage abnormalities (e.g. kyphoscoliosis)	Increased Pa_{CO_2}; increased FiO_2 abolishes fall in Pa_{O_2}, normal alveolar–arterial O_2 gradient
Impaired gas transfer in lungs	Pulmonary fibrosis	Decreased Pa_{CO_2}, increased alveolar–arterial O_2 gradient, increased FiO_2 corrects fall in Pa_{O_2}
Anatomical shunting	Extrapulmonary disorders (e.g. VSD) and intrapulmonary disease (e.g. consolidation)	Normal Pa_{CO_2}, increased alveolar–arterial O_2 gradient

FiO_2, inspired oxygen concentration; VSD, ventricular septal defect.

06

respiratory failure is defined as P_{ao_2} of 8.0 kPa (60 mmHg) or less. Cyanosis is usually apparent when P_{ao_2} falls below 7 kPa (53 mmHg), although may occur at a higher P_{ao_2} in a polycythaemic patient, or not at all in an anaemic patient.

Estimation of the alveolar–arterial O_2 difference $(P_{alv}o_2 – P_{ao_2})$ is a measure of the efficiency of the lung as a gas exchanger. $P_{alv}o_2$ is sometimes written as P_{Ao_2}. It can be determined from the alveolar air equation:

$$P_{alv}o_2 = P \text{ inspired } O_2 – (P_{aco_2} \div 0.8).$$

Normal P_{aCo_2} is 4.8–6.0 kPa (35–45 mmHg). A rising P_{aco_2} implies alveolar hypoventilation.

Oxygen intake. Measurement of O_2 intake during exercise breathing is particularly useful in the objective assessment of effort-related dyspnoea.

Immunology

Relevant immunological findings include:
- An elevated serum immunoglobulin E (IgE) level in allergic lung disease
- Non-specific elevation of serum immunoglobins in chronic suppurative lung disease (e.g. bronchiectasis)
- Elevated serum angiotensin-converting enzyme level serum (SACE) in sarcoidosis
- Low/absent α_1-antitrypsin in emphysema

Diagnostic imaging

Radiography

Chest radiography accounts for more than 50% of all radiological investigations. Interpretation of the chest radiograph is therefore an essential skill for everyone involved in clinical medicine, and a systematic method for examining the film is required (Fig. 6.12).

Computerized tomography of the thorax

Computerized tomography (CT) of the thorax has a number of advantages over chest radiography. It is more sensitive in demonstrating small lesions and in determining their relationship to other intrathoracic structures (Fig. 6.13). Indications for it are:
- *Bronchial carcinoma:* to assess operability from extent of the tumour and the presence of mediastinal lymphadenopathy
- *Mediastinal masses:* to determine their extent, relationship to other structures and density

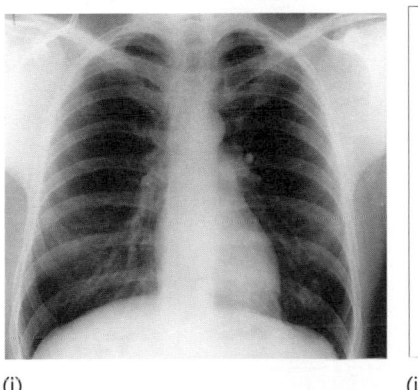

(i)

(a)

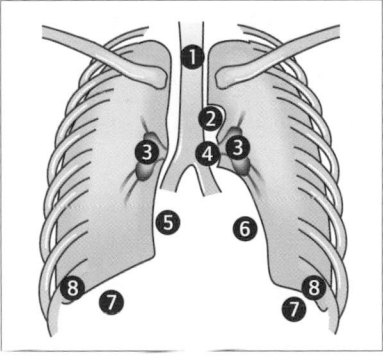

(ii)

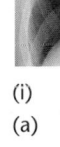

(i)

(b)

(ii)

Figure 6.12 (a) (i) Normal postero-anterior (PA) chest radiograph. (ii) Line diagram of a PA chest radiograph. 1, Trachea; 2, aortic arch; 3, hilar shadows (made up of bronchi, arteries and veins); 4, pulmonary artery trunk; 5, right atrium; 6, left ventricle; 7, diaphragms; 8, costophrenic recesses. (b) (i) Lateral chest radiograph. (ii) Line diagram of a lateral chest radiograph. 1, Trachea; 2, aorta; 3, pulmonary trunk; 4, heart; 5, scapulae; 6, thoracic vertebral bodies.

06

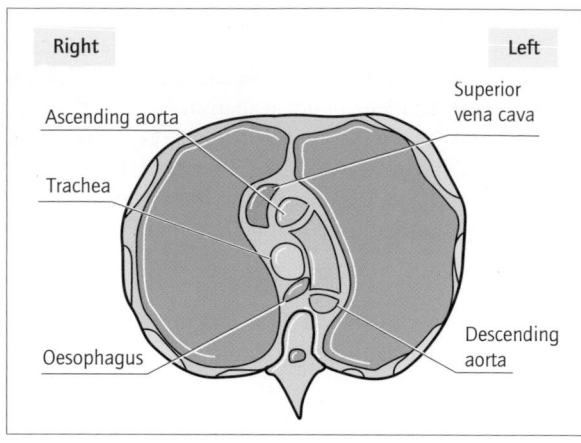

(a)

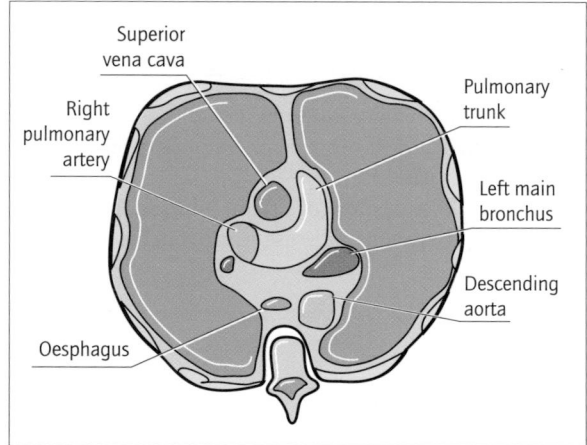

(b)

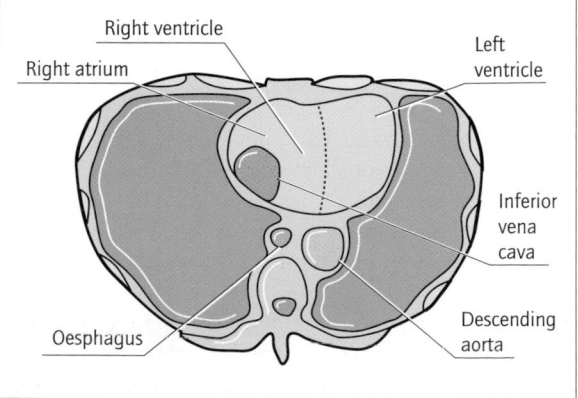

(c)

Figure 6.13 Computerized tomography (CT) and diagrams of the normal thorax: (a) the upper mediastinum; (b) the middle mediastinum; (c) the lower mediastinum.

• *Lung parenchymal disease:* to detect fibrosis, bronchiectasis and small tumours
• *Pleural diseases:* to detect asbestos-related plaques, and to determine the cause of pleural effusion

Bronchoscopy

The endobronchial tree can be directly visualized down to the fourth or fifth divisions of the bronchial tree using a bronchoscope (Fig. 6.14).

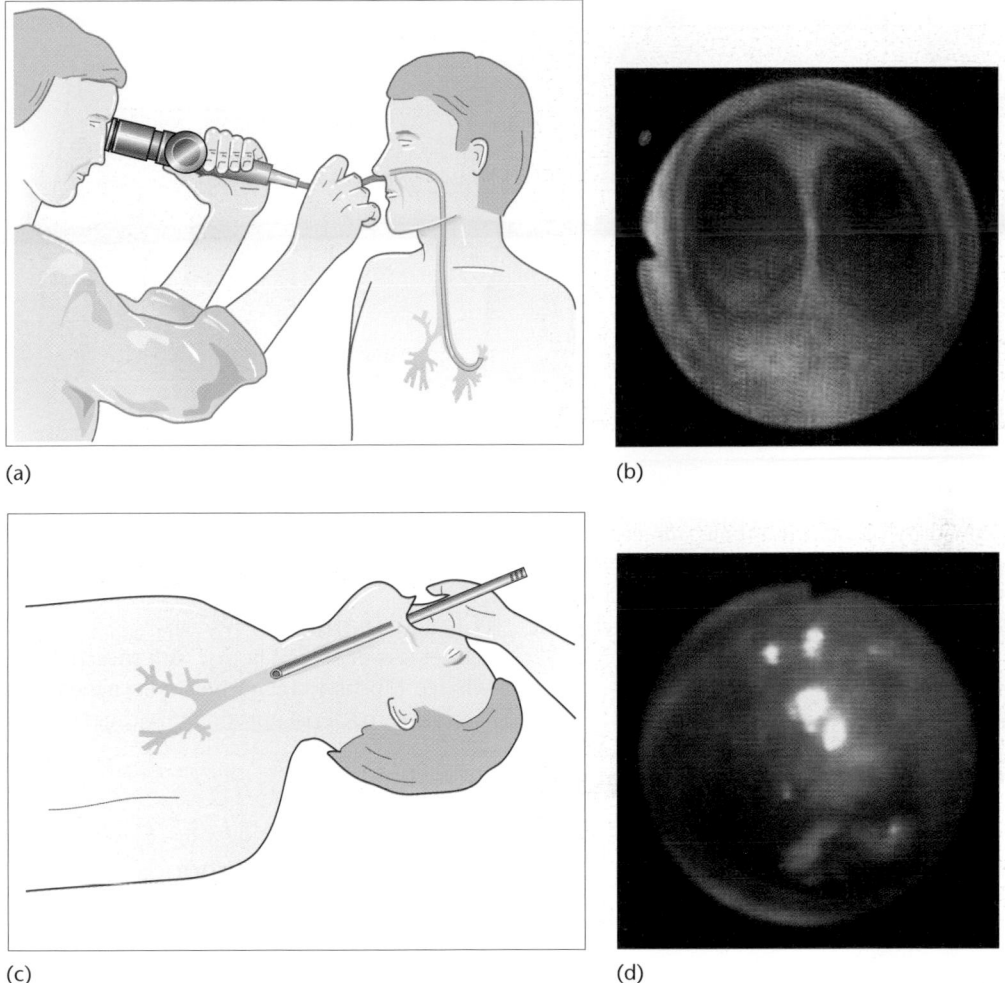

(a)

(b)

(c)

(d)

Figure 6.14 (a) Fibre-optic bronchoscopy. (b) Bronchoscopic view of normal trachea dividing into the main bronchi. (c) Rigid bronchoscopy. (d) Endoscopic view of a lung carcinoma.

Bronchoalveolar lavage. Fibre-optic bronchoscopy also allows collection of bronchoalveolar fluid (bronchoalveolar lavage) from segments of the lungs. This is particularly useful for determining the cause of parenchymal shadowing in immunosuppressed patients (see pp. 326–7).

Transbronchial biopsy. Blind biopsies of bronchial walls beyond the fifth division of the bronchial tree (transbronchial biopsies) include pieces of adjacent lung parenchyma. Such a technique can therefore be used to determine the cause of parenchymal lung disease (e.g. infection, fibrosis or granulomatous disease).

Bronchography. This technique outlines the bronchial tree by injecting dye down a bronchoscope, but is now seldom performed. It is sometimes used in bronchiectasis to determine the extent of disease before consideration for surgical resection of localized disease.

Microbiology and histopathology

Sputum culture and direct staining is invaluable in pneumonia, brochiectasis and tuberculosis. Pleural aspiration and biopsy are illustrated in Fig. 6.15.

For discrete lesions beyond bronchoscopic range, a percutaneous biopsy may be performed using conventional tomography or CT. Pneumothorax is the most common complication, occurring in 20–33% of cases.

Principles of management

The majority of patients with chronic respiratory diseases such as asthma, chronic bronchitis and emphysema are managed in the community. These conditions cause considerable morbidity and loss of time from work. Patient education is of increasing importance in asthma, with monitoring of the patient's own peak flow readings at

06

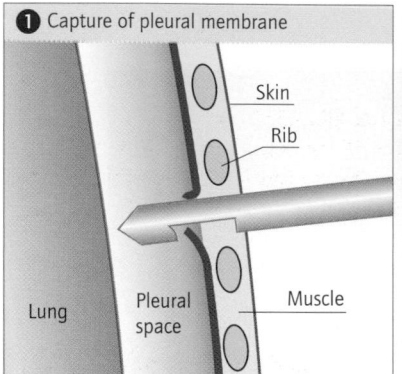 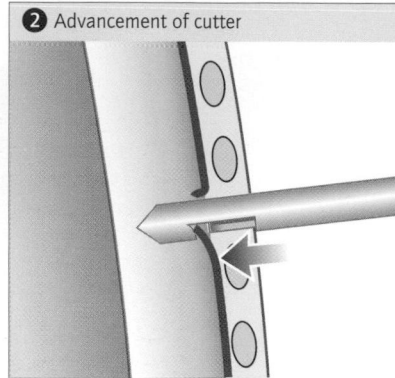 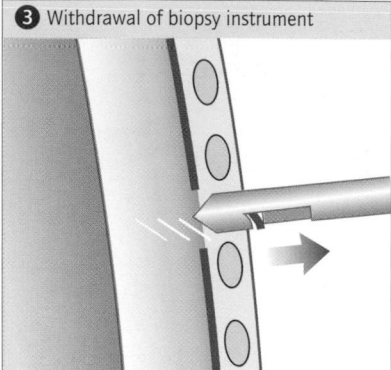

① Capture of pleural membrane

Skin

Rib

Lung   Pleural space   Muscle

Pleural space

② Advancement of cutter

③ Withdrawal of biopsy instrument

Figure 6.15 Three stages of closed pleural biopsy. Multiple samples are taken.

home. The majority of chest infections are also treated outside hospital.

Drugs are used to treat many respiratory diseases and are discussed in the appropriate sections of this chapter. Surgery is carried out primarily for cancer (see p. 362).

Physiotherapy

Physiotherapy is usually used in the hospital setting:
- To help clear secretions in postoperative patients
- For those recovering from pneumonia

Patients with bronchiectasis receive instruction for performing their own drainage at home.

Diseases and their management

Respiratory tract infections

These are a major cause of morbidity and mortality and account for 16% of all consultations with GPs. Infections of the upper respiratory tract and bronchitis are more common than lower respiratory tract infections, but the latter (e.g. pneumonia) account for the greater mortality (6%).

Upper respiratory tract infections

Coryza (the common cold)

Disease mechanisms

These are caused by a number of viruses including echo-, adeno-, parainfluenzae, rhino- and respiratory syncytial viruses. They are highly infectious and transmitted by droplet spread.

Clinical features

Onset is over several hours, with sneezing and nasal discharge. Mucosal swelling blocks the nasal air passages and secondary bacterial infection may cause sinusitis.

Investigation

Usually none.

Management and prognosis

Symptomatic only. Remits after 2–3 days if there are no complications. Immunity is short-lived.

Pharyngitis

Disease mechanisms

Infection of the pharyngeal lymphoid tissue (tonsils and adenoids). Infection is usually viral (adeno-, echo- or Coxsackie viruses), but can be caused by haemolytic streptococci.

Clinical features

Sore throat and constitutional upset; there may be an exudative tonsillitis. If severe, a peritonsillar abscess (quinsy) requiring surgical drainage may develop. Severe painful dysphagia (herpangina) with punched-out faucial ulcers can result from Coxsackie virus infection.

Investigation

Throat swab. Antistreptolysin-O (ASO) titres.

Management and prognosis

Antibiotics if bacterial. Remits in less than 1 week if caused by a virus.

Sinusitis
Disease mechanisms
Inflammation of the nasal sinuses.

Clinical features
Causes headache, facial pain and a blocked nose.

Investigation
Usually none. Sinus radiography.

Management and prognosis
Secondary bacterial infection requires treatment with an antibiotic. Chronic sinusitis may require sinus washouts and is difficult to treat. Remits if acute and treated with antibiotics. Chronic disease is problematic.

Laryngitis
Disease mechanisms
Infection of the larynx. Usually viral (influenza, para-influenza or respiratory syncytial viruses; RSVs), but can be caused by *Streptococcus pneumoniae* or *Haemophilus influenzae*.

Clinical features
Causes a hoarse voice, malaise and pyrexia. Because of the narrowness of the airway at this point, any swelling of the tissues can have serious consequences, especially in small children. Diphtheria can produce an acute epiglottitis in infants that threatens the airway.

Investigation
Throat swabs.

Management and prognosis
Antibiotics, humidification. Remits with treatment.

Lower respiratory tract infections

Tracheitis and bronchitis
Disease mechanisms
Most common in winter. Usually viral (adeno-, influenza and RSVs), but may be bacterial (commonly caused by *Streptococcus pneumoniae* or *Haemophilus influenzae*) if pre-existing airways disease (e.g. chronic bronchitis).

Clinical features
Dry tickly cough and retrosternal soreness. May be overlying bronchospasm. If there is a bacterial infection, purulent sputum is produced.

Investigation
Sputum culture.

Management and prognosis
Commonly resolves if untreated, but there is a risk of bronchopneumonia. Antibiotics are usually given for 5–7 days. Remits in less than 1 week if treated.

Bronchiolitis
Disease mechanisms
Usually occurs in young children, but also in adults in a chronic form associated with autoimmune disorders, particularly rheumatoid arthritis. It is usually caused by adenoviruses and RSV (which carries a significant morbidity in infants less than 2 years of age).

Clinical features
The child becomes markedly unwell, with cyanosis, tachypnoea and mild pyrexia. Chest auscultation reveals fine inspiratory crackles.

Investigation
Nasopharyngeal aspirate for virology. Viral titres.

Management and prognosis
There are no effective antibiotics or immunization against RSV; treatment is supportive. It carries significant mortality, and may cause lung hypoplasia.

Pneumonia

Pneumonia is an acute inflammation of the lung caused by invasion by micro-organisms. It may occur in a lobar or bronchopneumonic (patchy) distribution, and different organisms cause different types (Fig. 6.16). These vary according to where the infection was acquired (community or hospital, including aspiration), and whether the patient is immunocompromised, in which case a differentiation should be made between people with and those without AIDS. These factors determine the likely cause of the pneumonia, its clinical features and prognosis.

Community-acquired pneumonia
Disease mechanisms
This is a common disorder accounting for at least 1 million hospital admissions/year in the UK. Infection is spread by micro-organism droplet inhalation, which overcome the individual's pulmonary defence mechanisms and cause pneumonia. Several factors can impair

06

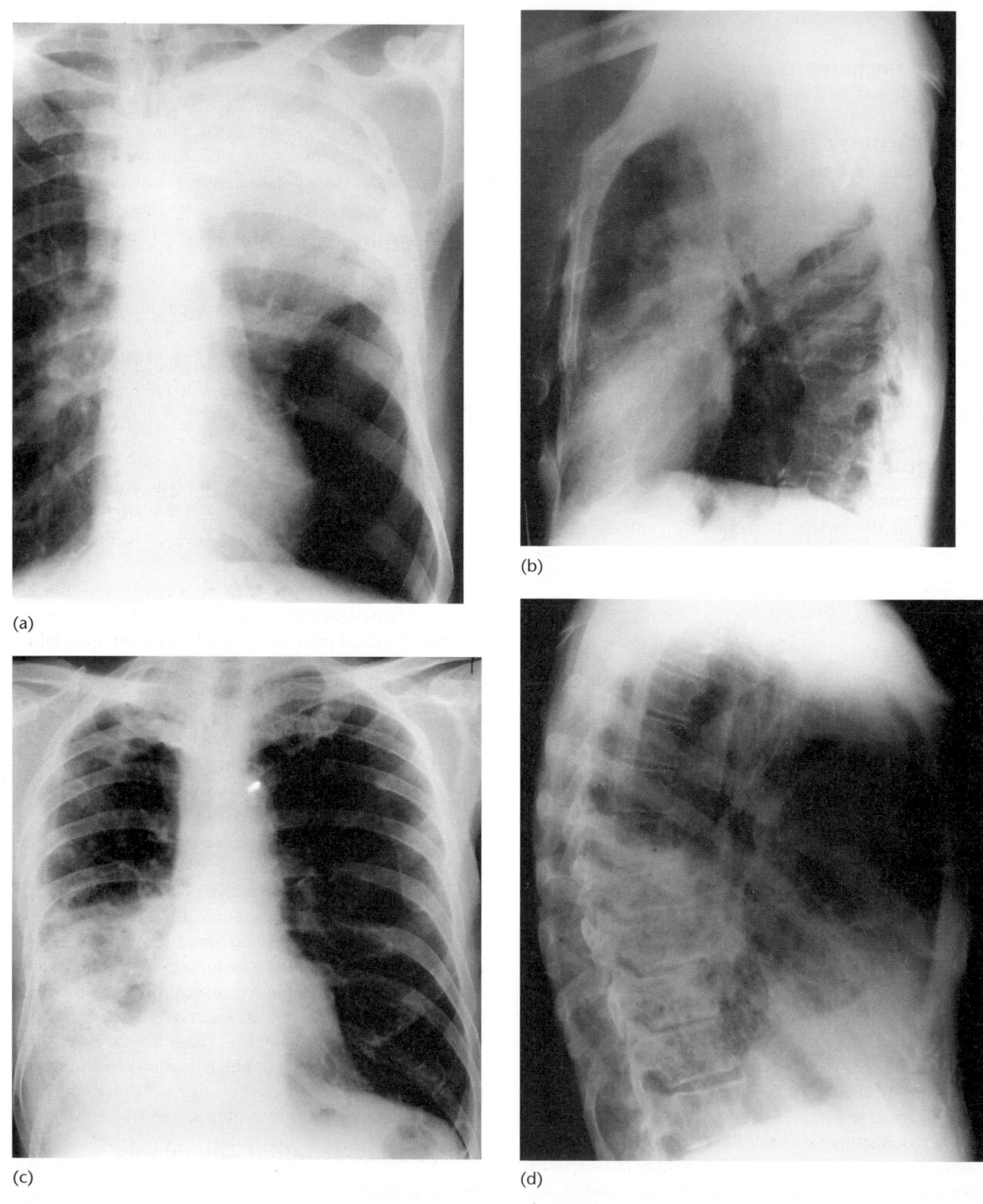

(a)

(b)

(c)

(d)

Figure 6.16 Chest radiographs in community-acquired pneumonia. (a) Posteroanterior chest radiograph showing lobar consolidation in the left upper lobe, caused in this case by infection with *Streptococcus pneumoniae*. (b) Lateral chest radiograph showing lobar consolidation in the left upper lobe, caused in this case by infection with *Streptococcus pneumoniae*. (c) Posteroanterior chest radiograph showing bronchopneumonia in the right lower lobe, caused in this case by *Mycoplasma pneumoniae*. (d) Lateral chest radiograph showing bronchopneumonia in the right lower lobe, caused in this case by *Mycoplasma pneumoniae*.

these mechanisms (cigarette smoke and alcohol depress ciliary function and phagocytosis; corticosteroid therapy depresses phagocytosis), explaining why pneumonia is more common in certain groups (e.g. smokers).

Lobar and bronchopneumonia

In lobar pneumonia, the colonizing organisms cause alveolar consolidation with fibrin and red blood cells (red hepatization). The overlying pleural surface is inflamed and a pleural effusion may develop. The red cells are resorbed and the alveoli are invaded by leucocytes (grey hepatization). Without treatment, resolution occurs by liquefaction of the consolidation, which is expelled by coughing.

In bronchopneumonia there is patchy alveolar consolidation and pus spills into the bronchi.

Pathogens

Streptococcus pneumoniae. The most common pathogen to cause lower respiratory tract infection (60–75% of cases) in all age groups. It can also cause acute bronchitis. It is often a commensal in the upper respiratory tract. Infection rates peak in the winter months.

Mycoplasma pneumoniae. Causes pneumonia in autumnal epidemics, usually every 3–4 years. It usually occurs in young adults and adolescents, particularly those living in close proximity.

Haemophilus influenzae. Usually produces bronchopneumonia in those with pre-existing lung disease (e.g. chronic bronchitis).

Viral pneumonia. Many viruses can cause respiratory tract infections, but they rarely produce pneumonia in the immunocompetent host:
• RSV can cause bronchiolitis and frank pneumonia and is an important cause of morbidity and mortality in children under 2 years of age
• Influenza, parainfluenza, measles and adenoviruses can all produce pneumonia and are more common in children and the elderly
• Chickenpox pneumonia occurs in adults and produces nodular miliary pulmonary shadows that later calcify

Legionella pneumophila. Frequently contaminates badly maintained air-conditioning systems. Outbreaks of Legionnaires' disease occur in fit individuals exposed to aerosols of infected water. Legionnaires' disease also occurs sporadically in immunocompromised individuals or in elderly patients with pre-existing lung disease. The disease is more common in autumn and in men.

Psittacosis. An ornithosis (an infection caught from birds) caused by *Chlamydia psittaci*. Chlamydia pneumonia (caused by *Chlamydia pneumoniae*) can also occur.

Coxiella burnetii. A rickettsial organism that causes Q fever, it is transmitted from cattle and sheep, and occurs in farmers and abattoir workers.

Staphylococcus aureus pneumonia. This is a rare pneumonia in previously well individuals, but commonly complicates viral pneumonia (particularly influenza A) in outbreaks.

Clinical features

While no symptoms or signs are unique, certain features suggest the microbiological aetiology:
• *Streptococcus pneumoniae*: a history of previous chest disease, pleural pain, rigors and labial herpes simplex I infection
• *Mycoplasma pneumoniae* infection: a 3-yearly cycle, and a younger fitter patient
• *Legionella pneumophila* infection: recent travel abroad (e.g. Spain), confusion, pyrexia (> 39°C), abnormal liver function tests, hyponatraemia and hypoalbuminaemia

Streptococcus pneumoniae pneumonia. An acute illness rapidly develops with a high pyrexia, rigors, a dry cough and pleuritic chest pain, and possibly herpes simplex labialis. As consolidation increases, there may be tachypnoea and cyanosis. Rusty sputum is produced after several days.

Mycoplasma pneumoniae pneumonia. This has an insidious onset (vague constitutional illness and headaches) over several days. Respiratory symptoms and signs are often sparse, but there may be cyanosis and a dry cough. Extrapulmonary manifestations may occur; erythema nodosum and skin rashes are common, myocarditis, pericarditis and meningoencephalitis or neuropathies are rare.

Haemophilus influenzae pneumonia. Symptoms of an acute infective bronchitis (a cough producing purulent sputum, and a mild pyrexia) worsen, with increasing pyrexia, dyspnoea, malaise and cyanosis.

Legionnaires' disease. An incubation period of 2–10 days is followed by a constitutional illness with headaches, malaise and myalgia. A dry cough and breathlessness are common. There is a spectrum of disease: severely ill patients have a high pyrexia, gastrointestinal symptoms, mental confusion and hepatitis.

Psittacosis. The onset of psittacosis is insidious over several weeks in individuals in close contact with infected birds; hence the name 'parrot fever'. There is a malaise and a low-grade pyrexia that can last for months.

06

Community-acquired pneumonia at a glance

Epidemiology
Prevalence
At least 1 000 000 admissions/year in UK

Age
• Respiratory syncytial virus pneumonia in children under 2 years of age
• Mycoplasmal pneumonia in children and young adults
• Chickenpox pneumonia in adults
• Influenza, parainfluenza, measles and adenoviral pneumonias in children and elderly
• Streptococcal pneumonia affects all age groups

Sex
Legionella pneumophila is more common in males

Findings on investigation
Haematology
Peripheral polymorph leucocytosis in streptococcal and mycoplasmal pneumonias
Leucopenia in *Staphylococcus aureus* pneumonia

Biochemistry
Hypoalbuminaemia, hyponatraemia and abnormal liver enzymes suggest *Legionella pneumophila*

Immunology
Antibody titres to distinguish organism
• Blood cold agglutinins for *Mycoplasma pneumoniae*
• Pneumococcal Ag in body fluids for *Streptococcus pneumoniae*
• Urinary Ag for early diagnosis of *Legionella pneumophila*

Microbiology
Sputum culture and Gram stain to confirm causative organism
Blood culture to detect bacteraemia

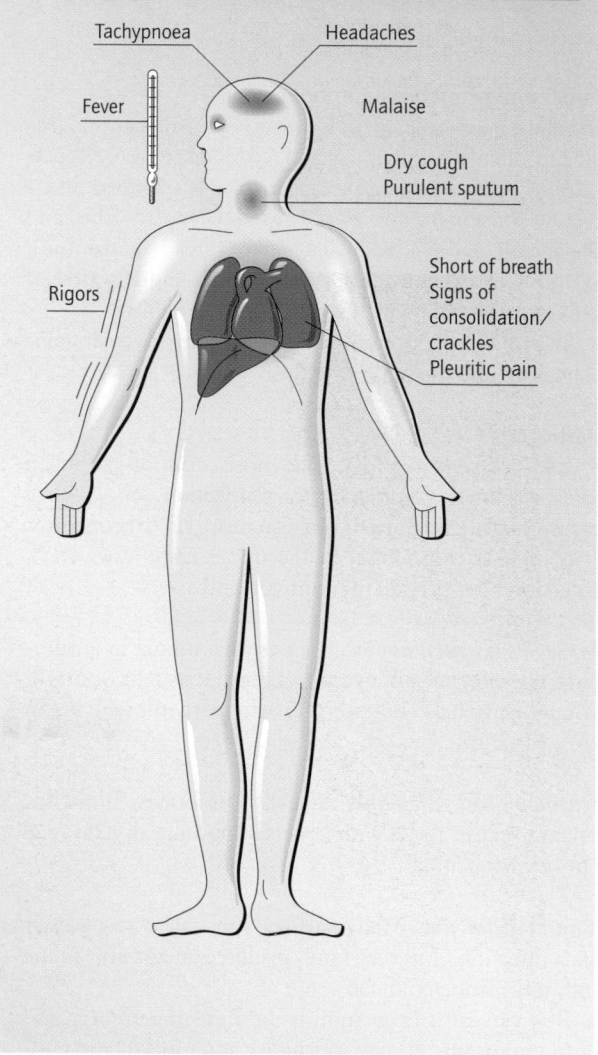

Coxiellá burnetii infection (Q fever). This has a chronic course with pyrexia, malaise, headaches and myalgia. Endocarditis may be a feature.

Staphylococcus aureus pneumonia. An apparently mild 'flu-like illness may rapidly worsen with a cough productive of foul yellow sputum. The patient then becomes severely ill with a high pyrexia, cyanosis and dyspnoea. Metastatic abscesses can develop in other organs as the disease becomes fulminant. Metastatic staphylococcal disease can occur in the lungs of intravenous drug abusers, and can also occur following vascular procedures.

Diagnosis
Microbiological confirmation of infection is obtained in only 50% of community-acquired pneumonias. The diagnosis is usually made on the history and examination, together with findings of consolidation on the chest.

Investigation
Tests other than chest radiography and sputum and blood culture are indicated if the clinical picture suggests a specific type of pneumonia as outlined below.

Haematology
Streptococcus pneumoniae pneumonia and *Mycoplasma pneumoniae* pneumonia may cause a peripheral polymorph leucocytosis. In psittacosis, the peripheral white cell count is often normal. In *Staphylococcus aureus* pneumonia the peripheral blood may show a relative leucopenia.

Diagnostic imaging
Chest radiography confirms diagnosis
• *Streptococcus pneumoniae:* patchy bronchopneumonia, lobar consolidation, pleural effusion
• *Mycoplasma pneumoniae:* lobar consolidation, patchy shadowing, sometimes normal
• *Haemophilus influenzae:* widespread inflammatory shadowing, scattered alveolar consolidation
• *Legionella pneumophila:* spreading inflammation

• *Coxiella burnetii:* patchy diffuse inflammation
• *Staphylococcus aureus:* spreading bronchopneumonia, patchy consolidation, abscesses (may cavitate)
• Persistent consolidation after 6 weeks suggests possible carcinoma

ECG
Myocarditis in *Coxiella burnetii*

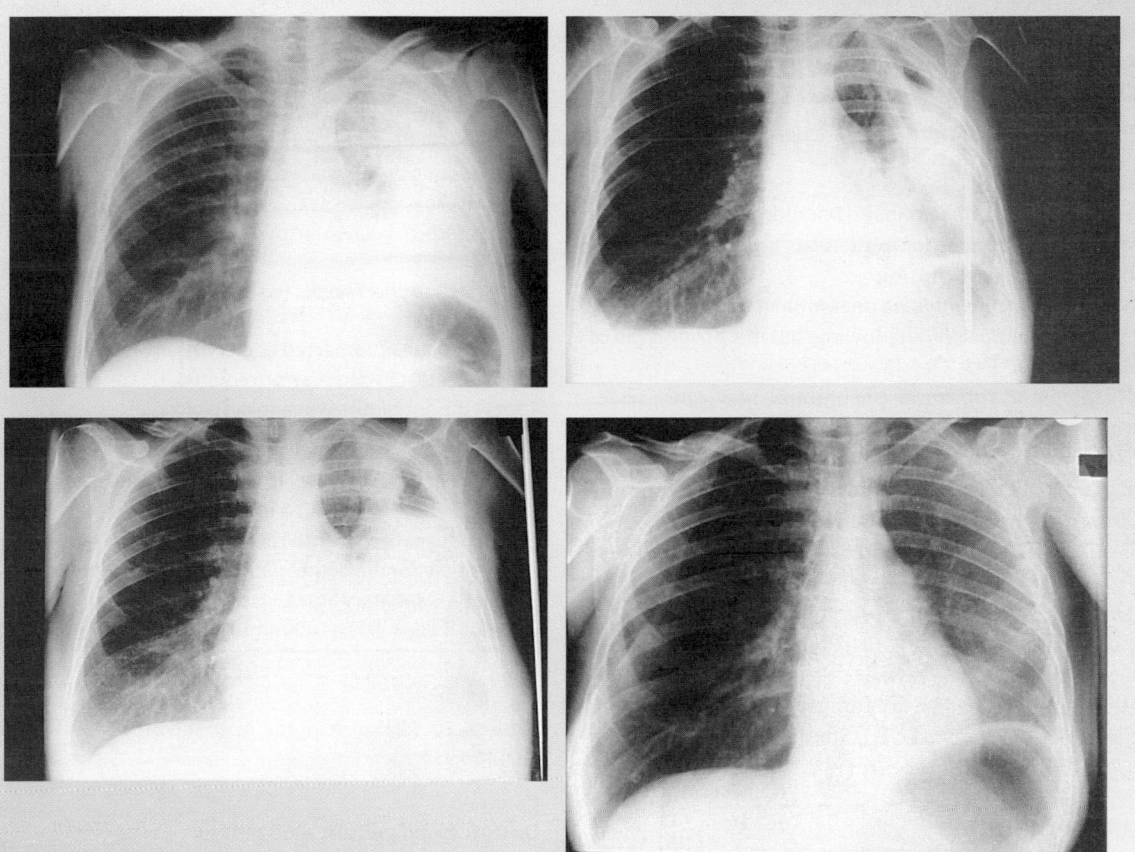

Fig. A (i)–(iv) Chest X-ray series showing management of pneumococcal empyema complicating lobar pneumonia. The empyema was first aspirated, but later required drainage with an indwelling catheter before resolution. Reproduced from Bannister *et al. Infectious Disease,* 1996 (Blackwell Science, Oxford) with the permission of the authors.

Biochemistry
Arterial blood gases of all patients admitted to hospital with pneumonia should be measured. Hypoxaemia is common.

Immunology
Blood cold agglutinins are present in 50% of patients with *Mycoplasma pneumoniae* pneumonia. **Antibody titres** confirm *Mycoplasma pneumoniae, Chlamydia psittaci,* *Legionella pneumophila* or *Coxiella burnetii.* **Countercurrent immune electrophoresis** (CIE) on sputum, blood and/or urine for *Streptococcus pneumoniae.* **Pneumococcal antigen** is present in most body fluids in *Streptococcus pneumoniae* pneumonia. **Rising antibody titre** allows a retrospective diagnosis of *Mycoplasma pneumoniae* pneumonia and confirms a diagnosis of Legionnaires' disease or psittacosis. **Urinary antigen detection** allows an early diagnosis of Legionnaires' disease.

Microbiology

Sputum and blood culture. Sputum should be sent for Gram staining and semiquantitative culture to identify the causal organism (e.g. *Streptococcus pneumoniae*) and to obtain antimicrobial sensitivities. Blood cultures should also be performed as bacteraemia occurs in 90% of patients with lobar consolidation. *Legionella pneumophila* can be isolated from sputum after up to 2 weeks' incubation.

Pleural aspiration for culture. Fluid aspiration for culture should be considered if pneumonia is complicated by pleural effusion, particularly if empyema is suspected.

Diagnostic imaging

Chest radiography:

- *Streptococcus pneumoniae* pneumonia: can cause patchy bronchopneumonia or lobar consolidation and sometimes a pleural effusion
- *Mycoplasma pneumoniae* pneumonia: may cause lobar consolidation or patchy shadowing, but in a proportion of cases is normal
- *Haemophilus influenzae* pneumonia: may cause widespread inflammatory shadowing, and scattered alveolar consolidation
- *Legionnaires' disease:* produces a spreading pneumonia
- *Psittacosis:* may show diffuse pneumonia
- *Coxiella burnetii* infection: causes a patchy diffuse pneumonia
- *Staphylococcus aureus* pneumonia: causes a spreading bronchopneumonia with patchy consolidation and abscesses, which may cavitate. Pleural effusions, pneumothorax and empyema are common complications.

Electrocardiogram (ECG) may show evidence of myocarditis in *Coxiella burnetii* infection.

Management

Specimens (e.g. sputum, blood) should be sent for culture before antibiotic treatment is given, but their collection should not delay treatment. The usual treatment is with a broad-spectrum penicillin antibiotic such as amoxicillin. Erythromycin is usually added if there is a suspicion of an atypical organism (Table 6.19). Oxygen therapy is usually given and in severe cases ventilation may be necessary. The clinical features used to distinguish a seriously ill patient are shown in Table 6.20.

Slow-to-resolve pneumonia

Pneumonia should rapidly respond to antibiotics, but the chest radiograph may take several weeks to clear. Failure to respond to therapy may be a result of the wrong antibiotic, poor compliance, mixed infection, bronchial obstruction (e.g. resulting from carcinoma or inhaled foreign body) or non-infective pneumonia (e.g. lipoid pneumonia, alveolar cell carcinoma, radiation pneumonitis).

Table 6.19 Management of community-acquired pneumonia

Supportive treatment
Rehydration
Physiotherapy
Oxygen as required
Ventilatory support as required

Specific treatment
Antibiotic therapy must be started immediately. Do not delay for results from microbiological specimens

If the patient is moderately ill
Most likely organism is *Streptococcus pneumoniae*; therefore, use amoxicillin or ampicillin. If there is allergy to penicillin, use erythromycin
Give the antibiotic intravenously at first
If *Haemophilus influenzae* suspected add erythromycin
If *Mycoplasma pneumoniae* suspected add erythromycin or tetracycline
If *Staphylococcus aureus* suspected add intravenous flucloxacillin
If *Chlamydia psittaci* suspected add erythromycin or tetracycline
If *Coxiella burnetii* suspected add erythromycin or tetracycline
Supplemental oxygen may be required
Review the antibiotics when microbiological results are available

If the patient is seriously ill
Give high-dose cefotaxime plus erythromycin plus flucloxacillin
Transfer the patient to intensive care unit as soon as blood gases deteriorate; do not wait until the patient is exhausted or has a respiratory arrest
Ventilate if $Po_2 < 8$ kPa (60 mmHg) on 60% oxygen

Table 6.20 Clinical features of a seriously ill patient with pneumonia

Confused
Diastolic blood pressure < 60 mmHg
Respiratory rate > 30/min
Lymphocytes $< 1 \times 10^9$/l
Urea > 7 mmol/l
$Po_2 < 6.6$ kPa on air
Chest radiograph shows multilobe involvement or rapid progression
Bacteraemia
± Antigenaemia

Complications of pneumonia

Lung abscess causes a swinging pyrexia and is treated with intravenous antibiotics. It may need surgical drainage. **Pneumothorax** is particularly associated with *Staphylococcus aureus* pneumonia and is treated with an intercostal tube and drainage. **Empyema** is treated with an intercostal tube and drainage and prolonged intravenous antibiotics. It may require surgical drainage. **Parenchymal organization** (ongoing alveolar inflammation and fibrosis in the absence of infection) is rare and is treated with oral corticosteroids.

Prognosis

Streptococcus pneumoniae pneumonia. Untreated, the disease resolves by crisis (by sudden resolution). An overwhelming pneumococcal septicaemia with circulatory collapse and rapid death can occur, particularly in splenectomized patients. With antibiotics, slow resolution (lysis) is usual. Although there is a significant mortality (5–7%), long-term morbidity is unusual.

Mycoplasma pneumoniae pneumonia. The illness can run a lengthy course (1 month), but recovery within 2 weeks is usual if treated.

Legionnaires' disease. Symptoms can last several weeks despite treatment with erythromycin and rifampicin. There is a high mortality in the elderly and in those with pre-existing lung disease.

Staphylococcus aureus pneumonia. This has a high mortality.

Chlamydia pneumoniae

Epidemiology

Large-scale epidemics are followed by periods of infrequent infection. Transmission is from person to person in schools and in the family. Infection starts in late childhood and the prevalence of seropositivity rises steadily with age (60% of individuals have evidence of past infection by 50 years of age).

Clinical features

- Atypical pneumonia (approximately 50% of cases)
- Acute bronchitis
- Sinusitis
- Pharyngitis
- Laryngitis
- Otitis media

Serological tests of pneumonia indicate that 5–10% are caused by *Chlamydia pneumoniae*. Primary infections are generally more severe and last longer than reinfections.

Patients often present with symptoms of the above infections, including fever and non-productive cough. Chest auscultation provides minimal findings.

Investigation

Haematology

Leucocytosis is frequently absent.

Biochemistry

Mild elevation of liver transaminases is common.

Microbiology

Chlamydia pneumoniae is more difficult to culture than other chlamydial infections, especially from clinical specimens. Particle agglutination tests indicate the presence of IgM and recent infection. Rises in titres of complement-fixing antibodies to whole cell preparations also indicates chlamydial infection. Species-specific antibodies that distinguish between *Chlamydia pneumoniae* and other *Chlamydia* are detected by microimmunofluorescence techniques.

Diagnostic imaging

Small segmental infiltrates on X-ray.

Management and prognosis

The antibiotics of choice are tetracycline, chloramphenicol or erythromycin given orally for 10–14 days in mild to moderate cases, or parenterally in severe and complicated cases. Hospitalization may be required in the elderly.

Chlamydia pneumoniae causes acute self-limiting respiratory infections that are often mild and patients rarely present to hospital.

Hospital-acquired pneumonia

Hospital-acquired (nosocomial) pneumonia is defined as a new episode of pneumonia occurring 48 h after a patient has entered hospital.

Epidemiology

It occurs in up to 5% of patients hospitalized for whatever reason. **Gram-negative bacterial pneumonia** accounts for about 50% of all hospital-acquired infections. *Klebsiella pneumoniae* pneumonia is rare. It is most common in the elderly and has an equal sex distribution.

Hospital- vs. community-acquired pneumonia

The pathogenic organisms causing hospital-acquired pneumonia and community-acquired pneumonia differ. Community-acquired pneumonia is caused by *Streptococcus pneumoniae*, *Haemophilus influenzae*, *Legionella pneumophila*, *Staphylococcus aureus* and *Mycoplasma pneumoniae*.

06

Hospital-acquired pneumonia is often caused by Gram-negative organisms but no pathogen may be identified. Secondary pneumonia can follow surgery or hypostasis from immobility in patients who are already colonized by potential pathogens. The nasopharynx of up to one-third of hospital patients is colonized by Gram-negative bacteria. If they are already receiving broad-spectrum antibiotics for infection elsewhere, such organisms are likely to be resistant strains.

General host defences are impaired in severely ill patients and the ability to clear respiratory tract secretions can be diminished by a variety of factors:
● Smoking
● Pre-existing lung disease
● General anaesthesia and/or sedation
● Poor hygiene amongst attendant staff
● Assisted ventilation
● Chest or upper abdominal surgery

Aspiration pneumonia. This occurs when commensal organisms (usually from the oropharynx) enter the lower respiratory tract. The organisms involved are varied, but anaerobic bacteria are common. Because of the anatomy of the bronchial tree, aspirated foreign bodies are most likely to pass into the basal segments of the right lower lobes. Risk factors associated with the development of aspiration pneumonia are:
● Poor dentition (caries)
● Sepsis of the oropharynx
● Bulbar palsy
● Vocal cord paralysis
● Achalasia of the oesophagus
● Hiatus hernia with severe reflux
● Binge drinking

Pathogens
Staphylococcus aureus pneumonia accounts for a significant proportion (30%) of hospital-acquired respiratory infections. Gram-negative organisms responsible are:
● *Escherichia coli* and *Proteus* species.
● *Pseudomonas aeruginosa* pneumonia occurs in outbreaks in some centres. *Pseudomonas* commonly colonizes the respiratory tract in patients with bronchiectasis and cystic fibrosis and in those ventilated on an intensive care unit. *Pseudomonas aeruginosa* pneumonia has a high mortality if it is a frank pneumonia.
● *Klebsiella pneumoniae* pneumonia occurs sporadically in the elderly and in people with pre-existing lung disease. It has a high mortality.

Clinical features
Similar to those of community-acquired pneumonia but patients tend to be more ill. However, *Klebsiella pneumo-niae* pneumonia is characterized by a sudden onset of a severe pneumonia, which is usually localized to one of the upper lobes. The patient is very ill and produces large amounts of gelatinous or frankly bloodstained sputum. The lesions tend to cavitate and may destroy the affected lobe. Aspiration pneumonia presents with an acute lobular pneumonia and there may be a history of alcohol abuse.

Investigation
The investigation of hospital-acquired pneumonia is the same as for community-acquired pneumonia.

Management
Empirical antibiotic therapy is started while awaiting microbiological guidance This will be based on local microbiological sensitivities and may be one of the following:
● Third-generation cephalosporin (e.g. cefotaxime, ceftazidine) plus an aminoglycoside (e.g. gentamicin)
● Carbapenem (e.g. imipenem)
● Monocyclic beta-lactam (e.g. aztreonam) plus flucloxacillin
● Quinolone (e.g. ciprofloxacin)
Vigorous physiotherapy is necessary.

Staphylococcus aureus pneumonia. Multiresistant strains of *Staphylococcus aureus* (e.g. MRSA) are becoming increasingly common and are difficult to treat. Flucloxacillin is usually part of the treatment.

Pseudomonas aeruginosa pneumonia. Treatment is with gentamicin, piperacillin or a quinolone antibiotic (e.g. ciprofloxacin).

Aspiration pneumonia. Treatment is usually with a third-generation cephalosporin, such as cefotaxime and metronidazole, to cover anaerobes.

Prevention
Measures to prevent hospital-acquired pneumonia include:
● Prevention of preoperative smoking
● Early postoperative mobilization
● Consideration of enteral sterilization in ventilated patients to prevent reflux (and aspiration) of gastric bacteria
● Awareness and careful monitoring of high-risk groups

Pneumonia in the immunocompromised

Patients with suppressed immune responses are more susceptible, not only to the usual pathogenic organisms but also to a variety of opportunistic organisms. More than

Table 6.21 Pulmonary disorders associated with acquired immune deficiency syndrome (AIDS)

	Uncommon	Common
Infections	Legionella	Pneumocystis carinii pneumonia
	Fungi	Mycobacterium tuberculosis
	Herpes viruses	Cytomegalovirus
	Toxoplasmosis	Mycobacterium avium-intracellulare complex
	Cryptococcus	Pyogenic bacteria
Tumours	Kaposi's sarcoma	
	Lymphoma	

one opportunistic infection can occur simultaneously, and there is often a lack of localizing clinical features. Invasive procedures (e.g. bronchoscopy) are required to obtain specimens for microbiological guidance. The 'pneumonia' can be mimicked by non-infective conditions (e.g. drug reactions, malignant pulmonary infiltration).

Pneumonia in HIV infection

An opportunistic lung infection should always be considered in any at-risk patient (male homosexual or bisexual, intravenous drug abuser, haemophiliac) with respiratory symptoms. A range of infections can occur (Table 6.21).

Disease mechanisms and epidemiology

Opportunistic lung infection in an HIV-positive person is the most common presentation of AIDS. The most common life-threatening opportunistic infection is *Pneumocystis carinii* pneumonia (PCP). The mode of infection with *Pneumocystis carinii* is unknown, but it causes an evolving interstitial pneumonitis. Other opportunistic pathogens include cytomegalovirus and *Mycobacterium tuberculosis*.

Clinical features

Pneumocystis pneumonia presents insidiously over 3–4 weeks, with a dry cough (80% of patients), dyspnoea (70% of patients) and pyrexia (80% of patients). On examination there is a pyrexia and some sparse crackles, but chest signs are absent in 70% of patients. Other signs such as associated oropharyngeal candidiasis, generalized lymphadenopathy or the skin lesions of Kaposi's sarcoma may be present.

Investigation

Haematology and immunology

There may be a lymphopenia (particularly affecting the CD4 count) in HIV infection.

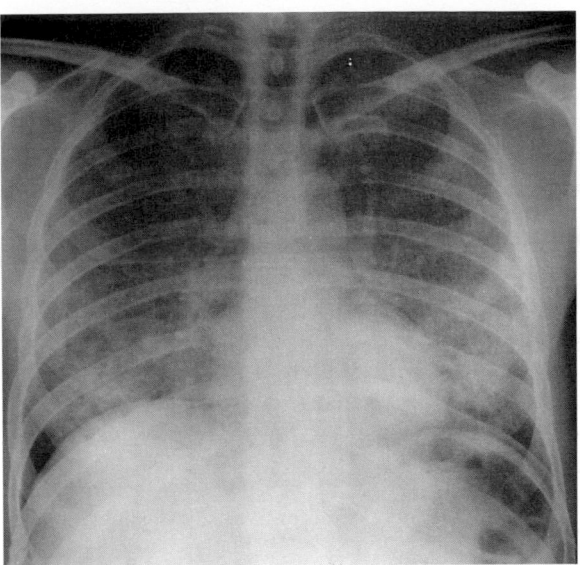

Figure 6.17 *Pneumocystis carinii* pneumonia (PCP). Chest radiograph from a patient with AIDS showing the typical features of PCP. There is bilateral diffuse alveolar shadowing spreading from the perihilar region into a butterfly pattern with relative sparing of the lung apices and bases. This pattern, however, is not unique to PCP and may also be seen in cytomegalovirus pneumonia, mycobacterial pneumonia and Kaposi's sarcoma.

Microbiology

Pneumocystis pneumonia can only be confidently diagnosed by identifying *Pneumocystis carinii* on direct examination of sputum.

Diagnostic imaging

Although many changes can be seen on the **chest radiograph** related to *Pneumocystis carinii* pneumonia, the typical change is that of spreading perihilar shadows (Fig. 6.17). **Fibre-optic bronchoscopy** is the procedure of choice for investigating possible *Pneumocystis* pneumonia if microbiological tests are negative. Bronchoalveolar lavage and transbronchial biopsy provide a diagnosis in 95–100% of patients. These techniques can also demonstrate evidence of other pathogenic or non-pathogenic conditions.

Histopathology

Examination of sputum samples induced by nebulized 5% saline may reveal *Pneumocystis carinii* cysts.

Management

Drug treatment is as follows:
- *Pneumocystis pneumonia:* oral or intravenous co-trimoxazole and intramuscular, intravenous or nebulized pentamidine with or without corticosteroids

06

- *Cytomegalovirus infection:* intravenous ganciclovir or foscarnet and sometimes hyperimmune gammaglobulin
- *Candida albicans:* amphotericin
- *Aspergillus fumigatus:* amphotericin
- *Mycobacterium tuberculosis:* antituberculous therapy

Prognosis

More than 80% of patients survive their first episode of *Pneumocystis* pneumonia, unless it is complicated by respiratory failure requiring assisted ventilation when the survival rate is 0–14%.

Pneumonia in immunosuppressed patients without HIV infection

Epidemiology

This is increasingly common with increasing immuno-suppression.

Disease mechanisms

There are many causes of immunosuppression and the increasing use of immunosuppressive drugs has led to an increase in opportunistic lung infections. Immunosuppressive treatment with corticosteroids and/or cytotoxic agents (e.g. azathioprine, methotrexate, vinca alkaloids) is used in acute leukaemia, lymphoma, organ transplantation, autoimmune diseases and solid tumours. Immunosuppression also occurs in the primary immunodeficiency syndromes and starvation. As with HIV infection, the spectrum of infective organisms is wide, but their relative incidence is determined by the nature of the immunosuppression.

Clinical features

The clinical picture is usually non-specific (cough, breathlessness, pyrexia, infiltrates on the chest radiograph).

Investigation

Haematology
There may be leucopenia.

Immunology
Immune studies may reveal a specific immune deficiency.

Microbiology
Sputum or **blood cultures** may reveal the infecting organism.

Diagnostic imaging
Fibre-optic bronchoscopy and bronchoalveolar lavage (with or without transbronchial lung biopsy) appears to be the best initial investigation and should be performed early in the course of the illness.

Histopathology
Histopathology may reveal *Pneumocystis* pneumonia, tuberculosis or cytomegalovirus infection.

Management and prognosis

Management of pneumonia is as for nosocomial pneumonia. Specific agents are added if certain organisms are suspected. Amongst immunocompromised patients with haematological disorders, 25–50% of all deaths are caused by infection from pulmonary sepsis.

Whooping cough

Disease mechanisms

Epidemics occur every 3 years, but sporadic cases are also common. The incidence is 25–60 cases/1000/year in the UK. The disease can occur at any time from birth to 5 years of age and is more common in girls.

Whooping cough is caused by *Bordetella pertussis* and *Bordetella parapertussis*, which are transmitted in respiratory droplets from convalescent and asymptomatic carriers or current cases. A number of toxins are made by the infecting organism, many of which have been shown to cause features of the disease.

Clinical features

The incubation period is 3–4 days. The symptoms are similar to those of an upper respiratory tract infection, with a cough and a nasal discharge that lasts for approximately 10 days. The cough then becomes more acute and spasmodic, and a deep intake of breath through a partially opened glottis at the end of a paroxysm of coughing results in the characteristic whoop (often absent in infants). Coughing continues for up to 3 months.

Physical signs are often few, but the spasmodic cough is always present, and patients may cough until they vomit. Constant coughing may produce an associated conjunctival haemorrhage.

Complications
Apnoea during coughing bouts can lead to cerebral anoxia and convulsions, with brain damage or death in extreme cases. Secondary bronchopneumonia is the most common complication and improvement in the management of this condition has resulted in the decrease in morbidity and mortality associated with whooping cough. Otitis media develops in about 10–15% of cases, while CNS abnormalities (fits and encephalopathy) occur in about 2% of children hospitalized with whooping cough. Fits are relatively common in severe whooping cough; encephalopathy is rare.

Investigation

Immunology
Serology. Rapid diagnosis can be achieved with antigen detection techniques.

Microbiology
Inoculation of a pernasal swab on Bordet–Gengou culture medium, when *Bordetella pertussis* can be grown, allowing a definitive diagnosis.

Management
Erythromycin may be beneficial if started during the catarrhal phase of the infection. It is also effective for the prophylaxis of close contacts. Secondary bronchopneumonia should be treated with amoxicillin, trimethoprim or erythromycin. Chlorpromazine may reduce the severity of the coughing spasms.

Hospital admission may be required if the illness is severe, usually for children under 1 year of age. Admission may be needed for patients with cyanosis or apnoeic attacks, severe secondary bronchopneumonia (rare) or parental exhaustion.

Prevention
The introduction of an effective vaccine in 1955 resulted in a steady decline in the number of cases, but worries about its safety reduced uptake. Because *Bordetella pertussis* continues to circulate in the community, epidemics continue to occur. The vaccine is contraindicated in children with a history of previous vaccine reaction and in those who have had an epileptiform seizure. It should not be given during a concurrent upper respiratory tract infection. The benefit of vaccination for children with cerebral damage in the neonatal period should be considered carefully. The risks of worsening cerebral function by vaccine should be weighed against the risk of disease.

Lung abscess

A lung abscess is a cavitating lesion within the lung parenchyma caused by infection.

Disease mechanisms
Lung abscesses are uncommon. Usually they occur secondary to bronchogenic infection, but can also arise from septic emboli (Table 6.22). They are more common in alcoholics, the elderly, intravenous drug abusers and people who are immunocompromised. A severe purulent reaction to an infection causes local alveolar necrosis and abscess formation.

Table 6.22 Causes of lung abscess

Primary infection
Pyogenic bacteria (e.g. *Staphylococcus aureus*, *Klebsiella pneumoniae*, *Pseudomonas* species)
Mycobacteria (e.g. *Mycobacterium tuberculosis*, atypical mycobacteria)
Fungi
Parasites

Cavitating tumours
Bronchogenic (usually squamous cell)
Secondary deposits

Pulmonary infarction
Thromboembolism
Septic emboli
Foreign body embolism (e.g. intravenous drug abuse)

Bronchial occlusion
Bronchial tumour
Inhaled foreign body (e.g. tooth, peanut)
Localized bronchial stenosis

Miscellaneous
Wegener's granulomatosis
Infected bullae
Pulmonary sequestration

Clinical features
The clinical picture is that of bronchopulmonary infection where the patient fails to respond to the usual antibiotic treatment. If the abscess connects with a bronchus (common when infection is brought about by pneumonia), large volumes of foul sputum may be expectorated. Sometimes the abscess will discharge entirely by this mechanism. If the abscess becomes chronic, the patient may develop finger clubbing and cachexia. In *Klebsiella* pneumonia the abscess is commonly large and may occupy most of an upper lobe; the patient is acutely unwell and coughs up bloodstained sputum. In tuberculous infection the onset is much more indolent. Amoebic abscesses sometimes affect the lung as well as the liver; in such cases the patient may cough up brown sputum ('anchovy paste').

Investigation

Haematology
There may be an increased white cell count.

Immunology
Immunoglobulins are increased in chronic disease.

Microbiology
Cultures of sputum or lung aspirate reveal the organism.

06

Diagnostic imaging

Chest radiography shows an area of cavitation within the lung parenchyma, which may contain an air–fluid level. In staphylococcal pneumonia, there may be multiple small thin-walled lung abscesses.

Management

Most respond to large doses of intravenous antibiotics to which the organism is sensitive, but drainage via needle aspiration or thoracotomy may be necessary. If there is an endobronchial foreign body, removal is essential. The prognosis is excellent if the lesion is drained and relevant antibiotics are given.

Cryptogenic organizing pneumonia

Cryptogenic organizing pneumonia (COP) is of unknown aetiology.

Disease mechanisms

This is an uncommon condition that can occur at all ages and is more common in women. The aetiology is unknown, but is probably not caused by infection. There is a progressive spreading patchy pneumonic reaction which organizes and impairs respiratory function.

Clinical features

There is a short history of malaise, pyrexia, weight loss, dry cough and increasing breathlessness.

Investigation

Haematology

The white cell count is usually normal; the erythrocyte sedimentation rate (ESR) is markedly raised.

Immunology

This is normal.

Microbiology

Sputum cultures are negative.

Diagnostic imaging

Chest radiography shows patchy alveolar shadows which wax and wane.

Diagnosis

Clinical, or by lung biopsy.

Management

Responds well to a prolonged course of oral steroids.

Mycobacterial lung diseases

There are several mycobacterial organisms that can cause

disease in humans. The most important of these is *Mycobacterium tuberculosis*, which causes tuberculosis (see Chapter 3).

Pulmonary tuberculosis

Epidemiology

Prevalence. Pulmonary tuberculosis is common world-wide (10 million cases and 3 million deaths/year), but now uncommon in the UK. It affects 1–2/1000 population in the UK. It is more common in the immunocompromised (especially with HIV infection) who may present with miliary disease.

Ethnicity. It is most common amongst Asians and Chinese people. Asians are 40 times and West Indians are four times more likely to develop tuberculosis than indigenous white people in the UK.

Geography. Most common in developing countries.
The infection is spread by close contact with an infected person. Pulmonary tuberculosis is most common amongst:
- Asians and West Indians
- people who are immunosuppressed because of HIV infection, diabetes mellitus, lymphoma, immunosuppressive steroid or cytotoxic therapy or alcoholism
- the elderly
- people who are malnourished

Disease mechanisms

Primary pulmonary tuberculosis

This is an inhaled disease. The infecting dose of the bacillus, *Mycobacterium tuberculosis*, is small and settles in well-ventilated but poorly perfused areas (usually a sub-pleural region in the upper or middle lobe). This causes an initial leucocyte inflammatory response. Macrophages then envelop the tubercle bacilli and die, and the sub-pleural lesion develops into a granuloma. This commonly contains a central necrotic area consisting of cheesy (caseous) material, surrounded by Langerhans' giant cells, all of which is known as the Ghon focus. The lymph nodes draining the affected lobe at the hilum of the lung enlarge. The combination of a Ghon focus with hilar lymph node enlargement is called the 'primary complex'.

The process from infection to development of the primary complex takes 3–8 weeks and is accompanied by the development of positive skin reactivity to tubercular protein (tuberculin). Occasionally, the tubercle bacilli overcome the host defences and spread, giving rise to tuberculous pneumonia and pleural effusion. Haemato-genous spread causes disease in other organs, and tuberculous meningitis is particularly serious. Where host defences are very poor, there can be widespread diffusion of tubercle bacilli via the blood (miliary tuberculosis). All these complications resulting from poor host defences and dissemination of the initial infection are potentially fatal. The primary complex usually heals completely. The Ghon focus fibroses and may later calcify.

Postprimary pulmonary tuberculosis
This occurs if the Ghon focus fails to heal or there is later reinfection or reactivation.

Clinical features
Primary pulmonary tuberculosis
The primary complex commonly develops at an early age with no specific symptoms, although there may be a mild illness with erythema nodosum. Usually there are no physical signs, but a small pleural effusion may develop on the affected side. If hilar lymphadenopathy compresses a major bronchus, there may be a fixed wheeze and collapse of the distal lobe. This is particularly common in the middle lobe, where failure of correct lung reinflation after healing can cause bronchiectasis (Brock's syndrome).

Postprimary pulmonary tuberculosis
This usually becomes manifest over several months, causing malaise, weight loss, anorexia, night sweats and a productive cough. There may also be haemoptysis, breathlessness and dull chest pain. Auscultation of the chest may reveal a pneumonia or a pleural effusion. Finger clubbing is unusual unless the onset is prolonged. Some patients present with tender enlarged lymph nodes in the neck, usually in the anterior triangle. Occasionally, these may be the only manifestation of postprimary disease. Indolent skin infection may occur (lupus vulgaris).

Miliary tuberculosis
Miliary tuberculosis is characterized by a non-specific pyrexial illness with malaise and weight loss. Physical signs are sparse, but there may be hepatosplenomegaly and choroidal tubercles in the retina.

Investigation
Haematology
There may be anaemia, but haematology is usually normal.

Biochemistry
Plasma sodium may be decreased; plasma calcium may be increased.

Immunology
Mantoux tests are usually strongly positive (at least 5 mm induration with 10 tuberculin units) in postprimary pulmonary tuberculosis, but are frequently negative in miliary tuberculosis because of a lack of host response. Mantoux tests may be negative in patients with HIV because of reduced cellular immunity.

Microbiology
Sputum microscopy and culture. Tubercle bacilli are slow growing and culture takes 4–6 weeks. In postprimary pulmonary tuberculosis the bacilli can be stained (Ziehl–Neelsen stain) and cultured from sputum or washings obtained from the lung at bronchoscopy.

Bone marrow culture. Bacilli can be cultured from the bone marrow in patients with miliary tuberculosis.

Diagnostic imaging
Chest radiography in postprimary pulmonary tuberculosis may demonstrate a pleural effusion or pneumonia. A soft spreading apical shadowing is strongly suggestive of tuberculosis. It is highly unusual for the chest radiograph to be clear. In miliary tuberculosis there is miliary shadowing (widespread small nodules 2–3 mm in diameter), which may easily be missed.

Histopathology
Pleural aspiration and biopsy when there is a pleural effusion usually provides a diagnosis of postprimary pulmonary tuberculosis and granulomas are seen. **Tissue biopsy** from the liver or from the lung transbronchially diagnoses miliary tuberculosis in 60% and 70% of patients, respectively.

Management
Drug treatment
Multidrug regimens are used to prevent the development of resistant strains (Tables 6.23 and 6.24, pp. 334 and 335). Uncomplicated pulmonary tuberculosis is treated with a relatively short course (6 months). If other organs are involved a longer course of treatment may be necessary (e.g. 18 months for bone disease).

Prevention
Vaccination. Vaccination with bacille Calmette–Guérin (BCG), a non-virulent strain of bovine tuberculosis, produces cellular immunity. It can reduce the risk of developing pulmonary tuberculosis by up to 70%, and reduces the risk of developing tuberculous meningitis and miliary tuberculosis. In some countries it is offered to school children at 12–13 years of age. Vaccination is offered in infancy to people in high-risk groups (e.g. Asian

06

Pulmonary tuberculosis at a glance

Epidemiology

Prevalence
Common worldwide. Affects 1–2/1000 population in the UK

Ethnicity
Most common amongst those of Asian, West Indian and Chinese ethnicity in the UK

Geography
Most common in developing countries

Findings on investigation

Haematology
FBC may show anaemia

Biochemistry
May be hyponatraemia and hypercalcaemia

Immunology
Tuberculin: Mantoux test positive

Microbiology
Sputum culture reveals *Mycobacterium tuberculosis* (takes up to 6 weeks), Ziehl–Neelsen stain microscopy reveals acid-fast bacilli

Histopathology
Pleural, lymph node or lung biopsy: histology reveals caseating granulomas (see Fig. D)

Diagnostic imaging
Chest radiography: upper zone soft shadowing, cavities

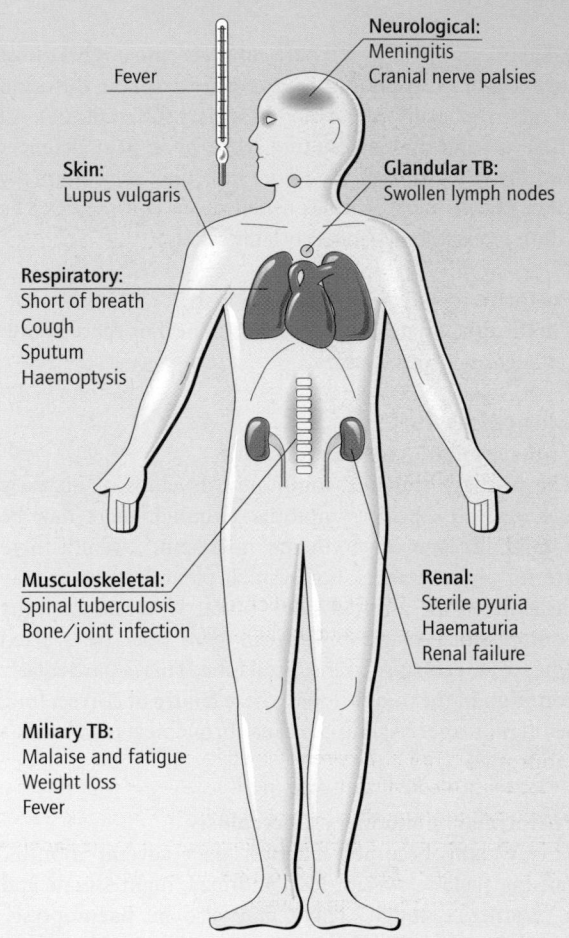

Fever

Neurological:
Meningitis
Cranial nerve palsies

Skin:
Lupus vulgaris

Glandular TB:
Swollen lymph nodes

Respiratory:
Short of breath
Cough
Sputum
Haemoptysis

Musculoskeletal:
Spinal tuberculosis
Bone/joint infection

Renal:
Sterile pyuria
Haematuria
Renal failure

Miliary TB:
Malaise and fatigue
Weight loss
Fever

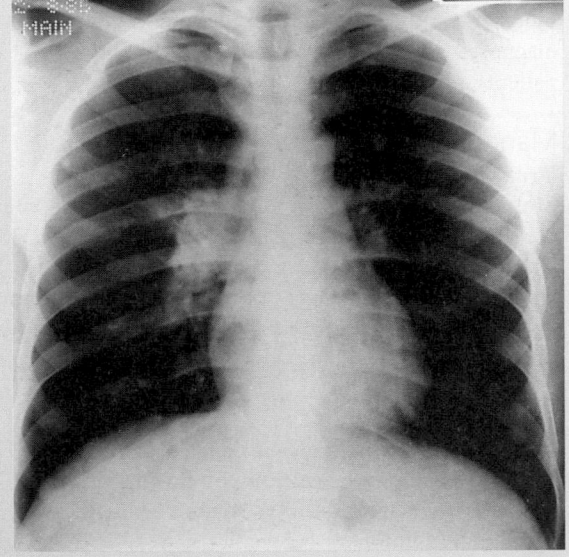

Fig. A Primary pulmonary TB. Chest radiograph showing unilateral hilar lymphadenopathy. The Ghon focus is often not visible on the radiograph.

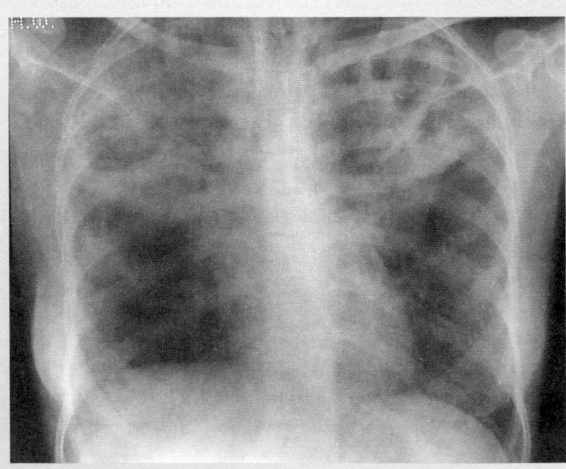

Fig. B Postprimary TB. Chest radiograph showing bilateral apical cavitating pneumonia.

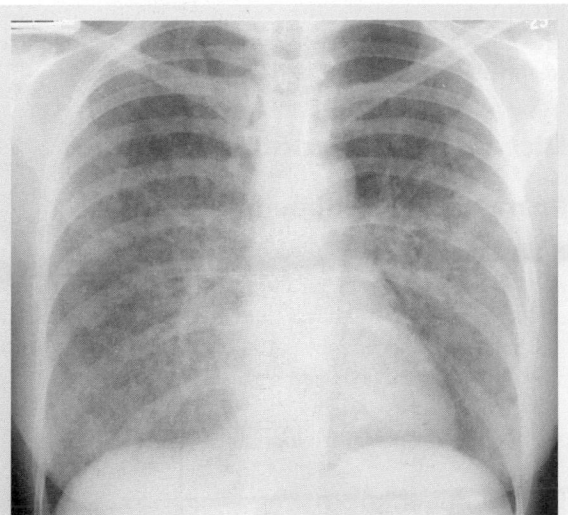

Fig. C Miliary TB. Chest radiograph showing widespread small nodules throughout the lung fields.

Fig. D (*right*) Ziehl–Neelsen-stained material obtained from a caseating mediastinal lymph node. Many acid–alcohol-fast bacteria are seen, with the typical red 'cording or clustering' appearance of *M. tuberculosis*. Reproduced from Bannister *et al. Infectious Disease*, 1996 (Blackwell Science, Oxford) with the permission of the authors.

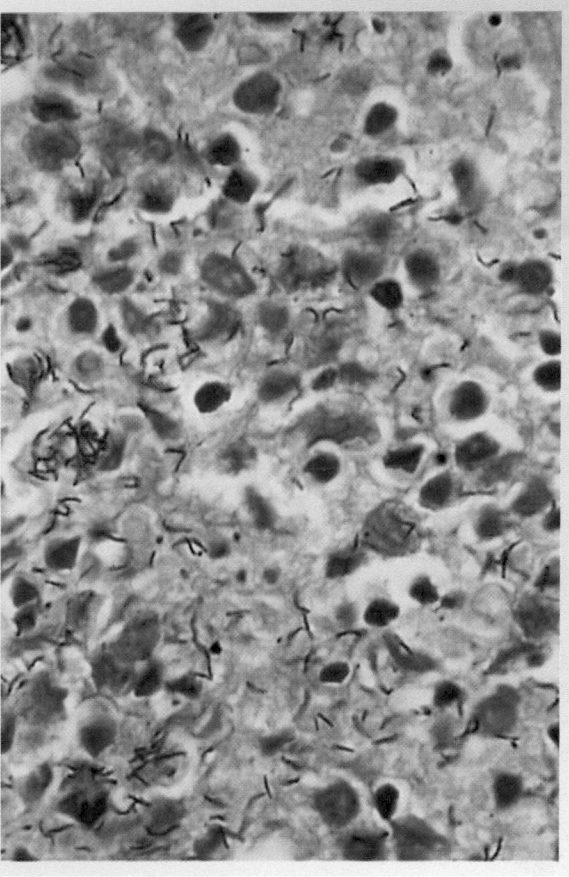

immigrants) and those in endemic areas. Only tuberculin non-responders are vaccinated. Tuberculin responders are screened with chest radiography to examine for pulmonary infection.

Contact tracing and screening. If a person with tuberculosis (the index case) is producing infected sputum (it is possible to culture tubercle bacilli from it), an important part in prevention of the spread of pulmonary disease is the screening and treatment of contacts (Table 6.25, p. 335). The local community medical service must be notified of people with tuberculosis for contact tracing.

Chemoprophylaxis. The presence of healed tuberculous scars, which can contain viable tubercle bacilli, and any procedure that diminishes cellular immunity (e.g. therapy associated with organ transplantation, cytotoxic chemotherapy) may cause a recrudescence of disease. People with such scars who are undergoing any treatment that reduces cellular immunity are therefore given chemoprophylaxis with isoniazid or rifampicin.

Prognosis

The prognosis is good if the patient is not immunosuppressed.

Infection with other 'atypical' mycobacteria

Epidemiology

Prevalence. This is sporadic, but in some areas can account for up to 30% of cases of pulmonary 'tuberculosis'. It usually occurs in elderly individuals with concurrent pulmonary disease.

Disease mechanisms

Mycobacterial organisms other than *Mycobacterium tuberculosis*, which causes pulmonary tuberculosis, can produce similar disease in humans. *Mycobacterium avium* and *Mycobacterium intracellulare* originate in birds and can cause pulmonary and lymph node disease. *Mycobacterium bovis* originates in cattle and can cause pulmonary, lymph node and gut disease. *Mycobacterium melitensis*

Table 6.23 Management of tuberculosis

Supportive treatment
Good nutrition
Reduce alcohol intake

Prevention
Vaccination of tuberculin non-responders with BCG for
school children at 12–13 years of age in the UK, and infants
in high-risk groups and endemic areas
Contact tracing and screening
Chemoprophylaxis for anyone with a primary complex scar
who is undergoing a procedure that reduces cellular
immunity

Drug treatment for pulmonary tuberculosis (fully sensitive
strains)
Multidrug regimens are used to prevent the development of
resistant strains
Uncomplicated pulmonary TB is treated with a relatively short
course (6–9 months)
TB in other organs may need a longer course of treatment
(e.g. 18 months for bone disease)

Regimen 1
Rifampicin plus isoniazid (+ pyridoxine) plus pyrazinamide†
for first 2 months. Then:
Rifampicin plus isoniazid (+ pyridoxine) for 4 months

Regimen 2
Ethambutol* or streptomycin* plus isoniazid (+ pyridoxine)
plus rifampicin for 2 months. Then:
Isoniazid (+ pyridoxine) plus rifampicin for a further
7 months

Surgery
To remove severely damaged bronchiectatic lobes

BCG, bacille Calmette–Guérin; TB, tuberculosis.
* Require more supervision, more toxic, less active.
† Ineffective after the first 2–3 months.

and *Mycobacterium kansasii* originate in river estuaries
and can cause pulmonary disease. People with these infections are not infectious even if sputum is positive.

Clinical features
As for tuberculosis (see p. 331).

Investigation
As for tuberculosis (see p. 331).

Management
In vitro studies suggest that the organisms are commonly
insensitive to standard antituberculous chemotherapy,
but such treatment often causes remission.

Prognosis
The infection sometimes becomes chronic and requires
treatment for years.

Disease of the pulmonary vessels

Pulmonary thromboembolic disease

Epidemiology
Prevalence. Prevalence is unknown because many are
undiagnosed. Although less than 10% cause death, in the
UK the autopsy incidence is 10–25% and there are probably more than 30 000 deaths/year.

Age. More common with increasing age.

Disease mechanisms
All the blood volume passes through the lungs with every
cardiac cycle and any emboli embed in the pulmonary
capillaries. Most pulmonary thrombi embolize from pre-
existing venous thrombi, usually in the pelvic (15%) and
femoral veins (70–80%). Thrombi in veins below the
knee rarely cause pulmonary thromboembolic disease.
Emboli can also consist of tumour, amniotic fluid, air,
parasites and material injected intravenously.
  Risk factors for thromboembolism are:
- immobility
- trauma
- surgery (particularly emergency)
- pregnancy
- high-oestrogen oral contraceptive pill
- indwelling venous catheters
- clotting abnormalities (antithrombin III deficiency,
lupus anticoagulant, etc.)
- myocardial infarction involving the right ventricle
- intravenous drug abuse
  Thrombi lodge in the muscular pulmonary arteries,
particularly in the basal segments of the lower lobes.
Infarction and necrosis of distal tissues is uncommon
(because of collateral circulation), unless the obstructed
vessel is large or the collateral supply is poor (e.g. in the
elderly). Vascular occlusion in the presence of normal
ventilation causes ventilation–perfusion mismatching,
and shunting occurs. With time, the emboli can organize
and recanalize.
- *Acute minor pulmonary embolism:* embolism obstructing less than 50% of the pulmonary circulation
- *Acute massive pulmonary embolism:* embolism
obstructing more than 50% of the pulmonary circulation
- *Chronic thromboembolic disease:* rare. Small pulmonary
emboli gradually occlude the pulmonary vascular tree
over a period of months or years to produce secondary
pulmonary hypertension

Table 6.24 Treatment of tuberculosis

Antituberculous drugs*

Rifampicin

Pharmacological action	Bactericidal
Indications	Treatment or prophylaxis
Side-effects	Induces liver enzymes, causes gastrointestinal upset, stains body secretions orange
Contraindications	Porphyria, jaundice
Monitoring of patients	Monitor liver function

Isoniazid

Pharmacological action	Bactericidal
Indications	Treatment or prophylaxis
Side-effects	Peripheral neuropathy, gastrointestinal upset, skin rashes, hepatitis. Pyridoxine is given to reduce the probability of peripheral neuropathy
Contraindications	Porphyria
Monitoring of patients	Not necessary if pyridoxine is given as well

Pyrazinamide

Pharmacological action	Bactericidal
Indications	Treatment
Side-effects	Liver failure, anaemia
Contraindications	Liver disease, porphyria
Monitoring of patients	Monitor liver function

Streptomycin

Pharmacological action	Bactericidal
Indications	Treatment. Parenteral administration only, which means that long-term use is difficult
Side-effects	Vestibular neuronitis, allergic reactions
Contraindications	Renal disease. Use with caution in renal failure
Monitoring of patients	Monitor serum drug levels

Ethambutol

Pharmacological action	Bacteriostatic
Indications	Treatment
Side-effects	Optic and peripheral neuritis
Contraindications	Renal disease, poor vision
Monitoring of patients	Monitor vision and renal function

* Most antituberculous drugs have significant side-effects and the patient must be warned of these before therapy is started.

Table 6.25 Screening and management of tuberculosis contacts

BCG	Tuberculin test*	Chest radiograph	Repeat tuberculin test at 6 weeks	Age (years)	Index smear	Action
Yes	0–2	Normal				Discharge
Yes	0–2	Abnormal				Treat
Yes	3–4	Normal		> 16	Negative	Discharge
				> 16	Positive	Periodic chest radiograph
				< 16		Chemoprophylaxis
Yes	3–4	Abnormal				Treat
No	2–4	Normal		> 16		Periodic chest radiograph
				< 16		Chemoprophylaxis
No	2–4	Abnormal				Treat
No	0–1	Normal	2–4			Chemoprophylaxis
			0–1	> 35		Discharge
				< 35		BCG. Discharge
				High risk		Chemoprophylaxis

* A negative tuberculin test in an immunocompromised individual does not exclude infection. Grade 0–2, negative or weakly positive; grade 3–4, strongly positive.

Pulmonary embolism at a glance

Epidemiology

Prevalence

Unknown. Could be as high as 1/500. Mortality is around 1/3000–5000/year

Age

More common with increasing age

Geography

More common in western countries where the incidence of medical and surgical procedures and higher survival in trauma patients creates a larger population at risk

Findings on investigation

Blood gas analysis

Hypoxia in acute massive pulmonary embolism (PE)

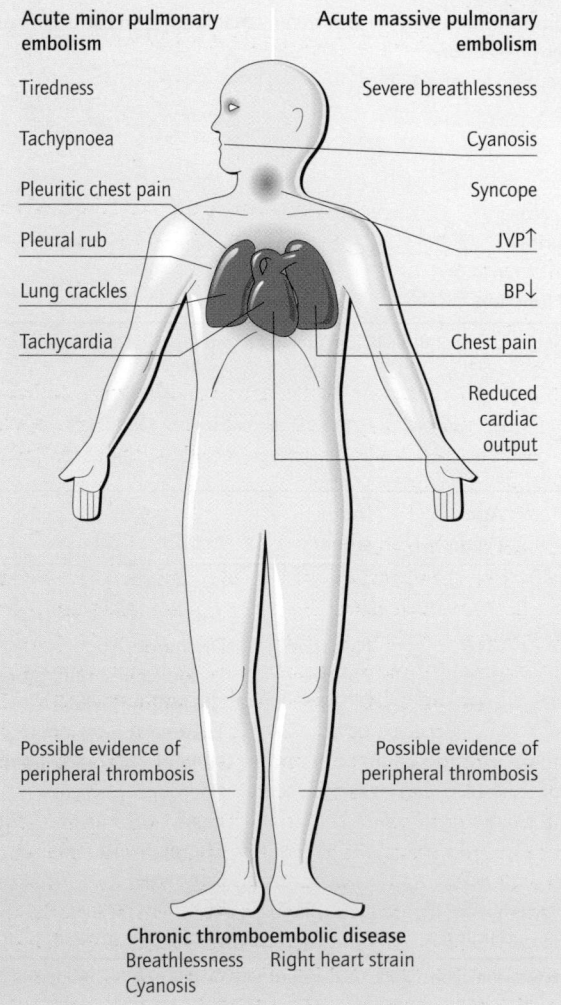

Acute minor pulmonary embolism	Acute massive pulmonary embolism
Tiredness	Severe breathlessness
Tachypnoea	Cyanosis
Pleuritic chest pain	Syncope
Pleural rub	JVP↑
Lung crackles	BP↓
Tachycardia	Chest pain
	Reduced cardiac output
Possible evidence of peripheral thrombosis	Possible evidence of peripheral thrombosis

Chronic thromboembolic disease
Breathlessness   Right heart strain
Cyanosis

Diagnostic imaging

Chest radiography

- Linear atelectases develop later in acute minor PE
- Area of pulmonary oligaemia in acute massive PE

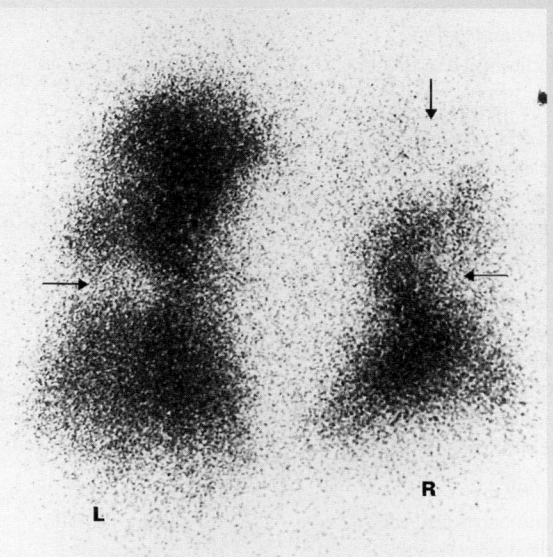

(i)

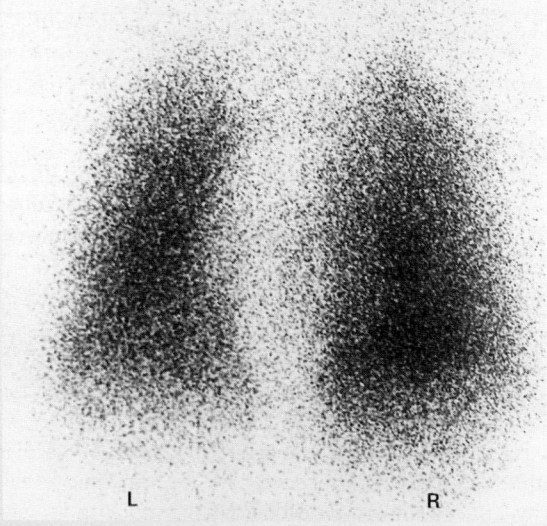

(ii)

Fig. A Mismatched ventilation/perfusion defects in pulmonary embolism (PE). (i) ^{99m}Tc macroaggregate perfusion scan showing multiple wedge-shaped defects (arrows). (ii) Normal ^{81m}Kr ventilation scan.

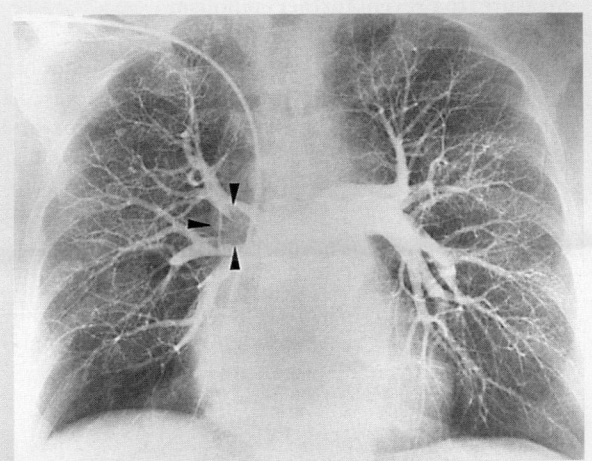

Fig. B Pulmonary arteriogram. Note: (i) a large embolus causing a filling defect at the bifurcation of the right pulmonary artery (arrows); (ii) reduction in branches of the lower lobe arteries due to obstruction of emboli; and (iii) catheter passing from the right arm into the heart. All figures reproduced from Armstrong & Wastie, *Diagnostic Imaging*, 3rd edn, 1992 (Blackwell Scientific Publications, Oxford) with the permission of the authors.

• Dilation of main pulmonary arteries in chronic thrombo-embolic disease

CT pulmonary angiogram
• Non-invasive contrast imaging is increasingly useful

Radionuclide lung scan (V/Q scan)
• Perfusion defects not matched by ventilation defects in acute minor PE
• Large perfusion defects in acute massive PE
• Widespread ventilation–perfusion (V/Q) mismatching in chronic thromboembolic disease

Pulmonary angiography. Requires definite indications
• Delineates the blocked arteries in acute massive PE
• Peripheral pruning of the arterial tree indicates chronic thromboembolic disease

ECG
• Acute right heart strain in acute massive PE (S1 Q3 T3 and right axis deviation)
• Right heart strain in chronic thromboembolic disease

Clinical features

These vary according to the timescale and degree of thromboembolism.

Acute minor pulmonary embolism. Young individuals (younger than 40 years of age) with small occlusions may have no symptoms or signs, or there is a sudden onset of pleuritic chest pain resulting from a pulmonary infarction involving the pleural surface. There may be an associated tachycardia and rapid shallow breathing because of pleuritic pain. Cyanosis is not usual because the disturbance to gas exchange is slight. Auscultation reveals crackles and perhaps a pleural rub. Only 20% of patients will have clinical signs of the deep venous thrombosis that produced the embolus.

Acute massive pulmonary embolism. The patient becomes acutely ill, with marked breathlessness and chest pain. There may be syncope because of a diminished cardiac output with right heart obstruction. Examination reveals tachycardia, cyanosis, reduced cardiac output and hypotension. There may be a right ventricular heave and a split second heart sound resulting from delayed closure of the pulmonary valve.

Chronic thromboembolic disease. This produces few symptoms until late in the disease and patients often present with increasing breathlessness or right heart failure. There may be cyanosis and evidence of right heart strain late in the disease.

Investigation
Blood gases

Blood gas analysis in acute massive pulmonary embolus reveals marked hypoxaemia. Chronic thromboembolic disease also causes hypoxaemia, which fails to correct with oxygen treatment.

Diagnostic imaging

• *Chest radiography* in acute minor pulmonary embolism is normal at first, but linear atelectases (from pulmonary collapse) develop later. In acute massive pulmonary embolism it may show an area of pulmonary oligaemia caused by obstructed pulmonary arteries. In chronic thromboembolic disease it shows dilatation of the main pulmonary arteries and possibly peripheral pruning of the pulmonary vascular tree.
• *Early ventilation–perfusion* lung scanning in acute minor pulmonary embolism reveals perfusion defects not matched by ventilation defects. Lung scanning in acute massive pulmonary embolism reveals large perfusion defects and in chronic thromboembolic disease demonstrates widespread ventilation–perfusion mismatching.
• *Pulmonary angiography* in acute minor pulmonary

06

embolism confirms the diagnosis. Pulmonary angiography in acute massive pulmonary embolism delineates the blocked pulmonary arteries. In chronic thromboembolic disease it reveals a typical appearance (peripheral pruning of the arterial tree). Conventional angiography of the bronchial tree is rarely carried out and is being replaced by spiral CT angiography.

ECG changes
Electrocardiogram in acute massive pulmonary embolism may show evidence of acute right heart strain ('S1 Q3 T3' and right axis deviation), while an ECG in chronic thromboembolic disease shows evidence of right heart strain.

Lung function
Spirometry in chronic thromboembolic disease demonstrates slightly lower than predicted lung values for volumes.

Management
General measures include pain relief and oxygen therapy.

Treatment of the embolus itself (Table 6.26)
Intravenous streptokinase or t-PA (tissue plasminogen activator) are reserved for massive pulmonary embolism because of their side-effects. They activate plasminogen and enhance the lysis of intravascular clots, but increase risk of bleeding elsewhere. Rarely, massive pulmonary embolization requires cardiothoracic surgery to remove the emboli.

Table 6.26 Management of pulmonary embolism

Supportive treatment
Pain relief
Oxygen therapy

Drug treatment
Thrombolysis
Intravenous streptokinase or t-PA is reserved for massive pulmonary embolism because of its side-effects

Anticoagulation
Used for all types of pulmonary thromboembolic disease to prevent the development of further intravascular thrombosis

Surgery
An inferior vena cava filter
To prevent emboli from reaching the pulmonary tree if thromboemboli are recurrent despite adequate anticoagulation

Measures to prevent further embolism
These include anticoagulation and surgery:
- *Anticoagulation:* used for all types of pulmonary thromboembolic disease. It prevents further intravascular thrombosis by inhibiting clotting factors. Heparin is used in the acute stage because it has an immediate effect and may be the only effective treatment when the thromboemboli are a manifestation of underlying malignancy. Longer term anticoagulation can be achieved with oral warfarin.
- *Surgery:* rarely, an inferior vena cava filter is inserted to prevent emboli reaching the pulmonary tree if thromboemboli are recurrent despite adequate anticoagulation.

Prognosis
Acute minor pulmonary embolism. The prognosis is good if the disease is recognized and treated in good time (before pulmonary infarction).

Acute massive pulmonary embolism. The prognosis depends on the size of embolus and the underlying health of the patient. Death is usually caused by obstruction of the pulmonary circulation by embolus or a fatal arrhythmia.

Chronic thromboembolic disease. Most of the damage to the pulmonary vascular tree is irreversible by the time the disease presents. Although adequate anticoagulation prevents the development of further emboli, pulmonary hypertension does not reverse once established and cor pulmonale eventually ensues.

Obstructive airways disease

Asthma/allergy

Asthma is defined as reversible partial obstruction to airflow in the intrathoracic airways.

Epidemiology
Prevalence. This is increasing; 10–15% of individuals will experience wheezing at some stage. The mortality rate in the UK is more than 2000/year.

Age. Most common in children.

Genetics. Associated with atopy.

Disease mechanisms
The bronchi are surrounded by smooth muscle, which normally reacts only slightly to stimuli. Asthmatics have an abnormally increased reaction to stimuli (bronchial hyper-reactivity), probably because of inflammatory

mechanisms. Repeated stimuli cause ongoing bronchial inflammation in predisposed individuals, and this sustains bronchial hyper-reactivity.

Specific bronchial stimuli include inhaled allergens (e.g. house dust mite, pollen, cat), occupational allergens and drugs (e.g. aspirin for 3% of the population). In general, they are more likely than non-specific bronchial stimuli to cause ongoing bronchial inflammation and result in lasting bronchial hyper-reactivity. Non-specific bronchial stimuli include viral infections, cold air, exercise, emotional stress and inhaled pollutants (e.g. perfume, dust).

Bronchial hyper-reactivity

The process that generates bronchial hyper-reactivity is highly complex and ill understood. It probably involves several pathways, and possible mechanisms include:
- *Immune reaction:* releasing inflammatory mediators
- *Imbalance:* between cholinergic and adrenergic airway control
- *Abnormal calcium flux:* across cell membranes, increasing smooth muscle contraction and mast cell degranulation
- *Leaky tight junctions:* between bronchial epithelial cells allow ingress of allergen

Atopic individuals have increased levels of circulating IgE (the reaginic antibody), which binds to mast cells in the bronchial mucosa and lumen. Inhaled allergen interacts with the bound IgE causing the mast cells to degranulate and produce histamine and neutrophil and eosinophil chemotactic factors. These and other cells release powerful mediators that cause the bronchial inflammatory reaction and increase bronchial hyper-reactivity.

Bronchial inflammatory mediators include:
- *Platelet activating factor:* causes inflammation
- *Leucotrienes, prostaglandins* and *thromboxanes:* cause bronchoconstriction and attract inflammatory cells
- *Eosinophilic major basic protein:* causes mucosal damage and shedding

The ongoing inflammatory reaction accounts for persistent asthmatic symptoms following allergen inhalation. Three types of asthmatic response are recognized (p. 341):
1 immediate
2 late reactive
3 recurrent

Classification of asthma

Asthma may be allergic or non-allergic.

Allergic asthmatics. These have high circulating levels of IgE and usually have positive skin-prick tests to common allergens (85% testing positive to house dust and house dust mite, 70% to pollens, 40% to cat epithelium and 20%

to fungi). They may also have eczema or hay fever, and usually give a family history of atopy. Asthmatic symptoms commonly occur in childhood, and there is a tendency for the symptoms to improve during adolescence. The symptoms may recur later in life or asthma may not be recognized until middle age. Allergen avoidance or hyposensitization can alleviate symptoms.

Non-allergic asthmatics. These are usually not atopic and often develop asthma in middle age. Their symptoms tend to be progressive and unremitting.

Severe asthma. This is life-threatening and can occur as a sudden deterioration in otherwise stable asthma (acute severe asthma) or as the end-stage of slowly deteriorating asthma (chronic worsening asthma). Acute severe asthma can be precipitated by emotional stress or a viral infection, but chronic worsening asthma usually develops over weeks with a gradual increase in symptoms and progressive failure to respond to inhaled β_2-agonists. A small group of patients have brittle asthma, where severe life-threatening attacks develop within minutes or hours when the symptoms are apparently otherwise well controlled.

Clinical features

Asthma usually presents as attacks of wheezing, which commonly occur following exercise and viral infections, and on exposure to cold air. Less severe symptoms are nocturnal coughing and wheezing. A cough producing small amounts of yellowish sputum or bronchial plugs (caused by eosinophils) is common. Some patients present with breathlessness alone, or in cor pulmonale.

Asthmatic symptoms can vary from the occasional wheezing spell every 2–3 months to severe chronic wheezing with little apparent reversibility.

Severe asthma

The features of severe asthma are:
- inability to talk in uninterrupted sentences
- Exhaustion
- Respiratory rate higher than 30/min
- Silent chest (severe bronchospasm prevents air entry)
- Cyanosis
- Tachycardia (faster than 120/min) in the absence of chronotropes
- Pulsus paradox (systolic blood pressure drops more than 15 mmHg during inspiration)

Diagnosis

This depends on the objective demonstration of reversible airflow obstruction by spirometry, but sometimes diagnosis is made on the symptom of episodic wheezing alone.

06

Asthma at a glance

Epidemiology
Prevalence
10–15% of the population

Age
Most common in children

Genetics
Associated with atopy

Findings on investigation
Haematology
FBC may show eosinophilia

Immunology
IgE may be increased in allergic asthma

Spirometry
An improvement in FEV_1 or PEFR of at least 15–20% following inhalation of a bronchodilator is consistent with a diagnosis of asthma

Bronchial provocation challenge
Using methacholine or histamine demonstrates bronchial hyper-responsiveness. This test is rarely used

Allergen provocation testing
May be of use in occupational asthma or food allergy, but must be carefully supervised because of the possibility of a late asthmatic reaction

Tests for allergy
Skin-prick tests and radioallergosorbent test (RAST) to demonstrate atopy

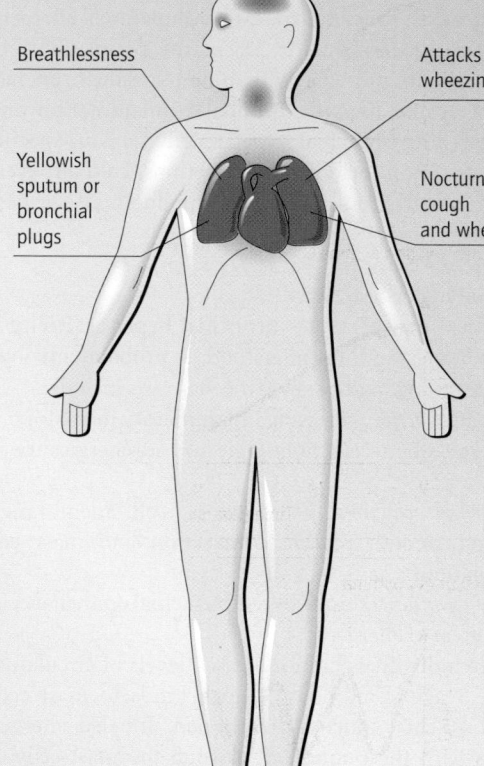

Breathlessness

Attacks of wheezing

Yellowish sputum or bronchial plugs

Nocturnal cough and wheeze

Differential diagnosis
People who have smoked cigarettes may have coexistent chronic bronchitis and emphysema, which may present with similar symptoms. Asthma is characterized by episodic breathlessness with wheezing. In contrast, a fixed localized obstruction in the extrathoracic airways such as a foreign body causes stridor.

Investigation
Haematology
There may be eosinophilia.

Immunology
IgE may be increased in allergic asthma.

Histopathology
Inflamed bronchi and hypertrophied smooth muscle.

Spirometry
1 Improvement in FEV_1 or PEFR of at least 15–20% after inhaling a bronchodilator provides a diagnosis of asthma.
2 A peak flow chart will show a diurnal variation in peak flow in asthma. This technique is also useful in the diagnosis of occupational asthma.
3 A corticosteroid challenge (prednisolone 30 mg/day for 2 weeks) given to patients with marked airflow limitation who do not respond to an inhaled bronchodilator may show a substantial improvement in FEV_1 or FVC.
4 Exercise and cold air challenge tests stimulate the bronchial mucosa by altering respiratory heat exchange and may demonstrate asthma. They are often used in children, but a negative test does not rule out the disorder.

Bronchial provocation challenge, using methacholine or histamine, demonstrates bronchial hyper-reactivity,

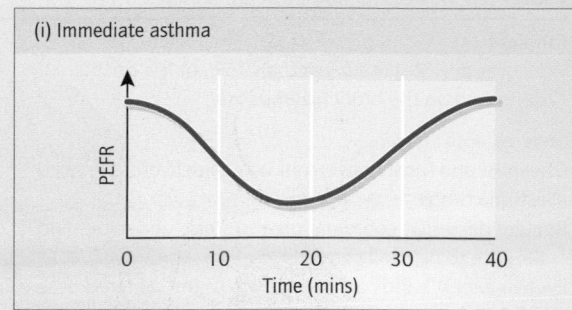

(i) Immediate asthma

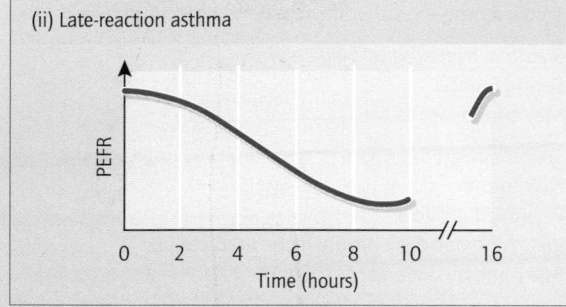

(ii) Late-reaction asthma

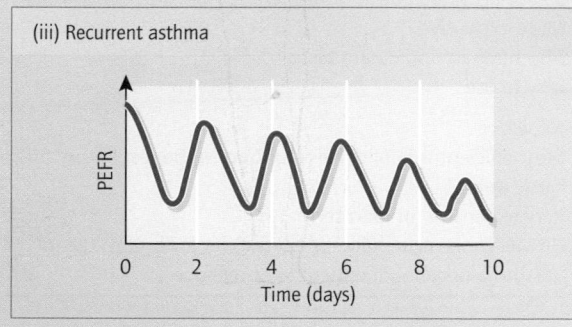

(iii) Recurrent asthma

Fig. A (*left*) Asthmatic responses and their modification by treatment. (i) Immediate asthma develops within a few minutes and lasts for less than 1 hour. It can be abolished by treatment. (ii) Late-reaction asthma occurs several hours after the first reactions. It can be reduced by treatment. The combination of (i) and (ii) is known as the dual response. If it occurs without the preceding immediate reaction it is known as the isolated late response, which is sometimes a feature of occupational asthma. (iii) Recurrent asthma is due to a worsening of bronchial hyper-reactivity (BHR), producing ongoing asthmatic symptoms for days after the initial challenge. It can be reduced by treatment. This response is typical of viral infections.

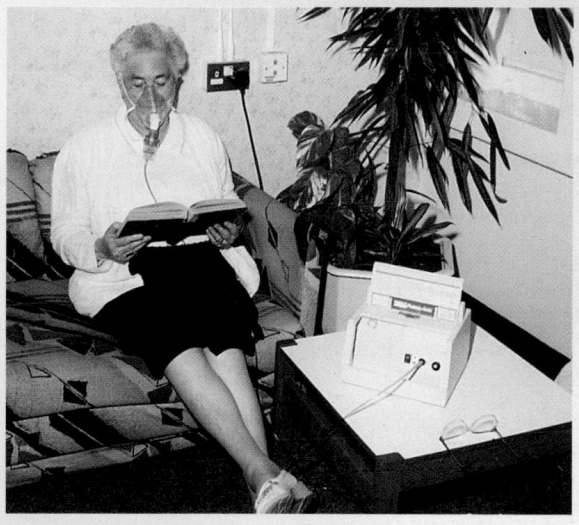

Fig. B Patient using home nebulizer.

which is a universal feature in asthma. Such testing is often not performed in a clinical setting. **Allergen provocation testing** in occupational asthma or food allergy must be carefully supervised because of the possibility of a late asthmatic reaction. **Tests for allergy** help demonstrate atopy, but do not make the diagnosis of asthma. They include skin-prick tests, which are cheap and easy to perform, looking for eosinophilia, which may occur in the sputum or peripheral blood; and a radioallergosorbent test (RAST), when elevated levels of allergen-specific IgE suggest sensitization.

Management

Avoidance of precipitating causes. Some patients show a marked improvement, but up to 50% of patients, particularly those with occupational asthma, continue to have severe symptoms. In addition, avoidance of major allergens (such as the house dust mite antigen) by people with allergic asthma may be difficult; removal of cats and dogs is less problematic.

Hyposensitization (giving small doses of allergen to build up tolerance) is not effective for house dust mite-sensitive asthma, but some people do benefit from hyposensitization to seasonal allergens (e.g. pollens).

Drug treatment

The British Thoracic Society has introduced guidelines on the management of asthma (Table 6.27; for details of drugs and delivery devices used in the treatment of asthma see Table 6.28 and Fig. 6.18). Leukotriene antagonists have only a mild anti-asthma activity. They are available in oral form and can be taken once (montelukast) or twice (zafirlukast) daily.

Severe asthma

Severe asthma warrants the following immediate management.
1 Treatment before admission to hospital
   • Nebulized salbutamol 5 mg 4–6 hourly and ipratropium bromide 500 µg 4–6 hourly

06

Table 6.27 Management of asthma

Supportive treatment
Avoid precipitating causes
Hyposensitization to seasonal allergens (e.g. pollens) for
    some people

Drug treatment
The British Thoracic Society has produced guidelines on
the drug management of asthma. Steps 1–3 apply to the
treatment of less severe asthma, in an attempt to control
symptoms. Steps 4 and 5 apply to the treatment of more
severe asthma, when it may not be possible to abolish
symptoms. Stepping down and up is recommended to
match therapy to need

Step 1
Inhaled short-acting β_2-agonist as required (not more than
    once daily). No prophylaxis

Step 2
Inhaled short-acting β_2-agonist as required
Regular low-dose inhaled steroids (e.g. 100–400 µg
    beclometasone or budesonide daily via large volume spacer)

Step 3
Inhaled short-acting β_2-agonist as required
Regular high-dose inhaled steroids (e.g. 800–2000 µg
    beclometasone or budesonide daily via large volume spacer)

Step 4
Inhaled short-acting β_2-agonist as required
Regular high-dose inhaled steroids (e.g. 800–2000 µg
    beclometasone or budesonide daily via large volume spacer)
Add in long-acting β_2-agonist or sustained release
    theophylline or inhaled ipratropium/oxtropium or
    cromoglycate or nedocromil or high-dose inhaled
    bronchodilators

Step 5
Inhaled short-acting β_2-agonist as required
Regular high-dose inhaled steroids (e.g. 800–200 µg
    beclometasone or budesonide daily via large volume spacer)
Add in one or more long-acting bronchodilators as in step 4
    plus regular oral prednisolone as a single daily dose

- • Oxygen
- • Steroids if the diagnosis of asthma is clear
2 Admission to hospital
    - • Hydrocortisone 200 mg intravenously followed by
    oral prednisolone 40 mg
    - • Blood gas analysis (consider ventilation if $Pao_2 < 7\,kPa$)
    - • A chest radiograph to exclude a pneumothorax
3 Further treatment
    - • Infusion of β_2-agonist or theophylline if there is
    no improvement. Intravenous theophyllines can cause
    toxic blood levels if the patient has been on oral

Table 6.28 Devices for administering inhaled drugs

Inhalers
Whatever device is used, less than 15% of the dose is
    deposited on the bronchial mucosa

Metered-dose inhaler
Cheapest and most convenient way of delivering inhaled
    asthma drugs
Require dexterity, coordination and some understanding if
    they are to be used correctly
Even in expert hands only about 8% of the metered dose will
    reach the respiratory tract
To overcome this other devices have been used (Fig. 6.18)

Breath-activated spray inhalers
Spring loaded
May be difficult to use

Spacer devices
Easy to use
Improved delivery
Ideal for twice daily prophylactic medication
Bulky and inconvenient

Breath-activated powder inhalers
More expensive
May have an unpleasant taste
Easy to use

Nebulizer
Most efficient way of delivering drug to the respiratory tract
Large dose
Very expensive for long-term use
Unwise (unless carefully supervised) for long-term use in
    asthma because of patient over-reliance

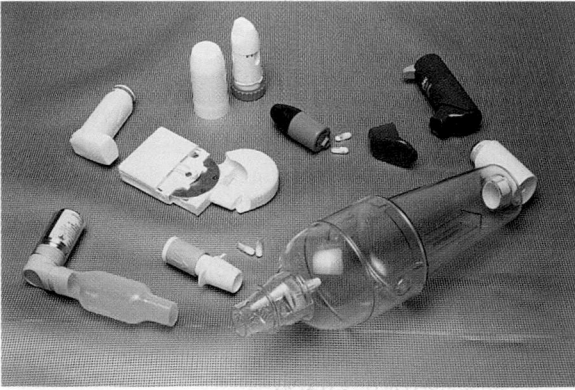

Figure 6.18 A range of inhaler devices are available for the
treatment of respiratory disease as shown. These include
sprays that deliver a fixed dose of aerosolized drug and devices
that deliver powdered drug. Plastic chambers, such as that
shown on the right of the image enable drug to be sprayed
into the chamber at one end and then inhaled by the patient
from the other end. This can increase drug delivery to the lung.

Emergency 6.1: Acute severe asthma

Diagnosis

The presence of one or more of the following features suggests acute severe asthma:

- Peak flow less than 40% of predicted normal of the patient's best obtainable result if known (< 200 l/min if not known)
- Inability to talk in uninterrupted sentences
- Respiratory rate > 30/min
- Tachycardia > 120/min

Specific treatment

At home

Assess airway/breathing/circulation

Oxygen—high flow

Nebulized β_2-agonists (e.g. salbutamol 5 mg, terbutaline 5–10 mg) or via a spacer

Prednisolone 40 mg orally

At hospital

Reassess airway/breathing/circulation

Oxygen—high flow

Nebulized β_2-agonists (e.g. salbutamol 5 mg, terbutaline 5–10 mg) 4 hourly

Chest X-ray to exclude pneumothorax

Hydrocortisone 200 mg 4 hourly intravenously

Intravenous bronchodilators

If there is no improvement or if obviously life-threatening features are present (see p. 339) give intravenous aminophylline (250 mg over 30 min) or an intravenous β_2-agonist (e.g. salbutamol 200 mg or terbutaline 250 µg over 10 min). A β_2-agonist is preferred if the patient is already taking oral theophylline.

Unhelpful treatment

Sedatives are absolutely contraindicated outside the intensive care unit

Antibiotics are not indicated unless there is radiological evidence of an infection

Indications for intensive care

Patients with features of life-threatening asthma require intensive monitoring by experienced staff. Patients with the following features require intensive care:

- hypoxia (Pao_2 < 8 kPa) despite 60% inspired oxygen
- hypercapnia ($Paco_2$ > 6 kPa)
- cyanosis
- exhaustion
- bradycardia
- hypotension
- confusion or drowsiness
- unconsciousness
- respiratory arrest

theophyllines or has already had a loading dose, so serum levels are measured

- Intravenous antibiotics if there is evidence of bacterial chest infection, which is an uncommon cause of severe asthma
- Consider the use of intravenous magnesium, which has been shown to have some effect in acute severe asthma

In severe asthma, larger doses of β_2-agonists can be self-administered by home nebulizer.

Prognosis

Acute severe asthma carries a significant mortality, but if asthma is treated adequately the prognosis is good. Chronic worsening asthma in middle age may progress slowly despite the best treatment.

Chronic obstructive airways disease (chronic bronchitis and emphysema)

These are separate diseases that coexist to some degree (along with asthma) in the same patients, and are referred to as chronic obstructive airways disease. They directly cause approximately 30 000 deaths/year in the UK, and both are strongly associated with cigarette smoking.

Chronic bronchitis

This is a clinical diagnosis, defined as a daily cough with sputum for at least 3 months of the year, for at least 2 consecutive years.

Epidemiology

Prevalence. Ten per cent in older people.

Age. More common in people over 50 years of age.

Geography. More common in industrialized countries.

Disease mechanisms

Causes are cigarette smoking, atmospheric pollution and respiratory infection (particularly in infancy).

Pathogenesis

Hypertrophy of the mucus-secreting glands in the bronchial mucosa causes increased mucus production, which overloads the mucociliary escalator and is expelled by coughing. Chronic mucosal inflammation causes mucosal hypertrophy and narrowing of the smaller airways, which obstructs airflow.

Clinical features

A chronic cough producing colourless or mucoid sputum is interspersed by acute infections when the sputum becomes frankly purulent. The disease progresses over

06

Chronic obstructive airways disease at a glance

Epidemiology
Prevalence
- Chronic bronchitis: 10% in older people
- Emphysema: 5% in older people

Age
More common over 50 years of age

Genetics
Emphysema associated with α_1-antitrypsin deficiency

Geography
Common in industrialized countries

Association
Chronic bronchitis is strongly associated with smoking

Findings on investigation
Haematology
May reveal secondary polycythaemia in chronic bronchitis and emphysema

---

many years from a troublesome cough (frequently early morning) with a little clear sputum, to marked wheezing and severe breathlessness leading to poor exercise tolerance and copious sputum production.

On examination there is poor chest expansion and there may be an auscultatory wheeze.

Investigation
Diagnostic imaging. Chest radiography is commonly normal. If there is significant airflow obstruction there may be signs of chest overexpansion (flattening of the diaphragms) and an enlarged retrosternal airspace. The angle of the ribs may be altered.

Histopathology. Mucus gland hyperplasia. Spirometry may show an obstructive picture.

Management
Precipitating factors should be avoided and bronchospasm and acute infections should be treated (Table 6.29).

Prognosis
Chronic bronchitis is slowly progressive unless the precipitating factors are avoided and it is treated.

Emphysema

Emphysema is characterized by histological dilatation of the air spaces, accompanied by destruction of the lung parenchyma.

Epidemiology
Prevalence. Five per cent in older people.

Age. More common in people over 50 years of age.

Genetics. Associated with α_1-antitrypsin deficiency.

Geography. More common in industrialized countries.

Disease mechanisms
There are two types of emphysema:
- *Generalized involvement* of lung tissue results in panacinar loss of tissue, which can lead to the formation of bullae
- *More localized centriacinar destruction* of lung tissue, which is common and present to some extent in most lungs at autopsy, results in less severe dysfunction

The cause of emphysema at a cellular level is poorly understood. There is probably an imbalance between proteolytic and antiproteolytic enzymes, allowing destruction of parenchymal elastic tissue and loss of the normal elastic recoil in the lung. This results in air-trapping and lung overinflation.

Causes of emphysema are:
- Cigarette smoking
- Exposure to heavy metal (e.g. cadmium)
- α_1-Antitrypsin deficiency (5% of cases)

α_1-Antitrypsin deficiency
This is an autosomal recessive disorder in which there is a failure to produce α_1-antitrypsin. The homozygous condition occurs in approximately 1/5000 live births and is associated with the early development (at less than 40 years of age) of basal emphysema, usually in smokers.

Clinical features
In pure emphysema the loss of lung tissue results in exertional dyspnoea, quiet breath sounds and overinflation of the chest. The patient may attempt to overcome air-trapping by increasing end-expiratory pressure by breathing through pursed lips.

Investigation
Biochemistry
α_1-Antitrypsin may be deficient. This can be assessed by genotyping or biochemically.

06

Blood gases
Hypoxia and hypercapnia can be present in chronic bronchitis and emphysema

Biochemistry
α_1-Antitrypsin deficiency in emphysema

Diagnostic imaging
Chronic bronchitis: commonly normal; may show flattened diaphragms, enlarged retrosternal space, altered rib angle
Emphysema: overinflation, loss of lung markings, flattened heart (in severe cases)

ECG
Right ventricular strain and 'pulmonale' in cases of cor pulmonale

Lung function
Spirometry: air-trapping, increased residual volume, airflow obstruction in emphysema
Transfer factor: markedly diminished in emphysema

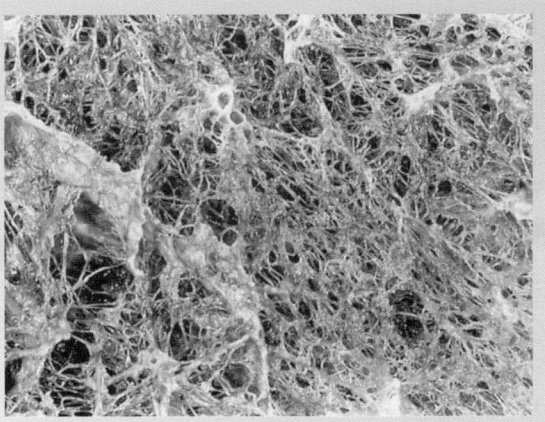

Fig. A Emphysema. Lung slice, inflated and fixed with formalin. Reproduced from Seaton *et al.*, *Crofton & Douglas's Respiratory Diseases*, 4th edn, 1989 (Blackwell Scientific Publications, Oxford) with the permission of the authors.

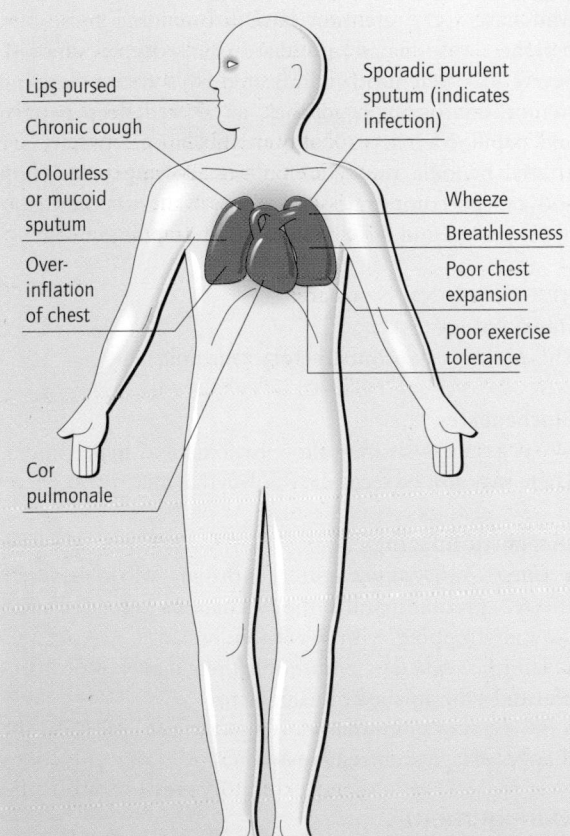

Lips pursed
Chronic cough
Colourless or mucoid sputum
Over-inflation of chest
Cor pulmonale

Sporadic purulent sputum (indicates infection)
Wheeze
Breathlessness
Poor chest expansion
Poor exercise tolerance

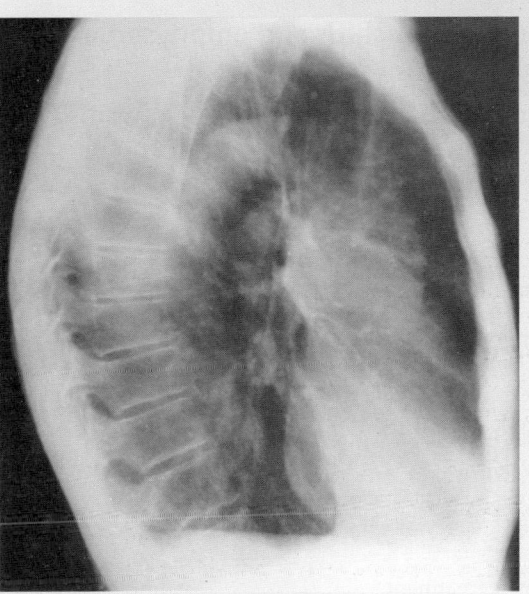

Fig. B Lateral radiography of severe emphysema showing over-inflation, flattened diaphragms and avascular lower zones. Reproduced from Seaton *et al.*, *Crofton & Douglas's Respiratory Diseases*, 4th edn, 1989 (Blackwell Scientific Publications, Oxford) with the permission of the authors.

06

Diagnostic imaging

Chest radiography shows signs of overinflation and a generalized loss of lung markings. These features can also occur in asthma. In severe emphysema the heart may be flattened by the distended lungs. If there is panacinar disease, bullae may be apparent.

Spirometry shows air-trapping, with an increased residual volume and airflow obstruction.

Lung function tests

Because of the loss of lung tissue, transfer factor is markedly diminished.

Management

Precipitating factors should be avoided and any causes should be treated (Table 6.29).

Prognosis

The prognosis is variable. Progression is slow only if it is treated.

Chronic bronchitis and emphysema (combined)

Epidemiology and disease mechanisms

As for chronic bronchitis and emphysema, presenting separately.

Table 6.29 Management of chronic bronchitis and emphysema

Supportive treatment

Physiotherapy
Little role unless there is an overlying infection or secondary bronchiectasis

Psychotherapy
Pulmonary rehabilitation classes can help severely affected individuals cope with their disability

Specific treatment
Remove causal agent (cigarettes or occupational exposure)

Drug treatment
Inhaled bronchodilators and inhaled corticosteroids if there is an asthmatic element

Antibiotics
Limited to the prompt treatment of acute infections
Sometimes long-term rotating antibiotics are used to prevent recurrent infections, but this is controversial
Main infecting organisms are *Streptococcus pneumoniae* and *Haemophilus influenzae*, which are usually sensitive to amoxicillin

Clinical features

Chronic bronchitis and emphysema produce a spectrum of disease, with two distinct types of patient at each end, referred to as blue bloaters and pink puffers.

● *Blue bloaters:* have cor pulmonale and are not unduly breathless. Their poor respiratory drive results in alveolar hypoventilation, arterial hypoxia, CO_2 retention and secondary polycythaemia.
● *Pink puffers:* have a strong respiratory drive and are breathless. They do not develop cor pulmonale or CO_2 retention until late stages. Arterial O_2 tension is relatively normal.

There is no correlation between blue bloaters and pink puffers or a predominance of emphysema or chronic bronchitis.

The clinical features of chronic bronchitis and emphysema usually include a productive cough, exertional dyspnoea and wheezing. Physical examination reveals use of the accessory muscles of respiration and a prolonged expiratory phase. The chest is overinflated and further chest expansion is poor. Lip pursing may be a feature. People who have CO_2 retention have a bounding pulse and peripheral vasodilatation, and are usually deeply cyanosed. Severe CO_2 retention is indicated by a coarse flapping tremor, confusion, headaches, an altered sleep pattern and papilloedema (CO_2 narcosis). Chronic pulmonary arterial hypoxia results in pulmonary vasoconstriction and can be complicated by polycythaemia, pulmonary hypertension and right heart failure (cor pulmonale).

Investigation

Haematology

This may reveal secondary polycythaemia.

Biochemistry

Blood gas analysis may show hypoxia and hypercapnia. There may also be secondary polycythaemia.

Diagnostic imaging

● *Chest radiography:* often normal. More severely affected, predominantly emphysematous individuals will show air-trapping, with or without bullae
● *Lung function tests:* commonly there is airflow obstruction and a diminished transfer factor
● *ECG:* as cor pulmonale develops the ECG will show the changes of right ventricular strain

Management

Removal of the causal agent is the most important factor in management (Table 6.29). Usually, the causal agent is cigarette smoking, cessation of which will slow the accelerated decline in lung function and prolong survival. If industrial agents are implicated (e.g. cadmium fumes), the patient should be removed from occupational exposure.

Drug treatment is aimed at achieving maximal bronchodilatation and treating infections. Airflow obstruction is commonly irreversible, but some patients have an asthmatic element, which can be diagnosed by a trial of oral corticosteroids (30 mg/day for 2 weeks). If the trial produces significant improvement (more than a 15% change in FEV_1 or FVC), inhaled corticosteroids should be substituted and inhaled bronchodilators prescribed.

Antibiotics are limited to the prompt treatment of acute infections. Long-term rotating antibiotics are sometimes used to prevent recurrent infections, but this practice is controversial. The main infecting organisms are *Streptococcus pneumoniae* and *Haemophilus influenzae*, which are usually sensitive to amoxicillin or trimethoprim.

Physiotherapy has little role, unless there is an overlying infection or secondary bronchiectasis (see p. 356). Pulmonary rehabilitation classes may help the individual to cope with their disability.

Influenza vaccine is recommended on a yearly basis because of tendency for secondary bacterial infection following viral respiratory infection.

Prognosis
The 5-year survival rate if there is severely impaired gas exchange ($Pao_2 < 8$ kPa or $Paco_2 > 7$ kPa) with complicating cor pulmonale is less than 50%.

Respiratory failure

Respiratory failure is defined as an inability of the lungs to exchange gases adequately ($Pao_2 < 8$ kPa or $Paco_2 > 7$ kPa).

Epidemiology
Prevalence. Uncommon.

Disease mechanisms
There are two main types of respiratory failure, depending on the underlying lung disease and the central response to hypoxaemia and hypercapnia (the causes are listed in Table 6.30):
• *Type 1:* low blood oxygen and low/normal blood carbon dioxide, implies a primary failure of gas exchange, and can be a result of an acute or chronic cause
• *Type 2:* low blood oxygen and elevated blood carbon dioxide, implies ventilatory failure, which may be primary or may complicate hypoxic respiratory failure
Respiratory failure results from a failure to exchange gases either because of lack of ventilation or a problem at the alveolar–capillary membrane.

Table 6.30 Causes of respiratory failure

Type 1. Hypoxia without hypercapnia
Acute causes
Pneumonia
Severe asthma
Pulmonary embolus
Pulmonary oedema

Chronic causes
Chronic bronchitis and emphysema (pink puffers)
Pulmonary infiltrations (e.g. lymphangitis)
Fibrosing alveolitis
Asbestosis

Type 2. Hypoxia with hypercapnia
Chronic bronchitis and emphysema (blue bloaters)
Obesity
Chest wall disease (e.g. thoracoplasty, kyphoscoliosis)
Postoperative hypoventilation
Obstructive sleep apnoea

Clinical features and investigation
The clinical features and investigation depend on the cause.

Management
Treatment of respiratory failure depends on whether there is hypercapnia:
• If $Pao_2 < 8$ kPa and $Paco_2 < 7$ kPa, the treatment is controlled oxygen therapy, and treatment of the underlying disease with appropriate use of diuretics, antibiotics, bronchodilators, corticosteroids and physiotherapy.
• If $Pao_2 < 8$ kPa and $Paco_2 > 7$ kPa, the treatment is controlled oxygen therapy, treatment of the underlying disease and respiratory stimulants. Ventilation should be considered. Patients who are not considered for intensive care unit ventilation may be suitable for nasal intermittent positive pressure ventilation (NIPPV) in a high-dependency unit setting.

Long-term or home oxygen treatment
Chronic hypoxaemia is lethal and treatment with controlled oxygen therapy improves survival. For such treatment, Pao_2 must be less than 7.3 kPa on air in a stable clinical state and the patient must not smoke. Home oxygen therapy needs to be given for at least 15 h/day and Pao_2 must be more than 8.0 kPa on treatment for it to be beneficial. Treatment is best given by nasal cannulae using an oxygen concentrator. Care must be taken not to remove the hypoxic drive and thereby worsen the respiratory failure.

06

Prognosis
The prognosis depends on the cause.

Obstructive sleep apnoea

Epidemiology
Prevalence. Unknown, but may be as high as 1% of the male population.

Sex. More common in males.

Disease mechanisms
Loss of muscular tone during rapid eye movement (REM) sleep allows the soft tissues of the oropharynx to obstruct the upper airway. This is common, normally after alcohol or sedatives, but arterial hypoxaemia is rare. Significant asphyxiation can occur if there is gross obesity or chronic bronchitis and emphysema, and the patient will rouse, perhaps many times each night.

Clinical features
Obstructive sleep apnoea should be suspected if a person snores or has a morning headache and/or daytime somnolence.

Investigation
Investigation involves overnight oximetry and sleep studies.

Management
Treatment includes weight reduction and avoidance of sedatives (including alcohol). Orolaryngopalatoplasty will not maintain the upper airway. Nasal positive airway pressure via a mask during sleep can help.

Prognosis
This is good if treated effectively.

Pleural disease

Pleurisy

Epidemiology
Prevalence. Common.

Disease mechanisms
Any process that inflames the pleural surface will cause the visceral and parietal pleura to come into direct contact with each other and cause pain. The causes of pleurisy are:
- Viral infection, which is the most common cause
- Pulmonary infarction
- Bronchial carcinoma
- Pneumonia
- Autoimmune multisystem disease (e.g. systemic lupus erythematosus, rheumatoid arthritis)

Viral infections causing pleurisy have a peak incidence in autumn. A particularly severe form is produced by Coxsackie B virus (epidemic myalgia).

Clinical features
Pleuritic pain is sharp (knife-like), severe and related to movement of the chest wall (e.g. deep inspiration or coughing). It is usually well localized to the area of the chest under which the pleural irritation lies. Irritation of the diaphragmatic pleura, however, causes pain sensation via the phrenic nerve and this is often referred to the tip of the shoulder. There may be an audible pleural rub related to respiration over the affected area.

Investigation
There may be an increased white cell count if there is infection. Chest radiography may reveal the underlying cause.

Management
This consists of analgesia and treatment of the underlying cause.

Prognosis
Pleurisy invariably settles with the correct treatment and analgesia.

Bornholm disease

Epidemiology
Prevalence. Uncommon.

Age. Typically occurs in young adults and children.

Disease mechanisms
Bornholm disease is caused by Coxsackie B virus and can occur in epidemics.

Clinical features
A short pyrexial upper respiratory tract illness culminates in severe chest wall pain, which inhibits all movement. There is often an associated overlying myositis (pleurodynia) and sometimes a pericarditis.

Investigation
Antibody titres
Diagnosis can be made from rising antibody titres to the virus.

Management
There is no specific treatment.

Prognosis
The condition usually resolves spontaneously over 1–2 weeks.

Pleural effusion

A pleural effusion is an excessive accumulation of fluid in the pleural space.

Epidemiology
Prevalence. Common.

Disease mechanisms
Causes of pleural effusion are listed in Table 6.31.

Pathogenesis
A pleural effusion may be a transudate or an exudate:

- *Pleural transudates:* clear watery fluids, low in protein (less than 30 g/l). They result because of an imbalance between the hydrostatic pressures across the pleural capillaries, which normally allow the continuing secretion (parietal pleura) and absorption (visceral pleura) of pleural fluid. For example, an increase in visceral pleural capillary pressure will impede the resorption of pleural fluid.
- *Pleural exudates:* rich in protein (more than 30 g/l) and usually dark amber in colour, although some may be milky because of chyle (chylothorax), bloodstained (haemothorax) or contain frank pus (empyema). Pleural exudates commonly occur as a result of primary disease of

Table 6.31 Causes of pleural effusion

Type of effusion	Prevalence	Mechanism	Example	Comment
Transudate (< 30g/l)	Most common cause	Haemodynamic failure	Cardiac failure	
	Common	Hypoproteinaemia	Nephrotic syndrome, starvation	
	Rare	Haemodynamic failure	Myxoedema	
	Rare	Haemodynamic failure	Constrictive pericarditis	
	Rare	Ascitic transfer	Meigs' syndrome	A rare syndrome of ovarian fibromas associated with a right-sided pleural effusion, which clears with removal of the tumour
Exudate (> 30g/l)	Common	Bacterial pneumonia	*Streptococcus pneumoniae* pneumonia	
	Common	Carcinoma	Bronchial carcinoma, metastatic carcinoma (e.g. breast carcinoma)	Often bloodstained
	Common	Pleural inflammation	Pulmonary infarction	Often bloodstained
	Rare	Pleural inflammation	Tuberculosis	
	Rare	Pleural inflammation	Autoimmune rheumatic disease (e.g. RA, SLE)	
	Rare	Pleural inflammation	Acute pancreatitis	Commonly left-sided, has a high amylase concentration, and may be bloodstained
	Rare	Pleural inflammation	Subphrenic or hepatic abscess	Right-sided
	Rare	Primary pleural tumour	Mesothelioma	
	Rare	Pleural inflammation	Benign asbestos-related pleural effusion	
	Rare	Blocked lymphatics	Yellow nail syndrome	Yellow nails, chronic lymphoedema and pleural effusions result from an abnormality of lymphatic drainage
	Rare	Fatty effusion	Chylothorax	Usually left-sided and results from disruption of the thoracic duct by tumour or trauma
		Pleural bleeding	Trauma to the chest wall resulting in haemothorax	

RA, rheumatoid arthritis; SLE, systemic lupus erythematosus.

06

Pleural effusion at a glance

Epidemiology

Prevalence

More than 1 million cases/year in USA

Pleural effusion is most commonly a complication of:

- left ventricular failure
- bacterial pneumonia
- malignancy

Fig. A Chest radiograph showing a small right-sided pleural effusion. Note the obliteration of the normal costophrenic angle.

Chest wall movement reduced on affected side

Stony dull on percussion

Absent/reduced breath sounds

Mediastinum shifted to opposite side

Bronchial breathing above the effusion (occasionally)

Reduced vocal resonance and vocal fremitus

the underlying lung or pleura. Fluid is actively secreted into the pleural cavity.

Clinical features

Typically, a patient with pleural effusion presents with increasing breathlessness, with or without symptoms of the underlying cause (e.g. haemoptysis in bronchial carcinoma). The most important physical sign is stony dullness on percussion over the fluid. This is associated with absent or reduced breath sounds and reduced tactile vocal fremitus. Bronchial breathing can be heard just above the effusion, and vocal resonance may be aegophonic ('bleating').

A pleural effusion can be detected clinically only when it is larger than 500 ml. Small effusions (220–500 ml) are revealed by chest radiography.

Investigation

Haematology, biochemistry, immunology and microbiology

Investigations are those for the underlying disease.

Diagnostic imaging

- *Chest radiography:* confirms the presence and site of the effusion (Figs A and B, pp. 350 and 351) and may suggest the underlying cause. CT scanning may provide further information.
- *Fibre-optic bronchoscopy:* forms part of the investigation of a pleural effusion when the diagnosis is not evident from pleural aspiration and biopsy.
- *Pleuroscopy:* direct examination of the pleura either through a thoracoscope or via a thoracotomy.

Findings on investigation

Haematology, biochemistry and immunology

As for the underlying disease (see Fig. C)

Microbiology

Sputum culture for infection

Diagnostic imaging

Chest radiography: confirms site of effusion and may suggest cause. Dense uniform opacity in lower and lateral parts of hemithorax

Diagnostic pleural tap, with:

Cytology: detects malignancy

Microbiology: Gram stain and culture detects infection

Biochemistry: protein content differentiates transudate (< 30 g/l) from exudate (> 30 g/l). Amylase high in pancreatitis. Glucose low in rheumatoid arthritis, tuberculosis and carcinoma

Histopathology and cytology

Sputum cytology: cytology for malignancy

Needle biopsy of pleura: detects malignant cells or *Mycobacterium tuberculosis*

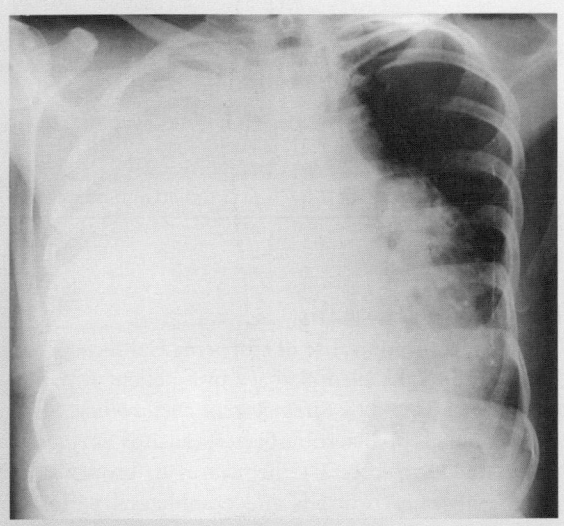

Fig. B Massive pulmonary effusion. Note how the mediastinal structures (trachea, heart) are pushed to the contralateral side.

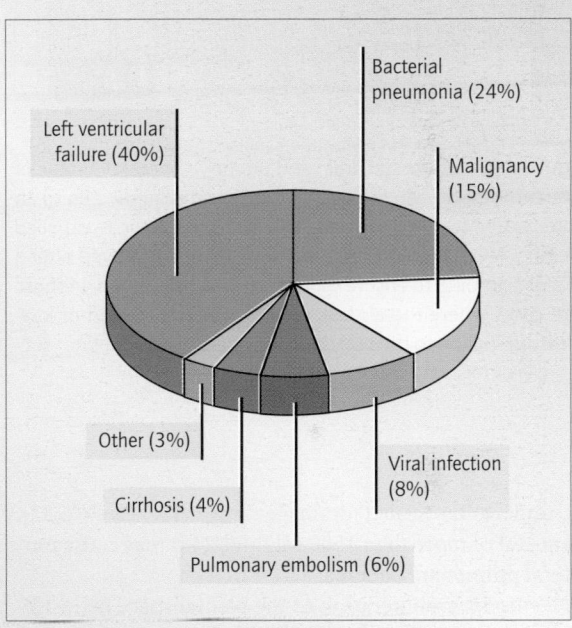

Fig. C Common causes of pleural effusion.

Histopathology

- *Needle biopsy of the pleura:* the detection of malignant cells or *Mycobacterium tuberculosis* in pleural fluid is not easy. In those cases in which the diagnosis is not evident on examination of the fluid, a needle biopsy of the pleura should be considered (Fig. 6.15).
- *Sputum examination:* for organisms and malignant cells.

Diagnostic pleural tap

A sample of pleural fluid (30 ml) is aspirated through the skin using a sterile approach, and examined. The macroscopic appearances in empyema, chylothorax and haemothorax are of obvious diagnostic importance, and the following investigations may be appropriate:

- *Cytology:* to detect malignancy

- *Gram stain and culture:* to detect infection
- *Protein content:* to differentiate between a transudate (protein < 30 g/l) and an exudate (protein > 30 g/l)
- *Amylase content:* high in pancreatitis
- *Complement level:* low in rheumatoid arthritis and systemic lupus erythematosus
- *Glucose level:* low in rheumatoid arthritis, tuberculosis and carcinoma

Management

- *Pleurocentesis:* patients with respiratory distress resulting from a large collection of pleural fluid are treated with pleurocentesis. A large amount (up to 1500 ml/24 h) of pleural fluid is removed either by a hand-operated syringe or by the insertion of an intercostal drain attached

06

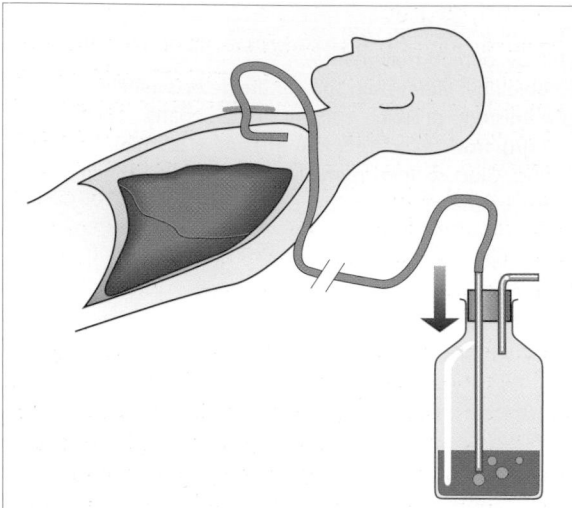

Figure 6.19 Intercostal drain and underwater seal drainage of a pneumothorax. An intercostal tube drain is connected to an underwater seal drainage. Usually the pleural air is expelled within a few days, and the tube drain can be removed after a trial of clamping to ensure that the air leak has settled. In those rare cases where the air leak persists, the application of low-pressure suction to the seal drain may help. If this does not succeed, pleurectomy may be required.

to underwater sealed drainage (Fig 6.19; Table 6.32). Removal of more than 1500 ml fluid/24 h may cause unilateral pulmonary oedema.
• *Pleurodesis:* obliteration of the pleural space by instilling chemicals (e.g. tetracycline, bleomycin and talc, which inflame the two pleural surfaces, encouraging them to stick together) through an intercostal drain. This often provides successful palliation for malignant effusions, which commonly reaccumulate soon after initial pleurocentesis.
• *Pleurectomy:* may be considered if pleurodesis is not successful.
   Specific treatment is aimed at the underlying cause.

Prognosis
The prognosis depends on the underlying cause.

Empyema

Empyema is a collection of pus in the pleural space.

Epidemiology
Prevalence. Five per cent of patients who are hospitalized with pneumonia.

Table 6.32 Management of pleural effusion

Pleurocentesis
Removal of a large amount (up to 1500 ml/24 h) of pleural fluid
For patients with respiratory distress resulting from a large collection of pleural fluid
Performed either by a hand-operated syringe or by the insertion of an intercostal drain attached to underwater seal drainage (Fig. 6.19)
Removal of more than 1500 ml fluid/24 h may cause unilateral pulmonary oedema

Pleurodesis
Obliteration of the pleural space by instillation of chemicals (e.g. tetracycline, bleomycin, talc) through the intercostal drain
Often successful palliation for malignant effusions

Pleurectomy
May be considered if pleurodesis is not successful

General measures
The underlying cause of the effusion should also be treated

Disease mechanisms
The most common cause of empyema is direct spread of infection into the pleural space in a patient with either pneumonia caused by *Streptococcus pneumoniae*, *Staphylococcus aureus* or anaerobic bacteria such as *Streptococcus milari*, or a lung abscess. Other causes are bronchiectasis, penetrating chest wounds and oesophageal perforation (*Escherichia coli*, anaerobes). Empyemas are often fibrinous and commonly become encysted and loculated.

Clinical features
A pleural effusion in a patient whose pneumonia is not responding to adequate antibiotic treatment suggests the presence of an empyema. **Chronic empyema** is rare and may result from inadequate treatment of acute empyema, indolent infection (e.g. tuberculosis, actinomycosis), bronchopleural fistula (e.g. following pneumonectomy) or a foreign body in the pleural space. It causes a debilitating illness with anaemia, weight loss, finger clubbing and persistent respiratory symptoms, and may be complicated by amyloidosis.

Investigation
Pleural tap confirms the diagnosis as the sample is often thick and purulent, and may be foul-smelling. **Pleural fluid cytology** reveals an exudate with pus cells and organisms.

Management
Treatment is drainage via an intercostal tube drain to

obtain satisfactory resolution. Rib resection may be necessary to gain adequate drainage if the effusion is very thick or loculated. Decortication of the thickened pleura may be indicated if the pus sets into a thickened fibrinous mass that undergoes fibrosis and restricts chest wall movement.

Prognosis
Good if treated early.

Pneumothorax

In pneumothorax, air collects between the visceral and parietal pleura, causing a real rather than potential pleural space. Air in the pleural space will allow the lung to move away from the chest wall and the lung will partially deflate.

Epidemiology
Prevalence. Prevalence of spontaneous pneumothorax is 1/10 000/year.

Age. Most common in young adults and in elderly people with chest disease.

Sex. More common in males (6 : 1).

Disease mechanisms
Pneumothorax can arise spontaneously either as a primary spontaneous pneumothorax, which is the most common type of pneumothorax, or secondary to underlying lung disease. Such underlying lung disease can result from:
- Airflow limitation from asthma or bullous emphysema
- Positive pressure ventilation in intensive care units
- Infections (e.g. staphylococcal pneumonia, tuberculosis)
- Inherited disorders (e.g. cystic fibrosis, Marfan's syndrome)
- Rare disorders (e.g. lymphangioleiomyomatosis, endometriosis externa)

   Alternatively, pneumothorax can arise following trauma, when it may be caused by:
- Penetrating injury to the chest wall (e.g. fractured rib following a road traffic accident, stab wound)
- Non-penetrating injury to chest wall (e.g. road traffic accident)
- Therapeutic procedures (e.g. insertion of subclavian venous line, surgery to chest wall, pleural aspiration or biopsy)

   Usually there is no obvious abnormality of the underlying lung (primary spontaneous pneumothorax). Typically, this occurs in tall fit young men and is thought to result from the rupture of small apical subpleural blebs.

Clinical features
A pneumothorax causes a sudden onset of sharp pleuritic pain and breathlessness. Most primary spontaneous pneumothoraces are small (defined as occupying less than 30% of the diameter of the hemithorax) and cause few symptoms other than the initial pain. The physical signs are summarized in Table 6.11. A pneumothorax should always be considered in any patient with known lung disease (e.g. asthma, bullous emphysema) who becomes more breathless for no obvious reason.

Tension pneumothorax. This occurs when a positive pressure builds up in the pleural space, leading to mediastinal shift, breathlessness, hypoxaemia and, eventually, shock secondary to impaired venous return to the heart. It is a medical emergency. Although rare, it is most commonly a complication of a traumatic pneumothorax, or of pneumothorax in a patient on a ventilator.

Recurrent pneumothorax. Twenty per cent of patients with primary spontaneous pneumothorax will have an ipsilateral recurrence. After a second and third episode the recurrence rates are over 65% and 85%, respectively.

Subcutaneous emphysema. At the time of the pleural air leak or following the insertion of an intercostal drain, air may track into the subcutaneous tissues of the back or mediastinum (pneumomediastinum). This is more commonly associated with traumatic rather than spontaneous pneumothorax. Subcutaneous air has a pathognomonic crackling sensation on palpation. Although dramatic in some cases, surgical emphysema does not cause respiratory embarrassment and eventually subsides completely (Fig. 6.20).

Investigation
Diagnostic imaging
Chest radiography confirms the diagnosis (Fig. 6.21). Inspiratory and expiratory radiographs help define the visceral pleura where there is a small pneumothorax.

Management
The management of a pneumothorax is outlined in the Emergency box on p. 355.

   A small (occupying less than 30% of the diameter of the hemithorax) primary spontaneous pneumothorax can usually be left to resorb naturally. If the pneumothorax is larger or if there are marked symptoms of breathlessness, aspiration of the entrapped air with a needle or cannula (16 G or less), syringe and three-way tap is usually successful (Table 6.33). Insertion of an intercostal drain is recommended for very large primary spontaneous pneumothorax or any size of secondary spontaneous

06

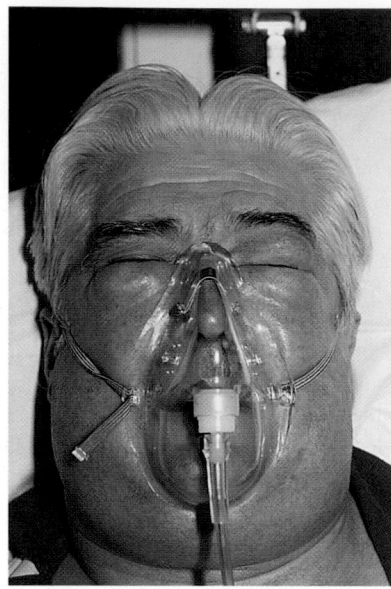

Figure 6.20 Surgical emphysema. Extensive surgical emphysema following insertion of an intercostal tube drain into a patient with a spontaneous pneumothorax secondary to bullous emphysema. Note the involvement of the eyelids with consequent complete closure of both eyes.

Table 6.33 Aspiration of a pneumothorax

Simple aspiration

Infiltrate local anaesthetic down to the pleura, in the second intercostal space in the mid-clavicular line. The cannula should be 16 G or less and at least 3 cm long

Having entered the pleural cavity, withdraw the needle

Connect a three-way tap to the cannula and a 50 ml syringe (Luer lock) and an exit tube, fed under water to ensure correct direction of airflow

Discontinue aspiration if:

- resistance is felt
- the patient experiences excessive coughing
- more than 2.5 l (50 ml removed 50 times) have been aspirated

Repeat chest X-ray

If the pneumothorax is now only small or resolved, the procedure has been successful

N.B. Failure to aspirate further may be a result of the cannula being inadvertently withdrawn from the pleural cavity, or becoming kinked

All patients in whom aspiration is attempted should be observed overnight

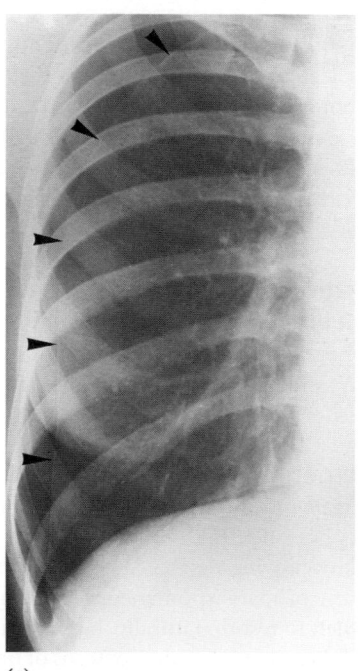

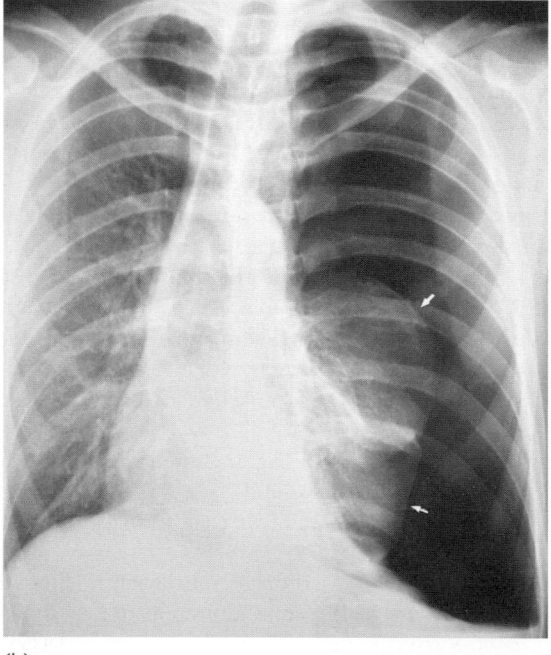

(a)   (b)

Figure 6.21 (a) Pneumothorax. The diagnosis of pneumothorax requires identification of the pleural edge (arrowed) and the clear space beyond it. (b) Tension pneumothorax. The left hemidiaphragm is depressed and the mediastinum shifted to the right. The left lung is substantially depressed (arrowed). Reproduced from Armstrong & Wastie, *Diagnostic Imaging*, 3rd edn, 1992 (Blackwell Scientific Publications, Oxford) with the permission of the authors.

Emergency 6.2: Pneumothorax

Diagnosis
Sudden pleuritic pain and breathlessness are the most common symptoms. A chest X-ray confirms the diagnosis (for a list of causes see p. 353)

Assessment
Airway
Breathing
Circulation

Supportive therapy
Oxygen
Analgesia

Specific therapy
Traumatic pneumothorax
All require formal drainage as there is an increased risk of tension pneumothorax

Tension pneumothorax
Rare. Clinical diagnosis in a patient with a pneumothorax with respiratory distress and cardiovascular compromise. Decompress with a 14 G needle in the second intercostal space/mid-clavicular line. Then insert a chest drain.

Other pneumothoraces
Treatment of other pneumothoraces depends upon:
- size
- symptoms of breathlessness
- whether there is underlying lung disease (secondary)

The following advice (Table A and Fig. A) is based upon the *British Thoracic Guidelines* for the treatment of a pneumothorax.

Table A Treatment of a pneumothorax

	Complete	Moderate	Small
Primary	Aspirate/chest drain	Aspirate	Observe
Secondary	Chest drain	Chest drain	Chest drain

Aspiration of a pneumothorax
Infiltrate local anaesthetic down to the pleura, in the second intercostal space in the mid-clavicular line. The cannula should be 16 G or less and at least 3 cm long. Having entered the pleural cavity, withdraw the needle. Connect a three-way tap to the cannula and a 50 ml syringe (Luer lock) and an exit tube, fed under water to ensure correct direction of airflow.

Discontinue aspiration if:
- resistance is felt
- the patient experiences excessive coughing
- more than 2.5 l (50 ml removed 50 times) have been aspirated

Repeat chest X-ray. If the pneumothorax is now only small or resolved, the procedure has been successful. (N.B. Failure to aspirate further may be because the cannula is being inadvertently withdrawn from the pleural cavity, or becoming kinked.) All patients in whom aspiration is attempted should be observed overnight.

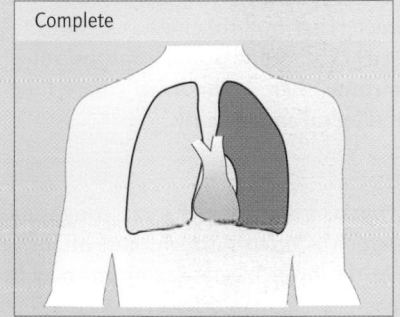 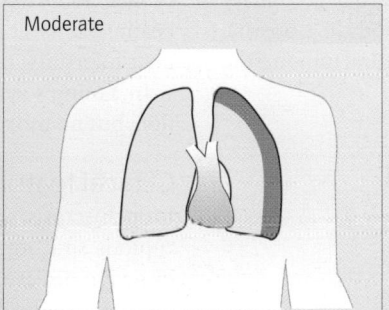 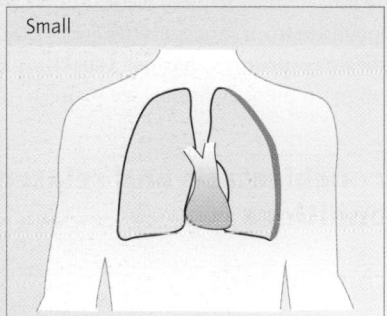

Complete — Moderate — Small

Fig. A Degree of collapse in pneumothorax.

or traumatic pneumothorax (Fig. 6.19). The increased pleural pressure of a tension pneumothorax must be reduced promptly by inserting a hollow syringe needle or an intercostal tube drain.

Surgical pleurectomy is indicated for recurrent pneumothorax.

Prognosis
The prognosis of pneumothorax is good.

Pleural thickening

Epidemiology
Prevalence. A common sequela to pleurisy.

Disease mechanisms

Pleural thickening can be a result of:

- Fibrosis following pleurisy
- Fibrosis following thoracotomy
- Fibrosis associated with asbestos exposure
- Asbestos-related pleural plaques
- Secondary tumour metastases
- Malignant mesothelioma

Chronic irritation of the pleura by asbestos will result in more marked fibrosis, which can inhibit chest wall movement. Plaques on the parietal pleura are a specific feature of asbestos exposure (see p. 379).

Clinical features

Usually of no consequence unless it is severe when it can cause pulmonary restriction.

Investigation

Chest radiography and CT scanning will show the extent of the disease.

Management

Surgical pleurectomy may be indicated if there is marked pulmonary restriction and the cause is benign.

Prognosis

Good if the cause is not malignant.

Pleural tumours

The most common pleural tumour is caused by secondary deposition from cancer elsewhere in the body (e.g. breast). Asbestos exposure can cause a specific pleural tumour: the malignant mesothelioma (see p. 366).

Bronchiectasis and related conditions

Bronchiectasis

Epidemiology

Prevalence. Approximately 1/1000.

Age. Any age. Usually starts in childhood.

Genetics. Usually an acquired condition. Common in patients with cystic fibrosis and IgA deficiency.

Geography. More common in developing countries.

Disease mechanisms

The most common cause of bronchiectasis is damage

Table 6.34 Causes of bronchiectasis

Localized bronchial obstruction
Inhaled foreign body (e.g. peanut, tooth)
Enlarged hilar glands (which can compress the right middle lobe bronchus)
Bronchial tumours

Generalized bronchial obstruction associated with reduced clearance of secretions
Slow-to-resolve pneumonia (e.g. resulting from whooping cough, measles)
Recurrent infections resulting from immune defects (e.g. hypogammaglobulinaemia)
Altered secretions (e.g. cystic fibrosis; see p. 357)
Ciliary dysfunction (e.g. Kartagener's syndrome or Young's syndrome)

---

to the bronchial tree after an infection (Table 6.34). Bronchiectasis may also complicate bronchial obstruction or a more widespread disorder (e.g. cystic fibrosis).

Bronchiectasis is chronic dilatation of the bronchi. It can be tubular, fusiform or saccular. Any condition that causes a chronic retention of bronchial secretions with subsequent infection can lead to bronchiectasis. The mucociliary transport mechanism is disrupted, secretions collect in the dilated bronchi and infection ensues. This damages the bronchi further, causing increasing sepsis, worsening bronchial inflammation and more secretion retention.

In **Kartagener's syndrome** ('immotile cilia' syndrome or primary ciliary dyskinesia), there is a congenital microtubular abnormality of the cilia that prevents normal cilial beating. It is characterized by bronchiectasis, sinusitis, male infertility, dextrocardia and visceral transposition.

In **Young's syndrome**, there is abnormal ciliary function, but no morphological abnormality.

Clinical features

Bronchiectasis is characterized by a chronic cough and copious sputum, which is often purulent and offensive in severe disease. In dry bronchiectasis, sputum may be produced only during a chest infection. Exacerbations of infection are common, and may be associated with haemoptysis.

Examination may reveal halitosis and coarse lung crackles that are widespread or localized to one area. Bronchospasm may be a feature, particularly in bronchopulmonary aspergillosis. **Other manifestations** include finger clubbing and manifestations of the predisposing disease, for example:

- enlarged hilar glands
- bronchial tumour
- slow-to-resolve pneumonia resulting from whooping cough or measles

- immune defects
- altered secretions
- sinusitis, male infertility, dextrocardia and visceral transposition of Kartagener's syndrome
- cystic fibrosis (see below)

Complications of bronchiectasis include:
- recurrent chest infections (common)
- haemoptysis (can be life-threatening and may require surgical resection)
- emphysema (rare)
- systemic amyloid (rare)
- cor pulmonale (commonly develops after years of pulmonary sepsis and arterial hypoxaemia)

Diagnosis
This is clinical if mild, but a definitive diagnosis requires further investigation, usually with CT or, rarely, bronchography.

Investigation
Haematology
Decreased haemoglobin in severe disease.

Biochemistry
No significant findings.

Immunology
Immunoglobulins. Usually a non-specific increase; however, immunoglobulin deficiency is a cause of bronchiectasis.

Microbiology
Sputum culture grows staphylococci and *Pseudomonas* spp.

Diagnostic imaging
- *Chest radiography:* may show bronchial wall thickening or cystic areas
- *CT scanning:* shows bronchial wall thickening
- *Bronchography:* reveals dilated bronchi, but is rarely performed

Histopathology
Histology reveals infected distorted bronchi and pulmonary fibrosis.

Management
The anatomical picture makes little difference to the treatment of the disease unless it is proximal bronchiectasis, which is likely to be caused by bronchopulmonary aspergillosis (see p. 368).

Postural drainage. This requires appropriate posture with associated percussion to drain affected lobes. To remove retained bronchial secretions is the most important step. Many people with mild disease can be managed in good health with postural drainage 2–3 times/day alone.

Antibiotic therapy. This, coupled with postural drainage, reduces bacterial load in the respiratory tree during acute infections. Intravenous treatment is indicated for severe infections. Inhaled (delivered by nebulizer) or continuous oral therapy can be used for chronic sepsis and more resistant pathogens (e.g. *Staphylococcus aureus*, *Pseudomonas aeruginosa*). A regular course of intravenous antibiotics is sometimes advocated for cystic fibrosis to reduce the bacterial load, but this can increase the probability of antibiotic resistance.

Bronchodilators. These are indicated for bronchospasm, which is often a concomitant feature.

Oral corticosteroids. These may be required during an acute exacerbation.

Surgery. In localized disease removal of a segment of lung can effect a cure, but when symptoms are severe enough to merit surgery, the disease is rarely localized.

Prognosis
Bronchiectasis is a chronic disease that can be controlled by effective treatment.

Cystic fibrosis
Epidemiology
Prevalence and ethnicity. Incidence is 1/2000 births in white people, 1/20 000 in Afro-Caribbeans and 1/100 000 in Asians.

Age. Patients usually present at less than 1 year of age.

Genetics. Autosomal recessive inheritance.

Disease mechanisms
The cystic fibrosis gene is found on chromosome 7. It is very large, and to date over 600 mutations causing cystic fibrosis have been described. The most common mutation, $\Delta F508$, is responsible for over 70% of cases of cystic fibrosis in the UK.

Pathogenesis
The gene product is the cystic fibrosis transmembrane regulator (CFTR) protein. This regulates the chloride channel in the cell at its luminal surface and its absence or dysfunction results in an abnormally high concentration of sodium in sweat and in a low water content in the

06

Bronchiectasis at a glance

Epidemiology

Prevalence
About 1/1000

Geography
More common in developing countries

Findings on investigation
Haematology
FBC: decreased haemoglobin in severe disease

Immunology
Immunoglobulins: usually a non-specific increase. Decreased immunoglobulins in hypogammaglobulinaemia

Microbiology
Sputum culture: often staphylococci and *Pseudomonas* spp.

Diagnostic imaging
Chest radiography: bronchial wall thickening, ring shadows
CT scanning: bronchial wall thickening
Bronchography: dilated bronchi

Histopathology
Infected distorted bronchi, pulmonary fibrosis

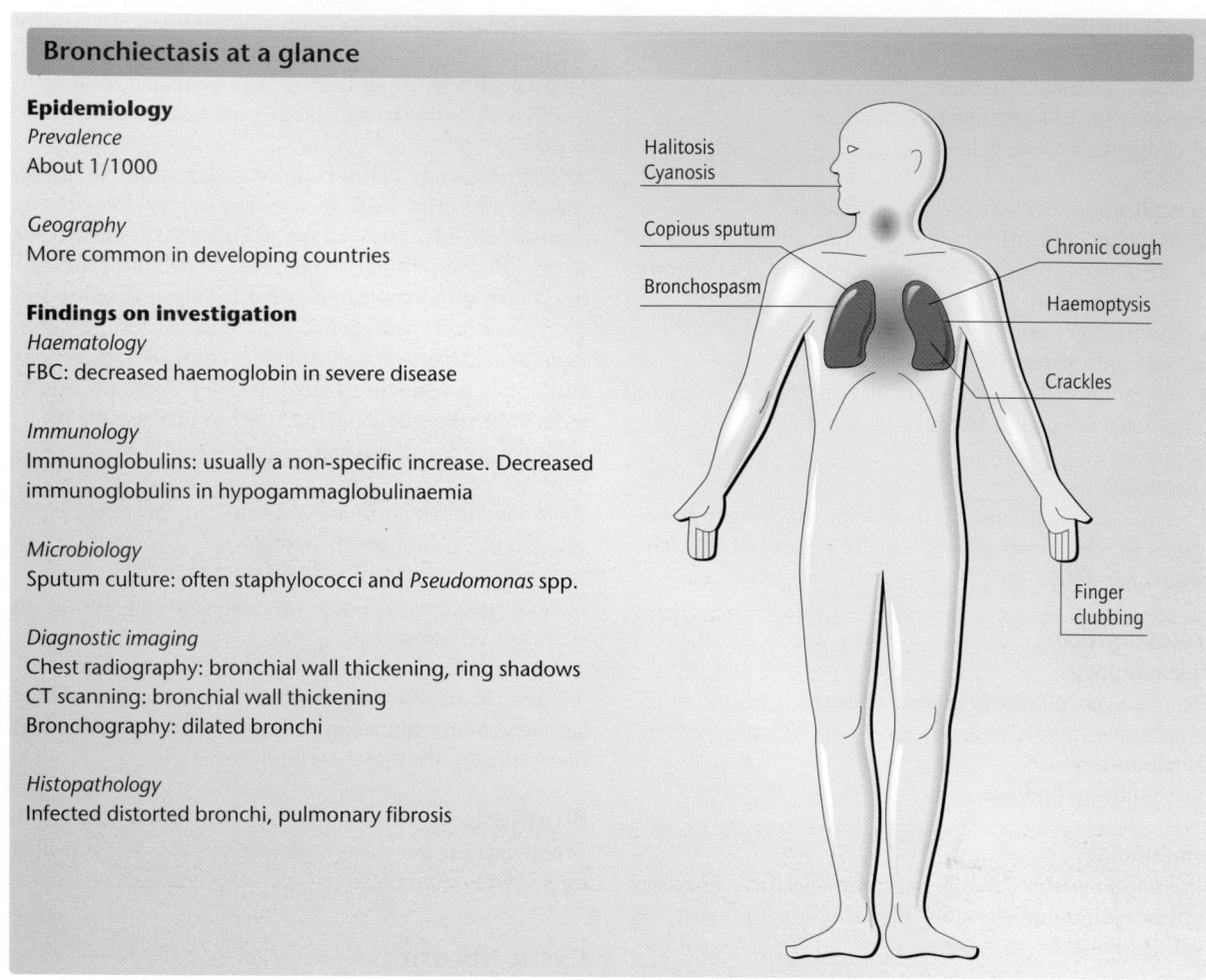

Halitosis
Cyanosis
Copious sputum
Bronchospasm
Chronic cough
Haemoptysis
Crackles
Finger clubbing

---

mucus produced by airways, pancreas and intestine. Different gene abnormalities can cause differing degrees of CFTR malfunction, and there is some correlation between genotype and manifestation of disease.

Clinical features

At birth the infant is normal, but symptoms of organ dysfunction can occur soon after birth. Presenting features vary widely. Manifestations include the following:

● *Meconium ileus:* 10% of infants present with this, caused by the abnormally viscid nature of the meconium causing obstruction of the terminal ileum.

● *Malabsorption and steatorrhoea:* resulting from secretory dysfunction of the exocrine pancreas.

● *Bronchiectasis:* associated with finger clubbing and haemoptysis and usually develops during childhood. Recurrent *Staphylococcus aureus* infections are common and *Pseudomonas* spp. colonize the respiratory tract. Most

patients reaching adulthood are colonized by multiresistant pseudomonads. Haemoptyses and pneumothoraxes are common.

● *Intrahepatic cholestasis and gallstones:* common. Secondary biliary cirrhosis develops in 5–10% of patients.

● *Delayed puberty and maturity:* common and probably brought about by chronic malnutrition.

● *Diabetes mellitus:* results from destruction of islet cells because of chronic pancreatitis.

● *Meconium ileus equivalent* (distal intestinal obstruction syndrome): a similar syndrome to meconium ileus presenting in adults.

● *Altered fertility:* ninety-seven per cent of males are infertile because the vas deferens fails to develop. Females may be fertile.

● *Finger clubbing and arthropathy:* finger clubbing is common and more significant arthropathy or even vasculitis can occur.

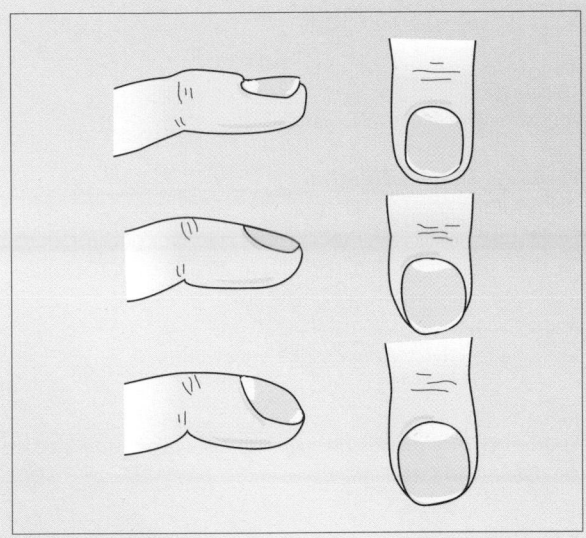

Fig. A Finger clubbing. The first sign of clubbing is loss of the angle between the nail and the nail bed. This is followed by increased fluctuation of the nail bed and an increased ability to rock the nail from side to side. In extreme cases there is an increased curvature of the nail, and an increase in the soft tissues in the ends of the fingers to form so-called 'drumstick' fingers.

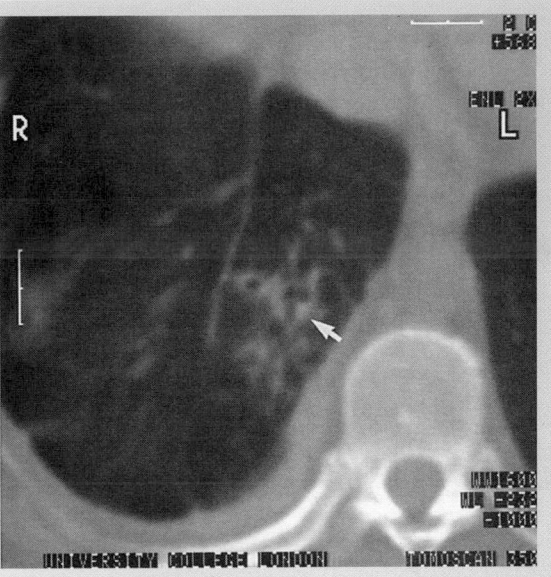

Fig. B CT scan of the thorax showing posterior right lower lobe. Note the bronchial wall thickening. Reproduced from Johnson, *Respiratory Medicine, Pocket Consultant*, 2nd edn, 1990 (Blackwell Scientific Publications, Oxford) with the permission of the author.

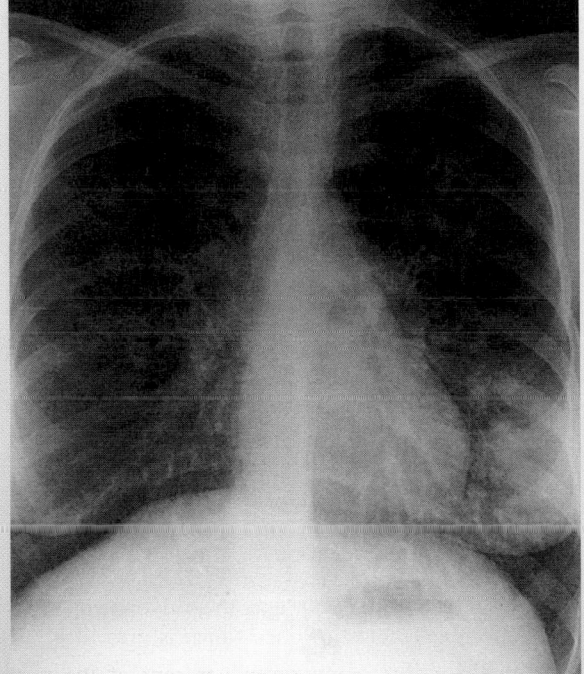

Fig. C Chest radiograph. In bronchiectasis the chest radiograph may be entirely normal in mild disease, but in more severe cases bronchial wall thickening or even cystic areas are visible.

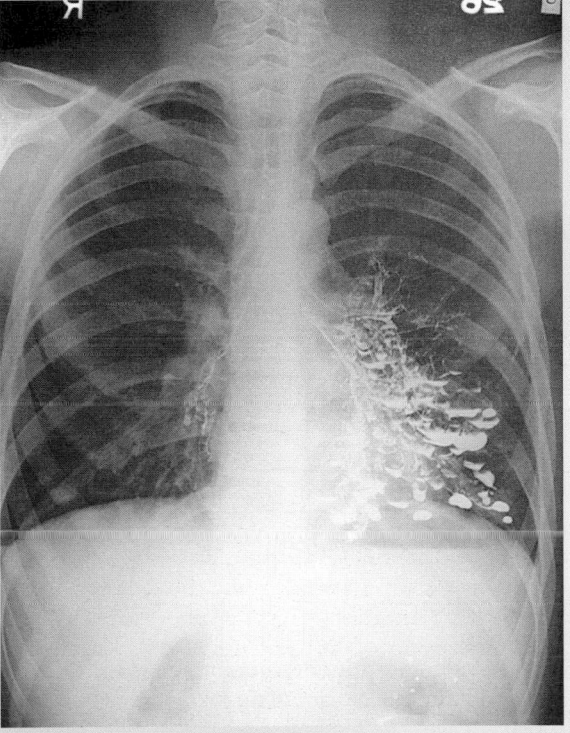

Fig. D Bronchogram demonstrating bronchiectasis in the left lower lobe.

06

Cystic fibrosis at a glance

Epidemiology
Prevalence
1/2500 in the UK

Age
Commonly presents in infancy

Race
Most common in white people

Genetics
Autosomal recessive inheritance

Findings on investigation
Biochemistry
Sweat test: raised sweat sodium and chloride concentrations
Tests for diabetes mellitus positive in 20% of adult patients

Immunology
Immune reactive trypsin positive in newborn

Microbiology
Sputum culture reveals *Haemophilus influenzae*, *Staphylococcus aureus* and *Pseudomonas*

Diagnostic imaging
Chest radiography shows bronchiectasis

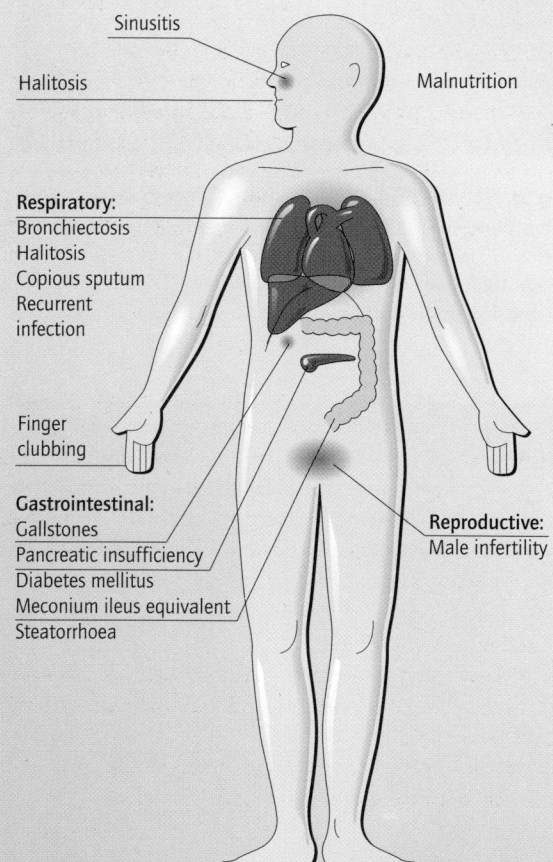

Sinusitis

Halitosis

Malnutrition

Respiratory:
Bronchiectosis
Halitosis
Copious sputum
Recurrent
infection

Finger
clubbing

Gastrointestinal:
Gallstones
Pancreatic insufficiency
Diabetes mellitus
Meconium ileus equivalent
Steatorrhoea

Reproductive:
Male infertility

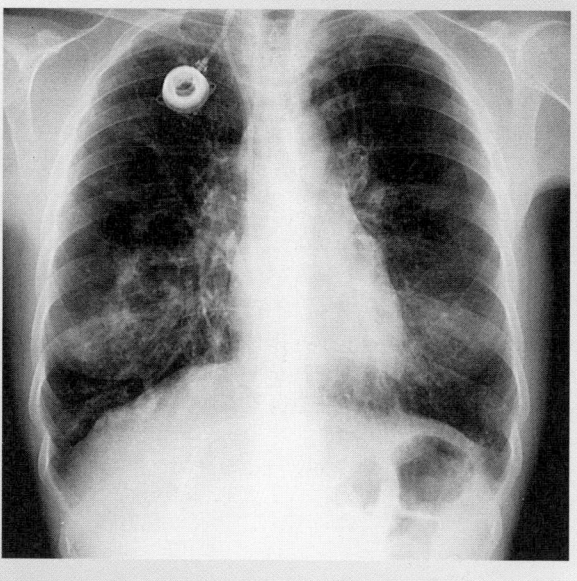

Fig. A Chest radiograph showing widespread bronchiectasis in cystic fibrosis. Note the implanted venous access device for repeated intravenous antibiotic treatment.

Investigation
Biochemistry
Sweat sodium and chloride concentrations are elevated (sweat sodium more than 70 mmol/l) in children over 10 years of age. The test is less reliable in older children and adults.

Glucose. With increasing age there is an increasing incidence of diabetes mellitus, which is present in 20% of adult patients.

Immunology
Immunoglobulins may be increased. Immune reactive trypsin positive in the newborn period.

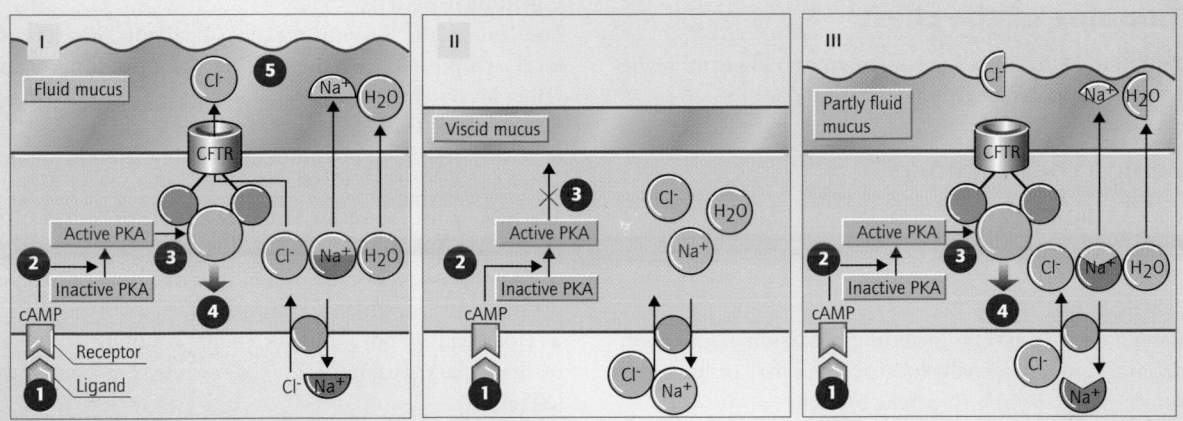

Fig. B Pathophysiology of cystic fibrosis. (I) Normal mucus-secreting epithelium. 1, Cell surface receptor stimulates cAMP production; 2, cAMP activates protein kinase (PKA); 3, PKA phosphorylates cystic fibrosis transmembrane receptor (CFTR); 4, ion channel opens; 5, chloride ions (Cl^-), sodium ions (Na^+) and water (H_2O) are secreted, yielding a well-lubricated and moist airway. (II) Severe cystic fibrosis: steps 1–2 occur normally but the CFTR protein is absent so secretion of Cl^-, Na^+ and H_2O is impossible. The result is a viscid (semi-viscous and sticky) mucus, salty sweat and severe clinical disease in 70% of cases. (III) Mild cystic fibrosis: steps 1–3 occur normally but the CFTR protein is abnormal and phosphorylation causes only partial opening of the channel. The secretion of Cl^-, Na^+ and H_2O is, therefore, reduced. The result is partly fluid mucus, mildly salty sweat and milder clinical disease.

Microbiology
Sputum culture and sensitivity often reveal *Staphylococcus aureus* and *Pseudomonas* spp.

Diagnostic imaging
- *CT scanning:* demonstrates bronchiectasis, pancreatitis and cirrhosis
- *Chest radiography:* demonstrates bronchiectasis with cystic changes
- *Ultrasound:* demonstrates liver disease
- *Gene typing:* can be carried out on a blood sample

Management
Cystic fibrosis is best treated in a recognized cystic fibrosis centre where staff are experienced in the special needs of the patient. Each feature is treated according to its severity. Most patients require regular pancreatic supplements and regular physiotherapy, with frequent courses of antibiotic.

Patients reaching maturity often have stunted physical development and psychological problems, which may require skilled help.

Treatment of bronchiectasis
More than 90% of patients survive into adult life, when bronchiectasis is the main feature. Most require regular courses of intravenous antipseudomonal antibiotics, and implanted lines for venous access are frequently necessary. Despite the best treatment, almost all develop progressive cardiorespiratory failure during early adult life, and heart–lung transplantation is the only solution. Organ replacement is being used with increasing success in such patients, none of whom have developed bronchiectasis in their donor lungs.

Further developments
1 Recombinant human deoxyribonucleic acidase (DNAase) to thin sputum and help expectoration has been developed.
2 Inhaled gene therapy to correct the underlying bronchial mucosal defect is being developed.

Genetic counselling
Parents of a child with cystic fibrosis have a 1 in 4 chance of producing another child with cystic fibrosis. The genetic status of the fetus can be assessed by chorionic villus sampling at amniocentesis. Work is progressing on routine screening tests to determine carrier status. Females with cystic fibrosis reaching maturity may be fertile, but their long-term survival may preclude the rearing of a family.

Prognosis
Median survival is now 31 years of age.

06

Tumours of the chest

Tumours of the chest can be benign or malignant; malignant tumours can be primary or secondary.

Benign chest tumours

Epidemiology
Prevalence. Rare.

Clinical features
Benign chest tumours (including hamartomas and chondromas) are rare, usually localized and may be incidental findings or present by blocking bronchi.

Investigation
Lung biopsy may be necessary to make a diagnosis.

Management and prognosis
Depends on the type. Surgical resection if at all possible.

Primary malignant chest tumours

Bronchial carcinoma

Epidemiology
Prevalence. Most common cause of death from cancer in men. Second most common cause of death from cancer in women (second to breast carcinoma, although it has overtaken it in some western cities). Causes more than 30 000 deaths/year in the UK.

Age. Peak incidence around 65 years of age.

Disease mechanisms
Cigarette smoking causes more than 90% of bronchial carcinomas; the risk depends on the number smoked, the age of starting and the total timespan of smoking. There is an increased incidence of bronchial carcinoma in passive smokers (those who live with heavy smokers) and in pipe and cigar smokers. Urban pollution, asbestos exposure and uranium mining are associated with an increased risk of bronchial carcinoma.

There is a spectrum of malignancy: small cell carcinoma rapidly divides, metastasizes early and is rarely amenable to surgical therapy, while adenocarcinoma grows slowly and tends not to metastasize until late.

The four main groups of bronchial carcinoma depending upon cell type are detailed in Table 6.35. Small cell lung cancer is treated differently because it metastasizes very early. The other types are commonly referred to together as non-small cell lung cancer.

Clinical features
Local symptoms. Seventy per cent of patients present with local symptoms. Haemoptysis is the most important. Other local manifestations include:
- A persistent cough
- Slowly resolving pneumonia resulting from bronchial obstruction
- Chest pain resulting from pleural or chest wall involvement
- Breathlessness because of collapse of a lung or lobe, or pleural effusion, which is common
- Hoarseness and a bovine cough resulting from left recurrent laryngeal nerve involvement by a tumour at the left hilum
- Stridor because of narrowing of trachea or main bronchus
- Diaphragm paralysis because of phrenic nerve palsy caused by a tumour at either hilum
- Superior vena caval obstruction because of invasion of the superior mediastinum
- Arm and shoulder pain resulting from tumour at the apex of the lung (Pancoast's tumour) invading the brachial plexus
- Horner's syndrome of ptosis, miosis, enophthalmos and anhidrosis resulting from involvement of the lower cervical sympathetic ganglion
- Cardiac arrhythmias, commonly intractable atrial fibrillation resulting from direct invasion of the pericardium

Metastases. Thirteen per cent of patients present with symptoms and signs of metastases. Patients with:
- Cerebral metastases present with stroke, headaches and epilepsy
- Bone metastases present with spinal cord compression, pathological fracture and bone pain
- Liver metastases present with jaundice and hepatomegaly
- Adrenal metastases caused by Addison's disease (rare)
- Skin metastases producing nodules (rare)

Non-metastatic manifestations. Twelve per cent of patients present with non-metastatic manifestations, which may be:
- *Cutaneous:* e.g. finger and toe clubbing, acanthosis nigricans, hypertrophic pulmonary osteoarthropathy, dermatomyositis
- *Endocrine:* e.g. hypercalcaemia, which is sometimes caused by excess production of a parathyroid hormone-like peptide, inappropriate antidiuretic hormone (ADH) secretion, ectopic adrenocorticotrophic hormone (ACTH) secretion
- *Neuromuscular:* e.g. subacute cerebellar degeneration, polymyopathy, pseudomyasthenia or Eaton–Lambert syndrome

Table 6.35 Classification of bronchial carcinoma

Histology	Proportion of bronchial cancers (%)	Comments
Squamous cell	50	Locally invasive, may cavitate
Oat/small cell	25	Small lung primary, rapidly dividing, metastasize early
Large cell	12	Intermediate between squamous and oat/small cell
Adenocarcinoma	12	Slow growing, metastasizes late, often peripheral lung tumours
Miscellaneous	1	e.g. alveolar cell carcinoma

● *Haematological:* e.g. thrombophlebitis migrans, thrombotic endocarditis, refractory anaemia, haemolysis or disseminated intravascular coagulation (DIC)

Routine chest radiography. Five per cent of patients present as a result of routine chest radiography.

Investigation
Biochemistry
Sodium may be decreased; calcium may be increased.

Diagnostic imaging
● *Chest radiography:* necessary for all patients with haemoptysis, and demonstrates over 90% of lung tumours at presentation. Small lesions (less than 1.5 cm in diameter) and those occurring centrally will be missed.
● *CT scanning:* sensitive and therefore used to identify smaller lesions. It is also used to assess suitability for surgery by demonstrating evidence of mediastinal gland spread or local invasion (e.g. chest wall, mediastinal structures). It is an essential investigation in the preoperative assessment of a patient.

Histopathology
● *Sputum cytology:* easy to carry out and may provide the diagnosis, especially for squamous carcinoma, which often desquamates. Three samples must be sent.
● *Bronchoscopy:* useful for obtaining material for histological diagnosis and for assessing operability. It should be considered for any smoker with haemoptysis, even if the chest radiograph is normal, to exclude the possibility of a central endobronchial tumour that might not be visible on radiography. The fibre-optic technique is simple to carry out and has low morbidity.
● *Percutaneous needle biopsy:* may be necessary for the histological diagnosis of peripheral lung lesions, or of central lesions that are not visible endobronchially.
● *Pleural aspiration and biopsy:* may be required for those presenting with an effusion.

Management
For most patients treatment is palliative.

Surgery. Lobectomy and pneumonectomy are potentially curative, but only 20% of patients are suitable (depending on cell type, general health, presentation time). The best results are obtained with peripheral adenocarcinomas. Preoperative checks for distant metastases and to ensure that the patient's cardiorespiratory system can cope are necessary.

Chemotherapy. This is the treatment of choice for small cell lung tumours. Combination chemotherapy is not curative and has unpleasant side-effects. Some patients gain a reasonable quality of life for several years, but median survival is less than 1 year from presentation. Increasingly, adjuvant chemotherapy is being given in patients with non-small cell lung carcinoma.

Radiotherapy. High-dose radiotherapy is rarely curative in squamous carcinoma. Low-dose radiotherapy provides palliation of bone pain, troublesome haemoptysis and superior vena cava obstruction.

Laser phototherapy, endobronchial radiotherapy or stenting. These can be used to treat persistent localized disease obstructing a major airway.

Terminal care. Most patients with lung cancer die from their disease. In the terminal stages attend to the patient's general well-being and mental state. Some patients benefit from hospice care. Adequate opiate analgesia is essential for pain, and severe cachexia may respond to prednisolone 10 mg/day.

Prognosis
The prognosis for lung cancer is poor, with an overall 5-year survival rate of less than 5% (Fig. 6.22).

Alveolar cell carcinoma
Epidemiology
Prevalence. Accounts for 1% of all malignant primary lung tumours.

Age. Most common in middle age.

Bronchial carcinoma at a glance

Epidemiology
Prevalence
30 000 deaths/year in the UK

Age
Commonly presents in late middle age

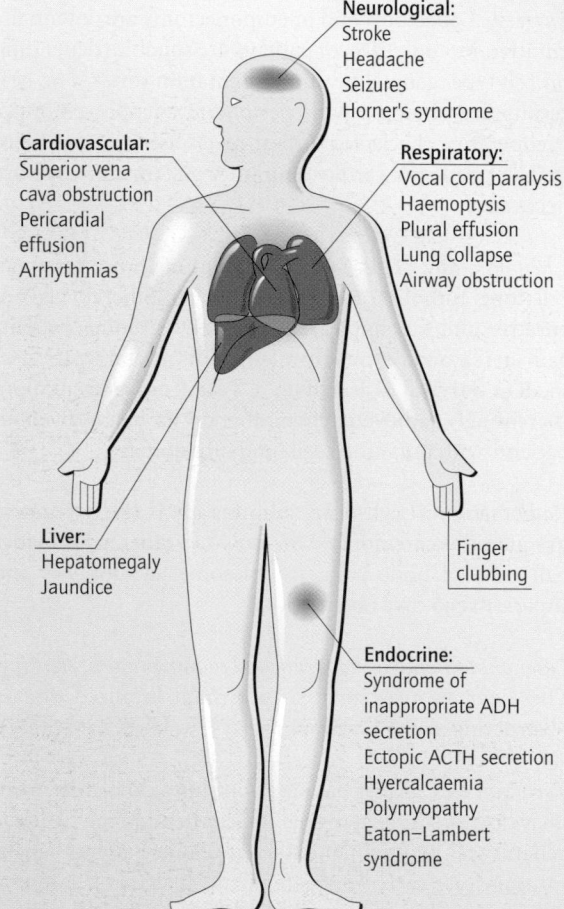

Neurological:
Stroke
Headache
Seizures
Horner's syndrome

Cardiovascular:
Superior vena
cava obstruction
Pericardial
effusion
Arrhythmias

Respiratory:
Vocal cord paralysis
Haemoptysis
Plural effusion
Lung collapse
Airway obstruction

Liver:
Hepatomegaly
Jaundice

Finger
clubbing

Endocrine:
Syndrome of
inappropriate ADH
secretion
Ectopic ACTH secretion
Hyercalcaemia
Polymyopathy
Eaton–Lambert
syndrome

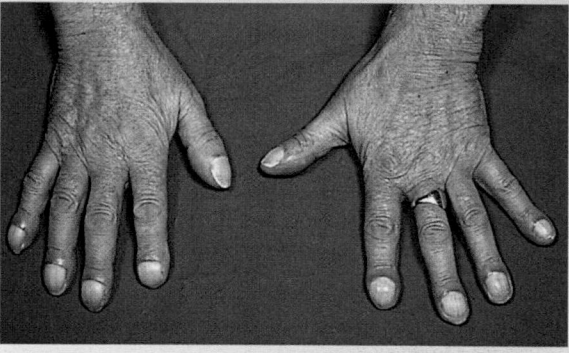

Fig. A Finger clubbing is a common manifestation of bronchial carcinoma. Smokers who present with clubbing should be carefully screened for the disease.

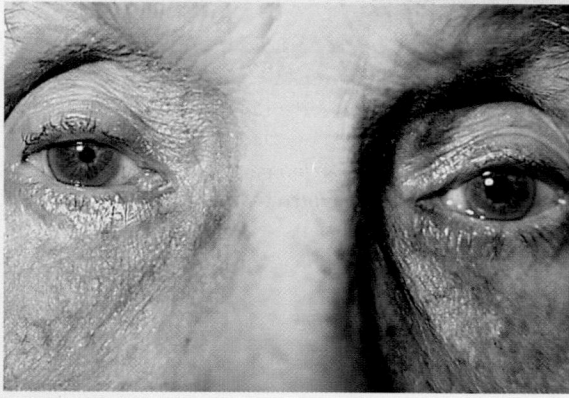

Fig. B Horner's syndrome: ptosis, miosis, enophthalmos and anhidrosis.

Disease mechanisms
Alveolar cell carcinoma arises from the bronchoalveolar lining cells. It is not related to smoking, but may be associated with previous lung disease. The tumour grows along the alveolar walls and may manifest as multiple foci of disease in more than one lung.

Clinical features
The patient usually presents with progressive breathlessness and commonly produces large volumes of pink pulmonary oedema-like fluid, which may have a salty taste.

Investigation
Chest radiography may show single or multiple nodules, or more diffuse confluent shadowing (Fig. 6.23). Sputum cytology or lung biopsy confirms the diagnosis.

Management
There is no effective treatment.

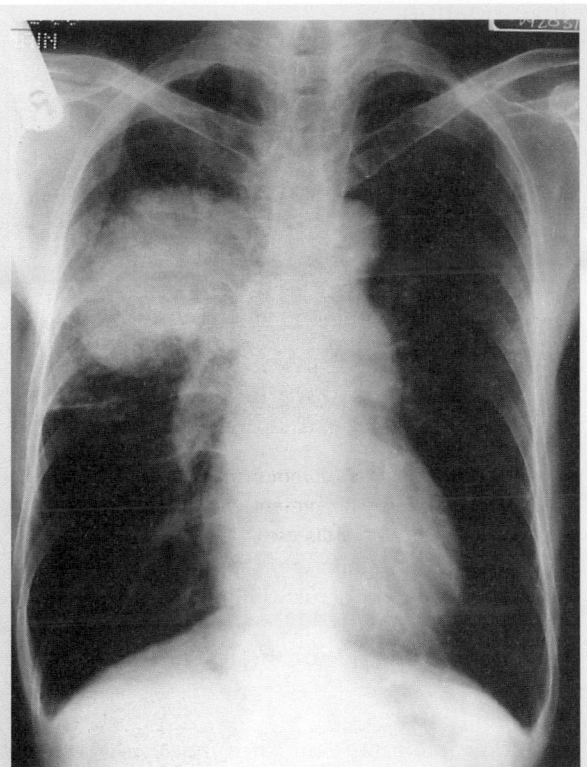

Fig. C Squamous cell carcinoma of the lung. Chest radiograph showing a large round mass in the right mid-zone.

Findings on investigation

Biochemistry
Serum calcium may be increased and there may be hyponatraemia

Diagnostic imaging
Chest radiography reveals a lung shadow
CT scanning reveals the extent of involvement of the lungs, lymph nodes and other structures

Histopathology
Sputum cytology and biopsy reveal cancer cells

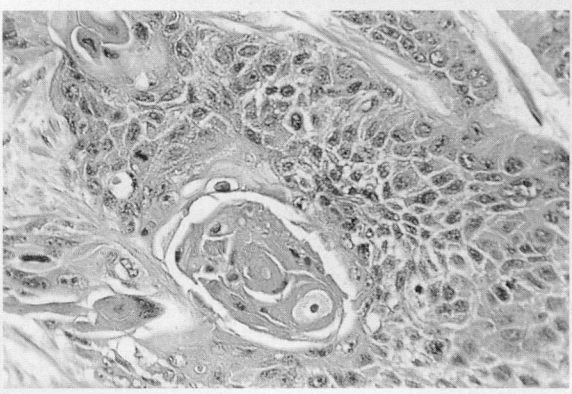

Fig. D Well-differentiated squamous carcinoma, showing keratin pearl formation and intracellular cytoplasmic bridges.

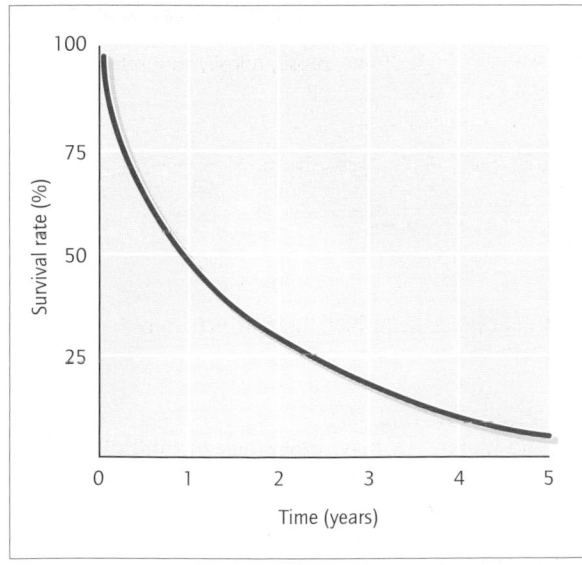

Figure 6.22 Prognosis in non-small cell lung cancer.

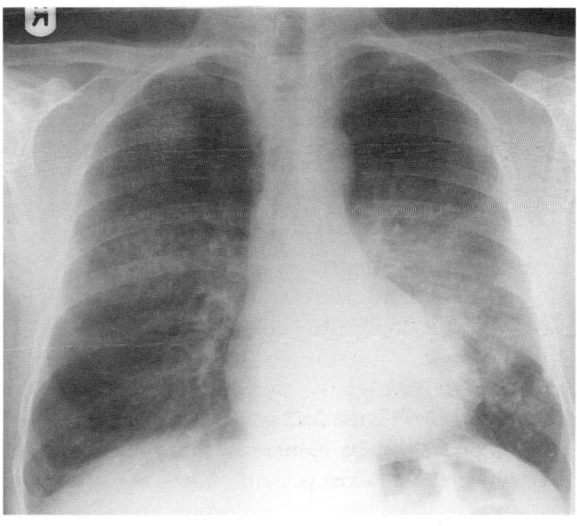

Figure 6.23 Alveolar cell carcinoma. Note the fluffy consolidation in both mid-zones.

06

Prognosis

Death usually occurs within 1 year of presentation.

Bronchial carcinoid tumour

Epidemiology

Prevalence. Uncommon.

Age. Younger adults.

Disease mechanisms

Bronchial carcinoid is only occasionally malignant. It resembles the intestinal carcinoid tumour, but rarely causes the carcinoid syndrome.

Clinical features

Bronchial carcinoids commonly cause bronchial obstruction and usually present with peripheral lung collapse. Haemoptysis and cough are also common.

Investigation

Bronchoscopy. Bronchial carcinoids are highly vascular and endobronchially appear as a cherry-red tumour growing into the lumen of the bronchus.

Management

Treatment is surgical resection, which is usually curative.

Prognosis

Excellent unless it is invasive, in which case 5-year survival is about 70%.

Investigation

Lung biopsy may be necessary to make a diagnosis.

Mesothelioma

Epidemiology

Prevalence. Rare.

Disease mechanisms

Most cases result from only limited inhalation of asbestos many years previously (more than 20 years).

Clinical features

Insidious onset of chest wall pain and weight loss. There may be breathlessness if there is an associated pleural effusion. Finger clubbing presents in 10% of cases. Examination reveals dullness to percussion and diminished breath sounds, with progressive cicatrization of one side of the chest.

Investigation

Chest radiography. CT scan shows a characteristic lobulated pleural tumour. Pleural biopsy at thoracoscopy confirms the diagnosis.

Management

The tumour is inoperable and insensitive to radio- or chemotherapy. Palliative treatments are offered.

Prognosis

Most patients die within 18 months of presentation.

Secondary malignant lung tumours

Epidemiology

Prevalence. Fifty per cent of cases of lung tumour.

Disease mechanisms

The lungs are a common site of spread for other tumours. The deposits usually occur within the lung parenchyma. Common primary sites are the prostate, breast, bone, kidneys, uterus, ovary and gastrointestinal tract.

Clinical features

Often asymptomatic, even when the deposits are quite large or multiple.

Investigation

Chest radiography. Metastases from the kidneys can be very large ('cannon ball' secondaries) (Fig. 6.24).

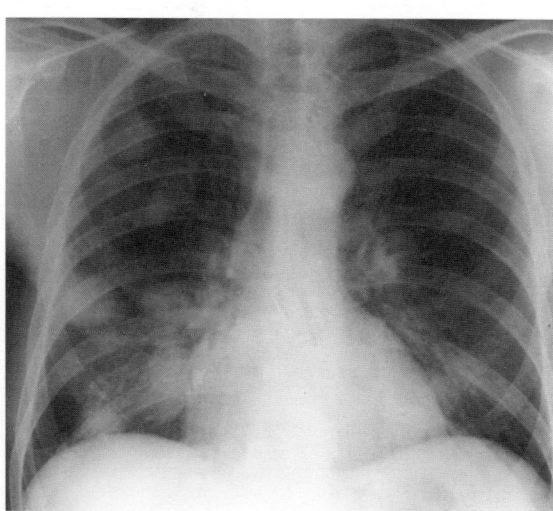

Figure 6.24 Pulmonary 'cannon ball' metastases from a renal cell carcinoma. Note the large round tumours in the right lung field.

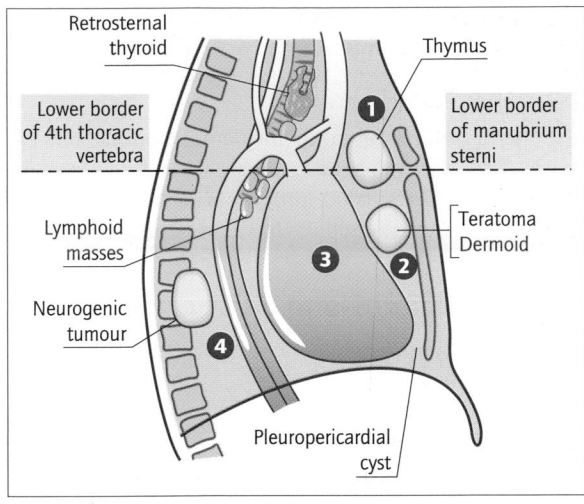

Figure 6.25 To help in the differential diagnosis of masses the mediastinum is divided into four regions: (1) superior mediastinum; (2) anterior mediastinum; (3) middle mediastinum; and (4) posterior mediastinum. The locations of the common mediastinal masses are shown.

Management
Treatment is usually that of the primary tumour.

Prognosis
Depends on the primary tumour.

Mediastinal masses

The mediastinum is divided up into different compartments (Fig. 6.25). Masses in each compartment are likely to have differing aetiologies. The vast majority are asymptomatic, and only 5% of these are malignant, but 50% of symptomatic masses are malignant.

Clinical features
These are usually caused by a compression on a vital structure and include the following.
- *Stridor or unilateral wheeze:* airway compression
- *Dysphagia:* oesophageal compression
- *Headache, facial plethora, distended arm/neck veins:* superior vena caval compression
- *Horner's syndrome, recurrent laryngeal nerve palsy:* nerve involvement
- *Scoliosis:* spine involvement

Investigation
- *Chest radiograph:* posteroanterior and lateral
- *CT scan*
- *Imaging:* may involve thoracoscopy, mediastinoscopy and thoracotomy

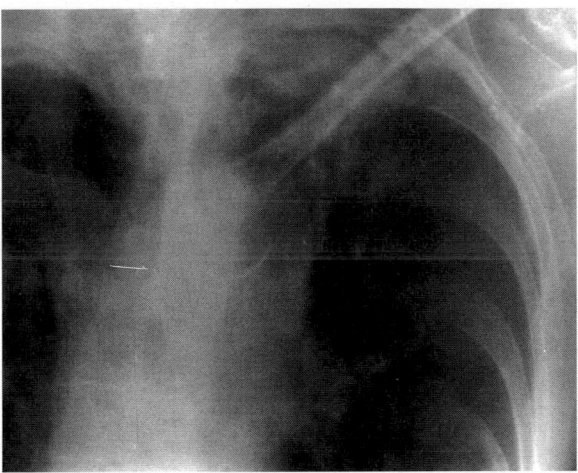

Figure 6.26 Aspergilloma. Chest radiograph showing a cavity in the upper zone containing a fungal ball surrounded by a crescent of air.

Management
Surgery is the preferred treatment for retrosternal or intrathoracic tumours and for thymic tumours. No treatment is required for pleuropericardial cysts, but patients should be monitored and enlarging cysts removed.

Fungal lung disease

Aspergillus lung disease

The fungus that most commonly produces lung disease is *Aspergillus fumigatus*.

Epidemiology
Prevalence. Uncommon.

Age. Most common in the elderly.

Disease mechanisms
Aspergillus fumigatus is ubiquitous and can be cultured from the sputum of many people in whom it is not pathogenic. There are three distinct patterns of disease that this organism can cause:
1 *Aspergilloma* (mycetoma; Fig 6.26) is a ball of fungal mycelia in a pre-existing lung cavity (e.g. following tuberculosis).
2 *Allergic bronchopulmonary aspergillosis* results when immune response to the *Aspergillus* fungus causes inflammation and swelling in the walls of the proximal bronchi.
3 In *invasive aspergillosis* the fungus invades the parenchymal lung tissue.

06

Clinical features

Aspergilloma is commonly an incidental finding, but is sometimes associated with haemoptysis, which can be massive and life-threatening.

Allergic bronchopulmonary aspergillosis presents acutely with episodes of cough, pyrexia and malaise. Asthma is a predominant feature. Yellowish sputum and brownish-yellow bronchial plugs in the form of small pellets may be expectorated. Repeated episodes cause permanent damage to the bronchi with proximal bronchiectasis, more common in the upper lobes.

Invasive aspergillosis is uncommon except in immunocompromised or neutropenic patients.

Investigation

Haematology
Normal.

Immunology
IgE is increased. *Aspergillus* precipitins (antibodies against *Aspergillus*) are increased.

Microbiology
Sputum culture. *Aspergillus fumigatus* can be cultured.

Diagnostic imaging
Chest radiography in allergic bronchopulmonary aspergillosis shows patchy transient consolidation, often in the upper zones, and proximal bronchial oedema results in a 'gloved fingers' appearance. Bronchial plugging can cause areas of lobar collapse.

Allergy tests
There is usually a peripheral blood eosinophilia, and skin-prick tests to *Aspergillus* spp. are positive. Specific serum IgE levels to the fungus are high, and serum precipitins are positive.

Histopathology
Sputum cytology reveals an excess of eosinophils, and mycelia may be seen on direct microscopy.

Management

Aspergilloma. Antifungal agents are ineffective, but newer agents (e.g. ketoconazole) may have a role. Life-threatening massive haemoptysis resulting from aspergilloma is treated by surgical removal, which is technically difficult, or by selective arterial embolization.

Allergic bronchopulmonary aspergillosis. This is treated with oral corticosteroids in the acute stage. Maintenance oral corticosteroids are usually required to prevent repeated episodes.

Invasive aspergillosis. This is treated with systemic antifungal agents (e.g. amphotericin or ketoconazole).

Prognosis

Aspergillomas are often an incidental finding, but can cause fatal haemoptysis. Allergic bronchopulmonary aspergillosis has a good prognosis if it is adequately treated. Invasive aspergillosis has a grave prognosis.

Candida albicans lung disease

Epidemiology
Prevalence. Uncommon.

Disease mechanisms
Candida albicans can cause both bronchial and pulmonary disease, and occurs as a superinfection following broad-spectrum antibiotic therapy or in severely ill or immunocompromised patients.

Clinical features and investigation
(See nosocomial pneumonia, p. 325).

Management
Intravenous amphotericin.

Prognosis
Poor.

Actinomycosis

Epidemiology
Prevalence. Uncommon. Five per year in the UK.

Disease mechanisms
Caused by *Actinomyces israelii*, a gut commensal and probably an anaerobic or microaerophilic bacterium. It is aspirated into a hypoxic area where it develops into a chronic inflammatory mass invading the chest wall.

Clinical features
Cough, weight loss and malaise.

Investigation
- *Chest radiography:* shows a mass, which may be thought to be cancer.
- *Pus aspiration:* reveals sulphur granules.

Management
Treatment is with high doses of intravenous penicillin, followed by a prolonged course of oral therapy.

Prognosis
Good if the disease is treated early.

Granulomatous lung disease

Sarcoidosis

This is a multisystem granulomatous disorder of unknown aetiology. It most commonly affects the lungs, mediastinal lymph nodes and skin.

Epidemiology
Prevalence. UK incidence is about 1/20 000 population.

Age. Peak incidence is in early adult life.

Sex. More common in women than in men.

Race. More severe and 16 times more common in Afro-Caribbeans. Also slightly increased incidence in young Irish women. Least common in Asians and people of Chinese extraction.

Geography. Most common in countries with large black populations.

Disease mechanisms
Unknown. It is possible that a causal agent is inhaled and that this is what induces the predominantly activated T-lymphocytic alveolitis. Activated T lymphocytes recruit monocytes and macrophages to form widespread non-caseating granulomas. Increased macrophage metabolic activity increases angiotensin-converting enzyme (ACE) levels in the lungs.

Clinical features
The most common presentation is an acute illness with a mild pyrexia, malaise, erythema nodosum and polyarthralgia, but it may present with symptomless bilateral hilar lymphadenopathy. Less commonly, chronic insidious disease presents with progressive breathlessness. Chronic skin infiltration, particularly on the face, gives a blue discoloration (lupus pernio).

Examination reveals restricted chest movement and respiratory crackles. Other features are:
- An abnormal chest radiograph (40%)
- Respiratory symptoms (e.g. dyspnoea) (25%)
- Erythema nodosum (15%)
- Hypercalcaemia (10%)
- Arthropathy (4%)
- Uveitis and keratoconjunctivitis (5%)
- Skin sarcoid (5%)
- Generalized lymphadenopathy (4%)
- Parotitis (< 1%)
- Hepatosplenomegaly (< 1%)
- Neuropathy and cranial nerve lesions (< 1%)

Differential diagnosis is tuberculosis, in which granulomas usually caseate and tubercle bacilli can be seen.

Investigation
Haematology
The full blood count is usually normal; the ESR is increased.

Biochemistry
Serum ACE is increased when there are extensive granulomas. Calcium is often increased because the macrophages in the granulomas make vitamin D.

Immunology
A Mantoux test is negative in most patients (80%), unlike tuberculosis.

Diagnostic imaging
Chest radiography usually shows bilateral hilar gland enlargement or, less commonly, parenchymal infiltration, and allows staging of the disease (Table 6.36).

Histopathology
Kveim test. This is no longer used because of the risk of transmitting infection.

Tissue biopsy. Biopsy from an involved organ may show granulomas (transbronchial biopsy at fibre-optic bronchoscopy, blind scalene node biopsy or mediastinal gland biopsy at mediastinoscopy).

Lung function tests. These reveal a decreased gas transfer factor (DLCO) in acute sarcoidosis and also a restrictive defect in chronic disease.

Management
Treatment of acute sarcoidosis is often unnecessary. Chronic pulmonary sarcoidosis and sarcoidosis involving other organs (e.g. skin) are treated with oral corticosteroids.

Prognosis
A young patient, an acute onset, erythema nodosum and hilar lymphadenopathy are good prognostic factors. An older patient, an insidious onset, extrapulmonary disease and pulmonary parenchymal involvement are poor prognostic factors. Acute sarcoidosis has a good prognosis.

06

Sarcoidosis at a glance

Epidemiology
Prevalence
Approximately 1/20 000 in the UK

Age
Early adult life

Sex
More common in women

Race
More severe and 16 times more common in Afro-Caribbeans than in white people. Least common in Asians and people of Chinese origin

Geography
Most common in countries with large black populations

Findings on investigation
Haematology
ESR may be increased

Biochemistry
Serum angiotensin-converting enzyme (ACE) and calcium may be increased

Immunology
Kveim test positive—but this test is no longer used

Table 6.36 Grading of pulmonary sarcoidosis according to its appearance on chest radiograph

Grade	Chest radiograph
Stage 0	Clear chest radiograph
Stage 1	Bilateral hilar lymphadenopathy
Stage 2	Bilateral hilar lymphadenopathy plus pulmonary infiltration
Stage 3	Pulmonary infiltration alone

Wegener's granulomatosis

Epidemiology
Prevalence. Rare.

Sex. More common in males.

Disease mechanisms
This is a systemic vasculitic disease characterized by necrotizing granulomas in the respiratory tract and focal necrotizing glomerulonephritis (see Chapter 8). In the lungs there are isolated or confluent areas of necrotizing granulomas that may cavitate. In the kidneys there is a focal necrotizing glomerulonephritis, often with crescents. Vasculitis lesions can occur in any tissue.

Clinical features
Patients typically present with a nasal discharge, respiratory symptoms (cough, pleurisy and perhaps haemoptysis) and general malaise. The lungs are involved in most cases, and other systems are involved as follows:
- kidneys (80%)
- joints (56%)
- skin (44%)
- eye (39%)
- middle ear (39%)
- heart/pericardium (28%)
- nervous system (22%)

Investigation
Chest radiography. Rounded opacities, which may cavitate. There may also be pleural effusions and areas of infiltration.

Serology. Antineutrophil cytoplasmic antibody (ANCA) may be positive.

Renal studies. If the kidneys are involved there is haematuria, proteinuria and rapidly progressive renal failure.

Biopsy. Biopsy reveals typical granulomatous lesions. Biopsy of the upper airway is a simple procedure if there are upper respiratory symptoms. Renal biopsy is necessary if renal involvement is apparent.

Management
Renal involvement is treated with high-dose prednisolone and cyclophosphamide. Respiratory disease is treated in the same way.

Prognosis
If the kidneys are involved, renal failure is common, but treatment improves the outcome. Respiratory disease usually responds to immunosuppressive therapy.

Histiocytosis X

Epidemiology
Prevalence. Very rare.

06

Diagnostic imaging
Chest radiograph is either normal or shows hilar lymphadenopathy and/or diffuse shadows.
CT scanning can be helpful

Histopathology
Lung biopsy: histology reveals non-caseating granulomas

Lung function
There may be a reduction in gas transfer and also a restrictive defect in chronic disease

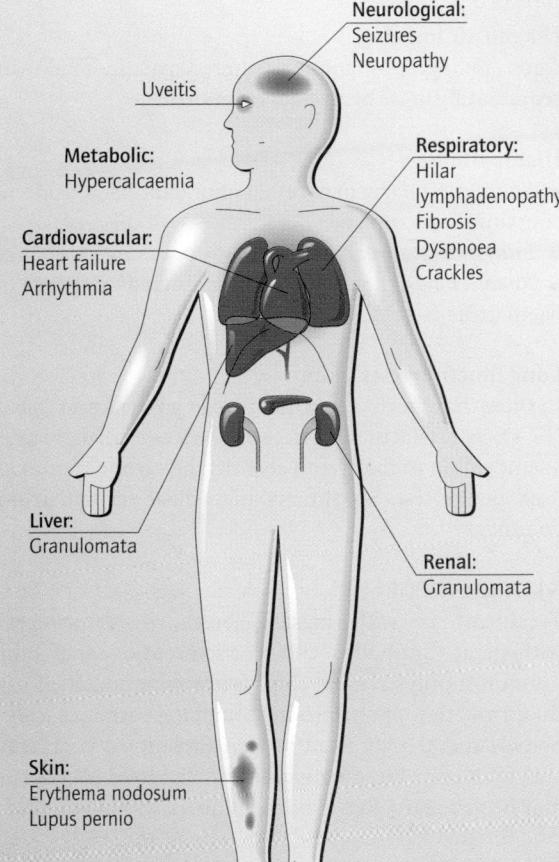

Neurological:
Seizures
Neuropathy

Uveitis

Metabolic:
Hypercalcaemia

Respiratory:
Hilar lymphadenopathy
Fibrosis
Dyspnoea
Crackles

Cardiovascular:
Heart failure
Arrhythmia

Liver:
Granulomata

Renal:
Granulomata

Skin:
Erythema nodosum
Lupus pernio

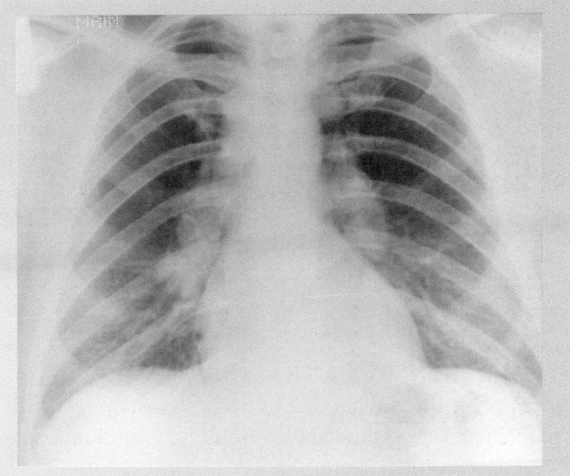

Fig. A Chest radiograph of stage 1 sarcoidosis showing bilateral hilar lymphadenopathy and clear lung fields.

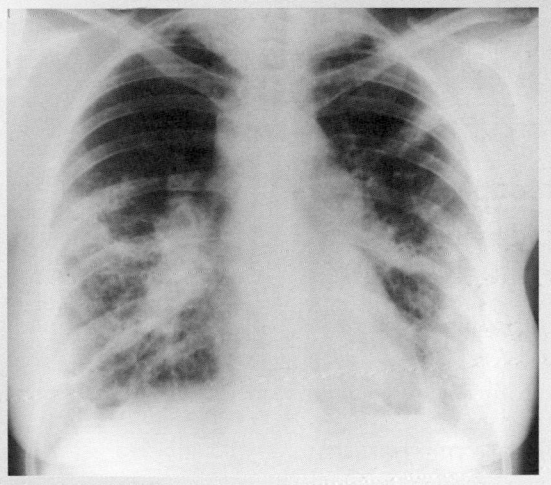

Fig. B Chest radiograph of stage 2 sarcoidosis showing bilateral hilar lymphadenopathy and pulmonary infiltrates, predominantly in the mid-zone.

Sex. More common in males.

Disease mechanisms

A condition in which granulomatous disease can occur in many organs, commonly the bones and lungs. There is an initial proliferation of histiocytes resulting in granulomas, followed by lipoid phagocytosis and the foamy cell formation. The process terminates with a variable amount of healing and scar tissue production.

Clinical features

Three types are recognized:

1 *Letterer–Siwe disease:* has an insidious onset, but is usually fatal before age 3 years. The lungs become voluminous and are filled with a honeycomb of cysts, with histiocyte infiltration and granulomas in the bronchi and perivascular tissue.

2 *Hand–Schüller–Christian disease:* begins in childhood with bone defects, exophthalmos and diabetes insipidus.

06

Granulomas develop in the bones which sclerose with healing. The lungs are involved in one-third of patients, who develop miliary or confluent shadowing on chest radiography and a defect in gas transfer.

3 *Eosinophilic granuloma:* occurs in young adults, often as a routine finding on chest radiography, which shows diffuse bilateral mottling. There may be 'punched-out' bone lesions. If there are respiratory symptoms, cough and dyspnoea are predominant. Pneumothorax is common in this group and may be the presenting feature.

Investigation
Biopsy of an affected organ. Electron microscopy of bronchoalveolar lavage fluid in eosinophilic granuloma may reveal characteristic 'tennis-racket' bodies.

Management
Treatment is with immunosuppressives.

Prognosis
Very variable. In general, the later the onset in life the more slowly progressive the disease process.

Vasculitic lung disease

Goodpasture's syndrome (see Chapter 8, p. 507)
Epidemiology
Prevalence. Rare.

Age. Young adults.

Sex. Much more common in males.

Disease mechanisms
There is pulmonary haemorrhage with associated nephritis. Pathogenic antibodies against the basement membranes in the lung and the kidney are found in the circulation and in the affected tissues.

Electron microscopy reveals widespread capillary damage in the kidney and lung; the endothelium is oedematous and there are basement membrane protein deposits. Specific stains for IgG reveal that these deposits are caused by antibasement membrane antibodies.

Clinical features
Often there is an initial upper respiratory tract infection and episodes of haemoptysis occur because of lung bleeding. This may be preceded by acute glomerulonephritis. Severe bleeding is uncommon.

Physical signs are few, but the patient may have a non-specific malaise resulting from renal disease or iron-deficiency anaemia. There may be clinical signs of anaemia.

Investigation
Haematology
There may be anaemia.

Biochemistry
May indicate renal disease.

Immunology
Antibasement membrane antibodies can be detected.

Diagnostic imaging
Chest radiography shows scattered patchy shadowing representing areas of alveolar haemorrhage.

Histopathology
- *Sputum cytology:* may reveal abundant haemosiderin-containing macrophages
- *Lung biopsy:* reveals characteristic pathological changes
- *Renal biopsy:* should be considered if there is haematuria

Lung function tests
If there has been an acute bleed, gas transfer factor (KCO) is artefactually increased because exsanguinated haemoglobin in the alveoli absorbs the carbon monoxide used in the test. Spirometry may show restricted lung volumes.

Management
Treatment is with plasmapheresis to remove the pathogenic antibody, and corticosteroids and other immunosuppressives (cyclophosphamide and then azathioprine) to suppress production of the pathogenic antibody. Patients may need oxygen therapy or ventilation and, if alveolar bleeding is substantial, blood transfusion may be necessary. Renal dysfunction may require dialysis.

Prognosis
Most patients survive if plasmapheresis is started early.

Idiopathic pulmonary haemosiderosis
Epidemiology
Prevalence. Rare.

Age. Children and young adults.

Disease mechanisms
The cause is unknown, but hypersensitivity to cow's milk and viral infections have been postulated.

06

Table 6.37 Pulmonary manifestations of autoimmune rheumatic diseases

Pulmonary manifestation	Comments
Rheumatoid arthritis	
Pleural effusion	The most common pulmonary manifestation of the disease. Usually unilateral, has a low glucose, high rheumatoid factor, and sometimes a green tinge
	Chronic, but may respond to oral corticosteroids
Bronchiolitis obliterans	Rare. Progressive small bronchiole obliteration causes increasing breathlessness, and irreversible airflow obstruction. Treatment is ineffective
Fibrosing alveolitis	Has the same features as CFA, runs a chronic indolent course, and shows little response to treatment
Rheumatoid nodules	Asymptomatic. May be single or multiple and up to several centimetres in size
	They frequently cavitate. The lesions are larger in association with pneumoconiosis (Caplan's syndrome)
Cricoarytenoiditis	Causes hoarseness and stridor, and may require tracheostomy
Systemic lupus erythematosus	
Pleurisy	A feature in 50% of patients. Often associated with small bilateral effusions. It responds to corticosteroids
Basal atelectases	Common and caused by restricted chest wall movement
Fibrosing alveolitis	An unusual manifestation. It has the same features as CFA and may respond to oral corticosteroids
Shrinking lung syndrome	Uncommon. There is a diminution in lung size, but no evidence of parenchymal disease. It is caused by chest wall or diaphragm malfunction, and shows little response to treatment
Systemic sclerosis	
Pulmonary fibrosis	There is some degree of pulmonary fibrosis in most patients with systemic sclerosis, and parenchymal disease may be severe, with restricted lung volumes and poor gas transfer. Cyclophosphamide and steroid may help
Aspiration pneumonitis	Common manifestation and is associated with oesophageal dysfunction
Chest wall restriction	Causes breathlessness and is a result of sclerosis of the chest wall

CFA, cryptogenic fibrosing alveolitis.

Clinical features

Idiopathic pulmonary haemosiderosis has similar features to Goodpasture's syndrome, but the pulmonary haemorrhages tend to be more serious and iron-deficiency anaemia is more common. Glomerulonephritis is not usually a feature.

Investigation

Antibasement antibodies are not detectable.

Management

Treatment is supportive. Corticosteroids are probably ineffective.

Prognosis

The disorder may run a chronic course, but 50% of patients die within 3 years.

Autoimmune rheumatic disease and the lung

Pulmonary involvement commonly occurs in rheuma-

toid arthritis, systemic lupus erythematosus and systemic sclerosis (Table 6.37).

Eosinophilic lung disease

There are a number of lung diseases associated with pulmonary eosinophilia.

Pulmonary eosinophilia

Pulmonary eosinophilia is characterized by pulmonary infiltration associated with a peripheral eosinophilia.

Epidemiology
Prevalence. Uncommon.

Disease mechanisms
The cause is unknown, but allergies to many common parasites and drugs have been implicated (Table 6.38). Rarer causes are:
- *Polyarteritis nodosa:* a rare necrotizing arteritis that affects many organs, but lung involvement is not usually marked.

06

Table 6.38 Causes of eosinophilia and pulmonary infiltration

Fungi
Aspergillus fumigatus
Candida albicans

Parasites
Ascaris lumbricoides
Strongyloides stercoralis
Trichuris trichiura
Wuchereria bancrofti (tropics)

Drugs
Aspirin
Penicillin
Para-aminosalicylic acid
Nitrofurantoin
Sulphonamides
Many others

Autoimmune
Polyarteritis nodosa
Churg–Strauss syndrome

● *Churg–Strauss syndrome:* associated with a high eosinophil count, asthma and the presence of allergic granulomas in most tissues. There is also a vasculitis affecting the small arteries and veins.
● *Hypereosinophilic syndrome:* a very rare eosinophilic infiltration of many organs associated with arteritis. It usually presents with pyrexia, weight loss, abdominal pain and congestive cardiac failure resulting from myocardial involvement.

Clinical features

Recurrent episodes of short-lived cough and mild pyrexia. There may be associated bronchospasm. The symptoms are more severe when the disease occurs in tropical countries and there is often a confluent pneumonia. In these circumstances, the causal agents are usually microfilarial species.

Investigation
Haematology
There is a peripheral eosinophilia, which is usually of the order of 10–20% of the total white cell count.

Immunology
IgE levels may be increased.

Microbiology
Sputum cytology reveals abundant eosinophils.

Diagnostic imaging
Chest radiography:
● *Polyarteritis nodosa:* pulmonary vascular abnormalities, causing haemorrhage or infarction with areas of patchy consolidation
● *Churg–Strauss syndrome:* pulmonary shadows similar to polyarteritis nodosa, but massive bilateral lesions are also seen
● *Hypereosinophilic syndrome:* 50% have pulmonary involvement, usually as pulmonary infiltrates or pleural effusion

Histopathology
The alveoli are full of eosinophils. In polyarteritis nodosa, Churg–Strauss syndrome and hypereosinophilic syndrome there is also evidence of vasculitis.

Management
Systemic corticosteroids shorten the duration of pulmonary eosinophilia and clear the pulmonary infiltrates. Polyarteritis nodosa and Churg–Strauss syndrome are treated with oral corticosteroids and other immunosuppressive drugs (azathioprine and cyclophosphamide). Hypereosinophilic syndrome is treated with oral corticosteroids.

Prognosis
In simple pulmonary eosinophilia and Churg–Strauss syndrome the prognosis is good. In polyarteritis nodosa the prognosis largely depends on other organ involvement.

Alveolitic diseases and pulmonary fibrosis

Alveolitic diseases are characterized by inflammatory changes, which often result in pulmonary fibrosis affecting the alveoli and lung parenchyma. Pulmonary fibrosis is the end-stage of many diseases that inflame the lung parenchyma. Diagnosis is often made by lung biopsy. There are a group of lung diseases caused by the inhalation of mineral (inorganic) dusts, termed pneuoconioses.

Cryptogenic fibrosing alveolitis (idiopathic pulmonary fibrosis)
Epidemiology
Prevalence. 3/100 000 in the UK.

Age. Usually older adults.

Aetiology. Usually idiopathic (cryptogenic fibrosing alveolitis; CFA), but sometimes it is associated with a specific disease (Table 6.39).

Table 6.39 Association of fibrosing alveolitis

	Cause
Idiopathic	Most cases
Autoimmune	Rheumatoid arthritis
	Systemic sclerosis
	Sjögren's syndrome
Gastrointestinal disease	Chronic active hepatitis
	Ulcerative colitis
	Coeliac disease
Renal tubular acidosis	Systemic sclerosis
	Sjögren's syndrome

Pathogenesis

Progressive fibrosis of the alveolar walls can eventually lead to respiratory failure. The alveolar walls become thickened, with an increase in type 2 pneumocytes and macrophages, and gradually fibrose and scarring spreads into the parenchyma. The cause is unknown.

Clinical features

An insidious onset of breathlessness is often associated with a cough productive of a little clear sputum. As it progresses there may be marked respiratory distress.

On auscultation, the typical sign is showers of mid- to late fine inspiratory crackles. As the disease progresses these may spread throughout inspiration. Many patients develop marked finger clubbing and cyanosis.

Hamman–Rich syndrome is an acute-onset fibrosing alveolitis characterized by predominant alveolar inflammation.

Investigation

Biochemistry

Blood gases reveal progressive hypoxia. Hypercapnia is a late phenomenon.

Immunology

Autoantibodies. Tests for rheumatoid factor and antinuclear factor are positive in 33–50% of patients, but these patients do not usually have any other stigmata of the diseases (rheumatoid arthritis or systemic lupus erythematosus).

Diagnostic imaging

Ground glass appearance on chest X-ray occurring mainly in the lower zones. As the disease progresses, this becomes more discrete and nodular.

Histopathology

Bronchoalveolar lavage may show a non-specific increase in neutrophils. Transbronchial or open lung biopsy shows interstitial and alveolar fibrosis.

Lung function tests

A restrictive deficit with reduced gas transfer factor.

Management

Hamman–Rich syndrome may respond to high doses of oral corticosteroids. Chronic forms are treated with high doses of oral corticosteroids, but their efficacy is not proven. Other immunosuppressive drugs (azathioprine, cyclophosphamide) are sometimes used as well.

Supportive treatment includes long-term oxygen therapy and prompt treatment of intercurrent chest infections. Heart–lung transplantation may be considered for younger patients.

Prognosis

The median survival of patients is less than 5 years, although some patients live for much longer. In general, the earlier the onset of disease, the worse the prognosis.

Extrinsic allergic alveolitis

Epidemiology

Prevalence. 1–2/100 in the UK.

Age. Peaks in middle age.

Disease mechanisms

Inhalation of a number of common antigens causes an acute inflammatory reaction in the bronchioles and alveoli (Table 6.40).

Table 6.40 Causes of extrinsic allergic alveolitis

Disease	Cause	Antigen
Bird fancier's lung	Pigeons	Proteins in the 'bloom' budgerigars, poultry
Farmer's lung	Mouldy hay	Thermophilic actinomyces, *Micropolyspora faeni*
Byssinosis	Cotton dust	Undefined contaminants
Humidifier fever	Contaminated humidifiers	A variety of bacteria and amoebae
Suberosis	Cork dust	Undefined moulds

06

Extrinsic allergic alveolitis at a glance

Epidemiology
Prevalence
1–2/100 in the UK. Most common in farmers throughout the world. Age, race and sex reflects the farming community

Genetics
No known predisposition other than occupation (see Table 6.40)

Geography
Especially common in poorer farming communities in wet areas

Findings on investigation
Haematology
Acute disease: neutrophil leucocytosis
ESR may be raised

Arterial blood gases
Hypoxia if severe acute episode or if progressive chronic disease

Immunology
Serum antibodies (precipitins) usually positive for the offending antigen

Diagnostic imaging
Chest X-ray may be normal or show varying degrees of fluffy nodular shadowing. Ground glass appearance in chronic cases CT scanning can be useful

Lung function tests
Reduced ventilatory capacity and restrictive ventilatory deficit. Reduced transfer factor

Histopathology and cytology
Bronchoalveolar lavage shows increased neutrophils and lymphocytes
Transbronchial or open lung biopsy
Acute disease: extensive lymphocyte and neutrophil infiltration of the alveoli
Chronic disease: classical granuloma and fibrosis

Pathogenesis
Following antigen inhalation, there is an inflammation of the bronchioles and alveoli with ingress of neutrophils and lymphocytes, followed by development of small non-caseating granulomas.

Clinical features
Malaise, cough, pyrexia and breathlessness develop several hours after exposure to antigen. In chronic long-term low-dose exposure, the patient may present with insidiously progressive breathlessness.

On examination, the patient may be cyanosed and pyrexial, and have mid- to late inspiratory crackles, heard mainly over the upper lobes. The presence of bronchiolar wall oedema may give rise to high-pitched mid-inspiratory monophonic wheezes (the 'squawk').

In chronic disease there may be cyanosis and persistent crackles, and considerable pulmonary fibrosis reduces respiratory capacity.

Investigation
Haematology
Patients with acute disease often have a polymorph leucocytosis.

Immunology
Serum precipitins (antibodies) are usually positive for the offending antigen.

Diagnostic imaging
Chest radiography may be normal or it may show a ground glass appearance throughout the lung fields. Sometimes there are more diffuse shadows.

Histopathology
Bronchoalveolar lavage may show a non-specific neutrophil infiltration. Transbronchial or open lung biopsy shows the classical granuloma.

Lung function tests
There is a restrictive ventilatory deficit and diminished gas transfer and there may be arterial hypoxaemia.

Management
Prevention of exposure to the antigen is the most important step. Oral prednisolone may improve symptoms of acute disease.

Prognosis
In acute disease the prognosis is excellent if the offending antigen is removed, but permanent pulmonary damage develops in chronic or recurrent disease.

Acute respiratory distress syndrome

Acute respiratory distress syndrome (ARDS) is defined by:
• Refractory hypoxia

Acute disease	Subacute disease to chronic disease

Heavy intermittent exposure to antigen mimicking recurrent chest infection

Mild continuous exposure causes subacute disease

Recurrent attacks or long-term exposure cause chronic disease

Breathlessness within hours of exposure

Slowly progressive breathlessness

Cough

Productive cough

Malaise

Decreasing exercise tolerance

Fever

Loss of weight

Fatigue

N.B.
Farmer's lung often recurs at end of winter when farmers handle contaminated hay indoors

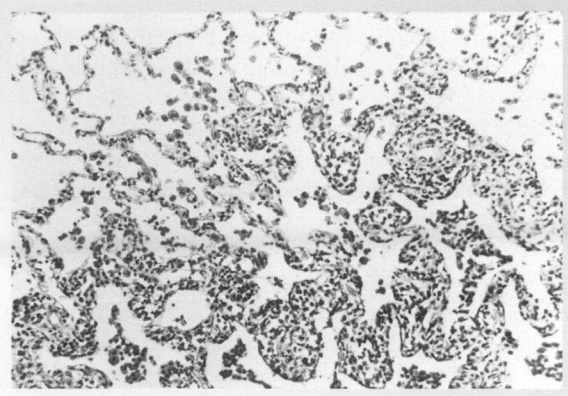

Fig. A Acute allergic alveolitis with lymphocyte infiltration of alveolar walls and peribronchial tissue. Reproduced from Mygind, *Essential Allergy*, 2nd edn, 1995 (Blackwell Science, Oxford) with the permission of the author.

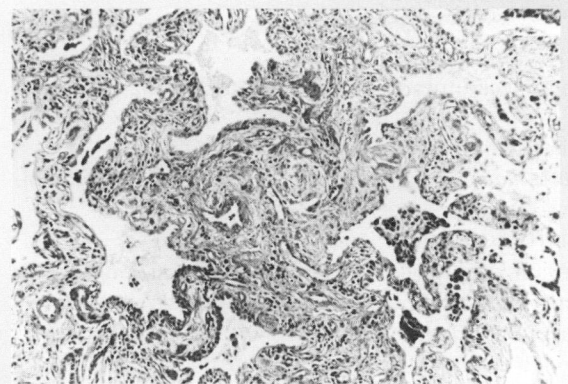

Fig. B Chronic allergic alveolitis with fibrosis and obliteration of many alveolar spaces. Reproduced from Mygind, *Essential Allergy*, 2nd edn, 1995 (Blackwell Science, Oxford) with the permission of the author.

- Pulmonary oedema on the chest radiograph
- Normal pulmonary capillary wedge pressure
- Normal intravascular osmotic pressure
- Low or normal respiratory compliance

It is a syndrome in which non-cardiogenic pulmonary oedema is associated with respiratory failure.

Epidemiology

Prevalence. At least 10 000 cases/year in the UK.

Disease mechanisms

It is a complication of serious acute pathologies that may affect the lung. A wide variety of illnesses can indirectly damage the pulmonary vascular endothelium and include pulmonary aspiration, severe burns, severe pneumonia,

DIC, severe trauma, septicaemia, cardiopulmonary bypass, pancreatitis, massive blood transfusion, pre-eclampsia and amniotic fluid embolism.

The principal underlying defect is increased permeability of the alveolar–capillary membrane, resulting in alveolar oedema and extravasation of inflammatory cells into the interstitium. The precise mechanisms are unclear, but activated neutrophils are thought to release vasoactive mediators that damage the integrity of the alveolar–capillary membrane.

As this acute phase progresses, there is increasing congestion in the lymphatics and capillaries, with hyaline membrane formation. The loss of functioning alveoli results in gradual hypoxaemia and respiratory failure.

06

If the patient survives the acute phase there may be healing with proliferation of type 1 pneumocytes and interstitial fibrosis, mainly around the alveolar ducts.

Clinical features

Increasing breathlessness is accompanied by a dry cough, crackles over both lung fields and spreading bilateral pulmonary infiltrates on the chest radiograph. The onset occurs several hours after the initial insult (e.g. amniotic fluid embolus during childbirth), and the radiographical changes progress over several days.

Continuing capillary leakage causes respiratory failure, and mechanical ventilation is required. The lungs become progressively stiffer, and adequate ventilation and oxygenation becomes more difficult.

Investigation

Biochemistry

Po_2 is reduced.

Microbiology

Sputum culture and sensitivity for underlying infection.

Diagnostic imaging

Chest radiography. Demonstrates alveolar consolidation.

Management

Any underlying cause is treated, and adequate oxygenation is provided by mechanical ventilation, increased inspired oxygen concentration and positive end-expiratory pressure to maximize alveolar recruitment (Table 6.41).

Swan–Ganz catheterization may be necessary to rule out cardiogenic pulmonary oedema, assist with appropriate fluid balance and assess cardiac output. The fluid load in the lungs is reduced without embarrassing the circulation and secondary infection is prevented.

Table 6.41 Management of adult respiratory distress syndrome

Supportive treatment
Resuscitative measures
Ensure adequate oxygenation using mechanical ventilation, increased inspired oxygen concentration and positive end-expiratory pressure
Swan–Ganz catheterization to monitor and optimize pulmonary artery wedge pressures
Reduce the fluid load in the lungs without embarrassing the circulation
Prevent secondary infection

Specific treatment
Treat any underlying cause

Prognosis

Mortality exceeds 60%, and if associated with other organ failure approaches 100%. Overwhelming secondary infection is the major cause of death. There is some evidence that early diagnosis and treatment improves mortality, and a small number of patients have undergone heart–lung transplantation.

Benign pneumoconioses

Epidemiology

Prevalence. Uncommon.

Age. More common with increasing age. Exposure related.

Sex. Mainly males.

Disease mechanisms

Common causes of benign pneumoconiosis are iron (siderosis), tin (stannosis), barium (baritosis), antimony, cerium (a rare earth metal) and chromium.

Clinical features

Benign pneumoconioses cause no symptoms or functional disability.

Investigation

Chest radiography shows a characteristic appearance, with 0.5–4.0 mm diameter nodules spread throughout the lung fields.

Management

No treatment is needed.

Prognosis

Benign pneumoconioses do not affect life expectancy.

Fibrogenic pneumoconiosis: asbestos-induced lung disease

Epidemiology

Prevalence. Common. Exposure related.

Age. More common with increasing age.

Sex. Mainly males.

Disease mechanisms

Asbestos is a fire-resistant mineral and is mined in Canada, Russia and South Africa. The three common types are chrysotile, amosite and crocidolite (blue asbestos). Because of its properties, asbestos was widely used in roofing materials, fireproofing and lagging, and so occupational exposure was common. Careful history taking is therefore essential in the diagnosis of asbestos-related diseases.

The fibres of blue asbestos are short and straight and are able to penetrate beyond the mucociliary escalator of the bronchial tree and into the alveoli. These fibres are the most important in the development of asbestosis and mesothelioma.

- *Asbestosis:* a progressive diffuse interstitial pulmonary fibrosis associated with exposure to asbestos. Asbestos fibres entering the alveoli are engulfed by macrophages, which become disrupted. This precipitates a fibrogenic process and progressive obliterative fibrosis, which mainly involves the lower lobes.
- *Pleural fibrosis and plaque formation:* an indication of asbestos exposure. Plaques are avascular hyaline collagen bundles that occur bilaterally and are best seen on the diaphragmatic and lower zone parietal pleural surfaces.
- *Malignant mesothelioma:* a tumour strongly associated with asbestos exposure (see p. 366).

Clinical features
Asbestosis. This results in an insidious onset of breathlessness associated with a dry cough, commonly 10–15 years after exposure to asbestos. Auscultation reveals persistent inspiratory crackles, which are fine early in the disease but later become more coarse and widespread. There is a strong association between asbestosis and lung cancer, and this is exaggerated in cigarette smokers.

Malignant mesothelioma. This presents insidiously, with dull chest pain and weight loss. Finger clubbing is a feature in 10% of patients, and examination of the chest reveals dullness to percussion and diminished breath sounds over the affected side. As the disease progresses, there is cicatrization of one side of the chest.

Pleural fibrosis and plaque formation. These do not usually give rise to symptoms. However, extensive pleural fibrosis can restrict chest wall movement and reduce spirometric lung volumes.

Asbestos-related pleural effusion. This is benign, but can be acute and associated with chest pain.

Investigation
Diagnostic imaging
Chest radiography in asbestosis shows progressive fibrotic changes, which start in the lower zones, often at the costophrenic angles. As the disease advances there may be widespread nodular shadowing and honeycombing. In malignant mesothelioma there are irregular lobulated masses on the chest wall, and there may be a pleural effusion.

Histopathology
Needle or open lung biopsy is necessary in suspected malignant mesothelioma to make a tissue diagnosis.

Lung function tests
Liver function tests in asbestosis show a gradual restriction of lung volumes and impairment of gas transfer as the fibrosis progresses.

Management
Asbestosis. Removal from exposure is mandatory. There is no specific treatment.

Prognosis
Asbestosis. Heavy asbestos exposure is associated with early onset of asbestosis. Usually the disease progresses to respiratory failure and cor pulmonale, but early detection and removal from exposure may halve the rate of pulmonary fibrosis.

Asbestos-related pleural effusion. This may leave pleural thickening after resolution. It is important to exclude an underlying mesothelioma.

Coalworker's pneumoconiosis
Epidemiology
Prevalence. Dose–response relationship with exposure to coal dust. More than 400 cases/year in the UK.

Age. More common with increasing age.

Sex. Mainly male.

Disease mechanisms
Coalworker's pneumoconiosis is caused by inhalation of coal dust. There are two types: simple and complicated. In simple pneumoconiosis, coal dust inhaled into the alveoli is engulfed by macrophages, which congregate around the respiratory bronchioles, chiefly in the upper lobes. These areas become fibrotic and centrilobular emphysema may develop in complicated disease. Coalescence of fibrotic lesions can lead to progressive massive fibrosis. The development of lesions appears to be related to the total amount of dust inhaled, and is said to be greater with anthracite coal.

Clinical features
Simple coalworker's pneumoconiosis produces no symptoms or signs. Progressive massive fibrosis causes increasing breathlessness, cough and sputum (which can be black).

06

Investigation

Chest radiography may show nodular opacities, which can be graded in simple disease. In progressive massive fibrosis, the nodules coalesce and occur predominantly in the upper and middle zones.

Lung function tests

In simple disease there may be minor abnormalities in lung spirometry and gas transfer. These changes are more marked in progressive massive fibrosis.

Management

There is no specific treatment. Affected individuals are usually entitled to industrial compensation.

Prognosis

Simple coalworker's pneumoconiosis does not cause disability or shorten life, whereas progressive massive fibrosis does. Eventually, progressive massive fibrosis can result in respiratory failure.

Silicosis

Epidemiology

Prevalence. Rare.

Age. More common with increasing age.

Sex. Mainly male.

Disease mechanisms

Silicosis is a fibrotic lung disease caused by inhalation of silicon dioxide. Exposure can occur during underground mining, stonemasonry, foundry work and sandblasting. Silicon dioxide is a potent tissue poison. Inhaled particles are ingested by macrophages, which then die and cause a vigorous local fibrous reaction.

An insidious onset of progressive breathlessness may continue even after exposure to silica dust has ceased. Concomitant tuberculosis is common because silicosis predisposes to this infection. If there has been an acute and intense exposure to silicon dioxide, there may be a rapid onset of breathlessness, cough and sputum (acute silicosis).

Investigation

Chest radiography in uncomplicated silicosis shows fine nodular opacities (1–3 mm in diameter), which are present mainly throughout the upper zones. As the disease progresses, these may coalesce into larger opacities. Commonly, the hilar lymph nodes calcify at their periphery, producing the classical 'eggshell calcification'.

Lung function tests

In early disease pulmonary function tests are normal, but as the disease progresses both lung volumes and gas transfer factor decrease.

Management

Remove the patient from exposure and regularly screen for tuberculosis.

Prognosis

Silicosis usually runs a benign course, but respiratory failure and cor pulmonale can result from acute silicosis or progressive massive fibrosis.

Berylliosis

Epidemiology

Prevalence. All forms of berylliosis are rare.

Age. More common with increasing age.

Sex. Mainly male.

Disease mechanisms

Berylliosis is a pneumoconiosis caused by beryllium. This rare metal is used in industry because of its lightness and strength. Acute berylliosis follows intense exposure to beryllium. Chronic berylliosis is associated with granulomatous lesions, which are similar in appearance and distribution to those of sarcoidosis.

Clinical features

Acute berylliosis is characterized by a rapid onset of breathlessness and is accompanied by the production of bloodstained sputum and respiratory failure. The main symptoms of chronic berylliosis are progressive breathlessness and lassitude, which may occur after only a brief exposure. The somatic changes are identical to those of sarcoidosis but ocular and bone lesions do not occur.

Investigation

Chest radiography in acute berylliosis shows patchy consolidation throughout the lung fields resulting from a chemical pneumonia.

Management

Treatment of acute berylliosis is oxygen and high-dose corticosteroids. Treatment of chronic berylliosis is long-term oral corticosteroids.

Prognosis

Acute berylliosis may progress to the chronic form.

! Must know checklist

- Diagnosis and treatment of asthma
- Diagnosis and treatment of chronic obstructive pulmonary disease
- Effects of smoking on the lung
- Diagnosis and treatment of community acquired pneumonia
- Clinical features and treatment of pneumothorax

- Causes, investigation and treatment of lung cancer
- Diagnosis and treatment of tuberculosis
- Types of and treatment for respiratory failure
- Treatment of adult cystic fibrosis
- Clinical features and treatment of sleep apnoea

Further reading

Books

Baum GL, Wolinsky E, eds. *Textbook of Pulmonary Diseases*, 6th edn. London: Lippincott, Williams & Wilkins, 1998.

Murray JF, Nadel JA. *Textbook of Respiratory Medicine*, 3rd edn. London: Harcourt, 2001.

Warrell DA, Cox TM, Firth JD, Benz EJ. *Oxford Textbook of Medicine*, 4th edn. Oxford: Oxford University Press, 2003.

Journals

Thorax http://thorax.bmjjournals.com/ BMJ Publishing

European Respiratory Journal http://www.ersnet.org European Respiratory Society

American Journal of Respiratory and Critical Care Medicine http://ajrccm.atsjournals.org/ American Thoracic Society

Websites

American Thoracic Society: www.thoracic.org

British Thoracic Society (for guidelines): www.brit-thoracic.org.uk

European Respiratory Society: www.ersnet.org

UK Cystic Fibrosis Trust: www.cftrust.org.uk

Heart Disease

Introduction

Cardiovascular disease is the most common cause of death worldwide, but the distribution of the various types of cardiac disease varies. Rheumatic heart disease remains common in countries with inadequate and overcrowded housing and poor hygiene, but is becoming much less common in the West. Hypertension is prevalent world-wide, but has an especially high prevalence in West Africa and the Caribbean and is a major cause of premature death from stroke. Hypertension is covered in detail in Chapter 8. In South America the most common heart disease is heart failure from Chagas' disease resulting from infection by *Trypanosoma cruzi*. In countries where malnutrition occurs, heart failure develops because of beriberi (vitamin B_1 deficiency) and protein deficiency (kwashiorkor and marasmus).

In the UK, approximately 30% of all deaths among men and 20% of deaths among women result from ischaemic heart disease. There is marked international variation in the occurrence of this disease (Table 7.1). In Japan, the incidence of new cases is 1.5/1000/year, but in Finland it is 20/1000/year. The main factors are almost certainly environmental, because people travelling from low- to high-risk areas tend to acquire the incidence of coronary disease of the host country. Because of the increasing understanding of factors involved in the causes of coronary artery disease, there appears to have been a reduction in its incidence in some countries. In the USA and Finland, the mortality from ischaemic heart disease has fallen, but the rate in the UK has remained unchanged.

Table 7.1 Death rates from coronary heart disease in males aged 55–64 years

Country	Death rates/100 000 population
Finland	997
Northern Ireland	925
Scotland	899
New Zealand	767
Australia	731
USA	715
England and Wales	710
Canada	697
Norway	570
Sweden	563
Austria	443
Japan	95

Structure and function

Myocardium

The heart beats at approximately 70 beats/min at rest, increasing to as many as 200 beats/min with exercise. It pumps 5 l blood/min, increasing to up to 20 l/min with exercise. Weighing 200–300 g, it is mainly composed of muscle cells and specialized conducting cells that initiate and coordinate contraction.

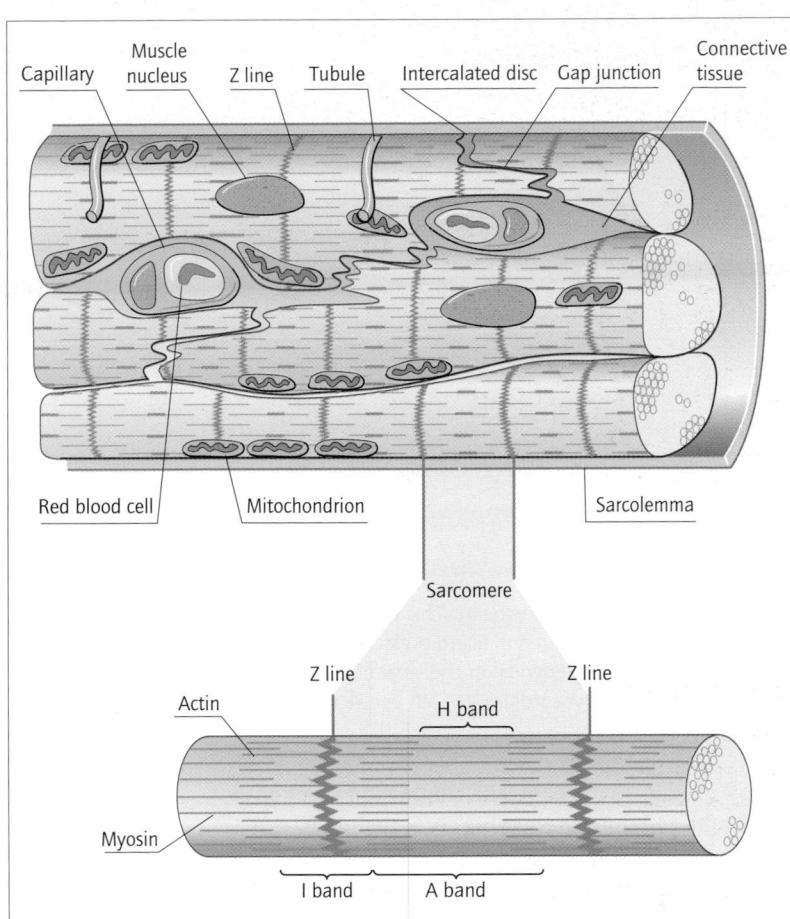

Figure 7.1 Diagram of myofibril showing the basic structure as repeated sections— known as sarcomeres—joined at the Z line. The contractile proteins actin and myosin overlap within the sarcomere.

Myocardial cells

Heart muscle (myocardial) cells are 100 μm in length and 15 μm wide. Each cell joins the next at an intercalated disc, which is a specialized area because it not only allows transmission of the electrical signal, but also transmission of force when the heart contracts.

Myocardial cells consist of myofibrils running the length of each cell. Each myofibril consists of repeating sections known as sarcomeres, which are the basic unit of contraction (Fig. 7.1). Each sarcomere is joined to the next at the Z line. The contractile protein actin is attached to the Z line and overlaps the filaments of the other contractile protein myosin. The two proteins are attached to each other by cross-bridges containing adenosine triphosphatase (ATPase). During systole, the actin filaments slide between the myosin filaments following breakdown of ATP by ATPase.

Contraction is normally inhibited by the protein troponin. During electrical depolarization, calcium enters the cell through slow channels and releases intracellular (sarcoplasmic) calcium. This then inactivates troponin,

allowing contraction to occur. During relaxation, calcium is taken up again by the sarcoplasmic reticulum. The flow of calcium is therefore a key factor in the force of contraction (inotropic state) of the heart.

The performance of the myocardium depends on four factors:

1 Filling pressure (venous pressure or preload)
2 Outflow resistance (afterload)
3 Heart rate
4 Myocardial contractility (inotropic state)

The relationship between the venous return to the heart and the cardiac output is defined by Starling's law of the heart (Fig. 7.2): 'When the pressure against which the heart has to beat (afterload) is kept constant, the force of contraction has a positive relationship to the end-diastolic fibre length.' Stroke volume therefore increases when end-diastolic volume increases as a result of increased filling of the heart because of increased venous return. Cardiac output also increases when the afterload is reduced.

The contractility of the heart is influenced by neurological and biochemical factors. Increased sympathetic

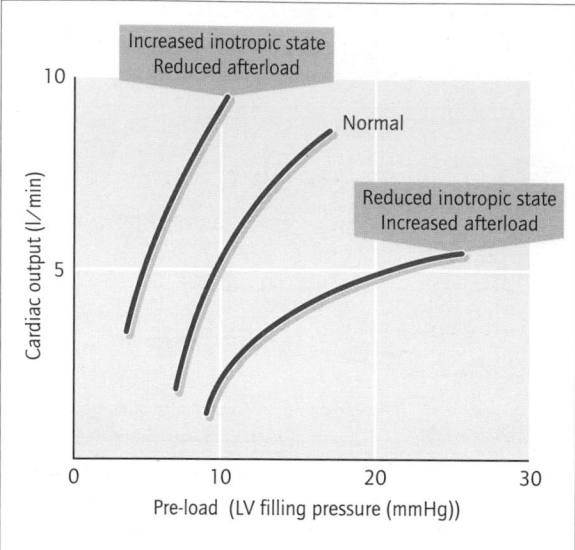

Figure 7.2 Starling's law of the heart. This shows the relationship between cardiac output and filling pressure. The position and shape of the curve depends on the level of afterload and inotropic state of the myocardium. LV, left ventricle.

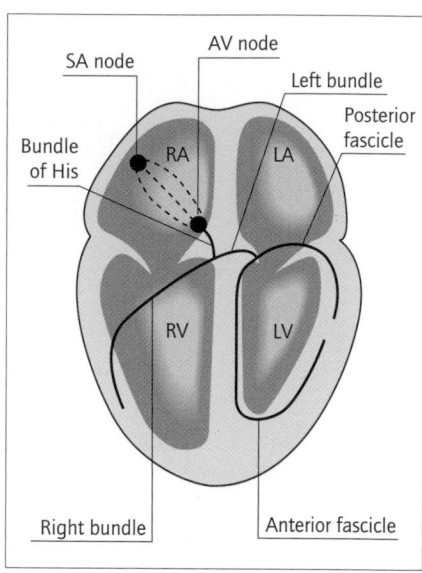

Figure 7.3 Conducting tissue of the myocardium. LA, left atrium; LV, left ventricle; RA, right atrium; RV, right ventricle.

outflow produces a more forceful contraction at any given fibre length and shifts the Starling curve to the left.

Nerve supply

The sympathetic nervous system supplies both the atria and the ventricles. There are more beta-1 receptors in the heart than in the peripheral arterioles, where the receptors are mainly beta-2.

The parasympathetic nervous system influences the heart through the vagus nerve, which supplies both the sinoatrial (SA) and atrioventricular (AV) nodes. The muscarinic effect on the SA node causes slower spontaneous depolarization of the heart and therefore a tendency to bradycardia. At rest, the influence of the vagus nerve on the heart rate is greater than that of the sympathetic nervous system.

Control of the peripheral circulation

The flow of blood to the peripheries is dictated by the resistance to flow generated by the arterioles. The higher the resistance (afterload), the higher the blood pressure. A high blood pressure therefore does not necessarily mean good tissue perfusion; conversely, too low a blood pressure can also mean inadequate tissue perfusion.

Vascular tone is determined by both hormonal and neural influences:

- *Adrenaline and noradrenaline:* high levels of circulating adrenaline or noradrenaline cause vasoconstriction and, independent of the effect on the heart, increased blood pressure.
- *Vagal tone:* in contrast, excessive vagal tone causes vasodilatation and, independent of its influence on heart rate, can cause hypotension. If severe, this can cause blackouts (hypervagotonic syncope).
- *Locally produced hormones:* include endothelial-derived relaxing factor (EDRF) and prostacyclin (PGI_2), both of which cause vasodilatation and therefore increase regional blood flow.

The conduction system of the heart
(Fig. 7.3)

The heart beat begins with the depolarization of the natural pacemaker of the heart. This is the SA node, which is located at the junction of the superior vena cava and right atrium, although its position can vary. The impulse is generated by progressive loss of the diastolic resting membrane potential until a threshold is reached when there is a sudden rapid depolarization of the sinus node tissue (Fig. 7.4). This triggers waves of depolarization throughout the atrial myocardium until it reaches the annulus fibrosis, which acts as a barrier separating the atrium from the ventricles.

The impulse then passes slowly through the AV node, which is located within the lower part of the atrial septum and is transmitted to the ventricles through the bundle of

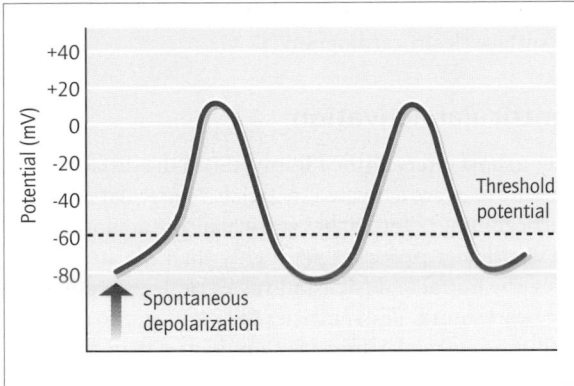

Figure 7.4 Action potential in the sinoatrial (SA) node giving rise to spontaneous depolarization.

His. The bundle of His subdivides into a right bundle to the right ventricle and a left bundle to the left ventricle:
● The right bundle passes down the right side of the interventricular septum and then spreads out in a fan of fibres spreading along the subendocardial surface of the right ventricle.
● The left bundle divides into two sub-branches (or fascicles). The anterior fascicle (or hemibundle) is relatively discrete, supplying the anterior myocardium; the posterior fascicle is more widespread and supplies the posterior and inferior surface of the left ventricle.

Depolarization of the AV node largely depends on action potentials produced by slow transmembrane calcium flux. In contrast, depolarization of the rest of the myocardium is caused by action potentials generated by rapid transmembrane sodium diffusion.

The coronary circulation (Fig. 7.5)

The two coronary arteries arise from the coronary sinus immediately above the aortic valve.

Right coronary artery

The right coronary artery passes down the right side of the AV groove, giving off vessels to both the right atrium and right ventricle. In 70% of people it continues along the inferior border of the left ventricle giving rise to the posterior descending branch which supplies the posterior part of the interventricular septum, and the left ventricular branches which supply the posterior left ventricular wall.

The sinus node and AV node are usually supplied by the right coronary artery. Acute ischaemia arising from this artery can therefore lead to sinus bradycardia and AV block.

Left coronary artery

The left coronary artery supplies blood to most of the left ventricle. It consists of a left main artery, which divides early into two main branches. Disease in the left main artery is therefore extremely dangerous.

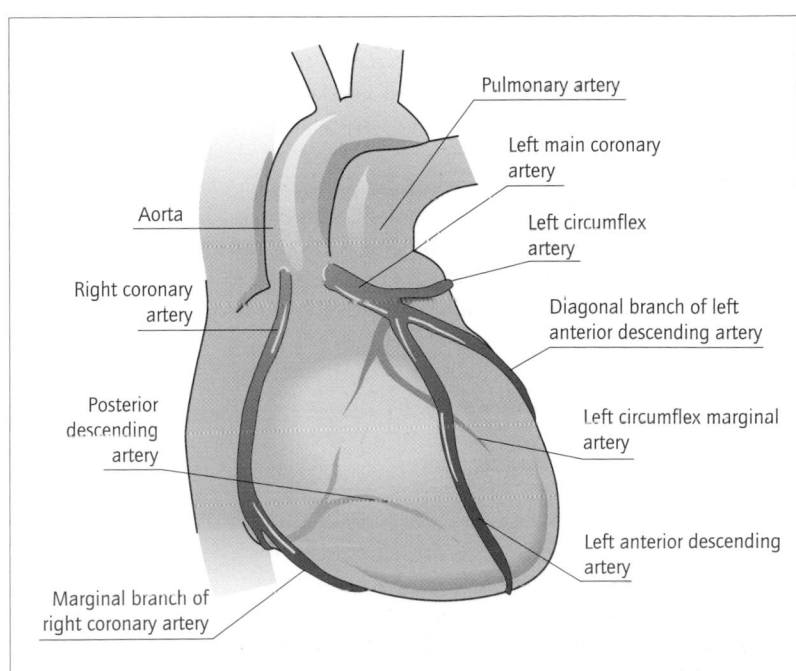

Figure 7.5 The coronary arterial tree.

- The left anterior descending branch descends in the interventricular groove supplying the anterior left ventricular wall, including the septum.
- The left circumflex branch descends in the left AV groove supplying blood to the left atrium and left ventricle. In 30% of patients it is extensive, giving rise to the posterior descending branch and therefore supplying blood to the inferior part of the left ventricle and posterior part of the interventricular septum.

Regulation of coronary blood flow

The coronary circulation receives about 5% of the cardiac output: 250 ml/min. Because the heart extracts most of the oxygen carried in the coronary circulation, increases in myocardial oxygen demand are met by increases in coronary blood flow. Coronary blood flow is determined by the transcoronary pressure gradient, myocardial metabolism and neurohumoral control:

- *Transcoronary pressure gradient:* the gradient between mean aortic pressure and the pressure in the left ventricle at the end of diastole. Coronary blood flow mainly occurs during diastole because the intramyocardial vessels are compressed during cardiac contraction. High end-diastolic pressures in the left ventricle reduce the transcoronary pressure gradient and so reduce flow, particularly to the endocardium.
- *Myocardial metabolism:* controls the coronary circulation by releasing vasodilator metabolites. The relationship between coronary blood flow and myocardial oxygen consumption is linear, but how this is achieved is not fully understood. It is thought that changes in the arterial levels of both oxygen and carbon dioxide are factors, together with local production of potassium and prostaglandin. Adenosine is possibly another important regulatory metabolite.
- *Neurohumoral control:* achieved through the sympathetic and parasympathetic nervous system. Stimulation of alpha adrenoreceptors results in vasoconstriction, and stimulation of the beta-2 receptors leads to vasodilatation. The parasympathetic coronary innervation is limited to the small vessels distal to the epicardial arteries; their activation produces vasodilatation, but the functional significance of this is currently unknown.

Cardiac cycle (Fig. 7.6)

Electrical depolarization of the sinus node leads to a coordinated sequence of electromechanical events (the cardiac cycle).

Atrial activation

Depolarization of the SA node leads to right atrial and then left atrial contraction and constitutes the P wave on the surface electrocardiogram (ECG).

Ventricular activation

After a short interval (the PR interval on the surface ECG) the ventricles are activated, with left ventricular contraction beginning before right ventricular contraction. When the ventricular pressures are higher than the atrial pressures, the mitral and tricuspid valves close generating the **first heart sound**. The ventricles then continue to contract until the ventricular pressures are higher than the pressures in the aorta and pulmonary artery, at which point the aortic and pulmonary valves open. This phase is known as **isovolumic contraction**.

At the end of systolic contraction, the ventricular pressures begin to fall and when the aortic and pulmonary artery pressures are higher than those of the ventricles, the aortic and pulmonary valves close, generating the aortic and pulmonary components of the **second heart sound**. When the ventricular pressures are lower than the atrial pressures, the tricuspid and mitral valves open. This phase is known as **isovolumic relaxation**. A period of rapid ventricular filling follows and coincides with the timing of the **third heart sound**.

Normal haemodynamics

Figure 7.7 shows the normal pressures measured with reference to a zero pressure set at 5 cm below the sternal angle with the patient recumbent.

The circulating blood volume is about 5 l, of which:
- 1.5 l is in the heart and lungs
- 3.5 l is in the systemic circulation (60% in the veins)

The left ventricular end-diastolic volume is about 150 ml with a stroke volume of 75–105 ml. The ejection fraction can therefore vary from 50 to 70%.

Cardiac output is the product of the heart rate and stroke volume. It is related to body size and is therefore more usefully presented as a cardiac index of litre/minute/metre^2 of body surface area. The range of values for normal cardiac indexes is 2–5 l/min/m^2.

Calculating vascular tone or vascular resistance

Vascular tone or vascular resistance can be calculated by dividing the pressure across the circulation by the cardiac output (Fig. 7.8):
- *Pulmonary vascular resistance* is calculated by subtracting mean left atrial pressure (or pulmonary capillary wedge pressure) from mean pulmonary artery pressure and dividing by cardiac output. Normally it is less than 2 mmHg/l/min.

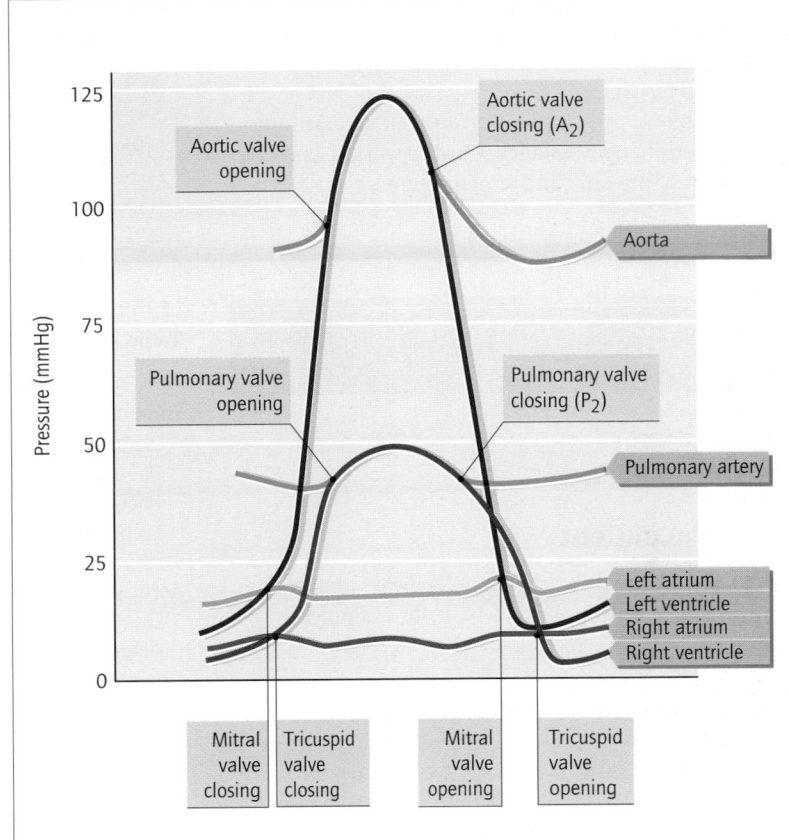

Figure 7.6 The cardiac cycle. The changing relationship of the pressures in the cardiac chambers and great vessels during systole and diastole which determines the opening and closing of the cardiac valves. (The interval between mitral and tricuspid valve closure and aortic and pulmonary valve opening is known as the *isovolumic contraction period*; the interval between aortic and pulmonary valve closure and mitral and tricuspid valve opening is known as the *isovolumic relaxation period*.)

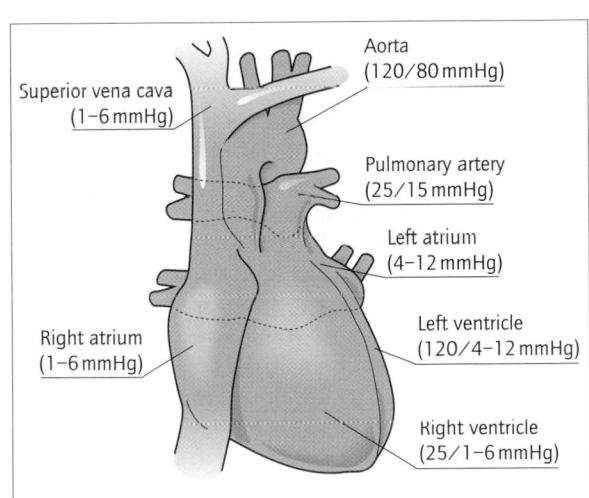

Figure 7.7 Normal pressures in the cardiac chambers and great vessels.

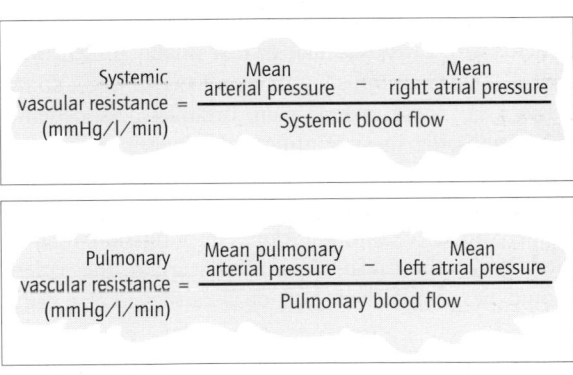

Figure 7.8 Formulae for measurement of systemic and pulmonary vascular resistance. To convert mmHg/litre/minute into dyne × second/centimetre^5 multiply by 80.

07

- *Systemic vascular resistance* is calculated by subtracting the right atrial pressure from the mean aortic pressure and dividing by the cardiac output. Normally it is between 10 and 20 mmHg/l/min.

Arterial blood pressure is a product of cardiac output and total peripheral resistance. Cardiac work is a product of mean aortic pressure and stroke volume.

Approach to the patient

History

About the patient

General information about patients is always important in putting their symptoms into context, for example:

- age
- sex
- work status (e.g. employed/unemployed) and the nature of their work
- whether they smoke

In contrast to a 55-year-old male smoker, a non-smoking female of 35 complaining of chest pain is unlikely to have obstructive coronary disease.

Symptoms

Patients with cardiovascular disease usually present with well-defined symptoms (HISTORY & EXAMINATION BOXES 7.1 & 7.2). These include pain, breathlessness, oedema, palpitations, dizziness, fainting and fatigue.

Pain

Chest pain is a common cause of admission to hospital. When the cause of pain is uncertain, the patient should be admitted to exclude a cardiovascular cause (Table 7.2).

Typical cardiac pain

Typical cardiac pain is centrally located and crushing in nature, and can radiate through to the back, up to the neck, or down one or both arms. It is commonly associated with exertion or emotional upsets and usually arises when myocardial oxygen demand exceeds oxygen supply as a result of a fixed coronary stenosis. Alternative causes are aortic stenosis, hypertrophic cardiomyopathy and pulmonary hypertension.

Angina has been categorized by the Canadian Cardio-

Table 7.2 Causes of chest pain

Pericarditis
Lung disease
Pleurisy
Pneumonia
Pneumothorax
Embolism
Oesophageal disease
Aortic pathology
Dissection
Aneurysm
Chest wall pain

Table 7.3 Canadian Cardiovascular Society grading of angina

Grade 1	Angina on strenuous physical activity
Grade 2	Angina on ordinary physical activity (e.g. walking uphill or climbing more than one flight of stairs)
Grade 3	Marked limitation on ordinary physical activity (e.g. angina on climbing one flight of stairs)
Grade 4	Angina on any physical activity and also at rest

vascular Society according to the exercise limitation it imposes on the patient (Table 7.3).

Atypical chest pain

Atypical chest pain does not fulfil the usual criteria for cardiac pain. It has a different character and occurs in any part of the chest or upper abdomen. It usually has no cardiac cause, but occasionally is caused by coronary spasm. Other cardiac causes of atypical pain are mitral valve prolapse and mitral stenosis, which may cause pain possibly because of expansion of the left atrium.

Hepatic angina

Hepatic angina is a right hypochondral pain induced by exercise and caused by increased venous congestion of the liver with exercise. It occurs in people with right atrial hypertension, and is usually caused by right ventricular failure.

History & Examination 7.2: Important questions to ask in cardiology

About the patient
How old are you?
What work do you do?

Symptoms
What symptoms do you get?

Chest pain
Where is it?
What does it feel like (a tight band, crushing, an ache, sharp)?
How long does it last?
Does it radiate into your arms, neck or back?
When do you get it (on exertion, at rest, when stressed)?
Is it painful to breathe deeply?
Do you have to take occasional deep breaths?

Breathlessness
When do you get it (on exertion, on lying flat, during the night)?
Is it painful to breathe deeply?
Do you have to take occasional deep breaths?

Ankle swelling
When do you get it (all the time, at the end of the day)?
What makes it worse?
What makes it better?

Palpitations
What are they like (fast or slow; regular or irregular)? Ask the patient to tap the beat onto the table
When do you get them?
What brings them on?
Do they stop suddenly or gradually?

Dizziness and fainting
Describe what happens

What brings it on?
Do you have any warning?
Do you fall and hurt yourself?
Are you incontinent?

Pattern of disease
Onset and progression
How long have you had these symptoms?
Are the symptoms getting better or worse?

Associated features
Have you noticed any other associated symptoms (e.g. sweating, tiredness, pins and needles)?

Drug history
What prescribed and non-prescribed medicines, pills and potions do you take (including all those bought from health food shops such as vitamins)?

Past medical history
What illnesses have you had other than the usual childhood infections?
Have you had rheumatic fever?
What operations have you had?

Family history
Does anyone in your family have (or has anyone had) a heart condition or high blood pressure? If so, what?

Social history
Do you smoke? If so, how much?
Do you drink alcohol? If so, what and how much?
Do you drink a lot of coffee?
How much exercise do you do?
What sort of foods do you eat (a lot of sausage, egg and chips, a lot of salads and low-fat foods)?

Breathlessness

Exertional dyspnoea

Exertional dyspnoea (or breathlessness) is a normal response to exercise. However, in heart disease it becomes exaggerated because of two mechanisms:

1 Increased pressure in the left atrium and pulmonary veins with exercise causes stiffness of the lungs

2 Inadequate cardiac output during exercise results in poor peripheral perfusion and an increased metabolic acidosis

Exertional dyspnoea can be an angina equivalent (global myocardial ischaemia giving rise to poor ventricular function on exercise without chest pain). Distinguishing a cardiac cause from a respiratory cause for breathlessness can be difficult. Exertional dyspnoea can be classified according to its effect on the patient's life (Tables 7.4 and 7.5).

Table 7.4 Differential diagnoses of exertional dyspnoea: distinction between cardiac and respiratory causes

If cardiac:
1 Dyspnoea is usually associated with chest tightness
2 Dypsnoea will usually be exertionally related
3 Chest X-ray will be normal
4 A stress test (exercise test or thallium scan or dobutamine echocardiogram) will be helpful

Table 7.5 New York Heart Association (NYHA) grading of dyspnoea

Grade 1	No breathlessness
Grade 2	Breathlessness on severe exertion
Grade 3	Breathlessness on mild exertion
Grade 4	Breathlessness at rest

Paroxysmal nocturnal dyspnoea

Paroxysmal nocturnal dyspnoea (PND) is usually a symptom of poor left ventricular function. The patient wakes from sleep acutely dyspnoeic because of a rise in left atrial pressure, and has to sit up or walk, the symptoms settling after a few minutes. This must not be confused with the nocturnal dyspnoea of asthma. (PND was first described in asthma when it is caused by the early morning reduction in peak expiratory flow, but it was then noticed that heart failure caused similar symptoms, often with a marked expiratory wheeze resulting from bronchial congestion; hence the term, cardiac asthma.)

Orthopnoea

Orthopnoea is a symptom of left ventricular failure or mitral stenosis, and is also caused by a rise in left atrial pressure. The patient is unable to lie flat because of breathlessness resulting from chronically raised left atrial pressure. Often patients report that they have increased the number of pillows they sleep on.

Oedema

Right heart failure is one of the many causes of dependent oedema, which is usually first visible at the ankles. If a patient is confined to bed, peripheral oedema usually occurs in the sacrum. Hepatomegaly and ascites develop in more severe right heart failure.

Palpitations

Palpitations is a term used by patients to describe an awareness of a disturbance in the rhythm of the heart (irregular and/or accelerated) or an awareness of the force of the heart beat without there necessarily being a disturbance in the rhythm. When a patient reports palpitations, it is important to establish precisely what sensation they are experiencing.

Dizziness and fainting

Cardiac causes of dizziness and fainting arise as a result of poor cerebral perfusion. The most common causes are postural hypotension and vasovagal syncope. Other cardiac causes include arrhythmias, aortic stenosis, hypertrophic cardiomyopathy and pulmonary hypertension.

Fatigue

Fatigue is a relatively non-specific symptom of heart disease. It is often reported by patients with coronary artery disease and is also a feature of poor peripheral perfusion in patients with heart failure or aortic stenosis.

Pattern of the disease

It is very helpful in diagnosis and management to establish whether the symptoms are getting better or worse, and over what period. Furthermore, how much the symptoms interfere with the quality of life is a useful guide to their severity. Patients with chest pain that has been present on and off for many years are unlikely to be as much at risk as patients presenting with a deteriorating and limiting chest pain of recent onset.

Beware of the patient who denies symptoms because they have adapted their way of life and take no exercise. A formal exercise test (or walk along the corridor with the patient) can be very helpful.

Drug history

Finding out whether the patient smokes, and his or her alcohol intake and use of other drugs is important, as illustrated by the following examples:
- *Smoking:* a risk factor for coronary artery disease
- *Alcohol:* can cause heart failure and arrhythmias (particularly atrial fibrillation)
- *Hallucinogenic drugs:* can cause severe disturbance in heart rhythm
- *Cardiac drugs:* can cause severe side-effects (e.g. beta-blockers can make patients breathless, dizzy and impotent, and digoxin can cause palpitations, nausea and anorexia).

Past medical history

A history of other vascular disease [e.g. a cerebrovascular accident (stroke) or peripheral vascular disease (intermittent claudication)] makes the presence of coronary disease more likely. Only about 50% of patients with rheumatic heart disease will give a history of rheumatic fever.

Family history

Some cardiac disorders have a clearly established pattern of inheritance [e.g. Marfan's syndrome (see p. 498) is an autosomal dominant condition, so 50% of the children of a patient with Marfan's syndrome are likely to inherit the disease]. Coronary artery disease can also be familial, even though there may be no inherited risk factor (e.g. hypertension or hypercholesterolaemia).

<table>
<tr><td>

History & Examination 7.3: Examination in cardiology

First impressions

Is the patient breathless at rest? (At rest 12–14 inspirations/min is normal)

Note how breathless the patient becomes on climbing onto the couch

Check the patient's pulse rate before and after climbing onto the couch. Has it accelerated inappropriately?

When the patient is relaxed and lying at 45° note any cyanosis, cachexia, obesity, anaemia, jaundice and features of thyroid disturbance (tremor, exophthalmos)

Look for signs of endocarditis: clubbing, splinter haemorrhages, Osler's nodes, skin rash, Roth's spots, splenomegaly, haematuria

Pulse

Feel the radial pulse and apex beat at the same time and note the rate and any apex : radial deficit

Note the character of the carotid pulse (normal, slow rising, collapsing, bisferiens, sharp)

Note the volume of the carotid pulse (normal, increased, decreased, alternans, paradoxus)

Blood pressure

Note the patient's blood pressure both lying and standing

Venous pressure

Palpate the precordium

● Note the position of the apex beat (normally in the fifth intercostal space and in the mid-clavicular line)

● Note the character of the apex beat (normal, double, tapping)

● Feel for a thrill to the right of the sternum when the patient sits forward

● Feel for a palpable component to the second heart sound in the second left intercostal space

Listen to the heart

First with the patient at 45°, then sitting forward, then lying on their left side

Note the intensity of the first heart sound (normal, loud, soft, variable)

Note the character of the second heart sound (normal, physiologically split, increased split, reversed split, increased aortic sound, softer aortic sound, increased pulmonary sound)

Listen for a third heart sound

Listen for a fourth heart sound

Listen for a systolic murmur (pansystolic, late systolic, ejection systolic, innocent benign systolic)

Listen for a diastolic murmur (early, mid-diastolic or presystolic)

Listen for a continuous murmur

</td></tr>
</table>

Social history

It is important to take account of the patient's background and lifestyle. Thus, a patient of African origin is less likely to have coronary artery disease than a patient from the Indian Subcontinent. Similarly, note the exercise capacity of the patient: do they play competitive sport and how far are their symptoms interfering?

Examination

When examining a patient, the following general points should be noted first (HISTORY & EXAMINATION BOX 7.3):

● How breathless is the patient climbing onto the couch?

● Does climbing onto the couch accelerate the heart rate inappropriately?

● When the patient is relaxed and sitting at 45°, note whether the patient is cachexic, obese, anaemic, jaundiced, or has features of thyroid disturbance or renal failure

Cardiovascular signs

Cyanosis. This is a blue discoloration of skin and mucous membranes that occurs when there is more than 5 g/dl of deoxygenated haemoglobin. It can either be central (with a blue tongue) caused by heart and lung disease, or peripheral because of poor peripheral perfusion. The signs of endocarditis are listed in Table 7.6 and those of rheumatic fever in Table 7.7.

Pulse

Identify all the pulses and note their rate, rhythm, character and volume.

Rate

Compare the pulse rate with that of the apex. A deficit in the radial pulse can occur in atrial fibrillation or if there

Table 7.6 Signs of infective endocarditis

Fever

Anaemia

Heart murmur—may change

Splenomegaly

Nail bed splinter haemorrhages

Clubbing of nail bed

Petechial rash

Osler's nodes—painful nodules on the finger pads

Janeway's lesions on hand—maculopapular rash caused by immune complex deposition

Roth spots in retina resulting from retinal microinfarcts

Weight loss leading to cachexia

Haematuria

07

Table 7.7 Features of rheumatic fever (Duckett–Jones criteria)

Major
Carditis
Polyarthritis
Chorea
Erythema marginatum
Subcutaneous nodules

Minor
Fever
Arthralgia
Previous rheumatic fever or rheumatic heart disease
Elevated ESR or CRP
Prolonged PR interval

CRP, C-reactive protein; ESR, erythrocyte sedimentation rate.

are ectopic beats. A **bradycardia** is a heart rate less than 60/min; a **tachycardia** is a rate more than 100/min.

Rhythm
The rhythm may be:
- *Regular:* there is a normal increase and decrease in the heart rate with respiration—sinus arrhythmia
- *Irregularly irregular:* as a result of atrial fibrillation or because of irregular atrial or ventricular ectopics or intermittent heart block
- *Regularly irregular:* because of regular atrial or ventricular ectopics

Character
The character of the pulse reflects the state of the outflow tract of the left ventricle (Fig. 7.9). It may be:
- *Normal*
- *Slow rising:* resulting from aortic stenosis and best felt at the carotid pulse
- *Collapsing:* resulting from aortic incompetence (or, very rarely, an arteriovenous fistula or patent ductus arteriosus) and best felt at both the radial pulse and the carotid pulse
- *Bisferiens:* resulting from a combination of a slow rising and a collapsing pulse in mixed aortic valve disease
- *Sharp:* resulting from the abrupt ending of systole as in hypertrophic cardiomyopathy or mitral regurgitation

Volume
The volume of the pulse may be:
- *Normal*
- *Increased:* as in high-output states such as anaemia, thyrotoxicosis and fevers
- *Decreased:* resulting from reduced cardiac output as in left ventricular failure, aortic stenosis and causes of reduced circulating blood volume such as haemorrhage

Pulsus alternans. This occurs when, in the presence of a regular rhythm, the systolic blood pressure varies from beat to beat. It gives rise to an alternating weak and strong ('thready') pulse and is caused by the variable recovery time of weak heart muscle. It indicates a poor prognosis from left ventricular failure.

Pulsus paradoxus. This is an exaggeration in the difference in pulse pressure during inspiration and expiration. Normally this difference is less than 15 mmHg. In severe asthma, constrictive pericarditis or pericardial tamponade, inspiration results in a greater fall in systolic pressure (sometimes the systolic pressure disappears). Right ventricular filling, which is normally increased by the negative intrathoracic pressure of inspiration, then compromises left ventricular filling because of the inability of the heart to expand in the fixed volume of the pericardium. Output from the left ventricle and blood pressure therefore fall on inspiration.

Blood pressure
The blood pressure is defined by the systolic pressure (when the pulse first becomes audible) and the diastolic pressure (when the pulse is no longer heard). A wide pulse pressure is typical of aortic incompetence, patent ductus arteriosus or a large arteriovenous fistula. A small pulse pressure can but usually does not occur in aortic stenosis.

Measurement
Blood pressure is measured as follows:
- The patient should be sitting and as relaxed as possible.
- Place the sphygmomanometer cuff above the brachial artery on either the left or right arm.
- Inflate the sphygmomanometer until the radial pulse is no longer palpable (too high an inflation can be very uncomfortable).
- Place the stethoscope over the brachial artery and lower the pressure until the pulse can be heard (*Korotkoff phase 1*). This is the systolic pressure.
- Continue to lower the cuff pressure until the sounds become muffled (*Korotkoff phase 4*) and disappear (*Korotkoff phase 5*). The latter is the diastolic pressure and correlates more closely than phase 4 to diastolic pressure measured intravascularly.

The sounds may disappear (*phase 2*) and reappear (*phase 3*) between the systolic and diastolic pressures, which can lead to phase 2 being mistaken for the diastolic pressure or phase 3 for the systolic pressure.

Venous pressure
There are two peaks and two troughs in a normal venous pressure in every cardiac cycle (Fig. 7.10):

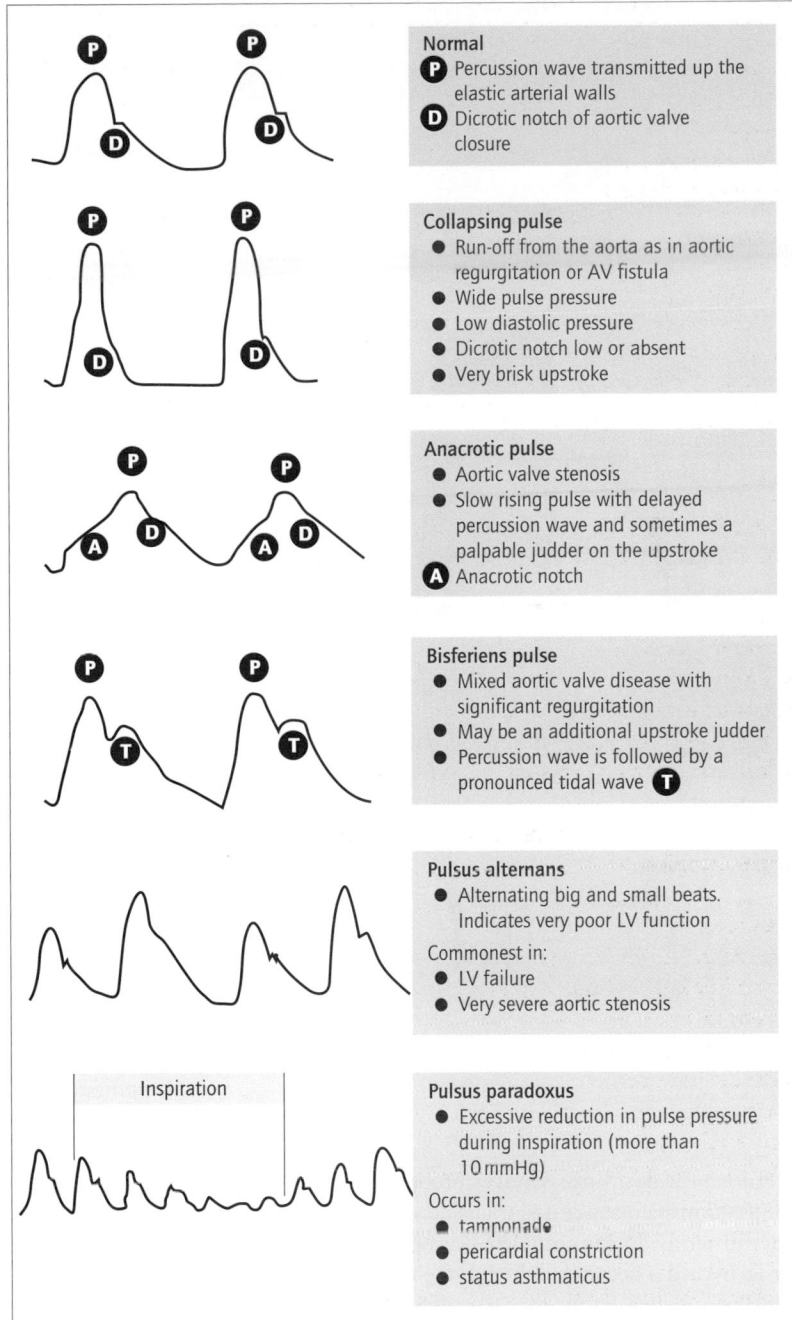

Normal
- **P** Percussion wave transmitted up the elastic arterial walls
- **D** Dicrotic notch of aortic valve closure

Collapsing pulse
- Run-off from the aorta as in aortic regurgitation or AV fistula
- Wide pulse pressure
- Low diastolic pressure
- Dicrotic notch low or absent
- Very brisk upstroke

Anacrotic pulse
- Aortic valve stenosis
- Slow rising pulse with delayed percussion wave and sometimes a palpable judder on the upstroke
- **A** Anacrotic notch

Bisferiens pulse
- Mixed aortic valve disease with significant regurgitation
- May be an additional upstroke judder
- Percussion wave is followed by a pronounced tidal wave **T**

Pulsus alternans
- Alternating big and small beats. Indicates very poor LV function

Commonest in:
- LV failure
- Very severe aortic stenosis

Inspiration

Pulsus paradoxus
- Excessive reduction in pulse pressure during inspiration (more than 10 mmHg)

Occurs in:
- tamponade
- pericardial constriction
- status asthmaticus

Figure 7.9 The types of arterial pulse which can be identified on clinical examination.

- a *wave:* brought about by atrial contraction
- x *descent:* brought about by movement of the base of the heart towards the apex in systole
- v *wave:* brought about by right atrial filling against a closed tricuspid valve
- y *descent:* brought about by opening of the tricuspid valve

Abnormalities

Abnormalities of the venous pressure are as follows:
- *Elevated venous pressure:* indicates increased right atrial pressure.
- *Large* a *waves:* occur when there is right ventricular hypertrophy, usually as a result of pulmonary hypertension or pulmonary stenosis.

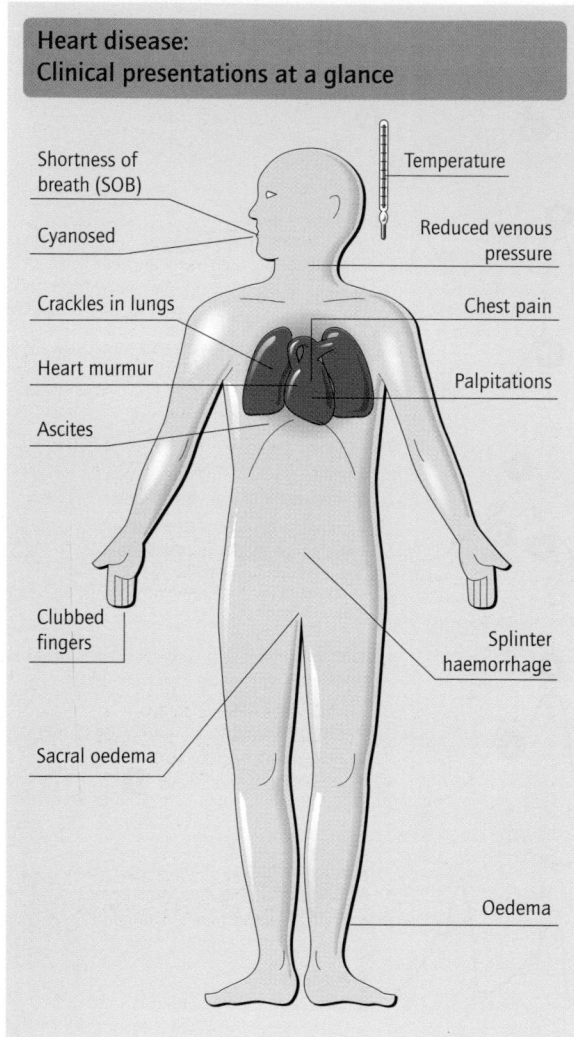

Heart disease:
Clinical presentations at a glance

Shortness of breath (SOB)

Cyanosed

Crackles in lungs

Heart murmur

Ascites

Clubbed fingers

Sacral oedema

Temperature

Reduced venous pressure

Chest pain

Palpitations

Splinter haemorrhage

Oedema

• *Cannon waves:* huge *a* waves brought about by atrial contraction against a closed tricuspid valve. They are seen intermittently during complete heart block and ventricular tachycardia because, although the atria and ventricles contract independently, they occasionally contract at the same time. Cannon waves occur regularly with junctional tachycardias when the atria and ventricles usually contract simultaneously.

• *Systolic v waves:* brought about by tricuspid incompetence when blood regurgitates into the atrium during systole and obliterates the *x* descent and normal *v* peak.

• *Slow* y *descent:* occurs when tricuspid stenosis delays right ventricular filling. This is difficult to see, but can be observed on a pressure monitor trace.

• *A* c *wave:* may occasionally be visible immediately

after the *a* wave during the *x* descent and is brought about by right ventricular contraction filling the right atrium before the tricuspid valve is closed.

Examination of the precordium

Palpation of the precordium
Four areas of the precordium should be palpated:
1 Apex beat
2 Left sternal edge
3 Aortic area
4 Pulmonary area

Apex beat
The apex beat is the most lateral and inferior pulsation of the left ventricle and is normally in the mid-clavicular line in the fifth intercostal space. It can be hypertrophied and displaced.

• *Displacement of the apex beat:* usually lateral and a result of either mediastinal shift or dilatation of a cardiac chamber. When displaced because of cardiac disease, there is either spontaneous dilatation of the ventricle as in cardiomyopathy, or dilatation because of volume load as occurs in mitral or aortic regurgitation.

• *Hypertrophy of the apex beat:* hypertrophy of an apex beat that is not displaced indicates a systolic pressure load on the left ventricle as a result of either systemic hypertension or aortic stenosis. When these conditions are advanced, the left ventricle begins to dilate.

Double apex beat. A palpable impulse additional to that of the apex beat can be caused either by atrial contraction as a result of atrial hypertrophy secondary to left ventricular hypertrophy, or late outward movement of a ventricular aneurysm.

Tapping apex beat. In mitral stenosis the first heart sound is loud and may occasionally be felt, producing a so-called tapping apex beat.

Left sternal edge
A palpable impulse at the left sternal edge indicates either right ventricular hypertrophy or systolic expansion of the left atrium as in mitral regurgitation.

Aortic area
In aortic stenosis it is possible to feel a thrill (palpable murmur) to the right of the sternum when the patient sits forward.

Pulmonary area
A palpable pulmonary component to the second heart sound in the second left intercostal space indicates pulmonary hypertension.

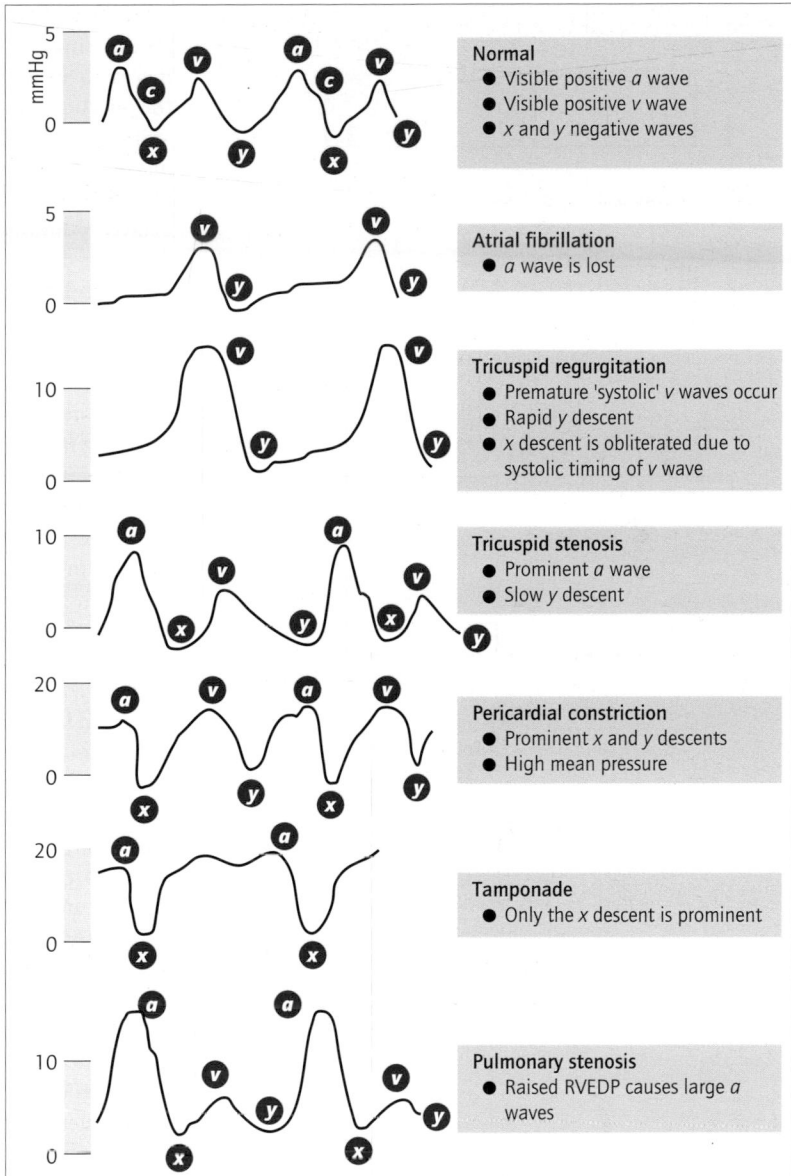

Figure 7.10 The types of venous pressure pulse which can be identified on clinical examination. RVEDP, right ventricular end-diastolic pressure.

Auscultation of the heart

Heart sounds (Fig. 7.11)

First heart sound

The first heart sound is caused by the consecutive closure of the mitral and tricuspid valves and is maximal over the apex beat. It is usually single but can be split, in which case the double click must be distinguished from either a fourth heart sound or an ejection click. Normally, the valves are beginning to close before the onset of systole. Abnormal findings include the following:

● *Loud first heart sound:* this results if ventricular systole

starts when the valve is fully open and occurs in mitral stenosis or when there is a short PR interval.

● *Soft first heart sound:* this results when the valve leaflets are immobile, as in advanced calcific mitral stenosis, or when the valve is already half shut before the onset of systole, as in a long PR interval. The first heart sound can also be soft when there is poor transmission of the sound because of a pericardial effusion, a barrelled chest or obesity.

● *Variable intensity:* the intensity of the first heart sound can vary when the relationship between atrial and ventricular systole varies, as in complete heart block.

07

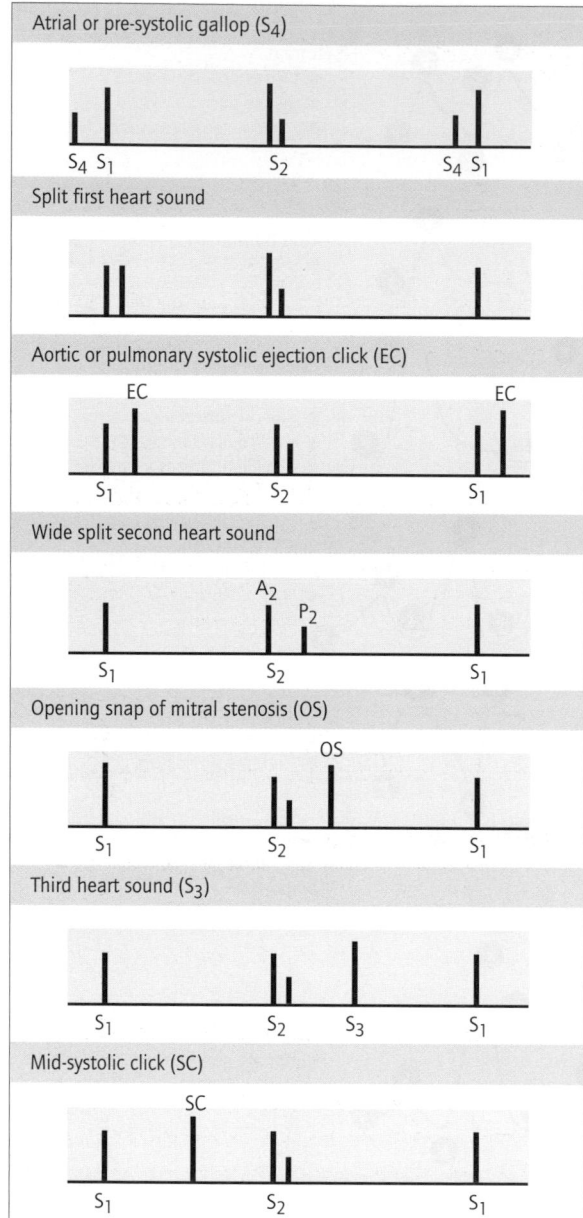

Figure 7.11 The timing of the heart sounds in the cardiac cycle. S_1, first heart sound, mitral and tricuspid valve closure; S_2 second heart sound, aortic and pulmonary valve closure. (When noting heart sounds in the patient's records, the full cardiac cycle should be described and the height of the sound relates to its intensity.)

Second heart sound

The second heart sound is caused by closure of the aortic and pulmonary valves and is best heard in the second left intercostal space (the pulmonary area):

- *Physiological splitting of the second heart sound:* the separation of the pulmonary component from the aortic component is increased by deep inspiration, which increases venous return to the right heart, leading to the ejection of more blood from the right ventricle and delaying pulmonary valve closure. This is known as physiological splitting.
- *Increased split of the second heart sound:* occurs with delayed pulmonary valve closure resulting from a pathology that delays emptying of the right ventricle, such as right bundle branch block or pulmonary stenosis.
- *Fixed splitting of the second heart sound:* an atrial septal defect delays pulmonary valve closure for two reasons: first, there is usually a degree of right bundle branch block and, secondly, there is increased right ventricular volume resulting from the flow of blood from the left atrium to the right atrium (left to right shunt). The splitting of the second heart sound is fixed and does not vary with respiration because the pressures between the right and left atrium during respiration are constantly equalized.
- *Reverse splitting of the second heart sound:* occurs when the aortic valve closes after the pulmonary valve because there is a delay in left ventricular emptying. This is caused by severe aortic stenosis, left bundle branch block or advanced left ventricular failure.
- *Increased aortic sound:* the aortic sound increases with systemic hypertension.
- *Softer aortic sound:* the aortic sound is softer in aortic stenosis.
- *Increased pulmonary sound:* the pulmonary component is louder in pulmonary hypertension.
- *Softer pulmonary sound:* the pulmonary sound is soft in pulmonary stenosis.

Third heart sound

A third heart sound occurs after the second heart sound and is produced by filling of a non-compliant ventricle. It indicates left ventricular failure, but can be a normal finding in children and young adults.

Fourth heart sound

A fourth heart sound occurs after the third sound and immediately before the first sound. It is brought about by atrial hypertrophy and indicates increased pressure in the atrium.

Ejection click

An ejection click occurs shortly after the first heart sound and indicates a bicuspid aortic valve. A pulmonary valve ejection click occurs in the pulmonary area in mild pulmonary stenosis.

Mid-systolic click

A mid-systolic click indicates mitral valve prolapse.

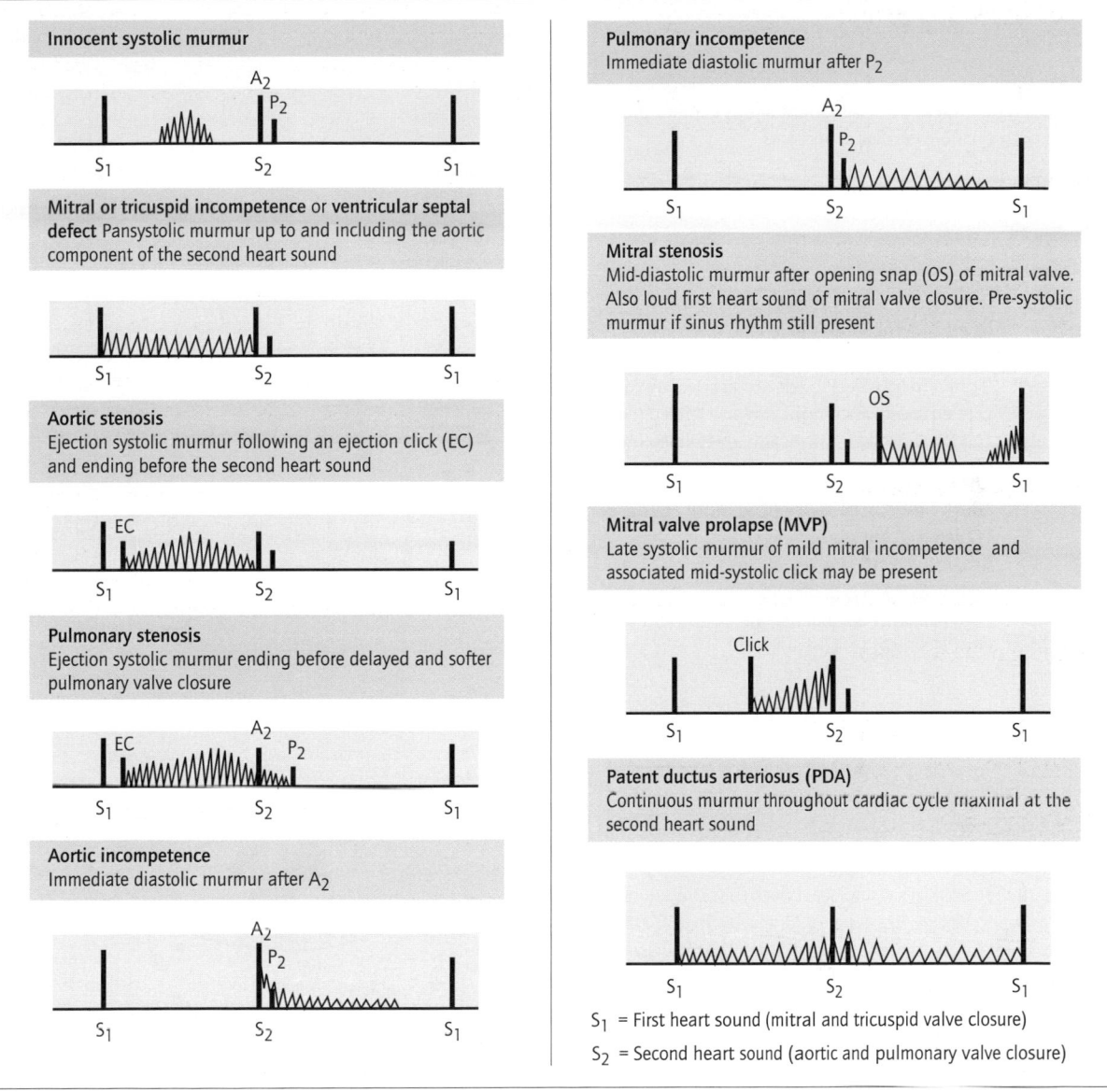

Figure 7.12 The timing of the various heart murmurs.

Pericardial click
A pericardial click in systole is rarely heard and is not pathological.

Heart murmurs (Fig. 7.12)
Heart murmurs are described according to their timing in the cardiac cycle.

Systolic murmurs
There are different types of systolic murmur:
• *Pansystolic murmur:* a sustained murmur throughout systole up to and including the aortic component of the second heart sound. It is a feature of mitral regurgitation, tricuspid regurgitation and ventricular septal defect (VSD).
• *Late systolic murmur:* a crescendo murmur in the latter part of systole. It is often preceded by a click and indicates mitral valve prolapse with regurgitation.
• *Ejection systolic murmur:* a crescendo/decrescendo systolic murmur caused by stenosis of the aortic or pulmonary valves.
• *Innocent (benign) systolic murmur:* particularly common in children and characteristically occurs early in systole. There is no underlying structural heart defect and it is of no importance.

Box 7.1: How to do an ECG

Indications
An ECG is needed in the assessment of any patient presenting with possible cardiac symptoms

Technique
Rest the patient at 45° having removed all clothing from
above the waist

Position the standard leads

Lead I	Right arm (negative) to left arm (positive)
Lead II	Right arm (negative) to left leg (positive)
Lead III	Left arm (negative) to right arm (positive)
Lead aVR	Right arm (positive) to left arm and left leg (negative)
Lead aVL	Left leg (positive) to right arm and left leg (negative)
Lead aVF	Left leg (positive) to right arm and left leg (negative)

Position the chest leads

V1	Fourth intercostal space (ICS), right sternal edge
V2	Fourth ICS, left sternal edge
V3	Between V2 and V4
V4	Fifth ICS, mid-clavicular line
V5	Fifth ICS, anterior axillary line
V6	Fifth ICS, mid-axillary line

Make the recording
One millivolt is represented as 10 mm on the paper.
This can be varied if large or small voltages are recorded,
but each recording must be calibrated: this is usually
performed automatically on modern ECG machines.
The paper is run at 25 mm/s

Measures against interference
When the recording is complete, check that there is no
interference either from mains AC electricity (50 Hz
waves) or by the patient's breathing. If there is, use
the electronic filter only as a last resort because this
can eliminate important diagnostic deflections on
the ECG

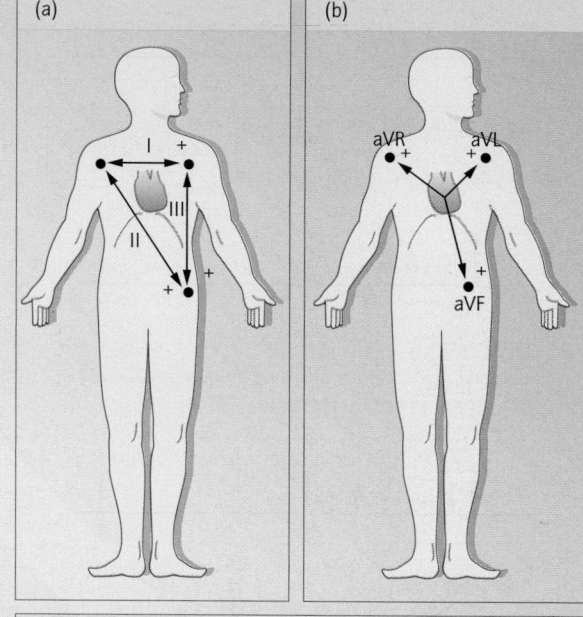

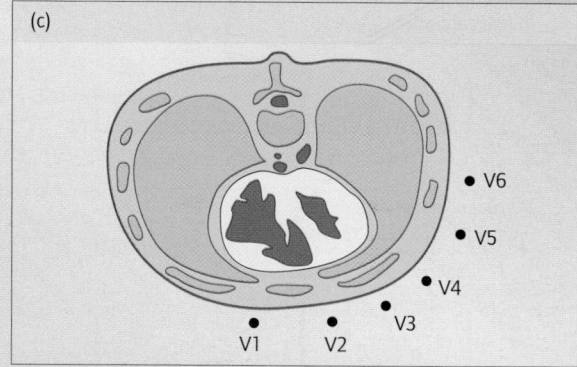

Fig. A The leads of the standard 12-lead ECG. (a) Bipolar
leads, (b) unipolar leads, (c) chest leads.

Diastolic murmurs

The different types of diastolic murmur are as follow:

- *Early diastolic murmur:* a decrescendo murmur in diastole that occurs immediately after the second heart
sound. It is caused by aortic or pulmonary regurgitation.
- *Mid-diastolic murmur:* a low-frequency rumble that
often follows an opening snap and indicates either mitral
or tricuspid stenosis.
- *Presystolic diastolic murmur:* a crescendo murmur
occurring immediately before the first heart sound. It
results from atrial systole accelerating blood flow through
a stenosed mitral or tricuspid valve.

Continuous murmur (Gibson's machinery murmur)

This is a continuous murmur throughout systole and
diastole, and results from continuous flow through a
patent ductus arteriosus.

Investigation

The electrocardiogram

The standard ECG consists of 12 leads that view the
electrical activity of the heart from different angles
(BOX 7.1; Fig. 7.13). The components of an ECG complex

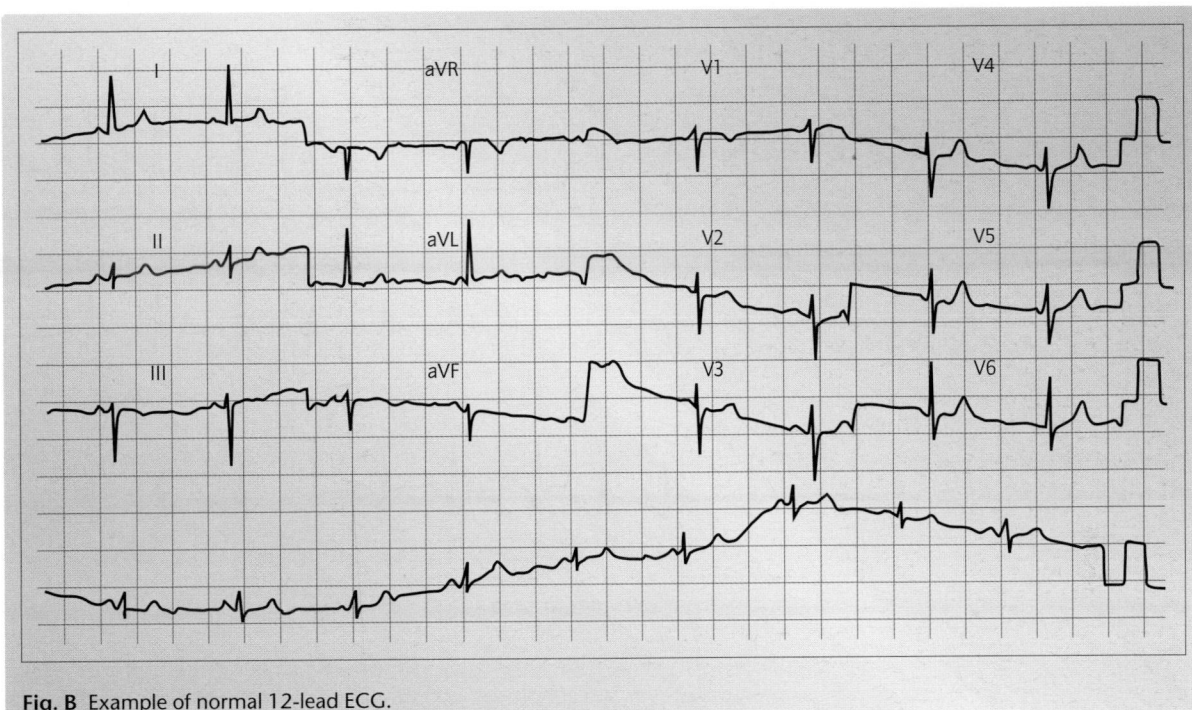

Fig. B Example of normal 12-lead ECG.

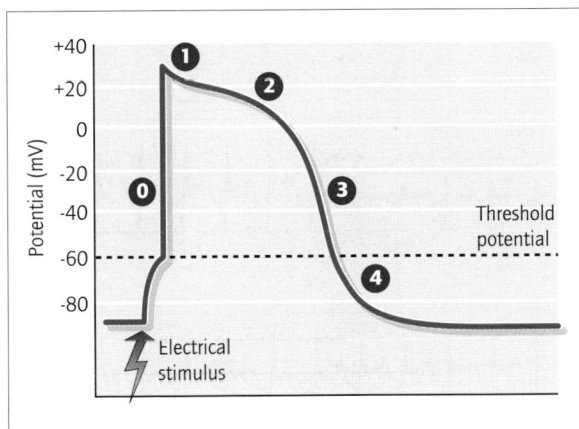

Figure 7.13 The different phases of the action potential of the myocardial cell.

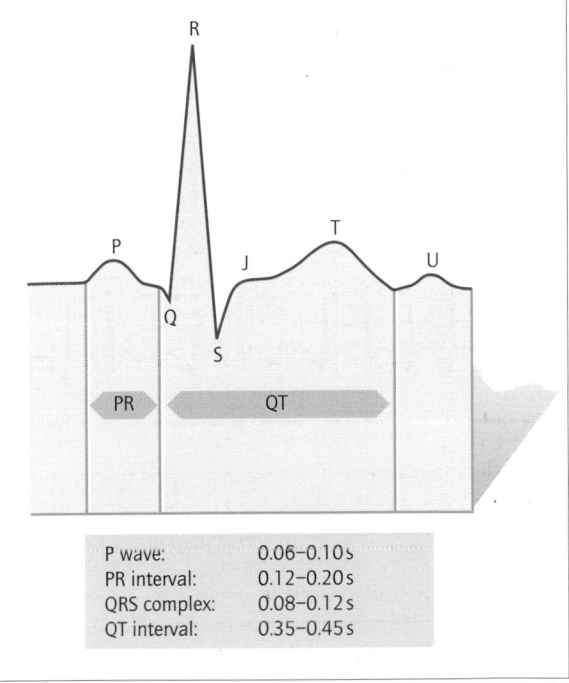

P wave:	0.06–0.10s
PR interval:	0.12–0.20s
QRS complex:	0.08–0.12s
QT interval:	0.35–0.45s

Figure 7.14 Components of the ECG complex. Note: J point, onset of ST segment; PR interval, onset of P wave to onset of QRS complex; QT interval, onset of QRS complex to end of T wave.

are the P wave, the PR interval, the QRS complex and the ST segment (Fig. 7.14).

• *P wave:* caused by atrial contraction and is best seen in standard lead II or V1.

• *PR interval:* the interval between the onset of the P wave and the onset of the QRS complex. It is usually 120–220 ms.

• *QRS complex:* results from ventricular depolarization with the wave of depolarization passing from the endocardium to the epicardium. It consists of the Q wave (the

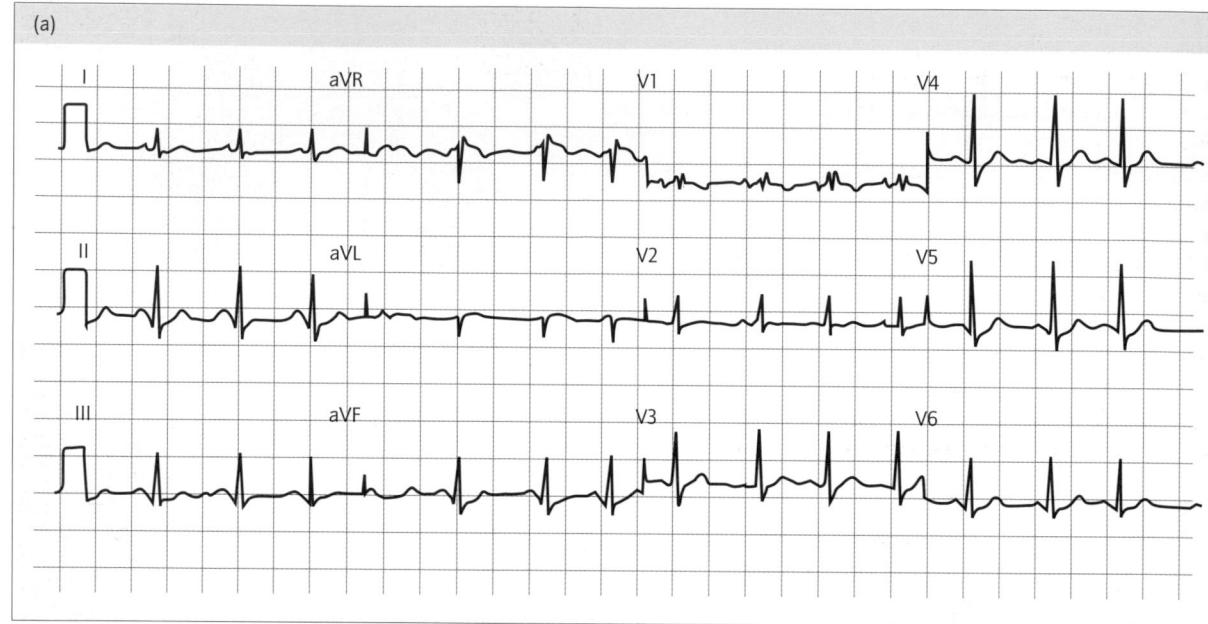

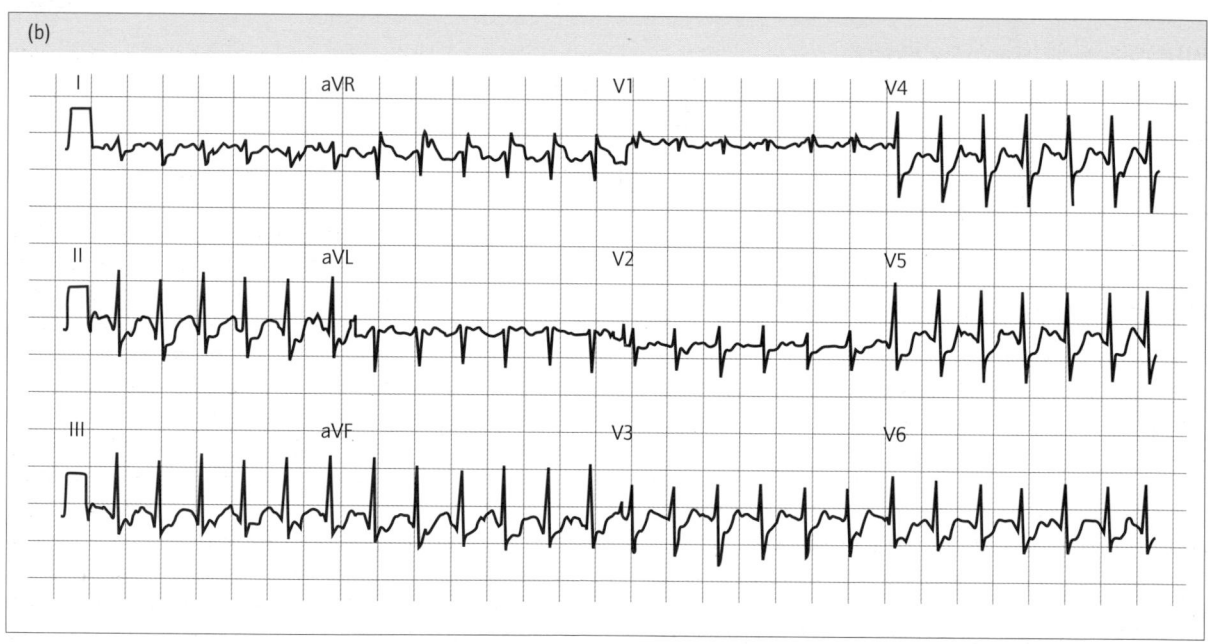

Figure 7.15 (a) The resting ECG and (b) peak exercise ECG of a patient with positive exercise test. Note the ST depression in the inferior and anterior chest leads. (This patient proved to have left main coronary artery disease.)

initial negative deflection), the R wave (the first positive deflection) and the S wave (the subsequent negative deflection). The normal width of the QRS complex is less than 120 ms.

● *ST segment:* normally isoelectric and with the T wave results from ventricular repolarization.

● *T wave:* usually in the same axis as the QRS complex because the wave of repolarization is usually in the opposite direction to depolarization (from the epicardium to the endocardium).

● *U wave:* can be prominent in hypokalaemia and myocardial ischaemia.

The exercise ECG

The exercise ECG is useful for:

- Diagnosing myocardial ischaemia
- Assessing exercise capacity in the context of ischaemic heart disease or heart failure
- Assessing prognosis in patients with ischaemic heart disease
- Promoting arrhythmias

It is usually performed according to a standard protocol (e.g. Bruce or Naughton).

A positive exercise test for myocardial ischaemia is defined by a 1–2 mm horizontal or downsloping ST-segment depression occurring in two or more leads (Fig. 7.15). Beware of the false-positives that can occur:

- In the presence of pre-existing repolarization abnormalities at rest
- In the presence of certain drugs, such as digoxin
- In pre-excitation syndromes, such as Wolff–Parkinson–White (WPW) syndrome
- If there is upsloping (as opposed to horizontal or downsloping) ST-segment depression

Analysis of cardiac rhythm

1 24 h Ambulatory ECG
2 Cardiac memo (as below)
3 'Reveal device', which is a long-term recorder implanted under the skin of the chest and then removed for analysis of the rhythm disturbances some time later

Diagnostic imaging

Chest radiography

A chest radiograph allows an assessment of heart size. The transthoracic cardiac diameter is normally less than 50% of the transthoracic diameter. The normal heart contour consists of the inferior vena cava, the right atrial junction, the right atrial border at the junction between the right atrium and the SVC, the aortic knuckle, the pulmonary artery, the left atrium and the left ventricular border (Fig. 7.16).

In older patients, the ascending aorta can extend to constitute part of the right heart border. A ring of calcium may be seen in the aortic knuckle, but this does not necessarily represent atherosclerosis.

Echocardiography

Echocardiography is a non-invasive technique for analysing cardiac structure and function. It creates a real-time image of the heart, which is displayed on a television screen, allowing analysis of blood flow through the heart and its connections. Abnormalities of the endocardium (including heart valves and tumours), pericardium and

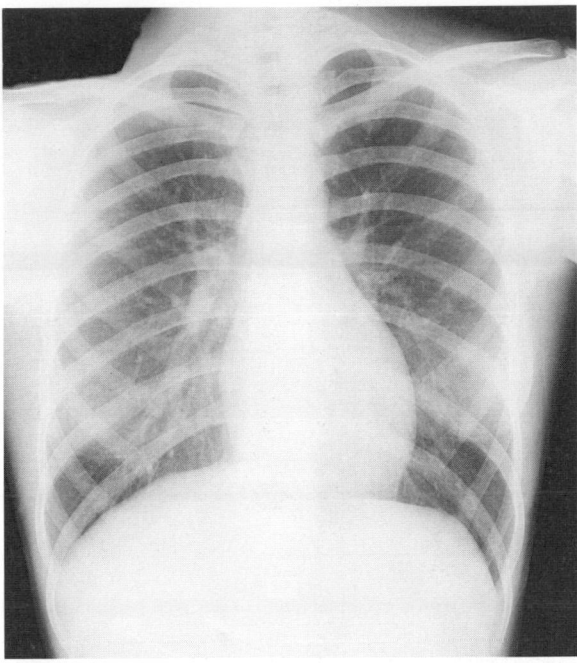

Figure 7.16 Normal cardiac contour on a posteroanterior (PA) chest radiograph.

myocardium can be identified, and chamber dimensions can be measured.

Ultrasound waves produced by electrically excited vibrating piezoelectric crystals on the head of a modern ultrasound transducer and received back by the same transducer visualize the heart. The higher the frequency of the ultrasound, the higher the quality of the image obtained. However, the higher frequencies do not penetrate far, so the higher frequencies (5–7 mHz; 1 mHz = 1 000 000 cycles/s) are used for neonates and children, and the lower frequencies (2–3 mHz) are used for adults.

As the ultrasound pulse enters the body it crosses tissue interfaces where some of the waves are reflected. Provided the angle of incidence of the wave to the tissue surface is approximately 90°, such reflected waves will return to the transducer. The distance of the tissue interface from the transducer can be estimated from the time delay between the generation of the pulse and the time of the arrival of the reflecting echo. The transducer head is kept stationary at any one time, but the ultrasound beam changes position, allowing analysis of all structures within a predetermined scanning arc.

The resultant electrical signals from the piezoelectric crystals are used to create a two-dimensional image of the heart on the television screen in real time, showing the structure of the heart and its movement. The images are recorded on videotape (Fig. 7.17).

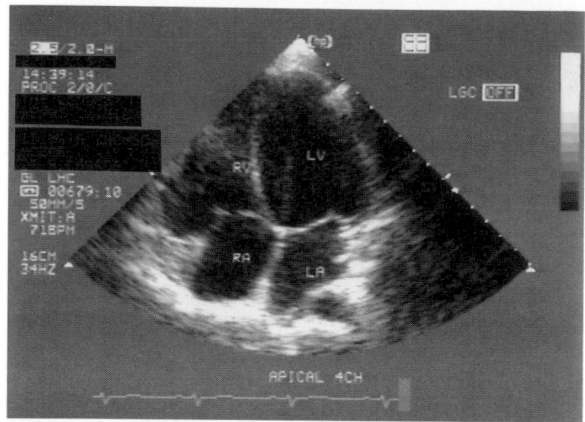

(a)

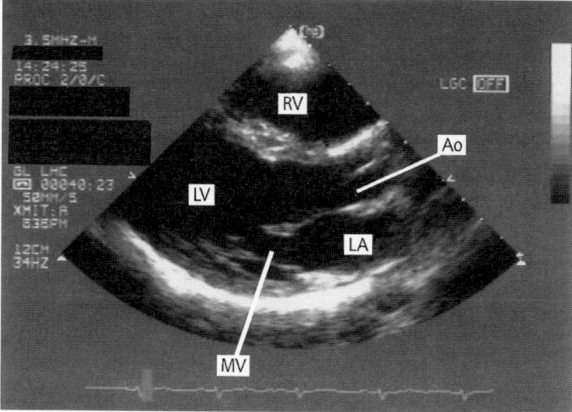

(b)

Figure 7.17 The normal two-dimensional echocardiogram. (a) Apical four chamber view; (b) normal long axis. Ao, aorta; MV, mitral valve.

M-mode recording

Ultrasound reflection from one particular beam direction can be processed onto paper moving at a particular speed. The movement of a structure of interest can therefore be carefully analysed: this is an M-mode recording (Fig. 7.18). Time markers and ECG signals are used to aid analysis.

Doppler techniques

The echo reflections described above are relatively strong and are used to produce images of the heart. If much higher amplification is used, the echo reflections detected are much weaker. This is useful for detecting echoes from red blood cells and allows the evaluation of blood flow through the heart.

The sound of a moving object changes as it passes a static listener. If an object produces a sound at a particular wavelength, it effectively catches up with the sound waves that it generates as it moves towards the listener, the wavelength shortens and the frequency of the sound appears higher than that originally generated. Similarly, when the object moves away from the listener, the wavelength lengthens and the frequency the listener hears is lower. The differences between the observed frequency and the original frequency is known as the Doppler shift (named after Christian Doppler) and is related to the speed of the object, the speed of sound and the generated frequency.

Two applications of the Doppler shift are used in investigating the heart:

1 Continuous wave Doppler
2 Pulse wave Doppler

Continuous wave Doppler ultrasound. In continuous wave Doppler ultrasound, the transducer continuously transmits sound waves into the tissue and another transducer continuously receives the reflected waves. The position of the blood flow under investigation cannot be localized because sound reflections from all depths are analysed simultaneously. However, this technique is extremely useful for measuring true velocity.

The velocity across a heart valve is related to the pressure difference across that valve. The Bernoulli equation describes this relationship and in practice this is modified to: pressure difference across the valve = $4 \times V^2$, where V is the velocity across the valve. Therefore, by measuring the velocity, the pressure gradient across the valve can be established (Fig. 7.19).

Pulse wave Doppler ultrasound. With pulse wave Doppler, a short burst of sound is emitted and a period of time is allowed to analyse the sound reflection. This technique is useful for localizing the depth of flow of interest, but cannot be used to measure high velocities. Computer technology in modern machines allows analysis of velocities at different depths.

Spectral tracings

Continuous wave Doppler signals or pulsed wave signals from distinct sample volumes at known depths can be displayed on paper in a similar way to M-mode echocardiograms. The velocity is plotted against time. By convention, velocities coming towards the transducer are plotted above the baseline and those away from the transducer are plotted below the baseline. These recordings are called spectral tracings and are used to measure the peak and mean velocities, and therefore the peak and mean pressure gradients across valves.

Transoesophageal echocardiography

The heart can be imaged from the oesophagus (transoesophageal echocardiography) to evaluate certain

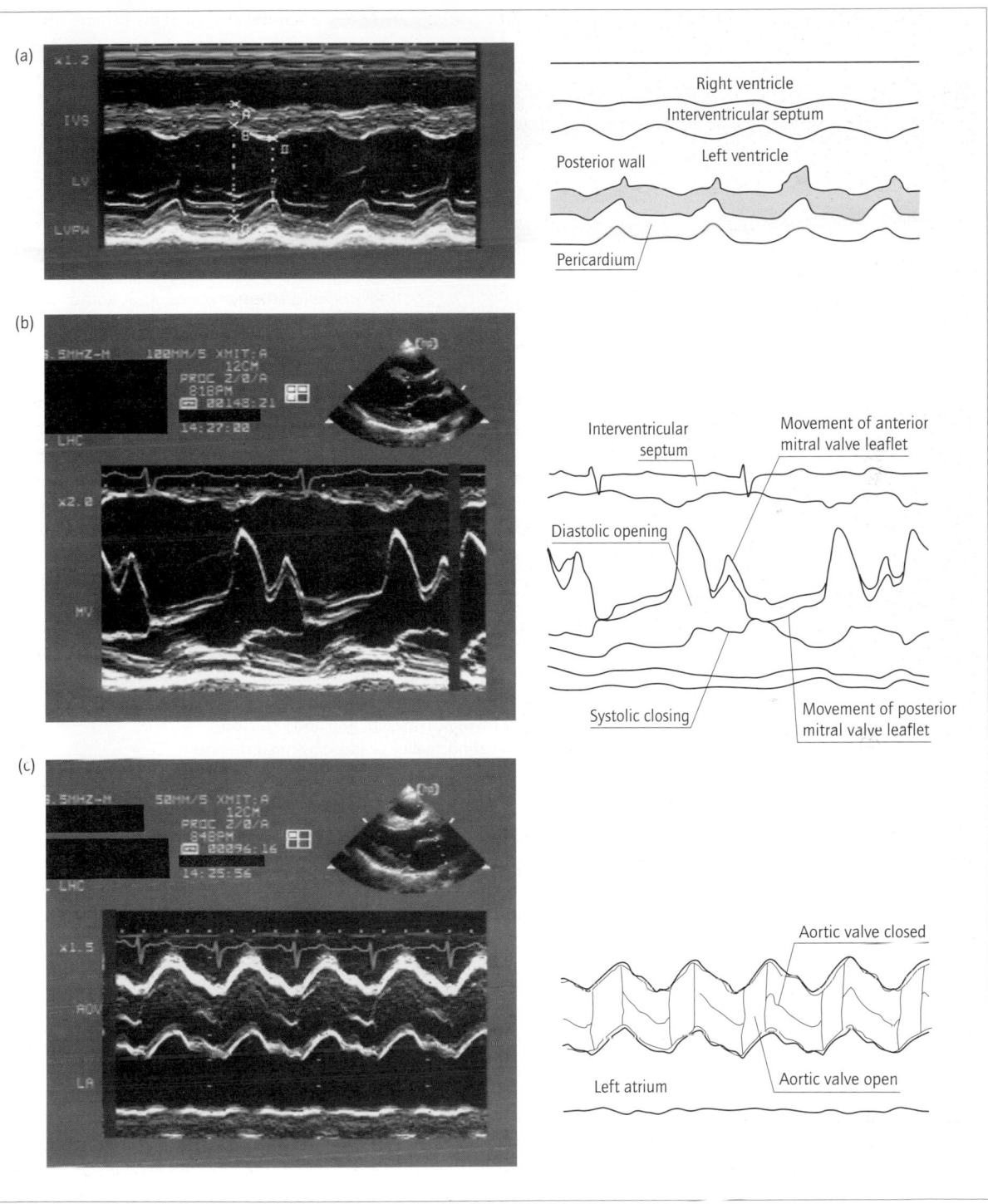

Figure 7.18 The normal M-mode echocardiogram. (a) Normal left ventricle; (b) normal mitral valve; (c) normal aortic valve and left atrium.

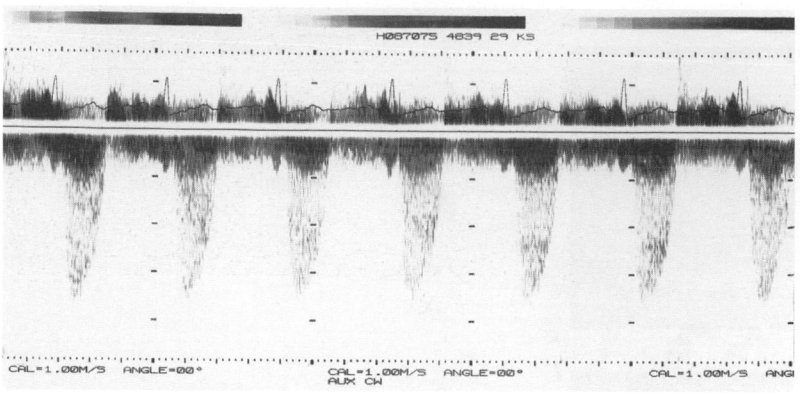

Figure 7.19 Measuring pressure gradients across valves using continuous wave Doppler ultrasound. The peak velocity is 3.5 m/s giving a pressure difference (gradient) across the aortic valve of 49 mmHg.

Table 7.8 Clinical applications of echocardiography

Type of disorder	Indication
Valvular heart disease	To diagnose the aetiology and severity of stenotic and regurgitant valves (e.g. mitral prolapse, rheumatic valvular heart disease, aortic stenosis)
	To diagnose endocarditis by the presence of vegetations (but the absence of vegetations on the echocardiogram does not exclude it)
	To estimate the peak pulmonary artery pressure by applying Bernoulli's equation to the velocity of the regurgitant jet in functional tricuspid regurgitation, which is often present on the right side of the heart
	To assess prosthetic valve function
	To locate regurgitant leaks
Heart muscle function	To assess the quality of myocardial systolic and diastolic function
	To diagnose ventricular hypertrophy
	To diagnose hypertrophic cardiomyopathy (see p. 486 and Fig. 7.66)
	To diagnose regional wall motion abnormalities caused by heart disease
	To diagnose ventricular thrombus
Aortic disease	To diagnose aortic aneurysms and dissections, particularly by the use of the transoesophageal approach
	To monitor the progression of aortic root dilatation in Marfan's syndrome
Congenital heart disease	To diagnose congenital heart disease in neonates, infants and children (has virtually replaced cardiac catheterization)
	To diagnose adult congenital heart disease
	To monitor adult congenital heart disease
Other lesions	To assess pericardial effusions and intracardiac tumours (see Fig. 7.68)

structures in more detail. A small transducer is placed on the tip of the standard gastroscope and is inserted into the oesophagus using standard endoscopic techniques. As with the gastroscope, its tip can be moved forward and backward and side to side, and modern probes have either two transducers (one to provide a transverse section and one to provide a longitudinal section) or a single rotating transducer. High-quality image acquisition in multiple planes is therefore possible with incorporated colour flow mapping and other Doppler techniques.

Clinical applications of echocardiography

Echocardiography is a safe and reproducible technique,

and is therefore often used to assess structural heart disease (Table 7.8).

● In non-ischaemic cardiac disease it is a valuable way of assessing structure and function, and repeated echocardiograms during the course of an illness provide objective measurements of the progress of the disease.

● Colour flow mapping is very useful for identifying abnormalities such as atrial and ventricular septal defects, patent ductus arteriosus (PDA) and other more complex abnormalities.

● A Doppler profile across a coarctation can establish the gradient across the lesion.

The transoesophageal technique is particularly useful in

adolescent and adult patients. At present, echocardiography is unable to visualize the coronary arteries to a clinically useful extent.

Colour flow echocardiography

Using continuous wave Doppler ultrasound, blood flow within the heart can be analysed and colour coded according to the direction within each sampling volume. The resulting colour flow map can then be superimposed on a two-dimensional image (colour flow mapping). This is an extremely useful technique for localizing the source of jets of blood and their spatial distribution. The images are created using the convention that blood flow towards the transducer is coded in hues of red and blood flow away from the transducer is coded in hues of blue.

Nuclear studies

Thallium and cardiolite scintigraphy

Myocardial perfusion can be assessed using the potassium analogue thallium-201. Thallium is taken up by viable perfused myocardium when given on exercise, or with the administration of the vasodilator, dipyridamole.

Scanning visualizes areas of myocardial ischaemia or permanent myocardial damage as cold unperfused spots. If a cold spot disappears on further scanning 3 h later it represents an area of reversible ischaemia (Fig. 7.20).

Multiple-gated acquisition scans (MUGA)

Technetium-99 can be injected into the blood where it is taken up by red cells. Imaging with a gamma camera then allows an assessment of:
- Ventricular function, including regional wall movement abnormalities
- Valve regurgitation
- Accurate measurements of the ventricular ejection fraction

Cardiac catheterization (Table 7.9)

Under radiographical control, fine-bore catheters can be introduced into the artery and veins of the elbow (brachial approach) or groin (femoral approach) and passed into all the chambers of the heart. Pressure measurements can be made and the shape and function of the chambers can be assessed by introducing a radio-opaque dye.

The left atrium is reached by a trans-septal puncture from the right atrium. Left atrial pressure can also be measured indirectly by wedging a catheter in the pulmonary arterioles (pulmonary wedge pressure). Various examples of abnormal haemodynamic data are given in Table 7.10.

Angiography

Angiography is a technique in which radio-opaque dye is

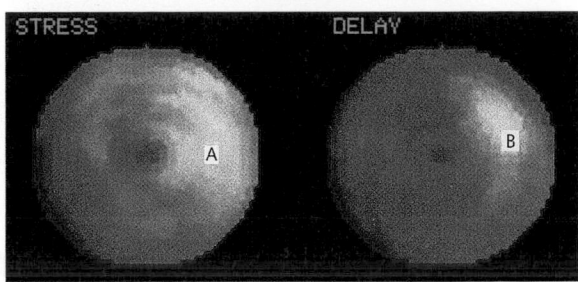

(a)

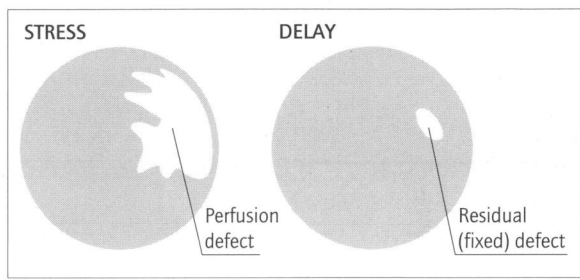

(b)

Figure 7.20 (a) Thallium scan visualizing myocardial ischaemia. A, a perfusion defect is seen on the stress image with reperfusion on the delayed image indicating reversible ischaemia. B, the residual defect on the delayed image indicates previous infarction. (b) Line representations of the scans.

Table 7.9 Indications for cardiac catherization

1	To assess presence and severity of coronary disease
2	Measure left ventricular function—when echo result is uncertain
3	Assess valvular disease
4	Measure intracardiac pressures and oxygen saturation

Table 7.10 Abnormal haemodynamic data

Disorder	Effect on haemodynamic data
Aortic stenosis	Higher peak systolic pressure in the left ventricle compared to the aorta
Pulmonary stenosis	Higher peak systolic pressure in the right ventricle than the pulmonary artery
Mitral stenosis	Higher pressure in the left atrium at the end of diastole than in the left ventricle
Tricuspid stenosis	Higher pressure in the right atrium at the end of diastole than in the right ventricle

injected either by hand or using a power injector into part of the circulation.

Aortogram

An aortogram demonstrates aortic regurgitation, aortic dissection and coarctation of the aorta.

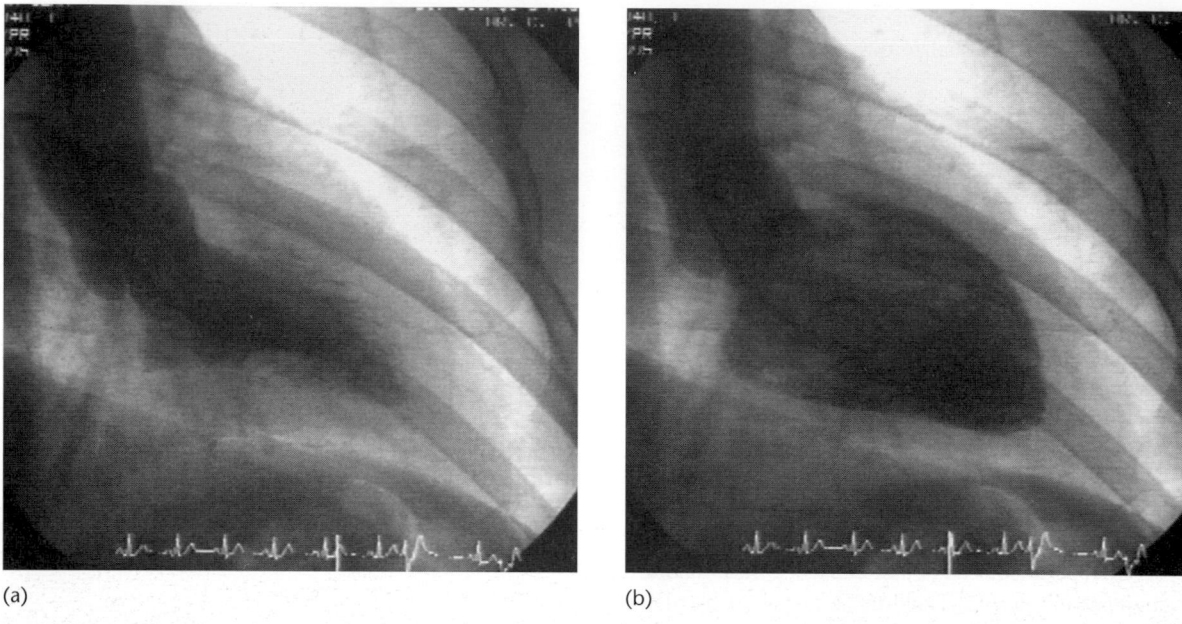

Figure 7.21 Normal left ventricular angiogram: (a) systole; (b) diastole.

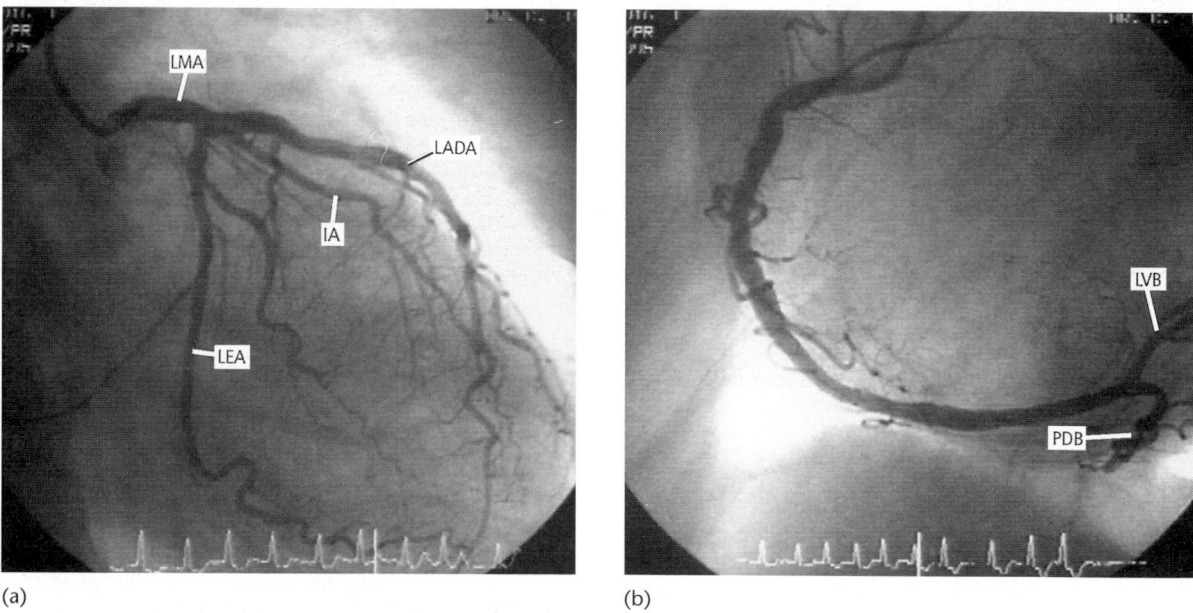

(a)   (b)

Figure 7.22 (a) Normal left and (b) right selective coronary arteriogram. IA, intermediate artery; LADA, left anterior descending artery; LCFA, left circumflex artery; LMA, left main artery; LVB, left ventricular branch; PDB, posterior descending branch.

Left ventricular angiogram

A left ventricular angiogram demonstrates the quality of left ventricular function, and allows identification and quantification of mitral regurgitation, a left ventricular aneurysm or a ventricular septal defect (Fig. 7.21).

Selective coronary arteriography (Fig. 7.22)

The origin of each coronary artery can be cannulated to allow visualization of coronary artery narrowings.

Measuring cardiac output

Cardiac output can be measured using a thermodilution technique with a Swan–Ganz catheter. This is advanced through a central vein into the pulmonary artery. Ice-cold saline is introduced at a standard rate into the right atrium through a proximal hole in the catheter, and its arrival in the pulmonary artery is detected by a thermistor at the distal end of the catheter.

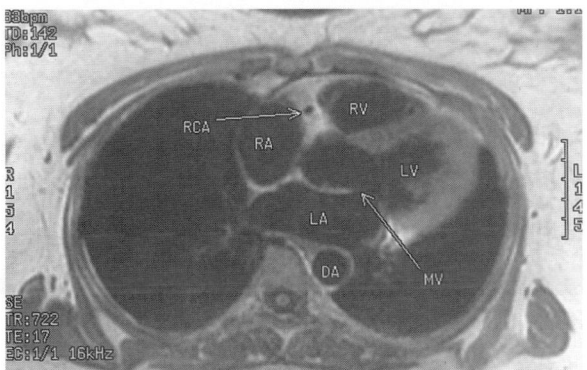 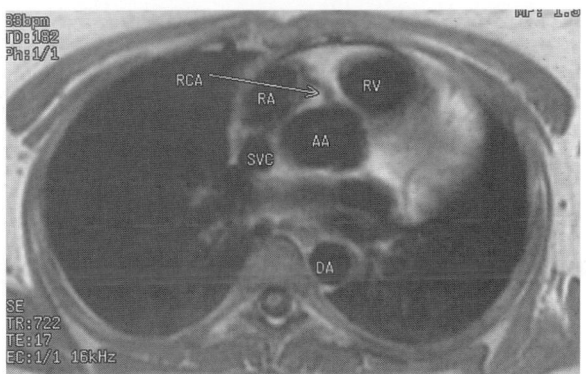

Figure 7.23 T1-weighted spin echo axial MRI scans of the chest. AA, ascending aorta; DA, descending aorta; RCA, right coronary artery; SVC, superior vena cava.

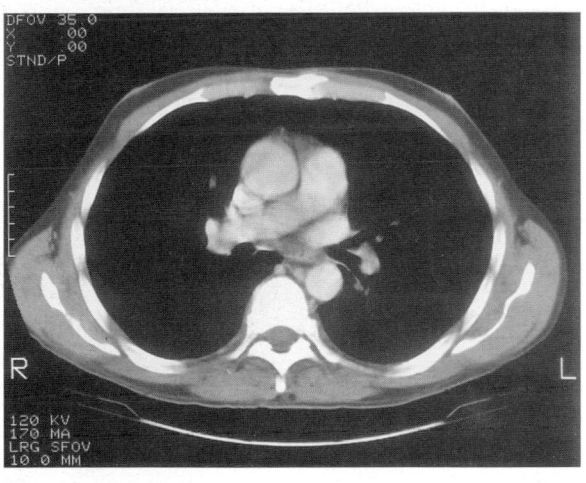 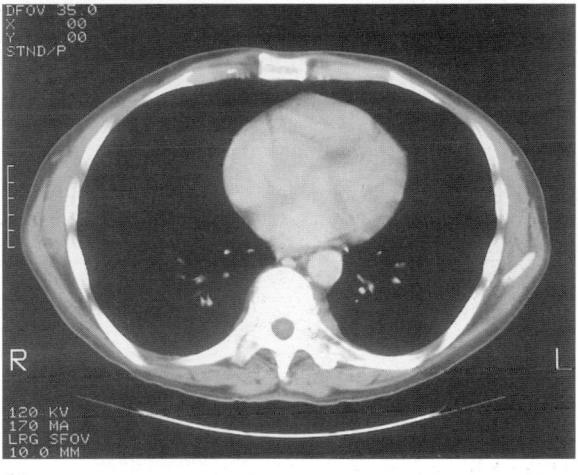

(a) (b)

Figure 7.24 Computerized tomography (CT) scan of the chest showing. (a) great vessels, ascending aorta, descending aorta, and right and left main pulmonary arteries; and (b) heart and descending aorta.

Measuring oxygen saturation and metabolites

Blood samples can also be taken for measuring oxygen saturations and metabolites (such as lactate) in the various chambers of the heart. This allows identification and quantification of intracardiac shunts.

Electrophysiological studies of the heart

Introducing electrodes into the right atrium, right ventricle and coronary sinus allows characterization of the electrical activity of the heart. The time delays in electrical activity of the heart can be measured and pathological arrhythmias can be stimulated.

Magnetic resonance imaging

Magnetic resonance imaging (MRI) is a relatively new non-invasive imaging technique that avoids the use of radiation (Fig. 7.23). A magnetic field influences the protons in the hydrogen atoms and then a radiofrequency emission distorts them. When the emission stops, the hydrogen atoms release energy, which can be reconstituted as an image. This technique is very useful for looking at the great vessels in the thorax, the pericardium and the lungs. Synchronization with the ECG allows cardiac images to be obtained in systole and diastole.

Computed tomography scanning

This can also provide good pictures of intrathoracic structures (Fig. 7.24).

Principles of management

The advice given to patients includes not only specific treatments such as drugs and surgery, but also more general advice as to how to adapt their lifestyle to accommodate their symptoms and to try to delay or prevent deterioration in the future. The object should be to get the patient's health

07

back to a state where they can lead the sort of life they wish. To tell a man whose angina is preventing him from working that he must find an alternative job is often unhelpful.

Advice about modifying risk factors is clearly important but should be given sympathetically to those who find it difficult to give up smoking, lose weight or change their diet. 'Healthy living' now involves:

- Not smoking
- Avoiding too much fat (especially saturated fat) and sugar in the diet
- Avoiding excessive weight
- Taking regular exercise
- Minimizing stress
- Occasional 'screening' measurement of blood pressure and cholesterol level

Specific treatment

Drug therapy

There are ever-increasing numbers of drugs available for treating heart disease. They can both improve symptoms and prolong survival. Examples of the latter are beta-blockers following myocardial infarction, and angiotensin-converting enzyme (ACE) inhibitors in heart failure. All drugs, without exception, can cause side-effects and so both the type of drug and its dosage should be tailored to the individual patient. This may require regular monitoring in the initial stages. The problem of drug compliance (the patient remembering or being prepared to take the drug) is underestimated. Therefore drugs that need only be taken once a day are desirable.

BOXES 7.2–7.7 present brief information relating to some of the commonly used drugs in heart disease. However, this information—especially that relating to side-effects and contraindications—is not complete. Fuller information is given in a formulary [e.g. *British National Formulary (BNF)*]. Dose regimens should also be checked in the *BNF*.

Surgical treatment

Cardiac surgery is now commonplace for both ischaemic

Box 7.2: Drugs for heart failure

(See pp. 425–433 for a general discussion)

Diuretics

Bendrofluazide (bendroflumethiazide)

Action. A thiazide diuretic. Inhibits sodium reabsorption at the beginning of the distal convoluted tubule. A moderately potent diuretic. Acts within 1–2 h of oral administration and duration of action is 12–24 h

Indications. Mild or moderate heart failure when the patient is not too ill and pulmonary oedema is not severe

Side-effects. Impotence (reversible on withdrawing the drug), hypokalaemia, hypomagnesaemia, hyponatraemia, hypochloraemic alkalosis, hyperuricaemia, gout, hyperglycaemia, increases in plasma cholesterol levels; rarely, rashes, photosensitivity, neutropenia, thrombocytopenia

Cautions. Aggravates diabetes mellitus and gout; pregnancy and breastfeeding; renal and hepatic impairment; porphyria.

Contraindications. Hypercalcaemia, severe renal and hepatic impairment, Addison's disease

Frusemide (furosemide)

Action. A loop diuretic. Inhibits resorption from the ascending loop of Henle. A powerful diuretic. Acts within

1 h of oral administration and diuresis is complete within 6 h. Peak effect within 30 min of intravenous administration

Indications. Pulmonary oedema caused by left ventricular failure and long-standing heart failure in patients who no longer respond to thiazides

Side-effects. Hyponatraemia, hypokalaemia, hypochloraemic alkalosis, increased calcium excretion, hypotension; less commonly, nausea, gastrointestinal disturbances, hyperuricaemia, gout, hyperglycaemia, temporary increase in plasma cholesterol and triglyceride levels; rarely, rashes and bone marrow depression, pancreatitis (with large parenteral doses), tinnitus and deafness (usually with large parenteral doses and rapid administration, and in renal impairment)

Cautions. Pregnancy; aggravates diabetes mellitus and gout; liver failure; prostatic enlargement; porphyria

Contraindications. Precomatose states associated with liver cirrhosis

Patient monitoring. Avoid hypotension. Watch out for urinary retention if the patient has an enlarged prostate

Spironolactone

Action. Potassium-sparing diuretic. Potentiates thiazide and loop diuretics by antagonizing aldosterone

Indications. Congestive heart failure, particularly when there is congestion of the liver

Side-effects. Gastrointestinal disturbances, gynaecomastia, hyperkalaemia, hyponatraemia

Cautions. Potential human metabolic products are carcinogenic in rodents; the elderly; hepatic impairment; renal impairment; porphyria

Contraindications. Hyperkalaemia, hyponatraemia, severe renal impairment, pregnancy and breastfeeding, Addison's disease

Patient monitoring. Monitor electrolytes. Discontinue if hypokalaemic

ACE inhibitors
Captopril
Action. Inhibits conversion of angiotensin I to angiotensin II

Indications. As an adjunct in congestive cardiac failure

Side-effects. Persistent dry cough, throat discomfort, voice changes, loss of taste, sore mouth, abdominal pain, rash, angioedema, hypotension; proteinuria, thrombocytopenia, neutropenia, agranulocytosis, hyperkalaemia (all more common in renal impairment); increases in liver enzymes, liver damage, cholestatic jaundice; renal impairment; pancreatitis

Cautions. Diuretics; first doses commonly cause a profound and potentially serious hypotension especially in those taking diuretics, on a low-sodium diet, on dialysis or dehydrated; avoid in dialysis patients using high-flux polyacrylonitrile membranes (associated with anaphylactoid reactions)

Contraindications. Hypersensitivity to ACE inhibitors; known or suspected renovascular disease; aortic stenosis or outflow tract obstruction; pregnancy; porphyria

Patient monitoring. Monitor initiation of treatment in hospital if first-dose hypotension is likely (e.g. if taking a large dose of diuretic, if hyponatraemic, if already hypotensive, if there is renal impairment, if on high-dose vasodilator therapy, if over 70 years of age); monitor renal function before and during treatment (reduce dose or avoid in renal impairment); white cell counts and urinary protein estimations in renal impairment

Positive inotropic drugs
Digoxin
Action. Increases the force of myocardial contraction and reduces conductivity of the heart. May improve heart failure because of changes in the availability of intracellular calcium

Indication. Heart failure. Can usually be withdrawn from patients with well-controlled heart failure unless needed to maintain a satisfactory rhythm (THERAPEUTICS BOX 7.4)

Side-effects. Usually associated with excessive dosage and include: anorexia, nausea, vomiting, diarrhoea, abdominal pain, visual disturbance, headache, fatigue, drowsiness, confusion, delirium, hallucinations, arrhythmias, heart block

Cautions. Recent infarction, hypothyroidism; reduce dose in the elderly and in renal impairment; avoid hypokalaemia

Contraindications. Supraventricular arrhythmias caused by the Wolff–Parkinson–White syndrome

Patient monitoring. Plasma digoxin (taken at least 6 h after a dose) and potassium concentration if there are any apparent side-effects

Dobutamine
Action. Acts on beta-1 receptors in cardiac muscle and increases contractility with little effect on rate

Indication. Cardiogenic shock

Side-effects. Tachycardia and a marked increase in blood pressure indicate overdosage

Cautions. Severe hypotension complicating cardiogenic shock

Vasodilators
Glyceryl trinitrate
Action. A potent vasodilator, but its main benefit results from a reduction in venous return, thereby reducing left ventricular work. Effect lasts 20–30 min

Indications. Left ventricular failure

Side-effects. Throbbing headache, flushing, dizziness, postural hypotension, tachycardia

Cautions. Hypotensive conditions (avoid intravenous administration); tolerance

Contraindications. Moderate–severe anaemia, head injury, cerebral haemorrhage, closed-angle glaucoma

Isosorbide dinitrate
Action. A vasodilator. Effect is slower in onset than that of glyceryl trinitrate, but may persist for several hours. Modified release preparations may act for up to 12 h

Indications. Left ventricular failure

Side-effects, cautions and contraindications. As for glyceryl trinitrate

Recommended adult doses
Bendrofluazide. Initially 2.5–10 mg/day or on alternate days, in the morning

07

Frusemide (furosemide). Oral, initially 40 mg in the morning. Maintenance, 20–40 mg, increased in resistant oedema to 80 mg/day. Intravenous injection (rate not exceeding 4 mg/min), initially 40–80 mg

Spironolactone. 50–200 mg/day, increased to 400 mg/day if necessary

Captopril. Initially 6.25–12.5 mg 3 times/day under close medical supervision. Usual maintenance dose, 25 mg 2–3 times/day

Digoxin. 125–250 µg twice daily for about a week, followed by a once-daily regimen

Dobutamine. Intravenous infusion, 2.5–20 µg/kg/min adjusted according to response

Glyceryl trinitrate. Sublingual: 0.3–1 mg, repeated as required. Oral: 2.6–6.4 mg as modified release tablets, 2–3 times/day. Intravenous infusion: 10–200 µg/min

Isosorbide dinitrate. Sublingual: 5–10 mg. Oral: 40–160 mg up to 240 mg/day in divided doses. Intravenous infusion: 2–10 mg/h

---

Box 7.3: Notes on drugs known to improve survival following infarction

Beta-blockers
Long-term use of beta-blockers, possibly for as long as 10 years, improves the prognosis. This is probably a generic effect of the drugs rather than specific to any one beta-blocker. The way this benefical effect is achieved is not clear because of the multiple effects of beta-blockers. It may be because they lower blood pressure or reduce ventricular arrhythmias or reduce myocardial ischaemia

Aspirin
Meta-analysis of studies evaluating aspirin following myocardial infarction shows an unequivocal improvement in prognosis, with mortality being reduced by 20%

ACE inhibitors
Studies of the use of these drugs in patients with reduced ejection fractions (below 45%) following infarction have shown an improved prognosis. The effect of offloading the damaged ventricle allows it to remodel and reduces the incidence of patients developing severe heart failure

Antiarrhythmic drugs
Although the beneficial effect of beta-blockers may be partly because of their antiarrhythmic effect, other antiarrhythmic drugs have not yet been shown to be of benefit. When patients present with malignant arrhythmias, their use may be indicated after careful evaluation by electrophysiological study. In patients who present with late ventricular fibrillation following myocardial infarction, an automatic implantable cardiac defibrillator may be indicated

---

Box 7.4: Diuretics

Loop diuretics (e.g. frusemide and bumetanide)
Block sodium resorption in the ascending loop of Henle and cause a brisk diuresis
The most powerful diuretics

Thiazide diuretics (e.g. hydrochlorothiazide)
Block sodium absorption in the proximal tubule
A less powerful effect and can cause greater potassium loss than loop diuretics
Metolazone is a particularly powerful thiazide diuretic when used in combination with a loop diuretic. It is, therefore, useful in refractory heart failure, especially if there is ascites

Potassium-sparing diuretics (e.g. spironolactone, triamterene, amiloride)
Weak diuretics and are usually used in combination with either thiazide or loop diuretics
Avoid in patients with renal failure because of their potassium-preserving effect

Spironolactone
An aldosterone antagonist and therefore has a potassium-sparing action
Useful if there is secondary hyperaldosteronism, which usually occurs in right heart failure

Amiloride and triamterene
Act on the distal tubule preventing potassium secretion

Box 7.5: Drugs for arrhythmias

(See pp. 448–454 for a general discussion)

Supraventricular arrhythmias

Digoxin

Action. Increases the force of myocardial contraction and reduces conductivity of the heart

Indication. Supraventricular arrhythmias, especially atrial fibrillation

Side-effects. Usually associated with excessive dosage and include anorexia, nausea, vomiting, diarrhoea, abdominal pain; visual disturbance, headache, fatigue, drowsiness, confusion, delirium, hallucinations; arrhythmias, heart block

Cautions. Recent infarction, hypothyroidism; reduce dose in the elderly and in renal impairment; avoid hypokalaemia

Contraindications. Supraventricular arrhythmias caused by the Wolff–Parkinson–White (WPW) syndrome

Patient monitoring. Plasma digoxin (taken at least 6 h after a dose) and potassium concentration if there are any apparent side-effects

Verapamil

Action. A calcium-channel blocker that reduces cardiac output, slows the heart rate and may impair AV conduction

Indications. Supraventricular arrhythmias

Cautions. First-degree AV block; acute phase of myocardial infarction (avoid if there is bradycardia, hypotension, left ventricular failure); concomitant administration of beta-blockers; reduce dose in hepatic impairment; children (seek specialist advice first); pregnancy and breastfeeding

Side-effects. Constipation. Less commonly, nausea, vomiting, flushing, headache, dizziness, fatigue, ankle oedema. Rarely, reversible impairment of liver function, allergic reactions (erythema, pruritus). Rarely after long-term treatment, gynaecomastia and gingival hypertrophy. After intravenous administration, hypotension, bradycardia, heart block and asystole

Contraindications. Hypotension, bradycardia, second- and third-degree AV block, sick sinus syndrome, cardiogenic shock, sinoatrial block, history of heart failure or significantly impaired left ventricular function (even if controlled by therapy), atrial flutter or fibrillation complicating WPW syndrome, porphyria. Do not use with beta-blockers, and do not inject into patients recently treated with beta-blockers because of the risk of hypotension and asystole. It may be hazardous to give verapamil and a beta-blocker together orally and this should only be contemplated if myocardial function is preserved. It should not be used for tachyarrhythmias where the QRS complex is wide unless a supraventricular origin has been established, and is also contraindicated in atrial fibrillation with pre-excitation (e.g. WPW syndrome), when amiodarone should be used instead

Patient monitoring. ECG monitoring during intravenous administration

Supraventricular and ventricular arrhythmias

Disopyramide

Indications. Ventricular arrhythmias, especially after myocardial infarction, supraventricular arrhythmias

Side-effects. Myocardial depression, hypotension, AV block, antimuscarinic effects (dry mouth, blurred vision, urinary retention)

Cautions. Glaucoma, heart failure (avoid if severe), prostatic enlargement, hepatic and renal impairment, elderly, pregnancy

Contraindications. Second and third degree heart block and sinus node dysfunction (unless a pacemaker is fitted); cardiogenic shock; severe uncompensated heart failure

Patient monitoring. ECG monitoring during intravenous administration

Ventricular arrhythmias

Lidocaine (lignocaine)

Indications. Ventricular arrhythmias, especially after myocardial infarction. Should be considered first in emergency use

Side-effects. Confusion, convulsions

Cautions. Lower dose in congestive cardiac failure, in hepatic failure, and following cardiac surgery

Contraindications. Sinoatrial disorders, all grades of AV block, severe myocardial depression, porphyria

Patient monitoring. ECG monitoring during administration

Sinus bradycardia

Atropine

Action. Antimuscarinic drug

Indications. Reversal of haemodynamically important bradycardia

Side-effects. Tachycardia

Cautions. Cardiovascular disease

Recommended adult doses

Digoxin. Rapid oral digitalization: 1–1.5 mg in divided doses over 24 h. Less urgent digitalization: 250–500 µg over 24 h, the higher dose in divided doses. Maintenance: 62.5–500 µg/day, the higher dose in divided doses. For atrial fibrillation the maintenance dose can usually be governed by the ventricular response, which should not fall below 60 beats/min except in special circumstances (e.g. with the concomitant administration of beta-blockers). Intravenous, for very rapid control. Give digitalizing dose of 0.75–1 mg, preferably as an infusion in a 50 ml volume, over 2 or more hours, followed by oral maintenance therapy

Verapamil. Oral: 40–120 mg 3 times/day. Slow intravenous injection over 2 min (3 min in the elderly), 5–10 mg

(preferably with ECG monitoring). A further 5 mg after 5–10 min if required for paroxysmal tachyarrhythmias

Disopyramide. Oral: 300–800 mg/day in divided doses. Slow intravenous injection: 2 mg/kg over at least 5 min to a maximum of 150 mg, with ECG monitoring, followed immediately by *either* 200 mg orally and then 200 mg every 8 h for 24 h; *or* 400 µg/kg/h by intravenous infusion. Maximum doses: 300 mg in the first hour and 800 mg/day

Lidocaine. Intravenous injection in patients who do not have gross circulatory impairment: 50–100 mg as a bolus over a few minutes, followed by an infusion of 2–4 mg/min

Atropine. Intravenous: initial dose of 600 µg, increasing to 1–2 mg if necessary

---

Box 7.6: Drugs for angina and ischaemic heart disease

(See pp. 414–419 for a general discussion)

Nitrates

Glyceryl trinitrate

Action. A potent vasodilator, but its main benefit results from a reduction in venous return, thereby reducing left ventricular work. Effect lasts 20–30 min

Indications. Prophylaxis and treatment of angina

Side-effects. Throbbing headache, flushing, dizziness, postural hypotension, tachycardia

Cautions. Hypotensive conditions (avoid intravenous administration); tolerance

Contraindications. Moderate–severe anaemia, head injury, cerebral haemorrhage, closed-angle glaucoma

Isosorbide mononitrate

Action. A vasodilator. Effect is slower in onset than that of glyceryl trinitrate, but may persist for several hours. Modified release preparations may act for up to 12 h

Indications. Prophylaxis and treatment of angina

Side-effects, cautions and contraindications. As for glyceryl trinitrate

Beta-blockers

Contraindications. The Committee on Safety of Medicines advises that beta-blockers, even those with apparent cardio-selectivity, should not be used in patients with asthma or a history of obstructive airway disease unless no alternative treatment is available. In such cases, the risk of inducing bronchospasm

should be appreciated and appropriate precautions should be taken

Atenolol

Action. A cardioselective beta-blocker

Indications. Angina; as a slow intravenous injection immediately following a myocardial infarction

Side-effects. Bradycardia, heart failure, bronchospasm, peripheral vasoconstriction, gastrointestinal disturbances, fatigue, sleep disturbances; rarely, rashes and dry eyes (reversible on withdrawal)

Cautions. Late pregnancy and breastfeeding; avoid abrupt withdrawal in angina; reduce dose in renal impairment; liver function deteriorates in portal hypertension; diabetes mellitus; myasthenia gravis; dangerous interaction with verapamil

Contraindications. Asthma or a history of obstructive airway disease, uncontrolled heart failure, sick sinus syndrome, second or third degree heart block, cardiogenic shock

Calcium antagonists

Nifedipine

Action. Relaxes vascular smooth muscle and dilates coronary and peripheral arteries

Indications. Prophylaxis and treatment of angina

Side-effects. Headache, flushing, dizziness, lethargy; also gravitational oedema, rash, nausea, increased frequency of micturition, eye pain, gum hyperplasia; reported depression, telangiectasia

Cautions. Withdraw if existing pain worsens shortly after starting treatment; heart failure or significantly impaired left ventricular function; severe hypotension; reduce dose in hepatic impairment; diabetes mellitus; may inhibit labour; breastfeeding

Contraindications. Cardiogenic shock, advanced aortic stenosis, pregnancy, porphyria

Antithrombotic drugs
Aspirin
Action. Reduces platelet stickiness

Indications. Prophylaxis of myocardial infarction

Side-effects. Bronchospasm, gastrointestinal haemorrhage (occasionally major), also other haemorrhages (e.g. subconjunctival)

Cautions. Asthma, uncontrolled hypertension, pregnancy

Contraindications. Breastfeeding and children under 12 years of age because of the risk of Reye's syndrome, active peptic ulceration, haemophilia and other bleeding disorders

Streptokinase
Action. Activates plasminogen to form plasmin, which degrades fibrin and so breaks up thrombi

Indications. Acute myocardial infarction. Acute pulmonary embolism

Side-effects. Anaphylactic reaction with hypotension and purpuric rash. Occasionally, severe myolysis and renal failure

Cautions. Known haemorrhagic diathesis (e.g. active peptic ulcer). Patients on oral anticoagulants. Hypotension

Contraindications. Previous treatment with streptokinase

Recommended adult doses
Glyceryl trinitrate. Sublingual: 0.3–1 mg, repeated as required. Oral: 2.6–6.4 mg as modified release tablets, 2–3 times/day; severe angina, 10 mg 3 times/day. Intravenous infusion: 10–200 µg/min

Isosorbide mononitrate. Oral, initially 20 mg 2–3 times/day *or* 40 mg twice daily (10 mg twice daily in those who have not had nitrates before), up to 120 mg/day in divided doses

Atenolol. Oral: 25–100 mg/day in 1 or 2 doses. Slow intravenous injection: 5 mg

Nifedipine. Oral: initially 10 mg (5 mg for the elderly) 3 times/day with or after food. Usual maintenance: 5–20 mg 3 times/day. For an immediate effect in angina, bite into capsule and swallow the liquid. Modified release, dose varies according to brand

Aspirin. Oral: 300 mg

Streptokinase. 1.5 million units intravenous infusion over 1 h

---

Box 7.7: Antiarrhythmic drugs

Vaughan Williams classification
Classification according to the effect on the action potential (Fig. 7.51a)

Class I drugs
Limit sodium entry into the myocardial cell and therefore reduce spontaneous discharge rate of the cells. Subdivided into those that lengthen the action potential (class Ia), those that shorten it (class Ib) and those that have no effect on its duration (class Ic)

Class II drugs
Beta-blockers inhibiting the effect of the circulating catecholamines on the action potential

Class III drugs
Prolong the action potential without affecting sodium transport through the cell

Class IV drugs: calcium antagonists
These reduce the plateau phase of the action potential by antagonizing calcium transport across the cell membrane and within the intracellular cytoplasmic reticulum. They particularly affect the SA and AV node. Not all calcium antagonist drugs have the same antiarrhythmic effect because their molecular structure is very different. Nifedipine has minimal electrophysiological effect, whereas verapamil has a powerful and important antiarrhythmic role. Diltiazem has a lesser electrophysiological effect and both it and verapamil have important negative inotropic effects

Classification according to the site of action
Antiarrhythmic drugs can be classified according to their site of action (Fig. 7.51b)

heart disese and valve disease and, like drugs, both relieves symptoms and prolongs survival. It is usual to delay surgery until drugs have been tried but there are certain situations where surgery should be offered because of its advantages over drugs (e.g. in left main coronary artery disease) in improving prognosis as well as symptoms.

Interventional techniques

Interventional techniques whereby therapeutic procedures can be carried out using long catheters have been introduced over the last 25 years. These include:

- Percutaneous transluminal coronary intervention (PCI) with or without stent insertion
- Mitral valvuloplasty
- Radiofrequency ablation

This is a fast moving area with frequent advances in the technology with more being achievable without resorting to open heart surgery.

Diseases and their management

Ischaemic heart disease

Epidemiology

Prevalence. Atherosclerosis of the coronary arteries is the main cause of death in developed countries. The incidence is highest in Finland and the UK. Although the incidence is falling in the USA, the reduction in the UK has been less, with 30% of men and 20% of women dying from ischaemic heart disease.

Sex. Premature coronary disease is more common in men, but after the menopause the incidence in women increases to approach that of men of the same age.

Age. The incidence of coronary heart disease rises with age, although atherosclerosis can be identified in autopsies on teenagers and young adults.

Genetics. Premature coronary artery disease undoubtedly runs in families, but there is no established pattern. In the absence of other risk factors, a history of ischaemic heart disease increases the risk of ischaemic heart disease in offspring by 20–30%.

Disease mechanisms

Myocardial ischaemia results from an imbalance between myocardial oxygen supply and demand. The causes of a reduced coronary blood flow, which leads to a reduced supply of oxygen and other essential substrates, are listed in Table 7.11. The most common cause of reduced coronary blood flow is atheroma. Coronary artery spasm is

Table 7.11 Causes of a reduced coronary blood flow

Atheroma
Spasm
Thromboembolism
Coronary arteritis (including coronary ostial arteritis caused by syphilis)

Ischaemic heart disease at a glance

Epidemiology

Prevalence
Main cause of death in developed countries. Incidence is falling in the USA, but less so in the UK, with 30% of men and 20% of women dying from ischaemic heart disease

Age
Incidence rises with age

Sex
Premature coronary disease is more common in men, but after the menopause the incidence in women increases to approach that of men of the same age

Genetics
Premature coronary artery disease runs in families, but there is

no established pattern. In the absence of other risk factors, a family history increases the risk in offspring by 20–30%

Geography
Highest in Finland and the UK

Risk factors
Hypercholesterolaemia
Hypertension
Cigarette smoking
Family history
Diabetes mellitus

Findings on investigation
Haematology
FBC to exclude anaemia

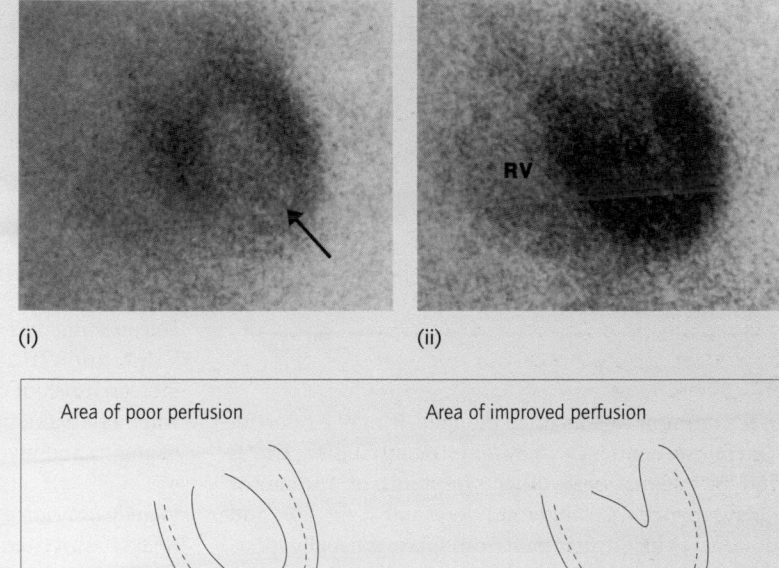

(i)   (ii)

RV

Fig. A Thallium-201 myocardial perfusion scans. (i) Exercise scan showing an extensive area of poor perfusion in the apical region of the left ventricle (arrow). (ii) The same patient, following surgical revascularization, showing a normal appearance. Both figures reproduced from Armstrong P, Wastie ML. *Diagnostic Imaging*, 3rd edn, 1992 (Blackwell Scientific Publications, Oxford) with the permission of the authors.

Area of poor perfusion   Area of improved perfusion

Biochemistry
- *Thyroid function tests:* to exclude thyroid dysfunction
- *Urea and electrolytes and glucose tests:* to diagnose renal failure and diabetes mellitus

Diagnostic imaging
- *Exercise thallium scintigraphy:* combined with exercise testing to improve the sensitivity and specificity of the exercise test
- *Cardiac catheterization and coronary aortography:* when the diagnosis of chest pain remains uncertain and when invasive treatment of coronary disease is contemplated
- *Multiple-gated acquisition scan (MUGA):* to assess ventricular contraction and provide a quantified measurement of the ejection fraction
- *Stress or dobutamine echocardiography:* to identify regional wall movement abnormalities caused by increasing the heart's work either by exercise or by dobutamine

Electrocardiology
- *ECG:* often normal between episodes of angina, but may reveal previous myocardial infarction
- *Exercise test:* to establish a diagnosis of angina and define the ischaemic threshold

Clinical features
Cardiovascular
Central chest tightness (sometimes described as crushing) that radiates through to the back and shoulder or down one or both arms or into the neck and jaw
Breathlessness with exertion
Hypercholesterolaemia
Hypertension
Reduced peripheral pulses
Carotid artery bruits
Signs of heart failure in severe cases

Skin
Xanthelasma resulting from hyperlipidaemia
Nicotine-stained fingers

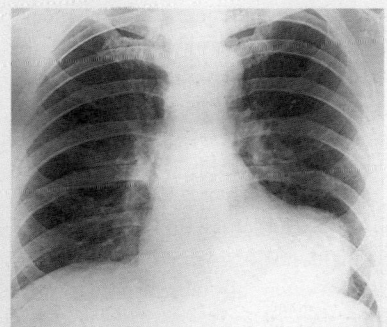

Fig. B Left ventricular aneurysm. The transverse diameter of the heart is moderately enlarged. There is a bulge of the lower half of the left heart border extending down to the apex. This bulge is caused by the aneurysm itself.

Table 7.12 Factors associated with the development of coronary artery disease

Strong association	Weak association
Increasing age	Gout
Male sex	Type A personality
Family history of coronary artery disease	Soft water
Hyperlipidaemia	Lack of exercise
Smoking	Contraceptive pill
Hypertension	Alcohol
Diabetes mellitus	
Haemostasis factors	

not as common as was once thought. It may be part of a generalized tendency to vasomotor instability, and is found in patients with other symptoms of vasomotor instability such as migraine, Raynaud's disease and abdominal pain. Cardiac pain from spasm is usually spontaneous, prolonged and worse in the morning (when vasomotor tone is highest). A hypertrophied myocardium (e.g. associated with hypertrophic cardiomyopathy, aortic stenosis or systemic hypertension) increases myocardial oxygen demand and leads to symptoms of myocardial ischaemia. These symptoms are worsened by any condition that increases cardiac output, such as anaemia or thyrotoxicosis.

A few people have typical ischaemic symptoms associated with an abnormal exercise test, normal coronary arteries and normal oxygen demand. The cause of this condition, known as syndrome X, is not understood, but it may be caused by abnormal myocardial metabolism or an inability to increase coronary flow on exercise (reduced coronary flow reserve).

Atherosclerosis

Atherosclerosis is thickening of the intima of the medium-sized arteries, and consequent narrowing of the artery because of lipid and fibrous tissue deposition.

Risk factors for coronary artery disease

Many factors have been associated with the development of coronary artery disease (Table 7.12).

Hyperlipidaemia. The higher the plasma cholesterol, the higher the incidence of coronary artery disease. The incidence rises exponentially above a plasma value of 5.2 mmol/l. The association is particularly strong when associated with low-density lipoprotein (LDL) cholesterol. High plasma triglycerides are also associated with premature coronary artery disease, probably because they inhibit natural tissue plasminogen activator (TPA).

Smoking. There is a direct link between the risk of coron-

ary artery disease and the number of cigarettes smoked. This risk declines to normal levels within 5 years of giving up smoking. The rise in the incidence of coronary artery disease in women is linked to the increased proportion of women who smoke.

Hypertension. Systolic and diastolic hypertension are associated with an increased risk of coronary artery disease, but this risk is not as high as it is for stroke (hypertension is covered in detail in Chapter 8).

Haemostatic factors. Increased plasma levels of factor VII, factor VIIIC and fibrinogen are associated with an increased risk of coronary artery disease. It is not known whether a reduction in these factors lowers the incidence of angina and myocardial infarction.

Weakly associated factors. There is no clear evidence that weakly associated factors can cause coronary artery disease. Physical activity may be beneficial on the coronary circulation, or merely indicate a healthy constitution in those who take exercise. Patients with type A personality (aggressive, restless, ambitious people who are constantly anxious about deadlines) have more coronary artery disease than others. This may be related to an increased level of circulating catecholamines. The risk from alcohol appears to be J-shaped: the more alcohol the higher the risk, but no alcohol is also thought to lead to a higher risk.

Angina

In developed countries most people develop some coronary artery disease. Symptoms of angina develop when the artery is too narrow to allow an adequate blood supply in the face of an increased demand for oxygen (e.g. during exercise or an emotional upset).

Clinical features

Characteristically, angina is a central tightness (sometimes described as crushing) in the chest. It radiates through to the back and shoulder or down one or both arms or into the neck and jaw. However, many patients do not describe such characteristic pain. Occasionally, the only symptom is breathlessness because of increased pulmonary venous pressure resulting from the left ventricle becoming stiff and failing to relax when ischaemic.

EXERTIONAL ANGINA

Exertional angina is the typical presentation of ischaemic heart disease. Pain develops with physical exertion, particularly in cold weather, after meals or with an emotional upset, and resolves rapidly on rest. Some patients experience 'a second wind', being able to undertake more

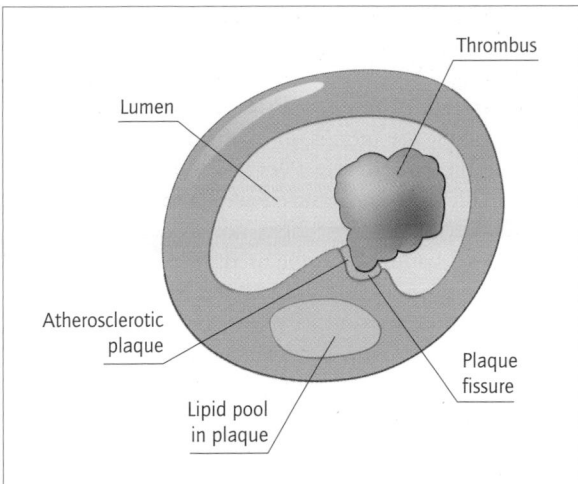

Figure 7.25 Cross-section of coronary artery in acute coronary syndrome.

exercise than at first after recovering from the initial pain because of metabolic adaptation in the myocardium.

VARIANT ANGINA

Originally described by Prinzmetal, variant angina is spontaneous severe angina occurring as a result of coronary artery spasm. It may occur in normal coronary arteries and in coronary arteries with eccentric plaques. It is more common in women and in the morning, and the pain can be prolonged and severe. The ECG characteristically shows S-T segment elevation. It is rarely induced by exercise.

Acute coronary syndromes

The atherosclerotic plaque can develop a fissure or rupture in its fibrous cap, exposing the lipid and collagen content of the plaque (Fig. 7.25). This causes platelets to accumulate on the surface of the plaque to rapidly reduce the diameter of the lumen or block it altogether. This results in unstable (unpredictable) cardiac pain that can take three forms:
1 Crescendo angina
2 Unstable angina
3 Myocardial infarction

Crescendo angina

Crescendo angina is either angina of recent onset or exertional angina with a deteriorating threshold. It implies that a coronary artery narrowing is becoming rapidly more severe.

Unstable angina

Unstable angina is angina occurring at rest. It can also occur at night when lying down (decubitus angina). It is caused by superimposed thrombus on a plaque, and up to 30% of people with this condition go on to have a myocardial infarction.

Myocardial infarction

This is defined as prolonged (more than 20 min) cardiac pain occurring at rest with characteristic ECG changes and the demonstration of measurable levels of troponin (T or I) in the blood. Paradoxically, the degree of arterial stenosis does not necessarily predict the likelihood of myocardial infarction. Plaque fissuring resulting in infarction can occur in relatively minor atherosclerotic plaques. The plaques can also be a site of platelet thrombosis with subsequent embolism causing patchy necrosis throughout the myocardium without causing complete transmural damage.

Sustained coronary artery spasm occasionally results in myocardial infarction. Similarly, prolonged periods of hypertension or relative underperfusion of the subendocardium in the presence of left ventricular hypertrophy can result in subendocardial infarction, even in the absence of coronary artery disease.

Diagnosis of ischaemic heart disease

Angina is diagnosed from the history. There are usually no physical signs unless there are identifiable risk factors such as hyperlipidaemia causing xanthelasma, smoking causing nicotine staining, or hypertension. Peripheral pulses in the feet may be reduced or there may be carotid artery bruits indicating widespread arterial disease.

Investigation

The investigation of angina involves two stages: (i) confirming the diagnosis, and (ii) assessing the severity of the ischaemia and its prognostic significance.

Electrophysiology

- *ECG:* often normal between episodes of angina, but may reveal previous myocardial infarction.
- *Exercise test:* the standardized treadmill exercise test according to a formal protocol is useful for establishing a diagnosis of angina and defining the ischaemic threshold. However, it is limited because it is neither totally specific nor sensitive, and there is a significant incidence of false-positive and false-negative results. The positive end-points to an exercise test are shown in Table 7.13.

Table 7.13 The positive end-points to an exercise test

Horizontal or downsloping ST-segment depression of at least
 1 mm in two or more adjacent leads
Development of angina
A fall in blood pressure with exercise
Development of ventricular arrhythmias

Diagnostic imaging

● *Exercise thallium scintigraphy:* thallium scintigraphy can be combined with exercise testing to improve the sensitivity and specificity of the exercise test. The intravenous potassium analogue is injected during exercise and a reduced area of uptake in the ischaemic myocardium is identified by a gamma camera. During recovery, thallium redistribution occurs in myocardium that has reversible ischaemia, but if the myocardium is infarcted there is no such redistribution.

● *Cardiac catheterization and coronary aortography:* indicated when the diagnosis of chest pain remains uncertain and when invasive treatment of coronary disease is contemplated.

● *Multiple-gated acquisition scan:* allows a radionuclide assessment of ventricular contraction and provides a quantified measurement of the ejection fraction.

● *Stress or dobutamine echocardiography:* identifies regional wall movement abnormalities caused by increasing the work of the heart, either by exercise or dobutamine.

Haematology

Full blood count. It is important to exclude anaemia, which can worsen angina.

Biochemistry

● *Thyroid function tests:* to exclude thyroid dysfunction
● *Urea and electrolytes and glucose:* both renal failure and diabetes mellitus can lead to premature coronary artery disease

Management

Angina is managed by:
● Modifying lifestyle
● Controlling risk factors
● Drug treatment
● Revascularization by balloon angioplasty
● Coronary artery bypass surgery

Modifying lifestyle

Many patients have stable symptoms from angina and it may be reasonable to treat these patients, particularly when elderly, by advising them to modify their lifestyle and their level of activity to accommodate their symptoms.

All patients should be advised to avoid factors known to worsen ischaemic heart disease. They should stop smoking, lose weight and eat a low-fat diet. They should exercise within the limitations of their symptoms and avoid, as far as possible, excessive stress or tiredness. Their blood pressure should be controlled. All patients should have their plasma cholesterol measured and if the level is over 5.2 mmol/l, dietary advice should be given in an attempt to reduce it. If after modifying their diet it remains above 5 mmol/l, lipid-lowering drugs are indicated.

Drug treatment

Nitrates. These are mono-, di- or trinitrates. They cause vasodilatation of both arterioles and veins, thereby reducing systemic arterial pressure and venous pressure. This reduces myocardial oxygen demand.

Sublingual trinitrate can be used for acute episodes of angina. The mononitrate preparation is preferred to the dinitrate because it avoids first-pass hepatic metabolism. Regular use of nitrates can result in tolerance because of the metabolism of sulphydryl groups. It is therefore recommended that each day there should be a nitrate-free period to allow the sulphydryl groups to regenerate. Nitrate can also be given as transdermal nitrate patches, but trials have not shown that this has any advantage over oral administration and it is more expensive.

Beta-blockers. Beta-blockers are a mainstay in the treatment of angina in patients for whom there is no contraindication. Cardioselective preparations with a long half-life (e.g. atenolol) are used first. They act by reducing myocardial oxygen demand. However, they can also increase peripheral resistance as a result of unopposed alpha tone in the peripheral arterioles and this can reduce their effectiveness. Theoretically they can also increase the tendency to coronary artery spasm.

Calcium antagonists. Calcium antagonists are a group of compounds with varying molecular structure, which inhibit the transfer of calcium into the cell and within the sarcolemma, thereby reducing myocardial oxygen consumption. They also reduce peripheral vascular resistance and therefore myocardial oxygen demand. These are the drugs of first choice for angina caused by coronary spasm. Some calcium antagonists also affect the SA node and AV conduction, and have useful antiarrhythmic properties.

Calcium antagonists have a spectrum of effect on ventricular contractility. The dihydropyridine calcium antagonists has a minimal effect on ventricular performance whereas verapamil and diltiazem have a significant negative inotropic effect.

Antithrombotic drugs. Aspirin, which reduces platelet stickiness, is the antithrombotic drug of choice in all patients with ischaemic heart disease, provided there is no contraindication. It may prevent the progression of underlying coronary narrowing and counteract the effect of hypercholesterolaemia. In patients with unstable angina it reduces the risk of infarction in the first 12 months by as much as 50%. Clopidogrel is also a powerful antiplatelet drug; but its role in clinical management is still being defined.

Lipid-lowering drugs. Every attempt must be made to reduce the plasma cholesterol towards 5.0 mmol/l or less. There is evidence that this delays the progression of the coronary narrowings and in some studies a reduction in the severity of the coronary narrowing has been demonstrated. The use of lipid-lowering drugs has been shown to reduce the incidence of fatal and non-fatal myocardial infarction.

Interventional treatment

Interventional treatment is conventionally offered to patients whose symptoms continue and are unacceptable despite medical therapy.

Percutaneous coronary artery intervention (PCI). Balloon dilatation of the coronary artery through guiding catheters introduced from the femoral or brachial artery has become an established technique for relieving discrete stenoses in the coronary ciculation. The initial success rate approaches 95%, but there is a 30–40% restenosis rate with a 20–25% symptomatic relapse rate within the first 6 months. The restenosis rate limits the effectiveness of angioplasty in multivessel disease. Introducing fine wire meshes (stents) to hold the artery open following balloon dilatation reduces the restenosis rate to 15–20%.

New drug eluting stents are reducing the incidence of restenosis significantly to less than 5%.

Coronary artery bypass surgery. Coronary artery bypass surgery is indicated when:
- Antianginal medication does not provide adequate symptomatic relief from angina, and the coronary stenoses are not suitable for PCI
- The pattern of narrowing suggests that the patient's prognosis can be improved by coronary surgery
  Such patterns of narrowing are:
- Left main stem coronary stenosis
- Proximal stenoses in all three coronary arteries in the presence of previous myocardial infarction

Arterial (internal mammary and radial arteries) are preferred to saphenous vein grafts to bypass the stenosis in the coronary circulation. It is now a safe operation with less than 2% perioperative mortality for elective (non-urgent) cases. The long-term patency of vein grafts is approximately 95% at 1 year, 70% at 5 years and 40% at 10 years. Arterial grafts have a much improved long-term patency rate of about 80% at 10 years.

The attrition rate of the bypass grafts means that many younger patients will require a second bypass operation. To reduce the frequency of this, many cardiologists carry out balloon angioplasty first where appropriate. The two treatments are therefore best regarded as complementary rather than competitive.

Unstable angina

Up to 30% of patients with unstable angina proceed to myocardial infarction and so all patients require immediate treatment as an inpatient. This involves pacifying the plaque on which thrombus is forming and is achieved by the use of antiplatelet drugs such as aspirin and glycoprotein inhibitors, subcutaneous low molecular weight heparin such as clexane, as well as the drugs available for angina. Most patients require intravenous nitrates until the symptoms settle. Diamorphine may be required for pain relief. Beta-blockers have been thought to be inappropriate because of their theoretical potential for increasing coronary artery spasm, but this is not an important consideration in clinical practice and beta-blockers should be used as they improve both the symptoms and the prognosis. Aspirin and clopidogrel have also been shown to improve prognosis.

Patients with unstable angina should undergo early coronary angiography with a view to revascularization either by PCI or coronary artery bypass surgery.

Myocardial infarction

Clinical features

Myocardial infarction usually consists of an episode of severe crushing chest pain, radiating into the jaw and into the arms or through to the back. The patient feels agitated or sweaty and is often breathless. The symptoms are unresponsive to glyceryl trinitrate (GTN). About 15% of patients, especially the elderly, do not have chest pain but have non-specific symptoms of malaise, tiredness and breathlessness.

Of people who have a myocardial infarction, 30–40% die suddenly and do not reach hospital. The majority are caused by ventricular arrhythmias, which could be treated effectively by people who have been properly trained in cardiopulmonary resuscitation (CPR; see pp. 449–451).

Diagnosis

A diagnosis of myocardial infarction is established if two of the following three criteria are present.
1 A characteristic cardiac pain lasting more than 20 min and unresponsive to GTN
2 The presence of troponin T or I in the blood 12 h after the onset of symptoms
3 Characteristic ECG changes in the infarct-related leads (see p. 421)

Differential diagnosis

The differential diagnosis of myocardial infarction must be considered because some of the treatments of infarction are specifically contraindicated if the symptoms result from an alternative cause. Conditions to consider include the following:

Table 7.14 The three phases in the ECG evolution of a Q-wave infarction. (Note that posterior infarcts cause ST depression in leads V1 and V2 (reciprocal of ST elevation) and R waves in these leads become more prominent, representing posterior Q waves.)

Phase	Features
Hyperacute	ST elevation in infarct-related leads
Acute	ST-segment elevation in infarct-related leads, development of Q waves, and the beginning of T-wave inversion
Chronic	Q waves, loss of R waves and T-wave inversion

● *Pericarditis:* can cause severe chest pain and ST-segment elevation on the ECG.

● *Aortic dissection:* also causes severe chest pain, often with non-specific ECG changes. Occasionally, the right coronary artery orifice is involved in the dissection and causes an inferior infarction. If it involves the left coronary orifice the patient will die, because too much heart muscle is jeopardized.

● *Spontaneous pneumothorax:* can cause collapse with chest pain, hypotension and breathlessness. A chest radiograph confirms the diagnosis.

● *Oesophageal rupture:* usually occurs with severe prolonged vomiting and causes chest pain radiating through to the back.

● *Pulmonary embolus:* usually clearly distinguishable from myocardial infarction by the different nature of the pain (pleuritic) and absence of troponin T. The ECG can be abnormal.

Investigation
Biochemistry
Cardiac enzymes. Troponin T or I is usually not present in the blood. It can be present in patients with renal failure. Normally the presence of troponin T indicates recent myocardial damage. It rises 12 h after the onset of symptoms and persists for up to 14 days. The assay of other enzymes such as creatinine phosphokinase, the transaminases (aspartate and alanine aminotransferase) and dehydrogenases (hydroxybutyrate dehydrogenase) has been largely discontinued.

Electrocardiography
The three phases in the ECG evolution of infarction are shown in Table 7.14 and Fig. 7.26.

Inferior infarcts are shown in leads II, III and aVF (Fig. 7.27); **anterior infarcts** in leads V2–V5 (Fig. 7.28); **lateral infarcts** in leads I, aVL, V5 and V6; and **true posterior infarcts** are seen in leads V1 and V2. A **non-Q-wave infarction** occurs if the infarct does not extend

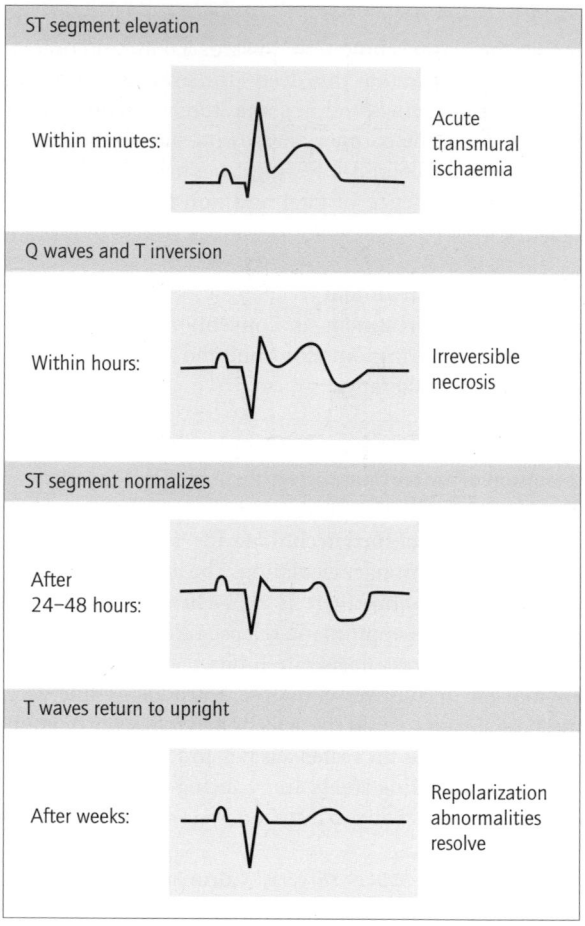

Figure 7.26 The changing pattern of the ECG in the affected leads during the evolution of a myocardial infarction.

ST segment elevation		
Within minutes:		Acute transmural ischaemia

| Q waves and T inversion | | |
| Within hours: | | Irreversible necrosis |

| ST segment normalizes | | |
| After 24–48 hours: | | |

| T waves return to upright | | |
| After weeks: | | Repolarization abnormalities resolve |

transmurally: Q waves do not develop and the changes are confined to the ST segment and T wave (Fig. 7.29).

Management
A fatal arrhythmia during myocardial infarction is most likely in the first 4 h after the onset of symptoms. This justifies immediate transfer to an accident and emergency department where resuscitation facilities are available (EMERGENCY BOX 7.1). Many ambulances now have paramedics equipped with defibrillators, and patients should therefore be transferred by ambulance to the hospital.

While a diagnosis of myocardial infarction is being established, the following treatment should be given (BOX 7.5, pp. 411–412):

● *Aspirin:* 300 mg orally.

● *Analgesia:* usually diamorphine 2.5 mg intravenously with a suitable antiemetic.

● *Oxygen:* by nasal cannulae if there are any features suggesting heart failure.

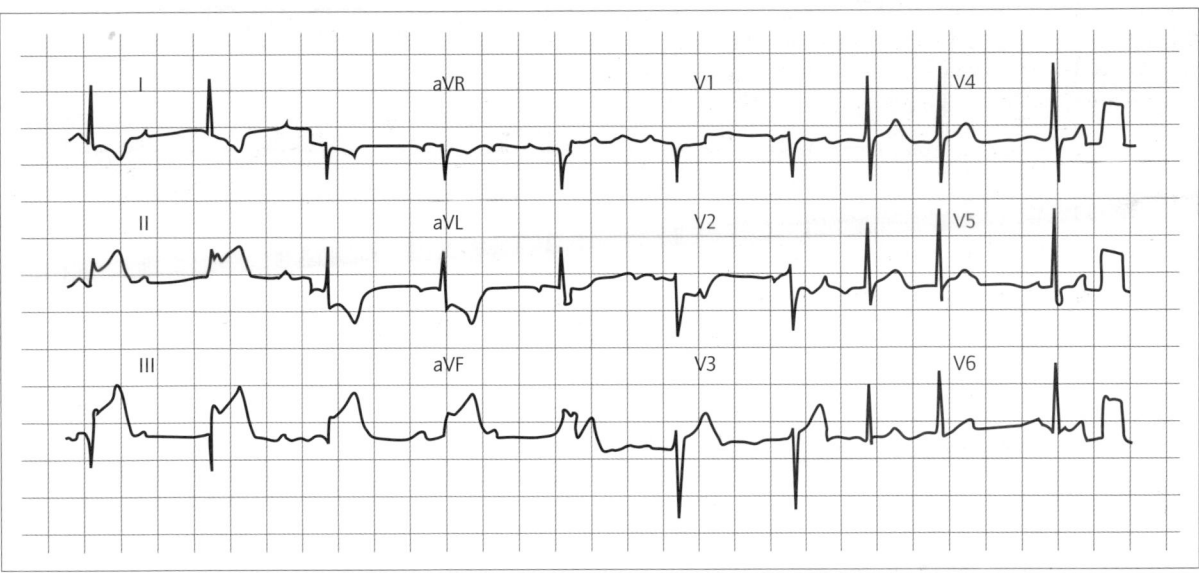

Figure 7.27 ECG showing acute inferior myocardial infarction.

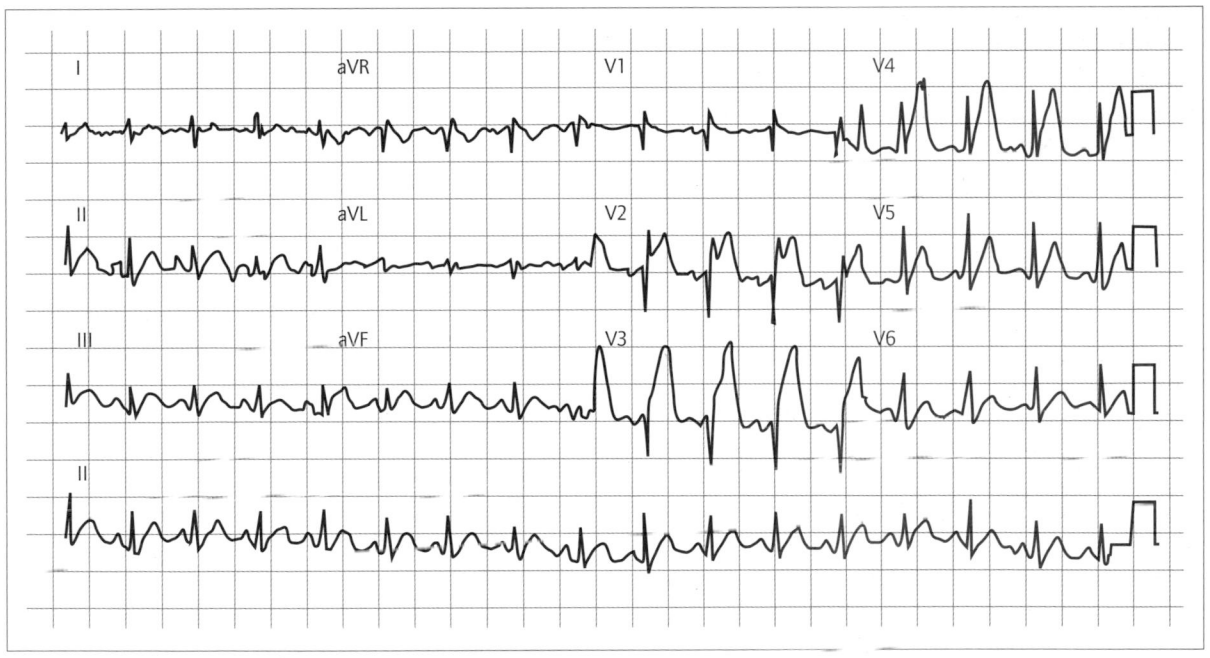

Figure 7.28 ECG showing acute anterior myocardial infarction.

● *Thrombolysis:* the earliest possible delivery of thrombolysis is mandatory. If the diagnosis can be confirmed by
the ambulance team, they should administer a thrombolytic agent. Ideally, tenecteplase should be given when
available. Alternatively, 1.5 million units of streptokinase
given over 1 h can be used (EMERGENCY BOX 7.2).

● *Intravenous nitrates:* in the presence of continuing
pain or evidence of heart failure, it is appropriate to give
intravenous nitrates provided the systolic blood pressure
does not fall below 100 mmHg.
● *Intravenous beta-blockers:* intravenous beta-blockers
are not yet standard practice, but trials have shown a small

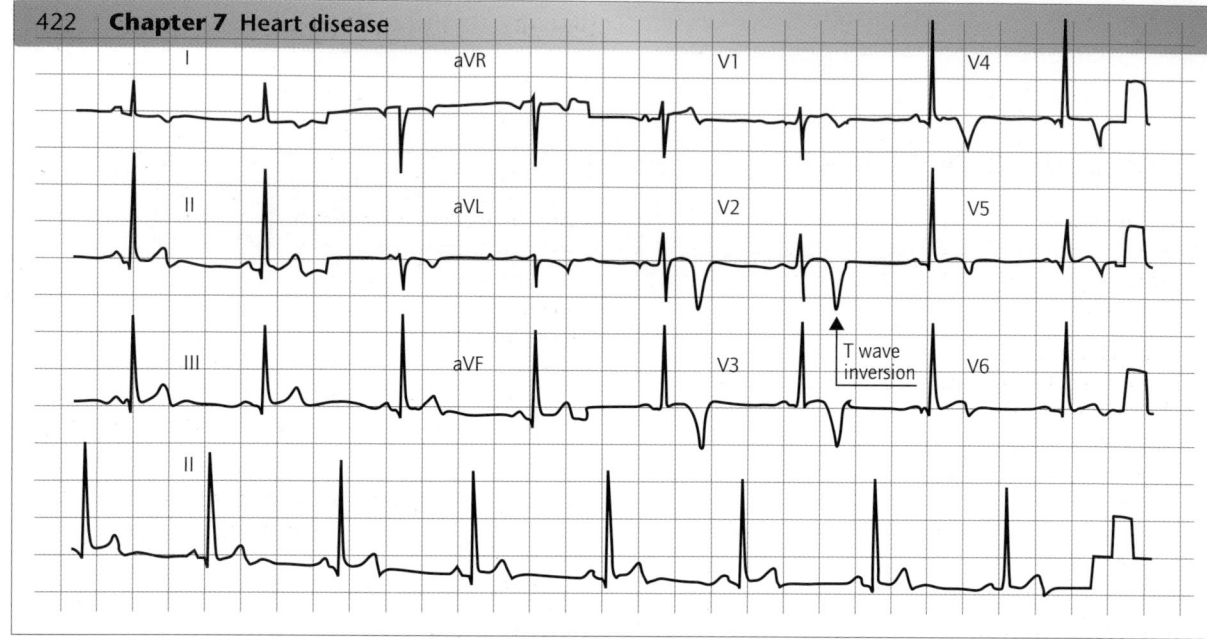

Figure 7.29 ECG showing non-Q-wave anterior myocardial infarction.

Emergency 7.1: Ischaemic heart disease

MYOCARDIAL INFARCTION

Diagnosis
Good history of cardiac pain with acute ST- or T-wave
changes on ECG

Resuscitative measures
Assess:
- *Airway* (oxygen)
- *Breathing* (cardiac monitor)
- *Circulation* (intravenous access)

Close, continuous observation is necessary for complications,
for example:
- Cardiac arrest
- Arrhythmias
- Heart failure

Specific treatment
Aspirin 300 mg (chewed)

Analgesia: diamorphine in increments of 2.5 mg intravenously as required with antiemetic (metaclopramide
10 mg intravenously)

Thrombolysis (EMERGENCY BOX 7.2)

Buccal or intravenous nitrates for continued pain or heart failure,
provided systolic blood pressure is higher than 100 mmHg

Intravenous beta-blockers for continued pain if no evidence
of heart failure, atenolol 5 mg bolus

UNSTABLE ANGINA
Requires immediate stabilization as an inpatient

Specific treatment
Drug treatment

Use the drugs available for angina, and most patients will
require intravenous nitrates until the symptoms settle

Diamorphine may be required for pain relief

Beta-blockers improve both the symptoms and the prognosis

Aspirin also improves prognosis

Surgery

If symptoms continue, refer early for coronary angiography
with a view to revascularization, by either balloon angioplasty or bypass surgery. Many of these patients will
require intravenous heparin until revascularization

ANGINA

Supportive treatment
Advise patients to avoid factors known to worsen ischaemic
heart disease: all patients should be advised to stop smoking, lose weight, eat a low-fat diet, exercise within the
limitations of their symptoms and avoid excessive stress
or tiredness as far as possible

Give dietary advice if plasma cholesterol is higher than
5.2 mmol/l

Specific treatment
Drug treatment

Nitrates

Beta-blockers for patients with no contraindications (e.g.
atenolol)

Calcium antagonists (e.g. nifedipine)

Antithrombotic drugs (e.g. aspirin)

Lipid-lowering drugs may be needed if plasma cholesterol
remains above 6 mmol/l after modifying diet

Surgery

Percutaneous coronary artery intervention

Coronary artery bypass surgery

Emergency 7.2: Thrombolysis

Tenecteplase

This is currently the drug of choice. Give 6000–10 000 units according to body weight as a single intravenous bolus over 10 s

Streptokinase

In some units streptokinase (1.5 million units dissolved in 100 ml 5% dextrose infused over 60 min)

Streptokinase is contraindicated in some patients:

- Has the patient received streptokinase in the last 4 years?
- Is the patient hypotensive (blood pressure below 100 mmHg)?
- Is the patient in cardiogenic shock?

Tissue plasminogen activator (TPA)

This is not recommended for routine use. Give to patients who:

- Have received streptokinase within the last 4 years
- Are hypotensive
- Are in cardiogenic shock

The usual dose of TPA is 100 mg with 50 mg given in the first hour, followed by 25 mg/h for the next 2 h

Indications for thrombolytic therapy

Within 12 h of onset of pain

ST elevation over 1 mm in the limb leads, or over 2 mm in the chest leads (two or more adjacent leads)

Contraindications to thrombolytic therapy

Absolute contraindications

Active gastrointestinal bleeding

Aortic dissection

Neurosurgery/head injury

Cerebrovascular accident (within last 2 months)

Intracranial neoplasm/aneurysm

Recent surgery (within last 4 weeks)

Relative contraindications

Traumatic cardiopulmonary resuscitation (CPR)

Diastolic blood pressure over 130 mmHg

Past history of gastrointestinal bleeding

Abdominal aortic aneurysm

Problems with thrombolysis

Allergic reactions

Recognized by fever, urticaria, back pain, hypotension

Stop thrombolysis and give chlorpheniramine 10 mg intravenously and hydrocortisone 100 mg intravenously. Consider restarting the infusion at a slower rate or changing to TPA if the reaction is severe

Bleeding

Oozing from puncture site is very common and is treated with direct pressure. If these measures fail to control the bleeding then stop the infusion and give tranexamic acid 1 g (10 mg/kg) intravenously over 10 min, and fresh frozen plasma

---

reduction in the mortality rate if they are given immediately. Therefore if there is a resting tachycardia and there are no signs of heart failure, and/or if the patient has continuing pain, it is appropriate to give intravenous atenolol, initially as a 5-mg bolus.

The patient should be transferred to the cardiac care unit for continuous monitoring. It is important to give sedation to relieve anxiety. Anticoagulants should be started 12–24 h after the thrombolytic therapy using subcutaneous low molecular weight heparin (enoxaparin for 7 days).

Complications

Arrhythmias

The most dangerous arrhythmia is ventricular fibrillation, which is treated by prompt direct current (DC) cardioversion. The treatment of an arrhythmia depends on its nature (e.g. ventricular ectopics or tachycardia). Ventricular tachycardia (VT) can be treated with intravenous lidocaine (lignocaine) or amiodarone. Atrial fibrillation can be treated with digoxin. In some patients with arrhythmias, intravenous magnesium proves to be valuable.

Heart failure

Signs of heart failure should be treated in the usual manner (see pp. 430–433). Studies have shown that aggressive treatment of early signs of heart failure in myocardial infarction, even when there are no symptoms, improves long-term survival.

Continuing angina

This has become more common since the introduction of thrombolysis because the latter limits the size of the infarct and continuing angina may indicate that the patient is at risk of extending the infarct. Coronary angiography with a view to revascularization either by PCI or coronary artery bypass surgery is indicated.

Systemic thromboembolism

It is not known whether oral anticoagulants reduce the risk of thromboembolism, but if thrombus is identified within the left ventricle anticoagulants are usually given.

Pulmonary embolism

This used to be a common complication of myocardial

Table 7.15 Investigations to identify those heart attack patients who have a high risk of further problems

To identify myocardial ischaemia

Pre-discharge submaximal treadmill exercise test

This exercise test is performed 5–10 days following the infarct, provided the patient is not experiencing continuing angina or is in heart failure, to ensure that it is safe for the patient to go home. It is limited to 6 min of the modified Bruce protocol

Cardiac catheterization with coronary angiography will probably be indicated if any of the standard end-points are reached within the first two stages of the protocol

Some centres prefer to use thallium or cardiolite treadmill exercise testing to improve the sensitivity of identifying myocardium at risk

To identify potential malignant arrhythmias

Signal average ECG

In patients more at risk of arrhythmias there may be a sudden dispersion of the electrical signal at the end of the QRS complex. This dispersion (or after-potential) can be identified using computer-aided ECG techniques

24-h Ambulatory ECG

Monitoring the patient's heart rhythm while mobilizing can identify arrhythmias, which may be markers of a predisposition to more serious arrhythmias. The ventricular arrhythmias have been classified into grades of increasing severity by Dr Bernard Lown

Grade 0   No ventricular premature beats (VPBs)
Grade 1   Occasional VPBs, less than 30/h, not more than 1/min
Grade 2   Frequent VPBs, more than 30/h
Grade 3   Multiform VPBs
Grade 4a   Couplets (two consecutive VPBs)
Grade 4b   Repetitive VPBs (three or more)
Grade 5   Early VPBs (the R wave of the ventricular ectopic occurs on the T wave of the previous beat)

Although it is possible to stratify patients according to their risk of either death or further myocardial infarction, there is no proven medication or surgical intervention that will unequivocally improve the prognosis of those most at risk

All trials of drugs aiming to improve the prognosis of infarct survivors have looked at all survivors of infarction. Therefore the value of the use of drugs in specific subsets of high-risk patients remains unproven. Although it is tempting to target such patients specifically, such targeting of at-risk patients with specific medication may be wrong. In one study of an antiarrhythmic drug treating patients with ventricular ectopics following myocardial infarction, the mortality of patients given the drug was higher than that of those given placebo

To identify patients with poor ventricular function

Although it is usually clinically evident at the bedside that a patient has ventricular dysfunction, it is useful to quantitate this by measuring the size of the infarct and ejection fraction. This is best done using a multiple-gated acquisition scan. ACE inhibitors have been shown to be of value in patients with poor left ventricular function, even in the absence of symptoms

---

infarction when patients were confined to bed without anticoagulants for long periods. Now, with the aggressive use of anticoagulants together with early mobilization (after 24 h in uncomplicated cases), the incidence is much less. All patients should be given subcutaneous heparin until mobilized, irrespective of whether they have been given thrombolysis or not, and they should wear stockings to prevent thromboembolic disease.

Ventricular septal defect, mitral regurgitation and cardiac rupture

If these complications occur, the patient's condition usually deteriorates suddenly. Cardiac rupture is usually fatal, but occasionally the leak of blood is contained in the pericardium without tamponade and a false aneurysm develops.

Dressler's syndrome

Dressler's syndrome usually develops 2–6 weeks after infarction and is characterized by pericarditis, pleurisy and malaise. Often the patient is febrile and anaemic, and has a high erythrocyte sedimentation rate (ESR). The condition usually settles with non-steroidal anti-inflammatory drugs (NSAIDs), but occasionally a short course of corticosteroids is required.

Prognosis
Angina

The prognosis in angina is worse when ischaemia is induced at low levels of exercise, when there is evidence of considerable ventricular damage, or when the angiogram shows a pattern of narrowing that is jeopardizing large amounts of the heart muscle.

Myocardial infarction

Approximately 10–15% of patients admitted to hospital with acute myocardial infarction die while in hospital. However, the majority will have an uncomplicated course and be fit for discharge after 7–10 days. Of patients who leave hospital, about 10% will die within the first 12 months. The strongest predictor of death is the size of the infarct. It is therefore important to minimize ischaemic damage with thrombolysis, and possibly subsequent percutaneous transluminal coronary angioplasty (PTCA) or coronary artery surgery. The mortality arises from heart failure, further infarction and malignant arrhythmias, which are often interrelated: tachycardia is more likely in patients with severe heart failure. Investigations are therefore undertaken to identify those patients at risk of further problems (Table 7.15).

Heart failure

Epidemiology

Prevalence. Heart failure is common, affecting approximately 1/100 people over the age of 65 years.

Disease mechanisms

Cardiac output is normally approximately 5 l/min and can increase to 25 l/min with heavy exercise. Heart failure occurs when the heart is unable to meet this demand. It can result from pathology affecting:

- *Endocardium and valves:* stenosis, regurgitation or endocardial fibroelastosis (EFE)
- *Myocardium:* ventricular failure
- *Pericardium:* constrictive pericarditis or tamponade

Left and right heart failure

Usually a distinction is made between left and right heart failure. Most commonly, right heart failure is a consequence of left heart failure and when the two occur together the condition is known as congestive cardiac failure.

Acute and chronic heart failure

It is also useful to distinguish between acute and chronic heart failure:

- *Acute heart failure:* symptoms result from a sudden rise in either right or left atrial pressure rather than as a result of excessive fluid retention, which develops later.
- *Chronic heart failure:* leads to fluid retention because of sodium retention by the kidney. Fluid (oedema) then accumulates in the lungs and in the periphery. Many litres may be retained over a long period as the patient develops ascites and swollen legs.

The causes of left and right, and acute and chronic heart failure are listed in Table 7.16. Acute heart failure most commonly results from myocardial infarction.

Cardiogenic shock. This specific syndrome occurs when the heart muscle is so weak that the patient is hypotensive,

Table 7.16 Causes of heart failure

Cause	Comment
Left heart failure	
Ischaemic heart disease	
Mitral valve disease	Mitral stenosis causes left atrial hypertension and pulmonary venous congestion, but does not cause left ventricular failure
Cardiomyopathy	Classically there are three types: dilated, hypertrophic or restrictive
Systemic hypertension	Because of left ventricular hypertrophy the ventricle is slow to relax in diastole (non-compliant). This restricts ventricular filling and causes left atrial hypertension
Aortic valve disease	
Right heart failure	
Chronic lung disease (cor pulmonale)	This causes pulmonary hypertension
Pulmonary hypertension	Caused by thromboembolism or primary pulmonary hypertension
Isolated right ventricular infarction	
Right ventricular cardiomyopathy	
Tricuspid valve disease	
Pulmonary valve disease	
Acute heart failure	
Myocardial infarction	
Sudden valve dysfunction caused by infective endocarditis	
Ruptured chordae tendineae	
Acute pericardial tamponade	

oliguric or anuric and confused because of poor central blood flow. The prognosis is very poor.

In heart failure renal perfusion is poor, resulting in salt and water retention through the renin–angiotensin system. This increases circulating blood volume. A normal heart can cope with an increased circulating blood volume by increasing contractility as the ventricular dimensions increase (Starling's law of the heart; Fig. 7.2). In a failing heart, however, the Starling curve is flatter, so there is less cardiac output for each unit increase in the venous pressure. As the circulating blood volume increases there is a compensatory release of atrial natriuretic peptides. These stimulate sodium excretion and are also potent vasodilators. They therefore counteract the consequences of heart failure, at least initially.

Pulmonary oedema

When the pulmonary capillary pressure rises above 24 mmHg, fluid filters first into the interstitial space of the lung (interstial oedema) and then, as the pressure rises, into the alveoli as well (alveolar oedema). If the oncotic pressure in the capillaries is low because of, for example, hypoalbuminaemia, pulmonary oedema will develop at a lower pulmonary capillary pressure.

Table 7.17 The symptoms and signs of left ventricular failure

Symptom/sign	Notes
Symptoms	
Exertional dyspnoea	Caused by increased pulmonary venous congestion and increased systemic acidosis (resulting from poor tissue perfusion during exercise)
Dyspnoea at rest, orthopnoea and PND	Caused by pulmonary venous congestion. When severe the patient is unable to lie down (orthopnoea) and can experience PND
Tiredness	Low cardiac output
Signs	
Resting tachycardia	
Pulsus alternans (see p. 393)	Occurs in severe left ventricular failure
Displaced apex beat	Left ventricular hypertrophy may develop as a result of systolic pressure overload (e.g. because of aortic stenosis or hypertension) or diastolic volume overload (e.g. mitral regurgitation or aortic incompetence). In dilated cardiomyopathy the ventricle is not hypertrophied and in restrictive cardiomyopathies the apex beat is not displaced
A third heart sound	Caused by blood filling a non-compliant (stiff) left ventricle
A fourth heart sound	Caused by an audible atrial systole filling the failing left ventricle (does not occur in atrial fibrillation)
Crepitations at both lung bases	Commonly caused by hypostatic pulmonary secretions and are particularly common in smokers Conversely, there may be no crepitations in severe pulmonary oedema
Pansystolic murmur of mitral regurgitation	As the left ventricle dilates, the mitral annulus is stretched causing functional 'mitral regurgitation'. It is a sign of severe ventricular dysfunction
Pulmonary oedema (usually acutely breathless, anxious, cold, clammy and cyanosed, and produce pink bloodstained sputum). Auscultation reveals crackles of alveolar oedema and the wheeze of bronchial congestion	Cold and clammy because of shut down of the peripheral circulation. Cyanosis caused by a fall in systemic oxygen, the $P\text{co}_2$ is also reduced because of the tachypnoea
Cardiogenic shock: cold, clammy and confused with hypotension and oliguria	The most severe form of ventricular failure: the cardiac output is so low that poor tissue perfusion leads to a systemic acidosis, oliguria and cerebral hypoperfusion, causing the patient to be confused. Sometimes, paradoxically, the pulmonary wedge pressure is not elevated, so the patient is not breathless from pulmonary congestion and may even require fluid to optimize the left atrial filling pressure and improve the output

PND, paroxysmal nocturnal dyspnoea.

Table 7.18 The symptoms and signs of right heart failure

Symptom/sign	Notes
Symptoms	
Breathlessness on exertion	Caused by reduced cardiac output causing poor peripheral tissue perfusion and metabolic acidosis
Tiredness	Caused by reduced cardiac output
Fluid retention	Such as ankle swelling and abdominal distension
Signs	
Elevated venous pressure	Caused by excessive systemic venous volume
	Often with tricuspid regurgitation because of functional tricuspid valve annulus dilatation
Ankle swelling	Can extend up the legs to the abdominal wall
Sacral oedema	
Hepatomegaly and ascites	
Pleural effusion	Most commonly on the right side
Resting tachycardia	May be present
Signs of tricuspid regurgitation (systolic murmur of tricuspid with a right ventricular third sound, systolic V wave in the neck, a pulsatile liver)	May be present

High output heart failure

Certain conditions generate a need for a cardiac output that the heart is unable to meet. These are:

- prolonged anaemia
- thyrotoxicosis
- beriberi
- septicaemia (sometimes)

Characteristically, the patient has a resting tachycardia and warm peripheries with dilated veins. Otherwise he or she has the usual features of left heart failure.

Clinical features

The main symptom of heart failure is shortness of breath, and the severity can be graded according to the classification of the New York Heart Association (NYHA; Table 7.4). Poor cardiac output causes skeletal muscle fatigue and generalized tiredness (Table 7.17). The principal symptoms of right heart failure are caused by fluid retention in the abdomen and peripheries (Table 7.18).

Investigation

The investigation of heart failure should be directed at identifying the cause.

Haematology

- *Full blood count (FBC):* to exclude anaemia
- *ESR*

Biochemistry

Routine biochemical screen of kidney and liver function.

Urea and electrolytes, creatinine and liver function tests.

Diagnostic imaging

- *Chest radiography:* often shows a large heart and increased pulmonary venous pressure (dilatation of the upper lobe veins and Kerley B lines), while pulmonary oedema causes a 'bat's wing' increase in shadowing around the hilum (Fig. 7.30)
- *Echocardiography:* identify disease of the valves and heart muscle

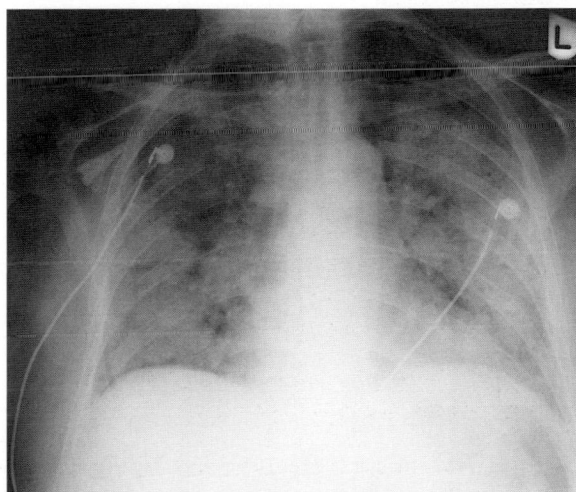

Figure 7.30 The chest radiograph in pulmonary oedema. Note extensive shadowing throughout both lung fields.

Left and right ventricular failure at a glance

Epidemiology

Prevalence
Heart failure affects between 1 and 2% of the population over 65 years of age; 10% of the population over the age of 75 years are on treatment for heart failure

Sex
Heart failure is more common in men in the UK, but in South America, where the trypanosomal infection Chagas' disease is a leading cause, this gender difference is not so marked

Genetics
In West Indian patients, heart failure is often a result of genetic predisposition to hypertension

Findings on investigation

Haematology
- *FBC:* to exclude anaemia
- *ESR*

Biochemistry
Routine biochemical screen of kidney and liver function

Diagnostic imaging
- *Chest radiography:* often shows a large heart and increased pulmonary venous pressure
- *Echocardiography:* may identify structural heart disease
- *Multiple-gated acquisition scan (MUGA):* quantifies the ejection fraction and locates regional wall motion abnormalities
- *Cardiac catherization:* to measure haemodynamic pressures in the cardiac chambers and to exclude significant coronary artery disease

Electrocardiology
- *ECG:* 24-h ambulatory ECG to identify any propensity for arrhythmias
- *Exercise test:* to provide a measurement of functional capacity

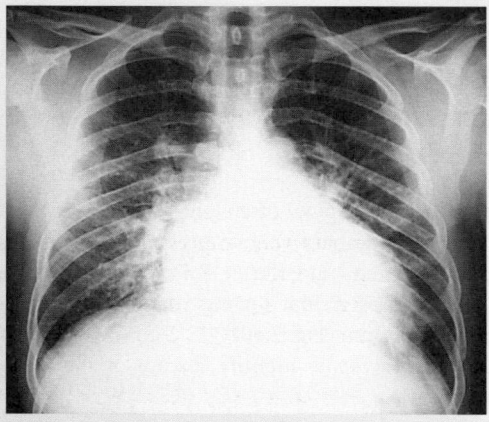

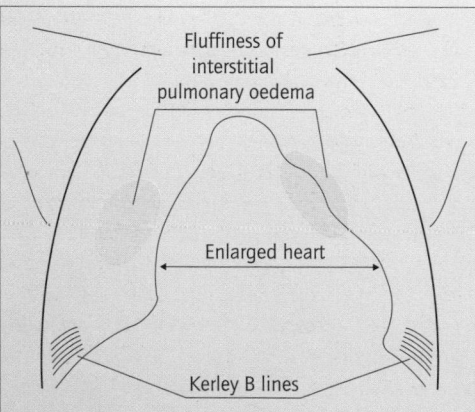

Fig. A Left ventricular failure. The chest X-ray shows cardiac enlargement, dilatation of the upper lobe veins and interstitial pulmonary oedema. Kerley B lines are seen in the right costophrenic angle.

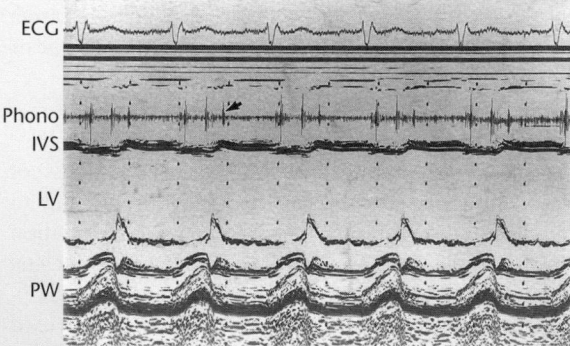

Fig. B Left ventricular failure. This M-mode echocardiogram shows considerable dilatation of the LV (the vertical dots are a 1-cm scale). Note that the IVS is almost akinetic, but the posterior wall (PW) is contracting normally. Regional contractile impairment of this type indicates coronary artery disease and must be distinguished from the global contractile impairment that occurs in cardiomyopathy. The phonocardiogram recorded simultaneously shows normal first and second heart sounds and also a third heart sound (arrowed). Both figures reproduced from Timmis AD, Nathan AW. *Essentials of Cardiology*, 2nd edn, 1992 (Blackwell Scientific Publications, Oxford) with the permission of the authors.

Clinical features	
Cardiovascular	Pansystolic murmur of mitral regurgitation
Exertional dyspnoea	Signs of tricuspid regurgitation (systolic murmur with a right
Dyspnoea at rest, othopnoea and paroxysmal nocturnal	ventricular third sound, systolic V wave in the neck, a pul-
dyspnoea	satile liver)
Tiredness	Pulmonary oedema
Resting tachycardia	Cardiogenic shock
Pulsus alternans	Elevated venous pressure
Displaced apex beat	Ankle swelling
A third heart sound	Sacral oedema
A fourth heart sound	Hepatomegaly and ascites
Crepitations at both lung bases	Pleural effusion, most commonly on the right side

- *Multiple-gated acquisition scan (MUGA)* (see p. 405): quantifies the ejection fraction and locates regional wall motion abnormalities
- *Cardiac catheterization:* probably justified in all patients with unexplained heart failure to measure haemodynamic pressures in the cardiac chambers, and to exclude significant coronary artery disease

Electrophysiology

- *ECG*
- *24-h Ambulatory ECG:* to identify any propensity for arrhythmias
- *Exercise test:* to provide a measurement of functional capacity

Management of heart failure

General measures

The majority of patients with heart failure can be managed as outpatients, but those with severe failure need to be admitted to hospital. While in hospital, the patient is usually most comfortable nursed in an upright position to reduce pulmonary venous congestion. Oxygen may be needed to maintain arterial oxygen saturation. Elastic stockings, and possibly low-dose anticogulation, may be required to prevent deep vein thrombosis. Dietary modifications including a reduced salt intake and eating small light meals are appropriate. Alcohol should be avoided because of its negative inotropic effect. Any readily remediable cause, such as pericardial tamponade or mitral regurgitation, should be relieved.

Drug treatment (Table 7.19)
Diuretics
Diuretics are a main treatment for heart failure, especially acute heart failure (BOX 7.3, p. 410), but nowadays are complemented by additional vasodilator drugs. By inhibiting sodium and chloride retention they promote

Table 7.19 Management of chronic heart failure

Drug treatment
Oral diuretics
Oral ACE inhibitors
Oral nitrates
Possibly antiarrhythmics
Oral anticoagulants
Possibly digoxin

See also text and BOX 7.1.

sodium excretion and therefore water loss through the kidneys. This reduces left and right atrial filling pressure and relieves the symptoms of heart failure.

All diuretics cause the following metabolic disturbances:
- Potassium loss (unless the diuretic is specifically potassium-sparing). This can be important in patients who have a tendency to arrhythmias. Potassium supplementation is therefore indicated for most patients.
- Glucose intolerance.
- Hyperuricaemia.
- Hypercholesterolaemia.
- Uraemia and hyponatraemia.

In severe heart failure, loop diuretics can reduce circulating blood volume enough to make the blood urea rise. In addition, the sodium loss can be out of proportion to the total volume of fluid lost, resulting in a dilutional hyponatraemia. However, the total body sodium still remains inappropriately high.

There are three types of diuretic: loop diuretics, thiazide diuretics and potassium-sparing diuretics (BOX 7.3).

Vasodilator drugs
The natural response in heart failure is vasoconstriction through a number of neural and hormonal mechanisms, including the renin–angiotensin system. Diuretics

07

increase the activity of these compensatory mechanisms, which are beneficial, but will eventually reduce cardiac output.

Vasodilating drugs are a group of drugs that act to reduce both **preload** (the atrial pressures) and **afterload** (the pressure against which the heart has to beat). Different vasodilators have different effects on the venous and arterial systems:

• Pure venous dilatation reduces left and right atrial pressure, but will not increase cardiac output and may possibly reduce it.
• Arteriolar dilatation increases cardiac output.

ACE inhibitors. These have a central role in treating heart failure, improving both symptoms and prognosis. They inhibit conversion of the vasoconstrictor peptide angiotensin 1 to angiotensin 2 and therefore lower systemic vascular resistance and venous pressure. They have a potassium-sparing effect and should be used with caution in patients who are also taking potassium-sparing diuretics. ACE inhibitors can cause significant hypotension, especially after the first dose. Treatment should therefore be started at the lowest dose available and increased according to their effect on blood pressure. The systolic pressure should not fall below 100 mmHg. Hypotension is particularly likely if diuretics have been used, so these should be temporarily discontinued as treatment with ACE inhibitors is introduced. Often the maintenance dose of diuretic can then be lowered.

ACE inhibitors should not be used in patients with renal artery stenosis because they can cause profound hypotension and renal failure. Even in the absence of renal artery stenosis, renal function can be compromised, particularly if NSAIDs are being used as well. Other side-effects of ACE inhibitors include an altered taste, rash, abdominal pain, angio-oedema and a dry cough. Because recent studies have shown that ACE inhibitors improve the prognosis of heart failure, they should be considered for all patients with heart failure.

Arteriolar vasodilators. Alpha-adrenergic blockers (e.g. prazosin) are effective arteriolar vasodilators and can therefore increase cardiac output. However, in clinical practice they are not as effective as ACE inhibitors in the treatment of heart failure.

Venodilators. Venodilators (e.g. isosorbide mononitrate) reduce left and right atrial pressure and can therefore relieve acute dyspnoea. However, long-term use can result in tolerance, and this limits their effectiveness.

Other vasodilators: phosphodiesterase inhibitors. Amrinone, milrinone and enoximone inhibit phosphodiesterase and thereby increase intracellular cyclic adeno-

sine monophosphate (cAMP). This increases myocardial contractility and peripheral vasodilatation. Their long-term pharmacological effect in improving heart failure probably relates to their vasodilator properties.

Antiarrhythmic drugs

At least 50% of patients with heart failure have evidence of ventricular arrhythmias. However, there is conflicting evidence about whether antiarrhythmic drugs have a role in reducing the incidence of sudden death in these patients.

Amiodarone. For patients with symptomatic arrhythmias, the class III antiarrhythmic drug, amiodarone, is probably the drug of first choice because it has the least negative inotropic effect of all the antiarrhythmic drugs. Type I drugs have a significant negative inotropic effect, and type Ic drugs have been shown to have a proarrhythmic effect in patients with a compromised myocardium, stimulating arrhythmias, which can worsen prognosis.

Beta-blockers. Despite their negative inotropic effect, these drugs can improve the symptoms and prognosis in patients with heart failure, especially if there is a resting tachycardia. Carvedilol, which has peripheral vasodilator properties, is particularly used in this context.

ACE inhibitors. These may exert their beneficial effect on prognosis in cardiac failure partly as a result of an indirect antiarrhythmic effect.

Device insertion

Permanent pacemaker insertion

In a few highly selected patients with widened QRS complexes on ECG and/or mitral regurgitation, biventricular pacing [one lead in the right ventricle and one lead in the coronary sinus (indirectly the left ventricle)] improves coordination of contraction and cardiac output.

Implantable cardiac defibrillator

An implantable cardiac defibrillator device improves the prognosis for patients with heart failure who have relatively infrequent life-threatening ventricular arrhythmias.

Management of acute heart failure

The treatment of sudden acute heart failure (BOX 7.9; EMERGENCY BOX 7.3), when the total circulating blood volume will not be increased, is directed at supporting the myocardium and encouraging blood flow with vasodilators, rather than using diuretics to achieve a diuresis. However, diuretics are often necessary to relieve acute pulmonary oedema, but may cause hypotension and compromise renal function.

Emergency 7.3: Acute heart failure

Diamorphine with an appropriate antiemetic
To reduce anxiety
To reduce vasomotor tone, so lowering both the filling
pressure (and therefore reducing breathlessness)
and offloading the heart (with a fall in systolic blood
pressure)

**Oxygen, 50% by face mask, unless the patient has a
chronic respiratory disease**
High oxygen concentrations in patients with obstructive
airway disease can precipitate carbon dioxide narcosis
by reducing the oxygen drive of the respiratory centre.
Occasionally the patient has to be ventilated

Intravenous frusemide (furosemide)
This produces both an immediate vasodilatation and
more prolonged diuresis
A pulmonary artery catheter (Swan–Ganz catheter) can
help guide fluid balance
Measuring pulmonary capillary wedge pressure provides
an indirect measurement of left atrial pressure, which
can be optimized at 18–22 mmHg

Venous dilatation
The acute reduction of atrial pressure with intravenous or
sublingual nitrates can rapidly reduce breathlessness,
but may cause significant hypotension

*Aminophylline 250–500 mg intravenously over 15 min (if
there is bronchospasm)*
Can vasodilate and bronchodilate, and is of value if there
is bronchospasm present. It is a phosphodiesterase
inhibitor and therefore improves myocardial contractility,
but can also precipitate serious arrhythmias

Beta-adrenergic agonists
e.g. dopamine, dobutamine

Intra-aortic balloon pump
(See p. 432)

Management of severe heart failure/cardiogenic shock

Cardiogenic shock is defined as heart failure with a BP of
less than 90 mmHg systolic, reduced urine output and
reduced central blood flow leading to confusion. The
patient should be nursed sitting up in bed or in a chair
with an oxygen mask to improve oxygen saturation. Mild
sedation with diamorphine or diazepam can be helpful,
provided it does not depress respiration.

Drug treatment
Inotropic agents
These drugs increase the contractility (force of contrac-

tion) of the myocardium. However, apart from digoxin,
they usually have to be given through a central venous line
and so their use is confined to the intensive care unit over
short periods.

Digoxin. Digoxin acts by inhibiting the sodium–
potassium ATPase pump. This leads to an accumulation
of intracellular sodium, which exchanges for extracellular
calcium. Increased cytosolic calcium increases contractility by inhibiting troponin and so stimulating the binding
of actin and myosin. Digoxin may have only a temporary
inotropic effect, but it is of particular value for patients
with heart failure and atrial fibrillation because it also
controls the heart rate.

Digoxin is protein bound and the binding proteins must
therefore be saturated by an initial digitilization dosage.
This is then followed by a lower daily dose. Digitilization
is achieved by giving 1.5 mg over 24 h in divided doses,
followed by 0.25 mg/day. Patients with a reduced glomerular filtration rate require a lower maintenance dose of
digoxin because 90% of digoxin is excreted by the kidneys,
but the same initial digitilization regimen will be required.

An alternative to digoxin is digitoxin, which is metabolized by the liver and may therefore be preferred for
patients with renal failure. It may also be preferred in
patients with an idiosyncratic sensitivity to digoxin. The
normal therapeutic level of digoxin is 1–2 ng/ml.

Digoxin toxicity: patients with hyperthyroidism or hypocalcaemia are particularly sensitive to digoxin. Features
of digoxin toxicity are:
● Nausea and vomiting
● Ventricular arrhythmias, particularly ventricular
ectopics and AV block
● Disturbance of vision, known as xanthopsia, when
everything looks yellowish
Toxicity is managed by stopping the digoxin, monitoring
the plasma potassium level and treating any arrhythmia.

Beta-adrenergic agonists
Adrenaline, dobutamine, dopamine and dopexamine are
adrenergic agonists that need to be given intravenously.
They all stimulate beta-1 receptors to a varying degree,
increasing intracellular cAMP and consequently increasing
contractility. Dopamine is less selective than dobutamine
and can therefore improve renal artery perfusion, which
acts synergistically with diuretics to improve urine output.

Patients with moderate to severe heart failure have high
levels of circulating endogenous catecholamines. This,
together with or without the long-term use of beta-1
agonists, can cause downregulation of beta receptors so
that the patient becomes less responsive to their actions.

Intra-aortic balloon pump
If surgery can improve the prognosis it is reasonable to

07

use an intra-aortic balloon pump to stabilize the patient until surgery can be carried out. A balloon is inserted into the femoral artery and advanced up the descending aorta to just below the aortic arch. It is timed to inflate during diastole and so provide additional mechanical support (counterpulsation) for the heart. It increases renal perfusion and diastolic coronary blood flow, and causes systemic vasodilatation.

Emergency balloon angioplasty

If a patient is in cardiogenic shock following a myocardial infarction, immediate restoration of coronary flow by balloon dilatation of the occluded artery can improve myocardial function.

Other measures

Other measures can be introduced to relieve catastrophic heart failure. These include:

● Venesection, which effectively reduces circulating blood volume

● Applying a sphygmomanometer cuff around both thighs at a pressure 10 mmHg below diastolic blood pressure to reduce venous return to the heart

Both these techniques are drastic measures and are now rarely used.

Prognosis

Whatever the cause, the prognosis of heart failure is poor, with 50% of patients who have severe heart failure dying within 5 years. The mortality rate of patients in cardiogenic shock who are not given a heart transplant is 90%.

Arrhythmias

An abnormal heart rhythm is one of the most common reasons for a patient to present to the cardiologist. The normal heart rhythm is controlled by the sinus node. It depolarizes spontaneously and its rate of discharge is influenced by the autonomic nervous system.

● *Increase in parasympathetic activity:* causes bradycardia, which, if severe, can result in a vasovagal episode; the patient becomes cold and clammy and feels nauseated. As the blood pressure drops, the patient feels faint and may black out.

● *Increase in sympathetic activity:* causes tachycardia.

Varying autonomic nervous activity during respiration causes a variation in normal sinus rhythm, known as sinus arrhythmia (Fig. 7.31a). The rate usually increases with inspiration. This is particularly common in children and young adults, but does not occur if there is an atrial septal defect. Bradycardia is a heart rate of less than 60 beats/min, and a tachycardia is a heart rate of more than 100 beats/min.

Bradycardia

Disease mechanisms (Table 7.20)

A sinus bradycardia results from a sinus rate of less than 60 beats/min and is common in athletes (Fig. 7.31b).

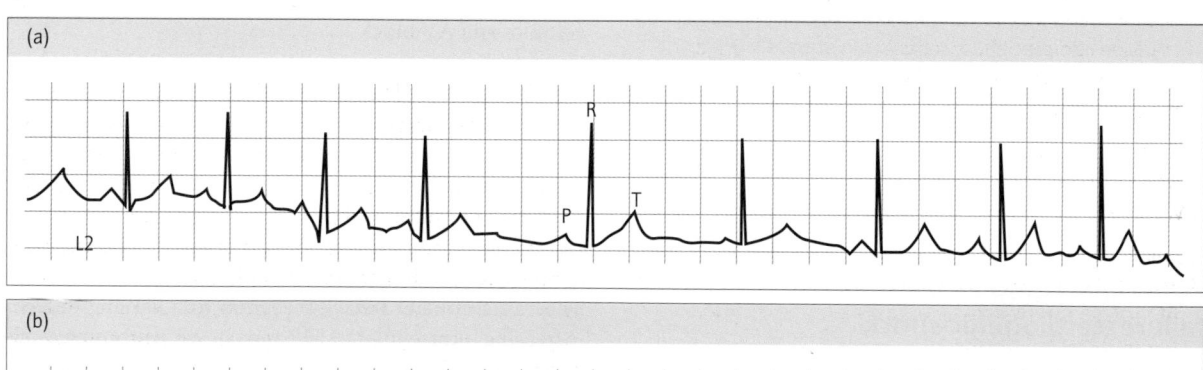

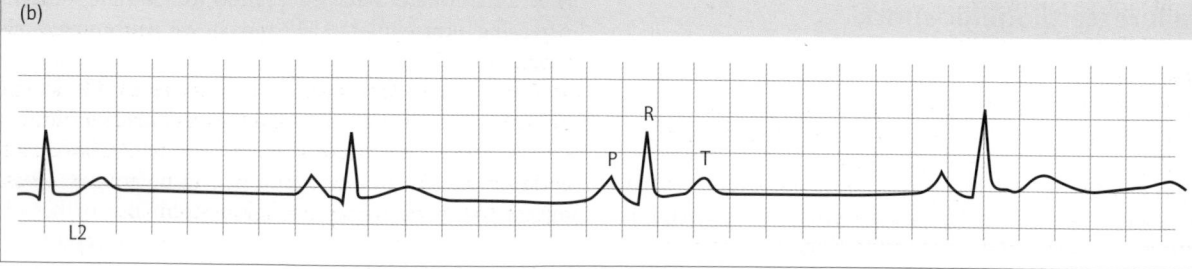

Figure 7.31 (a) Sinus arrhythmia: varying heart rate resulting from respiration. (b) Sinus bradycardia: P-wave rate less than 60 beats/min.

Table 7.20 ECG characteristics of bradycardias

Sinus bradycardia

Sinus node disease

P waves appear irregularly and the intervals between the P waves are either a multiple of the normal sinus rate (SA exit block), or more variable and unpredictable (sinus arrest)

AV block

First degree

Prolongation of the PR interval (beyond 220 ms) because of delayed conduction through the atria and/or AV node
Each P wave is followed by a QRS complex

Second degree

There are two forms:

Mobitz I Progressive prolongation of the PR interval (by decreasing amounts) until a P wave is not followed by a QRS complex. The PR interval of the beat following the blocked P wave is much shorter and then progressively prolongs again until the next dropped QRS complex (the Wenckebach phenomenon)

Mobitz II Intermittent or regular failure of the QRS complex to follow the P wave. 2 : 1 second degree heart block is conduction of every other P wave to the QRS, 3 : 1 second degree heart block is conduction of every third P wave to the QRS, and so on

Third degree

Failure of P-wave conduction to the ventricles. There is therefore no relationship between the P-wave rate and the QRS-complex rate. The QRS complex may be either narrow or wide. If it is narrow the escape rhythm is arising from the AV node or the proximal bundle and may have a rate that approximates that of the P wave. When the escape rhythm is a wide complex, the focus is in the distal His–Purkinje system or the ventricles, and the rate of the escape rhythm is usually slow

Bundle branch block

Incomplete bundle branch block

Widening of the QRS complex (up to 120 ms)

Complete bundle branch block

A wider QRS complex (longer than 120 ms). The morphology of the QRS complex depends on whether the right or left bundle branch is diseased

Left hemi-block

Left hemi-block shifts the axis of the QRS complex. A conduction delay in the anterior–superior fascicle causes left axis deviation (more than − 30°)
Conduction delay in the posterior–inferior fascicle causes right axis deviation (more than + 120°)

Table 7.21 Causes of sinus bradycardia

Sinus node disease (Table 7.20)

Infarction (particularly inferior infarction) involving the sinus node

Drugs (e.g. beta-blockers)

Degenerative changes in the sinus node (common in the elderly)

Non-cardiac (e.g. raised intracranial pressure, hypothermia, hypothyroidism)

Pathological causes of sinus bradycardia are listed in Table 7.21.

Bundle branch block

Delayed conduction through the bundle branches can result in incomplete or complete bundle branch block, but does not cause a bradycardia.

Right bundle branch block (Fig. 7.32). This is a normal finding in about 1% of the population. It is also found in association with other conditions. It delays depolarization of the right ventricle, delaying closure of the pulmonary valve and giving rise to wider splitting of the second heart sound.

Left bundle branch block (Fig. 7.33). This is much less common than right bundle branch block in healthy people and usually indicates severe disease of the left ventricle. It delays emptying of the left ventricle and closure of the aortic valve, leading to reversed splitting of the second heart sound.

Left hemi-block. This is delayed conduction in either the anterior (giving rise to left axis deviation) or posterior (giving rise to right axis deviation) fascicle of the left bundle. Left anterior hemi-block is more common because the anterior fascicle is more discrete than the posterior fascicle and can be affected by more localized damage (e.g. in ischaemic heart disease).

- *Bifascicular block:* occurs when conduction to both the right bundle and the left anterior or left posterior fascicle is delayed.
- *Trifascicular block:* results in complete AV block. The progression of bifascicular block to trifascicular block is uncommon, but is more likely if there is alternating left and right bundle branch block, or if there is right bundle branch block and right posterior hemi-block.

Atrioventricular block

There are three types of AV block: first, second and third degree AV block.

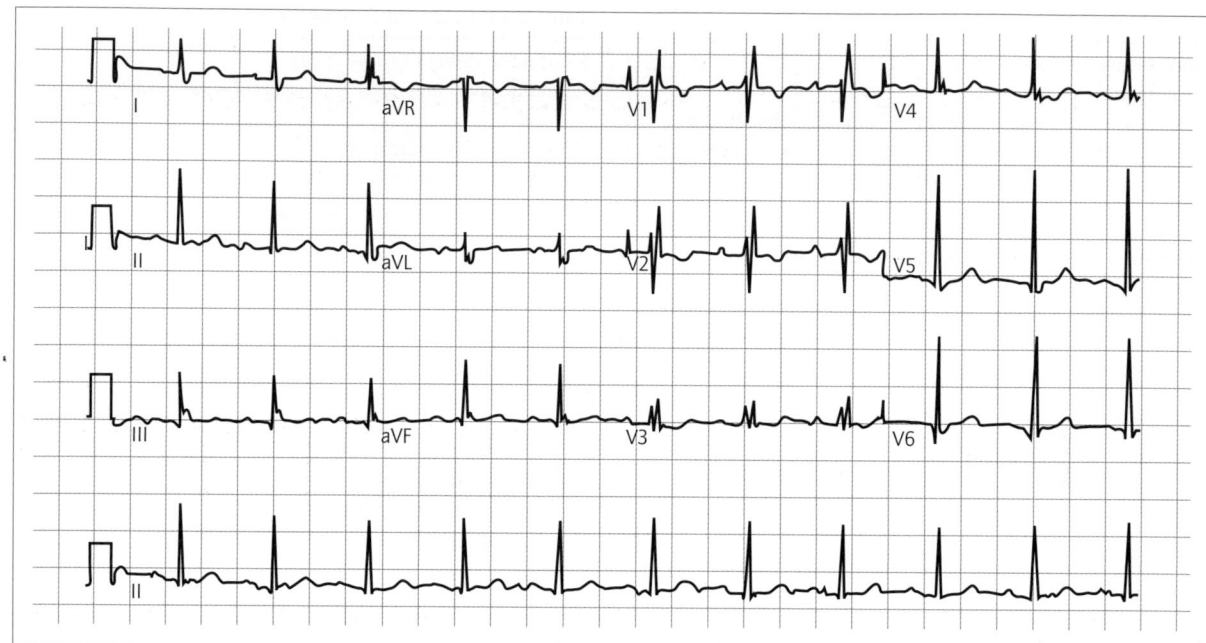

Figure 7.32 Right bundle branch block. Note: (i) QRS width more than 120 ms; (ii) RSR pattern in lead V1; (iii) late S wave in lead I.

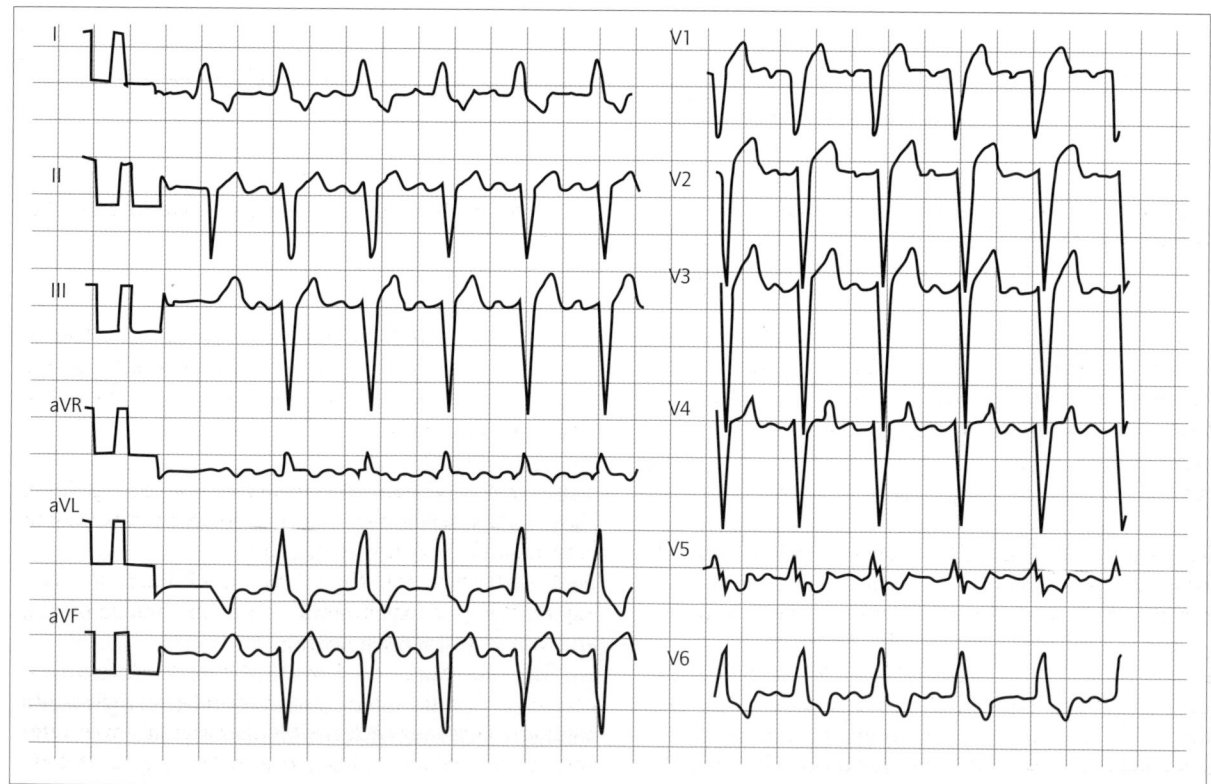

Figure 7.33 Left bundle branch block. Note: (i) QRS width more than 120 ms; (ii) ST depression and T inversion in leads I, aVL, V5 and V6; (iii) RSR pattern in left ventricular leads (e.g. lead V5 in this case).

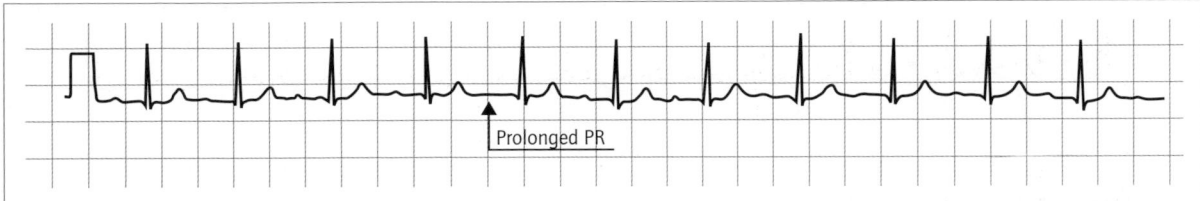

Figure 7.34 First degree heart block. Note long PR interval (more than 200 ms).

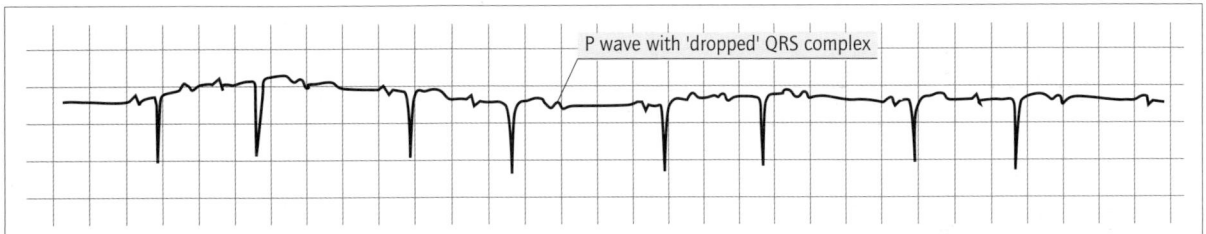

Figure 7.35 Second degree heart block. Mobitz type I (Wenckebach). Note the lengthening PR interval on each successive beat until a P wave is not followed by a QRS complex. The next PR interval returns to normal.

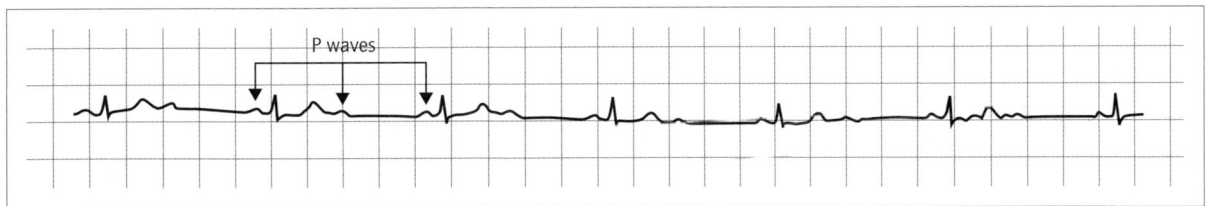

Figure 7.36 Second degree heart block. Mobitz type II. Note there is a fixed relationship between the P wave and the QRS complexes. In this case two P waves to one QRS complex (−2 : 1 AV block).

First degree AV block (Fig. 7.34). This is delayed conduction of the atrial impulse to the ventricles, usually within the AV node. It gives rise to a long PR interval (more than 220 ms), which can be a benign finding in young people with increased vagal tone. As with bundle branch block, this does not cause a bradycardia.

Second degree AV block. This occurs when intermittently the P wave is not followed by a QRS complex. The block to conduction occurs in the AV node and can be of two types:
• *Mobitz type I* (Wenckebach; Fig. 7.35): the PR interval increases with each beat until an atrial impulse is not conducted and then the PR interval returns to normal.
• *Mobitz type II* (second degree AV block; Fig. 7.36): the PR interval does not change, but the QRS complex fails to follow the P wave because of a regularly or intermittently occurring block, which is usually below the AV node in the

bundle branches or bundle of His. If there are two P waves to one QRS complex it is a 2 : 1 block, whereas if there are four P waves to one QRS complex it is a 4 : 1 block. The degree of block can vary.

Third degree AV block (complete heart block; Fig. 7.37). This occurs when there is a permanent dissociation between atrial and ventricular activity.
• *When the block is in the AV node:* a subsidiary and usually reliable pacemaker takes over in the bundle of His, and the QRS complex is narrow.
• *When the block is below the AV node:* the residual pacemaker is in the bundle branches and gives a wide QRS complex. These pacemaker sites discharge at slower rates and are less reliable, giving rise to fainting (a **Stokes–Adams attack**). Occasionally, a P wave can be transmitted to the ventricles in third degree block, when the P wave falls on the T wave. This can transiently improve AV

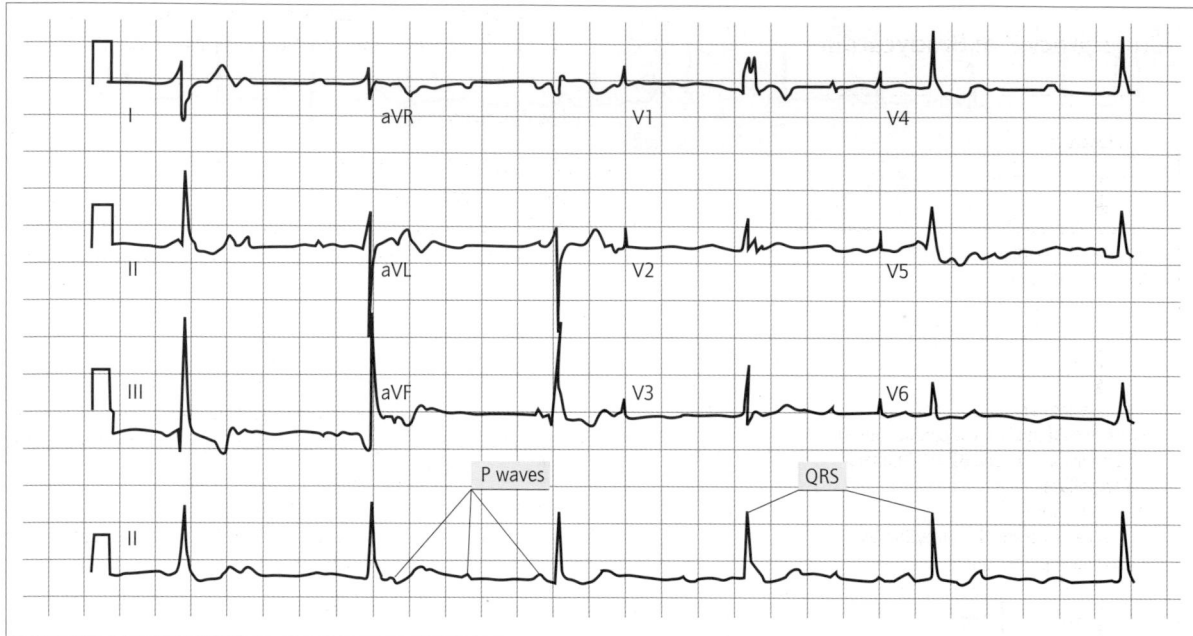

Figure 7.37 Complete heart block. Note that there is no relationship between P waves and QRS complexes.

conduction and give rise to an irregular ventricular rate. This is known as supernormal conduction.

Atrioventricular dissociation

In this type of dissociation of atrial and ventricular contraction, the ventricular rate is usually more than 60 beats/min and may be faster than the atrial rate. AV dissociation can also occur in ventricular tachycardia when the finding of 'independent' P waves can help in making the diagnosis.

The symptoms of AV dissociation depend on the ventricular rate and underlying cardiac pathology. The diagnosis is made on the 12-lead ECG, although the distinction between ventricular tachycardia and supraventricular tachycardia with aberrancy (when the QRS complex is widened) can be difficult (see Table 7.22, p. 439 below).

Management
Sinus bradycardia

Sinus bradycardia does not usually need treatment, except in the acute setting of a vasovagal attack (EMERGENCY BOX 7.4). Such haemodynamically important sinus bradycardias are treated with intravenous atropine. A pacemaker may be required for severe chronic sinus bradycardia.

Atrioventricular block

Both first and second degree AV block are usually asymp-

tomatic, but both can be markers of intermittent periods of third degree block, causing dizziness and blackouts. Patients with third degree AV block (complete heart block) usually require treatment with a pacemaker.

- *Temporary pacemaker:* used when complete AV block is brought about by a cause that is likely to resolve, such as an infarction. If the ventricular escape rhythm is fast enough, it may be possible to avoid a temporary pacemaker.
- *Permanent pacemaker:* usually required for chronic complete AV block or symptomatic second degree block. Types of pacemaker (BOX 7.8). A physiological rate responsive pacemaker system alters the heart rate in response to exercise and is appropriate except in very elderly patients. This involves a dual chamber system in which both an atrial and ventricular wire are implanted. The atrial wire can sense atrial activity and then coordinate ventricular systole sequentially (Fig. 7.38). If the atrial rate is slow, the atrial wire can stimulate the atrium at a preset interval before the ventricle is stimulated. This allows a normal cardiac activation sequence resulting in better cardiac output than occurs with simple single wire ventricular pacing. It also prevents retrograde activation of the atrium by ventricular pacing, which can give rise to a reflex reduction in blood pressure causing dizziness (known as the pacemaker syndrome).

Both dual chamber and single chamber systems can be rate responsive. This means that the generator senses the activity of the body, either by a movement-sensitive

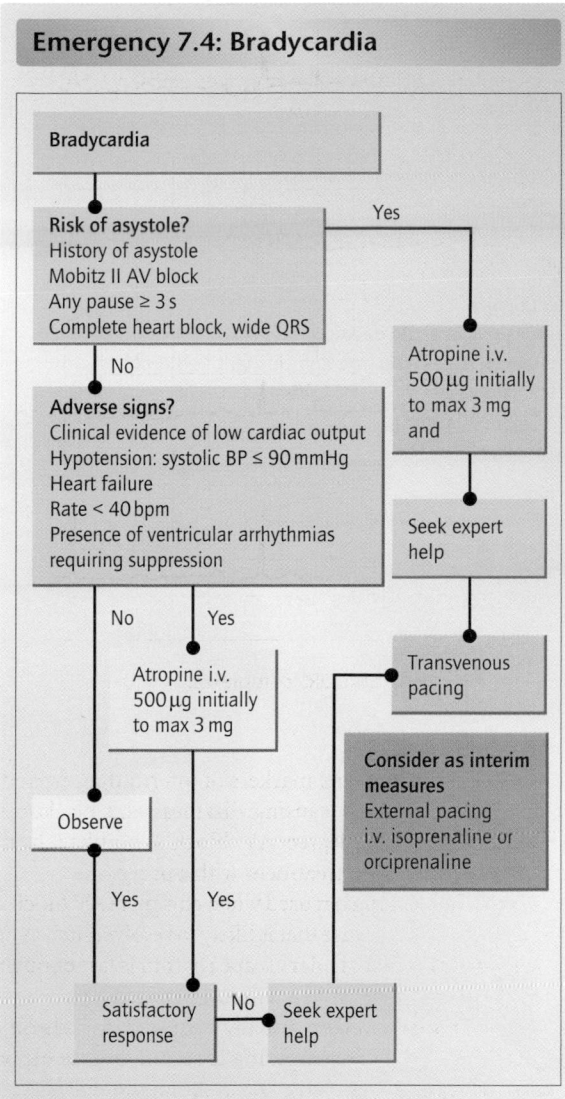

Bradycardia

Risk of asystole?
History of asystole
Mobitz II AV block
Any pause ≥ 3 s
Complete heart block, wide QRS

Yes

No

Adverse signs?
Clinical evidence of low cardiac output
Hypotension: systolic BP ≤ 90 mmHg
Heart failure
Rate < 40 bpm
Presence of ventricular arrhythmias
requiring suppression

Atropine i.v.
500 µg initially
to max 3 mg
and

Seek expert
help

No   Yes

Atropine i.v.
500 µg initially
to max 3 mg

Transvenous
pacing

Consider as interim measures
External pacing
i.v. isoprenaline or
orciprenaline

Observe

Yes   Yes

Satisfactory
response

No

Seek expert
help

Fig. A Approach to management of bradycardia. Doses based on adult of average body weight. In all cases give oxygen and establish intravenous access. BP, blood pressure

module within the generator, or by sensing the respiratory rate, and increases the heart rate appropriately.

Tachycardia

A tachycardia is defined as a heart rate of more than 100 beats/min, and can be subdivided into supraventricular and ventricular tachycardia. Pathological tachycardia can result from one of two mechanisms: automaticity or re-entry circuits (either macro or micro).

Automaticity

Automaticity describes normal depolarization of the transmembrane voltage during diastole until a threshold is reached and an electrical discharge occurs. The rate of discharge can be increased by:
- Reduced threshold potential
- Increased rate of diastolic depolarization, particularly in the presence of myocardial damage
- Increased circulating catecholamines or digoxin

Re-entry circuits

Re-entry circuits arise from different rates of repolarization in adjacent areas of myocardium.
- *Macro re-entry circuit:* a wave of depolarization travels in a circle of myocardial tissue. If the tissue in any part of the ring has recovered by the time the electrical impulse comes round to it again, it will depolarize and produce a circus movement resulting in a tachycardia. This mechanism is responsible for most paroxysmal tachycardias.
- *Micro re-entry circuit:* adjacent cells recover at different rates. Those that repolarize more rapidly are restimulated by adjacent cells, which have not yet repolarized. This is called cellular reflection.

Sinus tachycardia

Sinus tachycardia is defined as a sinus rate of more than 100 beats/min (Fig. 7.39). It is usually secondary to other causes (Table 7.22). Rarely, a primary sinus tachycardia can result from a sinus node re-entry mechanism.

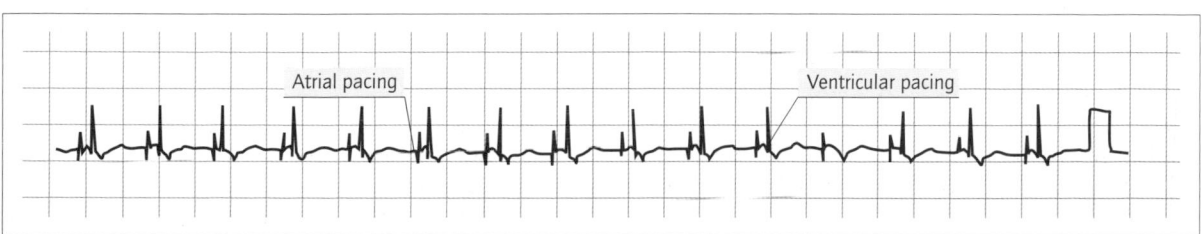

Atrial pacing   Ventricular pacing

Figure 7.38 ECG of AV pacing. Note the two pacing 'spikes': one initiating the P wave, the other initiating the QRS complex.

07

Box 7.8: Using pacemakers: what the student needs to know

Temporary pacemaker

This is inserted via the subclavian or internal jugular vein to pace the right atrium and/or the right ventricle. It is connected to an external box, which can be set to a predetermined rate. The output from the external generator can also be increased

Permanent pacemaker

This is implanted in the body, usually in the left prepectoral region, and is powered by a lithium battery which can last up to 10 years. The leads are introduced transvenously into the right atrial appendage and/or the right ventricular apex

Pacing threshold

Pacing threshold is the minimum voltage required by the pacemaker to depolarize the heart. It is assessed by reducing the energy of the external pacemaker until it fails to stimulate the myocardium. If this is more than 1 V, the pacemaker wire must be resited. For temporary pacemakers, the pacemaker output should be set at 2–3 times the pacing threshold in case it increases after insertion

Setting the pacemaker

The pacemaker is usually set on demand, so that it will only stimulate the myocardium when the spontaneous heart rate falls below a preset rate

Complications of pacemakers

Lead displacement

This results in a sudden intermittent or permanent loss of pacing and the recurrence of symptoms

Infection

This usually develops soon after pacemaker insertion and so prophylactic antibiotics are often used at implantation. If infection is established, the pacing system needs to be removed while the patient is maintained on a temporary pacing system. A new permanent pacing system can be installed when the infection is under control

Erosion

The generator or the pacing leads can erode through the skin, particularly in thin or cachexic patients

Pacemaker generator failure

This is uncommon but requires replacement of the generator

Lead fracture

This is rare, but if the pacing lead breaks symptoms will return. The lead fracture can be identified on chest radiography

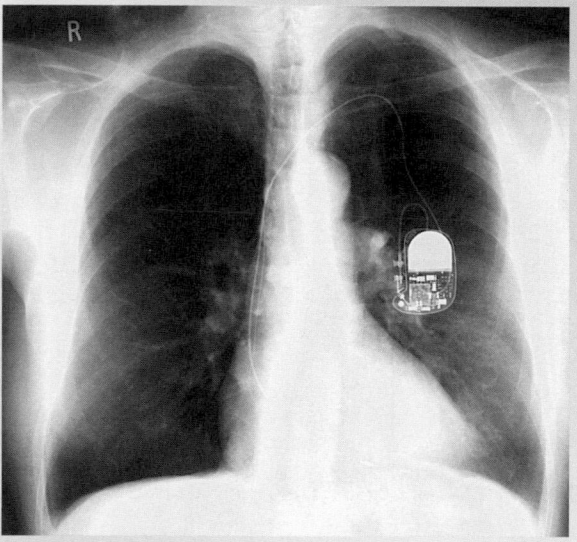

Fig. A Pacemaker lead and generator appearance on chest X-ray. Note old pacemaker lead which has been cut short in right cephalic vein.

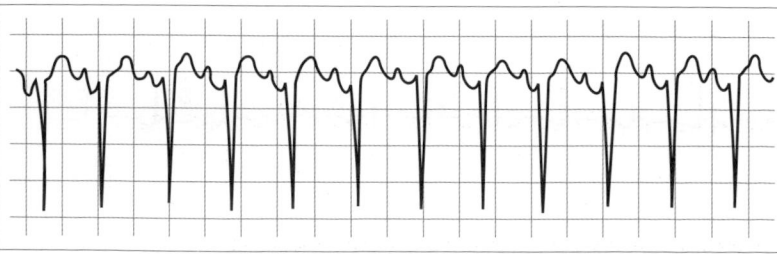

Figure 7.39 Sinus tachycardia.

Table 7.22 Causes of sinus tachycardia

Exercise
Thyrotoxicosis
Catecholamine stimulation (e.g. caused by emotion)
Fever
Anaemia
Cardiac failure
Hypovolaemia

Atrial tachyarrhythmias

Atrial ectopics, atrial flutter, atrial fibrillation and atrial tachycardia all arise from the atrial myocardium and all have similar aetiologies.

Atrial ectopic beats

Atrial ectopic beats can give rise to an awareness of a missed heart beat (Fig. 7.40).

Atrial flutter

Atrial flutter is a tachycardia in which the atrial rate is usually about 300 beats/min and there is a 2 : 1 AV block giving a ventricular rate of 150 beats/min (Fig. 7.41). Often the ECG appearance looks like sinus tachycardia unless the characteristic f (flutter) waves of the atrium are easy to see. They are usually most obvious in lead V1.

Atrial fibrillation

Atrial fibrillation is an irregularly irregular rhythm: atrial foci discharge at very high rates (Fig. 7.42). Not all impulses are transmitted by the AV node and so the ventricular rate is much slower and irregular. It is commonly caused by an associated cardiac abnormality, but there is no apparent cause in 40% of patients. A list of causes is given in Table 7.23.

Narrow QRS tachycardias

Two atrial tachycardias are caused by automaticity: atrial tachycardia and junctional tachycardia. The other narrow QRS tachycardias are caused by re-entry circuits, and are known as reciprocating tachycardias.

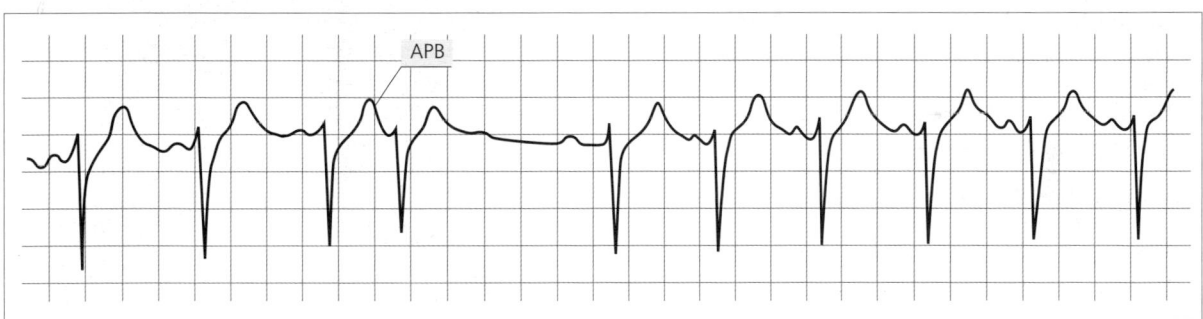

Figure 7.40 Atrial premature (ectopic) beat (APB). Note the compensatory pause.

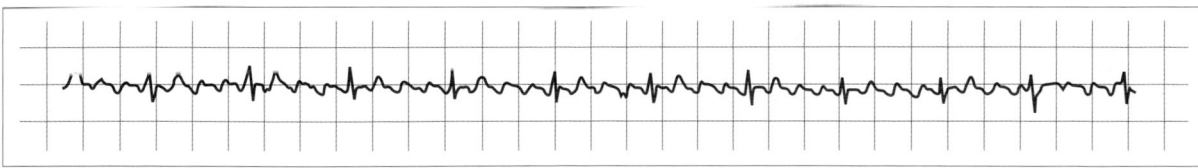

Figure 7.41 Atrial flutter. Carotid sinus massage or treatment with adenosine can increase the degree of AV block. Note saw-tooth pattern of baseline with atrial rate of 300 beats/min and ventricular rate of 75 beats/min.

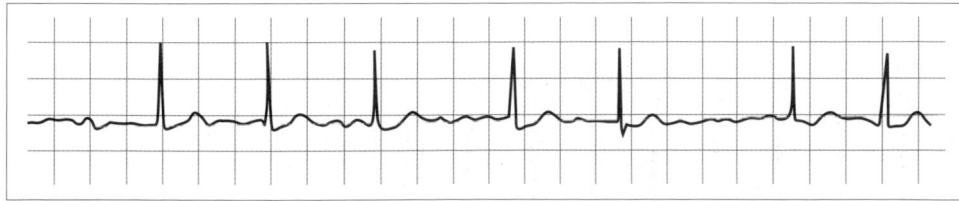

Figure 7.42 Atrial fibrillation. Note irregular ventricular response and absence of organized atrial activity.

07

Table 7.23 Causes of atrial fibrillation

Not known
Lone atrial fibrillation (no cause found)

Structural
Rheumatic heart disease
Ischaemic heart disease
Cardiomyopathy
Re-entry bypass tracts (Wolff–Parkinson–White syndrome)

Hormonal
Thyrotoxicosis

Metabolic
Acute and chronic alcoholism

Other
Carcinoma of the bronchus
Pneumonia
Pulmonary embolism

Atrial tachycardia (Fig. 7.43). This can be paroxysmal or chronic and is often associated with a degree of AV block. It is uncommon and is usually associated with underlying heart disease. The P-wave morphology is abnormal and AV block may be induced by carotid sinus massage. This will not stop the tachycardia, however, because the tachycardia is caused by automaticity rather than a re-entry circuit involving the AV node, where the effect of carotid sinus massage occurs.

Junctional tachycardia. This results from a junctional focus activating both atria and ventricles. It may be caused by digoxin toxicity or other forms of heart disease, such as coronary artery disease.

Pre-excitation syndromes
Atrial activity is usually conducted to the ventricles only via the AV node. In pre-excitation syndromes there is an extra connection between the atrium and the ventricles (Fig. 7.44). Because this accessory pathway does not delay conduction, an impulse via the accessory pathway depolarizes the ventricles before the impulse via the AV node.

There are two specific forms of AV electrical bypass tract that cause tachycardia: WPW syndrome and Lown–Ganong–Levine (LGL) syndrome. In these conditions, pulses from the atrium are rapidly transmitted through the bypass tract to the ventricle and therefore avoid delay at the AV node.

Wolff–Parkinson–White syndrome. The WPW syndrome is caused by a congenital accessory bundle (bundle of Kent) between the atrium and ventricular myocardium (Fig. 7.45). Early depolarization of the ventricular myocardium causes an initial deflection in the QRS complex, known as a delta wave. The location of the bundle of Kent in the AV groove defines the nature of delta wave on the ECG and the syndrome can be subdivided into either type A or type B. In type A the bundle of Kent is usually on the left side of the heart and in type B it is usually on the right side.

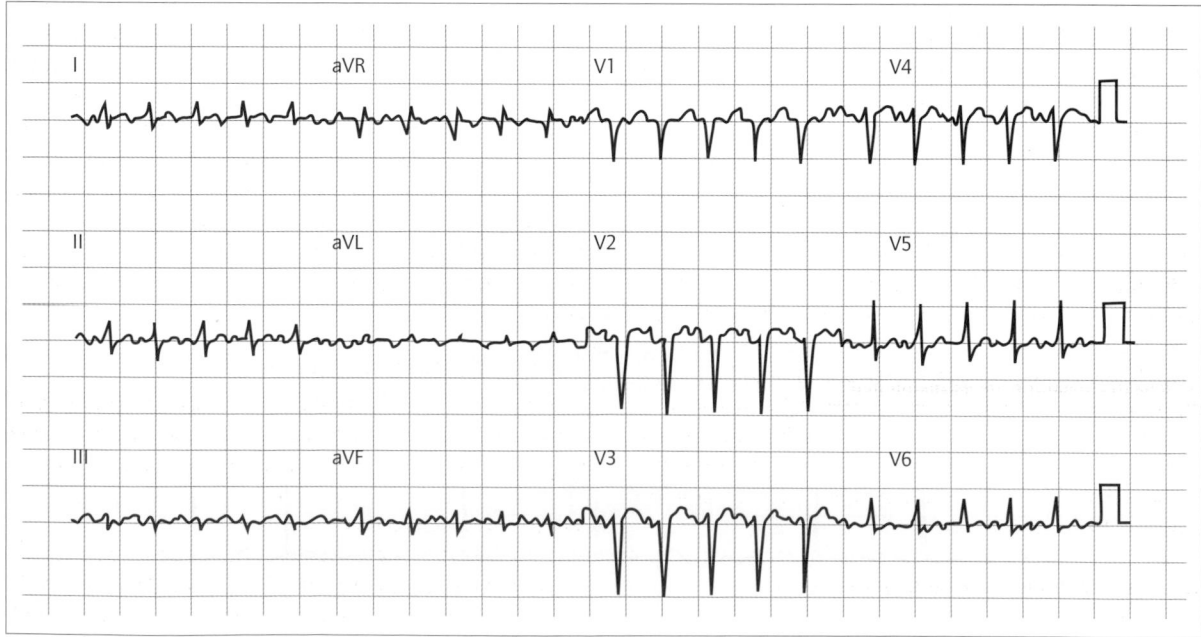

Figure 7.43 Atrial tachycardia.

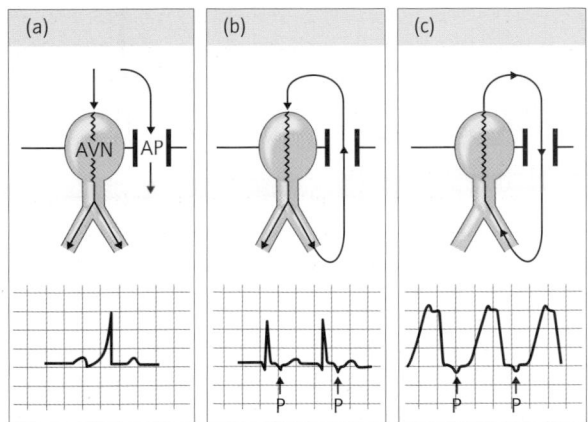

Figure 7.44 The pre-excitation syndrome. (a) Sinus rhythm with ventricular depolarization occurring because of impulses arriving via the AV node (AVN) and accessory pathway (AP). (b) Orthodromic AV re-entry tachycardia (AVRT) with narrow QRS complexes and retrograde P wave present in ST segment. (c) Antidromic AVRT with wide QRS complex and retrograde P wave present in ST segment.

The anatomical abnormality of WPW syndrome provides a substrate for two sorts of tachycardia: AV re-entry tachycardia (AVRT) and atrial fibrillation.
● *AVRT* occurs when the circus movement tachycardia starts in the atrium, travels to the ventricle through the AV node, and then returns to the atrium from the ventricle via the bundle of Kent. The QRS complex is narrow unless there is an associated intraventricular conduction abnormality and there is no delta wave.
● *Atrial fibrillation* impulses may be transmitted to the ventricles via both the AV node and the bundle of Kent. This can result in faster ventricular rates than usual in atrial fibrillation, and may lead to ventricular fibrillation and death.

Lown–Ganong–Levine syndrome. In LGL syndrome the additional AV connection is between the atrium and the bundle of His. The PR interval is short, but ventricular depolarization appears normal and there is no delta wave. Patients are prone to AVRT and should be treated appropriately.

A short PR interval does not always indicate an AV accessory bypass tract. Other causes of a short PR interval include small stature, increased sympathetic activity and a congenitally small AV node.

Atrioventricular re-entrant tachycardias (reciprocating tachycardias)
As well as the bundle of Kent, other types of extra connection can exist between the atria and ventricles. These pathways are not evident on the surface ECG and are called concealed pathways, which can only be identified by electrophysiological studies. Such concealed pathways can either be within or outside the AV node.

There are two types of reciprocating tachycardia: AV node re-entry tachycardia (AVNRT) and AV re-entry tachycardia (AVRT).
● *AVNRT* (Fig. 7.46a): a paroxysmal tachycardia where a circus of depolarization occurs within the AV node because of fast and slow conduction. This precipitates a tachycardia by simultaneously activating both the atrium and ventricle.
● *AVRT* (Fig. 7.46b): results from a larger circuit than that for AVNRT and includes the AV node, the bundle of His, the ventricles and an abnormal AV connection. Impulses travel from the atria to the ventricles via the AV node and then return to the atria via the abnormal conduction.

The two types of reciprocating tachycardia can usually be distinguished on the surface, especially when the tachycardia of AVRT is conducted through the concealed pathway and retrogradely through the AV node (antidiomic VRT), the QRS complexes are broad. If the tachycardia is atrial fibrillation then a characteristic broad comple tachycardia that is irregularly irregular develops (pre-excited atrial fibrillation). They can be provoked by specific stimuli such as exertion, caffeinated drinks and alcohol.

Ventricular ectopic beats
Ventricular ectopic beats are common, and may be present without evidence of underlying heart disease (Fig. 7.47). Sometimes they occur on a regular basis in relation to the normal beat. Alternation with a normal beat is ventricular bigeminy, occurrence every third beat is ventricular trigeminy, and so on. Occasionally, the timing is unrelated to the normal sinus rhythm, but is related to the interval between previous ventricular ectopic beats. As a result the ectopic beat can 'fuse' with the normal beat (so-called fusion beats). This phenomenon is known as parasystole, and is a feature of ischaemic heart disease.

Ventricular tachyarrhythmias
Ventricular tachyarrhythmias tend to be more serious than supraventricular tachyarrhythmias. They are usually a consequence of coronary artery disease or a cardiomyopathy.

Ventricular tachycardia
VT is a broad complex tachycardia of more than three consecutive ventricular beats (Fig. 7.48). Occasionally, it is well tolerated, but usually it causes hypotension and signs of cardiac decompensation. The ventricular rate is usually 120–250 beats/min. There may be signs of AV

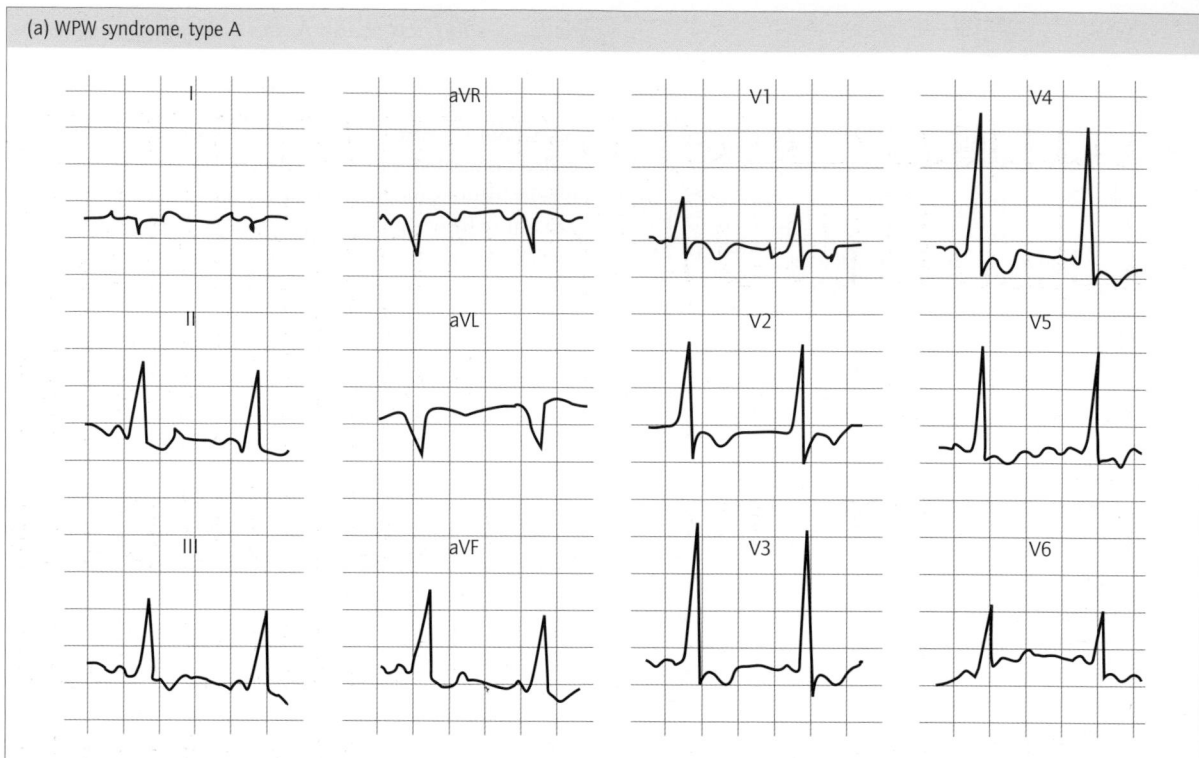

(a) WPW syndrome, type A

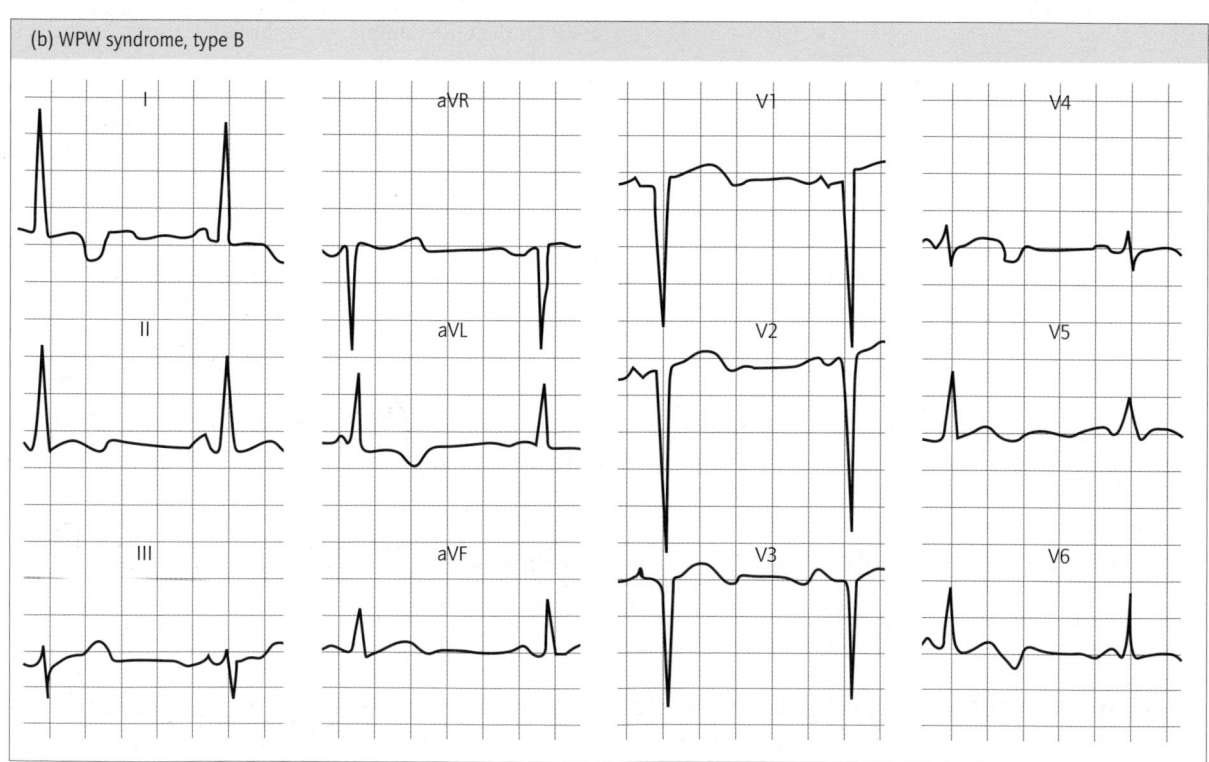

(b) WPW syndrome, type B

Figure 7.45 Wolff–Parkinson–White syndrome. (a) Type A. (b) Type B. Note: (i) short PR interval; (ii) delta wave giving widened QRS complex; and (iii) abnormal ST/T waves resulting from abnormal depolarization. In type A there is a predominantly positive complex in lead V1. In type B the QRS complex is predominantly negative in lead V1. The presence of the delta wave can give rise to misleading appearances. In type A, the ECG appearance can suggest right bundle branch block, right ventricular hypertrophy or true posterior infarction. In type B, the ECG appearance can look like left bundle branch block. A negative delta wave can mimic the Q wave of myocardial infarction.

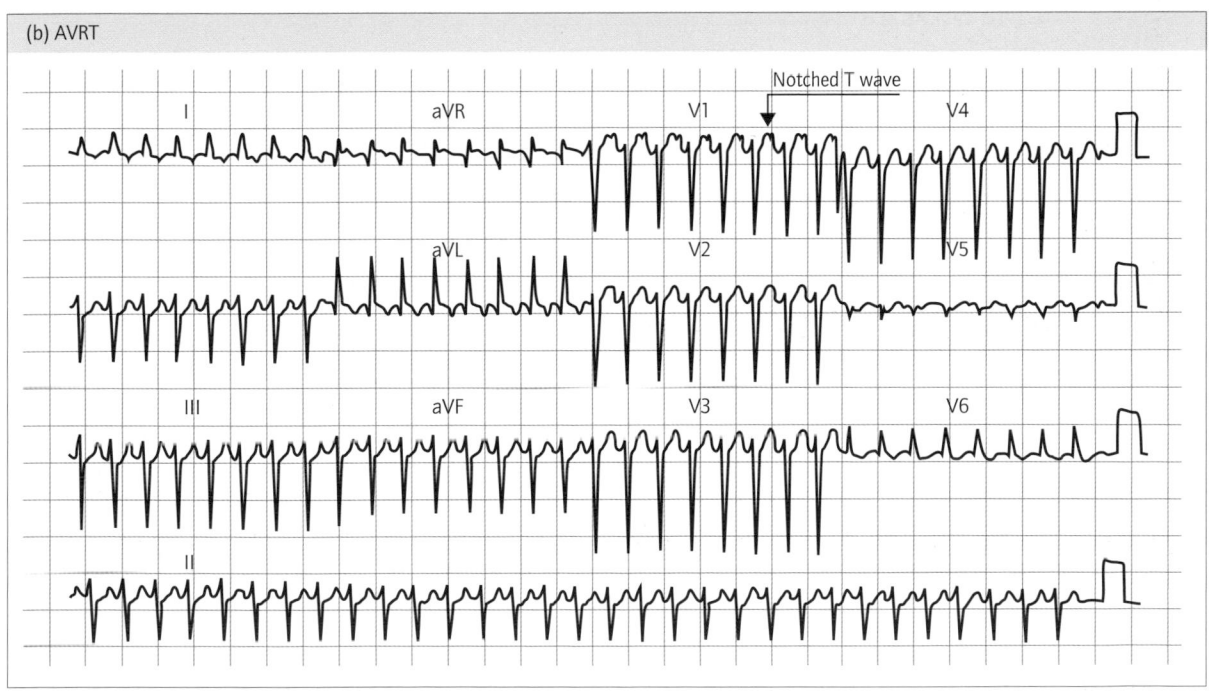

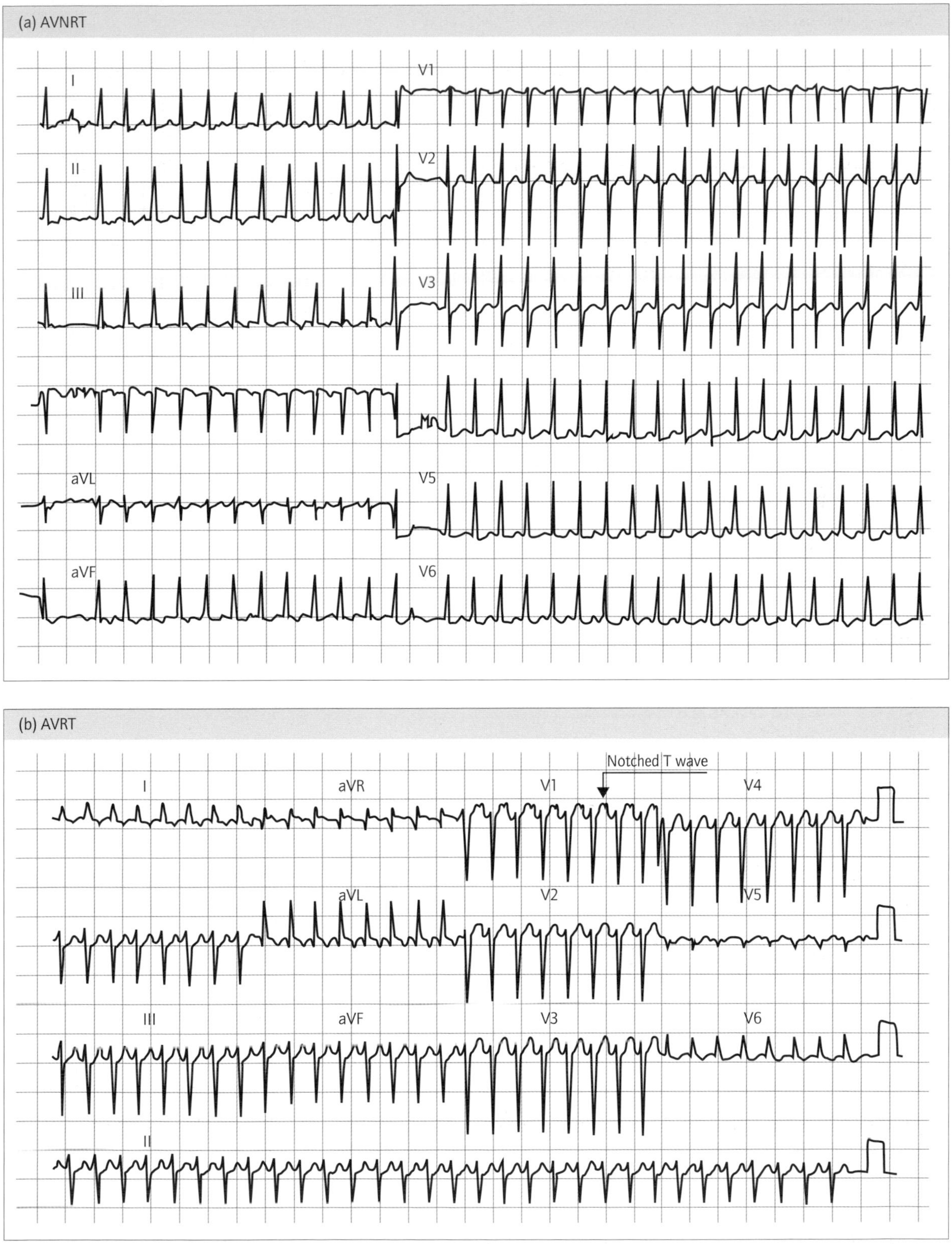

Figure 7.46 Reciprocating tachycardia: (a) AVNRT; (b) AVRT. Note the notched T wave in lead V1 in AVRT in contrast to AVNRT due to the atrium being activated after the QRS complex.

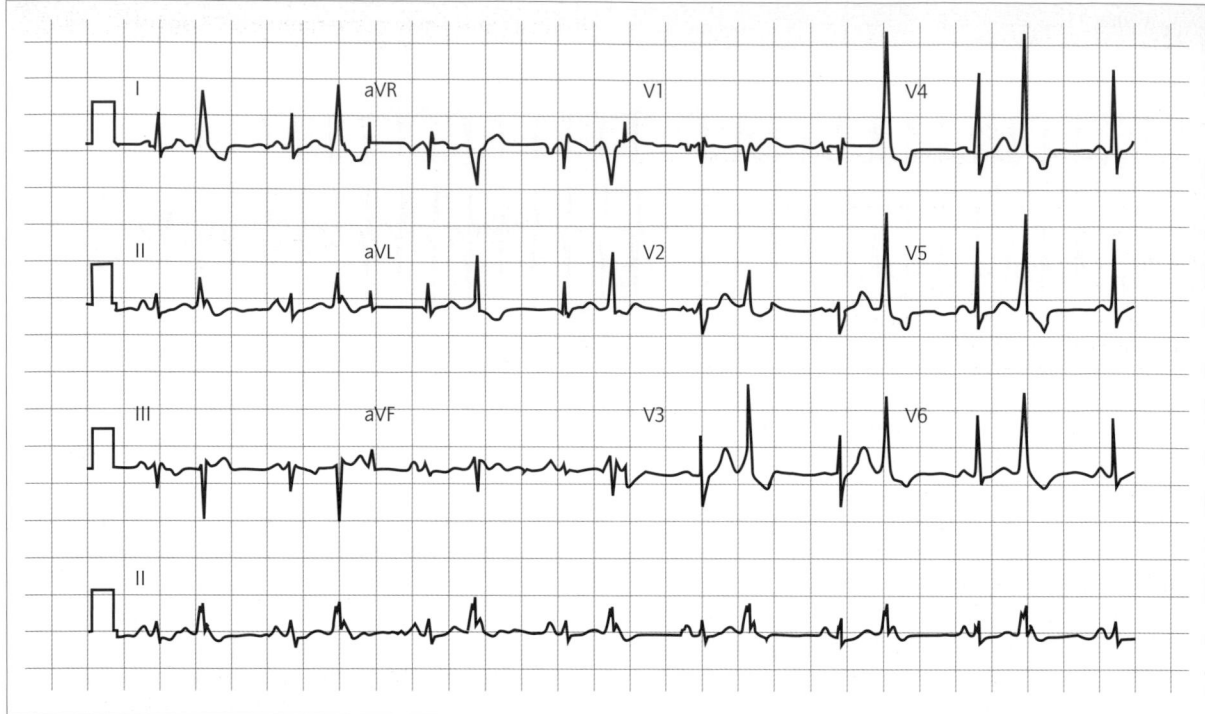

Figure 7.47 Ventricular ectopic beats. In this example note that the ectopic beats occur after each normal sinus beat, known as ventricular bigemin.

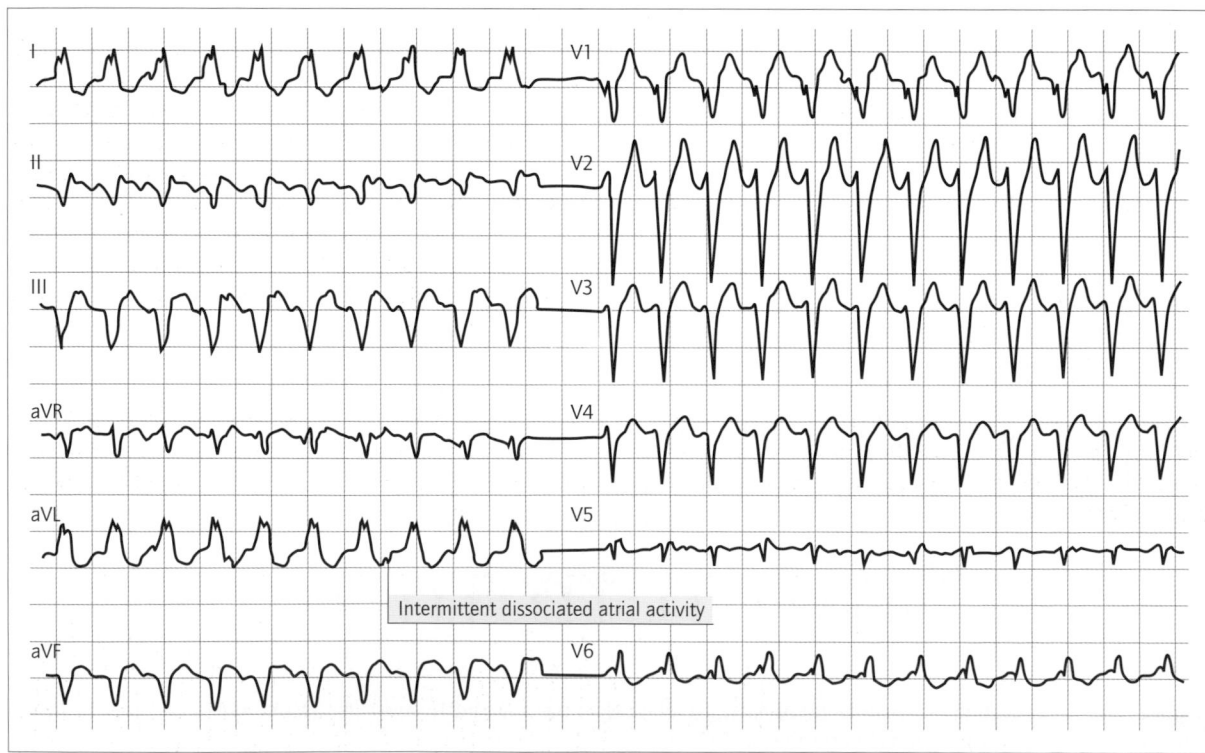

Intermittent dissociated atrial activity

Figure 7.48 Ventricular tachycardia. Note: (i) the QRS width; (ii) left axis deviation; (iii) the similarity of QRS morphology in leads V1–V5; and (iv) the dissociation of atrial and ventricular activity so independent P wave can occasionally be seen.

Table 7.24 Wide complex tachycardia: distinction of ventricular tachycardia (VT) from supraventricular tachycardia (SVT) with aberrant conduction

AV dissociation
QRS width >150 ms
History of ischaemic heart disease
Concordant QRS complexes in anterior leads (all QRS
    complexes in same direction)

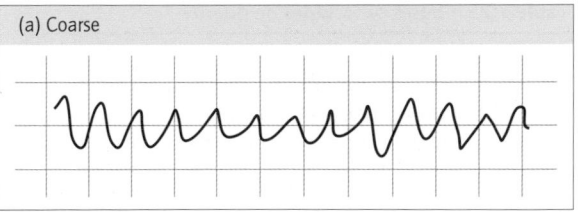

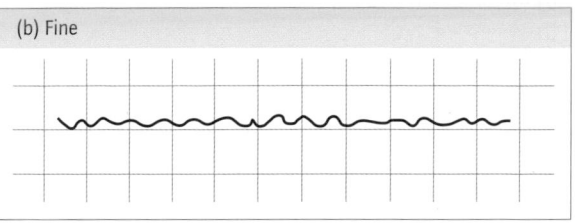

Figure 7.49 Ventricular fibrillation.

dissociation with intermittent cannon waves in the venous pressure pulse. The ECG shows a rapid heart rate with a QRS width of more than 140 ms.

A diagnosis of VT needs to be distinguished from that of supraventricular tachycardia (SVT) with bundle branch block resulting from blocked conduction down one of the bundles (aberrancy). The presence of dissociated P wave activity is extremely helpful in diagnosing VT. Other features that distinguish VT from SVT with aberration are listed in Table 7.24.

Ventricular fibrillation

Ventricular fibrillation (VF) is a disorganized rapid and irregular heart rhythm leading to no cardiac output (Fig. 7.49). The patient rapidly becomes unconscious and then stops breathing. The ECG shows no evidence of organized complexes. Only rarely will it reverse spontaneously.

VF most commonly occurs in the setting of acute myocardial infarction and therefore rarely recurs. If it is likely to recur, prophylaxis will be required. This is with either a beta-blocker and/or with amiodarone, but implantable defibrillators are now often indicated in this situation.

Torsade de pointes

On the ECG this tachycardia is characterized by wide complexes that change their axis from an upright to an inverted shape (Fig. 7.50). This causes syncope and sudden death. The QT interval on the ECG when in sinus rhythm is prolonged. It may be congenital, or brought about by metabolic disturbances, drug therapy or other causes (Table 7.25).

Clinical features of arrhythmias

Symptoms that can result from an abnormal heart rhythm are listed in Table 7.26. Some patients can be very aware of any change in rhythm, while others can have severe disturbances of rhythm without being conscious of any symptoms.

Investigation and management

The first step

The key to the management of cardiac arrhythmias is to identify their nature. The history may provide a clue; for example, the patient may be aware of an accelerated irregular rhythm suggesting atrial fibrillation, or report a diuresis in association with the symptoms which suggests a paroxysmal SVT. The diuresis is because the atrium is distended during the arrhythmia, leading to release of atrial naturietic peptide. Usually, however, a precise diagnosis can only be made by documenting the rhythm disturbance on an ECG.

Electrophysiology
● *Standard 12-lead ECG:* rarely helpful, although it may show the delta deflection of WPW syndrome. However, this can be intermittent and so a normal ECG does not exclude WPW.

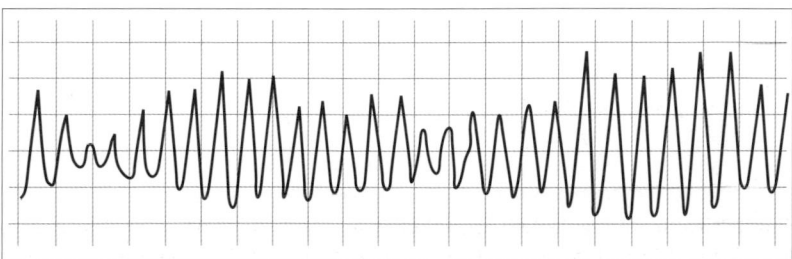

Figure 7.50 Torsades de pointes. Note the varying amplitude of the QRS complex as it changes its axis.

Table 7.25 Causes of torsades de pointes

Congenital syndromes
Jervell–Lange-Nielsen syndrome (autosomal recessive, associated with congenital deafness)
Romano–Ward syndrome (autosomal dominant)

Metabolic disturbances
Hypomagnesaemia
Hypokalaemia
Hypocalcaemia
Organophosphate insecticides
Prolonged dieting

Drugs
Class I drugs such as quinidine
Class III drugs such as amiodarone
Tricyclic antidepressants

Other
Bradycardia
Mitral valve prolapse
Acute myocardial infarction

Table 7.26 Symptoms that can result from an abnormal heart rhythm

Sudden death
Palpitations
Breathlessness
Presyncope and syncope
Chest discomfort

● *24-h ambulatory ECG:* the mainstay for identifying a rhythm disturbance. However, with intermittent symptoms, a 24-h tape is often negative, although occasionally asymptomatic markers of the rhythm disturbance may be present (e.g. a tendency to long pauses or occasional ventricular ectopics).

● *Cardiomemo:* a portable device that can be kept by the patient until symptoms develop. The device is then applied to the chest and records the rhythm disturbance. It is then possible to transmit the stored data on the device over the telephone to a centre where a printout on an ECG machine can be obtained. The memory on the cardiomemo can then be erased and used for a further episode if necessary.

● *Reveal device:* a long-term recorder implanted below the skin for months at a time. It is then removed for analysis.

● *Electrophysiological studies:* it is possible to provoke arrhythmias by electrically stimulating the atria and the ventricles, but unless there is a documented arrhythmia with which to compare the result, it is not possible to be confident that the arrhythmia provoked during the electrophysiological study is clinically relevant. Electrophysiological studies are more useful in monitoring the effect of treatment when the nature of the rhythm disturbance has been clearly defined.

The second step

The second step is to decide whether the arrhythmia is prognostically significant (is a marker of a life-threatening arrhythmia). If it is (e.g. if the patient is having episodes of VT), effective arrhythmia treatment is required (EMERGENCY BOX 7.5). If the arrhythmia does not have prognostic significance, management depends on whether the patient is prepared to tolerate the symptoms or wishes to have treatment to improve their quality of life.

Emergency 7.5: Cardiac resuscitation

All doctors should be able to perform efficient basic life support (BLS), the objective of which is to provide oxygen to vital organs (brain, heart) until spontaneous effective ventilation and circulation can be restored by definitive medical treatment (advanced cardiac life support). In England and Wales, more than 50 000/year sudden deaths occur in the community alone. Most of these deaths will be the result of ischaemic heart disease, and the preterminal arrhythmia in over 80% of these cases will be ventricular fibrillation. Studies from Seattle, where many of the local community can perform effective BLS, have shown that two factors determine survival when a patient collapses in the community with ventricular fibrillation:

■ the time elapsed before BLS is begun
■ the time elapsed before defibrillation (advanced cardiac life support)
Early intervention with BLS can therefore help to save lives

Basic life support
Whether confronted with a person who has suddenly collapsed, or on arriving at a scene where someone is unresponsive, the natural tendency is to panic. Panic can be minimized, and the chances of successful resuscitation maximized, if the ABC of resuscitation is adhered to:
■ *Assessment* and *Airway*
■ *Breathing*
■ *Circulation*

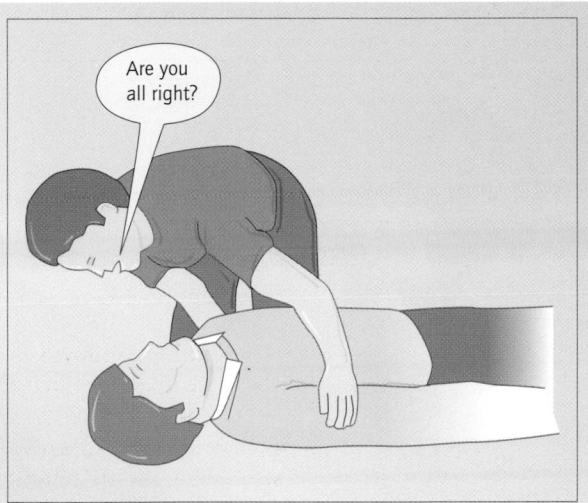

Fig. A Approach to the unconscious patient.

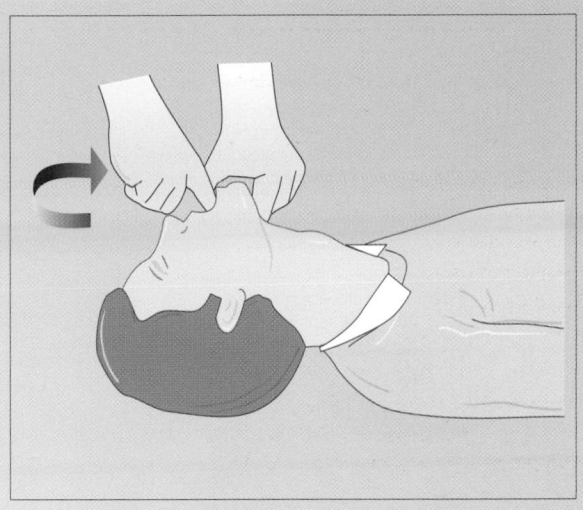

Fig. C Clearing the mouth and oropharynx.

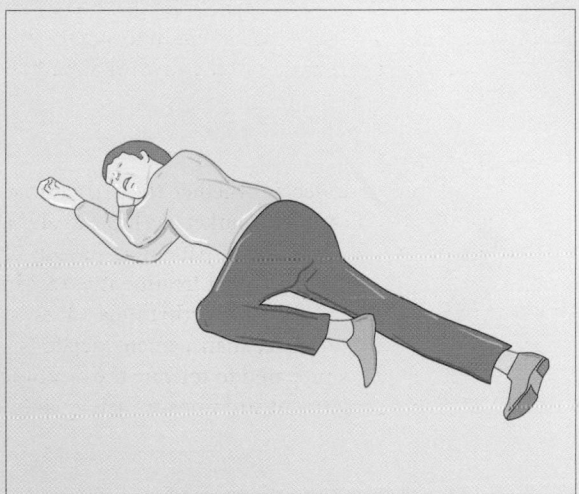

Fig. B The recovery position.

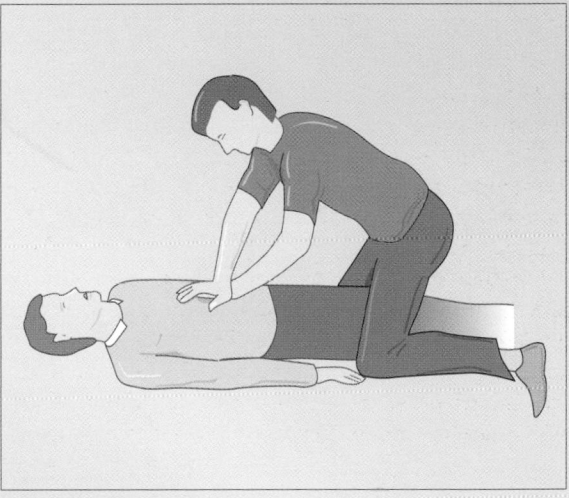

Fig. D The Heimlich manoeuvre.

Assessment

Assess the scene to ensure that you are not placing yourself in physical danger while caring for the patient. Minimize or remove any potential further risk to yourself, and instruct someone to call for help

Approach the patient and establish whether they are responsive by shouting 'Are you all right?', and gently shaking them by the shoulders, preventing movement of the head (Fig. A). Responsive but obtunded patients should be gently rolled over into the recovery position (Fig. B), care being taken not to exacerbate any injuries. With unresponsive patients, shout for help and then attend to the airway

Airway

The mouth and oropharynx should be cleared of any obvious foreign bodies, such as vomit or dislodged teeth, by sweeping an index finger around the oral cavity (Fig. C). Excess vomit should be allowed to drain from the mouth by turning the patient onto their side

Foreign bodies which are impacted can often be dislodged by the Heimlich manoeuvre (Fig. D). Kneeling astride the supine patient, a fist is placed in the epigastrium, with the other hand on top of the fist. Both hands are then thrust up beneath the costal margin in an attempt to raise the intrathoracic pressure suddenly, and thereby expel foreign bodies obstructing the upper airway

Continued on p. 448

07

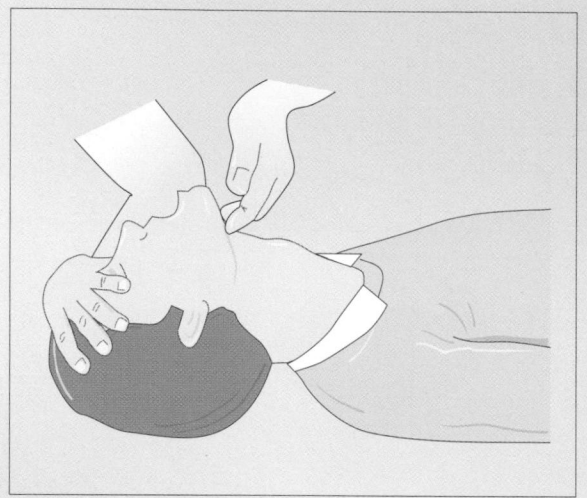

Fig. E The 'chin lift' manoeuvre.

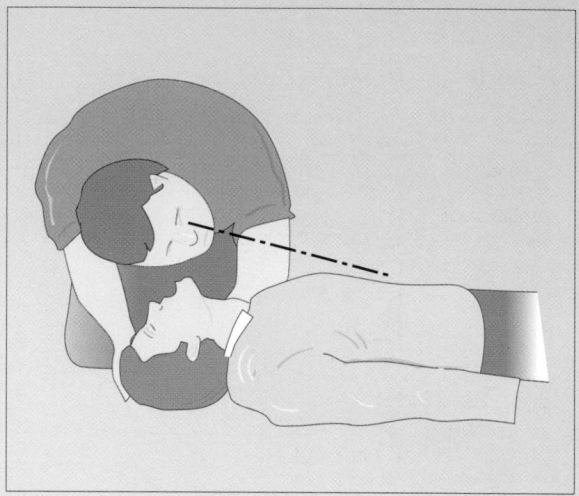

Fig. G Checking for spontaneous respiration.

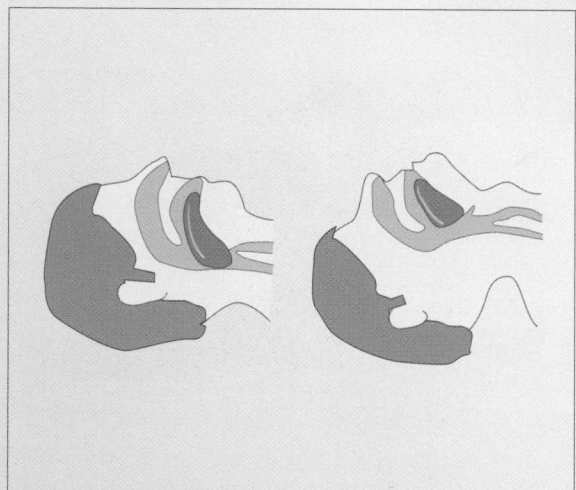

Fig. F Avoiding obstruction of the pharynx by the tongue.

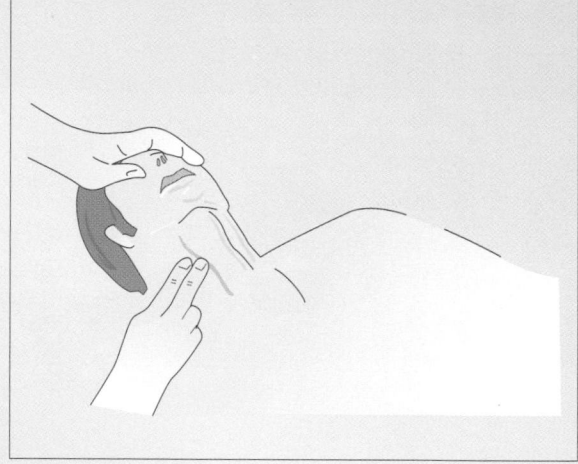

Fig. H Checking the carotid pulse.

When obstructions have been cleared, airway patency should be maintained by head tilt and the 'chin lift' manoeuvre (Fig. E). In the unconscious supine patient the tongue tends to flop back and obstruct the pharynx, and these two manoeuvres are designed to combat this (Fig. F)

Breathing
Having assessed and maintained the airway, evidence of spontaneous respiration should be sought. Place your cheek and ear over the patient's nose and mouth while watching the chest (Fig. G)

Look for chest wall movements, *listen* and *feel* for exhalations. This can be very difficult to do in some circumstances (e.g. beside a busy road in the dark)

If you are unsure that there are spontaneous respirations, assume that there are none. Having cleared and maintained the airway, and assessed breathing, the circulation should be assessed

Circulation
Feel for the carotid pulse (Fig. H). Pulse pressure may be low, so allow 5–6 s to ascertain whether it is present or not

Action
The sequence of resuscitation depends upon your assessment of the patient's *A*irway, *B*reathing and *C*irculation. Fig. I summarizes the suggested sequence
Note the importance of telephoning for help. It is essential to obtain a defibrillator as quickly as possible

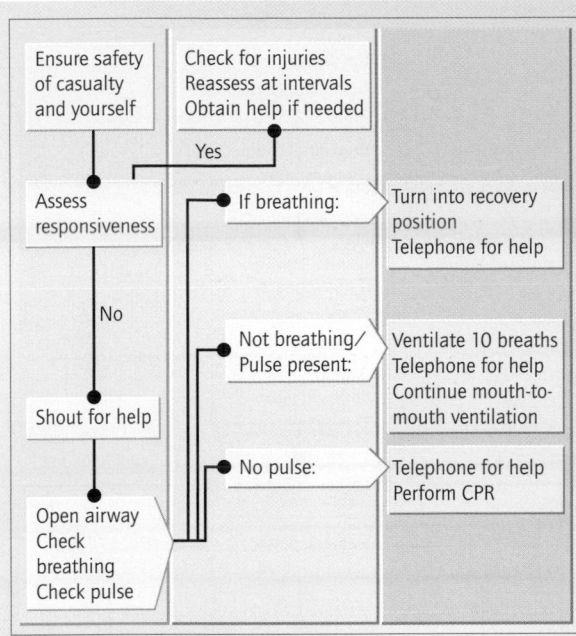

Fig. I The sequence of resuscitation.

Flowchart contents:

Ensure safety of casualty and yourself → Assess responsiveness → No → Shout for help → Open airway, Check breathing, Check pulse

Check for injuries, Reassess at intervals, Obtain help if needed → Yes

If breathing: → Turn into recovery position, Telephone for help

Not breathing/Pulse present: → Ventilate 10 breaths, Telephone for help, Continue mouth-to-mouth ventilation

No pulse: → Telephone for help, Perform CPR

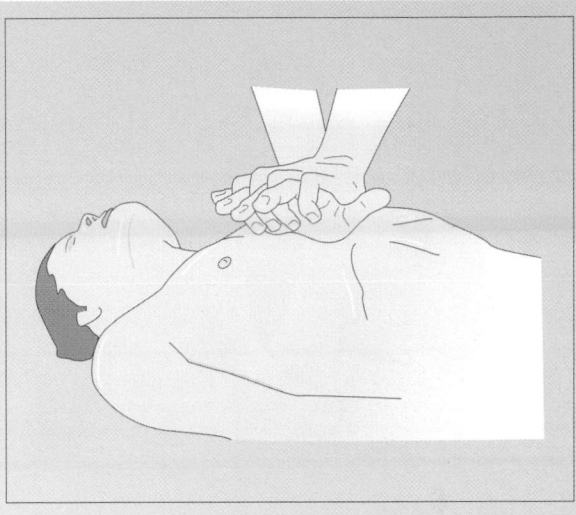

Fig. K Interlocking of fingers for CPR.

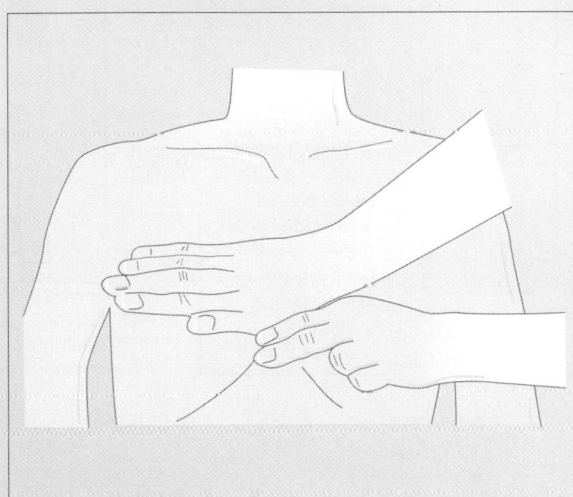

Fig. J Hand positioning for cardiopulmonary resuscitation (CPR).

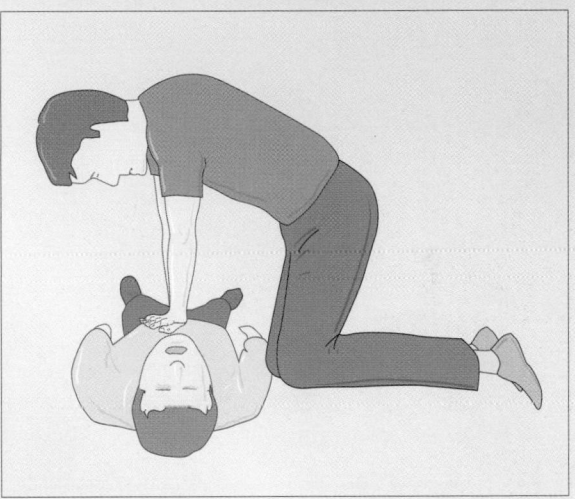

Fig. L Position for compression in CPR.

Cardiopulmonary resuscitation

The absence of breathing necessitates artificial ventilation, with mouth-to-mouth exhalations

With one hand performing the 'chin lift', the other hand pinches the nose and maintains slight extension of the neck by gentle pressure on the forehead. Take a deep breath and apply your lips firmly around those of the patient, creating an airtight seal. Breathe out, observing the chest for movement

Commence with two slow breaths, allowing the chest to deflate in between. If the chest does not rise, ventilation is inadequate and you will need to adjust your technique and try again. If your technique is good and the chest still does not rise, perform the Heimlich manoeuvre, as the upper airway is likely to be obstructed

In the absence of a pulse, external cardiac compression is necessary. Strict adherence to technique during this procedure allows maximum efficiency

Feel for the xiphoid sternum. Place the heel of one hand two fingers' breadth above this point in the midline (Fig. J). Place the heel of the other hand on the dorsum of the first and interlock the fingers (Fig. K)

Continued on p. 450

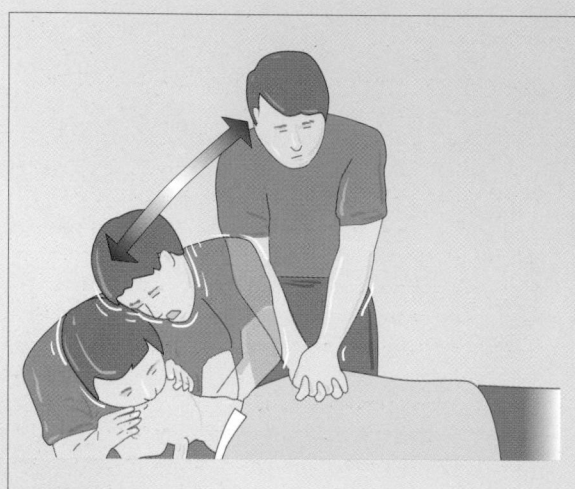

Fig. M Use a sequence of 15 compressions followed by two ventilations in CPR.

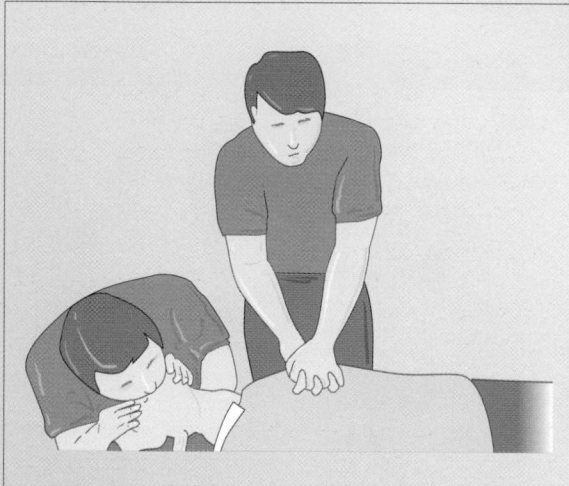

Fig. N CPR with two people.

Keeping your elbows firmly extended, position your shoulders directly over your hands so that the weight of your body, and not flexion/extension at the elbow, produces the compressions (Fig. L)

With a gentle rocking motion, depress the sternum 4–5 cm in a rhythmical fashion, counting 'one and two and three' for a total of 15 compressions. Then ventilate again with two breaths, followed by a further 15 compressions (Fig. M). Continue with this method until help arrives. (The rate of compressions should be 60–80/min)

If two people are available (Fig. N), the recommended sequence is one ventilation to every five compressions

The aesthetics of mouth-to-mouth resuscitation can be improved by an airway adjunct, such as a pocket face

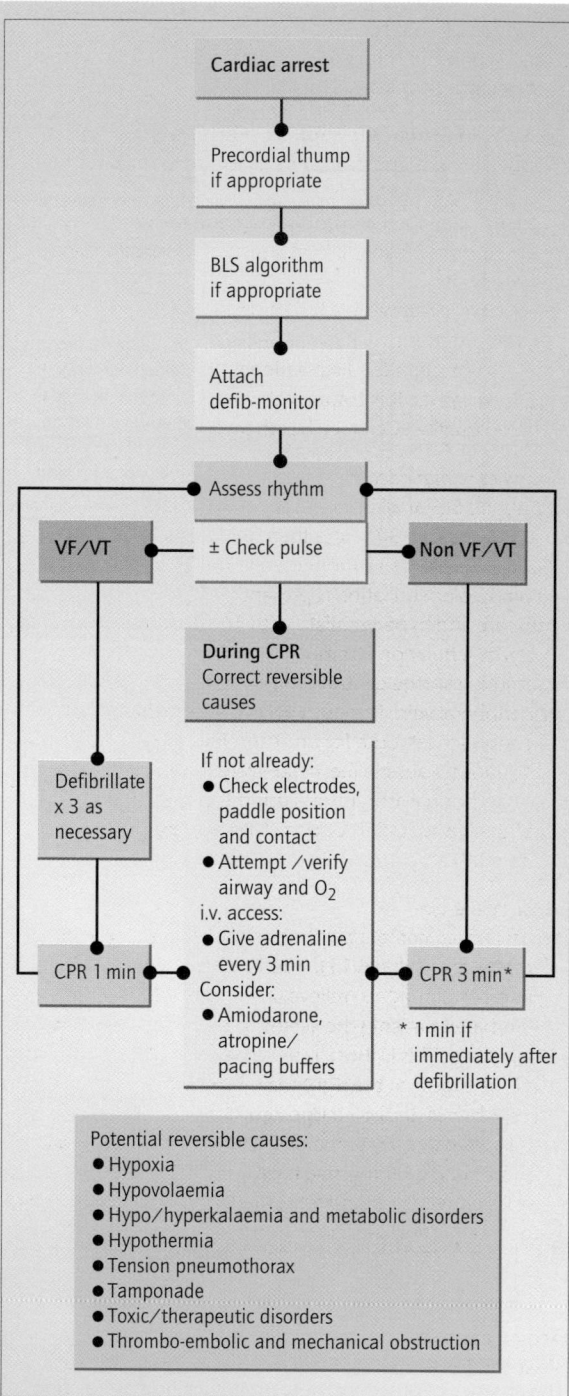

Fig. O Advanced cardiac life support.

mask, as long as an adequate flow rate is achievable. Such devices will also protect against disease transmission. There have been no documented cases of HIV transmission following mouth-to-mouth ventilation

The precordial thump
This manoeuvre should be employed only for witnessed or monitored arrests

Advanced cardiac life support (Fig. O)
Sudden cardiac arrests may be precipitated by one of the following arrhythmias
- Ventricular fibrillation/pulseless ventricular tachycardias are responsible for 80% of arrests and have the best prognosis
- Asystole is responsible for 12–15% of arrests and has a poor prognosis
- Electromechanical dissociation is responsible for less than 5% of arrests. It is diagnosed when the monitor shows a good quality ECG trace but there is no output

Priorities of management
Continue BLS at all times. At no time should it be interrupted for more than 30 s, and then only to allow intubation
Connect patient to a monitor, and defibrillate immediately if ventricular fibrillation is present
Intubate and hyperventilate with 100% oxygen. Hyperventilation attempts to correct the acidosis
Cannulate a large central vein, if this is not possible a large peripheral vein. If venous access is impossible, the endotracheal route for drug administration may be used. Administer adrenaline 1 mg every 2–3 min
Treat individual arrhythmias using the revised guidelines of the Resuscitation Council (UK) as stated below (BOX 7.9)

Specific therapy
Tension pneumothorax: If the patient has signs of a pneumothorax (Table 6.11), insert a cannula into the second intercostal space to relieve any tension. Beware the intubated patient who seems to be underventilating the left chest. This is most likely to be caused by the passage of the tube into the right main bronchus
Hypovolaemia: If this is suspected, continue BLS, give a 2 l fluid bolus, cross-match 10 units of blood and call the surgeon. Occult massive haemorrhage is the usual cause from either a leaking aortic aneurysm or an upper gastrointestinal lesion

Cardiac tamponade: In the absence of trauma this condition is uncommon. However, it can present acutely when associated with pericardial disease or dissection of the aorta. It should be considered in any patient with electromechanical dissociation who has full neck veins and in whom a tension pneumothorax has been excluded. Relief of the tamponade can buy valuable time while waiting for definitive intervention. Using a wide-bore needle attached to a 60 ml syringe, insert the needle just to the left of the xiphisternum at an angle of 30° to the skin, aspirating as you proceed. Aim the tip of the needle towards the tip of the left shoulder. When blood flushes back, aspirate 100 ml, if tamponade is present, this should lead to a clinical improvement
Pulmonary embolus: Without a thoracotomy this situation is rapidly fatal. However, an external cardiac massage may help to fragment the embolus so that it moves more peripherally and therefore does not produce such a profound effect

Recommended adult drug doses
- *Adrenaline (epinephrine):* 10 ml of 1 : 10 000 (1 mg) or 1 ml of 1 : 1000
- *Atropine:* 1 mg
- *Lidocaine:* 100 mg (up to a total of 3 mg/kg)
- *Calcium chloride:* 10 ml of 10% solution
- *Sodium bicarbonate:* 50 ml of 8.4% solution
- *Bretylium tosilate:* 500 mg
- *Amiodarone:* 5 mg/kg intravenously

Postresuscitation care
All patients should be managed in a high-dependency unit
Correct:
- Hypoxia
- Acid–base disturbance
- Electrolyte imbalance
Monitor all vital functions, including urine output
Perform:
- Chest X-ray to check position of endotracheal tube and central venous pressure lines, and to exclude a pneumothorax
- ECG for signs of acute ischaemia/myocardial infarction, etc.
- Continuous monitoring for arrhythmias

Drug treatment
Most arrhythmias can only be suppressed by drug therapy (BOX 7.10), and all antiarrhythmic drugs can cause serious side-effects. Some of them can also cause cardiac arrhythmias (so-called proarrhythmic effect). The need for treating an arrhythmia must therefore be carefully considered.

Radiofrequency ablation
This technique uses radiofrequency energy, delivered through electrodes introduced via the femoral vein, to destroy (ablate) targeted parts of the pathological electrical circuit. It is standard treatment for pre-excitation and reciprocating tachycardias, and atrial flutter. It is also being used for uncontrollable atrial fibrillation by destroying the AV node and inserting a pacemaker to maintain a ventricular rhythm.

Antiarrhythmic drug treatment
The number of antiarrhythmic drugs increases every

Box 7.9: Tachycardia

BRADYCARDIA

Sinus bradycardia
■ If haemodynamically important: intravenous atropine
■ If chronic: a pacemaker may be required

Sinus node disease
Chronic symptomatic sinoatrial disease
Permanent pacing
Antitachycardia drugs for any tachycardia
Anticoagulation with either aspirin or low-intensity warfarin
  (international normalized ratio 1.5–2.0)

AV block
Asymptomatic first and second degree
No treatment

Symptomatic first and second degree
Permanent pacing may be required

Stable third degree
Treatment is not usually necessary

Unstable third degree
A temporary wire may be appropriate until the AV block has
  resolved

Congenital complete heart block
Permanent pacing may be required
If the focus is in the distal His–Purkinje system or the ventricles, and the rate of the escape rhythm is slow and giving
  rise to dizziness and blackouts (Stokes–Adams attacks), a
  permanent pacemaker is indicated

Bundle branch block
Right bundle branch block
This is often an incidental finding so no treatment is required

Left bundle branch block
This is usually indicative of heart disease

Left hemi-block
Indicated by left axis deviation on the ECG

Bifascicular block
When associated with syncope, this may indicate intermittent
  conduction delay in the remaining fascicle, causing complete AV block; a permanent pacemaker may be required

Sinus tachycardia
Class II drugs

Atrial tachyarrhythmia
Atrial ectopic beats
Class II or IV drugs

Atrial flutter
Electrical cardioversion

Atrioventricular (AV) node-blocking drugs such as class II or
  IV antiarrhythmics, and digitalis if it is chronic
Prophylaxis against recurrent paroxysmal flutter with class I
  or III drugs

Atrial fibrillation
Treat any underlying cause (e.g. thyrotoxicosis)
Direct current (DC) cardioversion: patients undergoing
  elective DC cardioversion should be formally anti-
  coagulated for at least 2 weeks beforehand
Chemical cardioversion using class I or III antiarrhythmic
  drugs intravenously or orally
Class I or class III drugs as prophylaxis against recurrent
  paroxysmal atrial fibrillation
Control the ventricular rate in chronic atrial fibrillation with
  AV drugs
Anticoagulation (full-dose warfarin for mitral valve
  disease, otherwise low-intensity warfarin or aspirin
  probably provides sufficient protection)
Narrow QRS tachycardia/AV re-entrant tachycardia
Intravenous adenosine, verapamil or beta-blockers

Pre-excitation syndromes
Disopyramide and amiodarone for atrial fibrillation associated with Wolff–Parkinson–White (WPW) syndrome
  (verapamil or digoxin should *not* be used)
The preferred treatment of recurrent tachycardia caused by
  accessory pathways is to ablate the pathways between the
  atrium and the ventricle or within the AV node, using
  radiofrequency energy

Ventricular tachyarrhythmias
Ventricular ectopics
When no structural heart disease is present ventricular
  ectopic beats can be ignored
Treatment is indicated (with class I, II or III drugs) if they
  cause uncomfortable symptoms or predispose to a more
  serious ventricular arrhythmia, such as ventricular tachycardia or fibrillation

Ventricular tachycardia
Treatment is usually urgent, particularly if there is severe
  haemodynamic collapse
Immediate DC cardioversion (under short-acting general
  anaesthetic if the patient is still conscious)
If the patient's condition is stable lidocaine (bolus of
  50–100 mg intravenously initially followed by an
  infusion of 2–4 mg/min) may convert the rhythm
  back to sinus rhythm. If not successful, intravenous
  amiodarone (bolus of 300 mg over 1 h followed by
  700 mg over 24 h) may restore sinus rhythm
Avoid multiple intravenous drug administration because of the
  potentially proarrhythmic effects of antiarrhythmic drugs
Consider cardioversion early

Prevention of ventricular tachycardia
Document the effectiveness of prophylactic treatment
    by 24-h ambulatory ECGs or by demonstrating that
    provocative electrophysiological studies can no longer
    stimulate the tachycardia
Class I and II drugs are the first choice for prophylaxis. Beta-
    blockers are particularly appropriate when the arrhythmia
    is provoked by exercise. Class I drugs, particularly type Ic
    drugs, are potentially proarrhythmic and should be used
    with caution in patients with
    compromised ventricular function
Amiodarone (a class III drug) is the drug of choice if vent-
    ricular tachycardia is caused by severely compromised left
    ventricular function

Ventricular fibrillation
Rarely reverses spontaneously and immediate cardiopul-
    monary resuscitation is required until DC cardioversion
    can be carried out

Torsade de pointes
Correct any electrolyte disturbance and discontinue proar-
    rhythmic drugs
Overdrive pace the atrium and ventricles with temporary
    dual chamber pacing
Intravenous isoprenaline may be helpful in the acute situation
Beta-blockade is helpful if there is no congenital QT
    prolongation. This may require additional backup
    dual chamber pacing to prevent symptomatic bradycardia

year. They can be classified according to their effect on the action potential (Fig. 7.51a) or their site of action (Fig. 7.51b).

Sinus tachycardia. In the absence of contraindications, the most effective treatment for a sinus tachycardia is a small dose of a beta-blocker. Other drugs which affect the sinus node include calcium antagonists such as verapamil and diltiazem.

Atrial ectopic beats. These rarely require treatment, but, as with other atrial arrhythmias, they can be effectively controlled with type I, II or III drugs.

Atrial flutter. The most effective treatment is electrical DC cardioversion, where a small electric shock is given to the patient under general anaesthesia. AV node blocking drugs such as class II or IV antiarrhythmics and digoxin can be used either individually or together. Prophylaxis against recurrent paroxysmal flutter can be achieved with class I or III drugs.

Atrial fibrillation. Any underlying cause (e.g. thyrotoxicosis) should be treated. This may result in a spontaneous return to sinus rhythm, but if not DC cardioversion can be used. Chemical cardioversion can be achieved using certain antiarrhythmic drugs (e.g. class I or III), intravenously or orally. Class I and III drugs can also be used as prophylaxis against recurrent paroxysmal atrial fibrillation. The ventricular rate in chronic atrial fibrillation can be controlled by AV node-blocking drugs, such as digoxin and class II and IV drugs.

There is a significant risk of thromboembolism in patients with atrial fibrillation. Anticoagulation should therefore be considered for all patients, especially those over 65 years and those with an enlarged left atrium. Patients undergoing elective DC cardioversion should be formally anticoagulated for at least 4 weeks before it is carried out.

Narrow QRS tachycardia. Many patients have reported that their attacks can be aborted by specific vagotonic manoeuvres (e.g. carotid sinus pressure, induction of the diving reflex by immersing the face in water and the Valsalva manoeuvre; EMERGENCY BOX 7.6). Automatic tachycardias such as atrial and junctional tachycardias are difficult to treat, and class I or III drugs are usually used.

In reciprocating and pre-excitation tachycardias, drug treatment interrupts the electrical circus activity by blocking the AV node. Intravenous adenosine causes transient AV nodal block and is highly effective. It will also unmask an atrial tachycardia because it will not affect the atrial rate, but will slow the ventricular response. Alternatively, intravenous verapamil or beta-blockers will block the AV node. However, using both together intravenously should be avoided because it can cause severe haemodynamic depression.

If medical treatment fails, DC cardioversion or overdrive rapid atrial pacing can be used. Prophylactic radiofrequency ablation is the treatment of choice to prevent further episodes. Drugs can be used: class I and III drugs impair conduction in the abnormal AV connection; class II and IV drugs impair AV node conduction.

Pre-excitation syndrome. Neither verapamil nor digoxin should be used in the treatment of atrial fibrillation associated with WPW syndrome of a concealed pathway tachycardia. Drugs such as these, which depress transmission of the impulse through the AV node, may favour conduction through the abnormal pathway and give rise to a very fast ventricular rate which can be life-threatening. VF can develop. In contrast, disopyramide and amiodarone depress conduction through the abnormal pathway.

07

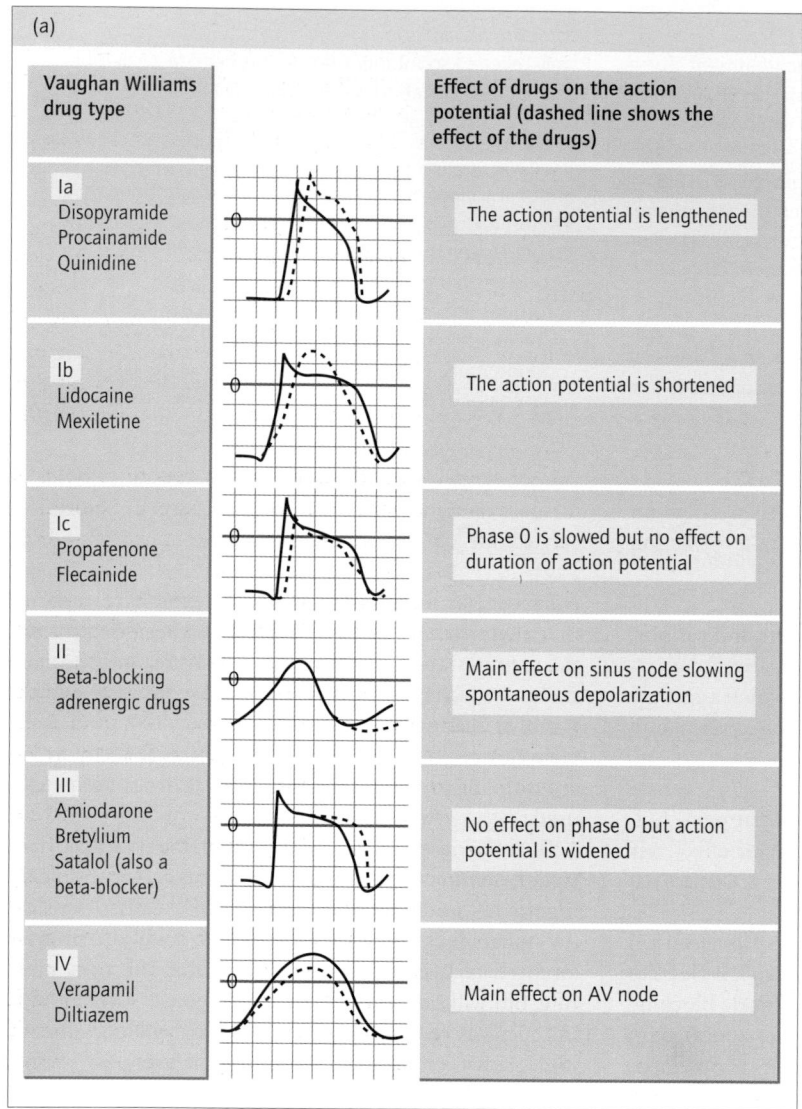

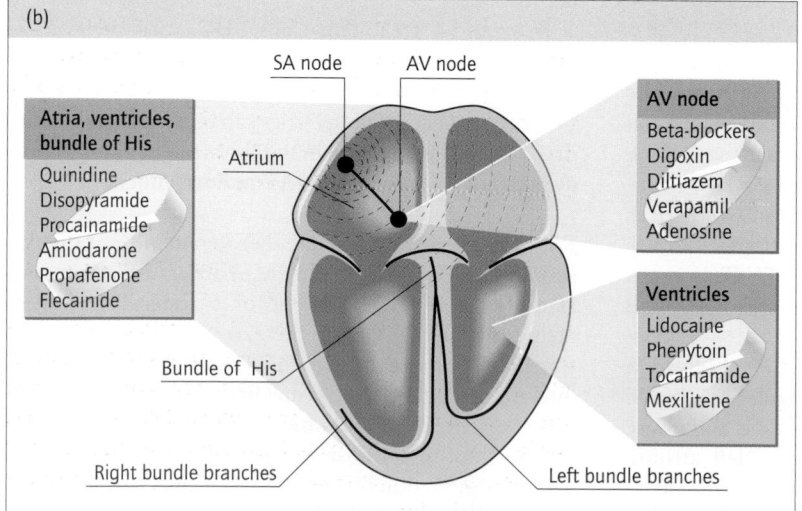

Figure 7.51 Antiarrhythmic drugs. (a) Vaughan Williams classification. (b) Sites of action.

Emergency 7.6: Narrow complex tachycardia (supraventricular tachycardia)

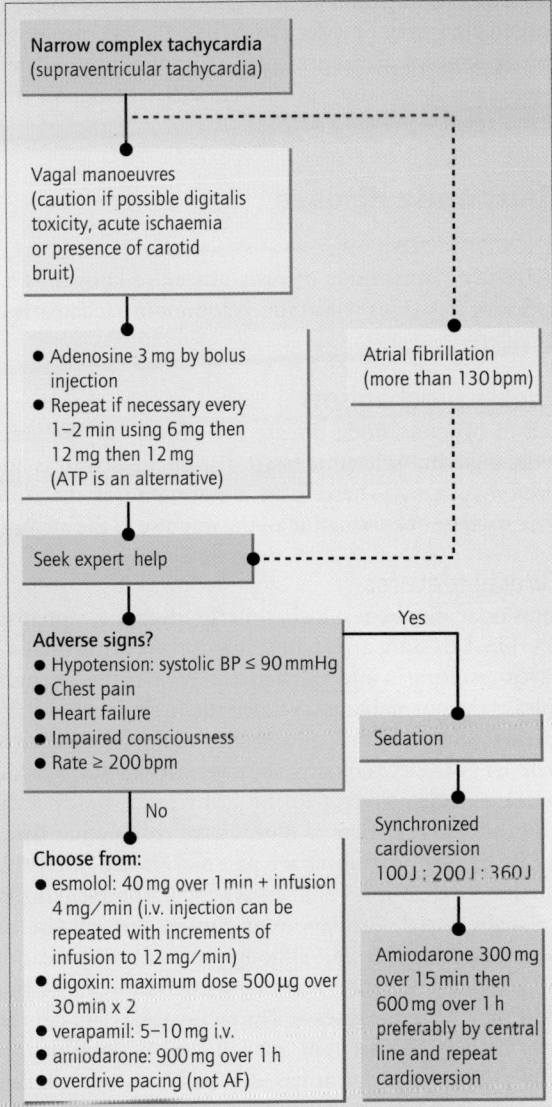

Narrow complex tachycardia
(supraventricular tachycardia)

Vagal manoeuvres
(caution if possible digitalis
toxicity, acute ischaemia
or presence of carotid
bruit)

- Adenosine 3 mg by bolus
  injection
- Repeat if necessary every
  1–2 min using 6 mg then
  12 mg then 12 mg
  (ATP is an alternative)

Atrial fibrillation
(more than 130 bpm)

Seek expert help

Adverse signs?
- Hypotension: systolic BP ≤ 90 mmHg
- Chest pain
- Heart failure
- Impaired consciousness
- Rate ≥ 200 bpm

Yes

No

Sedation

Choose from:
- esmolol: 40 mg over 1 min + infusion
  4 mg/min (i.v. injection can be
  repeated with increments of
  infusion to 12 mg/min)
- digoxin: maximum dose 500 μg over
  30 min x 2
- verapamil: 5–10 mg i.v.
- amiodarone: 900 mg over 1 h
- overdrive pacing (not AF)

Synchronized
cardioversion
100 J : 200 J : 360 J

Amiodarone 300 mg
over 15 min then
600 mg over 1 h
preferably by central
line and repeat
cardioversion

Fig. A Narrow complex tachycardia. Doses based on adult of average body weight. In all cases give oxygen and establish intravenous access.

The preferred treatment of recurrent tachycardia caused by WPW syndrome is to destroy the bundle of Kent between the atrium and ventricles by radiofrequency ablation. This is usually preferable to lifelong antiarrhythmic therapy.

Ventricular ectopics. If there is no structural heart disease, ventricular ectopic beats can be ignored. However, treatment is indicated when the patient experiences uncomfortable symptoms or when the ectopic beats are associated with more serious ventricular arrhythmias, such as VT or VF. The drugs of choice are those in class I, II or III.

Ventricular tachycardia. Treatment of VT is usually urgent, particularly if there is severe haemodynamic collapse (EMERGENCY BOX 7.7). Immediate DC cardioversion (under short-term general anaesthetic if the patient is still conscious) is required. If the patient's condition is stable, intravenous lidocaine with a bolus of 50–100 mg initially, followed by an infusion of 2–4 mg/min, may convert the rhythm back to sinus rhythm.

If treatment with lidocaine is not successful, a bolus of intravenous amiodarone of 300 mg over 1 h followed by 900 mg over 24 h, may restore sinus rhythm. Multiple intravenous drug administration should be avoided because of the potentially proarrhythmic effects of anti-arrhythmic drugs. Cardioversion should therefore be considered early.

Prevention of VT. Further attacks of VT must be prevented and the effectiveness of prophylactic treatment is best documented by 24-h ambulatory ECGs or by demonstrating that provocative electrophysiological studies no longer stimulate the tachycardia.

Class I and II drugs are the first choice of prophylaxis. Beta-blockers are particularly appropriate when the arrhythmia is provoked by exercise. Class I, particularly type Ic drugs, are potentially proarrhythmic and are used with caution in patients with compromised ventricular function. However, VT often arises as a result of severely compromised left ventricular function and class I and II drugs cannot be used because of their negative inotropic effect. Amiodarone, a class III drug, is then the drug of choice.

Ablative radiofrequency therapy. The ventricular endocardium can be mapped during an electrophysiological study to identify the focus of the VT, which can then be ablated by radiofrequency energy. This technique is still under evaluation and is not appropriate when there is more than one focus for the VTs.

Ventricular fibrillation. This rarely reverses spontaneously and immediate CPR is required until DC cardioversion can be carried out. An implantable cardiac defibrillator should be considered for patients who survive spontaneous VF not related to an acute myocardial infarct. This is a device buried below the skin of the chest connected to a transvenous wire which detects VT or VF. The heart is then defibrillated into sinus rhythm. This has been shown to improve survival compared to treatment with antiarrhythmic drugs.

Emergency 7.7: Broad complex tachycardia (sustained ventricular tachycardia)

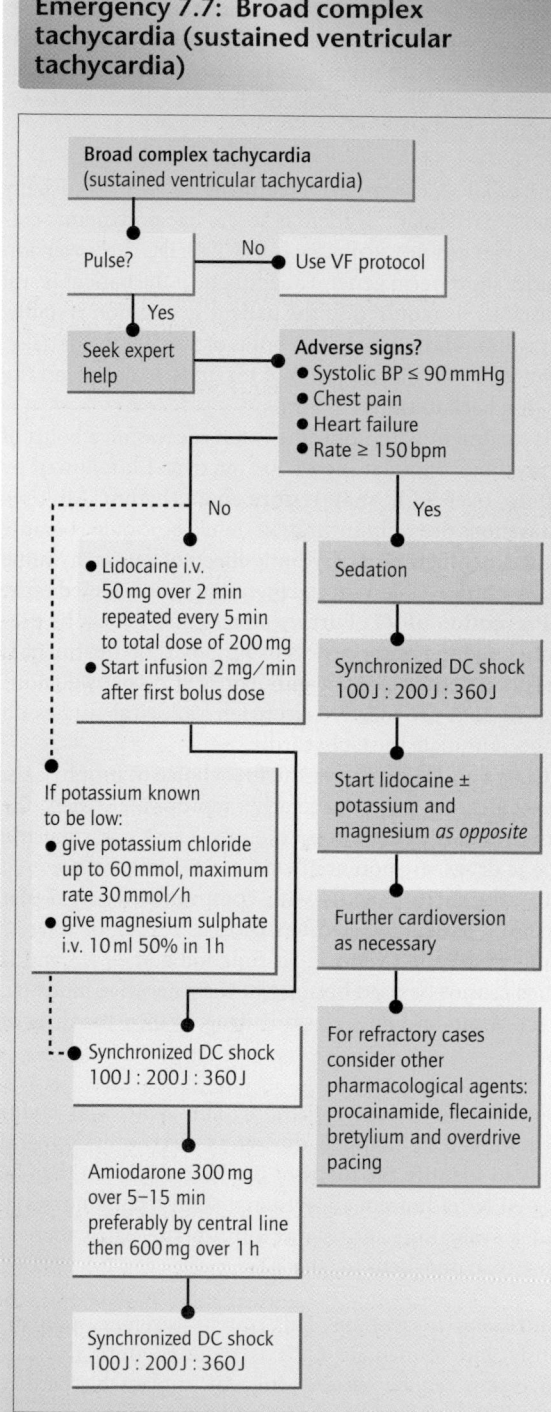

Fig. A Broad complex tachycardia. Doses based on adult of average body weight. In all cases give oxygen and establish intravenous access.

Torsade de pointes. The treatment of torsade de pointes involves correcting any metabolic disturbance and stopping potentially causative drugs. The heart rate must be maintained with atrial or ventricular pacing. In acquired prolongation of the QT interval, intravenous isoprenaline may be effective. When the QT prolongation is congenital, isoprenaline is contraindicated and β-blockade or ablation of the left stellate ganglion may be indicated.

Sinus node disease

Epidemiology

Prevalence. Sinus node disease, otherwise known as SA disease or sick sinus syndrome, is common, particularly in the elderly.

Disease mechanisms

Causes of sinus node disease are fibrosis of the sinus node, digoxin, ischaemic heart disease, myocarditis and cardiomyopathy. There is an abnormality of the sinus node itself or of conduction of the impulse to the atrium.

Clinical features

Sinus node disease results in sinus bradycardia, sinoatrial (SA) block or sinus arrest. In SA block there are dropped P waves, resulting in intervals between P waves that are multiples of the normal sinus cycle length. In sinus arrest there are no P waves and the pause is not a multiple of a normal cycle length. Occasionally, supraventricular tachycardia can also occur, leading to the tachycardia–bradycardia syndrome. Often there is more distal conducting tissue disease as well, so subsidiary pacemakers are unreliable and sinus arrest can result in syncope. The tachycardia is usually atrial fibrillation or flutter, but can be an automatic tachycardia, although not a reciprocating tachycardia. The ventricular rate is often slow, suggesting additional AV node disease. The tachycardias can depress sinus activity so that they are followed by long pauses; conversely, the tachycardias can be an escape rhythm from sinus arrest.

Patients present with palpitations, syncope or dizziness, and a significant number (15%) also develop systemic thromboemboli.

Investigation

Sinus node disease is most readily diagnosed on 24-h ambulatory ECG monitoring. Quite often it is an incidental finding.

Management

Treatment includes drugs to control the atrial arrhythmia. These can worsen the tendency to bradycardia, and so a

Table 7.27 The common lesions responsible for 70–80% of all congenital heart disease defects

Atrial septal defect
Ventricular septal defect
Persistent patent ductus arteriosus
Coarctation of the aorta
Pulmonary stenosis
Aortic stenosis
Tetralogy of Fallot
Transposition of the great vessels

Table 7.28 Congenital heart lesions causing left-to-right shunts

Level	Defect
Atrium	Atrial septal defect
Ventricle	Ventricular septal defect
Vessel	Patent ductus arteriosus
	Aortopulmonary window
Mixed	Aorta to atrium or ventricle (ruptured sinus of Valsalva aneurysm)
	Coronary artery to atrium or ventricle (coronary fistula)
	Ventricle to atrium (Garbode defect allowing shunting from the left ventricle to the right atrium)
Multiple	Atrioventricular septal defect

pacemaker is often needed. It is preferable to use a dual chamber pacemaker because the atrial wire may stabilize the atrial rhythm, but this is not always possible. Anticoagulants should be considered, especially for those with atrial fibrillation.

Congenital heart disease

Eight lesions are responsible for 70–80% of all congenital heart disease defects (Table 7.27).

Cyanotic and acyanotic congenital heart disease

It is conventional to subdivide congenital heart defects into cyanotic and acyanotic groups. Central cyanosis develops when the concentration of deoxygenated haemoglobin rises above 5 g/100 ml as a result of either mixing of systemic venous blood with systemic arterial circulation or a low pulmonary blood flow.

Differentiation between cyanotic and acyanotic conditions may be useful, although acyanotic congenital heart disease can progress to cyanotic heart disease when there is a defect allowing the flow of a large volume of blood from the left to the right ventricle. The increased flow in the pulmonary arteries leads to pulmonary hypertension, and when the pulmonary pressure and therefore the right ventricular pressure increases above the left ventricular pressure, blood will shunt from the right to the left ventricle. This is known as Eisenmenger's syndrome.

The most common left-to-right shunts are listed in Table 7.28.

Epidemiology

Prevalence of congenital heart disease is 8/1000 live births. Bicuspid non-stenotic aortic valves are present in 2% of the population; some of these will become stenotic. Mitral valve prolapse is found in 1% of males and 4% of females. Complications arise in only a very small percentage of these people.

Disease mechanisms

Congenital heart disease arises as a result of abnormal development of the circulation *in utero* or persistence of the remnants of the fetal circulation after birth (Fig. 7.52). The nature of the fetal circulation and changes at birth are listed in Table 7.29. It may be associated with other congenital defects, as in Down's syndrome and rubella syndrome. The aetiology may involve either genetic or extraneous influences (Table 7.30).

Clinical features

Depending on the defect, the major haemodynamic features are because of obstruction to flow and/or shunting of blood from one side of the heart to the other. Abnormal volume overloads or pressure loads on various chambers of the heart can ultimately cause heart failure, arrhythmias and sudden death. Patients with excessive pulmonary flow develop progressive pulmonary vascular disease.

Patients with shunts may develop paradoxical embolic events (passage of an embolus from the venous system across a shunt and into the systemic arterial circulation) and cerebral abscesses, which may be a terminal event. They risk developing endocarditis and many are prone to recurrent chest infections. The cyanotic group also have mild deficiencies of normal haemostasis and thrombocytopenia. They may also develop hyperuricaemia.

In cyanotic congenital heart disease, arterial blood is chronically desaturated because blood is shunted from the right to the left side of the circulation, bypassing the lungs. This desaturation leads to polycythaemia, the hyperviscosity syndrome (blurred vision, headaches, chronic fatigue), clubbing, small stature and poor dentition.

Management

Echocardiography of the fetus while *in utero* can allow early recognition of congenital heart disease, and may justify an elective termination of pregnancy.

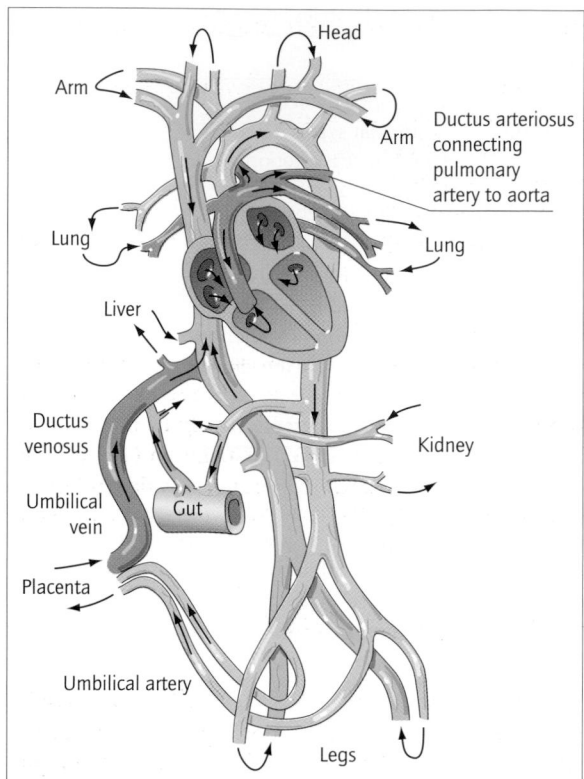

Figure 7.52 Fetal circulation *in utero*. The relative oxygenation of the blood is indicated by the colours and the direction of blood flow is indicated by the arrows. Note: (i) the ductus venosus carrying blood from the placenta; and (ii) the ductus arteriosus carrying blood from the pulmonary artery to the aorta and so bypassing the lungs.

Table 7.29 The fetal circulation

In the fetus

The pulmonary circulation is short circuited by the foramen ovale and a patent ductus arteriosus (oxygenation of fetal blood occurs at the placenta)

Systemic venous blood returns to the right atrium

Some crosses the foramen ovale into the left atrium, and then into the left ventricle and systemic circulation

Some crosses the tricuspid valve to enter the right ventricle and then the pulmonary artery, where it is diverted from the lungs through the PDA into the aorta (Fig. 7.52)

On delivery

The first inspiratory effort dilates the pulmonary arterioles causing a dramatic drop in pulmonary vascular resistance

The patent ductus arteriosus closes under the influence of a combination of oxygenated blood and lower levels of prostaglandins

The foramen ovale of the atrial septum is open as part of the normal fetal circulation and remains patent in all neonates. It closes because a rise in left atrial pressure and a fall in right atrial pressure allows the two edges of the atrial septum to oppose

It is only when the separation of the left and right heart circulation is achieved at birth that many fetal congenital abnormalities of the heart have an effect

Table 7.30 Causes of congenital heart disease

Chromosomal abnormalities
Down's syndrome (trisomy 21)
Turner's syndrome (45, X0)
Increased consanguinity (there is a 1–2% risk of congenital heart disease for siblings and a 5–10% risk for any offspring)
Rubella infection
Drugs (e.g. thalidomide, warfarin, phenytoin)
Irradiation
Maternal disease (e.g. diabetes mellitus, chronic alcoholism, systemic lupus erythematosus)

Atrial septal defects

Patent foramen ovale

The foramen ovale usually closes during infancy and childhood, but in 20–35% of adults closure is incomplete. In neonates there is a potential for early left-to-right shunting. In adults the hole is very small and because left atrial pressure is higher than right atrial pressure, the thin part of the septum acts as a flap valve and keeps the hole closed. However, under certain circumstances transient right-to-left shunting may occur. A patent foramen ovale has been implicated in paradoxical embolic events in adults and may also be involved in gas embolization and neurological bends in divers.

Atrial septal defect

There are three types of atrial septal defect (ASD).
1 *Ostium secundum defect:* the most common and occurs at the level of the foramen ovale.

2 *Sinus venosus defect:* occurs at the top of the atrial septum, is often associated with abnormal insertion of the right upper pulmonary vein into the lower end of the superior vena cava, and may cause partial anomalous pulmonary venous drainage to the right atrium.
3 *Ostium primum defect:* occurs at the lower end of the atrial septum and may be an isolated defect or part of a more complex lesion of the atrioventricular canal.
Partial anomalous pulmonary venous drainage may occur in isolation with no abnormality of the atrial septum.

The effects of all types of ASD vary considerably. Large defects cause little pressure gradient and the direction of flow depends on the relative compliance on the left and right side (resistance to filling). After birth, the pulmonary vascular resistance decreases, the right ventricle becomes more compliant, and left-to-right shunting occurs with right atrial and right ventricular volume overload.

Clinical features

Patients are often asymptomatic. Depending on the haemodynamic effects, children may be prone to recurrent chest infections and adults may develop atrial arrhythmias, decreased exercise tolerance and symptoms of right heart failure.

The venous pressure is usually normal, but tricuspid regurgitation may occur in the late stages. Other clinical signs include the following:

- *Parasternal heave:* if there is significant right ventricular overload.
- *Fixed splitting of the second heart sound:* right ventricular systole is delayed because of the increased volume of blood passing through the right ventricle. The ASD equalizes the pressure in the atria, and so the second sound is fixed and split (see p. 396).
- *Tricuspid and pulmonary flow murmurs:* may be audible and increase on inspiration.

Investigation

Electrocardiography

ECG may show right axis deviation and partial right bundle branch block (RBBB), and there may be features of right ventricular hypertrophy. An ostium primum defect causes left axis deviation as well as partial RBBB and possibly a long PR interval, with right ventricular hypertrophy.

Diagnostic imaging

- *Chest radiography:* shows large pulmonary arteries with increased pulmonary vascular markings and a prominent right heart border.
- *Echocardiography:* visualizes the defect and the shunt, and will show an enlarged right atrium and right ventricle with reversed motion of the ventricular septum. Doppler echocardiography also allows calculation of the pulmonary : systemic flow ratio.
- *Cardiac catheterization:* sometimes performed to measure pulmonary artery pressure and to calculate the ratio of blood flow through the pulmonary and systemic circulation.

Management

Surgical closure of the defect is considered if the pulmonary : systemic blood flow ratio is more than 2 : 1. It should be performed when the patient is young, when the risks of surgery are low and the longer term benefits are higher. The benefits of surgery may be considerably less for middle-aged and older patients (in some patients, the defect can be closed percutaneously using catheter techniques).

Potential benefits from closure include prevention of:
- Progressive pulmonary vascular disease
- Congestive failure
- Atrial arrhythmias
- Paradoxical embolic events

Antibiotic prophylaxis is not usually required for an isolated ASD.

Prognosis

Most patients develop atrial fibrillation in the fourth or fifth decade, and this can lead to systemic emboli. Other complications include progressive pulmonary vascular disease, which occurs in 10% of patients and can lead to left shunting of blood and systemic desaturation, infective endocarditis, which affects 0.5% of patients, and right ventricular dilatation and failure.

Ventricular septal defect

Epidemiology

Prevalence. Occurs in up to 2% of babies. It can be an isolated finding or part of a more complex congenital heart disease. Blood flows from the left ventricle to the right ventricle unless the pulmonary artery pressure is so high as to cause Eisenmenger's syndrome (see p. 458).

Disease mechanisms

Ventricular septal defects classically occur in three areas:
- *Perimembranous VSDs:* develop near the area of continuity between the tricuspid, aortic and mitral valves
- *Muscular VSDs:* have muscular margins that are away from the valves and there may be multiple defects
- *Supracristal VSDs:* the least common and are caused by a deficiency in the septum immediately below the aortic and pulmonary valve

Clinical features

The patient may be asymptomatic, but if the defect is large infants may fail to thrive and children may develop dyspnoea and recurrent chest infections.

The physical signs include:
- Parasternal and apical heaves
- Systolic thrill (small defects)
- Accentuated pulmonary component of the second heart sound
- Pansystolic murmur best heard at the lower left sternal edge (the murmur may disappear if Eisenmenger's syndrome occurs)

There may also be a mitral valve flow murmur, and subarterial defects may be associated with additional aortic regurgitation.

Investigation

Electrocardiography

ECG may show features of right ventricular hypertrophy.

Diagnostic imaging

● *Chest radiography:* the left- or right-sided chambers may be enlarged depending on the shunt, and the lungs may be normal (small VSD), plethoric (large VSD) or oligaemic (pulmonary vascular disease causing pulmonary hypertension)

● *Echocardiography:* visualizes the defect and the shunt, and allows calculation of the left : right ventricular pressure gradient and the pulmonary : systemic blood flow ratio

● *Cardiac catheterization:* sometimes carried out to confirm the diagnosis

Management

Most small restrictive membranous (maladie de Roger) defects close spontaneously. Surgery should be considered for larger defects to prevent heart failure and progressive pulmonary vascular disease.

Patients should be advised about antibiotic prophylaxis (see p. 482).

Patent ductus arteriosus

Disease mechanisms

The ductus arteriosus closes as a result of a prostaglandin-dependent mechanism at birth (Table 7.29; Fig. 7.52). Spontaneous closure is rare after 2 weeks unless the baby is premature. If it does not close and the pulmonary vascular resistance is low, aortic pressure is higher than the pulmonary pressures throughout the cardiac cycle. There is therefore a continuous flow of blood from the aorta to the pulmonary artery. This results in a high flow of blood through the lungs and left atrial and left ventricular volume overload.

Clinical features (Fig. 7.53)

Depending on the size of the shunt, premature babies may develop heart failure with tachypnoea and failure to thrive. Others may be asymptomatic, but have a continuous murmur. A patent ductus arteriosus (PDA) may occur as part of the rubella syndrome.

Physical signs include:
● Large pulse pressure
● Normal venous pressure
● Evidence of a dilated left ventricle
● A continuous murmur (Gibson's machinery murmur) under the left clavicle, although this may occur only in systole if the pulmonary vascular resistance is high, or not at all if pulmonary vascular resistance is very high because there is no shunt or it is reversed (blood flows from the

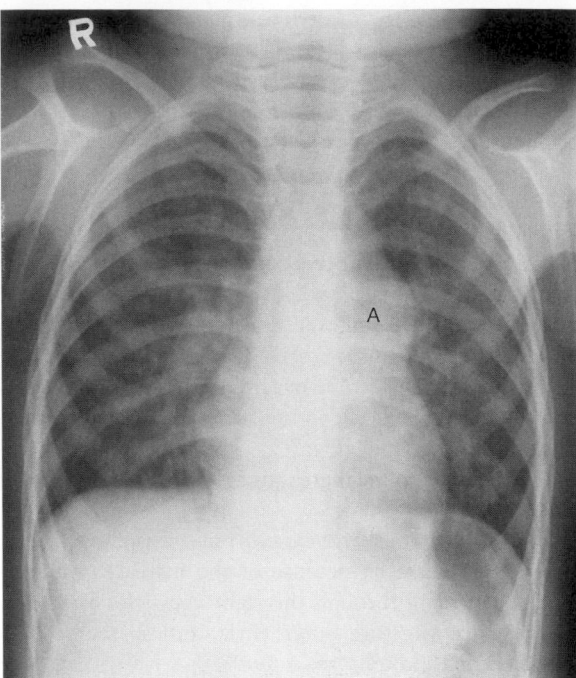

Fig. 7.53 Chest radiograph of patent ductus arteriosus (PDA). Note the enlarged pulmonary artery (A) and pulmonary plethora.

pulmonary artery to the aorta, which may be associated with toe clubbing and cyanosis)

● A mitral valve flow murmur (often present)

● A single second heart sound or a reversed split of the second sound if there is a large shunt because the aortic component of the second heart sound may be delayed

The differential diagnosis of a continuous murmur is given in Table 7.31.

Investigation

Electrocardiography

ECG may be normal or may show accentuated left ventricular voltages.

Table 7.31 Causes of a continuous murmur

Patent ductus arteriosus
Venous hum, which disappears when supine or with neck movement
Coronary fistula
Aortopulmonary window
Sinus of Valsalva fistula
Surgical systemic to pulmonary shunts (e.g. Blalock's, Waterston's, Pott's)
Aortopulmonary collaterals

Diagnostic imaging
- *Chest radiography:* may show an enlarged pulmonary artery with pulmonary plethora and evidence of an enlarged left atrium, left ventricle and aorta
- *Echocardiography:* visualizes the defect and Doppler techniques may be used to assess the shunt size

Management
In infancy indometacin promotes closure of a PDA. However, when indicated, occlusion can be achieved either surgically or by using a percutaneous approach. This involved introducing an occluder through the femoral vein and advancing it across the PDA.

Prognosis
The prognosis following succesful closure of a PDA is usually excellent.

Coarctation of the aorta
Epidemiology
Prevalence. This is a rare finding, occasionally not diagnosed until adult life. If untreated the majority of patients with severe coarctation will die in their mid-thirties.

Sex. Twice as common in men.

Genetics. Associated with Turner's syndrome.

Disease mechanisms
Coarctation of the aorta is a fibrous constriction in the aorta: 98% are distal to the origin of the left subclavian artery, but 2% may be abdominal or in the lower thoracic aorta. There are two types (COARCTATION OF THE AORTA AT A GLANCE):

Coarctation of the aorta at a glance

Epidemiology
Sex
Twice as common in men

Genetics
Associated with Turner's syndrome

Findings on investigation
Diagnostic imaging
- Chest radiography: shows a diminished aortic knuckle and dilatation of the left subclavian artery, and an indentation may be seen in the upper part of the descending aorta. Rib-notching may be seen and is a result of the formation of collaterals
- Echocardiography, CT, MRI and conventional or digital subtraction angiography: all useful for further evaluation of the coarctation and collaterals

Electrocardiology
ECG may show evidence of left ventricular hypertrophy

Clinical features (often asymptomatic)
Cardiovascular
Leg fatigue or claudication
Prominent upper limb pulses
Small femoral pulses with radial–femoral delay
Upper limb hypertension
Congenital berry aneurysms in the cerebral circulation
Bicuspid aortic valve (in 60%)
An ejection click (if the aortic valve is bicuspid)
An ejection systolic murmur
Asystolic murmur from the coarctation

Bruits over collaterals
Anomalous origin of the subclavian artery
Features of left ventricular hypertrophy
Palpable collaterals around the scapula

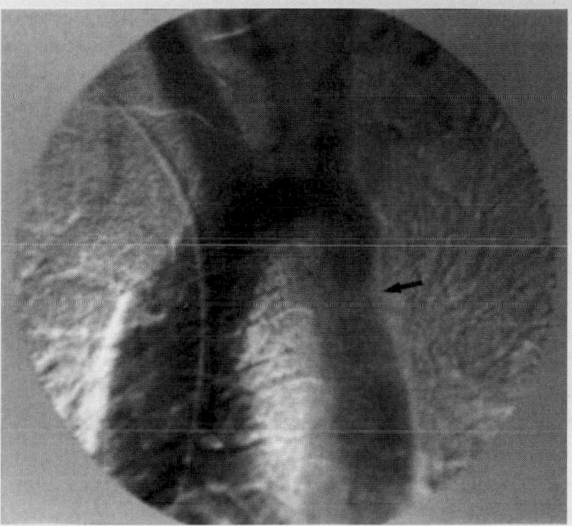

Fig. A Coarctation of the aorta: aortogram. This digital subtraction aortogram shows a discrete coarctation (arrowed) in the thoracic aorta just beyond the left subclavian branch. Reproduced from Timmis AD, Nathan AW. *Essentials of Cardiology*, 2nd edn, 1992 (Blackwell Scientific Publications, Oxford) with the permission of the authors.

• *Infantile type:* usually arises before the ductus arteriosus and blood passes to the lower body from the pulmonary artery via a PDA. The toes are therefore cyanosed while the hands are not (differential cyanosis). There is poor collateral development and it presents as heart failure in infancy.

• *Adult type:* arises after the ductus arteriosus and blood flows to the lower body via the coarctation and via collaterals involving the internal mammary arteries and scapular arteries.

Clinical features

Coarctation of the aorta usually presents as proximal hypertension caused by mechanical obstruction and a low renal perfusion pressure. It is associated with congenital berry aneurysms in the cerebral circulation, and 60% of patients have a bicuspid aortic valve. In some patients the subclavian artery has an anomalous origin. Patients are often asymptomatic, but may experience leg fatigue or claudication.

Clinical examination reveals:
• Prominent upper limb pulses
• Small femoral pulses with radial–femoral delay
• Upper limb hypertension
• Features of left ventricular hypertrophy
• Palpable collaterals around the scapula
• An ejection click (if the aortic valve is bicuspid), an ejection systolic murmur, a systolic murmur from the coarctation and bruits over collaterals

Investigation

Electrocardiography

ECG may show evidence of left ventricular hypertrophy.

Diagnostic imaging

• *Chest radiography:* shows a diminished aortic knuckle and dilatation of the left subclavian artery, and an indentation may be seen in the upper part of the descending aorta. Rib-notching may be seen and results from the formation of collaterals.

• *Echocardiography, CT, MRI and conventional or digital subtraction angiography:* all useful for further evaluation of the coarctation and collaterals.

Management and prognosis

In the infantile type, prostaglandin infusion may be required to keep the PDA open before surgical correction. Surgery for the adult type is usually best performed at 7–15 years of age or earlier if hypertension develops. The surgical risk increases thereafter with age. Hypertension, if present before surgery, does not always resolve.

Overall, without surgery, 90% of patients with coarctation of the aorta die before 40 years of age. If infancy is survived, about one-third die of aortic rupture, one-third die of endocarditis and one-third succumb to hypertension, left ventricular failure or cerebral haemorrhage.

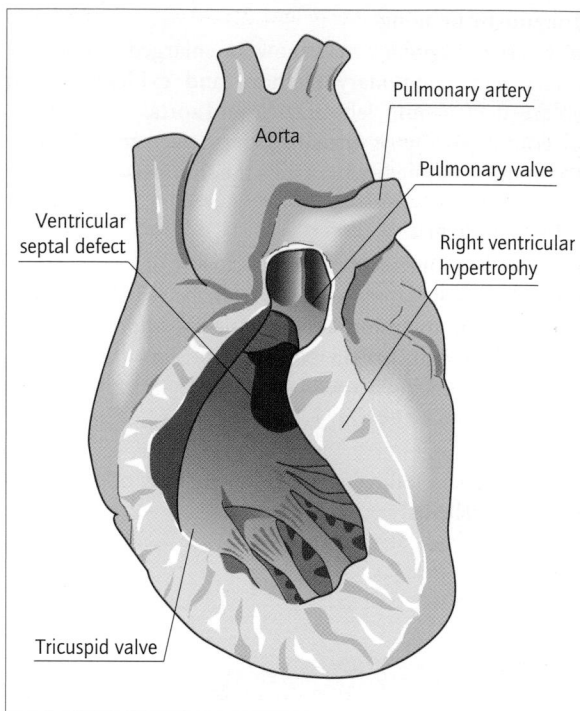

Figure 7.54 Fallot's tetralogy. Note: (i) VSD; (ii) overriding aorta; (iii) pulmonary stenosis; and (iv) right ventricular hypertrophy.

Congenital disease of the valves

Tetralogy of Fallot

Epidemiology

Prevalence. The most common cyanotic congenital heart defect.

Disease mechanisms

The abnormalities in Fallot's tetralogy (Fig. 7.54) are:
• Ventricular septal defect
• An aorta overriding the defect and therefore receiving blood from both the right and left ventricles
• Pulmonary stenosis (infundibular, valvar or supravalvar)
• Right ventricular hypertrophy

Right-to-left shunting increases with lowering of the systemic vascular resistance and increased infundibular obstruction. This may occur with exercise or emotional upsets. Children with Fallot's tetralogy often squat because this manoeuvre kinks the femoral arteries, increasing the systemic vascular resistance and decreasing the right-to-left shunt of blood through the VSD.

Clinical features

Depending on the severity of the defect, mild cyanosis may be apparent in infancy. Children have decreased exercise tolerance and occasional hypoxic crises.

Physical signs are:

- Variable cyanosis and clubbing
- Right ventricular hypertrophy
- A single second sound resulting from aortic closure (the pulmonary component is very late and too soft to hear)
- An ejection systolic murmur across the right ventricular outflow tract (the VSD is large and does not generate a murmur)

Investigation

Electrocardiography

ECG shows right axis deviation and evidence of right ventricular hypertrophy.

Diagnostic imaging

- *Chest radiography:* shows small pulmonary artery shadows and pulmonary oligaemia. Twenty-five per cent of patients have a right-sided aortic arch and there is a boot-shaped heart.
- *Echocardiography:* visualizes the defects.
- *Cardiac catheterization:* may be useful for evaluating the anomalies of the right ventricular outflow tract and the size of the pulmonary artery.

Management

In acute hypoxic crises, severe cyanosis can be treated with noradrenaline to increase systemic vascular resistance, and propranolol or morphine can be used to relax the infundibulum. Propranolol can be used to try to prevent cyanotic episodes.

All patients should be considered for surgery to increase blood flow to the lungs. Whether total correction is possible depends on the size of the pulmonary artery. A systemic to pulmonary artery shunt may be necessary for palliative surgery. The types most often used are:

- *Blalock–Taussig shunt:* an anastamosis of the subclavian artery with the ipsilateral pulmonary artery, which can also be achieved with a Gortex graft
- *Waterston's shunt:* from the ascending aorta to the right pulmonary artery
- *Pott's shunt:* from the descending aorta to the left pulmonary artery

Complex congenital heart disease

Other rare forms of complex congenital heart disease are

Table 7.32 Causes of acquired heart valve disease

Rheumatic fever
Valve calcification (in the elderly or congenitally abnormal valves)
Endocarditis
In association with other systemic disorders (e.g. ankylosing spondylitis, ischaemic heart disease, cardiomyopathy)

beyond the scope of this chapter and reference should be made to more specialist texts.

Valvular heart disease

Epidemiology

Prevalence and geography. Now that rheumatic fever is much less common, valve disorders are no longer the major cause of heart disease. However, the incidence of chronic rheumatic heart disease in the UK has not changed in recent years because of the postwar immigration of people from developing countries. Estimates of the prevalence of chronic rheumatic heart disease vary, but in the western world it is probably no more than 5/100 000 of the population, in contrast to 6/1000 in developing countries.

Age. The majority of patients are elderly and have degenerative disease of the heart valves.

Disease mechanisms

Table 7.32 lists causes of acquired heart valve disease.

Mitral valve disease

The mitral valve consists of two leaflets, the annulus (a muscular ring that contracts during systole to reduce the valve area), chordae tendineae and two papillary muscles. The cross-sectional area is 5 cm². The majority of ventricular filling occurs during early diastole and about one-third occurs during left atrial systole.

Mitral stenosis

Disease mechanisms

The main cause of mitral stenosis is rheumatic fever but it may be congenital. Occasionally, the physical signs of mitral stenosis occur in systemic lupus erythematosus, senile calcification of the valve ring and infective endocarditis with fleshy vegetations. Lutembacher's syndrome is the combination of mitral stenosis and an ASD.

In rheumatic heart disease the valve cusps become thickened and the commissures fuse. Similar thickening

07

of the subvalvar apparatus with contraction of the chordae tendineae leads to reduced ventricular filling. The left atrium increases in size and often develops mural thrombus.

Clinical features

Symptoms of mitral stenosis usually occur when the valve orifice is reduced to 1–2 cm^2. Breathlessness is caused by increased left atrial pressure and consequent pulmonary venous hypertension. Initially, the symptom is exertional dyspnoea but orthopnoea and PND develop with increasing stenosis, which eventually leads to pulmonary hypertension and signs of right ventricular failure (peripheral oedema and ascites).

Other symptoms include exertional fatigue, recurrent chest infections and haemoptysis. Palpitations are caused by atrial fibrillation, and occasionally the first symptom is caused by a systemic embolus, often arising at the onset of atrial fibrillation. They occur as a result of clot development in the left atrium, giving rise to a stroke or a loss of peripheral pulse.

Signs of mitral stenosis:

- A malar flush consisting of a dusky discoloration of the cheeks.
- The pulse is either normal or irregularly irregular because of atrial fibrillation.
- Venous pressure is raised if pulmonary hypertension has developed. Sometimes there is a systolic *v* wave of tricuspid regurgitation.
- The apex beat is not displaced because there is no load on the left ventricle. However, it has a tapping quality because of a palpable first heart sound. Because of the elevated left atrial pressure, which is always higher than the diastolic pressure in the left ventricle, the valve cusps are open to a maximum up to the onset of systole when they close abruptly, and this can be felt. A diastolic thrill may also be palpable. If pulmonary hypertension has developed, there is a palpable right ventricular heave and a palpable pulmonary component to the second heart sound in the second left intercostal space.
- A mid-diastolic murmur is the typical murmur. If the patient is in sinus rhythm atrial systole accentuates the diastolic murmur immediately before the first heart sound, giving rise to presystolic accentuation. As the mitral stenosis becomes more severe and the pulmonary artery pressure increases, the cardiac output falls and both the flow across the mitral valve and the loudness of the diastolic murmur decrease.
- There is a loud first heart sound and an opening snap in early diastole immediately before the mid-diastolic murmur if the valve cusps are mobile. The severity of the stenosis can be judged clinically by the interval

Table 7.33 Management of mitral stenosis

Specific treatment
Anticoagulation with warfarin
Essential as prophylaxis against thromboembolism

Lower left atrial pressure
Diuretics or nitrates

Atrial fibrillation
Digoxin (monitor plasma digoxin levels)
Additional antiarrhythmics (e.g. verapamil) if necessary

Surgery
To enlarge the mitral valve orifice as symptoms become more severe
Balloon valvotomy, closed mitral valvotomy, open mitral valvotomy or mitral valve replacement
Anticoagulation will almost certainly be indicated after all four procedures

between the second heart sound and the opening snap. The more severe it is the higher the left atrial pressure, and therefore the earlier the mitral valve opens in diastole bringing the opening snap closer to the second heart sound. As the mitral stenosis becomes more severe the valve cusps become immobile and the signs become less marked. The first heart sound and opening snap then disappear.

Differential diagnosis

The differential diagnosis of mitral stenosis is limited (Table 7.33):

- Left atrial myxoma (see p. 500)
- Austin Flint murmur (see p. 475)
- Cor triatriatum, a restrictive membrane above the mitral valve restricting blood flow

Investigation

Electrocardiography

While in sinus rhythm the left atrial component of the P wave of the ECG becomes more prominent, giving rise to the characteristically shaped P mitrale. Atrial fibrillation and the features of right ventricular hypertrophy (tall R waves in V1 and right axis deviation) develop as the condition progresses.

Diagnostic imaging

- *Chest radiography:* first the left atrium enlarges giving rise to a characteristic straight contour to the left heart shadow. As the condition becomes more severe, pulmonary hypertension develops and there is evidence of pulmonary venous congestion and enlarged pulmonary arteries. The transverse cardiac diameter then increases

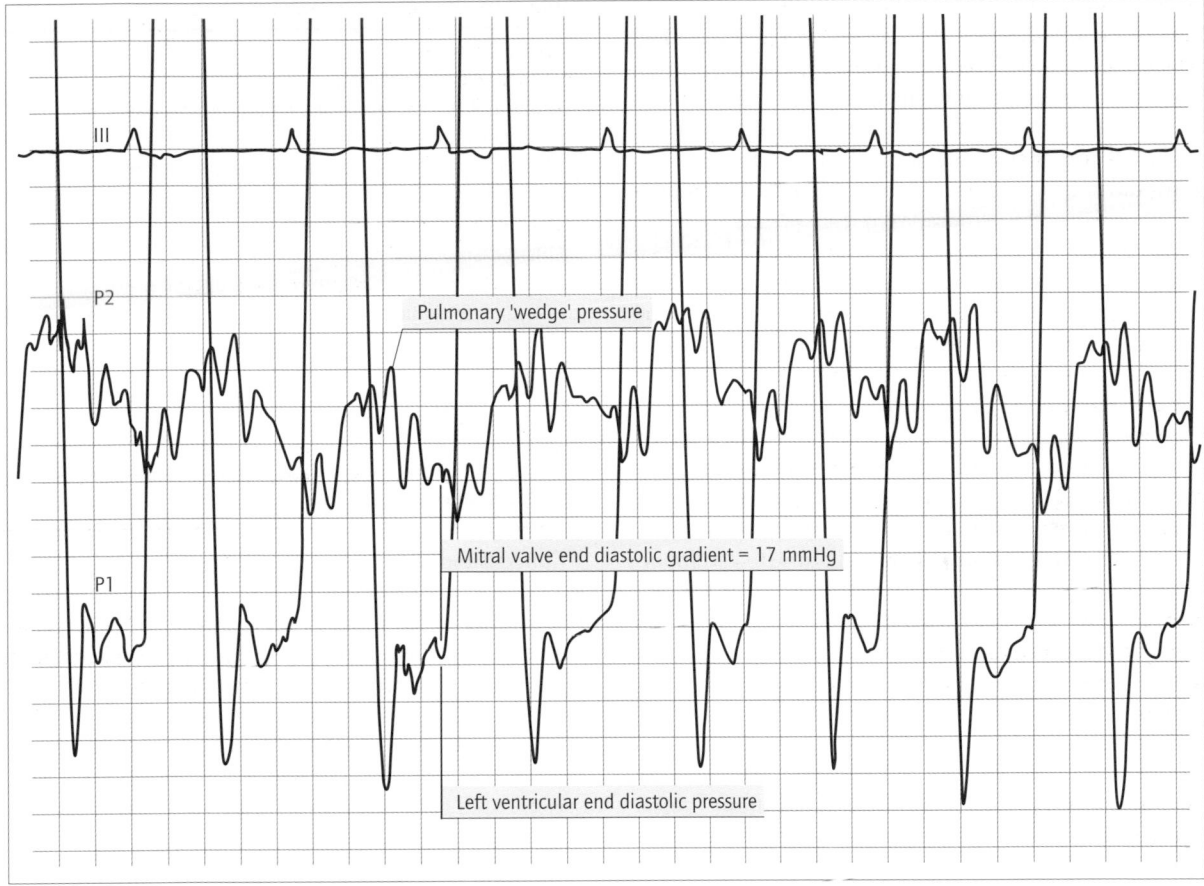

Figure 7.55 Haemodynamic assessment of mitral stenosis. Note the use of simultaneous intracardiac measurements of the pulmonary 'wedge' (indirect left atrial) pressure and left ventricular pressure.

because of right ventricular and right atrial dilatations. There may be calcification in the mitral valve.

• *Echocardiography:* shows a calcified valve with restricted cusp motion, an enlarged left atrium, and subsequently an enlarged right ventricle and right atrium. The Doppler signal allows assessment of the mitral valve orifice area and the maximum gradient across the mitral valve.

• *Cardiac catheterization:* often not required, particularly in young patients, because the echocardiogram provides enough information. However, it provides a haemodynamic assessment of the mitral stenosis, and should be performed if there is thought to be coexistent valvular or coronary artery disease (Fig. 7.55).

Management

Anticoagulation with warfarin is essential as prophylaxis against thromboembolism. This should be started early, and not only when atrial fibrillation has developed. Symptoms caused by fluid retention are helped by the addition of diuretics. However, the features of raised left atrial pressure are not helped by diuretics unless severe hypovolaemia is induced, which will reduce the cardiac output. This will cause symptoms from hypotension and is not desirable.

The onset of atrial fibrillation usually occurs in the third or fourth decade and is treated with digoxin. The exertional dyspnoea of mitral stenosis is often caused by uncontrolled atrial fibrillation on exercise, despite apparently well-controlled atrial fibrillation at rest. Plasma digoxin levels must be monitored and additional antiarrhythmics such as verapamil may be added to control the atrial fibrillation.

Surgery

As the symptoms become more severe, the mitral valve orifice will need enlargement. The four techniques available are:
1 Balloon valvotomy
2 Closed mitral valvotomy
3 Open mitral valvotomy
4 Mitral valve replacement

07

The first three techniques can produce good results for at least 10 years, but eventually cusp fusion will reoccur and further intervention becomes necessary. Anticoagulation will almost certainly be indicated after all four procedures because of the coexisting presence of atrial fibrillation, which will predispose to left atrial thrombus formation.

In **valvuloplasty**, a balloon or mechanical dilator is introduced via the femoral vein and passed by direct puncture across the atrial septum and mitral valve. When in position it is dilated for a few seconds. The advantage of this procedure is that it can be carried out under local anaesthetic and it is most suitable for young patients with no calcification in the valve and no mitral regurgitation.

Closed mitral valvotomy is carried out under general anaesthetic. A dilator is introduced via a left thoracotomy and passed across the mitral valve separating the valve commissures. This technique has now been superseded in the UK by open mitral valvotomy.

Open mitral valvotomy is carried out with cardiopulmonary bypass. This allows direct vision of the mitral valve and the cusps are separated by careful dissection. This reduces the likelihood of mitral regurgitation postoperatively.

Mitral valve replacement is required for patients with mitral stenosis if the valve is heavily calcified and the chordae tendineae are fibrosed and shortened by the rheumatic process, or if there is significant mitral regurgitation.

Prognosis

Without surgery, 70% of symptomatic patients will survive for 5 years. However, even with surgery the prognosis remains reduced. Following mitral valve replacement only 60–70% of patients survive for 10 years, because of problems with the prosthetic valve such as thromboembolism and endocarditis, and progressive left ventricular dysfunction.

Mitral regurgitation

Epidemiology

Because of its many causes, mitral regurgitation is common (Table 7.34).

Disease mechanisms

Because the pressure in the left atrium is much lower than that in the aorta, mitral regurgitation gives rise to a much greater stroke volume than normal. A significant volume of blood may regurgitate into the left atrium, even before the aortic valve has opened.

Pathogenesis

If the onset of mitral regurgitation is acute, the left atrium

Table 7.34 Causes of mitral regurgitation

Mitral valve prolapse
Rheumatic heart disease
Dilatation of the left ventricle (e.g. in cardiomyopathy or other causes of heart failure)
Ischaemic heart disease leading to a papillary muscle dysfunction
Collagen disorders such as Marfan's syndrome or Ehlers–Danlos syndrome
Hypertrophic cardiomyopathy
Infective endocarditis
Connective tissue disorders (e.g. systemic lupus erythematosus)

does not expand and the pressure wave is transmitted into the pulmonary veins. This causes acute breathlessness. However, if mitral regurgitation develops gradually, the left atrium expands and acts as a capacitance chamber absorbing the pressure wave generated by the regurgitant blood through the mitral valve. This causes only a small rise in pulmonary venous pressure and the patient is therefore not so breathless until the mitral regurgitation is very severe.

The left ventricular end-diastolic cavity does not increase in size early in the natural history of the condition, but the end-systolic size is considerably reduced because of the increased stroke volume.

Clinical features

Dyspnoea and orthopnoea are the typical symptoms of mitral regurgitation. When the onset is acute the initial symptoms can be severe, but as the left atrium expands the symptoms lessen. The reduced cardiac output can cause tiredness and fatigue.

As mitral regurgitation progressess, left ventricular failure and then pulmonary hypertension and right ventricular failure develop. Cardiac cachexia (loss of muscle mass because of the high-energy requirements of the myocardium) can be associated with congestive cardiac failure.

The physical signs of mitral regurgitation are as follows:
- *Peripheral pulse volume is reduced:* the character of the pulse is often jerky because of the abbreviated systole. In advanced disease, left atrial dilatation can cause atrial fibrillation.
- *Apex beat may be displaced laterally:* the impulse may be overactive because of increased volume load on the ventricle.
- *Murmurs:* on auscultation there is a pansystolic murmur, which is typically maximal at the apex and radiates to the axilla when the aetiology is rheumatic. However, in non-rheumatic mitral regurgitation, the radiation of the murmur is variable and may radiate to the neck. In mitral valve prolapse, the murmur may be late systolic and occur

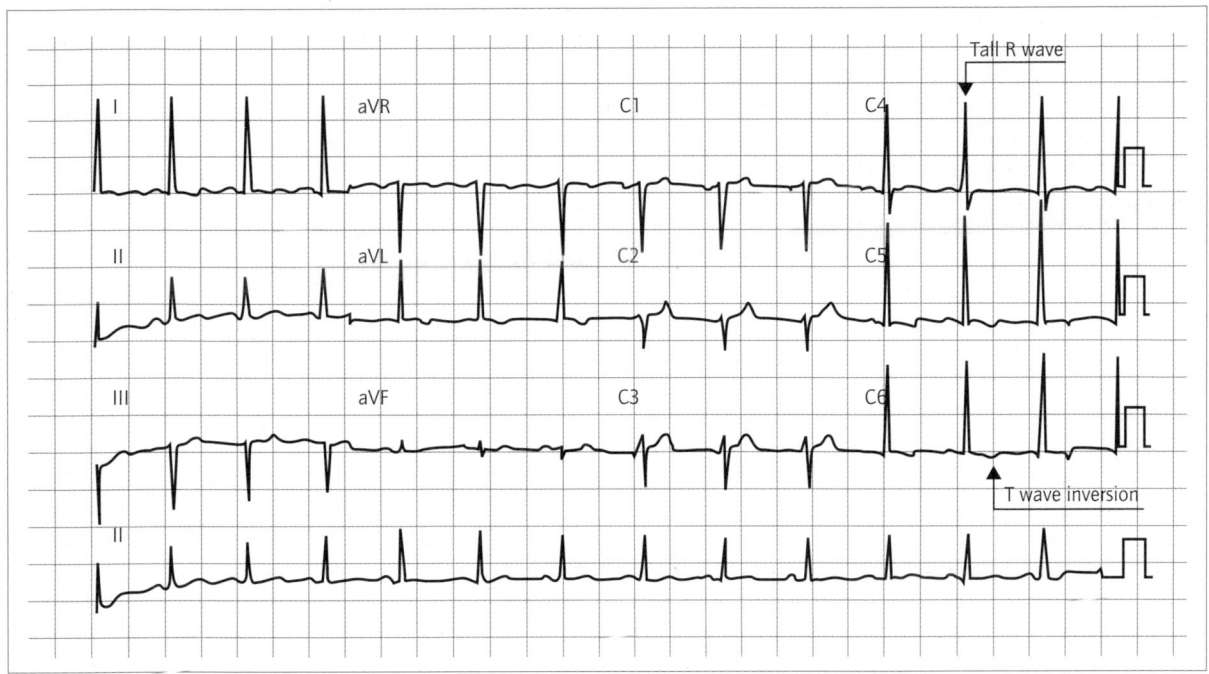

Figure 7.56 ECG showing counterclockwise rotation of the heart because of expansion of the left ventricle and features of left ventricular hypertrophy because of its volume load as in mitral or aortic incompetence. Note the increased amplitude of the R-wave and T-wave inversion (without the ST depression seen in left ventricular hypertrophy resulting from pressure load.

after a mid-systolic click. If the posterior leaflet is prolapsed, the regurgitant jet will be directed anteriorly and radiate to the left sternal edge.

● *The first heart sound is soft and there may be a third heart sound:* because of the increased volume of blood entering the left ventricle from the left atrium in diastole. Occasionally, this is followed by a mid-diastolic flow murmur.

Differential diagnosis

The differential diagnosis of mitral regurgitation includes the following:

● *Ventricular septal defect:* the murmur of a VSD classically radiates from the apex to the left sternal edge.
● *Aortic valve disease:* the ejection systolic murmur of aortic valve disease is often loudest at the apex and, if the aortic valve cusps are immobile, the second sound may be missing, giving the murmur a pansystolic quality.
● *Tricuspid regurgitation:* as with mitral regurgitation, tricuspid regurgitation gives rise to a pansystolic murmur and the distinction can be made by the presence of a systolic *v* wave in the neck.
● *Hypertrophic cardiomyopathy:* patients with hypertrophic cardiomyopathy frequently have a systolic murmur with characteristics that are difficult to distinguish from the pansystolic murmur of mitral regurgitation. Indeed, some patients with hypertrophic cardiomyopathy

have mitral regurgitation and the diagnosis is established by echocardiography.

Investigation
Electrocardiography

ECG may show an enlarged left atrium with P mitrale and bifid P waves in lead V1, and left ventricular hypertrophy from volume overload (increased voltages with T inversion in the lateral chest leads) (Fig. 7.56).

Diagnostic imaging

● *Chest radiography:* shows an increased transversed cardiac diameter with left atrial and left ventricular enlargement. Calcification in the mitral valve may be evident.
● *Echocardiography:* shows features of a volume-loaded left ventricle with vigorous systolic function of a dilated left ventricle and a dilated left atrium. The aetiology of the mitral regurgitation may be evident. The colour wave Doppler signal demonstrates the regurgitation, but is unreliable in assessing its severity.
● *Cardiac catheterization:* indirect measurement of left atrial pressure via a pulmonary artery wedge pressure catheter demonstrates a large atrial systolic *v* wave. The pulmonary artery pressure will probably be increased, and the left ventricular end-diastolic pressure will also be increased. The left ventricular angiogram shows reflux of

Table 7.35 Mitral regurgitation

Specific treatment
Antibiotic prophylaxis against endocarditis
When symptoms develop
Diuretics will reduce left atrial pressure
Vasodilators such as ACE inhibitors will encourage forward
   flow from the left ventricle

Atrial fibrillation
Digoxin
Anticoagulation with warfarin

Surgery
If the symptoms are inadequately controlled by medical
   therapy or there is evidence of left ventricular dysfunction
Either open mitral valve repair or valve replacement

blood across the mitral valve into the large left atrium. When there is associated left ventricular dysfunction it can be difficult to know whether the mitral regurgitation is the cause or result of the left ventricular dysfunction.

Management

When symptoms develop, diuretics reduce left atrial pressure and vasodilators such as ACE inhibitors encourage forward flow from the left ventricle. If atrial fibrillation develops, digoxin and anticoagulation with warfarin are required. Antibiotic prophylaxis against endocarditis is important (Table 7.35).

Surgery is required if the symptoms are inadequately controlled by medical therapy and can involve either open mitral valve repair or valve replacement. The major clinical dilemma is when to recommend surgical treatment if the patient apparently has no symptoms, as left ventricular dysfunction can progress in these patients. When the patient then complains of symptoms it may be too late for surgery to relieve all the symptoms, and the patient is left with compromised left ventricular function. It is therefore useful to monitor a patient's progress objectively with exercise testing and echocardiography.

Prognosis

Surgery has radically improved the prognosis of mitral regurgitation. Before surgery, however, approximately 80% of patients with severe regurgitation would survive for 5 years and 60% would survive for 10 years.

Mitral valve prolapse (floppy mitral valve)

Epidemiology

Prevalence. Up to 4% of women and 1% of men have mitral valve prolapse on routine echocardiography. In many ways mitral valve prolapse can therefore be considered a normal variant, but sometimes the associated regurgitation causes symptoms and treatment is necessary. It is most commonly identified in young women.

Disease mechanisms

Mitral valve prolapse is usually associated with myxomatous degeneration of either:
- *Mitral valve leaflet:* allowing the leaflet to billow into the left ventricle
- *Chordae tendineae:* which stretch and allow the leaflet to prolapse into the left atrium, resulting in mitral regurgitation

It is sometimes seen in association with an ASD, hypertrophic cardiomyopathy or Marfan's syndrome. Occasionally, there is a family history.

Clinical features

The most common symptom of mitral valve prolapse is palpitations, which on 24-h ambulatory monitoring are shown to be caused by atrial or ventricular ectopics. Patients also complain of stabbing-like atypical chest pain, which usually causes severe anxiety because of the associated palpitations.

In a small group of patients the degree of mitral regurgitation increases either gradually because of stretching of the chordae tendineae, or suddenly because of rupture of the chordae tendineae. This is a feature of connective tissue disorders such as Marfan's syndrome.

Typical signs are a mid-systolic click followed by a late systolic murmur. The click is caused by sudden tensing of the chordae tendineae during systole. The late systolic murmur can be variable and can become more evident with the Valsalva manoeuvre or on standing, both of which reduce ventricular filling and increase the degree of prolapse.

Investigation

Electrocardiography

ECG can show abnormal repolarization with inverted T waves in the inferior and lateral chest leads.

Diagnostic imaging

- *Chest radiography:* usually normal, but in patients with significant regurgitation there is an enlargement of both the left ventricle and left atrium
- *Echocardiography:* confirms the aetiology of the mitral regurgitation, demonstrating malposition of the mitral valve leaflets with prolapse of one or other of the cusps into the left atrium (Fig. 7.57)

Management and prognosis

Treatment is the same as for mitral regurgitation, but

Mitral regurgitation at a glance

Aetiology
Mitral valve prolapse
Rheumatic heart disease
Dilatation of the left ventricle
Ischaemic heart disease
Collagen disorders
Hypertrophic cardiomyopathy
Infective endocarditis
Connective tissue disorders

Findings on investigation
Diagnostic imaging
- *Chest radiography:* shows an enlarging heart with filling of left atrial bay. May be calcification in the mitral valve
- *Echocardiography:* colour Doppler gives a guide to the extent of regurgitation
- *Cardiac catheterization:* pulmonary artery wedge pressure catheter demonstrates a large atrial systolic *v* wave. Pulmonary artery pressure will probably be increased, and left ventricular end-diastolic pressure will also be increased. The left ventricular angiogram shows reflux of blood across the mitral valve into the large left atrium

Electrocardiology
ECG shows features of left atrial and/or left ventricular hypertrophy. Atrial fibrillation is common

Clinical features
Cardiovascular
'Sharp' low-volume pulse
Displaced palpable apex beat
Pansystolic or late systolic murmur
Third heart sound, occasionally followed by a mid-diastolic flow murmur
Dyspnoea
Orthopnoea
Tiredness and fatigue
Left ventricular failure
Right ventricular failure develops
Cardiac cachexia
Reduced peripheral pulse volume
Atrial fibrillation
Soft first heart sound

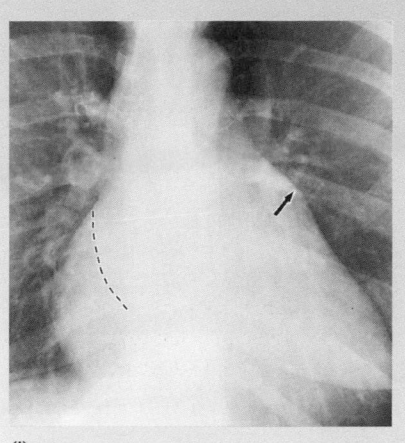

(i)

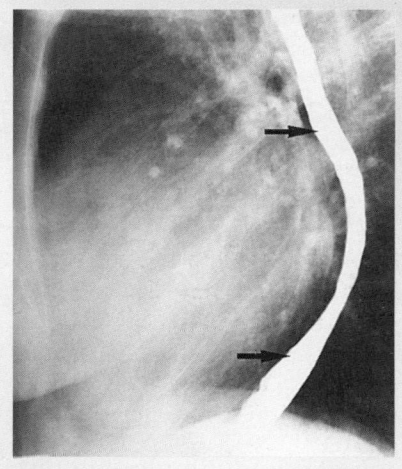

(ii)

Fig. A (i) Left atrial enlargement in a patient with MV disease showing the 'double contour sign' (the left atrial border has been drawn in) and dilatation of the left atrial appendage (LAA) (arrow). (ii) The lateral view shows how the enlarged left atrium displaces the barium-filled oesophagus between the two arrows. Reproduced from Armstrong P, Wastie ML. *Diagnostic Imaging*, 3rd edn, 1992 (Blackwell Scientific Publications, Oxford).

patients often present with atypical chest pain and palpitations, both of which can be difficult to control. Beta-blockers are the first drugs to try, but reassurance and an explanation of the benign nature of the condition is essential (Table 7.36).

Anticoagulation is required if atrial fibrillation develops. Prophylaxis against endocarditis is recommended. This is essential for the patient who has a murmur, but is probably not required for those who only have echocardiographical features of mitral prolapse.

For the great majority of patients, mitral prolapse is asymptomatic. For a small proportion (5%), haemodynamic problems develop, particularly as a consequence of either infective endocarditis or chordal rupture.

07

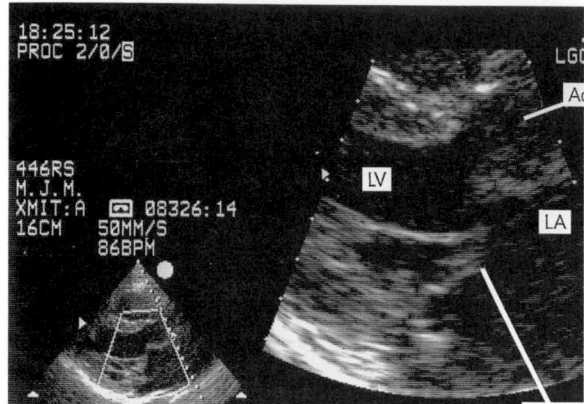

(a)

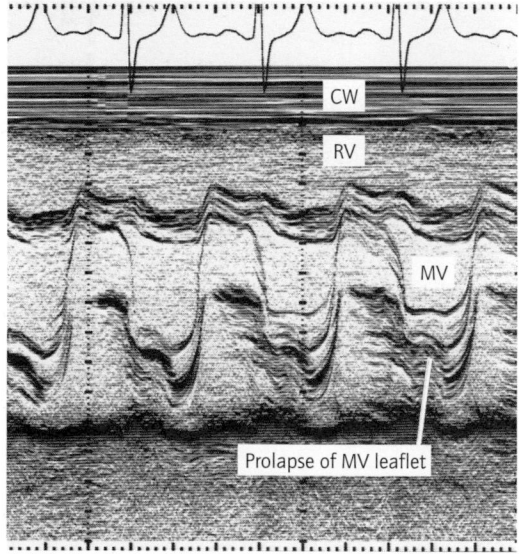

(b)

Figure 7.57 (a) Two-dimensional parasternal long axis view and (b) M-mode echocardiogram of mitral valve prolapse. Note the posterior leaflet of the mitral valve prolapsing into the left atrium on the two-dimensional long axis view. CW, chest wall; IVS, interventricular septum; MV, mitral valve; RV, right ventricle.

Tricuspid valve disease

Tricuspid valve disease (tricuspid stenosis or tricuspid regurgitation) is rare in isolation and is usually a result of rheumatic fever in which case left-sided valve disease is usually present. Carcinoid syndrome is another recognized cause, but tricuspid regurgitation is most commonly caused by dilatation of the tricuspid valve ring as a consequence of left ventricular dilatation brought about by pulmonary hypertension. Tricuspid regurgitation occurs in Ebstein's syndrome when there is congenital displacement of the valve into the right ventricle.

Table 7.36 Management of mitral valve prolapse

Specific treatment
Prophylaxis against endocarditis
As for all other valve diseases

Atypical chest pain and palpitations
Beta-blockers
Reassurance and explanation

When symptoms of breathlessness develop
Diuretics will reduce left atrial pressure
Vasodilators such as ACE inhibitors will encourage forward flow from the left ventricle

Atrial fibrillation
Digoxin
Anticoagulation with warfarin

Surgery
If the symptoms are inadequately controlled by medical therapy or there is evidence of left ventricular dysfunction
Open mitral valve repair or valve replacement

Clinical features

Both tricuspid stenosis and incompetence cause right atrial hypertension and reduced cardiac output leading to hepatomegaly, ascites and dependent oedema. The hepatomegaly can be painful because of stretching of the liver capsule. The reduced cardiac output leads to fatigue and exertional dyspnoea.

Signs of tricuspid valve disease:
1 Tricuspid stenosis
   ● Increased atrial component to the venous pressure pulse with a prominent A wave if the patient is in sinus rhythm
   ● Rumbling diastolic murmur
2 Tricuspid regurgitation
   ● Systolic V wave in the venous pressure pulse
   ● Pulsatile liver edge
   ● Pansystolic murmur at the right sternal edge
   ● Palpable right ventricle

Investigation
Electrocardiography

Tall peak P waves in lead 2 because of right atrial enlargement. Atrial fibrillation is common. If there is significant tricuspid regurgitation, right bundle branch block may develop.

Diagnostic imaging

● *Chest X-ray:* prominent right heart border and possible cardiomegaly.
● *Echocardiogram:* tricuspid stenosis; calcified immobile tricuspid valve. Tricuspid regurgitation, echo evidence

of volume load of the right ventricle with enlargement of the right ventricle and right atrium and paradoxical septal motion where the intraventricular septum contracts towards the free wall of the right rather than the left ventricle. (This is also seen in ASD and pulmonary regurgitation and is caused by increased right ventricular volume.)

● *Pulse Doppler:* detects a regurgitant jet from the right ventricle into the right atrium. This allows assessment of right ventricular and pulmonary artery systolic pressure, reverse blood flow in the inferior vena cava and hepatic veins can also be seen.

Management

For tricuspid stenosis, diuretics are the mainstay of medical therapy but valvotomy and, rarely, valve replacement may be necessary. For tricuspid regurgitation, treatment is as for congestive cardiac failure including the use of the diuretic spironolactone. Functional tricuspid regurgitation does not usually require surgery and can be managed medically but annuloplasty, where the tricuspid valve is repaired, is often carried out in association with surgery on left-sided heart valves.

Box 7.10: Tricuspid regurgitation

Specific treatment
Medical treatment
Treatment for congestive cardiac failure (see p. 429)

Surgery
Tricuspid valve repair by annuloplasty is often carried out in association with surgery on left-sided heart valves
In endocarditis it may be necessary to remove the tricuspid valve and leave severe tricuspid regurgitation or insert a prosthetic valve

---

Pulmonary valve disease

Pulmonary valve disease (pulmonary stenosis and pulmonary regurgitation) are uncommon. Pulmonary stenosis is either congenital or acquired as a consequence of rheumatic fever or carcinoid syndrome. Congenital pulmonary stenosis can be an isolated lesion found at a routine examination or be part of a more complex defect such as Fallot's tetralogy. It is a feature of Noonan's syndrome (phenotypically like Turner's syndrome but with normal chromosomes). Pulmonary stenosis may be either valvular, supravalvular or subvalvular and multiple stenoses in the pulmonary artery are a feature of rubella syndrome. Pulmonary regurgitation is most often seen following a valvotomy for pulmonary stenosis. The other cause is

pulmonary hypertension commonly resulting from left-sided valve disease, particularly mitral stenosis.

Clinical features

Pulmonary stenosis. Fatigue and syncope and symptoms of right ventricular failure. Often the murmur is heard as part of a routine medical examination without symptoms. Unless severe, pulmonary regurgitation causes no symptoms and then those symptoms are caused by right ventricular failure.

The clinical signs for pulmonary stenosis:
1 Ejection systolic murmur in the second left intercostal space
2 A delayed soft pulmonary component to the second heart sound
3 Pulmonary ejection click
4 Fourth heart sound
5 Prominent A wave in the venous pressure and right ventricular hypertrophy
Pulmonary regurgitation. An early diastolic murmur is heard immediately after the pulmonary component of the second heart sound (Graham Steell murmur).

Investigation

Electrocardiography

ECG shows evidence of right atrial and right ventricular hypertrophy with P pulmonale and prominent R waves in the anterior chest leads. For pulmonary regurgitation, the ECG may show an RSR pattern in V1, V2 compatible with right ventricular diastolic overload.

Diagnostic imaging

● *Chest X ray:* in pulmonary stenosis, poststenotic dilatation gives rise to a prominent pulmonary artery shadow. In pulmonary regurgitation there will be an enlarged heart and enlarged pulmonary arteries.
● *Echocardiogram:* pulse Doppler measures right ventricular systolic pressure and the gradient across the pulmonary valve. For pulmonary regurgitation, the echocardiogram shows a dilated right ventricle with reverse septal motion. Pulse Doppler detects a regurgitant jet.

Management

For pulmonary stenosis, antibiotic prophylaxis is required. If the right ventricular systolic pressure rises above 60 mmHg balloon dilatation and/or surgery of the valve is recommended (Table 7.37). No treatment is usually required for pulmonary regurgitation.

Aortic stenosis

Conditions that can obstruct the outflow of blood from the left ventricle include:

07

Table 7.37 Summary of valve defects, symptoms, signs and management

Valve	Defect	Symptoms	Murmur	Heart sounds	Management
Mitral valve	Stenosis	Breathlessness, palpitations	Mid-diastolic	Loud S_1 opening snap	Valvotomy
	Regurgitation	Breathlessness	Pansystolic	A_2 obscured	Diuretics, vasodilators, surgery
	Prolapse	Breathlessness, atypical chest pain, palpitations	Late systolic	Normal or mid-systolic click	Diuretics, vasodilators, surgery
Tricuspid valve	Disease	Swelling of ankles, swelling of abdomen (ascites), sacral oedema	Mid-diastolic	Opening snap	Diuretics
Aortic valve	Stenosis	Angina, syncope, breathlessness	Ejection systolic	Reduced A_2	Surgery
	Regurgitation	Breathlessness	Early diastolic		Vasodilators, diuretics, surgery
Pulmonary	Stenosis	Fatigue	Ejection systolic	Delayed P_2	Balloon dilatation

Table 7.38 Causes of aortic stenosis

Congenital, usually a bicuspid aortic valve (a bicuspid valve may not be stenotic, but may become so in later life because of calcification)

Rheumatic fever

Senile calcification of the aortic valve leaflets (does not usually cause severe aortic stenosis unless the valve is congenitally bicuspid)

- *Aortic valve stenosis*
- *Subvalvar aortic stenosis:* caused by a fibrous or muscular diaphragm situated below the aortic valve
- *Supravalvar stenosis:* caused by a fibrous band above the aortic valve, which may be part of Williams' syndrome (elfin-like facies, hypercalcaemia and mental retardation)
- *Hypertrophic cardiomyopathy*

Epidemiology
Aortic stenosis is the most common isolated single valve lesion. It is more common in men.

Disease mechanisms
The causes of aortic stenosis are shown in Table 7.38.

Clinical features
Aortic stenosis results in a reduction in cardiac output, especially on exercise, and left ventricular hypertrophy. As the hypertrophy increases the diastolic pressure in the left ventricle increases, reducing the transcoronary pressure gradient and increasing left atrial pressure and therefore pulmonary venous pressure. This pathophysiology gives rise to the three cardinal symptoms of aortic stenosis:

1 Angina
2 Breathlessness
3 Dizziness or syncope on exercise

The signs are:
- A slow rising carotid pulse.
- An ejection systolic thrill palpable at the right sternal edge.
- A thrusting apex beat from left ventricular hypertrophy.
- An ejection systolic murmur maximal at the left sternal edge and aortic area and radiating into the carotid arteries. It is sometimes associated with an ejection click from a bicuspid valve.

The second sound can become soft if the valve leaflets are immobile and reverse splitting can occur with A_2 following P2 caused by delayed emptying of the left ventricle.

Investigation
Electrocardiography
ECG shows the left ventricular hypertrophy and strain pattern of pressure overload (depressed ST segments and T-wave inversion in the left ventricular leads, with increased voltages) (Fig. 7.58).

Diagnostic imaging
- *Chest radiography:* shows a normal transverse cardiac diameter and a prominent left ventricular heart border.
- *Echocardiography:* demonstrates a calcified disorganized valve (Fig. 7.59). Doppler is used to measure the pressure difference across the valve. If ventricular function is normal a gradient up to 30 mmHg is considered to indicate mild aortic stenosis, while a gradient of 30–70 mmHg indicates moderate aortic stenosis, and a gradient greater than 70 mmHg indicates severe aortic stenosis. If left ventricular function is poor and cardiac output is reduced, the gradient will be less for each category.
- *Cardiac catheterization:* confirms the diagnosis and allows assessment of the coronary circulation (Fig. 7.60).

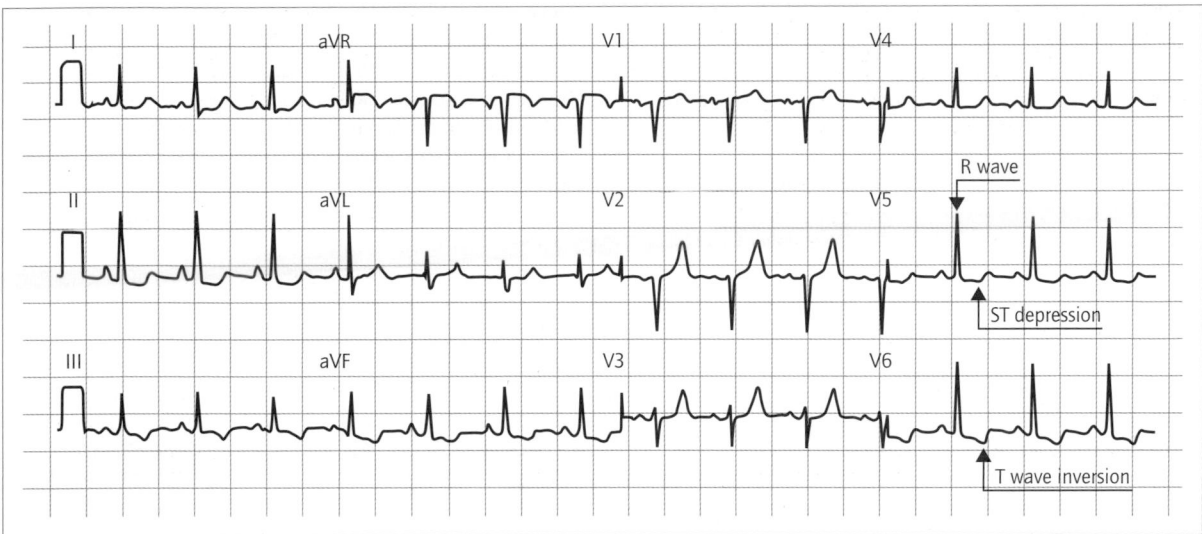

Figure 7.58 ECG showing left ventricular hypertrophy because of pressure load as in aortic stenosis or hypertension. Note the increased amplitude of the R waves and the ST depression and T inversion in leads I, II, III, aVF and V5–V6.

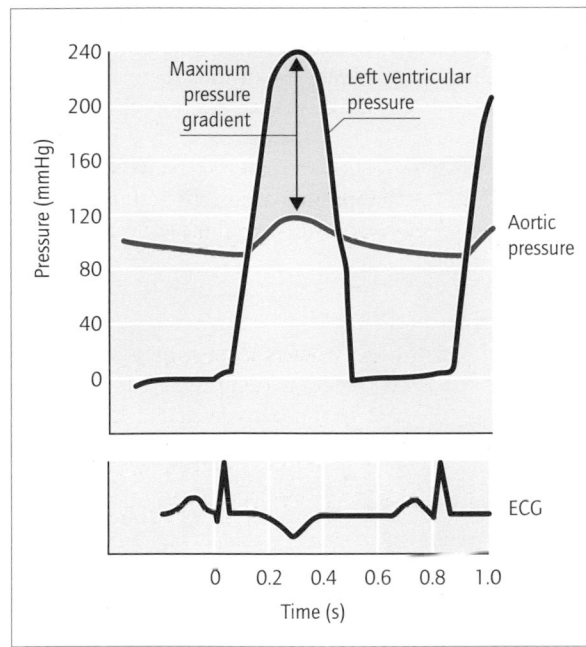

Figure 7.59 Haemodynamic assessment of aortic stenosis. The shaded area represents the pressure gradient across the aortic valve. Note the differences in left ventricular and aortic pressure during systole.

Management

Surgical aortic valve replacement is the only treatment, except in children when aortic stenosis can be treated by valvotomy when the valve cusps are split.

Prognosis

Severe aortic stenosis results in a very compromised prognosis with a significant risk of sudden death. Patients with left ventricular failure caused by aortic stenosis have a 50% mortality rate within 2 years without surgery.

Aortic regurgitation

Disease mechanisms

Blood leaking from the aorta into the left ventricle during systole leads to an increase in stroke volume and diastolic dimensions of the ventricle. Causes of aortic regurgitation are listed in Table 7.39.

As the degree of regurgitation increases, end-diastolic pressure in the left ventricle increases. Left atrial pressure is therefore increased, giving rise to pulmonary venous hypertension and exertional dyspnoea. Eventually, chronic left ventricular dysfunction develops and the symptoms of left ventricular failure occur at rest.

Clinical features

The symptoms are exertional dyspnoea first, and later the symptoms of left ventricular failure at rest (Table 7.17). Occasionally, coronary perfusion diminishes as the arterial diastolic pressure falls and the ventricular diastolic pressure rises, giving rise to angina.

Signs are:

- *Collapsing pulse in the arm:* with a wide pulse pressure
- *Early diastolic murmur:* maximal at the left sternal edge and towards the apex on auscultation. The regurgitant jet

Aortic stenosis at a glance

Epidemiology

Age
70 years of age and over

Sex
Male

Race
White people

Genetics
Often underlying valve abnormality—bicuspid

Findings on investigation

Diagnostic imaging
■ *Chest radiography:* shows a normal transverse cardiac diameter and a prominent left ventricular heart border
■ *Echocardiography:* demonstrates a calcified disorganized valve (Fig. A). Doppler is used to measure the pressure difference across the valve (Fig. B)
■ *Cardiac catheterization:* confirms the diagnosis and allows assessment of the coronary circulation (see Fig. 7.60)

Electrocardiology
ECG shows the left ventricular hypertrophy and strain pattern of pressure overload (depressed ST segments and T-wave inversion in the left ventricular leads, with increased voltages)

Clinical features

Cardiovascular
Angina
Breathlessness
Dizziness or syncope on exercise

Slow rising carotid pulse
Ejection systolic thrill palpable at the right sternal edge
Thrusting apex beat
Ejection systolic murmur maximal at the left sternal edge and aortic area, and radiating into the carotid arteries, sometimes associated with an ejection click
Soft and reversed split second sound if the valve leaflets are immobile

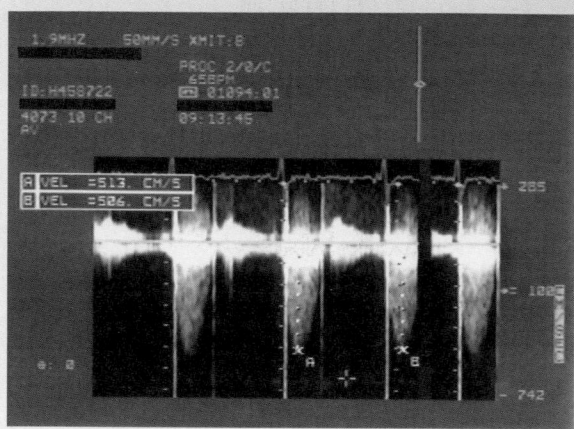

Fig. B Echocardiogram of aortic stenosis; Doppler estimate of velocity (>5 ms = >100 mmHg).

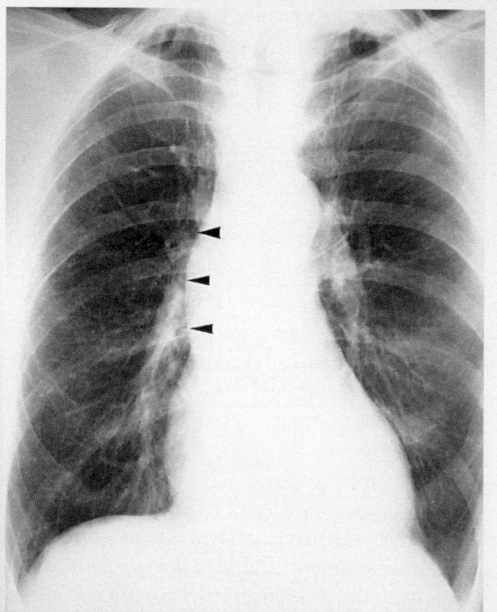

Fig. C Aortic stenosis showing poststenotic dilatation of the aorta (arrows). Note: there is little, if any, cardiac enlargement. Reproduced from Armstrong P, Wastie ML. *Diagnostic Imaging*, 3rd edn, 1992 (Blackwell Scientific Publications, Oxford) with permission of the authors.

Fig. A Severe aortic stenosis in parasternal long axis view showing calcified aortic valve and normal mitral valve. Left ventricle (LV) not enlarged, but very thick walls of interventricular septum (IVS) and posterior wall of LV (LVPW). RVOT, right ventricular outflow tract.

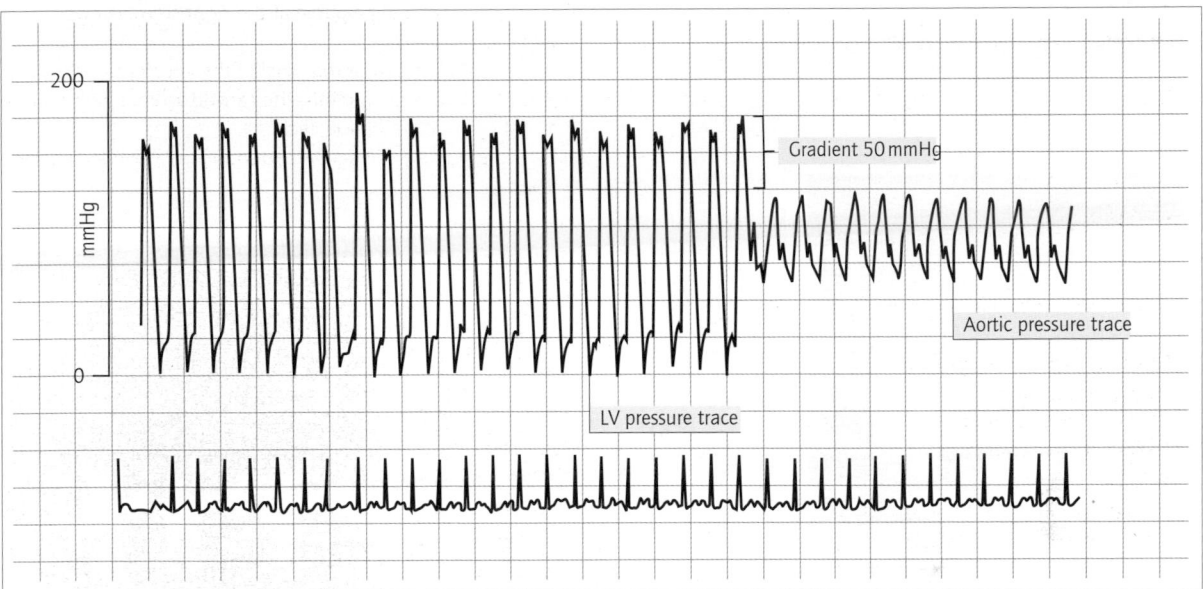

Figure 7.60 The pressure trace on catheter withdrawal across a stenosed aortic valve at cardiac catheterization.

Table 7.39 Causes of aortic regurgitation

Bicuspid aortic valve
Dilatation of the aortic valve ring
Hypertension
Rheumatic fever
Connective tissue disorders such as ankylosing spondylitis
Dissection of the aorta
Aneurysm of the aorta
Syphilitic aortitis

Table 7.40 Management of aortic regurgitation

Specific treatment
Offload the left ventricle
Vasodilators such as ACE inhibitors to reduce peripheral
   vascular resistance
Diuretics and nitrates to reduce the end-diastolic pressure in
   the left ventricle

Surgery (aortic valve replacement)
If symptoms are not satisfactorily controlled by medication
Indicated if there is evidence of ventricular decompensation
   such as an increase in the end-systolic dimension on
   echocardiography

of blood can cause the anterior mitral leaflet to vibrate, giving rise to a mid-diastolic (Austin Flint) murmur.

The apex beat may be displaced laterally and the impulse overactive. There may be an accompanying fourth heart sound indicating atrial hypertension because of raised left ventricular end-diastolic pressure.

Investigation
Electrocardiography
ECG may show counterclockwise rotation of the heart because of expansion of the left ventricle and features of left ventricular hypertrophy resulting from volume overload (increased voltages and T-wave inversion; Fig. 7.56, p. 467).

Diagnostic imaging
● *Chest radiography:* shows an enlarged transverse cardiac diameter and upper lobe blood diversion, indicating pulmonary venous hypertension.

● *Echocardiography:* shows a volume-loaded left ventricle. At first only the end-diastolic dimension is increased because compensatory increased systolic function preserves normal end-systolic dimension (Starling's law; Fig. 7.2, p. 384). If the condition deteriorates and the left ventricle begins to fail, the end-systolic dimension increases.
● *Cardiac catheterization:* aortography demonstrates regurgitation of the dye through the valve into the left ventricle.

Management
The aim of medical treatment is to offload the left ventricle. Peripheral vascular resistance is reduced with vasodilators such as ACE inhibitors. The end-diastolic pressure in the left ventricle is reduced using diuretics and nitrates (Table 7.40).

Aortic regurgitation at a glance

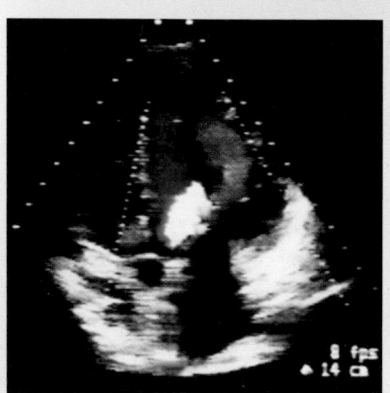

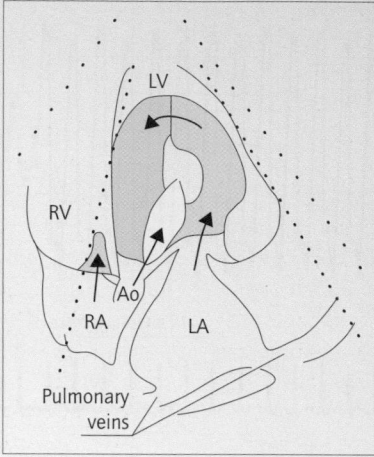

Fig. A Colour flow Doppler in a patient with aortic regurgitation. Apical four-chamber view showing turbulent jet (white) of regurgitant blood impinging on anterior leaflet of mitral valve to mix with the stream (red) passing from left atrium to left ventricle. Note change in colour to blue as the stream is directed by the ventricular apex towards the aortic valve. A small portion of right atrial to right ventricular flow is depicted in red.

Epidemiology and aetiology

Sex

75% of cases are men. Rheumatic aortic regurgitation is most common in women

Causes

Bicuspid aortic valve
Dilatation of the aortic valve ring (e.g. rheumatoid arthritis)
Hypertension
Rheumatic fever (particularly in developing countries)
Connective tissue disorders
Dissection of the aorta
Aneurysm of the aorta
Syphilitic aortitis

Findings on investigation

Diagnostic imaging

■ *Chest radiography:* shows an enlarging heart and an enlarging aortic root
■ *Echocardiography:* shows a volume-loaded left ventricle, often with 'fluttering' of the anterior mitral valve leaflet or intraventricular septum caused by the regurgitant jet
■ *Cardiac catheterization:* aortography demonstrates regurgitation of the dye through the valve into the left ventricle

Electrocardiology

ECG shows features of left ventricular volume load (increased voltages and T-wave inversion)

Clinical features

Cardiovascular

A collapsing pulse in the arm with a wide pulse pressure

Early diastolic murmur, maximal at the left sternal edge and towards the apex on auscultation
May be a third or fourth heart sound
Exertional dyspnoea
Later, the symptoms of left ventricular failure may develop
Apex beat may be displaced laterally and the impulse overactive

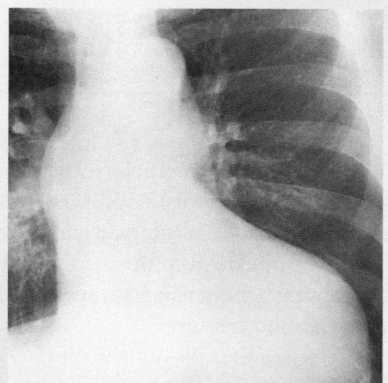

Fig. B Left ventricular enlargement in a patient with aortic incompetence. The cardiac apex is displaced downwards and to the left. Note also that the ascending aorta causes a bulge of the right mediastinal border—a feature that is almost always seen in significant aortic valve disease. Both figures reproduced from Armstrong P, Wastie ML. *Diagnostic Imaging*, 3rd edn, 1992 (Blackwell Scientific Publications, Oxford) with the permission of the authors.

If symptoms are not satisfactorily controlled by medication, aortic valve replacement is required. The timing of aortic valve replacement in patients who do not have symptoms is difficult. If it is delayed for too long the left ventricle can be irreversibly damaged. Aortic valve replacement is therefore indicated if there is evidence of ventricular decompensation such as an increase in the end-systolic dimension on echocardiography.

Prognosis

Moderate and even severe aortic regurgitation is often well tolerated for many years without symptoms. Without surgery, 75% of patients with severe aortic regurgitation survive for 5 years. Furthermore, offloading of the ventricle with vasodilators in aortic regurgitation can improve the prognosis by limiting the deterioration in left ventricular dysfunction.

Rheumatic fever

Epidemiology

Prevalence. Less than 0.1% of the population in the UK are now affected by rheumatic fever, whereas 50 years ago it affected more than 10% of the population.

Age. Rheumatic fever is an illness of childhood, usually occurring in 5–15-year-olds.

Geography. It is still common in developing countries, affecting about 1% of the population. It is unlikely to be brought about by a racial link, but rather because of the poorer living conditions in these countries where, in addition, antibiotics are used much less.

Disease mechanisms

Rheumatic fever results from a Lancefield group A streptococcal infection causing tonsillitis and scarlet fever. This gives rise to an autoimmune reaction with the development of antiheart antibodies and possibly an altered lymphocyte response.

The cardiac manifestations of rheumatic fever result in a pancarditis: a fibrinous pericarditis can develop. Aschoff nodules, which have a necrotic centre, develop in the myocardium. These nodules characteristically affect both ventricular and atrial muscle, with involvement of the latter predisposing to atrial fibrillation.

The endocardial lesions principally affect the valves, which become thickened and can stenose and regurgitate. This process occurs over many years and calcification can eventually develop. The mitral valve is more commonly involved than the aortic valve. The tricuspid valve can be affected, but tricuspid regurgitation in rheumatic heart disease usually results from pulmonary hypertension and consequent right ventricular dilatation. The pulmonary valve is rarely involved.

Clinical features

Rheumatic fever affects many systems, usually about 4 weeks after the history of sore throat.

Heart involvement

Heart involvement can lead to the development of a heart murmur. Both mitral regurgitation and aortic regurgitation can develop acutely and sometimes the leaflets thicken enough to give a diastolic murmur (a Carey Coombs murmur). Pericarditis with ST-segment elevation on the ECG can occur and myocarditis with inverted T waves on the ECG can develop, rendering the left ventricle hypocontractile, although this is only rarely severe. Dilatation of the mitral valve ring can lead to mitral regurgitation. There may be a pericardial effusion and arrhythmias, particularly first degree heart block, can occur. The heart involvement in the acute phase in rheumatic fever can be fulminant, leading to death, but this is rare in the UK.

About 50% of patients who have rheumatic valvular heart disease have no history of acute rheumatic fever.

Neurological involvement

Neurological manifestations include Sydenham's chorea or St Vitus' dance.

Skin involvement

Skin manifestations include erythema marginatum, which is an erythematous rash with a raised edge found mainly on the trunk. It may fade over 24 h, but keeps recurring. Nodules also develop over tendons and bony prominences. They are painless and can reach 1–2 cm in size.

Joint involvement

Joint involvement of the larger joints, such as knees and elbows, can manifest as a temporary polyarthritis that moves from one joint to another. The joints are red, swollen and tender, but there is no long-term damage.

Diagnosis

Diagnosis is based on the Duckett–Jones criteria (Table 7.41). Two or more major criteria, or one major plus two or more minor criteria must be fulfilled to make the diagnosis.

Investigation

Haematology

- *FBC:* a normochromic normocytic anaemia develops
- *ESR and C-reactive protein (CRP):* increased

Table 7.41 Duckett–Jones criteria for diagnosing rheumatic fever

Major
Polyarthritis
Carditis
Chorea
Erythema marginatum
Subcutaneous nodules

Minor
Previous rheumatic fever or scarlet fever
Arthralgia
Fever
Leucocytosis
Increased ESR or CRP
Increased ASO titre
Prolonged PR interval on the ECG

ASO, anti-streptolysin O; CRP, C-reactive protein; ECG, electrocardiogram; ESR, erythrocyte sedimentation rate.

Table 7.42 Management of rheumatic fever

Supportive treatment
Bed rest

Specific treatment
Drug treatment
Intramuscular or oral penicillin (or a sulphonamide if allergic to penicillin) for at least 1 week
Aspirin in high dose
Prednisolone (up to 120 mg/day) for 1 week until the ESR settles and then tail off over the next 2–3 weeks

Prophylaxis
Long-term penicillin until at least 25 years old

Immunology
● *Antistreptolysin O antibody titre:* raised
● *Anti-DNAase antibody and antihyaluronidase antibody:* raised

Microbiology
Throat swab cultures for group A streptococcus may be positive.

Management
The management of rheumatic fever involves bed rest, antibiotics, aspirin and corticosteroids (Table 7.42). Bed rest is required until the fever settles and the cardiac manifestations resolve.

Intramuscular or oral penicillin for at least 1 week treats a streptococcal infection. If the patient is allergic to penicillin, a sulphonamide should be used instead. This treatment should be given irrespective of whether the pharyngeal swabs grow streptococci. Aspirin is given in a dose sufficient to control pain and reduce the fever, but toxicity must be watched for. There is no evidence to suggest that aspirin reduces the long-term complications of rheumatic fever. Prednisolone (up to 120 mg/day) is given for 1 week until the ESR settles and is then tailed off over the next 2–3 weeks. However, the effectiveness of corticosteroids is questionable.

Surgery
Surgery to the valves may be necessary if severe heart failure develops because of valve regurgitation.

Prophylaxis
The need for prophylactic treatment against recurrences is clear. Preferably it should be with monthly injections of benzylpenicillin or a sulphonamide if the patient is allergic to penicillin. This should be increased to every 3 weeks if a recurrence has occurred. Prophylaxis with oral penicillin is less effective, with recurrence rates as high as 30%.

If the patient has no valvular heart damage the prophylaxis should be for a minimum of 10 years, or up to 25 years of age. If valvular damage has occurred, it should probably be continued until 40 years of age. Patients are often reluctant to continue with intramuscular injections and can be provided with oral antibiotics, but these are less effective.

Prognosis
About 5% of patients with rheumatic fever die during the acute episode. The subsequent prognosis is affected by the tendency to repeated attacks of rheumatic fever. Different strains of streptococcus can cause further damage to the valves and myocardial function. Patients are particularly vulnerable in the first few years after the initial attack.

Infective endocarditis

Infective endocarditis is a condition in which the cardiac valves or endocardium become infected. It is usually a chronic illness (subacute endocarditis), but it can pursue a fulminant course (acute endocarditis) when virulent organisms such as *Staphylococcus aureus* rapidly destroy the valves.

Epidemiology
Age. It used to affect the young with rheumatic valvular heart disease, but is now more common in older people with degenerative aortic and mitral valve disease.

Disease mechanisms
The infection is usually bacterial, but other organisms can be responsible (Table 7.43). The term infective

Table 7.43 Organisms causing infective endocarditis

Organism	Percentage of cases and notes
Streptococcus viridans	50%
Staphylococcus aureus	20% of cases, but a more common cause of fulminant acute endocarditis
Staphlylococcus epidermidis	Following valve replacement surgery
Gram-negative organisms (e.g. *Haemophilus influenzae*)	A much less common cause of endocarditis and usually occurs following heart valve surgery or in drug addicts
Coxiella burnetti (Q fever)	Rare
Chlamydiae	Rare
Fungi, especially in immunosuppressed patients	Rare

endocarditis is therefore preferred rather than subacute bacterial endocarditis.

Infective endocarditis usually occurs on abnormal valves, but the acute form can involve valves previously thought to be normal. It can also occur on the low-pressure side of shunts (e.g. VSDs, PDA, arteriovenous fistulae).

Over the last 30 years, intravenous drug abuse has led to a significant incidence of tricuspid valve endocarditis. Prosthetic valves are particularly vulnerable and, once established, the infection can be difficult to eradicate. Clumps of infecting organisms, fibrin and platelets develop on the affected valve. These vegetations can destroy the valve cusps, producing regurgitation and occasionally stenosis, and lead to systemic embolization.

Clinical features

Endocarditis should be suspected in any patient with a fever and a heart murmur. Anaemia, 'flu-like symptoms and weight loss are common and the patient has often been treated for influenza with antibiotics before a diagnosis of infective endocarditis is established.

There is often a heart murmur, but the diagnosis of infective endocarditis should be considered in appropriate circumstances, even if a murmur is absent. If a new murmur develops, or the character of a known heart murmur changes, endocarditis should be suspected.

Manifestations of infective endocarditis outside the heart result from systemic embolization and immune complex deposition:
- *Systemic embolization:* leads to splenic and renal infarcts, myocardial infarction, embolic strokes and loss of peripheral pulses. Mycotic aneurysms arise from weakening of the arterial wall by infected emboli and can cause subarachnoid haemorrhages (in the cerebral circulation).
- *Immune complex deposition:* gives rise to a vasculitis with manifestations in various parts of the body. These include small haemorrhages in the skin or mucosa (particularly the pharynx and conjunctiva), haemorrhages in the retina (Roth's spots) or in the nail beds (splinter haemorrhages), small red macules on the hands (rare and called Janeway's lesions) and Osler's nodes (rare, small painful subcutaneous swellings in the pads of the fingers and toes).

Haematuria is common. It is usually caused by acute glomerulonephritis if microscopic, or renal infarction as a result of emboli if macroscopic. As in any chronic infection, splenomegaly is common. If there is splenic infarction, the spleen will be painful and there may be a friction rub. Clubbing of the digits is rare, but can develop in the later stages of the illness. In right heart endocarditis, septic embolization to the lungs can cause pleuritic pain with haemoptysis. Pneumonia and lung abscesses can also develop.

Investigation
Haematology
- *FBC:* a normochromic normocytic anaemia is common, and there is usually only a modest increase in the white cell count
- *ESR and CRP:* raised

Biochemistry
Urea and creatinine may be raised.

Microbiology
Blood cultures are the key investigation. At least three sets of cultures should be taken over a 12–24-h period, before antibiotics are given. About 80% will prove to be positive, but 20% will be negative. Negative blood cultures are usually found in patients who have been exposed to antibiotics early on in the illness, or in those with a chronic history where high levels of antibodies have developed. Specific culture mediums and serological markers may be required for rarer organisms. Culture-negative endocarditis is associated with a poorer prognosis. Sensitivity should be performed to a range of agents, together with minimum inhibitory concentrations (MICs; see pp. 91–92) of the therapeutic agent to be used (e.g. penicillin for streptococcal infection).

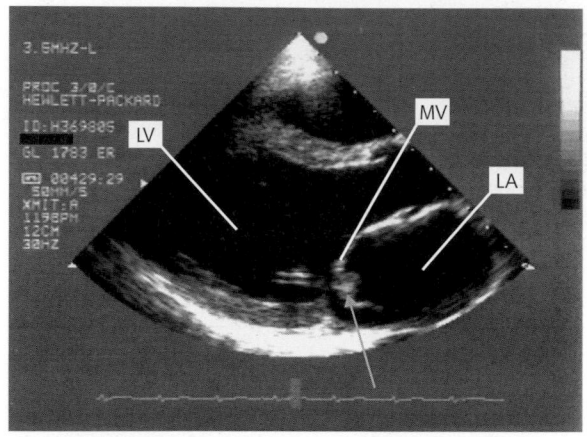

(a)

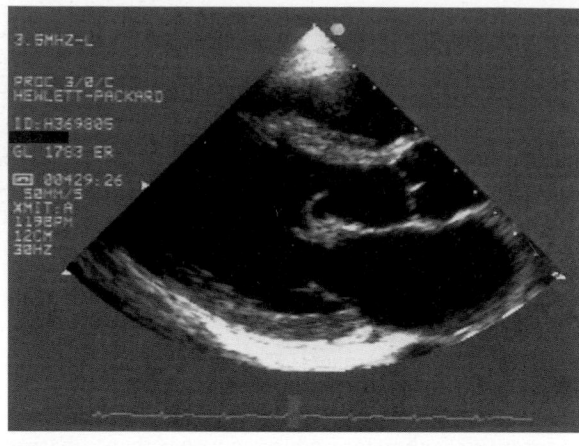

(b)

Figure 7.61 Two-dimensional echocardiograms showing parasternal long axis views of a vegetation (arrowed) attached to the anterior leaflet of the mitral valve in (a) systole and (b) diastole.

Diagnostic imaging
● *Chest radiography:* may show evidence of heart failure. If there is right-sided endocarditis there may be pulmonary emboli or an abscess.
● *Echocardiography:* may identify vegetations (Fig. 7.61). These have to be at least 2 mm to be seen, so the absence of vegetations on echocardiography does not exclude the diagnosis.
● *Transoesophageal echocardiography:* may be more sensitive than transthoracic echocardiography for identifying vegetations.

Electrophysiology
ECG is usually not altered in endocarditis. Involvement of the conducting tissue in aortic valve endocarditis results in a prolonged PR interval and indicates a severe infection, possibly with an aortic root abscess.

Management
Any underlying source of infection should be sought and treated; in particular, dental radiographs should be taken and tooth abscesses treated by immediate extraction (Table 7.44).

Table 7.44 Management of infective endocarditis

Specific treatment
Look for and treat any underlying infection
Take dental radiographs
Treat abscesses

Antibiotics
Give intravenous benzylpenicillin and gentamicin once the blood cultures have been taken and before the results are available, but avoid gentamicin toxicity (measure gentamicin levels frequently)
Change antibiotics according to the results of the blood cultures and sensitivities
Measure antibiotic levels and perform back titration against the bacteria to ensure dose is sufficient
If the blood cultures are negative give ampicillin instead of penicillin
Treat *Staphylococcus* endocarditis with three anti-staphylococcal antibiotics (e.g. flucloxacillin, fusidic acid and gentamicin)

Surgery
For worsening heart failure or uncontrolled infection or evidence of myocardial abscess

---

Infective endocarditis at a glance

Epidemiology
Prevalence
Incidence is about 5–10 cases/100 000 population/year in the UK

Age
Increases with age

Geography
Much more common in developing countries

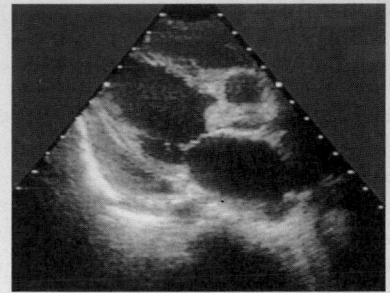

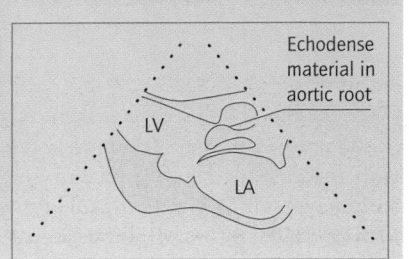

Fig. A Aortic root abscess: parasternal long axis view echocardiogram. Note the echodense material in the aortic root. Reproduced from Armstrong P, Wastie ML. *Diagnostic Imaging*, 3rd edn, 1992 (Blackwell Scientific Publications, Oxford) with the permission of the authors.

Findings on investigation

Haematology
- *Blood culture:* take three sets of blood cultures
- *FBC:* normochromic normocytic anaemia is common. Usually, only a modest increase in the white cell count
- *WBC, ESR and CRP:* raised

Biochemistry
- *Urea and creatinine:* may be increased
- *Liver enzymes:* may be increased, particularly alkaline phosphatase
- *Urinalysis:* usually reveals microscopic haematuria and sometimes proteinuria

Immunology
Antistreptolysin O antibody titre raised

Microbiology
A minimum of three sets of blood cultures should be taken. Specific serological and culture media may be required for the rarer organisms

Diagnostic imaging
- *Chest radiography:* may show heart failure or pulmonary emboli
- *Echocardiography:* may identify vegetations and allows assessment of valve regurgitation and ventricular function. Transoesophageal echocardiography to identify vegetations. Absence of vegetations does not exclude endocarditis

Electrocardiography
ECG is not altered, but involvement of conducting tissue in aortic valve endocarditis prolongs the PR interval

Clinical features

Constitutional
Fever
Malaise
Clubbing

Cardiac
Murmurs
Heart failure

Skin
Splinter haemorrhages
Nailfold infarcts

Vasculitic rash
Osler's nodes
Janeway's lesions

Other
Splenomegaly
Haematuria
Arthralgia
Roth's spots

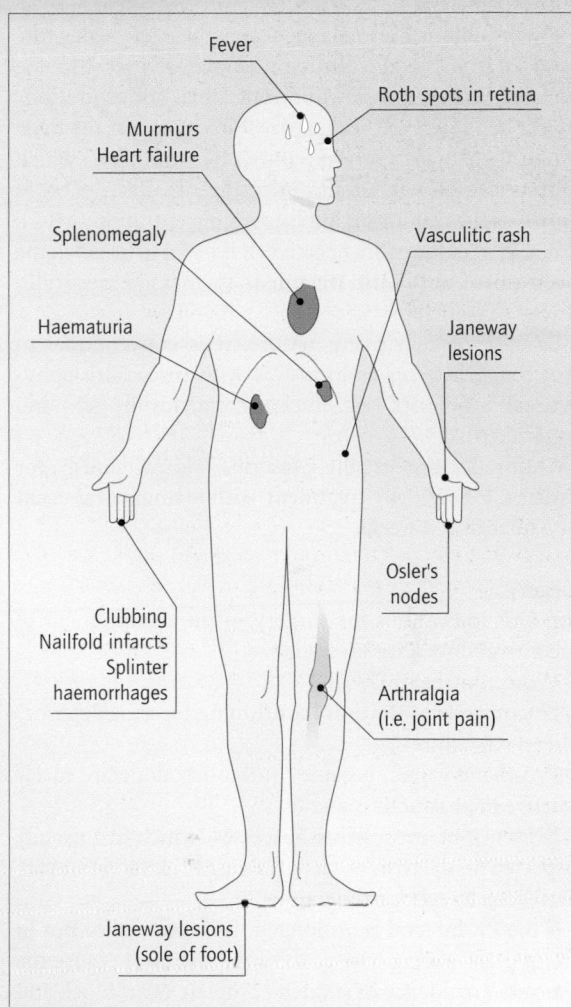

Fig. B Clinical features of infective endocarditis.

Antibiotics

Once the blood cultures have been taken and before the results are available, it is common practice to treat patients with intravenous benzylpenicillin and gentamicin. The aminoglycoside is given to provide synergy, and lower than usual blood concentrations are adequate. Aminoglycoside levels should be measured after the third dose and on alternate days.

The antibiotics are changed appropriately when the result of the blood cultures and sensitivities become available. Where possible, antimicrobial concentrations should be measured. Some microbiologists test the dilution of the patient's serum (containing antibiotic) which inhibits the growth of the infecting organism. This is known as the minimum inhibitory concentration (MIC). If the blood cultures are negative, it is usual to broaden the spectrum of antibiotic treatment to include ampicillin instead of penicillin.

Because of its virulent nature, it is conventional to treat *Staphylococcus* endocarditis with three antistaphylococcal antibiotics (e.g. flucloxacillin, fusidic acid and gentamicin).

Antibiotics are usually prescribed intravenously for 2 weeks, followed by treatment with a single oral agent for a further 2–4 weeks.

Surgery

The four indications for surgery in the management of infective endocarditis are:

- Worsening heart failure
- Uncontrolled infection (continuing fever or deteriorating renal failure)
- Prosthetic valves, because antibiotics alone are rarely effective in prosthetic material
- Evidence of myocardial abscesses, which are usually suspected on the basis of a lengthening PR interval and are rarely seen by echocardiography

If the PR interval is prolonged, it is essential to put in a temporary pacing wire as soon as possible, because the associated incidence of sudden complete heart block and death is high. The presence of large vegetations may indicate an increased risk of embolization, but the risk of embolization is very small once effective antibiotic treatment has been started.

Prognosis

The success of treatment can be measured by early normalization of the temperature, a fall in white blood cell count, and a reduction in ESR and CRP. This will be accompanied by an improvement in the patient's overall condition.

The continued high mortality of 20% associated with infective endocarditis in the UK is a result of the high incidence of prosthetic valve endocarditis, endocarditis in drug addicts and antibiotic-resistant organisms.

Antibiotic prophylaxis

Although there is no real evidence to support their use, antibiotics are now given prophylactically to patients with known valvular heart disease who are about to undergo dental or other potentially septic procedures.

The nature of the antibiotic depends on the nature of the procedure, but for dental treatment it is usual to give 3 g amoxicillin orally 1 h before the treatment is started. For patients with penicillin sensitivity, oral erythromycin is used instead. Intravenous antibiotic, usually vancomycin or clindamycin, is advised for people with prosthetic heart valves.

Myocardial disease

Myocarditis

Epidemiology

Prevalence. Viral myocarditis is probably underdiagnosed because evidence of a viral infection such as influenza has usually disappeared by the time cardiac symptoms develop. Many viral illnesses are associated with ECG changes suggesting cardiac involvement.

Disease mechanisms

Infections can damage the heart by direct infection of the myocyte (e.g. viruses) producing toxins (e.g. diphtheria), or inducing immune damage. Inflammation of the myocardium identified in biopsy has many causes (Table 7.45).

Clinical features

Myocarditis causes rapidly progressive heart failure, occasionally in association with a temperature. There

Table 7.45 Causes of inflammation of the myocardium

Cause	Example
Viruses	Coxsackie
	Influenza
	Mumps
	Epstein–Barr virus
Protozoa	Trypanosomiasis (endemic in Central and South America causing Chagas' disease; see p. 139), *Toxoplasma gondii*
Bacteria	Diphtheria
Rickettsia	*Coxiella* (causes Q fever)
Radiation	
Chemicals	Chloroquine
	Lead poisoning

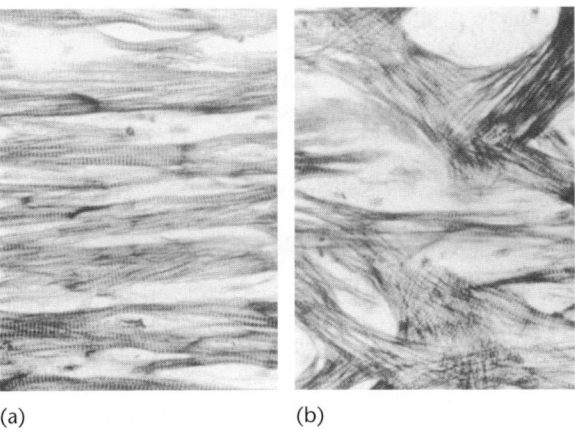
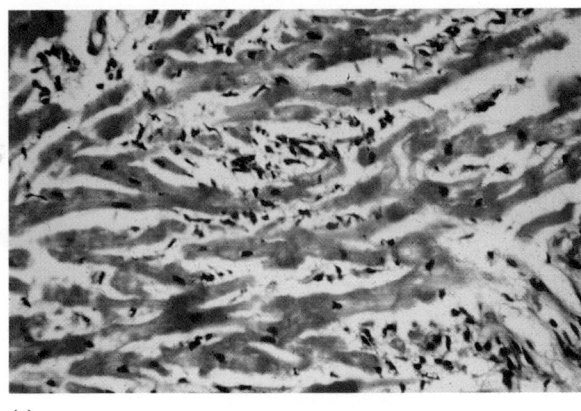

(a)   (b)   (c)

Figure 7.62 (a) Normal myocardium; (b) myocardium of hypertrophic cardiomyopathy; and (c) myocardium with inflammatory cells on biopsy.

may be history of a previous viral infection. The patient complains of fatigue, myalgia, shortness of breath and palpitations. Clinical examination reveals the signs of heart failure (raised venous pressure, bilateral basal crepitations and third and fourth heart sounds).

Investigation
Electrocardiography
ECG usually shows a tachycardia and non-specific ST waves, which are usually transient. Chagas' disease can cause heart block and ventricular arrhythmias. The ECG changes sometimes mimic those of myocardial infarction, with Q waves and loss of R waves in the anterior leads.

Diagnostic imaging
• *Chest radiography:* depending on the severity of the illness, the heart may be enlarged and the lungs may show venous congestion and alveolar oedema
• *Gallium-67 scintigraphy:* may show increased myocardial uptake, suggesting inflammation

Haematology
ESR may be elevated.

Biochemistry
Cardiac enzymes may be raised.

Immunology
Viral antibody titres may be raised and should be taken in the acute and convalescent phase to identify change.

Histology
Myocardial biopsy may show white cell infiltration (Fig. 7.62), and possible myocardial cellular death, but is

Table 7.46 Management of myocarditis

Supportive treatment
Bed rest
Specific treatment
Drug treatment
Heart failure
Diuretics and vasodilators
Arrhythmias
Digoxin for atrial fibrillation
Amiodarone for ventricular tachyarrhythmias
Anticoagulation
Immunosuppression
Corticosteroids and other immunosuppressive drugs, but there is no evidence that these are effective. Aciclovir or interferon may help if given early

often normal. At present there is probably no indication for routine biopsy in patients presenting with suspected myocarditis, although some clinicians use a positive biopsy to justify the use of immunosuppressive drugs.

Management
The treatment of myocarditis includes (Table 7.46):
• Bed rest
• Treatment of heart failure with diuretics and vasodilators
• Treatment of arrhythmias (atrial fibrillation with digoxin, ventricular tachyarrhythmias with amiodarone)
• Anticoagulation to prevent systemic and venous thromboembolism
• Corticosteroids and other immunosuppressive drugs—there is no evidence that these are effective, but they are often used
• Aciclovir or interferon may help if given early in the course of the illness

Table 7.47 Causes of cardiomyopathy

Mechanism	Condition
Dilatation	Idiopathic cardiomyopathy
	Alcohol
	Myocarditis
	Drugs (e.g. anthracyclines and cobolt)
	Iron overload
	Uraemia
	Phaeochromocytoma
	Deficiency states such as beriberi and selenium deficiency (Keshar disease)
	Sarcoid
	Dermatomyositis
	Anomalous coronary arteries
Hypertrophic	Idiopathic hypertrophic cardiomyopathy
	Friedreich's ataxia
	Glycogen storage diseases
	Muscular dystrophy
Restrictive	Radiation
	Amyloid
	Eosinophilic (Churg–Strauss syndrome)
	Pseudoxanthoma elasticum
	Carcinoid
	Methysergide

Prognosis

There may be complete resolution and a return to normal heart muscle function. However, in the long term there is usually evidence of chronic ventricular damage, and myocarditis is a common cause of cardiomyopathy.

Cardiomyopathy

Originally, cardiomyopathy was a term used to describe heart muscle disease of unknown cause, thereby excluding heart muscle diseases resulting from systemic or pulmonary hypertension, ischaemic heart disease, valvular disease and congenital abnormalities. Since then the aetiology of many causes of heart muscle disease originally termed cardiomyopathy has been identified (Table 7.47), and cardiomyopathies are now classified according to distinctive pathological and haemodynamic parameters affecting the ventricles.

● *Dilatated cardiomyopathy:* the most common and characterized by dilatation of the ventricle with systolic malfunction. This results in a reduction of the ejection fraction from a normal 60%. An ejection fraction of less than 40% usually causes symptoms.

● *Restrictive cardiomyopathy:* characterized by reduced ventricular filling and so there is diastolic dysfunction. The myocardium or endocardium may be involved and the ventricle does not dilate. Often there is an infiltration in the myocardium, which may be identified by myocardial biopsy (e.g. sarcoid).

● *Hypertrophic cardiomyopathy:* characterized by hypertrophied myocardium, giving rise to diastolic dysfunction.

Dilated cardiomyopathy

Epidemiology

Prevalence. Dilated cardiomyopathy is found worldwide, and estimates of its incidence vary from 10–50/1 000 000 of the population. This variation stems from the many subclinical cases found at postmortem and the absence of a gold standard diagnostic test.

Age and sex. Most common in middle-aged men.

Geography. Worldwide.

Disease mechanisms

There is characteristic dilatation of the cardiac chambers, although it can be confined to just the left or right ventricle. There is sometimes hypertrophy of the myocardium, suggesting a possible hypertensive aetiology, but the most favoured pathogenetic mechanism is a previous viral infection or cellular immune reaction, possibly precipitated by a viral infection, particularly a Coxsackie infection.

Clinical features

The symptoms and signs are those of progressive left and/or right heart failure. Dilatation of the annulus of both the mitral and tricuspid valves causing valve regurgitation may result from the ventricular dilatation. Atrial fibrillation can develop and lead to systemic thromboembolism.

Investigation

Electrocardiography

ECG shows non-specific ST- and T-wave changes. Arrhythmias are also seen, in particular atrial fibrillation and ventricular tachycardias.

Diagnostic imaging

● *Chest radiography:* shows cardiac enlargement with pulmonary venous congestion and possibly alveolar oedema

● *Echocardiography:* shows dilatation of the ventricles with poor systolic function (Fig. 7.63)

● *Cardiac catheterization:* excludes coronary artery disease and anomalies of the coronary circulation, which can be a rare cause of dilated cardiomyopathy.

● *Cardiac biopsy:* may identify a specific cause such as amyloid or sarcoid

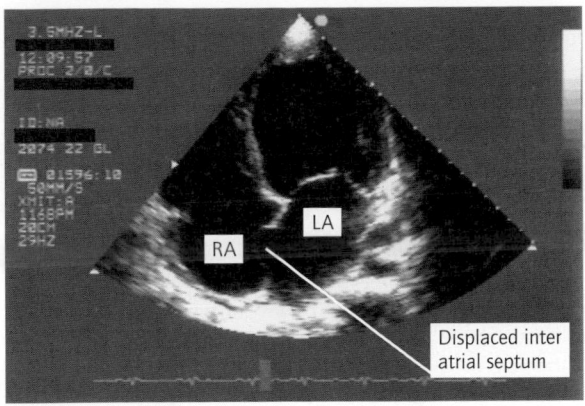

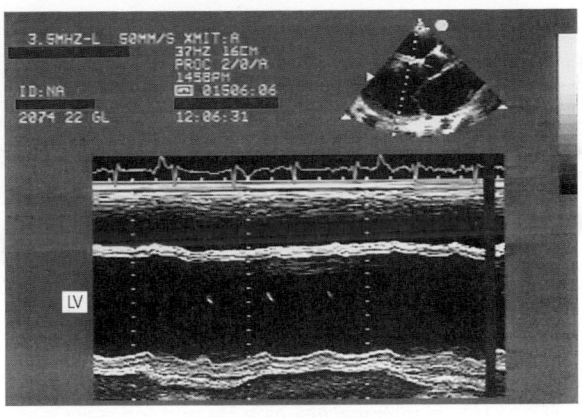

(a)   (b)

Figure 7.63 (a) Apical four-chamber view and (b) M-mode echocardiogram showing dilated left ventricle (LV) with reduced systolic motion of the septum and posterior wall. All chambers are enlarged, LV is globular with thin walls. Atrial septum is displaced showing raised left atrium (LA) pressure.

Management

As for other causes of heart failure, bed rest, diuretics, vasodilators and antiarrhythmic drugs are indicated. Anticoagulants should be given because of the risk of systemic thromboembolism. A heart transplant should be considered for patients under 60 years of age.

Prognosis

The prognosis is poor, with 70% of patients dying within 10 years of diagnosis.

Heart failure of pregnancy

It has long been recognized that heart failure can develop late in pregnancy or during the puerperium (KEYPOINTS BOX 7.1).

Disease mechanisms

Whether the cause is hypertension and haemodynamic problems or nutritional deficiency is not clear, but breastfeeding appears to be associated with its onset. The pathogenesis is not understood but even when there is a complete recovery further pregnancies may cause a relapse.

Management

The treatment is as for a dilated cardiomyopathy.

Endocardial fibroelastosis

Endocardial fibroelastosis (EFE) is a dilated cardiomyopathy that characteristically occurs during infancy and is caused by a diffuse endocardial thickening, which can affect the valves as well.

Disease mechanisms

It may result from intrauterine infections (the primary form) or in association with congenital cardiovascular abnormalities such as coarctation of the aorta (the dilated form).

Management and prognosis

Treatment includes digoxin, diuretics and vasodilators, but it carries a poor prognosis and few children survive to adulthood.

Hypertrophic cardiomyopathy

Epidemiology

Age. Usually presents by 30 years of age.

Genetics. A family history is common and the gene responsible has recently been identified. The gene is autosomally dominant with variable penetrance.

Disease mechanisms

Hypertrophic cardiomyopathy is characterized by spontaneous hypertrophy of the myocardium of either the right and/or left ventricle, and particularly in the septum. The hypertrophy can be global, obliterating the cavity, or focal, causing asymmetric septal hypertrophy (ASH). The myocardial hypertrophy restricts diastolic filling of the left ventricle. In many cases there is abnormal movement of the anterior leaflet of the mitral valve, which

07

Keypoints 7.1: Heart disease in pregnancy

Pregnancy may unmask asymptomatic cardiac disease

Cardiac output increases progressively during pregnancy reaching up to 50% higher than baseline at full term. This will unmask underlying heart disease (e.g. mitral stenosis) and patients who are asymptomatic before pregnancy may become symptomatic with breathlessness and pulmonary oedema

Mortality associated with heart disease in pregnancy

Five to 10% of maternal deaths in England and Wales during pregnancy are brought about by heart disease

Indications for terminating pregnancy

Significant pulmonary hypertension of whatever cause, because the mortality associated with pregnancy in this condition is very high (40–50%)

Advanced heart disease also justifies a consideration of termination of pregnancy because of the risk to the mother

Anticoagulants in pregnancy

Warfarin has a teratogenic effect but this is now considered to be sufficiently small for patients to be encouraged to remain on oral anticoagulation while attempting to become pregnant

Anticoagulation during pregnancy increases the risk of placental bleeding and fetal mortality

During the final trimester the risks of haemorrhage during labour justify transfer off warfarin onto chronic heparin therapy, usually given subcutaneously

Avoid endocarditis in patients with valvular heart disease

Bacteraemia during delivery can cause endocarditis in patients with underlying valvular heart disease. Prophylactic antibiotics are therefore required during the first stage of labour

Postdelivery cardiomyopathy

A rare form of cardiomyopathy can develop after delivery. It appears to be responsive to corticosteroids, sometimes with resolution of the condition

---

abuts against the septum. In many cases an outflow tract gradient can develop late in systole, and this may be an important cause of symptoms. There may be associated mitral regurgitation.

Clinical features

Symptoms include:

- *Syncope or presyncope:* often with exertion
- *Dyspnoea:* brought about by impaired filling of the left ventricle causing dilatation of the left atrium and raised pressure in the pulmonary veins
- *Angina:* resulting from inadequate perfusion of the hypertrophied myocardium because of obstruction of blood flow from the ventricle and increased diastolic pressure inside the ventricle (reduced transcoronary gradient)
- *Cardiac arrhythmias*
- *Sudden death:* commonly caused by ventricular arrhythmias, but it can be by asystole

Signs include:

- *Sharp carotid pulse:* caused by the sudden abbreviation of systole from outflow tract obstruction
- *An a wave:* in the venous pressure pulse
- *Forceful apex beat:* not displaced and which can be 'double' because of an independent palpable fourth heart sound of atrial contraction as well as ventricular contraction
- *Fourth heart sound*
- *Systolic murmur:* caused either by mitral regurgitation or outflow tract obstruction (this can be altered by the

Valsalva manoeuvre, which reduces venous return and ventricular filling and therefore increases outflow tract obstruction and the loudness of the murmur)

Investigation
Electrocardiography

- *ECG:* usually shows left ventricular hypertrophy and other repolarization abnormalities, but may be normal in children
- *Holter 24-h monitoring:* may reveal any type of atrial or ventricular arrhythmia

Diagnostic imaging

- *Chest radiography:* shows prominence of the left ventricular border, but can be normal.
- *Echocardiography:* usually diagnostic. The cardinal feature is a septal : posterior wall thickness ratio greater than 1.3 : 1 (Fig. 7.64a). Great care must be taken to exclude the normal hypertrophy that can develop in athletes. Other characteristic echo features are a systolic anterior movement of the mitral valve, premature closure of the aortic valve because of outflow tract obstruction, and diastolic dysfunction with a characteristic dip and plateau movement to the ventricular wall in diastole.
- *Cardiac catheterization:* angiography may show a characteristic banana-shaped left ventricle. In addition, there can be obliteration of the left ventricular cavity during systole with a tail of dye extending to the apex (Fig. 7.64b). The diagnostic haemodynamic features are the increase

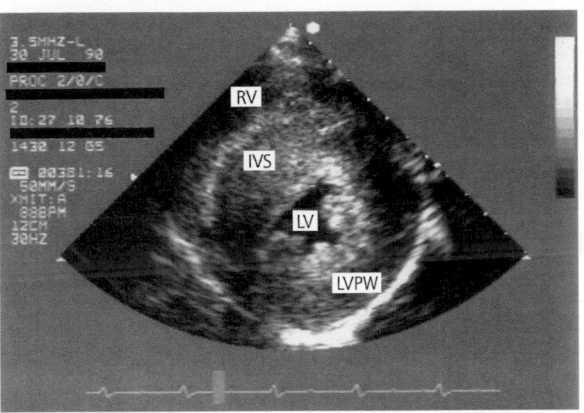

(a)

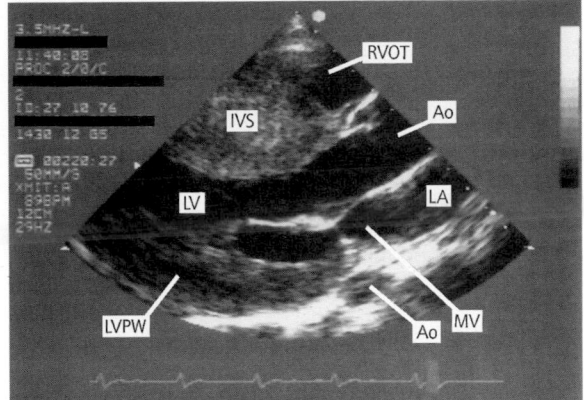

(b)

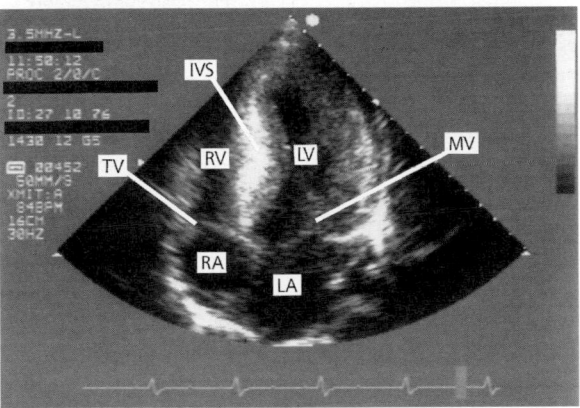

(c)

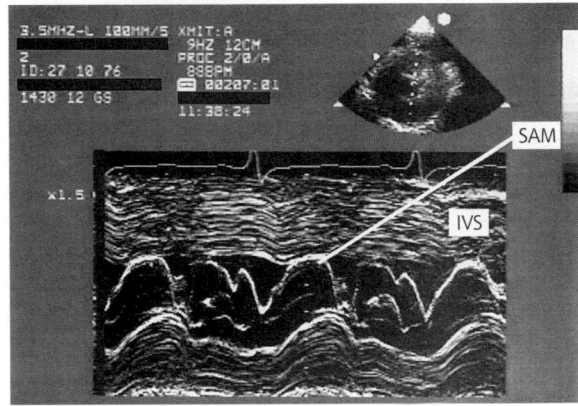

(d)

Figure 7.64 Echocardiograms of hypertrophic cardiomyopathy. (a) Parasternal short axis view at LV papillary muscle level. There is massive hypertrophy and reduction of the LV cavity. LVPW, posterior wall of LV. (b) Parasternal long axis view showing massive septal hypertrophy extending to RV outflow tract (RVOT). (c) Apical four-chamber view showing 'banana-shaped' interventricular septum and intense echoes from septum. IVS, interventricular septum; TV, tricuspid valve. (d) Asymmetrical septal hypertrophy, with systolic anterior motion (SAM) of mitral valve.

in outflow tract gradient seen after an ectopic beat, and the fall in aortic pressure; a similar increase in gradient occurs in aortic stenosis but there is also an increase in the aortic pressure.

Histology

Biopsy. Histology shows disarray of the myocardial fibres, giving a whorled appearance (Fig. 7.62b). This was originally thought to be specific to hypertrophic cardiomyopathy, but can be seen in secondary hypertrophy and congenital heart disease as well.

Management and prognosis

Treatment can be difficult and is often ineffective. There is no clear evidence that any particular drug reduces the incidence of sudden death (Table 7.48):

- Antiarrhythmic drugs can improve prognosis; in particular, long-term amiodarone
- Beta-blockers are indicated, particularly if there is angina

Arterial vasodilators should be avoided because they can increase the outflow tract obstruction by reducing arterial pressure. This will also reduce the transcoronary gradient further and exacerbate angina.

If severe outflow tract obstruction is demonstrated, removing a section of the myocardium can be helpful (Morrow resection). The outflow tract gradient can also be reduced by mitral valve replacement. Recently, the use of dual chamber pacing to alter the pattern of left ventricular depolarization has been found to be helpful in improving symptoms. An implantable cardiac defibrillator improves prognosis in selected cases.

Table 7.48 Management of hypertrophic cardiomyopathy

Specific treatment
Drug treatment
(There is no clear evidence that any particular drug reduces the incidence of sudden death)
Antiarrhythmic drugs may improve prognosis, in particular long-term amiodarone
Beta-blockers are indicated, particularly if there is angina
Avoid arterial vasodilators

Surgery
If severe outflow tract obstruction is demonstrated
  A section of the septal myocardium is helpful (Morrow resection)
  Mitral valve replacement to reduce the outflow tract gradient
End-stage hypertrophic cardiomyopathy
  Consider cardiac transplantation

Dual chamber pacing
Has been found to be helpful

A heart transplant can be considered for end-stage hypertrophic cardiomyopathy, which can progress to a dilated form.

Restrictive cardiomyopathy

Epidemiology
Prevalence. This is the rarest of the three types of cardiomyopathy. It is more common in countries such as equatorial Africa where it is acquired secondary to endomyocardial disease.

Disease mechanisms
Restrictive cardiomyopathies arise from loss of ventricular distensibility as a result of either myocardial or endocardial disease. The most common cause is endomyocardial fibrosis (EMF), which often occurs in association with eosinophilia (the hypereosinophilic syndrome). Other causes of restricted filling are amyloid disease and sarcoid. EMF usually affects both ventricular cavities, causing mitral and tricuspid regurgitation. Sometimes it can lead to the development of giant atria without the presence of mitral or tricuspid regurgitation.

Hypereosinophilic syndrome
An eosinophil count higher than 1.5×10^6/l can cause heart disease. Such eosinophilia can be idiopathic (this is much more common in men) or secondary to parasitic infections (especially in the tropics), malignancy, Churg–Strauss type of polyarteritis nodosa, asthma and drug reactions. Thromboembolism is common.

Amyloid heart disease
Amyloid is a fibrillar protein and can infiltrate the myocardium. It is produced either as a primary condition or secondary to other conditions such as multiple myeloma.

Deposits of amyloid can cause conduction disturbances and mitral or tricuspid regurgitation. Although it restricts ventricular filling, characteristically filling occurs throughout diastole (there is no dip and plateau movement to the ventricular myocardium in diastole) and the end-diastolic pressures can be very high, especially on the left side.

Clinical features
Shortness of breath is a predominant symptom associated with fatigue because of poor cardiac output. The elevated venous pressure on the right side gives rise to peripheral oedema, ascites and an enlarged liver, which can be painful. Signs include tachycardia, raised venous pressure with Kussmaul's sign (an increase in venous pressure on inspiration) and third and fourth heart sounds.

Investigation
Electrocardiography
ECG shows non-specific ST-segment and T-wave abnormalities.

Diagnostic imaging
● *Chest radiography:* usually there is no cardiac enlargement
● *Echocardiography:* shows restricted ventricular filling with the characteristic dip and plateau appearance of diastolic dysfunction except in amyloid disease

Histology
Myocardial biopsy is often indicated to establish a more precise diagnosis.

Management and prognosis
The treatment is as for cardiac failure. Systemic thromboembolism is common and anticoagulants are therefore required. A heart transplant may be considered.

Hypereosinophilic syndrome
Specific treatment of the hypereosinophilic syndrome includes cytotoxic drugs such as hydroxyurea and vincristine, together with anticoagulants.

Pericardial disease

The pericardium consists of two layers: a parietal layer and a visceral layer. The parietal layer is fibrous, protecting the heart with a potential space between it and the visceral layers.

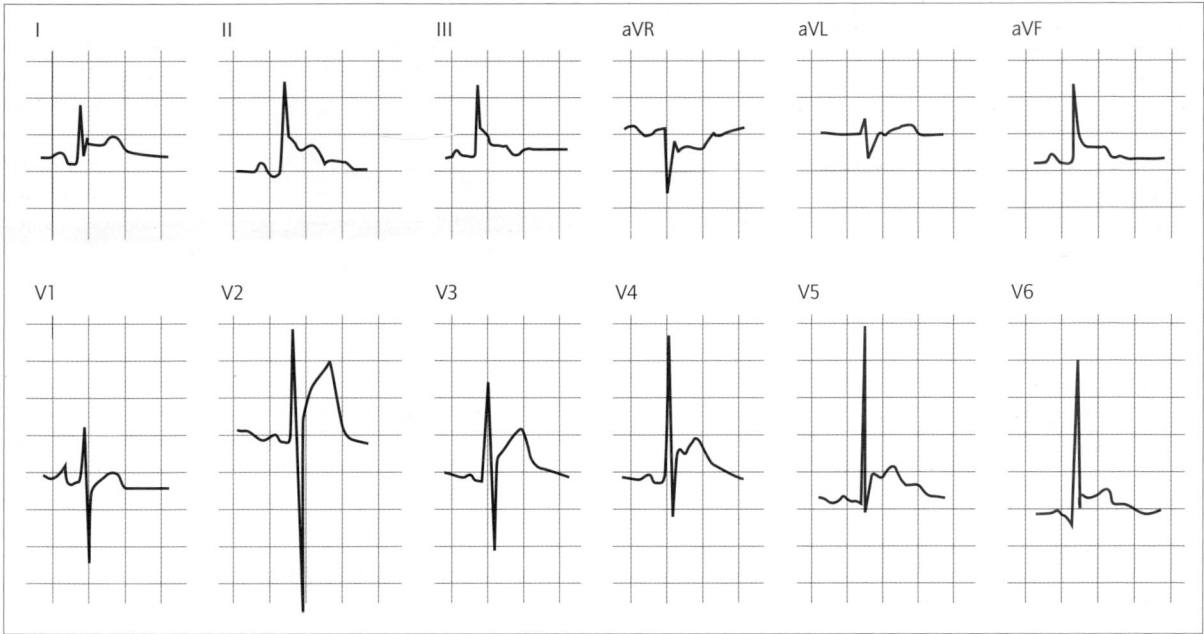

Figure 7.65 ECG of acute pericarditis. Note the widespread ST elevation affecting both inferior and anterior leads (often the ST segments are concave upwards which can distinguish them from the ST elevation of myocardial infarction).

Acute pericarditis

Epidemiology
Prevalence. Evidence of previous pericarditis is found in up to 6% of routine autopsies, suggesting that acute pericarditis occurs more commonly than its clinical presentation would suggest. Approximately 1/1000 hospital admissions are for acute pericarditis.

Disease mechanisms
Inflammation of the pericardium can arise from a number of causes. The most common is Coxsackie viral infection, which can occur in epidemics. Other causes include myocardial infarction, uraemia, connective tissue disorders (autoimmune rheumatic diseases), postpericardiotomy, postmyocardial infarction, trauma, tuberculosis and neoplasia.

Clinical features
The patient presents with severe substernal chest pain, which can radiate to the neck and shoulders and mimic the pain of myocardial infarction. It is characteristically worse on lying flat and on inspiration, and can be relieved by sitting forward. There may be a history of a recent viral infection, and the patient may have a fever, particularly when the pericarditis is caused by infection, rheumatic fever or myocardial infarction. The principal physical sign is a pericardial friction rub, which can be transitory.

Investigation
● *ECG:* shows characteristic concave upwards ST-segment elevation, usually in all leads, rather than localized as in myocardial infarction (Fig. 7.65). Later, the ST segments return to normal and P-wave inversion develops, but this eventually normalizes.
● *Cardiac enzymes:* may increase if there is associated myocarditis.

Management and prognosis
Bed rest is necessary, otherwise the illness can relapse. The cardinal treatment is anti-inflammatory medication with aspirin or indometacin. If pericarditis is severe or becomes recurrent, systemic corticosteroids may be required. Occasionally, colchicine is used in this situation.

Pericardial effusion

Epidemiology
Prevalence. Increased pericardial fluid above the normal 15–50 ml can occur with many conditions. Whether clinical symptoms develop depends on:

1 Volume of fluid
2 Rate of accumulation
3 Response of the pericardium to the fluid

Disease mechanisms

Fluid can accumulate in the pericardium following:

- Viral pericarditis
- Tuberculosis
- Uraemia
- Mxyoedema
- Neoplasia
- Myocardial infarction (Dressler's syndrome, myocardial rupture)
- Aortic dissection
- Radiotherapy
- Postpericardiotomy (heart surgery)
- Perforation of the heart during cardiac catheterization

Clinical features

When the pericardium cannot distend any further, ventricular filling is embarrassed, leading to a fall in cardiac output (**cardiac tamponade**). The main symptom is breathlessness, but the patient may present acutely unwell, collapsed and hypotensive. Signs include a paradoxical pulse (the blood pressure falls by more than 15 mmHg during inspiration) and a raised venous pressure with a further increase on inspiration (Kussmaul's sign; normally, inspiration reduces venous pressure but increases it if there is restricted ventricular filling). The heart sounds are soft and a friction rub is only rarely heard because the fluid separates the visceral and parietal pericardium.

Investigation

Electrocardiography

ECG shows reduced voltages with electrical alternans (varying amplitude of the QRS complex).

Diagnostic imaging

- *Chest radiography:* shows cardiomegaly with a globular cardiac outline.
- *Echocardiography:* identifies the pericardial effusion (Fig. 7.66). There may be collapse of the right ventricle in diastole if there is tamponade.

Management and prognosis

Pericardial drainage is required for tamponade. This can be carried out by direct puncture (pericardiocentesis), which can help in the diagnosis of a potentially infected pericardial effusion. Surgical drainage may be indicated for malignant pericardial effusions or when an effusion reaccumulates.

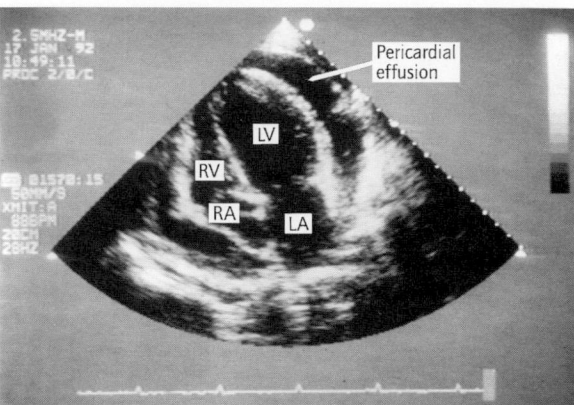

Figure 7.66 Four-chamber view of pericardial effusion.

Constrictive pericarditis

Epidemiology

Prevalence. In 50% of cases the cause of constrictive pericarditis is unknown and is presumed to be a consequence of viral pericarditis. The causes of constrictive pericarditis are:

- Presumed postviral
- Postcardiac surgery
- Postmediastinal radiotherapy
- Chronic renal failure
- Connective tissue disorders
- Pulmonary asbestosis
- Tuberculosis

With the advent of heart surgery, constriction resulting from surgery is now recognized. Only 15% of cases in developed countries are caused by tuberculosis—although this is much more common in developing countries.

Disease mechanisms

A thickened, fibrotic and calcified pericardium progressively embarrasses cardiac function, resulting in systemic venous congestion and reduced cardiac output. In developing countries, tuberculous pericarditis can present as early constriction especially after an effusion has been drained.

Clinical features

The patient presents with breathlessness, fatigue, dependent oedema, ascites and hepatomegaly. The physical signs are similar to those of tamponade (pulsus paradoxus and Kussmaul's sign). In addition, there may be a loud diastolic noise caused by rapid abbreviated ventricular filling (**pericardial knock**). Atrial fibrillation is common.

Table 7.49 Causes of pulmonary hypertension

Left-sided heart disease (causes pulmonary venous
 hypertension and secondary pulmonary arterial
 hypertension)
Pulmonary thromboembolism
Chronic lung disease
Congenital cardiac lesions causing left-to-right shunting of
 blood (increased pulmonary blood flow)
Primary pulmonary hypertension
Peripheral pulmonary artery stenoses (proximal to the
 stenoses pulmonary artery pressure is high, but distally
 pulmonary artery pressure will be normal)

Investigation
Electrocardiography
ECG shows low QRS voltages and T-wave abnormalities.

Diagnostic imaging
- *Chest radiography:* may show a normal-sized heart, and there may be calcification in the pericardium
- *Echocardiography:* may demonstrate thickened pericardium and restricted ventricular filling in diastole

Management and prognosis
Surgical removal of the pericardium is possible. However, it is often difficult to separate the pericardium from the myocardium, and the perioperative mortality can therefore be as high as 10%. When the myocardium is involved in this way, symptomatic improvement is often disappointing.

Pulmonary hypertension

Disease mechanisms
The normal pulmonary artery pressure is 25/15 mmHg (with a mean of 18 mmHg). The development of a raised pulmonary artery pressure (pulmonary hypertension: more than 30 mmHg systolic, with a mean of over 20 mmHg) has many causes (Table 7.49). Only rarely does the pulmonary artery pressure rise spontaneously without an apparent underlying cause (primary pulmonary hypertension) and this diagnosis is made only by exclusion.

The pulmonary artery pressure (P) is dependent on the cardiac output (Q) and the resistance (R) and, as with Ohm's law in electricity, $P = QR$. The resistance in the pulmonary arterioles arises as a consequence of:
- Alveolar hypoxia
- Pulmonary venous hypertension, as in diseases of the left side of the heart (e.g. mitral stenosis)
- Tissue destruction by chronic lung disease, but clinical cor pulmonale is only evident when 80% of the pulmonary circulation has been destroyed
- Vascular distension resulting from high blood flow, as in congenital left-to-right heart shunts

Initially, the pulmonary arteriolar muscle constricts leading to hypertrophy and subsequent irreversible changes including atheroma then develop.

Primary pulmonary hypertension

Primary pulmonary hypertension is a diagnosis arrived at by excluding other causes of pulmonary hypertension. It is much more common in women and usually presents at a relatively young age (in the thirties and forties). As knowledge increases, further causes for primary pulmonary hypertension become apparent (e.g. the so-called outbreak of primary pulmonary hypertension in the early 1980s that was attributable to the ingestion of rapeseed oil).

The natural history of primary pulmonary hypertension is variable, but the condition is usually progressive.

Clinical features
Exertional dyspnoea is the dominant symptom, but chest pain, syncope and sudden death can occur. The physical signs are those of right ventricular failure: there is sinus tachycardia, raised venous pressure, right ventricular heave, a loud pulmonary component to the second heart sound, a right atrial fourth heart sound and a right ventricular third heart sound. Rarely, there is a diastolic murmur of pulmonary regurgitation (Graham Steell murmur).

In advanced disease there is annular dilatation of the tricuspid valve with tricuspid regurgitation causing a pansystolic murmur and a systolic *v* wave in the venous pressure pulse.

Investigation
Electrocardiography
ECG shows the features of right ventricular hypertrophy (tall P waves of P pulmonale, tall R waves in lead V1, inverted T waves in the right precordial leads and right axis deviation; Fig. 7.67).

Diagnostic imaging
- *Chest radiography:* may show cardiac enlargement with prominence of the right heart border. The pulmonary arteries are enlarged and characteristically taper with peripheral pruning from reduced blood flow through the peripheral lung fields.
- *Echocardiography:* may identify the cause of the pulmonary hypertension, such as left or right trunks, or left-sided heart disease.

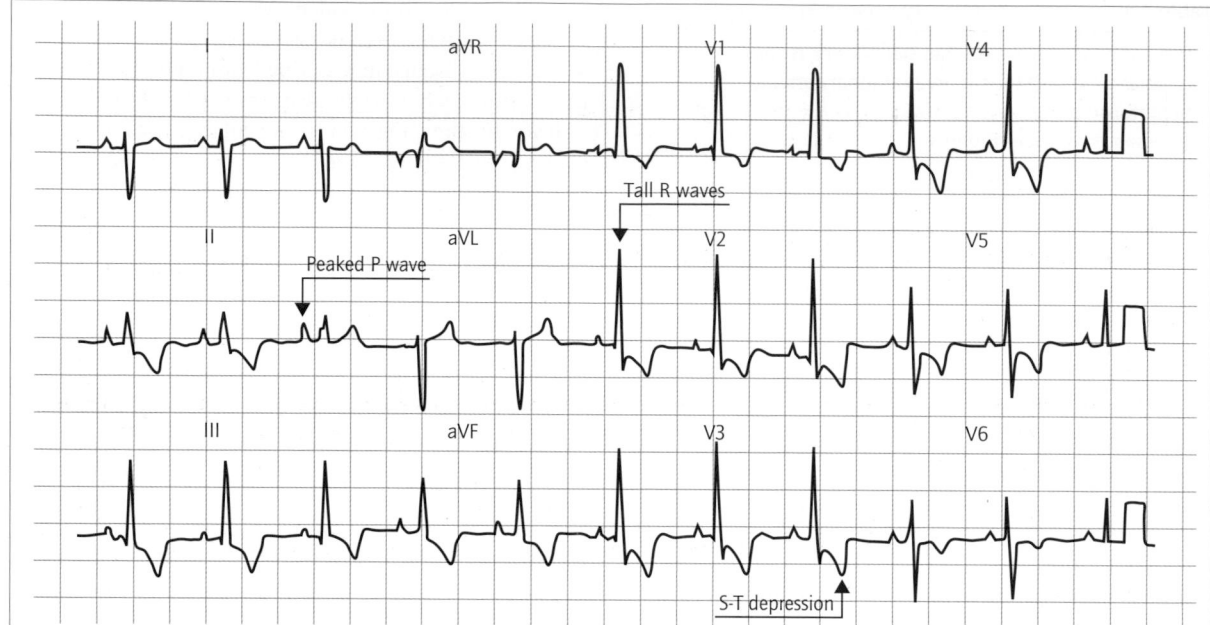

Figure 7.67 ECG of right ventricular hypertrophy secondary to pulmonary hypertension. Note: (i) right axis deviation; (ii) peaked P waves of P pulmonale; (iii) tall R wave in V1 and V2; and (iv) widespread ST depression with T-wave inversion.

● *Cardiac catheterization:* allows measurement of intracardiac and intrapulmonary pressures and oxygen saturations, and from these data the cardiac output and pulmonary vascular resistance can be measured. Pulmonary angiography carries a risk of causing severe right heart failure or VF when carried out in patients with severe pulmonary hypertension, but may identify pulmonary thromboembolic disease or pulmonary artery stenoses.

Management and prognosis

Treatment should be directed at the underlying cause of the pulmonary hypertension. Anticoagulants are indicated in pulmonary thromboembolic disease and primary pulmonary hypertension (Table 7.50).

Table 7.50 Management of pulmonary hypertension

Specific treatment

Treat underlying cause
Anticoagulants for pulmonary thromboembolic disease and
  primary pulmonary hypertension

Drug treatment
Diuretics can relieve the peripheral oedema, but can
  significantly reduce cardiac output

Surgery
Heart–lung transplantation

Diuretic therapy can relieve the peripheral oedema, but can also significantly reduce cardiac output by reducing filling of the left atrium and therefore left ventricular filling. Vasodilators can reduce pulmonary artery pressure, but usually reduce systemic blood pressure as well and no long-term benefit has been demonstrated. Heart–lung transplantation can be considered for younger patients. Anticoagulants are thought to be appropriate in case embolism is a factor, but otherwise no specific treatment is helpful other than heart–lung transplantation.

Pulmonary embolism

Epidemiology

Incidence. Approximately 1/1000, although many cases are undiagnosed.

Age. More common with increasing age.

Disease mechanisms

Thrombosis in the systemic veins can dislodge and embolize to the pulmonary arteries. Conditions predisposing to such clot formation are listed in Table 7.51. Embolism causes the lung to collapse and infarct, leading to hypoxaemia as a result of the mismatch between ventilation and perfusion of the affected lung.

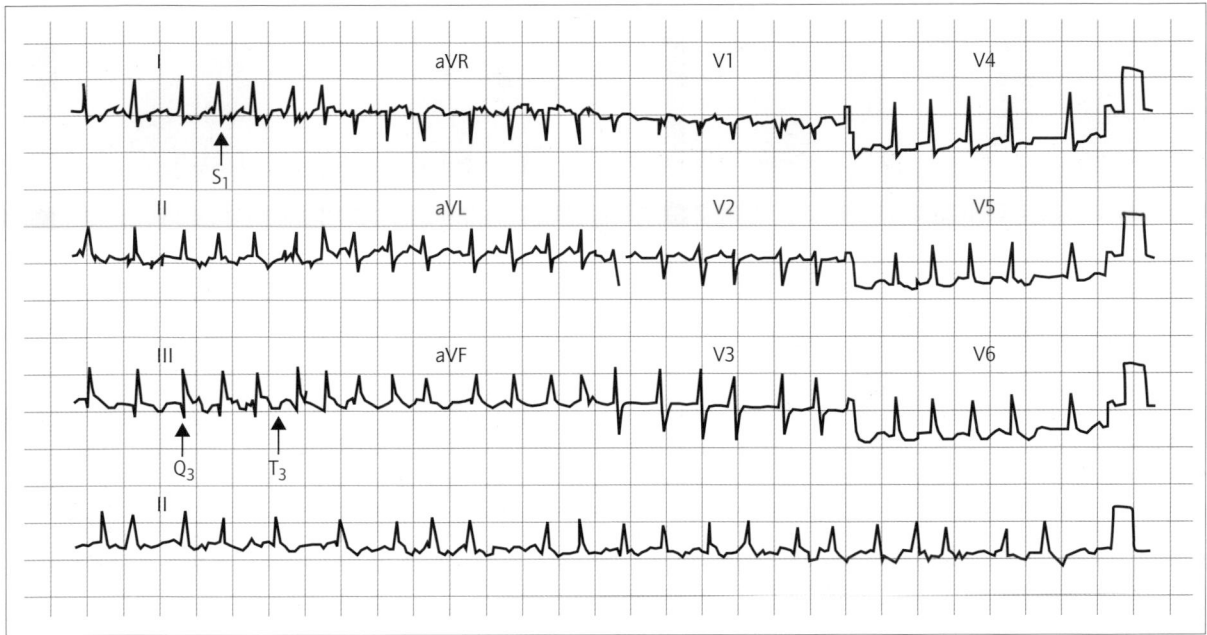

Figure 7.68 The ECG of acute pulmonary embolism. Note: (i) tachycardia and atrial fibrillation; (ii) S1 Q3 T3; although considered to be classical, these changes are not often seen in pulmonary embolism.

Table 7.51 Conditions predisposing to thrombosis in the systemic veins

Prolonged bed rest
Cardiac failure
Pelvic or orthopaedic surgery
Pregnancy and childbirth
Oral contraceptive pill
Malignancy
Hypercoagulable states
Prolonged air flights ('economy class syndrome')

Clinical features

Pulmonary embolism can either be acute or chronic. Chronic pulmonary emboli can present as gradual and insidious breathlessness, but acute pulmonary embolism presents with a sudden onset of symptoms, the nature of which depend on the size of the embolus:
- *Small pulmonary thromboembolus:* can lead to progressive shortness of breath and fatigue
- *Moderate-sized embolus:* presents with a sudden onset of pleuritic chest pain, cough with haemoptysis and shortness of breath
- *Large pulmonary embolus:* presents with sudden shortness of breath, chest pain and a compromised circulation
The physical signs depend on the size of the embolism. A small embolus may cause a tachycardia but no other signs.

A larger embolus causes a tachycardia and elevated venous pressure, a fall in blood pressure, a right ventricular third sound and a right ventricular heave. There may be a pleural rub. If severe, the patient can be cold and clammy, and unconsciousness and death can rapidly follow. There may be signs of a deep vein thrombosis.

Investigation
Haematology
Plasma D-dimer is usually raised above 0.3 mg/l. Arterial gases usually show arterial desaturation with a low P_{O_2} and P_{CO_2}.

Electrocardiography
ECG shows a sinus tachycardia, and the features of right ventricular hypertrophy may have developed, including partial right bundle branch block. In 50% of patients there is an S wave in lead I and a Q wave and inverted T wave in lead III (the classical 'S1 Q3 T3' change of pulmonary embolism; Fig. 7.68).

Diagnostic imaging
- *Chest radiography:* often normal. However, it can show underperfusion of the lung segment distal to the occluded artery, and there may be a pleural effusion and raised hemidiaphragm. A peripheral wedge-shaped opacity may indicate pulmonary infarction. Large pulmonary arteries

07

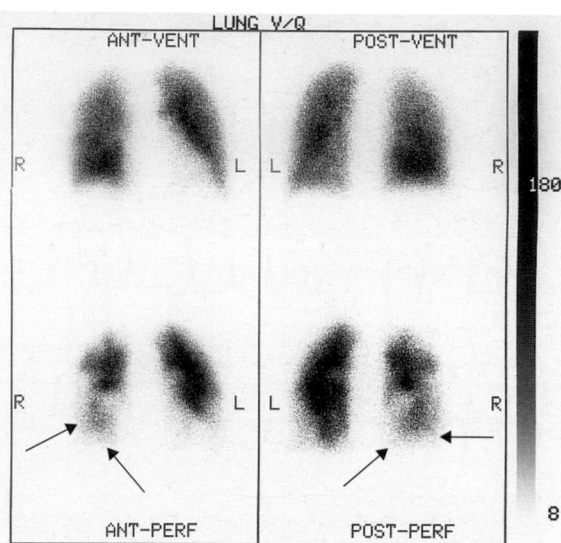

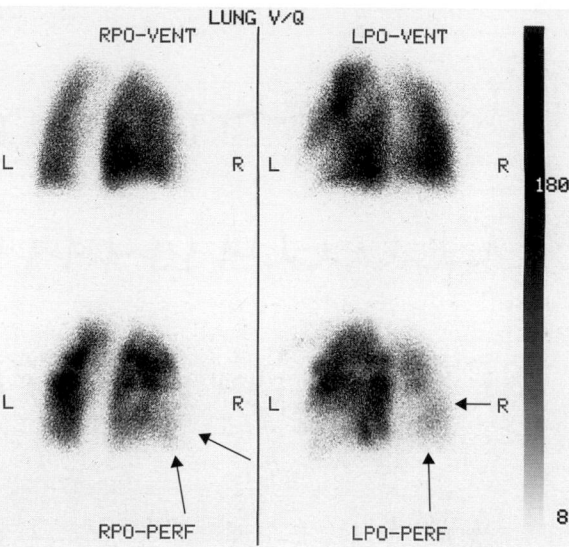

Figure 7.69 Ventilation–perfusion scan of pulmonary embolism. A mismatch of a non-perfused, but ventilated segment is highly diagnostic. Arrows indicate underperfused areas with ventilation mismatch. ANT-PERF, anterior perfusion view; POST-PERF, posterior perfusion view; RPO, right posterior oblique view; LPO, left posterior oblique view.

may develop in chronic pulmonary thromboembolic disease, because of pulmonary hypertension.

● *Lung scan:* a technetium-labelled lung scan demonstrates hypoperfused areas when combined with a ventilation scan (by inhalation of radioactive xenon); mismatch of a non-perfused, but ventilated segment is highly diagnostic of pulmonary embolism (Fig. 7.69).

● *Pulmonary angiography:* can precipitate acute right heart failure and circulatory collapse in acute severe pulmonary embolism, but demonstrates filling defects in the obstructed arteries (Fig. 7.70).

Management

The immediate management is to administer heparin to reduce the likelihood of further thromboembolism from the systemic veins. Therefore, subcutaneous low molecular weight heparin is started immediately on suspicion of the diagnosis. When the diagnosis is confirmed, 10 000 units of heparin are given as an immediate bolus, followed by a continuous infusion of 40 000 units in 24 h. The activated partial thromboplastin time should be kept at 160–200 s. Heparin may have some role in assisting lysis of the thrombus in the lungs (Table 7.52).

Oral anticoagulants are also started immediately and the heparin is tapered off as the oral anticoagulation results in an international normalized ratio (INR) of 2–3. Oral anticoagulants should be maintained for at least 3 months, but possibly longer if there is a risk of further venous thrombosis.

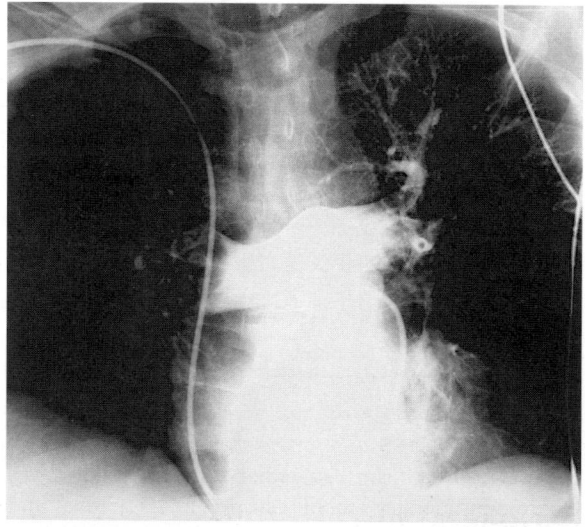

Figure 7.70 Pulmonary angiography can precipitate acute right heart failure and circulatory collapse in acute severe pulmonary embolism, but will demonstrate filling defects in the obstructed arteries. Note the 'meniscus' of dye in the right main coronary artery indicating thrombus obstructing blood flow. Additional thrombus present in left pulmonary artery.

Fibrinolytic therapy. The thrombus may be dissolved by infusing streptokinase into a vein or the pulmonary artery. It is often indicated when the circulation is clearly compromised but the patient is not *in extremis*. One million

Table 7.52 Management of pulmonary embolism

Supportive treatment
Pain relief
Oxygen therapy

Drug treatment
Anticoagulation (all cases)
10 000 units heparin as an immediate bolus, followed by a
    continuous infusion of 40 000 units in 24 h
The APTT should be kept at 160–200 s
Taper off as the oral anticoagulation results in an INR of 2–3
Start oral anticoagulants immediately and maintain for at
    least 3 months (possibly longer if there is a risk of further
    venous thrombosis)

Fibrinolytic therapy
Infusion of streptokinase into a vein or the pulmonary artery
1 million units are given over 1 h followed by an infusion of
    100 000 units/h for 5 h

Surgery
If there is severe haemodynamic collapse
Surgical embolectomy

If further pulmonary emboli occur despite anticoagulation
Filter in the inferior vena cava

APTT, activated partial thromboplastin time; INR, international
normalized ratio.

Table 7.53 Pathologies affecting the arterial system

Arteriosclerosis

Inflammatory disease
Thromboangiitis obliterans (Buerger's disease)
Takayasu's syndrome
Kawasaki's disease
Syphilis
Autoimmune rheumatic diseases

Vasomotor disease
Raynaud's disease

Atherosclerosis
Peripheral vascular ischaemia
Abdominal and thoracic aortic aneurysms

Connective tissue disease
Aortic dissection (Morton's syndrome)

units are given over 1 h followed by an infusion of 100 000
units/h for 5 h.

Surgical embolectomy. Surgical embolectomy is warranted when there is severe haemodynamic collapse. Embolectomy also reduces the risks from a further thromboembolism should it occur despite anticoagulation.

Inferior vena cava filters. It is occasionally necessary to introduce a venous filter into the inferior vena cava if further pulmonary emboli occur despite anticoagulation.

Peripheral vascular disease

The arterial system can be affected by different pathologies (Table 7.53).

Arteriosclerosis

Disease mechanisms

Otherwise recognized as 'hardening of the arteries', arteriosclerosis is an inevitable phenomenom of ageing. The media thickens as a result of smooth muscle hypertrophy, and there is additional intimal thickening in the smaller vessels. Superimposed atherosclerosis can occur in people with risk factors. In malignant hypertension there is fibrinoid necrosis in the arterioles. In diabetes mellitus there may be medial calcification (Mönckeberg's medial sclerosis).

Inflammatory disease

Thromboangiitis obliterans

Thromboangiitis obliterans (Buerger's disease) is an inflammatory disorder affecting both the arteries and veins of young men who smoke. Patients present with peripheral vascular disease.

Takayasu's syndrome

Takayasu's syndrome is a rare inflammatory vasculitis involving the aortic arch and occurs in young females, mainly in Japan. The aetiology is unknown and the patient presents with absent pulses and hypertension. There may be systemic symptoms such as fever, and the patient presents with stroke and heart failure.

Kawasaki's disease

This inflammatory vasculitis affects young children. They present with a febrile illness, and lymphadenopathy and microaneurysms of the coronary arteries are found.

Syphilis

The tertiary stage of infection with *Treponema pallidum* affects the cardiovascular system with the development of a characteristic aneurysm with linear calcification in the media in the ascending aorta and aortic regurgitation. There may be associated stenoses of the coronary ostia.

07

Autoimmune rheumatic diseases

Autoimmune rheumatic diseases can cause varying degrees of vasculitis (see p. 206).

Vasomotor disease (Raynaud's disease)

Epidemiology

Sex. Raynaud's disease characteristically affects young women who often have evidence of vasomotor instability elsewhere (e.g. migraine and coronary artery spasms causing angina-like symptoms).

Disease mechanisms and clinical features

Intermittent spasm of the digital arteries of both the hands and feet causes skin pallor and subsequent peripheral cyanosis. There is a characteristic clear demarcation of the affected area. The episodes are often precipitated by the cold and last for up to a few hours. Reactive hyperaemia during the recovery phase can cause intense pain.

Differential diagnosis

Raynaud's disease must be distinguished from Raynaud's phenomenon in which similar symptoms can be attributed to an underlying cause such as scleroderma, cryoglobulinaemia, drug therapy (e.g. beta-blockers) or the use of vibrating machinery.

Management and prognosis

Treatment includes keeping the hands and feet warm in cold weather. Vasodilators (e.g. nifedipine) can be beneficial.

Peripheral vascular ischaemia

Epidemiology

Prevalence. As with atherosclerotic disease elsewhere, peripheral arterial disease is common in industrialized countries. Smoking is a major cause.

Disease mechanisms

People with atherosclerosis of the aorta, iliac or femoral arteries may also have obstructive disease in the coronary and cerebral circulation. The presence of peripheral vascular disease in a patient with angina usually indicates widespread coronary artery narrowing.

Acute ischaemia can result from thromboembolism from the heart, or a more proximally located atherosclerotic plaque. Acute thrombosis *in situ* can also occur. The limb becomes acutely painful, pale, paralysed and pulseless.

Clinical features

The symptoms arising from peripheral vascular disease are:

- Intermittent claudication
- Pain at rest, particularly at night, in the feet and toes
- Ischaemic ulcers of the feet (in people with diabetes mellitus these can be painless, but at times can be intractably painful)

Intermittent claudication is a tightness in the calf on walking, particularly up hills, that makes the patient stop walking. The symptoms then settle and the patient can resume walking.

Examination reveals a cold limb with reduced peripheral pulses. The skin is dystrophic and sometimes there is a striking loss of hair (this is common in people without peripheral vascular ischaemia). Bruits may be audible over the abdominal aorta or femoral pulses. Elevation of the leg can cause venous guttering, indicating poor peripheral blood flow.

In **acute thrombosis** *in situ*, the limb becomes acutely painful, pale, paralysed and pulseless. **Leriche's syndrome** causes pain in the buttocks on walking and impotence, and is caused by complete obstruction of the aortoiliac bifurcation.

Investigation

Diagnostic imaging

- *Doppler ultrasound:* allows assessment of peripheral blood flow.
- *Aortography:* via the brachial or femoral route identifies the site of the stenosis. The recent introduction of digital imaging has improved the definition of the stenoses.

Haematology

- FBC and ESR
- Urea and electrolytes, creatinine, liver function tests

Management and prognosis

Management includes controlling risk factors and encouraging regular exercise to stimulate the development of collateral vessels. Low-dose aspirin should be prescribed. There is no evidence that vasodilators or anticoagulation are of benefit. Measures should be taken to care for the feet, including visits to the chiropodist. Such conservative treatment adequately controls the symptoms of many patients (Table 7.54).

Deteriorating symptoms. Despite conservative treatment, the symptoms of approximately 25% of patients worsen. Rest pain develops and the limb is at risk of gangrene. Relief of the obstruction should therefore be considered by either percutaneous balloon angioplasty, with or without additional laser treatment, or reconstructive surgery with bypass grafts. This is usually successful when used for the larger calibre vessels above the inguinal ligament, but

Table 7.54 Management of peripheral vascular ischaemia

Supportive treatment
Patient education
Control risk factors
Encourage regular exercise
Foot care

Specific treatment
Drug treatment
Low-dose aspirin
Acute ischaemia
   Thrombolytic drugs such as TPA with or without additional
      balloon angioplasty

Surgery
Deteriorating symptoms—rest pain develops and the limb is
   at risk of gangrene
   Consider relieving obstruction by either percutaneous
      balloon angioplasty with or without additional laser
      treatment or reconstructive surgery with bypass grafts
   Amputation
Acute ischaemia
   Thrombolytic drugs such as TPA with or without additional
      balloon angioplasty. Urgent surgical reconstruction may
      be required

TPA, tissue plasminogen activator.

there is a higher incidence of occlusion and restenosis of bypass grafts for more peripheral stenoses. Amputation may be necessary.

Acute ischaemia from thrombosis, or thromboembolism, is treated by identifying the location of the clot by angiography. The use of thrombolytic drugs such as TPA, with or without additional balloon angioplasty, is increasingly successful. Urgent surgical reconstruction may be required.

Disease of the aorta

Aneurysms can develop in any part of the aorta.

Abdominal aortic aneurysm

Epidemiology. The abdomen is the most common site for aneurysm formation.

Prevalence. This is the most common aortic aneurysm and routine screening by ultrasound is often recommended in people over 65 years.

Disease mechanisms

Abdominal aortic aneurysms result from atherosclerosis but evidence of an active inflammatory process may be found.

Clinical features

Abdominal aortic aneurysms present in one of three ways: as an asymptomatic finding on routine clinical examination, as a cause of epigastric pain or pain in the back, and a pulsatile mass found on examination, or if leaking, with pain, hypotension and a pulsatile mass in the abdomen. The pain characteristically radiates through to the back, but may radiate to the loin or into the testis, leading to a misdiagnosis of renal colic.

Investigation
Diagnostic imaging
● *Abdominal ultrasound and CT scan:* determines the size of the aneurysm and its relationship to branch vessels, particularly the renal arteries
● *Angiography:* occasionally helpful

Management and prognosis

Treatment is by surgery with resection of the aneurysm and insertion of a dacron prosthesis. This is indicated in asymptomatic patients with an aneurysm larger than 5.5–6.0 cm because of the risk of sudden rupture. The mortality rate of emergency surgery for a ruptured aneurysm is over 70%.

Thoracic aortic aneurysm
Disease mechanisms

Thoracic aortic aneurysms tend to arise in patients with hypertension and atherosclerosis. Occasionally, they are caused by chest trauma. Syphilis is now only a rare cause.

Clinical features

Commonly, patients are asymptomatic and the aneurysm is only revealed by a routine chest radiograph (Fig. 7.71). Symptoms may result from compression of the superior vena cava, oesophagus or bronchus. Pain may be a presenting symptom. Occasionally, patients are breathless because the aneurysm causes aortic incompetence. Very often, the first presentation is rupture and sudden death.

Investigation
Diagnostic imaging
● *Cardiac ultrasound, CT scan of the chest and angiography:* define the aneurysm
● *MRI:* proves valuable for defining the extent of the aneurysm
● *Coronary angiography:* often considered to be helpful for identifying coexistent coronary artery disease, which may require coronary artery bypass grafting at the time of surgery

07

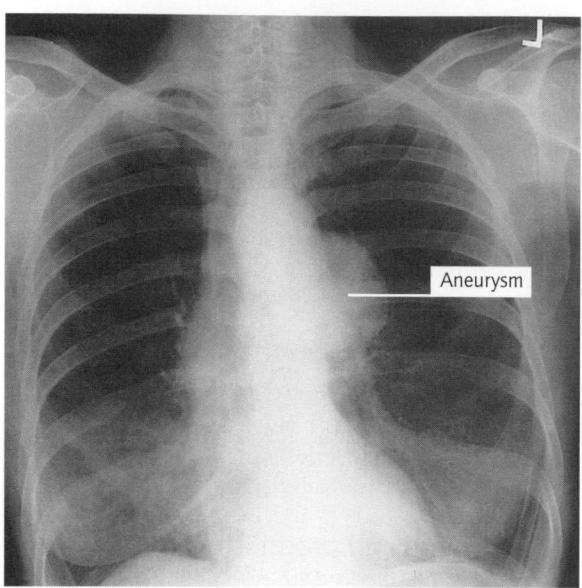

Figure 7.71 Incidental finding of thoracic aortic aneurysm on a routine chest radiograph.

Management and prognosis

Aneurysms larger than 5.5 cm are at risk of rupture and surgical reconstruction of the aorta is indicated.

Aortic dissection

Disease mechanisms

Dissection of the aorta arises as a result of a tear in the aortic intima. The subsequent dissecting haematoma can extend retrogradely towards the aortic valve. This can lead to aortic regurgitation and/or to the development of cardiac tamponade from blood leaking into the pericardium. The dissection can also extend progradely into the abdominal aorta and iliac vessels. The dissection can occur in aortic aneurysms and in aortas of previously normal size.

Classically, thoracic aortic aneurysms are subdivided into those in the ascending aorta (type I), those involving both the ascending and descending aorta (type II) and those confined to the descending aorta (type III). This classification is less useful than the classification which separates those involving the ascending aorta (type A), from those confined solely to the descending aorta (type B) (Fig. 7.72).

The main risk factors for aortic dissection are hypertension, Marfan's syndrome, pregnancy, a bicuspid aortic

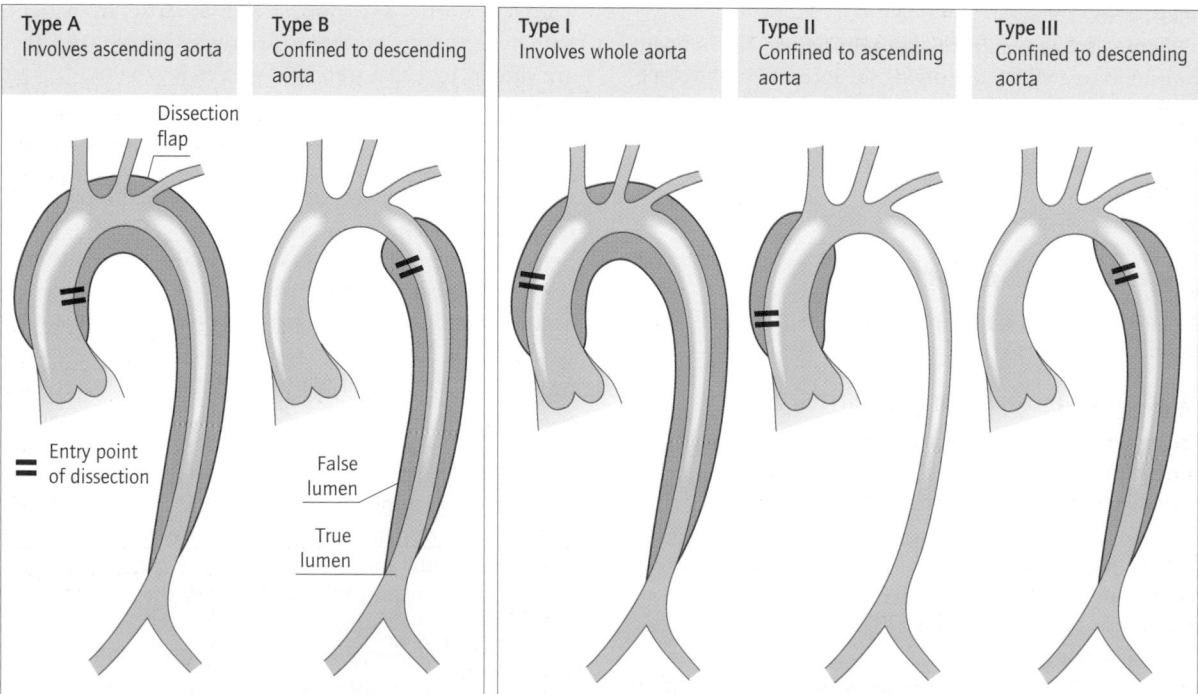

Figure 7.72 The two classification systems for dissection of the aorta.

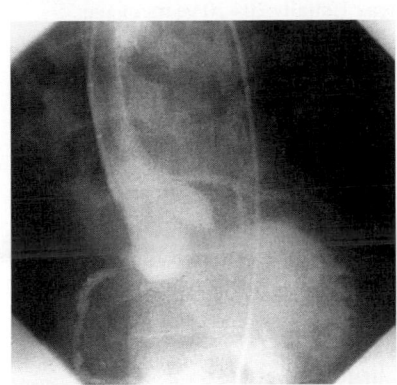 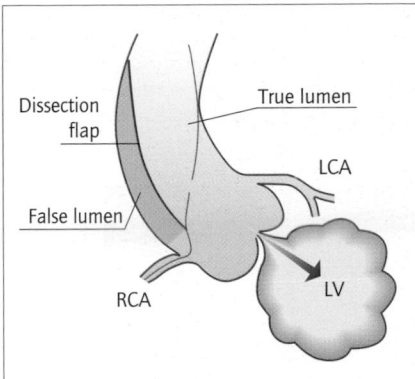

Figure 7.73 Aortography is helpful in defining the extent of the dissection and the site of the intimal tear. This aortogram of dissection in the ascending aorta shows the true and false lumen separated by the dissection flap, and aortic regurgitation. LCA, left coronary artery; RCA, right coronary artery.

valve and atherosclerotic disease (although the transmural nature of atherosclerosis is sometimes considered to protect against dissection).

Clinical features

The patient presents with acute chest pain often radiating through to the back. If there is extravascular bleeding into either the pleura or pericardium, the patient will be shocked, with a low blood pressure and tachycardia.

About 50% of patients lose peripheral pulses because the dissection occludes a branch artery. This can include the spinal arteries, so patients can present with paraplegia. There may be aortic regurgitation if the dissection dislocates the aortic valve ring, or myocardial infarction if it involves a coronary orifice.

Investigation

Diagnostic imaging
- *Chest radiography:* shows a widened mediastinum
- *Echocardiography and CT scanning:* confirm the diagnosis
- *Aortography:* helpful in defining the extent of the dissection and the site of the intimal tear (Fig. 7.73)

Management and prognosis

Treatment involves controlling the blood pressure, aiming for a systolic pressure of less than 110 mmHg, provided that the urine output is maintained.

Type A dissections. Surgery is required to prevent cardiac tamponade. The risks of surgery are great, with a perioperative mortality of more than 20%.

Type B dissections. The risk of paraplegia is high, and so attempts to stabilize the dissection with conservative treatment using hypotensive drugs are the preferred

Table 7.55 Types and relative incidence of benign cardiac tumours

Tumour	Relative incidence (%)
Myxoma	30
Lipoma	10
Fibroelastoma	10
Rhabdomyoma	8.5
Fibroma	4
Haemangioma	3.5
Other	34

option. However, if blood leaks into the pleura or symptoms continue, emergency reconstructive surgery may be required. If type B dissections are managed conservatively at first, an aneurysm may subsequently develop requiring elective surgery later.

Cardiac tumours

Cardiac tumours are rare. The different types are listed in Tables 7.55 and 7.56. The majority are secondary deposits involving the pericardium and occasionally the myocardium.

Table 7.56 Types and relative incidence of malignant cardiac tumours

Tumour	Relative incidence (%)
Angiosarcoma	10
Rhabdomyosarcoma	6
Fibrosarcoma	3.5
Malignant lymphoma	1.5
Other	79

07

Atrial myxoma

Epidemiology

Prevalence. The most common primary cardiac tumour, affecting 2/100 000 of the population.

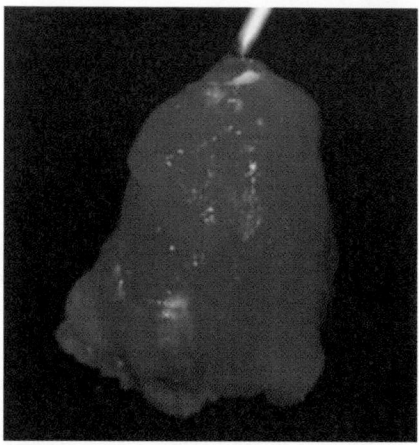

Figure 7.74 Atrial myxoma removed at surgery.

Age. Usually 20–70 years of age.

Sex. More common in women.

Disease mechanisms

An atrial myxoma consists of a gelatinous structure attached to the atrial septum (Fig. 7.74). Although usually occurring in the atrium, it can develop in any part of the heart. It may be a source of thrombus formation and can therefore lead to systemic embolization. It can also obstruct the mitral or tricuspid valve.

Clinical features

Left atrial myxoma can classically present in three ways:

1 *Systemic thromboembolism:* occurs in 40% of patients and the patient commonly presents with a stroke. All young patients with strokes should therefore undergo echocardiography. Occasionally, patients present with occlusion of a peripheral artery, such as an iliac artery. The thrombus removed at surgery should be sent for histological examination in case there is microscopic evidence of myxoma.

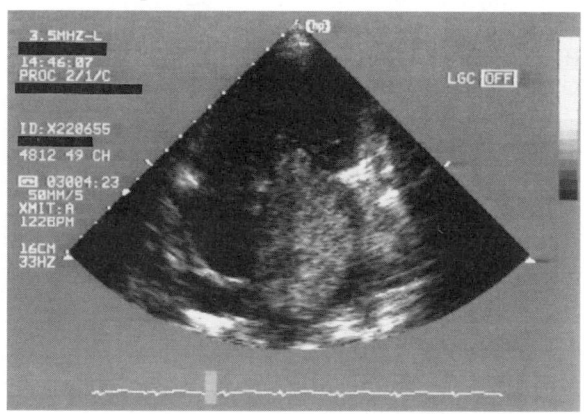

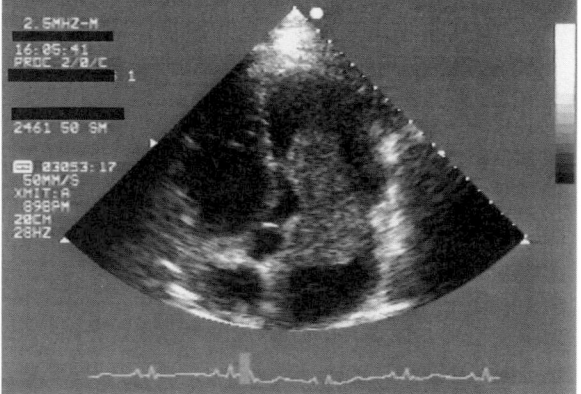

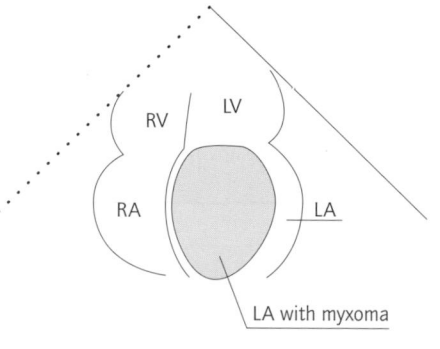

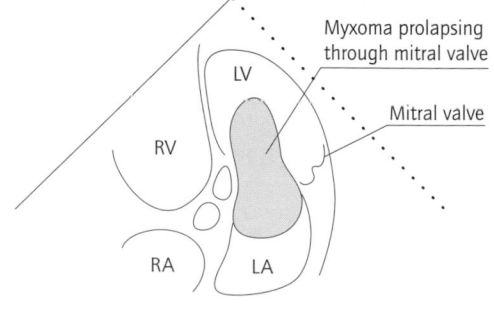

(a)   (b)

Figure 7.75 Echocardiogram of left atrial myxoma. Note prolapse of tumour through mitral valve in (b).

2 *Left atrial obstruction:* breathlessness together with paroxysmal nocturnal dyspnoea and atrial fibrillation can develop in about 50% of patients. This clinical course can closely mimic the natural history of mitral stenosis.

3 *Constitutional symptoms:* such as malaise, fever and weight loss occur in about 25% of patients and can be the first sign of a myxoma. About 60% of patients have a raised ESR and abnormal plasma electrophoresis.

Many patients have no specific signs to suggest a myxoma. In others, the physical signs are a loud first heart sound because of raised left atrial pressure and a tumour plop resulting from a loud third sound (caused by the tumour plopping through the valve).

Investigation

Haematology

- *FBC:* reveals a normochromic, normocytic anaemia
- *ESR:* may be increased

Diagnostic imaging

Echocardiography identifies the myxoma (Fig. 7.75).

Management and prognosis

The tumour should be removed surgically as soon as possible because of the risk of embolization. However, it recurs in 5% of patients over 5 years, particularly if the stalk is not fully removed from the atrial septum.

! Must know checklist

- Diagnosis of cardiac pain
- Diagnosis of heart failure
- Interpretation of an ECG
- Management of cardiac resuscitation
- Management of cardiac emergencies

- Management of acute chest pain
- Management of acute heart failure
- Management of acute arrhythmia
- Identification of heart murmurs
- How to exclude endocarditis

Further reading

Books

Braunwald E. *Heart Disease.* London: Harcourt, 1996.
Swanton RH. *Cardiology Pocket Consultant.* Oxford: Blackwell Publishing, 2003.

Journals

Journal of American College of Cardiology, American College of Cardiology Foundation/Elsevier. http://www.cardiosource.com/journal/journal?sdid=4884

Heart, Journal of British Cardiac Society. http://www.bcs.com/
European Heart Journal, Elsevier. http://www.escardiocontent.org/

Websites

www.ecglibrary.com
www.americanheart.org

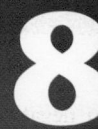

Renal Disease, Fluid and Electrolyte Disorders

Renal disease

Introduction

Overview

The kidney is an important organ with multiple functions. Without any renal function at all, death will usually occur in a matter of days. Fortunately, the kidney is the one organ for which medicine has an effective replacement in the form of dialysis. However, kidney failure is not the only result of renal diseases because the kidney is involved in many different types of disease processes. Understanding renal function in health and disease is important in many branches of medicine. This is because the renal system is central to some of the most common medical conditions; in particular, urinary tract infection, hypertension and the oedema caused by heart failure or liver disease. It is also important for all doctors to understand the kidney, because many renal problems result from the activities of doctors and health personnel. In particular, the kidney is vulnerable to damage from certain drugs or from inadequate hydration, especially in postoperative patients. It is vital that all doctors are aware of these pitfalls. Therefore, learning about the kidney and how to avoid damaging it are key objectives in medical training.

Scale of the problem

End-stage renal disease is defined as renal disease such that death would occur unless renal replacement therapy (a transplant or dialysis) is started. In the UK, there are over 500 patients per million of the population on some form of renal replacement therapy, including dialysis and transplantation. This number is currently increasing by about 5% each year. The prevalence of end-stage renal disease now exceeds 1000 cases/million in some developed countries and the incidence is around 70–120 new cases/million/year in Europe and the USA. Although transplantation can be cheaper than dialysis, the overall cost of the care of these patients is estimated at around one-quarter to one-half a billion UK pounds/year. This is a substantial portion of the total UK National Health Service budget and a very large portion of the total cost of hospital-based health care. A patient with such disease may live for many years on renal replacement therapy and will cost the health care system a great deal over these remaining years of their life. Unfortunately, in the poorer countries of the world the resources available for optimal treatment are not always available.

Preventing renal disease

Although we can keep people alive with dialysis and transplantation, renal disease can be unpleasant and can have a major negative impact on the lives of those who have it. The complications of long-term renal disease are serious and often debilitating. Sadly, much renal disease is preventable and whatever type of medicine they practise, all doctors should do everything they can to prevent renal disease. Often this requires only simple good quality medicine, such as the diligent care of children with urinary tract infections or the good control of blood pressure or of diabetes mellitus.

Patterns of renal disease

Age

Renal disease can occur at all ages. However, certain age-related diseases are well recognized. In small children, a key problem is reflex nephropathy (see p. 571). This arises when the entrance to the ureter allows backflow of urine up the ureter and can result in infection and damage to the kidney. Urinary tract infection in small children should always be investigated fully. Similarly, an abdominal mass in a child may represent the malignant Wilms' tumour.

The spectrum of renal disease in developed countries is changing. An emerging problem is that of impaired renal function in the **elderly**. The number of functional nephrons falls with age and the elderly are especially susceptible to damage to their kidneys. Many of the patients now on renal replacement therapy are elderly. In the elderly, most renal diseases are seen with greater frequency, partly because of the increased incidence of hypertension, diabetes mellitus, vascular disease and prostatic disease. Tumours are also more common in the elderly. Of the glomerular diseases, membranous nephropathy is more common in the elderly.

Gender differences

Urinary tract infection is much more common in women than men. Systemic lupus erythematosus is more common in women.

Pregnancy

Pregnancy is associated with an increased risk of upper urinary tract infection. In the final trimester, there is a significant risk of pre-eclampsia. Systemic lupus erythematosus can be exacerbated by pregnancy.

Diabetes mellitus

Diabetes mellitus is increasing in incidence. With this increase, principally of type 2 diabetes mellitus, especially in the elderly and obese, an increasing proportion of patients with end-stage renal disease are diabetic.

Ethnic differences

Ethnic differences have also been noted. In Western Europe and the USA, black patients and those with ethnic origins on the Indian subcontinent have been noted to have a significantly increased incidence of hypertension and renal disease, often with diabetes mellitus. Lupus erythematosus is also more common in black patients.

Geography

Geographical differences also arise in the distribution of renal diseases. Immunoglobulin A (IgA) nephropathy is more common in tropical climates than in Europe and the USA. Renal stone disease is more common in the drier climates (see map on p. 566). In those parts of the world where urinary tract schistosomiasis is prevalent (parts of Africa, especially East Africa), this can be a major problem and can cause bladder cancer and urinary tract obstruction (see p. 140). Urinary tract tuberculosis is more common in the poorer countries of the world.

08

Structure and function

Basic renal science

Structure

There are two kidneys, each weighing about 150 g, and they lie behind the peritoneum at the back of the upper abdomen. The right kidney lies below the liver and so is lower than the left kidney. Urine is formed in the kidneys and passes from each kidney down the ureters to the bladder (Fig. 8.1). Urine leaves the bladder through the urethra, which is shorter in women than in men. In men, the urethra passes through the prostate gland. The kidneys are supplied by blood from the renal arteries, which arise from the aorta. They are drained by the renal veins, which lead to the inferior vena cava. The **outer layer** of the kidney is the **renal cortex** and the inner layer is the **renal medulla**.

Development of the kidney and congenital anatomical abnormalities

The kidneys initially form in the pelvis and migrate up to their normal position during development. Sometimes one or both kidneys can remain in the pelvis. If both remain in the pelvis, they may fuse together to form a horseshoe kidney. It is relatively common for kidneys to have multiple renal arteries or veins, which often reflect persistent vessels from the developmental period when the kidneys were migrating from the pelvis. The ureters

08

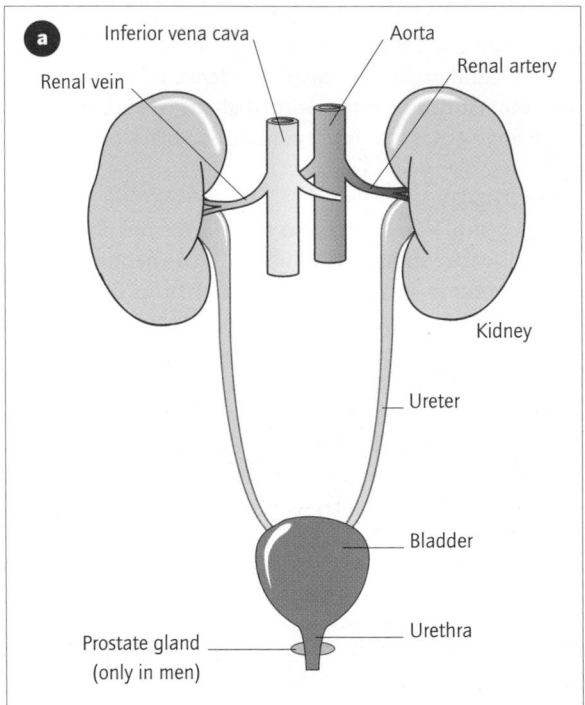

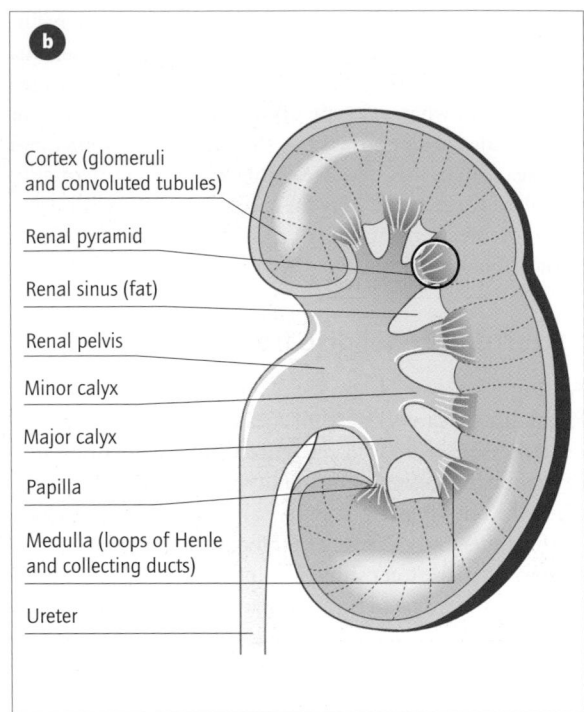

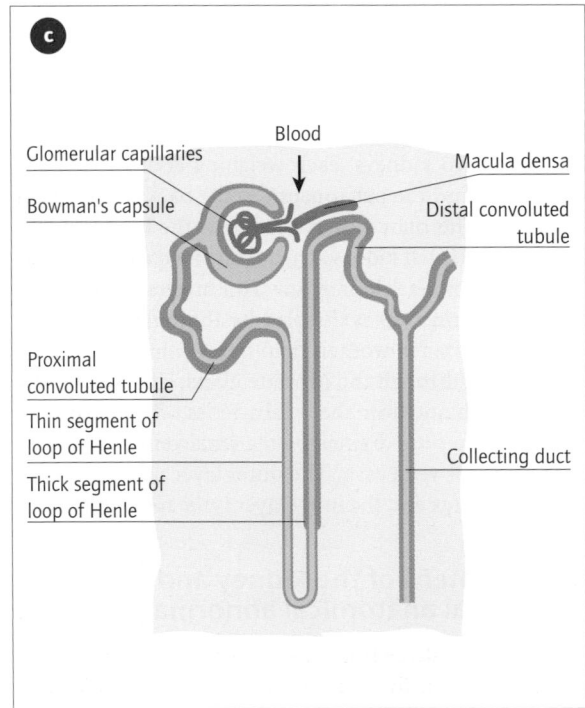

Figure 8.1 Renal structure and function. (a) Overview of the renal and urinary system. (b) Section through whole kidney. (c) A nephron.

are formed from a ureteric bud, which invades the developing kidney tissue. Common developmental variants include multiple ureters or one ureter that splits just before entering the kidney.

Functional overview

The kidney has several important functions:
1 The kidney has a critical **homoeostatic** function in

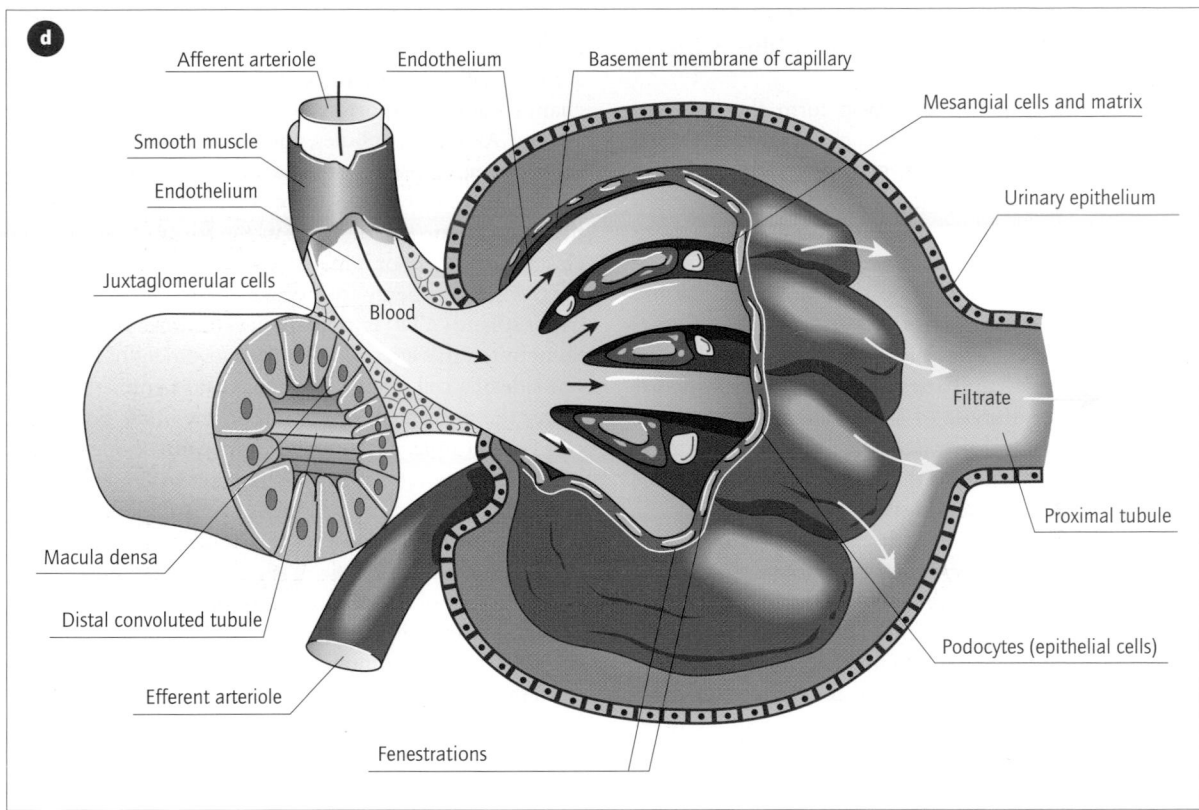

Figure 8.1(*cont'd*) (d) A glomerulus.

regulating a range of vital variables. These include the ionic composition and acid–base balance of body fluids and body water content, which dictates body fluid volume.

2 The kidney is an **excretory** organ that eliminates unwanted constituents of blood, such as metabolic products including urea, and unwanted water, ions and acid.

3 The kidney also has an **endocrine** function. It produces **erythropoietin**, which promotes red blood cell formation; **vitamin D**, which is involved in calcium and bone metabolism; and **renin**, which is involved in sodium and water regulation and blood pressure control. In addition, the kidney produces many compounds, such as prostaglandins, which are locally active.

4 The kidney also **responds** to a number of endocrine substances, including **aldosterone**, which promotes sodium retention; **antidiuretic hormone**, which promotes water retention; **parathyroid hormone**, which promotes calcium reabsorption and phosphate excretion; and **atrial natriuretic peptide**, which promotes some sodium excretion.

Structure and function of the nephron

The basic unit of the kidney is the **nephron**, which consists of the glomerulus, its blood vessels and the tubules, which run from the glomerulus to the urinary collecting system (Fig. 8.1c). Urine is first formed in the **glomerulus** by filtration and modified as it passes along the **tubules** by the reabsorption and secretion of solutes and of water.

Two types of nephron exist. Cortical nephrons are the predominant type of nephron and lie in the main part of the renal cortex, whereas juxtamedullary nephrons lie with their glomeruli close to the renal medulla.

Blood flow and filtration

Each kidney receives about 10% of the renal blood flow, which amounts to **500 ml/min for each kidney**. This blood passes through a branching system of arteries until it reaches the **afferent arterioles**. These small muscular vessels enter the glomerulus and carry arterial blood at high pressure. In the glomeruli, the blood enters the glomerular capillaries and the high pressure forces water and solutes, such as ions and other molecules, through the **glomerular filtration barrier**. This barrier is composed of three layers:

1 Endothelial cells lining the capillary

2 Basement membrane beyond these cells

3 Epithelial cells on the other side of this basement membrane

The tubular epithelial cells also form the lining of the urinary space, which in the glomerulus is known as Bowman's capsule. These epithelial cells are called **podocytes**, because they have highly developed foot processes, between which filtration occurs through an organized mesh of glycoproteins. Whether or not a substance is filtered depends on both its molecular size and its charge. Blood then leaves the glomerular capillaries through the **efferent arteriole**. This system is unique as blood usually leaves capillaries via a relatively unmuscular venule. However, the use of a muscular arteriole allows the kidney to control precisely the amount of filtration that occurs by controlling the muscle tone of both the afferent and efferent arterioles:

● Constriction of the afferent arterioles alters the amount of blood entering the glomerular capillaries

● Constriction of the efferent arteriole raises the pressure in the glomerular capillaries and increases filtration

After leaving the efferent arteriole, blood enters a second capillary bed surrounding the tubules. In those nephrons that lie near the medulla, the efferent arterioles lead into long deep vessels called **vasa recta** which descend and reascend with the loop of Henle. Eventually, all the blood vessels rejoin to form renal veins which leave the kidney.

Tubular function

The tubular system consists of several well-defined sections: the proximal tubule, loop of Henle, distal tubule and collecting tubule and ducts. The tubule walls are one cell thick and the cells have different sets of ion channels and transporters in the different sections of the system. Along the tubules, these cells act to modify the tubular fluid to produce the final urine.

Ions move only when there is an energetic reason for them to do so. This may be in the form of an ionic or electrical gradient or it may be in the form of active transport, whereby energy from the breakdown of adenosine triphosphate (ATP) is used to drive the movement of ions. Sometimes, this energy drives the movement of an ion on one side of a cell in the kidney to create a gradient, which drives the movement of the ion on the other side of the cell. For example, if sodium is pumped out of one side of a cell which has tight junctions separating the apical and basolateral faces of the cell, then the intracellular sodium level falls and this promotes the influx of sodium at the other side of the cell.

The details of the different ion movements are shown in Fig. 8.2. Initially, the glomerular filtrate is essentially similar to plasma, although some molecules are excluded from the filtrate by the filtration barrier.

Proximal tubule

In the **proximal tubule**, substantial active reabsorption takes place and the cells are well equipped with mitochondria to generate the energy necessary for this. Many substances are reabsorbed here, especially sodium, potassium, calcium, phosphate and glucose. Along with these substances, water moves by osmosis so that the filtrate is reduced in volume but the osmolality is unchanged.

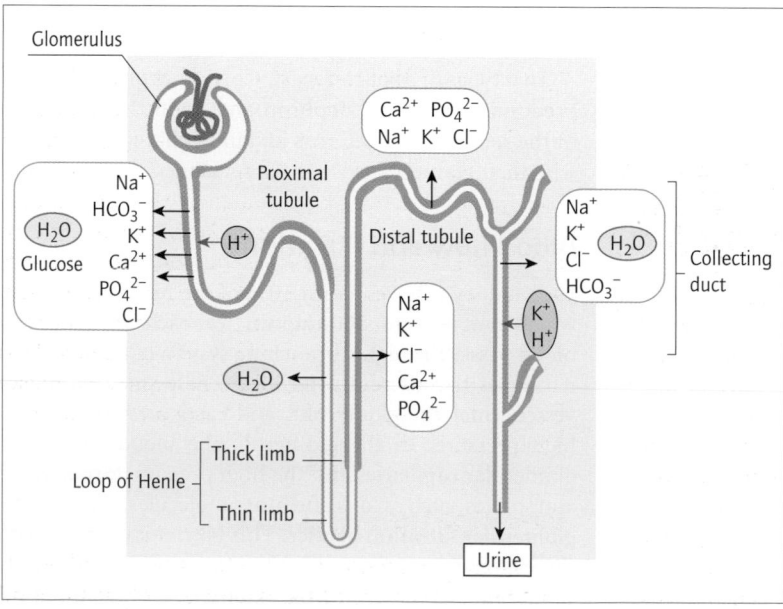

Figure 8.2 Overview of nephron function. The figure shows in schematic form the key ion movements along the nephron. Most reabsorption of water and electrolytes is performed in the proximal tubule. Urine is concentrated in the loop of Henle and then final adjustment of urine composition occurs in the distal tubule and collecting ducts.

Loop of Henle

The descending **loop of Henle** is permeable to water but not to ions, and water is removed by osmosis into the surrounding hyperosmotic medullary tissue. In the thick ascending loop of Henle, there is active movement of ions, especially sodium, out of the filtrate into the tissue. The ions pumped out of the ascending loop maintain the high osmolality of the medullary tissue.

Distal tubule

In the **distal tubule**, there is further active reabsorption of ions but no change in osmolality. By the time the filtrate reaches the collecting ducts, most of the ions and water have been reabsorbed. This segment of the nephron is able to **regulate** precisely how much of the various constituents of the filtrate will be excreted by making small adjustments to the filtrate. So, for example, there is a relatively constant reabsorption of around 95% of the sodium ions before the filtrate reaches the collecting tubules. The proportion of the remaining 5% which is or is not reabsorbed in the collecting tubules is accurately controlled by the effect of regulators such as **aldosterone** on the collecting duct cells.

Similarly, **water** reabsorption is regulated by the effects of **vasopressin** (antidiuretic hormone; ADH) on these cells. The loop of Henle makes the medullary interstitium hyperosmotic by pumping proportionately more ions into this tissue than water. The collecting ducts now pass down through this hyperosmotic medullary tissue and, as they do so, the osmotic gradient draws water out of the duct into the tissue. This process is controlled by vasopressin, which regulates the permeability of the duct to water. Vasopressin promotes water reabsorption by promoting the insertion of more aquaporin water channels in the membranes of collecting duct cells.

Approach to the patient

Renal disease can occur without any symptoms or signs, so the investigation of possible renal disease must always include the biochemical assessment of renal function. A general history is essential. Note the presence of pre-existing **diseases** that may predispose to renal disease, such as hypertension, diabetes or autoimmune disorders. The **drug history** may suggest the use of nephrotoxic drugs such as non-steroidal anti-inflammatory drugs. There may be a **family history** of a congenital renal disease. Chronic renal failure may be suggested by general malaise possibly including itching, muscle cramps, anorexia, nausea and confusion. Haemoptysis suggests a systemic vasculitis, especially Goodpasture's syndrome (HISTORY & EXAMINATION BOX 8.1).

History

Pain

Renal pain is not common. Pain from the kidneys can occur with renal obstruction or inflammation (usually resulting from infection). Very rarely, severe glomerular disease can cause lumbar pain. Urinary tract stones can also cause referred pain from the loin down to the external genitalia. Pain can also arise from infection or distension of renal cysts.

Urinary symptoms

Inflammation of the bladder, typically resulting from infection, can produce discomfort or burning on micturition, increased urinary frequency and offensive-smelling urine. Upper tract infection can produce loin pain, fever, flank tenderness and rigors. Prostatic disease can result in a poor urinary stream, hesitancy, terminal dribbling and urinary frequency. Incontinence can arise for mechanical reasons or as a result of neuromuscular instability and is usually investigated by urologists or in women by gynaecologists. Polyuria is an increase in total daily urine volume and is usually associated with a defect in the mechanism for controlling water excretion or, rarely, with excess water ingestion.

Urine appearance

Haematuria is the presence of blood in the urine and, when severe, the blood may be visible as frank haematuria. Bleeding can occur from anywhere along the urinary tract from the kidneys to the urethra. Common causes include renal stones, glomerulonephritis and urinary tract tumours. Typically, glomerular bleeding is present throughout the stream, whereas urethral bleeding may be present only at the beginning of the stream and prostate or bladder bleeding may be present only at the end of the stream. Frothy urine suggests a high protein content. Dark urine can occur with myoglobinuria because of muscle damage in rhabdomyolysis or haemoglobinuria when there is haemolysis.

Examination

A general examination should always be carried out. In particular, check the **blood pressure**, look at the **fundi**

08

History & Examination 8.1: Questions to ask if renal disease is suspected

Symptoms of kidney disease

Changes in urine
Is your urine ever discolored, red or frothy?
Have you ever seen any blood in your urine?
Have you ever passed a stone or any gravel?
Is your urine offensive smelling?

Changes in micturition
How often do you pass urine at night? During the day?
Do you pass urine more frequently than previously?
Do you pass normal amounts of urine?
Do you pass urine when you don't mean to?
Is it difficult to start or stop the flow of urine?
Does the urine come out in a normal stream or is the
 flow poor?
Do you have any pain, burning or discomfort when you
 pass urine?

Salt and water retention
Have your ankles or legs been swollen?
Have you noticed any shortness of breath? If so, is it worse
 when you lie flat?

Uraemia
Do you feel tired?
Do you feel generally weak?
Do you have difficulty sleeping?
Have you had any itching, muscle cramps or
 headaches?
Have you noticed any pins and needles, or numbness of
 your hands and feet?

Pain
Do you have loin pain or pain in the back, abdomen, pelvis
 or genitals?
When do you get this pain?
How severe is the pain?
What is it like?
Does it go anywhere else?

General questions
Do you have any other symptoms such as painful joints, a
 rash, indigestion, bowel disturbance or cough?
Have you travelled or lived abroad? If so, where?

Drug history
Have you taken any medications either prescribed by a
 doctor or bought from a chemist or health food shop in
 the last few years?
Have you taken painkillers, particularly non-steroidal anti-
 inflammatory drugs such as ibuprofen or indometacin?

Past medical history
Have you ever had an operation or been in hospital. If so,
 what for?
Do you have any other medical condition?
Are you diabetic?
Do you have high blood pressure?
Have you had any recent infections or a sore throat?

Family history
Does anyone in your family have kidney problems, kidney
 stones or high blood pressure or deafness (Alport's
 syndrome)?

---

and check for signs of dehydration or oedema. Check carefully for a distended and possibly obstructed **bladder**. In older men, examination of the **prostate** can be informative and **vaginal examination** may be necessary in women. Check for signs of systemic disease, such as joint problems or neurological abnormalities. Cardiac valve lesions may suggest glomerulonephritis associated with infective endocarditis. Vascular **bruits** may indicate vascular disease, which could also affect the renal arteries.

Carefully examine the patient's **fluid status**. Key signs include skin turgor, peripheral oedema—usually detectable at the ankles or sacrum, pulmonary oedema, the jugular venous pulse and the presence of a postural drop in blood pressure.

Examine the kidneys by **bimanual palpation**. From the patient's left side, the right hand is placed over the upper abdomen on one side and the left hand is placed in the renal angle on the same side. The **renal angle** is formed by the twelfth rib and the lumbar muscles. As the patient inspires, the left hand pushes into the renal angle and an enlarged kidney may be felt by the right hand as the kidney moves down the abdomen during inspiration and the left hand pushes it anteriorly (HISTORY & EXAMINATION BOX 8.2; Fig. 8.3).

Investigation

Bedside tests

Urine should be dipstick tested for **protein, blood and glucose**. There are various stick tests for infection. Positive tests for **nitrites** produced by Gram-negative bacteria and for **leucocytes** (the test usually measures esterases released by urinary white blood cells) indicate infection.

Microscopy

Microscopy of urine is easy to perform and can be very

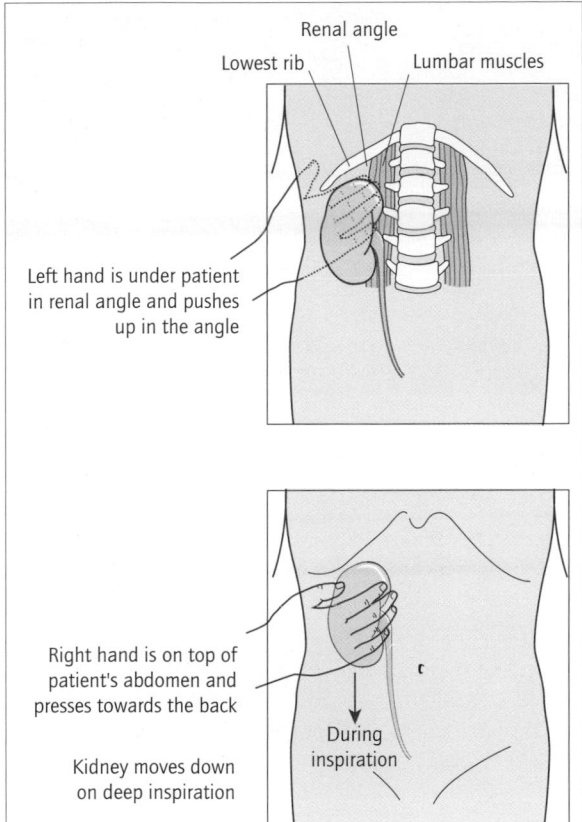

Renal angle

Lowest rib · Lumbar muscles

Left hand is under patient in renal angle and pushes up in the angle

Right hand is on top of patient's abdomen and presses towards the back

During inspiration

Kidney moves down on deep inspiration

Figure 8.3 Palpation of the kidneys. The upper panel shows the position of the left hand when palpating the right kidney. The lower panel shows the position of the right hand. On deep inspiration, the left hand pushes up in the renal angle and the kidney can be felt moving down by the right hand. The procedure is similar for the left kidney and the left hand is placed under the patient from the left side of the patient.

useful (Fig. 8.4). Fresh urine is ideally centrifuged to pellet any cells or casts and then the pellet is resuspended in a small volume, often with a dye. Uncentrifuged urine can also be used.

- *Red cells:* indicate bleeding.
- *White cells:* indicate inflammation, usually infection or the inflammation of interstitial nephritis.
- *Casts:* form in the nephron and are tube-shaped aggregations, usually containing protein, cells and sometimes lipid. **Red cell casts** indicate glomerular bleeding and so glomerulonephritis. **White cell casts** usually indicate acute infection. Some non-cellular casts such as granular casts can be normal findings.
- *Crystals:* can form after urine has been collected but, if present in fresh urine, they can suggest a stone-forming tendency.

History & Examination 8.2: Examination of a patient with renal disease

General appearance
Does the patient look well?
Does the patient look dehydrated or oedematous?
Do they have an unusual fishy smell (can occur in severe uraemia)?
Do they have a twitch, tremor or flap (check with the arms outstretched and wrists extended)?
Is there any lymphadenopathy?

Look at the skin
Look for any rashes, purpura, jaundice
Does the patient look pale or anaemic?
Are there any wounds, pressure sores or ulcers? If so inspect them for signs of infection

Look at the eyes
Look for signs of anaemia or jaundice
Look at the fundi, especially for hypertensive or diabetic changes

Cardiovascular system
Look for oedema
Feel the pulses
Measure the blood pressure
Listen for new murmurs or a pericardial rub
Listen for bruits (femoral, carotid, abdominal)

Respiratory system
Assess the breathing pattern. Is it laboured or rapid?
Listen to the chest for pulmonary oedema or other changes
Is the patient more breathless on lying flat?

Abdomen
Examine for enlarged or tender kidneys
Examine for a palpable bladder
Examine for hepatosplenomegaly
Inspect for the external genitalia for congenital abnormalities (e.g. hypospadias, phimosis) and testicular inflammation or tumour
Palpate the prostate in men
Consider the need for a vaginal examination in women if pelvic disease is suspected

Joints
Examine for evidence of arthropathy

Nervous system
Examine for evidence of peripheral neuropathy, focal neurological deficit and level of consciousness

Urine
Test the urine with a labstick for protein and blood
Examine the urine under a microscope

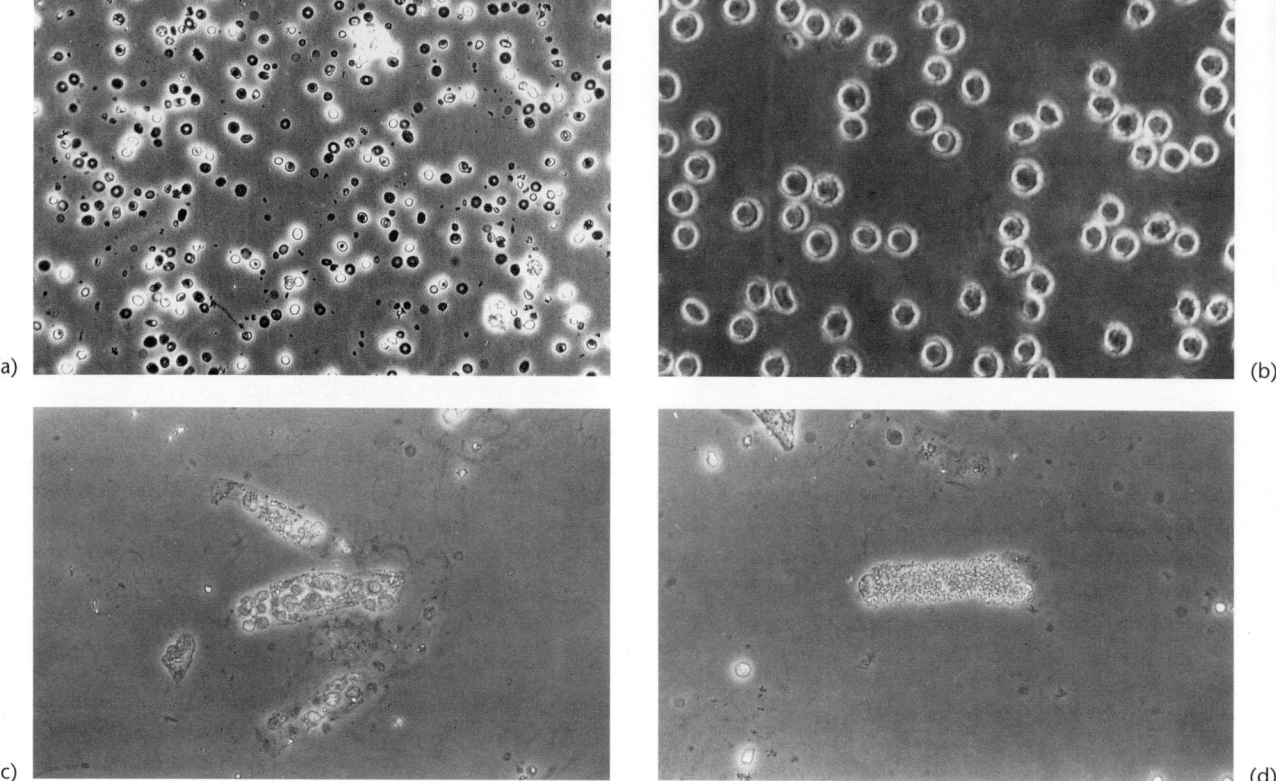

Figure 8.4 Appearances on phase contrast microscopy of red cells seen in urine: (a) dysmorphic red blood cells of glomerular bleeding; (b) non-dysmorphic red blood cells of lower urinary tract bleeding; (c) cellular casts; and (d) granular cast. Reproduced from Becker GJ, Whitworth JA, Kincaid-Smith P. *Clinical Nephrology in Medical Practice*. Oxford: Blackwell Scientific Publications, 1992 with the permission of the authors.

Tests of renal function

Both **urea** and **creatinine** are excreted by the kidney, so if renal function is impaired their concentrations in blood rise. However, there is normally excess renal excretory capacity, so the concentrations do not rise until there is a very substantial loss of renal function (Fig. 8.5). For this reason, normal urea and creatinine levels do not confirm that renal function is normal, but merely exclude severe renal impairment. Urea is a product of protein metabolism and urea levels rise after a protein meal.

More accurate estimations of glomerular filtration rate (GFR) can be made by comparing the amount of creatinine in the urine to that in blood. In practice, there is some tubular secretion of creatinine, but it is nevertheless a useful clinical test. In principle, a more accurate test is the calculation of **creatinine clearance** using plasma and urinary creatinine concentration and urine volume.

Often the urine collection is inaccurate because the patient may forget to collect all the urine. If the plasma

creatinine is known (or creatinine clearance measurements are suspect) the Cockcroft and Gault formula can be used to calculate creatinine clearance fairly accurately:

Creatinine clearance
= F (140 − age) × body weight (kg)/
plasma creatinine (μmol/l),

where F = 1.0 for females and 1.23 for males, and age is in years (KEYPOINTS BOX 8.1).

Other methods of estimating glomerular filtration rate rely on following the removal of injected radioactive markers such as ^{51}Cr-EDTA (ethylene diamine tetra-acetic acid) from blood by glomerular filtration.

Proteinuria

Normally, only a very small amount of **protein** (0.2–0.4 g/24 h) is excreted in the urine but with renal damage, especially to the glomeruli, this can increase substantially. This can be quantified by collecting all the urine passed in 24 h and assessing the total protein excretion. As this

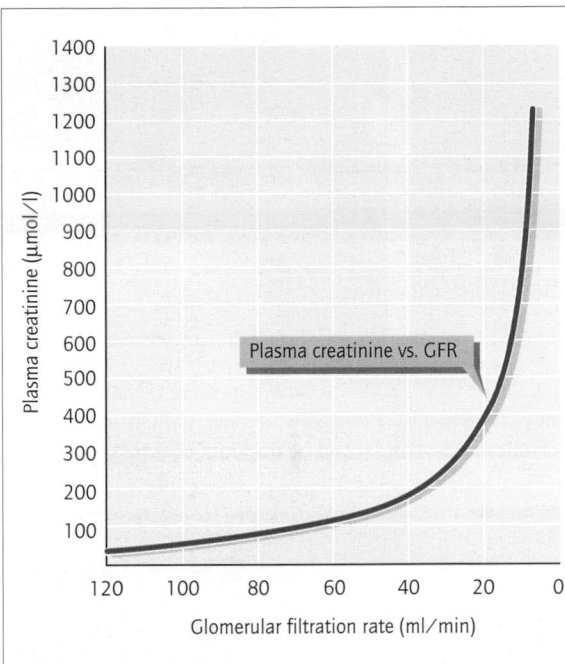

Figure 8.5 Graph of plasma creatinine vs. glomerular filtration rate (GFR).

08

Keypoints 8.1: Creatinine clearance

If a 24-h urine collection is made, then assuming that creatinine is neither reabsorbed nor secreted:

The amount of creatinine excreted in the urine per minute [the urine volume produced per minute (V) × the urine concentration (U)] equals the amount filtered [the plasma volume filtered per minute (C) × the plasma concentration (P)]

$$UV - CP$$

After rearranging the equation:

Clearance (C) = (U × V)/P

The plasma volume filtered per minute is called the clearance and is a measure of the glomerular filtration rate

The main problem lies in the human error involved in a 24-h urine collection

Clearance is measured in ml/min

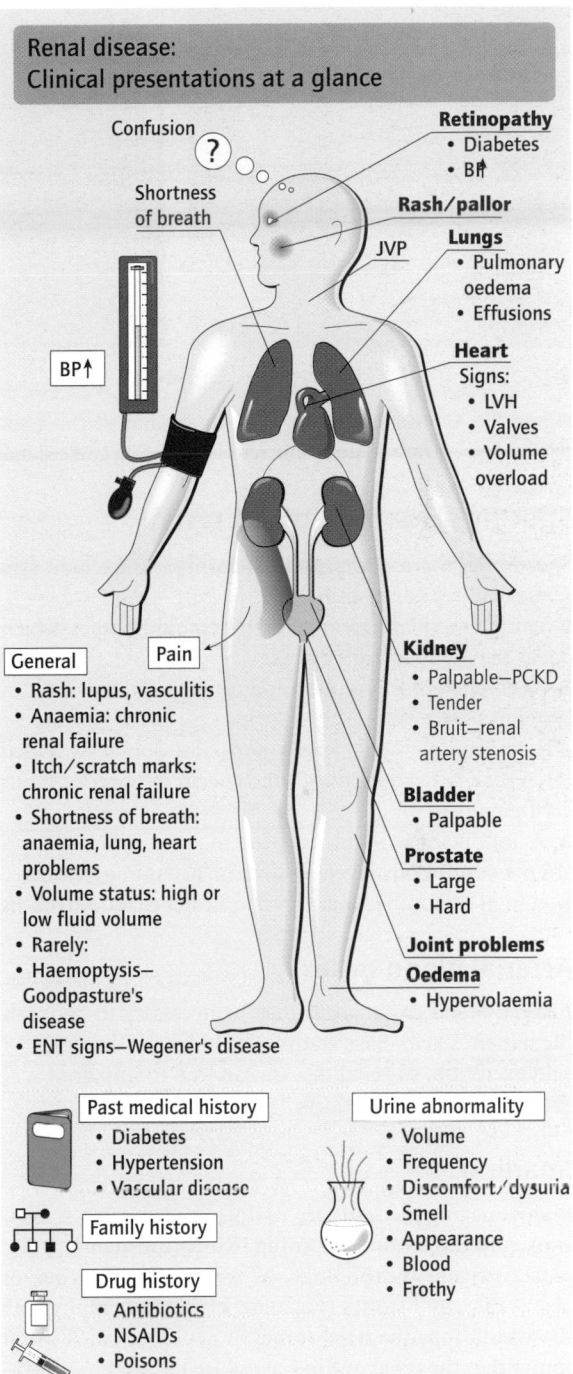

Renal disease: Clinical presentations at a glance

Confusion

Retinopathy
- Diabetes
- BP

Shortness of breath

Rash/pallor

JVP

Lungs
- Pulmonary oedema
- Effusions

BP↑

Heart
Signs:
- LVH
- Valves
- Volume overload

Pain

General
- Rash: lupus, vasculitis
- Anaemia: chronic renal failure
- Itch/scratch marks: chronic renal failure
- Shortness of breath: anaemia, lung, heart problems
- Volume status: high or low fluid volume
- Rarely:
- Haemoptysis— Goodpasture's disease
- ENT signs—Wegener's disease

Kidney
- Palpable—PCKD
- Tender
- Bruit—renal artery stenosis

Bladder
- Palpable

Prostate
- Large
- Hard

Joint problems

Oedema
- Hypervolaemia

Past medical history
- Diabetes
- Hypertension
- Vascular disease

Family history

Drug history
- Antibiotics
- NSAIDs
- Poisons
- ACEI

Urine abnormality
- Volume
- Frequency
- Discomfort/dysuria
- Smell
- Appearance
- Blood
- Frothy

---

depends on a reliably complete collection, it can also be useful to look at the ratio of protein : creatinine in a single random urine sample. Various tests are available to look for specific proteins in urine, in particular Bence Jones protein, which is the light chain of antibodies and occurs in the urine in some patients with myeloma. In diabetics, very sensitive tests are used to evaluate whether there is microalbuminuria, which is the excretion of very low levels of albumin in the urine. This is an early marker of diabetic renal damage.

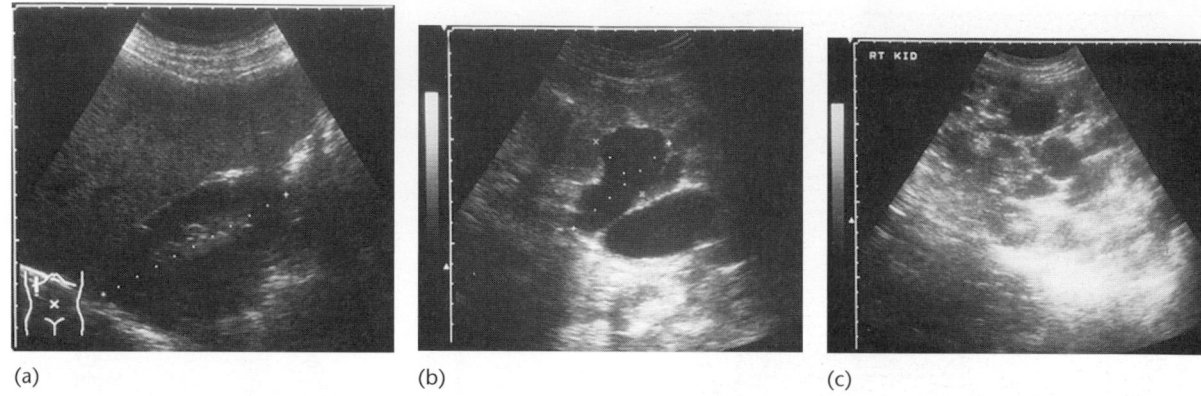

(a)   (b)   (c)

Figure 8.6 Ultrasounds of the kidney. (a) Normal. The length of kidney is marked by a dotted white line. (b) Obstructed. The dilated pelvicalyceal system appears black. (c) Polycystic kidney. Cysts of different sizes are scattered throughout kidney substance.

Specific diagnostic blood tests

Specific tests are commonly performed to exclude systemic disease. Key tests include:

- Antiglomerular basement membrane antibodies, which occur in Goodpasture's disease
- Antineutrophil cytoplasmic antibodies, which occur in systemic vasculitis
- Low complement levels and anti-double-stranded DNA (dsDNA) antibodies, which occur in systemic lupus erythematosus
- A monoclonal band on protein electrophoresis and abnormal antibody levels, which can occur in myeloma
- A high creatinine kinase level indicates rhabdomyolysis

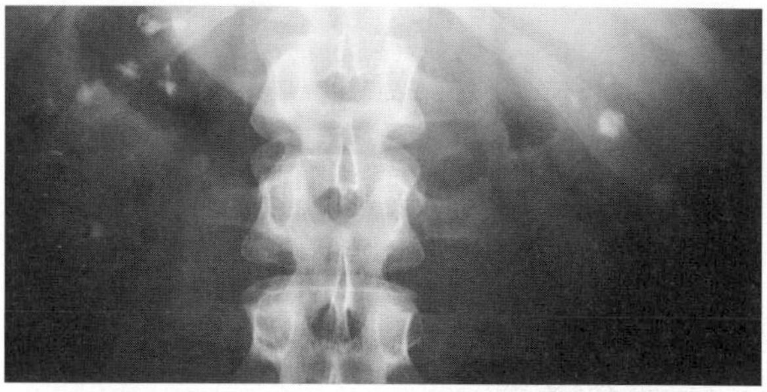

Arterial blood gases

Arterial blood gas analysis may be necessary to establish the patient's acid–base status. The kidney is the organ of acid excretion, so renal disease can lead to impaired acid excretion and so to acidosis.

Imaging

Many imaging methods are useful. The key investigation is usually **ultrasound scanning**, which can demonstrate renal size and morphology, as well as the presence of obstruction and stones (Fig. 8.6). Plain radiography may show radio-opaque renal stones or nephrocalcinosis, and sometimes the renal outline is visible (Fig. 8.7). An **intravenous urogram** (IVU) is performed by injecting the patient with an intravenous dye that is excreted by the kidneys and highlights the kidneys and urinary tract (Fig. 8.8). Alternatively, dye can be injected through the skin into the renal pelvis and followed down the ureter or injected up the ureter from the bladder by a perurethral approach. **Computerized tomography** (CT) and **magnetic resonance imaging** (MRI) are increasingly useful (Fig. 8.9).

Figure 8.7 Nephrocalcinosis on plain radiography. Calcification occurs first in the renal medulla. Calculi may also be present in the calyces or renal pelvis.

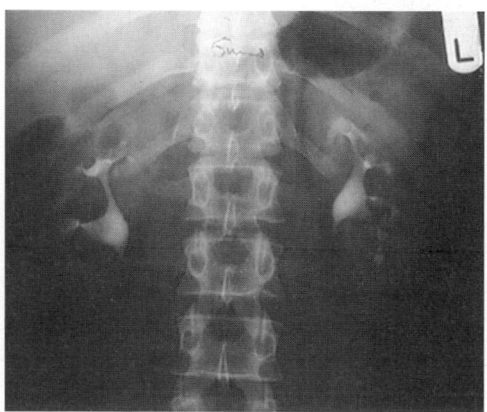

Figure 8.8 Intravenous urogram. Dye can be seen in the collecting systems of the kidneys. This examination shows the kidneys in a condition called medullary sponge kidney in which there are characteristic changes in the appearance of the collecting system in which dye accumulates.

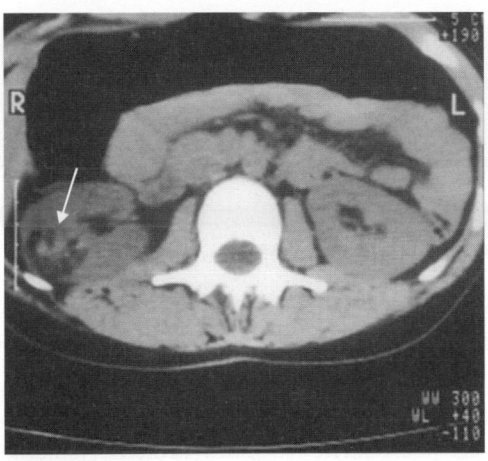

Figure 8.9 Computerized tomography (CT) scan of the kidney. A CT scan showing an angiomyolipoma in right kidney. Note the characteristic feature of fat within the lesion. This appears black (compare with subcutaneous fat in same picture).

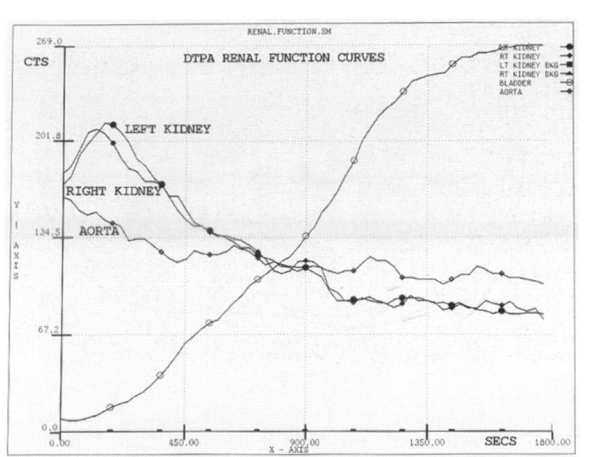

(a)

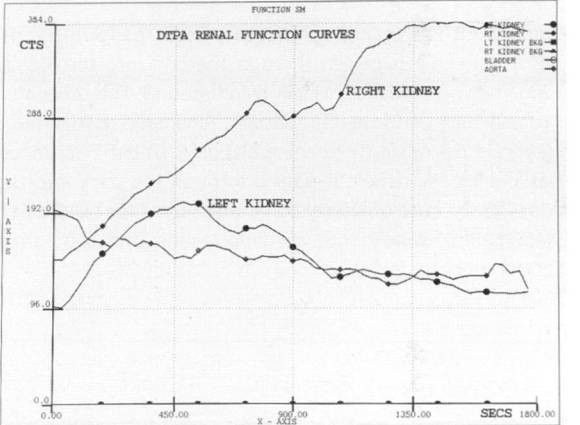

(b)

Figure 8.11 Isotope renogram of kidney (Tc-DTPA). (a) Normal. A sharp peak of activity on the graph is followed by a rapid fall as isotope is cleared from the kidney. (b) Obstruction of the right kidney. There is a continued rise of the right kidney graph as isotope is progressively trapped in the dilated kidney's collecting system.

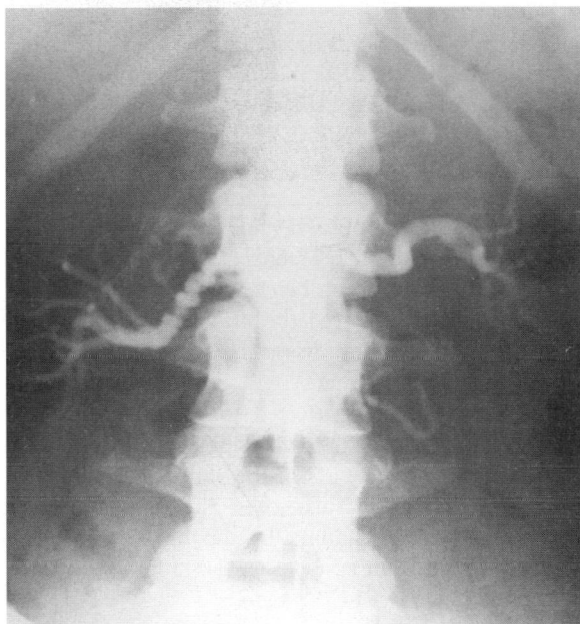

Figure 8.10 A renal angiogram showing fibromuscular hyperplasia of the right renal artery shown on the left side of the image. The right renal artery shows the characteristic beaded appearance of the condition. Reproduced from Becker GJ, Whitworth JA, Kincaid-Smith P. *Clinical Nephrology in Medical Practice*. Oxford: Blackwell Scientific Publications, 1992 with the permission of the authors.

Transcutaneous cannulation of large blood vessels, usually from the groin, can be used to inject radio-opaque dye down the renal arteries or veins to image these vessels as an **angiogram** (Fig. 8.10).

Nuclear tests

Injected radioactive markers can provide information about renal function. The markers are injected and gamma cameras read the radioactivity in the kidney over time. ^{99M}Tc-**DTPA** (diethylenetriamine penta-acetic acid) is rapidly excreted by the kidney and the kinetics of its renal handling provide information about renal blood flow and obstruction (Fig. 8.11). ^{99M}Tc-**DMSA** (dimercaptosuccinic acid) localizes in the proximal tubules and so gamma camera images of its distribution in the kidneys provide information about the function in each kidney and its localization within the kidneys.

The key test in many renal diseases is **renal biopsy** (Fig. 8.12). The appearances of a normal renal biopsy on light microscopy are shown in Fig. 8.13.

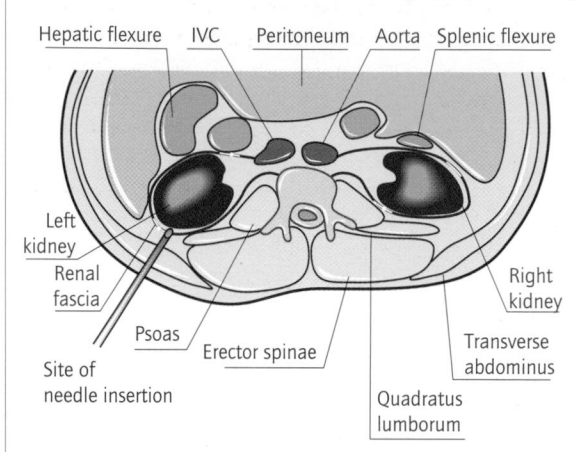

Figure 8.12 Percutaneous renal biopsy. To perform a renal biopsy a needle is placed through the skin into the kidney using imaging guidance, usually by ultrasound. This procedure is usually only performed in specialist renal units as it carries a significant risk of life-threatening bleeding. Under local anaesthesia, a biopsy needle is passed through the back into the kidney and a core of kidney tissue is removed for histological examination, usually with immunostaining and sometimes electron microscopy.

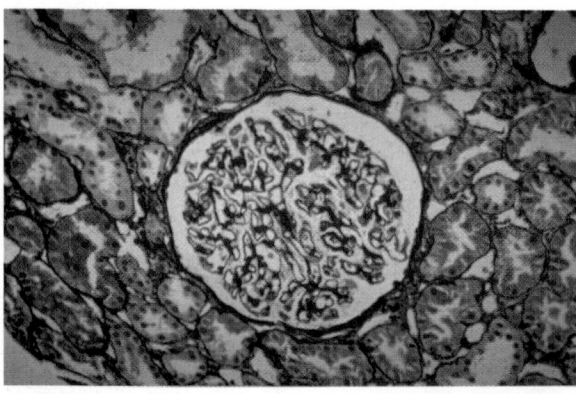

Figure 8.13 A normal renal biopsy. A section of normal kidney viewed through a light microscope. The large circular structure in the centre is a glomerulus, which contains glomerular capillary loops. Around these loops is Bowman's space, which is the space into which the filtrate passes. Outside the glomerulus are multiple smaller roundish structures, which represent cross-sections of different types of renal tubules. These tubules are lined by pink tubular epithelial cells and the nuclei of these cells have stained dark purple. The tissue section has been stained with a silver stain which makes basement membranes a blue colour.

Renal diseases and their management

Glomerular disease

Overview and classification of glomerular disease

Glomerular disease can often seem very confusing, largely because of the different ways it is classified. However, although many different diseases act on the glomeruli, the possible effects of glomerular damage are relatively similar whatever the cause. The effects include:

- Reduced glomerular filtration causing a rise in creatinine
- Proteinuria
- Haematuria
- Hypertension
- Sodium retention causing oedema

The clinical results of glomerular disease usually occur as one of several different **clinical syndromes** such as:

- Asymptomatic haematuria or proteinuria
- Nephritic syndrome
- Nephrotic syndrome
- Chronic slowly progressive renal damage
- Acute rapidly progressive renal damage

Glomerular disease can be classified according to the clinical syndrome produced, the histopathological appearance or the underlying disease. Glomerular disease is primary if there is no other system affected and secondary if there is another system affected (the renal disease is then considered secondary to the underlying systemic condition).

The glomerulus consists of the glomerular basement membrane, the glomerular cells, the intraglomerular vessels and the mesangium (the supporting connective tissue). Glomerular disease can affect one or more of these components:

- In **proliferative** glomerular disease, there is abnormal proliferation of cells within the glomerulus
- In severe cases, the proliferation of these cells, especially macrophages within Bowman's capsule, causes an appearance known as a **crescent**
- In **mesangial** disease, there is excess production of mesangial connective tissue matrix
- In **membranous** disease, there is no cell proliferation, but the glomerular basement membrane is damaged and thickened
- **Membranoproliferative** disease causes both thickening of the glomerular basement membrane and cellular proliferation, usually of mesangial cells

When viewed under the microscope, glomerular disease is described in the following way:

- **Focal** disease affects only some glomeruli
- **Diffuse** disease affects all the glomeruli
- **Segmental** disease affects only part of each affected glomerulus
- **Global** disease affects the whole of each affected glomerulus

Common clinical presentations of glomerular disease

In practice, there are a number of very well-defined clinical scenarios resulting from glomerular disease. Although not all disease conforms to these patterns, it is helpful to know them as they account for many cases that are encountered:

- A young person with nephrotic syndrome and no other disease is likely to have **minimal change nephropathy**
- A young person, typically male, with recurrent intermittent frank haematuria and sometimes hypertension or renal impairment will often be found to have **IgA nephropathy**
- An older person with nephrotic syndrome often has **membranous nephropathy**
- A young man with haemoptysis and renal failure is very likely to have **Goodpasture's disease**
- Someone with a recent history of a sore throat and renal disease may have **postinfective glomerulonephritis** (sometimes called poststreptococcal if the infection is a streptococcal infection)
- A young woman with joint pains, rashes, neurological or psychiatric problems and renal disease is likely to have glomerulonephritis associated with **systemic lupus erythematosus**
- Glomerular disease is often picked up when it is **asymptomatic** by routine urine or blood tests

Nephrotic syndrome

The nephrotic syndrome is one possible consequence of glomerular disease. The key features are:

- Heavy urine protein loss (e.g. 5 g/day)
- Low plasma albumin levels (e.g. 20 g/l)
- Oedema
- There is usually hypercholesterolaemia

The nephrotic syndrome can occur if there is damage to the glomerular filtration barrier resulting in heavy proteinuria. The loss of protein in the urine lowers the protein levels in the blood; in particular, the level of albumin is lowered in the blood. As a result of these changes the kidney retains sodium and water and peripheral oedema develops. There is debate about the exact pathogenesis of this oedema. It has been argued that the oedema arises because the low plasma albumin level results in a low osmotic pressure in blood vessels, which then allows water to leak out into the tissues. The nephrotic syndrome usually causes high lipid levels and predisposes the patient to venous thrombosis and infection, which are important complications. The precise diagnosis can be made by renal biopsy. The main causes are:

- Minimal change nephropathy
- Focal segmental glomerulosclerosis
- Membranous nephropathy
- Amyloidosis
- Diabetes mellitus
- Drugs
- Systemic lupus erythematosus

The nephrotic syndrome can be caused by non-steroidal anti-inflammatory drugs, which cause a minimal change nephropathy, or penicillamine, which causes membranous nephropathy. Systemic lupus erythematosus can cause a membranous nephropathy with nephrotic syndrome.

Treatment involves treatment of the underlying glomerular disease. In addition, diuretics are used to control the oedema and lipid levels may need controlling by lipid-lowering drugs, especially statins. In severe cases, anticoagulation is used to prevent venous thrombosis. The most likely cause of nephrotic syndrome in children is minimal change nephropathy, so they are often treated with steroids without a renal biopsy being performed.

Nephritic syndrome

This syndrome is caused by acute glomerular disease and results from aggressive inflammation in the glomeruli. The effects include:

- Hypertension
- Urine abnormalities: haematuria, often with red cell casts and usually proteinuria
- Oedema, caused by sodium and water retention
- Renal impairment, with reduced urine output and raised creatinine levels

Glomerular damage causes leakage of blood and protein into the urine. The damage also impairs kidney function so that urine output falls and there is an accumulation in plasma of substances such as creatinine that are normally excreted by the kidneys. Renal inflammation provokes the release of substances such as renin. Renin triggers angiotensin II and aldosterone production, which promote high blood pressure and sodium and water retention in the form of oedema.

Key causes include:

- Diffuse proliferative glomerulonephritis (or acute endocapillary glomerulonephritis), which often arises as a postinfective glomerulonephritis

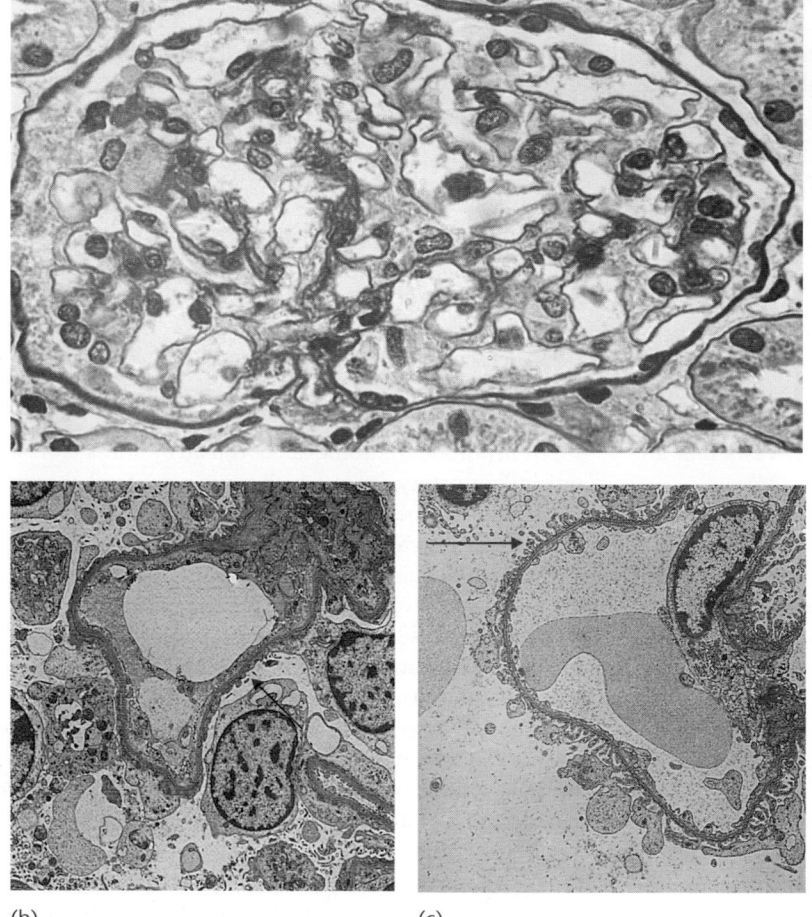

(a)

(b)   (c)

Figure 8.14 Minimal change nephropathy. (a) The appearance on light microscopy is normal. Reproduced from Kincaid-Smith P, Whitworth JA. *The Kidney: a Clinico-Pathological Study*, 2nd edn. Oxford: Blackwell Scientific Publications, 1987 with the permission of the authors. (b) The appearance on electron microscopy shows the characteristic fusion of the foot processes. Compare with (c) an electron micrograph of a normal kidney.

- IgA nephropathy
- Systemic lupus erythematosus
- Crescentic glomerulonephritis
- Systemic vasculitis
- Cryoglobulinaemia

Treatment of nephritic syndrome involves treatment of the underlying glomerular disease. Blood pressure should be controlled and diuretics may be necessary to control the oedema. In addition, renal replacement therapy may be necessary if the renal impairment is severe. Patients with postinfective glomerulonephritis should be given appropriate antibiotics to ensure that the infection is eradicated.

Primary glomerular disease

Minimal change nephropathy

Disease mechanisms

This condition is of unknown aetiology, but it is associated with atopy or an allergic tendency. Damage to the glomerular filtration barrier causes a protein leak and the nephrotic syndrome. Light microscopy and immunofluorescence are normal. Electron microscopy shows glomerular epithelial **podocyte foot process fusion** (Fig. 8.14). Disease associations are uncommon but include systemic lupus erythematosus and the use of non-steroidal anti-inflammatory drugs.

Epidemiology

The incidence is 2 per 100 000. The condition accounts for 80% of childhood nephrotic syndrome and 25% of adult nephrotic syndrome. The peak incidence is between the ages of 2 and 7 years, but all ages can be affected.

Clinical presentation

Typically, there is nephrotic syndrome, so patients may present with frothy urine caused by proteinuria or with swelling resulting from oedema. The condition often follows upper respiratory tract infection. Oedema is usually the only major physical sign and in children can take the form of facial swelling.

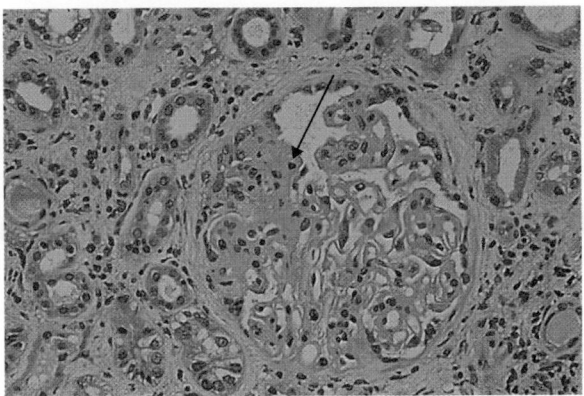
(a)

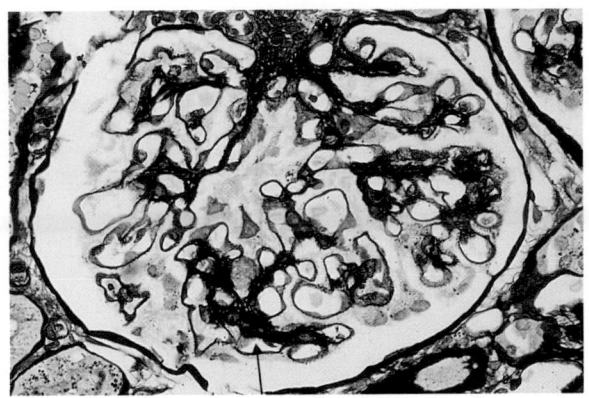
(b)

08

Figure 8.15 Focal segmental glomerulosclerosis (FSGS). (a) Affected capillary loops are necrosed and have been replaced by collagen. (b) Appearance on silver staining. Note segments of capillary loops being replaced by amorphous silver-positive sclerosis which appears black.

Investigation

Urinalysis demonstrates heavy proteinuria in the nephrotic range on a 24-h collection. However, GFR is usually normal and serum creatinine and urea are in the normal range. There is usually hypoalbuminaemia and often hyperlipidaemia, which arises in the nephrotic syndrome. In adults, renal biopsy may be performed to exclude other conditions, but children are usually treated with a trial of steroids without a biopsy.

Differential diagnosis

The differential diagnosis includes other causes of the nephrotic syndrome, especially focal segmental glomerulosclerosis and membranous nephropathy, amyloidosis, diabetic nephropathy, lupus and, rarely, a congenital nephrotic syndrome.

Management

The mainstay of treatment is steroids. Usually, they reverse the nephrotic syndrome, but sometimes the nephrotic syndrome relapses when they are stopped. If there are frequent relapses or a poor response to steroids, then cyclophosphamide or cyclosporin are useful. The oedema itself may require treatment with diuretics, such as frusemide (furosemide). Lipid-lowering drugs (usually a 'statin' hydroxymethyl glutaryl coenzyme A (HMG-CoA) reductase inhibitor) are necessary, if there is prolonged nephrotic syndrome with hyperlipidaemia. Penicillin prophylaxis can be given for streptococcal infection.

Prognosis and complications

The main complications are thrombosis, including renal vein thrombosis, and infection (especially streptococcal infection in children). The prognosis is that 98% of children and 94% of adults respond to steroids initially. In adults, 10–20% relapse several times and 40–50% relapse frequently.

Focal segmental glomerulosclerosis
Disease mechanisms

The aetiology is unknown, but minimal change nephropathy and focal segmental glomerulosclerosis (FSGS) share similarities and some clinicians consider them to be different points on the spectrum of a single or similar disease process. Damage to the glomerular filtration barrier causes renal protein leakage and the nephrotic syndrome. Light microscopy shows that there is focal and segmental glomerular sclerosis or scarring (Fig. 8.15). Immunofluorescence demonstrates IgM and C3 in the scars and on electron microscopy there is glomerular epithelial podocyte foot process fusion, like that seen in minimal change nephropathy.

Epidemiology

The condition accounts for 15% of adult nephrotic syndrome. FSGS occurs at increased frequency in black HIV-infected intravenous drug users.

Clinical presentation

The clinical presentation can be varied and may be with proteinuria, nephrotic syndrome, hypertension or chronic renal impairment. Physical signs may include hypertension and if there is nephrotic syndrome then there will be oedema.

Investigation

Investigation may reveal both blood and protein in the urine. There may be hypoalbuminaemia and renal impairment with elevated plasma urea and creatinine levels. Renal biopsy is necessary to make the diagnosis.

08

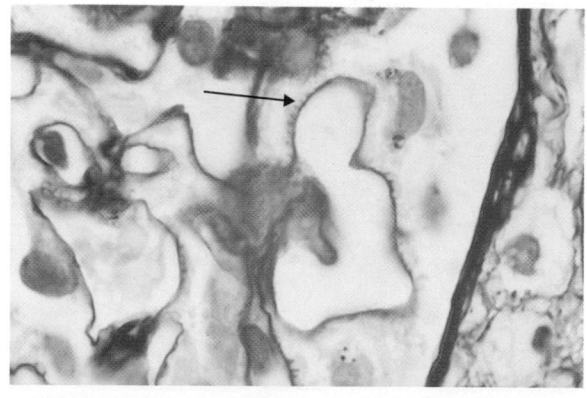

(a)

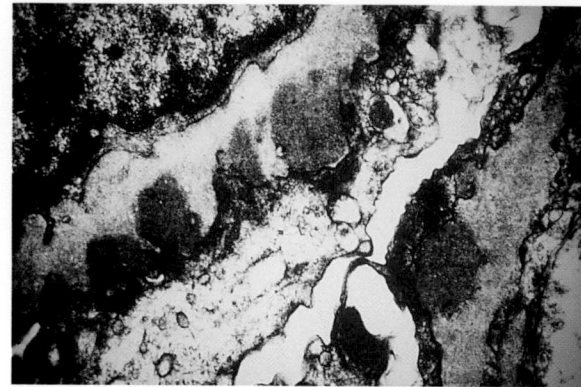

(b)

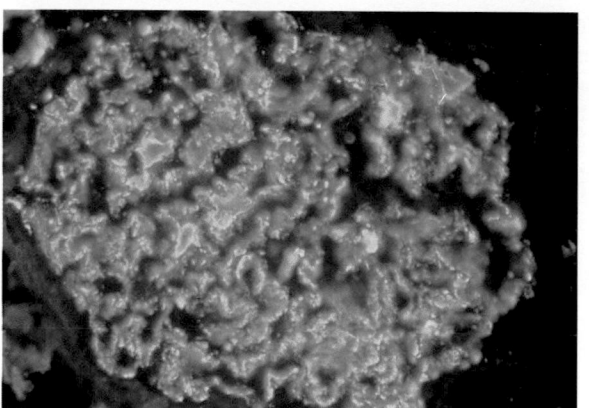

(c)

Figure 8.16 Membranous glomerulonephritis. (a) Silver stain. Note the appearance of 'spikes' on the outside of the capillary loop. The immune deposits between the 'spikes' of basement membrane do not stain with silver. (b) Electron microscopy. The immune deposits are electron dense and appear as black lumps in the basement membrane. (c) Fluorescence microscopy. IgG is shown by the fluorescence stain and is trapped in the basement membrane. The IgG appears as bright yellow-green spots and streaks.

Differential diagnosis

The differential diagnosis includes other forms of glomerulonephritis and other causes of nephrotic syndrome or renal impairment if present.

Management

Treatment can be of some use. Steroids are now thought to be of benefit and cyclophosphamide may be added as a means of reducing the steroid dose. Cyclosporin can also be beneficial. Blood pressure should be controlled. Angiotensin-converting enzyme (ACE) inhibitors help control blood pressure and have an antiproteinuric effect.

Prognosis and complications

The prognosis is not good, as 40–60% develop end-stage renal disease within 10 years of diagnosis. The nephrotic syndrome remits in up to 40% of both adults and children in response to steroids and those who do respond have a better renal prognosis. Complications that may arise include those of nephrotic syndrome (such as thrombosis and infection), of chronic renal impairment and of hyperlipidaemia if present. Unfortunately, FSGS can recur in a transplanted kidney from a donor who did not have the disease.

Membranous nephropathy

Disease mechanisms

The aetiology of membranous nephropathy is unknown. Damage to the glomerular filtration barrier causes a protein leak and the nephrotic syndrome. Light microscopy shows glomerular basement membrane thickening. Immunofluorescence shows immunoglobulin and complement deposition and electron microscopy shows subepithelial membrane deposits (Fig. 8.16). There are important disease associations with hepatitis B, malignancy, systemic lupus erythematosus, mercury exposure and the use of certain drugs (notably gold and penicillamine).

Epidemiology

This is the most common cause of adult nephrotic syndrome in the UK and the peak age incidence is between 30 and 50 years.

Clinical presentation

Clinical presentation may be with the nephrotic syndrome, chronic renal impairment, hypertension or asymptomatic microscopic proteinuria or haematuria. Physical signs may include hypertension or oedema if there is nephrotic syndrome.

Investigation

Investigation usually reveals protein, often with blood in the urine. There may be a low plasma albumin level as a result of the proteinuria and raised urea and creatinine levels. The diagnosis is made by renal biopsy.

Differential diagnosis

The differential diagnosis includes other forms of glomerulonephritis and other causes of nephrotic syndrome or renal impairment if present.

Management

Treatment is with steroids and chlorambucil (the 'Ponticelli regimen') and this can slow the loss of renal function. Cyclophosphamide has also been used instead of chlorambucil. Blood pressure should be controlled, as this may reduce the rate of deterioration of renal function. Complications include those of nephrotic syndrome, chronic renal impairment and hyperlipidaemia if present. The hyperlipidaemia can occur as part of the nephrotic syndrome caused by the protein leak.

Prognosis and complications

The prognosis is not good, as although 20–30% of cases remit spontaneously and 40% have a partial remission or remain stable, around 30% develop progressive renal failure.

IgA nephropathy

Disease mechanisms

The aetiology is unknown, although it has been suggested that it is related to aberrant switching of IgA subclasses during mucosal immune responses. Deposition of IgA

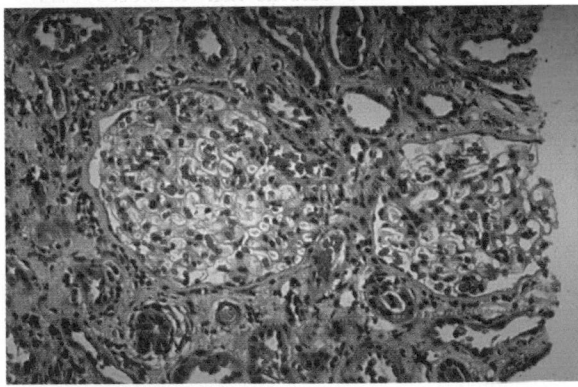

Figure 8.17 Light microscopy of IgA nephropathy. Two glomeruli are seen in this section of tissue which has been stained with haematoxylin and eosin. The increased amount of mesangial matrix is visible as bright pink material in the glomeruli. There is also an increase in the number of mesangial cells in the glomeruli.

in the kidney occurs and this may trigger complement-mediated damage. On light microscopy there is expansion of the mesangial matrix and proliferation of mesangial cells (see Fig. 8.17). Immunofluorescence shows **IgA deposits** in the mesangium (Fig. 8.18). There are associations with liver disease, alcoholic and viral hepatitis and coeliac disease, and a form of HIV-associated IgA nephropathy can occur.

Epidemiology

IgA is a relatively common form of glomerulonephritis

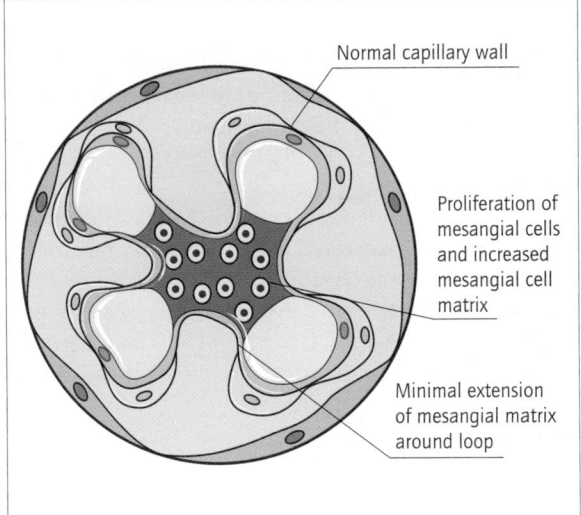

(a)

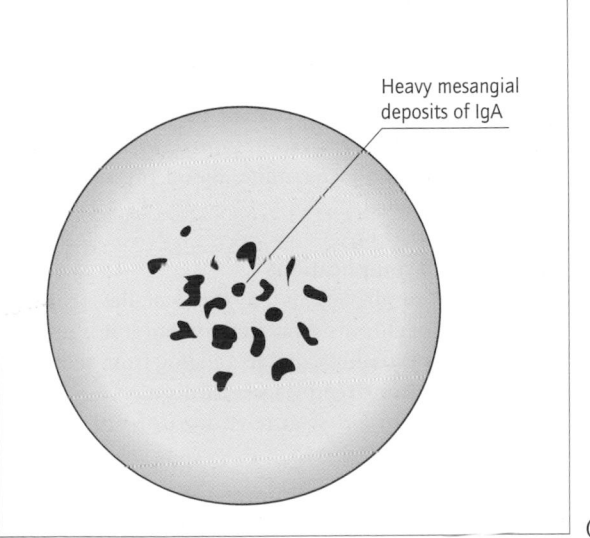

(b)

Figure 8.18 IgA nephropathy. (a) Light microscopy. A schematic view of the changes seen in IgA nephropathy. (b) Immunostaining. This is the pattern of IgA deposition that would be seen in the glomerulus shown in (a).

with a prevalence of 2 per 10 000. The peak incidence is in the second and third decades and the male : female ratio is 3.6 : 1. Curiously, postmortem studies have revealed similar renal changes in 2–5% of all postmortem cases. IgA nephropathy is more common in poorer countries.

Clinical presentation

The classic clinical presentation is with 'synpharyngitic' haematuria, which is macroscopic haematuria at the same time as, or 1–2 days after, a sore throat. However, IgA nephropathy can often come to clinical attention as asymptomatic microscopic haematuria, hypertension, renal impairment, the nephrotic syndrome or, rarely, as acute nephritic syndrome. There are no specific physical signs, although hypertension may be present or there may be signs of the complications of renal impairment or nephrotic syndrome if these are present.

Investigation

Investigations may demonstrate blood and protein in the urine. Blood tests may reveal evidence of renal impairment with raised urea and creatinine levels. In 50% of cases, serum IgA levels are elevated. A definitive diagnosis can only be made by renal biopsy (see Fig. 8.17). The differential diagnosis is of other forms of glomerulonephritis.

Differential diagnosis

The differential diagnosis includes other forms of glomerulonephritis and other causes of nephrotic syndrome or renal impairment if present.

Management

The role of treatment is unclear. Benefit is claimed for ACE inhibitors, fish oils and steroids. Steroids are usually given if there is severe persistent nephrotic syndrome. Aggressive disease with crescent formation is treated with steroids and cyclophosphamide. Blood pressure should always be controlled.

Prognosis and complications

The possible complications are those of the nephrotic syndrome or of chronic renal impairment if it is present. The prognosis is highly variable, ranging from remission to rapid progression to end-stage renal disease. Overall, 15% of patients develop end-stage renal disease by 10 years and 20–30% by 20 years.

Membranoproliferative or mesangiocapillary glomerulonephritis

Disease mechanisms

The aetiology of this condition is unknown, although if cryoglobulinaemia is present, hepatitis C is often the underlying cause. Light microscopy shows expansion of the mesangial matrix and proliferation of mesangial cells

as in IgA nephropathy. However, in addition there is thickening of the glomerular basement membrane. Two subtypes of this condition can be distinguished on the basis of immunofluorescence and electron microscopy. The most common form is **type I** disease in which immunofluorescence shows immunoglobulin and complement deposition and electron microscopy shows **subendothelial** deposits. In contrast, in the less common form or **type II** disease, immunofluorescence shows some C3 deposition and electron microscopy shows intramembranous deposits and **subepithelial** deposits. There are important disease associations; infection is commonly found, especially with the hepatitis viruses B and most importantly hepatitis C. Autoimmune disease can also be present, especially systemic lupus erythematosus. Other associations include complement deficiency syndromes and partial lipodystrophy, which is associated with type II disease. Hypogammaglobulinaemia has also been associated with the condition.

Epidemiology

Overall, the disease accounts for 10–20% of biopsies performed for presumed primary glomerulonephritis and 80% of cases are of type I disease. The disease appears to be declining in developed countries.

Clinical presentation

Clinical presentation can vary from symptomatic haematuria or proteinuria to acute nephritis or severe nephrotic syndrome. There are no specific physical signs, although hypertension and signs of renal impairment or the nephrotic syndrome may be present.

Investigation

Investigations typically reveal blood and protein in the urine. Blood tests can indicate renal impairment, hypoalbuminaemia and low complement levels, especially C3. In type II disease there may be antibodies to the C3 convertase C3bBb resulting in complement activation. Renal biopsy provides a definitive diagnosis.

Differential diagnosis

The differential diagnosis is of other forms of glomerulonephritis and causes of acute nephritis (the nephritic syndrome), chronic renal impairment and the nephrotic syndrome if they are present. Both postinfectious glomerulonephritis and systemic lupus erythematosus can also cause renal disease and hypocomplementaemia.

Management

Treatment must involve the treatment of any underlying cause. Although steroids and cytotoxic agents have been used, their benefit is unproven in adults. Blood pressure should be controlled.

Prognosis and complications

Complications include those of the nephrotic syndrome or of chronic renal impairment if present. There is a high recurrence rate after renal transplantation. The prognosis is that 50% of patients develop end-stage renal disease by 10 years and 90% by 20 years.

Diffuse proliferative glomerulonephritis (acute endocapillary glomerulonephritis)

Disease mechanisms

This type of glomerulonephritis can be idiopathic, secondary to infection (typically poststreptococcal infection) or associated with another condition such as IgA nephropathy or systemic lupus erythematosus. Light microscopy shows endothelial and mesangial cell proliferation and glomerular infiltration with neutrophils and monocytes. The increased cellularity can occlude the glomerular capillary loops and so contribute to a fall in GFR. Immunofluorescence shows complement and immunoglobulins and subepithelial deposits can be seen on electron microscopy.

Epidemiology

The condition is now declining in developing countries where it accounts for around 10% of glomerular disease, but is the most common histological presentation of intrinsic renal disease in developing countries. The peak age of incidence is 2–12 years and the male : female ratio is 2 : 1.

Clinical presentation

Clinical presentation is typically 1–2 weeks after a streptococcal throat infection or 3–6 weeks after a streptococcal skin infection. The presentation can vary from asymptomatic microscopic haematuria to acute nephritic syndrome with frank haematuria, oedema, hypertension and oliguria. There may be physical signs indicating the precipitating infection or signs consistent with the acute nephritic syndrome such as hypertension and oedema.

Investigation

Investigation shows blood in the urine in all cases and sometimes protein. Red cell casts are common. Blood tests may indicate impaired renal function with elevated plasma urea and creatinine. There may also be serological evidence of infection such as raised antistreptolysin O titres (ASOT), which indicate streptococcal infection. Low complement levels, especially C3, are often found. The differential diagnosis is of mesangiocapillary glomerulonephritis or systemic lupus erythematosus.

Management

Treatment is with antibiotics to ensure infection is eradicated. Blood pressure should be controlled and oedema treated with diuretics.

Prognosis and complications

The prognosis is good as only 0.1–1% have progressive renal impairment. Complications include those of any ongoing infection or of uncontrolled oedema or hypertension.

Antiglomerular basement membrane disease

Disease mechanisms

In this condition, there is tissue damage in the kidneys and the lungs caused by autoantibodies to the basement membrane in the glomeruli and in the alveoli. The antibodies are against an antigen that is usually part of the non-collagenous domain of the alpha-3 component of type IV collagen. Light microscopy shows focal segmental proliferative glomerulonephritis, often with necrosis and crescents (Fig. 8.19). Immunofluorescence shows antibody deposition (usually IgG) along the glomerular basement membrane—the antibody deposited is the antiglomerular basement membrane antibody. Electron microscopy is

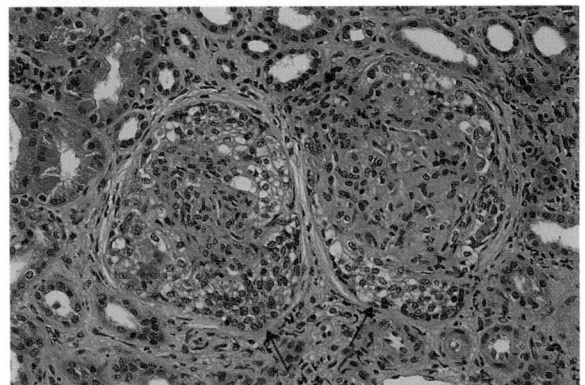

(a)

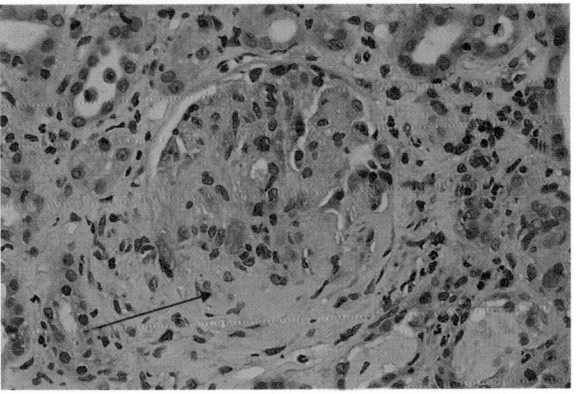

(b)

Figure 8.19 Crescentic glomerulonephritis (rapidly progressive glomerulonephritis). (a) Cellular crescents. The arrows indicate cellular crescents with active inflammatory cells within the glomerulus. (b) Collagenous crescents. Active cellular inflammation can lead to the laying down of collagen and in this specimen, large crescents can be seen which are formed by deposited collagen and which are now compressing and infarcting the glomerulus.

not usually necessary to make the diagnosis, but shows frequent breaks in a widened and damaged glomerular basement membrane with occasional deposits. The disease is strongly associated with HLA-DR15.

Epidemiology

The condition is rare, affecting only 0.5–1 per million, most of whom are white and male.

Clinical presentation

In 50–70% of cases, the presentation is with the features of lung haemorrhage causing cough, haemoptysis or shortness of breath. Renal involvement is initially asymptomatic, but can cause loin pain, frank haematuria, oliguria and acute renal failure. Pulmonary haemorrhage is more common if the patient is a smoker or has pulmonary infection or oedema, or if there is exposure to other inhaled toxins. Physical signs in the lung may resemble those of pulmonary oedema or infection.

Investigation

The urine may contain blood and protein and also red cell casts. Blood tests typically indicate acute renal impairment, with raised urea and creatinine levels. The key test is the detection of antiglomerular basement membrane antibodies in plasma. On a chest radiograph, diffuse pulmonary haemorrhage may resemble pulmonary oedema or infection. Lung function tests may show a raised gas transfer (KCO). This rise is an artefact caused by the absorption of carbon monoxide used in the test by blood that has leaked into the alveoli.

Differential diagnosis

The differential diagnosis is of systemic vasculitis, another glomerulonephritis with pulmonary oedema or pulmonary infection.

Management

Treatment is with plasma exchange to remove the pathogenic antibody and immunosuppression with steroids and cyclophosphamide to inhibit further antibody production and reduce inflammatory damage. Azathioprine may be substituted for cyclophosphamide in the later stages of treatment.

Prognosis and complications

Complications include respiratory failure, secondary pulmonary infection and toxicity from the treatment, especially infection or bone marrow suppression. The prognosis is that untreated, most patients will die. Patients who require dialysis before treatment is started do not usually recover renal function. If the plasma creatinine is less than 600 μmol/l before treatment, 80–90% of patients recover independent renal function.

Crescentic glomerulonephritis (rapidly progressive glomerulonephritis, focal necrotizing glomerulonephritis or renal microscopic polyangiitis)

Disease mechanisms

The aetiology of this condition varies and is often unknown. There are three types, caused by either:

1 Antiglomerular basement membrane antibodies (see p. 521).

2 Renal microscopic vasculitis, often but not always in the presence of systemic vasculitis. The systemic vasculitic diseases include microscopic polyangiitis, Wegener's granulomatosis, polyarteritis nodosa and Churg–Strauss syndrome.

3 A complication of a pre-existing glomerulonephritis, a systemic disorder or an infection. A crescentic glomerulonephritis can occur in association with lupus, Henoch–Schönlein purpura, IgA nephropathy, mesangiocapillary glomerulonephritis and postinfectious glomerulonephritis.

In all three types, light microscopy shows a small vessel vasculitis with fibrinoid necrosis in the glomeruli, often with crescent formation (crescents are inflammatory cells in Bowman's capsule; Fig. 8.19). If the cause is antiglomerular basement membrane antibodies, then these will usually be detectable in the blood and seen along the glomerular basement membrane on immunofluorescence studies. If the cause is renal microscopic vasculitis, then serum antineutrophil cytoplasmic antibody (ANCA) may be detectable and immunofluorescence shows scant or absent immunoglobulins. In this case there may be extrarenal manifestations. If the condition arises as a complication of a pre-existing glomerulonephritis, a systemic disorder or an infection, there is often immunoglobulin deposition on immunofluorescence.

Epidemiology

Crescentic glomerulonephritis accounts for around 2–5% of renal biopsies, and the male : female ratio is 2 : 1.

Clinical presentation

The renal disease is often asymptomatic but can result in oliguria and acute renal failure. More typically, the extrarenal manifestations of associated or underlying systemic diseases may be the presenting features. There may be systemic symptoms such as fever, weight loss and general malaise. Physical signs include manifestations of systemic disease, such as rashes or joint lesions.

Investigation

The urine may contain blood, protein and red blood cell casts. Blood tests may reveal evidence of renal impairment with raised urea and creatinine levels. There may also be raised inflammatory markers, such as C-reactive protein

(CRP), erythrocyte sedimentation rate (ESR) and elevated white cell and platelet counts. Immunological tests can indicate the cause of the renal disease and should include ANCA and antiglomerular basement membrane antibody. Renal biopsy is usually undertaken to make the diagnosis.

Differential diagnosis
The differential diagnosis is of other causes of acute renal failure (see p. 549).

Management
Treatment is with immunosuppression. Initially this is with prednisolone and cyclophosphamide, but later azathioprine may be substituted for the cyclophosphamide. Plasma exchange is used for antiglomerular basement membrane antibody disease (to remove the pathogenic antibodies) and sometimes for severe systemic vasculitis. Complications include those of immunosuppression and of acute renal failure. The prognosis is that less than 25% escape dialysis but, with treatment, the 5-year survival off dialysis is 60–80%.

Secondary glomerular disease

Glomerular disease can be secondary to many conditions and is considered under these conditions (see diabetes mellitus, hypertension, systemic lupus erythematosus, rheumatoid arthritis, systemic vasculitis). However, two conditions are discussed below because of their diagnostic importance.

Malignancy-associated glomerulonephritis
Disease mechanisms and epidemiology
The mechanism of this glomerulonephritis is unclear, but most patterns of glomerulonephritis can occur and the renal disease may improve with treatment of the malignancy. Approximately 15–60% of patients with malignancy have urinary abnormalities and up to 17% of patients with solid tumours have histologically evident glomerular changes. Membranous nephropathy is the most common histological type.

Clinical presentation
The presentation varies from an asymptomatic urinary or plasma abnormality to nephrotic syndrome or acute renal failure. Physical signs depend on the tumour and the renal pathology.

Investigation
Investigation is that of any glomerular disease and usually includes urine examination, plasma biochemistry and renal biopsy if necessary, as well as investigation of the malignancy itself.

Differential diagnosis
The differential diagnosis is that of other tumour-related causes of renal dysfunction including obstruction, invasion of the renal tract, renal vein thrombosis, urate nephropathy, hypercalcaemia and drug toxicity.

Management, prognosis and complications
Treatment is that of the malignancy. Complications are those of the malignancy and its therapy as well as nephrotic syndrome, hypertension or renal impairment if present. The prognosis depends on the malignancy, but generally renal involvement is associated with a worsened prognosis for the malignancy.

Infection-related glomerulonephritis
Disease mechanisms
The mechanism of this condition is usually unclear, but pathogen antigens may trigger an aberrant immune response causing renal damage. Most patterns of glomerulonephritis can occur (Table 8.1). Important problems are particularly associated with hepatitis C virus, hepatitis B virus, HIV, streptococcal infection and syphilis.

Clinical presentation
The clinical presentation and physical signs are highly variable, depending on the infection and its associated renal disease. Acute infections can cause a diffuse proliferative glomerulonephritis.

Investigation
Investigation is as for any glomerular disease and may include urine examination, plasma biochemistry and renal biopsy. Specific investigations should also aim to diagnose any suspected infection.

Differential diagnosis
The differential diagnosis should include AA amyloidosis, which can occur with chronic infection and drug toxicity, which may occur when infections are treated.

Management, prognosis and complications
The infection should always be treated where this is possible. The prognosis depends on the infection. Complications are those of the nephrotic syndrome, hypertension and renal impairment if present.

Hepatitis B virus-associated renal disease
Acute hepatitis B infection may be associated with microscopic haematuria, proteinuria and a mesangial proliferative glomerulonephritis. However, this type of acute renal pathology resolves with the acute hepatitis and with viral clearance in 90% of patients. The 10% of hepatitis B cases who become chronic carriers are

Table 8.1 Disease associations

Disease	Association
Hepatitis B	Membranous nephropathy
	Mesangiocapillary glomerulonephritis (type I)
	IgA nephropathy
Hepatitis C	Mesangiocapillary glomerulonephritis (type I)
	Mixed 'essential' cryoglobulinaemia type II (polyclonal IgG or monoclonal IgM)
HIV	Focal segmental glomerulosclerosis
EBV	Microscopic haematuria and proteinuria
Streptococcal infection	Poststreptococcal glomerulonephritis (diffuse proliferative glomerulonephritis)
Staphylococcal infection (endocarditis, shunt infections, general sepsis)	Diffuse proliferative glomerulonephritis or focal segmental proliferative glomerulonephritis, or type I mesangiocapillary glomerulonephritis
Salmonella infections	Mesangiocapillary glomerulonephritis
	IgA nephropathy
Tuberculosis	Amyloidosis
Leprosy	Amyloidosis
	Diffuse proliferative glomerulonephritis
	Mesangiocapillary glomerulonephritis
Syphilis	Nephrotic syndrome, usually caused by membranous nephropathy
E. coli and other enteric infections	Can cause haemolytic–uraemic syndrome (see p. 531)
Leptospirosis	Causes an acute tubulo-interstitial nephritis
Malaria	Associated with glomerulonephritis and the nephrotic syndrome

those in whom the syndromes of hepatitis B-associated glomerulonephritis and polyarteritis nodosa (PAN) occur.

Hepatitis B virus-associated glomerulonephritis. Patients present clinically with proteinuria and often renal dysfunction in association with a history or serological evidence of hepatitis B infection. The histological pattern is usually of membranous glomerulonephritis. Progressive disease does not respond to conventional therapy for membranous glomerulonephritis. Antiviral therapy with α-interferon may be beneficial.

Hepatitis B virus-associated polyarteritis nodosa. This is a vasculitis affecting small and medium-sized arteries. It usually presents within weeks to months of initial infection. Typical clinical features are rash, fever and arthralgia. The vasculitis can affect any organ, with renal involvement being common and associated with hypertension, proteinuria, haematuria and renal impairment. Diagnosis is made on the basis of hepatitis B serology, renal biopsy and angiography to demonstrate the medium-sized vessel vasculitis. Treatment with both steroids and cytotoxic agents improves long-term survival.

Hepatitis C virus-associated renal disease
Hepatitis C is the most common cause of cryoglobulinaemia with or without renal involvement. The renal lesion is usually a membranous glomerulonephritis. Some cases have remitted with antiviral therapy.

Human immunodeficiency virus-associated renal disease
A variety of renal disorders are described in HIV-infected patients. However, the clinically most significant form is an aggressive focal and segmental glomerular sclerosis characterized clinically by massive proteinuria and rapid progression to end-stage renal disease (within 3–4 months).

Malaria-associated renal disease
Plasmodium falciparum infection can be associated with a transient glomerulonephritis, which is rarely associated with renal impairment (blackwater fever). *Plasmodium malariae* infection can be associated with a chronic progressive glomerulonephritis, which usually presents with the nephrotic syndrome. Renal biopsy shows a mesangiocapillary glomerulonephritis, which does not respond to antimalarial therapy and often progresses to end-stage renal disease.

Tubulo-interstitial disease

The glomeruli act as sieves, producing 150 l of glomerular filtrate each day. The tubules, with their supporting interstitial structures, act on this filtrate to reabsorb vital nutrients, to concentrate the urine and to regulate its ion and water content. Diseases of the interstitium may present as:
- Acute or chronic renal failure
- Abnormalities of tubular function
- Proteinuria

Table 8.2 The differences between glomerulonephritis and interstitial nephritis

Feature	Glomerulonephritis	Interstitial nephritis
Proteinuria	Usually >1 g/day	Usually <1 g/day
Hypertension	Usually present	Usually absent
Urinary deposit	Casts, dysmorphic red blood cells, pyuria	Pyuria, white cell casts
Renal biopsy	Glomeruli primarily affected	Glomeruli spared

- Pyuria (pus in the urine)
- Haematuria

The differences between glomerulonephritis and interstitial nephritis are summarized in Table 8.2.

Acute interstitial nephritis

Acute interstitial nephritis is characterized by an acute usually reversible infiltration of inflammatory cells into the interstitium of the kidney. It represents an important cause of acute renal failure requiring identification and wherever possible elimination or treatment of any causative agent.

Disease mechanisms

Acute interstitial nephritis is thought to represent an induced hypersensitivity reaction or allergic reaction. The causative antigen can usually be identified and is typically a drug or infectious agent. Only a small percentage of patients treated with an implicated drug develop acute interstitial nephritis (usually approximately 3 weeks after commencing therapy) but the condition will recur if the individual is re-exposed to the drug or related compounds. Table 8.3 lists some of the agents most commonly implicated in acute interstitial nephritis.

Non-steroidal anti-inflammatory drugs (NSAIDs) cause acute tubular necrosis but they can also cause salt and water retention, hypertension and papillary necrosis. Rarely, they cause a minimal change-type nephrotic syndrome.

Epidemiology

Acute interstitial nephritis causes up to 10% of acute renal failure. There are no differences in age or sex, and neither ethnic nor genetic characteristics.

Clinical features

Typically, there is sudden renal impairment with proteinuria and abnormal urinalysis (particularly pyuria or eosinophiluria). Approximately half of all patients complain of flank pain. Non-renal manifestations complicate a significant percentage of cases with maculopapular rash, fever, arthralgia and eosinophilia.

Investigation

The urine usually contains protein and often contains white cells, especially eosinophils. There may also be a high plasma eosinophil count. Renal biopsy shows interstitial oedema, acute damage to tubular cells and a prominent interstitial infiltrate.

Management

If possible, the underlying cause should be removed. Idiopathic forms may respond to steroid therapy. The patient may need dialysis for acute renal failure.

Prognosis

Acute interstitial nephritis usually resolves completely unless there is papillary necrosis or it is caused by poisoning or drug toxicity. If damage is severe, it will heal by scarring rather than by regeneration of the tubules and interstitium. This results in a variable degree of impaired renal function in the long term. The efficiency of high-dose steroids in hastening clinical recovery is unproven.

Chronic interstitial nephritis

In chronic interstitial nephritis there is tubular atrophy, interstitial fibrosis and an infiltration with chronic

Table 8.3 Causes of acute interstitial nephritis

Antimicrobial agents	NSAID	Infections	Systemic disease	Other
Benzylpenicillin	Aspirin	HIV	Sarcoid	Phenytoin
Ampicillin	Naproxen	Hanta virus	SLE	Frusemide
Amoxicillin	Indometacin		Sjögren's syndrome	Allopurinol
Ciprofloxacin	Diclofenac			Cimetidine
Methicillin	Ibuprofen			Omeprazole
Sulphonamides				
Co-trimoxazole				
Rifampicin				

HIV, human immunodeficiency virus; NSAID, non-steroidal anti-inflammatory drug; SLE, systemic lupus erythematosus.

Table 8.4 Causes of chronic tubulo-interstitial nephritis

Drugs	Toxins	Systemic diseases	Other
Analgesics	Lead	Sarcoid	Obstructive nephropathy
Lithium	Mercury	SLE	Ischaemic nephritis
Ciclosporin	Cadmium	Tuberculosis	Myeloma
Cisplatinum	Other heavy metals	Sjögren's syndrome	Urate nephropathy
Aminoglycosides	Solvents		Hereditary nephritis (Balkan nephropathy)
			Radiation nephritis
			Chronic hypokalaemia

inflammatory cells (which is less marked than in acute interstitial nephritis) and proliferation of interstitial fibroblasts. It is an insidious process, which may lead to chronic and even end-stage renal failure.

Disease mechanisms

The tubules and interstitium can be directly injured by a variety of agents including drugs, toxins and infectious agents (Table 8.4). Tubular obstruction or ischaemia can also lead to typical histological change. The tubules and interstitium can also be injured in glomerular disease, presumably through the effects of cytokine release, ischaemia or proteinuria. Indeed, numerous studies have demonstrated a strong positive correlation between the degree of interstitial damage and a decline in renal function in a wide variety of primary glomerular diseases.

Chronic renal failure caused by analgesics mainly results from papillary necrosis, but NSAIDs can also cause chronic interstitial nephritis.

Epidemiology

Chronic interstitial nephritis is rare, but causes up to 10% of chronic renal failure.

Clinical features

There is usually low-level non-nephrotic range proteinuria with a relatively inactive urinary sediment (no cellular casts). The degree of renal impairment is variable. Damage to tubular function can result in a urinary concentrating defect, producing a dilute urine. There may also be other abnormalities of tubular function such as glycosuria, phosphaturia and bicarbonaturia (which causes renal tubular acidosis).

Investigation

Imaging of the kidneys can reveal macroscopic abnormalities in analgesic nephropathy or obstructive nephropathy, but where kidney size is normal renal biopsy is diagnostic.

Management

It is important to treat or remove the cause. This may involve antituberculous therapy in the presence of tuberculosis, or occasionally a trial of therapy if the diagnosis is unclear. In autoimmune disease steroids are usually given, and in the case of urate nephropathy allopurinol is given.

Prognosis

In chronic interstitial nephritis there is, by definition, irreversible structural damage and scarring. However, treatment of underlying hyperuricaemia, myeloma, tuberculosis or sarcoid may halt progression.

Papillary necrosis

This is a necrosis of the renal papillae involving the medulla and is often associated with cortical changes of chronic interstitial nephritis.

Disease mechanisms

Causes of papillary necrosis are:
- Analgesic abuse (more common in women), caused mainly by mixtures containing phenacetin, which is no longer available. High doses of other analgesics have also been implicated
- Sickle cell anaemia
- Severe pyelonephritis, especially in diabetes mellitus or in combination with urinary tract obstruction
- Liver disease, especially alcoholic liver disease

Epidemiology

It is most common in middle-aged women and usually occurs after many years of continued analgesic use. Papillary necrosis from other causes is uncommon.

Clinical features

Papillary necrosis may present with acute renal failure caused by ureteric obstruction by sloughed papillae or to severe interstitial inflammation. It may also present with chronic renal failure or a urine-concentrating defect. It may be complicated by the development of a urothelial tumour.

Investigation

Imaging with intravenous urography, CT scanning or a

Table 8.5 Tubular syndromes

Defect	Comment
Proximal tubule	
Aminoaciduria	Cystinuria (amino acids only): defective amino acid reabsorption causes excess urinary cystine which can form renal calculi (see p. 564)
Renal glycosuria	Defective glucose reabsorption causing glucosuria with a normal plasma glucose
Phosphaturia	e.g. hypophosphataemic rickets (see p. 590)
Bicarbonaturia	Defective proximal tubular bicarbonate reabsorption causing renal tubular acidosis type 2 (see p. 593)
Chloride leak	Bartter's syndrome (see p. 535)
Multiple abnormalities	Fanconi's syndrome (defective proximal tubular reabsorption of multiple substances causing glycosuria, phosphaturia and bicarbonaturia)
Distal tubule	
Nephrogenic diabetes insipidus	Impaired water reabsorption resulting from defects in collecting ducts (see p. 582)
Sodium-wasting nephropathy	e.g. chronic interstitial nephritis and any cause of interstitial damage
Bicarbonaturia	Defective distal tubular bicarbonate reabsorption causing renal tubular acidosis type 1 (see p. 593)

08

retrograde urogram may reveal the characteristic defects caused by sloughing of the papillae.

Management

Management involves stopping causative analgesics, treatment of any infection and the avoidance of sickle cell crises in patients with sickle cell disease. Sloughed papillae causing obstruction usually pass spontaneously, but occasionally surgical intervention is necessary to relieve the obstruction.

Prognosis

Prognosis depends upon the severity of damage at presentation (papillae cannot regenerate) and whether the underlying cause can be removed to prevent progression.

Abnormalities of tubular function

Diseases of the interstitium and renal tubules can present with renal impairment, proteinuria, pyuria, haematuria and urine-concentrating defects or specific wasting syndromes, with inappropriate loss of one or more ions or compounds.

Disease mechanisms

Syndromes of renal tubular dysfunction are usually caused by a genetic defect (usually a single gene disorder) or by a disease causing more general structural damage. One or more metabolic pathways can be affected, resulting in inappropriate loss of essential ions or nutrients (Table 8.5).

Epidemiology

The proximal tubular syndromes are congenital and rare (e.g. cystinosis has a prevalence of less than 1 in 20 000).

The distal tubular syndromes may be congenital (e.g. nephrogenic diabetes insipidus) or acquired as a result of tubulo-interstitial damage (e.g. sodium wasting or distal renal tubular acidosis). Distal tubular syndromes are most commonly seen as complications of chronic interstitial nephritis, reflux nephropathy or polycystic kidney disease. The various tubular syndromes are explained in Table 8.5.

Clinical features

The important syndromes are described in more detail in other sections (see cross-references in Table 8.5).

Fanconi's syndrome

The hallmark of Fanconi's syndrome is that it includes loss of more than one substance from the proximal tubules. Fanconi's syndrome can be caused by several different genetic defects (autosomal dominant, recessive or X-linked). It can also be secondary to many causes of interstitial damage including myeloma, heavy metal poisoning, inborn errors of metabolism or malignancy. Because there are many different causes, the manifestations and severity are variable. Typically, there is damage to several tubular pathways responsible for reabsorbing substances filtered by the glomeruli, such as amino acids, glucose, phosphate, bicarbonate, sodium, calcium and water. There may also be loss of potassium and proteinuria and the end results may include systemic acidosis, malnutrition, rickets, hypotension and dangerous episodes of hypokalaemia or dehydration. It can progress to chronic renal failure. Treatment is supportive. Any treatable cause should be treated.

Sodium wasting

Any cause of chronic interstitial nephritis can impair tubular reabsorption of sodium, chloride or bicarbonate

08

and result in sodium wasting. Even minor degrees of damage mean that patients are unable to conserve sodium in adverse circumstances and so any intercurrent illness such as diarrhoea can cause profound dehydration. Clinical features include hypotension, hypovolaemia and acute renal failure if dehydration is severe.

Renal glycosuria

In renal glycosuria the plasma glucose remains within the normal range. When this is an isolated defect it is a benign condition.

Systemic diseases affecting the kidney

Diabetes mellitus (see Chapter 11)

Disease mechanisms

Diabetic nephropathy is a glomerulonephropathy rather than a glomerulonephritis because it is not thought to be mediated by immunological mechanisms.

Type 1 diabetes mellitus nephropathy passes through five stages:
1 *Initial hyperfiltration:* with a raised glomerular filtration rate
2 *Microalbuminuria:* dipstick tests for protein are negative, but more sensitive radioimmunoassay tests for urinary albumin are positive, and the glomerular filtration rate falls to normal
3 *Glomerular proteinuria:* dipstick tests for protein are positive
4 *Substantial proteinuria:* more than 1 g/day and sometimes heavy enough to cause nephrotic syndrome, and diminishing glomerular filtration rate
5 *End-stage renal disease*
In type 2 diabetes, information on natural history is not as clear but appears similar, with 30–40% of newly diagnosed type 2 diabetics having an elevated glomerular filtration rate.

Epidemiology

Diabetic nephropathy is responsible for 30–50% of patients with end-stage renal disease in western societies. Type 2 diabetes mellitus is the fastest growing cause of patients entering dialysis programmes. The many other problems experienced by these patients consume a large percentage of the resources available on renal units and the need to prevent or delay the onset of end-stage renal disease is a significant public health challenge.

Clinical presentation

Hypertension is an early feature and accelerates the progression of renal failure. Salt and water retention may be

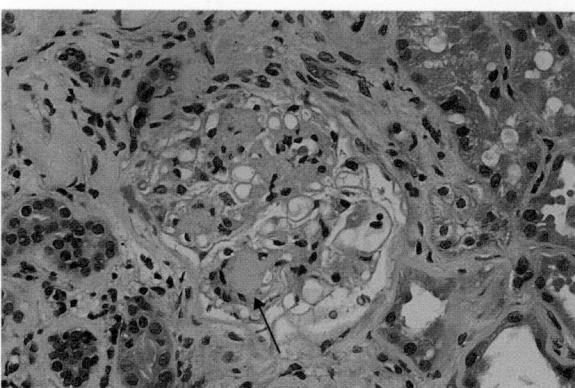

Figure 8.20 Diabetic nephropathy: appearance on light microscopy. Note the characteristic Kimmelstiel–Wilson nodules, which are rounded aggregations of the hyaline (structureless) red-staining material laid down within the glomerulus and occluding it.

marked and can cause oedema. The urine deposit may contain dysmorphic red blood cells and granular casts but does not usually contain cellular casts.

Investigation
Histopathology

Renal biopsy. Histology shows thickening of the glomerular basement membrane, the capillary wall and the mesangium, eventually resulting in glomerulosclerosis (Fig. 8.20). In a minority of patients the thickening looks like nodules within the glomerulus and these are **Kimmelstiel–Wilson lesions**, which are pathognomic of diabetic nephropathy.

Diagnostic imaging

Ultrasound should be used to check bladder emptying and exclude obstruction. **Intravenous urography** is generally avoided if possible, because diabetics are vulnerable to an acute deterioration in renal impairment caused by the nephrotoxicity of the radio-opaque dyes used.

People with diabetes mellitus may also develop hyper-reninaemia, hypoaldosteronism (presenting as hyper-kalaemia), pyelonephritis, papillary necrosis or bladder autonomic neuropathy.

Management

Strategies to prevent or delay the development and progression of diabetic nephropathy are as follows.

Intensive glycaemic control

Prospective randomized trials have shown that good glycaemic control reduces the rate of development of microalbuminuria in type 1 diabetics with normal albumin excretion. The rate of increase in albuminuria correlates with glycosylated haemoglobin in both type 1 and 2 diabetics. Although the best evidence for benefit from good glycaemic control is early in the history of diabetic nephropathy, there is now accumulating evidence that good glycaemic control can slow progression in established diabetic nephropathy (see p. 780).

Antihypertensive therapy

Hypertension is common in diabetic nephropathy and usually reflects salt and water retention. Good control of blood pressure has been shown to slow the progression of established nephropathy in type 1 diabetes. Target blood pressures have been set progressively lower, with a current suggested target of less than 130/85 mmHg in patients without proteinuria and less than 125/75 mmHg in patients with proteinuria. Additional renoprotective benefits from ACE inhibitors and angiotensin II receptor antagonists are discussed below.

Reduction in proteinuria

There is good evidence that ACE inhibitors and angiotensin II receptor antagonists have additional benefits to other antihypertensive agents in slowing the progression of diabetic nephropathy. This effect correlates with their ability to reduce proteinuria, possibly in part by relaxing the efferent arteriole and so lowering glomerular pressure. Up to 50% of diabetic patients treated with these agents show a reduction in proteinuria and the effectiveness of combination therapy with both types of drugs is yet to be established. In type 1 diabetes, captopril treatment for 5 years reduces the risk of death, dialysis or transplantation by 50%. Multicentre trials of angiotensin II receptor antagonist agents have also shown a significant reduction in the rate of progression of nephropathy in type 2 diabetes.

Other measures

In some studies, protein restriction has been shown to slow the rate of progression of nephropathy in type 1 diabetes. However, other studies have not shown any benefit and it is important to guard against severe protein restriction in patients whose diet is already limited by the demands of their blood sugar control. Protein restriction is not usually recommended. Treatment of raised plasma lipids is important to reduce the excess cardiovascular mortality these patients suffer. Evidence is now accumulating to indicate that HMG-CoA reductase inhibitors or statins may have an additional renoprotective effect.

Prognosis and complications

People with diabetes mellitus have a poorer prognosis on dialysis or after transplantation than non-diabetics because of the vascular disease and diabetic complications that they also suffer (see Chapter 11).

Systemic lupus erythematosus

Disease mechanisms

Renal involvement in systemic lupus erythematosus can vary from mild to severe. There is immune complex deposition in the glomeruli, which may in turn cause acute inflammation. On renal biopsy there are five recognized patterns of glomerulonephritis, all of which are associated with immunoglobulin and complement deposition. If a variety of immunoglobulins (IgG, IgM and IgA) are seen on immunostaining of a renal biopsy, this is suggestive of systemic lupus erythematosus. The five patterns are:

- *Type 1:* minimal change nephropathy with normal light microscopy
- *Type 2:* mesangial changes
- *Type 3:* focal proliferative glomerulonephritis
- *Type 4:* diffuse proliferative glomerulonephritis
- *Type 5:* membranous glomerulonephritis

Epidemiology

Prevalence. Renal involvement occurs in 35–75% of people with systemic lupus erythematosus.

Clinical presentation

Clinical features of renal involvement in systemic lupus erythematosus are asymptomatic proteinuria, haematuria, nephrotic syndrome, acute nephritic syndrome or more slowly progressive chronic renal failure. Very often the patient will have other features of the systemic disease, such as skin rashes, joint disease or neurological or psychiatric disturbances.

Investigation

Urine microscopy. There is usually a urine abnormality such as dysmorphic red cells and casts. The urine changes can indicate the severity of the glomerular lesion with macroscopic haematuria indicating severe type 4 disease.

Renal biopsy. The histology cannot always be accurately predicted from the clinical syndrome alone. The type of involvement is classified by the five histological patterns described above.

Management

Treatment depends on the histology and any evidence of progressing renal impairment. Corticosteroids alone do not usually halt the progression of the renal disease and need to be given in combination with a cytotoxic such as azathioprine or cyclophosphamide. Plasma exchange may be necessary for rapidly progressive glomerulonephritis.

Prognosis and complications

The most benign lesion is type 1, which does not normally

progress; types 2, 3 and 5 have an unpredictable course; type 4 usually results in end-stage renal disease if untreated. It must be remembered that renal lupus can transform spontaneously from a more benign to aggressive form and life-long monitoring is required. Resorting to repeat renal biopsy when necessary is essential for these patients' successful management.

Myeloma (see p. 1064)

Disease mechanisms

Common mechanisms of renal damage in myeloma are:

- *Hypercalcaemia:* inhibits tubular reabsorption of salt and water. This results in hypovolaemia and prerenal acute renal failure, and is the most common cause of acute renal failure in myeloma.
- *Hypovolaemia:* caused by reduced fluid intake as a result of vomiting.
- *Myeloma kidney (or cast nephropathy):* results from the formation of dense casts in the tubules, which contain antibody light chains (Bence Jones proteins). These light chains are toxic to the tubular cells and provoke tubulo-interstitial damage.
- *Light chain deposition disease:* a systemic disease that can cause renal failure because of deposition of light chains within the glomerular structures and tubular wall, rather than the formation of casts in the tubules. The deposits are only seen on electron microscopy, but can trigger mesangial proliferation producing the appearance of a nodular glomerulopathy. Light chains can also deposit and cause dysfunction in other organs such as the heart and liver.
- *Renal amyloid* (see below): can occur because of light chain deposition in amyloid fibrils.

Less commonly, renal damage is caused by hyperuricaemia following cytotoxic therapy; direct plasma cell invasion of renal tissue; hyperviscosity syndrome with IgM myeloma; or infection.

Clinical features

The usual presentation is with the features of myeloma such as bone pain or with renal impairment. The light chain deposition disease or renal amyloid may present with the nephrotic syndrome.

Management and prognosis

The treatment is that of the underlying myeloma plus supportive therapy (e.g. dialysis) as necessary. Vigorous treatment of hypovolaemia and hypercalcaemia often results in an immediate improvement of renal function. Light chain deposition disease is usually irreversible.

Fifty per cent of patients with multiple myeloma die of renal failure, but some patients may do well on dialysis for a few years while their myeloma is under control.

Amyloidosis

Disease mechanisms

Amyloidosis is characterized by the extracellular deposition of protein fibrils in many organs (see p. 814). The kidney is involved in up to 80% of patients. Amyloidosis may be primary or secondary and the fibril composition differs between the types, containing Ig light chains in AL amyloidosis associated with myeloma or a paraproteinaemia (see p. 1064) or the acute phase reactant protein serum amyloid A protein in AA amyloidosis associated with chronic inflammatory disease.

Clinical presentation

Proteinuria is common in patients with renal involvement and 25% of patients present with nephrotic syndrome. AL amyloidosis is associated with involvement of other systems (e.g. peripheral neuropathy, hepatomegaly, malabsorption). Patients with AA amyloidosis forms may present with features of the underlying disease.

Investigation

Renal biopsy. Amyloidosis is diagnosed by biopsy of affected tissues. Patients with amyloid have a greater than normal risk of haemorrhage because of the fragility of their blood vessels and renal biopsy carries an increased risk of significant bleeding. In the kidney there is a characteristic eosinophilic infiltration in glomeruli and around vessels. This amyloid infiltrate stains positively with Congo red stain and exhibits green birefringence under polarized light.

Management and prognosis

The prognosis for renal function of patients presenting with nephrotic syndrome and/or renal impairment is poor and the majority progress to end-stage renal failure. Any primary or secondary cause should be treated.

Systemic sclerosis

Systemic sclerosis is a disorder of unknown aetiology characterized by a progressive fibrosis affecting skin, blood vessels, gut, heart, lungs and kidneys (see p. 225).

Renal involvement

Renal involvement may present as proteinuria and hypertension, with a slow decline in renal function or, sometimes, a rapid decline in renal function with accelerated hypertension. Such a 'scleroderma renal crisis' is thought to result from renal arterial narrowing causing decreased renal perfusion and stimulating renin and subsequently angiotensin II production. Angiotensin II is then thought to aggravate the vascular lesion, leading to concentric intimal thickening within renal vessels and the characteristic 'onion skin' appearance. It may also cause acute vasoconstriction of the vessels, which causes further renal ischaemia and more renin production. Early recognition of a scleroderma renal crisis and treatment with ACE inhibitors may be helpful in preventing the otherwise inevitable progression to end-stage renal failure.

Sickle cell disease (see p. 1040)

Disease mechanisms

The normal renal medulla only receives blood flow from the vasa recta and may be relatively hypoxic. In sickle cell disease, hypoxia promotes sickling of the red blood cells (see Chapter 15). Therefore, sickling of red blood cells in patients with sickle cell disease is common in the medulla, and causes tubular dysfunction and interstitial damage.

Clinical features

Renal complications of sickle cell disease are:
- Minor tubular dysfunction (e.g. impairment of urine concentration and renal tubular acidosis)
- Papillary necrosis
- Frank haematuria resulting from rupture of vessels at the corticomedullary junction
- Focal segmental glomerulosclerosis and proteinuria

All these complications contribute to chronic renal failure. The glomerulonephritis often presents with nephrotic syndrome, but ends in glomerular scarring and chronic renal failure.

Management

Treatment of sickle cell disease is outlined in Chapter 15 (see p. 1041). Good medical care to limit the number of sickling crises will reduce renal damage.

Prognosis

Chronic renal failure occurs in 25% of people with homozygous sickle cell disease who reach 40 years of age and is the most common cause of death in that group.

Haemolytic–uraemic syndrome

Haemolytic–uraemic syndrome (HUS) predominantly affects children.

Disease mechanisms

There are epidemic and sporadic forms and an overlap between this condition and postpartum renal failure and thrombotic thrombocytopenic purpura, which affect adults.

Clinical features

Haemolytic–uraemic syndrome is characterized by the triad of:

- Intravascular haemolysis causing anaemia
- Thrombocytopenia
- Renal failure

In HUS, up to 75% of patients have had a preceding diarrhoeal illness, and the toxin-producing *Escherichia coli* strain 0157 has been implicated in its pathogenesis.

Investigation

The key investigation is a blood film, which shows fragmented red cells, characteristic of a haemolytic anaemia and thrombocytopenia. There may also be disseminated intravascular coagulation with raised fibrin degradation products, and a prolonged prothrombin time (PT) and activated partial thromboplastin time (APTT) are common. A renal biopsy shows fibrin thrombi occluding glomerular capillaries and sometimes there is glomerular crescent formation.

Management and prognosis

In children, the condition usually remits spontaneously, but a few children and most adults may become dialysis dependent. Plasma exchange, intravenous methylprednisolone and fresh frozen plasma have been used in adults, but their benefit is unproven.

Hereditary diseases

Polycystic kidney disease

Disease mechanisms

The genetic defect results in the formation of renal cortical cysts. The cysts may appear at any age, but are always present by the late teens or early adulthood and can be detected by ultrasound. As the cysts enlarge they compress and destroy normal renal tissue, resulting in a progressive decline in renal function. The cysts may bleed (into the cyst or urinary tract) and become acutely or chronically infected. This predisposes the patient to recurrent urinary tract infection, pyelonephritis and abscess formation.

Genetics. Adult polycystic kidney disease is usually caused by a defect in the *PKD1* gene on chromosome 16, which encodes the polycystin protein. The children of an affected parent have a 50% chance of inheriting the disease. New mutations in the gene are relatively common, so there may not be a family history. A minority of patients have mutations in the *PKD2* gene on chromosome 4 and generally have a milder form of the disease.

Epidemiology

Prevalence. 1 in 1000 live births. Adult polycystic kidney disease accounts for 8–10% of all end-stage renal disease.

08

Age. Autosomal dominant polycystic kidney disease (ADPKD) or adult polycystic kidney disease usually presents in early adult life, but it can be present at any age. A rarer autosomal recessive form presents in infancy.

Clinical presentation
Clinical features of polycystic kidney disease are haematuria, urinary tract infection and stones, renal abscess, hypertension and chronic renal failure. Subarachnoid haemorrhage can occur because of associated cerebral artery aneurysms. An association with mitral valve prolapse is described. Over time renal function deteriorates and end-stage renal disease usually occurs in later adult life.

Investigation
Ultrasound, CT or MRI scanning can all effectively diagnose the condition. Genetic diagnosis is possible within affected families.

Management
There is no treatment for the underlying disease. Good control of blood pressure, prompt treatment of infection and control of renal stones formation may help slow the progression to end-stage renal disease. Renal replacement therapy is indicated for end-stage renal disease. Families with a history of subarachnoid haemorrhage should be screened for the presence of dangerous aneurysms.

Alport's syndrome
Disease mechanisms
Alport's syndrome is an inherited disorder of basement membrane collagen (type 4 collagen). It is usually X-linked and causes severe disease in males and mild, if any, disease in females. There are abnormalities of the glomerular basement membrane, which has variable thickening, thinning and lamellations, that can only be seen with electron microscopy.

Clinical presentation
Presentation is in the first 10 years of life and affected males have persistent microscopic and sometimes macroscopic haematuria. Proteinuria and renal impairment develop later and progression to end-stage renal failure is usual in males. There is considerable variability in the rate of progression between affected families, but within each family a similar course is usually followed. Females typically have only intermittent microscopic haematuria and do not develop significant renal impairment.

Basement membrane defects outside the kidneys result in sensorineural **deafness** in over half of affected males and some affected females. One-third of patients have anterior lenticonus, which is an anterior protrusion of the lens in the eye.

Investigation
Diagnosis is based on clinical presentation, family history and renal biopsy.

Management
There is no treatment for Alport's syndrome. Patients who develop end-stage renal disease are treated with dialysis or transplantation. Male patients often require hearing aids.

Fabry's disease
Disease mechanisms
Fabry's disease is a limited genetic deficiency of the enzyme alpha galactosidase A (Gal A) resulting in intracellular accumulation of glycosphingolipid, which causes multisystem disease. The disease is X-linked, so males are severely affected and heterozygous females are mildly affected.

Clinical manifestation
The renal disease presents with proteinuria in the third decade of life. Renal impairment progresses to end-stage renal disease by the third to fourth decade of life. Systemic features include angiokeratomas of the skin, which appear as dark red papules. Coronary artery disease resulting from endothelial thickening and autonomic dysfunction are prominent features and are often the cause of death.

Investigation
Glycosphingolipid in the urine results in oval fat bodies exhibiting a characteristic 'Maltese cross' appearance under polarized microscopy. Both light and electron microscopy reveal cellular cytoplasmic vacuoles laden with glycosphingolipid and encouraging.

Management and prognosis
The prognosis is poor, but trials of regular infusions of synthetic Gal A are ongoing and encouraging.

Tuberous sclerosis (epiloia or Bourneville's disease)
Disease mechanisms
Tuberous sclerosis is characterized by multiple hamartomas. The disease is genetic and is caused by changes in the *TS* genes, which are growth regulating genes. Affected individuals have a germline defect in one of the pair of their *TS* genes in every (or most) cells in their body. The cells develop normally unless the second normal gene is damaged. If this second hit occurs in a cell, then the cell does not mature or migrate properly. Instead it forms a hamartoma and continues to proliferate while the organ

Adult polycystic kidney disease at a glance

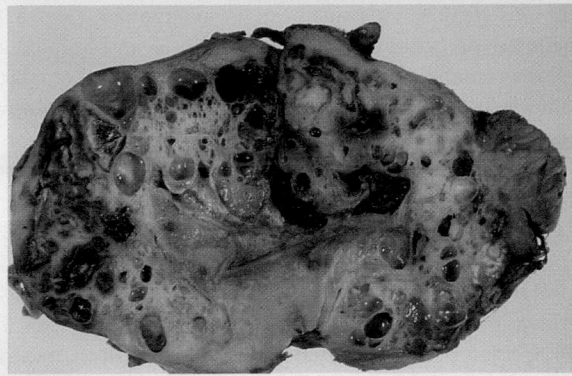

Fig. A A polycystic kidney. There are multiple cysts of different sizes, some filled with blood.

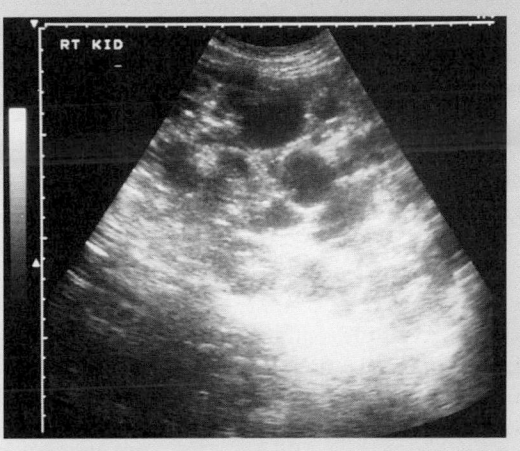

Fig. B Ultrasound of a polycystic kidney. Cysts of different sizes are scattered throughout the kidney substance and can be seen as round black shapes.

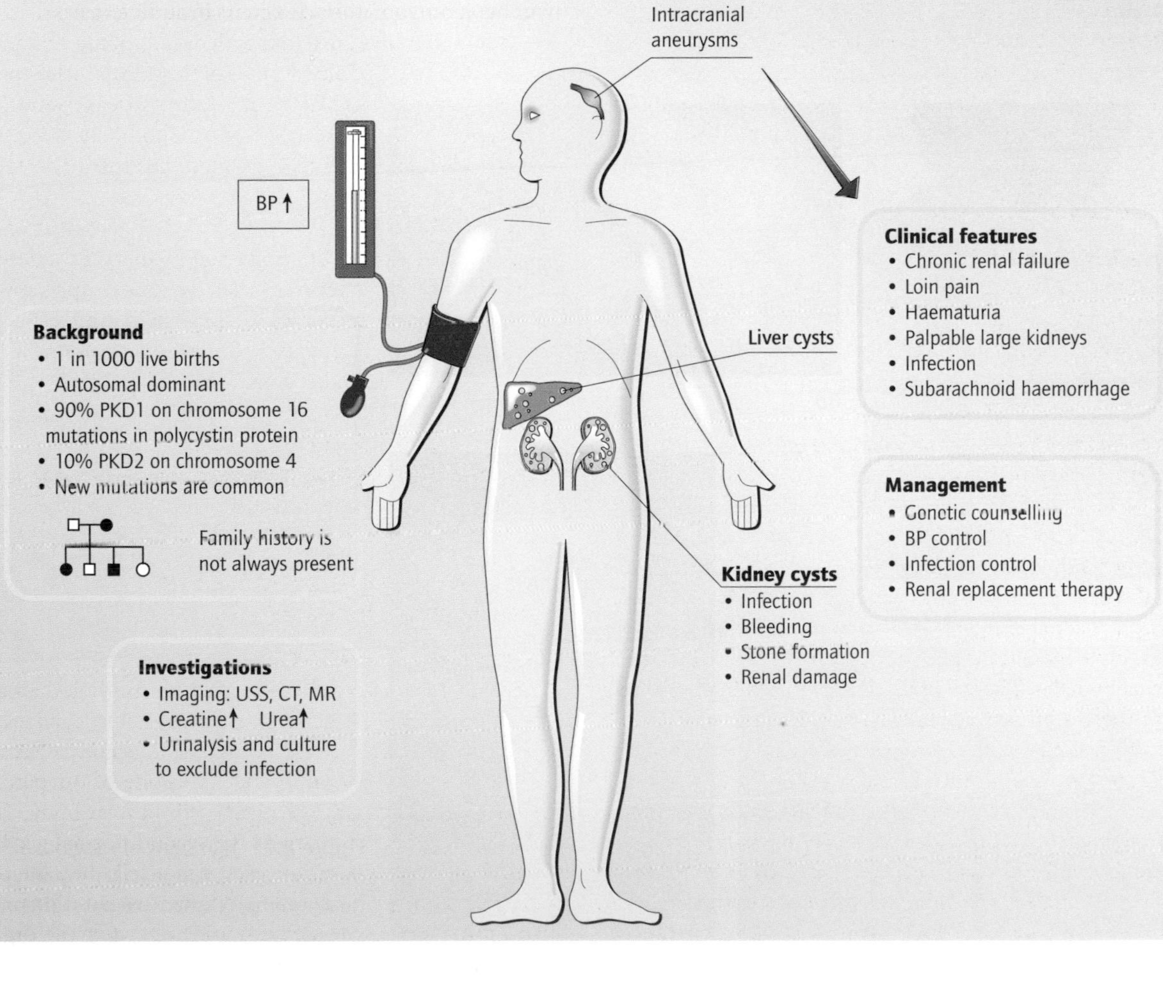

Intracranial aneurysms

BP ↑

Liver cysts

Background
- 1 in 1000 live births
- Autosomal dominant
- 90% PKD1 on chromosome 16 mutations in polycystin protein
- 10% PKD2 on chromosome 4
- New mutations are common

Family history is not always present

Clinical features
- Chronic renal failure
- Loin pain
- Haematuria
- Palpable large kidneys
- Infection
- Subarachnoid haemorrhage

Management
- Genetic counselling
- BP control
- Infection control
- Renal replacement therapy

Kidney cysts
- Infection
- Bleeding
- Stone formation
- Renal damage

Investigations
- Imaging: USS, CT, MR
- Creatine↑   Urea↑
- Urinalysis and culture to exclude infection

that it is in has growth potential. The hamartomas are thus clones from a single cell. The number of hamartomas and thus the severity of the disease depends upon the number of 'second hits'. This is random, which accounts for the variability of the condition. Occasionally, some cells suffer damage to other growth control genes and turn into benign or malignant tumours.

Epidemiology

Prevalence. 1 in 10 000 of the population.

Age. May present at any age.

Genetics. Sixty to 70% of the genetic defects are first gen-eration spontaneous mutations, the rest are autosomal dominant mutations with variable penetrance. Genetic markers have been found on chromosomes 9 and 16 (the latter is closely related to the marker for polycystic kidney disease). The affected gene on chromosome 16 has now been characterized.

Sex. Renal angiomyolipomas are more common in females.

Clinical features

The clinical features depend on the systems involved:

● *Renal involvement:* about 60% of patients have renal lesions, which are usually angiomyolipomas (Fig. 8.9, p. 513) or cysts, but occasionally focal and segmental glomerulosclerosis, renal carcinoma or urinary tract infections occur. Cysts are often few, but may be multiple or mimic polycystic kidney disease. Both angiomyolipo-mas and cysts may bleed. Renal failure may occur, and hypertension and hypercalcaemia have been reported.

● *Skin involvement* (Fig. 8.21): evident as hypomelanotic patches (white macules); angiofibroma (small red lesions in a butterfly distribution on face); shagreen patches (dark rough hands and feet).

● *Neurological manifestations:* include seizures, mental retardation, phakomas (retinal hamartomas), cortical tubers, subependymal glial nodules and giant cell astrocytomas.

● *Cardiac involvement:* cardiac rhabdomyomas in chil-dren and adults can occasionally cause obstructive symp-toms or arrhythmias. They tend to remit spontaneously.

● *Pulmonary involvement:* respiratory failure, haemopty-sis and pneumothorax can all be caused by pulmonary lymphangiomyomatosis. It occurs in adult females.

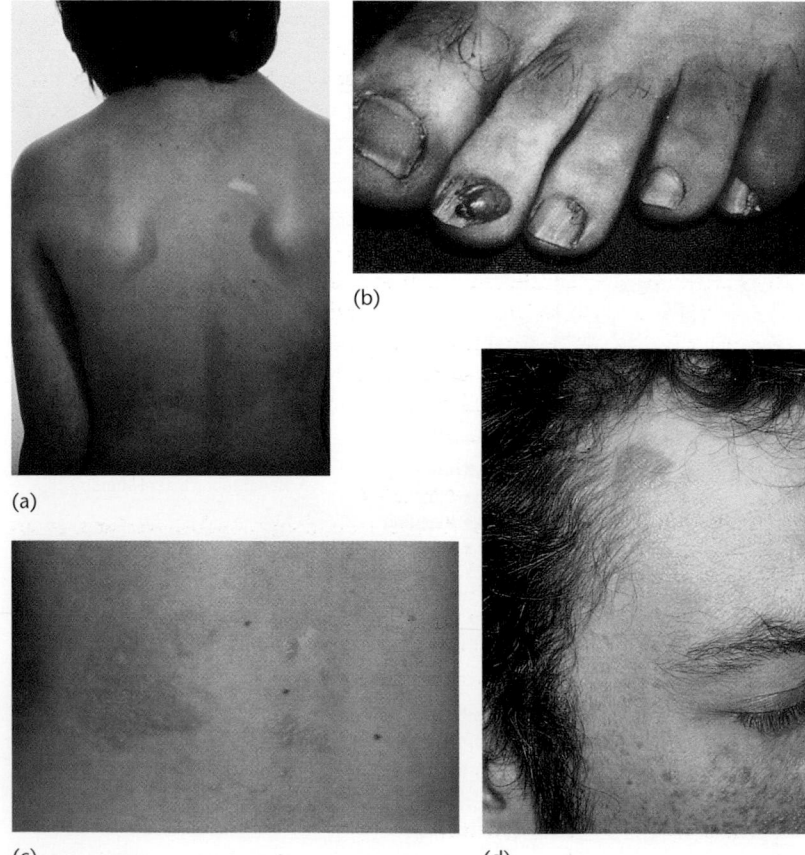

(a)

(b)

(c)

(d)

Figure 8.21 Skin signs of tuberous scle-rosis. (a) White skin macule; (b) periun-gual fibroma; (c) shagreen patch (fibrous skin plaque) on back; and (d) facial angiofibromas.

Careful clinical examination (including a skin inspection by ultraviolet light to show up hypomelanotic patches) confirms the diagnosis in most patients. Occasionally, signs may not appear until middle age (40–50 years of age).

Management and prognosis

Treat the associated problems. The angiomyolipomas that haemorrhage are almost always larger than 4 cm in diameter and may be treated by embolization of their blood supply or by surgery. The more conservative the surgery can be, the less likely renal failure is to occur.

The prognosis is very variable and, depending on the severity of clinical manifestations, ranges from death in infancy to normal adult life. For many patients the prognosis is for a normal lifespan, because the lesions are mainly hamartomas. Better understanding has markedly improved the prognosis. Dialysis and transplantation have both been used successfully in renal failure, which is rare.

Inherited tubular syndromes

Tubular epithelial cells are responsible for ion and water homoeostasis. They do this by tubular reabsorption and secretion, which is achieved by specialized channels and transporters in their cell membranes. Inherited defects of these mechanisms present clinically as disorders of ion and water handling with concomitant abnormalities of plasma electrolytes and acid–base status.

Bartter's syndrome

Bartter's syndrome is an autosomal recessive condition caused by a mutation in the NaK2Cl (NKCC2) transporter in the loop of Henle that reabsorbs sodium, potassium and chloride ions (Fig. 8.22). The effect is therefore similar to frusemide administration. The condition is characterized by sodium and chloride loss from the thick ascending loop of Henle and marked hypokalaemia. The diagnosis is made by identifying inappropriately raised urinary Na^+, K^+ and Cl^-. Plasma renin and aldosterone levels are elevated but hypertension is not a feature. Urinary calcium may be high and nephrocalcinosis may develop.

Treatment

In the acute situation, appropriate intravenous fluid and electrolyte replacement is indicated. Long-term potassium chloride supplementation is always necessary. Long-term prostaglandin synthetase inhibitors are beneficial, probably by decreasing Na^+ and Cl^- delivery to the distal tubule. ACE inhibitors, spironolactone and magnesium replacement may also be beneficial.

Prognosis

With therapy, most children develop normally although chronic interstitial fibrosis may develop, particularly in association with nephrocalcinosis.

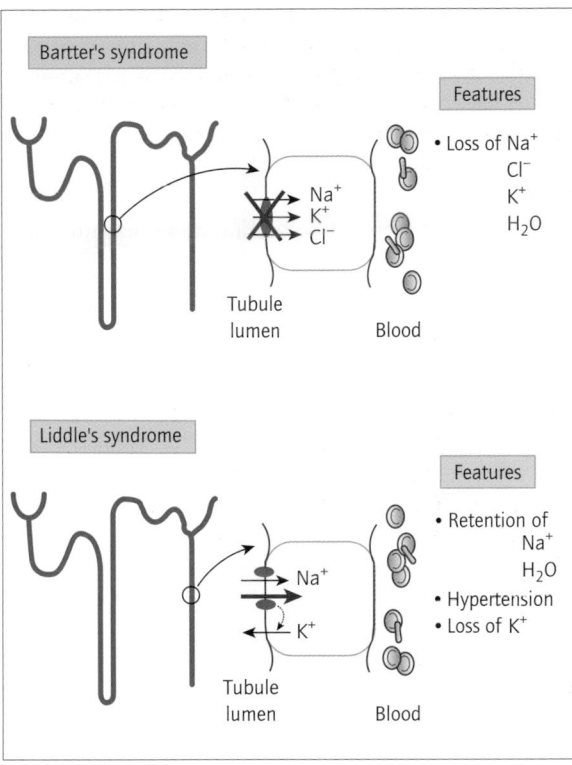

Figure 8.22 Bartter's syndrome and Liddle's syndrome. In Bartter's syndrome, the NaK2Cl cotransporter does not work properly. In Liddle's syndrome, the ENaC sodium channel is held open and the red arrow indicates the excessive sodium reabsorption that occurs.

Gitelman's syndrome

This is an autosomal recessive condition characterized by sodium and water loss as well as hypokalaemia. It is also associated with hypocalciuria and hypomagnesaemia. The condition results from a loss of function mutation in the sodium–chloride cotransporter in the distal tubule and so the effect is similar to that of thiazide administration.

Liddle's syndrome

Liddle's syndrome (pseudohyperaldosteronism) is an autosomal dominant condition characterized by increased reabsorption of sodium in the distal nephron (Fig. 8.22). This causes sodium and water retention with hypertension as well as hypokalaemia and metabolic alkalosis. The ENaC channel, which reabsorbs sodium, is inappropriately held open by the mutation. As this is one of the actions of aldosterone, the mutation mimics the effects of aldosterone.

Clinical features

The usual presentation is with polyuria, polydipsia and

failure to thrive, with significant hypertension in teenagers. The condition is distinguished from primary hyper-aldosteronism by normal or low levels of aldosterone. The sodium and water reabsorption inhibit aldosterone secretion.

Management
Management is with salt restriction and potassium supplementation. Triamterene and amiloride (which blocks the ENaC channel) are effective in increasing urinary sodium excretion and reducing blood pressure.

Prognosis
Life-long therapy is required.

Drugs and the kidney

Drugs and renal failure

Three questions need to be addressed when prescribing for a patient with renal impairment:

1 What is the effect of the renal impairment on the **drug level** (this is altered mainly by changes in renal excretion of the drug)?

2 What is the effect of renal impairment on the **drug action** (is there increased end-organ sensitivity)?

3 What is the effect of the **drug on the damaged kidneys**?

In the light of the answers to these questions, the clinician must alter the prescription appropriately (Table 8.6).

Most drugs, or their metabolites, are mainly excreted by the kidney if they are water soluble or by the liver if they are lipid soluble. Therefore, liver or renal impairment can reduce drug excretion allowing high drug levels to accumulate. For this reason, special regimens may be required if the patient has liver or renal impairment. For a drug that is renally excreted, smaller or less frequent doses may be required to keep the drug levels normal as glomerular filtration rate falls.

For some drugs, the actual level may not be such a problem and dosage adjustment is less of an issue. This depends on the **therapeutic ratio**, which is the concentration of the drug that is toxic divided by the minimum therapeutic concentration. A prescribing error for a drug with a wide therapeutic ratio, such as penicillin, does not usually result in a serious adverse effect. A prescribing error for a drug with a narrow therapeutic ratio, such as a cytotoxic drug, can be fatal.

Effects of renal impairment on drugs excreted by the liver
If a drug is metabolized by the liver, some of the active metabolites may be excreted by the liver. For example, diazepam is metabolized by the liver, but its active metabolite (desmethyldiazepam) is excreted by the kidney. Increased levels of this metabolite can accumulate and cause excessive sedation in renal failure if the dose is not lowered. A similar effect is seen with diamorphine, morphine and pethidine. Some drugs, such as gentamicin, are mainly excreted renally, but the non-renal excretion does increase in renal impairment. However, the dosage still needs to be lowered in renal impairment.

Mechanisms of renal excretion: glomerular filtration vs. tubular function
Glomerular filtration is the main mechanism of renal

Table 8.6 Renal damage caused by drugs

Damage	Drug
Idiosyncratic toxicity	
Allergic interstitial nephritis	Penicillins, rifampicin, cephalosporins, fluoroquinolones, aciclovir, NSAIDs, thiazides, frusemide, mesalazine
Glomerulonephritis	Penicillamine, gold, captopril, phenytoin, penicillins, sulphonamides, rifampicin
Analgesic nephropathy (papillary necrosis)	Phenacetin, other analgesics
Predictable toxicity	
Crystalluria	High-dose aciclovir, sulphonamides, methotrexate, acetazolamide
Renal calculi	Cytotoxics (urate release), possibly triamterene
Decreased creatinine secretion	Cimetidine, trimethoprim
Tubular damage	Lithium, ciclosporin, tacrolimus, gentamicin, foscarnet, amphotericin B, cisplatin, radiographical contrast
Bladder damage leading to obstructive uropathy	Cyclophosphamide
Exacerbation of renal ischaemia	ACE inhibitors, angiotensin II receptor antagonists, NSAIDs
Miscellaneous	Tetracycline, clofibrate, cefradine (combined with frusemide), ACE inhibitors

excretion for many drugs. However, tubular secretion can play a significant part in the renal excretion of certain drugs, such as sulphonamides. For such drugs, the dose adjustment cannot easily be calculated from first principles and in practice it is usual to follow the guidelines from *in vivo* pharmacokinetic studies. Furthermore, if the patient is on dialysis, this may not remove the drug well as dialysis membranes do not have any secretory functions.

Altered pharmacokinetics

Protein binding
Binding of drugs by plasma proteins is altered in uraemia. This arises mainly because of competition between drugs and uraemic toxins for the binding sites on proteins and sometimes because of changes in plasma pH. Altered binding becomes important if more than 90% of the drug is protein-bound in people with normal renal function. Renal impairment reduces this binding and the concentration of unbound or active drug is increased (e.g. benzodiazepines). An increased level of free drug can also have an opposing effect by enhancing excretion of the drug (e.g. phenytoin).

Volume of distribution
The volume of distribution depends upon:
- Patient's height, weight and obesity
- Drug's protein binding and its penetration into body spaces, which depends on its lipid and water solubility

Many of these variables can be altered in uraemia. The volume of distribution is important for calculating loading doses and is well established for most drugs in healthy individuals. Changes in the volume of distribution with renal failure are not easy to predict. Loading doses for patients with renal impairment are usually estimates based on the volume of distribution in people with normal renal function.

Blood levels
Measuring blood levels of drugs can make prescribing safer, but only if the results can be obtained quickly enough to make useful dosage changes. Remember that:
- If the assay measures the total blood level (protein-bound drug and free drug, e.g. digoxin assays) and protein binding is significantly altered, the results should be interpreted with caution.
- The assay may not measure active metabolites, which may also accumulate. For example, a renally excreted active metabolite of phenytoin can accumulate in renal failure. Therefore, the measured level of phenytoin, which is associated with a therapeutic effect, can be lower in renal failure than it is normally.

Effect of renal impairment on drug action

Uraemia may cause increased or decreased end-organ sensitivity.

Insulin
Uraemia decreases sensitivity, but also decreases excretion. The kidney is a major site of insulin metabolism. Starting dialysis increases the sensitivity to insulin, but does not increase its excretion and hypoglycaemia may occur if the dosage is not lowered.

Warfarin
An adequate therapeutic prothrombin time ratio (PTR) or international normalized ratio (INR) in people with uraemia is lower than in people with normal renal function (e.g. when an INR of 2.5–3.5 is necessary in people with normal renal function, an INR of 1.5–2.5 should be aimed for in uraemia). Uraemia causes other clotting defects, the results of which potentiate those of warfarin (and heparin).

Loop diuretics
Loop diuretics must be prescribed in much larger doses to obtain the same therapeutic effect in renal impairment. This is because they reach their tubular site of action by glomerular filtration which is impaired. Maintenance dosages of 250–500 mg/day frusemide are not unusual.

Potassium-sparing diuretics and potassium supplements
Potassium-sparing diuretics have a weak diuretic action, but are potent conservers of potassium. As the glomerular filtration rate falls, so does the ability of the kidney to excrete potassium, and potassium-sparing diuretics or potassium supplements can cause fatal hyperkalaemia. Blood potassium levels should be monitored very closely. Certain laxatives (e.g. Fybogel and Regulan) contain large amounts of potassium.

Vitamin D
The kidney is responsible for the 1-hydroxylation of vitamin D which converts 25-hydroxycholecalciferol to the more metabolically active 1,25-dihydroxycholecalciferol. This function declines with renal failure, so only vitamin D supplements that already have a 1-hydroxyl group (e.g. calcitriol or 1-alphacalcidol) have an effect in severe renal impairment (see p. 562).

Non-steroidal anti-inflammatory drugs
About 90% of people with renal impairment have difficulty excreting sodium and water once the glomerular filtration rate drops below 60 ml/min. The toxicity of drugs that enhance sodium and water retention, such as NSAIDs,

08

is therefore increased in renal impairment. These drugs can also lower glomerular filtration rate by opposing tonic prostaglandin-induced renal vasodilatation (see p. 551).

Sodium content

Certain proprietary antacids and magnesium and magnesium trisilicate, as well as some antibiotics such as carbenicillin, contain a large amount of sodium. The electrolyte content of a drug is recorded in its data sheet and should be considered in a patient with renal impairment who may have difficulty excreting electrolytes such as sodium or potassium.

Effect of the drug on damaged kidneys

Drugs can damage kidneys *de novo* by idiosyncratic toxicity, often at no more than the therapeutic dosage.

Alternatively, they can cause predictable renal damage because of high blood levels. In both cases, if kidneys are already damaged, they may be more susceptible to further damage (Tables 8.7 and 8.8).

Prescribing in renal impairment

Prescribing drugs for patients with renal disease requires special care, particularly if the drug is toxic and has a narrow therapeutic ratio. Information is given in formularies such as the *British National Formulary* (*BNF*), which contains a detailed appendix of drugs that require care in renal disease. More detailed information can be obtained from specialized renal formularies, your local pharmacy drug information service or the drug companies themselves. Tables 8.7 and 8.8 list drugs to be avoided or used only with special care.

Table 8.7 Drugs to avoid in renal impairment

Drug	Reason
Chlorpropamide	Risk of prolonged hypoglycaemia
Lithium	Narrow therapeutic ratio, severe toxicity, causes nephrogenic diabetes insipidus with polyuria and dehydration
Metformin, phenformin	Increased risk of lactic acidosis
Nitrofurantoin	Renally excreted metabolites cause peripheral neuropathy
Tetracyclines	Can precipitate acute-on-chronic renal failure (except doxycycline and minoxycycline)
Acetazolamide	Metabolic acidosis
Phenylbutazone	Increased risk of toxicity
Procainamide	Increased risk of toxicity
Thiazides	Ineffective with GFR less than 30 ml/min
Bismuth	Danger of bismuth poisoning
Clofibrate	Renally excreted metabolites are toxic to skeletal muscle
Sodium aurothiomalate	Increased risk of gold toxicity

GFR, glomerular filtration rate.
Note that doxycycline and minocycline are safe in renal impairment because they are excreted by metabolism in the liver.

Table 8.8 Drugs to be used only with special care in renal impairment. Enhanced effects and increased toxicity are a result of retention of renally excreted drug or active metabolite in renal impairment

Drug	Reason
Potassium-sparing diuretics	Danger of hyperkalaemia
Gentamicin, tobramycin and aztreonam	Increased toxicity
Nadolol	Enhanced effects
Vancomycin	Increased toxicity
Digoxin	Enhanced effects
Many cytotoxic agents	Enhanced effects
Ethambutol	Increased risk of optic neuritis and peripheral nephropathy
Allopurinol (especially in combination with azathioprine)	Enhanced bone marrow suppression
Sulphonamides	Increased prevalence of side-effects, and crystalluria if low urine flow
Diazepam	Active metabolite causing enhanced effect
Opiates	Active metabolite causing enhanced effect
Sucralfate and other aluminium-containing antacids	Risk of aluminium toxicity
Sulphonylureas (except gliclazide)	Retained metabolites cause prolonged hypoglycaemia

Loading dose

Because of our lack of knowledge of volumes of distribution in patients with renal disease, this is virtually the same as in people without renal impairment (loading dose = volume of distribution × desired steady state concentration).

Repeat dose adjustment

The half-life $(t_{1/2})$ of any renally excreted drug is prolonged in renal failure. Half-lives for various degrees of renal impairment are available for most drugs from tables. They can be used to calculate the adjustment of either the dose (D) or the dose interval using the following formulae:

Dose in renal failure
= normal dose × ($t_{1/2}$ normal renal function/
$t_{1/2}$ renal failure),

Dose interval in renal failure
= normal dose interval × ($t_{1/2}$ for renal failure/
$t_{1/2}$ normal renal function).

Standard tables give the dose or dose interval adjustments for a range of creatinine clearances. There is a comprehensive table in the *BNF* and a fuller table produced by Aronoff *et al.* (see Further reading on p. 595).

Adjusting the dose or the dose interval

The choice between adjusting dose or interval is usually arbitrary. However:

● If it is important to keep the drug level constant (e.g. digoxin), the dose should be reduced, keeping the interval the same
● If it is necessary to maintain peaks and troughs (e.g. with some antibiotics), the interval between doses should be increased

Calculation of creatinine clearance to estimate drug half-life

The patient's glomerular filtration rate or creatinine clearance must be known in order to be able to check the drug's half-life in renal failure in pharmacological tables. If only the plasma creatinine is known (or creatinine clearance measurements are suspect) the Cockcroft and Gault formula can be used to calculate creatinine clearance fairly accurately (see p. 510).

Creatinine clearance

$$= \frac{F\,(140 - age) \times body\ weight\ (kg)}{plasma\ creatinine\ (\mu mol/l)}$$

where F = 1.0 for females and 1.23 for males, and age is in years.

Prescribing for people receiving dialysis

It is essential to know whether a drug is removed by dialysis before prescribing it to patients on such treatment. In practice, water-soluble drugs are removed by dialysis. New compounds are often researched in people on dialysis so pharmaceutical companies are able to provide relevant information.

Difference between haemodialysis and peritoneal dialysis

Haemodialysis is fast, intermittent and of short duration; peritoneal dialysis is slow and continuous. When a constant blood level is required (e.g. digoxin) it is necessary to give an extra dose post haemodialysis to replace the drug lost by dialysis. People on peritoneal dialysis are sometimes given drugs intraperitoneally (e.g. insulin, potassium and antibiotics for the treatment of peritonitis). Haemofiltration is continuous and may require altered dosage. Most dialysis patients take phosphate binders. These bind other drugs and inhibit their absorption. Ideally, other drugs should be taken no less than 2 h before or after phosphate binders.

Transplantation patients

Transplantation recipients can be treated in the same way as patients with renal failure who have a similar glomerular filtration rate. However, there are many interactions with immunosuppressive agents. Allopurinol inhibits the oxidative metabolism of azathioprine and so enhances its bone marrow suppressive effect. Many drugs that affect the hepatic p450 cytochrome system raise or lower cyclosporin or tacrolimus levels (details on drug interactions are given in an appendix of the *BNF*).

Anaesthesia in renal impairment

Certain drugs used for anaesthesia have particular unwanted effects in renal impairment (see Table 8.9; KEYPOINTS BOX 8.2).

Table 8.9 Anaesthetic agents that have unwanted effects in renal impairment

Drug	Effect
Gallamine	Prolonged action
Succinyl choline	Prolonged action and muscular fibrillation leading to hyperkalaemia
Pancuronium	40% renally excreted. Prolonged action may cause delayed neuromuscular blockade after patient recovery

Note: Aminoglycosides potentiate the actions of muscle relaxants.

08

Keypoints 8.2: Drugs and the kidney

Do not prescribe any drug until you know how it is handled in renal failure

Use a source of drug information, e.g. *British National Formulary*

Reduce the dose or increase the dose interval for renally excreted drugs

Be extra careful with drugs having a narrow therapeutic ratio

In unexplained renal damage, always consider drug toxicity as a cause

Renal vascular disease

Disease of the renal arteries can cause hypertension, renal impairment from ischaemic nephropathy or, rarely, flash pulmonary oedema from sodium and water retention. Disease of the renal veins causes renal impairment because of renal vein thrombosis.

Ischaemic nephropathy

Disease mechanisms

Ischaemic nephropathy occurs when the kidney is chronically ischaemic, usually as a result of renal artery stenosis or of small artery disease caused by hypertension. Sometimes, small fragments of cholesterol may be dislodged from atherosclerotic plaques, usually in the aorta, and these can lodge in small renal vessels causing ischaemia or provoking an inflammatory response. This is known as cholesterol embolization. Ischaemic nephropathy causes approximately 10–20% of end-stage renal failure and is one of the most common causes of renal failure in people over 55 years of age.

Clinical features

Ischaemic nephropathy presents with acute or chronic renal failure, and sometimes with the features of hypertension (see p. 542). Some patients present with a clinical picture resembling that of chronic interstitial nephritis (see p. 525).

Investigation

Investigation is the same as that for any cause of renal failure, hypertension or suspected renal artery stenosis. It is essential to exclude other causes of renal failure, document the severity of the renal damage and assess risk factors for cardiovascular disease.

Renal histology may show glomerular shrinkage, glomerulosclerosis and chronic interstitial nephritis, as well as arterial changes.

Management

The management of ischaemic nephropathy involves treating any hypertension and modifying risk factors for cardiovascular disease (lipids and smoking). Renal artery stenosis should be actively sought and considered for treatment (see below).

Prognosis

Successful treatment of hypertension, modification of cardiovascular risk factors and treatment of any renal artery stenosis may halt the progression of renal failure, but the damage already done is often advanced and irreversible.

Renal artery stenosis

Renovascular disease may present with impaired renal function, hypertension, or both. There are two main types: fibromuscular dysplasia and atheromatous renovascular disease.

Fibromuscular dysplasia

Disease mechanisms

Fibromuscular hyperplasia affects any or all of the three layers of the vessel wall.

Epidemiology

Prevalence. Rare.

Age. Peak incidence is in the fourth decade.

Gender. More common in women.

Clinical presentation

The usual presentation is with hypertension.

Investigation

Angiography shows a beaded appearance of the renal artery in 75% of patients with fibromuscular dysplasia (Fig. 8.10, p. 513).

Management

The disorder responds well to angioplasty or surgery, but may recur or occur *de novo* elsewhere. Life-long follow-up is necessary.

Prognosis

The prognosis is excellent provided that the hypertension is diagnosed and treated before end-organ damage occurs. Hypertension is often cured by treatment.

Atheromatous renovascular disease

Disease mechanisms

The aetiology, pathogenesis and risk factors for atheromatous renovascular disease are the same as those for atheromatous vascular disease elsewhere, which is usually also present (e.g. peripheral vascular disease, coronary artery disease). The proximal part of the renal arteries is most commonly affected, possibly because the high pressure blood flow and 90° angle to the aorta causes more hydraulic trauma to the vessel wall at this position.

Epidemiology

Prevalence. Much more common than fibromuscular dysplasia. It is probably frequently missed and so left untreated. It is one of the most common causes of renal failure in the elderly, when hypertension may be absent.

Age. Peak incidence is in the fifth and sixth decades, in common with atheroma in the rest of the vascular tree.

Sex. Occurs earlier in males.

Geography. Most common in countries where atherosclerosis is prevalent.

Clinical features

The degree of hypertension may be variable, but it is often moderate to severe. Unlike the hypertension of fibromuscular dysplasia, hypertension caused by atheromatous renovascular disease often fails to improve when the stenosis is dilated by angioplasty.

Diagnosis. Features that suggest a diagnosis of renovascular disease:
- Severe hypertension *de novo* (blood pressure greater than 170/110 mmHg)
- Sudden deterioration in blood pressure or loss of therapeutic control
- Renal bruit
- Difference in renal size greater than 2 cm
- Renal impairment
- Deterioration in renal function following treatment with ACE inhibitors
- No family history of essential hypertension
- Episodes of pulmonary oedema not explained by ischaemic heart disease
- Severe atherosclerosis elsewhere in the vascular tree

Investigation

Biochemistry
- Plasma creatinine, urea and electrolytes to assess renal function
- Plasma lipids

Diagnostic imaging
- *Arterial angiography:* with digital subtraction is the gold

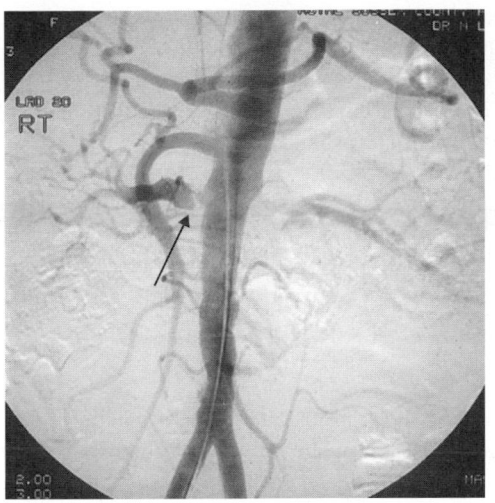

Figure 8.23 Renal angiogram showing bilateral atherosclerotic renal artery stenosis. The stenosis of the right renal artery, seen on the left of the image, is over 75% and there is post-stenotic dilatation; the left renal artery is completely occluded.

standard for diagnosing renal artery stenosis (Fig. 8.23). The reliability of magnetic resonance angiography (MRA) is currently being evaluated.
- *DTPA renograms* (see p. 513): can be used to assess the differential function of each kidney.
- *Pre- and postcaptopril renograms:* sensitive and specific. If renal artery stenosis is present, then the renogram shows a fall in renal perfusion with captopril. Pre- and post-captopril renograms may be the best method of predicting the response to surgery or angioplasty.
- *Ultrasound:* performed to measure renal size.

Management

The possible treatments for renal artery stenosis:
- *Conservative management:* treatment of hypertension and risk factors for cardiovascular disease
- *Percutaneous transluminal angioplasty:* usually with placement of an intra-arterial stent
- *Surgical revascularization:* aortorenal bypass; spleno-, hepato- or iliorenal bypass; autotransplantation

Revascularization by angioplasty and/or stenting in atherosclerotic disease cures hypertension in 30% of patients and improves it in 30%, but has no effect in the rest. In atherosclerotic renal artery stenosis, angioplasty or surgery is indicated to prevent progression to end-stage renal failure (if there is significant renal impairment), but it is not justified for treatment of hypertension alone unless difficult to control.

Complications of angioplasty:
- Rupture or dissection of the renal artery
- Thrombosis of the renal artery

- Peripheral artery embolization
- Haemorrhage at the puncture site
- Renal artery spasm
- Contrast- or ischaemia-induced acute renal failure, which may require dialysis
- Mortality of 1% or less

Long-term follow-up is needed for both types of renal artery stenosis. If it recurs, repeat angioplasty is usually the best treatment for fibromuscular dysplasia and surgery or conservative management for atheromatous disease.

Prognosis

Untreated, at least 30% of stenosed renal arteries progress towards complete occlusion. Atherosclerotic renovascular disease is responsible for renal failure in up to 14–20% of patients who need renal replacement therapy (mostly presenting with interstitial nephritis caused by ischaemia). This group of patients, who already have generalized atherosclerosis, have a much poorer prognosis on dialysis than the average dialysis patient. The main benefit of the treatment of renal artery stenosis is that when successful it prevents renal failure and markedly improves prognosis for this reason.

Renal vein thrombosis

Epidemiology and disease mechanisms

The most common cause of renal vein thrombosis is the nephrotic syndrome, which predisposes to venous thrombosis (see p. 515). Other causes include hyperviscosity syndromes such as that caused by an IgM myeloma, malignancy (when there may also be direct infiltration of the renal vein) and general thrombophilic disorders such as the antiphospholipid syndrome or antithrombin 3 deficiency.

Clinical features

Presentation may be insidious with increasing proteinuria and/or pulmonary emboli resulting from partial occlusion of one or both renal veins. There will be leg oedema if the clot extends into the inferior vena cava. If there is an acute complete occlusion, the patient will have flank pain, haematuria and a dramatic rise of urea, creatinine and lactate dehydrogenase (LDH), which is released from infarcted renal cells.

Investigation

Renal function tests may show a deterioration and LDH levels may rise. CT or MRI can be used to image the renal veins. Ultrasound sometimes gives useful information but often the renal veins cannot be clearly seen. Venography has been superseded by CT and MRI.

Treatment and prognosis

Anticoagulation should be continued as long as the underlying cause is still present. Thrombolysis may be needed for complete occlusion.

Hypertension

Hypertension is a systemic condition that can cause damage to many different parts of the body. The kidney has a key role in the maintenance of normal blood pressure and many drugs used to treat hypertension act through the kidneys or through the renin–angiotensin system. Most renal diseases can cause hypertension and hypertension itself can cause renal damage. Hypertension is important because it can directly damage the heart, the kidneys and the eyes and because it is a major risk factor for vascular disease (Fig. 8.24), especially cerebrovascular disease. The identification and treatment of hypertension is important because it improves the prognosis for these conditions.

Hypertension is referred to as '**essential**' if no obvious cause is identified and '**secondary**' if the cause is known; most cases are essential. The definition of hypertension is arbitrary and is usually considered to be above **140/90 mmHg**. The 140 refers to the systolic blood pressure resulting from contraction of the left ventricle and the 90 refers to the diastolic blood pressure present during ventricular relaxation when the aortic valve is closed.

Epidemiology

Hypertension is common, affecting 5–10% of the population in western countries (Fig. 8.25). The prevalence is similar in men and women. The prevalence is higher in black people of African origin. Large epidemiological studies, such as the Framingham study in Massachusetts, have determined that hypertension is a major risk factor for stroke and ischaemic heart disease. Risk factors for hypertension include a high alcohol intake and obesity. There is an association between hypertension and impaired glucose tolerance or diabetes, often with hyperlipidaemia. This has been termed the metabolic syndrome. Sodium chloride intake has been correlated with blood pressure and this effect may vary in different ethnic groups. Lowering sodium chloride intake is difficult because most ingested salt is in manufactured foods, including staple items such as bread.

Essential hypertension

Disease mechanisms

The causes of essential hypertension have not been well defined. However, systemic vascular resistance is usually increased and it is common to find a high level of renin production by the kidney. The main factors that influence

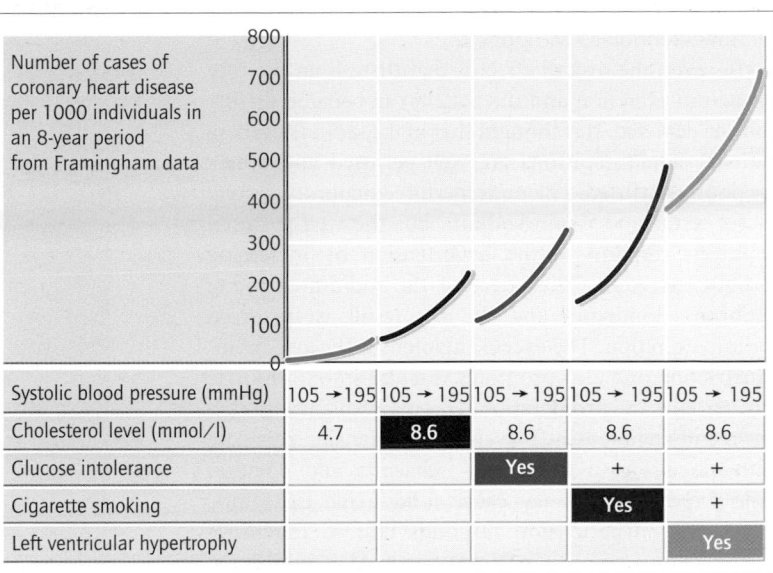

Systolic blood pressure (mmHg)	105 → 195	105 → 195	105 → 195	105 → 195	105 → 195
Cholesterol level (mmol/l)	4.7	8.6	8.6	8.6	8.6
Glucose intolerance			Yes	+	+
Cigarette smoking				Yes	+
Left ventricular hypertrophy					Yes

Number of cases of coronary heart disease per 1000 individuals in an 8-year period from Framingham data

Figure 8.24 The effect of blood pressure and other risk factors on the incidence of coronary heart disease. The incidence of stroke is affected in a similar way. The green line in the graph shows how the incidence of coronary heart disease rises as systolic blood pressure rises from 105 to 195 in people with no other risk factors. The other curves show how this incidence rises even further with each additional risk factor. However, even with multiple risk factors, systolic blood pressure itself still has a major effect.

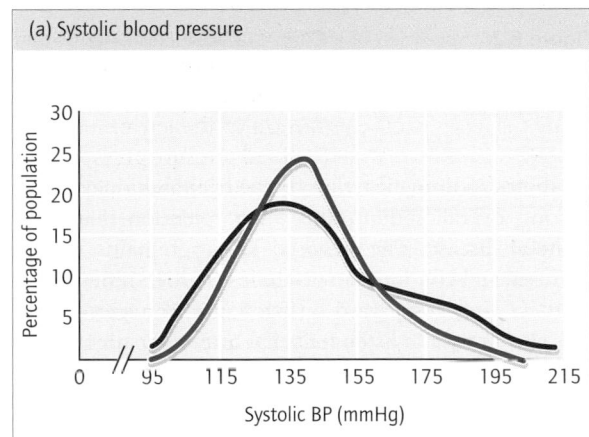

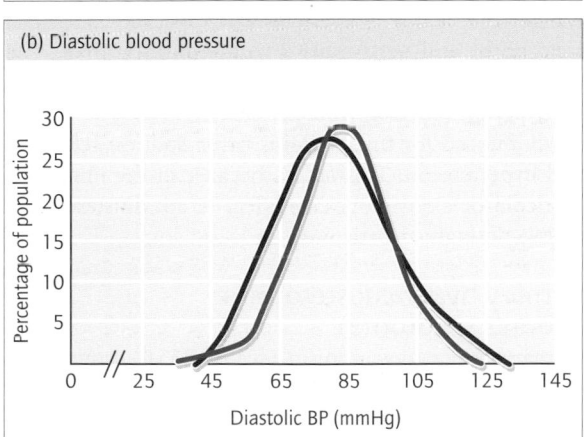

Figure 8.25 Normal distribution of: (a) systolic; and (b) diastolic blood pressure (BP) in a white population (males, blue; females, red).

blood pressure are cardiac output, systemic vascular resistance and circulatory volume. The key determinant of systemic vascular resistance is vasoconstriction of arterioles and the key determinant of circulatory volume is renal sodium excretion. Blood pressure rises:

- If the heart pumps more and cardiac output increases
- If systemic vascular resistance increases because of arteriolar constriction
- If there is an increase in the intravascular volume because of sodium and water retention by the kidney

The kidney has a key role in regulating systemic vascular resistance through the production of renin and the subsequent generation of angiotensin II. Drugs that block this pathway are highly effective in many cases of hypertension. Similarly, the kidney plays a key part in regulating body sodium and water content by altering urine output and concentration. Drugs such as diuretics that block this action can also be effective in hypertension.

Essential hypertension is characterized by an increase in peripheral resistance. This is caused by two mechanisms. The first mechanism operates in the 20% of patients with a high plasma renin level, whereas the second mechanism operates in the 30% of patients with a low plasma renin level. Both mechanisms probably operate in the 50% of patients with an intermediate plasma renin level.

High renin salt-resistant dry essential hypertension
These patients have a raised plasma renin level for their body sodium content. The hypertension is 'salt-resistant' because salt excretion is not impaired. The excess renin production by the kidneys causes angiotensin II production, which in turn causes vasoconstriction and aldosterone

08

secretion by the adrenal gland. Aldosterone promotes sodium retention by the kidney.

However, the overall effect is that there is an increase in sodium excretion and the patient can become slightly volume depleted. It is thought that in the kidneys of these patients, some nephrons are well perfused and others are poorly perfused. The underperfused nephrons secrete excess renin and retain sodium, but the well-perfused nephrons respond to the hypertension by increasing sodium excretion. The effect of the sodium-excreting nephrons dominates and the net result is increased sodium excretion. The **excess angiotensin II causes vasoconstriction** and also promotes vascular smooth muscle hypertrophy and proliferation. This may explain why high renin and angiotensin II levels in hypertension correlate with vascular and end-organ ischaemia and damage. Mild hypovolaemia may cause mild tissue ischaemia. High renin hypertension responds best to inhibition of the renin–angiotensin II axis with **ACE inhibitors, angiotensin II antagonists or beta-blockers** (which inhibit renin secretion).

Low renin salt-sensitive wet essential hypertension

These patients have **renal sodium and water retention**, which suppress renin secretion. The hypertension is therefore 'salt-sensitive' and worsens with a high salt intake as they retain more salt and retain water with it to maintain normal osmolarity. The reason for the sodium retention that can cause hypervolaemia and hypertension is not well understood, but may be caused by increased sympathetic adrenergic activity or a defect in sodium-coupled calcium transport. Excess sodium can cause vasoconstriction by altering smooth muscle calcium transport. There is less vascular and end-organ damage than with high renin salt-resistant hypertension. This is probably because angiotensin II levels are lower and there is no hypovolaemia. Patients response to **sodium restriction, diuretics and vasodilators such as alpha-1 adrenergic blockers and calcium-channel antagonists.**

Causes of secondary hypertension

Renal artery stenosis

Renal artery stenosis (see p. 540) reduces renal blood flow and glomerular filtration rate. This stimulates renin release and subsequent angiotensin II production. Angiotensin II causes hypertension by vasoconstriction and by stimulation of aldosterone release from the adrenal cortex, which promotes sodium retention by the kidney. If both kidneys have renal artery stenosis, the hypervolaemia and hypertension eventually restore renal perfusion and renin levels fall slightly. If only one kidney is normal, the hypertension increases its glomerular filtration rate. This

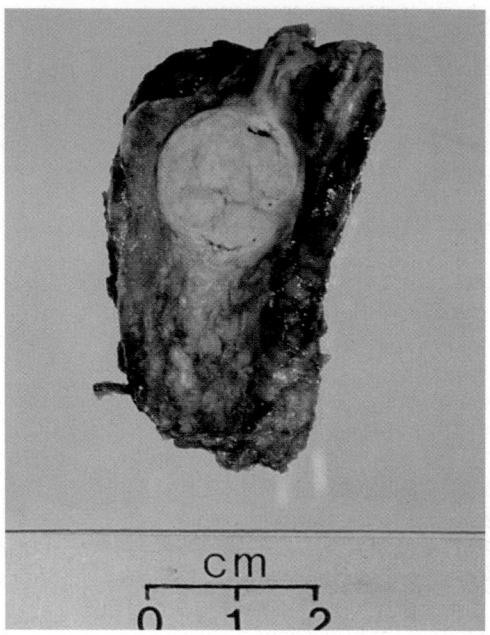

Figure 8.26 Specimen of a Conn's tumour contained within an excised adrenal gland. Note the characteristic yellow surface of the cut section of the tumour.

promotes sodium excretion by the healthy kidney, causing less overall sodium and water retention than with bilateral disease. The stenosed kidney remains underperfused and continues to produce very high renin levels, so there is ongoing vasoconstriction and hypertension. It is always wise to listen for renal bruits in patients with hypertension.

Drugs

Drugs can cause hypertension, especially steroids, ciclosporin and oestrogens in oral contraceptives. The oral contraceptive pill is an important potential cause of hypertension and women who are using it should be monitored for this. Steroids cause sodium retention and hypertension. This occurs because of the mineralocorticoid or aldosterone-like effect of administered and endogenous glucocorticoids.

Primary hyperaldosteronism (Conn's syndrome)

Primary hyperaldosteronism (see p. 855) accounts for 1–2% of all hypertension. Excess aldosterone increases renal sodium retention and potassium secretion. As sodium is retained, water is retained with it to maintain normal osmolarity and the resulting hypervolaemia causes hypertension. The cause may be a primary adrenal tumour secreting aldosterone (Fig. 8.26).

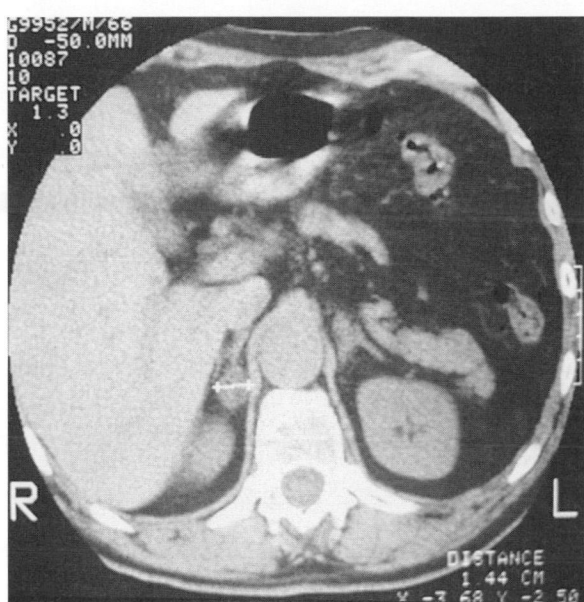

Figure 8.27 CT scan of a right adrenal tumour (marked with a white line) in a patient with phaeochromocytoma.

Intrinsic renal disease

Any renal disease can cause hypertension. **Severe renal impairment** reduces the capacity of the kidney for sodium excretion and sodium retention causes hypervolaemia and hypertension. This type of hypertension is 'salt-sensitive', because it is made worse if the patient ingests more salt. With **milder renal impairment**, the kidney may produce renin in response to its perceived renal hypoperfusion. This promotes renin secretion and angiotensin II-mediated vasoconstriction. This type of hypertension is not 'salt-sensitive' and is termed 'salt-resistant'. Severely damaged kidneys, even in patients with end-stage renal disease, sometimes continue to produce excess renin, which promotes this type of salt-resistant hypertension.

Other causes of hypertension

- *Coarctation of the aorta:* causes narrowing of the aorta which reduces renal perfusion and so triggers renin secretion. Characteristically, pulses are weaker in the legs than the arms.
- *Catecholamine:* release by a phaeochromocytoma causes systemic vasoconstriction and so hypertension (Fig. 8.27).
- *Acromegaly and hyperparathyroidism:* both associated with hypertension.

Clinical presentation

Hypertension is usually asymptomatic and is typically detected when a patient has his or her blood pressure measured for a routine health check or during evaluation for another clinical problem.

- Hypertension is usually diagnosed if blood pressure is equal to or above 140/90 mmHg (World Health Organization/International Society of Hypertension criteria) on three separate occasions.
- Sometimes it is unclear whether patients have genuine hypertension or are just anxious. When there is doubt, the diagnosis can be confirmed by 24-h ambulatory blood pressure monitoring.
- Evidence of end-organ damage from hypertension, such as retinopathy or left ventricular hypertrophy, demonstrates unambiguously that the patient is hypertensive.

The history and examination may indicate whether the hypertension is secondary and whether complications have developed. The patient may be taking drugs that are causing hypertension. Hypertensive retinopathy confirms the presence of hypertension and may indicate malignant hypertension. For this reason, **fundoscopy** is mandatory in all cases of hypertension and all clinicians should be familiar with the technique. Hypertension is often associated with obesity, excess alcohol intake, insulin resistance and gout. Examine carefully for peripheral **bruits**, which could indicate vascular disease, and could also affect the renal arteries and cause renal artery stenosis. Renal artery stenosis can cause renal artery bruits. Examine the **heart** for signs of left ventricular hypertrophy such as a left ventricular heave.

How to measure blood pressure

Blood pressure is usually measured with a sphygmomanometer, which uses an inflatable cuff around the arm. Good automatic devices are available, but it is still important to be able to check the action of these devices with a manual sphygmomanometer.

1 Choose a cuff of the right size. If the patient has a large arm, use a large cuff or the reading will be falsely high.
2 Wrap the cuff around the patient's arm and place a stethoscope over the brachial artery at the elbow.
3 Inflate the cuff until no sound is heard and then slowly deflate it.
4 When the first sounds start to be heard, this is the systolic pressure as indicated on the sphygmomanometer.
5 When the sounds finally disappear, this is the diastolic pressure.

If the patient is tense, allow them to relax and repeat the measurements a few times. In a well patient, elevated blood pressure is not an emergency and treatment should not be commenced until you are sure that the blood pressure is truly elevated.

When blood pressure is low in very sick patients, it can be difficult to hear the sounds and the systolic pressure can be approximately determined with a finger on the pulse instead of a stethoscope. No pulse will be felt when the cuff is inflated above systolic pressure and the pulse will reappear when the cuff is deflated to the systolic pressure. In acutely and severely sick patients, arterial blood pressure is measured directly by placing a catheter in the artery and connecting it to a pressure transducer.

Investigation

Key initial investigations:
- Urinalysis
- Serum electrolytes
- Urea and creatinine
- Lipids
- Glucose
- Electrocardiography, ideally with echocardiography to identify left ventricular hypertrophy

Urinalysis may indicate renal damage or disease. Protein in the urine can suggest hypertensive damage to the kidney. Renal damage or disease can also cause renal impairment with raised serum urea and creatinine values. Hypokalaemia suggests primary hyperaldosteronism. Other cardiovascular risk factors should be assessed, including lipids and plasma glucose to exclude diabetes mellitus.

Further investigations include plasma and urine catecholamines or vanillylmandelic acid (VMA) levels to exclude phaeochromocytomas, adrenal function tests to check for steroid excess and renal angiography to exclude renal artery stenosis.

Management

Unless there is severe hypertension, end-organ damage or malignant hypertension, treatment is not urgent and can await full evaluation. Blood pressure can be improved by exercise, reduced alcohol consumption and correction of obesity. Reducing salt intake will help salt-sensitive hypertension, especially if there is renal impairment. Other risk factors for vascular disease, including smoking, should be modified to reduce vascular complications.

The commonly used antihypertensives are diuretics, beta-blockers, ACE inhibitors, angiotensin II receptor blockers, calcium-channel blockers and alpha-blockers. Various trials have compared the different therapies. However, one of the most important is the very large ALLHAT (antihypertensive and lipid-lowering treatment to prevent heart attack) trial, which compared four classes of drug. The diuretic used was a thiazide diuretic. Doxazosin was less effective at reducing cardiovascular deaths, but the other three classes of drug had similar beneficial effects at reducing fatal coronary heart disease, non-fatal myocardial infarction and stroke. In practice, tailored therapy with the minimum number of drugs is increasingly popular and most patients in this trial required

two or more drugs to control their blood pressure. Often therapy is influenced by coexistent conditions so, for example, beta-blockers may be ideal for a patient who also has angina.
- **High renin** hypertension responds best to renin axis inhibition with ACE inhibitors, angiotensin II antagonists or beta-blockers
- **Low renin** hypertension with salt sensitivity, especially in black patients, responds best to calcium-channel blockers, alpha-1 adrenergic blockers and diuretics

Beta-blockers suppress renin secretion, reduce cardiac output and may have a centrally mediated effect. Lowering cardiac output can worsen the symptoms of peripheral vascular disease. Beta-blockers blunt the catecholaminergic effects, which normally warn diabetics of hypoglycaemia. Beta-1 selective blockers avoid the bronchospasm of beta-2 blockade.

ACE inhibitors inhibit angiotensin II production. They cause more dilatation in efferent arterioles than in afferent arterioles and this reduces the intraglomerular pressure. This reduces proteinuria and glomerulosclerosis. Complications include hyperkalaemia caused by reduced aldosterone production and renal impairment if renal artery stenosis is present. ACE degrades bradykinin, so ACE inhibitors cause high bradykinin levels, which can make patients cough.

Angiotensin II receptor antagonists such as losartan have the same effect as ACE inhibitors. Cough is not a problem.

Calcium-channel blockers cause vasodilatation. In salt-sensitive hypertension, they also increase sodium excretion by poorly understood mechanisms. Verapamil and diltiazem reduce atrioventricular nodal conduction and should not be given with beta-blockers. Nifedipine only dilates afferent arterioles, allowing systemic hypertension to cause intraglomerular hypertension.

Diuretics (see p. 578), mainly thiazides, are used in hypertension, but these are ineffective if glomerular filtration rate is low. Frusemide may then be beneficial.

Alpha-1 antagonists, such as doxazosin, block catecholaminergic vasoconstriction and can cause postural hypotension. However, they improve insulin sensitivity, lipid profiles and sometimes erectile function. They can increase urine flow rates when there is prostatic hypertrophy.

Direct vasodilators, such as sodium nitroprusside, intravenous nitrates, hydrallazine, diazoxide and minoxidil cause peripheral vasodilatation directly. This usually causes reflex tachycardia. Prolonged intravenous sodium nitroprusside administration causes toxic thiocyanate concentrations and after 48 h levels should be monitored.

Centrally acting drugs such as clonidine, methyldopa and guanethidine are seldom used because of multiple side-effects.

Hypertension at a glance

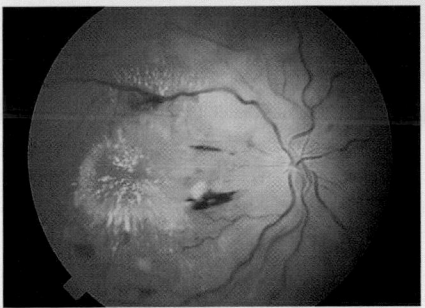

Fig. A Grade 4 hypertensive retinopathy with exudates, flame haemorrhages and papilloedema.

Background
- Affects 5–10% of western populations
- BP $\geq \frac{140}{90}$ mmHg on 3 separate occasions
- Can cause end organ damage
- Increases with:
  - Age
  - Obesity
  - Alcohol intake
- Secondary causes
  - Renal artery stenosis
  - Renal disease
  - Primary hyperaldosteronism
  - Phaeochromocytoma
  - Drugs: contraceptive pill
    steroids

Key questions
1. Is the patient truly hypertensive?
2. Is there end organ damage?
3. Is there a treatable cause?
4. Will lifestyle changes help?
5. Is urgent treatment required?
6. Which drug is most appropriate?

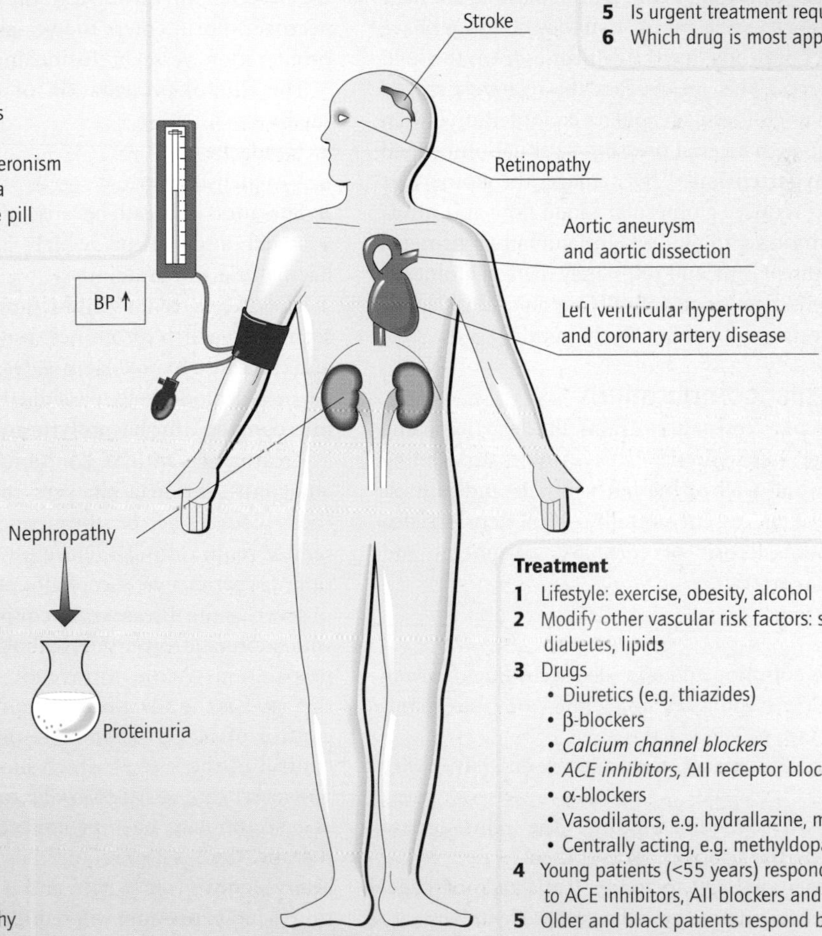

Stroke

Retinopathy

Aortic aneurysm
and aortic dissection

Left ventricular hypertrophy
and coronary artery disease

BP ↑

Nephropathy

Proteinuria

Treatment
1. Lifestyle: exercise, obesity, alcohol
2. Modify other vascular risk factors: smoking, diabetes, lipids
3. Drugs
   - Diuretics (e.g. thiazides)
   - β-blockers
   - *Calcium channel blockers*
   - *ACE inhibitors,* AII receptor blockers
   - α-blockers
   - Vasodilators, e.g. hydrallazine, minoxidil
   - Centrally acting, e.g. methyldopa
4. Young patients (<55 years) respond better to ACE inhibitors, AII blockers and β-blockers
5. Older and black patients respond better to calcium channel blockers and diuretics

Basic investigations
- Electrolytes
- Urea, creatinine
- Lipids, glucose
- ECG ± echocardiography
- Urinalysis

Complications of hypertension

Renal complications of hypertension

Essential hypertension seldom causes renal disease unless there has been malignant or accelerated hypertension. The occurrence of very low levels of albumin in the urine (microalbuminuria) or heavier levels of proteinuria that can be detected by standard dipsticks are both signs of hypertensive nephropathy. At this stage in the condition, blood pressure control will slow the rate of renal damage. The groups most likely to develop renal damage from hypertension are the elderly, the obese, black patients and those from the Indian subcontinent, especially if they have diabetes. In the long term, hypertension can damage the kidney so badly that end-stage renal disease results, but this is uncommon with simple essential hypertension.

The primary insult is **damage to renal vessels** from the raised pressure. The muscle in the interlobular artery walls is replaced by fibrotic tissue. The afferent arteriole walls undergo hyalinization—the subintimal deposition of lipids and glycoproteins exuded from plasma. Damage to these resistance vessels means that they no longer have the usual effect of protecting the capillaries from the high arterial pressures. This means that the relatively fragile and unmuscular glomerular capillary endothelium is then exposed to the high arterial pressure—a situation termed '**glomerular hypertension**'. This damages the glomerular capillaries and reduces glomerular blood flow and filtration and promotes proteinuria. Inflammatory proteins exude out of the plasma and ultimately there is **glomerular sclerosis** or ischaemic atrophy. The glomerulosclerosis is focal—it affects some but not all glomeruli.

Cardiovascular complications

The high vascular resistance strains the heart, causing left ventricular hypertrophy. This involves thickening of the myocardial wall of the left ventricle and is itself an indicator of increased mortality. Hypertension also increases atherosclerosis of coronary, peripheral and cerebrovascular arteries.

Eyes

Retinopathy is common and is graded according to severity. Grade 3 or 4 indicates accelerated or 'malignant' hypertension (see p. 547, Fig. A).
- *Grade 1:* Arterial spasm, tortuous arteries, silver wire appearance.
- *Grade 2:* Arteriovenous nipping. The veins appear narrowed where the arteries pass over them.
- *Grade 3:* Haemorrhage, including flame haemorrhage. Lipid extravasation causes exudates; hard exudates are old, but soft exudates or cotton wool spots indicate acute severe hypertension. Exudates are visible as whitish patches or spots on the retina.
- *Grade 4:* Papilloedema. A swollen optic disc.

Malignant or accelerated hypertension

Malignant hypertension is characterized by severe hypertension with grade 3 or 4 retinal changes and renal damage. It can occur *de novo* or as a complication of essential or secondary hypertension:
- The central feature is **renal vessel damage**, usually caused by hypertension
- This damage **reduces renal blood flow** and the reduction triggers renin secretion
- **Renin secretion** promotes **hypertension** and sodium retention

However, as the renal vessels are damaged, the increase in blood pressure does not result in the restoration of normal renal blood flow, so renin secretion stays high and the vicious cycle of damage to the kidney, increasing renin output and increasing blood pressure goes on. Damage to the endothelium throughout the body can cause **fibrinoid necrosis**—fibrin enters the vessel wall, triggering cellular proliferation, vessel occlusion and ischaemia.

The clinical presentation of malignant hypertension can be:
- Headache
- Visual disturbance
- Shortness of breath because of cardiac problems
- Renal impairment, which is common, often with haematuria and proteinuria

The excess renin production promotes aldosterone secretion, which promotes renal potassium excretion and can cause **hypokalaemia**. Damaged blood vessels can harm red blood cells passing through them, causing a **microangiopathic haemolytic anaemia**.

Treatment is with ACE inhibitors, angiotensin receptor antagonists or beta-blockers to block the renin cycle (beta-blockers act on the juxtaglomerular apparatus to reduce renin output). Diuretics promote sodium excretion. Hypertensive encephalopathy, pulmonary oedema or severe acute disease may require intravenous treatment with sodium nitroprusside, hydralazine, labetalol or a nitrate preparation. Acute intravenous sodium nitroprusside therapy has the advantage that precise minute-by-minute control of blood pressure is possible, allowing careful control of the rate at which blood pressure is reduced. However, care is necessary as toxic cyanide metabolites can accumulate over prolonged sodium nitroprusside therapy. Care is also required as patients may have renal artery stenosis (see p. 540) and if so then a sudden reduction in blood pressure will reduce renal perfusion and may cause an acute deterioration in renal function.

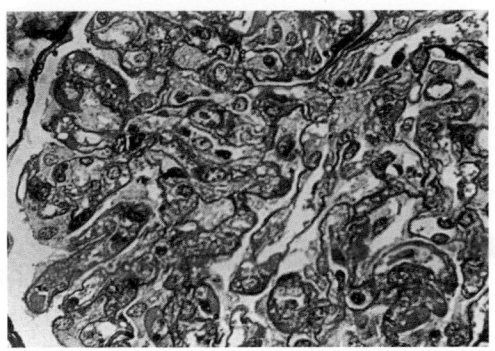

Figure 8.28 Light microscopy of a renal biopsy from a patient with severe pre-eclampsia. There is endothelial cell swelling and vacuolation. Reproduced from Kincaid-Smith P, Whitworth JA. *The Kidney: a Clinico-Pathological Study*, 2nd edn. Oxford: Blackwell Scientific Publications, 1987 with the permission of the authors.

Hypertension in pregnancy and pre-eclampsia

Pre-eclampsia

Hypertension complicates 5–10% of all pregnancies and pre-eclampsia occurs in up to 15% of first pregnancies. As pre-eclampsia (or pre-eclamptic toxaemia) can lead to fatal eclampsia, blood pressure is monitored carefully in pregnant women. Pre-eclampsia is a condition of the third trimester or final 3-month period of pregnancy and only occurs **after 20 weeks of gestation**. It is usually associated with **proteinuria and/or oedema**. The incidence is higher with multiple pregnancies such as twins or triplets. The cause is unknown but may relate to prostaglandin metabolism during pregnancy.

Untreated, it can lead to seizures (eclampsia), coagulopathy and acute liver and renal failure (Fig. 8.28). The condition is unlikely to arise in women who have already had a baby or in the second trimester. Apparent pre-eclampsia in these groups suggests intrinsic renal disease. Pre-eclampsia should always be managed with advice from an obstetric team. Women with signs indicating pre-eclampsia are usually admitted to hospital for closer monitoring and bed rest. If necessary the hypertension is treated with a drug that is safe in pregnancy. Hydralazine and labetalol can be used intravenously if necessary. If hypertension cannot be controlled and other complications arise such as liver dysfunction, thrombocytopenia or seizures, the fetus is delivered immediately.

Eclampsia

The mortality of eclampsia is around 3–4% for the mother and 30–40% for the fetus. The management of full-blown eclampsia involves immediate delivery of the baby, treatment of the hypertension and anticonvulsant therapy. The anticonvulsants used include diazepam to stop seizures, phenytoin to prevent further seizures and magnesium sulphate.

Other causes of hypertension in pregnancy

Hypertension in pregnancy can also result from essential hypertension, intrinsic renal disease or another disease process such as lupus erythematosus, which may be exacerbated by pregnancy. Hypertension that is not related to pre-eclampsia is treated with drugs that are known to be safe in pregnancy. Typically, these are methyldopa, hydralazine and labetalol, although there is some use of calcium antagonists such as nifedipine (always check a formulary such as the *BNF*).

Acute renal failure

Acute renal failure is an acute fall in glomerular filtration rate that causes an acute loss of renal function, often leading to the need for renal replacement therapy such as dialysis or haemofiltration. It is relatively common in hospital and is an important cause of morbidity and carries a **high mortality** (30–70%). Of those who survive, 60% regain normal function but 15–30% have significant renal impairment and approximately 5–10% will have permanent end-stage renal disease requiring dialysis or transplantation.

Disease mechanisms

It is important for all doctors in hospital or in the community to know about acute renal failure as unfortunately, much of it results from medical or surgical manoeuvres. In some cases this may be unavoidable, but in other cases it is clearly preventable and it is vital that all doctors fully understand the causes of renal failure so that they take appropriate action not to cause it. Acute renal failure can be caused by three types of problem: **prerenal, renal and postrenal**. Prerenal causes account for around 60% of cases, renal causes for 25% and postrenal for around 15%.

Prerenal. This refers to acute renal failure where the kidney itself is not initially diseased but is injured by inadequate perfusion. This can happen when there is a low intravascular volume and a low blood pressure, which can result from haemorrhage caused by trauma, gastrointestinal bleeding or sometimes even surgery. Poor renal perfusion can also arise as a result of impaired myocardial function with a reduced cardiac output or perfusion pressure. In addition, mechanical damage to or obstruction of the aorta or renal arteries will reduce renal perfusion. This can happen if the renal arteries are damaged during vascular surgery. The kidney is especially sensitive to ischaemia as it is a highly metabolically active organ because of all the tubular transport processes.

Renal. This refers to acute renal failure caused by a disease process that directly affects the kidney (e.g. glomerulonephritis).

Postrenal. This refers to acute renal failure where the kidney itself is not initially diseased but problems are caused by an obstruction to urine flow. The obstruction may be partial or complete, but it increases the back pressure in the kidney. As the pressure builds up, swelling occurs and this can impair blood flow through the kidney causing ischaemic damage. Overall, acute renal failure will only occur if both kidneys are affected, or if the non-obstructed kidney is already non-functional or absent. For both kidneys to be obstructed, the obstruction must affect either both ureters, the urethra or bladder outflow. The causes of obstruction can be subdivided into:

- Those that arise outside the wall of the urinary system
- Those that arise within the wall itself
- Those that arise within the lumen of the system

Causes from outside the wall include compression by an external mass such as a tumour or retroperitoneal fibrosis (see p. 562). Causes within the wall include tumours of the wall itself or strictures. Causes inside the lumen include stones, blood clots and pieces of detached tissue such as sloughed renal papillae or fragments of tumours.

Intrinsic renal diseases

There are many disease processes that can result in acute renal failure. Broadly, they can be divided into those processes that affect the glomeruli and those processes that affect the tubules. In some circumstances, both glomeruli and tubules are affected. Important causes of damage include drugs and toxins.

Glomerular damage. In acute renal failure this usually arises from glomerulonephritis (see p. 514). The most common types in this setting are diffuse proliferative glomerulonephritis (the pattern typically associated with poststreptococcal glomerulonephritis) and rapidly progressive glomerulonephritis (the pattern typically associated with Goodpasture's syndrome and the vasculitic diseases). Acute hypertension can also cause acute renal failure (see p. 548). Showers of cholesterol emboli can arise from atherosclerotic plaques in the aorta or renal arteries, especially after surgery or instrumentation such as radiological procedures. The multiple small fragments of organized lipid material can deposit in the kidneys, causing renal injury (see p. 540).

Table 8.10 Drugs implicated in acute renal failure

Drug	Renal effect
Aminoglycosides	Tubular toxin
NSAIDs	Inhibit prostaglandin-mediated vasodilatation
ACE inhibitors	Reduce efferent arteriole tone and glomerular filtration rate
Cephalosporins	Tubular toxins
Amphotericin	Vasoconstrictor, causes membrane damage
Aciclovir	Precipitates in tubules and can form crystals in urine
Ciclosporin/tacrolimus	Indirect vasoconstriction
Radiocontrast	Vasoconstriction

Tubular damage. In acute renal failure this can arise from **ischaemia** and is usually the basis of acute tubular necrosis. The other main causes of tubular damage are **toxins**, which poison the tubular cells. Some toxins are directly secreted into the tubules and others are concentrated in the tubules, making tubular cells especially vulnerable to their effects. Toxins can be exogenous, for example arising from drugs, heavy metals or contrast media. The major drugs implicated in acute renal failure are listed in Table 8.10 (see also Table 8.6, p. 536). An important exogenous toxin is the toxin produced by the *Escherichia coli* serotype 0157, which can cause a combination of haemolysis and acute renal failure. However, there are important endogenous toxins, principally:

- Myoglobin
- Haemoglobin
- Light chains of antibodies
- Calcium (although not strictly a toxin, calcium has deleterious effects at high concentration)

Normal plasma does not usually contain either of the pigmented oxygen-binding proteins, myoglobin or haemoglobin. However, if they are released from damaged cells and are present in plasma, free myoglobin or haemoglobin will be filtered in the glomerulus and both proteins are toxic to tubular cells. Muscle cell damage or **rhabdomyolysis** releases myoglobin into plasma and this can occur from trauma, severe exercise or other forms of muscle injury. Similarly, damage to red cells or **haemolysis** releases free haemoglobin from red cells into plasma. Myeloma causes the production of excess antibody protein and the **light chains** enter the glomerular filtrate and can precipitate in the tubules, causing inflammation and toxicity to the tubular cells (see p. 530). Very high levels of **calcium** can have a number of effects including renal vasoconstriction and calcium phosphate precipitation in the tubules. The vasoconstriction can contribute to tubular ischaemia and the precipitation to tubular injury. Tubular injury can occur with **acute interstitial nephritis** (see p. 525).

Drugs

Drugs can have a number of different effects (Table 8.10). Of these, **NSAIDs** are an important cause of renal problems. There is normally tonic prostaglandin-induced renal vasodilatation. NSAIDs reduce this by inhibiting prostaglandin synthesis. The result is renal vasoconstriction, which reduces renal blood flow and glomerular filtration rate. In situations where there is already a vasoconstrictive drive, such as occurs with volume depletion, then the combined vasoconstriction can be severe and results in a major fall in glomerular filtration rate. NSAIDs should therefore be used with extreme care, or not at all, in those patients who are likely to have such a vasoconstrictive drive already present. Risk factors for NSAID-induced renal disease are volume depletion, diuretic use, pre-existing renal disease and one of the oedema states (congestive heart failure, liver cirrhosis or nephrotic syndrome).

Aminoglycosides such as gentamicin are direct tubular toxins and cause acute tubular necrosis. With renal artery stenosis (see p. 540), renin levels are raised and this causes high levels of the vasoconstrictor angiotensin II. The vasoconstriction acts predominantly on the efferent arterioles in the kidney to maintain glomerular filtration rate. If an **ACE inhibitor** is administered, this vasoconstriction is removed and so glomerular filtration rate can fall.

Multifactorial acute renal failure

Multiple renal insults are often found to contribute to the acute renal failure, especially **fluid depletion, sepsis and drug toxicity** after surgery, trauma or burns. Such a combination may arise in a patient who has a major haemorrhage requiring surgery, resulting in low blood volume and blood pressure during the surgery, and who then develops infection and is given nephrotoxic antibiotics to treat the infection and NSAIDs as analgesics. Patient who are very sick from any cause, especially infection but also other conditions such as acute myocardial infarction with impaired cardiac contractility, are at substantial risk of acute renal failure, which is therefore common on intensive care units.

Epidemiology

The annual incidence of acute renal failure is around 180/million population in the UK. In developing countries the incidence is probably higher and obstetric complications and infections such as malaria are important causes of acute renal failure.

Clinical presentation

The most typical presentation is of a patient already in hospital who now has a rise in urea and creatinine and/or a fall in urine output. Probably the most common cause is simple fluid depletion because of mismanaged fluid replacement (see p. 579). Rarely, patients may present with frank haematuria, which suggests glomerulonephritis or urinary tract stones. In some cases, a patient may even notice that their urine volume has diminished and this has been documented with Goodpasture's syndrome.

A number of well-recognized scenarios can occur and it is important to be aware of these and to ask about them in the history:
- **Haemoptysis** suggests a pulmonary renal syndrome such as Goodpasture's syndrome or systemic vasculitis
- A recent **sore throat** or infection suggests postinfective glomerulonephritis (acute diffuse proliferative glomerulonephritis)
- In men, a history of **urinary symptoms** such as a poor urinary stream, dribbling, hesitancy, nocturia and urinary frequency suggests prostatic disease, which can cause obstruction as well as urinary tract infection
- A history of recent **trauma** or very heavy exercise, especially if associated with muscle pain, raises the possibility of rhabdomyolysis
- Recent **gastroenteritis** may indicate infection with *E. coli* serotype 0157 and the presence of the haemolytic–uraemic syndrome (see p. 531)

The **past medical history** may highlight an underlying multisystem disease associated with renal disease such as:
- Systemic lupus erythematosus
- Vascular disease, which is associated with renal artery stenosis
- Malignancy, which may be associated with hypercalcaemia
- Chronic infection such as osteomyelitis, which can be associated with amyloidosis affecting the kidney
- Abnormal or artificial heart valves, which are vulnerable to infection associated with glomerulonephritis

Any underlying renal disease increases the risk of acute renal failure from a relatively minor insult that might be of little consequence in a fit young person. In your history, ask about symptoms such as joint pains or a rash that might suggest an underlying disease such as systemic lupus erythematosus. Enquire about any prescribed or recreational **drugs** that the patient may have taken and ask about self-poisoning with drugs or other toxic substances.

Special considerations in hospitalized patients

In many cases, patients with acute renal failure are very sick or already in hospital and, under these circumstances,

Table 8.11 Renal causes of acute renal failure

Diagnosis	Clinical features	Investigations
Rhabdomyolysis	Muscle pain	CK ↑, myoglobulinuria
Glomerulonephritis		Red cell casts
Goodpasture's disease	Pulmonary haemorrhage	Anti-GBM antibodies ↑
Vasculitis	± Systemic features, sinusitis, rash	ANCA ↑
SLE	Joint/neurological signs, rash	Anti dsDNA ↑, antinuclear antibodies
Interstitial nephritis	Drug cause	Eosinophils ↑ (in blood and urine)
Haemolytic–uraemic syndrome	Diarrhoea	Hb ↓, haemolysis, platelets ↓
Acute tubular necrosis	Multiple factors, especially in hospitals	Granular tubular casts

ANCA, antineutrophil cytoplasmic antibodies; CK, creatinine kinase; GBM, glomerular basement membrane; Hb, haemoglobin; SLE, systemic lupus erythematosus.

the history must also include a careful search through their hospital records for evidence of renal insults. These are sometimes easy to identify, such as the prescription of a nephrotoxic drug, but sometimes they may be less obvious. Aim to look at all the relevant charts, remembering that if a patient was only home for a few days before the admission you may need to scrutinize the relevant documents from previous admissions.

• Check all operation notes and anaesthetic charts to establish whether there was a period of profound hypotension during an operation.

• Check all drug charts, including perioperative and radiological charts, for potentially toxic drugs or dyes.

• Check all blood pressure and pulse charts to identify a period of hypotension.

• Check all temperature charts for a fever, which may indicate infection.

• Check all blood tests to establish the previous level of renal function before the deterioration.

• Check all the weight charts or fluid balance charts to identify fluid depletion. Fluid balance charts may be unreliable, but if the patient's weight has fallen significantly over a few days this is likely to represent fluid loss rather than solid body mass loss.

The key aspect of examination is the assessment of **fluid status**. Is the patient dehydrated? Check the skin turgor and jugular venous pressure, examine the heart, check for peripheral and pulmonary oedema and measure the pulse and the blood pressure lying down and standing up if possible. Examine carefully for possible clues to the cause of the renal failure. Look for a focus of current or previous **infection**—this will involve looking at every part of the patient's skin and under all bandages and dressings. Check all surgical or traumatic **wounds** and examine any bed sores on the buttocks, legs, feet and back and head. Examine **muscles** for any tenderness or swelling that might suggest rhabdomyolysis.

Examine the **eyes** for diagnostic changes of hypertension, diabetes mellitus or other disease. Examine the

chest for pulmonary oedema and signs of pulmonary haemorrhage. Upper airway disease or **ear, nose and throat** problems may indicate Wegener's vasculitic disease. Polycystic **kidneys** may be palpable and a large palpable **bladder** suggests obstruction. A **rectal** examination may indicate prostatic or pelvic disease.

Check carefully for other signs of systemic disease, of cholesterol emboli and of intravenous drug use.

Investigation

Some investigations are useful in monitoring and treating acute renal failure, such as electrolytes, but a range of useful tests also provides diagnostic information such as antibody tests (Table 8.11).

Biochemistry

Plasma **urea and creatinine** levels are elevated. **Potassium and acid**, which are excreted by the kidneys, can accumulate causing dangerous hyperkalaemia and metabolic acidosis, which both carry a serious risk of cardiac arrhythmias and cardiac arrest. Rhabdomyolysis usually causes a major increase in **creatinine kinase** in the blood. **Arterial blood gases** must be checked to assess the extent of any metabolic acidosis.

Haematology

Anaemia may be present from blood loss, haemolysis, impaired erythropoiesis or low erythropoietin levels. A high **eosinophil** count can occur with acute interstitial nephritis. In haemolytic–uraemic syndrome (HUS), there may be **haemolysis**, causing anaemia with damaged red blood cells on a blood film and a low platelet count.

Urine

Urine dipstick analysis, microscopy and culture should all be performed. Although **haematuria** could indicate renal or postrenal disease, it can also be caused by urinary catheterization. Heavy **proteinuria** usually indicates a glomerular disease. Both myoglobin and haemoglobin can be measured in urine and indicate rhabdomyolysis and haemolysis, respectively. On microscopy, red cell **casts** are diagnostic of glomerulonephritis and white cells indicate infection or interstitial nephritis. **Eosinophils** in the urine are indicative of interstitial nephritis.

Imaging

The kidneys should be imaged, usually with ultrasound, to exclude urinary tract obstruction and to establish the renal sizes. If the kidneys are small then chronic renal failure is likely. Other abnormalities such as polycystic kidney disease will also be identified. If it is necessary to monitor renal perfusion, Doppler studies or radioisotope studies (e.g. DTPA scans) may be helpful, although ultimately it may be necessary to perform renal angiography. CT, MRI or renal venography exclude renal vein thrombosis.

Immunology and microbiology

High levels of antiglomerular basement membrane (AGBM) antibodies indicate Goodpasture's syndrome and high levels of antineutrophil cytoplasmic antibodies (ANCA) indicate vasculitis (see p. 522). Antibodies to double-stranded DNA are present in systemic lupus erythematosus. Low complement levels (usually C3 and C4 are measured) occur in systemic lupus erythematosus and postinfectious glomerulonephritis.

Microbiological tests should exclude current infection and rule out recent infection. High levels of antistreptolysin O may indicate recent streptococcal infection.

Histology

If the aetiology of the renal disease is unclear, then renal biopsy should be undertaken to exclude a treatable intrinsic renal disease. The renal histology may reflect whatever disease process is involved. If the main effect is acute tubular necrosis, then the tubular cells are usually seen to be swollen and the tubules may be filled with cellular debris. In the later stages, the tubule cells become flattened.

Differential diagnosis

The key differential diagnosis is of chronic renal failure. In chronic renal failure there may be complications such as anaemia and bone disease, but the most obvious difference is that the kidneys are usually small on ultrasound or other imaging in chronic renal failure (see p. 555).

Management

Acute renal failure is a medical emergency as the patient can die from a cardiac arrest if there is severe hyperkalaemia or acidosis. In its early stages, especially when caused by acute tubular necrosis, it may be reversible if appropriate measures are taken rapidly and further problems are not allowed to develop. Such measures may be as simple as rehydrating the patient and should not be delayed until specialist help can be arranged. It may be helpful and sensible to speak to a specialist at an early stage, but doctors should be aware of the basic general measures that relate to acute renal failure. Obviously, any cause of the renal failure should be corrected. This applies especially to pre- and postrenal causes.

General management

General measures apply, regardless of the aetiology of the condition, and their aim is to prevent life-threatening complications such as cardiac arrest and to optimize the chances of the kidney recovering. Sometimes this will require treatment on a **high dependency or intensive care unit**:

- If the patient is hypoxic, this should be corrected with oxygen therapy and **ventilation** if necessary.
- Cardiac output should be maintained with **inotropic** drugs and adequate circulatory volume maintained by **fluid** management.
- If the patient is anaemic, he or she should be transfused to ensure adequate oxygen delivery. Generally, a **haemoglobin** of 10 mg/dl or greater is considered appropriate.
- If the patient is not able or motivated to eat properly, he or she should be **fed** nasogastrically or parenterally.
- Any **hypertension** should be controlled to avoid further renal damage.

Specific issues in management

The absolute and immediate priorities in acute renal failure are to ensure that plasma potassium levels do not rise too high and that plasma pH does not fall too low; both are strong risk factors for cardiac arrest. Electrolytes should be measured daily, or more frequently if the patient is very sick or unstable.

Potassium. The kidney normally excretes potassium from the body, so when renal function is impaired, potassium accumulates. Potassium intake should therefore be restricted. In the short term, the standard methods of treatment for hyperkalaemia (see p. 585) may be of some help, but if renal function is substantially impaired, dialysis or haemofiltration is required to remove the potassium from the body.

Acid. The kidney normally excretes acid from the body, so acid accumulates when renal function is impaired. Acid can impair many metabolic processes and must be corrected. The only way to remove acid if the kidneys are not working is by dialysis or haemofiltration.

Acute renal failure at a glance

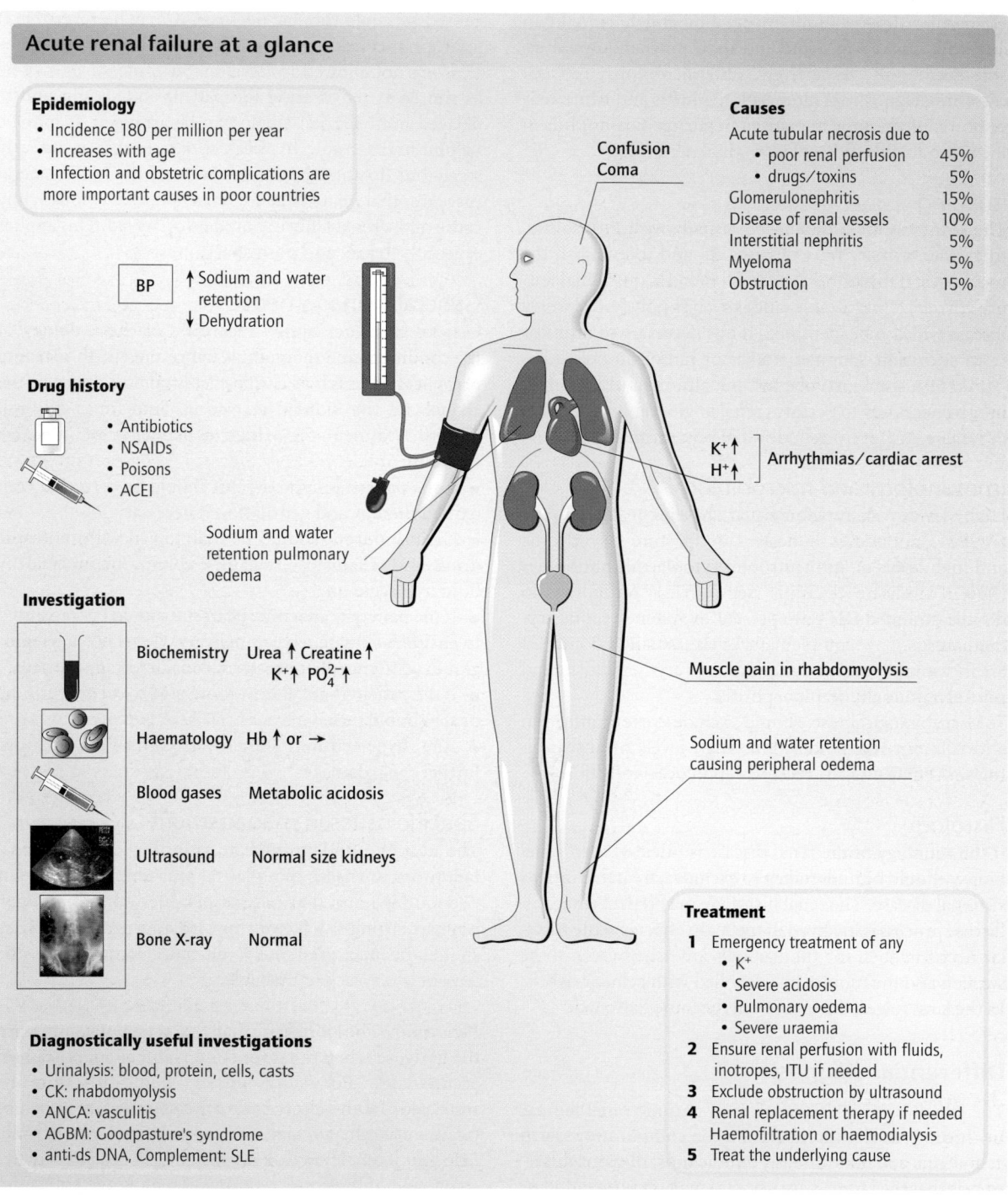

Epidemiology

- Incidence 180 per million per year
- Increases with age
- Infection and obstetric complications are more important causes in poor countries

BP   ↑ Sodium and water retention
      ↓ Dehydration

Confusion
Coma

Causes

Acute tubular necrosis due to
- poor renal perfusion   45%
- drugs/toxins   5%
Glomerulonephritis   15%
Disease of renal vessels   10%
Interstitial nephritis   5%
Myeloma   5%
Obstruction   15%

Drug history

- Antibiotics
- NSAIDs
- Poisons
- ACEI

Sodium and water retention pulmonary oedema

K^+ ↑
H^+ ↑   } Arrhythmias/cardiac arrest

Investigation

Biochemistry	Urea ↑ Creatine ↑ K^+↑ PO_4^{2-}↑	
Haematology	Hb ↑ or →	
Blood gases	Metabolic acidosis	
Ultrasound	Normal size kidneys	
Bone X-ray	Normal	

Muscle pain in rhabdomyolysis

Sodium and water retention causing peripheral oedema

Treatment

1 Emergency treatment of any
- K^+
- Severe acidosis
- Pulmonary oedema
- Severe uraemia
2 Ensure renal perfusion with fluids, inotropes, ITU if needed
3 Exclude obstruction by ultrasound
4 Renal replacement therapy if needed Haemofiltration or haemodialysis
5 Treat the underlying cause

Diagnostically useful investigations

- Urinalysis: blood, protein, cells, casts
- CK: rhabdomyolysis
- ANCA: vasculitis
- AGBM: Goodpasture's syndrome
- anti-ds DNA, Complement: SLE

Volume. Maintaining the patient's fluid status correctly helps prevent further renal damage in a patient who has not lost all their renal function:

- Regular clinical assessment of fluid status is essential at least once or twice daily (see pp. 579–80)

- A reliable index of fluid replacement is daily weighing of the patient when possible
- Fluid balance charts documenting all input and output should be kept, but are subject to human error
- When the patient is properly rehydrated, volume

replacement should match output and insensible losses, which are usually approximately 500 ml (or greater if there is fever)

- If necessary, insert a central venous catheter and measure central venous pressure to aid fluid replacement
- Urinary catheterization may be helpful to monitor urine output, but always carries the risk of infection

Pulmonary oedema. If the patient has excess body water, he or she may develop pulmonary oedema. In renal failure this is particularly dangerous because the kidneys may not be able to excrete the excess water in response to diuretic therapy:

- Sit the patient up and give him or her oxygen
- If there is any renal function, or even the suspicion of any, give diuretics
- If there is very poor renal function, arrangements must be made for urgent renal replacement therapy with dialysis or haemofiltration
- In the meantime, intravenous nitrates and opiates will provide vasodilatation
- If necessary and if renal replacement therapy cannot be arranged in time, venesect 200–500 ml blood and ventilate the patient with positive end-expiratory pressures (this opposes the entry of fluid into the alveoli)

Renal replacement therapy
There are certain absolute indications for starting renal replacement therapy in the presence of acute or chronic renal failure:

- Acute hyperkalaemia
- Severe metabolic acidosis
- Pulmonary oedema
- Severe uraemic complications (e.g. pericarditis; see p. 562)

Haemodialysis or haemofiltration may be used. Haemofiltration is slower, but may be better tolerated in haemodynamically unstable patients. Peritoneal dialysis has been used, but haemodialysis and haemofiltration are preferred.

Chronic renal failure

End-stage renal disease or end-stage renal failure occurs when the glomerular filtration rate is so low that life cannot be sustained without some form of renal replacement therapy, such as dialysis or transplantation. The clinical syndrome of **chronic renal failure** is caused by the long-term absence of normal kidney function and can occur both in patients who have reached end-stage renal disease and also in those patients who have just enough renal function to maintain life but not enough to prevent the syndrome and its complications from developing. In these cases, chronic renal failure is usually a deteriorating condition that eventually leads to end-stage renal disease. End-stage renal disease can also follow acute renal failure if there is acute irreversible renal damage of sufficient severity. Severe symptomatic untreated chronic renal failure is often termed the 'uraemic syndrome'.

Disease mechanisms

The syndrome of chronic renal failure consists of various features, but the key features reflect the different functions of the kidney. In both acute and chronic renal failure, the ability of the body to eliminate excess **potassium, acid and water** is impaired and hyperkalaemia, metabolic acidosis and hypervolaemia, which can cause systemic or pulmonary oedema, are all well-recognized features. However, in addition to these features, over a long period of renal failure, a number of other features also become important and characterize chronic renal failure compared to acute renal failure:

- The kidney makes **erythropoietin**, which promotes red blood cell formation. In chronic renal failure, there is inadequate erythropoietin and so anaemia is brought about by inadequate red blood cell formation.
- The kidney produces vitamin D and so helps regulate calcium and phosphate metabolism, so in chronic renal failure abnormalities of this metabolism occur and can cause **bone disease**.
- The kidney is an excretory organ for many molecules, so in chronic renal failure **excretion products can accumulate** in the plasma. Some of these excretion products can be toxic and may be the cause of itching, pericarditis, neuropathy and other problems that can arise in chronic renal failure.

The common causes of end-stage renal failure are shown in CHRONIC RENAL FAILURE AT A GLANCE on p. 558. The key point to note is that diabetes mellitus is an increasingly important cause and is especially prevalent in black patients and in those with an ethnic origin in the Indian subcontinent. Overall, there is a slight male predominance, with 60% of cases being male. The challenge for medicine is to reduce the amount of end-stage renal failure by early intervention in potentially treatable conditions such as diabetes mellitus, hypertension, glomerulonephritis and obstruction, especially prostatic obstruction.

Distinguishing acute and chronic renal failure

On investigation, patients with chronic renal failure have a range of abnormalities that are not usually seen in acute renal failure:

- They may be anaemic with no other obvious cause for the anaemia.

- Typically, they have a high plasma phosphate level and a low plasma calcium level. Occasionally, calcium levels may be high if tertiary hyperparathyroidism is present (see p. 290).
- Bone X-rays may show signs of bone disease caused by aberrant vitamin D, calcium and phosphate metabolism in chronic renal failure.
- They may have symptoms such as itch, tremor or pericarditis caused by accumulation of toxic substances.
- The key investigation is renal ultrasound or other imaging to examine the **renal size**. If the patient has normal-sized kidneys with normal morphology, then the renal failure is acute. If the patient has small shrunken kidneys, then the renal failure is chronic.

Clinically, patients with acute renal failure do not typically display the features of chronic renal failure such as anaemia, bone disease, itch, tremor and pericarditis.

Acute on chronic renal failure

This term describes the situation in a patient who has had chronic impairment of renal function, but whose renal function suddenly undergoes an acute further deterioration. In practice, the investigation and management of this situation is the same as that of acute renal failure. However, in some cases, no obvious cause will be found for the deterioration and it simply reflects an ongoing renal disease process. Sometimes an obvious cause is identified, such as obstruction, drug toxicity or fluid depletion. The discussion below relates principally to chronic renal failure without any acute deterioration.

Epidemiology

The exact incidence is difficult to determine, but around 80–200 people/million start renal replacement therapy each year in the developed world. Although this may seem a small number, these patients require this therapy for life and, with their many other complications, require a substantial amount of health care resources. There are some regional variations in the causes, e.g. schistosomiasis can cause renal obstruction and so chronic renal failure in those areas of the world where it is prevalent (see p. 140). With the increasing numbers of patients on renal replacement therapy, care is shared between GPs and hospital practitioners and patients are often dialysed at home or in small satellite dialysis units that do not usually have specialist doctors on site.

Clinical presentations

The clinical presentation of chronic renal failure is very variable. Often it is detected as a biochemical abnormality on routine blood testing. Rarely, full-blown chronic renal failure can present with the 'uraemic syndrome' consisting of the many clinical abnormalities that arise when renal function is impaired over a long period, including confusion, tremor, itch and pericarditis. Otherwise, the condition can present with any of the features of an underlying disease such as polycystic kidney disease, glomerulonephritis or diabetes mellitus.

Clinical assessment issues

There are several key questions to be answered about patients with suspected renal failure of any type:

1 *Does the patient have renal failure?* This question can be answered by plasma biochemistry.

2 *Does the patient have a potentially acute life-threatening disorder?* Hyperkalaemia, severe acidosis and pulmonary oedema are medical emergencies and must be dealt with immediately. Do not waste time at this stage trying to establish the cause of the renal failure or whether it is acute or chronic. In any patient with renal failure, you must rapidly determine the plasma potassium to ensure that they are not at imminent risk of cardiac arrest and death.

3 *Is there an acute and reversible cause for the patient's current condition that should be urgently corrected to prevent further renal damage?* In other words, is there an element of acute renal failure or acute on chronic renal failure? If there is acute on chronic renal failure, you may still be able to salvage some renal function by prompt action. If there appears to be acute damage, then investigate the condition as you would for acute renal failure. Even if the patient's underlying renal function is not good, giving a patient an extra year or two of life in which they do not need dialysis or transplantation is of great value.

4 *If the patient has chronic renal failure, what is the cause?* Assess the patient as described below to establish the cause if possible.

5 *Is renal replacement therapy necessary?* This depends on the level of renal function and the presence of unacceptable complications such as pericarditis. In general, renal replacement of some form is likely to be necessary for hyperkalaemia, acidosis or pulmonary oedema and when the patient is beginning to feel unwell because of accumulating uraemic toxins.

History

If the patient is not acutely unwell, the aim of the history is to establish:

1 The cause of the renal disease

2 What complications of chronic renal failure are present

Key questions are whether the patient has any **past medical history** of conditions that will predispose them to renal disease, especially diabetes mellitus, hypertension or an autoimmune condition such as systemic lupus erythematosus, or a malignancy, especially myeloma. As most causes of glomerulonephritis can cause chronic renal failure, consider whether there are any previous conditions consistent with a diagnosis of glomerulonephritis, such as episodes of haematuria. Ask also about a **family history** of renal disease, especially polycystic kidney disease and Alport's syndrome of deafness and renal failure.

Ask about the **general symptoms** of chronic renal failure:

- Tiredness
- Confusion
- Itch
- Tremor
- Loss of energy
- Shortness of breath (from anaemia or acidotic breathing)
- Nausea and vomiting
- Pain from bone disease
- Chest pain from pericarditis

Examination

- Check for signs of anaemia, scratch marks from itching, uraemic discoloration (a tanned/greyish colour to the skin). The patient's breath may smell 'uraemic' with a fishy urine smell somewhat like that of ammonia. 'Uraemic frost' is the precipitation of urea crystals on the skin and occurs rarely in severe uraemia.
- Check the patient's **blood pressure** and assess their **fluid status** carefully to exclude dangerous fluid overload with pulmonary oedema and to exclude fluid depletion that will worsen any remaining renal function.
- Examine the **heart**, listening carefully for the scratching sound that can occur with pericarditis.
- Palpate the **kidneys** to exclude large polycystic kidneys, kidneys that are enlarged by tumours and large obstructed kidneys.
- Check that the **bladder** is not palpably obstructed and in men exclude an enlarged **prostate** by rectal examination.
- Check for **neurological** signs such as brisk reflexes and check the **fundi** for signs of hypertension or diabetes mellitus.

Investigations

As in acute renal failure, some investigations are aimed at diagnosis and others are aimed at the more immediate care and monitoring of the patient.

Biochemistry

Plasma urea and creatinine levels are both elevated. Potassium and acid that are excreted by the kidneys accumulate and can cause dangerous hyperkalaemia and metabolic acidosis, each of which carries a serious risk of cardiac arrhythmias and cardiac arrest.

Arterial blood gases should be checked to assess the extent of any metabolic acidosis.

Measure plasma glucose levels to exclude hyperglycaemia. Plasma calcium and phosphate levels should be checked and the usual pattern in chronic renal failure is of a raised plasma phosphate (phosphate is usually excreted by the kidney) and a lowered plasma calcium. If there is tertiary hyperparathyroidism then the calcium level may also be raised (see p. 290). Measure plasma lipids to exclude hyperlipidaemia, which is common.

Haematology

Anaemia may be present and, unless there is another disease process or a deficiency of iron, folate or vitamin B_{12}, the anaemia is likely to result from erythropoietin deficiency. A raised ESR is a relatively normal finding in chronic renal failure and usually of no significance.

Urine

Dipstick analysis, microscopy and culture can help to make a diagnosis if some renal function remains. In a new patient it is usually sensible to exclude urinary tract infection.

Imaging

The kidneys should be imaged, usually with ultrasound to exclude urinary tract obstruction and to establish the renal sizes. If the kidneys are small, chronic renal failure is likely. Other abnormalities such as polycystic kidney disease can also be identified.

Bone X-rays may show signs of renal bone disease (see p. 561 and Fig. A on p. 558).

Immunology and microbiology

Immunological tests are principally of use in monitoring any underlying disease such as systemic lupus erythematosus.

Histology

Even if the aetiology of the renal disease is unclear, renal biopsy is not usually undertaken if the kidneys are small. This is for two reasons: first, the biopsy can be dangerous because of bleeding and, secondly, it is unlikely to yield much information as the kidneys are usually very badly damaged and fibrosed.

Management

If there is any component of acute on chronic renal failure, it should be managed in the same way as acute renal failure. If there is renal damage, but there is still a useful amount of renal function, then it is important to try to preserve that renal function for as long as possible. This is because end-stage renal disease has substantial morbidity and mortality and dialysis or transplantation can be

Chronic renal failure at a glance

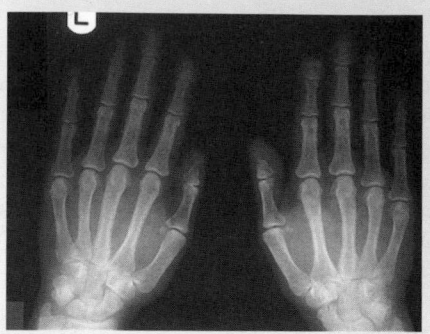

Fig. A Renal osteodystrophy with hyperparathyroidism. Erosion of the terminal phalanges is accompanied by a loss of cortical structure and cyst formation, most marked on the radial sides of other phalanges.

Epidemiology

- Prevalence >500 per million
- M>F 1.5:1
- Increased in black/Indian subcontinent ethnic groups
- Increased with age

General

- Itch
- Lethargy
- Bleeding
- Lowered immunity

Neurological

- Confusion
- Seizures
- Coma

Causes

- Diabetes mellitus   40%
- Hypertension   25%
- Glomerulonephritis   15%
- Polycystic kidney disease   4%
- Urological causes   6%
- Miscellaneous/unknown   10%

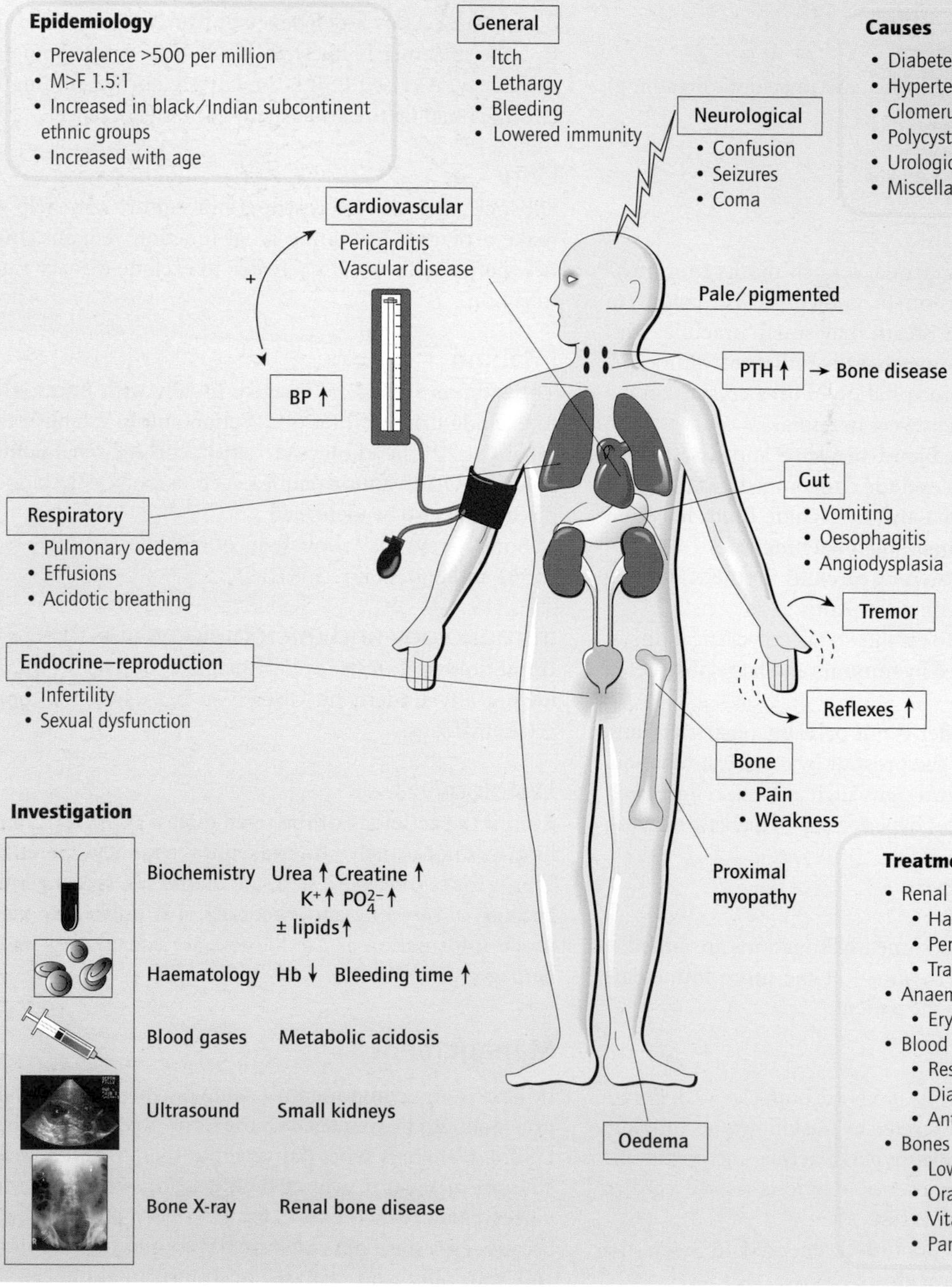

Cardiovascular

Pericarditis
Vascular disease

BP ↑

Pale/pigmented

PTH ↑ → Bone disease

Respiratory

- Pulmonary oedema
- Effusions
- Acidotic breathing

Gut

- Vomiting
- Oesophagitis
- Angiodysplasia

Tremor

Reflexes ↑

Endocrine–reproduction

- Infertility
- Sexual dysfunction

Bone

- Pain
- Weakness

Proximal myopathy

Oedema

Investigation

Biochemistry	Urea ↑ Creatine ↑ K^+↑ PO_4^{2-}↑ ± lipids↑	
Haematology	Hb ↓ Bleeding time ↑	
Blood gases	Metabolic acidosis	
Ultrasound	Small kidneys	
Bone X-ray	Renal bone disease	

Treatment options

- Renal function
  - Haemodialysis
  - Peritoneal dialysis
  - Transplantation
- Anaemia
  - Erythropoietin
- Blood pressure
  - Restrict fluid intake
  - Dialysis to remove fluid
  - Antihypertensive drugs
- Bones
  - Low phosphate diet
  - Oral phosphate-binders
  - Vitamin D
  - Parathyroid surgery

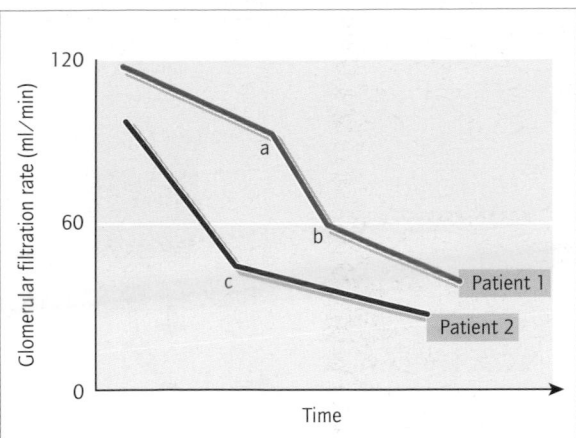

Figure 8.29 Plots of change in renal function (glomerular filtration rate) with time. Patient 1 suffered a sudden accelerated decline of renal function at point a (resulting from a urinary tract infection and hypovolaemia) with recovery at point b because of their correction. Patient 2 enjoyed a deceleration in decline because of control of hypertension at point c.

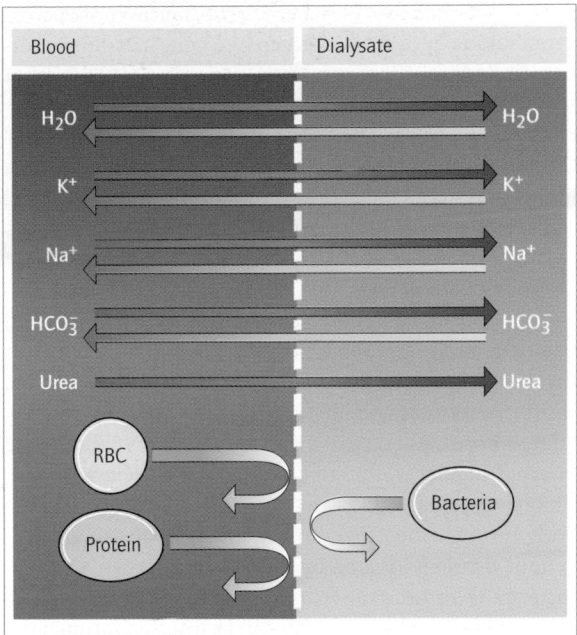

Figure 8.30 The principles of dialysis across a semipermeable membrane. The semipermeable dialysis membrane is shown as white dashes. Small molecules pass through the membrane along a concentration gradient. Larger molecules (e.g. proteins) and cells cannot do so. RBC, red blood cell.

disruptive to the patient's lifestyle. Any underlying disease causing renal damage, such as systemic lupus erythematosus, should be treated. However, for all patients, careful control of blood pressure and the avoidance of urinary tract infection, obstruction, nephrotoxic drugs and dehydration can slow the rate of progression (Fig. 8.29).

The management of established end-stage renal disease involves replacing the functions of the kidney to restore normal homoeostasis. The best way of doing this is to transplant a new kidney into the patient, but this is limited by the number of available organ donors. More commonly, renal replacement therapy entails a combination of:
- Dialysis to replace the excretory function of the kidney
- Erythropoietin administration to replace the erythropoietic synthetic function of the kidney
- Vitamin D administration to replace the vitamin D synthetic function of the kidney
- Various measures such as the restriction of water, sodium, potassium and phosphate intake to reduce the need for excretory function

Although haemodialysis can take over the function of the kidneys to some extent and certainly enough to maintain life, it is intermittent and is usually only performed for around 4 h about three times a week. In between dialysis sessions, steps are taken to reduce the amount of renal replacement therapy that is required by restricting intake of substances such as sodium, potassium, water and phosphate that the kidney would usually excrete. If

a haemodialysis patient with no renal function were to drink 4 l of fluid on the day between dialysis sessions, he or she could develop severe pulmonary oedema as they have no way to excrete the excess fluid. Peritoneal dialysis is more continuous, so less stringent fluid restriction is necessary.

Haemodialysis

In this procedure, blood is removed from the body and pumped past a semipermeable membrane. On the other side of the membrane, fluid is pumped in the opposite direction. Water, ions and small molecules move across the membrane from the blood into the dialysis fluid (Fig. 8.30). The dialysis fluid typically consists of the essential components of plasma including water, sodium, potassium, chloride, calcium, magnesium, glucose and a buffer such as bicarbonate, lactate or acetate. By controlling the composition of this fluid, it is possible to control the removal of substances from the blood. In practical terms, the membrane is usually in the form of small hollow fibres in a large cartridge, which maximizes the surface area for exchange. During haemodialysis **heparin** is usually given to prevent blood clotting in the dialysis machine.

Dialysis is the process whereby substances move across a membrane by diffusion driven by a concentration gradient. In addition to this process, it is possible to subject blood to **ultrafiltration** in a similar way to what happens in the glomerulus. This can be performed in a 'dialysis' machine if the blood is forced past the membrane at a higher pressure. Under these conditions, water and small molecules are forced through the pores in the membrane by the pressure gradient. This is a very effective way of removing fluid quickly.

To perform haemodialysis, blood must be removed from the body, pumped past the dialysis membrane in the dialysis machine and then returned to the body. In the short or intermediate term this can be carried out using a **large-bore catheter** with two lumens inserted into the internal jugular vein, subclavian vein or femoral vein. Blood leaves the body by one lumen and is returned to the body through the other. In the longer term, an **arteriovenous fistula** is created by joining an artery to a vein in the arm. Over time the fistula dilates and at each dialysis session two large bore needles can be inserted through the skin; blood is removed through one and returned through the other. In some cases, an artery and a vein can be joined together using a piece of synthetic (Gore-tex™) tubing to create a **synthetic fistula**.

Complications of haemodialysis

Acute removal of blood from the circulation can cause hypotension. Furthermore, exposure of blood to the dialysis membrane can cause allergic reactions. Various symptoms such as headache, itch and muscle cramps can also occur during dialysis and may reflect rapid changes in blood volume or plasma electrolyte concentrations. **Infection** can also be a problem and may be introduced at the site of access, especially with central venous catheters or acquired from the dialysis circuit—such infections include bacterial and viral infections such as hepatitis B and C. Arteriovenous fistulas can become blocked by **clot formation**. Haemodialysis is poor at removing very large molecules and beta-2 microglobulin protein can accumulate and form amyloid-like deposits, resulting in carpal tunnel syndrome and cystic bone lesions.

Peritoneal dialysis

The peritoneal membrane is a semipermeable membrane. Therefore, if fluid is placed in the peritoneal cavity, substances can diffuse from the blood across the peritoneal membrane into the fluid. This is the principle of peritoneal dialysis.

In practice, a soft synthetic tube is inserted permanently through the anterior abdominal wall, tunnelled through the skin and then into the peritoneal cavity (Fig. 8.31). Approximately every 4 h, the patient connects a bag of

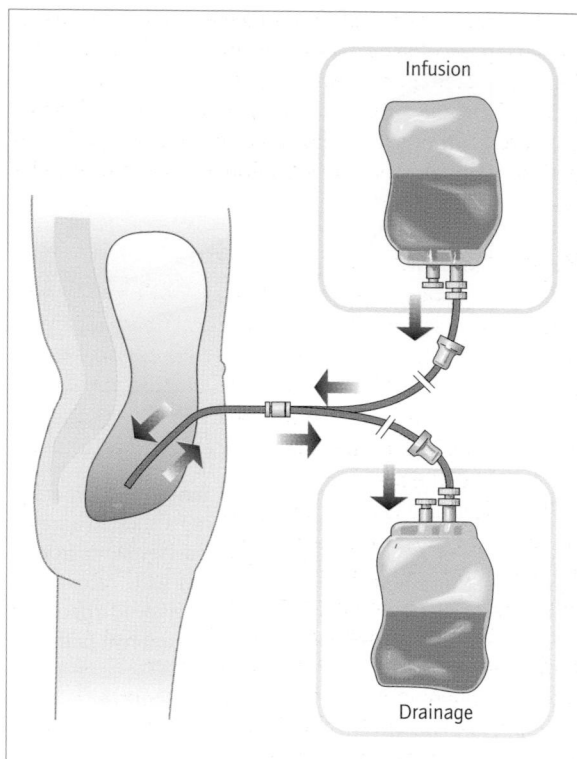

Figure 8.31 Continuous ambulatory peritoneal dialysis. The patient's peritoneum acts as the semipermeable membrane between the dialysate and the plasma. A bag of fluid is allowed to drain into the peritoneal space, left there for several hours and then drained out.

about 2 l of fluid to the tube and, by holding the bag above the abdomen, allows the fluid to flow into the peritoneal cavity. At the end of the 4 h, the fluid is removed by placing the bag below the abdomen. While the fluid is in place, the patient can go about their normal activities. By altering the composition of the bags, it is possible to control the removal of substances by diffusion. By altering the osmotic strength of the fluid it is possible to control the amount of fluid that is removed from the blood. The usual osmotic component in the bags is glucose. Patients can use a 'strong' bag of high osmotic strength to remove fluid more efficiently.

Complications of peritoneal dialysis

The major problem with peritoneal dialysis is **infection**, either of the skin and tissues around the tube or of the peritoneal cavity, causing peritonitis. This type of **peritonitis** is treated by repeated washing out of the peritoneum and by giving the patient antibiotics, often in the dialysis fluid itself. To avoid infection, care should always be taken when handling the peritoneal tube.

Most patients can only last for a few years on peritoneal dialysis. If they have a very small amount of residual renal function, then peritoneal dialysis can provide enough artificial renal function to keep a patient relatively healthy. However, without any renal function whatever, peritoneal dialysis is not always capable of doing this and haemodialysis may be necessary.

Renal transplantation

In this procedure, a kidney is taken with its attached artery, vein and ureter from a brain-dead donor or a living donor. Rarely, kidneys are removed from donors who are recently dead. The kidney is transplanted into the pelvis of the recipient outside the peritoneal cavity. The blood vessels are attached to the iliac vessels and the ureter is implanted in the bladder.

To reduce the chances of rejection of the kidney, the donor and the recipient are matched whenever possible for their HLA types, especially HLA-A, -B and -DR. In addition, the recipient is given immunosuppressive treatment. The drugs usually used are steroids, azathioprine and ciclosporin, but the use of tacrolimus, sirolimus and mycophenolate is increasing. In some cases, antibody therapy against white blood cells is given to provide increased immunosuppression.

A transplanted kidney can work very well and last for 20–30 years or sometimes more. However, many do not work so well and over several years their function deteriorates. In some cases, this has been shown to be because of a combination of low-grade rejection and of toxicity from the immunosuppressive drugs.

Immunosuppressive drugs used in transplantation

Steroids such as prednisolone bind nuclear steroid receptors and inhibit gene transcription and normal functioning in various immune cells. They have multiple side-effects, including infection, peptic ulceration, osteoporosis, hypertension, hyperglycaemia and hyperlipidaemia.

Azathioprine is metabolized to 6-mercaptopurine which inhibits purine metabolism and so nucleic acid synthesis and cell proliferation, especially in immune cells. Side-effects include bone marrow suppression with low white cell counts and pancreatitis.

Ciclosporin inhibits calcineurin, which disrupts the transcription of various T-cell components including interleukin 2 and so inhibits T-cell activation. Side-effects include renal toxicity, hypertension and electrolyte disorders such as hyperkalaemia.

Tacrolimus (FK506) and **sirolimus** (rapamycin) have similar activities to ciclosporin. Side-effects of tacrolimus include hypertension, nephrotoxicity and impaired glucose tolerance.

Mycophenolate has an analogous action to azathioprine as it inhibits inosine monophosphate dehydrogenase and so nucleic acid synthesis and cell proliferation. Side-effects are mainly gastrointestinal, including gastritis, oesophagitis and diarrhoea, but not bone marrow suppression.

Specific complications of renal transplantation

Immunosuppression carries two major risks: those of an increased tendency to infection and of an increased incidence of tumours. Cytomegalovirus infection is a major hazard in the early post-transplantation period. Skin cancer is a common late complication that is worsened by sun exposure. The different immunosuppressive agents each have their own adverse effects.

Complications of chronic renal failure

Anaemia

Anaemia arises because the damaged kidney fails to produce adequate erythropoietin. An exception to this occurs with polycystic kidney disease where erythropoietin production is often preserved. **Recombinant erythropoietin** is usually given 1–3 times weekly by subcutaneous injection. Complications of this therapy include hypertension and polycythaemia. The response to erythropoietin is poor in the presence of inflammation or deficiencies of iron, folate or vitamin B_{12}, so these situations should be excluded and treated if present. Obviously, blood loss should always be excluded in any case of anaemia.

Renal bone disease

The kidney excretes phosphate and synthesizes vitamin D. For this reason, chronic renal failure causes a rise in plasma phosphate and a reduction in renal vitamin D synthesis. The rise in plasma phosphate lowers plasma calcium by causing the precipitation of calcium phosphate in the tissues. The low calcium level then triggers parathyroid hormone (PTH) secretion from the parathyroid glands. There are vitamin D receptors on parathyroid gland cells and vitamin D normally suppresses PTH secretion. Therefore, the loss of renal vitamin D synthesis removes this suppression and so contributes to the high level of PTH. The high PTH level stimulates bone destruction or resorption and the new bone that replaces it is of poorer quality with disordered collagen. X-rays show subperiosteal resorption in the fingers, erosion of the phalangeal tufts and erosion of the heads of the clavicles (see p. 558).

Treatment is multiple:
- Dietary phosphate intake is reduced.
- Phosphate-binding salts such as calcium salts are used to bind dietary phosphate in the gut and prevent its absorption in the gut.
- Dialysis also removes some phosphate.

08

● Vitamin D can be given as 1,25-dihydroxy-vitamin-D_3 (calcitriol) or 1-hydroxy-vitamin-D_3 (alphacalcidol). This inhibits PTH secretion and bone turnover and raises plasma calcium by promoting gut calcium absorption. Vitamin D therapy can also help the proximal myopathy that may develop because of vitamin D deficiency.

Other complications of chronic renal failure

Bleeding time (the time for bleeding from a cut to stop) is increased, although clotting times are usually normal. This can be temporarily improved by administering synthetic vasopressin (desmopressin), which increases clotting factor VIII levels, and by correcting any anaemia, ensuring adequate dialysis and in some cases by the administration of conjugated oestrogens.

Endocrine complications include growth retardation in children and loss of fertility and libido in adults. Dry, itchy and sometimes pigmented **skin** is common. Itch may reflect calcium phosphate precipitation in the skin. **Nausea, anorexia, heartburn and angiodysplasia** are common. **Fatigue and peripheral neuropathy** can arise. Patients may have **muscle cramps or restless legs**. **Depression and anxiety** are common and the risk of suicide is increased. Immune function is impaired and **infection** is common, even in the absence of immunosuppressive drugs. **Pericarditis** can occur in untreated or undertreated chronic renal failure. Patients with chronic renal failure have an increased incidence of **vascular disease**. Various factors contribute to this. Hypertension is common as is hyperlipidaemia, especially hypertriglyceridaemia.

Hypertension can often be controlled by removing more fluid at dialysis sessions to reduce the patient's circulatory volume. However, the damaged kidneys sometimes secrete excess renin and in such cases therapy to block the effects of this is helpful. Such therapy includes ACE inhibitors, angiotensin II antagonists, beta-blockers and, in extreme cases, surgical nephrectomy to remove the source of the renin.

Postrenal problems

Obstructive uropathy

Obstruction to the flow of urine can arise at any point along the urinary tract (Fig. 8.1a, p. 504). Obstruction can arise from within the lumen of the collecting system (e.g. stones), from within the wall of the system (e.g. urothelial tumours) or from outside the system (e.g. pressure from a pelvic tumour). If pressure rises proximal to the obstruction, then glomerular filtration rate will fall because of this back pressure and renal damage may occur (see p. 550).

Lower tract obstruction is common in the elderly, mainly in older men with prostatic disease. The main causes of obstruction are benign or malignant prostatic disease, other tumours, stones, blood clots and retroperitoneal fibrosis.

Clinical presentation

Acute obstruction, especially with stones, can cause severe pain in the areas to which the urinary tract refers pain, which is from the loin down to the external genitalia. Chronic obstruction is often asymptomatic until there is substantial renal impairment. If there is prostatic disease in older men, there may be symptoms of this. A poor urinary stream suggests significant obstruction in prostatic disease. In addition, prostatic disease can cause hesitancy, terminal dribbling and urinary frequency.

The main physical signs to look for are prostatic enlargement on rectal examination and a large palpable bladder that does not empty properly and contains a significant residual volume.

Investigation

The renal tract should be imaged to identify whether obstruction is present and, if so, at what level. Ultrasound is good for this purpose. Blood tests should also be conducted to determine whether there is any renal impairment. If a particular cause is identified, further investigations may be necessary such as prostate-specific antigen.

Management and prognosis

The treatment of obstruction is the relief of the obstruction. In some cases this will require surgery. However, increasingly, radiologists are able to place percutaneous drains into the urinary system to relieve the obstruction. Ureteric stents can be helpful in conditions such as retroperitoneal fibrosis. Any specific cause of obstruction, such as prostatic disease, should be treated. If left untreated, obstruction can cause end-stage renal disease in the obstructed kidney and infection and stone formation can occur in the static urine. The renal outlook depends on the amount of renal damage caused by the obstruction before it is relieved.

Pelviureteric junction obstruction

This is a condition in which a ring of fibrous tissue occurs where the renal pelvis joins the ureter. This can obstruct the renal pelvis and calyces. The condition can correct spontaneously but, if there is pain or evidence of declining renal function, surgery can be helpful.

Retroperitoneal fibrosis or periaortitis

This is thought to be an autoimmune condition in which

there is inflammation around the aorta or periaortitis. This inflammation may be triggered by material leaking out of atheromatous plaques and there is usually thinning of the media of the aortic wall and increased adventitia with inflammatory infiltration of the vessel wall. The lower and mid-thirds of the ureters become embedded in fibrous tissue and can become obstructed.

Epidemiology

The condition is most common in people in their fifties and sixties and the male : female ratio is 3 : 1. Cases have been documented in which the condition was triggered by the drug methysergide, and possibly by beta-blockers and methyldopa.

Clinical presentation, investigation and differential diagnosis

The clinical presentation can be with occasional flank or abdominal pain, but the condition is often an incidental finding made during the investigation of impaired renal function or vascular disease. Physical signs include hypertension and signs of vascular disease. The condition can be diagnosed by imaging, usually by CT or MRI. Intravenous urography or retrograde contrast studies may show characteristic medial deviation of the ureters. A raised ESR and a normochromic normocytic anaemia are common. The differential diagnosis is of other causes of urinary tract obstruction.

Management and prognosis

Treatment is with steroids to reduce inflammation and, if still necessary, the ureters can be stented or surgically freed from the fibrotic tissue (ureterolysis). The prognosis for renal function is good with treatment.

Urinary tract stones

Urinary tract stones are common and affect up to 10% of men and 5% of women. Stones form if stone-forming substances in the urine reach high enough concentrations to exceed their solubility and to crystallize out of solution. If stones form from two substances this happens when the product of their concentrations (e.g. $[Ca^{2+}] \times [PO_4^{2-}]$) exceeds a certain value. However, debris or other crystals can promote crystal growth at lower concentrations. Conditions that raise urinary concentrations of stone-forming substances or that lower urinary levels of stone-inhibiting compounds cause stone formation. If urine volume is reduced, the concentration of stone-forming substances rises and stone formation increases. In addition, urinary stasis, infection and indwelling catheters all promote stone formation. For this reason, anatomical abnormalities, including polycystic kidney disease, are also associated with an increased risk of stone formation. Citrate, which is present in urine, inhibits stone formation by forming a soluble complex with calcium and so preventing calcium from becoming part of a crystal. Urinary proteins such as nephrocalcin inhibit crystal growth by binding calcium on the crystal surface. Rare renal chloride channel mutations can cause changes that promote stone formation.

Stones that have formed in the bladder may lodge at the junction with the urethra. Renal stones have a tendency to lodge in one of three sites within the ureters (see p. 566):

- at the junction of the renal pelvis with the ureter—the pelviureteric junction
- at the point in the lower ureter where it passes over the rim of the pelvic bones
- at the point where the ureter enters the bladder—the vesicoureteric junction

Nephrocalcinosis describes diffuse renal calcium deposition, mainly in the medulla (Fig. 8.7, p. 512). Causes include hyperparathyroidism, distal renal tubular acidosis and medullary sponge kidney.

Disease mechanisms

Stone types (see Table 8.12)
Calcium stones

The most common type of stones are **calcium stones**, which contain calcium oxalate or calcium phosphate or both. Factors that promote their formation include low urine volume, high urine calcium, high urine oxalate and low urine citrate levels. These factors should be addressed if present to prevent future stone formation.

Hypercalciuria occurs in 65% of all stone patients and is usually idiopathic and associated with increased intestinal calcium absorption, obesity and hypertension. For these patients, fluid intake should be increased and calcium, sodium and animal protein intake reduced. If hypercalciuria persists, **thiazide diuretics** can be useful as they inhibit calcium excretion. **Potassium citrate** may be a useful supplement, because it replaces any potassium that is lost as a result of the diuretic and it increases urine citrate levels, which inhibits stone formation.

Hypercalciuria can also be caused by other conditions including excess calcium intake and any cause of hypercalcaemia. High levels of PTH in primary hyperparathyroidism drive vitamin D synthesis, which promotes intestinal calcium absorption, hypercalcaemia and hypercalciuria. Excess dietary sodium can raise urine calcium levels by lowering proximal tubule sodium reabsorption and thereby lowering the usual cotransport of calcium. Animal protein intake also increases urine calcium levels for reasons that are not fully understood.

Table 8.12 Major causes of stone formation

Calcium stones (80%)	
Hypercalciuria	Causes of hypercalcaemia, especially primary hyperparathyroidism
	Idiopathic
Hyperoxaluria	Primary hyperoxaluria
	Excess intake
	Ileal disease and ileal bypass
Hypocitraturia	Distal tubular disease
Uric acid stones (10%)	
Acid urine causes uric acid precipitation	
High urate intake	
High cell turnover—tumours and tumour lysis	
Cystine stones (2%)	
Cystinuria	Autosomal recessive defect in dibasic amino acid transporter
Infection stones (5%)	
(Magnesium ammonium phosphate and calcium phosphate)	
Chronic infection with urea-splitting organisms	
Other stones (3%)	
Xanthine stones in xanthinuria	
Rare renal chloride channel mutations can cause stone formation	

Oxalate is a metabolic end product excreted in urine. Hyperoxaluria can arise when there is excess dietary oxalate intake in foods such as spinach, rhubarb and chocolate. Primary hyperoxaluria is an inborn error of metabolism that causes excess metabolic oxalate production, with calcium oxalate deposition in the kidney and often childhood renal failure. Ileal disease can cause fat malabsorption, which allows excess fatty acids to bind dietary calcium. Dietary oxalate that would normally be bound to calcium is left free and available for colonic absorption and subsequent renal excretion. This can result in renal calcium oxalate deposition.

Hypocitraturia can be idiopathic or can result from distal renal tubular acidosis, which causes excess mitochondrial metabolism of citrate. A low citrate level contributes to stone formation.

Urate stones

Sodium urate is relatively insoluble at acid pH and forms **radiolucent stones**. Most cases are idiopathic with normal blood and urine urate levels. However, it is common to find that the urine in these patients is acidic and this is likely to make stone formation more common.

Treatment involves reducing dietary purine intake (urate is a product of purine metabolism), increasing urine volume and making the urine more alkaline with **sodium bicarbonate or potassium citrate**. The drug **allopurinol** can be useful as it inhibits urate production.

Secondary causes of urate stones include excess urate production from rapid cell turnover or death, especially during cancer chemotherapy. Stone formation in these circumstances can usually be prevented by good hydration and sometimes alkalinization. High urate levels can also arise from inborn errors of purine metabolism. Diseases that cause very acidic urine will promote the formation of urate stones. Such a situation arises when there is acidosis brought about by loss of alkaline bowel contents because of diarrhoeal disease, an ileostomy or laxative abuse.

Cystine stones

An **autosomal recessive** defect in a renal amino acid transporter reduces tubular cystine reabsorption and therefore causes increased levels of cystine in the urine. Cystine consists of two disulphide-bonded cysteine amino acid molecules and is relatively insoluble, especially at acid pH.

Prophylaxis consists of a good fluid intake and alkalinization with sodium bicarbonate. Sulfhydriles such as dimethylcysteine (D-pencillamine) can be used to cleave cystine into soluble components and so reduce the chance of cystine stone formation in cystinuria.

Infection stones

These stones are often large staghorn calculi containing magnesium ammonium phosphate and calcium phosphate. Infection, usually with **Proteus** species, produces the enzyme urease, which splits urea to produce ammonium ions. The rise in pH promotes calcium phosphate crystallization and the ammonium crystallizes with magnesium and phosphate.

Treatment involves removal of the stones, antibiotics to eradicate infection and screening for an underlying stone-forming predisposition. If left untreated, infection stones can cause substantial renal damage and ultimately renal failure.

Epidemiology

Urinary tract stones are common and their incidence is increasing in industrialized countries where they affect up to 10% of men and 5% of women. Moreover, 50% of patients have a recurrence and there is often a metabolic or anatomical predisposition. For this reason, understanding the reasons why stones form and how their formation can be prevented is important.

Clinical presentation

Urinary tract stones can present in a number of different ways:

- Acute obstruction
- Recurrent infection
- Renal impairment
- Haematuria
- Uncomplicated passage of stones or gravel

Acute obstruction of a ureter by a stone causes the syndrome of **renal colic**, characterized by acute and intense flank pain, often radiating to the groin, and sometimes nausea, vomiting, abdominal discomfort, dysuria, renal tenderness and haematuria. As urine builds up because of the obstruction, the renal capsule is stretched causing severe pain with increased renal prostaglandin E2 production. Therefore, if there is good renal function, NSAIDs, which inhibit prostaglandin synthesis, are good analgesics.

There are three principal sites where stones can lodge in the ureter (see p. 566):
- Pelviureteric junction
- Pelvic brim, where the ureters cross over the rim of the pelvic bones
- Entry site of the ureter into the bladder

Sensory nerves from the ureter and renal pelvis enter the spinal cord at T11, T12, L1 and L2 and pain from the ureter and renal pelvis is referred to these dermatomes:
- Renal pelvis usually refers pain to the loin and back
- Lower ureter usually refers pain to the testis or labium majus
- Lowest pelvic part of the ureter usually refers pain to the tip of the penis or perineum

Bladder stones can halt urine flow suddenly, with penile or perineal pain that may be relieved by lying down. On examination, there may be renal tenderness on palpation if there is urinary tract obstruction.

Acute investigation of suspected stones

With an acute presentation, urine should be examined for bleeding by dipstick analysis for blood and microscopy for red blood cells. Urine should also be cultured to exclude infection. Imaging should be conducted to locate the stones. Plain radiography may show radio opaque stones in the ureters. However, not all stones show up on radiographs:
- Calcium and infection stones are clearly radio-opaque
- Cystine stones are weakly radio-opaque
- Urate stones are not radio-opaque

Ultrasound detects all stone types and can also give useful information about any gross anatomical abnormalities that may be contributing to stone formation, such as polycystic kidney disease. In some cases, precise localization may require an intravenous urogram or even the injection of radio-opaque dye down or up the ureter. Further investigation may identify a predisposing metabolic disorder and includes biochemical analysis of stones, urine and plasma.

Differential diagnosis

The differential diagnosis of an acute episode is obstruction by a clot (clot retention), papillary necrosis, or obstruction by a tumour or tumour fragment.

Management of an acute stone

Obstruction must always be relieved as it can cause renal damage and can be life threatening if the obstructed urine becomes infected. Small stones of less than 6 mm diameter usually pass spontaneously, but stones more than 1 cm will not. Stones can be broken up by extracorporeal shock wave lithotripsy (ESWL) or removed endoscopically, percutaneously or by conventional surgery. ESWL aims shock waves at the stone through the skin, but can be complicated by bleeding and sepsis.

Complications

The key complications of renal stone disease are infection and urinary obstruction, which can both lead to permanent renal damage.

Management: investigation of patients with stones

A full history and clinical examination should exclude bowel disease, diarrhoea and the use of antacids and diuretics. **Diet** should be assessed for fluid, protein, sodium, calcium, oxalate, purine and vitamin D intake and a family history taken. When available, the stones should be **analysed** to determine their constituents. Baseline investigations include:
- Urinalysis
- Serum calcium
- Phosphate
- Urate
- Creatinine and urea

Recurrent stone formation merits 24-h urine collections for volume, osmolality, calcium, phosphate, oxalate, citrate, urate, sodium creatinine and pH as well as serum sodium potassium, chloride and bicarbonate.

Prevention

The key to prevention of all stone formation is to increase fluid intake because this dilutes urine and so reduces the probability of stone-forming substances crystallizing and forming stones. Dietary changes can help by reducing the intake of relevant substances such as purines.

08

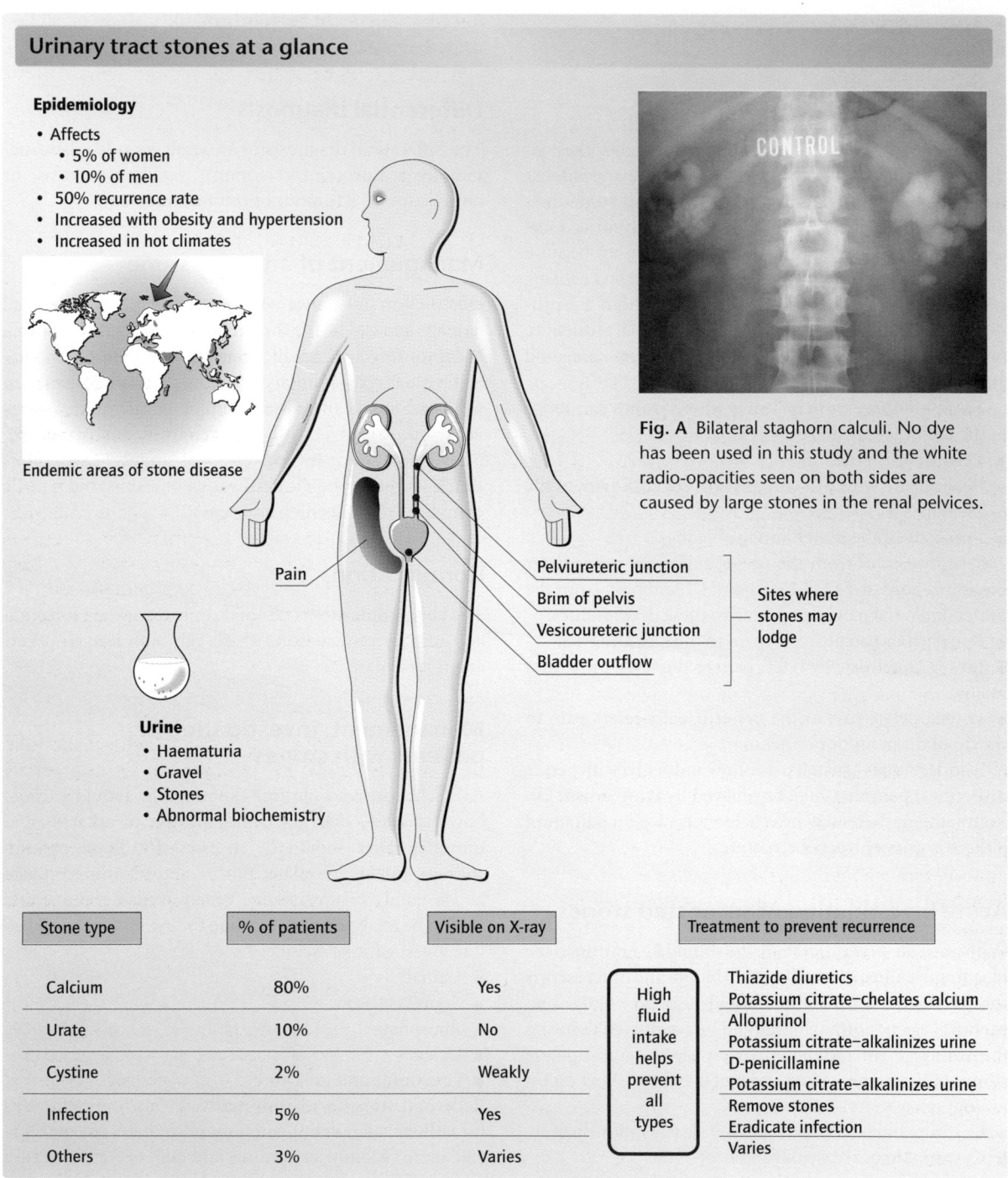

Urinary tract stones at a glance

Epidemiology

- Affects
  - 5% of women
  - 10% of men
- 50% recurrence rate
- Increased with obesity and hypertension
- Increased in hot climates

Endemic areas of stone disease

Fig. A Bilateral staghorn calculi. No dye has been used in this study and the white radio-opacities seen on both sides are caused by large stones in the renal pelvices.

Pain

Pelviureteric junction
Brim of pelvis   Sites where
Vesicoureteric junction stones may
                         lodge
Bladder outflow

Urine

- Haematuria
- Gravel
- Stones
- Abnormal biochemistry

Stone type	% of patients	Visible on X-ray		Treatment to prevent recurrence
Calcium	80%	Yes	High fluid intake helps prevent all types	Thiazide diuretics Potassium citrate–chelates calcium
Urate	10%	No		Allopurinol Potassium citrate–alkalinizes urine
Cystine	2%	Weakly		D-penicillamine Potassium citrate–alkalinizes urine
Infection	5%	Yes		Remove stones Eradicate infection
Others	3%	Varies		Varies

Any metabolic defect, such as hyperparathyroidism, should be treated. Alkalinization of urine with potassium citrate or sodium bicarbonate may help prevent urate stone formation. Cystine stones are also prevented by alkalinization and by D-penicillamine, which cleaves cystine to soluble cysteine products. Eradicate any chronic infection. Potassium citrate is helpful in most stone-forming situations because, as well as alkalinization, the citrate chelates calcium. Thiazide diuretics can inhibit calcium excretion.

Urinary tract tumours

Different tumours can arise at different sites along the renal tract. All these tumours can bleed into the renal tract and cancer should always be considered if there is haematuria or altered urinary flow, although in young adults it is unlikely to be present.

Renal carcinoma

In adults, renal cancer usually arises in the proximal tubules and is known as renal carcinoma, renal cell carcinoma or hypernephroma. The tumour spreads locally or via the lymphatics to the renal hilum, retroperitoneum and para-aortic lymph nodes. It often invades the renal veins and inferior vena cava. The left testicular vein drains into the left renal vein and so blockage of this vein by tumour can cause a left-sided varicocoele (dilated varicose vessels in the scrotum). Metastases typically arise in the lungs, liver, bones and brain.

Epidemiology
This is an uncommon malignancy and accounts for only 2% of adult malignancies. Most patients are over 50 years of age. The risk is increased in men and smokers.

Clinical presentation
The clinical presentation is usually with haematuria, but patients can also present with loin, back or abdominal pain. Haematuria is often frank visible haematuria and is uniform throughout the stream because the blood comes from high in the renal tract. On examination, there may be an abdominal mass, groin or neck lymphadenopathy, skin metastases or a large liver or spleen. Renal tumours commonly cause systemic effects including weight loss, night sweats, fever, anaemia, nausea, malaise, polyneuritis and myositis. Renal tumours also commonly produce excess hormones such as erythropoietin which can cause erythrocytosis, renin which can cause hypertension, or PTH-related protein (PTHrP) which can cause hypercalcaemia.

Investigation
Investigations include urinalysis and urine cytology looking for malignant cells and imaging by ultrasound, CT or MRI and, if possible, percutaneous biopsy.

Management
Treatment is surgical removal of the tumour and often the entire kidney. Immunotherapy with α-interferon and interleukin 2 can be of benefit.

Other renal tumours in adults
Secondary renal tumours can arise from lung or breast tumours, melanomas or lymphomas. Von Hippel–Lindau disease is an autosomal dominant condition caused by mutations in a gene on chromosome 3. It causes tumours in the kidneys, eyes, central nervous system, gonads, adrenals and pancreas.

Wilms' tumour in children

This accounts for 8% of childhood cancers, with a peak incidence at 2–3 years of age. It occurs alone or as part of a syndrome such as the WAGR syndrome (*W*ilms' tumour, *a*niridia, *g*enitourinary malformations and mental *r*etardation). Presentation is usually with an abdominal mass, although haematuria, pain or fever can occur. A cure is usually achieved with nephrectomy and chemotherapy.

Wilms' tumour arises from primitive renal stem cells and is caused by mutations in the *WT-1* gene on chromosome 11. Most patients just have mutations in tumour cells, but children with predisposing syndromes have germline mutations in all cells. The gene product is a transcription factor, which may regulate renal growth and developmental genes.

Urothelial tumours

Transitional epithelial cells form the lining of the renal tract from the tips of the renal papillae to the proximal urethra. Squamous epithelial cells line the distal urethra. Most transitional epithelial tumours arise in the bladder. The occurrence of tumours in the urethra is uncommon and can be a result of the spread of bladder cancers or to primary urethral squamous cell carcinomas, particularly following chronic inflammation.

Bladder cancer

Tumours are usually transitional cell tumours, but 5% are squamous cell tumours, which usually follow chronic inflammation. Tumours are staged according to the extent of invasion through the bladder wall. There may be local spread into the pelvis, but distant metastasis is uncommon.

Epidemiology
Bladder cancer accounts for 7% of malignancy-related deaths and is more common in men than women. The peak incidence of bladder cancer is around 65 years of age. Recognized risk factors include smoking, chronic bladder inflammation (especially that resulting from schistosomiasis infection; see p. 140) and exposure to industrial toxins from the dye industry.

Clinical presentation and investigation

The typical presentation is with painless haematuria. A bladder mass or obstructed kidney may be palpable. Investigation includes urine analysis and urine cytology, imaging using ultrasound, CT, MRI and cystoscopy and, if necessary, examination under anaesthesia. Contrast studies may show a filling defect. Sterile pyuria (pus cells such as polymorphonuclear leucocytes in the absence of infection) can occur.

Management

If a bladder tumour is superficial, it can usually be resected endoscopically and then followed up with repeated cystoscopic surveillance to detect recurrence. Deeper tumours may require total cystectomy, sometimes with removal of other pelvic contents. Radiotherapy or chemotherapy may be added. If the bladder is removed, an artificial bladder may be constructed from small intestine.

Carcinoma *in situ* describes malignant change over most of the surface epithelium. It causes similar symptoms to cystitis, and is treated with intravesical chemotherapy or intravesical bacille Calmette–Guérin (BCG) to trigger inflammation and promote tumour regression.

Prostate cancer

Prostate cancer is the third most common cancer in men. Most cancers are adenocarcinomas arising in the posterior outer zone of the prostate. They initially spread by local invasion and then involve pelvic lymph nodes, metastasizing to bone, especially the lumbar spine and pelvis, and less commonly metastasizing to lung and liver. Bone metastases are typically denser than normal bone tissue on plain radiography.

Clinical presentation

Presentation is usually with the symptoms of bladder outflow obstruction:

● Hesitancy
● Poor stream
● Terminal dribbling
● Frequency
● Nocturia
● Urinary retention or obstruction

The tumour is usually hard and irregular on rectal examination. The main differential diagnosis is benign prostatic hypertrophy.

Investigation

Prostatic cells secrete prostate-specific antigen (PSA) and acid phosphatase and plasma levels are usually elevated in the presence of a tumour. Transrectal ultrasound can be used to identify and biopsy tumours.

Management

Early tumours are treated with transurethral resection of the prostate (TURP) and regular follow-up. Advanced tumours may require radical prostatectomy and radiotherapy. Tumour growth may be promoted by testosterone. Hormonal therapy of metastatic disease includes orchidectomy, synthetic oestrogens, androgen receptor antagonists such as cyproterone acetate or flutamide and gonadotrophin-releasing hormone analogues such as buserelin.

Urinary tract infection

Although most urinary tract infections are self-resolving, ascending urinary tract infection can lead to acute septicaemia and permanent renal damage. Infection usually enters the urinary tract through the urethra, but blood-borne infection can deposit in the kidney. The usual organisms are the Gram-negative bacteria, *Escherichia coli*, *Klebsiella* and *Proteus* species.

● *Lower urinary tract infection:* restricted to the bladder and urethra. It usually involves only the superficial mucosa, is easily treated with a short course of antibiotics and has no long-term effects.
● *Upper urinary tract infection:* affects the kidney or ureters, involves the deep renal medullary tissue and can permanently damage the kidney. It is difficult to eradicate infection from the deep tissue and up to 6 weeks of antibiotic therapy may be necessary.

Infection of the urinary tract by *Mycobacterium tuberculosis* is uncommon in the UK, but is a cause of sterile pyuria (white cells in the urine, but no organism grown in standard culture conditions). Early morning urine samples should be cultured specifically for mycobacteria.

Risk factors for urinary tract infection

Urinary tract infection is more common in women than in men and the peak incidence is during the childbearing years. In women, the **shorter female urethra** provides easier access to the bladder for organisms that colonize the perineum from the bowel and genital tract. During micturition, there may be turbulence and backflow in the short female urethra, which does not occur in the longer male urethra. **Sexual activity** in women, especially initially or with a new partner, is associated with infection. It has been suggested that this occurs because bacteria in perineal secretions can be massaged up the urethra. It has certainly been observed that voiding before and after sexual activity reduces infection.

If there is urinary tract obstruction or incomplete bladder emptying, static urine can accumulate and become infected. Infection can also spread from a focus such as a chronically infected prostate gland or a urinary stone (typically *Proteus mirabilis* infection). Instrumentation or catheterization of the urinary tract can introduce infection and indwelling catheters pose a continued risk of infection. Diabetes and immunosuppression, especially in renal transplant recipients, predispose to urinary infection.

During **pregnancy**, endocrine changes, especially the high progesterone level, cause dilatation of the ureters and reduce the normal ureteric tone, which makes reflux of urine up the ureters more likely. This increases the risk of upper tract infection.

Epidemiology

Urinary tract infection is very common in all societies and is an important cause of morbidity. In the UK it accounts for 1–2% of all general practice consultations.

Clinical presentation

The clinical presentation of urinary tract infection can vary greatly and includes asymptomatic bacteriuria, acute uncomplicated lower urinary tract infection and acute pyelonephritis. Physical signs can include fever and tenderness over the kidneys or bladder:

- Lower urinary tract infection can produce discomfort or burning on micturition, increased urinary frequency and cloudy offensive-smelling urine
- Upper tract infection or pyelonephritis can produce loin pain, fever, flank tenderness and rigors

Investigation

Urine can be dipstick tested for nitrites which indicate the presence of bacteria in the urine, and for leucocyte esterases which indicate the presence of white blood cells. A mid-stream urine sample should be viewed under a microscope and cultured. In small children it may be necessary to perform suprapubic aspiration to obtain a clean urine sample. Organisms may not be seen, but white cells suggest infection and white cell casts suggest upper tract infection because the casts are formed in the tubules.

Urinary tract infection is diagnosed when there are **more than 100 000 organisms of the same bacterial species per millilitre of urine**. If upper tract infection is suspected, blood cultures should be taken and the urinary tract should be imaged, usually using ultrasound to exclude obstruction, stones or an anatomical abnormality.

Management

A key aspect of management is to maintain a high fluid intake, preferably more than 3 l/day of fluid. Drug therapy may not be necessary for lower urinary tract infection, but may help symptoms and should always be based on microbiological sensitivities, if available.

- For lower tract infection, eradication should be achieved with a short course of the locally recommended antibiotic, usually amoxicillin or trimethoprim
- For upper tract infection, courses lasting up to 6 weeks may be necessary to eradicate infection because the bacteria can be deep within the renal tissue

Prevention of recurrent urinary tract infection is important. In both sexes, any underlying cause should be treated. Women with recurrent infection and no obvious underlying cause should be encouraged to void frequently and to void before and after sexual activity.

Investigation of predisposing factors

A single urinary infection in a woman of childbearing age requires no investigation. In other groups and women with recurrent or severe infection, a predisposing condition should be sought. Useful investigations include plain radiography and ultrasonography to exclude stones, obstruction and anatomical anomalies. In men, the prostate should be assessed by rectal examination and investigated further if indicated.

Differential diagnosis

The differential diagnosis of acute upper tract infection or pyelonephritis is of renal colic resulting from stones or renal infarction causing pain.

Complications can include septicaemia, renal damage, stone formation and papillary necrosis.

Specific clinical syndromes or urinary tract infection

Asymptomatic bacteriuria

When routine screening is attempted, asymptomatic bacteriuria can be detected in approximately 5% of women, especially during pregnancy. Approximately 30% of patients progress to symptomatic infection within a year. Given the changes that occur to the ureters in pregnancy (see above), this infection is often upper tract infection. For this reason, pregnant women are screened and treated to prevent severe illness and renal damage.

Acute uncomplicated lower urinary tract infection

This is the most common presentation of lower urinary tract infection and mainly affects women of childbearing age.

Urinary tract infection at a glance

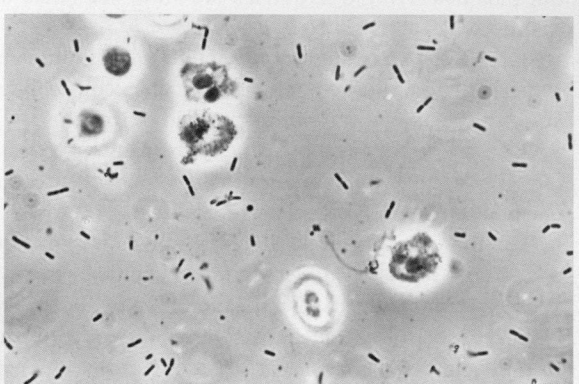

Fig. A White blood cells and bacteria in urine from a patient with bacterial cystitis. Reproduced from Becker GJ, Whitworth JA, Kincaid-Smith P. *Clinical Nephrology in Medical Practice*, Oxford: Blackwell Scientific Publications, 1992 with the permission of the authors.

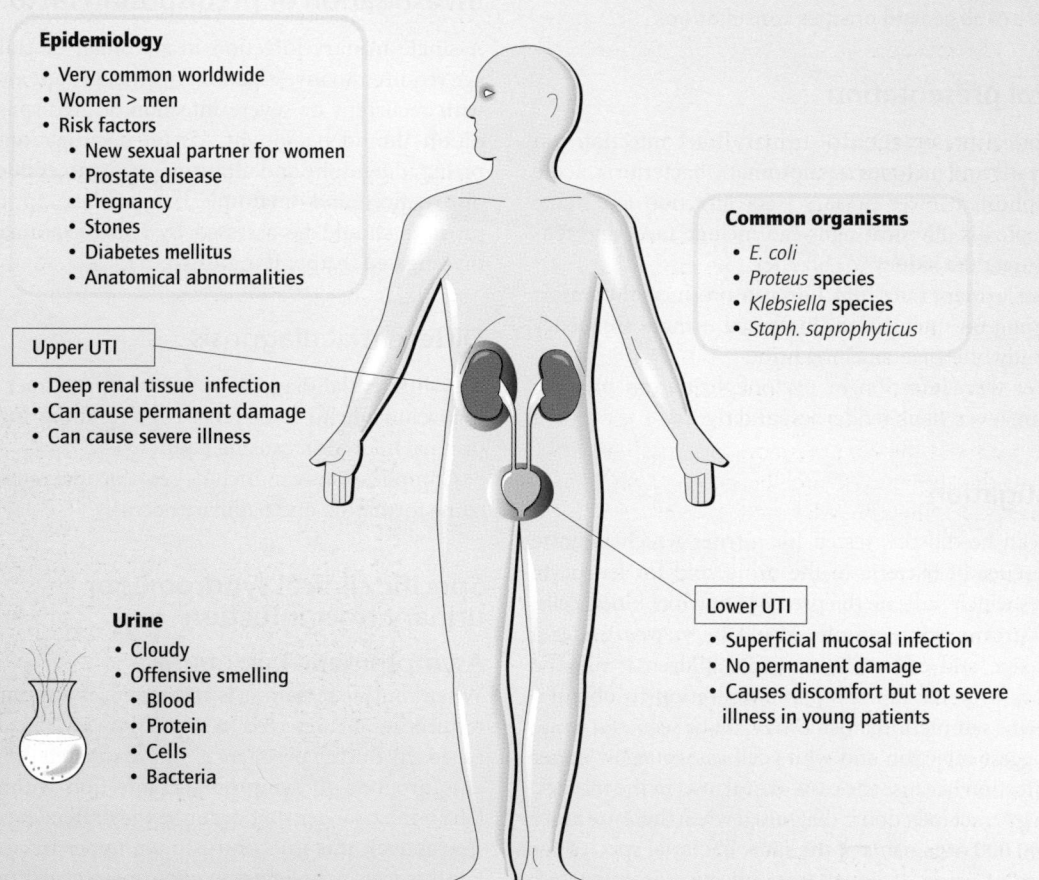

Epidemiology

- Very common worldwide
- Women > men
- Risk factors
  - New sexual partner for women
  - Prostate disease
  - Pregnancy
  - Stones
  - Diabetes mellitus
  - Anatomical abnormalities

Common organisms

- *E. coli*
- *Proteus* species
- *Klebsiella* species
- *Staph. saprophyticus*

Upper UTI

- Deep renal tissue infection
- Can cause permanent damage
- Can cause severe illness

Lower UTI

- Superficial mucosal infection
- No permanent damage
- Causes discomfort but not severe illness in young patients

Urine

- Cloudy
- Offensive smelling
  - Blood
  - Protein
  - Cells
  - Bacteria

Recurrent urinary tract infection

This term refers to repeated episodes of symptomatic infection, separated by symptom-free periods, which are often simply periods of asymptomatic infection. A predisposing risk factor should be sought, although in women it is uncommon to find one. Failure to eradicate organisms in the deep tissues in upper urinary tract infection can allow relapse of infection that may be mistaken for recurrent lower urinary tract infection. In men, chronic prostate infection can cause recurrent infection.

Acute pyelonephritis

This is the typical presentation of upper urinary tract infection.

Acute complicated urinary tract infection

This term refers to infection with a predisposing risk factor such as a stone or obstruction. Antibiotics are usually only effective if the complicating factor is treated.

Urinary tract infection in children and chronic pyelonephritis

Any childhood urinary tract infection must be investigated to exclude an underlying risk factor. The most important risk factor is vesicoureteric reflux caused by an abnormal entrance of the ureter into the bladder (Fig. 8.32). During voiding, bladder wall contraction normally closes the ureteric orifice and the angle of the ureter in the bladder wall creates a flap valve preventing reflux. However, if the ureter does not pass diagonally through the bladder wall and the orifice is enlarged, voiding causes reflux up the ureter and into the renal pelvis. Within the renal pelvis, there may be intrarenal reflux into the medulla.

The reflux usually resolves by adulthood, so the aim of therapy is to prevent renal damage from ascending infection. Unfortunately, most damage occurs before the age of 5 years and reflux nephropathy may account for 10–15% of end-stage renal failure. The renal damage caused by reflux is termed **chronic pyelonephritis** and is diagnosed radiologically with clubbing of the renal calyces and cortical scarring (Fig. 8.33). Vesicoureteric reflux is best diagnosed by a micturating cystourethrogram—contrast medium is placed in the bladder via a suprapubic or urethral catheter and images taken during voiding to see if the medium goes up the ureters.

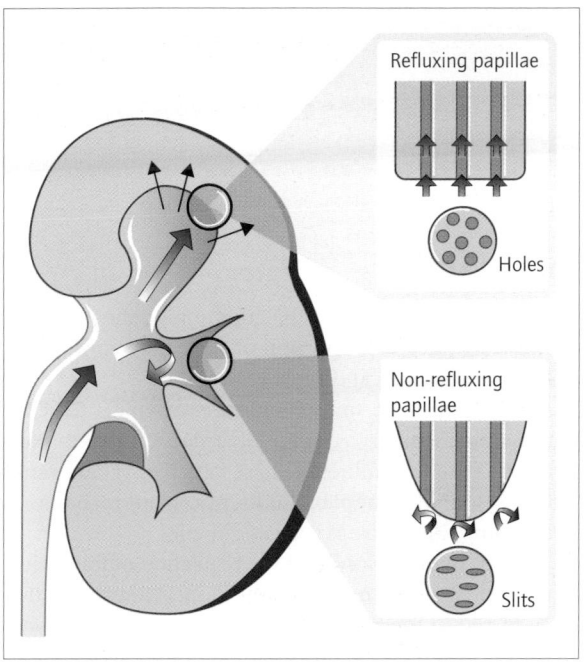

Figure 8.32 The pathogenesis of reflux nephropathy. Infected urine refluxes up the ureter and within the kidney can enter affected papillae causing damage. The result can be enlarged club-shaped calyces with overlying cortical thinning at refluxing (or compound) papillae.

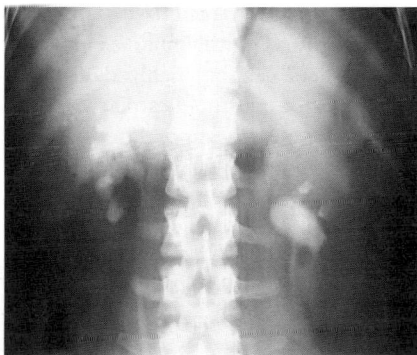

Figure 8.33 Chronic pyelonephritis. This is an intravenous urogram and dye can be seen in the collecting systems. There is chronic pyelonephritis on the right side of the image. There is dilatation of the collecting system on this side and this can cause urinary stasis and predispose to further infection.

Fluid, electrolyte and acid–base disorders

Introduction

Whether in hospital or in the community, most doctors spend a significant proportion of their time considering their patients' fluid and biochemical status. At the most basic level, this may simply involve reviewing a patient's routine biochemistry results. Most doctors make interventions that can influence these variables. These range from prescribing complex fluid replacement regimens to prescribing simple drugs such as diuretics.

The key organ involved in the regulation of fluid, electrolyte and acid–base status is the kidney. Renal function is discussed in the first section of this chapter. The focus of this section is on the normal and disordered fluid, electrolyte and acid–base situations. It is necessary to understand the normal situations because in sick patients, you may have to take over the functions that are normally regulated by homoeostatic mechanisms, such as the control of plasma electrolytes and body fluid volume. Understanding the basic mechanisms is essential to understanding how the abnormal situations can arise and so how rational therapy can be used to correct them. The mechanisms are mostly well characterized and understanding of them will last you a clinical lifetime. Finally, electrolyte and fluid disorders can be highly **dangerous**—a high potassium level can cause rapid cardiac arrest and death. You need to know how to respond to these situations as there may not be time to seek specialist advice.

Structure and function

Body fluid

When clinicians refer to body fluid, they mean body water content. Sometimes, the term body volume is used instead (e.g. 'volume contracted' or 'volume overloaded'), but the meaning is the same.
- Body water consists of the water that is in cells (intracellular fluid) and the water that is outside cells (extracellular fluid)
- The extracellular fluid consists of the water that is out-

Table 8.13 Normal constituents of body fluid compartments in mmol/l

	Extracellular fluid	Intracellular fluid
Na	141	10
K	4.1	120
Cl	113	3
HCO_3^-	26	10
Phosphate	2.0	140 (organic phosphate)

Table 8.14 The volumes of fluid in each fluid compartment and the percentage of body weight in each compartment

	Volume, in a 70-kg man (l)	Percentage of body weight
Total body fluid	45	60
Intracellular fluid	30	40
Extracellular fluid	15	20
Interstitial fluid	12	16
Plasma fluid	3	4
Total blood volume (plasma and blood cells)	5	7

side cells and in the circulation or vascular compartment (intravascular fluid) and the water that is outside cells and in the tissues or interstitial or extravascular compartment (extravascular fluid) of the body
- Intravascular extracellular fluid is plasma

In some situations, fluid can accumulate in spaces such as the peritoneal cavity or the pleural space. Such spaces are sometimes referred to as 'third compartments'.

Much confusion is generated by excessive attention to where the fluid is. The key issue is usually whether total body water content is too high or too low, rather than what is happening in the different compartments. The normal constituents of the different fluid compartments are shown in Tables 8.13 and 8.14.

Distribution of water and electrolytes

Unlike many ions and molecules, water cannot be pumped directly by any biological process. However, water will move between two sites by osmosis if there is a suitable osmotic gradient and if the barrier separating the two sites contains pores or channels through which water can move passively. Most cell membranes contain water channels in the form of aquaporin molecules. The distribution of water within the body depends on the distribution of osmotically active substances and the permeability of barriers between the different compartments.

A key difference between the extracellular and intracellular fluids is caused by the activity of the Na^+/K^+ATPase, which pumps sodium out of cells and potassium into cells. The end result is that:

- Intracellular fluid has high potassium and low sodium concentrations
- Extracellular fluid has low potassium and high sodium concentrations

Normally, the intra- and extracellular fluid compartments are in approximate osmotic equilibrium.

Body fluid composition is tightly regulated. Any regulatory mechanism requires some form of afferent or input system that detects changes in the variable (such as potassium concentration) and some kind of efferent or output system that acts to change the variable (such as renal tubular potassium reabsorption). The different body compartments interact and changes in one compartment often affect those in another. Together, the two kidneys receive around 20% of the renal blood flow or 1000 ml/min. Changes in how the kidney excretes or conserves water, ions or molecules will have a rapid effect on the composition of plasma (intravascular extracellular fluid). Plasma is in approximate equilibrium with the extravascular extracellular or interstitial tissue fluid, so changes in plasma will cause changes in the fluid bathing cells and this will influence the cells themselves.

Osmotic effects

An **osmole** of a substance is the amount of that substance that dissolves in solution to produce a mole of osmotically active species (ions or molecules). When 1 mole of glucose is dissolved in 1 litre of water, the water contains 1 osmole of solute:
- The **osmolarity** of a solution is the number of osmoles in 1 litre of the solution
- The **osmolality** of a solution is the number of osmoles in 1 kilogram of the solvent

In practice, the distinction between osmolarity and osmolality is usually not important under most circumstances in the body.

Regulation of body sodium and water

Because sodium is the major extracellular ion, it is the key ion that is regulated by the kidney and the major determinant of body water content. For this reason, the regulation and metabolism of sodium is inextricably linked to that of water and this relationship can at first seem confusing. The key thing to remember is that unless there is a massive body fluid volume change such as an acute bleed, **the body will tend to maintain osmolality, even at the expense of volume changes**. This makes sense, as a smallish change in body water content is easily tolerated by changes in vessel tone, but a change in the osmotic gradient across cells can have profound effects causing cellular dysfunction, such as seizures in the brain.

Control of osmolality. Osmoreceptors in the anterior hypothalamus detect changes in osmolality and trigger changes in water intake by thirst and in water excretion by altering vasopressin (ADH) secretion. This system **maintains normal osmolality by changing water handling** but does not control body water content.

Control of volume. Various volume receptors detect the stretch of different parts of the circulation including the low-pressure venous system, the high-pressure arterial system and the heart. The effector mechanisms regulating body volume include the many influences that act on renal sodium handling, especially angiotensin II and aldosterone. Because osmolality will always be regulated under normal conditions, the total body water **volume is controlled by changing the amount of sodium in the body**.

This is done by altering renal sodium excretion. For example, if body volume is low, angiotensin II and aldosterone levels rise and cause the kidney to retain sodium. The retained sodium will begin to increase plasma osmolality, so the osmolality regulating system will then kick in and cause more water to be drunk and less to be excreted. The end result is an increase in total body water.

Renal sodium handling

Plasma sodium is freely filtered in the glomerulus and then reabsorbed along the tubules. Most sodium is reabsorbed in the proximal tubule and the loop of Henle and then there is fine tuning of sodium excretion by control of the lesser amount of reabsorption in the distal tubule. The reabsorption is tightly controlled by different influences on the kidney, but especially by the action of angiotensin II and aldosterone, both of which promote sodium reabsorption.

Regulation of body potassium

Body potassium is regulated by the adrenal gland and the kidney. An increase in the potassium concentration of the extracellular fluid of the adrenal cortex stimulates aldosterone release. In the kidney, aldosterone acts on the tubular cells in the collecting duct to promote potassium secretion (and sodium reabsorption). Other influences can affect renal potassium handling such as pH changes—a high pH promotes potassium secretion. A high urine flow rate also promotes potassium loss from the kidneys.

Renal potassium handling

In the kidney, potassium is freely filtered and most potassium is reabsorbed in the proximal tubule and loop of Henle. Net potassium excretion is then controlled by the regulated secretion of potassium by collecting duct cells under the control of aldosterone.

Regulation of body calcium, phosphate and magnesium

The regulation of calcium and phosphate and magnesium is interlinked because they are all components of bone. Calcium and phosphate metabolism are very closely interrelated at all levels, but the detection and regulation of calcium levels appears to be the regulatory priority. The chief cells in the parathyroid gland have calcium-sensing proteins on their surface and the concentration of calcium surrounding these cells influences the amount of PTH that these cells secrete. PTH acts on bone and on the kidney. PTH acts on bone to causes bone resorption (destruction) with the release of calcium and phosphate into the plasma. PTH acts on the kidney to increase phosphate excretion, to increase calcium reabsorption and to increase vitamin D synthesis. Vitamin D is synthesized in the kidney. Vitamin D acts on the gut, on bone and on the kidney and the different actions all serve to increase calcium and phosphate levels in plasma. In the gut it promotes calcium and phosphate absorption, in bone it enhances the bone-resorbing effects of PTH and in the kidney it stimulates renal calcium and phosphate reabsorption. PTH secretion by the parathyroid gland is inhibited by vitamin D or hypercalcaemia (Fig. 8.34).

Renal calcium, phosphate and magnesium handling

In the kidney, calcium that is not protein-bound is freely filtered in the glomerulus. Most calcium is reabsorbed in the proximal tubule and the loop of Henle. The final small amount of calcium absorption in the distal tubules is controlled by PTH and vitamin D, which both increase this absorption.

In the kidney, phosphate that is not protein-bound is freely filtered in the glomerulus. Most phosphate is reabsorbed in the proximal tubule and loop of Henle, but further phosphate is reabsorbed in the distal tubules and collecting ducts.

Magnesium that is not protein-bound is freely filtered in the glomerulus. There is reabsorption along most of the nephron, but most reabsorption takes place in the loop of Henle. PTH also increases magnesium reabsorption.

Regulation of acid–base metabolism

Acids dissociate to produce hydrogen ions and the acidity of a solution is a measure of the number of free hydrogen ions in the solution. The pH is the negative logarithm of the hydrogen ion concentration. If the hydrogen ion concentration is 10^{-9} mol/l, the pH is 9 and if the hydrogen ion concentration is 10^{-3} mol/l, the pH is 3. A buffer is a substance that can accept and associate with hydrogen ions, so reducing the number of free hydrogen ions in solution.

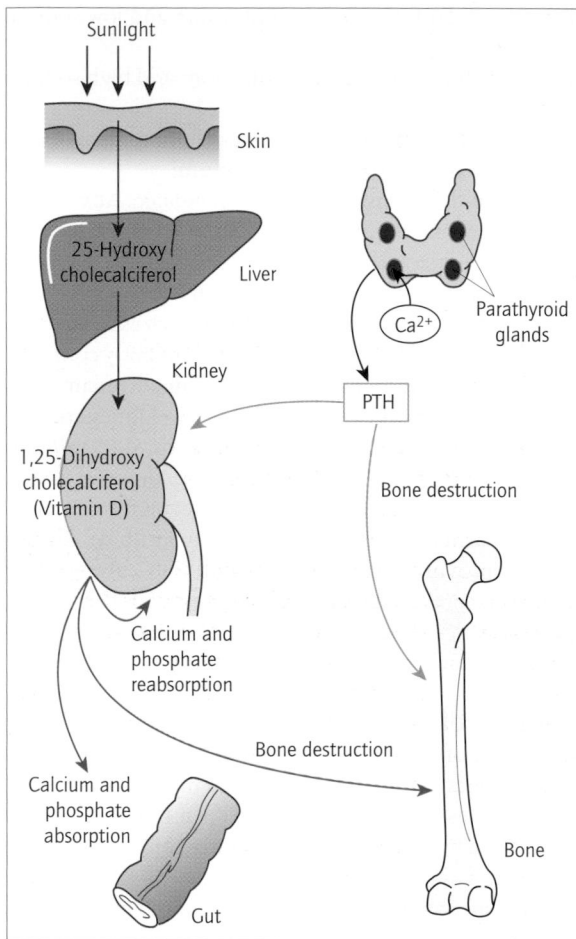

Figure 8.34 Calcium metabolism. The basic actions of parathyroid hormone and vitamin D are shown.

Large amounts of acids are produced by normal metabolism. However, small fluctuations in the acidity or alkalinity of the body can produce very serious problems for cells. For this reason, the body must do two things: buffer the acid as soon as it is produced and then excrete it. Excretion of acid from the body is performed by the kidney. However, acid is highly toxic and could cause problems before it can be excreted. To prevent this, a series of buffers reduce the effect of the acid on the actual pH of body fluids. Although buffers alter the pH of the body, they do not alter the total load of hydrogen ions that must be excreted.

Buffers. The major soluble buffers are **bicarbonate, phosphate ions and ammonia**, which combine with free hydrogen ions. Proteins can also act as buffers, as can bone. The buffer systems are all in equilibrium with each other. To understand medical acid–base problems it is important to understand how the bicarbonate buffer system

Figure 8.35 The carbonic anhydrase reaction. This is reversible, but dissociation of H_2CO_3 to carbon dioxide and water is speeded up by the enzyme carbonic anhydrase.

Figure 8.36 The Henderson–Hasselbalch equation. α is the solubility coefficient of carbon dioxide in plasma, where pK is the dissociation constant for the $HCO_3^- - P_{CO_2}$ system in plasma.

08

works. In essence, water and carbon dioxide can combine to form carbonic acid. Carbonic acid dissociates into hydrogen ions and bicarbonate ions as shown in Fig. 8.35.

The chemistry underlying the conversion of water and carbon dioxide to hydrogen ions and bicarbonate ions is catalysed by the enzyme carbonic anhydrase, which is expressed in various locations including the kidney. The significance of the system is that carbon dioxide is one of its components. Carbon dioxide is produced by aerobic metabolism and is normally removed by the lungs, and the amount removed depends on the amount of ventilation taking place.

Respiratory effects on acid–base balance

● If ventilation is reduced, carbon dioxide accumulates and the reaction shifts to the right. This will produce hydrogen ions and the body will become more acidotic. This is a respiratory acidosis.
● Similarly, if ventilation is increased, more carbon dioxide is removed from the body and the reaction shifts to the left. This results in fewer hydrogen ions and the body becomes more alkalotic. This is a respiratory alkalosis.

The corollary of this situation is that if there is an excess of acid in the body (an acidosis), then if ventilation is increased, this will remove some carbon dioxide, which will reduce the acidity of the solution back towards normal. This is **respiratory compensation for metabolic acidosis**. The opposite situation can happen if there is an alkalosis: a reduction in the acidity of the blood. Then, if ventilation is reduced, carbon dioxide builds up and the acidity shifts back towards normal. This is **respiratory compensation for metabolic alkalosis**.

Metabolic effects on acid–base balance

Bicarbonate ions are excreted by the kidney and so bicarbonate levels can be controlled by the kidney. Changes in bicarbonate concentration will alter the number of free hydrogen ions in body fluids. If the acidity of plasma is increased, then renal bicarbonate excretion is reduced, which increases the plasma bicarbonate level. This shifts the reaction to the left, which reduces the number of hydrogen ions. This is **renal compensation for acidosis**. Any extra carbon dioxide that is formed will be breathed away by the lungs. Conversely, if the acidity of plasma is reduced (an alkalosis), then decreasing the amount of bicarbonate in the plasma, by increasing its renal excretion, will shift the reaction to the right, which increases the number of hydrogen ions. This is **renal compensation for alkalosis**.

Regulating plasma pH

These relationships are expressed by the Henderson–Hasselbalch equation (Fig. 8.36) and the effects are shown in Fig. 8.37. In essence, this equation means that if the

Disorder	pH	P_{CO_2}	HCO_3-
Respiratory acidosis			
Acute	↓	⬆	↑
Chronic	N	⬆	⬆
Respiratory alkalosis			
Acute	↑	⬇	↓
Chronic	N	⬇	⬇
Metabolic acidosis			
Acute	↓	N	⬇
Chronic	N	⬇	⬇
Metabolic alkalosis			
Acute	↑	↑	⬆
Chronic	N	↑	⬆

Figure 8.37 The main changes in the different types of acid–base disturbance. N, normal; blue arrows indicate the first change causing the disturbance; red arrows indicate the change in pH that this causes; small black arrows indicate a small compensatory change; large black arrows indicate a large compensatory change. This may not normalize pH.

carbon dioxide concentration increases, the hydrogen ion concentration rises (Fig. 8.35) and the pH falls. If the bicarbonate concentration increases, the hydrogen ion concentration falls and the pH rises.

The body pH can be altered by regulating the ratio of carbon dioxide (acid) : bicarbonate ions (base):
- Carbon dioxide levels can be controlled by altering ventilation
- Bicarbonate levels can be controlled by the kidney

All the different buffer systems are in equilibrium, so a change in one affects the other buffer systems. Normally, both carbon dioxide and bicarbonate levels are carefully maintained in the normal ranges by homoeostatic mechanisms.

Acid–base disturbances

In an acid–base disorder, the problem can arise either:
- Because ventilation is abnormal and there is too little or too much carbon dioxide, in which case it is termed a **respiratory acid–base disturbance**

or

- Because bicarbonate levels are abnormal, which can arise through a direct effect on the bicarbonate level itself (such as failure of the kidney to reabsorb bicarbonate or loss of bicarbonate in the gut) or by the addition of an acid or a base to the body. In such cases, the disturbance is termed a **metabolic acid–base disturbance**

The terms respiratory and metabolic refer to the original cause of the acidosis. However, ultimately, the body responds to these changes by compensation. So, for example, poor breathing results in a build-up of carbon dioxide and a 'respiratory' acidosis. To compensate for this, the kidney then retains bicarbonate ions and so there is a 'metabolic' compensation. The respiratory compensations are triggered by arterial chemoreceptors, especially in the carotid body. Acidosis increases respiration to ventilate away carbon dioxide. Alkalosis reduces respiration, allowing some carbon dioxide to accumulate.

The anion gap

The anion gap is the difference between the positively charged measured cations ($Na^+ + K^+$) and the negatively charged measured anions ($HCO_3^- + Cl^-$). The body is electrically neutral, so this difference or gap is always filled with other anions, which are not measured. There is a normal anion gap of 6–16 mmol/l, which is made up of various anions such as organic acids, sulphate ions, phosphate ions and proteins:

$$\text{Anion gap} = (Na^+ + K^+) - (HCO_3^- + Cl^-).$$

The anion gap is useful because it can help in the diagnosis of a metabolic acidosis. If a new acid such as sulphuric acid or a metabolic acid is added to the body, the acid dissociates into hydrogen ions and anions, which contributes to the anion gap. The hydrogen ions (H^+) combine with bicarbonate to form carbon dioxide and water, so the bicarbonate level is lowered and body pH shifts downwards. In this situation, bicarbonate levels are low, but chloride levels are normal. The new anions contribute to the anion gap but are not measured so **the measured anion gap increases**. Examples include salicylic acid in aspirin overdose, lactic acid in lactic acidosis and ketoacids in ketoacidosis.

If there is just simple loss of bicarbonate (e.g. if the kidney cannot reabsorb bicarbonate or the gut is losing bicarbonate), then bicarbonate levels fall, but chloride levels rise to maintain electroneutrality and so the **measured anion gap is still normal**. This is because there is no addition of anions that are not measured by the standard test. In this situation, bicarbonate levels are low, but chloride levels are high.

Renal acid handling

The kidney can only move acid into the urine against a limited hydrogen ion concentration, so to excrete the amount of acid that is produced by metabolism every day, there must be buffers in the urine. These buffers mop up the hydrogen ions secreted into the tubules and reduce the hydrogen ion gradient that would otherwise build up between the urine and the renal tubular cells. The higher the level of the buffers in the urine, the higher the amount of acid that can be excreted. The excretion of hydrogen ions by the kidney can seem difficult to understand, partly because some of the secreted hydrogen ions are used to reabsorb bicarbonate and this does not cause net acid excretion.

Bicarbonate reabsorption. Bicarbonate ions are freely filtered in the glomerulus. When hydrogen ions are secreted into the tubules, where there is carbonic anhydrase, they interact with bicarbonate to form carbon dioxide and water (Fig. 8.38). These can both diffuse inside the cell where there is also carbonic anhydrase and where they form bicarbonate ions and hydrogen ions. The bicarbonate is reabsorbed into the blood and the hydrogen ions are secreted again. Thus, the hydrogen ions cycle in and out of the cell, but there is no net loss of hydrogen ions. However, this allows bicarbonate to be reabsorbed from the urine into the blood. Clearly, the amount of this reabsorption will affect the plasma bicarbonate level and so the pH of blood.

Acid excretion. When bicarbonate reabsorption is complete, the hydrogen ions that are secreted interact with buffers and are excreted in this form (Fig. 8.39). This results in net acid excretion and the key urinary buffers

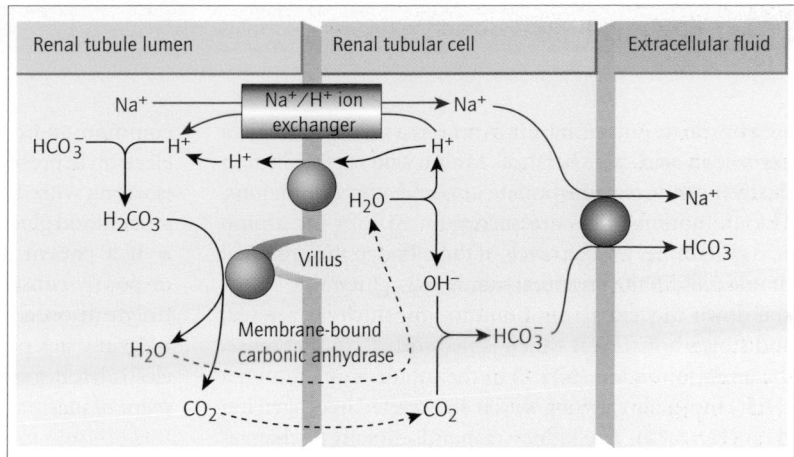

Figure 8.38 Bicarbonate reabsorption. Filtered bicarbonate is reabsorbed to maintain normal plasma bicarbonate levels and so pH. This process depends on the secretion of H^+ ions into the tubular lumen. There is no net loss of H^+ ions as the H^+ ions are recycled as shown.

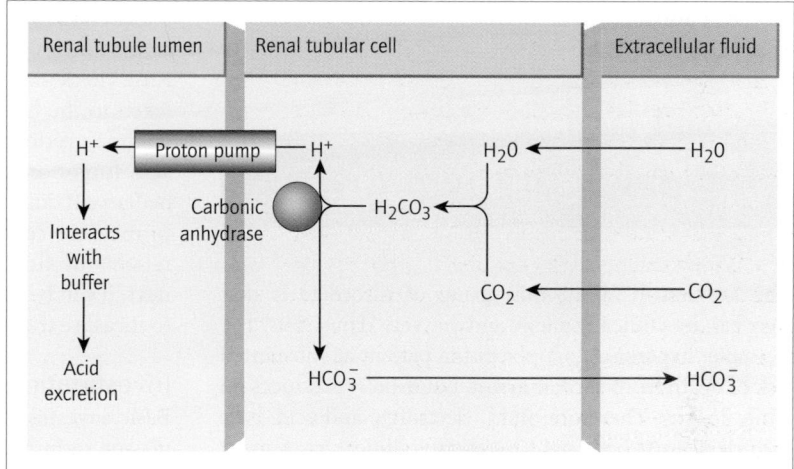

Figure 8.39 Acid excretion. When secreted H^+ ions interact with a urinary buffer such as phosphate, the H^+ ions are not recycled and are excreted with the buffer in the urine. These excreted H^+ ions do not contribute to bicarbonate reabsorption. Under these conditions, bicarbonate produced within the renal cell is added to the body without H^+, so the net effect is acid secretion and bicarbonate generation. This process occurs mainly in the distal tubule.

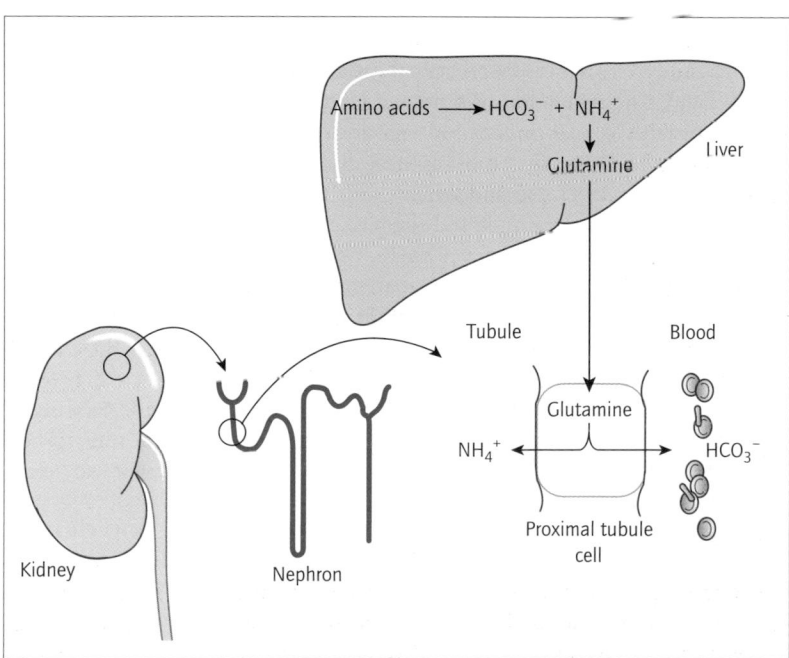

Figure 8.40 Ammonia metabolism. Glutamine is produced in the liver and transported by blood to the proximal tubular cells. Here it is converted into ammonium ions which are excreted and bicarbonate ions which are returned to the blood.

are phosphate and ammonia. Ammonia metabolism has a key role in acid–base balance. Amino acid metabolism in the liver produces bicarbonate ions and ammonium ions. The ammonium ions are incorporated into the amino acid glutamine, which travels in the blood to the proximal tubule cells. In the proximal tubule cells, glutamine is broken down to yield an ammonium ion which is excreted, and a bicarbonate ion which is reabsorbed. In that sense, the ammonium ion (NH^{4+}) in the tubule is an ammonia (NH^3) molecule carrying with it an excreted hydrogen ion (H^+) (Fig. 8.40). The kidney responds directly to changes in pH. Acidosis directly stimulates proximal tubule cells to break down glutamine to form ammonia for excretion and bicarbonate for reabsorption. Acid secretion into the tubules is also increased. Alkalosis has the opposite effects.

Approach to the patient

The key lesson about this group of disorders is that they can be clinically silent and yet very dangerous. For example, hyperkalaemia places the patient at substantial risk of death from cardiac arrest, but usually produces no clinical signs. Therefore, fluid, electrolyte and acid–base disorders must be sought by careful clinical assessment and appropriate investigation. If you do not consider a particular disorder, you may not order the right investigation and the disorder will be missed with potentially serious consequences.

Fluid and electrolyte disorders are common and can be rapidly fatal. The regulation of fluid and electrolyte and acid–base status is well understood and doctors can act rationally to prevent or treat most of these disorders. The diagnostic tests are simple and reliable and the actions required are also usually simple and effective. So acute are many of the scenarios, that you will see the results of your actions very quickly. For example, in a patient with hyperkalaemia and a dangerous cardiac rhythm, if calcium is administered intravenously, you may see the dangerous cardiac rhythm change to normal on a cardiac monitor as you are injecting the calcium.

Clinical considerations
A few key clinical points are worth bearing in mind in any clinical assessment of a fluid, electrolyte or acid–base disorder:
● Always ask about and consider the drugs the patient is using. Common drugs, such as diuretics, can cause profound disturbances.
● Always consider diabetes and ask about it. It is

common and causes some of the most severe fluid and electrolyte problems. If you suspect it or are not sure what is wrong with the patient, always measure a formal laboratory blood glucose, even if bedside stick tests are normal.
● If a patient seems vague, confused, irritable, sleepy or poorly conscious, always exclude acid–base and electrolyte disorders including hypercalcaemia.
● In any sick patient, always exclude acid–base, fluid and electrolyte disorders by clinical assessment and the measurement of plasma biochemistry and arterial blood gases.

Examination
This should always include blood pressure as a crude measure of fluid volume status. However, if you think that the patient has a low fluid volume, check for postural hypotension by measuring the lying and standing blood pressure. Also check the pulse and jugular venous pressure and listen to the heart for added sounds that might indicate volume overload such as a third heart sound. Also check skin turgor and examine for peripheral and pulmonary oedema. If doubt remains, insert a central venous catheter to measure central venous pressure. In the presence of relative dysfunction of one ventricle compared to the next, it can be helpful to use a pulmonary artery catheter to measure the filling pressure of the left side of the heart.

Investigations
Basic investigations should screen for abnormalities of plasma sodium, potassium, calcium and phosphate and, sometimes, magnesium. Renal function and plasma glucose are usually checked at the same time. Sometimes it is helpful to assess plasma osmolality. To exclude acid–base disorders, it is necessary to measure arterial blood gases.

Diuretics

Diuretics are commonly prescribed for hypertension and for heart failure with oedema. They act on the kidney to promote an increased urine output. Typically, they inhibit the reabsorption of electrolytes from the glomerular filtrate as it passes down the tubules. Water reabsorption is also inhibited as water is normally reabsorbed by osmosis with these ions. Therefore, most diuretics also cause ion or electrolyte loss from the body. The combination of fluid and electrolyte loss can result in fluid and electrolyte disorders. The key types of diuretics in clinical use are discussed below.

Loop diuretics
(principally frusemide and bumetanide)
These are strong diuretics, which inhibit the NaK2Cl (NKCC2) cotransporter in the loop of Henle. This causes loss of sodium, potassium and chloride as well as water. They are potent diuretics and are secreted into the tubule

by the organic anion transporter molecules in the proximal tubule. A secondary effect is a fall in the reabsorption of calcium and magnesium. In the long term, plasma urate levels rise, which can cause gout.

Thiazide diuretics
(such as bendrofluazide/bendroflumethiazide)

These are weak diuretics, which inhibit the NaCl (NCC) cotransporter in the distal tubule. This reduces the reabsorption of sodium and chloride and therefore water. In addition, some of the sodium is exchanged in the collecting ducts for potassium, so potassium loss also occurs. Calcium reabsorption is increased, so thiazides can be used to treat hypercalciuria. In the long term, plasma urate levels rise, which can cause gout, and lipid levels can rise, promoting vascular disease.

Potassium-sparing diuretics

Amiloride-type diuretics
(amiloride and triamterene)

These are weak diuretics, which inhibit the ENaC epithelial cell sodium channel in the principal cells of the collecting tubule. This blocks sodium reabsorption and, as sodium reabsorption in these cells is mechanistically linked to potassium secretion, potassium secretion is reduced. The end result is a weak loss of sodium and water and conservation of potassium. These agents are usually used in combination with a loop or thiazide diuretic to reduce potassium loss.

Aldosterone antagonist-type diuretics
(principally spironolactone)

Aldosterone promotes sodium reabsorption and potassium secretion. It does this in part by increasing the number of ENaC molecules in the tubular cells. Therefore blocking this has a similar effect to the amiloride-type diuretics and reduces sodium secretion and potassium reabsorption. Side-effects include gynaecomastia.

Less important diuretics

Osmotic diuretics (mannitol)

Water is normally reabsorbed from the tubules by osmotic movement with reabsorbed ions. An osmotically active substance that is filtered, but not reabsorbed, will osmotically oppose this reabsorption of water from the renal tubules. Mannitol is a substance with these properties and is sometimes used to promote a diuresis. In the body, it also has an osmotic effect in the circulation and draws water from cells. It is sometimes used to dehydrate brain cells if there is cerebral oedema. A high plasma glucose level will have the same effect and this is the basis of the fluid loss in uncontrolled hyperglycaemia.

Carbonic anhydrase inhibitors (acetazolamide)

Carbonic anhydrase is necessary for the reabsorption of bicarbonate ions. If carbonic anhydrase is inhibited, bicarbonate reabsorption is inhibited and bicarbonate ions in the renal tubules have an osmotic effect, like osmotic diuretics, which opposes the reabsorption of water from the tubules by osmosis. This increases urine volume.

Prescribing fluids

Fluids can be prescribed as oral fluids, nasogastric or other tube-feeding fluids, or intravenous fluids. It is often forgotten that it may be safer and easier to give simple fluids or even just water orally or nasogastrically. Intravenous lines are a significant infection risk and may well be unnecessary.

Using the gut

In some cases it is quite enough just to ensure that the patient drinks the right amount of fluid. It is often the case with the elderly that patients do not drink a lot of fluid, but this is not usually a reason for intravenous fluids. The doctors' and nurses' time is much better spent sitting down every so often and watching the patient drink a glass or two of water or a cup of tea than setting up and administering intravenous fluids under such circumstances. If a patient can be given fluid orally or via a nasogastric or enteral (enteral means in the gut) tube, then it is almost always possible to feed them in this way and prescribing fluids and electrolytes intravenously is unnecessary. The patient can absorb what they need from the food and water in their gut and their kidneys can regulate this in the normal way.

Using the intravenous route

When a patient is not able to drink properly and cannot be given fluids or food via a feeding tube, they must be given intravenous fluids and electrolytes. Usually, this is a short-term measure, especially around the time of surgery. However, in some cases it may go on for many days, weeks or longer. Before prescribing fluids, you need to know why you are prescribing them and whether it is really necessary. If a patient is nil-by-mouth for just a few hours and was normally hydrated beforehand, then there is no need for intravenous fluid therapy. If a patient is basically well and is just nil-by-mouth for reasons such as recent elective surgery, then the main issue is the provision of water and the replacement of any electrolytes that will have been excreted in urine or in faeces or lost in other body fluids such as sweat. However, in some circumstances, a sick patient may be found to have significant electrolyte abnormalities, or to be dehydrated or overhydrated. In these circumstances, more care and thought is required.

What fluids to use?

For the most part, fluid and electrolyte prescribing is restricted to giving either 5% dextrose, normal saline or one of these solutions to which potassium chloride has been added:

● 5% Dextrose is a solution of glucose in water such that there is 5 g of dextrose (dextrose is glucose) per 100 ml of solution, which is equivalent to a 278-mmol solution. This is approximately iso-osmotic with plasma.

● Normal saline is a 154-mmol solution of sodium chloride in water (9 g of sodium chloride per litre) and is also approximately iso-osmotic with plasma because there are both sodium and chloride ions in solution.

The difference between the two solutions is that with 5% dextrose the glucose is metabolized and so the end result is merely the addition of water to the body. Therefore, if the patient only needs water, give them 5% dextrose. In contrast, with normal saline, the patient also acquires 9 g or 154 mmol of sodium per litre of fluid administered. If the patient is given several litres of this a day, this can be a substantial sodium load for the kidney to excrete. In some diseases (e.g. heart failure, renal failure and liver failure), sodium excretion by the kidney may be reduced. The sodium will then accumulate and retain with it water, resulting in an abnormal increase in body fluid volume resulting in oedema. However, there are occasions when the patient has lost both sodium and water and in these circumstances it would be highly appropriate to replace their fluid losses with normal saline.

Prescribing potassium

Potassium chloride can be added to these fluids to replace any potassium loss. The kidney excretes a certain amount of potassium each day, so if a patient is on intravenous fluid therapy for several days it will be necessary to start replacing this urinary potassium loss. However, care is necessary as rapid infusion of large amounts of potassium can cause fatal cardiac arrest. Usually, 20–40 mmol of potassium are added to 1 litre of normal saline or 5% dextrose and this is given over 4–8 h. However, in cases of severe potassium deficiency, larger amounts are sometimes given more quickly with careful monitoring.

How much fluid to give?

The amount of fluid required depends on the exact circumstances. If a patient is essentially well, but simply cannot take fluids orally, nasogastrically or enterally, then the fluid regimen has to keep the patient in normal fluid balance. To do this, it is necessary to replace all the losses that will occur. This means replacing the urine output (and the output of any tubes, fistulae or drains) as well as the insensible losses. The insensible losses are mainly those from water vapour that is exhaled from the lungs and sweat. Typically, these are around 500 ml/day, but can rise significantly if the patient has a fever, a rough guide being that an extra 500 ml may be lost per degree centigrade of fever per day. Note that if you wish to replace fluid losses, you must measure them in the first place to know what they are. This can be easier said than done and, obviously, there is substantial potential human error in the measurements, so careful assessment of fluid status remains essential. However, daily weights can be particularly useful as they are less prone to error.

Usually, patients receive about 2–3 litres per day of maintenance fluid. Typically, this would be around 2 litres of 5% dextrose and 1 litre of normal saline with around 20–40 mmol/day of potassium. In a well patient with normal renal function, it is safer to give more rather than less fluid as the patient's kidneys will excrete any excess fluid that is administered.

In some cases it is necessary to provide long-term feeding through a central vein. In this case, the metabolic requirements are calculated according to standard guidelines and usually prescribed by senior doctors in liaison with a multidisciplinary team. However, the basic rules still apply to the volume of liquid required by the patients.

How to judge body fluid volume?

This is topic is discussed above (see p. 578). Key features to pay attention to are blood pressure (especially a postural drop), the jugular or central venous pressure and the presence of oedema in the lungs or the periphery. As part of a patient's fluid assessment, always listen to the bases of the lungs as severe pulmonary oedema can easily kill an elderly patient before you have time to treat it and is best detected early. There is no excuse for giving a litre of normal saline to a patient with early pulmonary oedema.

Always judge the amount of fluid to give first and then work out what type of fluid is needed. The amount of fluid is based purely on your assessment of the patient's body fluid volume and this assessment also includes information about the patient's fluid losses, temperature, etc. The composition of the fluid will depend principally on the patient's blood results, but also to some extent on the clinical situation (e.g. the patient may be known to be losing potassium because they are on diuretics and so be likely to need more potassium each day for that reason).

Any patient on intravenous fluids should have standard biochemistry (sodium, potassium and renal function) measured every day and should have their fluid volume status assessed clinically every day. Other electrolytes such as calcium, phosphate and magnesium should be assessed at least twice a week and preferably daily in sick patients.

Fluid, electrolyte and acid–base disorders and their management

Understanding disorders of body fluid volume, osmolality and sodium

Disorders affecting sodium and water

Sodium and water disorders are qualitatively different from other electrolyte disturbances because sodium is the major extracellular electrolyte and so the metabolism of sodium and water are closely interlinked (see p. 573). Always remember that osmolality is controlled at the expense of volume. This means that the kidney can alter fluid volume by retaining or excreting salt. Water moves with the salt. The mechanism that regulates osmolality will usually signal to the kidney to retain or excrete water to make the plasma osmolality normal, even if this will cause an abnormal body volume. Thus, in heart failure the kidney retains sodium and the osmolality regulation system triggers the retention of water with it to maintain normal osmolality.

Disorders of body fluid volume

Changes in body sodium content cause changes in body volume. Changes in body sodium can arise if there is a loss of body sodium from tissue fluids or if there is abnormal handling of sodium by the kidney. This may reflect a primary kidney disorder or a disorder of the regulatory mechanisms such as the adrenal gland, which influence renal sodium excretion. Because osmolality is usually maintained, the measured plasma sodium concentration may be normal.

Low body fluid volume—dehydration

Aldosterone deficiency. The usual cause in adults is Addison's disease (see p. 856) in which damage to the adrenal cortex reduces the amount of aldosterone released by the adrenal gland. Aldosterone normally causes the kidney to retain sodium and excrete potassium. The adrenal gland damage may also cause deficiency of glucocorticoids and pigmentation can also occur because of excess ACTH. The damage is usually caused by tuberculosis or an autoimmune process. In children, inborn errors of metabolism can cause similar problems.

Diuretics. These directly cause renal sodium excretion and with it water loss.

Renal disease. Damage to tubular function can impair the ability of the kidney to reabsorb sodium from the tubules. This can be hereditary, such as with Bartter's syndrome (see p. 535), or acquired, such as with a tubulo-interstitial nephritis.

Treatment is with fluid and electrolyte therapy to replace losses. Any underlying disease should be treated and any causative drug removed or the dosage decreased. Withhold diuretics until the patient is rehydrated. There is no point administering fluid at the same time as giving a diuretic to remove it. If there is a deficiency of aldosterone then this should also be replaced with synthetic mineralocorticoid in the form of fludrocortisone.

High body fluid volume—oedema

Aldosterone excess. Excess aldosterone promotes excess sodium retention by the kidney and can be caused by adrenal hyperplasia or a tumour or can occur in the oedema states as a result of excess renin and angiotensin. Renal failure also impairs the ability of the kidneys to excrete sodium, water or other electrolytes.

Oedema states. There are three main oedema states:
1 Congestive heart failure
2 Liver failure
3 Nephrotic syndrome

In all three conditions, the kidney retains sodium and water inappropriately, causing oedema. All three conditions are characterized by a regulatory response that would be appropriate if the body was hypovolaemic (e.g. if there was acute haemorrhage). However, in all three cases, there is excess body fluid. The body seems to 'perceive' that body fluid volume is low, generally because arterial blood pressure is low. In congestive heart failure (see p. 425) cardiac output is low and so arterial blood pressure is low. In liver failure (see p. 618) arterial blood pressure is low, because there is widespread vasodilatation as a result of accumulating vasoactive substances and the opening of multiple arteriovenous shunts (including cutaneous spider naevi). In nephrotic syndrome (see p. 515) the reasons are less well understood. The leak of protein from the kidney lowers plasma albumin levels, which may allow a leak of fluid into the tissues, which would lower circulatory volume.

The response to this perceived low body fluid volume is a regulatory response that includes high levels of renin–angiotensin II and aldosterone (promoted by the high angiotensin II levels), antidiuretic hormone and sympathetic nervous system activity. These three key factors act on the kidney to promote sodium and water retention, which causes a rise in body fluid volume and oedema.

08

08

Treatment is with diuretics to cause excretion of the sodium by the kidney. ACE inhibitors or angiotensin II antagonists block the effects of angiotensin II. Spironolactone is used, especially in liver disease, to directly block the effects of aldosterone. In these conditions, fluid restriction and sodium restriction are also helpful. Any underlying disease should be treated and any causative drug removed or the dosage decreased.

Disorders of osmolality

The key disorders of osmolality:
- Syndrome of inappropriate vasopressin secretion, in which there is too much vasopressin
- Diabetes insipidus, in which there is a deficiency of vasopressin or an inability of vasopressin to act on the kidney

Low osmolality

This arises if there if excess water retention compared to sodium. It is usually caused by an inappropriately high vasopressin level (syndrome of inappropriate ADH secretion; SIADH) causing the kidney to reabsorb more water than it otherwise would. The most common cause is vasopressin secretion from a lung cancer or a postoperative rise in vasopressin as part of the stress response. In the postoperative setting, the hypo-osmolality may be exacerbated by the administration of excess water in the form of 5% dextrose (see p. 580). **Urine osmolality is abnormally high compared to the low plasma osmolality.**

Treatment is with fluid restriction and sometimes demeclocycline, which causes a mild compensatory nephrogenic diabetes insipidus.

Very rarely, psychological disturbances can make a patient drink such vast quantities of water that they lower their plasma osmolality and this is termed psychogenic polydipsia.

High osmolality

This arises if there is inadequate water reabsorption by the kidney from the glomerular filtrate, compared to that of sodium. **Urine osmolality is abnormally low compared to the high plasma osmolality.** It is usually caused by diabetes insipidus as a result of inadequate vasopressin action. Clinically, there is usually dehydration and polydipsia. This can be because of:
- Failure of vasopressin secretion from the posterior pituitary gland (cranial diabetes insipidus)
or
- Failure of the kidney to respond to vasopressin (nephrogenic diabetes insipidus)
Nephrogenic diabetes insipidus is usually caused by

genetic defects or as a side-effect of a drug such as lithium, amphotericin or gentamicin. Treatment of cranial diabetes insipidus is with intranasal desmopressin (DDAVP), a vasopressin analogue. Note that osmolality can be high if there is excess ingestion or production of an osmotically active substance. The most common occurrence of this is in diabetes mellitus with excess glucose (see pp. 785, 788).

Disorders of plasma sodium

The normal plasma sodium concentration is 135–145 mmol/l. As sodium is the major extracellular electrolyte, hyponatraemia is usually associated with hypo-osmolality and hypernatraemia is usually associated with hyperosmolality. Both plasma hypo-osmolality and hyperosmolality can have adverse effects on cells, especially neural cells. In each case, the diagnosis and treatment depend on an assessment of body fluid volume.

Hyponatraemia
Disease mechanisms
The plasma hypo-osmolality causes the osmotic entry of water into cells, especially brain cells which swell.

Pseudohyponatraemia. It is always important to exclude pseudohyponatraemia, which occurs when another non-water substance, such as lipid, has accumulated in plasma. Although the amount of sodium per 100 ml of plasma water is normal, there is less sodium than normal per 100 ml of plasma volume as some of that 100 ml of plasma volume is not water. It is the amount of sodium per unit of plasma water that matters and this is normal—the **osmolality of plasma water remains normal in pseudohyponatraemia.**

It is also important to exclude an excess of another osmolyte. If another substance is present at high levels, the body compensates by lowering sodium levels to maintain **normal osmolality**. This can occur if the plasma glucose level is very high.

Hyponatraemia with low osmolality and low body volume
This is caused by fluid loss, with a greater loss of sodium than of water. The loss may be from the kidneys because of diuretics, tubular disease or inadequate aldosterone production in Addison's disease. Alternatively, the loss may be from outside the kidneys, usually from the gut or the skin.

Hyponatraemia with low osmolality and high body volume
This is caused by both sodium and water retention, such

that there is more water retained than sodium. This can commonly arise and is usually a result of:

- Renal failure
- One of the oedema states (congestive heart failure, liver failure or nephrotic syndrome)
- Excess water intake, usually in the form of excess administration of intravenous fluids

A common scenario in which hyponatraemia can easily arise is as follows. First, there is loss of both sodium and water, which promotes vasopressin secretion and then this is incorrectly replaced with intravenous 5% dextrose, which is essentially the same as giving water (see p. 580). The water dilutes the sodium that is present. Young menstruating women are particularly likely to retain water in this way and dangerous hyponatraemia can occur—especially postoperatively—if such women are given excess intravenous water in the form of 5% dextrose.

SIADH can cause a low sodium with a body fluid volume that is either normal or sometimes high (see p. 582). This is because of excess vasopressin secretion causing inappropriate renal water retention.

Clinical presentation

Typically, neurological function appears depressed with lethargy, confusion, cramps, reduced tendon reflexes and, ultimately, seizures and coma. It is important to remember that initially there may be no symptoms or signs.

Investigation

Check plasma sodium and osmolality and relate these to your clinical assessment of body volume.

Management

Any underlying cause should be corrected if possible. If the patient is basically well and there is no acute neurological change then treatment is not urgent:

- If body volume is high, then treatment is usually to restrict fluid intake
- If body volume is low, then the missing sodium and water should be replaced, usually with intravenous normal saline

However, plasma osmolality should not be corrected too quickly and plasma sodium should be monitored regularly to check this. This is because compensatory mechanisms alter intracellular osmolality, so that a sudden change to normality outside the cells can itself cause problems. If there is acute neurology, such as fitting, then it is important to correct the sodium concentration by giving normal saline (0.9% saline) or sometimes even twice normal saline (1.8% saline) and aim to increase plasma sodium concentration by around 1–2 mmol/l/h (and by a maximum of 25 mmol/l/24 h) until it is above 125 mmol/l.

Hypernatraemia

Disease mechanisms

Hypernatraemia always causes hyperosmolality because sodium is the major extracellular cation.

Hypernatraemia with low body volume

This arises because there is loss of both water and sodium, but a proportionately greater loss of water. As with hyponatraemia, the loss can be from the kidneys, because of diuretics, or resulting from tubulo-interstitial diseases that reduce the kidney's ability to produce a concentrated urine. Alternatively, as with hyponatraemia, the loss may be from outside the kidneys, usually from the gut or the skin. Normally, thirst corrects fluid intake, but in the sick and elderly this may not be possible. The hyperosmolality causes the osmotic exit of water from the cells, especially brain cells which may shrink. There may even be tearing of blood vessels as a result of this shrinkage.

Diabetes insipidus (see p. 836) can cause a high sodium with a body fluid volume that is either normal or sometimes low. This is because of inadequate vasopressin secretion or action causing inappropriate renal water loss.

Hypernatraemia with high body volume

This can arise with renal sodium retention in primary hyperaldosteronism when excess aldosterone promotes renal sodium retention in excess of water retention. Alternatively, it can be produced by excess administration of both sodium and water with relatively more sodium in intravenous fluids.

Clinical presentation

Typically, neurological function appears initially increased with irritability, muscle twitches, brisk tendon reflexes and spasticity, but ultimately seizures and coma can occur. It is important to remember that initially there may be no symptoms or signs.

Investigation

Check plasma sodium and osmolality and relate these to your clinical assessment of body volume.

Management

Any underlying cause should be corrected if possible. Water deficits should be replaced. Depending on the severity, this may be with oral water or intravenous 5% dextrose. However, plasma osmolality should not be corrected too quickly and plasma sodium levels should be regularly checked to monitor this. A rate of fall or no more than 0.5 mmol/l/h is usually considered acceptable. This is because compensatory mechanisms alter intracellular osmolality so that a sudden change towards normality can itself cause problems.

Disorders of plasma potassium

The normal plasma potassium concentration is 3.5–5.0 mmol/l. Most potassium in the body is inside cells. For this reason, relatively small changes in cellular potassium content can cause large changes in plasma potassium. Abnormalities of plasma potassium levels can arise from changes in the total body potassium content or from shifts of potassium in or out of cells. Potassium is the main ion affecting the resting membrane potential of nerve and muscle cells. Therefore, changes in plasma potassium levels can have serious effects on cardiac rhythm and even cause cardiac arrest. Abnormal plasma potassium values can be life-threatening and should always be treated promptly.

Hypokalaemia

Disease mechanisms

Hypokalaemia is usually caused by loss of potassium from the kidneys or the gut, or by a shift of extracellular potassium into cells. Potassium can be lost directly from the gut as a result of diarrhoea or vomiting.

Renal loss

By far the most common cause of renal potassium loss is the use of diuretics, especially loop or thiazide diuretics.

- *Aldosterone:* if levels of aldosterone are high, as happens in primary or secondary hyperaldosteronism, potassium excretion is increased
- *Magnesium* depletion can alter renal potassium handling and may need correction before it is possible to correct the hypokalaemia
- *Drugs* such as penicillin, aminoglycosides and amphotericin affect renal tubular function and can cause potassium loss
- *Genetic defects* in transporter channels can cause hypokalaemia (e.g. Bartter's syndrome; see p. 535)
- *Hypokalaemic periodic paralysis* is a rare autosomal dominant genetic disorder of intermittent paralysis and hypokalaemia
- *Renal tubular acidosis* can arise if there is abnormal tubular function and can also cause hypokalaemia

Gut loss

Any loss of potassium from the gut can cause hypokalaemia. In addition, with severe persistent vomiting, potassium may be lost from the kidney as well as from the gut. The loss of acid in the gastric contents that are vomited causes a metabolic alkalosis (see p. 591) and causes potassium depletion. Potassium and hydrogen ion excretion are to some extent linked and can appear to compete for the same excretory mechanism. With alkalosis, hydrogen ion excretion is reduced and, to some extent, potassium ions take their place. In part, this is because with a metabolic alkalosis, serum bicarbonate levels are elevated and more bicarbonate is filtered and reaches the distal tubule as sodium bicarbonate. In the distal tubule, the excess sodium is exchanged for potassium. A further mechanism is that vomiting can cause volume depletion and aldosterone release, which promotes both sodium retention to restore lost body fluid volume and potassium secretion.

Shifts into cells

Insulin, beta-2 adrenergic agonists and metabolic alkalosis can all cause a shift of potassium into cells. Acute stress such as that of a myocardial infarction or acute surgery is often associated with catecholamine release and a shift of potassium into cells, causing some hypokalaemia.

Clinical presentation

There are usually no symptoms, although occasionally there may be general lethargy, muscle weakness or reduced bowel activity causing constipation or symptomatic ileus of the bowel. Sometimes, the effect of hypokalaemia on the renal tubules can cause a resistance to the effects of vasopressin and so a mild diabetes insipidus-like effect can arise with polydipsia and polyuria. The cardiac arrhythmias that can arise include ectopic beats, atrioventricular block and atrial and ventricular fibrillation. Hypokalaemia can predispose patients to the toxic effects of digoxin on cardiac rhythm.

Investigation

It is usually clear what the cause of the problem is, which in most cases is potassium loss from the gut because of loss of gut fluids, or from the kidney, usually because of diuretics. If there is doubt, exclude magnesium deficiency and consider drug effects other than those of diuretics. If the problem seems likely to have been present since birth then specialist tests of renal function may be merited. In the presence of hypertension, hypokalaemia should raise the possibility of a high aldosterone level. This may be caused by a primary adrenal disorder (primary hyperaldosteronism) or it may result from another factor driving the aldosterone level high. This can happen with renal artery stenosis (see p. 540), where the high renin level promotes aldosterone secretion. In the oedema states, diuretics can cause hypokalaemia but, even in the absence of therapy, the high aldosterone levels (see p. 581) can cause hypokalaemia.

ECG changes

The classic changes of hypokalaemia on an electrocardiogram (Fig. 8.41):

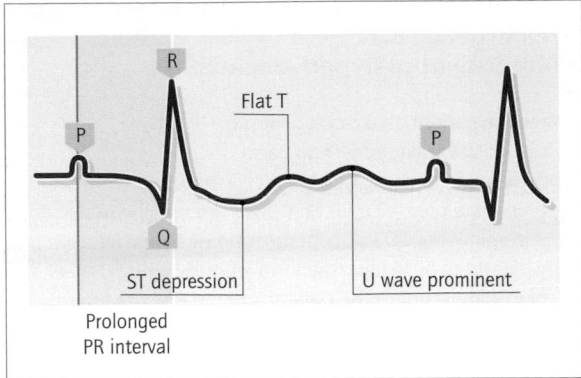

Figure 8.41 ECG changes in hypokalaemia. Hypokalaemia is first evident as ST-segment sagging, T-wave depression and U-wave prominence. The QT interval remains normal. As hypokalaemia progresses the T and U waves fuse.

- Prolonged PR interval
- ST depression
- Flattened T waves and sometimes enhanced U waves

Management

Any underlying condition causing hypokalaemia should be treated:

- If there is severe hypokalaemia or the patient is considered to be at high risk of a cardiac arrhythmia (such as in a patient with digoxin toxicity or congestive heart failure), they should be placed on a **cardiac monitor** while the risk is minimized by the correction of the hypokalaemia and any other reversible factors.
- Potassium levels should be corrected using oral or intravenous therapy. Oral therapy is fine if the risk of arrhythmias is low, otherwise it may be better to correct the potassium level more rapidly with intravenous therapy using potassium chloride.
- If a diuretic is causing the problem, but is necessary for the patient's underlying condition, then adding a potassium-sparing diuretic such as amiloride is helpful, sometimes with regular oral potassium supplements. Diuretics can often cause magnesium depletion, which can make it difficult to replace the potassium because of continued renal loss. If hypokalaemia persists in the face of treatment, check and correct the magnesium level.

Hyperkalaemia

Disease mechanisms

A trivial and artefactual cause of an elevated measured plasma potassium level is haemolysis of red cells in the blood sample, which releases the potassium from the cells. This will often be noted by the laboratory personnel and a fresh sample should be taken to establish the correct plasma potassium concentration.

- The kidneys normally excrete potassium, so **renal failure**, either acute or chronic, will cause a rise in plasma potassium.
- Various **drugs** can impair renal potassium excretion including the potassium-sparing diuretics, ACE inhibitors, angiotensin II receptor antagonists, trimethoprim, pentamidine and NSAIDs.
- Aldosterone normally promotes sodium reabsorption and potassium excretion, so a **deficiency of aldosterone** can cause a rise in plasma potassium levels. This can happen with adrenal disease, or with the drug spironolactone, which is an aldosterone antagonist, or with ACE inhibitors and angiotensin II antagonists, which both block the effect that angiotensin II has on the adrenal gland to promote aldosterone release.
- Potassium can **leak out of cells** when there is cellular injury, as can occur with the muscle damage of rhabdomyolysis (see p. 550). Insulin promotes the movement of potassium into cells, so in diabetic ketoacidosis the deficiency of insulin can contribute to hyperkalaemia. Similarly, catecholamines promote the entry of potassium into cells, so beta-blockers can cause hyperkalaemia. In metabolic acidosis, hydrogen ions enter cells to be buffered and potassium ions leave the cells to maintain electroneutrality.

Clinical presentation

Usually there are no symptoms, but there may be weakness and the effects of cardiac arrhythmias. Ultimately, ventricular fibrillation can cause a cardiac arrest.

Investigation

Check the drugs the patient is taking for possible causes. Check the renal function and plasma glucose levels. If muscle injury is suspected, plasma levels of the muscle enzyme creatinine kinase will probably also be elevated.

ECG changes

Initially, the P wave is narrow and peaked, then the QRS complex widens to meet the T wave (Fig. 8.42). The typical changes are:
- Loss of the P waves
- Widening of the QRS complex
- Loss of the ST segment
- Tall wide T waves

Ultimately, a sine wave appearance may be seen and ventricular fibrillation may occur.

Management

Place the patient on a cardiac monitor, on an intensively nursed coronary or high dependency unit. If there are

08

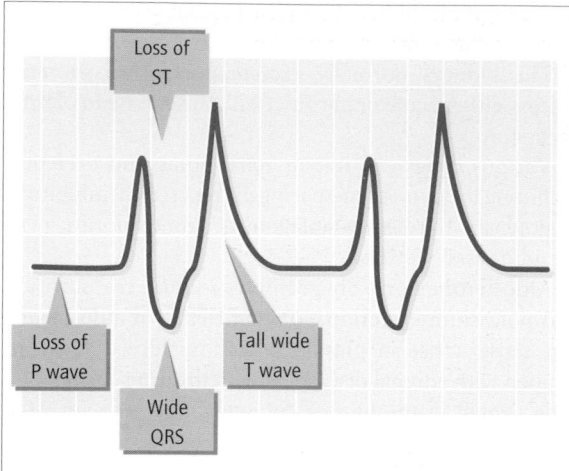

Figure 8.42 ECG changes in hyperkalaemia. This is a very important and potentially dangerous rhythm with the characteristics shown.

ECG changes, urgent treatment is required. In the immediate term, calcium chloride or calcium gluconate will antagonize some of the dangerous effects of the potassium on the heart and may reverse the ECG changes but the effect is short-lived. Plasma potassium can be lowered by giving intravenous insulin, which promotes the movement of potassium into cells. Glucose is given with the insulin to prevent hypoglycaemia. This effect is also relatively short-lived.

Ultimately, the potassium must be removed from the body. If the patient's kidneys are functioning, this can be achieved by the administration of diuretics such as frusemide with adequate hydration. If renal function is impaired, dialysis or haemofiltration can be used to remove the potassium. Oral or rectal administration of cation exchange resins is of some benefit as these bind potassium in the gut in exchange for sodium (EMERGENCY BOX 8.1).

Disorders of plasma magnesium

The normal range of serum magnesium is 1.4–1.75 mmol/l. Approximately 20% is protein-bound, and 98% of magnesium in the body is intracellular, mainly in bone and muscle. Most of this magnesium is not quickly exchangeable (nor acutely replaceable). Excess magnesium is excreted principally by the kidney. Magnesium has an inhibitory effect on nervous tissue, increasing the depolarization threshold, and so is useful as an anticonvulsant, especially in eclampsia. It is also involved in regulating the intracellular content of other ions (e.g. Ca^{2+} and K^+).

Emergency 8.1:
Treatment of hyperkalaemia

Place the patient on a cardiac monitor and have resuscitation equipment to hand

If there are ECG changes, give 10 ml of 10% calcium gluconate over 10 min. This dose can be repeated in 3–5 min if the ECG appearances do not improve

Give 50 ml of 50% dextrose intravenously with 10 units of insulin. Monitor the patient's blood glucose after this as hypoglycaemia can occur and may require further glucose infusion

If the patient has good renal function, then a loop diuretic such as frusemide will promote potassium excretion and this can be given with intravenous fluid to enhance the diuresis

Ion exchange resins are not of much use acutely, but are often given with some oral fluid

If the patient is acidotic, it may be necessary to give bicarbonate to correct the pH

If the patient has poor renal function then dialysis or haemofiltration are likely to be necessary

In the event of a cardiac arrest in a hyperkalaemic patient, give calcium intravenously

---

Hypomagnesaemia
Disease mechanisms
The main causes of magnesium depletion leading to a low plasma magnesium level are associated with loss of potassium by kidneys. Most patients with hypomagnesaemia also have a total body potassium deficit because hypomagnesaemia prevents potassium entry into cells.

Renal loss. The most common renal causes of hypomagnesaemia are diuretics and conditions such as diabetic ketoacidosis associated with a high urine output. A number of rare renal conditions such as Bartter's syndrome can also cause renal magnesium loss.

Gut loss. Prolonged diarrhoea, steatorrhoea or large-volume gut fistulae or ileostomies can be associated with gut loss of magnesium.

Reduced intake. Alcoholism, anorexia or starvation are associated with reduced magnesium intake.

Clinical presentation
Clinical features of hypomagnesaemia include tremors, Chvostek's and Trousseau's signs, tetany and convulsions, muscle weakness and fasciculation. There may also be a change of personality, anxiety, delirium and psychosis.

ECG changes include a **prolonged QT interval** and ventricular arrhythmias.

Investigation

Plasma magnesium levels are low and investigation should be focused on identifying one of the possible causes listed above. Also check for hypokalaemia, which is often present.

Management

The treatment is with oral magnesium trisilicate, intravenous magnesium chloride or magnesium sulphate and it is usual to replace magnesium over approximately 3 days or faster if the clinical situation is urgent. Measure plasma magnesium and potassium daily and give potassium chloride if plasma potassium is low.

Hypermagnesaemia

Disease mechanisms

Hypermagnesaemia is rare. It is sometimes seen in patients with end-stage renal disease on dialysis, in Addison's disease, in association with the use of magnesium-containing antacids or phosphate binders, or after intravenous magnesium therapy for pre-eclampsia. The effects of a chronic lower level of hypermagnesaemia (2–3 mmol/l), which is more common in dialysis patients, are unknown, but there are concerns that it may enhance vascular calcification and atherogenesis.

Clinical presentation

Hypermagnesaemia causes **neurological depression**. Tendon reflexes are reduced and the patient may develop flaccid quadriplegia, difficulty swallowing and talking and respiratory depression. There may also be bradycardia and hypotension. ECG changes mimic hyperkalaemia.

Investigation

Plasma magnesium levels are high. Check for hyperkalaemia—if the kidney has failed to excrete magnesium, it may also be unable to excrete potassium.

Management

The cause should be removed. Hydration and frusemide will promote renal excretion of magnesium, but if renal function is poor, dialysis may be required to remove the magnesium. Calcium can reverse some of the dangerous cardiac effects.

Disorders of plasma calcium

Disorders of calcium metabolism are common and important. Hypercalcaemia is the third most common electrolyte disturbance after hypokalaemia and hyponatraemia.

Table 8.15 Causes of chronic hypocalcaemia

With high phosphate level
1 Chronic renal failure
2 Acute renal failure
3 Hypoparathyroidism
4 Postparathyroidectomy

With normal or low phosphate levels
1 Disorders of vitamin D metabolism
   - Vitamin D deficiency
   - Decreased 25-hydroxy-vitamin D production (liver disease, anticonvulsants)
   - Decreased 1,25 hydroxy-vitamin D production (renal failure)
2 Acute pancreatitis
3 Magnesium deficiency
4 Postparathyroidectomy (hungry bone syndrome)

Hypocalcaemia

Hypocalcaemia may be acute or chronic. Much of the calcium in plasma is bound to albumin, but it is the level of free unbound ionized calcium (Ca^{2+}) that is important. For this reason, calcium values must always be corrected for the amount of albumin in plasma (sometimes biochemistry laboratories do this in their reporting) or else the free ionized calcium must be measured directly.

Disease mechanisms

Acute hypocalcaemia. This develops with hyperventilation. Hyperventilation reduces the level of carbon dioxide causing a respiratory alkalosis. Hydrogen ions leave proteins to buffer the pH of the plasma and calcium then binds to the sites on proteins that the hydrogen ions have just left. The result is a fall in free ionized calcium levels in plasma.

Chronic hypocalcaemia. This may be associated with high or normal or low phosphate levels (Table 8.15).

Clinical presentation

In acute hypocalcaemia, paraesthesia, particularly perioral and of the extremities, is common. More severe cases may be associated with tetany, laryngeal stridor and convulsions. Chvostek's and Trousseau's signs are often positive in both acute and chronic hypocalcaemia. Chronic hypocalcaemia may be associated with central nervous effects of confusion, depression or an acute brain syndrome.

Investigation

Plasma calcium and albumin levels must be measured to calculate the corrected calcium concentration (KEYPOINTS

08

Keypoints 8.3: Calculating corrected calcium levels

50% of plasma calcium is bound to plasma albumin, but it is the free calcium that is metabolically active and dangerous in hypercalcaemia

Total plasma calcium should therefore be corrected, taking into account the concentration of albumin to assess this danger

The calculation

Corrected calcium
= measured total calcium + $0.02 \times (40 - \text{plasma albumin g/l})$

A corrected calcium greater than 3.5 mmol/l is a medical emergency

---

BOX 8.3). If there is ambiguity, the laboratory can measure the free ionized calcium concentration. Levels of phosphate and PTH as well as vitamin D and urinary calcium levels may be useful in establishing the cause. Check renal function.

ECG changes include a **prolonged QT interval**.

Management

In acute hyperventilation with a respiratory alkalosis and hypocalcaemia, the respiratory alkalosis is corrected by simple rebreathing (usually into a paper bag), which elevates carbon dioxide levels and so corrects the alkalosis.

Emergency treatment of seizures or tetany requires prompt intravenous calcium gluconate, usually as a bolus of 10 ml of 10% calcium gluconate, followed by an infusion. Subsequently, or in less severe or chronic cases, identification and correction of the underlying cause is indicated.

Chronic hypocalcaemia is usually treated with oral calcium salts with or without vitamin D. In renal failure, activation of vitamin D is deficient and the active metabolite, calcitriol or its analogue 1-hydroxy-vitamin D_3, is given (see p. 562). This therapy can cause hypercalciuria promoting nephrocalcinosis and worsening renal function, so calcium levels and renal function must be monitored. Treatment of hypocalcaemia caused by hypoparathyroidism can have a similar effect. Urinary calcium excretion can be reduced by salt restriction and thiazide diuretics, which inhibit renal calcium excretion.

Hypercalcaemia

Disease mechanisms

Hypercalcaemia increases intracellular calcium. This inhibits muscle relaxation, disturbs neurone function and impairs renal tubular function. In addition, it may cause calcification in tissues (including the gastric lining and pancreas) and hypercalciuria causing urinary tract formation. The causes of hypercalcaemia are listed in Table 8.16.

Clinical presentation

The signs and symptoms of hypercalcaemia include:

Table 8.16 Causes of hypercalcaemia

Hyperparathyroidism
Primary (adenoma, multiple endocrine neoplasia syndrome)
Tertiary: one or more glands may become autonomous

Malignancy
Metastatic resorption of bone (especially common in myeloma)
Ectopic PTH production by tumour
Non-metastatic effects (e.g. by tumour secretion of osteoclast activation factors)

Vitamin D overdosage

Milk–alkali syndrome
Consumption of excess milk or antacids that promote enhanced calcium absorption from the gut

Immobilization
Promotes bone demineralization

Paget's disease of bone

Endocrine disorders
Thyrotoxicosis
Addison's disease

Granulomatous disorders
Commonly, sarcoid
Rarely, tuberculosis, berylliosis, histoplasmosis

Postrenal transplant
Resulting from tertiary hyperparathyroidism

- *Gastrointestinal disturbance:* anorexia, nausea, vomiting, constipation, peptic ulceration and pancreatitis
- *Other muscular dysfunction:* hypertension, ECG changes (shortened QT interval) or cardiac arrest (if plasma calcium is more than 4 mmol/l)
- *Neurological dysfunction:* psychosis, confusion, stupor, coma
- *Renal dysfunction:* polyuria, nocturia, polydipsia, acute or chronic renal failure, renal calculi
- *Calcification:* in other tissues (e.g. cornea)

All these symptoms and signs are increasingly likely to occur as plasma calcium increases above 3 mmol/l.

Serious complications arise if calcium is higher than 3.5 mmol/l. Hypercalcaemia often causes mild to severe renal failure because of dehydration secondary to polyuria. This dehydration and renal impairment usually exacerbates the hypercalcaemia.

Investigation

Calcium levels need to be corrected for the plasma albumin concentration (KEYPOINTS BOX 8.3). Renal function should be checked. A raised plasma alkaline phosphatase level may indicate bone disease. Parathyroid hormone levels should be measured to exclude hyperparathyroidism. A raised serum ACE level may indicate sarcoidosis. Myeloma is an important cause of hypercalcaemia in older patients and blood and urine should be checked for the presence of a monoclonal antibody band. Investigations, such as imaging by radiography or isotope scans, should be performed in the light of any clinical clues to exclude sarcoidosis, tuberculosis, Paget's disease and any suspected malignancy.

ECG changes include a **shortened QT interval**.

Management

Acute hypercalcaemia

When hypercalcaemia is severe, either because of its symptoms and signs or if the corrected plasma calcium is more than 3.5 mmol/l, emergency measures should be taken (EMERGENCY BOX 8.2). Aggressive hydration may not be possible if there is cardiac or renal failure and dialysis may be necessary. Bisphosphonates, such as sodium pamidronate or sodium alendronate are useful, especially in hypercalcaemia associated with malignancy. They may be administered orally or intravenously. Calcitonin may be beneficial in achieving rapid treatment of hypercalcaemia, but its effectiveness tends to decline rapidly and this limits its prolonged use.

Hypercalcaemia resulting from hyperparathyroidism is usually treated surgically by parathyroidectomy. Hyperparathyroidism in renal failure may respond to regular or pulsed vitamin D therapy but concomitant hyperphosphataemia must be controlled. Tertiary hyperparathyroidism in renal failure often requires parathyroidectomy. Calciphylaxis, where subcutaneous calcific deposits develop rapidly with associated soft tissue ischaemia, is a surgical emergency requiring parathyroidectomy.

Chronic hypercalcaemia

The degree of hypercalcaemia is usually less severe, but if calcium is initially more than 3.5 mmol/l, treatment is the same as for acute hypercalcaemia. Treat the underlying cause if possible. Increasingly, the mainstay of therapy in malignancy-related hypercalcaemia is the use of **bisphosphonates**.

> ## Emergency 8.2:
> ## Management of acute hypercalcaemia
>
> *If plasma calcium is more than 3.5 mmol/l or there are serious clinical complications*
> Insert central venous pressure line if fluid balance is critical or there is cardiac disease
> Give 1–5 l 0.9% saline intravenously to restore plasma volume
> Add frusemide 40–80 mg/h intravenously
> Measure urine volume, Na^+, K^+, Mg^{2+} and replace losses
>
> *If plasma calcium is still more than 3.5 mmol/l*
> Add 20 mmol magnesium chloride and infuse over 12 h
>
> *If plasma calcium is still more than 3.5 mmol/l*
> Give a bisphosphonate (e.g. pamidronate 15–60 mg as an intravenous infusion)
> (Can also use calcitonin 4 units/kg intramuscularly or intravenously every 12 h for up to 3–5 days, but the action is short-lived)
>
> *If plasma calcium is still more than 3.5 mmol/l or patient cannot tolerate fluid load of above*
> Commence dialysis (preferably haemodialysis)
>
> In desperate situations when immediate dialysis is not available, consider trisodium edetate 70 mg/kg body weight intravenously over 3 h

08

Oral phosphate therapy can be useful for primary hyperparathyroidism and malignancies. It inhibits calcium absorption by the gut and bone resorption, but should never be used when plasma phosphate is higher than normal because this will lead to metastatic calcification in the soft tissues. It often causes diarrhoea. Calcium levels fall within 1–2 days.

Glucocorticoids are sometimes useful for sarcoidosis, myeloma, some tumours, vitamin D intoxication and immobilization. They inhibit calcium absorption by the gut, especially when stimulated by vitamin D. They also inhibit bone resorption by tumours. Their onset of action is within 2–3 days.

Oestrogens blunt the tissue effects of PTH and are used for postmenopausal women with primary hyperparathyroidism who are awaiting surgery.

Plicamycin (mithramycin) is a cytotoxic that was useful in hypercalcaemia caused by malignancy. Repeated doses may cause fatal bone marrow suppression and it is seldom used.

Prognosis

The prognosis of hypercalcaemia is less favourable than

08

that of other electrolyte abnormalities because serious complications often occur before presentation and the underlying cause is commonly untreatable. However, in some conditions (e.g. hyperparathyroidism, vitamin D intoxication, immobilization and sarcoidosis) complete recovery is possible.

Disorders of plasma phosphate

Hypophosphataemia

Disease mechanisms

Phosphate is needed to make ATP, which maintains the integrity of plasma membranes and is an essential component of many enzyme systems. Severe hypophosphataemia (serum phosphate less than 0.5 mmol/l) indicates phosphate deficiency, but moderate hypophosphataemia (serum phosphate 0.5–0.8 mmol/l) may result merely from a shift of phosphate into cells. Hypophosphataemia is rare. **Alcohol** is the most common cause of severe hypophosphataemia.

● Contributory factors in alcoholics include a poor dietary phosphate intake, phosphate malabsorption because of vomiting and the use of antacids, and magnesium deficiency, which causes renal phosphate wasting
● Refeeding any malnourished patients can cause substantial hypophosphataemia because of a shift of phosphate into the cells
● Other causes include respiratory alkalosis, acute insulin therapy in diabetic ketoacidosis and excess parathyroid hormone
● Familial hypophosphataemic rickets is a rare genetic disorder of renal phosphate wasting

Clinical presentation

The symptoms and signs of severe hypophosphataemia can be widespread:
● Red cell, white cell and platelet dysfunction
● Cardiomyopathy
● Acute respiratory insufficiency because of weakness of the diaphragm
● Encephalopathy
● Rhabdomyolysis
● Metabolic acidosis
● Osteomalacia

It has been suggested that liver and renal dysfunction, ketoacidosis and peripheral neuropathy can also be caused by severe hypophosphataemia. Severe hypophosphataemia affects red blood cell metabolism so that the oxygen dissociation curve is shifted and oxygen is released less readily. This can be disastrous in the sick patient in intensive care in whom oxygen delivery is essential. Impaired integrity of the red blood cell membrane can

---

> ### Emergency 8.3:
> ### Treatment of hypophosphataemia
>
> **Severe hypophosphataemia**
> *Either*
> Oral phosphate; 1–2 g/day
> *or*
> Intravenous phosphate; 40 mmol/day added to parenteral nutrition
> (Monitor plasma values to ensure that the plasma $[Ca^{2+}] \times [PO_4^{2-}]$ product does not exceed 5 mmol/l because this is associated with a risk of tissue calcification)
>
> **In an emergency**
> Dilute one ampoule of Addiphos in 500 ml dextrose or 0.9% saline and give over 3–6 h
> Oral Sandoz phosphate: each effervescent tablet contains 16 mmol of phosphate
> Addiphos: each ampoule contains 40 mmol of phosphate, 30 mmol K^+ and 30 mmol Na^+
>
> **Mild to moderate hypophosphataemia**
> Remove cause
> Increase phosphate content of diet

---

also cause haemolysis. The neurological effect is similar to a metabolic encephalopathy, and osteomalacia is a longer term effect because of the mobilization of phosphate—and therefore calcium—from bones.

Investigation

Plasma phosphate is low. Check parathyroid hormone levels, and monitor and correct other electrolytes. A full blood count should exclude haemolysis, and liver and renal function should be checked. Creatinine kinase levels may indicate muscle damage.

Management

Intracellular stores of phosphate cannot easily be assessed. If hypophosphataemia is likely, it is safest to administer phosphate supplements orally or, in an emergency, intravenously (EMERGENCY BOX 8.3). Phosphate should be given prophylactically in intravenous nutrition.

Hyperphosphataemia

Hyperphosphataemia can result from phosphate release from damaged cells. This can occur with rhabdomyolysis or tumour lysis. However, the most common cause is renal failure which is discussed elsewhere (see pp. 549–55).

Table 8.17 Causes of respiratory alkalosis

Respiratory disease
Asthma
Emphysema
Pneumonia
Pulmonary emboli

Central nervous system
Midbrain lesion
Psychogenic

General
Fever
Early stages of shock

Metabolic
Liver disease
Aspirin poisoning

Pregnancy

Table 8.18 Causes of metabolic alkalosis

Prerenal causes
Extrarenal loss of acid
Vomiting
Nasogastric suction
Congenital alkalosis

Ingestion of alkali
Sodium bicarbonate as an antacid

Deficiencies affecting renal tubular function
Potassium or chloride deficiency
Hypovolaemia

Other causes of renal tubular dysfunction
Hyperaldosteronism
Bartter's syndrome
Diuretics

Iatrogenic
Overcorrection of respiratory or metabolic acidosis

Acid–base disorders

Alkalosis

Respiratory alkalosis

Respiratory alkalosis is caused by hyperventilation, which removes carbon dioxide (Table 8.17). It is usually asymptomatic but may cause dyspnoea, dizziness, palpitations, sweating, carpopedal spasm, chest pain and fainting. Some of these symptoms result from hypocalcaemia (see p. 587).

Metabolic alkalosis

Metabolic alkalosis is rare and the causes are listed in Table 8.18.

Chloride deficiency in adults causes renal bicarbonate wasting because chloride is reabsorbed in preference to bicarbonate.

Potassium deficiency causes excess H^+ wasting in the distal tubule as potassium ions are reabsorbed instead of H^+.

Increased distal renal tubular sodium delivery enhances potassium and acid excretion, possibly by causing excess potassium secretion and potassium deficiency. Diuretics increase distal renal tubular sodium delivery and can have this effect.

In **hyperaldosteronism**, aldosterone also stimulates distal tubular sodium reabsorption and potassium loss and directly stimulates acid secretion by the medullary collecting ducts. Hypovolaemia also stimulates aldosterone production.

Clinical presentation

Severe alkalosis causes cardiac arrhythmias, hypoventilation leading to hypoxia, especially if there is respiratory disease, and increased neuromuscular irritability (tetany, hyper-reflexia and epileptic fits). Rarely, coma, respiratory depression and death can occur.

Investigation

Most causes are obvious from the history and examination.

Arterial blood gas analysis will determine the pH, P_{CO_2}, P_{O_2} and HCO_3^-, allowing definition of the severity and type of alkalosis. Measure sodium, potassium and chloride to confirm the cause. Check plasma calcium and magnesium, because hypocalcaemia or hypomagnesaemia can also cause tetany. Check **salicylate levels** if aspirin overdose is suspected. If there is a metabolic alkalosis, hypertension and hypokalaemia, **check plasma renin and aldosterone** levels.

Management

Treatment of the underlying cause is usually the most effective and rapid way of correcting an alkalosis (EMERGENCY BOX 8.4).

In severe metabolic alkalosis, the retained bicarbonate prolongs the condition even after the cause has been removed. Intravenous sodium chloride and potassium chloride will speed up renal excretion of bicarbonate by providing volume and aiding H^+ ion retention.

Carefully supervised rebreathing or inhalation of 5% carbon dioxide will raise P_{CO_2} and can be used as a temporary emergency measure to stop cardiac arrhythmias. Dialysis is very effective in severe alkalosis (pH over 7.6) using either haemodialysis with a low bicarbonate or acetate buffer, or haemodiafiltration against a solution

08

Emergency 8.4: Treatment of alkalosis

Cardiac arrhythmias
Rebreathing (using a face mask or paper bag) or
   inhalation of 5% carbon dioxide

Drug treatment
H_2-antagonists or proton pump inhibitor if loss of gastric
   juice is part of the aetiology
Intravenous 0.9% sodium chloride with potassium
   chloride to speed excretion of retained bicarbonate

Other treatment
Haemodialysis if an emergency (e.g. cardiac arrhythmias,
   fits, coma)

Specific treatment
Stop diuretics if they are the cause
Increase dietary potassium

---

with no buffer at all (e.g. Hartmann's solution or normal saline).

H_2-antagonists or omeprazole block gastric acid secretion and are used when alkalosis is caused by vomiting or loss of nasogastric aspirate.

Acidosis

Respiratory acidosis

Any cause of hypoventilation that increases P_{CO_2} will lead to respiratory acidosis (Table 8.19).

Metabolic acidosis

This is the most common and most dangerous form of acid–base disturbance. Its classification and causes are listed in Tables 8.20 and 8.21.

Disease mechanisms

Metabolic acidosis

Metabolic acidosis is classified according to whether it causes a pathological increase in the anion gap or not (Table 8.20). Diseases that cause a metabolic acidosis by adding more anions to the plasma (or extracellular fluid volume) increase the anion gap (see p. 576). All the other diseases cause an acidosis indirectly by loss of bicarbonate from the body. Lost bicarbonate is replaced by chloride ions to maintain electroneutrality. The resultant acidosis is therefore known as **hyperchloraemic acidosis or normal anion gap acidosis**.

THE USE OF THE ANION GAP (Table 8.20)
All the major causes of an increased anion gap can be

Table 8.19 Causes of respiratory acidosis

Neurogenic
Drugs
Cerebrovascular accident
Motor neurone disease

Neuromuscular
Myasthenia gravis
Guillain–Barré syndrome

Respiratory
Any severe diffuse respiratory disease

Table 8.20 Classification of a metabolic acidosis

Increased anion gap—gain of acid
Renal failure
Lactic acidosis
Diabetic ketoacidosis
Poisoning (e.g. aspirin, ethylene glycol or methanol)

Hyperchloraemic or normal anion gap—loss of HCO_3^-
Renal tubular acidosis
Gastrointestinal HCO_3^- loss
Hyperparathyroidism
Hypoaldosteronism

Table 8.21 Causes of metabolic acidosis

Renal
Renal impairment
Renal tubular acidosis

Extrarenal bicarbonate loss
Severe diarrhoea
Small bowel fistula
Pancreatic drainage
Ureterosigmoidostomy
Long ileal loop urinary conduit

Ingestion of acid
Ingestion of mineral acids or rhubarb leaves (containing
   oxalic acid) or aspirin (salicylic acid)

Acid metabolized from exogenous substances
Ammonium chloride (forming hydrochloric acid)
Methanol (forming formic acid)
Ethylene glycol (forming oxalic acid)

Disturbances of endogenous acid–base metabolism
Lactic acidosis
Diabetic ketoacidosis

Endocrine
Hypoaldosteronism
Hyperparathyroidism

Table 8.22 Causes of lactic acidosis

Increased rate of lactate production by anaerobic tissues
Any cause of decreased tissue perfusion
Hypoxia
Increased skeletal muscle activity (e.g. status epilepticus or
    marathon runners)
Destruction of large tumour masses (e.g. lymphoma or
    leukaemia)
Poisoning (e.g. carbon dioxide or cyanide)

Decreased lactate transport
Decreased cardiac output resulting from any cause

Decreased lactate metabolism
Liver failure (any cause)
Intoxication (metformin or alcohol)
Diabetes mellitus
Liver hypoxia

Miscellaneous
Haemofiltration or dialysis with lactate buffer
Pregnancy

---

diagnosed easily from the history and a few simple blood tests (e.g. plasma urea, creatinine, glucose) except lactic acidosis and acid ingestion (e.g. salicylate poisoning). If salicylate poisoning is suspected, salicylate levels should be measured. If an increased anion gap exists with no obvious explanation, measure lactate levels. Lactic acidosis is the likely explanation and it is a dangerous and potentially treatable condition.

LACTIC ACIDOSIS
The end product of glycolysis is pyruvate. When oxygen is available, this is metabolized in the tricarboxylic acid or Krebs' cycle, but under anaerobic conditions it is converted to lactic acid. Lactic acid is almost completely dissociated at physiological pH to lactate and H^+ ions and causes a metabolic acidosis. The serum lactate level is normally ≤ 1 mmol/l and is regulated by the rate of lactate production, the rate of lactate transport from the tissues to the serum and then to the liver and the rate of lactate metabolism in the liver. The causes of lactic acidosis involve disturbances to these three main regulating factors (Table 8.22).

Carbon monoxide and cyanide poisoning cause tissue hypoxia. Phenformin—and, very rarely, metformin—and alcohol can cause lactic acidosis in the absence of other manifestations of severe liver dysfunction. The precise mechanisms are unknown. Metformin-associated lactic acidosis is associated with renal or liver failure, and metformin is therefore contraindicated in these conditions.

Alcohol intoxication often causes a modest rise in serum lactate, but occasionally in the presence of protein malnutrition it causes lactic acidosis. The liver is one of the first organs affected in the intensive care unit syndrome of multiple organ failure. This is because a major source of oxygen delivery to the liver is the portal (venous) circulation in which the Po_2 is low even in normal health. This organ is therefore particularly vulnerable to hypoxia.

Haemofiltration or dialysis with a lactate buffer can result in increased serum lactate levels if there is liver dysfunction. The patient becomes unexpectedly and increasingly acidotic and has an enlarging anion gap. A dialysate with acetate or bicarbonate buffer should be substituted.

OTHER TYPES OF INCREASED ANION GAP ACIDOSIS
Renal impairment reduces the acid-excreting capacity of the kidneys and results in an increase in organic acids.

The acidosis in **diabetic ketoacidosis** results from the accumulation of acidic ketone bodies and renal bicarbonate wasting secondary to the glucose-induced osmotic diuresis. Diabetes mellitus can also cause **lactic acidosis**, but the mechanism is unknown.

Salicylate poisoning or poisoning with other acids.

Normal anion gap or hyperchloraemic acidosis
Bicarbonate loss. The major cause of a normal anion gap metabolic acidosis is loss of bicarbonate from the gastrointestinal tract, usually through vomiting or severe diarrhoea. Loss of bicarbonate can also occur from the kidneys in renal tubular acidosis. Other causes include hypoaldosteronism and, rarely, hyperparathyroidism.

Renal tubular acidosis
Renal tubular acidosis may be congenital or acquired and is caused by a renal tubular defect in acid secretion causing bicarbonate loss and so a metabolic alkalosis. There are two broad groups of renal tubular acidosis:
- In the more common **distal** (type 1) renal tubular acidosis, bicarbonate losses are minor (less than 100 mmol/day) and can be replaced by oral therapy. Drug toxicity and diabetes mellitus can cause distal renal tubular acidosis.
- In the rarer **proximal** (type 2) renal tubular acidosis, bicarbonate losses are much greater and cannot be replaced. In proximal renal tubular acidosis there is usually evidence of other renal tubular defects, e.g. glycosuria, aminoaciduria, phosphaturia (together these defects form Fanconi's syndrome; see p. 527). Often the cause of proximal renal tubular acidosis is genetic.

Clinical features of acidosis
Severe acidosis affects cardiovascular, respiratory, neurological and skeletal function:

● *Cardiovascular manifestations* include decreased myocardial contractility and decreased peripheral vascular resistance, both leading to tissue hypoxia and hypotension; venoconstriction, which causes a falsely elevated central venous pressure; pulmonary oedema; and ventricular fibrillation.

● *Other manifestations* include rapid deep respiration (Kussmaul's breathing), confusion, fits and coma caused by neurological osmotic changes. If the acidosis is chronic and less severe, osteoporosis and osteomalacia can occur.

Investigation

Most causes are obvious from the history and examination.

Blood gas analysis will determine the pH, $P\text{CO}_2$, $P\text{O}_2$ and HCO_3^-, allowing definition of the severity and type of acidosis. Measuring sodium, potassium, chloride and bicarbonate levels will allow calculation of the anion gap. Measure plasma creatinine and urea, liver function and glucose to determine the cause. If relevant, check plasma lactate and salicylate levels.

Management of metabolic acidosis
General measures

Treatment is urgent if the plasma pH is less than 7.2 (EMERGENCY BOX 8.5). It is best to give intravenous bicarbonate

---

Emergency 8.5: Treatment of acidosis

Resuscitative measures
If plasma pH is less than 7.2
Intravenous sodium bicarbonate 8.4% in 50 ml aliquots until the pH is higher than 7.2

Cardiogenic shock
Intravenous fluids and inotropes if necessary

Pulmonary oedema
Diuretics or dialysis

Severe acidosis
Artificial ventilation may be needed and bicarbonate dialysis or haemofiltration

Specific measures
Respiratory failure
Ventilation

Myasthenia
Specific neuromuscular therapy

Renal tubular acidosis
Oral sodium bicarbonate (800–3600 mg/day)

Ethylene glycol or methanol poisoning
Dialysis if severe (against bicarbonate buffer)

---

as an 8.4% solution, which contains 1 mmol/ml in 50 ml aliquots, and to recheck the pH every 30 min until satisfactory. This avoids the danger of rebound alkalosis, and by using the 8.4% solution rather than the lower concentration the total amount of fluid that needs to be given is reduced. Although the patient is hypotensive with a low peripheral resistance, large amounts of fluid may precipitate pulmonary oedema because of the myocardial impairment caused by the acidosis.

The correct treatment for hypotension is to increase pH towards normal and to increase the central venous pressure (or pulmonary wedge pressure) to the normal range, and then to use inotropes. The venoconstriction that accompanies severe acidosis may mask a volume deficit by falsely elevating the central venous pressure. The central venous pressure then drops precipitously as bicarbonate is administered. It may not be possible to give a patient with renal failure any bicarbonate without dialysis because he or she is already fluid overloaded. In such patients a pH of less than 7.2 is an indication for dialysis. Milder degrees of acidosis can be corrected using either isotonic sodium bicarbonate intravenously or oral sodium bicarbonate.

In renal tubular acidosis, potassium citrate mixture is effective in restoring plasma potassium levels to normal and helping to prevent renal calculi.

Specific treatment of lactic acidosis
Correct the cause. Under aerobic conditions lactate is oxidized in the liver to bicarbonate. If liver function is impaired, haemofiltration or haemodialysis with a bicarbonate buffer may be necessary.

Lactic acidosis caused by poor peripheral perfusion, hypoxia or decreased oxygen delivery to the liver (reduced cardiac output). The underlying condition is obvious and needs urgent treatment, which should reverse this type of lactic acidosis.

Lactic acidosis not caused by simple hypoperfusion or hypoxia. This type of lactic acidosis is more difficult to treat. Any underlying cause should be treated as far as possible, but the acidosis itself also needs treatment because it is severe, dangerous and likely to persist. Bicarbonate is given in sufficient dosage to increase plasma pH to more than 7.2. This may mean giving a large amount of bicarbonate (e.g. 100–300 mmol) over 2–6 h. If the cause cannot be quickly identified and treated, this dosage may need to be continued or haemodialysis or haemofiltration started.

Patients with renal impairment are unable to tolerate the osmotic and fluid load of this treatment. Haemodialysis or haemofiltration without lactate is then necessary. A bicarbonate-buffered dialysate is preferred.

Prognosis

The general prognosis for acidosis is good if it is treated before there are cardiovascular or neurological complications and if the underlying disease is amenable to therapy.

The prognosis for lactic acidosis is worse because it presents at a more advanced stage and the underlying cause may have a poor prognosis.

! Must know checklist

- Always measure the blood pressure in any patient in any context—this is the only way to determine whether they are hypertensive

- In renal failure of any form—acute or chronic—always check the potassium and acid–base status to exclude severe hyperkalaemia or acidosis that could lead to a cardiac arrest

- In any case of acute renal failure, always exclude dehydration

- In any case of acute renal failure, always exclude obstruction

- In any patient with a renal problem, always dipstick the urine and, if possible, view under a microscope and culture

- In severe hyperkalaemia, give calcium chloride or calcium gluconate intravenously

- Consider renal artery stenosis in any case of renal failure

- Type 2 diabetes mellitus is the fastest growing cause of renal disease

- Nephrotic syndrome in children is usually caused by minimal change nephropathy

- Non-steroidal anti-inflammatory drugs are the most common drug cause of renal impairment

08

Further reading

There are a number of good sources of information on the conditions covered in this chapter.

A key problem for clinicians is knowing whether a drug is safe to use in a patient with renal disease. The *British National Formulary* is an excellent source of information about this and has an appendix that details which drugs are and are not safe in this situation.

Books

Aronoff GR, Berns JS, Brier ME *et al*. *Drug Prescribing in Renal Failure: Dosing Guidelines for Adults*, 4th edn. Philadelphia: American College of Physicians, 1999.

Brenner B, ed. *The Kidney*, 6th edn. Philadelphia: WB Saunders, 2000.

Davey A, Cameron JS, Grunfeld J-P, Kerr DNS, Ritz E, Winearls CQ, eds. *The Oxford Textbook of Clinical Nephrology*, 2nd edn. Oxford: Oxford University Press, 1997.

Greenberg A *et al*., eds, for the National Kidney Foundation. *Primer on Kidney Diseases*. San Diego, CA: Academic Press, 1998.

O'Callaghan CA, Brenner BM. *The Kidney at a Glance*. Oxford: Blackwell Science, 2000. [This covers all the key topics of this chapter.]

Journals

The key journals in the field are *Kidney International, American Journal of Kidney Disease, Journal of the American*

Society of Nephrology, Nephrology, Dialysis and Transplantation, Nephron, Transplantation and *Hypertension*. They can all be accessed to some extent through the PubMed Journal Browser at http://www.ncbi.nlm.nih.gov/entrez/jrbrowser.cgi

As regards EBM, the standard sources (e.g. Bandolier, etc.) are good on topics such as hypertension and diabetic nephropathy. However, for some of the rarer renal disorders, the clinical trials are necessarily smaller and clinicians do not have the luxury of huge studies with highly robust statistics based on well-defined populations. Nevertheless, a number of bodies have produced clinical guidelines such as the Renal Association in the UK (www.renal.org.uk).

Websites

A number of very useful sites are available on the web. These include the website for The Kidney at a Glance at www.learndoctor.com which also includes self-assessment and revision summaries of the key topics.

In addition, there is a good atlas of renal diseases at http://www.kidneyatlas.org/

An atlas of renal pathology is available on the web at http://ajkd.wbsaunders.com/atlas/

The American Society of Nephrology and the International Society of Nephrology have good sites at www.asn-online.org and www.isn-online.org

Liver, Biliary Tract and Pancreatic Disease

9

Introduction

The spectrum of liver disease varies from asymptomatic disease to jaundice and liver failure. The diagnosis and management of patients with liver disease or with only abnormalities of liver tests requires a full understanding of the various synthetic, metabolic, storage, immunological and excretory functions of the liver. In the West, alcoholic liver disease and chronic infection with hepatitis C virus account for most cases of cirrhosis. Disease of the gall bladder is common and is usually related to stones and infection. Pancreatic disease, whether from inflammation, cancer or obstruction, may result in failure of the exocrine or endocrine function.

Structure and function

Structural features of the liver, biliary tree and pancreas

The anatomical structure of the liver, biliary tree and pancreas is shown in Fig. 9.1.

Liver. The basic structural unit of the liver is the lobule (Fig. 9. 1). The lobule is made up of several cell types:
- *Hepatocytes:* make up 70% of the liver and are responsible for the majority of the liver's functions (see Table 9.1)
- *Biliary epithelial cells:* line the bile ducts
- *Stellate cells* (also known as Ito cells, fat-storing cells or myofibroblasts): closely involved in fibrosis

- *Kupffer cells:* the liver's tissue macrophages

The liver receives its blood supply from the hepatic artery (25%) and the portal vein (75%). The blood drains via the hepatic veins into the inferior vena cava.

Gall bladder. The gall bladder connects to the biliary tree and has a capacity of 50 ml (Fig. 9.2).

Pancreas. The pancreas contains cells involved in exocrine and endocrine function (Fig. 9.3).

Functions

Liver
The various functions of the liver are listed in Table 9.1.

Biliary tree
The main function of the biliary tree is to allow the passage of bile from the liver to the small bowel, where it contributes to digestion. The liver excretes about 1 litre bile per day but 90% of the water is absorbed in the gall bladder, which stores the concentrated bile until it is required.

Pancreas
The pancreas has both endocrine and exocrine functions:
1 **Endocrine functions** include the secretion of insulin and glucagon to maintain glucose homoeostasis:
- alpha cells secrete glucagons
- beta cells secrete insulin
- D cells secrete somatostatin
- PP cells secrete pancreatic polypeptide
2 **Exocrine functions** include:
- secretion of lipases and proteases for the digestion of food

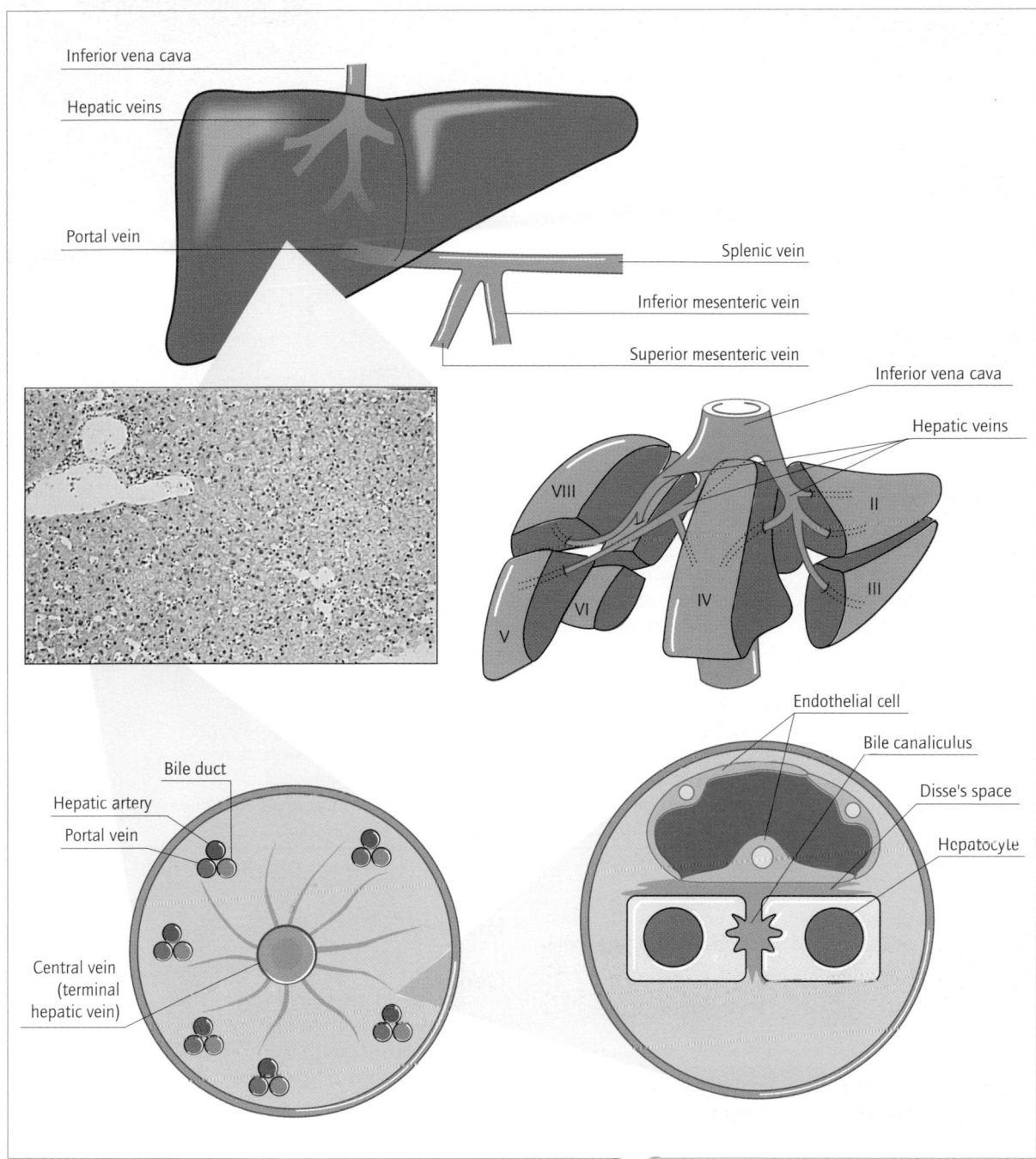

Figure 9.1 Structure of the liver and segmental anatomy of the liver showing the eight liver segments. I, caudate lobe; II–IV, left hemiliver; V–VIII, right hemiliver.

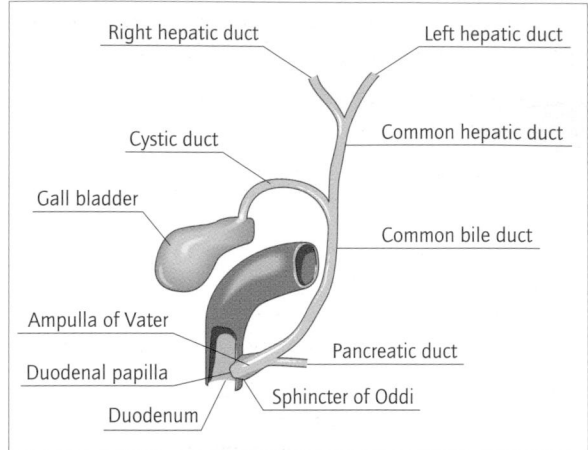

Figure 9.2 Structure of the biliary tract.

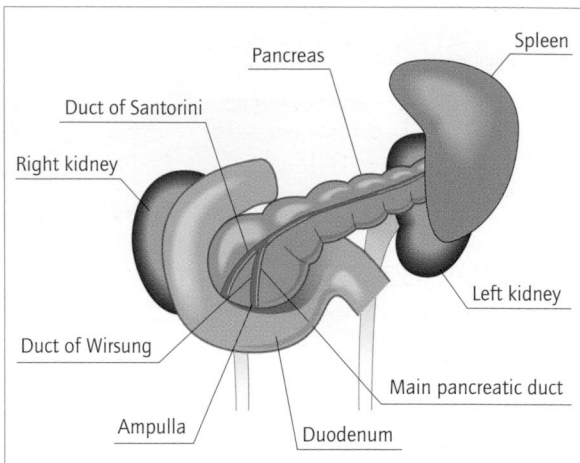

Figure 9.3 Structure of the pancreas.

Table 9.1 Liver functions

Type	Function
Metabolic	Carbohydrate metabolism (gluconeogenesis, glycolysis)
	Lipid metabolism (see Chapter 11, p. 800)
	Protein metabolism (synthesis of most plasma proteins, including albumin, most clotting factors, binding proteins)
	Bilirubin metabolism
	Bile acid metabolism
	Storage of glucose (as glycogen), fat, some vitamins
Immunological	The liver reticuloendothelial system acts as a barrier to infection
Toxicological	Metabolism and excretion of drugs and other xenobiotics
Hormonal	Synthesis of hormone-binding proteins and inactivation of hormones
Nutritional	Bile is important in digestion and absorption of fat-soluble vitamins

• secretion of bicarbonate, which neutralizes the acidic mixture leaving the stomach, creating the optimal pH for digestion

Approach to the patient

As for diseases of other systems, it should be possible to reach a diagnosis for most patients from a well-taken history. In the developed world, alcohol and fatty liver are the most common causes of liver disease, whereas in the developing world viral hepatitis and its consequences are a major cause of mortality. Diseases of the liver, biliary system and pancreas can present with a range of problems.

History

General

In the history, it is important to ask background questions about the factors outlined below, as these may suggest the cause of liver or pancreatic disease (HISTORY AND EXAMINATION BOX 9.1).

• *Age:* liver disease is most commonly caused by the syndrome of neonatal hepatitis in babies; metabolic disease in infants; viral hepatitis in adolescents; obstructive jaundice and gallstones, alcohol and other toxins in middle-aged adults; and infiltration and malignancy in the elderly. However, there is considerable overlap and this brief list is only a guide

• *Occupation:* may suggest exposure to known toxins, including alcohol

• *Obesity:* obesity is associated with fatty liver and non-alcoholic steatohepatitis

History & Examination 9.1

Symptoms of liver and pancreatic disease
Have you or has anyone else noticed any jaundice (yellowing of the whites of your eyes and skin)?
What colour are your stools?
Have you noticed any change in their colour and consistency?
Do they flush easily?
What colour is your urine?
Have you noticed any change in its colour?

Do you have any pain?
Where?
What is it like?
Does it radiate anywhere?
Did it occur before or after the jaundice developed?

Have you, or have you had recently, symptoms of 'flu or headaches?
Have you noticed any fever?
If so, what is your temperature?
Have you had any shivers or shakes (rigors)?
Do you have any bruising?
Have you noticed any increase in the size of your abdomen—do your clothes still fit around the waist?
How well do you sleep?
How much do you weigh?
Have you lost or gained weight recently?
If so, how much and over what time?
What is your appetite like?

Do you have any itching?
Any other symptoms?

Past medical history
Have you ever had a liver disorder in the past?
Have you ever had surgery?
If so, what and when?
Have you ever had a general anaesthetic?
Have you had any falls or broken bones?
Have you ever had a transfusion of blood or blood products?

Social history
What is your age and occupation?
How much alcohol do you drink each week?
Does anyone in your family have similar symptoms or any history of liver disease?
Have you been in contact with anyone with liver disease?
Have you been travelling abroad? Where? When?
Have you had any exposure to blood or blood products?
What drugs, tonics and herbal remedies are you taking, including those that are prescribed for you and those that you buy without prescription from the chemist, health food shops and elsewhere?
Are your symptoms long-standing or have they started recently?
Do your symptoms recur?

Family history
Has anyone in your family had liver disease?

- *Ethnicity:* chronic viral hepatitis B and C infection is particularly common in people of Afro-Caribbean or Asian origin
- *Sexual activity:* heterosexual or homosexual, current and/or past sexual activity is a risk factor for hepatitis B virus (HBV) infection
- *Pregnancy:* acute fatty liver and cholestasis of pregnancy may occur
- *Travel:* particularly to those countries where viral hepatitis is endemic, travel suggests the possibility of viral hepatitis.
- *Alcohol consumption:* exceeding 14 units/week in women or 21 units/week in men is associated with alcoholic liver disease
- *Drugs:* ask about all drugs taken prior to the onset of symptoms. Include those prescribed or bought over the counter; vitamins and 'health foods' can result in liver disease, as can 'recreational' drugs, especially Ecstasy and injected drugs (Table 9.2)
- *Intimate contact or needle-sharing:* with people at high risk of viral hepatitis, such as intravenous drug abusers or those in prisons or mental institutions, can result in viral hepatitis

- *Exposure to contaminated blood:* e.g. as a result of a needlestick injury, blood transfusion, visit to a tattoo artist or a dentist, or inoculation, is a risk factor for hepatitis B or C virus infection
- *Possible exposure to contaminated water and dietary exposure to shellfish:* associated with hepatitis A virus infection
- *Past medical history:* ask about a past history of liver disease, previous surgery on the biliary tract, anaesthetics, falls or fractures suggesting alcohol abuse, and blood or blood product transfusion
- *Family history of liver disease:* a family history of liver disease raises the possibility of α_1-antitrypsin deficiency, Wilson's disease or hereditary haemochromatosis. Alcoholic liver disease is also increased in family members

Symptoms of liver disease

Prodromal symptoms. 'Flu-like symptoms before the onset of jaundice suggest a viral hepatitis.

Jaundice (see Fig. 9.6). This arises when the plasma bilirubin level is high and strongly suggests liver disease or biliary

Table 9.2 Hepatic drug reactions

Hepatic disorder	Drug causes
Hepatitis	Paracetamol, analgesics, antibiotics (penicillins, sulphonamide, isoniazid), anticonvulsants, halothane, antidepressants
Fibrosis	Methotrexate, azathioprine
Fatty liver	Tetracycline
Cholestasis	Contraceptives, anabolic steroids, phenothiazines
Cholestatic hepatitis	Phenothiazines, non-steroidal anti-inflammatory drugs, carbimazole
Granulomas	Allopurinol, sulphonamides
Chronic active hepatitis	Methyldopa, sulphonamides
Liver tumours (benign and malignant)	Contraceptive steroids, anabolic steroids
Hepatic vein thrombosis	Contraceptive steroids
Veno-occlusive disease	Azathioprine

09

outflow obstruction, but may be caused by haemolysis. Bile is required for normal fat digestion, so if it does not reach the gut then fat is retained in the stools causing them to be pale, bulky and offensive. Bile originates as a breakdown product of haemoglobin, so haemolysis will cause a rise in bilirubin levels. However, this bilirubin is not conjugated and so is not very water soluble, and is not well excreted in the urine. The liver converts this unconjugated bilirubin to conjugated bilirubin, which is highly water soluble (Fig. 9.4). Therefore, haemolytic jaundice does not cause dark urine because the excess unconjugated bilirubin is not water soluble and so is not excreted in the urine and does not cause malabsorption because the liver is still producing conjugated bilirubin which is reaching the gut. In contrast, hepatic damage or biliary obstruction blocks the flow of conjugated bilirubin to the gut causing fat malabsorption and the excess conjugated bilirubin leaks into the blood and is excreted by the kidneys, producing dark urine:

● **Hepatic and obstructive** causes of jaundice are associated with dark urine and pale stools, which may be bulky, offensive or difficult to flush
● **Haemolytic disease** may lead to jaundice, which is associated with non-pigmented urine as unconjugated bilirubin is water insoluble

Abdominal pain. Hepatitis can cause right upper quadrant pain because of rapid distension of the liver capsule. Severe pain, usually colicky in nature, is associated with gallstones or cholecystitis (infection or inflammation of the gall bladder).

Pruritus. Pruritus is a feature of cholestatic disease, obstruction to the biliary tree and drug toxicity, even in the absence of jaundice. The cause is not known, but it may be related to retained endogenous opioid-like substances.

Bruising. Bruising results from a lack of clotting factor synthesis. This may be caused by impaired synthesis (the liver makes all clotting factors except factor VIII) or deficiency of the fat-soluble vitamins, which can arise with prolonged cholestasis or pancreatic disease) leading to inadequate synthesis of the vitamin K-dependent factors, factors II, VII, IX (XII).

Skin pigmentation. This is also seen in association with chronic cholestasis of any cause and is maximal around the face. A slate-grey appearance suggests hereditary haemochromatosis.

Ankle swelling. This may be caused by hypoalbuminaemia in liver disease.

Abdominal swelling. This may be caused by hepatomegaly, splenomegaly or ascites.

Haematemesis and/or melaena. This may be associated with impaired clotting, gastric erosions, variceal haemorrhage and peptic ulcer.

Symptoms of biliary tract disease

Many of the signs and symptoms of biliary tract disease are similar to those of liver disease discussed above.

Biliary tract obstruction is suggested by:
● Pain, which may be severe and colicky in nature, and may radiate to the back, shoulder or epigastrium
● Jaundice
● Pale stools
● Dark urine
● Fevers and rigors

Gallstones may be associated with fat intolerance, nausea and 'indigestion'.

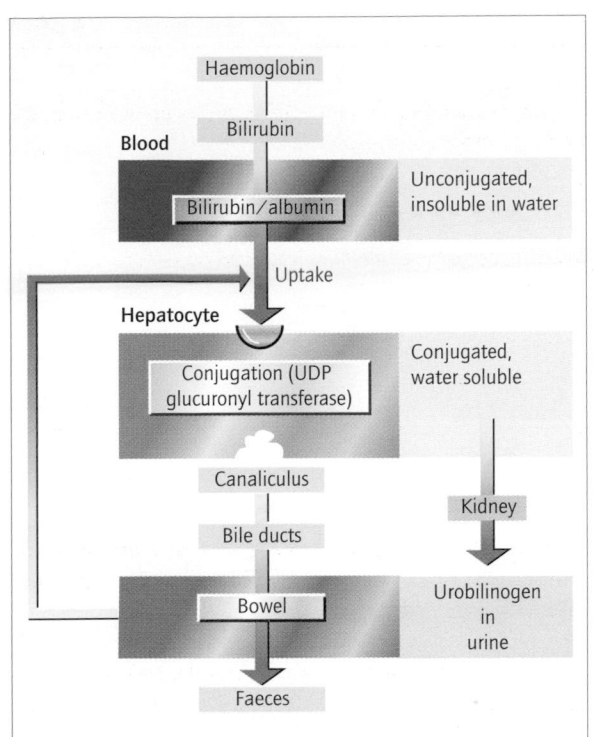

Figure 9.4 Metabolism of bilirubin.

Features of **chronic biliary obstruction** include pruritus, pigmentation, xanthoma and the consequences of malabsorption of the fat-soluble vitamins A, D, E and K.

Symptoms of pancreatic disease

The main symptoms of pancreatic disease are pain, weight loss, diarrhoea (or sometimes steatorrhoea) and jaundice:
- *Pain:* can be very severe, and is typically central and epigastric with radiation to the back. There is often associated nausea and vomiting
- *Weight loss:* despite an increased appetite, this can be profound and is caused by malabsorption
- *Diarrhoea:* pale, bulky and offensive (because of methane, not fat), and often contains undigested food
- *Jaundice:* obstructive in nature (stools are pale, urine is dark)

Examination

Although many signs are associated with liver disease, very few are specific (HISTORY & EXAMINATION BOX 9.2; Fig. 9.5).

General appearance

On examination, there may be jaundice, pigmentation,

spider naevi, telangiectasia, central cyanosis, loss of body hair and scratch marks:
- *Jaundice:* the classic sign of liver disease and first noticeable in the conjunctivae because bilirubin binds avidly to

09

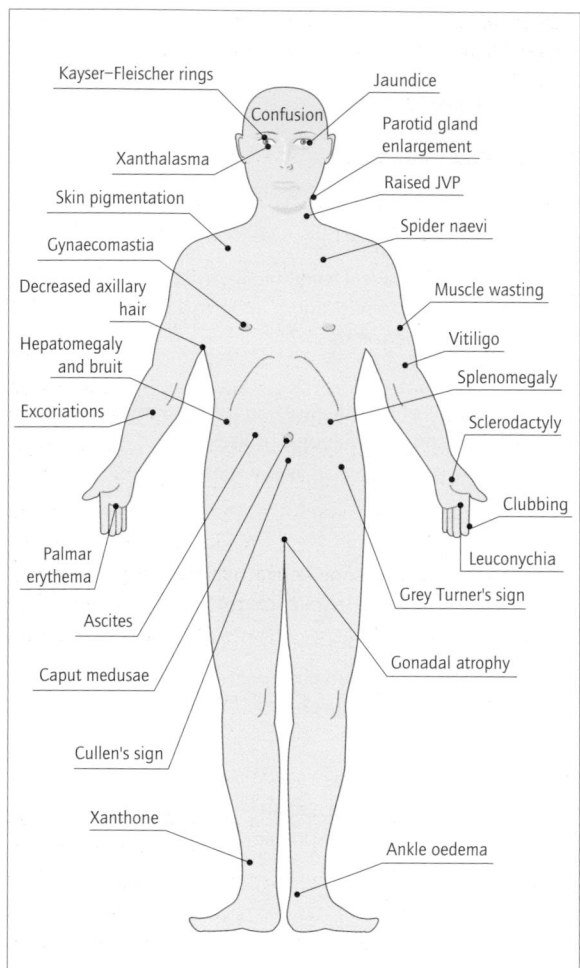

Figure 9.5 Signs of liver, biliary and pancreatic disease.

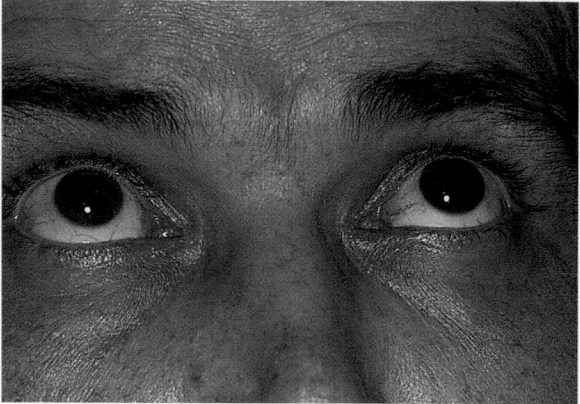

Figure 9.6 Jaundice.

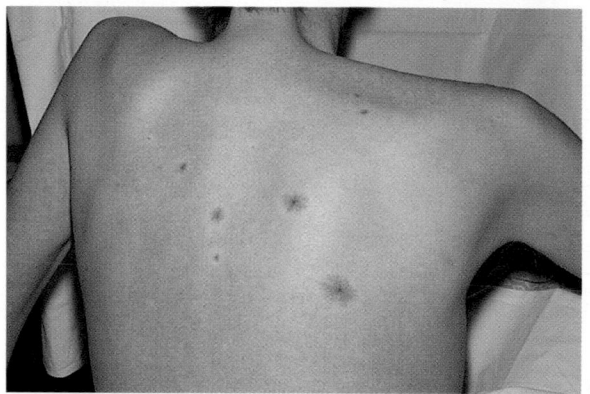

(a)

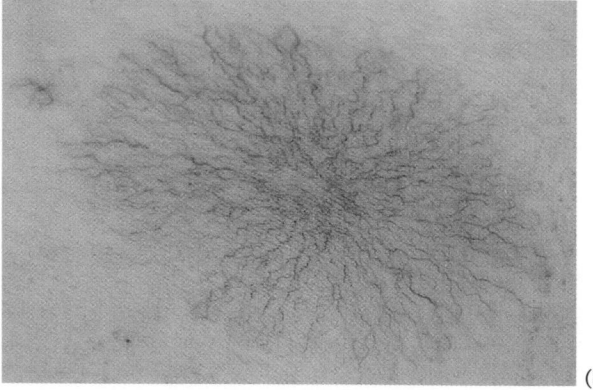

(b)

Figure 9.7 (a) Spider naevi on the back of a patient with cirrhosis. (b) Close-up view of a spider naevi.

elastin (Fig. 9.6). It is evident clinically when serum bilirubin exceeds 30–50 µmol/l

● *Increased pigmentation:* marked in biliary cirrhosis, especially over the temporal areas, the back and the chest. A more general slate-like discoloration suggests hereditary haemochromatosis

● *Spider naevi:* arterial dilatations on the skin are found in the area drained by the superior vena cava (Fig. 9.7). They are not specific for liver disease and may be found in other conditions, such as pregnancy or with oral contraceptive use. A few spider naevi may be normal

● *Telangiectasia:* may be present around the mouth or on the hands

● *Central cyanosis:* may indicate intrapulmonary shunting.

● *Loss of body hair:* most noticeable in men, especially in the axillae and pubic region

● *Excoriations:* indicate severe pruritus

● *Feminization in men:* may arise with altered body hair distribution, gonadal atrophy and gynaecomastia

● *Kayser–Fleischer rings* (Fig. 9.8): rings of brown pigment just internal to the rim of the iris. They are best seen using a slit lamp and indicate Wilson's disease or, rarely, chronic severe cholestasis

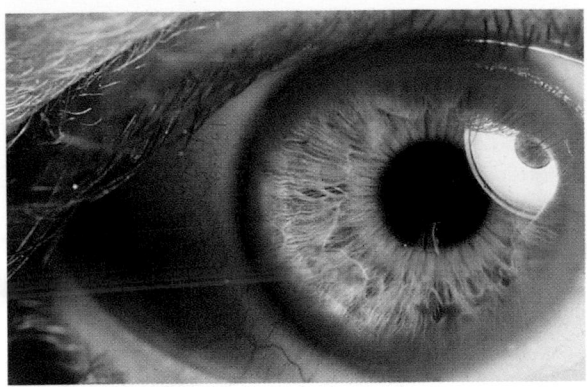

Figure 9.8 Photograph of the eye of a patient with Wilson's disease showing the brown Kayser–Fleischer ring.

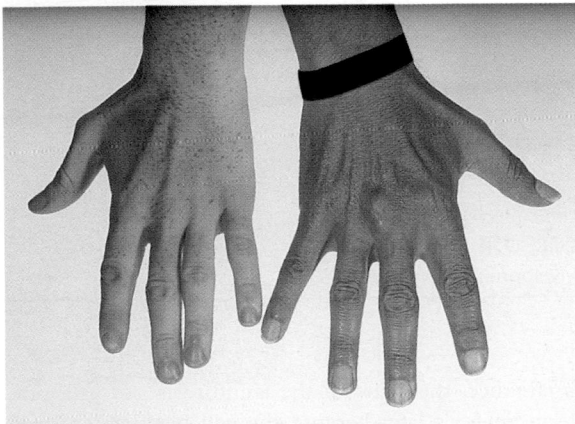

Figure 9.9 Hands of a patient with cirrhosis demonstrating clubbing and leuconychia.

- *Xanthelasmas and xanthomas:* yellowish deposits around the eye or tendons, and a feature of chronic cholestatic diseases
- *Generalized muscle wasting:* associated with advanced liver disease
- *Leuconychia* (Fig. 9.9): white pigmentation of the nails is associated with hypoalbuminaemia (from any cause)
- *Clubbing* (Fig. 9.9)
- *Dupuytren's contracture:* said to be associated with alcoholic liver disease, but the association is probably no more than a coincidence

Cardiovascular examination

Because of a generalized peripheral vasodilatation, there may be warm peripheries, tachycardia and low blood pressure. A raised jugular venous pulse (JVP) may suggest fluid overload, or cardiac or pericardial disease, which may cause or be associated with liver disease. Peripheral oedema can occur as a consequence of a low serum albumin.

Neurological examination

Hepatic encephalopathy is associated with a characteristic fetor and its manifestations may range from a mild disturbance of sleep pattern and apraxia to coma. Mild encephalopathy may cause difficulty in performing simple tasks such as doing up buttons or tying laces.

The Wrighton Trail test (the test measures the time taken for the subject to link a series of randomly placed numbered points) is a simple quantifiable measure of encephalopathy, but the ability to draw a five-pointed star better than the doctor is a more traditional test.

A liver flap is evident when the arms are extended forward and the hands are fully dorsiflexed. It can be differentiated from essential tremor because a liver flap is a coarse movement in which the hands do not 'flap' together. A similar flap may also be a feature of carbon dioxide retention.

Peripheral neuropathy may also occur.

Abdominal examination

The abdomen may be distended because of ascites. Mild to moderate ascites is evident clinically as dullness to percussion in the flanks and suprapubically when the patient lies supine. When the patient rotates onto his or her side, the ascites moves, resulting in shifting dullness. Ascites may result from causes other than liver and pancreatic disease, such as malignancy. There may be an associated para-umbilical hernia.

Dilated veins around the umbilicus (**caput medusae**) suggest portal hypertension. Ascites is revealed by percussion. Small amounts (less than 500 ml) are difficult to detect clinically.

Normally, the upper border of the liver in an adult lies at the fifth intercostal space and has a span in the mid-axillary line of 15 cm.

Use fingertips to feel for hepatomegaly while the patient lies supine and breathes quietly. If the liver edge is felt below the costal margin, percuss the upper border of the liver to differentiate hepatomegaly from downward displacement of the liver by overinflated lungs or sub-diaphragmatic fluid.

In cirrhosis, the liver may be enlarged, normal in size or shrunken. Sometimes, the right lobe is atrophied and the left lobe hypertrophied so that the liver is felt in the epigastrium rather than in the right upper quadrant.

In hepatitis, the liver may be slightly enlarged and tender. A small and shrinking liver indicates a poor prognosis.

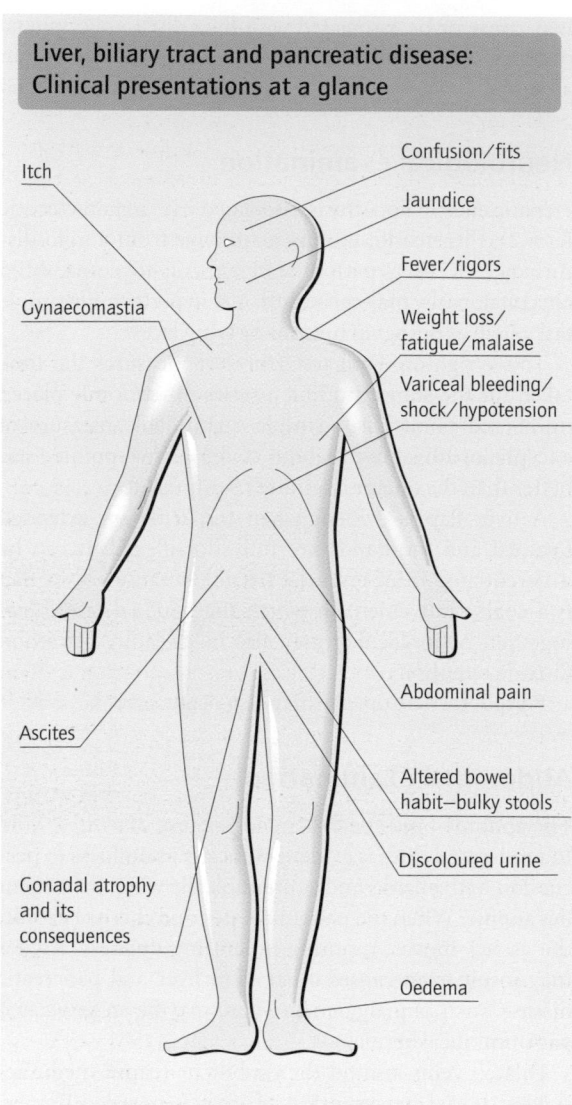

Liver, biliary tract and pancreatic disease:
Clinical presentations at a glance

- Itch
- Gynaecomastia
- Ascites
- Gonadal atrophy and its consequences
- Confusion/fits
- Jaundice
- Fever/rigors
- Weight loss/fatigue/malaise
- Variceal bleeding/shock/hypotension
- Abdominal pain
- Altered bowel habit—bulky stools
- Discoloured urine
- Oedema

Table 9.3 Causes of hepatomegaly. Common causes are in capital letters

Inflammation
HEPATITIS (alcoholic, viral or autoimmune)
Abscesses (pyogenic or amoebic)
Schistosomiasis

Tumours
Primary or SECONDARY CARCINOMA
Haematological malignancy

Cysts
Hydatids
Polycystic liver disease

Biliary obstruction
Extrahepatic causes (e.g. carcinoma of head of pancreas)

Venous congestion
CONGESTIVE CARDIAC FAILURE
Hepatic vein occlusion

Metabolic
Fatty liver
Amyloid
Glycogen storage diseases

Other mechanisms
CIRRHOSIS
Myeloproliferative disorders

The presence of a bruit over the liver suggests a tumour. The causes of hepatomegaly are listed in Table 9.3.

The spleen is not normally palpable, and it is usually about three times larger than normal before it can be tipped by the finger. The spleen can be differentiated from the left kidney because it:

- Has a notch
- Moves with respiration
- Enlarges towards the left iliac fossa

Signs of pancreatic disease

The patient with pancreatic disease often has a thin and wasted appearance. If the gall bladder is palpable and there

is jaundice, the cause of the jaundice is not gallstones (Courvoisier's law) because the gall bladder is usually fibrotic and shrunken if it contains gallstones.

Investigation

Haematology

Full blood count and erythrocyte sedimentation rate (ESR). A full blood count may show an anaemia with a macrocytosis caused by abnormal membrane lipids, or because of malabsorption of folate or vitamin B_{12} caused by pancreatic disease. A pancytopenia may be caused by hypersplenism as a result of portal hypertension. The ESR may be elevated. Haemolysis may accompany some liver diseases. Spur cells are found in some patients with alcoholic liver disease. The serum B_{12} may be elevated in cases of hepatitis because the hepatocytes store this vitamin.

Prothrombin time

In the absence of vitamin K deficiency, the prothrombin time (PT) is a sensitive marker of hepatocyte synthetic function because the liver synthesizes all the major clotting factors (except factor VIII). The short half-life (6–8 h) of these clotting factors means that the PT is a valuable guide to the severity of an acute hepatitis and acute liver failure. In some patients with prolonged jaundice, the PT may be prolonged because of malabsorption of the fat-soluble vitamins; intramuscular or water-soluble vitamin K will rapidly correct the abnormal PT (see Chapter 15, p. 1012).

Biochemistry

Urea and electrolytes

The urea may be low in liver disease because of impaired hepatic synthesis or poor protein intake. Serum sodium is also sometimes low as a result of impaired renal water excretion (see Chapter 8, p. 581).

Liver function tests

The conventional 'liver function' tests are not specific for liver disease and do not really assess liver function. A better term is 'liver tests'. Commonly used tests and their interpretation are as follows:

● *Serum bilirubin:* elevated in most forms of liver disease. Bilirubin is derived primarily from the destruction of haemoglobin (see Fig. 9.4, p. 601). The unconjugated form, which is water insoluble, is transported loosely bound to albumin to the liver, where it is conjugated by the enzyme UDP-glucuronyl transferase in the hepatocyte. This enzyme adds a water-soluble group to the bilirubin and so makes it water soluble. The conjugated bilirubin, which is water soluble, is excreted in the biliary system. The jaundice occurring as a result of increased red cell destruction is associated with unconjugated bilirubin and so the urine is not pigmented

● *Serum aminotransferases* (ALT and AST): aminotransferases are intracellular enzymes. Aspartate aminotransferase (AST) is primarily a mitochondrial enzyme, whereas alanine aminotransferase (ALT) is mainly found in the cytosol. Increased serum levels indicate liver cell damage with leakage of the enzymes into the plasma. In liver disease, the concentration of ALT is usually higher than that of AST (except in alcoholic liver disease); both enzymes are found in other cells, especially cardiac and skeletal muscle. The level of transaminases reflects the rate and extent of hepatocyte damage

● *Serum albumin:* albumin is synthesized by hepatocytes, so liver disease can result in a low serum albumin level. It has a long half-life (14–20 days), so low levels imply long-standing disease. Serum albumin may be low from non-hepatic disease, such as poor intake, malabsorption (such as coeliac disease), or increased loss through the skin (as in extensive burns), loss from the kidneys (as in nephrotic syndrome) or loss from the bowel (as in protein-losing enteropathy). Albumin synthesis is downregulated when there is an acute phase response or chronic inflammation

● *Serum alkaline phosphatases:* these enzymes are located in the canalicular and sinusoidal membrane of the hepatocyte and in biliary epithelium. Alkaline phosphatase is also found in the gut, bone and placenta, so increased levels of other isoforms occur during growth spurts, bone fractures (e.g. some bone diseases) and pregnancy. Increased levels of hepatic isoforms are a feature of obstructive jaundice, space-occupying lesions in the liver and direct damage to the bile ducts

● *Serum gamma-glutamyl transferase* (GGT or gamma-GT): the distribution of this enzyme within the liver is similar to that of alkaline phosphatase. However, unlike alkaline phosphatase, it is not increased in bone disease. It is readily inducible and increased levels are therefore detected in people taking drugs such as alcohol and phenytoin

● *Serum 5′-nucleotidase:* this enzyme is similar in distribution to alkaline phosphatase in the liver, but is not inducible

● *Serum α-fetoprotein:* levels are normally less than 10 ng/ml, but may increase up to 500 ng/ml if there is liver regeneration. High levels are associated with hepatocellular carcinoma

● *Iron status:* high iron saturation (iron : total iron binding capacity higher than 70%) suggests primary hereditary haemochromatosis. A high serum ferritin indicates iron overload or hepatocellular disease

● *Copper studies:* low serum copper and caeruloplasmin associated with high urine copper excretion suggest Wilson's disease

● *Serum α_1-antitrypsin levels:* low levels suggest α_1-antitrypsin deficiency, but serum levels in those with congenital deficiency may be within the normal range because it is an acute phase protein. Phenotyping is required to diagnose deficiency. The ZZ phenotype is associated with liver disease

Urine tests. The urine can be tested for bilirubin and urinobilinogen.

Biochemistry of biliary tract disease

● *Serum bilirubin, alkaline phosphatase, 5′-nucleotidase and GGT:* increased in biliary tract obstruction
● *Aminotransferases:* may be elevated in acute cholecystitis

Biochemistry of pancreatic disease

Conventional blood tests such as a full blood count and biochemical profile are non-specific, but may reveal consequences of malabsorption:

● *Serum glucose:* in pancreatic insufficiency insulin levels fall, so glucose levels may rise

- *Serum levels of insulin, glucagon and pancreatic polypeptide and glucose tolerance tests:* provide an assessment of pancreatic endocrine function
- *Serum amylase, fat absorption tests* (faecal fat, breath tests) and *tests of secretion* (collection and measurement of duodenal enzymes after hormone stimulation, food stimulation; *Lundh test*) or indirectly with the *para-amino benzoic acid (PABA) test* allow assessment of pancreatic exocrine functions
- *PABA test:* PABA is formed by the action of chymotrypsin on orally administered *N*-benzoyl-L-tyrosyl PABA; PABA is absorbed and excreted in the urine; thus, urine excretion is a good guide to pancreatic function
- *Faeces:* tests on faeces may be helpful in diagnosing pancreatic disease, but are usually unwelcome in the laboratory! Estimation of faecal fat content will document steatorrhoea; measurement of faecal elastase and chymotrypsin may help establish a diagnosis of pancreatic insufficiency

Immunology

Immunoglobulins (Ig) are often polyclonally raised in liver disease, but:
- IgG elevation is particularly associated with autoimmune hepatitis
- IgA elevation is particularly associated with alcoholic liver disease
- IgM elevation is associated with primary biliary cirrhosis
  Autoantibodies may help in the diagnosis of liver disease:
- *Antinuclear antibodies:* associated with autoimmune hepatitis
- *Antimitochondrial antibodies:* diagnostic of primary biliary cirrhosis
- *Antiliver/kidney microsomal antibodies:* associated with some forms of autoimmune hepatitis and drug-related liver damage
- *Antineutrophil cytoplasmic antibodies (ANCAs):* have been associated with primary sclerosing cholangitis

Microbiology

Microbiology is needed to identify causes of viral hepatitis (see p. 609), hydatid and amoebic infection (antibody tests), and sepsis.

Diagnostic imaging

Ultrasound, endoscopic retrograde cholangiopancreatography (ERCP) and magnetic resonance cholangiopancreatography (MRCP) are the principal imaging investigations in the liver and biliary tract.

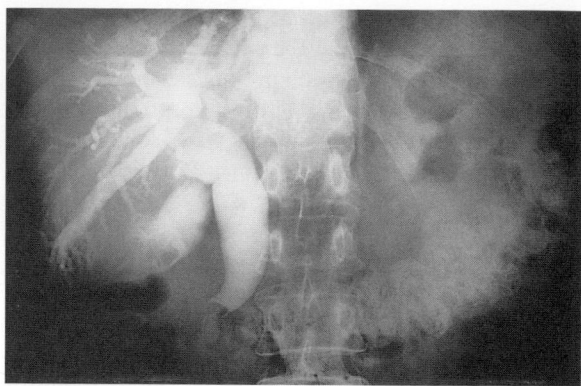

Figure 9.10 Endoscopic retrograde cholangiopancreatography (ERCP) showing a local stricture at the lower end of the common bile duct because of pancreatic cancer. There is dilatation above the stricture (the endoscope has been removed).

Ultrasound

Ultrasound is a non-invasive method of examining the liver, biliary tree, pancreas, spleen and blood vessels. It is useful for detecting:
- Alterations in parenchymal consistency, tumours, cysts and dilatation of the intrahepatic biliary tree within the liver
- Dilatation of the biliary tree and stones within the gall bladder
- The pancreas can be obscured by overlying gas in the bowel, so visualization is often poor but pancreatic tumours and cysts may be visualized
- The patency and direction of blood flow in all major arteries and veins
- Ascites

Visualization of tumours allows targeted biopsies.

Endoscopic ultrasound allows closer evaluation of the lower end of the common bile duct and is very helpful in the diagnosis of stones in the common bile duct and abnormalities of the head of the pancreas.

Endoscopic retrograde cholangiopancreatography

ERCP allows both visualization and therapeutic intervention of the biliary or pancreatic ducts after they have been cannulated using an endoscopic duodenoscope and injected with contrast (Fig. 9.10). It allows biopsy or cytology of the pancreatic ampulla and some bile duct lesions. Diagnostic ERCP is being replaced by MRCP.

Therapeutic manipulations include cutting the sphincter of Oddi, dilatation and stenting of biliary strictures and tumours (see Fig. 9.30), removal of gallstones (see Fig. B, p. 637) and obtaining material for histology or cytology.

Complications of ERCP are:
- Hyperamylasaemia (50%)
- Pancreatitis (mild 25%, severe 5%)
- Cholangitis (3%)
- Perforation (2%)
- Bleeding, after sphincterotomy (3%)
- Death (1%)

Plain abdominal radiography

Plain abdominal radiography is of limited value and rarely indicated. However, it may reveal some gallstones; calcification within the liver, gall bladder or pancreas (e.g. caused by hydatid disease); amoebic abscesses; haemangiomas; hepatomas; and infections (e.g. histoplasmosis, tuberculosis and *Brucella*).

Oral cholecystogram

An oral cholecystogram provides useful information about the function of the gall bladder (poor opacification in chronic cholecystitis) and may reveal the presence of gallstones. It has been largely superseded by ultrasound.

Percutaneous transhepatic cholangiography

Percutaneous transhepatic cholangiography (PTC) is used to visualize the biliary tree. A fine needle is passed through the liver and contrast is injected into the biliary tree. This approach allows therapeutic intervention such as dilatation of strictures, insertion of stents or local irradiation.

Computerized tomography

Computerized tomography (CT) gives higher resolution than ultrasound, and the use of intravenous contrast allows better visualization of vascular lesions (see Figs 9.31 and 9.32, p. 641).

Magnetic resonance imaging

Magnetic resonance imaging (MRI) is increasingly used to supplement other imaging techniques. Using appropriate techniques, arterial and venous vessels and bile ducts can be readily demonstrated.

Radioisotope scanning

Isotope scanning has been largely superseded by ultrasound, CT and MRI. Different isotopes are used to assess different aspects of liver structure and function:
- *Technetium sulphur colloid:* taken up primarily by the reticuloendothelial cells of the liver and spleen, and to a lesser extent by the bone marrow and lungs. It therefore allows an assessment of the general shape of the liver. Absent uptake indicates either Wilson's disease or alcoholic hepatitis
- *Gallium:* taken up in areas of inflammation and has been used to localize abscesses

- *Hepato-iminodiacetic acid (HIDA):* taken up by hepatocytes and excreted like bile
- *75-selenium homocholic acid taurine (SeHCAT) scanning:* assesses bile acid metabolism

Angiography

Angiography demonstrates the hepatic arterial and venous anatomy. It is useful for visualizing tumour circulation, which can be embolized, either with material to interrupt the arterial supply or with drugs for chemoembolization. It also allows venous sampling for abnormally high levels of pancreatic hormone.

Endoscopy

Upper gastrointestinal endoscopy is used to detect the presence of oesophageal and gastric varices and, where appropriate, to treat oesophageal varices by injection or banding.

Histopathology

Liver biopsy

Liver biopsy is used to confirm the nature and severity of liver disease. If there is focal disease, the biopsy can be targeted after visualization with ultrasound or CT scanning. A needle is passed through the skin into the liver (Fig. 9.11).

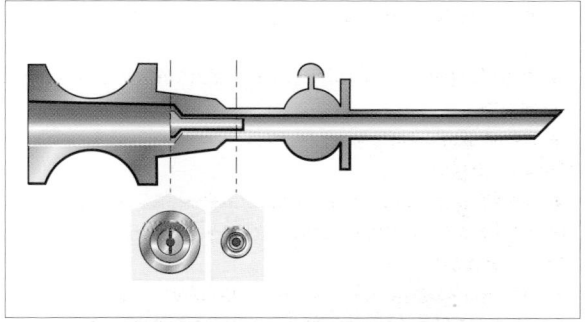

(a)

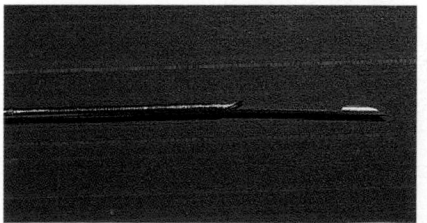

(b)

Figure 9.11 (a) Menghini liver biopsy needle. Note the oblique and slightly convex tip, and the blunt nail in the shaft to prevent fragmentation or distortion of the biopsy. (b) Trucut liver biopsy needle. Note the outer cannula and inner cutting needle.

After a liver biopsy, the patient must lie on their side for 2 h and remain in bed for 6 h. Their pulse and blood pressure should be monitored. The procedure is not without risk and complications include:

- Pain (up to 30%)
- Bleeding (moderate, requiring transfusion: 3%; severe, requiring surgery: less than 1%)
- Haemobilia (1%)
- Perforation of other organs (less than 1%)
- Tumour seeding (2%)
- Death (0.15%)

Contraindications for percutaneous liver biopsy include:

- Inability to cooperate with the clinician
- Abnormal blood clotting (PT more than 4 s or platelets less than 40×10^9/l)
- Difficulty in targeting the liver (small liver or ascites present)
- Abnormal anatomy
- Amyloidosis (increased risk of bleeding)
- Possible hydatid cyst (risk of shock)

If there is abnormal clotting, then a transjugular or plugged biopsy may be performed. A transjugular biopsy can be taken through the transjugular route when a flexible needle is passed, under radiological imaging, through from the internal jugular vein to the hepatic vein and then into the liver (Fig. 9.12). Any bleeding then occurs into the hepatic vein. Complications of transjugular liver biopsy include liver perforation, sepsis, perforation of vessels and pneumothorax.

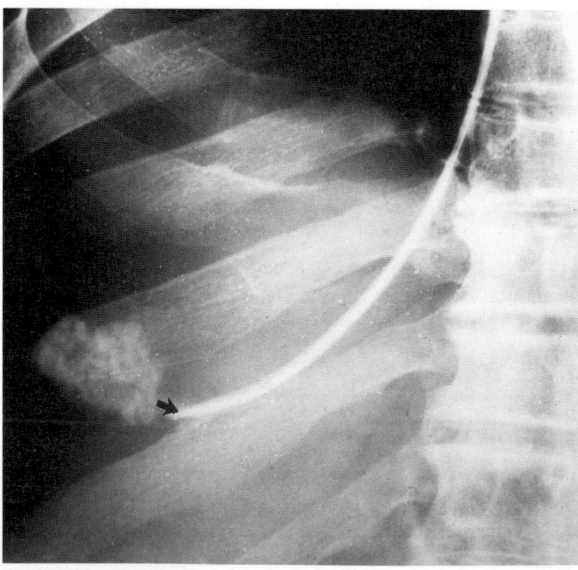

Figure 9.12 Transjugular liver biopsy. The catheter is in the hepatic vein and contrast has been injected to show the wedged position. The Trucut needle is taking the liver biopsy (arrow). Contrast is present to identify the location of the catheter.

Management

The general principles of management of a patient with liver, pancreatic or biliary tract disease are as follows:

- Make the diagnosis
- Consider specific treatment
- Treat complications
- Advise on social aspects
- Give prophylactic therapy when indicated

Diet

No specific dietary restrictions are required in liver disease unless there is:

- *Ascites:* restrict dietary sodium
- *Hyponatraemia:* restrict water intake
- *Encephalopathy:* protein may be restricted
- *Steatorrhoea:* restrict fat (but can be supplemented by medium-chain triglycerides)

Drug prescribing

Drug treatments are discussed with the diseases for which they are used. Drug pharmacokinetics and dynamics may be altered in patients with liver disease:

- *Absorption:* may be affected by a reduced amount of bile in the bowel
- *First pass metabolism:* may be affected in cirrhosis where portal blood may bypass the liver
- *Metabolism:* may be affected by reduced hepatocyte number or function
- *Drug levels:* may be affected by acidosis and reduced levels of the proteins that would normally bind the drug
- *Drug distribution volume:* may be increased if there is ascites
- *Excretion:* may be reduced in the presence of cholestasis

Because of the complexity of drug handling in liver disease, prescribing must be performed with care and should always be checked in a formulary (e.g. *British National Formulary; BNF*).

Diseases and their management

Jaundice (non-hepatitic, non-obstructive)

In the absence of hepatitis or obstruction, jaundice can be caused by congenital abnormalities or can be acquired. Congenital non-haemolytic jaundice can be:

- *Unconjugated:* e.g. Gilbert's syndrome, common; Crigler–Najjar syndrome, very rare

● *Conjugated:* Dubin–Johnson syndrome and Rotor's syndrome, both rare
    Acquired causes of jaundice include:
● Drugs
● Sepsis
● Enteral nutrition
● Some leukaemias
Cholestasis of pregnancy is discussed below (see p. 618).

Benign recurrent cholestasis is characterized by episodes of acute cholestasis, with jaundice, pruritus, steatorrhoea and weight loss.

Gilbert's syndrome
Disease mechanisms
The defect is complex and is characterized by low levels of UDP-glucuronyl transferase. Serum bilirubin rarely exceeds 75 µmol/l. The bilirubin is unconjugated and is therefore insoluble and not excreted by the kidneys.

Epidemiology
Prevalence. Common. Affects 3–5% of the population.

Age. Usually presents at 10–25 years of age.

Sex. Both males and females are affected.

Genetics. Autosomal dominant.

Clinical features
Jaundice is exacerbated by stress, illness and fasting. The urine is not pigmented.

Investigation
The diagnosis is made by demonstrating an unconjugated hyperbilirubinaemia in the absence of haemolysis. If the diagnosis is in doubt, a stress test such as intravenous nicotinic acid or a 3-day fast will lead to a twofold rise in unconjugated bilirubin in people who have the syndrome.

Management
No treatment is required.

Prognosis
Normal.

Crigler–Najjar syndrome
This is a very rare cause of unconjugated hyperbilirubinaemia. Treatment is with liver transplantation:
● *Type I:* seen in neonates. It is autosomal recessive and is brought about by an absence of UDP-glucuronyl transferase

● *Type II:* seen in younger adults. It is autosomal dominant and is associated with a decrease of UDP-glucuronyl transferase

Acute hepatitis
Acute hepatitis is a syndrome with many causes. The symptoms and signs are usually similar irrespective of the cause. However, it is important to establish the cause of the hepatitis to exclude treatable causes and to ensure resolution. In some cases, acute hepatitis may be the herald of chronic liver disease.

Viral hepatitis
The viruses that commonly cause hepatitis are:
● *Hepatitis viruses:* hepatitis virus A (HAV), B (HBV), C (HCV), D, E and others, termed non-A non-B
● *Other viruses:* cytomegalovirus, Epstein–Barr virus, adenovirus
Toxoplasmosis (a protozoal infection) is clinically similar to viral hepatitis.

The clinical pattern of viral hepatitis is broadly similar for all viruses (although HCV rarely causes an acute illness). There is a prodromal period of 'flu-like symptoms, anorexia, nausea and muscular aches. This is followed by the appearance of dark urine, pale stools and clinical jaundice.

Usually, the symptoms resolve after 2–6 weeks and recovery is uneventful. Treatment is symptomatic. Avoidance of fatty foods and bed rest are often advocated, but have no proven value.

Hepatitis A virus hepatitis
Disease mechanisms
Hepatitis A virus is an RNA virus spread by the orofaecal route. Infection is therefore highest where sanitation is poor. Epidemics may be water- or food-borne. Shellfish are a particularly potent source of transmission, because they may ingest sewage. Blood transmission is rare. The incubation period of HAV infection is 3–5 weeks, and the virus is shed faecally until the jaundice stage.

Epidemiology
Prevalence. Accounts for 30–40% of acute hepatitis.

Age. More common in younger people, but occurs at all ages. Mortality is higher (but still less than 0.5%) in older patients.

Sex. Equal sex distribution.

Geography. Endemic in all parts of the world.

09

Clinical features
Infection may be subclinical. Fulminant disease is rare.

Investigation
- *Serology:* IgM antibodies to the virus indicate recent infection and IgG antibodies indicate past infection
- *Liver tests* (see p. 605): show a hepatitis with a high serum AST and ALT
- *Prothrombin time:* a useful marker of disease severity

Management
Prevention involves careful attention to hygiene.

Normal human immunoglobulin containing at least 100 IU/ml anti-HAV can be given at a dosage of 2 IU/kg to people at risk. It is not always protective and is effective for only a few months. Prophylaxis with immunoglobulin should be considered for:
- Close contacts of patients
- Controlling epidemics in institutions

Vaccination should be considered for non-immune people (especially those over 40 years of age) who are travelling to endemic areas. The vaccine is prepared from formaldehyde-inactivated virus.

Prognosis
Nearly all patients make an uneventful recovery, and there are no long-term consequences. In older patients, the disease is more severe.

Hepatitis B virus hepatitis
Disease mechanisms
The hepatitis B virus is a DNA virus that may give rise to an illness clinically similar to that caused by HAV. However, there are important differences in the mode of transmission and the long-term effects.

The incubation period of HBV infection is 3–6 months. The time course leading to acute and chronic hepatitis B

Acute viral hepatitis at a glance

Epidemiology
Prevalence
Very common worldwide, exact figure unknown
Hepatitis A: 30–40%
Hepatitis B: 0.2% in UK
Hepatitis C: 15–20%

Age
Hepatitis A mostly affects children 5–14 years of age and young adults

Geography
Worldwide
Hepatitis B: estimated 350 million carriers of hepatitis B virus with prevalence reaching 10–15% of acute hepatitis infections in parts of Africa and Middle and Far East
Hepatitis C: more common in Southern Europe and Japan

Transmission
Hepatitis A: via faecal–oral route and contaminated food; overcrowding and poor sanitation facilitate spread
Hepatitis B and C: from mother to child at birth, or via blood transfusion, contaminated needles, sexual intercourse (particularly homosexuals)

Clinical features
Hepatitis A and B (C is rarely symptomatic)
Nausea
Vomiting
Diarrhoea
Anorexia
Headaches
Malaise
Jaundice (after 14 days)

Incubation
Hepatitis A: 3–5 weeks
Hepatitis B: 1–4 months
Hepatitis C: 2 weeks to 2 months

Hepatitis B
Mainly:
- Fever
- Rashes

Hepatitis C
Often asymptomatic then mild jaundice and late complications of chronic liver disease become apparent, including:
- Fever
- Spider naevi
- Palmar erythema
- Hepatomegaly
- Gynaecomastia or testicular atrophy

Investigation
Haematology
Hepatitis A: leucopenia with lymphocytosis is typical
Hepatitis B and C: no specific changes

Prothrombin time
Prolonged in severe cases. Useful marker of severity of infection

Biochemistry
Elevated aspartate aminotransferase (AST) and alanine aminotransferase (ALT)

Immunology
Serology:
• Hepatitis A: anti-HAV IgM antibodies indicate acute infection, anti-HAV IgG antibodies indicate past infection
• Hepatitis B: anti-HBsAg, anti-HBcAg, anti-HbeAg; HBV DNA for active infection
• Hepatitis C: anti-HCV and HCV RNA (RNA or ELISA)

Diagnostic imaging
Ultrasound to exclude bile duct obstruction

Histopathology
Biopsy: only when doubt over diagnosis. Ground glass cells may be present, suggesting HBsAg. Specific stains for core and surface antigens in hepatocytes

Management
Hepatitis A
Prophylactic vaccination or specific immunoglobulin

Hepatitis B
Prophylactic vaccination or specific immunoglobulin
Interferon-α
Lamivudine

Hepatitis C
Prophylactic vaccination or specific immunoglobulin
Interferon-α
Ribavirin

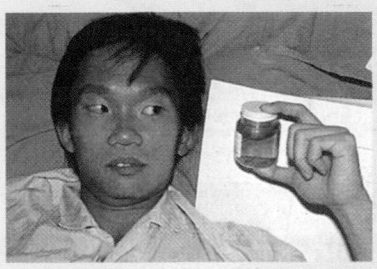

Fig. A Hepatitis A. Typical appearance of jaundice and dark urine in viral hepatitis. Reproduced from Bannister B, Begg N, Gillespie S. *Infectious Disease*. Oxford: Blackwell Science, 1996 with the permission of the authors.

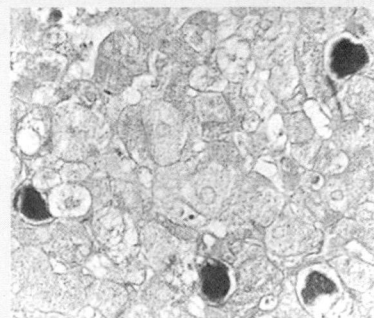

Fig. B Orcein staining shows brown liver cells containing HBsAg. Reproduced from Sherlock S, Dooley J. *Diseases of the Liver and Biliary System*, 9th edn. Oxford: Blackwell Scientific Publications, 1992 with the permission of the authors.

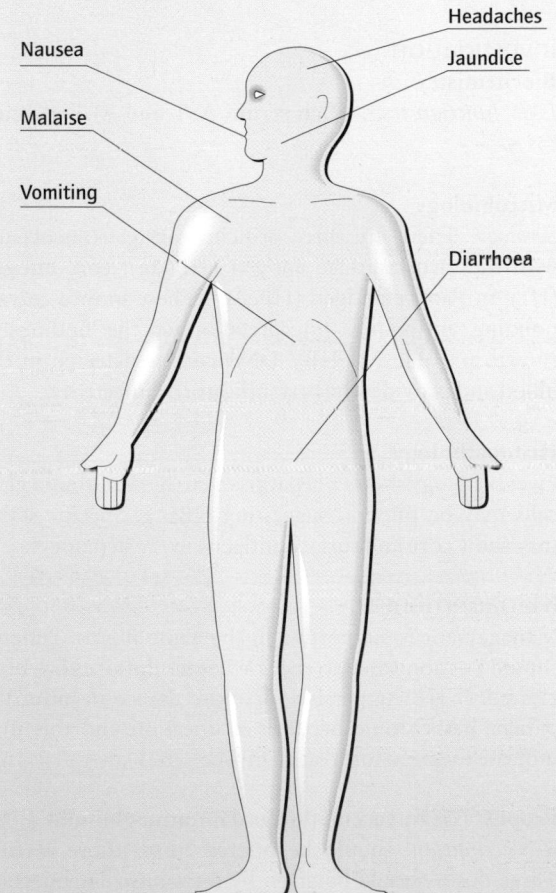

Headaches
Jaundice
Nausea
Malaise
Vomiting
Diarrhoea

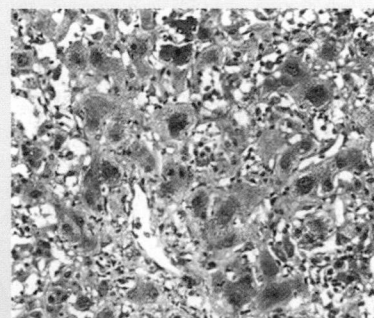

Fig. C Viral hepatitis. There is marked necrosis, swollen cells and necrophilic bodies.

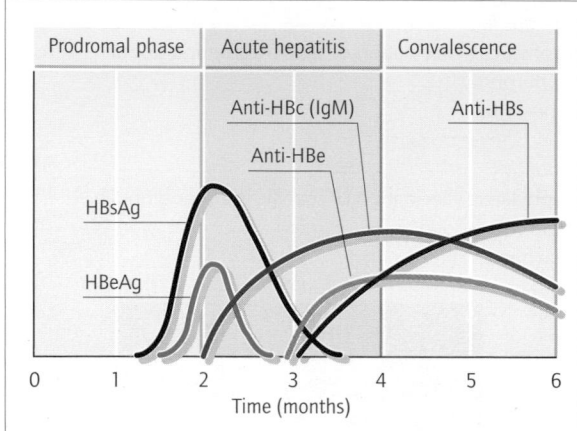

Figure 9.13 Time course of events in acute hepatitis B infection.

Table 9.4 Interpretation of hepatitis B virus (HBV) serology

Antibody/antigen	Interpretation
Anti-HBsAg	Past history of infection or vaccinated
Anti-HbcAg (IgG)	Infected with HBV in past
Anti-HbcAg (IgM)	Recent history of HBV infection
HBsAg present	Currently infected with HBV
HBeAg present	Active viral replication
Anti-HBeAg	Little viral replication unless infected with a mutant virus
HBV-DNA	Active HBV replication

An increasing number of mutant HBVs have been described in which the HBeAg is altered (and is very similar to the core antigens); hence anti-HBeAg antibodies may not be detected.

infection is shown in Fig. 9.13. HBV spreads parenterally by blood and blood products and, rarely, by mouth-to-mouth contact. It is excreted in body fluids such as saliva, serous exudates, vaginal and menstrual discharges, and seminal fluid, and can be spread by:
- *Horizontal transmission* (subject to subject): by inoculation of minute amounts of contaminated blood such as by vaccination or needles, or sexually
- *Vertical transmission* (from mother to baby)

Epidemiology
Prevalence. 0.2% in the UK, 0.5% in the USA, and up to 15% in the Far East and parts of Africa.

Age. All ages.

Sex. Chronic carriage is more common in males.

Ethnicity. More common in people of Asian and Afro-Caribbean ethnicity.

Geography. Prevalence of HBV is highest in the Far East and Africa. High-risk groups in the UK include:
- Immigrants from countries with a high prevalence
- Intravenous drug abusers
- People who frequently change sexual partners
- People in closed institutions, especially if mentally handicapped

Clinical features
Subclinical infection occurs in less than 5% of those infected. Other patterns of illness are:
- *Acute viral hepatitis:* with resolution in 80% of those infected
- *Chronic liver disease:* in 20%

- *Fulminant hepatic failure:* in less than 0.5%
Chronic liver disease often progresses to cirrhosis and liver cell cancer.

Diagnosis
It is important to establish a diagnosis of HBV serologically and to follow the patient to ensure clearance of the virus.

Investigation
Biochemistry
Liver function tests. High serum AST and ALT in acute cases.

Microbiology
Serology. There are three principal antigens associated with the virus: surface antigen (HBsAg); core antigen (HBcAg); and e antigen (HBeAg). These induce corresponding antibodies. Interpretation of the findings is shown in Table 9.4. HBV DNA can be detected in the blood and provides the best indicator of infectivity.

Histopathology
Liver histology shows a hepatitis or cirrhosis. Ground glass cells may be present, suggesting HBsAg. Specific stains may show core and surface antigens in the hepatocytes.

Management
Management is supportive in the acute illness. Patients should be monitored to check whether the virus has been cleared. If HBsAg persists for more than 6 months, the patient has chronic hepatitis B infection and this may indicate the need for treatment (see p. 621).

Prophylaxis by vaccination and immunoglobulin
- *Vaccination:* should be offered to all those at risk. Three doses should be given by intramuscular injection into the arm at 0, 1 and 3 months. Levels of anti-HBsAg

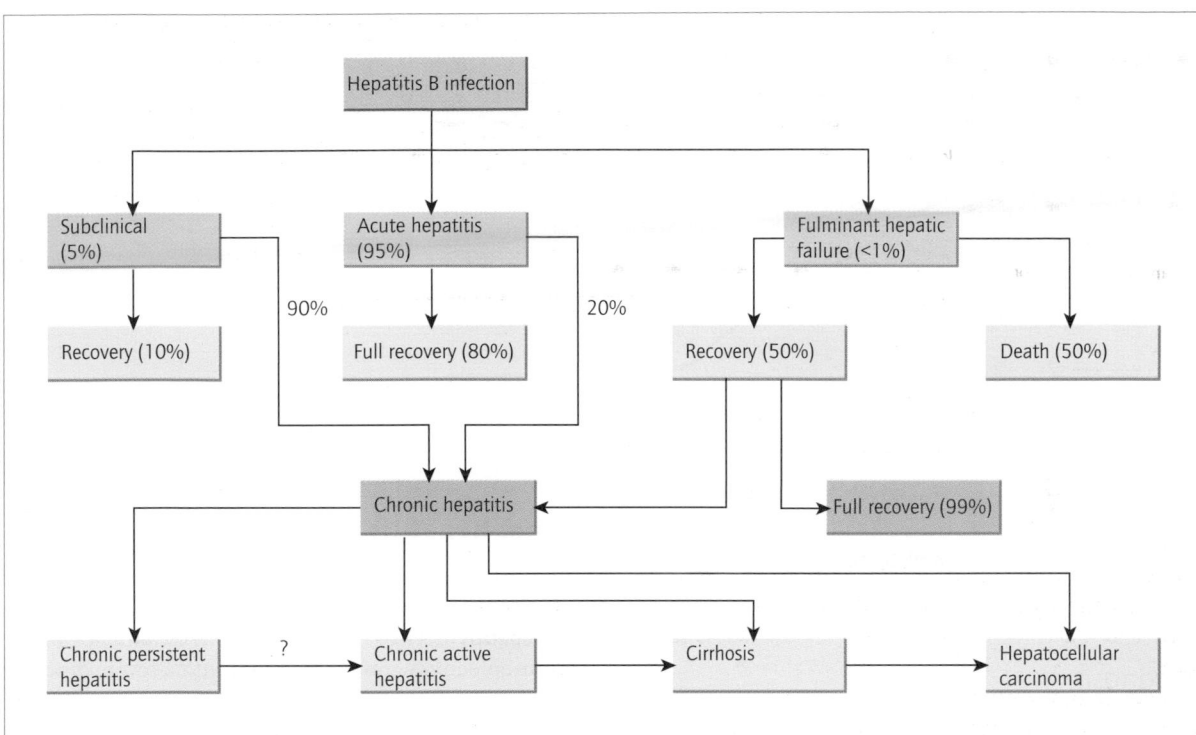

Figure 9.14 Outcomes of hepatitis B infection.

antibodies above 100 IU/ml imply good immunity. Levels should be checked after vaccination and, if adequate, repeated every 3–5 years thereafter. Vaccination should also be given for postexposure protection (in conjunction with immunoglobulin)

• *Immunoglobulin* (passive immunity): should be given to anyone who has a needlestick injury or who requires immediate protection. Babies born to mothers who are chronic carriers or who have HBV in the third trimester should be given immunoglobulin at birth and should be vaccinated

Prognosis

Hepatitis B virus hepatitis usually resolves completely (Fig. 9.14). About 10–20% of patients become chronic carriers. Of these, about 20% develop chronic hepatitis, ultimately leading to cirrhosis and, later in some cases, to hepatocellular carcinoma. The other 80% of carriers remain healthy for many years, although an unknown number may convert to chronic hepatitis.

Hepatitis C virus hepatitis

Disease mechanisms

Hepatitis C virus, an RNA flavivirus, is the main agent in post-transfusion hepatitis. There are several subtypes (main genotypes 1–4); there is significant geographical variation and differences in the response to therapy. Type 1b is thought to be the most virulent.

Epidemiology

Prevalence. Accounts for a minority of cases of acute hepatitis and nearly all cases of post-transfusion hepatitis.

Clinical features

Symptomatic acute hepatitis is rare. More commonly, HCV causes chronic liver disease, often leading to cirrhosis (Fig. 9.15).

Investigation

Diagnosis is made by demonstrating the antibody in the serum using an enzyme-linked immunosorbent assay (ELISA) or the polymerase chain reaction (PCR) method on either serum or liver tissue to detect viral RNA.

Management

For patients with acute HCV infection, treatment is with interferon-α. For those with chronic HCV infection, the treatment of choice is pegylated interferon-α in combination with ribavirin. The dose and duration of therapy will

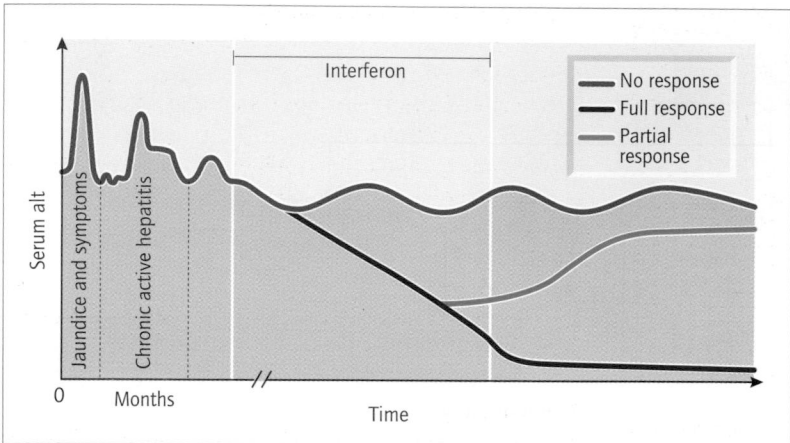

Figure 9.15 Time course of events in chronic hepatitis C infection and possible responses to interferon.

depend on the viral genotype, with non-type 1 responding well to a 6-month course of treatment; non-responders will have a benefit with less fibrosis and a lower probability of developing hepatocellular cancer.

Prognosis

Most patients (over 80%) become chronic carriers and develop cirrhosis over 20 years or more. Older patients have a more aggressive course. The virus rarely, if ever, causes fulminant hepatic failure (Fig. 9.16).

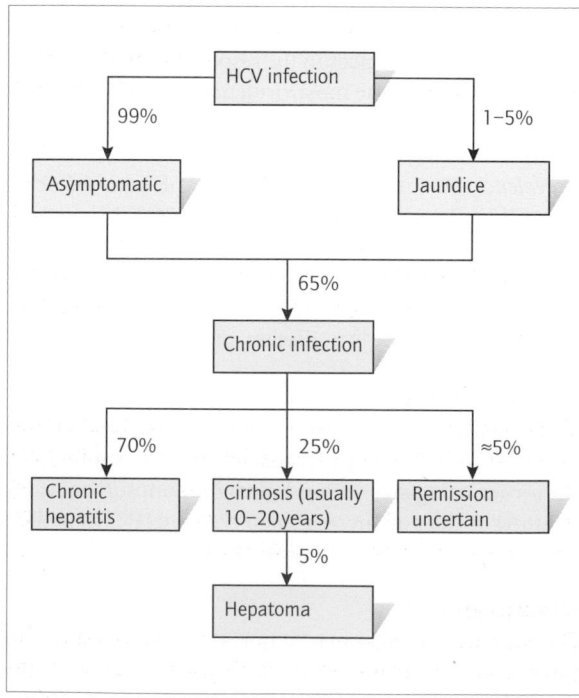

Figure 9.16 Prognosis in hepatitis C infection.

Other hepatitis virus infections

Hepatitis D virus can infect the liver only in association with HBV.

Hepatitis E virus, an RNA calcivirus, induces waterborne epidemics and is associated with a severe outcome in older people and during pregnancy.

Hepatitis viruses F and G have recently been identified. Hepatitis F virus, like HCV, is a flavivirus, which is present in less than 1% of the general population and accounts for about one in eight cases of non-A non-B non-C acute hepatitis. The pathogenicity of hepatitis G virus is not yet clear.

Other viral causes of hepatitis

Hepatitis may result from systemic infection with adenovirus, herpesvirus or Epstein–Barr virus.

Acute liver failure

This is an acute syndrome resulting from liver failure. If encephalopathy develops, the syndrome is termed fulminant hepatic failure (FHF); this is associated with a high mortality. Early recognition is important as specialist management is essential and if transplantation is a possibility patients should be transferred early. The interval between the onset of symptoms and the development of encephalopathy is of prognostic importance: the shorter the interval, the better the prognosis:

- *Hyperacute:* 2 weeks
- *Acute:* 2–8 weeks
- *Subacute:* 8–26 weeks

Fulminant hepatic failure is defined as hepatic encephalopathy occurring within 8 weeks of the onset of symptoms in a person with a previously normal liver.

These terms subacute or late-onset hepatitis apply to hepatitis with encephalopathy where the interval between

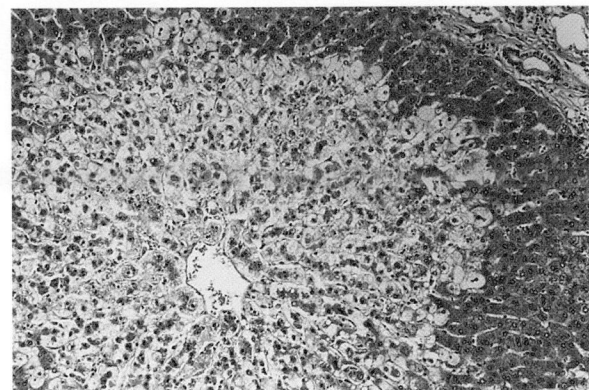

Figure 9.17 Zonal necrosis of hepatocytes associated with paracetamol toxicity.

Table 9.5 Causes of fulminant hepatic failure in the UK

Cause	Proportion of cases
Paracetamol overdose	45%
Viral hepatitis	55%
Drug induced (such as halothane)	
Wilson's disease	<5%
Other causes including sepsis, pregnancy, malignancy	

symptoms and jaundice exceeds 8 weeks. This illness runs a fluctuating course where encephalopathy tends to be mild and there is early development of ascites. The prognosis, in the absence of transplantation, is very poor.

Disease mechanisms
The major causes of FHF in the UK are paracetamol overdose (Fig. 9.17) and viral hepatitis. A fuller list is given in Table 9.5.

Clinical features
Confusion, drowsiness and coma follow a prodromal illness with non-specific symptoms. There are usually no cutaneous stigmata of chronic liver disease. The liver is slightly enlarged at first, but gradually shrinks. Ascites is uncommon. Hypoglycaemia may occur as the condition progresses and liver glucose-producing capacity declines. In the later stages, there is multisystem failure with cerebral oedema, renal failure, vasomotor disturbances, adult respiratory distress syndrome and often sepsis.

It may sometimes be difficult to distinguish between encephalopathy and alcohol withdrawal. In general, hepatic encephalopathy is associated with depression of cerebral function, whereas alcohol withdrawal is associated with excitation. Hepatic encephalopathy has been classified into four grades.

Grading of hepatic encephalopathy
1 Mild or episodic drowsiness; impaired concentration, rousable and coherent
2 Increased drowsiness; confusion and disorientation, rousable and conversant
3 Very drowsy, disorientated, response to simple commands
4 Response to painful stimuli only

Investigation
Haematology
Prothrombin time and clotting factor 5 levels are the best indicators of progression.

Biochemistry
Standard liver tests reveal severe hepatitis. Serum transaminases are often higher than 5000 IU/l. A low serum alkaline phosphatase raises the possibility of Wilson's disease.

Management
Management includes:
- Careful monitoring and early treatment of sepsis and hypoglycaemia
- Avoidance of factors precipitating cerebral oedema such as stress and fluid overload
- Prompt treatment of cerebral oedema
- Supportive treatment, particularly for renal and cardiovascular manifestations
- Antibiotics and antifungal prophylaxis should be given early as these patients are at high risk of infection
- A proton pump inhibitor or H_2 receptor blocker should be given to reduce the risk of gastric erosions and bleeding
- Nutritional support should be instituted early
- If there are features suggestive of a poor prognosis, consideration should be given to transfer of the patient to a specialist unit where transplantation is available
- There is increasing interest in the use of molecular adsorbent recirculating systems (MARS) to help support the patient

Paracetamol overdose
If an overdose has been taken 4–24 h before presentation, blood paracetamol levels should be estimated. If they are in the 'toxic' range, the antidote, N-acetyl cysteine, should be given immediately. If there is any doubt, N-acetyl cysteine should be administered anyway.

Prognosis
The mortality approaches 90% if there is a coma in the absence of transplantation. Death usually results from cerebral oedema, sepsis (bacterial or fungal) or cardiovascular instability.

09

Markers of a poor prognosis indicating the need for transplantation

1 Paracetamol-associated liver failure

either

- pH less than 7.3 after volume repletion *and* more than 24 h postoverdose

or a combination of:

- grade 3–4 encephalopathy
- *and* serum creatinine more than 300 µmol/l
- *and* prothrombin time more than 100 s

or

- lactate more than 3 mmol/l after adequate resuscitation

2 Other aetiologies

- pH less than 7.3

or

- prothrombin time more than 100 s

or

- three of the following in association with hepatic encephalopathy
  - age under 10 years or over 40 years
  - bilirubin more than 300 µmol/l
  - interval from jaundice to encephalopathy over 7 days
  - prothrombin time over 50 s
  - aetiology: seronegative hepatitis or drug associated

Seronegative hepatitis is defined as hepatitis without any identifiable cause. Although it is sometimes termed non-A non-B hepatitis, this term is inappropriate as there is rarely any evidence to incriminate a virus.

Drug reactions and the liver

The diagnosis of drug hepatotoxicity depends on taking a good drug history and always considering it as a possibility. Other causes for liver damage must be excluded and there must be a temporal relationship between starting the drug and the appearance of liver damage. Drug withdrawal is usually associated with an improvement in the symptoms and signs of liver disease.

The 'golden rules' for diagnosing drug reactions affecting the liver are:

- Any drug or medicinal compound should be considered as a potential cause of hepatotoxicity
- Any type of liver disease can be caused by drugs
- The diagnosis is one of exclusion

Obtain details of all medications used by the patient—not only drugs prescribed by a doctor, but also non-proprietary medicines and any other possible hepatotoxins, including herbal remedies.

Hepatic drug reactions may be classified as predictable or idiosyncratic (Table 9.2):

- *Predictable drug reactions:* dose dependent and host independent. The probability of a reaction may be modified by age, sex, disease and other drugs (enzyme inducers such as alcohol or phenobarbital increase susceptibility, and enzyme inhibitors reduce susceptibility)
- *Idiosyncratic drug reactions:* dose independent and host dependent. They may occur as a result of a metabolic idiosyncrasy (e.g. metabolism of a drug through a usually minor pathway) or an immunological idiosyncrasy (e.g. involvement of allergic mechanisms)

Vascular abnormalities of the liver

Budd–Chiari syndrome

Disease mechanisms

Budd–Chiari syndrome results from thrombosis of the hepatic veins. Causes include hypercoagulable states (polycythaemia, protein C or S deficiency, lupus anticoagulant, factor V Leiden mutation (see p. 1075), malignancy, cysts, congenital webs, trauma, drugs (especially oral contraceptives) and idiopathic mechanisms.

Clinical features

Presentation may be acute or chronic. If it is acute, there is right upper quadrant pain, diarrhoea and rapid abdominal distension with ascites. Encephalopathy may ensue. Chronic disease presents with ascites and complications of portal hypertension. On examination there is hepatomegaly and ascites.

Investigation

- *Doppler ultrasound:* shows no flow in the hepatic veins, and may reveal a blood clot or tumour
- *CT examination or angiography:* confirms a thrombosis
- *Ultrasound or technetium scan:* in 70% of patients the caudate lobe, which has a separate venous drainage, is hypertrophied and this can be visualized by ultrasound or technetium scanning

Management

In the acute stage, clot lysis with streptokinase or recombinant tissue plasminogen activator (TPA) may be successful. Otherwise, a portocaval (portal vein to inferior vena cava) or peritoneovenous or transjugular intrahepatic portosystemic shunt (TIPS) is usually successful. Transplantation should be considered if there is fulminant hepatic failure.

Prognosis

The prognosis varies: patients with fulminant hepatic failure or bleeding varices do badly; in a few the hepatic veins recannulate spontaneously. The prognosis depends on the extent of thrombosis and the nature of the underlying disease.

Veno-occlusive disease

Disease mechanisms

In contrast to Budd–Chiari syndrome, the sites of damage and venous obstruction in veno-occlusive disease are the smaller intrahepatic veins. Common causes include cytotoxic agents, hepatic irradiation and Jamaican bush tea, which contains toxic alkaloids.

Clinical features

The clinical presentation of veno-occlusive disease is similar to that of Budd–Chiari syndrome.

Investigation

- *Liver biopsy:* diagnosis is made by liver biopsy, which shows features of venous outflow obstruction
- *Angiography:* shows no block in the main hepatic vein

Management

Management is symptomatic.

Prognosis

Prognosis partly depends on the underlying cause.

Haemangiomas

These benign vascular malformations occur in about 7% of the population.

Clinical features

Small lesions are commonly revealed on screening for other conditions and are of no significance. Lesions larger than 10 cm may cause pain and carry a small risk of haemorrhage (Fig. 9.18).

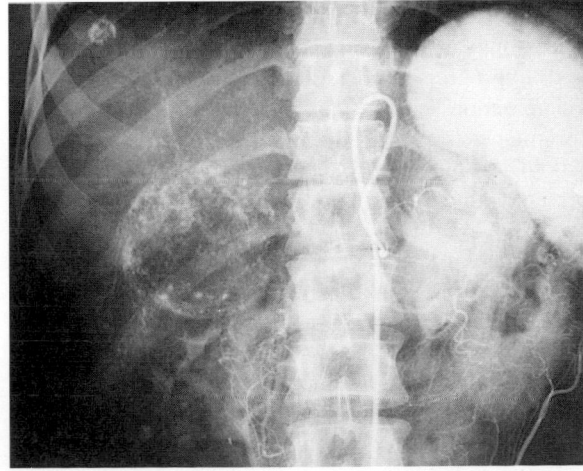

Figure 9.18 Hepatic angiogram showing a vascular haemangioma.

Investigation

- *Ultrasound:* most haemangiomas have a characteristic appearance on ultrasound
- *CT scanning with intravenous contrast or radiolabelled red cell scanning:* confirms the diagnosis. Both ultrasound and CT scanning show slow 'emptying' of the lesion
- *Angiography or biopsy:* rarely required to exclude a malignant process

Management

Treatment is not required unless the haemangiomas are very large.

Prognosis

Usually excellent.

Liver abscesses

Disease mechanisms

Pyogenic liver abscesses are caused by infection, commonly with *Streptococcus milleri*, *Streptococcus faecalis* and *Escherichia coli*. Infection may arise from umbilical sepsis, biliary sepsis, abdominal sepsis (e.g. diverticular disease) or bacteraemia (often caused by dental sepsis).

Amoebic abscesses usually result from spread of amoebic dysentery from *Entamoeba histolytica* (see Chapter 3). Hydatid cysts are caused by the larvae of animal tapeworms of *Echinococcus* species (see Chapter 3).

Clinical features

Pyogenic liver abscesses present with fever, anorexia, vomiting and abdominal pain. On examination there is hepatomegaly and commonly a right pleural effusion. The signs and symptoms of an amoebic abscess are similar.

Investigation

Haematology

FBC shows a neutrophil leucocytosis.

Biochemistry

- *Serum albumin:* low
- *Alkaline phosphatase:* elevated

Immunology

Antibody and antigen detection ELISAs are available for diagnosis.

Diagnostic imaging

Ultrasound will confirm the abscess. Calcification is common in the wall of a hydatid abscess.

Aspiration

Aspiration confirms the diagnosis, shows the organism and guides the choice of antibiotic. However, because of

09

the risk of anaphylaxis, amoebic abscesses should not be aspirated.

Management

Pyogenic liver abscesses. Treatment is percutaneous aspiration and drainage with systemic antibiotics for up to 3 months. Do not aspirate if there is a possibility of hydatid disease. Surgery may be required if there are multiple abscesses.

Amoebic abscess. Treatment is metronidazole 800 mg three times daily for 10 days.

Other infections of the liver

Hydatid cysts and schistosomiasis (see Chapter 3).

Liver diseases of pregnancy

Recurrent intrahepatic cholestasis

Disease mechanisms

Recurrent intrahepatic cholestasis is closely associated with oral contraceptive-associated jaundice.

Epidemiology

Prevalence. Most common in Chileans and Scandinavians.

Clinical features

Usually presents in the third trimester with pruritus followed 6–8 weeks later by mild jaundice. The condition usually recurs in subsequent pregnancies.

Management

Treatment is symptomatic. Ursodeoxycholic acid (UDCA) 10–15 mg/kg/day is helpful but is not licenced for this indication.

Prognosis

The disorder resolves spontaneously after delivery, but can recur in subsequent pregnancies. There is no adverse effect on the mother, but there is an increased incidence of premature delivery.

Acute fatty liver of pregnancy

Disease mechanisms

The cause of this rare but serious condition is unknown. The liver cells become full of fat (Fig. 9.19).

Clinical features

Presents in the last trimester with vomiting, abdominal pain and jaundice, and may rapidly progress to fulminant hepatic failure.

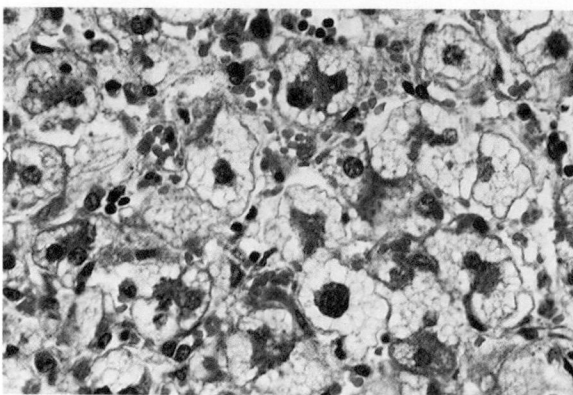

Figure 9.19 Acute fatty liver of pregnancy. The liver cells are filled with fat.

Investigation

- *FBC:* may show an increase in normoblasts (see Chapter 15)
- *Serum urate:* high
- *Ultrasound:* shows a bright liver
- *Liver biopsy:* shows fatty liver

Management

Treatment is supportive, with rapid delivery of the fetus.

Prognosis

If severe, there is a high maternal and fetal mortality. It does not necessarily recur in subsequent pregnancies.

Chronic liver disease

Chronic liver disease is usually defined as liver disease, of any cause, that lasts for more than 3 months (although definitions vary). The ongoing liver inflammation usually leads to progressive fibrosis and eventually cirrhosis. The inflammation may be mild or severe (hence the terms chronic persistent and chronic active hepatitis). A single aetiological factor, such as a hepatitis B infection, may present with either acute or chronic liver disease and the severity of liver disease depends on several factors, including host factors (such as host genes, alcohol abuse, obesity, other comorbid conditions) and disease factors (such as the genotype of the virus).

Chronic liver disease is associated with both hepatic complications and systemic disease. In considering the patient with chronic liver disease, it is important to consider several aspects:

- *Cause of the liver disease:* specific treatment may be indicated and family screening may be required. It may be necessary to advise changes in behaviour (e.g. because

Table 9.6 The Child–Pugh classification of cirrhosis

Parameter	Points		
	1	2	3
Encephalopathy grade	Nil	1–2	3–4
Ascites	Nil	Slight	Moderate–severe
Serum albumin (g/l)	>35	28–35	<28
Prothrombin (s prolonged)	1–4	4–6	>6
Serum bilirubin (μmol/l)			
Non-cholestatic	<35	34–50	>50
Cholestatic	<70	70–170	>170

A score of 5–6 is classified as Child–Pugh A, 7–9 as B and 10–15 as C.

of the risk of infection) or change in alcohol intake or patterns of drug use or abuse.

• *Presence of portal hypertension:* may lead to ascites and the development of varices that require screening and treatment
• *Possibility of developing liver cancer:* and so the need for screening
• *Effect on management of the patient:* such as lifestyle, drug treatment, nutrition

Cirrhosis

Cirrhosis is a syndrome that is defined pathologically and characterized by fibrosis and nodule formation. There are several guides for the severity of cirrhosis, of which the most commonly used is the Child–Pugh classification. Six factors are assessed and a score given (Table 9.6). There are many causes of cirrhosis (Table 9.7), but the main causes are:
1 Chronic viral infection (HBV, HCV)
2 Alcohol
3 Autoimmune diseases
   • primary biliary cirrhosis
   • primary sclerosing cholangitis
   • autoimmune hepatitis
4 Metabolic diseases
   • Wilson's disease
   • α_1-antitrypsin deficiency
   • haemochromatosis

Chronic hepatitis

A diagnosis of chronic hepatitis is based on the presence of abnormal liver tests for more than 3 months and a liver biopsy showing the characteristic features of a mixed portal tract infiltrate and piecemeal necrosis.

Causes of chronic active hepatitis include:
• Autoimmune hepatitis
• Chronic HBV infection
• Chronic HCV infection
• Wilson's disease
• α_1-Antitrypsin deficiency
• Drugs such as methyldopa

Table 9.7 Causes of cirrhosis

Viruses
Hepatitis B virus
Hepatitis C virus

Toxins
Alcohol
Drugs

Immune
Autoimmune hepatitis
Primary biliary cirrhosis

Metabolic
Wilson's disease
Haemochromatosis
α_1-Antitrypsin deficiency
Fibrocystic disease
Storage disorders (glycogen storage disease, galactosaemia, tyrosinaemia)

Biliary disease
Primary sclerosing cholangitis

Outflow obstruction
Cardiac cirrhosis
Budd–Chiari syndrome
Veno-occlusive disease

Autoimmune hepatitis

Disease mechanisms

There is an autoimmune attack on the hepatocyte.

Epidemiology

Age. The two peak age ranges are 20–30 and 55–65 years.

Sex. In younger patients it is more common in females.

Genetics. Associated with the HLA phenotype B8, DR3 and DR4.

Cirrhosis at a glance

Causes of cirrhosis

Cirrhosis is a syndrome, with many causes including:
- *Toxins:* alcohol and drugs
- *Chronic viral infection:* HBV, HCV
- *Autoimmune:* autoimmune hepatitis, primary biliary cirrhosis, primary sclerosing cholangitis
- *Metabolic:* Wilson's disease, haemochromatosis, some glycogen storage diseases
- *Chronic venous outflow obstruction:* heart failure, Budd–Chiari syndrome, portal venous thrombosis

Epidemiology

Sex
Both sexes

Genetics
Some causes are genetic

Geography
Worldwide

Investigation

Haematology
FBC reveals anaemia and an increased mean corpuscular volume
Prothrombin time is increased

Biochemistry
Albumin is decreased
Alkaline phosphatase, gamma-glutamyl transferase, AST, ALT and bilirubin are increased
To look for causes:
- Iron, total iron-binding capacity (TIBC), ferritin and *HFE* (haemochromatosis gene) genotype if appropriate
- α_1-Antitrypsin phenotype
- Copper, caeruloplasmin, 24-hour urine copper
- Alpha-fetoprotein to look for evidence of hepatocellular cancer

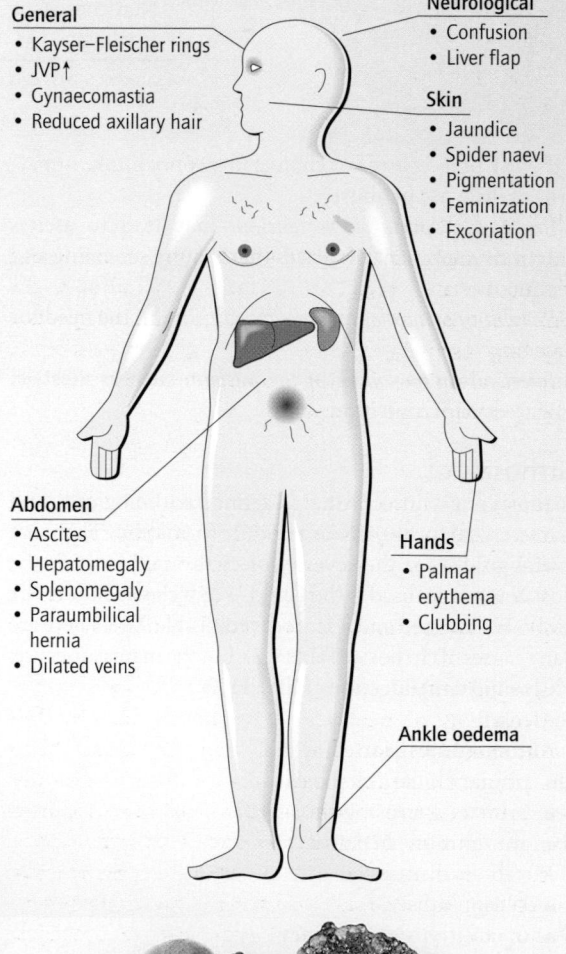

General
- Kayser–Fleischer rings
- JVP↑
- Gynaecomastia
- Reduced axillary hair

Neurological
- Confusion
- Liver flap

Skin
- Jaundice
- Spider naevi
- Pigmentation
- Feminization
- Excoriation

Abdomen
- Ascites
- Hepatomegaly
- Splenomegaly
- Paraumbilical hernia
- Dilated veins

Hands
- Palmar erythema
- Clubbing

Ankle oedema

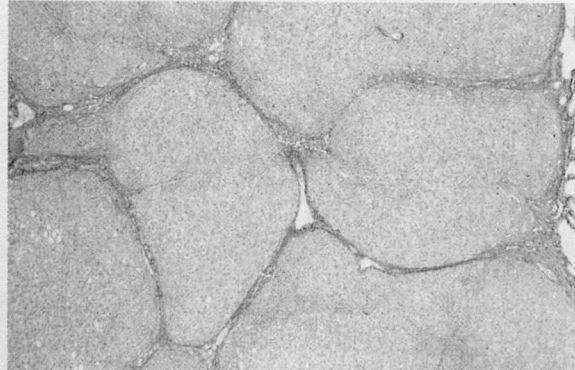

Fig. A Cirrhotic liver showing nodules of liver parenchyma surrounded by a border of fibrous connective tissue.

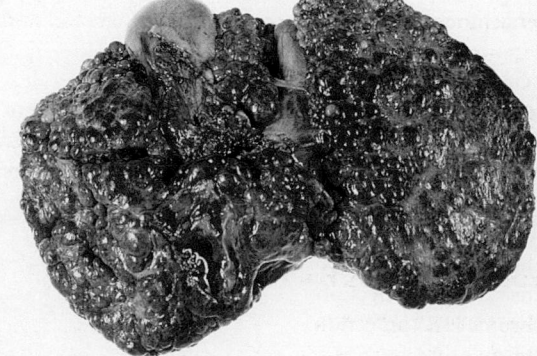

Fig. B Macronodular cirrhosis.

Immunology
Immunoglobulins may be increased depending on the cause
Autoantibodies may be present according to cause

Microbiology
HBV, HCV, HDV status should be checked

Diagnostic imaging
May reveal abnormalities
• Ultrasound
• CT scan (if indicated)
• MRI (if indicated)

Histopathology
Shows cirrhosis

Complications
Portal hypertension
Bleeding varices or ascites
Liver cell cancer (especially in males)
Liver failure
Osteoporosis

Management
Control of the complications
Transplantation if suitable

Clinical features

Autoimmune hepatitis presents with jaundice, an episode of acute hepatitis that fails to resolve, arthralgia or the complications of liver disease. Other autoimmune diseases may be present or develop, including thyroid disease, fibrosing alveolitis and glomerulonephritis. Examination reveals multiple spider naevi.

Investigation

• *Serum aminotransferases:* elevated
• *Serum immunoglobulins:* especially IgG, increased
• *Serum autoantibodies:* present in increased titres. These include antinuclear antibody, antiliver/kidney microsomal antibody and antismooth muscle (actin) antibody

Management

The mainstay of treatment is corticosteroids. Prednisolone should be started at 30–60 mg/day and reduced when the serum aminotransferases are within the normal range. Azathioprine should be introduced when the prednisolone dose is 20 mg/day if liver tests are normal. In some cases it is possible to withdraw the steroids completely, but life-long treatment is usually necessary. Withdrawal of the treatment may lead to a relapse. Other drugs that are effective include mycophenolate and ciclosporin.

Prognosis

Without treatment the 5-year survival rate is 50%. If treatment is started before cirrhosis has occurred, the prognosis is good (90% 5-year survival).

Chronic hepatitis B virus infection

Disease mechanisms

Fewer than 5% of people with acute HBV infection develop chronic liver disease and remain HBsAg positive (unless perinatal transmission occurs). Failure to clear the virus correlates with a poor cell-mediated immune response to the virus.

Epidemiology

Prevalence. Varies from less than 0.1% in the UK to 15% in the Far East and Africa.

Sex. More common in males than in females.

Clinical features

The condition may be detected at routine screening, such as during pregnancy or in a genitourinary medicine clinic. Alternatively, it may present with jaundice, pruritus or complications of liver disease. Examination is the same as for autoimmune hepatitis.

Investigation

• *Liver tests:* may be normal or show non-specific changes such as elevations in serum aminotransferases, alkaline phosphatase and bilirubin
• *HBV serology:* essential to determine the treatment options
• *Liver biopsy:* may be performed to confirm the diagnosis, exclude other coexisting causes of liver disease and monitor the response. Histopathological findings range from minimal changes to a chronic persistent hepatitis, a chronic active hepatitis or cirrhosis. The presence of 'ground glass hepatocytes', orcein-positive cells (HBsAg-containing hepatocytes) and positive viral immunostaining are all useful confirmatory findings

Management

Treatment with interferon-α given subcutaneously three times a week for 3 months is effective only if there is active viral replication (HBeAg or HBV DNA positive). The response is characterized by a hepatitis and an initial conversion from HBeAg status to anti-HBe antibody positive and a later loss of HBsAg. This occurs in about 30–50% of patients. Lamivudine is an alternative treatment for those with active viral replication.

Prognosis

Without treatment, 3–5% of patients spontaneously seroconvert with loss of antigenaemia each year. This compares with 50% seroconversion among patients who are treated. Without treatment or spontaneous seroconversion, the disorder progresses to cirrhosis and hepatocellular carcinoma.

Predictors of a good response to treatment include adult onset, a defined history of hepatitis, hepatitis within 2 years of treatment, high serum transaminases and low serum HBV DNA level. Males have a poorer prognosis than females. People who are HIV positive and those with established cirrhosis are least likely to respond to treatment.

Chronic hepatitis C virus infection

Disease mechanisms

Those with additional causes for liver disease (such as chronic HBV infection or chronic alcohol abuse) and those who acquire the infection at an older age have a more rapid progression.

Epidemiology

Prevalence. Accounts for about 50–70% of cases of what was previously termed cryptogenic cirrhosis.

Clinical features

Disease progression is insidious and the patient remains well and asymptomatic until there are complications of cirrhosis or abnormal liver tests are detected incidentally.

Investigation

• *Liver tests:* as with chronic HBV, there is a great range of liver test abnormalities in chronic HCV infection. Serum aminotransferases usually show a fluctuating course.
• *HCV serology:* detects antibodies to structural and non-structural viral proteins. As with human immuno-deficiency virus (HIV), the presence of antibodies indicates active infection. This can be confirmed using an adaptation of the PCR to detect viral RNA.
• *Liver biopsy:* histology usually reveals a mild active hepatitis or lobular hepatitis, but there are no specific histological features. There may be fatty change and lymphoid aggregates.

Management

Treatment includes symptomatic support and interferon-α and ribavirin for 6–12 months, depending on viral genotype and the response during treatment.

Prognosis

A response to treatment is characterized by a fall in serum transaminases, which occurs in about 50% of patients. About 33% of these patients will relapse.

Primary biliary cirrhosis

Disease mechanisms

Unknown—possibly autoimmune.

Epidemiology

Prevalence. One in 5000 women in Europe. Less common in Africa and India.

Age and sex. Predominantly occurs in middle-aged women.

Clinical features

Primary biliary cirrhosis (PBC) may present in several ways:
• Progressive pruritus followed by jaundice
• Asymptomatic incidental finding
• With complications such as ascites, jaundice, gastrointestinal bleeding

Associated diseases include sicca syndrome with dry mouth and eyes, thyroid disorders, pancreatic insufficiency, vitiligo, coeliac disease, Raynaud's phenomenon, scleroderma, arthralgia and osteoporosis.

On examination, there is pigmentation and there may be xanthomas around the eyes. Hepatosplenomegaly is common even in the early stages. Palmar erythema (liver palms) may also be seen (Fig. 9.20).

Investigation
Biochemistry

Serum liver tests reveal an elevated serum alkaline

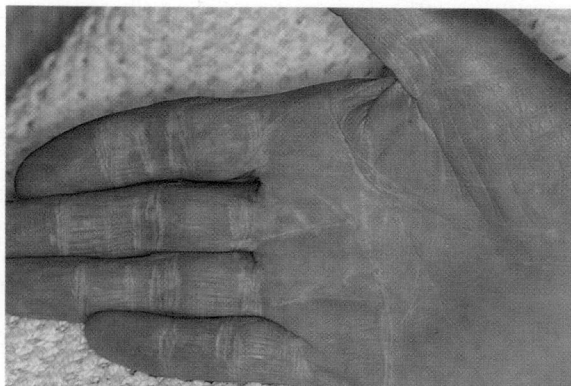

Figure 9.20 Hand of a patient with primary biliary cirrhosis showing palmar erythema and xanthoma.

phosphatase. As the disease progresses, serum bilirubin increases.

Immunology
- *Serum immunoglobulins:* increased, especially serum IgM.
- *Autoantibodies:* antimitochondrial antibodies are diagnostic of the disease. In addition, antinuclear antibodies are often present.

Histopathology
Liver histology shows a lymphocytic infiltration around damaged middle-sized intrahepatic bile ducts or their remnants.

Management
There is no effective treatment that alters the prognosis, although many drugs have been evaluated. UDCA has been shown to produce an improvement in biochemical tests and possibly a delay in progression, but a clear effect on survival has not been demonstrated.

Pruritus, possibly caused by increased endogenous opioids rather than retained bile acids, is best treated with colestyramine (cholestyramine) (4–28 g/day as required).

Prognosis
The prognosis of primary biliary cirrhosis varies, but the median survival is about 10 years from diagnosis. Serum bilirubin is the best prognostic marker.

Metabolic liver diseases

Metabolic liver diseases are uncommon, but their diagnosis is important because:
- Early diagnosis and institution of specific therapy can prevent irreversible complications
- They are inherited and there is a need for genetic counselling
- Family members must be screened

Wilson's disease
Disease mechanisms
Wilson's disease is a disorder of copper metabolism. There is a defect in copper transport with copper deposition in various organs, most importantly the liver and the brain.

Epidemiology
Genetics. Autosomal recessive. Too many genetic abnormalities have been determined to allow for routine use of genetic markers in making the diagnosis.

Clinical features
The disorder presents in childhood or young adulthood with either neurological or hepatic manifestations.
- *Neurological signs:* caused by copper deposition in the basal ganglia. They may be subtle, such as a progressive decline in mental function, or more obvious, such as a tremor, dysarthria, involuntary movements or dementia
- *Hepatic features:* range from mildly elevated liver tests to a chronic active hepatitis or fulminant hepatitic failure, which is often complicated by haemolysis
- *Kayser–Fleischer rings:* caused by copper deposition on Descemet's membrane in the eye and characteristic of the disease. They are best seen with a slit lamp

Investigation
- *Liver tests:* variable, but in the fulminant presentation there is a low serum alkaline phosphatase
- *Serum copper and caeruloplasmin:* low
- *24-h urine copper levels:* elevated
- *Liver biopsy:* shows few diagnostic features, but allows the assessment of liver copper levels
- *Liver copper levels:* very high

Management
Copper chelation with D-penicillamine reverses many of the complications and prevents progression. However, the introduction of treatment is associated with a deterioration in neurological function that is not always reversible.

Screening. All the relatives of a patient must be screened so that specific treatment can be started early.

Prognosis
Excellent if treatment is instituted before the development of irreversible organ damage

Hereditary or primary haemochromatosis
Disease mechanisms
Haemochromatosis results from iron overload, which may be:
- *Primary:* genetic
- *Secondary:* caused by repeated blood transfusions as in thalassaemia, sickle cell disease or alcohol excess

The defect in primary haemochromatosis is thought to lie partly within the enterocyte, where the mutation causes increased iron absorption. Hereditary haemochromatosis is an autosomal recessive disease with mutations in the HFE protein, which binds to the transferrin receptor and plays a part in iron metabolism. Ninety-five per cent of patients are either homozygous for a point mutation

09

at amino acid position 262 (C → Y) or compound hetero-zygotes with one C262Y mutation and one mutation at point 63 (H → D). Only a small proportion of those with genetic haemochromatosis (less than 5%) will develop disease.

Epidemiology
Prevalence. The genotype for hereditary haemochromatosis has a prevalence of 0.4% in the UK, but the disease is less common.

Age. Hereditary haemochromatosis usually presents between 40 and 60 years of age.

Sex. Males with hereditary haemochromatosis usually present at a younger age than females.

Clinical features
Hereditary haemochromatosis. Iron is deposited in various tissues, resulting in a variety of clinical presentations. Deposition in:
- *Liver:* manifests as the complications of cirrhosis
- *Skin:* leads to a slate-grey discoloration
- *Pancreas:* results in diabetes mellitus
- *Pituitary:* manifests as gonadal atrophy and impotence
- *Heart:* leads to arrhythmias and heart failure
- *Joints:* associated with chondrocalcinosis, which may cause arthritis similar to osteoarthritis or a distinctive erosive arthropathy; however, the relationship to iron overload is not clear

Investigation
Biochemistry
- *Liver tests:* may be normal
- *Serum ferritin:* increased, often exceeding 1000 µg/l
- *Serum iron:* high
- *Iron saturation* (serum iron : total iron binding capacity): exceeds 75%
- *Liver iron:* exceeds 180 µg/g liver (dry weight)

Histopathology
Liver biopsy may reveal established cirrhosis, and there is excess iron deposition in the hepatocytes and biliary epithelial cells.

Management
The treatment of choice is venesection. One unit of blood should be removed once or twice weekly until the haematocrit falls and weekly venesection should be continued until the serum ferritin is normal. Serum ferritin levels must then be monitored and venesection restarted when the serum ferritin rises.

Screening. Relatives should be screened by genotyping.

Prognosis
Without treatment there is progressive damage because of continuing iron deposition, and many patients die from hepatocellular carcinoma.

α_1-Antitrypsin deficiency
Disease mechanisms
α_1-Antitrypsin is a protease inhibitor and deficiency is associated with emphysema because of unchecked protease activity and chronic liver disease because the hepatocyte fails to excrete α_1-antitrypsin from the liver.

Epidemiology
Genetics. Autosomal dominant inheritance.

Clinical features
α_1-Antitrypsin deficiency may present with neonatal hepatitis or with complications of cirrhosis.

Investigation
- *Serum α_1-antitrypsin levels:* usually, but not always, low
- *Phenotype measurement:* the diagnosis is confirmed by measuring the α_1-antitrypsin phenotype. The MM phenotype is normal, the Z or S phenotypes are associated with disease
- *Liver biopsy:* may reveal a chronic active hepatitis or cirrhosis. Periodic acid–Schiff (PAS)-positive, diastase-resistant globules in the hepatocytes containing α_1-antitrypsin are characteristic

Management
There is no specific treatment.

Prognosis
Varies; only 25% with the ZZ phenotype will develop liver disease.

Alcoholic liver disease

Excess alcohol consumption has major social, economic and medical consequences, including alcoholic liver disease. Alcohol consumption is rising in the UK and people are starting to drink at an earlier age. It is important that a full alcohol history is obtained and, where appropriate, multidisciplinary support given to encourage abstinence.
   Liver damage associated with alcohol includes:
- Fatty liver
- Fibrosis
- Alcoholic hepatitis
- Alcoholic cirrhosis

Primary haemochromatosis at a glance

Epidemiology
Prevalence
0.4%, but the prevalence of identified cases is much less

Age
Usually 40–60 years of age

Sex
Males usually present before females

Genetics
Autosomal recessive
Fewer than 5% with genetic haemochromatosis develop iron overload

Investigation
Biochemistry
Liver tests may be normal
Serum ferritin is increased, often exceeding 1000 µg/l
Serum iron is high

Iron saturation (serum iron : total iron binding capacity) exceeds 75%
Liver iron exceeds 180 µg/g liver (dry weight)
Genetics: shows *HFE* genes in >95% cases

Genetics
Recognized mutations in *HFE* are C282Y and H63D

Histopathology
Liver biopsy may reveal an established cirrhosis. There is excess iron deposition in the hepatocytes and biliary epithelial cells

Management
Venesection

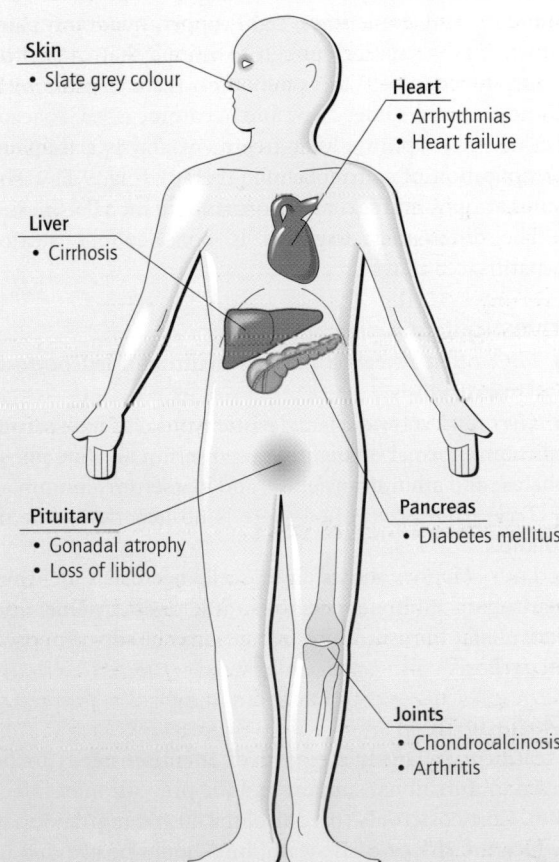

Skin
• Slate grey colour

Heart
• Arrhythmias
• Heart failure

Liver
• Cirrhosis

Pituitary
• Gonadal atrophy
• Loss of libido

Pancreas
• Diabetes mellitus

Joints
• Chondrocalcinosis
• Arthritis

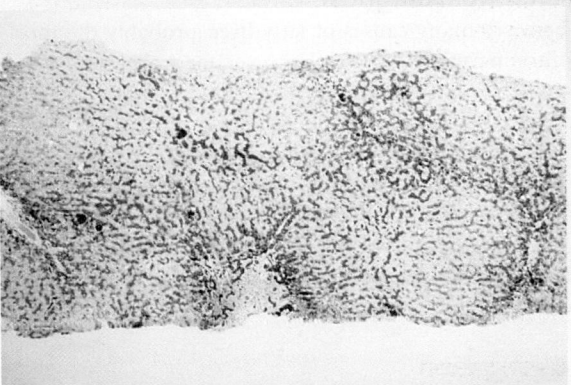

Fig. A Perls' stain showing grade 4 siderosis with normal architecture.

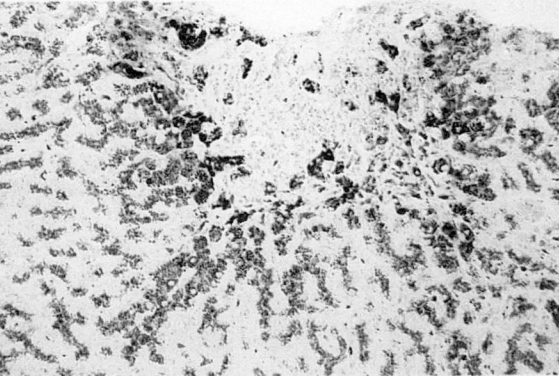

Fig. B Perls' stain showing periportal deposits, heavier pigment and biliary epithelium.

09

Disease mechanisms

The hepatotoxic effects of alcohol are brought about largely by the main metabolite of ethanol, which is acetaldehyde (ethanal). There is a close relationship between the amount of ethanol consumed and the probability of developing severe liver damage. However, there is great variation. Women are more susceptible than men. A weekly consumption of more than 21 units for men and 14 units for women is associated with an increasing risk of liver disease. One unit is equal to approximately half a pint of beer, a 'pub measure' of spirits or a glass of wine.

Fatty liver and steatohepatitis

Clinical features

Clinically, the patient may be asymptomatic and the only abnormality on examination is hepatomegaly.

Differential diagnosis

There are many causes of fatty liver: probably the most common cause is alcohol. However, there are many other causes of a fatty liver. The clinical, biochemical and histological pattern of alcoholic fatty liver and non-alcoholic fatty liver disease (NAFLD) are very similar.

The differential diagnosis of alcohol-induced fatty liver includes diabetes mellitus, hyperlipidaemia, obesity, starvation and drugs or NAFLD. The increasing prevalence of obesity in western populations is likely to be associated with an increase in fatty liver.

Investigation

Investigations are not specific and blood tests may be normal.
- *Red cell mean cell volume:* often increased
- *Gamma-glutamyl transferase:* often elevated
- *Carbohydrate-deficient transferrin:* a marker of recent alcohol consumption
- *Ultrasound:* shows an echobright liver
- *Liver biopsy:* shows fatty infiltration of the liver with ballooning of the cells and nuclei

Management

This involves treating the causes, so alcohol should be withdrawn and weight reduced as appropriate. There have been encouraging reports about the effect of metformin in NAFLD.

Prognosis

The prognosis of simple fatty liver is very good. However, where there is evidence of a superimposed hepatitis, there is a high probability of progression to fibrosis and cirrhosis.

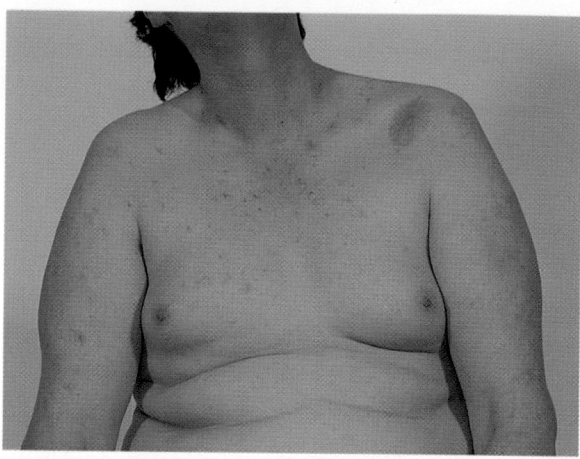
Figure 9.21 Gynaecomastia in alcoholic cirrhosis.

Alcoholic hepatitis

Clinical features

Alcoholic hepatitis is much more severe than fatty liver, but its clinical spectrum varies from a mild non-specific illness to a progressive fatal disease. It presents with jaundice and sometimes right upper quadrant pain, which may be severe enough to mimic that caused by acute cholecystitis. On examination there is prominent jaundice, fever, spider naevi and hepatomegaly. Gynaecomastia often appears after treatment and is a frequent complication of spironolactone therapy (Fig. 9.21). The testes atrophy and sexual performance in men declines.

The differential diagnosis is non-alcoholic steatohepatitis (see above).

Investigation

- *FBC:* often reveals a marked neutrophil leucocytosis and macrocytosis
- *Liver tests:* show a characteristic pattern of high serum bilirubin, normal or slightly raised serum alkaline phosphatase and aminotransferase, and low serum albumin
- *Technetium scan:* often there is no hepatic uptake of colloid
- *Liver biopsy:* shows liver cell necrosis, a heavy neutrophil infiltrate, steatosis, Mallory's hyaline and perivenular fibrosis. These features may be superimposed on cirrhosis

Management

Treatment is largely supportive: attention needs to be given to nutritional support and the prevention of infection. Corticosteroids (prednisolone 40–60 mg/day) may reduce the risk of early death, but should be avoided in those with encephalopathy.

Alcoholic liver disease at a glance

Epidemiology

Most common cause of liver disease in UK with rising incidence

Risk depends on:

• Amount and duration of alcohol consumed (safe limits of 14 units/week for females and 21/week for males are only a general guide)

Other risk factors are:

• Gender (females more susceptible)
• Chronic viral infection
• Obesity
• α_1-Antitrypsin deficiency
• Hereditary haemochromatosis

Symptoms

Range from nil to severe liver disease

May present with extrahepatic manifestations, such as fits, neuropathy, pancreatitis

Examination

Ranges from normal to signs of decompensated liver disease

Note alcohol on breath

Investigation

No specific liver tests

Raised gamma-glutamyl transferase and mean corpuscular volume are suggestive but not diagnostic

Serum IgA is high

Carbohydrate-deficient transferrin may be a useful marker of excess alcohol intake

Alcoholic hepatitis

Typical pattern with high WBC, very high serum bilirubin with alkaline phosphatase and transaminases rarely twice the upper limit of normal

Consider blood/urine/breath alcohol testing

Carbohydrate-deficient transferrin levels indicate chronic alcohol use (but are not totally specific)

Treatment

Non-specific

Alcohol withdrawal may precipitate fits so give chlordiazepoxide

Give vitamin replacement (especially thiamine)

Supportive therapy as appropriate (addiction counselling, Alcoholics Anonymous or other)

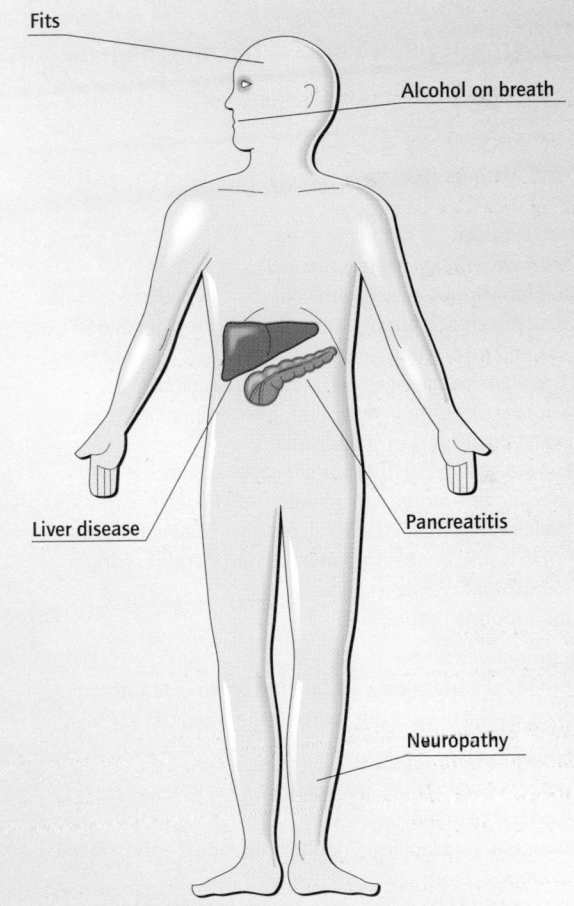

Fits

Alcohol on breath

Liver disease

Pancreatitis

Neuropathy

09

Prognosis

The prognosis is poor if alcohol consumption continues. In severe cases, renal failure, increasing jaundice and prolonged clotting usually herald death. The severity is assessed by Maddrey's Discriminant Factor:

(4.6 × prothrombin time – control PT) + serum bilirubin (mg/dl).

Values greater than 32 imply a poor prognosis.

Alcoholic cirrhosis

Clinical features

Alcoholic cirrhosis may present with any of the complications of cirrhosis. **Diagnosis** is made on the history and confirmed by liver biopsy.

Investigation

Liver biopsy shows features such as Mallory's hyaline,

fatty infiltration and perivenular fibrosis, which are suggestive but not diagnostic of alcoholic cirrhosis.

Management
Treatment is largely supportive. Alcohol must be avoided.

Prognosis
The prognosis is greatly improved by abstinence from alcohol. One study revealed a 50% median survival of 3 years for those who continued to drink alcohol after

diagnosis compared with more than 10 years for those who were abstinent.

Complications of cirrhosis

Variceal haemorrhage
Disease mechanisms
Varices are at risk of bleeding when the portal pressure exceeds 12 mmHg (EMERGENCY BOX 9.1). Portal hypertension has various causes (Table 9.8), but in the UK most cases are caused by cirrhosis. Portal hypertension in the absence of cirrhosis ('non-cirrhotic' portal hypertension) may be caused by:
- Idiopathic portal hypertension
- Portal vein thrombosis
- Early biliary disease (such as precirrhotic PBC)
- Schistosomiasis
- Nodular regenerative hyperplasia

Epidemiology
Prevalence. About 50% of patients with cirrhosis have varices and about 30% of these bleed from the varices.

Disease mechanisms
Varices may occur anywhere in the gastrointestinal tract and can all bleed, but those that bleed are usually in the distal oesophagus or stomach.

Clinical features
Clinically the patient presents with haematemesis, melaena or both. The clinical picture is that of shock with hypotension, tachycardia and cold clammy skin. In portal venous obstruction and inferior vena caval obstruction, some blood from the left branch of the portal vein may be

---

Emergency 9.1: Variceal haemorrhage

Presentation
Haematemesis
Melaena
Shock

Resuscitation
Check airways, breathing circulation
Establish venous access with wide-bore cannula
Cross-match at least 10 units of blood; check full blood count and clotting
If hypotensive, give colloid until blood available
If variceal bleeding is suspected, give terlipressin 2 mg every 6 h (if no contraindications)
Start antibiotics (such as ciprofloxacin, co-amoxiclav)
If clotting abnormal, correct with fresh frozen plasma
If platelets less than 20×10^9/l, consider platelet transfusion
If drowsy and unable to protect airway, consider early ventilation
Monitor urine output

Diagnosis
Confirm at early endoscopy as 10% of patients with varices will bleed from sources other than the varices

Management
If oesophageal varices are bleeding, sclerotherapy or variceal banding
If this controls bleeding, monitor and repeat endoscopy in 1 week
If no control of bleeding, pass Sengstaken–Blakemore tube to control bleeding and repeat endoscopy 24 h later to band/inject varices
If no control, urgent shunting by transjugular intrahepatic shunt or mesocaval shunt to a mesenteric vein
If this fails, consider oesophageal transection
If gastric varices are present, either injection with Histoacryl or thrombin or proceed to shunt (as above)

Once bleeding controlled
Look for precipitating causes: portal vein thrombosis, hepatoma development
Consider patient for prophylaxis with either propranolol or a banding programme

---

Table 9.8 Causes of portal hypertension

Prehepatic
Portal vein thrombosis
Hepatic
Cirrhosis*
Idiopathic non-cirrhotic portal hypertension
Nodular regenerative hyperplasia
Schistosomiasis
Congenital hepatic fibrosis
Severe hepatitis (rare)
Posthepatic
Veno-occlusive disease
Budd–Chiari syndrome
Inferior vena caval obstruction
Constrictive pericarditis

* Cirrhosis is the most common cause by far in the UK.

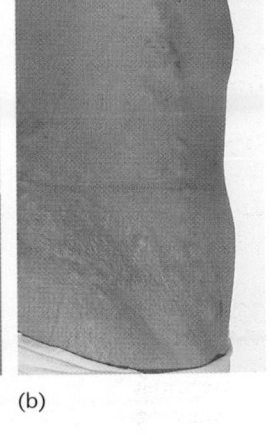

Figure 9.22 (a) Abdomen of a patient with cirrhosis showing dilated veins (caput medusae). (b) Dilated veins in a patient with inferior vena caval obstruction. Note the different distribution of veins.

(a)

(b)

09

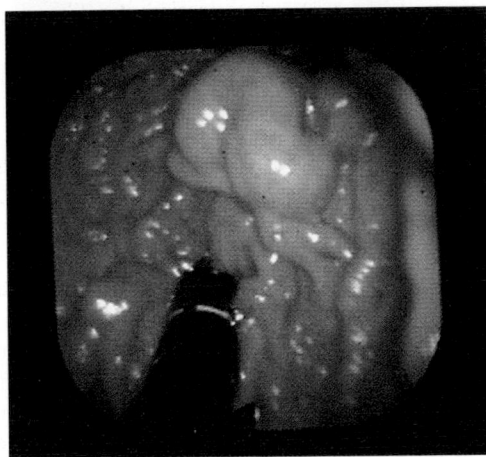

Figure 9.23 Gastric varices seen through the endoscope.

diverted to the umbilicus. From there it reaches the veins of the vena caval system. A number of prominent collateral veins radiating from the umbilicus is termed caput medusae (Fig. 9.22). In inferior vena caval obstruction, the collateral venous channels carry blood upwards to reach the superior vena caval system.

Management

The immediate need is resuscitation. Antibiotics reduce the mortality and should be given early, even in the absence of overt infection. Once stability is achieved, endoscopy should be performed without delay to determine the cause and site of bleeding (Fig. 9.23). Endotracheal intubation is necessary if the patient is drowsy (bleeding may precipitate hepatic encephalopathy). Early endoscopy is important as up to 20% of patients with varices bleed from sources other than varices (such as portal hypertensive gastropathy or peptic ulcers). It also allows therapeutic intervention (Fig. 9.24).

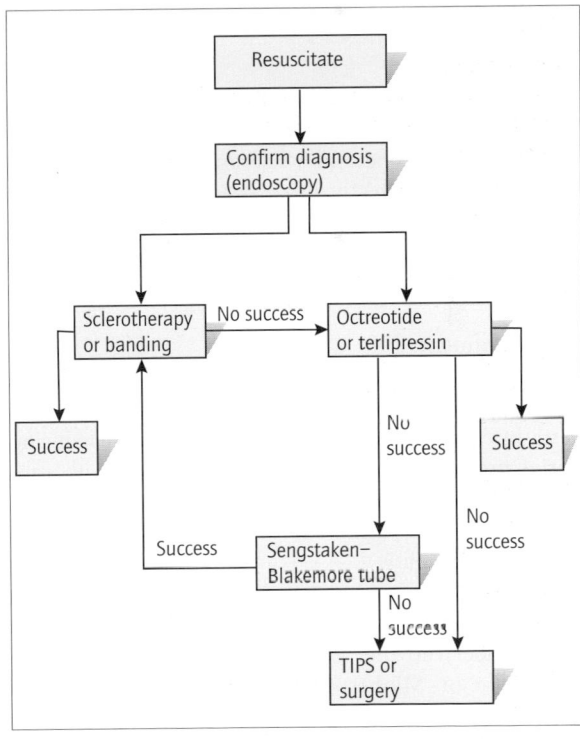

Figure 9.24 Management of variceal haemorrhage. TIPS, transjugular intrahepatic portosystemic shunt.

Specific treatment includes variceal sclerotherapy or band ligation. Vasopressin or synthetic analogues such as terlipressin also reduce the portal pressure and reduce variceal bleeding. If these measures fail to control bleeding, a Sengstaken–Blakemore tube will give temporary relief until definitive therapy (surgical or radiological shunt) can be achieved.

09

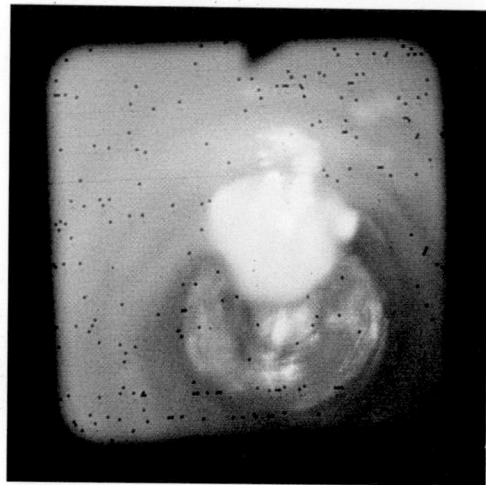

Figure 9.25 Injection of an oesophageal varix.

Variceal sclerotherapy or banding
- *Injection:* the varices are injected via a needle passed down the endoscope and a sclerosant such as ethanolamine is injected directly into the varix (Fig. 9.25)
- *Banding:* a small band is used to thrombose the varix. Complications include ulceration and stricture formation

Drug treatment
Portal pressure can be lowered using vasopressin or a longer acting analogue such as terlipressin. These act partly by causing splanchnic vessel constriction, so reducing portal pressure. These drugs must be given with care to patients over 50 years of age because they can induce coronary artery spasm. Use of antibiotics reduces the associated mortality.

Direct pressure
Tamponade can be achieved using a Sengstaken–Blakemore or Minnesota tube (Fig. 9.26). The tube is passed into the stomach and the gastric balloon is inflated. The tube is then withdrawn and traction is applied. The compression of the gastric fundus will stop most variceal bleeding but, if not, the oesophageal balloon can be inflated. The pressure in the oesophageal balloon must be carefully monitored and must not exceed 40 mmHg because higher pressures can cause mucosal damage. The balloon must not remain inflated for more than 24 hours.

Transjugular intrahepatic portosystemic shunt
More recently great success has been achieved by the use of TIPS. From a transjugular route a wire is passed through the hepatic vein, through the liver substance

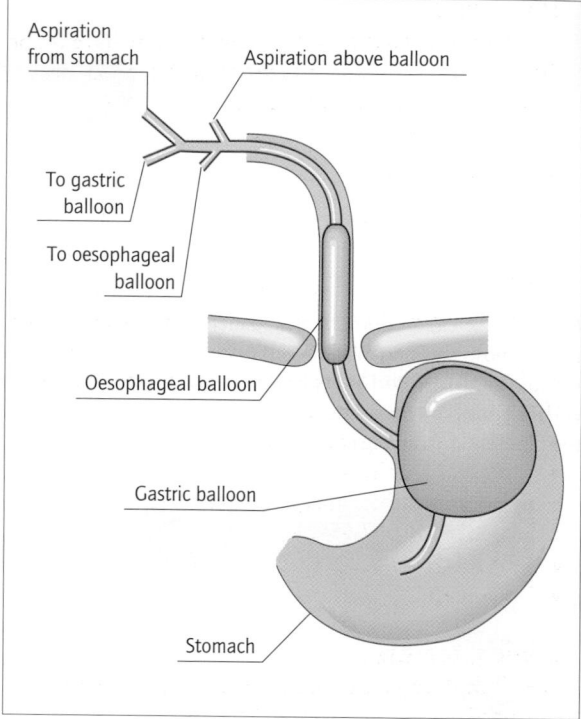

Figure 9.26 Sengstaken–Blakemore tube.

into the portal vein. Over the guide wire a self-expanding stent is passed which will allow for a decompression of the portal vein without the need for surgery. Encephalopathy may occur, especially in older patients.

Surgery
Portal decompression is required in a small minority of patients. There are several different operations, all of which may induce encephalopathy.

Measures against rebleeding
The risks of rebleeding can be reduced by prophylactic sclerotherapy or banding or by pharmacological treatment. Prophylactic banding or sclerotherapy involves regular endoscopy until all the varices at the gastro-oesophageal junction have been obliterated. Six-monthly checks are required to treat newly formed varices. Alternatively, propranolol has been shown to reduce portal pressure and the frequency and severity of the rebleeds. Surgical shunting or a TIPS is rarely required, but should be considered if there is excellent liver function (such as in portal vein thrombosis) or if there is delayed access to medical attention.

Propranolol is effective as both primary and secondary prophylaxis. The dose should be adjusted to maintain portal pressure below 12 mmHg.

Prognosis

The mortality after a first variceal haemorrhage is about 40%. Gastric varices are usually difficult to treat medically and early TIPS is often indicated.

Encephalopathy

Disease mechanisms

The cause of hepatic encephalopathy is not understood, but it is related to failure of the liver to remove toxic substances from the blood, absorption of nitrogen from the bowel and stimulation of the gamma-aminobutyric acid (GABA)–benzodiazepine receptor in the brain. **Precipitating factors** include:

- Sepsis (including spontaneous bacterial peritonitis)
- Drugs (especially sedatives or narcotics)
- Portal and/or hepatic vein thrombosis
- Gastrointestinal bleeding
- Electrolyte disturbances
- Constipation

Clinical features

The clinical features of hepatic encephalopathy have been described above (see p. 603). The diagnosis is confirmed by electroencephalogram (EEG) and/or a number connection test (where the time taken to connect a series of numbered spots is measured).

Investigation

EEG shows a classical triphasic pattern.

Management

Treatment comprises a search for and correction of any precipitating factors, a low-protein (40 g/day) diet and lactulose. Oral neomycin may have a short-term benefit and reduces gut bacterial populations, but is not significantly absorbed. Unproven treatments include bromocriptine and flumazenil (benzodiazepine antagonist).

Prognosis

Depends on the underlying cause and the extent of liver damage.

Ascites

Disease mechanisms

The cause of hepatic ascites is not clear, but portal hypertension and a low serum albumin are necessary (Fig. 9.27).

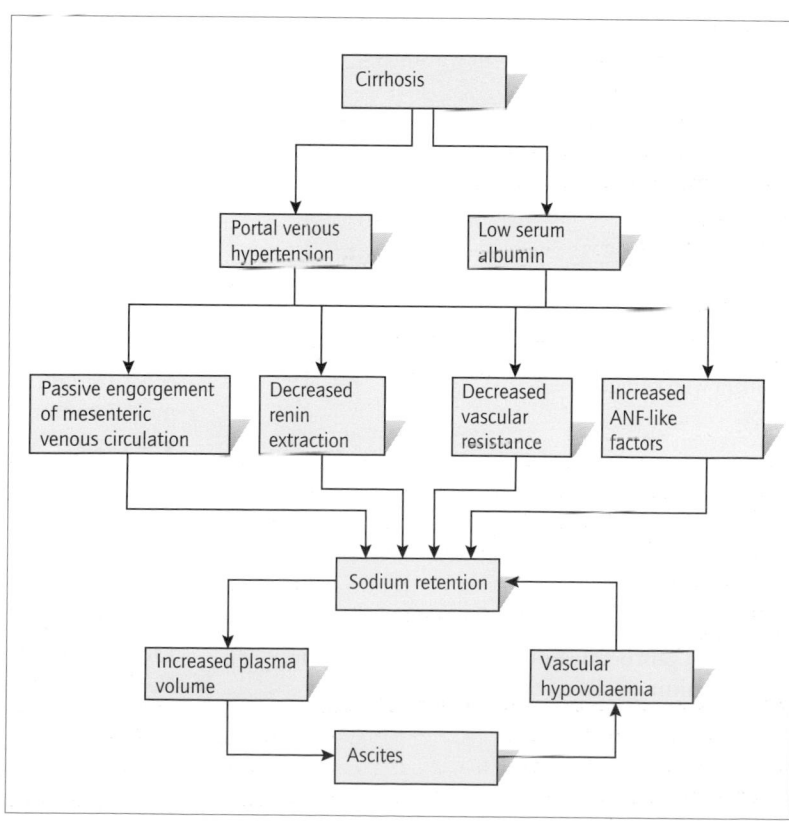

Figure 9.27 Causes of ascites. ANF, antinaturetic factor.

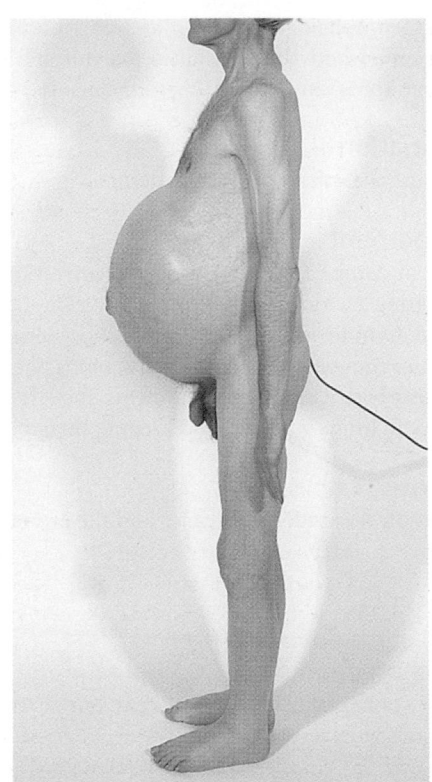

(a)

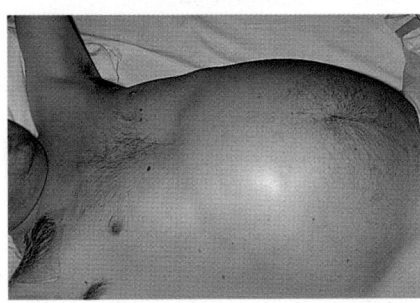

(b)

Figure 9.28 (a) Gross ascites and muscle wasting caused by cirrhosis. (b) Ascites, muscle wasting and scanty axillary hair in a patient with cirrhosis.

The aetiology relates to peripheral and splanchnic vasodilatation associated with liver disease, resulting in splanchnic hypoperfusion.

Clinical features

Clinically ascites causes increasing abdominal distension and weight gain because of fluid accumulation (Fig. 9.28). There is shifting dullness to percussion.

Investigation
Diagnostic imaging
Ultrasound will confirm ascites.

Management

Patients with ascites should be given prophylactic antibiotics (long-term treatment with ciprofloxacin, norfloxacin, co-trimoxazole or co-amoxiclav) which reduce the risk and mortality of bacterial infection.

Treatment includes:
- *Salt restriction:* water restriction is required only if there is hyponatraemia as well
- *Diuretics* (e.g. spironolactone up to 800 mg/day with frusemide): renal function must be closely monitored. A rising serum urea indicates prerenal failure and the need to reduce medication

Most patients will respond to these two measures. The most common cause for failure is not complying with salt restriction.

Paracentesis. Ascites is directly drained from the abdomen; albumin should be given intravenously (8 g albumin per litre of ascites removed) to prevent the associated hypovolaemia.

Transjugular intrahepatic portosystemic shunt. Recurrent ascites can also be treated by the formation of a TIPS (see p. 630).

Bacterial peritonitis may be fatal and should be considered in any patient who develops encephalopathy. It is diagnosed by removing 10 ml ascites: the presence of organisms or a white cell count greater than 250/ml indicates peritonitis requiring immediate antibiotic therapy. The most common organisms are *Escherichia coli*, *Klebsiella* and *Enterococcus* species.

Prognosis
Ascites usually indicates deteriorating liver function.

Liver tumours

Most tumours in the liver are secondary tumours. The most common primary liver tumours can be classified as:
- *Benign:* adenoma, focal nodular hyperplasia, haemangioma
- *Malignant:* hepatocellular carcinoma, cholangiocarcinoma

Benign adenoma
Disease mechanisms
Benign adenomas are associated with prolonged use of the oral contraceptive and other sex steroids.

Epidemiology
Age. Most common age of presentation is 30–40 years.

Sex. Female.

Clinical features

The tumour may present as an incidental mass, with abdominal pain or with bleeding.

Investigation

Ultrasound and liver biopsy usually confirm the diagnosis.

Management

If associated with pregnancy or sex steroids, a benign adenoma may regress when the drug is withdrawn or after the pregnancy. Surgery is indicated if the adenoma does not regress.

Prognosis

Usually excellent.

Hepatocellular carcinoma

Disease mechanisms

Hepatocellular carcinoma usually arises in a cirrhotic liver and may be solitary or multiple. Risk factors for hepatocellular carcinoma include a long history of cirrhosis, male sex, chronic infection with HBV or HCV, drugs (especially anabolic or contraceptive steroids), exposure to aflatoxin (a fungal metabolite found on mouldy ground nuts) and smoking.

Epidemiology

Prevalence. One of the most common cancers worldwide, but relatively rare in the UK.

Sex. About 75% of patients are male.

Clinical features

Hepatocellular carcinoma is often asymptomatic, but its presence should be considered in any patient with cirrhosis who decompensates or if there is increasing hepatomegaly.

Investigation

- *Liver tests:* not specific
- *Serum alpha-fetoprotein* (AFP): usually raised
- *Ultrasound, CT scanning or radioisotope scanning:* shows a filling defect
- *Angiography:* may show a tumour circulation
- *Liver biopsy:* confirms the diagnosis, but carries the risk of tumour dissemination (2%). It should be avoided if transplantation is considered and the diagnosis can be confirmed by other means (e.g. a rising serum AFP in a known cirrhotic with a space-occupying lesion on ultrasound)

Management

Small tumours or tumours in non-cirrhotic livers may be suitable for resection. Chemotherapy is helpful in a minority. Radiotherapy is ineffective. Arterial embolization, direct ethanol injection, cryotherapy or radiofrequency ablation may improve symptoms such as pain or bile duct obstruction, but an effect on survival has yet to be shown.

Prognosis

The median survival of patients with cirrhosis and hepatocellular carcinoma is 12 months.

Hepatorenal syndrome

Disease mechanisms

Hepatorenal syndrome consists of functional renal failure in patients with advanced liver disease. The aetiology is not clear, but endotoxaemia and renal arterial vasoconstriction have been implicated. The urine sodium is very low.

Management

Hypovolaemia should be corrected, but treatment is otherwise directed at maintaining renal function. Intravenous terli-pressin is of help but dopamine is usually of little value. A TIPS may be helpful.

Prognosis

Renal failure caused by liver disease carries a poor prognosis. It is often associated with a terminal illness.

Liver transplantation

Liver transplantation is now the treatment of choice for patients with end-stage disease. The 1-year survival rate for elective liver transplantation exceeds 90% and 10 year rates are in excess of 70%. Most patients require long-term immunosuppression to prevent rejection of the graft. Many autoimmune diseases (such as primary sclerosing cholangitis, primary biliary cirrhosis and autoimmune hepatitis) can recur in the graft. In patients with HCV, reinfection is almost invariable and may lead to graft failure over 10 years. The main causes of graft loss are recurrent disease (viral hepatitis or cancer) in about 50%, and other causes such as *de novo* malignancy, sepsis and cardiovascular disease caused by the immunosuppressive drugs used. Most centres use a combination of corticosteroids, azathioprine and a calcineurin inhibitor (such as ciclosporin and tacrolimus); newer drugs being used include mycophenolate and leflunomide.

Indications for liver transplantation
The indications for transplantation are:

09

09

Hepatocellular carcinoma at a glance

Epidemiology

Prevalence
One of the most common cancers worldwide but rare in UK

Sex
75% male

Age
Varies with cause

Geography
Most common in Africa and South East Asia (probable association with incidence of chronic hepatitis B infection). Rare in Western hemisphere

Investigation

Biochemistry
Serum α-fetoprotein is raised
Liver tests are not specific

Diagnostic imaging
- *Ultrasound:* hypoechoic (or mixed) shadow
- *CT:* hypodense lesions which do not enhance with contrast
- *Radioisotope scanning:* shows a filling defect
- *Angiography:* shows tumour circulation
- *MRI scan:* space-occupying lesion

Histopathology
Biopsy, under ultrasonic guidance, confirms diagnosis but risks tumour dissemination and is only performed if resection or transplantation is not planned

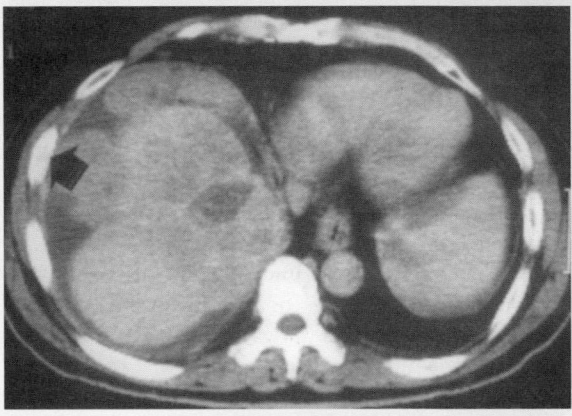

Fig. A CT scan shows a low density tumour bursting through capsule (arrow). Ascites is also present.

Fever

Large irregular liver

Abdominal mass

Ascites

Anorexia

Weakness

Weight loss

Abdominal pain

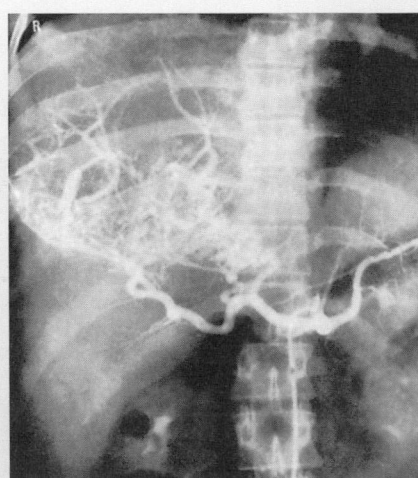

Fig. B Hepatic angiography showing catheter in the bottom right-hand corner. The tumour is supplied by the hepatic artery and the lesion is an abnormal pattern.

Management

Resection for small tumours or tumours in non-cirrhotic livers
Chemotherapy
Embolization, ethanol injection, cyrotherapy, radiofrequency ablation

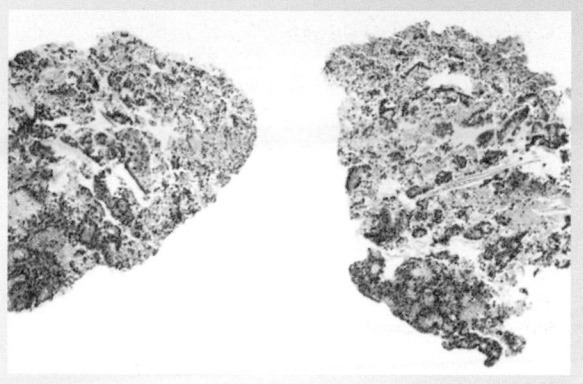

Fig. C Fine needle aspiration under ultrasound guidance yielded a clump of hepatocellular carcinoma. All figures reproduced from Sherlock S, Dooley J. *Diseases of the Liver and Biliary System*, 9th edn. Oxford: Blackwell Scientific Publications, 1992 with the permission of the authors.

Table 9.9 Features of liver disease suggesting a limited survival (less than 1 year)

Serum bilirubin > 200 µmol/l in cholestatic disease
Serum albumin < 28 g/l
Systemic hypotension
Low urine sodium excretion
Spontaneous encephalopathy
Recurrent episodes of bacterial peritonitis
Increasing ascites

- Estimated survival in the absence of grafting of less than 1 year (Table 9.9)
- Intolerable quality of life because of the liver disease or its consequences (such as lethargy, intractable pruritus, encephalopathy, severe ascites)

Contraindications for liver transplantation

Contraindications to transplantation include:
- Primary liver cancer with extrahepatic spread
- Metastatic liver disease (except carcinoid)
- Advanced cardiac, pulmonary or cerebral disease
- Active sepsis
- Continued alcohol abuse
- Significant psychiatric disease

Any patient who may be a potential candidate for transplantation should be discussed with the local transplant centre before the condition becomes terminal. Therapies continue to evolve.

Gall bladder diseases

Gallstones

Disease mechanisms

About 15% of gallstones are composed of bile pigment and 80% are composed of cholesterol. Mixed gallstones contain bile salts and calcium:

- *Bile pigment stones:* composed of calcium bilirubinate, phosphate and carbonate. They are commonly associated with haemolysis
- *Cholesterol gallstones:* most of the cholesterol in the bile is derived from the diet, but some is synthesized in the liver, small intestine and other organs. Cholesterol is secreted into the bile and, because it is esterified, it is insoluble in water. It is kept in solution by the formation of micelles with bile salts and lipids. Cholesterol stones form when there is a relative excess of cholesterol to bile salts and phospholipids. Subclinical infection is an important precipitating factor. Cholesterol stones are more likely to form when there is reduced gall bladder motility and this may explain the increased incidence in pregnancy and diabetes.

Risk factors include:
- Female gender
- High cholesterol diet
- Use of the oral contraceptive pill
- Obesity (body mass index over 30 kg/m^2)
- Ileal resection or disease
- Diabetes mellitus
- Rapid weight loss
- Positive family history
- Some drugs (such as lipid-lowering agents)
- Gall bladder hypomobility

Epidemiology

Prevalence and geography. Gallstones are present in 15% of people in Europe and North America and are more common in the elderly (40% of people aged over 70 years). Mixed cholesterol stones are the most common.

Age. The prevalence increases with age.

Sex. In the younger age group (under 45 years of age), gallstones are more common in females.

Gallstones at a glance

Epidemiology
Prevalence
Affects 15% of people

Age
More common in older age

Sex
More common in women (male : female 1 : 2)

Stone types
Cholesterol stones (80%)
Usually in gall bladder
Risk factors: female sex, oral contraceptives, obesity, rapid weight loss, some drugs, diabetes mellitus, gall bladder hypomotility

Brown pigment stones (10%)
Usually in bile duct
Usually following surgery to biliary tree

Black pigment stones (10%)
Gall bladder (or bile duct)
Risk factors include chronic haemolysis

Clinical features
Significant pain lasting more than 15 min to 5 h
Epigastric or right upper quadrant site; radiation to back
Often occurs at night
Recurrence at irregular intervals
Jaundice, fever and rigors may be present
Tenderness in the right upper quadrant

Investigation
Blood tests may show leucocytosis and obstructive patterns of liver tests
Ultrasound for gall bladder stones
Endoscopic ultrasound, ERCP or MRCP for bile duct stones

Treatment
General
Analgesia and antibiotics (if evidence of infection)

Specific
Gall bladder stones: if symtomatic: usually surgery (occasionally extracorporeal shock wave lithotripsy and gallstone dissolution). Asymptomatic stones usually no treatment required
Bile duct stones: stone extraction at ERCP
If obstructive and infected biliary tree, the bile duct must be decompressed (endoscopically or percutaneously as an emergency)

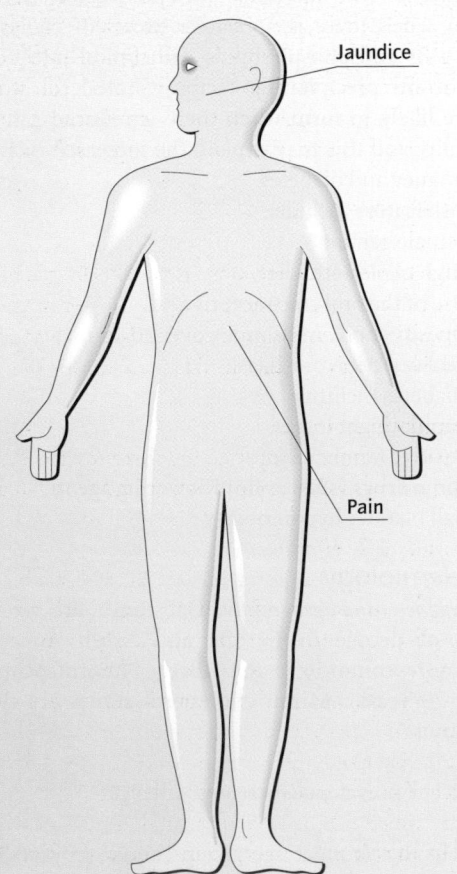

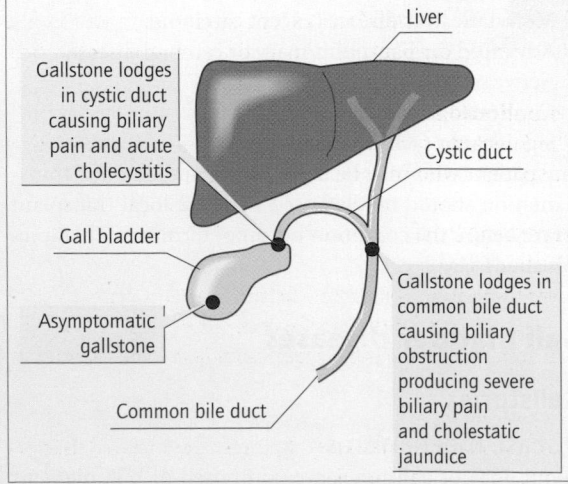

Fig. A Gallstones.

Complications
Pain and infection
Perforation
Pancreatitis
Biliary obstruction
Rarely, bowel obstruction
Pancreatitis

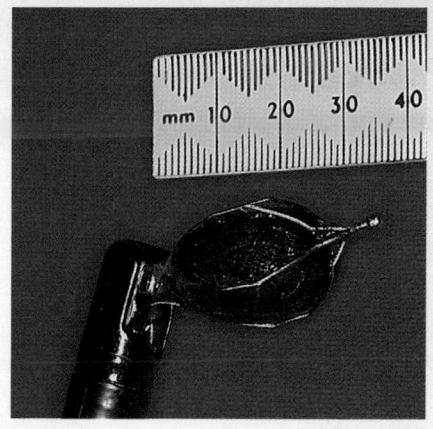

Fig. B Stone removed from the common bile duct using a basket at ERCP.

Clinical features

The clinical presentation of gallstones is characterized by right upper quadrant or epigastric pain which may radiate to the back. The pain usually lasts for more than 15 min, occurs mainly in the evening or night and recurs at irregular intervals. The association with fatty meals is less clear than previously thought.

If the stone impacts in the biliary tree, the pain becomes more severe and is associated with nausea and vomiting. Impaction outside the gall bladder results in the symptoms and signs of obstructive jaundice. Superadded infection is associated with fevers and rigors.

On examination, there is right upper quadrant tenderness and guarding in acute cholecystitis. Pain over the gall bladder on respiration is common.

Common bile duct stones

Stones in the common bile duct can present in association with gallstones, following cholecystectomy, or on their own. The clinical features are similar to those of acute cholecystitis, but pain, jaundice and rigors are more marked.

Complications of gallstones

These include pancreatitis, empyema, bowel obstruction and biliary–enteric fistula formation.

Investigation
Biochemistry

Liver tests show obstructive features (high serum alkaline phosphatase and bilirubin) in complicated cases if a stone has impacted in the biliary tree outside the gall bladder.

Microbiology

- *Blood culture:* necessary to detect associated bacteraemia and/or septicaemia
- *Urine culture:* needed to exclude urinary tract infection and pyelonephritis from the differential diagnosis, but in gallstone cholangitis, bacteria are sometimes also isolated from urine

Diagnostic imaging

Only 10% of stones are detectable on plain abdominal radiography:
- *Ultrasound:* confirms the presence of gallstones, but provides unreliable images of the lower end of the bile duct and stones in the common bile duct may be missed
- *ERCP:* allows visualization of stones in the common bile duct. After sphincterotomy, the stones can be removed if not too large (usually less than 1 cm diameter) or a nasobiliary drain can be placed to decompress the biliary tree

Management
Acute cholecystitis

This is usually caused by obstruction of the gall bladder by a stone. The management of acute cholecystitis involves analgesia, fluid replacement and antibiotics. Surgical advice should be sought on the need for and timing of surgery.

Chronic cholecystitis

Cholecystectomy is required for chronic cholecystitis and can be performed either laparoscopically or at laparotomy.

Common bile duct stones

An obstructed biliary tree is associated with a high risk of biliary sepsis and renal failure. Unless the biliary system is urgently decompressed either surgically, by percutaneous drainage, or at ERCP (see p. 606), the mortality is high. If the bile duct is not obstructed, the stones should be removed either surgically or at ERCP.

In most cases, cholecystectomy is the treatment of choice for all patients with symptomatic gallstones. Depending on the health of the patient, the location of the stone and risk factors such as previous surgery, the cholecystectomy may be performed laparoscopically.

09

Medical dissolution of gallstones

There are several possibilities for medical dissolution of stones in the gall bladder:

● Oral therapy with UDCA (ursodeoxycholic acid) and chenodeoxycholic acid may be effective if the stones are small and non-calcified, and the gall bladder is functioning
● The gall bladder can be punctured and the stones perfused with solvents such as mono-octanoin or methyl tert-butane ether (MTBE)
● Extracorporeal shock wave lithotripsy (ESWL) can be effective for single larger non-calcified stones

These methods can also be used for bile duct stones, but are less effective.

Prognosis

Asymptomatic gallstones may be discovered accidentally and should be left alone; over a 15-year period, only 20% become symptomatic. The risk of gall bladder cancer is low.

Extrahepatic biliary cysts and Caroli's syndrome

Disease mechanisms

Extrahepatic biliary cysts (choledochal cysts) and Caroli's syndrome (intrahepatic biliary cysts) form a spectrum of disease characterized by cystic dilatation of the intra- or extrahepatic biliary tree.

Caroli's syndrome is characterized by intrahepatic biliary cysts and is associated with congenital hepatic fibrosis. This is a rare syndrome in which the normal architecture of the liver is disrupted by broad bands of fibrous tissue, leading to portal hypertension. It is often sporadic, but may be inherited as an autosomal recessive condition.

Epidemiology

Age. Extrahepatic biliary cysts usually present in childhood.

Clinical features

Extrahepatic biliary cysts usually present in childhood with fever, abdominal pain and cholangitis. Caroli's syndrome may be asymptomatic, being diagnosed at a routine examination. Infection of the cysts results in fever, rigors and jaundice. Congenital hepatic fibrosis presents with the complications of portal hypertension.

Investigation

Ultrasound is required to diagnose extrahepatic biliary cysts or Caroli's syndrome. MRCP will confirm the diagnosis, but ERCP should be avoided because of the risks of infection.

Management

Treatment of extrahepatic biliary cysts is surgical excision. Caroli's syndrome does not need treatment if the patient is asymptomatic. Antibiotics are required if the cysts are infected. Treatment of congenital hepatic fibrosis is symptomatic.

Primary sclerosing cholangitis

Disease mechanisms

Primary sclerosing cholangitis affects both the intra- and extrahepatic biliary tree. There is diffuse inflammation, leading to stricture and dilatation. There is a strong association with inflammatory bowel disease, especially ulcerative colitis, but the extent of inflammation in one condition does not parallel the other. There is an increase in the probability of developing colon cancer, especially on the right side. Primary sclerosing cholangitis, like ulcerative colitis, is more common in non-smokers.

Epidemiology

Age. Any age.

Sex. About 67% of patients are male.

Genetics. Associated with HLA DR3.

Clinical features

Primary sclerosing cholangitis may be asymptomatic, or may cause pruritus, jaundice or complications of cirrhosis. Examination usually reveals hepatomegaly in the early and later phases. There is a significant risk of cholangiocarcinoma (see p. 639), which should be considered in all patients with primary sclerosing cholangitis who suddenly deteriorate.

Investigation

● *Liver tests:* show an obstructive pattern; serum alkaline phosphatase is elevated and, in the later stages, serum bilirubin is also increased
● *Autoantibodies:* antineutrophil cytoplasmic antibodies may be present but are not specific
● *MRCP and/or ERCP:* confirm the diagnosis, showing beading and dilatation throughout the biliary tree (Fig. 9.29)

Management

Treatment is symptomatic. UDCA (15–20 mg/kg/day) may slow progression.

Prognosis

Prognosis is variable with progression usual.

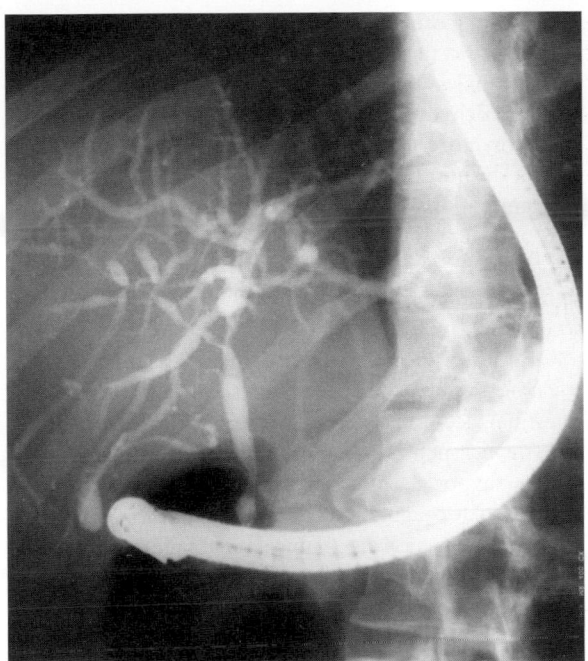

Figure 9.29 ERCP of primary sclerosing cholangitis, showing beading and dilatation in the biliary tree.

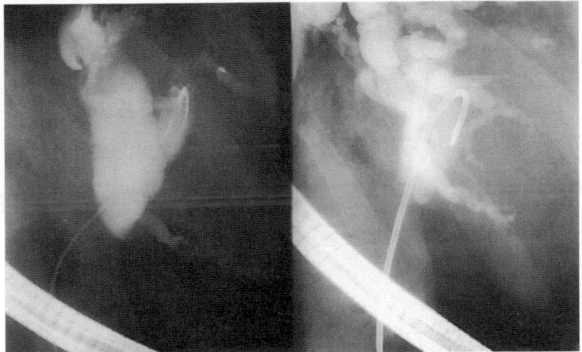

Figure 9.30 Endoscopic stenting of a bile duct tumour resulting in palliative relief. There is gross dilatation of the intrahepatic ducts.

Management

There is usually local spread by the time the diagnosis is made and so treatment is largely palliative, consisting of stenting or bypass surgery (Fig. 9.30).

Prognosis is poor, with a 1-year survival of less than 20%.

Gall bladder cancer

Gall bladder cancer is very rare. It is most common in people with gallstones.

Other disorders of the biliary tree:
- *Cholesterosis of the gall bladder:* characterized by deposits of cholesterol in the gall bladder wall. It is asymptomatic and no treatment is required
- *Adenomyomatosis of the gall bladder:* an incidental finding on cholecystography. There is thickening of the muscle layers and the gall bladder mucosa. Usually no treatment is indicated
- *Acalculous cholecystitis:* may occur in association with systemic diseases such as infection, polyarteritis nodosa and diabetes mellitus

Diseases of the pancreas

Overview of pancreatitis

Pancreatitis may be classified as:
- Acute pancreatitis
- Recurrent acute pancreatitis
- Chronic pancreatitis
- Chronic relapsing pancreatitis

Acute and recurrent acute pancreatitis are associated with a full recovery, but chronic pancreatitis is associated with inflammation and fibrosis.

Tumours of the biliary tree

Cholangiocarcinoma

Disease mechanisms

Cholangiocarcinoma can occur anywhere in the biliary tree. Histology shows an adenocarcinoma. Risk factors include primary sclerosing cholangitis and infestation with the liver fluke or trematode worm, *Clonorchis sinensis,* which is common in the East (see Chapter 3).

Clinical features

Patients present with features of obstructive jaundice or a sudden deterioration in primary sclerosing cholangitis.

Investigation

- *Serum carcinoembryonic antigen and carbohydrate antigen (CA19-9):* elevated in about 20% of patients
- *Ultrasound or CT scanning:* commonly fail to reveal these tumours
- *Angiography:* tumours are usually hypovascular and cannot therefore be seen on angiography
- *ERCP, bile cytology and brushings of the stricture:* may provide the diagnosis

09

Table 9.10 Causes of acute pancreatitis

Mechanical obstruction
Gallstones

Toxic effect
Alcohol

Iatrogenic
Post-ERCP
Surgery

Drugs
Azathioprine
Corticosteroids

Infections
Mumps
Coxsackie

Autoimmune

Metabolic
Hyperparathyroidism
Hyperlipidaemia

Ischaemia

Trauma

Idiopathic

Acute pancreatitis

Disease mechanisms
The causes of acute pancreatitis are listed in Table 9.10. Gallstones and alcohol are the leading causes of acute pancreatitis in the UK.

Clinical features
Acute pancreatitis presents with central or epigastric abdominal pain, radiating to the back or to between the shoulder blades. The pain may be mild or severe, and is associated with nausea and vomiting. In severe acute pancreatitis the patient may be in shock. Markers of severe acute pancreatitis include:

- Age
- Obesity
- Multiorgan dysfunction syndrome

There are several systems for assessing the severity of the attack; the Ransom system was developed for patients with alcohol-related pancreatitis; the APACHE system is also helpful. The Glasgow scoring system is based on eight factors:

1 Low Pao_2, less than 8 kPa (less than 60 mmHg)
2 Albumin less than 32 g/l
3 White blood cells more than 15×10^9/l
4 AST/ALT more than 200 µ/l

5 Blood glucose more than 10 mmol/l (non-diabetic)
6 Blood urea more than 16 mmol/l
7 Calcium less than 2.0 mmol/l
8 Lactic dehydrogenase more than 600 IU/l

Three or more factors indicates severe pancreatitis; the greater the number of factors, the poorer the prognosis.

Examination may reveal shock, with abdominal tenderness and guarding. There may be bruising in the loins (Grey Turner's sign) and around the umbilicus (Cullen's sign). Jaundice and respiratory failure are features of severe inflammation.

Complications may be:

- *Local:* such as pseudocysts, abscesses, ascites, gastrointestinal bleeding, ileus and portal vein thrombosis
- *Systemic:* such as shock, respiratory failure, acute renal failure, hypocalcaemia, hyperglycaemia, disseminated intravascular coagulation (DIC) and fat necrosis
- *Early:* such as cardiac failure, renal failure, respiratory failure, DIC and venous thrombosis
- *Late:* such as pseudocyst, abscess, diabetes mellitus, fistula, ascites and stricture

Investigation

Haematology
FBC may show evidence of complications such as DIC.

Biochemistry

- *Serum or urine amylase:* raised and confirms the diagnosis. These levels may be increased in any cause of an acute abdomen, and must therefore be considered in conjunction with the history and other tests. However, a serum amylase five times the normal upper limit is highly suggestive of acute pancreatitis
- *Serum lipase:* may be increased but is less specific
- *Biochemical profile:* may reveal features of complications, such as hypocalcaemia, hypoglycaemia, hypoalbuminaemia or uraemia

Diagnostic imaging
Ultrasound, CT scanning and MRCP are helpful for following progression of the disease and detecting some of the complications such as pseudocyst formation (Fig. 9.31).

Management
Management is largely supportive. The patient is kept nil-by-mouth and a nasogastric tube is inserted. Fluid and electrolyte balance must be maintained, usually by intravenous administration. In order to maintain adequate nutrition, a nasojejunal tube is also passed; intravenous or parenteral nutrition, while effective, is associated with a high risk of sepsis. Arterial blood gases should be measured.

Some antibiotics (third generation cephalosporins)

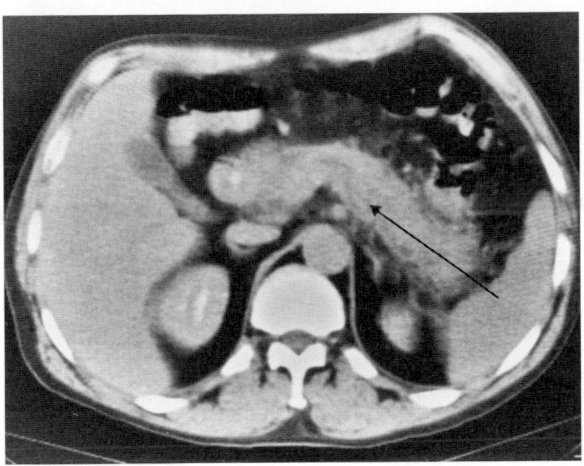

Figure 9.31 Acute pancreatitis. CT scan showing diffuse enlargement of the pancreas with ill-defined edges.

improve outcome. It may be difficult to achieve analgesia, but opiates should be avoided as they are reputed to worsen the illness by increasing the tone of the sphincter of Oddi.

If there is good evidence that gallstones are the cause, ERCP and sphincterotomy are indicated in selected patients.
- *Pseudocysts:* usually develop late and no treatment is required if they are small. Large and recurrent collections need drainage or surgical excision
- *Pancreatic abscess formation:* suggested by fever, neutrophil leucocytosis and deterioration about 1–2 weeks after the initial presentation. Intensive treatment with antibiotics and either surgical or percutaneous drainage is required

Prognosis
The prognosis varies with the severity of the attack. Old age, a neutrophil leucocytosis, low serum albumin, hypocalcaemia, hypoxia and uraemia suggest a poor outcome (Table 9.11).

Chronic pancreatitis
Disease mechanisms
Causes of chronic pancreatitis are:
- Alcohol (over 60% of cases)
- Hyperlipidaemia
- Malnutrition
- Cystic fibrosis
- Hypercalcaemia
- Hereditary (autosomal dominant)
- Idiopathic causes

Table 9.11 Markers of severe acute pancreatitis

Age >55 years
WBC >16 × 10^9/l
Hypocalcaemia (calcium <2.2 mmol/l)
Renal impairment (urea increase >2 mmol/l
Hypoxaemia (Po_2 <8 kPa/60 mmHg)
Acidosis (base deficit >4 mmol/l)

WBC, white blood cell count.

Clinical features
The cardinal features of chronic pancreatitis are abdominal pain, weight loss and steatorrhoea. Less common presentations include jaundice, diabetes mellitus or portal hypertension. Examination is often unhelpful, revealing no specific physical signs.

Complications are chronic abdominal pain, malabsorption, diabetes mellitus, pseudocyst, common bile duct strictures, intestinal obstruction, ascites, pleural effusions, aneurysm of arteries around the pancreas and splenic vein thrombosis.

Investigation
Blood tests are helpful for detecting early consequences of malabsorption:
- *Serum amylase:* usually normal
- *Plain abdominal radiography:* reveals pancreatic calcification
- *Ultrasound, CT scanning and ERCP:* show an irregular fibrosed gland. Calcification in chronic pancreatitis is mainly caused by small calculi within the pancreas that are obvious on CT scanning (Fig. 9.32)

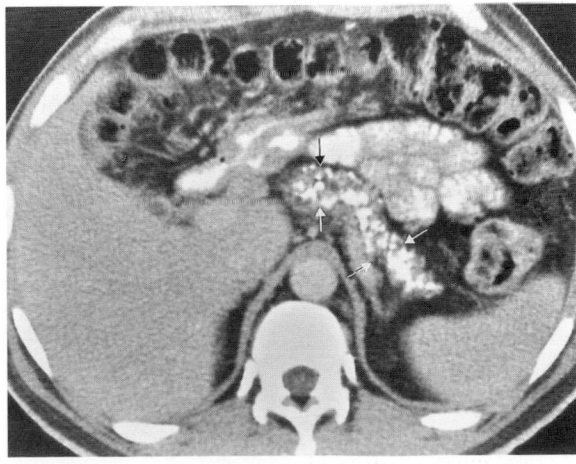

Figure 9.32 Chronic pancreatitis. CT scan showing numerous small areas of calcification within the pancreas (arrows).

• *Pancreatic function tests:* raised faecal fat levels (higher than 6 g in 72 h), reduced faecal chymotrypsin, or an abnormal Lundh test (which measures duodenal trypsin after a standard meal) can all be used to assess pancreatic function

Management

There is no specific treatment. Alcohol must be avoided. It may be very difficult to achieve pain relief and, in extreme cases, surgical removal of some or all of the pancreas may be necessary. Treatment of complications is symptomatic. Pancreatic enzyme supplements (such as Creon or Pancrex) may help relieve symptoms of pancreatic exocrine insufficiency. Insulin may be required for diabetes mellitus.

Pancreatic carcinoma

Disease mechanisms

The aetiology is not clear, but pancreatic carcinoma is more common in smokers and alcoholics.

Most pancreatic cancers are adenocarcinomas arising from the ductal. Other tumours include sarcomas, cystadenomas, insulinomas and lymphomas.

Epidemiology

Prevalence. The incidence of pancreatic cancer is increasing. There has been a threefold increase in the UK in the last 30 years. Certain occupations (e.g. metal working) and smoking are associated with an increased risk. Chronic pancreatitis may predispose to pancreatic cancer.

Age. Usually over 60 years of age.

Sex. More common in males (about two-thirds).

Clinical features

The presentation of tumours in the body and tail of the pancreas differs from that of tumours at the ampulla or in the head of the pancreas:

• *Tumours in the body and tail:* present with abdominal pain and weight loss and, rarely, with diabetes mellitus. The pain is central and classically relieved by sitting forward

• *Tumours in the head and ampulla:* present earlier with obstructive jaundice and weight loss and, in the early stages, without severe pain

Examination reveals few clinical signs, but there may be evidence of weight loss, jaundice, hepatomegaly and a palpable gall bladder.

Investigation

Biochemistry

Serological tests are rarely helpful. Serum markers have been proposed to differentiate pancreatic cancer from inflammation and include CA19-9, carcinoembryonic antigen and immunoreactive elastase. None of these markers, however, is of adequate sensitivity or specificity to be diagnostic alone.

Diagnostic imaging

Ultrasound (percutaneous and endoscopic), CT scanning, MRCP and ERCP are helpful in defining the extent of the abnormality, but will not confidently differentiate malignant disease.

Histopathology

Fine needle aspiration and biopsy of the gland may lead to

Pancreatic carcinoma at a glance

Epidemiology

Prevalence

15 in 100 000 males in USA. Increasing in many Western countries, now the fourth most common cause of cancer death in the UK and USA

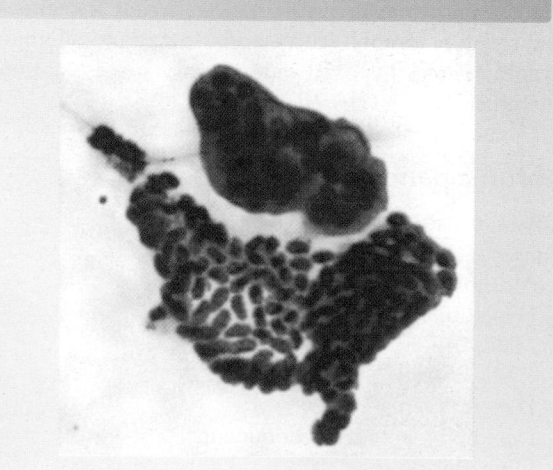

Fig. A Brush cytology taken from a low common bile duct stricture. There is a sheet of benign biliary epithelial cells and above this a small group of large polymorphic cells characteristic of adenocarcinoma. (Reproduced from Sherlock S, Dooley J. *Diseases of the Liver and Biliary System*, 9th edn. Oxford: Blackwell Scientific Publications, 1992 with the permission of the authors.)

Age
Especially over 60 years of age

Sex
More common in males (2 : 1)

Investigation
Biochemistry
Serum alkaline phosphatase may be raised

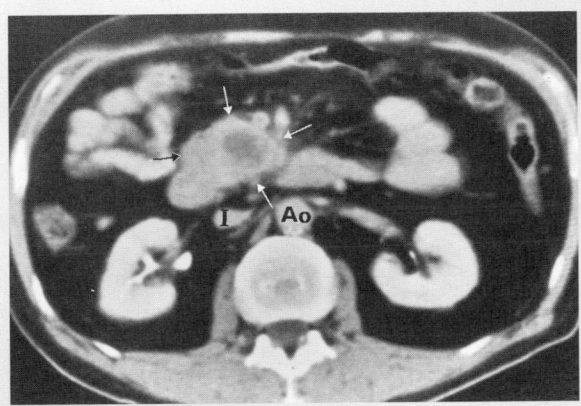

Fig. B CT scan showing focal mass in head of pancreas (arrows). Ao, aorta; I, inferior vena cava. Reproduced from Armstrong P, Wastie M. *Diagnostic Imaging*, 3rd edn. Oxford: Blackwell Scientific Publications, 1992 with the permission of the authors.

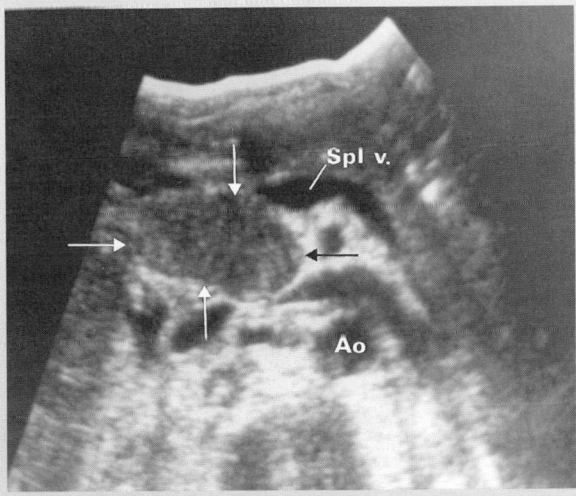

Fig. C Ultrasound, transverse scan (different patient), showing a similarly situated mass (arrows). Ao, aorta; Spl v., splenic vein. Reproduced from Armstrong P, Wastie M. *Diagnostic Imaging*, 3rd edn, Oxford: Blackwell Scientific Publications, 1992 with the permission of the authors.

Diagnostic imaging
CT or MRI may confirm diagnosis and define extent of malignancy
Ultrasound is useful for initial screening test
Duodenoscopy with ERCP may detect tumours at head of duct of the pancreas

Histopathology
Fine needle aspiration biospy (guided by ultrasound, CT or ERCP) distinguishes from chronic pancreatitis
Note risk of dissemination

Treatment
Surgical: curative resection is rarely possible
Good palliation
Drug therapy: gemcitabine may help

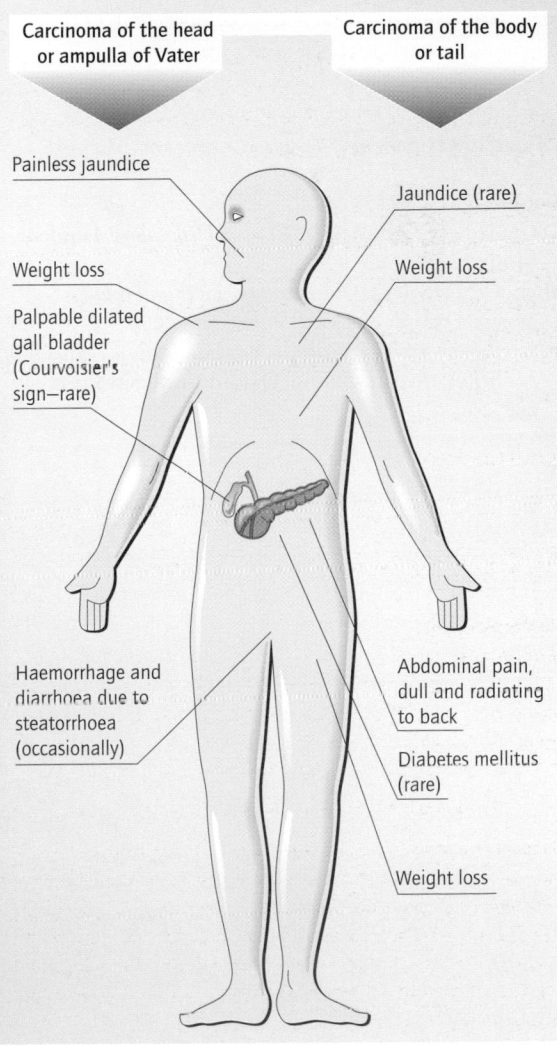

Carcinoma of the head or ampulla of Vater

Carcinoma of the body or tail

Painless jaundice

Jaundice (rare)

Weight loss

Weight loss

Palpable dilated gall bladder (Courvoisier's sign—rare)

Haemorrhage and diarrhoea due to steatorrhoea (occasionally)

Abdominal pain, dull and radiating to back

Diabetes mellitus (rare)

Weight loss

09

tumour dissemination along the track and development of a fistula, and have a high false-negative rate; for this reason, histology is rarely taken.

Management

In the elderly, treatment should be symptomatic. Obstructive jaundice can be relieved by stents. Surgical treatment is indicated in selected patients with limited disease. The cytotoxic agent gemcitabine is proving useful.

Prognosis

Ampullary tumours carry a better prognosis, possibly because they present earlier and are therefore amenable to excision. About 85% of patients with pancreatic cancer die within 1 year. Around 10% are amenable to surgery and the 5-year survival is about 25%.

Endocrine tumours of the pancreas

Gastrinomas, insulinomas, glucagonomas and VIPomas are rare tumours that may arise in the pancreas.

! Must know checklist

- Causes, signs and symptoms of acute hepatitis
- Diagnosis and early treatment of paracetamol overdosage
- The causes, signs and symptoms of cirrhosis
- Prevention and management of complications of cirrhosis

- Serology and treatment of hepatitis viruses (A, B, C)
- Investigation and management of gallstones
- Diagnosis and management of acute pancreatitis

Further reading

Books

O'Grady JG. *Comprehensive Clinical Hepatology*. London: Mosby, 2000.

Sherlock S, Dooley J. *Diseases of the Liver and Biliary System*. Oxford: Blackwell Publishing, 2002.

Warrell DA, Cox TM, Firth JD, Benz EJ. *Oxford Textbook of Medicine*, 4th edn. Oxford: Oxford University Press, 2003.

Journals

Current Opinion in Gastroenterology, Lippincott, Williams & Wilkins. www.co-gastroenterology.com

Journal of Hepatology, European Association for the Study of the Liver/Elsevier. http://www.jhep-elsevier.com/

Hepatology, American Gastroenterological Association.

Websites

www.gastrohep.com

Gastrointestinal Disease

Introduction

Gastrointestinal disorders are common, accounting for up to 20% of consultations in general practice. The most common chronic symptoms are dyspepsia, abdominal pain and change of bowel habit. Other common problems leading to referral for gastroenterological investigation are weight loss and anaemia.

Approximately half of the patients referred to hospital clinics with gastroenterological symptoms will have no disease found using conventional diagnostic tests. These patients are labelled as having functional symptoms. Functional disease occurs in every specialty: in gastroenterology common diagnostic labels used are 'non-ulcer dyspepsia' for upper gastrointestinal, and 'irritable bowel syndrome' for lower gastrointestinal symptoms where no 'organic' disease (e.g. peptic ulcer, cancer) is found to explain them. 'Functional' does not mean that the patient's symptoms are imagined or have no physiological basis—just that we are unable as yet to define with routine tests the abnormality present. Patients whose primary problem is a psychological condition such as anxiety or depression frequently present to gastroenterologists with somatic symptoms such as dyspepsia, which are labelled as 'functional' disease after normal investigations. However, their symptoms may well have an 'organic' basis: for example, specialized research techniques demonstrate disordered gastrointestinal motility patterns in volunteers subjected to stress. Conversely, some 'organic' disease detected may be symptomless and completely coincidental to symptoms (e.g. gallstones or chronic gastritis). Thus, while the terms organic and functional are in common use in gastroenterology, be aware of the imprecision of these terms, and avoid a pejorative approach to patients whose symptoms are not explained by an 'organic' diagnosis with conventional tests.

The most frequent organic diagnoses are reflux oesophagitis, gastritis, peptic ulceration and diverticular disease. Patients with haemorrhoids, another common gastrointestinal diagnosis, usually present to surgical clinics. The most frequently occurring gastrointestinal malignancy in developed nations is colorectal cancer. Cancers of stomach and oesophagus are regularly seen in hospital practice. Chronic conditions that commonly require prolonged hospital clinic follow-up are inflammatory bowel disease and malabsorption syndromes including coeliac disease.

Most gastroenterology in hospitals takes place on an outpatient basis: patients are often discharged back to their general practitioner (GP) after a diagnosis and management plan have been made. Inpatient gastroenterology is typically concerned with management of gastrointestinal bleeding, cancer and inflammatory bowel disease, in close cooperation with specialities such as surgery, radiology and histopathology. Management of liver, pancreatic and biliary disease and ascites is discussed in Chapter 9.

Structure and function

Structure

The structure of the alimentary tract is similar throughout its length, comprising a tube of three main layers (Fig. 10.1):

1 *Inner:* mucosa (squamous in the oesophagus, columnar elsewhere). The surface area of the small intestinal mucosa is enormously increased by **mucosal folds**, **villi** and **microvilli** (Fig. 10.2).

2 *Middle:* circular and longitudinal muscle fibres, with an additional transverse muscle layer in the stomach. The longitudinal muscles run in three discrete bands (taenia

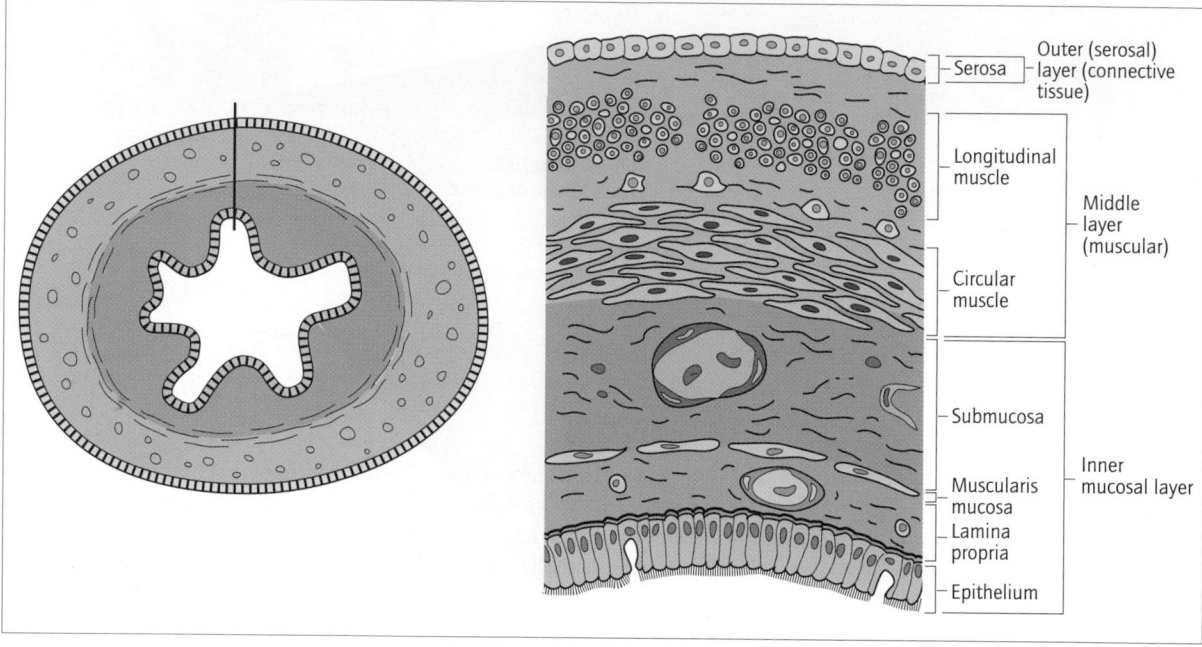

Figure 10.1 Overview of the three-layered structure of the gastrointestinal tract.

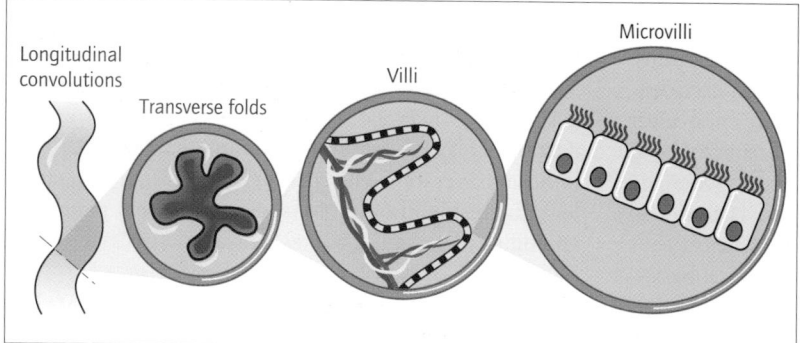

Figure 10.2 Factors increasing the surface area of the small intestine.

coli) in the colon. The muscle layer thickens at various points and, through neuronal control, can act as a valve (e.g. upper and lower oesophageal sphincters, pylorus, ileocaecal valve).

3 *Outer:* serosa (a layer of connective tissue).

Arterial blood supply

The upper oesophagus is supplied by branches of the thoracic aorta. The rest of the gut is supplied by branches of three arteries arising from the abdominal aorta:

1 *Coeliac axis:* lower oesophagus, stomach and duodenum.
2 *Superior mesenteric artery (SMA):* duodenum, small bowel, colon as far as the proximal two-thirds of the transverse colon.
3 *Inferior mesenteric artery (IMA):* distal one-third of

transverse colon, descending and sigmoid colon, rectum and upper two-thirds of the anal canal.

The watershed between SMA and IMA supplies, near the splenic flexure, is particularly susceptible to ischaemia.

Venous drainage

The majority of the gut circulation drains via the portal venous system through the liver, returning to the inferior vena cava via the hepatic veins. Haematogenous spread of gastrointestinal malignancies to the liver via this route is common. At the proximal and distal ends of the portal supply (Fig. 10.3), venous drainage becomes direct to the systemic system. This allows formation of portosystemic anastomoses (Table 10.1). The dilated veins that result at these anastomotic sites (oesophageal and rectal varices)

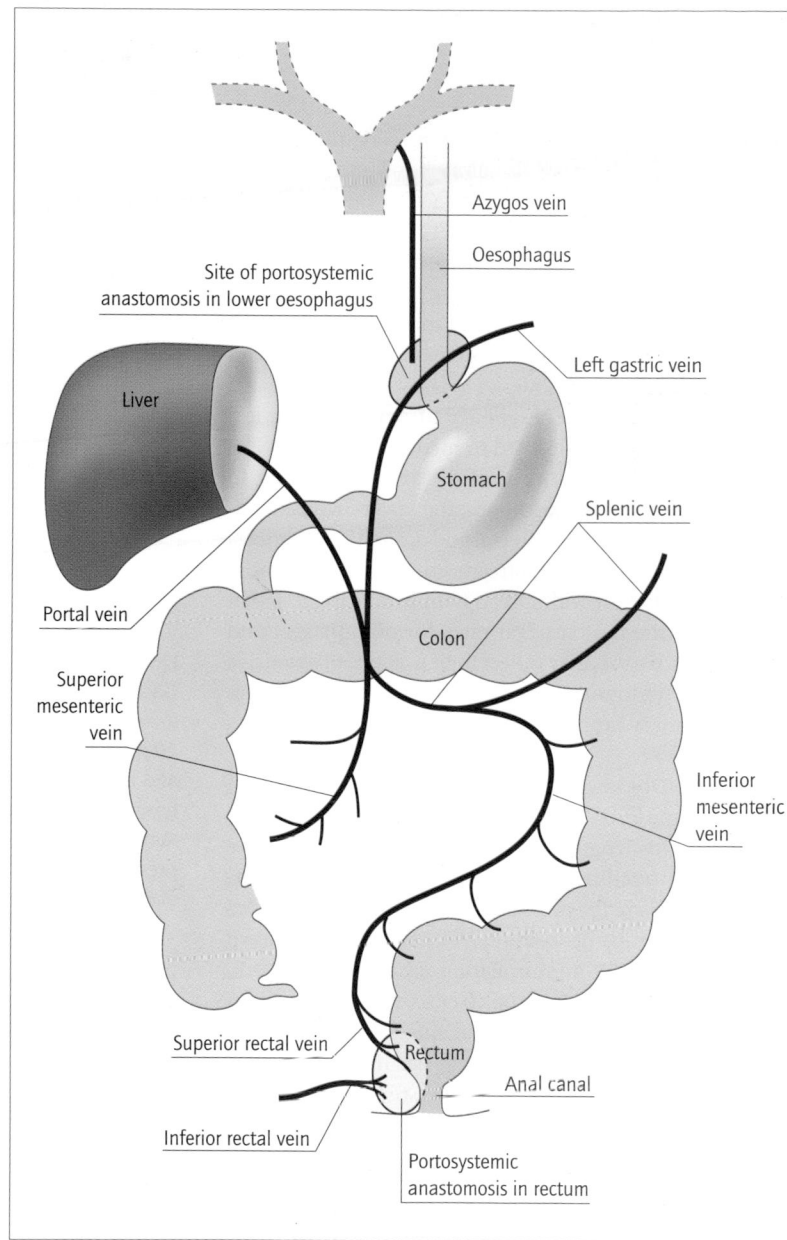

Figure 10.3 Venous drainage of the gastrointestinal tract showing clinically important sites of portosystemic anastomoses.

Table 10.1 Details of the anastomoses between the portal and systemic veins draining the gastrointestinal tract

Site	Portal vessel	Systemic vessel	Clinical manifestation
Lower oesophagus	Left gastric vein	Azygous vein	Oesophageal varices
Rectum	Superior rectal vein	Inferior rectal vein	Rectal varices

may rupture, causing potentially life-threatening gastro-intestinal bleeding (see Chapter 9, p. 628).

Lymphatic drainage

The mucosa of the gastrointestinal tract is richly supplied with lymphatics, draining via submucosal and subserous plexuses to local nodes on the surface of the gut. These then drain to nodes beside arteries, eventually back to one of three groups of preaortic nodes around the origins of the three main arteries of the gut (see p. 646). The lymphatic supply follows the arterial supply (e.g. the stomach is supplied by the coeliac axis vessels, and so its lymphatics drain to the coeliac axis nodes).

The upper third of the oesophagus drains to the cervical lymph nodes; the middle third to mediastinal nodes. The rectum and upper two-thirds of the anal canal drain to internal and common iliac nodes; the lower anal canal to superficial inguinal nodes. Rectal and oesophageal cancers pose special problems in gastrointestinal surgery because of their potential for widespread lymphatic spread. Japan has some of the best survival rates for oesophageal and gastric cancers—this may reflect their practice of extensive resection of abdominal, mediastinal and cervical nodes with the primary cancer.

Nerve supply

The gastrointestinal tract receives autonomic efferents throughout its length. Parasympathetic supply causes increased contractility and reduced sphincter tone; sympathetic effects are the opposite. The vagus nerve provides the main parasympathetic supply. Although it is best known for its efferent role in stimulating gastric acid output, 90% of vagal fibres are afferent (sensory). Abnormalities of sensory feedback from the gut may be important in functional bowel disorders. The gut has its own intrinsic neural network, 'the enteric nervous system', which allows for coordination of gastrointestinal motility and secretions independent of central nervous control.

Function

Oesophagus

During the first phase of swallowing, the cricopharyngeal and upper oesophageal sphincter muscles relax, and the epiglottis and soft palate seal off trachea and nasopharynx, respectively. In the second phase, the bolus is propelled by peristalsis to the lower oesophageal sphincter (LOS), an anatomically indistinct high pressure area, which relaxes to allow the bolus to enter the stomach. One of the most common problems in gastroenterology is gastro-oesophageal reflux disease (GORD), caused in part by failure of LOS competence. Other factors normally preventing gastro-oesophageal reflux are shown in Fig. 10.4.

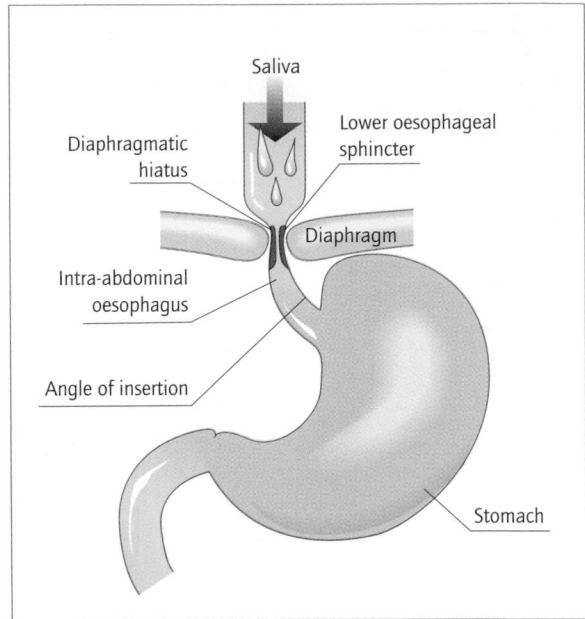

Figure 10.4 Factors preventing gastro-oesophageal reflux. Gastro-oesophageal reflux is prevented by the action of: (i) the lower oesophageal sphincter, the pressure of which is normally 20 mmHg and is increased by cholinergic stimulation, gastrin and food in the stomach; (ii) the acute angle of entry of the oesophagus into the stomach; (iii) compression of the intra-abdominal segment of the oesophagus by intra-abdominal pressure; (iv) the diaphragmatic hiatus; and (v) neutralization of any acid reflux by swallowed saliva (approximately 1 l/day).

Stomach

The stomach mixes and begins digestion of food. **Gastric secretions** include:

• *Hydrochloric acid:* produced by parietal (oxyntic) cells in the gastric body in response to three stimuli: the vagus nerve; gastrin (released from cells in the antrum); and histamine (Fig. 10.5). The acid breaks down and sterilizes food

• *Pepsinogen:* released from chief cells and converted by acid to the active protease, pepsin, which begins protein digestion

• *Intrinsic factor:* a glycoprotein secreted by parietal cells under similar control mechanisms as hydrochloric acid. It binds vitamin B_{12} for later absorption in the terminal ileum

To defend itself from these digestive secretions, and from exogenous agents (e.g. food, drink, heat, cold, bacteria, drugs), the gastric mucosa secretes **mucus**, and **bicarbonate** to neutralize acid (Fig. 10.6). These defences are stimulated by prostaglandins and cholinergic agonists, and decreased by alcohol and non-steroidal anti-inflammatory drugs (NSAIDs).

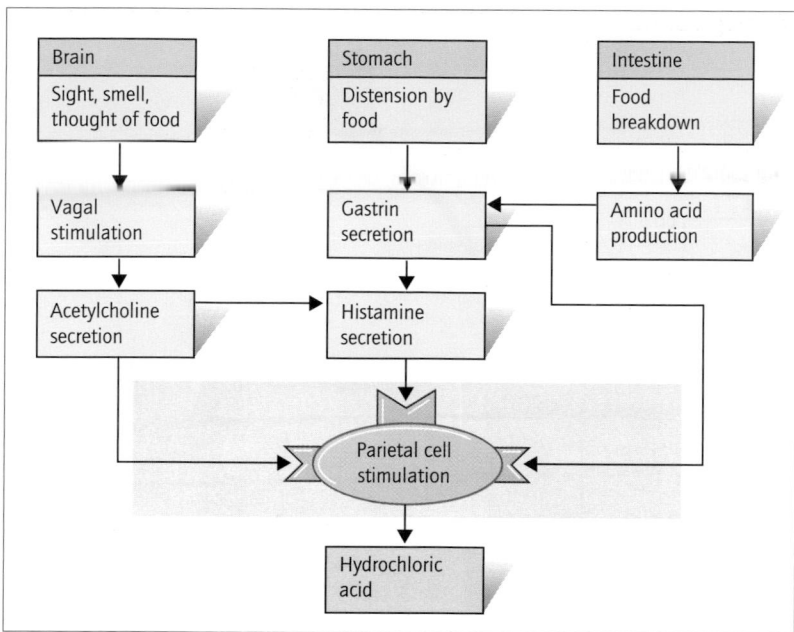

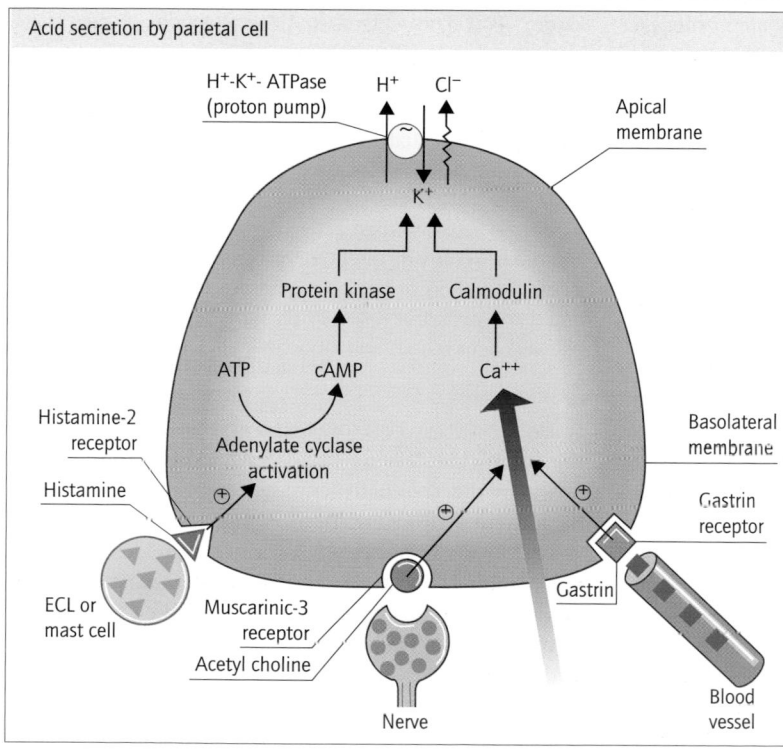

Figure 10.5 Control of gastric acid secretion. Secretion of gastric acid is controlled by: (i) a cephalic phase, mediated via the vagus nerve; (ii) a gastric phase, mediated by gastrin released in response to the presence of food and a rising pH in the gastric lumen, and gastric distension following a meal; and (iii) an intestinal phase, caused by further gastrin release stimulated by amino acid production from protein digestion in the small intestine. Note the negative feedback loops, as stimuli that trigger gastrin release also trigger D-cell activation, resulting in inhibitory influences on gastrin-producing cells and parietal cells. The receptors and pathways for parietal cell activation and hydrogen ion secretion are shown.

Small intestine

The most important functions of the small intestine are digestion and absorption; immunological protection against entry of antigens and/or micro-organisms; neuroendocrine; and movement of digestive contents.

Digestion and absorption

Fat. Fatty acids are the main and most efficient fuel store of the body. Dietary fat consists mainly of triglycerides, which are molecules in which three fatty acid molecules are linked to a glycerol molecule with ester bonds. The

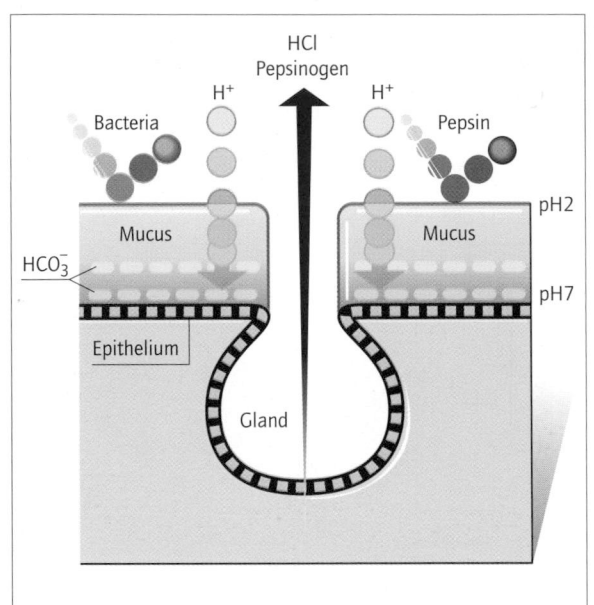

Figure 10.6 The protective mucus–bicarbonate barrier. A layer of mucus slows the diffusion of H⁺ ions back towards the epithelium, and allows their progressive neutralization by bicarbonate ions trapped in it. The mucus also protects the epithelium from bacteria and pepsin. The production of both mucus and bicarbonate is increased by prostaglandins, and reduced by alcohol and non-steroidal anti-inflammatory drugs (NSAIDs).

length of the carbon chain of the fatty acids occurring naturally in animal diets varies from 12 to 24, with 16–18 carbon ('long-chain') fatty acids being the most common. Dietary fat is almost completely absorbed in the proximal small bowel: on a diet containing 100 g/day fat, more than 6 g/day appearing in the stool indicates malabsorption.

Fat absorption requires solubilizing lipids in an aqueous environment. The actions of chewing and gastric mixing convert fats into a coarse emulsion (a suspension of fat droplets in water, exposing a large surface area to lipolytic enzymes). This emulsion empties slowly into the duodenum, triggering pancreatic secretion and gall bladder contraction. Dietary and bile juice-derived phospholipids coat the fat droplets, stabilizing the emulsion. Pancreatic lipase degrades triglycerides to monoglycerides and free fatty acids. These water-insoluble molecules then combine with conjugated bile salts, forming small aggregates known as micelles or larger aggregates known as liposomes. Bile salts, which have both water- and lipid-soluble domains, permit migration of micelles across the unstirred water layer lining the mucosal surface. The lipid contents of the micelles then pass by passive and active uptake mechanisms through the lipid-rich membrane of

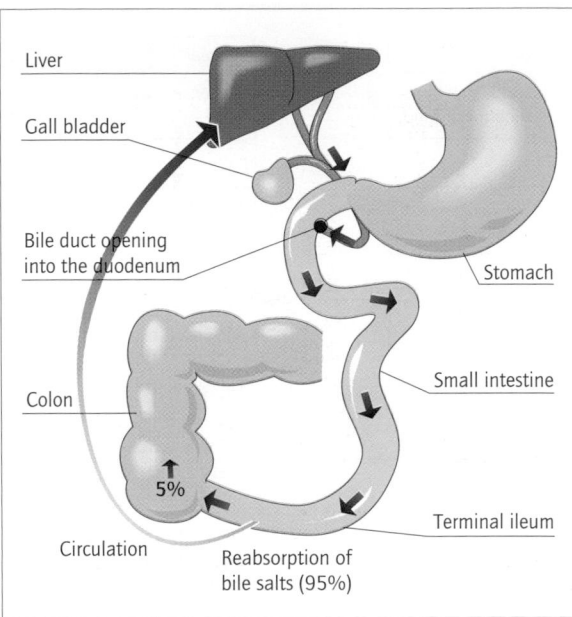

Figure 10.7 The enterohepatic circulation of bile salts. The primary bile salts cholic and chenodeoxycholic acid are synthesized in the liver from cholesterol. They are then conjugated with glycine and taurine to make them water-soluble, and stored in the gall bladder. Conjugated cholic and chenodeoxycholic acid are secreted into the small bowel after a meal to aid in fat absorption. Ninety-five per cent of conjugated bile salts are then actively reabsorbed in the terminal ileum and return to the liver for recirculation. The normally small proportion of bile salts entering the colon is deconjugated and dehydroxylated by bacterial flora to the secondary bile salts deoxycholic and lithocholic acid, respectively.

the enterocyte, leaving the conjugated bile salts to pass down to the terminal ileum for reabsorption (enterohepatic circulation; Fig. 10.7).

Within the enterocyte, triglycerides are resynthesized and combine with cholesterol, apoproteins and phospholipids to form chylomicrons, which are then transported to the intestinal lymphatics and eventually to the general circulation.

A small proportion of medium-chain (8–12 carbon atoms) triglycerides are absorbed intact by and hydrolysed within enterocytes, then passing directly into the portal venous system.

Carbohydrate. Dietary carbohydrate is mainly starch, accompanied by sugars such as sucrose and lactose. Pancreatic amylase breaks down starch to the disaccharide maltose (a glucose dimer) and other small carbohydrate molecules (oligosaccharides). Digestion is completed by

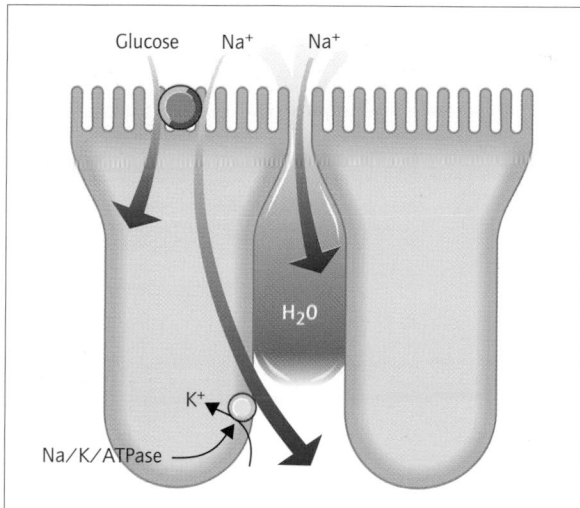

Figure 10.8 Glucose-stimulated sodium absorption in the jejunum. Glucose and sodium are transported into the cell on a 'common carrier' and the sodium is actively extruded at the basolateral membrane. Water flowing through the tight junctions in response to the osmotic pressure gradient created by solute movement sweeps more sodium up by 'solvent drag'.

di- and oligosaccharidases in the microvilli to produce the monosaccharides glucose, galactose and fructose, which are then transported into the enterocytes.

Protein. Polypeptides, produced by gastric secretions acting on protein, are further broken down to release free amino acids and oligopeptides by peptidases (e.g. trypsin, chymotrypsin and elastase) secreted by the pancreas. These protein breakdown products are then actively transported across the mucosa.

Water and electrolytes. In the jejunum, **sodium** absorption occurs by:
● Solvent drag (water flow-mediated) secondary to monosaccharide absorption (Fig. 10.8)
● Glucose- and amino acid-stimulated active absorption (Fig. 10.8)
● Bicarbonate-stimulated sodium–hydrogen exchange
● Electrogenic active transport

Chloride is absorbed passively down electrical potential and concentration gradients. In the ileum, electroneutral sodium–chloride absorption results from parallel ion exchanges (sodium–hydrogen and chloride–bicarbonate).

Water and electrolyte transport are normally controlled by local neural and paracrine factors (see p. 652) as well as luminal fatty acid and bile salt concentrations. In inflammatory diseases, soluble mediators such as prostaglandins become important in inducing diarrhoea, which

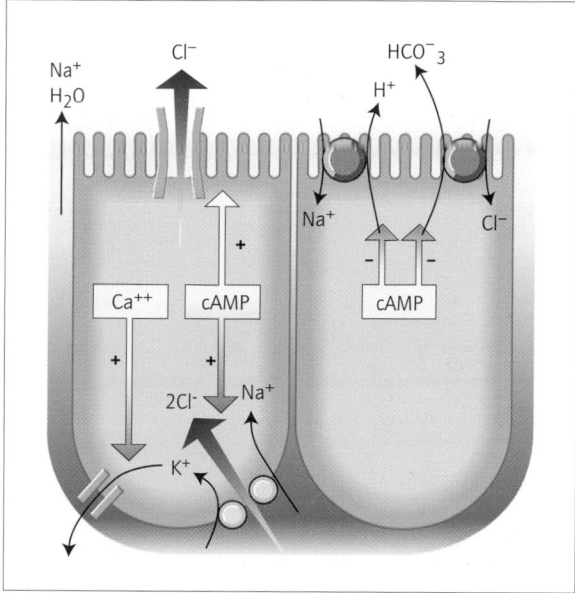

Figure 10.9 Ionic basis of secretion. Three events occur during secretion: (i) sodium chloride uptake (via double ion exchangers) is inhibited (right-hand epithelial cell); (ii) a chloride conductance (anion channel) is opened in the apical membrane; and (iii) chloride uptake at the basolateral side of the cell is stimulated via a triple Na, 2Cl, K uptake process. The opening of a K^+ channel in the basolateral membrane allows K^+ to escape and enhances uptake via the Na, 2Cl, K cotransporter. Na^+ and water accompany the Cl^- by passing between enterocytes down the electrochemical gradient.

occurs when there is either reduced intestinal water and electrolyte absorption or active secretion (Fig. 10.9).

Calcium is absorbed both actively and passively throughout the small intestine.

Miscellaneous. Folic acid, iron and vitamins A, B, C and D are absorbed mainly by the jejunum and proximal ileum. Vitamin B_{12} and conjugated bile salts are absorbed only by the terminal ileum: surgery or pathology (e.g. Crohn's disease) affecting this part of the gut (Fig. 10.10) may lead to:
● Vitamin B_{12} malabsorption
● Reduced bile recycling, leading to steatorrhoea and reduced absorption of fat-soluble vitamins (A, D, E and K)
● Diarrhoea caused by the secretory effect of unabsorbed bile salts on colonic mucosa
● Oxalate renal stones, because unabsorbed bile salts increase colonic absorption of dietary oxalate

Immunological protection

Gut-associated lymphoid tissue provides local and sys-

10

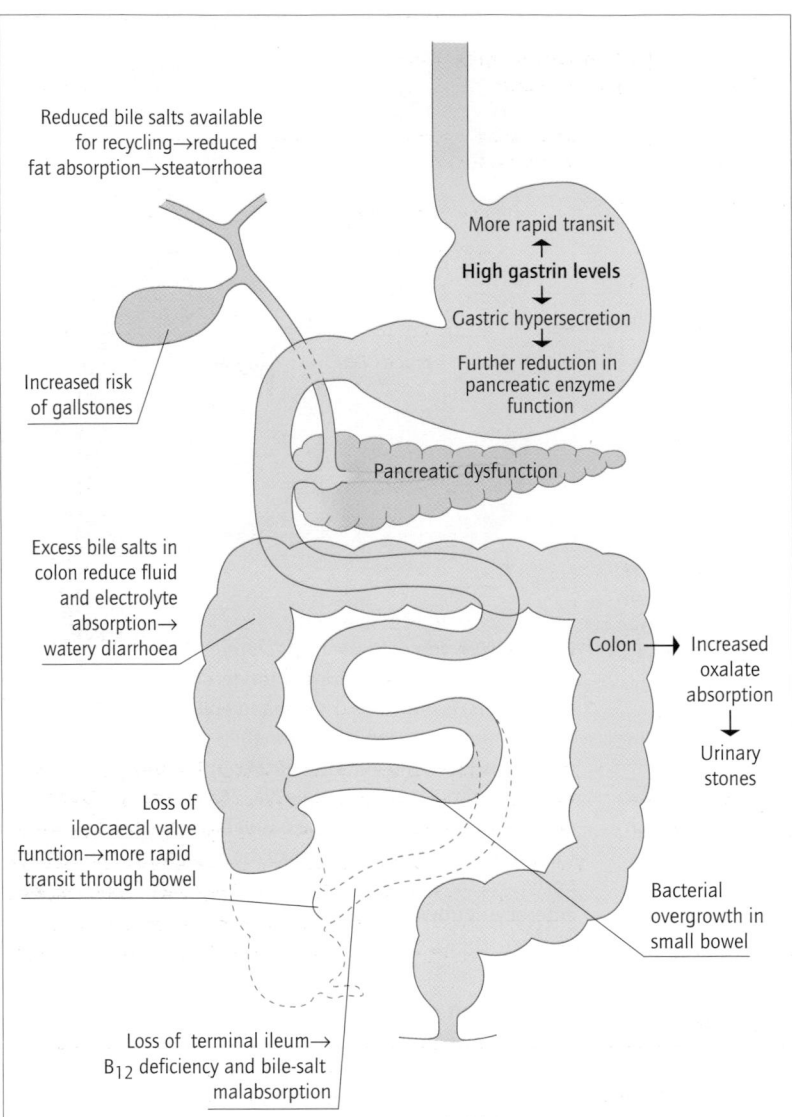

Reduced bile salts available for recycling→reduced fat absorption→steatorrhoea

More rapid transit
↑
High gastrin levels
↓
Gastric hypersecretion
↓
Further reduction in pancreatic enzyme function

Increased risk of gallstones

Pancreatic dysfunction

Excess bile salts in colon reduce fluid and electrolyte absorption→ watery diarrhoea

Colon → Increased oxalate absorption
↓
Urinary stones

Loss of ileocaecal valve function→more rapid transit through bowel

Bacterial overgrowth in small bowel

Loss of terminal ileum→ B_{12} deficiency and bile-salt malabsorption

Figure 10.10 Consequences of surgery or disease affecting the terminal ileum. Terminal ileal disease (e.g. Crohn's disease) or resection leads to bile-salt malabsorption. This results in steatorrhoea (because of bile-salt deficiency in the small bowel), diarrhoea (because of colonic secretion of water and electrolytes), gallstones (because of bile-salt deficiency) and hyperoxaluria (because of bile-salt-induced colonic hyperabsorption of dietary oxalate).

temic protection against luminal antigens and microorganisms (Fig. 10.11).

Local immunity is provided by secretory immunoglobulin A (IgA) and, to a lesser extent, by IgM, IgG and IgE, together with lamina proprial macrophages, neutrophils, mast cells, eosinophils and Paneth cells (Fig. 10.12). These cells are situated at the base of the small intestinal crypts and secrete antibacterial substances (e.g. defensins and phospholipase A_2).

Neuroendocrine function

Regulatory peptides are present in the gut and brain and are involved in endocrine (systemic), paracrine (local intercellular) and neurocrine (synaptic, peptidergic)

transmission, which modify gut function (Table 10.2). These peptides are secreted by 'apud' (amine precursor, uptake and decarboxylation) cells, which share a common embryological origin in the neural crest.

Motor function

Movement of chyme in the small bowel results from cyclical contractions of smooth muscle initiated by depolarization of the muscle membrane (slow waves). Motility is under neural and humoral control (Table 10.2), being influenced, for example, by meals. Abnormal motility patterns can be induced in volunteers by stress, and may be one factor in the aetiology of symptoms in functional bowel conditions such as irritable bowel syndrome.

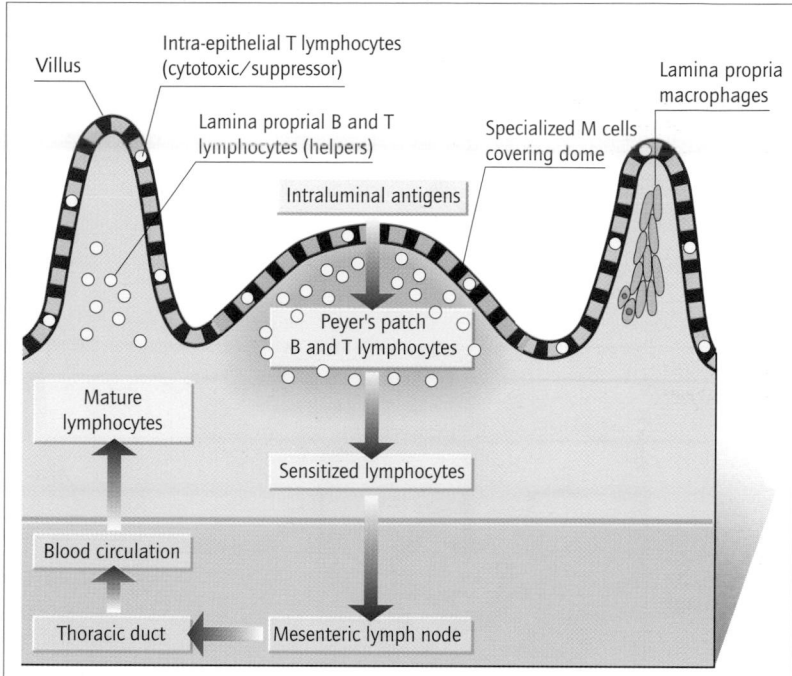

Figure 10.11 Gut-associated lymphoid tissue. Lymphocytes are found mainly in the epithelium, lamina propria and Peyer's patches. Peyer's patches are covered by specialized flattened M cells containing pinocytic vesicles to facilitate transfer of antigen from the gut lumen to sensitize lymphocytes. These lymphocytes migrate to the local lymph nodes and then return via the systemic circulation to the gut mucosa as mature lymphocytes and IgA-secreting cells.

Large intestine

The large intestine has special absorptive and motor mechanisms to enable it to form a soft stool for controlled evacuation.

Absorption of water and electrolytes

Sodium is absorbed actively against a concentration gradient, creating an electrical potential difference across the mucosa of −40 mV (lumen negative). **Chloride** is absorbed in a neutral anion exchange process for bicarbonate. **Potassium** accumulates in the lumen by passive movement down the electrical gradient, some active secretion, and loss in mucus and desquamated cells. **Water** is absorbed passively with sodium as for the small

Table 10.2 Examples of gastrointestinal regulatory peptides

Peptide	Locations	Function	Conditions associated with raised levels
Gastrin	Antral G cells, duodenum, pancreas	Stimulates acid release and gut hypertrophy, inhibits small gut absorption. Promotes gut motility	*Very high*—gastrinoma, pernicious anaemia *Moderately raised*—renal failure, vagotomy, proton pump inhibitors
Cholecystokinin, pancreozymin	Upper small gut, colon, brain	Stimulates pancreatic enzyme secretion and gall bladder contraction	
Secretin	Upper small gut	Stimulates pancreatic bicarbonate secretion	
Vasoactive intestinal polypeptide (VIP)	Throughout gut, brain	Stimulates small gut secretion	VIPoma (WDHA syndrome*)
Somatostatin	Upper gut, pancreas	Inhibits gastrin, insulin, and growth hormone release. Inhibits gut motility	Somatostatinoma

* WDHA, watery diarrhoea, hypokalaemia and achlorhydria.

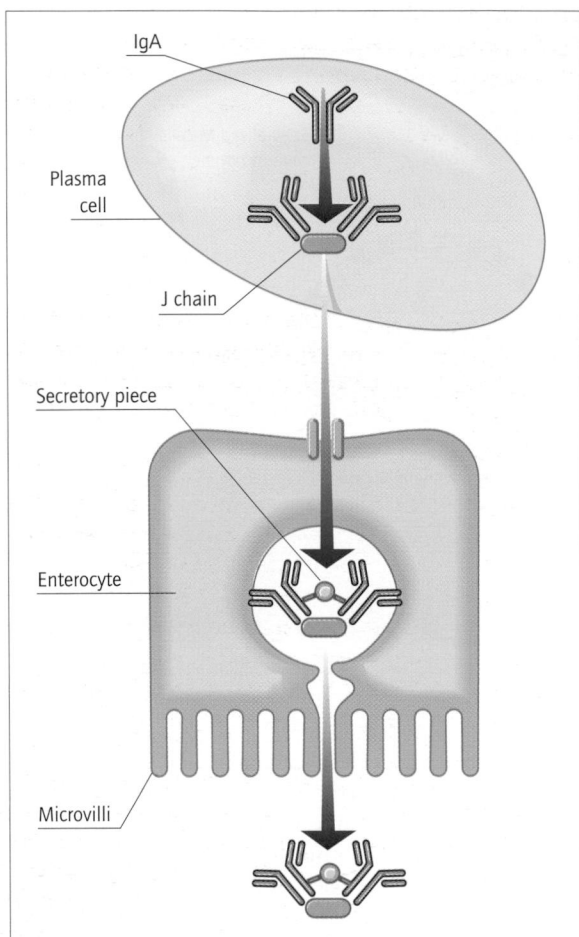

Figure 10.12 Secretory IgA. In plasma cells two molecules of monomeric IgA are joined together by a J chain to form a dimer. This enters enterocytes through gaps in the basement membrane. Within enterocytes secretory piece is added to form secretory IgA. Secretory IgA then enters the gut lumen by pinocytosis. Secretory piece facilitates transepithelial transfer of dimeric IgA and prevents its intraluminal proteolysis. Secretory IgA has an important role in local immunity to bacteria and viruses, and in regulating antigen absorption, but the precise mechanisms are unclear. Secretory IgA is later reabsorbed for recirculation via the bile, where it may help to maintain sterility.

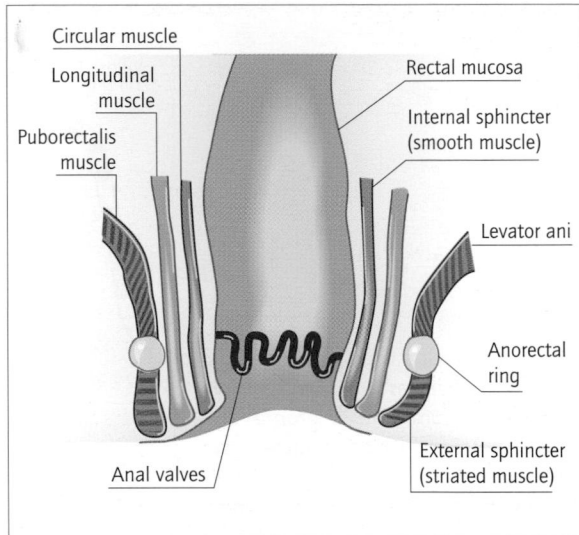

Figure 10.13 Functional anatomy of the anus and rectum. Continence depends on: (i) sustained voluntary contraction of the external sphincter and levator ani; (ii) involuntary maintenance of internal sphincter tone to keep the anal canal closed; (iii) maintenance of the anorectal angle by puborectalis; and (iv) the creation of a flap valve by the intra-abdominal pressure exerted on the anterior rectal wall.

Motor function

Colonic contractions are either segmental, in which mixing of contents but no forward flow occurs, or propulsive. Contractions are stimulated by the entry of ileal effluent into the caecum, which in turn is controlled by a high-pressure zone at the ileocaecal valve. The time taken for material to pass from caecum to anus normally varies from 12 to 48 h, depending on a number of factors including dietary fibre intake, absorptive and motor function, and drugs. Fast transit times from caecum to rectum reduce the amount of fluid that can be reabsorbed and predispose to diarrhoea. Conversely, slow colonic transit times predispose to constipation. Continence is maintained by a number of factors, which are illustrated in Fig. 10.13. The processes involved in normal defecation are complex, involving a sequence of events that are initiated by the entry of stool into the rectum. Usually the rectum is empty. After meals, the sigmoid colon contracts (gastrocolic reflex), pushing its contents into the rectum, and stimulating stretch receptors in the levator ani. Defecation occurs by:

- Conscious relaxation of levator ani and the external anal sphincter
- The Valsalva manoeuvre to increase intra-abdominal pressure
- Reflex relaxation of the internal sphincter

intestine. Factors modulating colonic salt and water transport resemble those in the small bowel (see p. 651). The normal large bowel has a remarkable reserve capacity, being able to absorb up to 4000 ml/day ileal effluent. This illustrates the critical role of the colon in the pathogenesis of diarrhoea and maintenance of continence.

Roles of colonic bacteria

These include:

- Metabolism, for example of ammonia, bile salts (see Fig. 10.7) and drugs e.g. activation of sulfasalazine (see p. 739)
- Synthesis of vitamin K
- Fermentation of dietary fibre to short-chain fatty acids—these are absorbed passively, stimulating sodium absorption, and providing an energy source for the colonic mucosa
- Modulation of colonic mucosal function. Changes in colonic flora may lead to altered fibre digestion and possibly in some patients to symptoms of irritable bowel syndrome; they may also provoke subtle changes in mucosal immunology. The oral administration of 'probiotic' bacteria such as *Lactobacillus*, which are thought to have a beneficial effect on colonic function, is currently under evaluation for the treatment of both irritable bowel syndrome and inflammatory bowel disease

Approach to the patient

The overall aims of the history and examination in gastroenterology are shown in HISTORY & EXAMINATION BOX 10.1.

History & Examination 10.1:
Questions to be addressed by the history and examination in gastroenterology

What are the symptoms?
What are the signs?
What is the differential diagnosis?
What is the site, extent and severity of the problem?
Are there any complications?
What are the appropriate investigations?
What is the appropriate treatment?
Are unnecessary investigations and treatments being avoided?
What is the prognosis?
What is the patient's understanding of his or her symptoms?
What are the patient's expectations of treatment?

History

As in other areas of medicine, the history is the most important factor in achieving a diagnosis. Taking into account the factors below, the aim is to formulate a differential diagnosis and avoid unnecessary investigations. It is important to consider why the patient is presenting at a particular time. Because many symptoms in gastroenterology may have no specific cause or 'curative' treatment, it is important to reassure patients about what their symptoms mean, and address any concerns they may have about their illness and its investigation. Patients are often happy to live with their symptoms if the physiological basis of them is explained, and specific fears (often of underlying cancer) addressed.

General features in the structured history of particular relevance to gastrointestinal disease are presented first, followed by a specific approach to common presenting symptoms.

About the patient

Age

Knowing the typical age of presentation of common gastrointestinal conditions helps in producing a sensible differential diagnosis (Table 10.3). Some congenital conditions present exclusively in the first few weeks of life (e.g. pyloric stenosis) while others may also present later (e.g. cystic fibrosis, Hirschsprung's disease). With the exception of some specific familial conditions (e.g. polyposis coli; see p. 729), gastrointestinal cancers are extremely rare in patients under 45 years. This fact underpins many management strategies in gastroenterology, such as recommending early endoscopy for investigation of uncomplicated dyspepsia only in those over 45 years (see p. 660).

Sex

Irritable bowel syndrome, slow transit constipation, inflammatory bowel disease and gastric ulcer are more common in women, duodenal ulcer and Barrett's oesophagus in men. However, the ratios are insufficient to allow a different approach to symptoms based on the patient's gender.

Ethnicity

Some disorders are more common in certain ethnic groups:

- *Gastric cancer:* more common in Japanese people than in white people
- *Inflammatory bowel disease:* more common in Jews than in other white people
- *Lactose intolerance:* more common in non-whites
- *Coeliac disease:* more common in Celts (the highest worldwide incidence is in Ireland)

Some geographical variations in disease prevalence are caused by local environmental factors such as diet, rather

Table 10.3 Relative incidence* of common gastrointestinal disorders by age group

	Children	Adults		
		20–40 years	40–60 years	60+ years
Appendicitis	+ +	+		
Coeliac disease	+ + +	+ +	+	+
Inflammatory bowel disease	+	+ + +	+	+ +
AIDS		+ +	+	
Peptic ulcer		+ +	+ + +	+ + +
Gastro-oesophageal reflux		+ +	+ + +	+ + +
Irritable bowel syndrome	+	+ + +	+ +	+
Upper gastrointestinal cancer			+	+ +
Lower gastrointestinal cancer			+	+ +
Diverticular disease			+	+ +
Drug side-effects				+

* NB, these relativities only apply *within* each disease row, not *between* different diseases (e.g. appendicitis is more common in children than appendicitis in 20–40-year-olds; however, in children coeliac disease is not more common than appendicitis).

than ethnicity *per se* (e.g. tuberculosis in Asia and squamous oesophageal cancer in parts of China)

History of the presenting complaint

Attempt to build a picture of how the symptoms have evolved with time. Rapid or steady progression of a symptom (e.g. dysphagia) fits with an underlying malignancy, whereas recurrent symptoms with periods of normality in between, or symptoms stable over many years argues for functional or benign disease. Establish how symptoms relate to daily activities: to timing and content of meals, posture (for reflux symptoms), timing of defecation or to external stresses. Assess the onset in relation to any changes in job, lifestyle, diet or medication.

Past medical history

Many gastrointestinal diseases chronically relapse and remit. Patients may present with new symptoms 10 years or more after a previous diagnosis of peptic ulceration or Crohn's disease. A past history of any malignancy may be relevant. Symptoms from recurrence of gastrointestinal cancers typically occur in the first few years after treatment. Additionally, previous abdominal surgery may explain new presenting symptoms:

- Dyspepsia in a person who has had a gastrectomy may be caused by recurrent ulceration or cancer
- Diarrhoea or steatorrhoea may be caused by previous gastrectomy, vagotomy, small bowel resection or pancreatectomy
- Abdominal pain may be caused by adhesions

Social history

This may be directly relevant to specific gastrointestinal symptoms (e.g. dyspepsia to smoking, alcohol or caffeine, and diarrhoea to caffeine or alcohol). Stresses of home and work life commonly have a role in the cause of functional gastrointestinal symptoms. Patients may be stressed by specific symptoms (e.g. fear of incontinence in conditions associated with diarrhoea and/or urgency), and so addressing these specific concerns is useful in management. Traumatic childhood events may underlie functional symptomatology—successful exploration of such areas requires advanced consultation skills; conversely, unskilled questioning in this area can destroy the doctor–patient relationship. Patients may not talk about such areas during initial consultations, and information from the patient's GP can be vital in highlighting these elements of the history. Patients, particularly those with inflammatory bowel disease and gastrointestinal cancers, are often concerned about the effect of disease on sexual function. Embarrassment on both sides may inhibit discussion of these issues—use of specific questioning, provision of written information, and input from suitably trained gastrointestinal nurse specialists can be helpful.

Diet

A dietary history is important. Anaemia and weight loss can result from a poor intake (e.g. vegetarians, the elderly living alone, rejection of food in institutions). A diet high in cereal, fruit or vegetable fibre may provoke symptoms in patients with mechanical bowel obstruction or the irritable bowel syndrome. Carbonated drinks, diet products and health products (e.g. multivitamins with iron) are amongst many dietary factors that may provoke gastrointestinal symptoms. The use of specific diets in managing gastrointestinal disease is discussed below.

Gynaecological and obstetric history

Symptoms from some gynaecological conditions (e.g. pelvic inflammatory disease, endometriosis) overlap with gastrointestinal problems and, in particular, the irritable bowel syndrome—often dual investigation is indicated. Traumatic labour can cause pelvic muscle and nerve injury and lead to problems with defecation (especially faecal incontinence). A history of gynaecological and obstetric interventions should be taken, and any relationship of symptoms to menstrual cycle noted.

Drug history

Common drug-induced gastrointestinal problems:
- *Dyspepsia, nausea, vomiting* (hundreds of drugs implicated; common culprits shown in Table 10.4)

Table 10.4 Causes of dyspepsia (most common causes in capital letters)

Oesophageal
OESOPHAGITIS, carcinoma, motility disorder

Gastric
ULCER, GASTRITIS, motility disorder, carcinoma

Duodenal
ULCER, DUODENITIS

Gall bladder
Gallstones

Pancreas
Pancreatitis, carcinoma

Liver
Hepatitis, metastases

Intestine
Irritable bowel syndrome, ischaemia, transverse colon carcinoma

Lifestyle
Certain foods (e.g. fatty, spicy), alcohol, smoking, coffee

Metabolic
Hypercalcaemia

Psychogenic
Stress, depression, anxiety

Drugs
NSAIDs, corticosteroids, anticholinergics, antiparkinsonian drugs, antidepressants, antidiabetics, antibiotics, iron, potassium, digoxin

Other
FUNCTIONAL*

* No disease found to explain the symptoms—will include patients with unrecognized psychogenic problems (see discussion of functional vs. organic gastrointestinal symptoms on p. 645).

- *Peptic ulcer:* aspirin, NSAIDs
- *Gastrointestinal bleeding:* aspirin, NSAIDs, warfarin
- *Vomiting:* opiates, digoxin, NSAIDs
- *Diarrhoea:* NSAIDs, antibiotics, statins, laxatives, colchicine, magnesium-containing antacids
- *Constipation:* opiates, iron, antidepressants, anticholinergics, aluminium-containing antacids

Family history

The risk of peptic ulceration, inflammatory bowel disease or coeliac disease is increased if the patient has an affected family member. The risks of developing colorectal cancer are directly linked to the number of close relatives with the disease, and the age they developed the disease (see p. 733).

Approach to common gastrointestinal symptoms

The important questions to ask in response to specific gastrointestinal symptoms are listed in HISTORY & EXAMINATION BOX 10.2. The causes of and general approach to each of these common symptoms are discussed below.

Dysphagia

Dysphagia is difficulty in swallowing; odynophagia means painful swallowing. The patient's perception of the level of obstruction to swallowing is often inaccurate. Dysphagia is highly predictive of oesophageal disease, and urgent investigation by barium swallow (see p. 675) or gastroscopy (see p. 670) is required to exclude cancer.

Causes
Dysphagia has many causes (Table 10.5), as swallowing can be affected by disorders of the central nervous system (CNS), mouth, pharynx, neck and mediastinum as well as oesophagus and stomach. The most common causes are severe reflux oesophagitis, peptic stricture and malignancy. A history of ingested foreign body is important because if impaction in the oesophagus is the cause of the dysphagia, urgent endoscopy is indicated. Left untreated, impacted foreign bodies may erode through the wall of the oesophagus.

Difficulty with solids more than liquids suggests a mechanical cause, a progressive story pointing to neoplasia. In neurological and motility disorders, there may be more trouble with liquids, and regurgitation into the back of the nose is often a feature. Associated symptoms often give a clue to the diagnosis (e.g. chronic heartburn suggests a peptic stricture).

Heartburn

Heartburn is a burning substernal discomfort, sometimes radiating to the epigastrium, jaws, arms and back. When

Gastrointestinal symptoms

Dysphagia

Do you have difficulty swallowing?

How long has this been going on for?

Is it worse for liquids or solids?

Is it getting worse?

Does liquid run up the back of your nose?

Do you have heartburn?

Is your weight steady?

Heartburn

Is it worse after heavy meals, fatty foods, alcohol, in bed at night or on bending down?

Does fluid regurgitate into your mouth?

Do you vomit?

Has your weight increased recently?

Do you have any difficulty swallowing?

Dyspepsia

How long have you had the pain?

Where do you feel it?

Does it go into your chest or back?

Is it intermittent or always present?

When do you get it?

For how long does it last?

How severe is it?

Is it related to eating?

Does it wake you at night?

Does anything make it better or worse?

Do antacids make any difference?

Do you have any associated symptoms, such as loss of appetite, difficulty in swallowing, vomiting, weight loss or change of bowel habit?

Acute (recent onset) severe abdominal pain

Where is the pain?

Does the pain radiate anywhere?

Did the pain start suddenly or develop over a few hours?

Is the pain constant and does it make you want to keep still, or is it colicky, making you restless?

Have you vomited?

Have you had diarrhoea or are you constipated?

Have you noticed any rectal bleeding?

Are you menstruating regularly?

Do you have a vaginal discharge?

Do you have any pain on passing urine or have you noticed any blood in your urine?

Chronic abdominal pain

How long have you had pain?

Where is the pain?

Does it radiate anywhere?

Is the pain moderate or severe?

Is the pain intermittent or continuous?

Is the pain constant or colicky?

Does the pain wake you at night?

Is it related to meals, defecation or menstruation?

Is your weight steady, increasing or decreasing?

How is your appetite?

Have you had any vomiting?

How are your bowels—have you had any constipation or diarrhoea, or noticed any blood?

Are there any relieving factors?

Vomiting

What does the vomit look like?—undigested food, blood, coffee grounds, green bile, yesterday's food, faeculent material?

How much do you vomit?—an eggcup, a teacup, a bucket?

Is the vomit projectile?—does it shoot out vigorously?

How long did the vomiting last?—a few hours, days, weeks?

Do you vomit at particular times of the day?

Do you have any associated symptoms?—dyspepsia, weight loss, diarrhoea, chest pain, headache, vertigo, deafness, depression, anxiety?

Diarrhoea or steatorrhoea

How often are your bowels open?

How long have you had the diarrhoea?

Did it start suddenly or gradually?

Is the stool watery or mushy?

What colour is the stool?

Does it flush easily?

Is there blood, pus or mucus with the stool?

Do any family members or friends have diarrhoea?

Do you have any eye, skin or joint problems?

Have you had any fever or weight loss?

Constipation

How often are your bowels open?

For how long have you been constipated?

Are there any accompanying symptoms?—anal pain, rectal bleeding, diarrhoea?

Is your weight steady?

What do you eat normally? Do you eat wholemeal bread, cereal, vegetables and fruit?

Past medical history

Have you had any similar symptoms in the past?

Have you had any abdominal surgery?

Do you have any other illnesses (e.g. diabetes)?

Personal history

Do you smoke?

How much alcohol do you drink?

Drug, family and social history

What medication do you take?

Has any family member had or got a similar illness?

What is your job?

Do you have any work and/or domestic problems? —unemployment, bereavement, divorce?

Have you been abroad recently?

What is your sexual preference?

10

Table 10.5 Causes of dysphagia (most common causes in capital letters)

Type of disorder	Examples
Oral disorders	Ulcers, stomatitis, neoplasm
Pharyngeal disorders	Pharyngitis, pouch, neoplasm
Disorders causing extrinsic oesophageal compression	Lymphadenopathy (usually neoplastic), aortic aneurysm, neoplasms (usually carcinoma of the bronchus), left atrial enlargement
Mechanical oesophageal disorders	OESOPHAGITIS, PEPTIC STRICTURE, CARCINOMA, foreign body impaction
Motility disorders of the oesophagus	Achalasia, spasm
Disorders of the stomach	CARCINOMA OF THE GASTRIC CARDIA

associated with regurgitation of gastric contents and relief with antacids, a diagnosis of gastro-oesophageal reflux disease (GORD; see p. 692) is extremely likely. Symptoms are often worsened by anything that increases the intragastric pressure (stooping, lying down, straining, tight clothing and weight gain) and by fatty foods, smoking, spirits, caffeine and hot drinks.

Dyspepsia

The symptom is extremely common, occurring in approximately 25% of the population each year, although most do not consult their doctor. Definitions of dyspepsia (or indigestion) are vague (e.g. food- or drink-related upper abdominal or lower chest pain or discomfort). While usually associated with oesophageal, gastric or duodenal disease, symptoms that could be classed as 'dyspepsia' can arise from the colon, biliary system, pancreas and small bowel: thus, there is an extensive differential diagnosis (Table 10.3). Symptoms triggered during or soon after eating and/or relieved by antacids or acid-suppressant medication suggest a cause in the upper gastrointestinal tract.

Causes

The mechanisms causing dyspepsia are multifactorial and include mucosal damage (e.g. peptic ulcer, cancers); mucosal inflammation (e.g. caused by *Helicobacter pylori* infection, drugs, acid, bile); disordered motility and distension; food intolerance; and increased visceral sensitivity (which can be caused by stress) leading to perception of normal events in the gastrointestinal tract as painful. Apart from features associated with GORD (see p. 692), dyspeptic symptoms are non-specific for particular diagnoses. An empirical approach to diagnosis and treatment is therefore taken, investigating patients aged over 45 years by gastroscopy and managing those under 45 years initially on the basis of their *H. pylori* status (Fig. 10.14). The exceptions to this approach are patients with 'alarm symptoms', where urgent investigation is warranted whatever the patient's age. Recent evidence suggests that some of the traditional 'alarm' symptoms are strongly predictive of significant upper gastrointestinal pathology

(dysphagia, haematemesis, melaena and anaemia), while others are not (weight loss, anorexia and vomiting). Intermittent attacks of severe pain lasting a few hours, radiating to the back and associated with vomiting and sweating suggest biliary colic (see p. 635) and abdominal ultrasound is required.

Abdominal pain

The 'acute abdomen' is easy to identify, with a recent onset of severe continuous or colicky pain in a sick patient, often associated with vomiting, guarding, pyrexia, leucocytosis and raised inflammatory markers such as C-reactive protein. The condition requires urgent admission for prompt surgical assessment. Questions to ask the patient with acute abdominal pain are listed in HISTORY & EXAMINATION BOX 10.2, while Table 10.6 shows how these points in the history help to differentiate between the most common causes of the acute abdomen.

Chronic abdominal pain is a frequent presenting complaint to hospital gastrointestinal clinics. It can be difficult to diagnose, with no organic illness found in a high proportion of cases. The possible differential diagnosis is wide (Tables 10.7 and 10.8). The site and nature of the pain often give little discriminatory diagnostic information (Table 10.9). Common diagnostic clues are onset during or soon after meals, suggesting a gastric or biliary cause; response to antacids or acid-suppressant medication, suggesting oesophageal, gastric or duodenal disease; periods of constant right upper quadrant pain lasting several hours with long symptom-free periods, suggesting biliary colic caused by gallstones; and altered defecation pattern or relief of pain with defecation, suggesting a colonic cause. Continuous pain, night waking, weight loss, anaemia and raised inflammatory markers suggest serious underlying organic disease. Abdominal pain may be visceral, parietal, referred or psychogenic in origin.

Visceral abdominal pain. This can result from obstruction, distension, inflammation, ischaemia or neoplastic infiltration of a viscus. It is poorly localized and of variable character. Obstructive pain is characteristically colicky

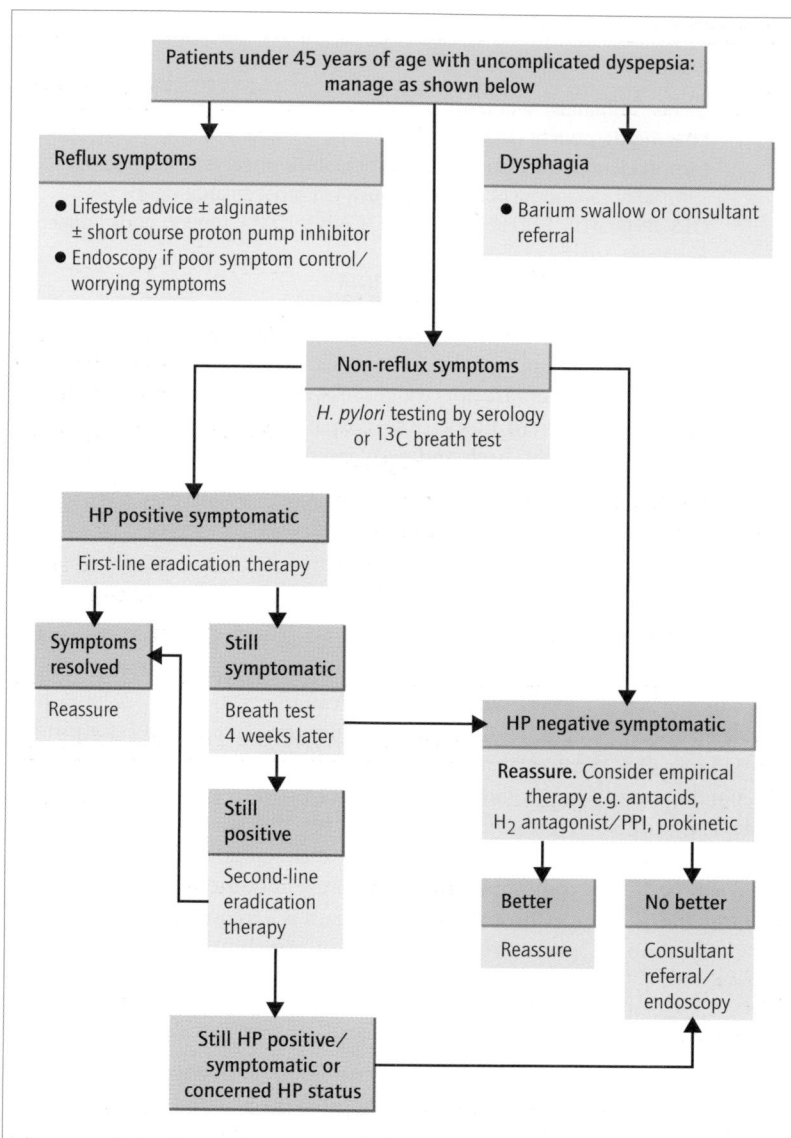

Figure 10.14 Example of a management algorithm provided for GPs to help with management of dyspepsia in patients under 45 years of age. Risk of cancer is very low, and initial treatment is empirical based upon the results of *Helicobacter pylori* testing.

(cramping, coming in waves) and causes the patient to be restless. The common surface area markings for visceral pain from various organs is shown in Fig. 10.15—however, there is a wide variation in practice.

Parietal abdominal pain. This is sharp and discrete, and worse on moving. It is accompanied by rebound tenderness and guarding. It results from involvement of the parietal peritoneum, usually by inflammation. Causes include appendicitis, a perforated viscus and pancreatitis.

Referred pain. This is felt in skin or muscles supplied by the same segment of the spinal cord as that receiving the sympathetic afferents from a diseased abdominal viscus.

Examples of this are pain between the shoulder blades in biliary colic, and thigh pain caused by colonic distension.

Psychogenic/functional abdominal pain. This is variable in character and site. There is no structural abnormality of the gut detectable by standard tests. Likely mechanisms include disordered gastrointestinal motility, hypersensitivity of visceral pain pathways and altered central processing of signals from the gut. Each of these mechanisms has been demonstrated in research settings, and shown to be influenced by physical and emotional stress.

Vomiting

Vomiting is forceful ejection of gastric contents, usually

Table 10.6 Diagnostic features of acute abdominal pain

	Site	Radiation	Intensity	Character	Exacerbating factors	Onset	Other symptoms
Acute appendicitis	Central abdomen then right iliac fossa	No	Moderate	Constant	Movement, coughing	Gradual	Anorexia, fever
Acute diverticulitis	Lower abdomen, usually left iliac fossa	No	Moderate	Constant	Movement, coughing	Gradual	Fever, change in bowel habit
Perforated intestine	Upper abdomen, then generalized	No	Severe	Constant	Movement, coughing	Sudden	Shock, fever
Intestinal obstruction	Central abdomen	No	Severe	Colicky	Food	Gradual	Vomiting if high small bowel, constipation
Acute pancreatitis	Upper abdomen, then generalized	Back	Severe	Constant	Movement, coughing	Sudden	Vomiting, shock
Acute cholecystitis	Right upper quadrant	Between the scapulae	Moderate/ severe	Constant	Inspiration, coughing	Gradual	Vomiting, fever, jaundice
Acute salpingitis	Lower abdomen	Back, groin	Moderate	Constant	Movement	Gradual	Fever, vaginal discharge
Renal colic	Unilateral loin	Ipsilateral groin	Severe	Colicky	None	Sudden	Vomiting

Table 10.7 Causes of abdominal pain caused by disease of intra-abdominal organs (most common causes in capital letters)

Type of disorder	Cause
1 *Distension/tension*	
Obstruction	
Intestinal	TUMOUR, HERNIA, ADHESIONS, volvulus, intussusception, faecal impaction
Biliary	GALLSTONE, TUMOUR, stricture, haemobilia
Ureteric	RENAL STONE
Motility	IRRITABLE BOWEL SYNDROME
Hepatic capsule distension	HEPATITIS, Budd–Chiari syndrome
Gynaecological	Ectopic pregnancy
2 *Inflammation*	
Generalized peritonitis	PERFORATED VISCUS (peptic ulcer, diverticulum, gall bladder), ruptured ovarian cyst
Localized peritonitis	APPENDICITIS, DIVERTICULITIS, PANCREATITIS, CHOLECYSTITIS, SALPINGITIS, abscess
Other infection	ASCENDING URINARY TRACT INFECTION, abdominal tuberculosis
Inflamed viscus	PEPTIC ULCER, NSAID or other drug-induced mucosal injury, INFLAMMATORY BOWEL DISEASE
Mesenteric adenitis	
3 *Ischaemia*	
Mesenteric angina/infarction	Atheroma (thrombosis, embolus), arteritis
Splenic infarction	
Torsion	Ovarian cyst, testicle
Tumour necrosis	Hepatoma, fibroid/liver metastases

preceded by nausea. The vomiting centre is the medulla, which controls the integrated reflex of vomiting.

Causes

Causes are listed in Table 10.10. Drug-induced vomiting may be caused by direct gastric irritation, or the effects of drugs on the CNS pathways (vomiting centre and the chemoreceptor trigger zone in the floor of the fourth ventricle). Non-gastrointestinal causes are likely to induce vomiting through CNS effects alone.

10

Site/type of disorder	Cause
Retroperitoneal	Aortic aneurysm, neoplasia
Thoracic	Basal pneumonia, myocardial infarction
Neurological	Herpes zoster, spinal arthritis, tabes dorsalis
Metabolic	Diabetic ketoacidosis, hypercalcaemia, hypoadrenalism, uraemia, porphyria, hypertriglycerideraemia, familial Mediterranean fever
Haematological	Sickle cell disease, paroxysmal nocturnal haemoglobinuria, haemorrhagic diathesis
Immunological	Angioneurotic oedema
Toxins	Lead poisoning
Drugs	Chronic high dose usage of opiate drug, part of acute opiate withdrawal syndrome
Psychogenic	Depression, anxiety, Munchausen's syndrome, hypochondriasis

Table 10.8 Causes of abdominal pain referred from sites outside the abdominal cavity, or caused by systemic medical disease

Table 10.9 Typical features of some conditions that cause chronic or recurrent abdominal pain

	Reflux oesophagitis	Gastric carcinoma	Peptic ulcer	Biliary colic
Site	Retrosternal, epigastrium	Epigastrium	Epigastrium	Epigastrium/right upper quadrant
Radiation (sometimes)	Neck, back, arms	Back	Back	Back, T7 dermatome on right
Intensity	Moderate	Moderate	Moderate	Moderate to severe
Character	Burning, rising up	Constant	Constant	Constant, lasting several hours
Exacerbating factors	Lying, stooping	Food	Food or fasting	
Relieving factors	Antacids	Antacids (sometimes)	Antacids	Potent analgesics
Natural history	Bouts and remissions	Progressive	Bouts and remissions	Bouts and remissions
Associated features	Nausea, regurgitation	Weight loss, vomiting, anorexia, anaemia	Vomiting	Vomiting, sweating

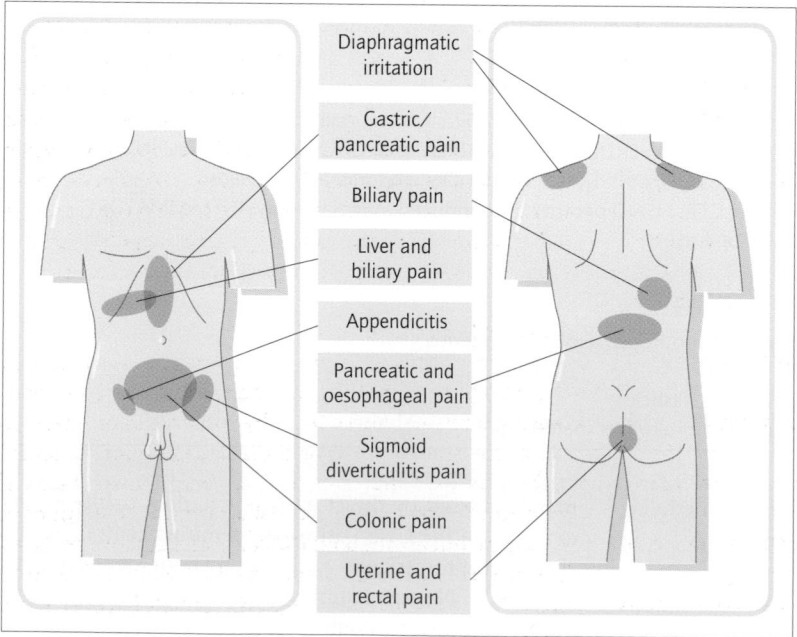

Figure 10.15 Surface markings of radiation of pain from abdominal viscera.

Table 10.10 Causes of vomiting

Gastrointestinal
Disorders of oesophagus, stomach, duodenum (see Table 10.4, p. 657)
Pyloric obstruction, intestinal obstruction, peritonitis, other intra-abdominal causes (see Table 10.7, p. 661)

Iatrogenic
Opiates, anaesthetics, digoxin, cytotoxic drugs, radiotherapy

Metabolic
Diabetic ketoacidosis, uraemia, hypoadrenalism

Vestibular
Ménière's disease, motion sickness, labyrinthitis

Cerebral
Raised intracranial pressure, meningism, migraine

Psychogenic
Anorexia nervosa/bulimia, emotional shock

Other causes
Pregnancy (hyperemesis gravidarum), alcohol, severe pain (e.g. myocardial infarction), poisons

Clues from the history
- *Undigested food:* if vomiting results from regurgitation resulting from achalasia, oesophageal stricture or a pharyngeal pouch
- *Blood or coffee grounds:* results from upper gastrointestinal bleeding; however, bleeding may itself be induced by vomiting (Mallory–Weiss tear)
- *Yesterday's food:* vomited if there is pyloric obstruction
- *Faeculent vomit:* results from a gastrocolic fistula or low intestinal obstruction
- *Large volumes of vomit:* suggest intestinal obstruction
- *Projectile vomiting:* caused by pyloric stenosis or raised intracranial pressure
- *Short-lasting self-limiting vomiting:* characteristic of acute gastroenteritis
- *Early morning vomiting:* a feature of pregnancy, alcohol and raised intracranial pressure
- *Cyclical vomiting:* with normal digestion in between attacks, in an otherwise well patient, suggests a functional cause, as does a history of unexplained vomiting in childhood

Other symptoms which may be present in patients with vomiting:
- *Chest pain:* if the underlying cause is myocardial infarction or oesophagitis
- *Diarrhoea:* if the cause is gastroenteritis or subacute obstruction
- *Early morning headache:* if vomiting is caused by raised intracranial pressure or migraine

- *Vertigo and deafness:* if caused by a labyrinthine disorder
- *Psychiatric symptoms and signs:* if the underlying cause is anorexia nervosa or bulimia

Anorexia

Anorexia is diminution or loss of appetite. It probably results from interference with appetite control centres in the hypothalamus.

Common causes of anorexia:
- *Psychiatric:* depression, anorexia nervosa
- *Neoplastic:* carcinoma of stomach or oesophagus, metastatic cancer
- *Iatrogenic:* drugs, radiotherapy
- *Metabolic:* uraemia, hypercalcaemia, hypopituitarism
- *Infective:* many infections including viral hepatitis, tuberculosis
- *Lifestyle:* excess alcohol, smoking, stress
Other causes are those of dyspepsia (Table 10.3).

Diarrhoea

Diarrhoea is defined as a stool output of more than 200 g/day on an average Western diet, or more than 400 g/day on a high-fibre diet. However, patients' definitions of diarrhoea vary greatly. Diarrhoeal stool is loose and either mushy or watery. It is usually passed more often than usual, the normal range of bowel habit being three times a day to three times a week. People who pass frequent small hard pellets do not have diarrhoea.

An increased faecal weight is caused by an increased water content resulting from either increased secretion (secretory diarrhoea) or reduced absorption of water and electrolytes by the small and/or large intestines. In some patients, the diarrhoea is caused by an excess of osmotically active small molecules in the gut lumen (e.g. malabsorbed lactose in lactase deficiency; see p. 682) and is termed osmotic diarrhoea. In many diseases the mechanism is either poorly understood, or mixed. However, in cases where the cause of diarrhoea is hard to establish, investigations to determine whether a predominant secretory or osmotic mechanism is occurring can be useful to narrow down the diagnostic possibilities (Table 10.11).

Causes of diarrhoea
These are listed in Table 10.12. Diarrhoea caused by altered intestinal motility may be as a result of conditions causing intestinal hurry (e.g. thyrotoxicosis) or intestinal stasis (e.g. systemic sclerosis, diabetic autonomic neuropathy), as the latter can lead to small bowel bacterial overgrowth and subsequent malabsorption. Questions to ask to find out more about the cause of diarrhoea are listed in HISTORY & EXAMINATION BOX 10.2 while Table 10.13 shows how these features help differentiate between some common causes.

10

Table 10.11 Osmotic and secretory diarrhoea—pathophysiology, features and causes

	Osmotic diarrhoea	Secretory diarrhoea
Mechanism	Osmotic action of ingested and/or malabsorbed solutes in the gut lumen prevents absorption of fluid	Intestinal secretion of salt and water, caused by activation of mucosal adenyl cyclase (see Fig. 10.9, p. 651)
Effect of fasting	Stops diarrhoea	Diarrhoea persists
Stool analysis	Osmolality $\geqslant 2 \times$ plasma ($[Na^+] + [K^+]$)	Osmolality $= 2 \times$ plasma ($[Na^+] + [K^+]$)
Causes	Magnesium-containing antacids and lactase deficiency, malabsorption syndromes	Toxin-producing bacteria (e.g. cholera), endocrine tumours (e.g. carcinoid, VIPoma), certain laxatives (e.g. phenolphthalein), bile-salt malabsorption (e.g. ileal resection)

Table 10.12 Causes of diarrhoea (most common causes in capital letters)

Acute
Infective
FOOD POISONING (see p. 751)
VIRAL GASTROENTERITIS (see p. 746)
TRAVELLER'S DIARRHOEA (see p. 746)

DRUG-INDUCED
NSAIDs
Antibiotics (including *Clostridium difficile* causing pseudomembranous colitis)
Cytotoxics

Chronic
Infective
Parasitic/fungal infections
Giardiasis
AIDS ± opportunistic infection

Inflammatory
ULCERATIVE COLITIS
CROHN'S DISEASE

Neoplastic
CARCINOMA OF THE COLON
Endocrine tumours (carcinoid)
Lymphoma

Iatrogenic
Bowel surgery (vagotomy, ileal resection)
Radiation enteritis

Metabolic
Thyrotoxicosis
Diabetic autonomic neuropathy

Other
IRRITABLE BOWEL SYNDROME
ANXIETY
COELIAC DISEASE
SEVERE CONSTIPATION WITH OVERFLOW DIARRHOEA
Laxative abuse
Lactase deficiency

The nature of diarrhoea and associated features may indicate its cause:
- *Watery diarrhoea, particularly with blood:* usually indicates colonic inflammation or cancer
- *Mushy stools:* often indicate a small intestinal disorder
- *Pale, difficult to flush, greasy and particularly smelly stools:* suggest steatorrhoea
- *Family history:* suggests inflammatory bowel disease, coeliac disease or lactase deficiency
- *Associated eye, skin or joint problems:* features of inflammatory bowel disease, Whipple's disease or Behçet's disease
- *Long history over many years:* suggests irritable bowel syndrome
- *Short history over a few days, with sudden onset:* indicates infection
- *Too much alcohol or caffeine:* may cause diarrhoea
- *Weight loss:* suggests an organic cause, and makes diagnoses such as irritable bowel unlikely
- *Drug use* (e.g. laxatives, NSAIDs, antibiotics, iron, statins): may explain diarrhoea
- *Foreign travel:* suggests infection
- *Homosexuality:* associated with an increased risk of HIV infection, which may cause diarrhoea directly or by predisposing to AIDS-related enteral infections (see p. 170).
- *Previous gastrointestinal surgery:* suggests possible malabsorption

Steatorrhoea

Steatorrhoea is stool containing excessive fat (more than 5 g/day on standardized (100 g/day) fat intake). Classically, steatorrhoea is pale, floats, smells offensive and is difficult to flush; however, in practice, inspection is an unreliable way of assessing stool fat content. Causes of steatorrhoea are listed in Table 10.14.

Constipation

Constipation is defined as the passage of hard stools, with

Table 10.13 Typical clinical features of some common conditions associated with diarrhoea

	Irritable bowel syndrome	Ulcerative colitis	Acute infective enteritis	Coeliac disease
Duration	Chronic (intermittent)	Acute or chronic	Acute	Chronic
Stool consistency	Variable	Watery	Watery or mushy	Mushy
Stool volume	Normal	<500 g	<500 g	<500 g
Blood or pus present	No	Yes	Yes or no	No
Mucus present	Yes	Yes	No	No
Urgency/incontinence	Maybe	Yes	Maybe	No
Nocturnal diarrhoea	No	Maybe	Maybe	Maybe
Other features	Abdominal pain, bloating, constipation, psychiatric symptoms	Weight loss, pain, family history, skin/eye/joint symptoms	Weight loss, abdominal pain, vomiting, contact with *Salmonella* infection, foreign travel	Weight loss, bloating, steatorrhoea

Table 10.14 Causes of steatorrhoea (more common causes in capital letters)

	Cause
Luminal factors	
Reduced bile salts	Obstructive jaundice, parenchymal liver disease (cirrhosis)
Reduced pancreatic lipase	CHRONIC PANCREATITIS, CARCINOMA OF THE PANCREAS, cystic fibrosis, pancreatectomy
Bacterial overgrowth	Blind loops (e.g. Billroth II), fistulae, strictures (e.g. Crohn's disease), jejunal diverticulosis, reduced motility (e.g. pseudo-obstruction, radiotherapy, old age), achlorhydria (vagotomy, pernicious anaemia)
Mucosal factors	
Disease	COELIAC DISEASE, CROHN'S DISEASE, tropical sprue, giardiasis, intestinal lymphangiectasia
Surgery	Gastrectomy, intestinal resection
Systemic factors	
Drugs	Colestyramine, Orlistat*

* A drug for weight reduction that inhibits pancreatic lipase and thus reduces digestion and absorption of dietary fat—patients who consume excessive fat while on this treatment will develop steatorrhoea.

straining. It is extremely common, with 1% of the population consulting their doctor about it each year. Women and the elderly are most commonly affected.

Causes of constipation

These are listed in Table 10.15 and the important questions to ask about it are given in HISTORY & EXAMINATION BOX 10.2. Certain features may suggest the cause of constipation:

- *Onset in early childhood:* suggests Hirschsprung's disease (diagnosis, however, may be delayed to adulthood; see p. 734)
- *History of traumatic labour* (e.g. forceps delivery): may indicate damage to anorectal neuromusculature
- *Anal pain:* suggests a local anorectal cause
- *Bleeding:* indicates colorectal cancer, proctitis, piles or anal fissure
- *Alternating diarrhoea and constipation:* suggests colonic cancer, irritable bowel syndrome or faecal impaction
- *Weight loss:* suggests cancer, a reducing diet or poorly controlled diabetes mellitus

- *Weight gain:* suggests hypothyroidism
- *Low dietary fibre intake or certain drug treatments:* may be directly responsible

The complications of constipation include haemorrhoids, anal fissures and, rarely, stercoral perforation (in the elderly), as well as the side-effects of chronic laxative use (see p. 753).

Examination

General examination

Examination of the alimentary system begins with general observations (HISTORY & EXAMINATION BOX 10.3).

Is the patient ill or well?

- Cachexia suggests advanced cancer or malabsorption
- Signs of volume depletion (tachycardia, hypotension, postural drop in blood pressure) may indicate gastrointestinal bleeding, severe diarrhoea or intra-abdominal

Large bowel disease	CARCINOMA, perianal pain (haemorrhoids, fissures, abscess, fistula)
Abnormal motility	
Idiopathic	IRRITABLE BOWEL SYNDROME, pseudo-obstruction, severe idiopathic constipation (also known as slow transit constipation)
Structural	DIVERTICULOSIS, Hirschsprung's disease
Neurological disorders	Autonomic neuropathy, spinal cord disease, Parkinson's disease, multiple sclerosis
Metabolic disorders	Hypercalcaemia, hypothyroidism
Other	Pregnancy, anorectal dysfunction
Dietary	LOW FIBRE DIET, WEIGHT-REDUCING DIETS, FASTING, DEPRESSION, DEMENTIA, anorexia nervosa, parenteral nutrition
Lifestyle	Unaesthetic lavatory, too busy, inactivity, fluid depletion
Drugs	OPIATES, iron, anticholinergics, antidepressants
Old age	

Table 10.15 Causes of constipation (common causes in capital letters)

History & Examination 10.3

General examination

Appearance

Does the patient look ill or well?

Is the patient fluid-depleted, cachexic, shocked or feverish?

Observe the patient's mood

Inspect the conjunctivae of the lower eyelids: look for anaemia

Inspect the eyes: look for iritis, conjunctivitis, jaundice, and around the eyes for xanthelasma

Inspect the hands: look for clubbing, leuconychia, koilonychia, palmar erythema, Dupuytren's contracture and liver flap

Inspect the mouth: look for ulcers, candidiasis, glossitis and cheilitis

Inspect the skin: look for reduced turgor, rashes and telangiectasia

Inspect the joints: look for arthropathy

Lymph nodes

Feel for lymphadenopathy: palpate the neck, axillae and groins

Pulse

Note any tachycardia or atrial fibrillation

Blood pressure

Note any hypotension

Abdominal examination

Inspection

Look for:
• Distension and exaggeration of the normal lumbar lordosis
• Masses
• Visible peristalsis
• Striae
• Scars

Palpation

Feel for:
• Masses in each quadrant—define the mass by its size, shape, consistency, site, movement with respiration, tenderness and resonance to percussion
• Local or generalized tenderness, rebound tenderness, guarding and rigidity

Examine the hernial orifices

Percussion

Percuss for:
• Shifting dullness, indicating ascites
• Hyper-resonance, suggesting intestinal ileus or obstruction

Auscultation

Listen for:
• Arterial bruits
• Bowel sounds, which are increased in intestinal obstruction and absent in ileus

Rectal examination

Examine the perineum for tags, fistulae, external piles, fissures and excoriation

Examine the rectum digitally for masses, oedema, induration or stool abnormalities (e.g. constipation, diarrhoea)

Palpate the prostate in men and the cervix in women

Feel for localized tenderness to the palpating finger if the patient has abdominal pain

Inspect the glove for blood, pus or melaena

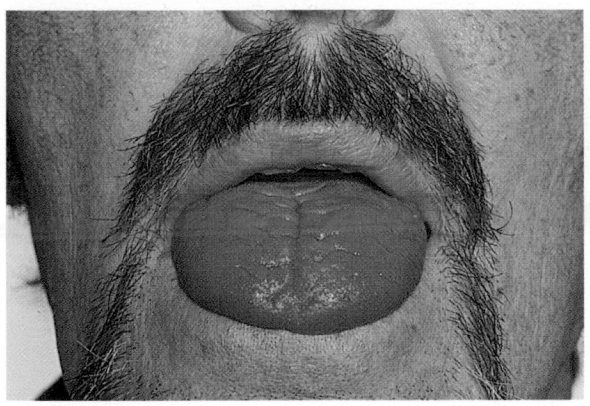

Figure 10.16 Glossitis (smooth, red, raw tongue—causes include iron deficiency and B_{12} deficiency).

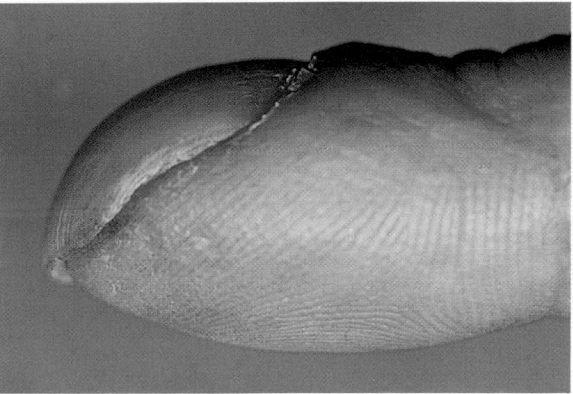

Figure 10.17 Clubbing.

inflammation such as pancreatitis: urgent admission is required
- Fever with abdominal symptoms suggests inflammation or infection, and often the need to admit acutely
- A depressed or anxious mood may be obvious, and indicate functional gastrointestinal symptoms
- Look for anaemia and jaundice
- Lymphadenopathy, particularly in the neck, may be caused by metastatic malignancy

Mouth
Examination of the mouth may reveal:
- *Oral ulceration:* usually idiopathic, but may also be a feature of Crohn's, coeliac or Behçet's disease, or of ill-fitting dentures
- *Candidiasis:* suggesting immunosuppression, effects of oral or inhaled steroids, recent antibiotic treatment or diabetes mellitus
- *Telangiectasia:* suggesting hereditary haemorrhagic telangiectasia (Osler–Rendu–Weber syndrome)
- *Cheilitis or glossitis:* suggesting vitamin deficiencies (Fig. 10.16)
- *Erosions on the posterior surface of incisors:* suggest frequent vomiting (e.g. bulimia) or severe gastro-oesophageal reflux

Hands
Inspect the hands, looking for the following signs:
- *Clubbing:* indicating inflammatory bowel or chronic liver disease (Fig. 10.17)
- *Leuconychia:* indicating hypoalbuminaemia (Fig. 10.18)
- *Koilonychia:* indicating severe iron deficiency
- Stigmata of chronic liver disease (Fig. 10.19) and liver flap (see p. 603; Fig. 9.5)

Feel the radial pulse—atrial fibrillation should alert you

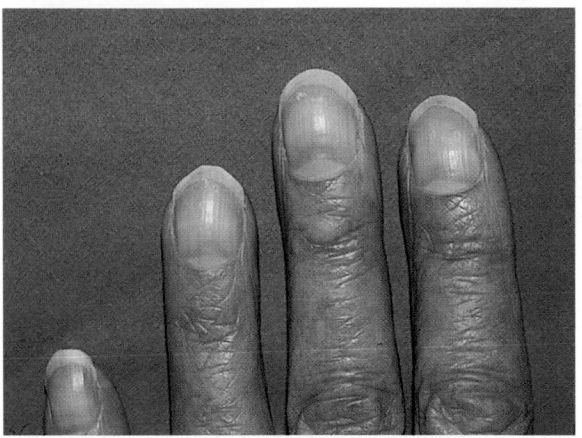

Figure 10.18 Leuconychia.

to the possibility of emboli and bowel ischaemia in patients with acute abdominal pain.

Eyes, skin and joints
Examination of the eyes, skin and joints may reveal extra-abdominal manifestations of inflammatory bowel disease such as iritis, erythema nodosum, pyoderma gangrenosum (Fig. 10.20) and arthritis.

Abdominal examination
To examine the abdomen, the patient should be comfortable and lying flat with just one pillow and their arms by their sides (HISTORY & EXAMINATION BOX 10.3). The abdomen should be uncovered from the pubis to the xiphisternum. Subsequent exposure and examination of the upper half of the body is important: signs related to gastrointestinal diagnoses may be found by examination of the chest (e.g. pleural effusion), breasts (e.g. primary

10

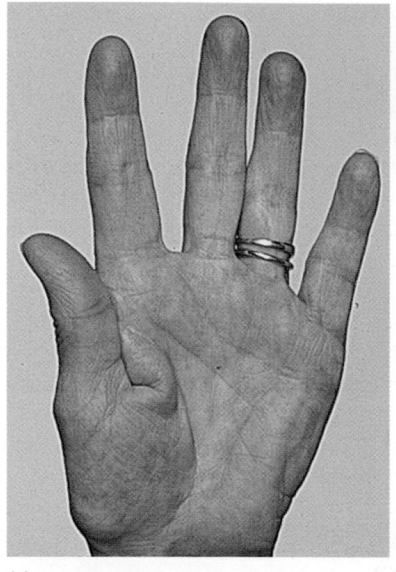 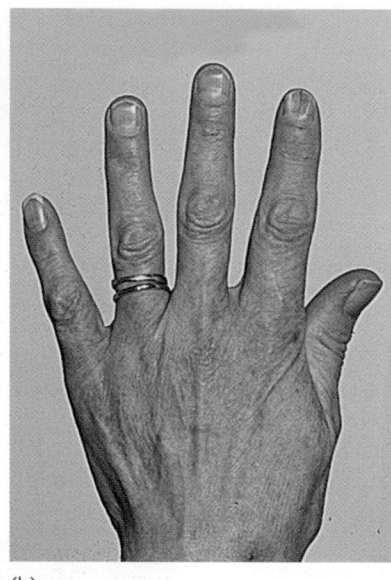

(a)   (b)

Figure 10.19 Signs of chronic liver disease in the hand. Note the large spider naevus on the dorsum of the wrist, leuconychia and palmar erythema.

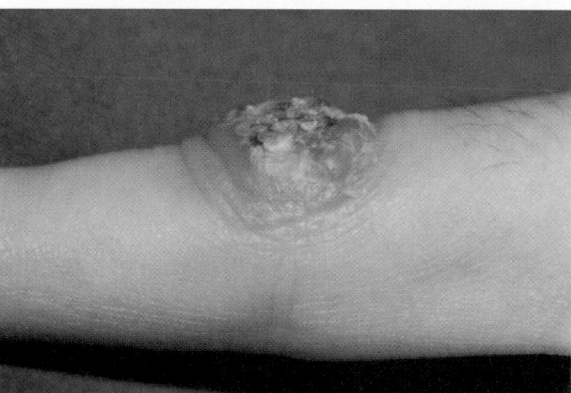

Figure 10.20 Pyoderma gangrenosum over a knuckle in a patient with ulcerative colitis.

malignancy presenting as weight loss, ascites or enlarged liver from metastases), supraclavicular region and neck (enlarged lymph nodes from primary gastrointestinal malignancies), arms (e.g. spider naevi in chronic liver disease), and cardiovascular system (e.g. heart failure as the cause of hepatomegaly or ascites, and endocarditis as the cause of weight loss).

Inspection

Look for distension, masses, visible peristalsis, striae and scars:

- *Distension:* suggests fat, fluid (ascites, large ovarian cyst or bladder), fetus, flatus (intestinal obstruction or ileus) or faeces. Bulging of the umbilicus may occur in ascites
- *Visible peristalsis:* indicates intestinal obstruction

- *Striae:* indicate recent change in abdominal size because of pregnancy, ascites or cachexia. Purple striae are a feature of Cushing's syndrome
- *Scars:* indicate previous surgery

Palpation

Ensure your hands are warm. Ask the patient if they have any pain, and avoid these areas at first. Feel with the flat of the hand using 4–6 movements to cover the abdomen. Begin lightly—watch the patient's face all the time; do not palpate deeply until you are sure that light palpation is not painful. Feel specifically for the liver, spleen, kidneys and aortic aneurysm. In patients with pain, examine the hernial orifices carefully for a strangulated hernia. Decide on the origin of any mass by its size, shape and consistency, site, movement with respiration and resonance to percussion.

If an area is tender, note if there is resistance to pressure (guarding) or if pain increases when the hand is lifted (rebound tenderness)—both indicating peritoneal inflammation. In chronic abdominal pain, if tenderness to palpation stays the same or worsens when the abdominal muscles are tensed voluntarily (ask the patient to lift their legs a few inches off the couch), it is evidence in favour of abdominal wall damage rather than visceral pain.

Percussion

The liver and spleen, if palpable, are dull to percussion as they lie anteriorly in the abdomen, while there is usually resonance over the kidneys as they lie retroperitoneally with overlying loops of gas-filled bowel. Percussion is painful in peritonitis.

Ascites produces **shifting dullness**—an area dull to percussion in the flank becomes resonant when the patient rolls to put that side uppermost, as the ascitic fluid sinks and gas-filled bowel rises. Abdominal percussion may be tympanic (**hyper-resonant**) when the bowel is distended with gas, as in intestinal ileus or obstruction.

Auscultation

Auscultation is of limited value in the diagnosis of gastrointestinal disease.

In thin people, an aortic bruit may be heard in the epigastrium and does not necessarily denote aortic disease. Bowel sounds may be accentuated in volume, pitch and frequency in intestinal obstruction, and diminished or absent in paralytic ileus. Occasionally, acute or chronic abdominal pain is a result of bowel ischaemia—the presence of abdominal and femoral bruits suggest underlying arteriopathy.

Rectal examination

In patients presenting with abdominal pain, colorectal symptoms or gastrointestinal bleeding, rectal examination is absolutely mandatory. It is also important prior to colonoscopy, as disease near the anal verge can easily be overlooked during insertion and withdrawal of the instrument.

Explain what you are going to do. Ask the patient to lie on their left side with the hips flexed. Look first for perianal disorders (tags, fistulae, external piles, fissures, excoriation). Then gently insert your lubricated gloved finger into the anal canal. Feel for mass lesions (e.g. cancer, polyp), oedema or induration (inflammatory bowel disease) or abnormalities of the stool (constipation, diarrhoea). In men, palpate the prostate anteriorly, and in women the cervix.

Fresh blood or pus may be seen on the glove after its withdrawal in patients with cancer or mucosal inflammation, and melaena (see p. 714) in patients with upper gastrointestinal bleeding.

In patients with abdominal pain, localized tenderness to the palpating finger may help in diagnosing appendicitis and pelvic inflammatory disease.

Investigation

Blood tests rarely indicate a specific diagnosis in gastroenterology, although several help in assessing the severity of established disease. The implications of abnormalities in the standard full blood count and biochemistry tests are listed below. Other test findings are discussed in the context of specific symptoms or diagnoses.

Haematology

Full blood count

Haemoglobin. Anaemia is common in patients with digestive disease:

- *Microcytic anaemia:* caused by iron deficiency may be a feature of patients with poor nutritional intake, malabsorption (e.g. coeliac disease) or chronic intestinal blood loss (gastrointestinal malignancies, peptic ulceration, use of NSAIDs, inflammatory bowel disease)
- *Normocytic anaemia:* suggests recent bleeding or can be a response to chronic active inflammation (e.g. inflammatory bowel disease)—known as 'anaemia of chronic disease'
- *Macrocytic anaemia:* may be found in patients with malabsorption of folate (e.g. coeliac disease) and/or vitamin B_{12} (e.g. pernicious anaemia, Crohn's disease

**Gastrointestinal disease:
Clinical presentations at a glance**

Iritis, conjunctivitis
Anaemia
Cheilitis, glossitis, ulceration, Candida
Dermatitis herpetiformis
Other rashes
Increased or absent bowel sounds
Distension
Ascites
Abdominal pain
Bloating
Masses
Clubbing
Leuconychia
Koilonychia
Hernial orifices
Scar
Diarrhoea
Constipation
Bleeding
Bruising
Arthropathy
Arthritis
Oedema

Anorexia
Mood
Temperature
Pigmentation
Telangiectasia
Lymph nodes
Heartburn
Dysphagia
Fluid depletion
Weight loss
Dyspepsia
Nausea
Vomiting
Succusion splash
Tenderness
Guarding rigidity
Visible peristalsis
Rectal examination
Erythema nodosum
Pyoderma gangrenosum

10

affecting terminal ileum). Other causes of macrocytosis include alcohol, chronic liver disease and treatment with sulfasalazine or the immunosuppressive drug, azathioprine

White cell count. A neutrophil leucocytosis is common in patients with acute inflammatory or ischaemic abdominal conditions (Table 10.6, p. 661) and is also provoked by steroids. Patients taking immunosuppressives as steroid-sparing agents may have low leucocyte counts as a consequence of treatment, and their blood count should be monitored regularly to pick up bone marrow suppression.

Platelet count. Raised platelet counts may occur in patients with gastrointestinal bleeding; they may also indicate active inflammation (e.g. in inflammatory bowel disease). A low platelet count of whatever primary cause (see p. 1046) predisposes to gastrointestinal haemorrhage.

Blood film. Howell–Jolly inclusion bodies suggest hyposplenism (e.g. coeliac disease).

Acute phase markers

The acute phase protein C-reactive protein and the erythrocyte sedimentation rate (ESR) and plasma viscosity are raised in infection (e.g. bacterial gastroenteritis), in inflammation (particularly if chronic, such as Crohn's disease) and sometimes in gastrointestinal cancer, especially if disseminated.

Prothrombin time

A prolonged prothrombin time is much more often brought about by warfarin or liver disease than malabsorption of vitamin K.

Biochemistry

Urea and electrolytes

Severe diarrhoea and/or vomiting may increase blood urea and decrease serum sodium and potassium concentrations. Hypokalaemia and hypomagnesaemia, of whatever cause, may produce paralytic ileus. A raised blood urea, out of proportion to any rise in serum creatinine concentration, often occurs in upper gastrointestinal bleeding. This is because of the breakdown of blood proteins in the gut and their conversion by the liver to urea.

Diagnostic imaging

Flexible endoscopy

Introduced in the early 1970s, flexible endoscopy is now the major diagnostic tool in gastroenterology (Fig. 10.21). The ability to detect flat mucosal lesions and take biopsies are clear advantages over barium techniques. The possibilities for delivering therapy for gastrointestinal diseases endoscopically are increasing. Informed consent is essential before endoscopy, and the person obtaining consent should have a good understanding of the risks and benefits. These procedures are best appreciated by a visit to the endoscopy unit. Most units now use video technology (Fig. 10.21), with endoscopic images displayed on monitors as the procedure is taking place.

Upper gastrointestinal endoscopy (also known as gastroscopy or oesophagogastroduodenoscopy)
Oesophagogastroduodenoscopy (OGD) is the most commonly used special investigation technique to assess upper gastrointestinal symptoms. It is now often performed without sedation, using lidocaine to numb the back of the throat, and is extremely safe (mortality 0.01%). If sedation is used, the most common agent is an intravenous benzodiazepine (e.g. midazolam). These drugs have a useful amnesic effect when given intravenously; however, their main side-effect is respiratory depression, which is a leading cause of complications associated with OGD (see p. 673). Increasingly, diagnostic OGDs are being carried out by specialist nurses.

Diagnostic indications. These include dyspepsia, dysphagia, nausea and vomiting, haematemesis and melaena, weight loss and iron-deficiency anaemia. Duodenal biopsies may be taken to look for coeliac disease (see p. 722), gastric biopsies to determine the cause of diffuse mucosal abnormalities (e.g. *Helicobacter pylori*; see p. 706) or to exclude malignancy in gastric ulcers or other localized oesophageal and gastric lesions.

Therapeutic indications and techniques. These include treatment of bleeding peptic ulcer by thermal coagulation or local injection methods; banding or sclerosant injection for oesophageal varices (see p. 630); dilatation of oesophageal strictures using mechanical or balloon devices (Fig. 10.22); and placement of feeding tubes directly into the stomach through the overlying abdominal wall (percutaneous endoscopic gastrostomy—PEG; Fig. 10.23).

Contraindications and precautions. These are all relative —in the emergency situation it may be appropriate to carry out OGD in high-risk patients (e.g. to diagnose and treat a cause of upper gastrointestinal bleeding), as any other approach (surgery, doing nothing) may be even more dangerous. Ideally, patients with acute upper gastrointestinal bleeding should be endoscoped within 24 h of admission. Patients who are haemodynamically shocked should be resuscitated first.

In the routine diagnostic setting, care is needed with

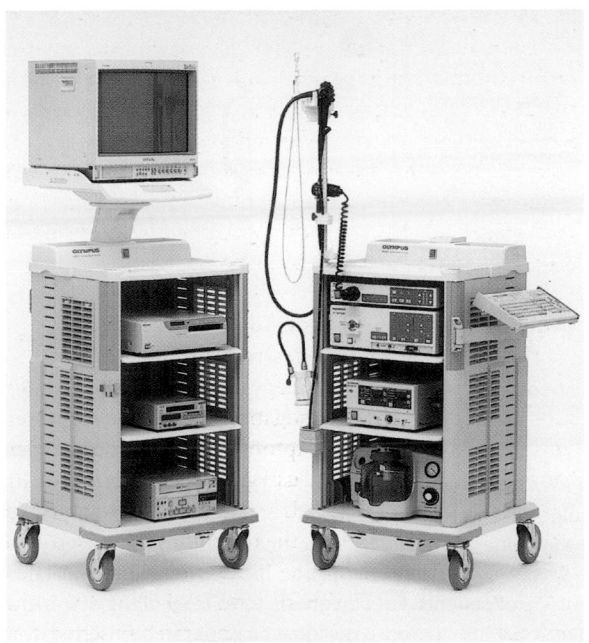

(a)

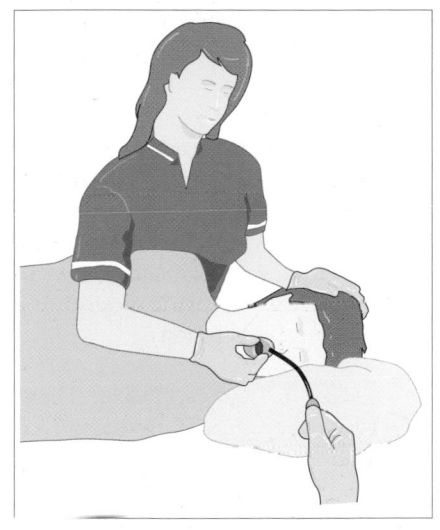

(d)

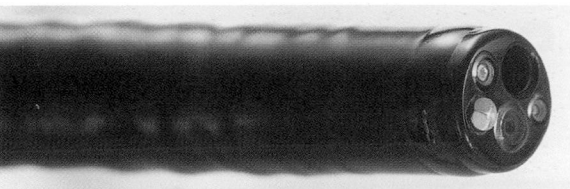

(b)

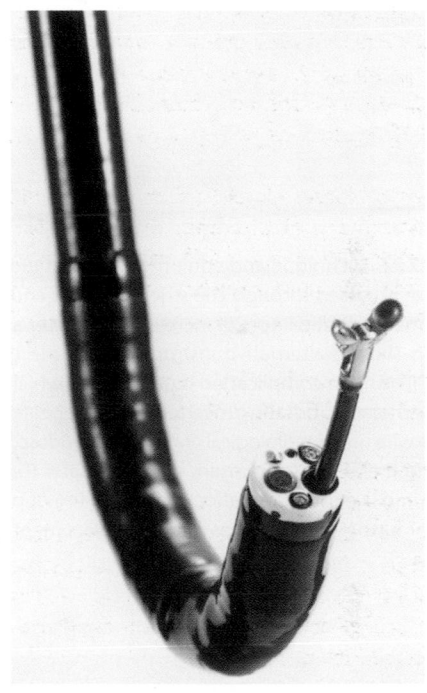

(c)

Figure 10.21 Fibre-optic endoscopy. (a) General view of endoscope and video image processing unit. Equipment for producing hard copy photographs or video recordings of endoscopic views is shown under the monitor. (b) End view of endoscope. (c) Biopsy forceps exiting the endoscope's biopsy channel. (d) Patient position for the procedure—the nurse holds the mouthguard, aspirates the oral cavity as necessary and monitors the patient's overall condition.

10

sedation in the elderly and patients with severe chest disease; patients with atlantoaxial subluxation (usually caused by rheumatoid arthritis) should have their neck supported in a hard collar, and the procedure should not be performed in those with a recent myocardial infarction or high risk of bleeding. Patients at high risk of bacterial endocarditis (prosthetic valves, significant valve lesions, previous endocarditis) need prophylactic antibiotics. Each hospital should have its own guidelines for antibiotic use in this setting: in the absence of local advice, amoxicillin 1 g intravenously + gentamicin 80–120 mg intravenously (depending on weight) immediately pre-

procedure, with amoxicillin 500 mg oral 6 h postprocedure can be used. Teicoplanin as a 400-mg intravenous bolus or vancomycin 1 g intravenous infusion are alternatives to amoxicillin in penicillin-allergic patients.

Preparation and technique. Preparation consists of a 6-h fast, although sips of water may be allowed until shortly before the procedure, and essential medication should be given. Proton pump inhibitors (PPIs) should be avoided, ideally for 4 weeks before the procedure, as they may mask pathology and invalidate urease-based tests for *Helicobacter* (see p. 706).

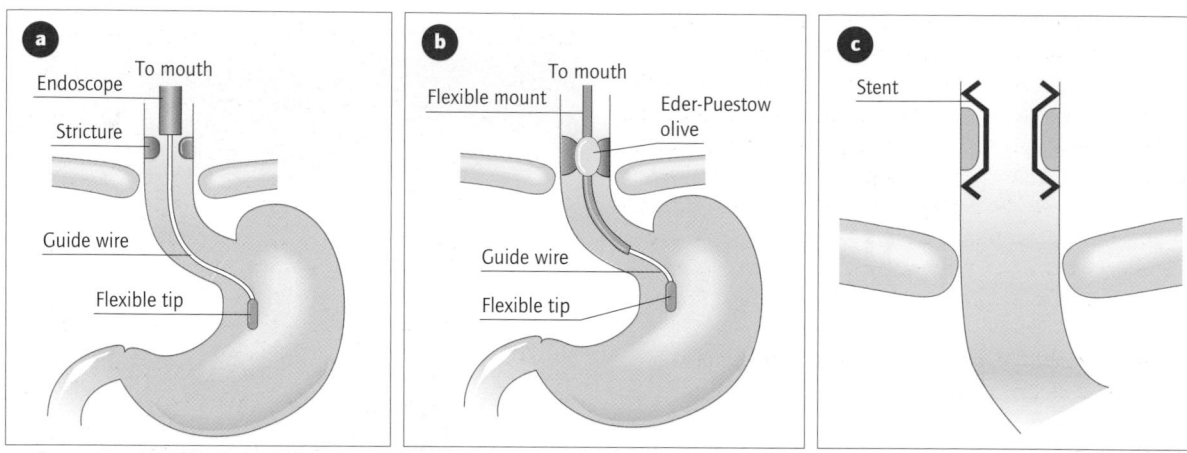

Figure 10.22 Technique and equipment for dilatation and intubation of oesophageal strictures. (a) The patient is sedated and a guide wire is passed through the stricture under endoscopic ± radiological control. (b) The endoscope is then withdrawn and a series of mechanical dilators of increasing diameter are passed over the guide wire. A metal 'olive'-shaped dilator (Eder–Puestow system) is shown; alternative instruments include the Celestin or Savery dilators (flexible plastic tapered tubes) or inflatable balloons. The main complication is perforation, which occurs in about 2% of patients. For benign strictures relief of the dysphagia is often permanent, but the procedure can be repeated when necessary. (c) If the stricture is malignant a stent can be inserted over the guide wire under radiological control, after endoscopic dilatation. The patient can then swallow liquid and soft foods. Increasingly, expanding metal stents are used, which are safer than fixed diameter plastic stents (see p. 699). The most common immediate complication is perforation, affecting up to 10% of patients. Later problems include aspiration pneumonia, blockage of the tube by food or further tumour growth, and displacement or disintegration of the tube.

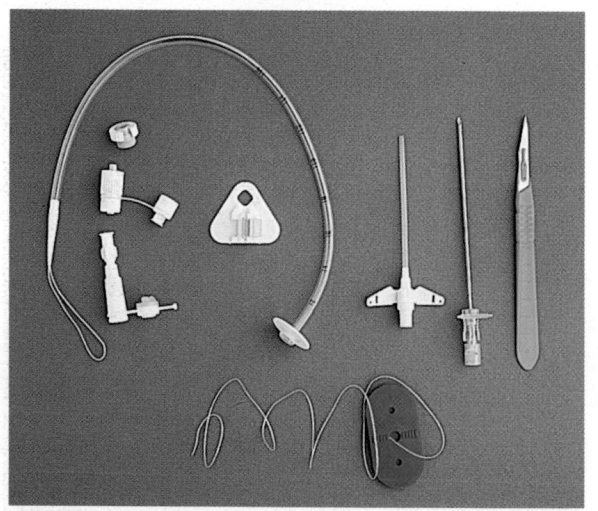

(a)

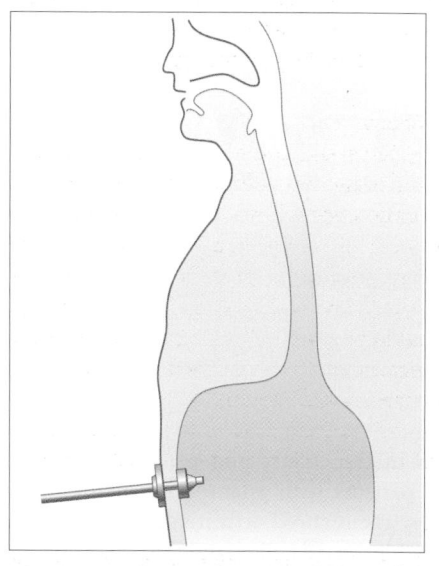

(b)

Figure 10.23 Percutaneous endoscopic gastrostomy (PEG). (a) A kit for placement of a PEG tube. A cannula (right of figure) is introduced into the stomach—the site of puncture of the abdomen being guided by the prepositioned gastroscope. A nylon or metallic 'string' (bottom of picture) is passed through the cannula, grasped by a snare passed down the biopsy channel of the gastroscope, and pulled up out of the patient's mouth. The string is then attached to a loop on the end of the PEG tube (left of figure) and the tube pulled back down the oesophagus and out through the abdominal wall. A hard taper helps the leading end of tube pass through the abdominal wall, while a circular buffer stops the back end of the tube when it reaches the stomach wall. Once pulled through, the tapered end of the tube is cut off, and a valve attached to allow delivery of enteral feed. (b) Diagram showing the final position of a PEG tube.

Serious complications. These are extremely rare, with an overall incidence of 1 in 2000, confined mainly to therapeutic procedures in the acute setting, where it is the underlying condition (e.g. liver disease) rather than the OGD procedure *per se* that is the cause of the complication or death. Problems may arise because of the respiratory depression caused by benzodiazepine sedation—an effective reversal agent, flumazenil, is available. Oesophageal dilatation techniques for strictures (especially malignant ones), or for achalasia, may result in oesophageal perforation.

Endoscopic retrograde cholangiopancreatography

This is discussed in detail on p. 606.

Enteroscopy

Recently introduced long upper gastrointestinal endoscopes allow visualization, biopsy and treatment of lesions in the distal duodenum and proximal jejunum (e.g. angiodysplasia and tumours; Fig. 10.24). The technique and complications resemble those for OGD described above.

Specialist centres are developing techniques that can view the whole of the small bowel mucosa directly. In 'sonde' enteroscopy, a 2.5-m ultraflexible endoscope is pulled through the small bowel by peristalsis (Fig. 10.24). Miniaturization techniques have allowed the development of wireless image-transmitting video capsules, whose data output can be analysed by computer. Neither of these techniques offers therapeutic capability.

Colonoscopy

Barium enema and colonoscopy are currently the main tools for investigating colonic symptoms. In colonoscopy, a 1.5-m endoscope is introduced via the anus, and manipulated under direct vision around the colon. The bowel is prepared prior to the procedure using a strong laxative and restricted low-residue diet. Iron-containing preparations should be avoided for at least a week as they impair bowel cleansing. Computerized tomography (CT) and magnetic resonance imaging (MRI) techniques for colonic imaging are evolving, and may have a particular role in the frail elderly, where conventional methods may be

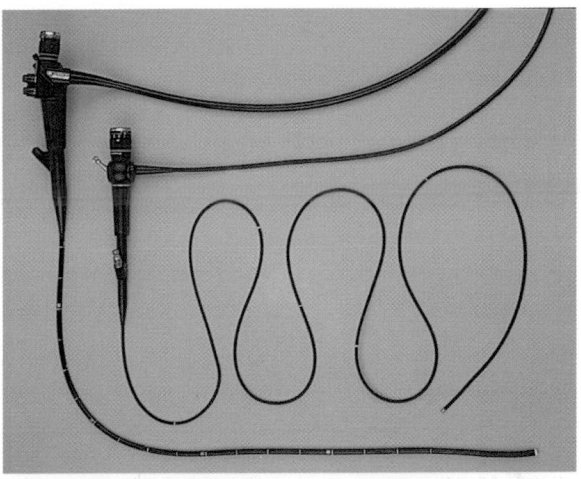

(a)

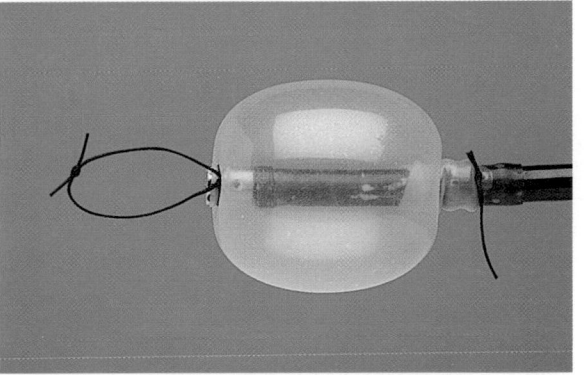

(b)

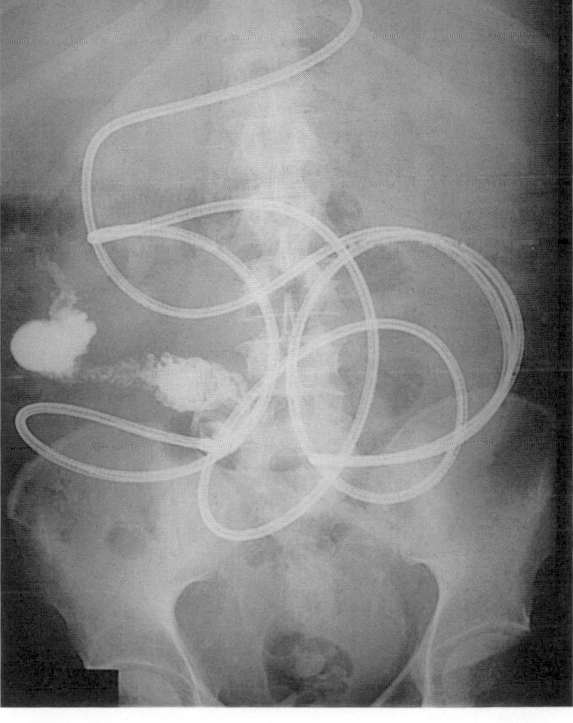

(c)

Figure 10.24 (*right*) Examples of 'push' and 'sonde' type enteroscopes for examination of the small bowel beyond the duodenum. (a) The 'push'-type enteroscope is a slightly longer (1.7 vs. 1.2 m) and slightly stiffer version of a conventional endoscope; the 'sonde' enteroscope is thinner, more flexible and much longer (3 m) than a conventional endoscope. (b) The tip of the 'sonde' enteroscope, showing the balloon that is inflated once the tip is in the duodenum. (c)The instrument is then pulled down the small bowel by peristalsis.

10

considered too invasive, and where sufficient information can often be obtained by a plain abdominal CT without bowel preparation. To obtain the detail equivalent to colonoscopy, the bowel needs laxative preparation and insufflation with gas prior to the CT scanning. Software programmes allow three-dimensional reconstructions of the colon to be made, and for the radiologist to view the

result in the form of a 'virtual' colonoscopy. If these techniques are being considered, it is best to discuss individual cases with the local radiologist.

Diagnostic indications. These include anaemia; investigation of a change in bowel habit—particularly diarrhoea, where mucosal biopsies may reveal colitis in an otherwise

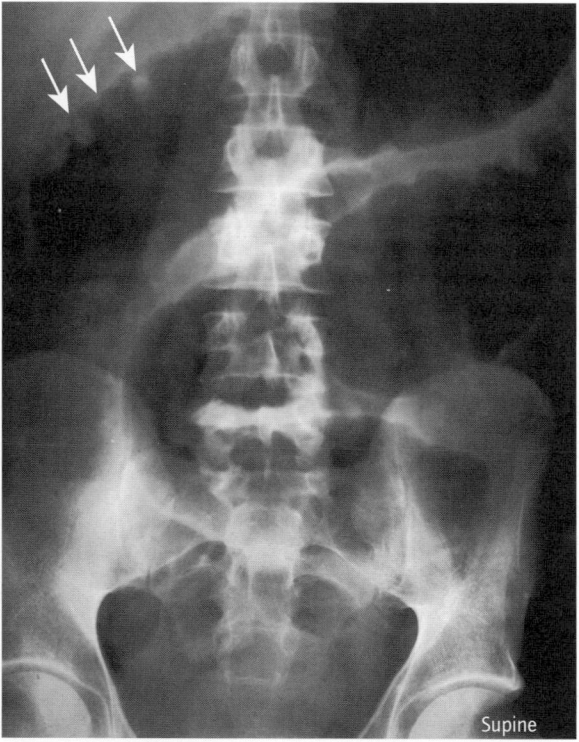

(a)

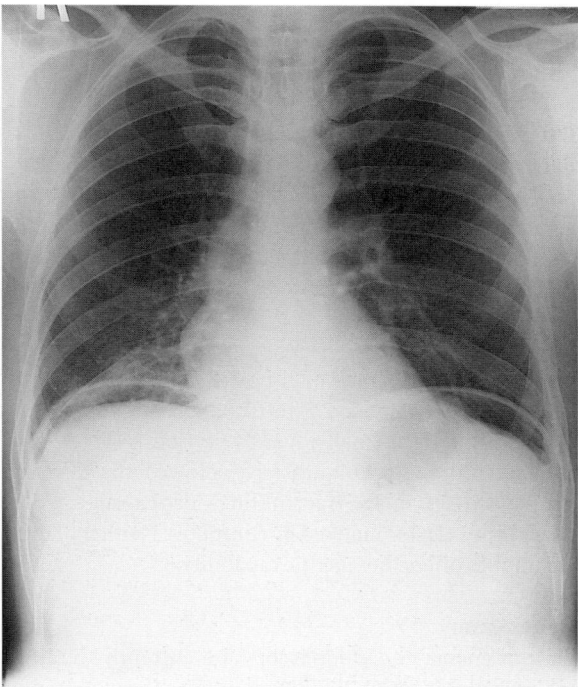

(b)

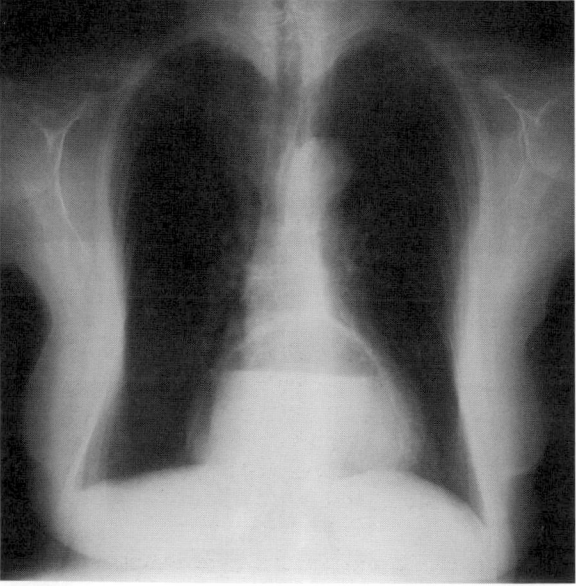

(c)

Figure 10.25 Plain radiographs of the chest and abdomen revealing gastrointestinal disorders. (a) Toxic megacolon. The colon is dilated throughout. Mucosal islands are visible (arrows): nodules of oedematous mucosa protruding into the dilated lumen, surrounded by ulcerated mucosa (e.g. at hepatic flexure). (b) Intra-abdominal perforation. Note the air under both diaphragms. (c) Hiatus hernia. Note the air–fluid level in the gastric lumen behind the cardiac shadow.

normal-looking bowel; rectal bleeding; and further invest-igation and biopsy of abnormalities found with barium enema. In inflammatory bowel disease, the technique is frequently used to assess disease extent and response to treatment (see p. 738). 'Screening' colonoscopy is used in asymptomatic patients known to be at increased risk of colon cancer, particularly those with sporadic adenomatous polyps or other premalignant polyposis syndromes (see p. 729), a strong family history of colon cancer or with extensive inflammatory colitis present for over 8 years.

Common therapeutic indications. These are the removal of polyps and thermal treatment of angiodysplasia. Benign strictures can be dilated using inflatable balloons, malignant strictures treated with expanding metal stents, and a colon obstructed by twisting (volvulus) or invagina-tion into the adjacent colonic segment (intussusception) mechanically reduced endoscopically.

Contraindications. Similar to those for OGD above.

Complications. These include perforation and bleeding, and are more common if therapy such as polypectomy has been undertaken.

Colonoscopy vs. barium enema

Colonoscopy is more dangerous than barium enema (perforation rate 1 in 2000 vs. 1 in 25 000), less successful at imaging the right colon, and requires senior medical staff and nurses as opposed to radiographers alone. The main advantages of colonoscopy are the ability to diag-nose lesions such as angiodysplasia and flat polyps that are undetectable by barium enema; the ability to biopsy both normal-looking mucosa and lesions; greater accuracy for imaging the sigmoid colon (where overlapping loops frequently make barium interpretation difficult); and the ability to deliver therapy.

Rigid endoscopy

Rigid sigmoidoscopy remains a useful, quick, cheap, safe, outpatient technique for the initial endoscopic examina-tion of patients with diarrhoea, constipation, rectal bleed-ing and inflammatory bowel disease. Despite the name, the sigmoid colon is rarely reached, and visualization and biopsy by this technique are unsafe alone to exclude organic causes of these symptoms, unless the clinical sus-picion is extremely low (e.g. young patients with classic irritable bowel symptoms).

Radiology

The best results are obtained when the clinical problem is discussed with the radiologist.

Plain radiography

Plain radiography of the chest and abdomen helps in the diagnosis of many gut disorders (Fig. 10.25), especially in the acute setting. **Chest radiography** may show features of relevance to gastrointestinal disease (e.g. metastases, which can originate from gastrointestinal sites including oesophagus, stomach and pancreas); tuberculosis as a clue to the presence of abdominal involvement with the infec-tion, or pleural effusions which may be linked to gastroin-testinal disease such as perforation of the oesophagus, pancreatitis or any malabsorption state with low albumin (see p. 720).

Barium swallow

This shows both **structure and function** of the oeso-phagus. It is particularly useful in patients with dysphagia possibly caused by neurological disease, because move-ments of the pharynx can be analysed and aspiration into the trachea and nasopharynx assessed. Motility dis-orders of the oesophagus may be demonstrated (although manometry is the 'gold standard'; see p. 677).

Barium meal

Because of the ease and technical advantages of gastro-scopy (see p. 670), barium meals are now used infrequently. Indications include assessment of gastric function (e.g. delayed emptying), complex anatomy (e.g. postoperative stomachs, volvulus), gastro-oesophageal reflux and lesions in the proximal small bowel beyond the reach of the gastroscope (Fig. 10.26a).

Barium follow-through and small bowel enema

Films are taken as barium flows down the small intestine. The barium is either swallowed (barium follow-through) or introduced directly into the small bowel via a nasogas-tric tube (small bowel enema, also known as enteroclysis). The latter may be slightly more accurate but is more uncomfortable for the patient and less commonly used. The tests are used in the investigation of steatorrhoea; abdominal pain thought to be caused by a structural disorder of the small bowel; diarrhoea; and chronic gastro-intestinal bleeding where first-line tests have proved negative.

Barium enema

Films are taken as barium and air (introduced into the rectum through a soft cannula) are passed retrogradely through the colon (Fig. 10.26d). A barium enema should not be carried out unless digital and sigmoidoscopic rectal examinations have been performed, as the procedure can easily miss rectal lesions.

Indications. Indications for a barium enema include a

10

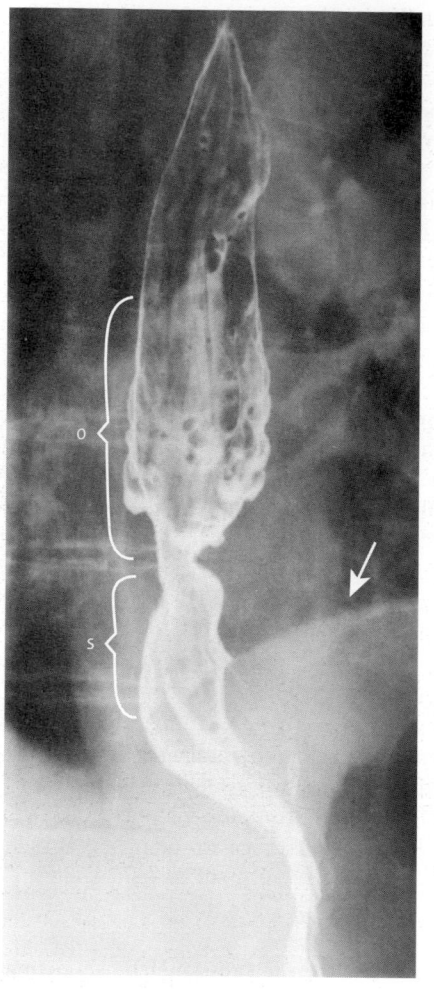

(a)

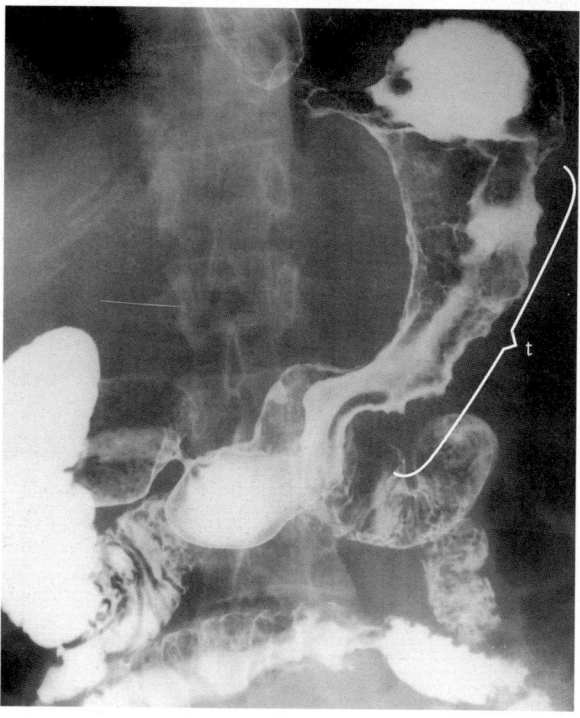

(b)

Figure 10.26 Contrast radiology of the gastrointestinal tract. (a) Barium swallow showing an hiatus hernia. Stomach (s), lying above diaphragm (arrow), and reflux oesophagitis, with irregularity of distal oesophageal mucosa (o) because of ulceration. (b) Contrast study showing advanced gastric carcinoma. Note the irregularity caused by tumour and ulceration along the greater curve (t).

change of bowel habit, microcytic anaemia, abdominal pain and weight loss. Minor rectal bleeding is best investigated by immediate digital rectal examination and rigid sigmoidoscopy or proctoscopy, followed by flexible sigmoidoscopy in the endoscopy unit if these are negative; major bleeding requires urgent full colonoscopy often with gastroscopy (see p. 719).

Common findings are carcinoma, polyps and inflammatory bowel disease (all of which usually need subsequent colonoscopy to obtain tissue for histology) and diverticulosis.

Contraindications. Frail patients with poor anal sphincter function are often unable to retain barium sufficiently. Barium enema may be dangerous in patients with sus-

pected perforation or acute severe ulcerative colitis. If in doubt, discuss the individual case with the radiologist.

Gastrointestinal angiography
Indications. The most common indication for this difficult technique is active obscure gastrointestinal bleeding (see p. 720).

Selective catheterization of the coeliac axis, or superior and inferior mesenteric arteries may be necessary to show angiomatous malformations and bleeding from ulcers, tumours or Meckel's diverticulum (Fig. 10.27).

Ultrasound, CT and MRI scanning
Indications. Ultrasound and cross-sectional imaging techniques of CT and MRI scanning are most commonly used

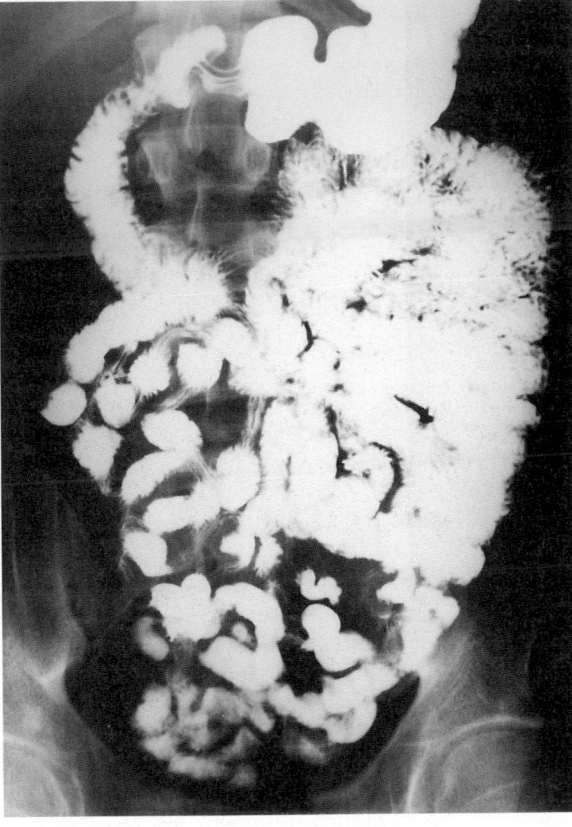

(c)

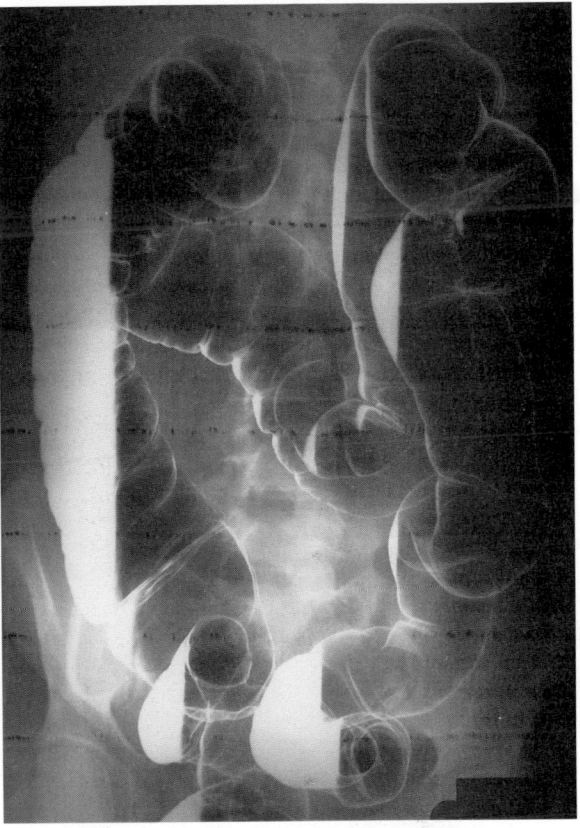

(d)

10

Figure 10.26 (*Cont'd*) (c) Normal double-contrast barium meal. The lumen is distended with gas (introduced as an effervescent CO_2-releasing agent) while the mucosa is lined by a thin coating of barium. (d) Normal barium enema. After preparation of the bowel as for colonoscopy (see p. 673), barium suspension is run into the rectum and around the colon as air is insufflated. Muscle relaxants are injected and the patient is positioned as required, for this film in the right lateral decubitus position. Both parts reproduced from Misiewicz JJ, Pounder RE, Venables CW. *Diseases of the Gut and Pancreas*, 2nd edn. Oxford: Blackwell Scientific Publications, 1994 with the permission of the authors.

in assessment of pancreatic, biliary and liver disease, including biopsy of suspected liver metastases (see Chapter 9). Other common uses include evaluation and/or biopsy of:

- Intra-abdominal and pelvic masses and abscesses
- Abdominal pain
- Weight loss

It is possible to detect thickened bowel wall (e.g. because of malignancy or inflammation), but endoscopy and/or contrast radiology are more sensitive and specific. These techniques are complementary, and all three may be required in some cases—some liver lesions may be 'invisible' to one technique yet show up on another.

A promising recent development is endoluminal ultrasound. The transducer is either incorporated into the end of the endoscope or passed down the biopsy channel, giving high-resolution views of the gut wall (e.g. for tumour staging in oesophageal cancer) and nearby structures (e.g. the pancreas).

Radioisotope tests

Radioisotope tests are sometimes helpful in the diagnosis of gastrointestinal disorders (Table 10.16).

Oesophageal function tests

Oesophageal pH testing

To help in the diagnosis of GORD (see p. 692), distal oesophageal pH over 24 h can be measured using a pH-sensitive electrode introduced via the nose and positioned above the lower oesophageal sphincter. A representative result is shown in Fig. 10.28.

Oesophageal manometry

This test is performed by inserting a thin flexible catheter down the oesophagus, which can measure pressure at several points. This allows recording of the amplitude and coordination of peristalsis, and assessment of lower oesophageal sphincter function.

10

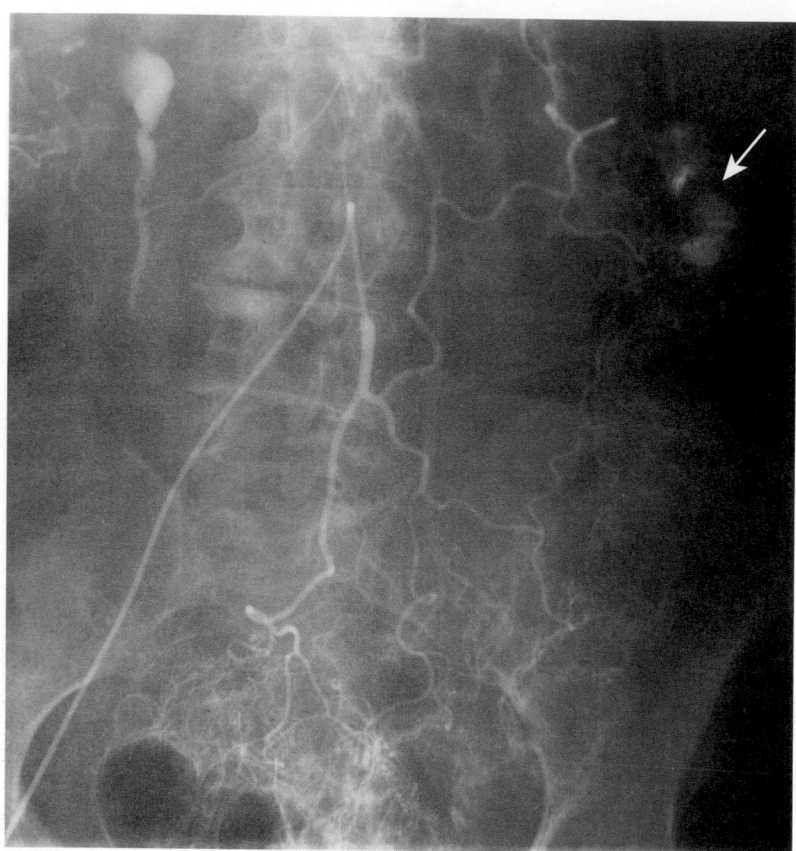

Figure 10.27 Angiography of the mesenteric circulation in the investigation of obscure gastrointestinal bleeding. The film shows contrast injected into the inferior mesenteric artery. An angiodysplasia has been demonstrated in the region of the splenic flexure. Bleeding from the lesion shows as a 'blush' of contrast pooling in the lumen (arrow).

Table 10.16 Radioisotope tests in gastrointestinal disease

Disorder	Scan/count	Isotope	Comments
Obscure bleeding	Abdomen Blood, faeces	^{99m}Tc-sulphur colloid, i.v. ^{51}Cr-labelled erythrocytes, i.v.	Labelled erythrocytes or colloid suspended in plasma are lost into bowel lumen at point of bleeding—if blood loss is rapid enough it will show as a 'hot spot', helping to locate site of bleed
Meckel's diverticulum	Abdomen	^{99m}Tc-pertechnetate, i.v.	Taken up exclusively by acid-secreting cells, thus any activity away from stomach uptake indicates ectopic gastric mucosa
Inflammatory bowel disease	Abdomen	^{111}In- or ^{99}Tc HMPAO-labelled leucocytes, i.v.	Radiolabelled leucocytes accumulate in areas of inflamed bowel/or abdominal abscesses
Intra-abdominal abscess	Abdomen	^{111}In- or ^{99}Tc HMPAO-labelled leucocytes, i.v.	
Bile acid malabsorption	Abdomen, faeces	^{75}Se-homocholyl taurine (SeHCAT), orally	The total amount of isotope retained in the body at 5 days is measured: low levels indicate reduced absorption by the terminal ileum and loss of the radiolabelled bile marker in faeces
Vitamin B$_{12}$ malabsorption	Urine, blood (sometimes body)	^{57}Co-B$_{12}$, orally, with or without intrinsic factor	(See Schilling test, p. 1032)
Apudoma metastases	Abdomen	^{131}I-meta-iodobenzyl guanidine (MIBG), i.v.	Taken up by neuroendocrine tumours—used both to localize and treat (by administering radiotherapeutic doses)

HMPAO, hexamethylpropylene amine oxime; i.v., intravenous.

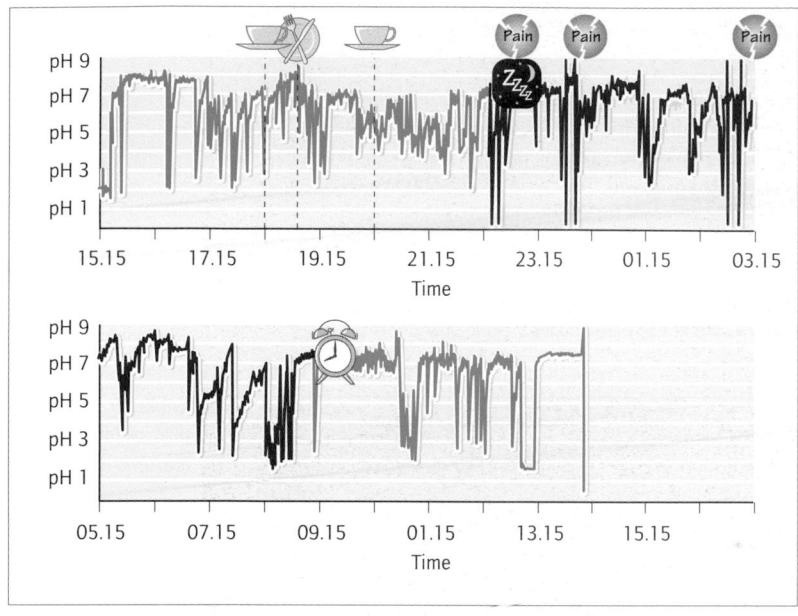

Figure 10.28 24-h Oesophageal pH study result. The *x* axis shows time: this study was started at 15.15 in the afternoon and continued until the same time the following day. The *y* axis shows the pH recorded in the distal oesophagus during the 24-h period. The patient records major events as shown by the self-explanatory cartoons at the top of the trace, indicating drinking, eating, pain, going to bed and waking. The red trace shows the period the patient was supine in bed, the green period the awake and upright period. The greater the amount of time the trace dips below pH 4, the greater the potential for acid-induced damage to the oesophageal mucosa. This cumulative time where this patient's pH dropped below 4 was only marginally above the normal range at 4.7% of the 24-h period. However, there is a strong symptom correlation. The patient awoke three times during the night as a result of reflux-type pain, clearly corresponding to periods of marked oesophageal acidification. The trace probably underestimated the normal situation, as this patient found the presence of the monitoring tube so uncomfortable he could only manage one light meal during the monitoring period. Oesophageal manometry showed him to have a grossly lax lower oesophageal sphincter. His symptoms were abolished by surgery to repair the valve.

10

Surgery

Conventional surgery, often involving resection of diseased bowel, continues to have a major role in the management of the acute abdomen, persistent acute gastrointestinal bleeding, gastrointestinal neoplasia and inflammatory bowel disease. However, its indications are being eroded by the rapidly advancing capabilities of less invasive techniques, such as endoscopy and laparoscopy. These can often be carried out with intravenous sedation rather than general anaesthesia, require a much shorter stay in hospital and are cheaper.

Laparoscopy

Laparoscopy is usually undertaken in the UK by surgeons and gynaecologists. It can provide both visual and histological evidence of malignancy, tuberculosis or cirrhosis when the diagnosis remains obscure after other investigations. The increasing capability of CT, MRI and abdominal ultrasound is reducing the diagnostic role of laparoscopy outside gynaecology, but its therapeutic capabilities are steadily increasing. It is now used routinely in preference to open abdominal surgery (laparotomy) for cholecystectomy and for hiatus hernia repair (see p. 696) and its role in appendicectomy and limited colectomy is being evaluated.

Indications. Indications in gastroenterology:
- Investigation of obscure ascites (allowing biopsy of intra-abdominal masses, peritoneal nodules and liver)
- Assessment of operability of known cancer
- Evaluation and biopsy of intra-abdominal masses (e.g. of the pancreas)
- Occasionally, evaluation of patients with abdominal pain

Contraindications. Relative contraindications to laparoscopy include previous abdominal surgery (adhesions increase the risk of intestinal perforation on insertion of the trochar), and coagulation disorders.

Clinical features	Steatorrhoea, diarrhoea, weight loss
*Non-specific tests**	
Haematology	Haemoglobin and MCV, iron, TIBC, ferritin, vitamin B_{12}, folate, prothrombin time (indirect marker of vitamin K levels)
Biochemistry	Calcium, phosphate, alkaline phosphatase, vitamins A, D and E, magnesium, zinc, albumin, globulin
Tests specifically measuring absorptive function	
Dynamic tests	Xylose absorption, Schilling test, lactose tolerance test
Faecal tests	Faecal fat

* The many other causes of low values of these parameters include poor intake.

Table 10.17 Features suggesting malabsorption is occurring

Clinical feature	Malabsorbed nutrient
DIARRHOEA and/or fluid depletion	Water and electrolyte
Steatorrhoea	Fat
ABDOMINAL DISTENSION, PAIN and BORBORYGMI	Carbohydrate, leading to colonic bacterial fermentation
WEIGHT LOSS	Calories
ANAEMIA	Folate, iron, vitamin B_{12}
Bleeding, bruising	Vitamin K, vitamin C
Rickets, osteomalacia, tetany	Vitamin D, calcium
Peripheral neuropathy	Vitamin B_{12}, vitamin E, thiamine, folate
Oedema, ascites	Protein
Rash	Essential fatty acid, zinc
Night blindness, keratitis	Vitamin A
Amenorrhoea	Multifactorial
Mouth ulcers, glossitis, stomatitis	Vitamin B, vitamin C, folate, iron
Urinary tract oxalate stones	Hyperabsorption of dietary oxalate
Failure to thrive (children)	Multifactorial
Short stature (children)	Multifactorial

Table 10.18 Clinical features of malabsorption of fat and other nutrients (common features in capital letters)

Investigations for assessment of malabsorption

Malabsorption means impaired absorption of nutrients. The term is applicable whether or not there are overt clinical manifestations such as steatorrhoea, diarrhoea and weight loss (Table 10.17), and whether there are multiple deficiencies because of generalized involvement of the absorption process (e.g. reduced fat, carbohydrate, iron and folate absorption in severe coeliac disease), or just an isolated deficiency (such as low serum B_{12} in pernicious anaemia; see p. 1031).

Systemic levels of nutrients, proteins, haemoglobin, vitamins, etc., are relatively easy and accurate to test for (Table 10.18), but are not diagnostic of 'malabsorption' in themselves, as reduced intake or other disease may explain low values. Specific tests for malabsorption include those demonstrating abnormal faecal loss of an administered nutrient (e.g. faecal fat assay), or reduced absorption of an administered test substance (e.g. lactose tolerance test;

Table 10.17). These specific tests are technically hard to perform, and many factors such as age and comorbidity affect results.

Thus, in practice, the diagnosis is often based on non-specific markers of malabsorption (Table 10.17); establishing a cause for the malabsorption (Table 10.19); and exclusion of poor intake or other disease to explain the abnormality(ies).

Tests for fat malabsorption
Faecal fat
In practice, if the stool looks overtly steatorrhoeic, formal confirmation is often unnecessary. The patient is then investigated to find out the extent and cause of the malabsorption (Tables 10.17 and 10.19).

To confirm suspected fat malabsorption, all stool passed over 3 days is collected while the patient eats a diet containing 100 g/day fat. Values above 5 g/day (20 mmol/day) suggest fat malabsorption from any cause. Incidentally useful information is a measurement of faecal

Table 10.19 Tests to investigate the cause of malabsorption

Test	Comments
Biochemistry	
Thyroid function tests, blood sugar	Exclude hyperthyroidism, diabetes as cause of weight loss
	Diabetes may be secondary to chronic pancreatitis
Gut hormones	Zollinger–Ellison syndrome may present with fat malabsorption
Immunology	
Gammaglobulins, immunoglobulins	Rarely, immunodeficiency syndromes may cause malabsorption
Microbiology	
Stools, jejunal aspiration, HIV	Exclude giardiasis, small bowel bacterial overgrowth, AIDS
Diagnostic imaging	
Barium follow-through/small bowel enema	May show Crohn's disease, other structural damage to small bowel, such as lymphoma
Plain abdominal radiography, ultrasound, CT scan, MRI, ERCP	Particularly to exclude structural changes indicating chronic pancreatitis
Pancreatic function tests	
Pancreolauryl test	Assessment of pancreatic exocrine function
Gastroscopy	
Small bowel biopsy	Gold standard test for coeliac disease
Breath tests	
Lactose	To look for lactase deficiency as cause of malabsorption
Lactulose	To look for small bowel bacterial overgrowth
Sweat test	To exclude cystic fibrosis, younger patients only (see p. 357)

AIDS, acquired immune deficiency virus; CT, computerized tomography; ERCP, endoscopic retrograde cholangiopancreatography; HIV, human immunodeficiency virus; MRI, magnetic resonance imaging.

10

weight, which gives a measure of the severity of diarrhoea. This procedure is tedious and unpleasant for the patient and the nursing and laboratory staff. The results are also unreliable, usually as a result of incomplete faecal collection.

^{14}C-triolein breath test
As faecal fat analysis is unpopular and inaccurate, alternative methods have been tried to quantify fat malabsorption. The general principles of breath tests are shown in Fig. 10.29. In the ^{14}C-triolein breath test, a triglyceride radiolabelled with ^{14}C is administered. If fat digestion and absorption is impaired, less of the triglycerides will be broken down, and thus less labelled $^{14}CO_2$ exhaled during the test. Unfortunately, many factors independent of fat absorption may influence the result (e.g. age), and the radiation dose precludes its use in children and women of childbearing age.

Pancreatic function test
Pancreatic exocrine dysfunction is the usual cause of very severe fat malabsorption. Assays such as the pancreolauryl test measure indirectly the activity of fat-digesting enzymes such as lipase, and thus the exocrine function of the pancreas. Abnormal tests confirm that fat absorption is impaired and point to reduced secretion of pancreatic enzymes because of pancreatic disease as the cause.

Tests for carbohydrate malabsorption
Xylose tolerance test
Xylose is a pentose sugar that is both passively and actively absorbed by the upper small bowel. It is not metabolized, and thus excreted unchanged in urine. Because the majority of active and passive carbohydrate absorption occurs in the upper small bowel, xylose malabsorption is a good marker for disease that is likely to affect this process.

An oral dose of 25 g is given after an overnight fast, and all urine collected for the next 5 h. A 1-h blood sample may also be taken. Diffuse mucosal disease of the upper small bowel (e.g. coeliac disease) impairs absorption, and reduced urinary excretion (less than 17% dose administered) and 1 h serum levels of xylose are found. Bacterial overgrowth may also cause reduced urinary excretion, because of microbial breakdown of the xylose in the gut lumen. Falsely low urinary xylose excretion occurs in the elderly and in patients with renal failure, ascites or delayed gastric emptying.

Lactose tolerance test

This test measures the activity of the enzyme lactase, located in the brush border of the upper small bowel. Serial measurements of blood glucose are made for 2 h after an oral dose of 50 g lactose—an increase of less than 1.1 mmol/l suggests a deficiency of the enzyme (hypolactasia). There will usually be accompanying bloating and diarrhoea driven by the osmotic effects of the unabsorbed disaccharide load. A positive test indicates either an isolated lactase enzyme deficiency or diffuse mucosal disease affecting the upper small bowel (e.g. coeliac disease). A positive test requires further investigation, in particular small bowel biopsy.

Another form of the test is measurement of breath hydrogen following the oral lactose challenge. Normally, oral ingestion of lactose produces no change in expired breath hydrogen concentration: gut mucosal lactase splits the lactulose into its constituent monosaccharides, glucose and galactose, which are rapidly absorbed by active transport mechanisms. If lactase activity is reduced, undigested lactose passes on into the colon, where its metabolism by faecal flora results in release of hydrogen. An increase in breath hydrogen by more than 20 p.p.m. following a 50-g lactose load is diagnostic.

In everyday practice, the quickest and most convenient test is the symptomatic response to 50 g oral lactose or, more simply, 500–1000 ml milk (which contains 25–50 g lactose)—patients with significantly reduced lactase activity develop transient abdominal pain, borborygmi and diarrhoea.

Other tests for malabsorption

Hydrogen breath tests

Breath tests can also be used to detect small bowel bacterial overgrowth. Lactulose is a sugar that is not absorbed by or metabolized in the normal small intestine. In the normal subject, it is metabolized by colonic bacteria, with release of hydrogen. A peak in exhaled hydrogen concentration thus occurs in normal subjects corresponding to the time taken for the lactulose to pass from mouth to colon (usually 70–90 min). If there are high levels of

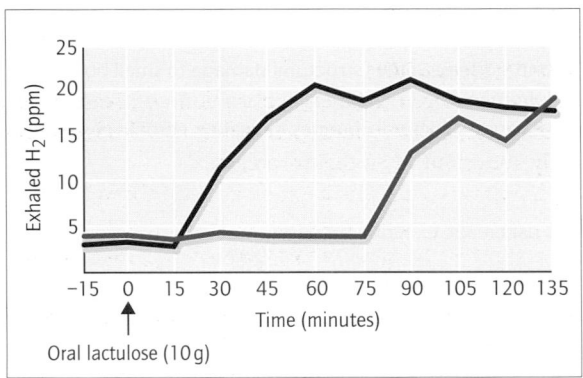

(a)

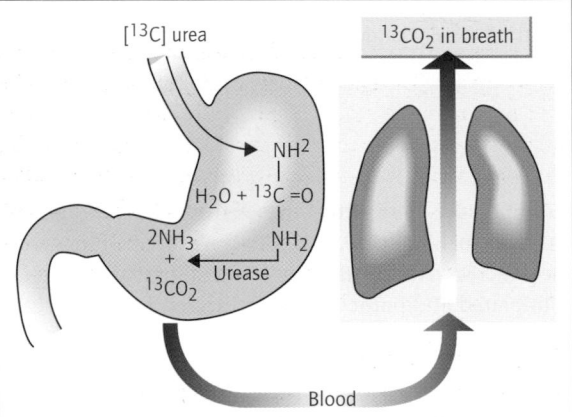

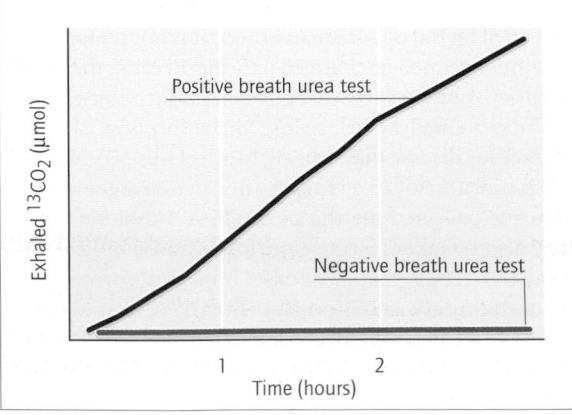

(b)

Figure 10.29 (*left*) Examples of breath tests used in gastroenterology. (a) Lactulose breath test to determine orocaecal transit time and detect small bowel bacterial overgrowth. The diagram shows normal exhaled hydrogen curve (blue)—orocaecal transit time is about 75–90 min; exhaled hydrogen curve of a patient with bacterial overgrowth (red)—the diagnosis is revealed by the early (at 15–30 min) rise of breath hydrogen concentration as lactulose is metabolized to hydrogen by bacteria in excess in the small intestine. (b) Urea breath test for the diagnosis of *Helicobacter pylori* infection. Urea labelled with carbon-13 is ingested and hydrolysed by urease, present in *H. pylori*. Hydrolysis of urea produces labelled CO_2 which is absorbed rapidly into the bloodstream and detected in expired air.

bacteria in the small bowel, then the hydrogen peak will be very early (Fig. 10.29). A positive lactulose breath test thus suggests small bowel bacterial overgrowth as the cause of malabsorption.

Unfortunately, like all hydrogen-based breath tests, this basically simple technique can be confounded by a high-fibre meal the night before the test, metabolism of the lactulose or other substrate by oral flora, vagaries of gastric emptying and intestinal flora that are unable to break down the substrate.

Tests for diarrhoea

The list of possible tests for diarrhoea is extensive, reflecting the differential diagnosis. A selective approach is used, based on clinical suspicion. Essential initial tests for troublesome diarrhoea include haemoglobin, mean corpuscular volume, ESR and C-reactive protein, coeliac serology, thyroid function tests, stool microscopy and culture, sigmoidoscopy and rectal biopsy. The clinical assessment may allow for prioritization of further specialized tests if these initial tests are negative. For example, a family history of coeliac disease would lead to duodenal biopsy early in the investigation cycle; a young patient with right iliac fossa pain and weight loss would have a small bowel study early on to look for Crohn's disease; a patient with culture-negative bloody diarrhoea would have colonoscopy as the next step. Tests are otherwise best performed in a staged manner (Fig. 10.30). Therapeutic trials may also be useful, e.g. of broad-spectrum antibiotics (for small bowel bacterial overgrowth); pancreatic enzyme supplements (for chronic pancreatitis) or colestyramine (for bile salt malabsorption).

Tests for constipation

In young patients with an obvious reversible cause (e.g. low-fibre diet, drugs, anal fissure), no investigations other than sigmoidoscopy are necessary. When a metabolic disorder is suspected, appropriate blood tests are undertaken (Table 10.15, p. 666).

A barium enema or colonoscopy, to look for structural disease of the large bowel, is usually only necessary in older patients. Transit studies, using plain X-rays to monitor passage of radio-opaque markers through the colon, are useful in this situation: they may show delayed transit throughout the bowel, indicating a diffuse motility disorder; accumulation of markers in the distal colon, suggesting a problem with defecation rather than motility in general (e.g. constipation because of pelvic nerve injury); or that the markers have passed out of the bowel, showing there is in fact no delay in oroanal transit, despite the patient's symptoms.

In refractory cases, other tests can be of use (e.g. defecating proctography, anorectal manometry and neurophysiology, anorectal ultrasound); however, these are rarely available outside specialist centres.

Management

Management of digestive disease may have general, dietary, pharmacological, endoscopic, surgical and laparoscopic components. The different tests available are discussed above, while the strategy for use of tests is discussed under individual conditions.

Communication

All patients need detailed explanation and reassurance, where appropriate, about their condition. This is particularly important when their problem:

- *is chronic:* coeliac disease, inflammatory bowel disease
- *is potentially fatal:* cancer
- *is complex to treat:* eradication of *H. pylori*, inflammatory bowel disease
- *involves a major psychological component:* irritable bowel syndrome

Such information may not only help patients cope with their disorder, but also alleviate symptoms, as in the irritable bowel.

Information to patients often needs to contain specific advice about changes in lifestyle (e.g. stopping smoking and avoidance of NSAIDs in peptic ulcer and inflammatory bowel disease, postural measures in reflux oesophagitis). For certain diseases, information leaflets and patient support groups (e.g. Coeliac Society, National Association for Colitis and Crohn's Disease) provide invaluable educational and practical support, for example with information about diet.

Dietary treatment

Supportive dietary treatment is often helpful:

- A high-fibre diet for constipation
- Low-residue diet for Crohn's disease complicated by small bowel stricturing
- Low wheat/fibre diet in irritable bowel syndrome, particularly with bloating
- Protein supplements for malnourished patients
- Enteral feeding for patients with deficient oral food intake (see p. 688)
- Parenteral nutrition for patients with such severe gastrointestinal dysfunction that oral or enteral feeding are precluded (see p. 689)

In some cases, diet is used as a primary therapeutic manoeuvre (e.g. a gluten-free diet in coeliac disease and specifically formulated feeds for some patients with active Crohn's disease).

10

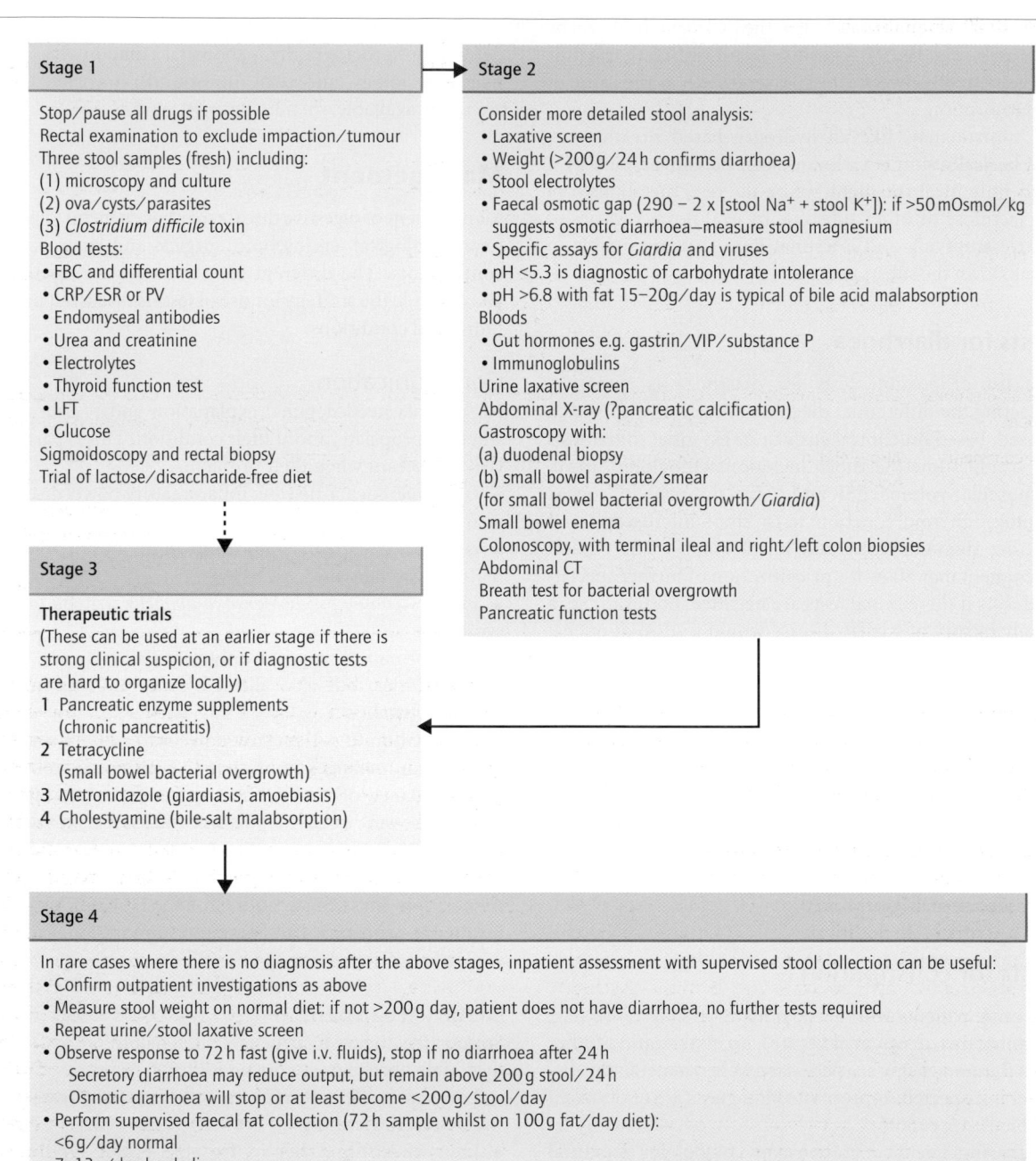

Stage 1

Stop/pause all drugs if possible
Rectal examination to exclude impaction/tumour
Three stool samples (fresh) including:
(1) microscopy and culture
(2) ova/cysts/parasites
(3) *Clostridium difficile* toxin
Blood tests:
• FBC and differential count
• CRP/ESR or PV
• Endomyseal antibodies
• Urea and creatinine
• Electrolytes
• Thyroid function test
• LFT
• Glucose
Sigmoidoscopy and rectal biopsy
Trial of lactose/disaccharide-free diet

Stage 2

Consider more detailed stool analysis:
• Laxative screen
• Weight (>200 g/24 h confirms diarrhoea)
• Stool electrolytes
• Faecal osmotic gap (290 − 2 x [stool Na$^+$ + stool K$^+$]): if >50 mOsmol/kg suggests osmotic diarrhoea—measure stool magnesium
• Specific assays for *Giardia* and viruses
• pH <5.3 is diagnostic of carbohydrate intolerance
• pH >6.8 with fat 15–20g/day is typical of bile acid malabsorption
Bloods
• Gut hormones e.g. gastrin/VIP/substance P
• Immunoglobulins
Urine laxative screen
Abdominal X-ray (?pancreatic calcification)
Gastroscopy with:
(a) duodenal biopsy
(b) small bowel aspirate/smear
(for small bowel bacterial overgrowth/*Giardia*)
Small bowel enema
Colonoscopy, with terminal ileal and right/left colon biopsies
Abdominal CT
Breath test for bacterial overgrowth
Pancreatic function tests

Stage 3

Therapeutic trials
(These can be used at an earlier stage if there is strong clinical suspicion, or if diagnostic tests are hard to organize locally)
1 Pancreatic enzyme supplements
   (chronic pancreatitis)
2 Tetracycline
   (small bowel bacterial overgrowth)
3 Metronidazole (giardiasis, amoebiasis)
4 Cholestyamine (bile-salt malabsorption)

Stage 4

In rare cases where there is no diagnosis after the above stages, inpatient assessment with supervised stool collection can be useful:
• Confirm outpatient investigations as above
• Measure stool weight on normal diet: if not >200 g day, patient does not have diarrhoea, no further tests required
• Repeat urine/stool laxative screen
• Observe response to 72 h fast (give i.v. fluids), stop if no diarrhoea after 24 h
    Secretory diarrhoea may reduce output, but remain above 200 g stool/24 h
    Osmotic diarrhoea will stop or at least become <200 g/stool/day
• Perform supervised faecal fat collection (72 h sample whilst on 100 g fat/day diet):
<6 g/day normal
7–13g/day borderline
>14 g/day, clear fat malabsorption
>20 g day usually indicates pancreatic disease

Figure 10.30 Stages in the investigation of chronic diarrhoea.

Table 10.20 Drugs used in nausea and vomiting

Drug class	Prokinetics	Antihistamines	Anticholinergics	Phenothiazines	5-HT3 antagonists
Example	Metoclopramide Domperidone	Cyclizine	Hyoscine	Prochlorperazine	Ondansetron
Pharmacological action	Central and peripheral dopamine antagonists	Centrally acting antihistamine	Central and peripheral anticholinergic actions involved	Centrally acting dopamine receptor antagonist	Centrally acting 5-HT3 receptor antagonist
Side-effects	Extrapyramidal effects (young people), hyperprolactinaemia	Drowsiness, dry mouth, blurred vision, potentiation of alcohol	Dry mouth, blurred vision, constipation, urine retention, confusion in the elderly	Drowsiness, postural hypotension, dry mouth, extrapyramidal effects	Constipation, headache, flushing
Contraindications/ cautions	Chronic administration	Glaucoma, prostatism	Glaucoma, prostatism	Parkinson's disease, glaucoma, prostatism	Lactation and special care with pregnancy
Uses/comments	Also useful in heartburn and irritable bowel syndrome	Vomiting caused by vestibular disease, pregnancy, radiotherapy	Vomiting caused by vestibular disease or postanaesthesia	Vomiting caused by vestibular disease, anaesthesia, chemotherapy, radiotherapy	Prophylaxis and treatment of post-operative nausea and vomiting and caused by chemotherapy and radiotherapy

Drugs

Common symptomatic treatments are reviewed below and in Tables 10.20 and 10.21. For full information on dosage and side-effects, refer to local or national formularies (e.g. *British National Formulary*).

Drugs for treating nausea and vomiting (Table 10.20)
All have some action on the vomiting centre and/or chemoreceptor trigger zone, located in the floor of the fourth ventricle. In addition, metoclopramide and domperidone have prokinetic activity, promoting gastric emptying and stimulating gastrointestinal motility in general. This prokinetic property leads to additional uses for these drugs, such as oesophagitis (more rapid clearance of acid from the oesophagus), and the irritable bowel syndrome (reducing abnormal gastrointestinal motility). Maxolon, and to a lesser extent domperidone, can provoke an acute extrapyramidal syndrome in young people (which can be rapidly terminated using intravenous antimuscarinics, e.g. benzatropine). They may also cause hyperprolactinaemia.

Phenothiazines (e.g. prochlorperazine—Stemetil) are widely used in the treatment of drug-induced nausea and vomiting, such as that resulting from opiate use. However, care is needed, particularly in the elderly, because of side-effects such as postural hypotension, confusion and parkinsonism.

Drugs for treating diarrhoea
Most diarrhoea is self-limiting after a few days, and antidiarrhoeals are best avoided. Non-specific treatment with antidiarrhoeal drugs is indicated while awaiting diagnosis and definitive treatment of more persistent diarrhoea, where a diagnosis cannot be achieved, or where symptoms cannot be controlled despite a known diagnosis and resultant specific treatment. The main contraindication is patients admitted with acute severe colitis, where antidiarrhoeals may precipitate toxic megacolon. Most antidiarrhoeals are opioid drugs. Loperamide is widely used as a first-line agent, and rarely causes CNS side-effects. Co-phenotrope combines an opiate and an anticholinergic. More potent opiates such as codeine or even morphine preparations are occasionally required for troublesome chronic diarrhoea, such as that associated with the short bowel syndrome (see p. 724). Side-effects are those of any opiate, such as drowsiness, confusion and nausea.

Colestyramine is an ion exchange resin that can bind bile salts, reducing diarrhoea from disease or the effects of surgical resection on the terminal ileum (see p. 652). This drug can interfere with the absorption of fat-soluble vitamins and many drugs, thus it is advisable to take concomitant medication well before or after the colestyramine dose.

Drugs for treating constipation
Faecal impaction should be excluded by rectal examination, and suppositories (e.g. glycerol) and/or enemas (e.g. Micralax) used as part of the treatment if present. If diet is low in fibre, supplements such as ispaghula, sterculia and

Table 10.21 Inhibitors of gastric acid secretion

Cimetidine	Ranitidine	Proton pump inhibitors
		PPI drugs available (full/'step down' dose*)
		Omeprazole (20/10 mg)
		Esomeprazole† (40/20 mg)
		Lansoprazole (30/15 mg)
		Pantoprazole (40/20 mg)
		Rabeprazole (20/10 mg)
Pharmacological action		
H_2 receptor blockade	H_2 receptor blockade	Inhibit hydrogen/potassium exchange pump on mucosal surface of parietal gastric cells ('proton pump')
Main indications		
Non-ulcer dyspepsia	Non-ulcer dyspepsia	Non-ulcer dyspepsia
Reflux oesophagitis	Reflux oesophagitis	Reflux oesophagitis
Peptic ulcer healing	Peptic ulcer healing	Peptic ulcer healing
Peptic ulcer prophylaxis	Peptic ulcer prophylaxis	Peptic ulcer prophylaxis
Prophylaxis against bleeding in intensive care	Prophylaxis against bleeding in intensive care	Prophylaxis against bleeding in intensive care
		Zollinger–Ellison syndrome
		Treatment/prophylaxis of NSAID-induced gastroduodenal injury
		Component of many *H. pylori* eradication regimens
Side-effects		
As for ranitidine, plus gynaecomastia	Headache	Diarrhoea
Drug interactions	Confusion in the elderly	Nausea
Loss of libido		Headaches
Raised serum creatinine		Rashes
		Blurred vision
		For omeprazole and lansoprazole only: inhibition of drug metabolism—enhanced effects (e.g. of anticoagulants, phenytoin)
Contraindications/cautions		
Elderly, renal failure, use of other drugs	None	Potential drug interactions as above

PPI, proton pump inhibitor.
*Because of the high cost of PPI drugs, the lower 'step down' dose should be used where possible in long-term prescribing.
†A preparation of omeprazole s-isomer, with the inactive r-isomer removed.

methylcellulose may be of use. Adequate fluid intake must be encouraged. These bulking agents are contraindicated if there is known or suspected mechanical obstruction of the bowel (e.g. by cancer)—they simply aggravate the problem. Impacted stool proximal to a mechanical obstruction may result in bowel perforation, particularly in the thin-walled right colon.

Faecal softeners can be effective alone, or in conjunction with colonic stimulants. Magnesium hydroxide and docusate sodium are relatively gentle and inexpensive first-line agents. Lactulose is a commonly prescribed softener, but is expensive and often causes uncomfortable bloating. Both these sugar-based osmotic softeners have a specific additional role in the treatment of hepatic encephalopathy (see p. 615). Magnesium sulphate is a more potent osmotic agent, usually for short-term use.

Movicol is a preparation of polyethylene glycol, and a potent if expensive faecal softener. It does not cause bloating, is useful in resistant cases, and is well tolerated in the long term.

Drugs to suppress gastric acid production (Table 10.21) Strategies for the use of these drugs are discussed under individual diseases below. PPIs are more potent than H_2 receptor antagonists (H$_2$RAs), but considerably more expensive. In both primary and secondary care they are amongst the top few drugs for annual costs, because of the large number of patients using them long term. The main indications where PPIs significantly outperform H$_2$RAs in clinical trials are reflux oesophagitis (see p. 692) and prophylaxis and treatment of NSAID-induced upper gastrointestinal injury (see p. 705). They have a specific role in *H. pylori* eradication regimens (see p. 709). Other indications such as peptic ulcer healing and prophylaxis (see p. 706), and non-specific dyspepsia (see p. 659) may be adequately dealt with by the cheaper H₂RAs. It is important periodically to review the need for PPI prescription in long-term users, and explore whether a lower dose of the same PPI, a cheaper PPI alternative, or alternative drug class would deal with the condition.

PPIs inhibit urease enzyme activity. *Helicobacter pylori* has very high urease activity, and several tests for its detection make use of this fact (breath tests and biopsy urease tests; see Fig. 10.29, p. 706). PPIs should be avoided for at least 4 weeks before these tests to avoid false-negative results. They are also best avoided prior to endoscopy as they may mask pathology, including causing temporary healing of mucosal ulceration resulting from gastric malignancy.

Enteral and parenteral nutrition

Nutritional depletion

Nutritional depletion can result from:
- Poor appetite
- Inability to assimilate food
- Increased catabolic rate (e.g. sepsis, cancer)
- Excessive loss of nutrients from the body (e.g. diarrhoea, steatorrhoea)

Malnutrition is common in patients admitted to hospital (KEYPOINTS BOX 10.1) where too often there is a failure to record and respond to the above factors, or to make basic assessments of nutritional status using the body mass index (BMI; weight in kilograms divided by height in metres squared). Not infrequently, patients become nutritionally depleted as a result of the above factors even while in hospital. This is sometimes compounded by the misapprehension that malnutrition can be averted by using intravenous glucose solutions.

> ### Keypoints 10.1: Nutrition
>
> Undernutrition is common in patients admitted to hospital
> Malnutrition delays recovery from most illnesses and after surgery
> Unless gut function is severely impaired, nutritional replacement should be given enterally rather than intravenously

The main gastrointestinal causes of undernutrition are listed in Table 10.22. Malnutrition has clinical, haematological and biochemical consequences:
- *Clinical consequences:* include weight loss, apathy, weakness, decreased resistance to infection, delayed wound

Table 10.22 Main gastrointestinal causes of nutritional depletion and indications for nutritional support

Loss of appetite
Non-specific anorexia, nausea, vomiting, anorexia nervosa

Oropharyngeal disease
Neoplasms, trauma

Oesophageal disorders
Strictures (neoplastic, peptic), motility disorders (achalasia, bulbar palsy)

Gastric disorders
Neoplasms, pyloric stenosis

Malabsorption
Crohn's disease, small bowel resections, fistulae, pancreatitis

Intestinal obstruction/ileus

Increased catabolism
Active inflammatory bowel disease, sepsis, neoplasia, surgery, trauma

healing, specific nutritional deficiencies as for malabsorption states (Table 10.18, p. 680) and death
- *Haematological consequences:* include anaemia, lymphopenia and low folate, serum iron and ferritin
- *Biochemical consequences:* include low serum levels of albumin, calcium, magnesium, zinc and fat-soluble vitamins

Nutritional support

Nutritional support should be considered for anyone who has lost, or is likely to lose, more than 10% of his or her normal body weight, whose BMI is less than 20 or in whom abnormalities in laboratory tests are thought to be brought about by malnutrition.

Often, deficits can be replaced by attention to food intake, supplemented if necessary by specially prepared high-protein and/or calorie drinks. Sometimes, however, nutrition needs to be introduced artificially, usually via pumps, directly into the gastrointestinal tract (enteral nutrition) or intravenously (parenteral nutrition).

Note, however, that patients who are *severely* malnourished may have significant and even fatal complications if nutrients are replaced too quickly. These complications, which together are known as the refeeding syndrome, include salt and water retention, excess CO_2 production with acidosis, hypokalaemia and hypophosphataemia. Providing increased calories without appropriate vitamins and trace elements can precipitate deficiency syndromes as the increased cellular activity in response to refeeding places increased demand on limited micronutrient supplies.

10

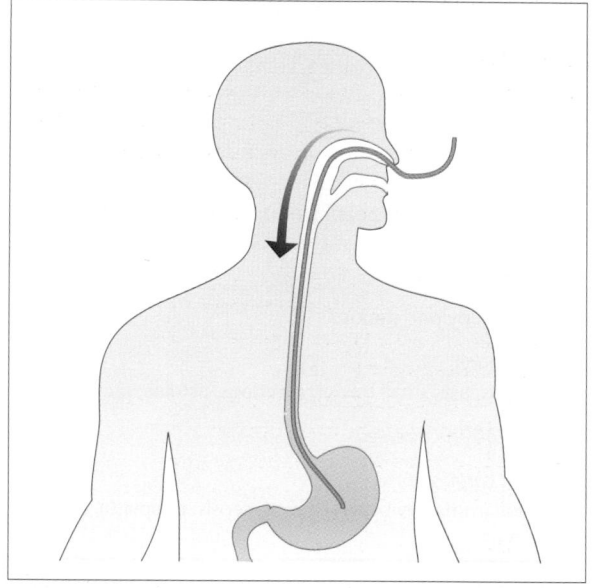

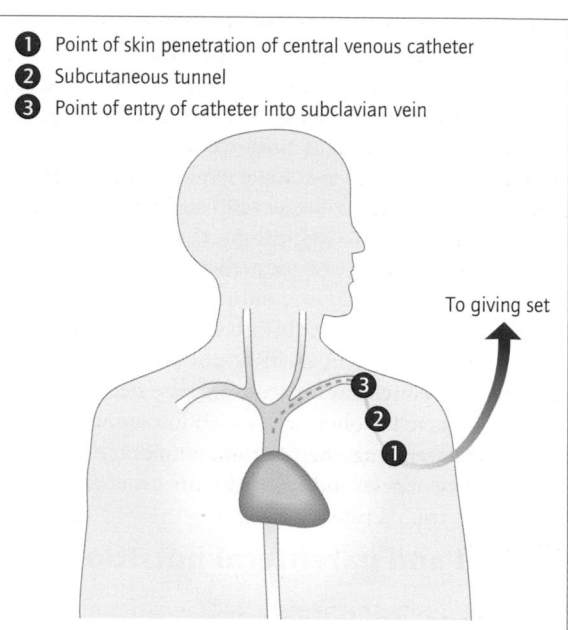

① Point of skin penetration of central venous catheter
② Subcutaneous tunnel
③ Point of entry of catheter into subclavian vein

To giving set

(a)

(b)

Figure 10.31 (a) Inserting an enteral feeding tube. A lubricated fine-bore polyvinyl or polyurethane tube stiffened by a guide wire is inserted through the nostril and passed gently down the oesophagus to the stomach; the guide wire is then removed. Its position in the stomach is checked by auscultation below the left costal margin while injecting 10 ml of air down the tube with a syringe, by testing aspirate for acidity using litmus paper or by plain radiography. (b) Inserting a parenteral feeding line. The silastic feeding catheter is aseptically introduced via the subclavian vein into the superior vena cava. Its proximal end is brought out through a subcutaneous tunnel to reduce the risk of infection, and connects via a Luer lock, with an extension tube, which is attached to the giving set. The rate of flow of feed from the 3-l bag is controlled by a volumetric pump.

10

Choice of route

Enteral should always be used in preference to parenteral nutrition if intestinal function is not severely impaired. This is because it is safer, simpler and cheaper.

Enteral nutrition

Inserting the feeding tube

Nasogastric tube

A lubricated fine-bore polyvinyl or polyurethane tube is inserted through the nostril and passed gently down the oesophagus to the stomach (Fig. 10.31). Its position is checked by a combination of auscultation below the left costal margin while 10 ml of air is injected down the tube, by plain radiography and by checking the acidity of aspirate. If there is an obstructing lesion of the oesophagus or stomach, the fine-bore tube can often be passed using endoscopic or guide wire techniques.

Fine-bore tubes can be left *in situ* for several weeks. Larger bore tubes should not be used for enteral feeding for more than a week because they cause nasal discomfort, oesophagitis and peptic stricture.

Gastrostomy or gastrojejunostomy tube

If long-term enteral feeding is required, it is often preferable to insert a percutaneous gastrostomy or gastro-jejunostomy tube using an endoscopic (PEG) or radiological technique (see p. 672).

Choice of enteral feed

There is a wide variety of nutritionally complete proprietary preparations available (e.g. Fresubin, Ensure). They are based on milk, soya or beef protein, with a calorie source of glucose polymer or vegetable oil and additional vitamins and minerals. Most hospitals will have a local formulary choice—hospital dietitians are best placed to advise on when and which to use. These provide a flexible prescription for:

- *Catabolic states:* e.g. sepsis
- *Metabolically compromised patients:* e.g. diabetics requiring close monitoring and frequent adjustment of regimen
- *Non-catabolic states:* e.g. stroke

These products, which contain whole protein, are referred to as **polymeric** feeds. **Peptide** feeds contain the protein source as polypeptides, and **elemental feeds** deliver protein as free amino acids. The more 'pre-digested' the protein source, the less potential it has for inducing immune reactions in the gut. For this reason, elemental feeds were used in early trials comparing exclusive enteral feeding against steroids in the treatment of active Crohn's disease. Elemental diets appeared as effective as steroids in those who could tolerate them. Subsequent trials have suggested polymeric and peptide feeds are as effective in Crohn's disease. Elemental feeds are used in some centres for direct infusion into the jejunum in the treatment of severe pancreatitis, which seems to have advantages over the traditional approach of keeping such patients nil-by-mouth. In patients who are thought to have problems absorbing fat, **medium-chain triglyceride** feeds may be tried—this lipid is less reliant on pancreatic lipase and bile salts for absorption than long-chain triglycerides, which are the fat source in standard oral supplemental feeds (see p. 649). In almost all other settings, where nutritional support is required by mouth, the polymeric-type feeds are the appropriate first choice.

Administration and monitoring of enteral feeding

Enteral feeds can be administered continuously. Alternatively, they can be taken at night only. Because of the discomfort and awkwardness of nasogastric tubes, patients who need enteral feeding for more than 2 weeks should be considered for percutaneous gastrostomy as the feeding route (see p. 672). Enteral feeding rarely precludes the consumption of at least small amounts of ordinary food and drink to add to quality of life. Progress should be monitored with a fluid balance chart and twice weekly measurements of weight, urea, electrolytes, glucose and albumin.

Complications of enteral feeding

- *Diarrhoea:* from the use of antibiotics or hyperosmolar, too cold or infected feed, fast administration of feed, or lactose intolerance. 'Half-strength' (low osmolality) and smaller volumes are used initially to minimize this problem
- *Pulmonary aspiration:* because the tube finds its way into the pharynx or trachea, or because rapidly administered feed is regurgitated
- *Inflammation of the nose or oesophagus*
- *Metabolic problems:* from fluid overload or depletion, and glucose and electrolyte disturbances

Parenteral nutrition

Because of its complexity, potential hazards and expense, patients requiring parenteral nutrition should be man-

aged by a specially trained and experienced nutrition team composed of clinicians, nurses, pharmacists and dietitians.

Indications

Intravenous feeding should be restricted to the few patients whose gastrointestinal function is so severely impaired that they are unable to absorb enough enterally administered nutrients to maintain or replace their requirements. Placement of lines, choice of feed and patient monitoring should be under the supervision of the local nutrition team.

The most common indications are:

- Prolonged ileus or obstruction
- Massive intestinal resection
- Proximal enterocutaneous fistula
- Severe inflammatory bowel disease
- Intra-abdominal sepsis and pancreatitis
- Perforated oesophagus

Technique

Intravenous nutrient solutions are usually hypertonic and are most safely given slowly into a large central vein where they are rapidly diluted with blood. Because these catheters are often used long term, they are best placed under strict aseptic conditions in theatre. The distal end of the line is 'tunnelled' under the skin, reducing the chance of systemic infection resulting from pathogen entry around the exit site of the line (Fig. 10.31b). In the absence of complications and with scrupulous care, the catheter can be left in place for many months.

Occasionally, it is appropriate to feed patients parenterally for a short period through a peripheral vein. A less hypertonic feeding solution is used and the drip site should be rotated every 24–48 h to prevent irreversible venous damage.

Choice of parenteral feed

There is a wide range of intravenous feeds available, their selection for individual patients depends on the indication and whether the patient is catabolic or has a particular problem such as diabetes or renal, hepatic or cardiac failure. Nitrogen (usually 9 g/day) is supplied as synthetic amino acids, and calories (200 kcal/g N) as glucose and fat emulsion; electrolytes, trace elements and vitamins are also added. The feed is aseptically prepared, usually in 3-l bags, for administration over 18–24 h.

Complications of parenteral feeding

Complications of intravenous feeding include those related to the line and problems related to the feed. They are best prevented by limiting use of lines to feeding alone (they are not used for central venous pressure measurement, blood transfusion, blood sampling or drug administration) and confining line management to specially trained nutrition nurses.

Complications of parenteral feeding:

- *Local trauma:* pneumothorax, haemothorax, subclavian artery puncture or brachial plexus damage caused by insertion of the catheter
- *Air embolism:* resulting from negative intrathoracic pressure or catheter disconnection or fracture
- *Infusion of fluid into the mediastinum or pleural cavity:* because of perforation of the vein by the catheter
- *Thrombosis of the vein:* resulting from the presence of the catheter
- *Infection:* as a result of failure of aseptic technique or use of the line for purposes other than feeding
- *Metabolic problems:* hyperglycaemia; reactive hypoglycaemia; hypophosphataemia or refeeding syndrome; electrolyte or acid–base imbalance; deficiencies of trace elements, essential fatty acids, folate and vitamins; lipaemia; and jaundice

The most serious and frequent complication is infection. Central intravenous feeding often has to be discontinued as a result.

Discontinuing parenteral feeding

Patients on long-term intravenous feeding tend to have a reduced appetite and decreased small intestinal absorptive capacity because of mucosal atrophy. Such patients should be encouraged to eat and drink when possible, but conversion from parenteral to enteral or oral nutrition should be gradual.

Diseases and their management

Diseases of the oesophagus

Gastro-oesophageal reflux disease (GORD) is extremely common, particularly in affluent societies. The condition overlaps with the topics of hiatus hernia, Barrett's oesophagus and oesophageal adenocarcinoma, and an overview is presented here before considering the individual components.

A hiatus hernia is one of several factors that can reduce the mechanical competence of the lower oesophageal sphincter (LOS; Fig. 10.4). The LOS is the main barrier to reflux of gastric contents into the oesophagus. Many patients with hiatus hernia do not reflux gastric contents to an abnormal degree and, conversely, many patients with significant GORD do not have an hiatus hernia. In general, however, the larger the hiatus hernia, the more defective the antireflux mechanism. Whenever the pressure in the gastric lumen exceeds that generated by the LOS, gastric contents can be refluxed into the oesophagus. The refluxate contains hydrochloric acid, bile and pepsin —all of which can injure the squamous mucosa of the oesophagus. Some gastro-oesophageal reflux occurs in normal subjects; however, as long as the events are short-lived, with the refluxate rapidly cleared or neutralized (e.g. by oesophageal peristalsis or swallowing of saliva), no symptoms occur and no mucosal injury results. If oesophageal exposure to the gastric refluxate is too prolonged, typical GORD symptoms (heartburn and acid reflux to the mouth) and/or mucosal injury may result (typically, linear erosions in the lower oesophagus—reflux oesophagitis).

The correlation between degree of oesophageal injury and reflux symptoms is poor. Some patients with severe reflux oesophagitis have no or few symptoms. Conversely, half of patients with classic heartburn symptoms and/or abnormal oesophageal pH studies have no visible oesophagitis if endoscoped.

When gastro-oesophageal acid reflux is severe and prolonged, the lower oesophageal mucosa may undergo a defensive metaplastic change from squamous to columnar epithelium, called Barrett's oesophagus. Barrett's mucosa is unstable, and in some cases progresses through dysplasia to adenocarcinoma. The acid reflux events that stimulate the development of Barrett's often cause no symptoms in themselves. Thus, the first symptom some patients may have is dysphagia from oesophageal carcinoma, arising in Barrett's mucosa.

Most cases of oesophageal adenocarcinoma develop in Barrett's oesophagus. The incidence of this tumour is rising rapidly, particularly in the developed world. This observation is thought to reflect the adverse effect of an affluent lifestyle (obesity, large fat-rich meals) on the competence of the LOS, and thus on the propensity for development of GORD and Barrett's oesophagus.

The significance of GORD is therefore much greater than was previously recognized. A recent large study highlighted this, showing that patients with severe and long-standing GORD symptoms had over 40 times the risk of developing oesophageal cancer than matched controls.

Hiatus hernia

A hiatus hernia is defined as the presence of part of the stomach in the chest. There are two types (Fig. 10.32a):

- *Sliding hiatus hernia:* protrusion of the proximal stomach through the diaphragm in continuity with the oesophagus

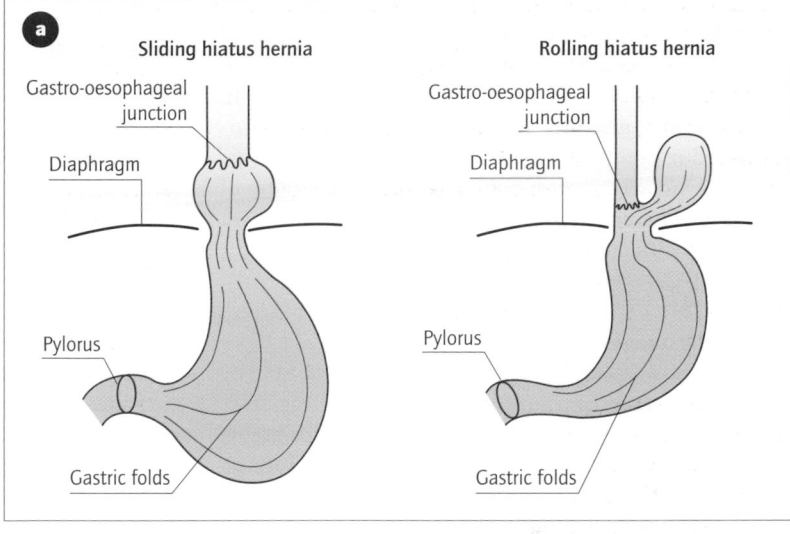

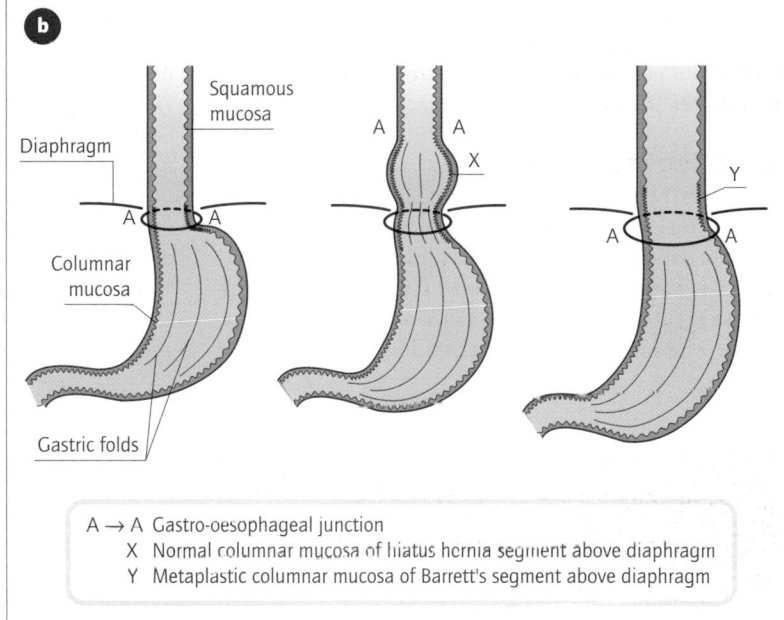

A → A Gastro-oesophageal junction
X Normal columnar mucosa of hiatus hernia segment above diaphragm
Y Metaplastic columnar mucosa of Barrett's segment above diaphragm

Figure 10.32 (a) Different types of hiatus herniae. (b) Differentiation of Barrett's columnar lined oesophagus and a hiatus hernia. Note the presence of gastric folds in continuity with the columnar mucosa above the diaphragm in hiatus hernia.

• *Rolling or para-oesophageal hiatus hernia:* the presence of part or all of the proximal stomach in the chest lateral to the gastro-oesophageal mucosal junction because of failed closure of one of the two pleuroperitoneal canals. The presence of gastric folds within the segment of columnar type mucosa in the chest helps differentiate hiatus hernia from Barrett's oesophagus (Fig. 10.32b)

Disease mechanisms

Contributory factors to a sliding hiatus hernia include a lax hernial orifice and increased intra-abdominal pressure (e.g. through weight gain).

Epidemiology

Prevalence. Occurs in 30% of people over 50 years old. The sliding is much more common than the rolling type.

Age. Incidence increases with age.

Sex. More common in women than in men.

Geography. Affluent societies.

Clinical features

A hiatus hernia can occur without any significant

disruption to the antireflux mechanism or symptoms, or it may contribute to gastro-oesophageal reflux and its complications. There may be occult bleeding or ulceration within the hiatal constriction, leading to iron-deficiency anaemia as well as bleeding from associated reflux oesophagitis. Occasionally, a rolling hernia presents with severe chest pain and vomiting because of gastric volvulus and strangulation, with dysphagia or with respiratory difficulties.

Investigation
Diagnostic imaging
- *OGD:* shows gastric mucosa above the diaphragmatic orifice (see REFLUX OESOPHAGITIS AT A GLANCE, Fig. A)
- *Barium swallow and meal:* a small sliding hiatus hernia with reflux can be produced temporarily by pressure on the abdomen in many normal people in the supine position during a barium swallow. Thus, there is a tendency to over-report the presence of hiatus herniae radiologically (Fig. 10.26a)
- *Chest radiography:* may reveal a large hiatus hernia as an incidental finding as a retrocardiac gas-filled shadow, sometimes containing a fluid level (Fig. 10.25c)

Management
No treatment is required for asymptomatic hiatus hernia. The main complications are not of the hiatus hernia *per se*, but of the reflux oesophagitis and Barrett's oesophagus that may subsequently develop (see p. 696). Rolling herniae producing obstructive symptoms require surgery.

Gastro-oesophageal reflux disease/reflux oesophagitis

The term GORD is applied to patients with symptoms suggestive of reflux (heartburn, acid reflux, rapid relief of symptoms with antacids, symptoms provoked by posture and postprandially), but not necessarily with oesophageal inflammation. A diagnosis can be made if these features are present, even in the face of a normal gastroscopy. A 'gold standard' diagnosis can be achieved through 24-h ambulatory pH monitoring (Fig. 10.28), and this technique can be extremely useful when the diagnosis is unclear.

Some patients with GORD have reflux oesophagitis, which is defined as inflammation of distal oesophageal mucosa because of reflux of gastric contents. Half of patients with GORD symptoms have no macroscopic reflux oesophagitis when examined endoscopically. A proportion of these 'normal' cases will have histological features of reflux-induced mucosal inflammation if the normal-looking distal oesophageal mucosa is biopsied. However, a large proportion of patients with significant GORD symptoms have a completely normal oesophagus macroscopically and microscopically. Conversely, some patients with typical reflux oesophagitis have no GORD symptoms. Variable oesophageal sensitivity to mucosal acid exposure inflammation explains this poor correlation between symptoms and pathology.

Where reflux oesophagitis occurs, the chief injuring agent is acid, as demonstrated by the response of most

---

Reflux oesophagitis at a glance

Epidemiology
Prevalence
Affects 30% of the population

Geography
Affluent societies where obesity is common

Causes
Hiatus hernia
Obesity
Drugs
- NSAIDs
- Antidepressants
- Anticholinergics
- Calcium-channel blockers
Reflux is not always associated with either hiatus hernia or symptoms

Investigation
Most patients need none

Endoscopy
Hyperaemia, erosions, ulceration, with or without hiatus hernia and/or stricture
Of those with reflux symptoms, only 50% will have an abnormal gastroscopy

Barium meal
Rarely necessary
Reflux, with or without hiatus hernia and/or stricture

Oesophageal function tests
Rarely necessary
Episodic acidification (pH < 4) of distal oesophagus, lax lower oesophageal sphincter on manometry

Management

Treatment of reflux comprises dietary and postural measures, with inhibition of acid production

General advice

Avoid stooping
Elevate bed head 10–15 cm
Stop smoking
Avoid causative drugs (see above)

Diet

Lose weight
Avoid fatty and spicy foods
Avoid late-night meals
Avoid alcohol
Avoid hot drinks (especially coffee and tea)
Avoid large meals

Medical treatment

Antacids: magnesium and aluminium hydroxide mixture
Inhibitors of acid secretion: proton pump inhibitors (e.g. omeprazole) are superior in this disease to H_2 receptor antagonists (e.g. ranitidine)
Prokinetic agents: metoclopramide, domperidone

Surgery or laparoscopy

Antireflux operation: fundoplication
Rarely, surgery for complicating peptic stricture

Treatment of complications

Endoscopic dilatation for peptic stricture
Endoscopic surveillance for early diagnosis of adenocarcinoma if there is Barrett's metaplasia of the epithelium
Chronic reflux predisposes, through Barrett's metaplasia, to adenocarcinoma of the oesophagus

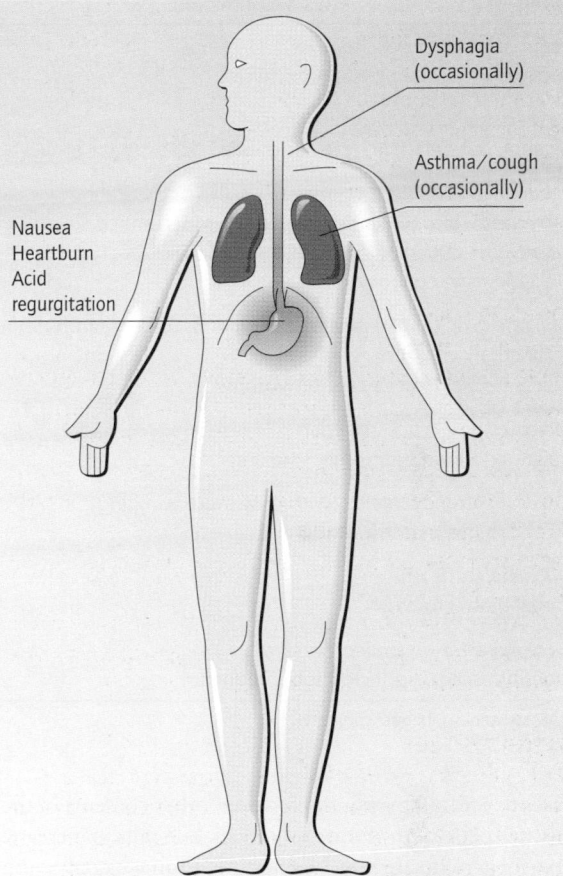

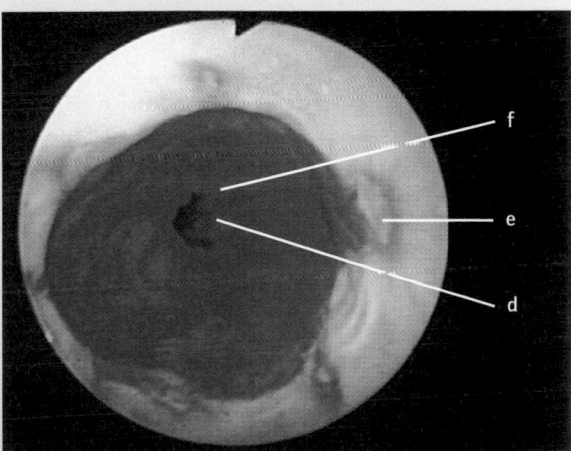

Fig. A Reflux oesophagitis with typical linear erosions of the squamous mucosa (e). Note small hiatus hernia in this case, shown by gastric folds (f) above the diaphragmatic constriction (d).

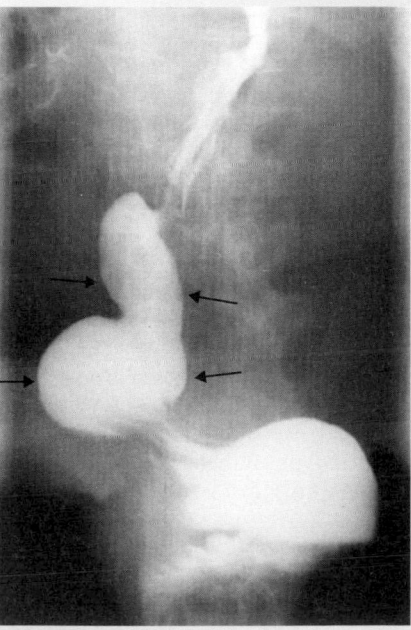

Fig. B Hiatus hernia and reflux oesophagitis. Note the barium-filled hiatus above the diaphragm (arrowed).

Table 10.23 Causes of reflux oesophagitis

Reduced oesophageal clearance
Recumbent posture, systemic sclerosis

Direct oesophageal mucosal damage
Alcohol, hot drinks, NSAIDs, acid, bile

Reduced LOS pressure
Fatty foods, alcohol, coffee, smoking, drugs (anticholinergics, calcium-containing antacids, nitrates, calcium-channel blockers), pregnancy

Damage to or loss of antireflux mechanisms (other than LOS function)
Hiatus hernia, Heller's cardiomyotomy

Increased gastric acid secretion
Zollinger–Ellison syndrome, smoking

Increased gastric contents (with or without vomiting)
Pyloric stenosis, gastric atony

Duodenogastric reflux
Partial gastrectomy

Increased intra-abdominal pressure
Obesity, ascites, tight clothing, pregnancy

LOS, lower oesophageal sphincter.

cases to acid suppression. However, other contents of the gastric (pepsin) or duodenal (alkali, bile salts, pancreatic enzymes) refluxate may be relevant in some patients, and may explain the 5–10% of patients not helped by acid suppressants.

Disease mechanisms

The causes and pathogenesis of GORD/reflux oesophagitis are listed in Table 10.23.

Pathology

The macroscopic appearance of the lower oesophagus ranges from normal, through diffuse or linear hyperaemia with superficial erosions (Fig. 10.33) to frank ulceration. Histologically, hypertrophy of the basal epithelial layer with elongation of the rete papillae is followed by exudation, ulceration and chronic inflammatory cell infiltration. Healing by fibrosis can cause stricture (Fig. 10.33b).

Prolonged acid exposure can lead to metaplasia to columnar gastric-type epithelium (Barrett's oesophagus; see p. 696 and Fig. 10.33c).

Epidemiology

Prevalence. About one-third of the normal population experiences monthly episodes of heartburn.

Geography. Affluent societies.

Clinical features

Symptoms arise both from the injured oesophageal mucosa, and from the effects of refluxate passing up into the pharynx and mouth (Table 10.8, p. 662; REFLUX OESOPHAGITIS AT A GLANCE, pp. 692–3):
- Heartburn
- Dysphagia (caused by oesophageal ulceration, spasm or stricture)
- Regurgitation of gastric contents into the throat, resulting in a bitter or acid taste
- Bleeding (rarely)

Other symptoms include nausea, vomiting, epigastric and back pain, odynophagia and aspiration of refluxed gastric contents (coughing, asthma, chest infections). There are commonly no clinical signs.

Differential diagnosis

Includes other causes of dyspepsia (Tables 10.4, p. 657, and 10.8, p. 662). Additional features favouring GORD include:
- A postural component
- Provocation by large and/or fatty meals, posture, tight clothing
- Rapid, if temporary, relief of symptoms with use of antacids

Symptoms of GORD overlap with those of angina, particularly if there is associated oesophageal spasm. To add to the confusion, acid reflux may be worsened by exercise and oesophageal spasm relieved by antianginal therapies such as glyceryl trinitrate spray. If there is doubt it is safest to assume the pain is cardiac initially (EMERGENCY BOX 10.1). A response to a therapeutic trial of PPIs, and the results of gastroscopy and 24-h pH studies are helpful in differentiating between oesophageal and cardiac pain.

Emergency 10.1: Reflux oesophagitis

Beware: the pain of myocardial ischaemia and oesophageal reflux and/or spasm may be indistinguishable. When there is diagnostic uncertainty, treat as myocardial ischaemia initially

---

Complications. Complications of reflux oesophagitis include peptic strictures (Fig. 10.33c), bleeding, Barrett's epithelium (Fig. 10.33d) and lung disorders (asthma and pneumonia).

Investigation
Haematology
FBC. Rarely, there is a microcytic anaemia.

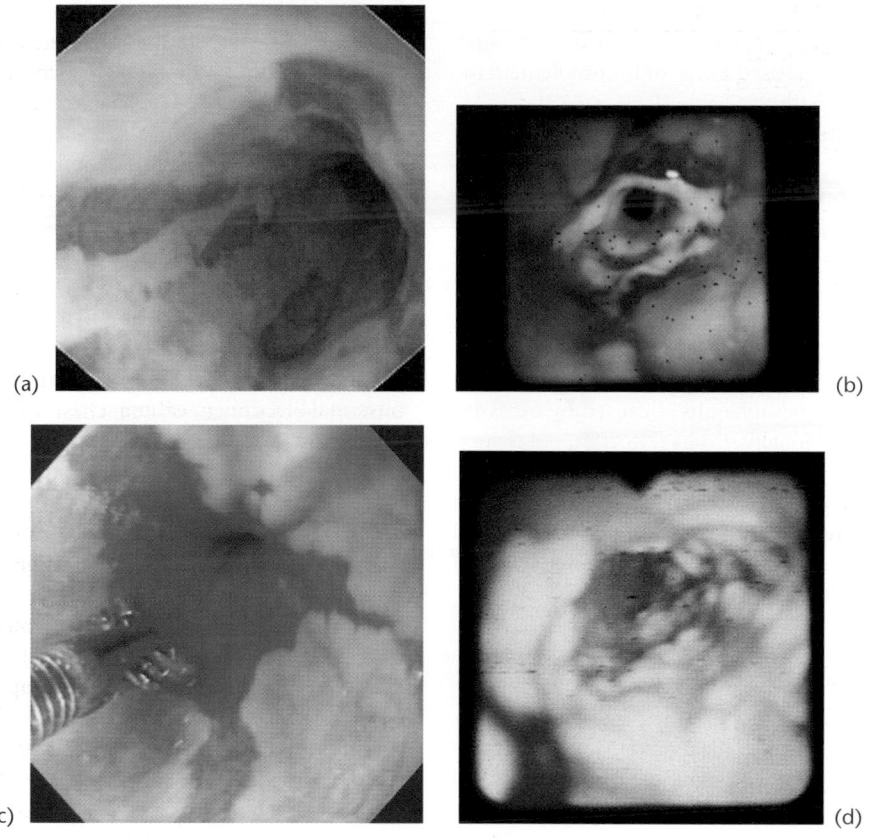

(a)

(b)

(c)

(d)

Figure 10.33 Endoscopic views of the distal oesophagus. (a) Linear hyperaemia with erosions: reflux oesophagitis. (Reproduced from Cotton PB, Williams CB. *Practical Gastrointestinal Endoscopy*, 3rd edn. Oxford: Blackwell Scientific Publications, 1990 with the permission of the authors.) (b) Benign peptic oesophageal stricture. (c) Barrett's oesophagus. Note the tongues of orange–red columnar-type mucosa extending proximally up the distal oesophagus. The biopsy forceps are positioned at the junction of Barrett's mucosa and normal oesophageal mucosa. (Reproduced from *Slide Atlas of Gastroenterology* with the kind permission of the author and Times Mirror International Publishers.) (d) *Candida* oesophagus. Note ulceration and pseudomembranes.

10

Diagnostic imaging

● *Gastroscopy:* may show the typical features of reflux oesophagitis (Fig. 10.33), but is normal in 50% of patients with GORD

● *Barium swallow and meal:* shows gastro-oesophageal reflux in many normal asymptomatic subjects and is an insensitive method of detecting oesophageal mucosal inflammation (Fig. 10.26)

Other

Oesophageal pH measurement. In patients with equivocal or refractory symptoms, or where there are typical GORD symptoms but a normal endoscopy, oesophageal pH studies allow continuous 24-h assessment of the total oesophageal acid exposure, and of the relationship between lower oesophageal pH and symptoms (Fig. 10.28).

Management

The general and dietary measures shown in REFLUX OESOPHAGITIS AT A GLANCE are important in all cases. If a patient has mild symptoms that do not respond to dietary changes, postural measures and simple antacids, then gastric acid secretion should be inhibited pharmacologically. Some patients respond to minimal therapy with intermittent treatment with H$_2$ receptor antagonists, whereas others require maximal acid suppression with long-term high-dose PPIs. For patients with mild or intermittent symptoms, a 'step-up' approach is often used, working up from minimal to maximal options as above. For patients with more severe symptoms or oesophagitis at OGD, or complications such as stricturing, the reverse approach ('step-down'), starting with PPIs, is recommended. Alginate (which forms a raft on the surface of the gastric contents) and dimeticone (an antifoaming agent) are no more effective than simple antacids. Prokinetic agents such as domperidone may be used alone, or to complement the actions of acid suppressants (Table 10.20, p. 685).

A minority of patients fail to respond to these measures and require surgery, usually a laparascopic Nissen fundoplication, in which the gastric fundus is sutured around the distal oesophagus to create a lower oesophageal high-pressure zone to resist reflux (for treatment of peptic strictures see Fig. 10.22).

Other causes of oesophagitis

The vast majority of oesophagitis is caused by excessive acid exposure. Occasionally, drugs (NSAIDs, potassium, bisphosphonates), corrosives or previous radiation can cause similar appearances. *Candida* oesophagitis is seen in immunocompromised patients (e.g. AIDS, steroid use—including inhalers) and has a typical appearance of easily detached white plaques (Fig. 10.33d).

Barrett's oesophagus

In Barrett's oesophagus, the stratified squamous epithelium that normally lines the distal oesophagus undergoes metaplastic change (where one type of fully differentiated cell replaces another) to columnar epithelium. It is a highly detrimental consequence of chronic gastro-oesophageal reflux as it predisposes to oesophageal carcinoma.

Disease mechanisms

The development of Barrett's mucosa is probably a defensive response of the oesophagus to excessive reflux of caustic gastric contents. Thus, the condition is always acquired, and commences in the lower oesophagus. Traditionally, at least 3 cm of the distal oesophagus needs to be affected to make the diagnosis. Although there may be clinical consequences of shorter segments of Barrett's metaplastic change, the lower oesophagus is often lined for 1–2 cm by normal gastric mucosa, as a congenital variant, so diagnosis is more difficult. The discussion below refers to the 'classic' type of Barrett's, with at least 3 cm of distal oesophagus affected.

The most important feature of Barrett's mucosa is its instability—up to 25% of cases have dysplasia present on histological analysis. A proportion of these will progress through severe dysplasia to invasive adenocarcinoma. Overall, about 0.5–1% of patients with Barrett's will develop adenocarcinoma each year. It has been estimated that Barrett's cases have a 30–50 times increased risk of oesophageal adenocarcinoma compared to matched controls.

Epidemiology

Epidemiology mirrors that of reflux oesophagitis, being more common in developed countries, white people, smokers and males. Typical age at diagnosis is 50–60 years. True prevalence is difficult to assess, but may be around 1–2% in high-risk populations.

Clinical features

Barrett's oesophagus itself is usually symptomless, although there may be reflux symptoms from oesophagitis, which can coexist. Rarely, the Barrett's mucosa may become severely inflamed or ulcerate, and present with retrosternal pain, odynophagia (pain on swallowing), upper gastrointestinal bleeding or anaemia.

Investigation

The diagnosis is usually made by gastroscopy. The different colours of squamous (pink) and columnar (orange) mucosa allow differentiation by the endoscopist (Fig. 10.33c). Usually, the change from squamous to columnar epithelium occurs at a sharply demarcated margin at the distal end of the tubular oesophagus. If columnar-type mucosa is seen within the distal tubular oesophagus for longer than 3 cm, and if biopsies confirm specialized columnar mucosa with intestinal metaplasia, then the diagnosis can be made.

Management

Associated reflux oesophagitis usually warrants treatment with PPIs—the lowest dose necessary to control symptoms is recommended. Standard doses of PPIs do not cause regression of Barrett's mucosa (Table 10.21, p. 686).

Because the condition is premalignant, surveillance by gastroscopy has been recommended; however, the evidence in the literature is conflicting, and consequently some specialists do not think surveillance is justified. The recommended screening interval varies widely, with every 1–2 years being typical. The aim is to detect premalignant changes with a view to treatment before invasive cancer develops. If severe dysplasia is seen in biopsy samples from a Barrett's oesophagus, there is often a focus of adenocarcinoma somewhere else in the segment. However, progression to cancer is not inevitable, and in less fit patients it may be appropriate to shorten the surveillance interval and consider non-surgical treatment. Options include thermal ablation or endoscopic resection of macroscopically evident malignant areas, or photodynamic therapy (PDT). In PDT the patient is first given a drug that becomes concentrated in adenocarcinoma cells and can be activated by light, producing cytotoxic products intracellularly. Light of the appropriate wavelength is then delivered by a probe placed down the oesophagus, beside

Table 10.24 Contrasting features of squamous and adenocarcinoma of oesophagus

	Squamous carcinoma	Adenocarcinoma
Incidence	Wide variation between countries, 5–260/100 000/year, but stable within countries	9 per 100 000/year, increasing rapidly in developed countries
Age	Rare before 50 years	Rare before 50 years
Sex	M > F	M > F
Aetiology	Smoking, alcohol, dietary factors	Barrett's oesophagus
Site	Mid oesophagus	Lower oesophagus

the Barrett's segment. The long-term success of these local methods has not been established and, if the patient is fit enough, oesophageal resection remains the treatment of choice for high-grade dysplasia.

Carcinoma of the oesophagus

Primary carcinoma of the oesophagus has two main forms: adenocarcinoma, associated strongly with Barrett's oesophagus, and squamous carcinoma, associated with environmental carcinogens (Table 10.24). Together, they comprise over 90% of oesophageal malignancies (KEY-POINTS BOX 10.2). Although, very rarely, a site of distant metastases from other primary sites, the oesophagus may be invaded by direct extension of mediastinal tumours, particularly carcinoma of the bronchus.

Disease mechanisms

Squamous carcinoma is strongly associated with smoking, alcohol and dietary factors as discussed above. Oesophageal damage, particularly from ingestion of caustic substances, and the presence of achalasia predispose to squamous carcinoma (see p. 701). By contrast, there is no association between alcohol and adenocarcinoma. Chronic severe iron deficiency is associated with squamous carcinoma—in the postcricoid region only. The majority of adenocarcinomas arise in Barrett's oesophagus and the

aetiological factors are those of the Barrett's itself—mainly excessive gastro-oesophageal reflux.

Pathology
Squamous carcinoma occurs most commonly in the mid-oesophagus, while adenocarcinoma, because of the association with Barrett's, arises mainly in the distal oesophagus. Otherwise, the macroscopic appearances are similar: shouldered strictures and ulcerated or polypoid tumours.

Both tumour types invade the submucosa at an early stage and extend locally. Local lymph node invasion occurs early and quickly because the lymphatics in the oesophagus are located in the lamina propria, in contrast to the rest of the gastrointestinal tract, in which they are located beneath the muscularis mucosa. Mediastinal and cervical nodes are more commonly involved with squamous carcinoma, and coeliac axis and porta hepatis nodes more common with adenocarcinoma. Squamous carcinoma can invade local structures, resulting in fistula formation to the trachea or aorta. Distant metastases are common at presentation.

Epidemiology
Prevalence and geography. The incidence of squamous carcinoma is relatively stable over time in any one geographical area: however, there are dramatic differences between areas, from 5 in 100 000 in the UK to 260 in 100 000 in northern Iran. This reflects varying exposure to carcinogens rather than effects of race. Smoking and alcohol consumption are major risk factors. Several dietary factors have been implicated, including betel nut chewing (common in parts of Asia), consumption of *N*-nitrosamines (e.g. in foods produced by pickling techniques, found in high-risk areas) and consumption of food and drink at high temperatures.

Adenocarcinoma used to be uncommon, but has shown the greatest rate of increase in incidence of any cancer over the last few decades. The increase in incidence is most marked in developed countries (e.g. at 20% per annum in the UK) where the rates of 5–9 in 100 000

Keypoints 10.2: Oesophageal cancer

Cancer of the oesophagus is either squamous or adenocarcinoma

Adenocarcinoma can arise from Barrett's mucosa and is the cancer with the most rapidly rising incidence in the West

All patients with dysphagia should undergo prompt gastroscopy to exclude oesophageal cancer

A few patients have resectable tumours but, for most, palliation with radiotherapy, chemotherapy and/or endoscopic techniques is the only option

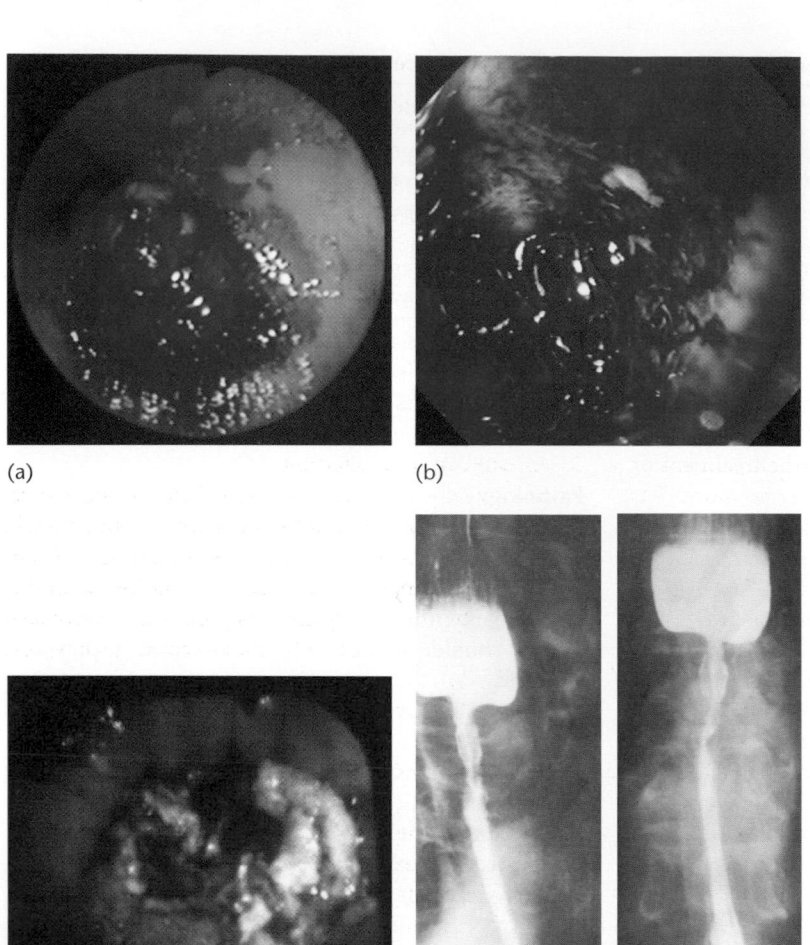

(a)

(b)

(c)

(d)

Figure 10.34 Endoscopic views of oesophageal carcinoma. (a) Polypoidal oesophageal carcinoma. (b) Haemorrhagic oesophageal carcinoma. (c) Ulcerating oesophageal carcinoma. The blackened areas are caused by palliative laser therapy, which debulks the tumour improving swallowing, and reduces bleeding from the ulcerated mucosa. (d) Barium swallow showing a 10-cm irregular stricture produced by a carcinoma. Inoperability is inferred by the length of the lesion. Malignant strictures are usually longer than peptic ones and may show shouldering (an 'apple-core appearance'). Reproduced from Misiewicz JJ, Pounder RE, Venables CW. *Diseases of the Gut and Pancreas*, 2nd edn. Oxford: Blackwell Scientific Publications, 1994 with the permission of the authors.

now exceed those of squamous carcinoma—a complete reversal of the situation 30 years ago.

Age. The incidence of both types increases with age, being rare before age 50.

Sex. Both types are more common in men.

Clinical features

Patients with oesophageal carcinoma present with progressive dysphagia, initially to solids and then to liquids, of rarely more than a few months' duration. Other symptoms include acute obstruction by a bolus of food, regurgitation, weight loss, haematemesis, anaemia, hoarseness (because of recurrent laryngeal nerve involvement) and chest pain (because of infiltration of intercostal nerves, pleura, pericardium and other mediastinal structures).

Patients with oesophagotracheal fistulas present with coughing on swallowing and, if untreated, death from aspiration results rapidly. Oesophagoaortic fistulas may result in massive and almost universally fatal gastrointestinal bleeding. Often there are no signs. The patient may be cachexic and anaemic, and have cervical lymphadenopathy.

Investigation
Haematology
FBC. There may be a microcytic anaemia.

Diagnostic imaging
● *Endoscopy or barium swallow:* reveal the lesion (Fig. 10.34)
● *Chest radiography, CT scan and endoluminal and hepatic ultrasound:* subsidiary investigations, when surgery is contemplated

Histopathology

Endoscopic biopsy and brush cytology confirm the diagnosis.

Management

The success of treatment for oesophageal cancer depends mostly on the disease stage. Treatment decisions are complex, and are best carried out in specialist units by multidisciplinary teams managing a high caseload. The usual approach is to begin with cross-sectional imaging (usually CT scanning) to detect distant metastases or extensive local disease, either of which precludes a surgical approach. Unfortunately, the majority of tumours are unresectable at presentation, and treatment is palliative in this situation. Occasionally, cases appearing inoperable because of local disease spread respond sufficiently to chemotherapy, with or without radiotherapy, to be offered potentially curative surgery. Long-term responses have been achieved through radiotherapy and/or chemotherapy.

Many methods are available for palliation of the main symptom of dysphagia, and some are discussed below. Supportive measures include an explanation of the situation to the patient and relatives, pain control (e.g. with opiates), nutritional replacement when appropriate, often by percutaneous gastrostomy (see p. 672), and arrangements for terminal care.

Surgery

If the tumour is operable on CT grounds, an endoluminal ultrasound should be performed to assess local spread. Radical resection offers the best chance of long-term cure. A combined thoracoabdominal procedure is used to resect the tumour and restore gut continuity, if necessary with a colonic interposition. Pre- and postoperative nutritional support is usually needed and immediate mortality is high.

Radiotherapy

Radiotherapy can provide effective palliation when given by external beam, or by a radioactive source placed within the tumour via a nasogastric tube (brachytherapy) positioned across the tumour. It is particularly useful for tumours in the upper third of the oesophagus where surgery is often impracticable, and where there may not be room for placement of an endoluminal stent. Also, this site is away from more radiosensitive structures, in particular the small bowel, allowing higher doses to be given.

Radiation alone can result in long-term survival in a minority of patients with apparently localized disease. However, current evidence demonstrates better long-term survival rates for chemotherapy alone or chemoradiotherapy.

Chemotherapy and chemoradiotherapy

Currently emerging data suggest that preoperative chemotherapy improves outcomes in patients with localized disease, and that combined chemoradiotherapy regimens alone may give results equivalent to surgery. Many single-agent and multiagent palliative chemotherapy regimens have been assessed for patients with metastatic disease, or advanced local disease that is inoperable. The median survival rates for multiagent therapy are typically better (around 12 months vs. 6 months for single agents); however, this has to be balanced against the greater toxicity.

Endoscopic tumour ablation

Endoscopically delivered intralesional alcohol injections, laser, argon beam and diathermy methods are available to reduce tumour bulk and improve swallowing. All can be (and usually have to be) repeated on multiple occasions to achieve best initial stabilization, and when dysphagia recurs. This compares with radiotherapy techniques, which usually require a single treatment to achieve similar palliation of dysphagia.

Endoscopically assisted tumour intubations

These provide a good palliative solution. Dysphagia can be relieved rapidly by inserting a prosthetic stent under radiological control, usually over a guide wire positioned endoscopically (Fig. 10.22). If available, expanding metal stents are superior, as when introduced they are less than 1 cm wide and far less likely to perforate the oesophagus than plastic prostheses, which are around 2 cm wide when pushed though the tumour.

Prognosis

Overall prognosis is very poor. Five-year survival rates are 30% for patients with well-localized disease, 10% for those with regional metastases or locally advanced disease, and almost zero for those presenting with distant disease.

Trauma-induced oesophageal disorders

Mallory–Weiss syndrome

Mallory–Weiss syndrome is haematemesis caused by a mucosal tear in the distal oesophagus or gastric fundus as a result of vomiting.

Disease mechanisms

Retropulsion of the cardia into the chest during repeated vomiting (e.g. because of alcohol excess or pregnancy) can cause one or more short linear mucosal tears.

Epidemiology

This is one of the most common causes of minor upper

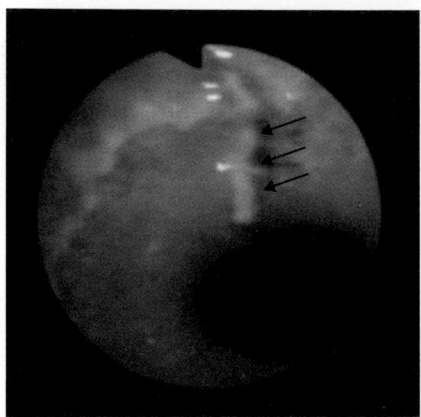

Figure 10.35 Mallory–Weiss tear in the distal oesophagus. Note the linear tear (arrows) in the proximal gastric mucosa immediately distal to the gastro-oesophageal mucosal junction.

gastrointestinal bleeding (see p. 713) and occurs mainly in young adults.

Clinical features
Patients usually present with a small fresh haematemesis.

Investigation
Endoscopy. The diagnosis is confirmed endoscopically (Fig. 10.35). The mucosal tears heal rapidly and may not be visible if endoscopy is delayed.

Management
Usually no treatment is necessary. Exceptionally, bleeding is massive and surgical intervention is required.

Acute oesophageal perforation
Disease mechanisms
The most common cause of acute oesophageal perforation is endoscopy, especially during dilatation and intubation (Fig. 10.36). Oesophageal perforation rarely occurs spontaneously during vomiting (Boerhaave's syndrome) or secondary to chest trauma, or ingestion of corrosives or foreign bodies.

Clinical features
Presentation depends on the size and site of the rupture. It includes pain in the chest, neck, back and upper abdomen with fever, cyanosis, shock and surgical emphysema. Mediastinitis is the main complication.

Investigation
The diagnosis is confirmed by chest radiography and/or contrast radiology. Early diagnosis is important, so

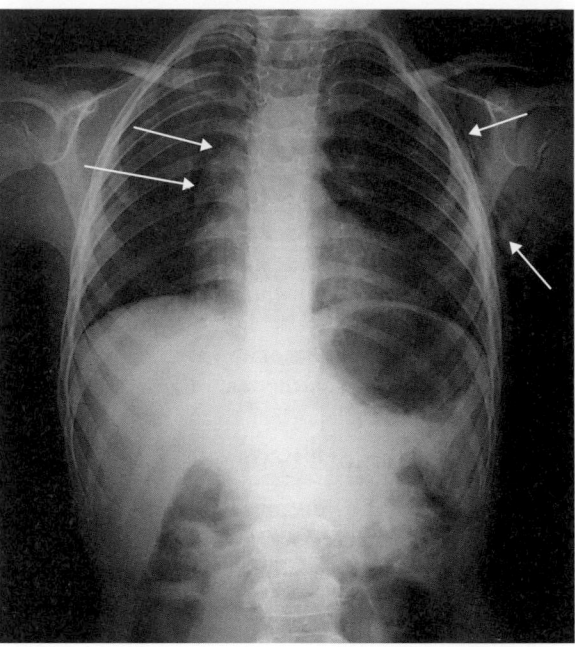

Figure 10.36 Chest radiograph showing oesophageal perforation in a 5-year-old child (after rigid oesophagoscopy). Note the mediastinal air on the right and subcutaneous air, particularly on the left.

patients undergoing oesophageal dilatation or intubation should be assessed clinically and have a chest radiograph immediately after the procedure.

Management
Large defects require early surgical repair. Smaller ones often heal spontaneously if the patient is kept nil-by-mouth and maintained on antibiotics, endoscopically introduced nasogastric feeding or parenteral nutrition, and analgesia.

Foreign bodies
Disease mechanisms
Coins, safety pins, batteries and other objects may be swallowed by children and the mentally handicapped or disturbed. Those not passing into the stomach tend to impact at the cricopharyngeal level or in the distal oesophagus.

Epidemiology
This scenario arises mainly in children.

Clinical features
Impaction at cricopharyngeal level or in the distal oesophagus results in dysphagia, often with chest pain. Perforation is a risk.

Investigation

Plain neck and chest radiography and, if necessary, contrast radiology along with the history will reveal the diagnosis.

Management

Impacted food boluses may pass spontaneously into the stomach, but other foreign bodies in the oesophagus need prompt endoscopic removal. Objects already in the stomach usually pass through the rest of the bowel without further trouble; however, sharp objects and batteries should be removed endoscopically to reduce the chance of damage to gastrointestinal mucosa.

Oesophageal motility disorders

Oesophageal motility disorders may be primary or secondary. All are rare, but are important to consider as causes of dysphagia and chest pain when common oesophageal and cardiac conditions have been excluded. Primary disorders include achalasia and diffuse oesophageal spasm. Secondary motility disorders occur in scleroderma (see p. 225), Chagas' disease and diabetes (because of autonomic neuropathy).

Achalasia

In achalasia of the cardia there is loss of oesophageal peristalsis and failure of lower oesophageal sphincter relaxation after a swallow, as a result of degeneration of ganglion cells of the myenteric plexus and in the dorsal vagal nucleus in the medulla.

Disease mechanisms

A functionally identical abnormality is seen in Chagas' disease (see p. 139), and it is possible that achalasia is also caused by an infective agent.

PATHOLOGY

Initially, the oesophagus is macroscopically normal, but later it becomes dilated. Occasionally, carcinoma develops, perhaps as a result of food stasis above the LOS. Microscopy of autopsy specimens shows reduced numbers of intramural ganglion cells.

Epidemiology

The incidence is 1 in 100 000 in the UK and the condition is rare in children.

Clinical features

Dysphagia may be intermittent at first and relieved by drinking, changes in position or regurgitation. Later, more persistent dysphagia, which is often worse for liquids than for solids, may cause nutritional deficiencies and weight loss. Other features include occasional retrosternal chest pain from oesophageal spasm, and respiratory symptoms including cough and nocturnal wheezing. Recurrent chest infections may occur.

There are usually no signs other than those of malnutrition and pulmonary complications.

Complications. These include an increased risk of oesophageal carcinoma, and aspiration can cause pneumonia.

Differential diagnosis. This is as for dysphagia (see p. 659).

Investigation

Oesophageal manometry. The gold standard for diagnosis of achalasia is oesophageal manometry, which usually shows raised resting pressure (higher than 30 mmHg) in the LOS and failure of LOS relaxation on swallowing; there is always a lack of peristalsis in the body of the oesophagus.

Diagnostic imaging

- *Chest radiography:* may show the right wall of a dilated oesophagus lying to the right of the mediastinum. There may be an oesophageal air–fluid level, and the normal gastric air bubble may be absent (Fig. 10.37a).
- *Barium swallow:* shows reduced peristaltic contractions and a poorly relaxing LOS. There is often a smooth tapering down to the LOS and, in late cases, a dilated oesophagus containing food residue (Fig. 10.37b).
- *OGD:* normal in the early stages, but important for the evaluation of the differential diagnosis (see p. 659), the detection of complications (particularly carcinoma of the oesophagus) and treatment (see below).

Histopathology. Biopsies are taken to exclude carcinoma.

Management

Smooth-muscle relaxing agents (e.g. nifedipine, verapamil and isosorbide) provide temporary relief for a few patients but most require more invasive therapy. The standard current treatment is endoscopic dilatation of the LOS with a pneumatic balloon. This has an 80% success rate but may cause perforation. When dilatation fails, surgical procedures such as Heller's cardiomyotomy (in which the muscle at the lower end of the oesophagus is incised longitudinally to weaken it) can be performed laparoscopically. Sometimes, Heller's cardiomyotomy is combined with an antireflux procedure. Recent data suggest that surgery as an initial treatment is superior in patients under the age of 40 years at presentation. Endoscopic injections into the LOS of botulinum toxin,

10

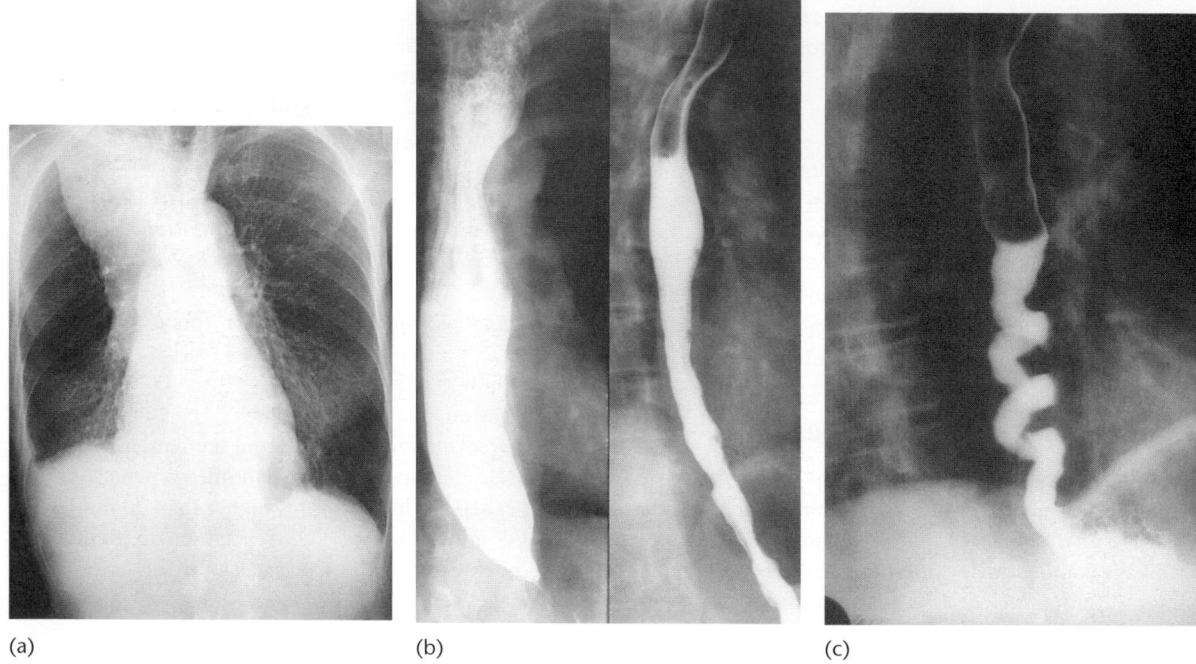

(a)   (b)   (c)

Figure 10.37 Radiological appearances of oesophageal motility disorders. (a) Chest radiograph in achalasia showing the dilated oesophagus and loss of the gastric air bubble. (b) Achalasia. Barium swallow showing excess food residue and dilated oesophagus tapering smoothly down to the cardia before (left) and after (right) pneumatic dilatation. Reproduced from Misiewicz JJ, Pounder RE, Venables CW. *Diseases of the Gut and Pancreas*, 2nd edn. Oxford: Blackwell Scientific Publications, 1994 with the permission of the authors. (c) Oesophageal spasm. The tertiary contractions in a normal calibre oesophagus give a corkscrew appearance. Reproduced from *Slide Atlas of Gastroenterology* with the kind permission of the author and Times Mirror International Publishers.

a specific neuromuscular transmission blocker, have recently been used; however, the long-term outcome of this approach is unclear.

Oesophageal spasm

Oesophageal spasm is an idiopathic motility disorder.

Epidemiology

Age. Usually at least middle-aged.

Clinical features

Chest pain and sometimes dysphagia are associated with intermittent non-propulsive repetitive oesophageal contractions. Main differential diagnoses are cardiac ischaemia, achalasia and gastro-oesophageal reflux.

Investigation

● *Barium swallow* (Fig. 10.37): often helpful, as is *oesophageal manometry*
● *Endoscopy and resting and exercise ECG:* needed to exclude reflux oesophagitis and angina

Management

Treatment can be difficult. If smooth-muscle relaxants such as nitrates and nifedipine, or low-dose tricyclic antidepressants (e.g. amitriptyline 25 mg at night) do not help, balloon dilatation and even surgical cardiomyotomy may be necessary. Some attacks appear to be precipitated by gastro-oesophageal reflux and measures to prevent this may be beneficial (see p. 695).

Oesophageal strictures

Disease mechanisms

Most benign oesophageal strictures are caused by acid. The aetiology is thus as for reflux oesophagitis discussed above. Stricturing, usually of the lower oesophagus, is one consequence of severe and prolonged reflux. Benign strictures may also complicate severe forms of any other cause of oesophagitis (see p. 696), with the exception of *Candida*.

Clinical features

The presenting symptom is usually dysphagia, and there is often weight loss.

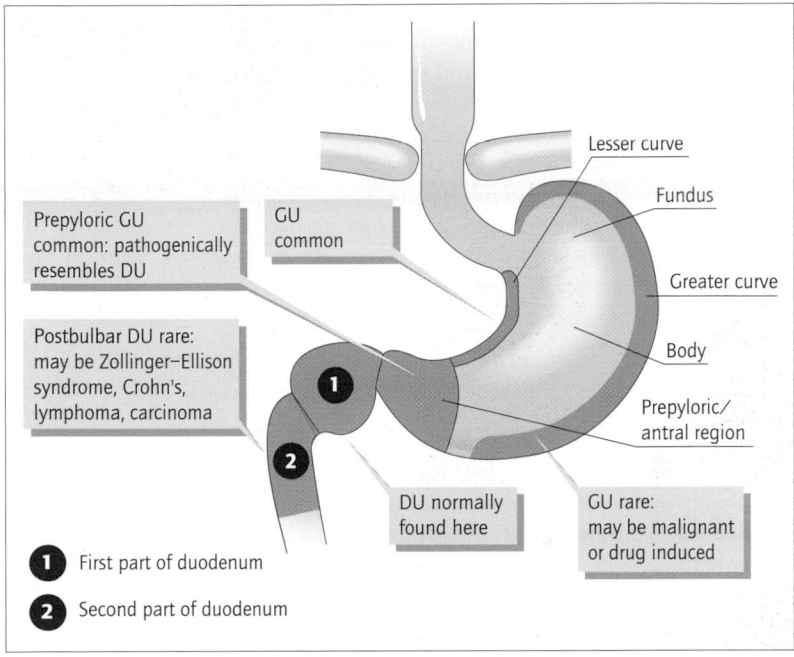

Prepyloric GU
common: pathogenically
resembles DU

GU
common

Lesser curve

Fundus

Greater curve

Body

Postbulbar DU rare:
may be Zollinger–Ellison
syndrome, Crohn's,
lymphoma, carcinoma

Prepyloric/
antral region

❶

❷

DU normally
found here

GU rare:
may be malignant
or drug induced

❶ First part of duodenum

❷ Second part of duodenum

Figure 10.38 Sites of chronic peptic ulceration.

Investigation

Contrast radiology and/or endoscopy with biopsy and cytology are necessary to reveal the cause (Fig. 10.33).

Management

If the stricture is symptomatic, it is usually treated by endoscopic dilatation and/or intubation (Fig. 10.22). If the cause is reflux oesophagitis, long-term high-dose PPIs should be prescribed, as these have been shown to prevent restricturing.

Oesophageal varices

(See p. 628.)

Diseases of the stomach and duodenum

Peptic ulcer

A peptic ulcer is a break in the mucosa within or close to acid-secreting areas of the gastrointestinal tract. This occurs most commonly in the stomach (gastric ulcer, GU) or proximal duodenum (duodenal ulcer, DU) (Fig. 10.38). The term is technically inaccurate, as the most important aetiological factors for ulcers in these sites are *Helicobacter pylori* infection and NSAIDs, not a primary disturbance of acid or pepsin secretion. Other aetiological factors associated with gastric or duodenal ulceration are all uncommon (Table 10.25). The clinically important uncommon cause is gastric malignancy, which may present as a

Table 10.25 Factors causing breakdown of gastroduodenal mucosal integrity and thought to predispose to peptic ulceration or gastritis/duodenitis (most important factors shown in capital letters)

Increased mucosal attack
HELICOBACTER PYLORI, ACID, BILE SALTS

Reduced mucosal defence
Mucus deficiency, bicarbonate deficiency

Lifestyle
SMOKING, alcoholism, stress

Drugs
Aspirin, NSAIDs

Other benign diseases (mainly for DU)
Zollinger–Ellison syndrome, renal dialysis, primary hyperparathyroidism, lymphoma

Malignant disease
Primary adenocarcinoma, lymphoma

benign-looking ulcer. Rarely, ulceration occurs in other sites exposed to gastric acid, such as the oesophagus, the jejunum distal to a gastrojejunal anastomosis or a Meckel's diverticulum containing ectopic gastric acid-secreting mucosa (see p. 725). At these sites, excessive acid exposure *is* usually the major aetiological factor. The term 'stress ulceration' refers to lesions developing in severely ill patients, usually in the intensive care unit setting. They are typically multiple small superficial ulcers of the gastric

10

mucosa. Prophylaxis against stress ulceration—for example, using ranitidine or enteral feeding—is now part of standard intensive care unit practice and this type of ulcer will not be considered further here.

Although the epidemiology and aetiology of NSAID- and *H. pylori*-related peptic ulcers are different, their clinical presentation and complications are similar. This section focuses on the features of benign gastric and duodenal ulcers associated with these two main factors, highlighting differences where relevant. Malignant gastric ulcers are considered separately (see p. 711). Malignant duodenal ulceration is very rare, and not discussed here.

Disease mechanisms

In peptic ulceration, the balance between factors attacking and defending gastroduodenal mucosa is disturbed. Attacking factors may predominate in DU, and failed defence mechanisms in GU. NSAID toxicity is largely exerted through inhibition of gastroduodenal mucosal prostaglandin synthesis: prostaglandins are central to mucosal defence, for example by stimulating mucosal blood flow and mucus secretion, and duodenal bicarbonate secretion.

Attacking factors in the aetiology of peptic ulcer

Attacking factors include *H. pylori*, acid and bile salts.

Helicobacter pylori. *H. pylori* gastritis is found in 70% of patients with GU and 95% of patients with DU (PEPTIC ULCER DISEASE AT A GLANCE, Fig. C); in *H. pylori*-negative patients there is almost always another explanation for ulceration (e.g. NSAIDs, malignancy). This is not in itself proof that *H. pylori* is involved with ulcerogenesis; however, studies of peptic ulcer relapse rates provide strong evidence that *H. pylori* is a causal factor. If ulcers are healed (e.g. with cimetidine) but *H. pylori* not eradicated, a relapse rate around 70–90% within 1 year is observed. If the ulcer is healed and *H. pylori* eradicated, a relapse rate of less than 5% is usual. Healing of uncomplicated duodenal ulcers can be achieved through *H. pylori* eradication alone (using no acid-suppressant therapy). *H. pylori* eradication leads to regression of gastritis and restitution of normal gastric acid and pepsin secretory responses.

However, any aetiological link must explain why the majority of *H. pylori*-infected patients do not have gastric or duodenal ulceration. This observation is partly explained by different serotypes of *H. pylori* having different pathogenicity, and partly by different genetic and acquired host factors allowing variable resistance to the effects of infection.

The pathogenic mechanisms by which *H. pylori* leads to peptic ulceration are multifactorial, and likely to differ between DU and GU. In DU the disturbance of gastric acid secretion (see below) is likely to be of major importance, while in GU direct toxicity of bacterial products (e.g. cytotoxin) and the effects of stimulation of a mucosal immune and inflammatory response may predominate.

Acid. The variable disturbances of gastric acid secretion found in peptic ulcer patients can be explained through the effects of *H. pylori* infection. There are two patterns of distribution of *Helicobacter* infection within the stomach:

1 *Antrum-predominant* H. pylori *gastritis:* in some patients, the infection remains confined to the gastric antrum, leaving the acid-secreting cells of the gastric body unharmed. The antral mucosal damage seems to preferentially damage 'D' cells (responsible for negative feedback inhibition of antral gastrin secretion, and thus of the gastric acid secretion; Fig. 10.5). The effect is to increase gastric acid secretion, particularly in response to normal physiological stimuli. This pattern of *H. pylori* distribution is associated with development of DU. The pathogenesis is probably not dependent on *Helicobacter* infection *per se*, just the secondary disturbance of acid secretion, as increased gastric acid output from any cause can lead to DU (e.g. Zollinger–Ellison syndrome; see p. 759). When the duodenal mucosa is exposed to excessive acidity, foci of gastric metaplasia develop and it is thought that these may be areas of reduced mucosal defence, which mark the first stage in the process that leads to DU. Foci of duodenal gastric metaplasia can be colonized by *H. pylori*, and this may further reduce the mucosal defence in these sites.

2 *Diffuse* H. pylori *gastritis:* in other patients, infection spreads to involve both gastric antrum and body (pangastritis). Varying severities of chronic gastritis result with time, causing reduced function of gastric parietal cells and reduced gastric acid output—this pattern is associated with gastric ulceration. The situation is reversible at first, as eradication of *H. pylori* can lead to restitution of normal gastric acid output. Untreated, this pattern of infection eventually progresses to irreversible mucosal atrophy. Mucosal atrophy and reduced gastric acid secretion, whether through *H. pylori* pangastritis or other factors (e.g. gastric surgery, autoimmune gastritis), increases the risk of gastric carcinoma. Reduced gastric acid secretion allows colonization by bacteria capable of converting dietary nitrates to potent mutagenic *N*-nitroso compounds. Chronic gastritis and/or atrophy also leads to a reduction in luminal vitamin C levels (a potent antioxidant and thus anticarcinogenic agent). In response to the reduced gastric acid output there is increased gastrin secretion. Gastrin induces gastric epithelial cell proliferation, and thus potentially contributes to the premalignant risk in this setting as an initiator of carcinogenesis.

Bile salts. Duodenogastric bile reflux appears to be a pathogenic factor for GU and chronic gastritis.

Failed mucosal defence in the aetiology of peptic ulcer

Defects in mucosal defence are less well defined than aggressive factors. NSAID-induced damage is primarily related to reduced mucosal defences through inhibition of cyclo-oxygenase (COX) enzyme, which exists in two forms. COX-1, the constitutive 'housekeeping form', contributes to mucosal defence in the upper gastrointestinal tract through mucus production, improved blood flow and bicarbonate production in the duodenum. The other isoenzyme, COX-2, is inducible and responsible for prostaglandin production and associated pain in inflamed tissues. The therapeutic role of NSAIDs relates to COX-2 inhibition, whereas concurrent COX-1 inhibition (a feature of most NSAIDs), leads to reduced gastrointestinal mucosal defence, and thus increased risk of gastroduodenal ulceration. Some recently developed NSAIDs are relatively COX-2 specific, and have been shown to cause less gastrointestinal mucosal injury. NSAIDs also reduce the capacity of the mucosa for repair, through mechanisms independent of prostaglandin synthesis inhibition.

Other factors

Other factors predisposing to peptic ulceration are shown in Table 10.25.

Pathology

Histologically, there is necrotic granulation tissue with chronic inflammatory cell infiltration and endarteritis at the base of a peptic ulcer. Healing by fibrosis leads to scarring. At the pylorus this can result in stenosis and obstruction to gastric outflow.

Epidemiology

These diseases are common: the 1-year prevalence of peptic ulcer is nearly 2 in 100, and the condition affects approximately 10–15% of people at some stage in their lives. These epidemiological data tend to include NSAID- and non-NSAID-related ulcers. In studies focusing specifically on NSAID users, point prevalence of peptic ulcer is much higher at 10–30%. In NSAID users, gastric ulcers are far more common (around 10 times) than duodenal ulcers.

Age. Duodenal ulcer is most common in people aged 20–60 years. Gastric ulcer is most common in the elderly.

Sex. Duodenal ulcer is slightly more common in men than women. Gastric ulcer is more common in women.

Genetics. Duodenal ulcer is occasionally associated with a positive family history, but there is no clear-cut inheritance.

Trends over time. The incidence of all forms of ulcer disease increased during the early 20th century then declined after the 1950s. The epidemiology of peptic ulcer shows a marked birth cohort effect: the pattern of disease varies not just with age, but also with the period of birth. For example, people aged 40 born in 1900 have a different pattern of disease to people aged 40 born in 1940. The birth cohort effect for peptic ulcer strongly suggests an environmental aetiological factor, and would be entirely compatible with a primarily infective aetiology and childhood acquisition, as proposed for *H. pylori* (see below).

Clinical features

The clinical features are similar for GU, DU and other causes of dyspepsia (Table 10.4, p. 657). Epigastric pain when the patient is hungry and in the middle of the night are, however, characteristic of DU. Vomiting may relieve the pain. If vomiting is persistent, copious and/or contains old food, pyloric stenosis should be suspected. Episodes of pain brought about by recurrent ulceration often occur over many years. Usually the only sign is epigastric tenderness.

Differential diagnosis

This is shown in Table 10.4 (p. 657).

Complications

Complications of peptic ulceration are haemorrhage, perforation and pyloric stenosis. Some gastric ulcers will turn out to be malignant, and it is believed that they may develop both *de novo* and from pre-existing benign peptic ulcers. Very rarely, an ulcerated duodenal lesion will turn out to be malignant.

Haemorrhage (see p. 713): the most common complication, occurring in about 15% of patients. Many will have been taking NSAIDs, and will have had no pain.

Perforation. The incidence of perforation has fallen dramatically since 1950. Patients present with sudden severe upper abdominal pain and signs of peritonitis (see p. 668). Perforation is confirmed by the presence of air under the diaphragms on a chest radiograph (Fig. 10.25).

Pyloric stenosis. Oedema and abnormal motility during acute exacerbations, or fibrosis during healing in patients with prepyloric and duodenal ulcers can lead to gastric outflow obstruction. Its incidence is falling. Patients present with large-volume stale vomiting, dyspepsia and weight loss. Examination reveals a succussion splash and fluid depletion.

Complex metabolic changes occur if the history is prolonged:

- Plasma HCO_3^-, pH and urea increase and K^+ and Cl^-

10

decrease because of loss of H^+, Cl^-, Na^+, K^+ and H_2O in vomit
● Urine is alkaline in early pyloric stenosis as a result of urinary excretion of HCO_3^-. Later it is paradoxically acidic because of urinary excretion of H^+ and K^+ because of insufficient Na^+ for excretion with HCO_3^-

Carcinoma. Some GUs (but not DUs) are malignant. The risk of gastric cancer is increased in patients with benign gastric ulcer. Gastric ulcers therefore require endoscopic inspection with biopsy with or without cytology every 2 months until fully healed.

Investigation
Dyspepsia is very common. Most peptic ulcers are benign and caused by factors identifiable without endoscopy (*H. pylori*, NSAID use). Most malignant ulcers occur in patients over 45 years of age. Thus, if the patient has no symptoms to suggest complications of peptic ulcer (e.g. vomiting, weight loss, anaemia), management is as for other causes of dyspepsia (Fig. 10.14). Patients under 45 years should generally not be endoscoped, but tested for *H. pylori* and treated if positive. If symptoms persist after treatment, the patient should be endoscoped. NSAIDs should be stopped if possible. Endoscopy is indicated if patients with dyspepsia are unable to manage without use of NSAIDs. Patients over 45 years with new onset dyspepsia should be endoscoped, partially in order to exclude gastric cancer, and not go through the 'blind' test and treat strategy.

Haematology
Occasionally, occult blood loss causes a microcytic anaemia.

Biochemistry
In the rare patient with DU refractory to treatment, **serum gastrin** and **calcium** should be checked to look for Zollinger–Ellison syndrome (see p. 759) and hyperparathyroidism, respectively.

Detection of *Helicobacter pylori*
If peptic ulcer is diagnosed endoscopically, it is usual to test for *H. pylori* using biopsy methods, either by histology (most sensitive but expensive) or by a biopsy urease test such as the 'CLO' (*Campylobacter*-like organism) test. These latter tests are based on the strong urease enzyme activity of *H. pylori*. The test gel contains urea, which will be converted to ammonia by urease activity if *Helicobacter* are present in the biopsy. A pH-sensitive indicator changes colour if the gel becomes more alkaline because of ammonia production (PEPTIC ULCER DISEASE AT A GLANCE). *H. pylori* can be also cultured from biopsy samples, and antimicrobial sensitivities established.

Helicobacter can be detected without endoscopic biopsies by a serological blood test (*H. pylori* ELISA) or by a breath test. In breath testing, urea labelled with ^{13}C (a stable non-radioactive carbon isotope) is ingested. If *H. pylori* are present, the urea is broken down into ammonia and $^{13}CO_2$, the latter being detected by collection of breath samples (Fig. 10.29). The serological test is used as the first-line diagnostic test in young (under 45 years) dyspeptic patients. Although breath testing is more accurate, it is far more inconvenient for the patient, because the test is usually performed in hospital departments. Kits have been developed that allow the breath test to be performed in a primary care setting, which reduces the inconvenience factor. If *H. pylori* testing is being performed to confirm the success of treatment, then a breath test should be used, as serology may remain positive for many months following *H. pylori* eradication. Endoscopy should not be requested simply to obtain biopsies to confirm *H. pylori* eradication; however, if a follow-up endoscopy is required for another clinical reason (most commonly confirmation of gastric ulcer healing), then success of eradication can be checked by biopsy methods at the same time. It is vital that the patient does not take PPI drugs (substituting H_2 receptor antagonists if required for symptom control) for 4 weeks prior to breath or biopsy tests.

Diagnostic imaging
Endoscopy is preferable to a barium meal because it allows biopsy and cytology of a GU and biopsy for *H. pylori*, and can distinguish between active DU, and scarring and deformity from a previous ulcer.

Histopathology
Biopsy. If a GU is found on endoscopy or barium meal (PEPTIC ULCER DISEASE AT A GLANCE), endoscopic biopsies and cytology are essential to exclude malignancy. Duodenal ulcers require biopsy only when refractory to treatment, to exclude carcinoma, lymphoma, Crohn's disease and tuberculosis.

Management
The aims of treatment are to heal the ulcer and prevent relapse.

Specific treatment
The majority of peptic ulcers are now treated by drugs that reduce gastric acid secretion, with eradication of *H. pylori* if present. The drugs listed in Table 10.21 (p. 686) are all effective in healing peptic ulcers. They differ in their price, side-effects, convenience to take and ability to prevent relapse.

Proton pump inhibitors. These are extremely potent and

specific inhibitors of acid secretion, acting by blocking parietal cell $H^+/K^+/ATPase$. They heal peptic ulcers more quickly than H_2 receptor antagonists, but are currently more expensive. They are the most common acid suppressant used in *H. pylori* eradication regimens, usually in combination with two antibiotics. They are also useful in refractory peptic ulceration, reflux oesophagitis and Zollinger–Ellison syndrome.

H_2 receptor antagonists (e.g. ranitidine, cimetidine). The management of peptic ulceration was revolutionized in the 1970s by drugs that inhibit acid and pepsin secretion by blocking gastric histamine (H_2) receptors (Fig. 10.5). The side-effects of H_2 receptor antagonists are few, and rarely serious (Table 10.21, p. 686). Cimetidine potentially has the most adverse effects and drug interactions, and is best avoided in the elderly, patients with renal failure and those taking other drugs.

Antacids. High doses of antacids taken regularly heal ulcers, but at considerable inconvenience and at the risk of side-effects. Their main use is for symptomatic relief. The preparation selected should be cheap and potent, and a mixture of magnesium and aluminium salts to minimize any disturbance of bowel habit.

Helicobacter pylori *eradication.* *H. pylori* eradication using a PPI and two antibiotics together for a week is now the first-line treatment (for common regimens see PEPTIC ULCER DISEASE AT A GLANCE).

Treatment strategies
Duodenal ulcer. For patients with *H. pylori*-positive DU, the infection should be eradicated using one of the triple therapy regimens shown in PEPTIC ULCER DISEASE AT A GLANCE. It is not necessary to give additional acid-suppressant therapy for management of uncomplicated DU. Success of treatment is best assessed using the ^{13}C breath test; however, this is unnecessary for uncomplicated DU cases who become asymptomatic after treatment. Where the DU has led to a serious complication (e.g. bleeding, perforation), long-term maintenance with a PPI or H_2 receptor antagonist is given.

   H. pylori-negative patients taking NSAIDs should stop the drug, and take a PPI for 4–8 weeks to heal the ulcer. Occasionally, patients feel their musculoskeletal symptoms are unmanageable without NSAIDs. Ulcers can be healed if the NSAID is continued with coprescription of a PPI. In this situation, healing of any lesion should be confirmed endoscopically. *H. pylori*-negative DU in patients not on NSAIDs is treated initially with a PPI for 2 months, with avoidance of aggravating factors such as smoking. Very occasionally, the patient's symptoms

persist or recur despite removal of the causative factor (*H. pylori* and/or NSAIDs). In this situation, re-endoscope to check for ulcer healing, take biopsies from ulcer margins to exclude rare ulcer types (lymphoma, Crohn's disease, etc.) and from the gastric antrum to confirm *H. pylori* eradication, and check serum calcium (to exclude primary hyperparathyroidism) and gastrin (to exclude Zollinger–Ellison syndrome). If the ulcer is still present and biopsies unhelpful as to aetiology, long-term PPI or H_2-blocker treatment can be used. Surgery may be indicated for the small number of patients who do not respond to these measures.

Gastric ulcer. A similar scheme is adopted for GU, except that repeat OGD is necessary in all patients to check for healing and to take further biopsies and cytology to exclude carcinoma (see p. 711), even if the patient is asymptomatic after initial treatment. Additionally, 6–8 weeks treatment with a PPI is given (including the initial week of *H. pylori* eradication therapy if indicated).

Peptic ulcers in patients taking NSAIDs who are *H. pylori*-positive
The interaction between *H. pylori* and NSAIDs is unclear. Both are proven aetiological factors for peptic ulceration, through different mechanisms. Surprisingly, the risk of peptic ulcer in patients taking NSAIDs does not differ between *H. pylori*-infected and -uninfected patients. Studies to date have also found no consistent reduction in ulcer incidence if *H. pylori* is eradicated prior to starting NSAID therapy.

   For patients who are *H. pylori*-positive *and* taking NSAIDs, it is not possible to say which is the main aetiological factor when peptic ulceration is found. A pragmatic approach is therefore to assume both are relevant, stop the NSAID therapy *and* eradicate *H. pylori*. Even if it were not relevant to the ulcer formation in such situations, eradicating *H. pylori* would have the advantage of reducing the longer term complications of infection, especially gastric atrophy and increased risk of gastric cancer.

Surgery. The efficacy of modern medical treatment has reduced the need for surgery. Indications for its use in peptic ulceration are:
- Failure to respond to adequate medical treatment
- Complications (haemorrhage, perforation, stenosis)
- Malignant GU

Supportive treatment
Smoking retards healing and increases relapse rates and should be stopped. Patients should be encouraged to eat what they want.

10

Peptic ulcer disease at a glance

Epidemiology

Prevalence
2% of the population per year; 10–15% lifetime prevalence

Age
Commonly 20–60 years for duodenal ulcers and over 60 years for gastric ulcers

Sex
Gastric ulcers are more common in women, duodenal ulcers in men
Gastric ulcers are more common in women over 60 years and in NSAID users
Duodenal ulcers are more common in male smokers. Most duodenal ulcers result from *Helicobacter pylori* infection or NSAIDs

Geography
Worldwide, areas of social deprivation (higher *H. pylori* prevalence)

Causes
H. pylori: 90% of duodenal ulcers; 70% of gastric ulcers

NSAIDs
Gastric atrophy (gastric ulcers)

Investigation
Non-invasive testing for H. pylori
^{13}C-urea breath test, serology

Haematology
FBC and iron studies: iron-deficiency anaemia (occasionally)

Biochemistry
In duodenal ulcers there may be a raised calcium if the cause is hyperparathyroidism or raised gastrin in Zollinger–Ellison syndrome (both rare)

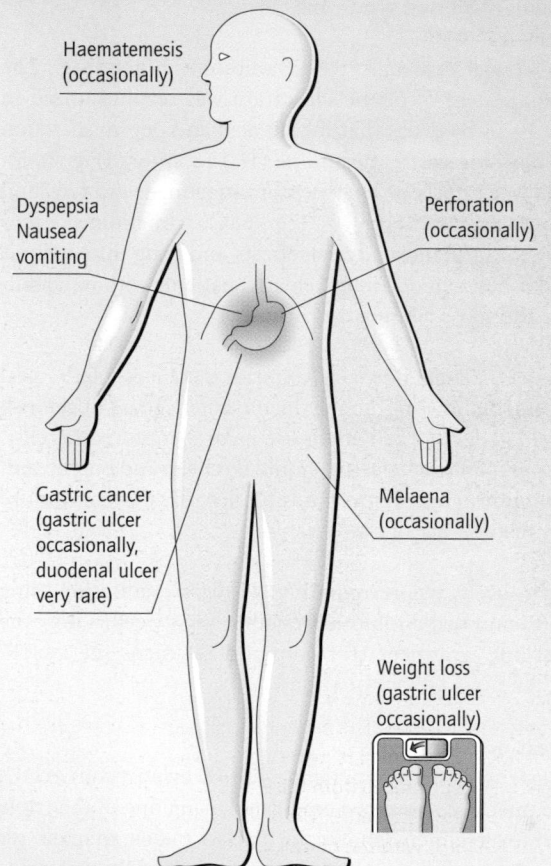

Haematemesis (occasionally)

Dyspepsia Nausea/ vomiting

Perforation (occasionally)

Gastric cancer (gastric ulcer occasionally, duodenal ulcer very rare)

Melaena (occasionally)

Weight loss (gastric ulcer occasionally)

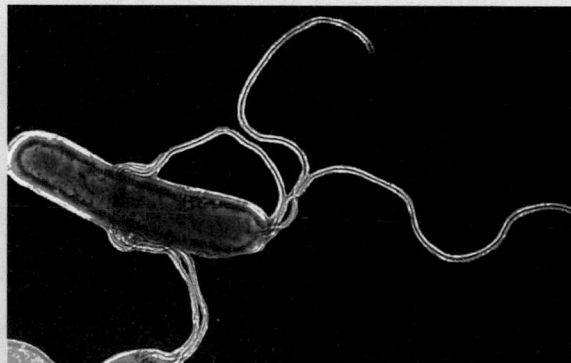

Fig. A *H. pylori* is a spiral urease-containing bacterium which can be identified histologically and biochemically in 90% of patients with duodenal ulcer.

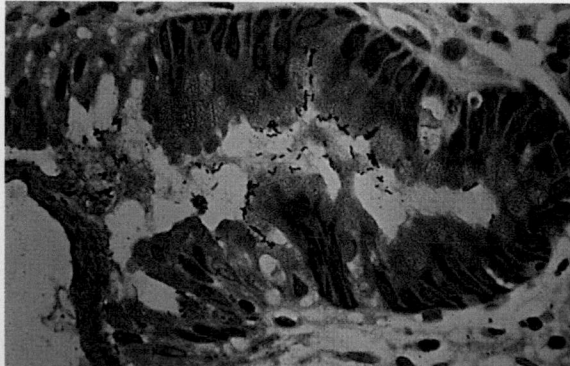

Fig. B Antral gastric epithelium colonized with *H. pylori*, shown as black rods apposed to epithelial surface.

Endoscopy

Endoscopy reveals the ulcer and allows biopsy and/or cytology
Biopsy for histopathology
Brushings for cytology mandatory in gastric ulcers to exclude malignancy
Biopsies can be taken to detect *H. pylori* by urease test, formal histological analysis or culture

Management

Gastric ulcers can be malignant, but duodenal ulcers almost never are

Most ulcers can be cured by *Helicobacter* eradication with a proton pump inhibitor and two antibiotics
The most common and serious complications of peptic ulceration are haemorrhage and perforation

Supportive treatment

General advice
- Stop smoking
- Stop aspirin or NSAIDs
- Avoid stress

In the long term, NSAIDs should be avoided in patients with previous or present peptic ulceration
Avoid specific foods that provoke symptoms

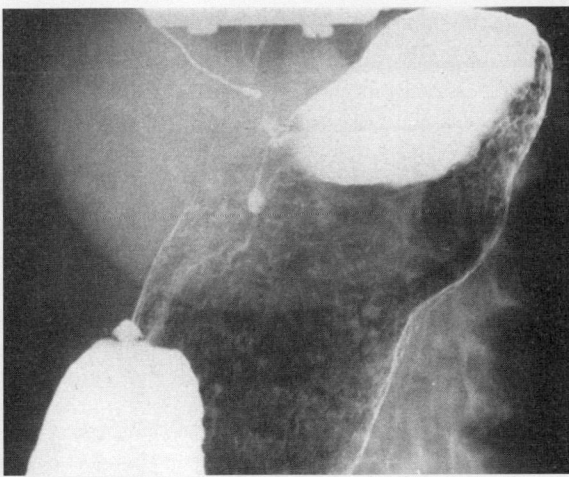

Fig. C Barium meal showing a benign gastric ulcer. Note the barium collection close to the cardia with mucosal folds radiating from its edge. The patient also has a cardiac pacemaker, the bottom of which is just visible at the top of the picture (centre). Reproduced from Misiewicz *et al.*, *Diseases of the Gut and Pancreas*, 2nd edn, 1994 (Blackwell Scientific Publications, Oxford) with the permission of the authors.

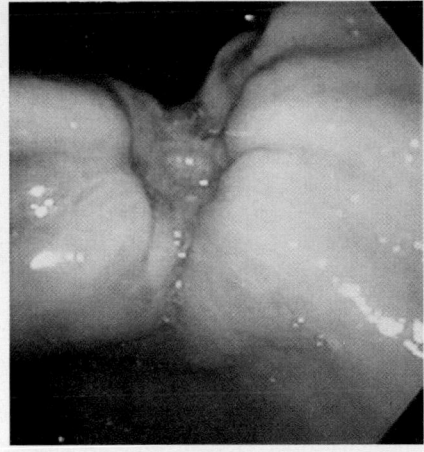

Fig. D Endoscopic view of a gastric ulcer at the angulus. The pylorus is seen at the bottom of the image. Reproduced from Cotton & Williams, *Practical Gastrointestinal Endoscopy*, 3rd edn, 1990 (Blackwell Scientific Publications, Oxford) with the permission of the authors.

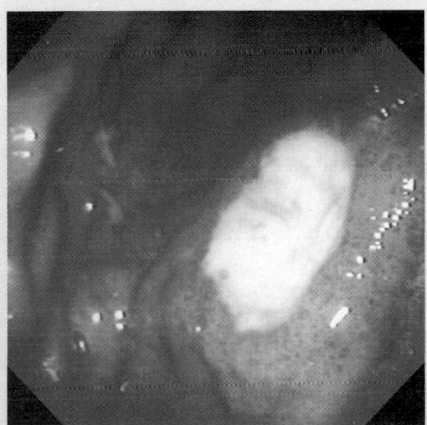

Fig. E Endoscopic view of a duodenal ulcer.

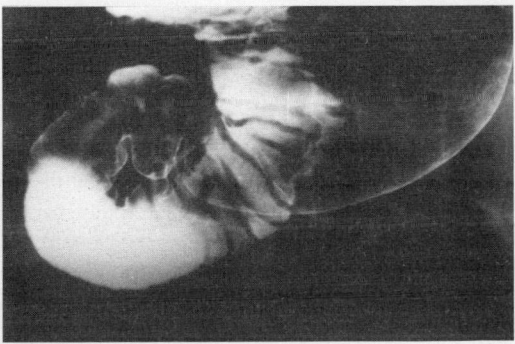

Fig. F Barium meal showing a duodenal ulcer. Note the large crater in the duodenal bulb, which is otherwise only slightly deformed. Reproduced from Misiewicz *et al.*, *Diseases of the Gut and Pancreas*, 2nd edn, 1994 (Blackwell Scientific Publications, Oxford) with the permission of the authors.

Continued on p. 710

10

Specific treatment

Drugs (Table 10.20)

• Antacids
• H$_2$ receptor antagonists (e.g. ranitidine)
• Proton pump inhibitors (e.g. omeprazole, lansoprazole) to inhibit mucosal attack; omeprazole or lansoprazole with antibiotics to eradicate *H. pylori*

Suggested regimens are:

• Lansoprazole 30 mg twice daily, amoxicillin 1 g twice daily (tetracycline 500 mg four times daily if allergic) and metronidazole 400 mg three times daily, altogether for 1 week
• Lansoprazole 30 mg twice daily, amoxicillin 1 g twice daily (tetracycline 500 mg four times daily if allergic) and clarithromycin 500 mg twice daily, altogether for 1 week

Surgery

For refractory ulcers or complications (Fig. 10.34)

• Partial gastrectomy
• Truncal vagotomy and drainage
• Highly selective vagotomy

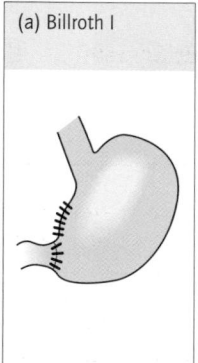 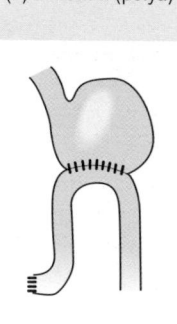 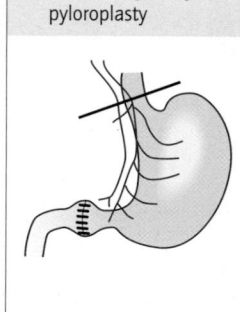 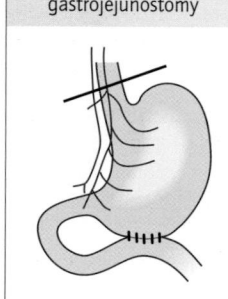 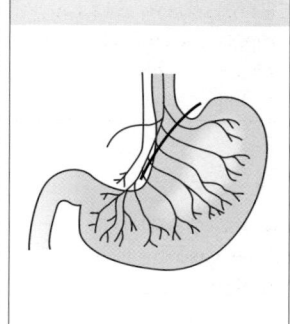

(a) Billroth I | (b) Billroth II (polya) | (c) Truncal vagotomy and pyloroplasty | (d) Truncal vagotomy with gastrojejunostomy | (e) Highly selective vagotomy

Figure 10.39 Operations for peptic ulceration. (a) Partial gastrectomy with Billroth I anastomosis. The ulcer and the ulcer-bearing portion of the stomach are resected. (b) Partial gastrectomy with creation of a duodenal loop (Billroth II, polya). (c) Truncal vagotomy and pyloroplasty. The main nerves are divided to eliminate nervous stimulation of the stomach, reducing the acid secretory capacity, and gastric emptying is maintained with pyloroplasty. (d) Truncal vagotomy with gastrojejunostomy. The main nerves are divided and gastric emptying maintained with gastrojejunostomy. (e) Highly selective vagotomy. Innervation of the acid-producing area of the stomach is interrupted, leaving the nerve supply to the antrum and pylorus intact. This does not affect gastric emptying so a drainage procedure is not required.

Treatment of complications of peptic ulcer

Haemorrhage (see p. 713).

Perforation. Half are associated with NSAID use. All patients require urgent resuscitation, intravenous fluids, nasogastric suction, a nil-by-mouth regimen, antibiotics and antisecretory agents (e.g. PPIs). Although perforations can heal spontaneously, early surgical closure is the treatment of choice, unless the patient's general condition and comorbidity are very poor. The simplest form of surgery is to close the defect and clean out the peritoneal cavity. This approach is effective and probably the best option when the patient is shocked, frail and presenting late with considerable peritoneal soiling, or where the surgeon is inexperienced. In fit patients, being operated upon by an experienced surgeon, a surgical procedure that both closes the defect and provides a definitive long-term treatment to prevent ulceration (such as truncal vagotomy and pyloroplasty for perforated DU) will give better long-term results (Fig. 10.39).

Pyloric stenosis. Initial treatment is restoration of fluid and electrolyte deficiencies. Gastric outlet obstruction may respond to medical treatment or endoscopic balloon dilatation, but surgical drainage and vagotomy may be necessary.

Carcinoma (see p. 711).

Prognosis

Before the role of *H. pylori* was recognized, relapse of peptic ulcer disease after a course of healing treatment was extremely common (up to 90%), and most patients had recurrent episodes of pain over many years. Now, *H. pylori* eradication usually leads to lasting cure, with annual recurrence rates as low as 2% reported.

Table 10.26 Chronic gastritis–classification, histology, clinical features and treatment

Pathology	Clinical features/associations	Treatment
Type A: autoimmune Chronic atrophic gastritis: reduced parietal and chief cells, mucosal thinning	Pernicious anaemia (achlorhydria, hypergastrinaemia, antibodies to gastric parietal cells and intrinsic factor, and malabsorption of vitamin B_{12}; increased risk of autoimmune thyroiditis, Addison's disease, vitiligo, gastric carcinoma)	Vitamin B_{12} for pernicious anaemia
Type B: bacterial Chronic gastritis mainly affecting antrum: *H. pylori*, chronic inflammatory cell infiltration	*H. pylori*, peptic ulceration	Eradication of *H. pylori*
Type C: chemical Chronic superficial gastritis: lymphocytic and plasma cell infiltration, sometimes intestinal metaplasia	Alcohol, smoking, NSAIDs, previous gastrectomy (bile reflux)	Avoid cause, bind bile salts with colestyramine

Gastritis

Acute gastritis

Acute gastritis is defined as acute inflammation of the gastric mucosa.

Disease mechanisms

Helicobacter pylori, other infections, alcohol and drugs (e.g. aspirin, NSAIDs), and severe systemic illness are the most common causes.

Epidemiology

This is a common condition and occurs mainly in adults.

Clinical features

Drug- and alcohol-induced gastritis is often asymptomatic. Bleeding from extensive acute erosive gastritis in patients with serious illnesses (e.g. shock, sepsis, major trauma) can be severe and is often the terminal event.

Investigation

Endoscopy shows multiple superficial erosions and/or submucosal oedema and erythema. Changes may heal rapidly, particularly if caused by NSAID use, and can be missed if OGD is delayed by more than 24 h.

Management

The main indication for treatment is bleeding. Apart from general measures (see p. 715), the underlying cause will need treatment or removal. Drug treatment (e.g. with PPIs or H_2-blockers), is of dubious efficacy. Surgery should be employed only as a last resort because it may involve total gastrectomy. Drugs used to prevent bleeding in patients at risk, such as those in intensive care units, include H_2-blockers, PPIs and/or sucralfate; reversal of shock, hypoxia and sepsis is also important.

Chronic gastritis

Chronic gastritis is chronic inflammation of gastric mucosa. It can be classified and treated according to its aetiology (Table 10.26). Most chronic gastritis is asymptomatic and requires no treatment.

Gastric neoplasms

Gastric carcinoma

Gastric carcinoma is a primary malignant tumour of the stomach (KEYPOINTS BOX 10.3). The discussion below focuses on gastric adenocarcinoma, which accounts for the vast majority of cases. Lymphomas and malignant smooth muscle tumours (leiomyosarcomas) are occasionally found. Presentation is usually late, and survival rates poor.

Disease mechanisms

- For non-cardia gastric cancer, *H. pylori* infection has been identified as an aetiological factor. The relative risk in infected vs. uninfected patients varies widely between studies; it is around fourfold overall, but much higher in Japan. At present it remains speculative as to whether the link is causal or coincidental; it is possible that *Helicobacter* infection is simply a passive marker for other, perhaps dietary, risk factors
- Because many 'gastric' cardia cancers are in fact distal oesophageal adenocarcinomas, they share the same

10

Keypoints 10.3: Gastric cancer

Distal gastric adenocarcinoma is strongly associated with *Helicobacter* infection

Adenocarcinoma at the gastric cardia is usually a complication of Barrett's oesophagus

Patients whose dyspepsia is accompanied by 'alarm' symptoms (e.g. weight loss, vomiting, melaena, anaemia) need prompt gastroscopy to exclude gastric cancer

Less than one-quarter of patients with gastric cancer have resectable disease; palliation with radiotherapy, chemotherapy and/or endoscopic procedures is used in the remainder

aetiological factors, with Barrett's mucosa being the most important

● Carcinogenic nitrosamines are formed intragastrically from dietary nitrate, particularly when hypochlorhydria allows the proliferation of bacteria that reduce it to nitrite

● A strong correlation exists between the widespread use of refrigeration and the declining incidence rates of gastric cancer in developed countries. This may reflect reduced usage of salt and/or pickles for preservation, which may be directly carcinogenic, and reduced contamination of food with micro-organisms

● Dietary salt intake, particularly in Japan
● Atrophic gastritis
● Intestinal metaplasia of the gastric mucosa
● Gastric ulceration
● Previous partial gastrectomy
● Smoking

Pathology

Microscopically, the vast majority are adenocarcinomas, subdivided into intestinal and infiltrative types. When contrasted with the infiltrative type, intestinal tumours are more common in men, tend to affect older patients, have a better prognosis and are often preceded by a prolonged precancerous state (e.g. atrophic gastritis, benign gastric ulcer). Macroscopically, tumours may be flat, depressed, ulcerating or polypoid. In some cases, the cancer spreads widely in superficial and/or submucosal planes, causing a rigid stomach (linitis plastica). Local invasion is common, with early spread to regional and distant lymph nodes, liver, lungs, brain and bones.

Early gastric cancer describes a curable stage of the tumour in which involvement is limited to the mucosa and submucosa.

Epidemiology

Prevalence. Previously one of the most common cancers, the incidence of gastric cancer has fallen since 1950, particularly for distal gastric cancers in developed nations. Explanations for this include reduced prevalence of *Helicobacter* infection and improved methods of food preservation, reducing the exposure of the gastric mucosa to potential carcinogens. In contrast, there has been a rise in the incidence of cancer affecting the gastric cardia—many of these tumours are in fact oesophageal adenocarcinomas arising in Barrett's mucosa, growing downwards to involve the proximal stomach (see p. 697).

Age. Gastric cancer is rare below the age of 55 years (8% of cases), and in virtually all younger patients there are features other than simple dyspepsia at presentation (e.g. weight loss, dysphagia). Incidence rises sharply after age 65, peaking around age 80.

Sex. More common in men than women.

Genetics. Associated with blood group A. There is a very small increased incidence in first-degree relatives.

Geography. The annual incidence varies widely between and within countries. Mortality varies from 70 in 100 000 in Japan to 10 in 100 000 in the USA. In the UK, incidence is about 30 in 100 000.

Clinical features

Presentation is late because small and potentially curable cancers are usually asymptomatic. The common features, in order of frequency, are weight loss/anorexia, abdominal pain, nausea/vomiting, dysphagia and features of gastrointestinal blood loss (e.g. haematemesis, melaena, iron-deficiency anaemia). Occasionally, patients present with features relating to metastatic disease such as jaundice, a palpable abdominal mass, supraclavicular lymphadenopathy or ascites; these indicate inoperability.

Differential diagnosis. This is as for dyspepsia (Table 10.4, p. 657).

Investigation
Haematology
FBC. There may be a microcytic anaemia.

Biochemistry
Liver function tests suggest metastatic disease if abnormal.

Diagnostic imaging
● *Endoscopy with biopsy and cytology* (Fig. 10.40): the main diagnostic method. To minimize the chance of obtaining false-negative histology, multiple (e.g. 6–8) biopsies should be taken from the edge and base of any ulcerating lesion in the stomach

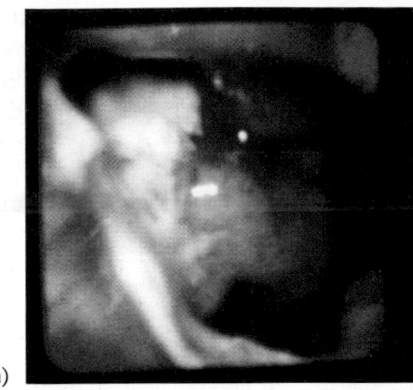

(a)

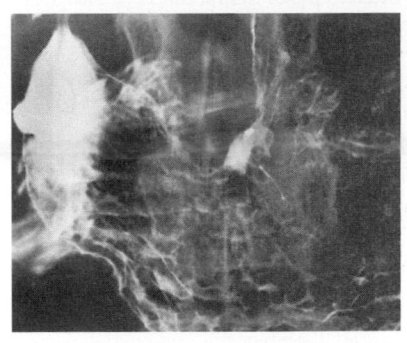

(b)

Figure 10.40 (a) Endoscopic appearance of gastric carcinoma. Note the ulcerating nodular friable mass. (Reproduced from *Slide Atlas of Gastroenterology* with the kind permission of the author and Times Mirror International Publishers.) (b) Double contrast barium meal demonstrating a neoplastic ulcer at the angulus surrounded by blunted mucosal folds. (Reproduced from Misiewicz JJ, Pounder RE, Venables CW. *Diseases of the Gut and Pancreas*, 2nd edn. Oxford: Blackwell Scientific Publications, 1994 with the permission of the authors.)

- *A barium meal* (Fig. 10.26b and 10.40b): shows gastric mucosal lesions, and differentiation between benign and malignant ulceration is often possible radiologically. However, gastroscopy is generally more sensitive, particularly for early gastric cancers, and is required in all cases for confirmatory biopsy diagnosis. The linitis plastica variety may spread largely submucosally, and endoscopic biopsies can fail to detect the tumour. In this situation, the barium meal can be superior, demonstrating an abnormally indistensible stomach
- *Chest radiography, ultrasound, CT scan and/or laparoscopy*: required to detect distant metastases and assess resectability

Management

As for people with other cancers, supportive measures include an explanation of the situation to the patient and relatives, pain control (e.g. with opiates), nutritional replacement when appropriate, making contact with support services such as specialist cancer nurses, liaising early with the primary care team and arranging, as necessary, for terminal care.

Surgery. This offers the only chance of a cure. Unfortunately, only a minority (approximately 25%) present with potentially resectable disease. The operation performed ranges from subtotal or total gastrectomy for potentially curable lesions, to local resection, gastroenterostomy and intubation for palliative purposes. For patients who have had a potentially curative disease, recent studies show a significant survival advantage if postoperative (adjuvant) chemoradiotherapy is given. Giving radio- and/or chemotherapy before surgery (neoadjuvant therapy) has not yet shown convincing benefits.

Endoscopic palliative intubation and tumour destruction using diathermy or laser can be helpful for inoperable disease. Chemotherapy (e.g. 5-fluorouracil, cisplatin) can produce temporary tumour regression in patients with advanced disease.

Prognosis

The overall 5-year survival rate in the UK is less than 10%. This dismal figure is related mainly to late presentation. In Japan, where population screening programmes are in place, gastric cancer is more commonly detected at an early stage, and its surgical treatment is followed by a 90% 5-year survival rate.

Gastrointestinal bleeding

The principles of investigation, resuscitation and treatment are similar in patients with upper and lower gastrointestinal bleeding.

Acute upper gastrointestinal bleeding

Acute upper gastrointestinal bleeding (EMERGENCY BOX 10.2; ACUTE UPPER GASTROINTESTINAL BLEEDING AT A GLANCE) is defined as acute bleeding from the gut proximal to the junction between the duodenum and the jejunum.

Disease mechanisms

In the UK, the most common cause of acute upper gastrointestinal bleeding is peptic ulcer, which accounts for 50% of episodes. Gastric ulcers and duodenal ulcers are equally responsible. Other common causes are oesophagitis (7%), gastritis (7%) and Mallory–Weiss syndrome

10

Emergency 10.2: Upper gastrointestinal bleeding

Diagnosis
Usually manifested by haematemesis and melaena.
Commonly caused by peptic ulceration (for a full list of causes see Table 10.27)

Supportive treatment
Assess
Look for signs of shock, anaemia, chronic liver disease

Resuscitate
Oxygen, intravenous fluid, then blood
Platelets or fresh frozen plasma if thrombocytopenic or prothrombin time is prolonged
Treat in intensive care or high dependency unit with a central venous pressure (CVP) line if there are signs of shock or if there is associated serious cardiac, renal or liver disease

Reassess and monitor
Stool chart, pulse, blood pressure, blood count and/or CVP and urine output, to detect continued bleeding or rebleed
Frequent joint review by physician and surgeon
Always consider—could this patient have oesophageal varices (as treatment options differ; see p. 630)?

Specific treatment
Drugs
Oral proton pump inhibitor as soon as peptic ulceration has been diagnosed endoscopically

Early endoscopy, if necessary repeated
Injections, ligation, electrocoagulation or laser for bleeding peptic ulcers, varices, ligation, erosions, tumours and vascular anomalies

Surgery
For persistent bleeding

Angiography
Arterial embolization for vascular malformations

Table 10.27 Common causes of upper gastrointestinal bleeding (most common causes are given in capital letters). A, characteristically bleeds acutely; C, tends to cause chronic, usually minor or occult bleeding; AC, causes either A or C

Location	Cause
Oesophagus	OESOPHAGITIS (AC)
	MALLORY–WEISS TEAR (A)
	VARICES (A)
	Neoplasia (C)
Stomach	GASTRIC ULCER (AC)
	GASTRITIS (AC)
	NEOPLASIA (AC)
	NSAIDs
	Aspirin
	Alcohol
	Hereditary haemorrhagic telangiectasia and other vascular malformations (AC)
	Haemorrhagic diathesis (AC, anticoagulants, thrombocytopenia)
Duodenum	DUODENAL ULCER (A)
	Duodenitis (A)

Acute tubular necrosis, shock lung, myocardial infarction, cerebral infarction and death may ensue. In self-limiting episodes, fluid transfers over a few hours from the extravascular to the intravascular compartment. Haemoglobin concentration and the haematocrit therefore fall.

Epidemiology
This is one of the most common medical emergencies.

Clinical features
Patients present with haematemesis and/or melaena (stool that is tarry because of the presence of a black pigment derived from haemoglobin by the action of colonic bacteria). The haematemesis may consist of either fresh or altered blood. Altered blood resembles coffee grounds. Patients with marked bleeding may have symptoms of shock, including light-headedness, fainting and sweating. Diagnostically useful information includes:
• A history of dyspepsia (suggesting peptic ulcer) or heartburn (oesophagitis), repeated vomiting (Mallory–Weiss syndrome) or concurrent liver or other disease associated with bleeding
• Recent drug ingestion (aspirin, NSAIDs, anticoagulants)
• Alcohol consumption
Signs of shock include cold clammy peripheries, pallor, tachycardia and supine or postural hypotension. A rectal examination will confirm melaena. The underlying diagnosis may be suggested by:
• Epigastric mass (gastric carcinoma)

(5%) (Table 10.27). The incidence of bleeding caused by oesophageal varices varies widely between centres, but may approach 10% of cases; its management is discussed in Chapter 9. No cause is found in 20% of patients. Aspirin and NSAIDs appear to precipitate bleeding from established peptic ulcers, as well as from gastritis.

Acute blood loss results in a fall in blood volume. This leads to:
• Decreased venous return, cardiac output and blood pressure
• Peripheral vasoconstriction
• Oliguria

- Signs of chronic liver disease (see p. 667)
- Telangiectasia on the tongue, lips and fingers (hereditary haemorrhagic telangiectasia)
- Aortic stenosis: an association with intestinal angiodysplasia has been reported

Differential diagnosis

The causes of upper gastrointestinal bleeding are shown in Table 10.27. Melaena without haematemesis may be caused by a lesion of the jejunum, ileum, caecum or upper alimentary tract. Darkening of the stool by oral iron may be mistaken for melaena.

Investigation

Haematology

- *Urgent blood-grouping and cross-matching:* necessary
- *FBC:* the initial haemoglobin is not helpful for assessing the extent of blood loss because haemodilution does not occur for several hours. A low value, microcytosis or hypochromia may suggest chronic bleeding before the acute episode, while the platelet count may rise after a major haemorrhage. Thrombocytopenia may indicate an underlying bleeding diathesis or portal hypertension
- *Prothrombin time:* check clotting if the patient is shocked or bleeding or has liver disease

Biochemistry

- *Urea:* an elevated blood urea soon after admission indicates substantial upper (in contrast to lower) gastrointestinal blood loss rather than renal failure if the serum creatinine is normal. This is because after absorption the digestive products of blood are metabolized by the liver to urea
- *Liver function tests:* useful for revealing hepatic disorders

Diagnostic imaging

- *OGD:* should be performed immediately after haemodynamic stabilization for shocked patients, and otherwise within 24 h. After a longer delay, minor lesions such as a Mallory–Weiss tear, acute gastritis and duodenitis may not be detectable. OGD is used to detect the site of bleeding and to assess the chances of rebleeding of ulcers from the presence or absence of stigmata of recent haemorrhage (fresh blood or visible vessel in the ulcer base). It is also used therapeutically (see below). About 20% of patients will remain undiagnosed after OGD. The cause for most of those who have no further trouble is a small and/or superficial lesion that has healed. No further action is required, except in patients with melaena without haematemesis in whom a lower alimentary source should be considered (see p. 718). A few of those who are undiagnosed rebleed. OGD should then be repeated, particularly if it was first carried out by an inexperienced endoscopist

- *Arteriography:* indicated if OGD is again negative. The diagnostic rate of arteriography is highest when the patient is actively bleeding more than 0.5 ml/min. It is particularly useful for identifying small vascular malformations (and for their embolization; see below) and haemobilia

Other

Exploratory laparotomy is very occasionally necessary if profuse upper gastrointestinal bleeding continues and OGD and arteriography are non-diagnostic.

Management

Management of upper gastrointestinal bleeding should be modified according to the patient's haemodynamic state and local facilities (e.g. availability of endoscopic therapy). It is usually managed first by physicians, but early involvement of the surgical team is essential (EMERGENCY BOX 10.2).

Supportive treatment

Resuscitation. If the patient is shocked, start resuscitation with plasma expanders (e.g. Gelofusine), blood, platelets and fresh frozen plasma as necessary before obtaining a detailed history and examination. Patients with signs of shock and/or associated serious cardiac, renal or liver disease are best treated in an intensive care or high dependency unit with a central venous pressure line so that transfusion requirements can be monitored and rebleeding can be detected early.

Reassessment. Monitor the patient with a stool chart and frequent measurement of pulse, blood pressure, blood count and/or CVP to detect continued bleeding or rebleeding promptly. Risk factors for rebleeding are age (over 60 years), peptic ulceration (particularly gastric) with stigmata of recent haemorrhage, oesophageal varices and accompanying serious medical conditions.

Specific treatment

Drugs. Intravenous high-dose omeprazole (80 mg bolus followed by 8 mg/h for 72 h) has been shown to reduce the risk of peptic ulcer rebleeding following endoscopic therapy. Oral PPIs are unlikely to add to the efficacy of endoscopic haemostasis methods in the prevention of recurrent upper gastrointestinal bleeding during the first few days after hospital admission. However, where endoscopic therapy has not been used, high-dose omeprazole (40 mg b.d.) is superior to placebo in preventing ulcer rebleeding. Even though oral PPIs do not unequivocally decrease rebleeding rates, it is appropriate to give them orally to start healing as soon as possible after peptic ulceration has been diagnosed endoscopically (following

Acute upper gastrointestinal bleeding at a glance

Epidemiology

Incidence
50–150 in 100 000. The mortality is about 10%

Age
70% of patients are over 60 years of age

Sex
No significant difference

Genetics
No association

Geography
Wide variation between countries

Causes

The most common causes are:
- Peptic ulceration
- Oesophagitis

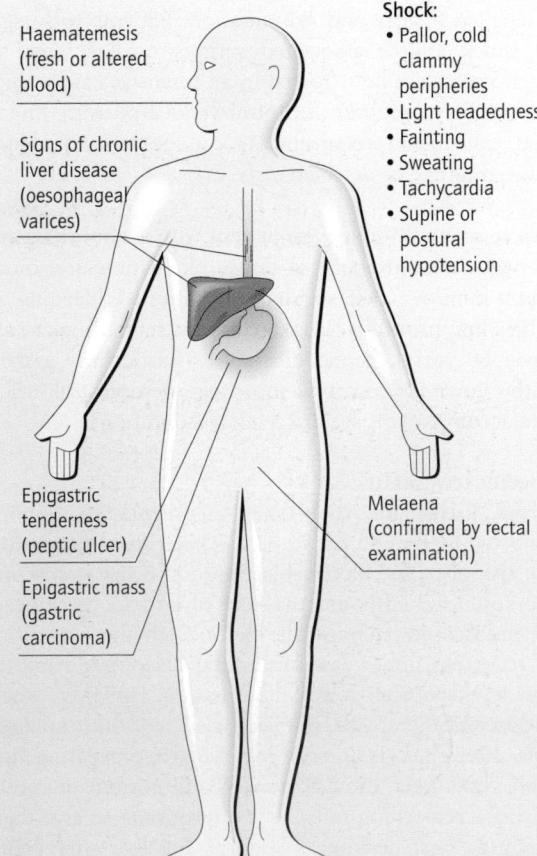

Haematemesis (fresh or altered blood)

Signs of chronic liver disease (oesophageal varices)

Epigastric tenderness (peptic ulcer)

Epigastric mass (gastric carcinoma)

Shock:
- Pallor, cold clammy peripheries
- Light headedness
- Fainting
- Sweating
- Tachycardia
- Supine or postural hypotension

Melaena (confirmed by rectal examination)

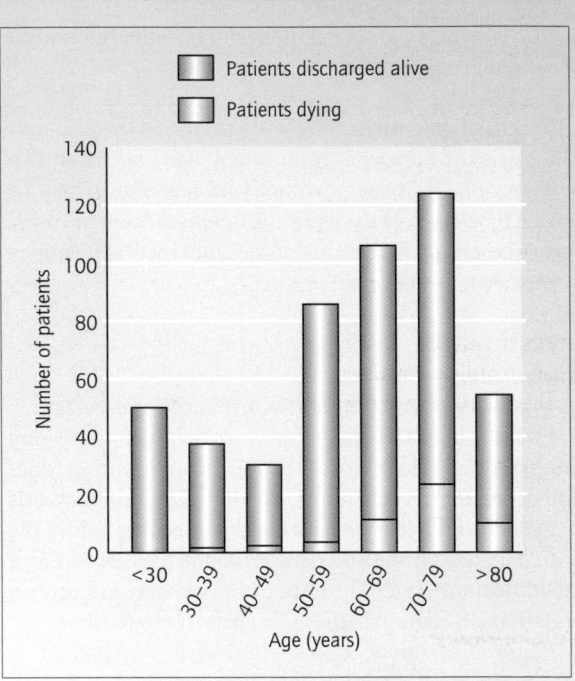

Fig. A Age distribution of patients admitted with, and dying from, acute upper gastrointestinal bleeding.

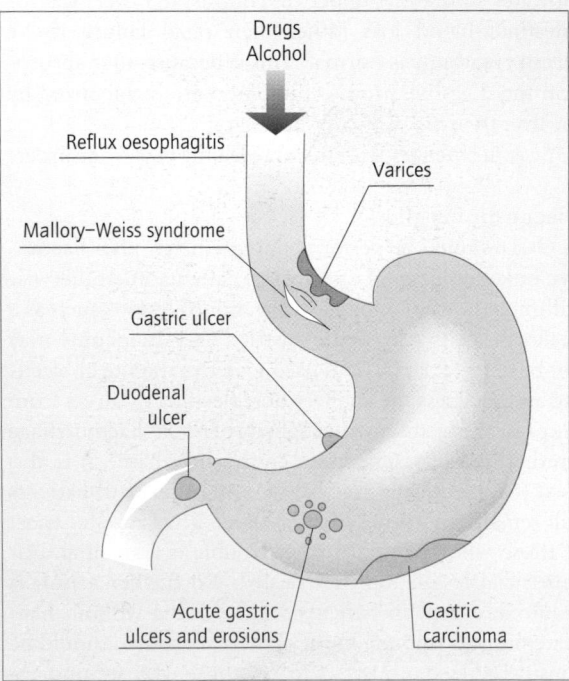

Drugs
Alcohol

Reflux oesophagitis

Varices

Mallory–Weiss syndrome

Gastric ulcer

Duodenal ulcer

Acute gastric ulcers and erosions

Gastric carcinoma

Fig. B Common causes of acute upper gastrointestinal bleeding.

- Gastritis
- Mallory–Weiss tears
- Oesophageal varices
- Aspirin and NSAIDs are contributory factors

Investigation
Haematology
- *Blood grouping and cross-matching:* urgent
- *FBC, microcytic or hypochromic anaemia:* suggest chronic bleeding before acute episode. Acute haemoglobin does not reflect blood loss
- *Prothrombin time:* check clotting in cases of shock or liver disease
- *Urea:* may be elevated, and distinguishes from lower gastrointestinal bleeding
- *Liver function tests:* reveal hepatic disorders if abnormal

Endoscopy
OGD may be able to detect site of bleeding and likelihood of rebleeding from ulcers in 80% of cases
Therapeutic management by electrocoagulation, injections, banding or laser

Angiography
If OGD is negative and bleeding severe
Good for identifying vascular tumours, malformations and haemobilia

Management
Patients with haematemesis and/or melaena need urgent resuscitation with intravenous volume expanders and blood transfusion
The next step is urgent gastroscopy for diagnosis and endoscopic therapy; further definitive therapy depends on the cause

Supportive treatment
Assess. Look for signs of:
- Shock
- Anaemia
- Chronic liver disease
Resuscitate
- Oxygen, intravenous fluid, then blood
- Platelets or fresh frozen plasma if clotting abnormal
- Treat in intensive care or high dependency unit with central venous pressure (CVP) line if patient shocked or has serious cardiac, renal or liver disease (remember possible oesophageal varices)
Reassess and monitor
- Stool chart
- Pulse
- Blood pressure
- Blood count and/or CVP to detect continued bleeding or rebleed
- Urine output
Frequent joint review by physician and surgeon

Specific treatment
- *Drugs:* oral proton pump inhibitor if peptic ulceration or oesophagitis diagnosed
- *Early endoscopy:* if necessary repeated. Injections, ligation, electrocoagulation or laser for bleeding peptic ulcers, varices, erosions, tumours and vascular anomalies
- *Surgery:* for persistent bleeding
- *Angiography:* arterial embolization for vascular malformations

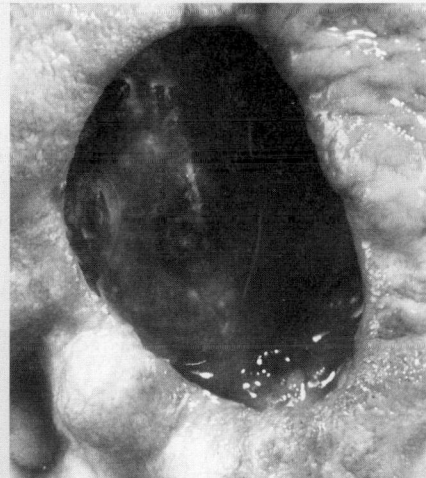

Fig. C Post-mortem specimen. The patient was thought to have expired from bleeding varices but in fact exsanguinated from a gastric ulcer. Reproduced from Misiewicz JJ, Pounder RE, Venables CW. *Diseases of the Gut and Pancreas*, 2nd edn, 1994 (Blackwell Scientific Publications, Oxford) with the permission of the authors.

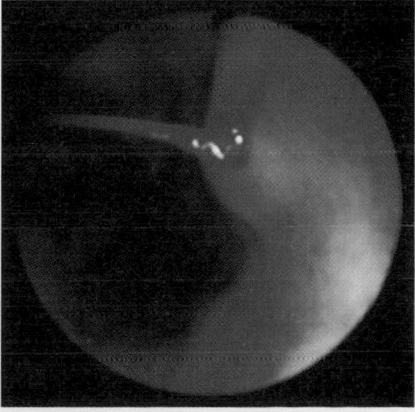

Fig. D Endoscopic view of an actively bleeding oesophageal varix.

10

Table 10.28 The Rockall Scoring system: a means of assessing risk of rebleeding and mortality following non-variceal upper gastrointestinal bleeding

Points allocated	0	1	2	3
Age	<60	60–79	≥80	
Shock indices (blood pressure and pulse)	Systolic >100 Pulse <100	Systolic >100 Pulse >100	Systolic <100	
Comorbidity	None		Heart failure IHD Major comorbidity	Renal failure Liver failure Disseminated malignancy
Diagnosis	Mallory–Weiss tear Normal (and no blood seen)	All other diagnoses	Upper gastrointestinal malignancy	
Stigmata of haemorrhage	None (or dark spot only)		Fresh blood seen; adherent clot; visible vessel; spurting vessel	

on from intravenous PPI therapy if given). Coagulopathy (raised prothrombin time, low platelet count) should be corrected if present.

Endoscopy. Varices are injected or ligated (see p. 630). Bleeding peptic ulcers, erosions, tumours and vascular anomalies can also be treated endoscopically using electrocoagulation, injections or laser.

Surgery. Profuse bleeding or rebleeding usually requires prompt surgery. The timing of operative intervention, which carries a significant mortality in sick elderly patients, remains controversial.

Arteriography. Arteriography can have therapeutic as well as diagnostic uses (see above). In particular, arterial embolization can be effective for vascular malformations.

Prognosis

Despite improved diagnostic and therapeutic methods in the last 20 years, mortality remains at about 10% because of the increasing incidence of haemorrhage in elderly patients. Risk factors for a poor prognosis include age, serious comorbid disease, shock on admission, rebleeding and transfusion requirement exceeding 3 units.

Various scoring systems have been devised to try to predict patients at greatest risk of rebleeding and death. One such is the Rockall system, which integrates information from examination and endoscopy (Table 10.28). Points are allocated for each variable such as age, blood pressure and pulse, and then totalled, to predict the risk of bleeding and death (Table 10.29).

Table 10.29 The Rockall Scoring system: the risk of rebleeding and death

Total score	Death (95% CI)	Rebleeding (95% CI)
8+	40% (30–51%)	37% (27–47%)
7	23% (15–31%)	37% (28–46%)
6	12% (6.3–17%)	27% (20–34%)
5	11% (6.3–15%)	25% (19–31%)
4	8.0% (4.0–12%)	15% (10–21%)
3	1.9% (0.0–3.9%)	12% (6.8–17%)
0–2	0.0% (0.0–0.93%)	5.9% (3.3–8.5%)

CI, confidence interval.

Acute lower gastrointestinal bleeding

Acute lower gastrointestinal bleeding is defined as acute bleeding from the gut distal to the ligament of Treitz (junction of duodenum and jejunum). Major bleeding from the lower bowel is less common than from the upper bowel and its cause is more difficult to diagnose.

Disease mechanisms

Causes of lower gastrointestinal bleeding vary with age (Table 10.30).

Clinical features

Acute lower gastrointestinal bleeding presents with either frank rectal bleeding or melaena, with or without symptoms of shock. (If rectal bleeding results from upper gut pathology, the haemorrhage is profuse and the patient is usually shocked.) The patient may be shocked, or anaemic if there have been previous episodes. Abdominal examination may reveal a mass (suggesting neoplasia) or tenderness and a bruit (suggesting ischaemia).

Table 10.30 Common causes of painless lower gastrointestinal bleeding (most common causes are in capital letters). A, characteristically bleeds acutely; C, tends to cause chronic or recurrent, usually minor or occult bleeding; AC, either A or C

Children
Meckel's diverticulum (A)
Haemangiomas (C)
Intussusception (A)
Inflammatory bowel disease (AC)
Infections (A)

Young adults
INFLAMMATORY BOWEL DISEASE (AC)
HAEMORRHOIDS (C)
Meckel's diverticulum (A)
Vascular malformations (AC)
Benign solitary rectal ulcer (C)

Elderly
CARCINOMA (C)
POLYPS (C)
INFLAMMATORY BOWEL DISEASE (AC)
HAEMORRHOIDS (C)
DIVERTICULOSIS (A)
Vascular malformations (especially angiodysplasia) (AC)
Ischaemia (A)
Radiation enterocolitis (AC)

Bleeding from anal pathology such as haemorrhoids or anal fissures is usually obvious from the history (e.g. anal pain on defecation because of an anal fissure, haemorrhoids noticed by the patient), or on rectal examination. It is rarely of significant volume, and is usually managed in surgical outpatient departments.

Investigation
Haematology
As for upper gastrointestinal bleeding (see p. 715):
- Blood grouping and cross-matching
- FBC to identify chronic bleeding
- Prothrombin time

Biochemistry
A normal blood urea suggests a lower bowel source for melaena (see p. 715).

Diagnostic imaging
- *Sigmoidoscopy:* often shows simply melaena or bleeding from above, but the cause of minor rectal bleeding is sometimes obvious (e.g. anal disorders, rectal carcinoma, proctitis)
- *OGD:* should be performed to exclude an upper gastrointestinal cause if there is melaena or substantial rectal bleeding and shock

- *Colonoscopy:* if OGD is negative, the next step is colonoscopy, preferably after adequate bowel preparation because large amounts of blood in the colonic lumen impair visualization
- *Urgent mesenteric arteriography:* the next investigation if colonoscopy is inconclusive and bleeding continues (see p. 676)
- *Exploratory laparotomy:* necessary if profuse undiagnosed bleeding persists. Peroperative colonoscopy and/or enteroscopy may be helpful
- *Isotopic bleeding and Meckel's scans* (Table 10.16, p. 678) *and barium studies of the small bowel:* further investigations for patients who are undiagnosed after colonoscopy, but in whom the acute bleeding has settled. Using these techniques, the cause of bleeding is identified in about 80% of patients

Management
The steps taken depend on the haemodynamic state of the patient and local expertise (EMERGENCY BOX 10.3).

Emergency 10.3: Lower gastrointestinal bleeding

Diagnosis
Self-evident with either fresh blood or melaena per rectum (for causes see Table 10.30)

Supportive treatment
Assess
Look for signs of shock, anaemia

Resuscitate
Oxygen, intravenous fluid, then blood
Platelets or fresh frozen plasma if clotting abnormal
Treat in intensive care or high dependency unit with CVP line if patient shocked or has serious cardiac, renal or liver disease

Reassess and monitor
Stool chart, pulse, blood pressure, respiration, blood count and/or CVP to detect continued bleeding or rebleed
Frequent joint review by physician and surgeon

Specific treatment
Endoscopy
Colonoscopic electrocoagulation or laser for bleeding from a polyp, angiodysplasia or telangiectasia, as well as for recurrent bleeding from colorectal carcinomas in patients too frail for surgery

Angiography
Selective embolization of vascular malformations

Surgery
For some causes of acute lower bowel haemorrhage (e.g. haemorrhoids, carcinoma)

10

Supportive treatment

Monitor, and if necessary resuscitate as for upper gastro-intestinal bleeding. As with upper gut bleeding, blood loss from the lower bowel usually stops spontaneously.

Specific treatment

Endoscopy. Colonoscopic electrocoagulation or laser can stop bleeding from a polyp, angiodysplasia or telangiectasia, as well as from recurrently bleeding colorectal carcinomas in patients who are too frail for surgery.

Surgery. Treatment for many of the causes of acute lower bowel haemorrhage is elective surgery.

Arteriography. Vascular malformations can be selectively embolized.

Iron deficiency caused by occult gastrointestinal bleeding

Many patients have chronic and recurrent minor, often occult, gastrointestinal haemorrhage rather than a single major acute episode.

Disease mechanisms

The causes of chronic and recurrent gastrointestinal haemorrhage are shown in Tables 10.27 (p. 714) and 10.30 (p. 719).

Clinical features

Patients present with iron-deficiency anaemia. Differential diagnosis of non-gastroenterological causes of iron-deficiency anaemia is discussed on p. 1020.

Investigation

- *Faecal occult blood tests:* can be used to direct investigation of patients with iron-deficiency anaemia and no other digestive symptoms. When positive, they point to investigation of the alimentary tract, but low sensitivity tests (e.g. haemoccult) may give a false-negative result
- *OGD:* carried out in patients with iron-deficiency anaemia to look for peptic ulcer and gastric neoplasia in particular; if negative, distal duodenal biopsies should be taken to look for coeliac disease
- *Colonoscopy:* preferred to barium enema because it allows instant treatment of some causes (e.g. polyps, angiodysplasia)
- *Enteroscopy* (see p. 673): may show proximal small intestinal causes of blood loss
- *Arteriography, isotope bleeding scan, and/or small bowel radiology:* may be necessary for the rare patient eluding diagnosis after being investigated as outlined above

Management

Treatment is of the underlying cause. Oral iron therapy is often required.

Diseases of the small intestine

Malabsorption syndromes

The causes and investigation of patients with malabsorption syndromes are described on pp. 680–3 and in Tables 10.18 and 10.19 (pp. 680–1). The clinical features common to all full-blown malabsorption syndromes are shown in Table 10.17 (p. 680).

Certain signs sometimes indicate the diagnosis:
- An abdominal mass suggests Crohn's disease or lymphoma
- Erythema nodosum and/or arthritis suggest Crohn's disease
- Dermatitis herpetiformis suggests coeliac disease
- Mouth ulcers suggest coeliac or Crohn's disease
- An abdominal scar suggests blind loop or short bowel syndrome
- Jaundice suggests cancer of the pancreas
- Anxiety, tremor, warm skin and tachycardia suggest hyperthyroidism

Coeliac disease

Coeliac disease is malabsorption caused by gluten-induced small intestinal damage, which is reversed when gluten is removed from the diet. Synonyms include idiopathic steatorrhoea, gluten-sensitive enteropathy and non-tropical sprue. Highly accurate non-invasive antibody-based tests are now available for diagnosis (see below).

Disease mechanisms

Gluten is the water-insoluble protein fraction of cereal grain (wheat, barley, rye and, possibly, oats). The toxic constituent of gluten appears to be α-gliadin, but whether the harmful effects are mediated by an immunological mechanism, or a mucosal enzyme defect or have a different explanation is not clear.

Pathology

The small bowel mucosa shows subtotal or total villous atrophy on dissection and light microscopy. Other features are increased intraepithelial lymphocytes, which may reflect the immune pathogenesis, and a chronic inflammatory cell infiltrate in the lamina propria, which is much less specific.

Epidemiology

Prevalence. In the UK, about 1 in 500 of the population

has positive serology for coeliac disease but most cases are not clinically apparent.

Age. Any age, but presentation in childhood is most common.

Genetics. First-degree relatives have a 10% chance of developing the disease. HLA B8 is found in 85% of people with coeliac disease compared with 20% of controls.

Geography. Varies geographically. It is very common in Galway, Ireland but is rare in Africa and China.

Clinical features

Children present with failure to thrive, with or without other features of malabsorption (Table 10.18, p. 680). Adults most commonly present with anaemia caused by iron and/or folate deficiency.

Dermatitis herpetiformis is associated with coeliac disease, and anyone with this skin disorder should be referred for small bowel biopsy. The rash responds to a gluten-free diet.

Coeliac disease is also associated with:
- Hyposplenism
- Infertility
- Occasionally, autoimmune disorders (e.g. adrenal insufficiency) and immunoglobulin deficiency (see p. 726)

Complications. Coeliac disease is associated with an increased risk of small intestinal T-cell lymphoma and carcinoma of the oesophagus and small bowel. A strict gluten-free diet reduces this risk.

Differential diagnosis. This includes other causes of diarrhoea (Table 10.12, p. 664), steatorrhoea (Table 10.14, p. 665) and malabsorption (Table 10.19, p. 681).

Investigation
Haematology
- *FBC:* there may be anaemia because of iron or folate deficiency
- *Blood film:* Howell–Jolly bodies indicate associated hyposplenism; dimorphic red cells indicate iron and either folate or vitamin B_{12} deficiency
- *Prothrombin time:* rarely prolonged

Biochemistry
- *Serum calcium, phosphate:* may be low and *alkaline phosphatase* may be raised indicating biochemical osteomalacia because of vitamin D deficiency and calcium malabsorption (see p. 280)
- *Serum albumin:* may be reduced as a result of protein malabsorption

Immunology
While circulating antibodies to gliadin and reticulin are often found in patients with coeliac disease, neither is adequately specific or sensitive for diagnosis or screening. By chance, coeliac patients have been found to have antibodies to endomysium (a component of the smooth muscle of monkey oesophagus); they also have antibodies to tissue transglutaminase, with high specificity (nearly 100%) and sensitivity (90%) for the disease. In those with positive antibody testing, small bowel biopsy should be requested to confirm the diagnosis. Despite the near 100% specificity, the occasional patient will have normal duodenal mucosa despite positive endomyseal antibodies. More commonly, the biopsy adds important information by quantifying the mucosal lesion, which may vary from a slight increase in lymphocytes in the epithelial layer to complete villous atrophy. This then provides an important baseline for assessing response to diet by rebiopsy (see below).

Histopathology
The diagnosis is confirmed on endoscopic duodenal biopsies (see p. 670).

Management
The cornerstone of treatment is a gluten-free diet with lifelong avoidance of products containing wheat, rye or barley flour. Expert dietary advice is essential, and joining a local or national support group (e.g. the Coeliac Society) helps long-term compliance. Patients should be screened for osteoporosis at diagnosis, and followed up in a specialist clinic at least annually, and assessed for nutritional deficiencies (e.g. iron, folate, calcium and vitamin D). In many centres, duodenal biopsies are taken after 6 months on the diet to confirm an adequate response.

In rare patients not responding to a gluten-free diet, remission can be induced using oral corticosteroid therapy after ensuring that the non-response is not caused by non-compliance with the diet or to a complication of coeliac disease (see above).

Prognosis
Symptoms usually respond rapidly. Reasons for failing to respond to a gluten-free diet include incorrect diagnosis, non-compliance with diet, secondary hypolactasia and small bowel neoplasia such as lymphoma.

Small bowel bacterial overgrowth

Bacterial counts in the small bowel are normally very low (e.g. less than 10^4/ml aspirated jejunal fluid). Conditions where small bowel bacterial overgrowth occurs usually present with malabsorption.

10

Coeliac disease at a glance

Epidemiology
Prevalence
1 in 500 in the UK

Age
Childhood, any age

Genetics
Associated with HLA B8, DR3/DQW2 and DR7/DQW2

Geography
Most common in Galway, Ireland

Cause
Immunologically mediated mucosal sensitivity to gluten-containing cereal products (wheat, barley, rye, possibly oats)

Investigation
Haematology
- *FBC:* anaemia (because of iron or folate deficiency)
- *Film:* dimorphic red cells, Howell–Jolly bodies

- *Ferritin, folate:* low
- *Calcium and phosphate:* low
- *Alkaline phosphatase:* raised
- *Albumin:* low
- *Antibodies:* to gliadin, reticulin, endomysium

Histopathology
Biopsy (usually endoscopic) of proximal small intestine. Subtotal or total villous atrophy

Management
Supportive treatment
Explanation
Patient support group (e.g. Coeliac Society)
Restore nutritional deficiencies (e.g. iron, folate, calcium, vitamin D)

Specific treatment
Gluten-free diet
Drugs
- Prednisolone
- Azathioprine (rarely, for refractory disease)

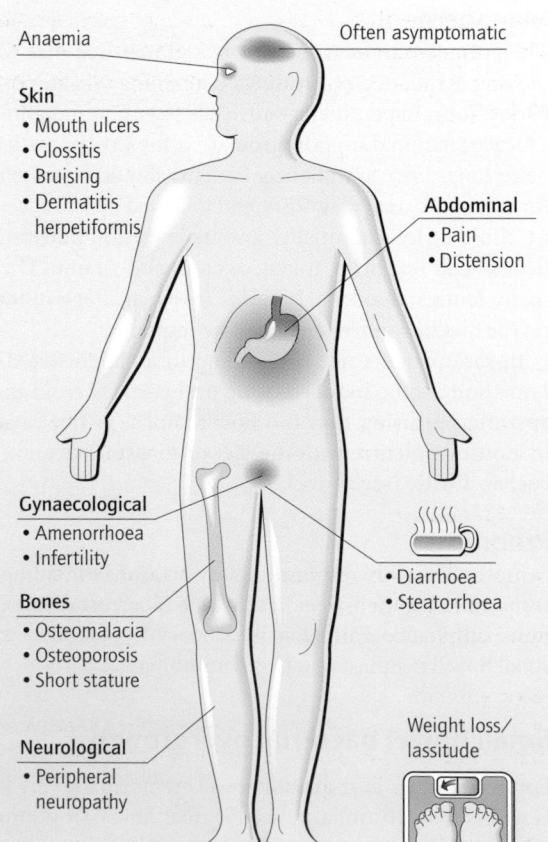

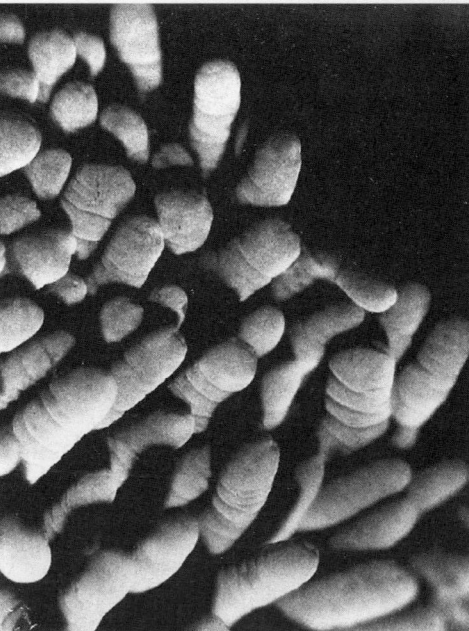

Fig. A Dissecting microscope appearance of normal jejunal mucosa showing finger-shaped villi.

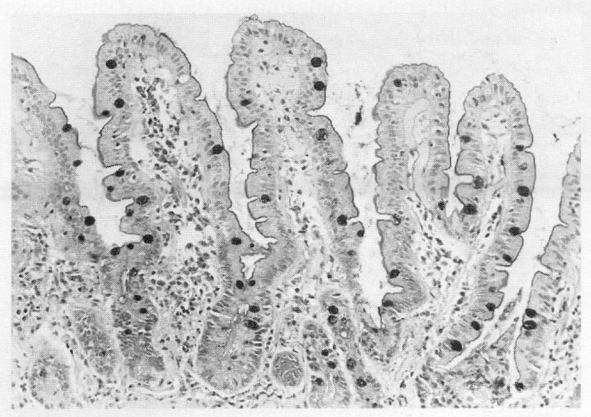

Fig. B Histological appearance of normal jejunal mucosa (PAS; magnification ×50).

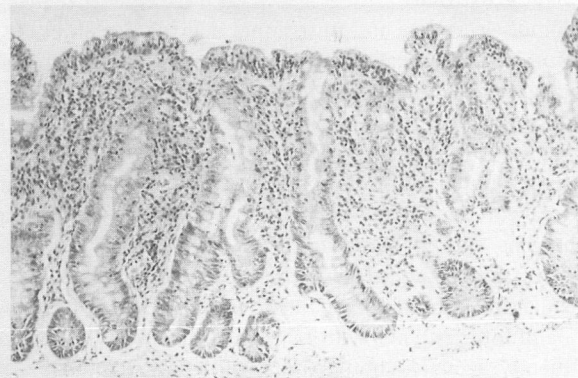

Fig. C Histological appearance of coeliac disease (H&E; magnification ×50) showing absent villi, elongated crypts and cellular infiltration.

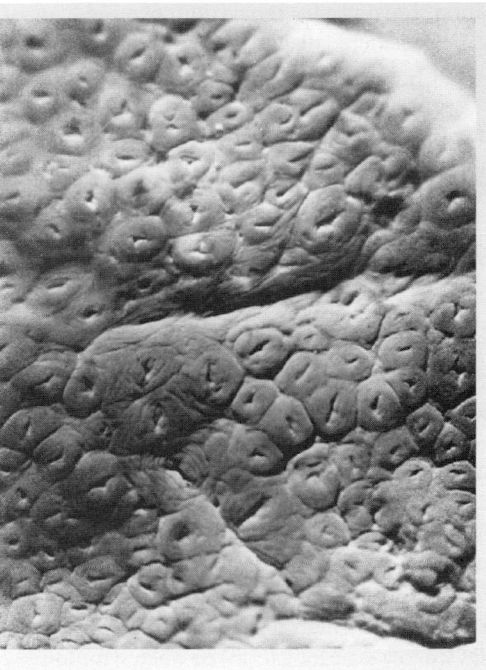

Fig. D Dissecting microscope appearance of untreated coeliac disease showing subtotal villous atrophy. All photographs reproduced from Misiewicz JJ, Pounder RE, Venables CW. *Diseases of the Gut and Pancreas*, 2nd edn, 1994 (Blackwell Scientific Publications, Oxford) with the permission of the authors.

10

Disease mechanisms

Small intestinal blind loops, fistulae, strictures, diverticula, abnormal motility, achlorhydria or hypogammaglobulinaemia all predispose to bacterial overgrowth. An excessive small bowel bacterial population:

- Deconjugates bile salts, causing steatorrhoea because micelle formation is defective, and diarrhoea because terminal ileal bile-salt absorption is reduced (presence of excess bile in the colon promotes water secretion; Fig. 10.7)
- Synthesizes folate, sometimes increasing serum folate
- Binds vitamin B_{12}, reducing serum vitamin B_{12}

Clinical features

Diarrhoea and/or steatorrhoea and macrocytic anaemia may be accompanied by other clinical or laboratory features of malabsorption (Table 10.18, p. 680) and a history of previous surgery or bowel disorder.

Investigation

Haematology

- *FBC:* commonly reveals a macrocytic anaemia
- *Serum vitamin B_{12}* is often low; *folate* is often high because bacteria synthesize it

Biochemistry

- *Serum calcium, phosphate and alkaline phosphatase:* may reveal biochemical osteomalacia (see p. 280)
- *Serum albumin:* may be low

Microbiology

Quantitative (anaerobic) bacteriology of a small bowel

aspiration showing a bacterial count of more than 10^6/ml would be considered diagnostic, but this test is not always available.

Diagnostic imaging
Barium study of the small bowel may show a blind loop, diverticula, fistula, stricture or reduced motility.

Other
- *Hydrogen (lactulose) breath test:* usually positive (Fig. 10.29)
- *Antibiotic test:* often the simplest test to see whether the steatorrhoea and/or diarrhoea resolves promptly on administration of an oral antibiotic (see below)

Management
Nutritional deficiencies should be rectified and, when feasible, the underlying cause should be corrected (e.g. a fistula or stricture should be surgically excised). Otherwise, antibiotics (e.g. tetracycline, amoxicillin, trimethoprim or metronidazole) are given as rotating courses (in low dose long term) or when symptoms recur. Non-specific antidiarrhoeal agents are often required (see p. 685).

Short bowel syndrome

Short bowel syndrome is malabsorption brought about by small intestinal resection. The type and severity of malabsorption is variable. In many patients, excessive fluid and electrolyte losses are the main problem (especially if the colon is not in continuity with the shortened small bowel). In others, protein or other major nutrient, or individual mineral and vitamin deficiencies may predominate.

Disease mechanisms
The most common indications for extensive small bowel resection are Crohn's disease, mesenteric vascular occlusion, trauma and neoplasia. Factors affecting symptomatology after intestinal resection include:
- *Extent of the resection:* removal of more than 50% of upper small bowel causes malabsorption
- *Site of resection:* terminal ileal resection causes vitamin B_{12} deficiency and bile salt-induced diarrhoea, steatorrhoea, gallstones and hyperoxaluria, while removal of the colon with small bowel causes severe diarrhoea because of loss of colonic absorptive capacity
- *Intestinal adaptation:* mucosal hyperplasia in the residual small bowel in response to stimuli such as local luminal factors (e.g. food, secretions) and hormones (e.g. enteroglucagon) results in a functional improvement over several months
- *Retention of the ileocaecal valve:* slows small bowel

transit and inhibits colonization of the distal small bowel by colonic flora
- *Disease of residual small bowel:* increases the risk of malabsorption (and of further resection)
- *Colonic function:* the ability of the colon to help regulate fluid and electrolyte losses means that patients can usually manage with only 1 m of bowel remaining if the colon is present and in continuity, but need at least 2 m if the shortened small bowel is discharging directly into a stoma.

Clinical features
Watery diarrhoea develops immediately after resection. It may then improve as the intestine adapts, or may progress to steatorrhoea as bile-salt deficiency develops.

Complications may occur later and include gallstones and urinary oxalate stones.

Investigation
Fluid, electrolyte and nutritional deficiencies, stool output, bile-salt malabsorption, vitamin B_{12} absorption and urinary oxalate excretion should be quantified.

Management
Intravenous restoration of fluid and electrolytes and total parenteral nutrition may be necessary at first. Enteral feeding should be started early to promote intestinal adaptation using lactose-free, iso-osmolar solutions. Later, small frequent meals are introduced, a low-fat diet being helpful for patients with marked steatorrhoea. Excessive dietary oxalate should be avoided as hyperoxaluria and renal oxalate stones can result. Specific nutritional deficiencies (calcium, magnesium, zinc, folate B_{12}, vitamins A, D and E) should be tested for and replaced as necessary.

Drugs that slow intestinal transit (e.g. loperamide, codeine phosphate) improve absorption and reduce stool output. Patients with more than 200 cm of small bowel remaining, and the colon in continuity, can usually be managed by oral fluids and feed alone. At the other end of the spectrum, patients with less than 100 cm of small bowel, and no colon in continuity, are very unlikely to manage without long-term intravenous nutrition and fluids.

Patients without a colon in continuity with the faecal stream are at great risk of dehydration and salt depletion. It is vital to avoid such patients trying to rehydrate themselves orally with water or hypotonic solutions. As the small bowel mucosa is relatively impermeable to water, drinking hypotonic liquids will cause sodium to be lost as it moves down the concentration gradient into the bowel lumen. Normally, the colon reabsorbs water and sodium; thus, without it, salt and water loss with subsequent dehydration and prerenal failure, are likely. If these patients are taking liquid by mouth, it should be as near iso-osmolar with tissue fluids as possible—the World Health Organization (WHO) formula is commonly used.

● *After ileal resection:* colestyramine binds bile salts and reduces diarrhoea, sometimes at the expense of worsening steatorrhoea. Vitamin B_{12} is replaced intramuscularly

● *After more extensive small gut resections:* treatment includes dietary calorie supplementation with medium-chain triglycerides, H_2 receptor antagonists to reduce the gastric hypersecretion that can follow major resections and inactivates pancreatic enzymes, and antibiotics if there is small bowel bacterial overgrowth

● *Patients with massive resections:* need to be referred to specialist centres. They may need regular parenteral supplements of calcium, magnesium, trace elements, essential fatty acids and vitamins, or even total parenteral nutrition organized for home administration (see p. 689). Small bowel transplantation offers a potential method for these patients to avoid lifelong parenteral nutrition. It has been undertaken in a small number of centres worldwide, but is not yet established clinical practice

Disaccharide malabsorption

Deficiency of intestinal mucosal disaccharidases can be either primary (congenital or acquired) or secondary to extensive mucosal pathology.

Disease mechanisms
Disaccharide malabsorption may result from lactase deficiency, sucrase isomaltase deficiency, or glucose–galactose malabsorption. The undigested sugars draw fluid osmotically into the intestinal lumen, and are degraded by colonic bacteria to hydrogen, carbon dioxide and short-chain fatty acids.

Epidemiology
Prevalence. Primary acquired alactasia is the most common disaccharidase deficiency worldwide.

Age. Rare congenital varieties present in childhood. In primary acquired alactasia, the enzyme disappears soon after weaning, but symptoms do not usually occur until the teenage years.

Race. Primary acquired alactasia is normal in over 70% of non-white people.

Genetics. Congenital varieties are autosomal recessive.

Clinical features
These are abdominal distension, pain and diarrhoea after consumption of the relevant sugar. In lactase deficiency the symptoms are worsened; for example, by drinking a pint of milk.

Investigation
Diagnosis can be confirmed by appropriate breath test (see p. 682).

Management
Treatment is avoidance of the offending sugar. In alactasia, restriction of cow's milk intake, its replacement by lactose-free preparations or its treatment before drinking with an exogenous lactase (Lactaid) are the therapeutic alternatives. Lactose-containing medication should be avoided.

Prognosis
Primary alactasia persists throughout life. The symptoms of the secondary variety gradually remit if the underlying cause (e.g. an acute infective enteritis) is itself reversible.

Meckel's diverticulum

Meckel's diverticulum is 5 cm long, and is situated about 0.6 m from the ileocaecal valve. It is a congenital anomaly.

Disease mechanisms and clinical features
Meckel's diverticulum is usually asymptomatic, but may present with bleeding from local ulceration because of acid secretion by ectopic gastric mucosa within it, Meckel's diverticulitis or intestinal obstruction caused by an associated band. Meckel's diverticulitis resembles appendicitis except in its localization to the left iliac fossa.

Epidemiology
Prevalence. In 2% of the population.

Sex. Male : female ratio is 2 : 1.

Investigation
● *Barium radiology:* sometimes reveals a Meckel's diverticulum
● *^{99}Tc pertechnetate scan:* the intravenously injected isotope is preferentially taken up by the ectopic gastric mucosa
● *Laparoscopy:* allows visualization and resection of the diverticulum

Management
Treatment is surgical (open or laparoscopic) if the diverticulum causes symptoms.

Small intestinal neoplasms

Small intestinal tumours are rare—most are lymphomas

10

or adenocarcinomas. There are some established risk factors that help with detection (see below). They are often asymptomatic, but may present with bleeding, intussusception, obstruction or perforation. Treatment is generally surgical.

Small intestinal lymphoma

Small intestinal lymphoma is a primary tumour of the small bowel arising as a result of malignant proliferation of either B or T cells.

Disease mechanisms
Coeliac disease is a risk factor for T-cell lymphoma.

Pathology
Macroscopically, the lymphomas can be annular, ulcerative, infiltrative or polypoid. They are sometimes multiple. Spread is to local lymph nodes and mesentery. Immunohistochemistry is used to identify whether the tumour is of B- or T-cell origin.

Epidemiology
This condition is rare and occurs mainly in people over 45 years of age.

Clinical features
Early symptoms include malaise, anorexia, vomiting, diarrhoea and weight loss. Later there is bleeding, obstruction or perforation. There may be a palpable mass.

Investigation
- *Barium follow-through meal:* shows non-specific ulceration, stricturing or mass lesions
- *Laparotomy:* usually required to establish the diagnosis and stage the tumour

Management
If possible, the lesion should be resected surgically. Chemotherapy and radiotherapy are alternative treatments.

Prognosis
The overall survival rate is poor (20% at 5 years).

Immunodeficiency syndromes
Primary immunodeficiency syndromes
Selective IgA deficiency affects 1 in 700 of the population and is the least rare of the primary immunodeficiency syndromes, which are listed in Table 10.31.

If possible, the primary deficiency is treated (e.g. immunoglobulin deficiency is treated with immunoglobulin injections). Identified gastrointestinal complications (e.g. giardiasis) also need treatment.

Table 10.31 Primary immunodeficiency disorders and their intestinal manifestations

Immune deficiency
B-cell defects
Selective IgA deficiency
Common variable acquired immunoglobulin deficiency
T-cell defects
DiGeorge's syndrome (congenital thymic hypoplasia)
Combined defects
Wiskott–Aldrich syndrome
Severe combined immunodeficiency

Secondary immunodeficiency syndromes
The most important secondary immunodeficiency syndrome affecting the bowel is now **AIDS** (see p. 170). Its multiple gastrointestinal effects include:
- *Candida*, cytomegalovirus and herpes simplex infection of the oropharynx and oesophagus
- *Cryptosporidia, Giardia, Entamoeba histolytica, Isospora, Microsporidia, Mycobacterium* (*avium-intracellulare* and *tuberculosis*), *Campylobacter, Salmonella, Shigella* spp. and cytomegalovirus infections of the small and large intestines
- *Cryptosporidia, Giardia, Entamoeba histolytica*, gonorrhoea, syphilis, *Chlamydia*, cytomegalovirus and herpes simplex infections of the anus and rectum
- Kaposi's sarcoma and non-Hodgkin's lymphoma throughout the bowel

Food allergy

Adverse reactions to food are listed in Table 10.32. Only about 20% of patients who present with food-induced symptoms have true food intolerance, which can be confirmed by double-blind challenge. For 10% of these the mechanism is immunological.

Two main types of immunological reaction occur: type I immediate hypersensitivity reactions; and type II delayed hypersensitivity reactions.

Type I immediate hypersensitivity reactions
Within a few minutes or hours, small quantities of antigen (e.g. shellfish or nut) produce a variety of gastrointestinal symptoms (e.g. swelling of the lips, vomiting, diarrhoea, abdominal pain) and remote effects (e.g. rhinorrhoea, urticaria, angioedema, migraine, asthma, eczema, anaphylaxis).

People with this type of food allergy have elevated serum IgE and positive radioallergosorbent (RAST) and skin-prick tests.

Table 10.32 Classification of adverse reactions to food

Pharmacological
Tyramine in cheese and wine, caffeine in coffee, histamine in mackerel

Toxic
Glutamates in Chinese food, acetanilide in rapeseed oil

Irritant
Alcohol, very hot or cold drinks, curry

Enzyme deficiencies
Alactasia

Immunological
Allergy

Psychiatric/psychological
Many 'allergic' patients, anorexia nervosa, bulimia

The treatment is avoidance of the incriminated food. Rarely, corticosteroids, adrenaline and/or antihistamines are required.

Type II delayed hypersensitivity reactions

Cow's milk protein allergy in young children causes vomiting, diarrhoea, proctocolitis, failure to thrive, eczema, asthma and, possibly, irritability. Allergy to egg, chicken, rice and soya proteins produces similar symptoms. In adults, the foods and their allergic consequences are less clear-cut, and are likely to explain only a tiny minority of cases of irritable bowel syndrome or migraine.

There are no simple confirmatory tests. The only way to investigate is by instituting tedious and expensive exclusion diets with rechallenge. Treatment is avoidance of implicated foods. Some patients gain relief from oral disodium cromoglycate. There is no place for desensitization.

Diseases of the large intestine

Colonic diverticulosis

Colonic diverticulosis is an acquired disease with mucosal and submucosal protrusions through the bowel wall at points of weakness where blood vessels enter (Fig. 10.41). Like gallstones, this gastrointestinal disease is extremely common, but usually asymptomatic and coincidental to the patient's symptoms.

Disease mechanisms

There is an inverse correlation between the prevalence of diverticulosis and dietary fibre intake. Low fibre consumption may predispose to mucosal herniation through the colonic wall by causing high intracolonic segmental pressures.

Diverticulosis in the UK usually affects the sigmoid

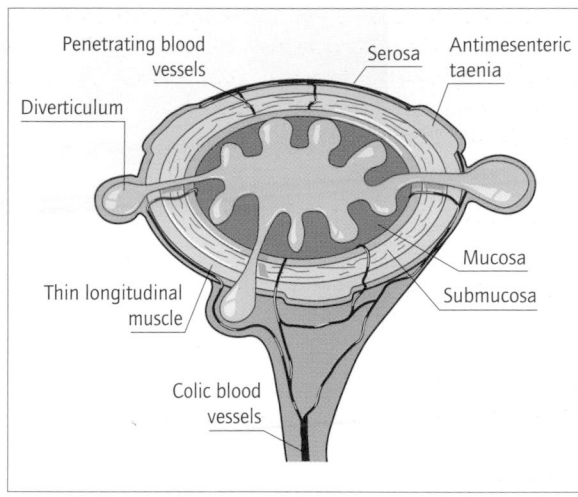

Figure 10.41 Colonic diverticula. Diagram showing the appearance of colonic diverticula. Note protrusion of the diverticula close to the blood vessels.

colon, but in Africa and Japan it is usually right-sided. Macroscopically, diverticula and thickening of the sigmoid circular muscle are seen.

Diverticulitis causes local inflammatory changes that are sometimes associated with perforation, abscess formation, obstruction, peritonitis, bleeding and/or fistulae to the small bowel, bladder or vagina.

Epidemiology

Prevalence. Increases with age, affecting about 50% of 70-year-olds in the West.

Sex. Women are affected more frequently than men.

Geography. Rare in Africa.

Clinical features

Most people with diverticulosis are asymptomatic, but some have symptoms resembling the irritable bowel syndrome, perhaps because of abnormal segmental contractions. In severe cases there may be stricturing of the colon, which may cause colicky abdominal pain and altered bowel habit.

Occasionally, patients present with profuse rectal bleeding. Diverticulitis causing left iliac fossa pain, fever and a tender mass is more common, and may be accompanied by clinical features of any of the complications listed above.

Investigation
Haematology
FBC. There may be a neutrophil leucocytosis in acute diverticulitis.

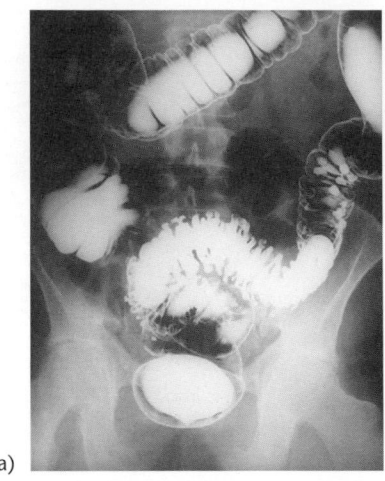
(a)

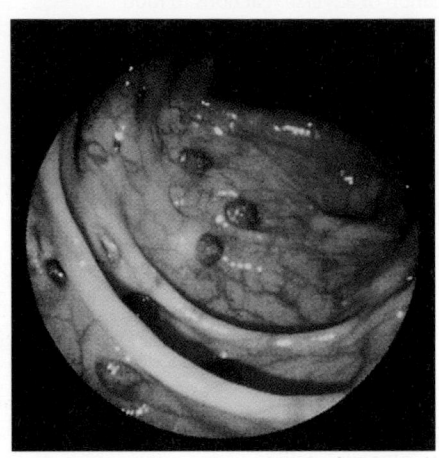
(b)

Figure 10.42 Colonic diverticulosis. (a) Barium enema showing multiple diverticula throughout the colon. (b) Colonoscopic view showing multiple diverticula in sigmoid colon. (Reproduced from *Slide Atlas of Gastrointestinal Endoscopy* with the kind permission of the author and Times Mirror International Publishers.)

Table 10.33 Classification of colonic polyps

	Associated disorder	**Malignant potential**
Neoplastic		
Adenoma (tubular, tubulovillous, villous)	Usually none, sometimes as in Table 10.34	High (especially if larger than 1 cm, villous, multiple)
Non-neoplastic		
Metaplastic	Nil	
Inflammatory	Inflammatory bowel disease	Nil*
Hamartomas	Juvenile polyps	Low
	Peutz–Jeghers syndrome	Low

*The inflammatory polyps themselves are not premalignant, but the underlying colitis is (see Table 10.35).

Diagnostic imaging

● *Barium enema:* the easiest way to visualize diverticula (Fig. 10.42a). However, when diverticular disease is severe, it can be impossible for the radiologist to exclude small polyps in the affected segment

● *Colonoscopy* (Fig. 10.42b): can be awkward and dangerous because of spasm and distortion, but is necessary in patients with rectal bleeding, where stricturing is seen on the barium, or where the exclusion value for coexistent cancer or polyps on a barium study is low because of the severity of the diverticular disease

Management

Asymptomatic diverticulosis. This requires no treatment. Pain and/or variable bowel habit usually respond to a high-fibre diet with additional bulking agents (e.g. ispaghula husk) and antispasmodics (mebeverine, cyclomine) if necessary.

Acute diverticulitis. This is treated with fluids and antibiotics.

Surgical resection. This may be necessary for refractory cases and those with complications such as fistula.

Colonic tumours

Colorectal tumours comprise both polyps, themselves of various different types (Table 10.33), and adenocarcinomas.

Colonic polyps

A colonic polyp is a tumour that projects into the colonic lumen and is of variable clinical significance. One third are non-neoplastic and two-thirds are neoplastic. The different types of polyp are shown in Table 10.33. The most common non-neoplastic type is metaplastic—they are usually multiple, small (less than 5 mm) and in the

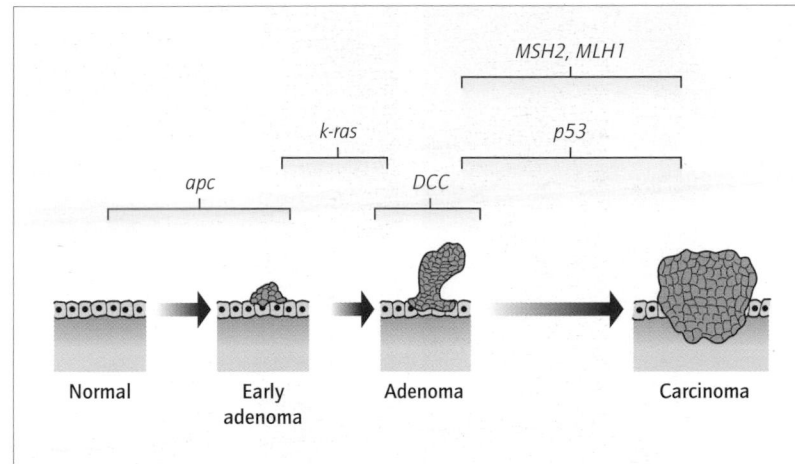

Figure 10.43 The adenoma–carcinoma sequence for colonic neoplasia, showing the points at which associated gene mutations occur (see text for explanation).

Table 10.34 Multiple adenomatous polyposis syndromes (all are premalignant)

Syndrome	Associated clinical features
Familial polyposis coli	Polyps in stomach and small bowel
Gardner's syndrome	Osteomas, epdermoid cysts, soft tissue tumours, congenital hypertrophy of retinal pigment epithelium
Turcot's syndrome	Glioblastomas or medulloblastoma

Table 10.35 Risk factors for colorectal carcinoma (the factors in capital letters warrant colonoscopic screening; see below)

Predisposing disorders
ADENOMATOUS POLYPS
FAMILIAL POLYPOSIS COLI
PREVIOUS COLORECTAL CANCER
EXTENSIVE ULCERATIVE COLITIS
EXTENSIVE CROHN'S COLITIS

Genetics
FIRST-DEGREE RELATIVES
HNPCC*

Diet
Excess animal fat and refined carbohydrate
Low fruit, vegetable, calcium and vitamin D intake

*See p. 731.

rectum. The most common neoplastic polyps are adenomatous: their importance lies in their tendency to transform into invasive adenocarcinoma (Fig. 10.43).

Adenomas
Disease mechanisms
Adenomas may be single, multiple or part of a polyposis syndrome (Tables 10.33 and 10.34). Possible aetiological factors are shown in Table 10.35. The risk of malignant transformation in individual polyps is increased by size (1% if less than 1 cm, 50% if larger than 2 cm), by villous rather than tubular histological type and by the presence of severe dysplasia.

Epidemiology
Adenomas are common, affecting 30–40% of the population in developed countries over 60 years of age.

Clinical features
Most polyps are asymptomatic and are found incidentally at colonoscopy when patients are investigated for change in bowel habit, abdominal pain or bleeding piles. Some bleed or intussuscept. Villous adenomas may present with profuse loss into the lumen of clear mucus with secondary hypokalaemia and protein-losing enteropathy. Too often, polyps present after malignant transformation.

External examination is usually negative.

Investigation
Colonoscopy is preferred to barium enema, particularly if there is rectal bleeding, because it is more sensitive and allows for definitive treatment by polypectomy.

Management
Treatment is colonoscopic polypectomy. Very large or sessile polyps may require formal surgical removal. Thereafter, surveillance for recurrences using total colonoscopy is required every 3–5 years.

Familial polyposis coli (familial adenomatous polyposis)
Disease mechanisms
One hundred to 5000 polyps appear in the colon in the

10

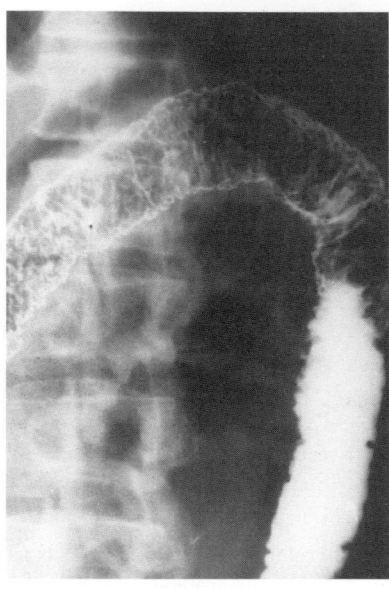
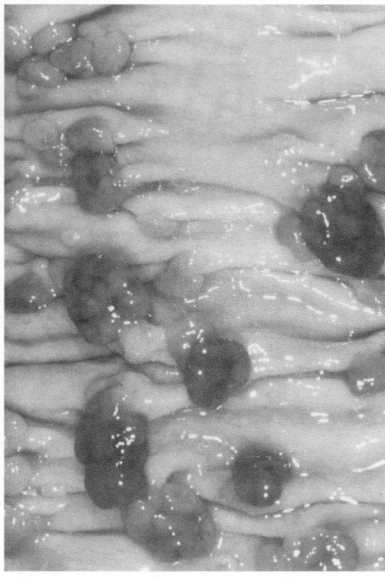

(a)   (b)

Figure 10.44 Familial polyposis coli. (a) Barium enema showing multiple very small adenomatous polyps. (b) Colonic resection specimen showing multiple small adenomatous polyps. Both reproduced from Misiewicz JJ, Pounder RE, Venables CW. *Diseases of the Gut and Pancreas*, 2nd edn. Oxford: Blackwell Scientific Publications, 1994 with the permission of the authors.

second decade (Fig. 10.44). They may also occur in the stomach and small bowel. Colonic cancer, which is often multiple, develops at an average age of 40 years.

Epidemiology
Prevalence. Rare.

Age. Usually presents in early adulthood.

Genetics. Autosomal dominant familial disorder. The gene responsible (the *APC* gene) has been localized to chromosome 5 and has been cloned.

Clinical features
Patients may present with rectal bleeding or overt cancer, or be detected by a family screening programme (see below). Associated manifestations may include sebaceous cysts, mandibular osteomas, desmoids and pigmented hypertrophic lesions of the retina (congenital hypertrophy of retinal pigment epithelium): these features constitute Gardner's syndrome.

Investigation
● *Colonoscopy and biopsy:* confirm the diagnosis
● *OGD:* necessary to look for and remove upper gastrointestinal polyps

Management
Early colectomy is required to prevent the development of carcinoma. Colonoscopic screening of family members from their teens onwards is mandatory; methods involving genetic analysis will soon be available.

Other polyposis syndromes
Features of other polyposis syndromes are given in Table 10.34.

Colorectal carcinoma

Colorectal carcinoma is a malignant tumour—usually an adenocarcinoma—of the large intestine.

Disease mechanisms
Prevalence. There are wide geographical variations in incidence, ranging from less than 10 in 100 000 in Nigeria, through 40 in 100 000 in the UK to 60 in 100 000 in New Zealand. In the West, colorectal carcinoma is one of the most common cancers, with a lifetime risk of 1 in 20.

Age. Most common in people over 60 years of age.

Environmental and other risk factors. The major risk factors for colorectal carcinoma are listed in Table 10.35.

GENETICS
● *Sporadic colorectal carcinoma:* most colorectal carcinomas result from a stepwise progression from normal mucosa through adenomatous polyps to carcinoma. This progression is associated with serial mutations in several growth regulating genes (Fig. 10.43). These cause activation of proto-oncogenes such as k-*ras* and c-*myc* oncogene and, conversely, inactivation of tumour suppressor genes such as the *p53* gene, the *DCC* gene (gene deleted in colorectal cancer) and the *apc* gene (responsible for familial polyposis coli; see above)

Table 10.36 Staging and prognosis of colorectal carcinoma: the TNM (Tumour, Nodes, Metastases) classification has largely superseded Dukes'

TNM classification	Modified Dukes' staging	5-year survival (%)
Stage 0: carcinoma *in situ*		
Stage I: no nodes or metastases, tumour invades submucosa (T1, N0, M0); tumour invades muscularis propria (T2, N0, M0)	A	90
Stage II: no nodes or metastases (T3, N0, M0); tumour invades other organs (T4, N0, M0)	B	80
Stage III: regional lymph nodes involved (any T, N1, M0)	C	30
Stage IV: distant metastases	D	<5

- *Cancer family syndromes:* there is a slightly increased risk of developing colorectal carcinoma if one first-degree relative is affected, but this increases substantially with the number of relatives affected. A particularly high risk occurs in patients with hereditary non-polyposis colon cancer syndrome (HNPCC), which accounts for approximately 5% of all colorectal carcinoma
- *Hereditary non-polyposis colon cancer syndrome:* this is an autosomal dominant syndrome giving affected patients a lifetime risk for colorectal carcinoma (usually right-sided) of 80%; these usually occur before the age of 50, making early screening essential (see below). Affected patients are also at risk of other cancers, including endometrial, ovarian, upper gastrointestinal, pancreatic, biliary, genitourinary and cerebral. HNPCC is almost always caused by a mutation affecting one of the two DNA mismatch repair genes, *MSH2* and *MLH1*; these lead to widespread microsatellite instability

Pathology

Macroscopically, the tumour may be ulcerating, polypoid or annular; 60% occur in the rectosigmoid area and 25% in the right colon. Spread is to local lymph nodes, into the peritoneal cavity and via the portal vein to the liver and beyond. Microscopically, most tumours are adenocarcinomas. Adenomatous polyps (see p. 729) and epithelial dysplasia are often found elsewhere in the colon. Staging of resected tumour determines the prognosis (Table 10.36).

Clinical features

Patients with right colon cancers typically present with an iron-deficiency anaemia caused by occult bleeding. Those with left-sided and rectal tumours present with a change in bowel habit, obstruction and overt rectal bleeding. There is weight loss in advanced disease. Dyspepsia may be a feature of lesions of the transverse colon. Occasionally, patients present late with perforation, hepatic metastases and ascites.

Examination may reveal anaemia, cachexia and an abdominal mass, or nothing. Rectal examination is essential to check for low rectal tumours.

Differential diagnosis

Differential diagnosis of colorectal carcinoma depends on the clinical presentation:
- *Other causes of an abdominal mass:* include an appendix abscess, a diverticular inflammatory mass, Crohn's disease, other neoplasms (of the stomach, pancreas, omentum, kidney, lymphoma, etc.), an ovarian cyst, torsion, tumour or uterine fibroid
- *Other causes of abdominal pain:* listed in Tables 10.7 and 10.8 (pp. 661–2)
- *Other causes of constipation and diarrhoea:* listed in Tables 10.12 and 10.15 (pp. 664 and 666)
- *Other causes of obstruction:* include adhesions, hernia, volvulus, intussusception, Crohn's disease, small intestinal neoplasm, faecal impaction and pseudo-obstruction
- *Other causes of rectal bleeding:* listed in Table 10.30 (p. 719)

Investigation

Haematology

FBC. There may be a microcytic anaemia.

Biochemistry

Liver function tests may be abnormal if there are hepatic metastases.

Diagnostic imaging

- *Sigmoidoscopy with barium enema and/or colonoscopy:* the key tests, with biopsy of any lesions seen
- *Chest radiography, ultrasound and/or CT scanning:* to look for metastases

Histopathology

Biopsy to confirm the diagnosis.

Management

Established colorectal carcinoma. Potentially curable lesions

10

Colorectal carcinoma at a glance

Risk factors

These include:

- Adenomatous polyps
- First-degree relatives
- Hereditary non-polyposis coli
- Familial polyposis coli
- Extensive ulcerative or Crohn's colitis for more than 10 years

Most colorectal cancers develop from sporadic adenomatous polyps, but a minority occur in association with genetic disorders such as familial adenomatous polyposis

Investigation

Haematology

- *FBC:* iron-deficiency anaemia
- *Faecal occult blood:* positive
- *Liver function tests:* abnormal if hepatic metastases present

Diagnostic imaging

- *Colonoscopy, sigmoidoscopy or barium enema:* 'apple-core' stricture
- *Ultrasound/CT scan:* evaluation of spread prior to surgery

Histopathology

Biopsy: adenocarcinoma

Management

Older people presenting with rectal bleeding should have colonoscopy performed promptly to exclude colorectal cancer

Therapy of established colorectal cancer is primarily surgical, but adjuvant radiotherapy and chemotherapy have an increasingly important role

The value of preventive screening programmes, including faecal occult blood tests, flexible sigmoidoscopy and colonoscopy, is under intense evaluation

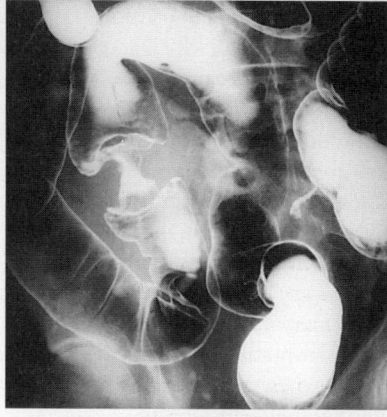

Fig. A Barium enema showing annular colonic carcinoma in the sigmoid colon. Note the shouldered margin giving the characteristic 'apple-core' appearance. Reproduced from *Slide Atlas of Gastroenterology* with the kind permission of the author and Times Mirror International Publishers.

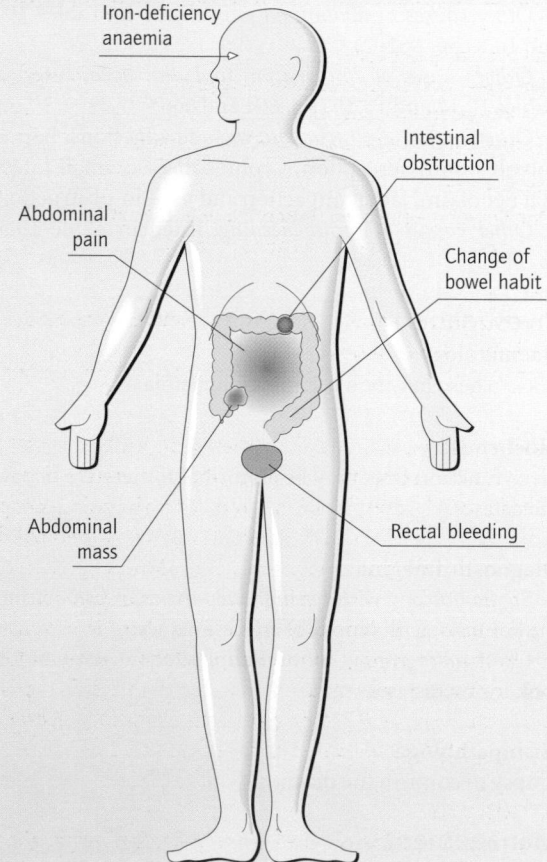

Iron-deficiency anaemia

Intestinal obstruction

Abdominal pain

Change of bowel habit

Abdominal mass

Rectal bleeding

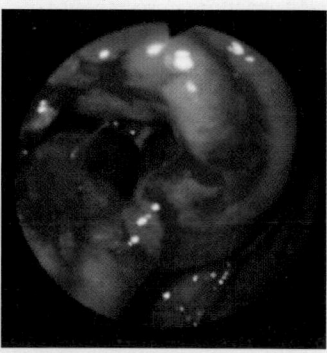

Fig. B Colonoscopic view of caecum showing annular ulcerated bleeding carcinoma.

Supportive treatment
Explanation
Terminal care when necessary

Specific treatment
- *Surgery:* resection for potentially curable lesions; resection of both a solitary hepatic metastasis and the primary; pan-procto- or total colectomy for multiple polyposis or chronic extensive ulcerative colitis
- *Drugs and radiotherapy:* palliative and adjuvant radiotherapy and chemotherapy (5-fluorouracil, levamisole)
- *Endoscopy:* colonoscopic stenting, laser therapy or electrocoagulation for obstructive symptoms or bleeding in the frail

Prevention
Endoscopy: colonoscopic screening for predisposing disorders (Table 10.37)

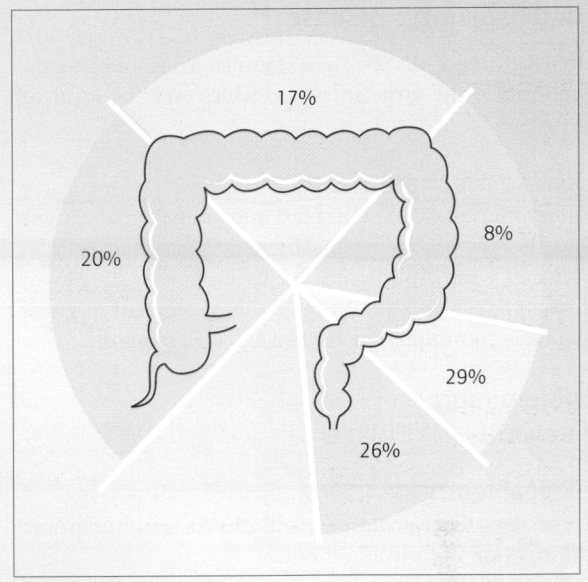

Fig. C Distribution of colorectal cancer.

are resected. A temporary defunctioning colostomy may be necessary for patients presenting with obstruction. Occasionally, prolonged survival can be achieved by resection of both a solitary hepatic metastasis and the primary. Palliative and adjuvant radiotherapy and chemotherapy are often used. Obstructive symptoms or bleeding in people who are very frail can be relieved by colonoscopic stenting, laser therapy and/or electrocoagulation.

Prevention
Lifestyle measures. Knowledge of the environmental risk factors for colorectal carcinoma (Table 10.35, p. 729) means that individuals may be able to reduce their chances of getting the disease by eating more fruit, vegetables and calcium and less animal fat; taking more exercise may also help. They should see their doctor promptly in the event of an unexplained change in bowel habit or rectal bleeding, with a view to early investigation by flexible sigmoidoscopy or colonoscopy (see above).

Population screening programmes. Population screening techniques include annual faecal occult blood testing, leading to colonoscopy if positive; or once-only flexible sigmoidoscopy at age 55. These programmes have been shown to increase detection and survival of colorectal carcinoma. As yet, however, they have not been widely introduced for patients at low risk of colorectal carcinoma (Table 10.37). Screening based on detecting genetic abnormalities will probably be possible within the next 10 years.

Table 10.37 Colorectal cancer (CRC): who should be screened?

High risk
Familial polyposis coli
Hereditary non-polyposis colon cancer
Previous adenomatous polyps
Chronic extensive ulcerative or Crohn's colitis

Medium risk
One first-degree relative presenting with CRC at age < 45
Two or more first-degree relatives with CRC

Low risk
One first-degree relative with CRC presenting at age > 55
No family history of CRC

Patients at increased risk. Patients at medium risk of colorectal carcinoma because of their family history (Table 10.37) should be offered 5-yearly colonoscopy, starting 5 years before the youngest relative developed the disease. More regular (e.g. 2-yearly) colonoscopic screening is advised for those at high risk; for example, previous adenomatous polyps, HNPCC and chronic extensive ulcerative or Crohn's colitis. Panproctocolectomy or total colectomy is performed for patients with familial polyposis coli (see p. 729) or total long-standing ulcerative colitis complicated by dysplasia (see p. 734).

Prognosis
The spread and histological grading determine prognosis (Table 10.36).

Hirschsprung's disease

Hirschsprung's disease is a familial congenital aganglionosis of the large intestine, which may be local or diffuse.

Disease mechanisms

Embryonic failure of neuroblast migration from the vagus into the gut results in an absence of ganglion cells in Meissner's and Auerbach's plexuses and hypertrophy of the nerve trunks. Usually, only a short segment of gut is involved, commonly the rectum and lower sigmoid.

Epidemiology

Rare: about 1 in 5000 births.

Clinical features

These vary from acute neonatal obstruction to chronic constipation in early adulthood.

Investigation

- *Barium enema:* may show dilatation above the narrowed segment
- *Full-thickness biopsy:* shows aganglionosis and hypertrophied nerve trunks
- *Acetylcholinesterase:* increased in the nerve fibres histo- and biochemically
- *Anorectal manometry:* shows an absent rectosphincteric inhibitory reflex

Management

Varies with age and the length of the involved segment. Usually, a decompressing colostomy is followed at a later date by resection of the aganglionic segment.

Miscellaneous disorders of the small and large intestine

Inflammatory bowel disease

Ulcerative colitis (UC) and Crohn's disease (CD) are idiopathic chronic inflammatory diseases of the gastrointestinal tract (KEYPOINTS BOX 10.4). They have much in common and may be at opposite ends of a single spectrum, but their differences make it convenient to describe them separately.

Ulcerative colitis

Disease mechanisms

The primary cause of UC remains unknown. It may result from an abnormally prolonged inflammatory host response, determined by genetic and/or environmental

---

Keypoints 10.4: Inflammatory bowel disease

Inflammatory bowel disease comprises ulcerative colitis and Crohn's disease; two related chronic inflammatory diseases with peak onset at 20–40 years of age

Inflammatory bowel disease appears to be caused by abnormal stimulation of the gut mucosal immune response by luminal bacterial flora in genetically predisposed individuals

Patients present with abdominal pain, malaise, weight loss and diarrhoea that is often bloody; the course is characterized by relapses and remissions

The main treatments of active disease are corticosteroids, aminosalicylates and, in refractory disease, azathioprine

Aminosalicylates and azathioprine are also used to maintain remission

Patients not responding to medical treatment require surgical resection of involved bowel

---

factors, to bacteria or dietary products in the bowel lumen.

Postulated (but unproven) aetiological factors include:

- Infection
- Psychosocial factors
- Immunological abnormalities
- Defective mucus
- Not smoking cigarettes

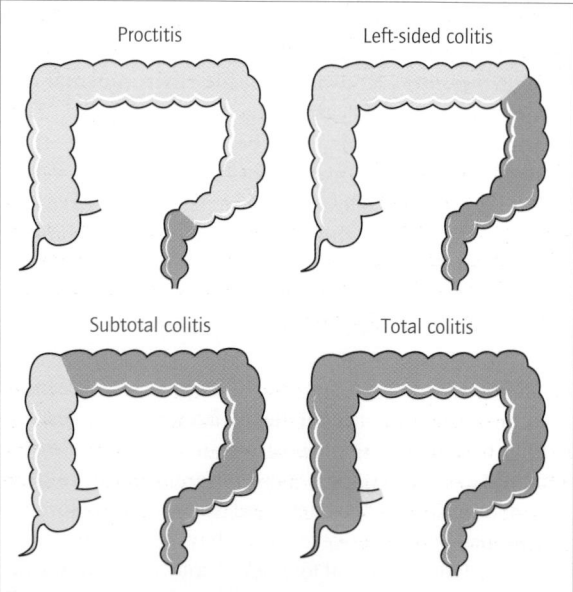

Figure 10.45 Distribution of large intestinal involvement in ulcerative colitis.

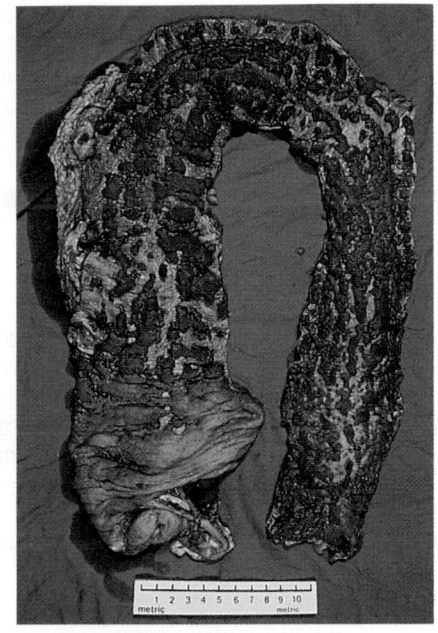

(a)

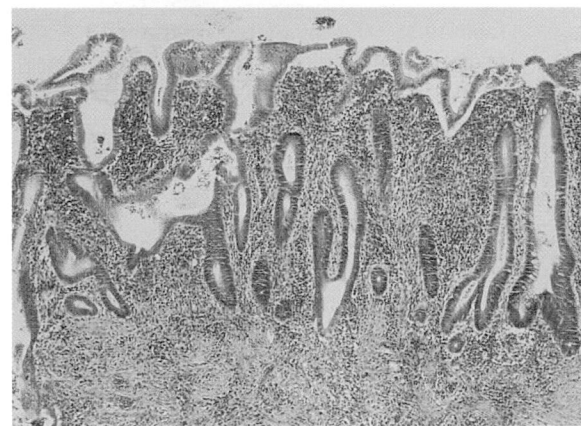

(b)

Figure 10.46 (a) Colonic resection specimen from a patient with ulcerative colitis (UC). Note subtotal involvement with areas of ulceration and pseudopolyps. (b) Histopathology of UC showing epithelial cell loss, inflammatory cell infiltrate in the lamina propria, separation and distortion of crypt architecture, and goblet cell depletion.

Whatever the primary stimulus, activated mucosal leucocytes produce an excess of pro-inflammatory cytokines (e.g. interleukin-1 and tumour necrosis factor alpha; TNF-α) and soluble mediators (eicosanoids, reactive oxygen metabolites), which amplify and perpetuate the inflammatory response.

Pathology

The disease usually begins in the rectum, and either remains there or spreads proximally (Fig. 10.45). There

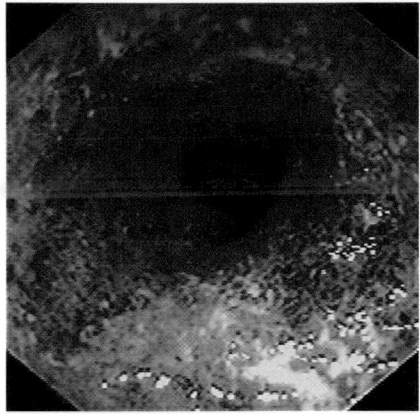

Figure 10.47 Colonoscopic view of moderately severe UC, showing diffuse mucosal bleeding, oedema, granularity and ulceration.

is diffuse inflammation of affected mucosa with hyperaemia, granularity, and surface pus and blood, leading in severe cases to extensive ulceration (ULCERATIVE COLITIS AT A GLANCE). The pathological appearance of UC is shown in Figs 10.46(a) and 10.47. This heals by granulation to form multiple pseudopolyps.

Microscopically, acute and chronic inflammatory cells infiltrate the lamina propria and crypts (crypt abscesses), and goblet cells lose their mucus (goblet cell depletion; Fig. 10.46b). There is epithelial ulceration. Biopsies from people with long-standing total colitis may show dysplastic changes in which epithelial cell nuclei are enlarged and crowded and lose their polarity; frank carcinoma may supervene.

10

Epidemiology

Prevalence. Appears to be more common in developed countries, where the prevalence is approximately 70 in 100 000, and incidence is about 5/100 000/year, than in Africa and Asia.

Age. Incidence shows a bimodal age distribution, with a major peak at 20–40 years of age, and a lesser peak at 60–80 years of age.

Sex. More common in women.

Race. Most common in white people, particularly Jews.

Genetics. There is an increased incidence of about 10% of either UC or CD in first-degree relatives, but no simple Mendelian inheritance or clear HLA association. About 66% of HLA B27 positive individuals with UC have associated ankylosing spondylitis, compared with only 5% of

HLA B27 people without UC. There appear to be susceptibility loci on chromosomes 2 and 6.

Clinical features

The onset of UC is usually gradual, and its severity varies with activity and extent of disease. The natural history is chronic, with relapses and remissions over many years. Between attacks, there are usually no symptoms.

Emotional stress, intercurrent infection, acute gastroenteritis, treatment with drugs such as antibiotics and NSAIDs, and discontinuation of prophylactic treatment (see below) may all precede a relapse.

Features of active UC depend on the extent of the disease:

- *Proctitis:* causes rectal bleeding and a mucous discharge. Sometimes there is tenesmus and pruritus ani. The stool is usually well formed. Well-being is maintained and external examination is normal
- *Proctosigmoiditis:* causes rectal bleeding and mucus discharge accompanied by diarrhoea, urgency and sometimes abdominal pain. There may be malaise, but examination is usually normal
- *Extensive colitis:* causes profuse frequent diarrhoea with blood and mucus, fever, malaise, anorexia and weight loss, sometimes with extraintestinal manifestations. On examination, the patient is thin, anaemic, fluid-depleted and febrile, and has a tachycardia.

Local complications

Complications may be local or systemic. Local complications include the following:

- *Toxic megacolon:* occurs rarely in fulminating colitis. The patient deteriorates with tachycardia, fever and pain, and there is increasing abdominal distension, tenderness and loss of bowel sounds. The diagnosis is confirmed on plain abdominal radiography
- *Colonic perforation:* may occur in very active UC with or without preceding toxic megacolon. Corticosteroids can mask the signs of the resultant peritonitis (see p. 668).
- *Haemorrhage:* massive haemorrhage necessitating urgent colectomy is very rare. Iron deficiency because of chronic minor blood loss is common
- *Carcinoma:* there is an increased incidence of colonic carcinoma in patients who have had extensive disease for more than 10 years. The cumulative risk is about 20% at 30 years. Other risk factors are onset in childhood and continuous activity

Systemic complications

Systemic complications are many and varied and are summarized in ULCERATIVE COLITIS AT A GLANCE.

Differential diagnosis

Differential diagnosis of bloody diarrhoea in association with inflamed rectal mucosa on sigmoidoscopy is listed in Table 10.38.

Investigation

Haematology

- *FBC:* anaemia with a raised white cell count is common
- *ESR and CRP:* often increased

Table 10.38 Differential diagnosis of bloody diarrhoea in association with inflamed rectal mucosa on sigmoidoscopy (common causes given in capital letters)

Inflammation
ULCERATIVE COLITIS
CROHN'S DISEASE
Behçet's disease
Infection
CAMPYLOBACTER
SALMONELLA
Cl. difficile
Shigella
Escherichia coli 0157:H7
Iatrogenic
Irradiation
Drugs (NSAIDs)

Ulcerative colitis at a glance

Epidemiology
Prevalence
70 in 100 000

Age
Peak is 20–40 years of age

Sex
Slightly more common in women

Race
Most common in white people, particularly Jews

Genetics
Increased prevalence (10%) in first-degree relatives. Susceptibility loci on chromosomes 2 and 6

Geography
Developed countries

Cause
Unknown. Abnormal mucosal immune response to luminal flora in genetically predisposed people

Investigation
Haematology
- *FBC:* iron-deficiency anaemia
- *ESR:* increased
- *Albumin:* low

Microbiology
- *Stool microscopy:* white and red blood cells
- *Stool culture:* negative

Imaging
- *Plain abdominal radiography:* may show mucosal oedema, toxic megacolon
- *Sigmoidoscopy/colonoscopy:* oedema, hyperaemia, ulceration, bleeding, pseudopolyps
- *Radiolabelled leucocyte scan:* positive colonic uptake

Histopathology
- *Biopsy*: epithelial ulceration, acute and chronic inflammatory cell infiltration in lamina propria, crypt abscesses, goblet cell depletion. Beware dysplasia; it is precancerous

Management
Supportive treatment
Explanation
Nutritional support
Long-term specialist follow-up
Patient support groups (e.g. National Association for Colitis and Crohn's Disease)

Specific treatment
Modify according to the clinical presentation (Table 10.39)
Drugs (Table 10.40)
- *Corticosteroids:* to induce remission
- *Aminosalicylates:* to maintain remission
- *Azathioprine:* to maintain remission in refractory disease

Surgery
Panproctocolectomy with ileoanal pouch
Panproctocolectomy with ileostomy
Colectomy with ileorectal anastomosis

Preventive treatment
Endoscopy: surveillance colonoscopy to prevent cancer in patients with chronic extensive ulcerative colitis

Eyes:
- Episcleritis
- Uveitis

General:
- Weight loss
- Malaise
- Growth retardation in children

Liver and biliary tree:
- Fatty change
- Sclerosing cholangitis
- Bile duct carcinoma

Blood:
- Arterial and venous thrombosis

Gut:
- Diarrhoea
- Rectal bleeding and pus
- Tenesmus

Joints:
- Arthropathy (asymmetrical, large joints)
- Sacroiliitis
- Ankylosing spondylitis

Skin:
- Erythema nodosum
- Pyoderma gangrenosum

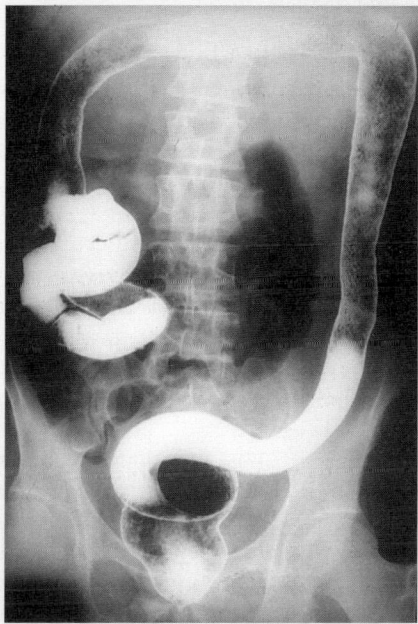

Fig. A Barium enema showing subtotal disease. Note the superficial ulceration and loss of haustrations extending from the rectum to the hepatic flexure. Reproduced from *Slide Atlas of Gastroenterology* with the kind permission of the author and Times Mirror International Publishers.

Table 10.39 Treatment of ulcerative colitis

Clinical features	Treatment
Proctitis	*Supportive.* Treat proximal constipation with a high-fibre diet and/or lactulose *Specific.* Aminosalicylate orally or rectally (enemas or suppositories) and rectal corticosteroid

More extensive colitis:
  mild–moderate attack
  —well with less than
  six stools daily
	Supportive. Haematinics (iron, folate) if necessary
	Specific. Aminosalicylate and prednisolone 40 mg orally and corticosteroid enemas daily, as outpatient. Prednisolone is tailed off as remission is achieved. Aminosalicylate is continued indefinitely

More extensive colitis:
  severe—ill with more
  than six bloody
  diarrhoeal stools daily
	Supportive. Hospital admission, close observation by physician and surgeon, intravenous fluids and electrolytes, blood transfusion, prophylactic subcutaneous heparin
	Specific. Methylprednisolone or hydrocortisone intravenously, oral aminosalicylate. Surgery or intravenous ciclosporin if no response in 5–7 days

Toxic megacolon	*Supportive.* Intravenous fluids, nasogastric suction, antibiotics *Specific.* Medical treatment as for severe UC. If no improvement in 12–24 h, colectomy
Colonic perforation	*Supportive.* Antibiotics, intravenous fluids *Specific.* Immediate colectomy and peritoneal toilet
Massive haemorrhage	*Supportive.* Blood transfusion *Specific.* Urgent colectomy sometimes necessary
Extensive UC for >10 years (to prevent carcinoma)	Surveillance colonoscopy every 1–2 years with multiple biopsies and colectomy if histology shows persistent dysplasia

Biochemistry

Serum albumin is often low.

Microbiology

● *Stool microscopy:* shows white and red blood cells
● *Stool culture:* necessary to exclude infective diarrhoea (Table 10.38)

Diagnostic imaging

● *Sigmoidoscopy:* shows inflamed rectal mucosa (Fig. 10.47)
● *Plain abdominal radiography:* may reveal the extent of disease by the distribution of gas and faeces. In proctitis, there may be proximal faecal loading. In acute total UC, colonic dilatation (Fig. 10.20), mucosal oedema (islands) and submucosal and intraperitoneal gas should be sought
● *Colonoscopy* (Fig. 10.47): indications for colonoscopy are to define the extent of disease (microscopically as well as macroscopically); to distinguish UC from Crohn's colitis and other diagnoses by multiple biopsies; and to screen for dysplasia and carcinoma. It should not be performed in acute UC because of the risk of causing perforation

Histopathology

Rectal or colonic biopsy confirms the diagnosis and degree of activity (see p. 735).

Management

The aim of treatment is to induce and maintain remission.

People with UC are best managed by specialist medical and surgical staff with access to a dietitian and stoma therapist. The wide variety of treatments and the recommended treatment programmes for different manifestations of UC are summarized in Table 10.39.

Supportive treatment

A full explanation of the disease to the patient and their relatives is essential. Patient support groups can provide additional help. Haematinic, electrolyte and nutritional deficiencies should be rectified. In patients admitted to hospital with severe attacks of UC, but without extensive rectal bleeding, it is advisable to give subcutaneous heparin to reduce the risk of vascular thrombosis (ULCERATIVE COLITIS AT A GLANCE).

Specific dietary advice is not usually needed, but a small minority of patients may improve if they avoid cow's milk.

Specific treatment

Drugs. The drugs available for management of UC and CD are shown in Table 10.40. Strategies for their use in UC are included in Table 10.39:
● *Corticosteroids:* given topically (as enema, foam or suppository), orally or intravenously, for a few weeks, to abort an acute attack. They have no prophylactic role. Their mode of action is unknown, but may involve

Table 10.40 Drugs most commonly used for treatment of inflammatory bowel disease

	Corticosteroids	Aminosalicylates	Thiopurines
Example	Prednisolone	Mesalazine (Asacol, Pentasa)	Azathioprine
Formulations	Oral Intravenous Enema, suppository	Oral Enema, suppository	Oral
Mechanism of action	Anti-inflammatory	Anti-inflammatory	Immunosuppressive
Indications	Active IBD	Active and inactive UC; active Crohn's	Refractory IBD
Side-effects	Facial mooning, diabetes, hypertension, hypokalaemia, osteoporosis, psychosis, myopathy	Rash, headache, diarrhoea, interstitial nephritis (all rare)	Nausea, rash, headache, bone marrow depression, pancreatitis, hepatitis
Contraindications	Uncontrolled diabetes or hypertension	Salicylate sensitivity	Sepsis
Monitoring	Blood pressure, blood sugar, bone density	Serum urea and creatinine	Blood count, liver function tests

IBD, inflammatory bowel disease; UC, ulcerative colitis.

immune suppression and inhibition of the production of inflammatory mediators

● *Sulfasalazine:* consists of 5-aminosalicylic acid (5-ASA) and sulfapyridine linked by an azo-bond. Sulfapyridine acts as a carrier molecule to take the active ingredient, 5-ASA, to the colon, where it is released by colonic bacterial action to exert its therapeutic effect. The sulfapyridine element of the drug causes most of the adverse effects, which range from minor rashes, headaches and dyspepsia through to life-threatening blood dyscrasias. Diarrhoea is a paradoxical side-effect of sulfasalasine and newer 5-ASA-containing drugs, whose primary role is the treatment of a diarrhoeal illness. The possibility of a drug-induced diarrhoea should be considered in patients not responding to standard therapy

Because of the side-effects of sulfapyridine, other methods have been devised to deliver 5-ASA to the colon. These include delayed-release (Asacol) or slow-release (Pentasa) 5-ASA tablet formulation; linking two molecules of 5-ASA by an azo-bond that is broken down by gut bacteria (olsalazine), and linking 5-ASA to the inert carrier aminobenzoylalanine (balsalazide) again by an azo-bond, leading to release of active drug by the action of colonic bacteria. Sulfasalazine, and these newer derivatives, have a minor role in the treatment of acute episodes. Taken long-term, they all reduce frequency of relapse. Sulfasalazine and 5-ASA may act by modifying the production of inflammatory mediators (see p. 735)

● *Azathioprine* (or its active metabolite, 6-mercaptopurine): reduces relapse rate and is occasionally used for its corticosteroid-sparing effect. Its side-effects necessitate regular FBC and liver function tests. It acts as an immunosuppressive

● *Ciclosporin:* given first intravenously then orally, it is an immunosuppressive drug used in combination with further corticosteroids in patients with acute severe UC who fail to improve within 5 days and may avert the need for urgent colectomy in this situation. Ciclosporin has serious side-effects that include renal damage, hypertension, electrolyte disturbances, opportunistic infections and epileptic fits. Frequent monitoring of blood levels is required

Surgery. A minority of patients need total colectomy. Preoperative counselling about ileostomy or its alternatives is mandatory.

● *Elective surgery:* may be indicated for chronic intractable UC, carcinoma and its prevention and prevention of growth retardation in childhood

● *Urgent surgery:* may be required for fulminant colitis, toxic megacolon, perforation or massive haemorrhage

Preventive treatment

Surveillance colonoscopy with multiple biopsies to look for epithelial dysplasia is carried out every 1–3 years in patients who have had total UC for more than 10 years to minimize the risk of colonic cancer. Colectomy is recommended if histology shows severe dysplasia. However, the efficacy of surveillance colonoscopy in reducing mortality from cancer in patients with UC has not yet been proved.

Prognosis

Most people with UC experience recurrent episodes of acute colitis, but their mortality rate is similar to that of the general population. The main risks to life are severe attacks of acute colitis and colonic cancer in people with chronic extensive UC.

10

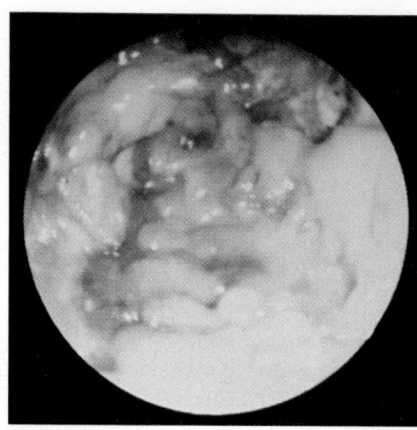

Figure 10.48 Colonoscopic appearance of active Crohn's disease showing cobblestoning and ulceration. Reproduced from *Slide Atlas of Gastroenterology* with the kind permission of the author and Times Mirror International Publishers.

Crohn's disease

Disease mechanisms
As for UC, the cause of CD is unknown. However, it seems likely that the disease is triggered by genetically determined abnormal mucosal immune responses to postulated (but unproven) aetiological factors such as the luminal gut flora, specific infections (measles, *Mycobacterium paratuberculosis*), diet and smoking. As in UC, mucosal inflammation is cytokine-driven, TNF playing a central part.

Pathology
Crohn's disease can affect any part of the gut from the mouth to the anus—most frequently the anus, ileocaecum, small bowel and colon. Typically, there are discontinuously affected gut segments (skip lesions). The first abnormality is aphthoid ulceration, which progresses to deep fissuring ulcers with cobblestoning, fibrosis, stricturing and fistulation (Fig. 10.48). Histologically, there is transmural chronic inflammatory cell infiltration with ulceration, microabscesses and pathognomonic non-caseating epithelioid granulomas.

Epidemiology
Prevalence. Like UC, CD is most common in developed countries, where it has a prevalence of about 50 in 100 000 and an incidence of about 5/100 000/year. Unlike UC, the incidence of CD has risen rapidly since 1960, but may now be reaching a plateau.

Age. A biphasic age incidence, as for UC. Older patients tend to have colonic disease rather than small bowel disease.

Sex. More common in women.

Race. Most common in white people, particularly Jews.

Genetics. There is an increased incidence in first-degree relatives and, through HLA B27, of ankylosing spondylitis (see p. 228). Linkage studies have identified a region on chromosome 16 (IBD-1) associated with susceptibility to inflammatory bowel disease. The specific genes involved with inflammatory bowel disease pathogenesis within this area have not been confirmed. However, one gene (*NOD2*) and its product from this region may be of particular relevance. The wild-type, or 'normal' protein encoded by the *NOD2* gene is involved in interactions between macrophages and bacterial antigens. There are polymorphisms of this gene in a proportion of patients with CD. There is good evidence that a disordered gut immune response to gut bacterial and dietary antigens is involved in the pathogenesis of inflammatory bowel disease; thus it is entirely plausible that an abnormal *NOD2* gene product is of causal relevance.

Clinical features
The clinical features vary depending on the site of disease (CROHN'S DISEASE AT A GLANCE). The history is often chronic with remissions and exacerbations. Common symptoms are diarrhoea, weight loss, abdominal pain (sometimes obstructive) and fever. People with small bowel disease may have steatorrhoea, and those with colitis, rectal bleeding. Chronic perianal symptoms are common.

Examination may show features of malabsorption (Table 10.18, p. 680), perianal disease (skin tags, fissures, fistulae, abscesses), an abdominal mass and/or clubbing.

Complications
Complications may be local or systemic (CROHN'S DISEASE AT A GLANCE). **Local complications** include:
- *Strictures:* commonly present with obstruction and sometimes with malabsorption caused by proximal small bowel bacterial overgrowth
- *Perforations:* common, contained locally and produce abscesses (see below). Free perforation is rare
- *Abscess and fistula:* usually form close to inflamed bowel and later discharge through fistulae into the skin, gut, bladder, vagina and, rarely, other sites
- *Anal fissure, fistula and abscess:* common
- *Haemorrhage:* usually minor and recurrent from inflamed mucosa and results in anaemia
- *Toxic megacolon:* rarer in CD than in UC
- *Carcinoma:* small bowel and colorectal carcinoma are slightly more common among people with CD than among the general population

Table 10.41 Causes of a mass in the right iliac fossa

Ileocaecal
Crohn's disease
Appendix mass
Carcinoma
Lymphoma
Tuberculosis
Yersiniosis
Amoebiasis
Actinomycosis

Other
Ovarian, tubal or renal mass

The many **systemic complications** are summarized in CROHN'S DISEASE AT A GLANCE.

Differential diagnosis
Differential diagnosis of bloody diarrhoea with inflamed rectal mucosa is given in Table 10.38 (p. 736), that of a mass in the right iliac fossa in Table 10.41.

Investigation
Investigations are similar to those for UC, but also include small bowel radiology and tests for malabsorption (see p. 680) in patients with suspected small bowel involvement.

Haematology
● *ESR, CRP and/or platelet count:* can be used to assess disease activity
● *Iron, folate and vitamin B$_{12}$ deficiencies causing anaemia:* common, vitamin B$_{12}$ deficiency suggesting terminal ileal disease

Biochemistry
Serum albumin can be used to assess disease activity, undernutrition and malabsorption.

Microbiology
Stool microscopy and culture to exclude infection in patients with diarrhoea.

Diagnostic imaging
● *Sigmoidoscopy:* may show perianal disease. Rectal CD is suggested by patchy inflammation with cobblestoning
● *Barium studies of small bowel:* often necessary. They may show strictures, local dilatation and/or fistulae; aphthoid, linear, collar-stud or rose-thorn ulcers, oedematous folds, cobblestoning and inflammatory polyps may also be seen (Fig. 10.49)
● *Sinograms:* may be necessary if there are enterocutaneous fistulae to delineate involved bowel prior to surgery

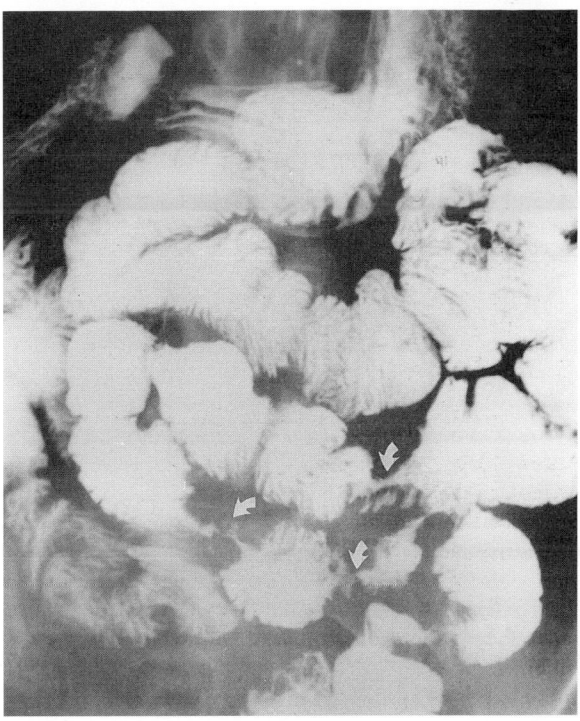

Figure 10.49 Small bowel barium meal showing Crohn's disease of the small intestine with areas of stricturing (arrowed) and dilatation. (Reproduced from Misiewicz JJ, Pounder RE, Venables CW. *Diseases of the Gut and Pancreas*, 2nd edn. Oxford: Blackwell Scientific Publications, 1994 with the permission of the authors.)

10

● *Colonoscopy:* useful for defining the extent of disease and distinguishing it from UC
● *Ultrasound and CT scan:* may help in the diagnosis of suspected intra-abdominal abscess, while *MRI* is excellent for delineating pelvic anatomy in patients with perianal fistulae

Histopathology
Colonic or rectal biopsy is necessary to confirm CD. Even if the mucosa looks normal, biopsy may show diagnostic granulomas.

Management
Treatment in CD is aimed at inducing remission. Unlike UC, prophylactic therapy is not yet well established.

Supportive treatment
Supportive treatment includes an explanation of the nature of CD and its prognosis. Long-term specialist follow-up, joining patient support groups, and nutritional support and advice are at least as important as in UC.

Crohn's disease at a glance

Epidemiology

Prevalence
50 in 100 000

Age
Peak is 20–30 years

Sex
More common in women

Race
Most common in Jews

Genetics
Increased prevalence of 10% in first-degree relatives. *NOD2* gene mutation on chromosome 16

Geography
Developed countries

Cause

Unknown. Abnormal mucosal immune response to luminal flora in genetically predisposed people

Investigation

Haematology
- *FBC:* anaemia resulting from iron, vitamin B_{12} or folate deficiency, increased platelet count
- *ESR:* increased
- *Albumin:* low
- *C-reactive protein:* increased

Microbiology
- *Stool culture*: negative

Diagnostic imaging
- *Barium follow-through:* may show stricture, fistula, abscess
- *Sigmoidoscopy:* perianal disease, patchy inflammation, cobblestoning
- *Colonoscopy:* patchy inflammation, aphthoid ulcers, cobblestoning
- *Ultrasound/CT scan:* intra-abdominal abscess, mass
- *Radiolabelled leucocyte scan:* positive uptake by inflamed bowel or abscess

Histopathology
- *Biopsy*: transmural and patchy inflammation, granulomas

Management

Supportive treatment
Explanation
Nutritional support and advice
Long-term specialist follow-up
Patient support groups (e.g. National Association for Colitis and Crohn's Disease)
Drugs: antidiarrhoeals (loperamide, codeine phosphate)

Specific treatment
Modify according to the clinical presentation (Table 10.42)
Drugs (Table 10.40)

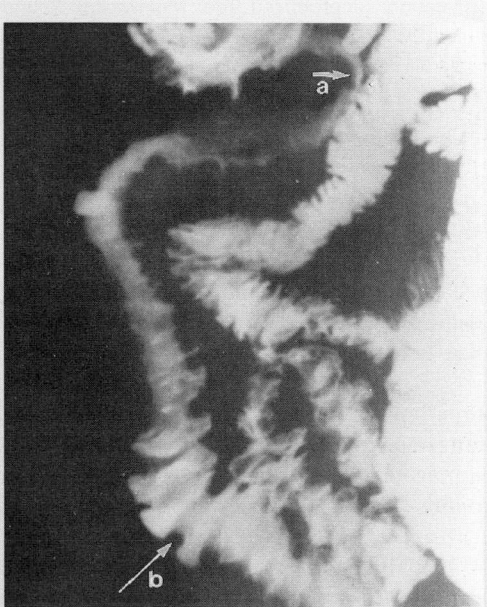

Fig. A Barium follow-through showing stricturing of the small intestine (a) and oedematous small bowel with thickening of the valvulae conniventes (b). Reproduced from Misiewicz *et al.*, *Diseases of the Gut and Pancreas*, 2nd edn, 1994 (Blackwell Scientific Publications, Oxford) with the permission of the authors.

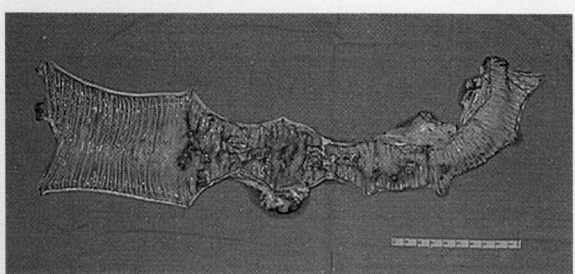

Fig. B Resected small bowel showing segmental stricture with patchy deep ulcers and proximal intestinal dilatation (left). The patient presented with subacute small bowel obstruction.

- Corticosteroids
- Aminosalicylates (active disease)
- Metronidazole and ciprofloxacin
- Azathioprine
- Methotrexate (rarely)
- Infliximab (rarely)

Diet: liquid formula diet

Surgery
- Depends on indication
- Local resection for strictures, abscesses and fistulae
- Stricturoplasty for strictures
- Colectomy for fulminant or intractable colitis

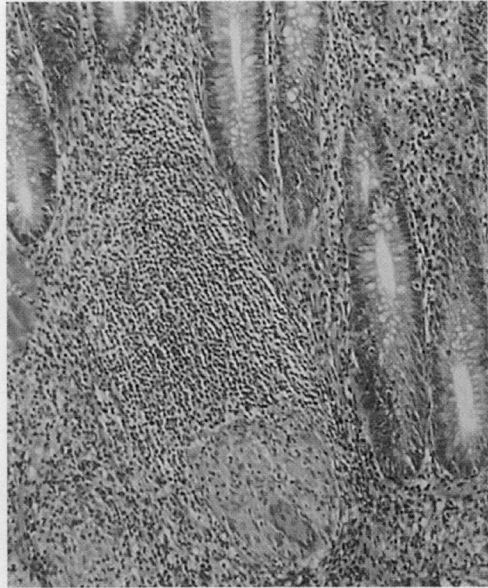

Fig. C Histopathology of Crohn's colitis showing intense mucosal inflammatory cell infiltration and an epithelioid granuloma containing a giant cell (centre, bottom).

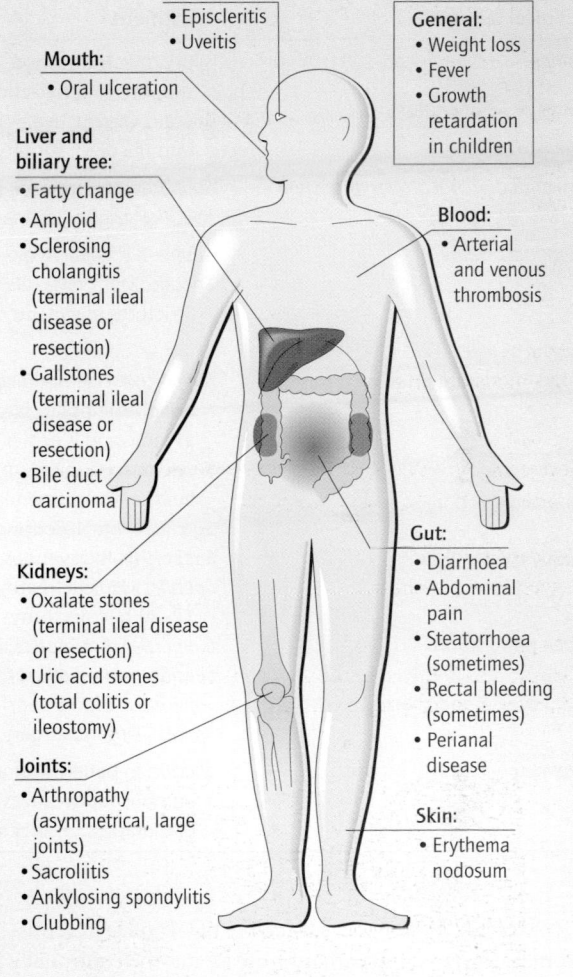

Eyes:
- Episcleritis
- Uveitis

Mouth:
- Oral ulceration

General:
- Weight loss
- Fever
- Growth retardation in children

Liver and biliary tree:
- Fatty change
- Amyloid
- Sclerosing cholangitis (terminal ileal disease or resection)
- Gallstones (terminal ileal disease or resection)
- Bile duct carcinoma

Blood:
- Arterial and venous thrombosis

Kidneys:
- Oxalate stones (terminal ileal disease or resection)
- Uric acid stones (total colitis or ileostomy)

Joints:
- Arthropathy (asymmetrical, large joints)
- Sacroliitis
- Ankylosing spondylitis
- Clubbing

Gut:
- Diarrhoea
- Abdominal pain
- Steatorrhoea (sometimes)
- Rectal bleeding (sometimes)
- Perianal disease

Skin:
- Erythema nodosum

Diet. People with CD often ask about the need for changes in their diet. Those with small bowel strictures should avoid high-residue foods (e.g. citrus-fruit segments, sweetcorn, uncooked vegetables, nuts), which might cause bolus obstruction. Nutritional deficiencies (e.g. iron, folate, magnesium, zinc and vitamins B_{12} and D) are common and should be corrected as necessary. Very sick inpatients may need enteral or total parenteral nutrition (see p. 687).

Drugs. Diarrhoea is often relieved by loperamide and codeine phosphate (see p. 685). Prophylactic subcutaneous heparin should also be given to reduce the risk of vascular thrombosis.

Specific treatment

Drugs. The main drugs available for treatment of inflammatory bowel disease are shown in Table 10.40 (p. 739). The strategies for their use in CD depend on the individual's clinical problem, and are discussed below and summarized in Table 10.42.

- *Oral steroids*: of proven value in active CD. For patients with ileocaecal CD, oral budesonide CR provides local topical release of a steroid that is effectively anti-inflammatory in the ileocaecal mucosa but, because of rapid first-pass hepatic metabolism, produces much less adrenal suppression and fewer systemic side-effects than conventional preparations such as prednisolone. As for

Table 10.42 Treatment of Crohn's disease

Clinical features	Treatment
Stricture	*Supportive.* Intravenous fluids if total obstruction; low residue diet if subacute. Nutritional support. Prophylactic subcutaneous heparin *Specific.* Obstructive episodes may settle with medical treatment (corticosteroids or liquid formula diet); surgery (resection or stricturoplasty) often necessary
Intra-abdominal abscesses, fistula	*Supportive.* Nutritional support, prophylactic heparin, antibiotics *Specific.* Surgical drainage/resection
Perianal disease	*Supportive.* Local hygiene, salt baths *Specific.* Metronidazole/ciprofloxacin or azathioprine. Abscesses require surgical drainage. Strictures may need dilatation
Crohn's colitis Mild–moderate attack	*Supportive.* Haematinics (iron, folate) if necessary *Specific.* Aminosalicylate and prednisolone orally, as an outpatient. Prednisolone tailed off as remission is achieved
Severe attack	*Supportive.* Hospital admission, close observation by physician and surgeon, intravenous fluids and electrolytes, blood transfusion, prophylactic heparin *Specific.* Methylprednisolone or hydrocortisone intravenously, oral aminosalicylate
Toxic megacolon	*Supportive.* Intravenous fluids, nasogastric suction, antibiotics *Specific.* Medical treatment as for severe Crohn's colitis. If no improvement in 12–24 h, colectomy
Free perforation	*Supportive.* Antibiotics, intravenous fluids *Specific.* Immediate surgery for resection and peritoneal toilet
Massive haemorrhage	*Supportive.* Blood transfusion *Specific.* Urgent surgery sometimes necessary
Refractory Crohn's disease	*Specific.* In patients refractory to or dependent on corticosteroids, consider immunosuppressives (azathioprine, methotrexate); if still unresponsive to or intolerant of therapy, consider infliximab

UC, steroids do not prevent relapse of CD once in remission; however, some patients' disease may be continually active, and thus the patient can be dependent on continuous steroids for continuous disease control.

● *Sulfasalazine* (see p. 739): effective in active Crohn's colitis and less so in active small bowel CD. Slow-release mesalazine (Pentasa), in which 5-ASA is released in greater amounts in the small bowel, is of value in the treatment of active ileocaecal Crohn's, but not in the prevention of relapse. ·

● *Azathioprine* (or its metabolite, 6-mercaptopurine): can be used as corticosteroid-sparing agents as in UC. Both drugs may be useful for perianal CD.

● *Methotrexate:* given intramuscularly or orally in low doses once a week, as an alternative to azathioprine in patients unresponsive to or intolerant of this drug. Its potential side-effects include bone marrow depression, pneumonitis and hepatic fibrosis, and patients taking methotrexate require FBC and liver function tests at least monthly.

● *Metronidazole and other antibiotics such as ciprofloxacin:* often used in active CD, and may have a specific role in perianal disease.

● *Infliximab:* a recently introduced monoclonal antibody to TNF. It can sometimes induce remission in patients with severe active CD refractory to all other therapies, but needs to be given by single or repeated intravenous infusion. It is also of specific benefit in patients with perianal CD. Its side-effects include infusion reactions, infections (including exacerbation of intra-abdominal sepsis and tuberculosis), serum sickness-like reactions and possibly lymphoma. Its side-effects and expense mean that its use is confined to very sick patients with otherwise unresponsive disease in specialist centres.

Diet. Enteral feeding with a chemically defined liquid formula diet treats active CD nearly as effectively as corticosteroids. Its disadvantages include its unpalatability and expense, and the rapid rates of relapse after it is discontinued. Possible modes of action are improved nutrition, hypoallergenicity, low residue and avoidance of trigger factors in ordinary food.

Surgery. About 80% of people with CD require surgery eventually, and 50% of these will need a second operation

Table 10.43 Inflammatory bowel disease (IBD) in pregnancy

Fertility
Female fertility is impaired
Male fertility may be impaired as a result of azoospermia in patients on sulfasalazine, but this reverses on changing to an alternative aminosalicylate

Outcome of pregnancy
Normal in quiescent IBD
Increased spontaneous abortion, premature delivery and stillbirth rates in active IBD

Effect of pregnancy on IBD
None

Treatment
Corticosteroids and aminosalicylates have no adverse effects on the fetus or baby during lactation
Azathioprine theoretically contraindicated in pregnancy although the outcome is usually satisfactory
Ciclosporin, methotrexate and infliximab should be avoided because of teratogenicity

---

Table 10.44 Inflammatory bowel disease (IBD) in childhood

Prevalence
Ulcerative colitis may occur at any age; allergy to cow's milk protein produces a similar syndrome and needs to be excluded
Crohn's disease is rare in children under 8 years of age

Growth
Active IBD and its long-term treatment with corticosteroids impair growth in childhood
A liquid formula diet usually induces remission and a growth spurt

---

for a recurrence within 10 years of the first. Because CD tends to recur, surgery should be as conservative as possible:
• Strictures require either minimal resection or strictureplasty
• Colitis may require colectomy with ileorectal anastomosis if the rectum is spared, or ileostomy. Pouch procedures are contraindicated because they are associated with a high rate of breakdown and sepsis in CD
• Abscesses are drained and enteric fistulae are resected

Special problems in inflammatory bowel disease
The particular problems of pregnancy and childhood in relation to inflammatory bowel disease are outlined in Tables 10.43 and 10.44, respectively.

Prognosis
Most patients experience recurrent morbidity throughout

their lives from CD and its treatment. The risk of death is about twice normal.

Irritable bowel syndrome

Irritable bowel syndrome (IBS) is a very common syndrome of abdominal pain and disordered bowel habit for which there is no organic explanation. Unsatisfactory and obsolete synonyms are nervous dyspepsia, irritable colon, spastic colon and mucous colitis.

Disease mechanisms
Possible aetiological factors include anxious or depressed personality and food intolerance. In some patients the syndrome is a consequence of an acute gastrointestinal infection.

Abdominal pain is often associated with abnormal intestinal motility. In some patients, symptoms seem to be caused by heightened perception of normal intestinal activity, 'visceral hypersensitivity'. Intestinal transit times are reduced in people with IBS complaining of diarrhoea and increased in those with constipation. How these abnormalities arise is unclear.

Epidemiology
Prevalence. Twenty per cent of normal adults have symptoms of IBS intermittently, but only one-quarter of these consult a doctor. About 50% of referrals to UK gastroenterological clinics have IBS.

Age. Peak age at presentation is 20–30 years.

Sex. Three times as common in women as in men.

Clinical features

Key symptoms
Irritable bowel syndrome should be a positive diagnosis, not one of exclusion. To facilitate this, an international working party has laid down the following 'ROME II' diagnostic criteria:
1 At least 12 weeks, which need not be consecutive, in the preceding year of abdominal discomfort or pain that has two of the three features:
  • Relieved by defecation
  • Onset with a change in stool frequency
  • Onset with a change in form (appearance) of stool
2 Supportive symptoms are:
  • Hard or lumpy stools
  • Loose or watery stools
  • Straining during a bowel movement
  • Urgency of defecation
  • Feeling of incomplete defecation

10

- Passing mucus (not pus) rectally
- Abdominal bloating

Other gastrointestinal symptoms

These include nausea, vomiting, heartburn, dyspepsia, dysphagia (globus hystericus) and proctalgia fugax (lancinating rectal pain caused by spasm of levator ani).

Symptoms arising from other systems

- *Psychiatric symptoms:* including anxiety, depression and a preoccupation with bowel habit
- *Gynaecological symptoms:* including dyspareunia, dysmenorrhoea and bowel symptoms related to menstrual cycle
- *Urinary symptoms:* including frequency and urgency
- *Constitutional symptoms:* including lassitude and headaches

   Examination may reveal no abnormality, anxiety, diffuse or localized abdominal tenderness, a squelchy caecum, a tender palpable descending colon, loud borborygmi and/or reproduction of the patient's symptoms on insufflation of air at sigmoidoscopy.

Differential diagnosis

Differential diagnosis in young adults includes coeliac disease, lactase deficiency, Crohn's disease, giardiasis, pelvic inflammatory disease and thyrotoxicosis. Colorectal carcinoma, diverticulosis, peptic ulcer and gallstones should also be considered in older people.

Investigation

Avoid overinvestigating young patients with typical symptoms; sigmoidoscopy and rectal biopsy, FBC and ESR, if normal, suffice.

Management

Explanation. First reassure the patient that he or she has no serious organic disorder, and explain that the pain and altered bowel habit are caused by spasm in the muscle of the bowel or by increased perception of normal gut activity. This approach helps break the vicious circle of anxiety about the possible cause of the symptoms causing more symptoms. Nevertheless, in patients with continuing symptoms and psychological disturbance, psychiatric referral may be appropriate.

   Management otherwise depends on the predominant symptoms in each patient:

- *Pain-predominant:* antispasmodics such as mebeverine and cyclomine may help, as may low doses of tricyclic antidepressants (e.g. amitriptyline) and selective serotonin reuptake inhibitors (paroxetine), the latter perhaps acting directly on gut receptors rather than in the brain. Dietary factors (e.g. wheat) identified by the patient as causing symptoms should be avoided, but there is usually no place for a formal exclusion regimen

- *Diarrhoea-predominant:* antidiarrhoeal agents such as loperamide (see p. 685) may decrease bowel frequency and improve stool consistency

- *Constipation-predominant:* people with constipation may benefit from a high-fibre diet and/or bulking agents (see p. 685). Warn them that a sudden increase in fibre intake will temporarily increase abdominal distension and flatus

Prognosis

The short-term prognosis for symptom relief is poor, but most people are asymptomatic 5 years later.

Infective diarrhoea

Disease mechanisms

Common causes of infective diarrhoea are shown in Table 10.45 (see also Chapter 3). The effects of enteric infection depend on host defences and microbial virulence.

Host defences. The risk of getting infective diarrhoea is increased by:

- Poor socioeconomic conditions
- Early childhood and old age, probably as a result of reduced immune defences
- Malnutrition
- Immunocompromise (e.g. AIDS)
- Reduced gastric acid secretion (e.g. gastrectomy or PPI)
- Impaired intestinal motility

Microbial virulence. This depends on:

- Adherence of the organism to surface enterocytes
- Production of enterotoxins
- Invasion of the intestinal mucosa

Surface expression of adhesive proteins facilitates adherence of the organism to the enterocyte and subsequent mucosal secretion and/or invasion (Fig. 10.50).

   Various organisms produce **enterotoxins** that, by inducing small intestinal secretion of water and electrolytes (Figs 10.50 and 10.9) through activation of adenyl or guanyl cyclase, lead to profuse watery diarrhoea. There are two main types of such toxins, which are either heat labile or heat stable:

- *Heat-labile toxins:* complex macromolecules. Cholera toxin is the classic example, but some strains of enterotoxigenic *E. coli* (ETEC) produce closely related toxins (Fig. 10.50)

- *Heat-stable toxins (ST):* low molecular weight peptides. The best understood is STa, which causes a reversible activation of guanyl cyclase. STa-type toxins are found in ETEC and some strains of *Yersinia*

   Other organisms (e.g. *Clostridium difficile, Shigella*

Irritable bowel syndrome at a glance

Disease mechanisms and epidemiology

Irritable bowel syndrome is very common, accounting for up to 50% of patients referred to gastrointestinal outpatient clinics

The cause is unknown

Trigger factors include acute enteritis, stress, anxiety and food intolerance

The pain is caused by abnormal gut motility and, in some patients, visceral hypersensitivity

Investigation

The diagnosis is made positively when there is at least a 3-month history of defecation-related abdominal pain with a change in stool frequency or stool form

Supporting features include a sensation of incomplete evacuation of stool, and bloating relieved by defecation

Haematology

- *FBC:* normal
- *ESR:* normal

Diagnostic imaging

Sigmoidoscopy: normal

Management

Therapy includes explanation, dietary modification, antispasmodics and antidiarrhoeals

In some cases antidepressants, alternative medicine approaches and other treatments aimed at underlying psychological problems are successful

Supportive treatment

Reassurance and explanation

Specific treatment

Diet

- Avoid dietary precipitants, but there is usually no place for a formal exclusion regimen
- High-fibre diet for constipation

Drugs (avoid if possible)

- Antispasmodics (e.g. mebeverine, cyclomine)
- Antidiarrhoeals (e.g. loperamide)
- Antidepressants (e.g. amitriptyline) if necessary

Other

Psychiatric referral occasionally

Hypnosis if refractory

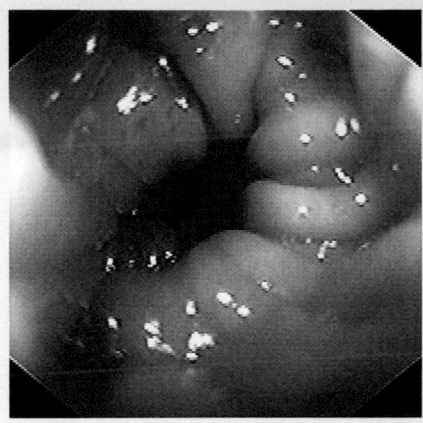

Fig. A Sigmoidoscopic appearance in IBS. Note the normally glistening mucosa with some spasm in sigmoid colon.

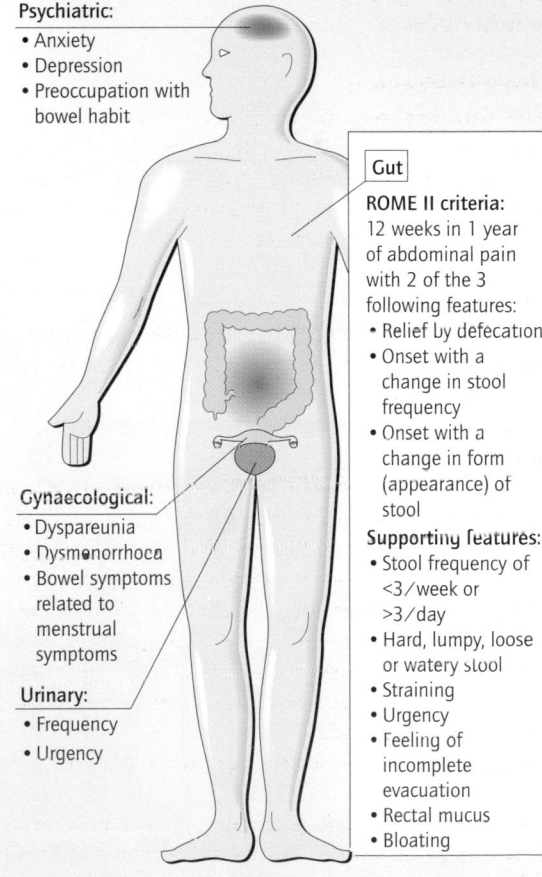

Psychiatric:
- Anxiety
- Depression
- Preoccupation with bowel habit

Gut

ROME II criteria: 12 weeks in 1 year of abdominal pain with 2 of the 3 following features:
- Relief by defecation
- Onset with a change in stool frequency
- Onset with a change in form (appearance) of stool

Supporting features:
- Stool frequency of <3/week or >3/day
- Hard, lumpy, loose or watery stool
- Straining
- Urgency
- Feeling of incomplete evacuation
- Rectal mucus
- Bloating

Gynaecological:
- Dyspareunia
- Dysmenorrhoea
- Bowel symptoms related to menstrual symptoms

Urinary:
- Frequency
- Urgency

10

Table 10.45 Common causes of infective diarrhoeal syndromes (infections marked with an asterisk are uncommon in developed countries except in returned travellers or immunocompromised patients)

	Acute watery diarrhoea	Dysentery (bloody diarrhoea, systemic upset)	Chronic diarrhoea
Major site	Jejunum	Colon	Small (S) and/or large (L) intestine
Toxigenic bacteria			
*Vibrio cholerae**	+		
Enterotoxigenic *E. coli* (ETEC)	+		
Invasive bacteria			
Shigella spp.	+	+	
Salmonella spp.	+	+	
Enteroinvasive *E. coli* (EIEC)		+	
Campylobacter jejuni		+	
Viruses			
Rotavirus	+		
Norwalk virus	+		
Adenovirus	+		
Protozoa			
*Entamoeba histolytica**		+	+L
*Giardia lamblia**	+		+S
Cryptosporidium parvum	+		
Schistosoma spp.*		+	+L
Strongyloidosis*			+S, L

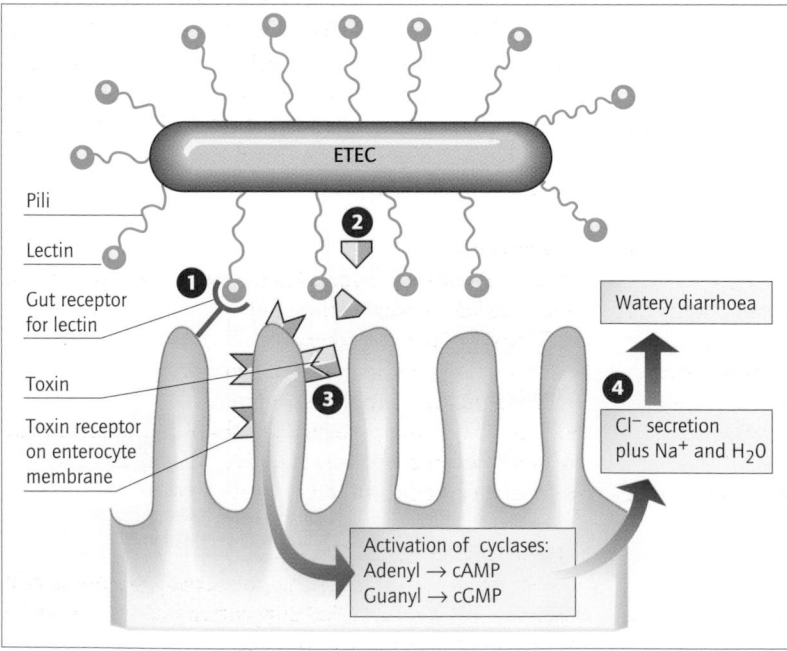

Figure 10.50 Pathogenesis of watery diarrhoea caused by enterotoxigenic *Escherichia coli* (ETEC). ETEC attaches to receptors (1) on the intestinal epithelium by a lectin, which is a specific sugar-binding protein. ETEC then secretes a toxin (2) or toxins that bind to another receptor (3), which activates adenyl and guanyl cyclase to produce the second messengers cyclic adenosine monophosphate (cAMP) and cyclic guanosine monophosphate (cGMP). cAMP and cGMP cause chloride, sodium and water secretion (4), resulting in watery diarrhoea.

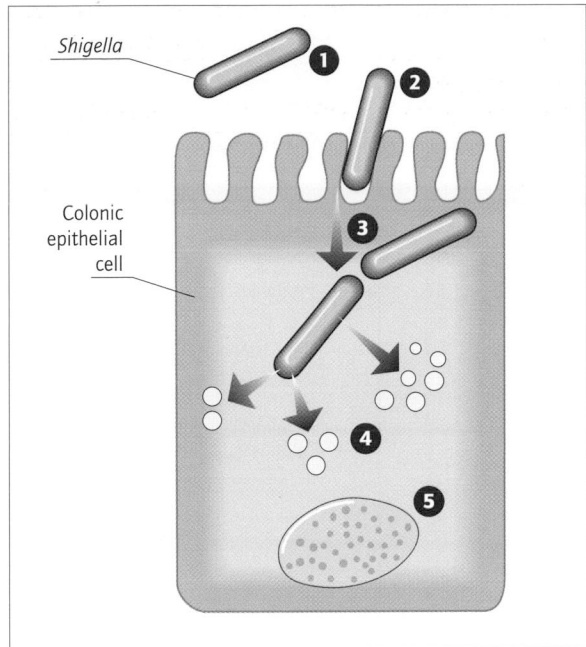

Figure 10.51 Pathogenesis of *Shigella* dysentery. (1) *Shigella* multiplies within the intestinal lumen and directly invades (2) epithelial cells of the colon. After intracellular multiplication (3) the organism produces a cytotoxin (4) that inhibits protein synthesis (5), ultimately leading to cell death, epithelial cell loss and ulceration.

spp.) produce **cytotoxins**, which probably contribute to mucosal damage and inflammation.

Inflammatory dysentery is usually a response to colonization of the colon by invasive organisms such as *Shigella*, *Salmonella* and *Campylobacter* spp. and amoebae (Fig. 10.51).

Epidemiology
Prevalence and geography. Common, although often trivial, in developed countries. In contrast, infective diarrhoea is a major killer in developing countries, particularly of children. Predisposing factors include poor hygiene and sanitation, overcrowding, malnutrition caused by poor diet and/or recurrent diarrhoea, international travel and immunocompromised patients.

Age. Most common and most dangerous in young children and the elderly.

Clinical features
There are three main clinical presentations (Table 10.45):
1 Acute watery diarrhoea
2 Dysentery
3 Chronic diarrhoea

Acute watery diarrhoea. This is the most common presentation. The onset is characteristically sudden, and the severity varies from a mild looseness of stools to profuse watery diarrhoea with rapid progression of fluid depletion, leading to reduced skin turgor, sunken eyes, hypotension and peripheral vasoconstriction. Systemic symptoms are unusual and the illness is self-limiting, with complete resolution within a week.

Dysentery. This is characterized by bloody diarrhoea, often preceded by a constitutional upset. Abdominal pain, tenesmus and fever are common. Although toxic megacolon and septicaemia are rare, the illness can be severe and prolonged.

Chronic diarrhoea. This may be watery or mushy, sometimes causes malabsorption, and may last for weeks and occasionally years. The symptoms may be intermittent, and abdominal pain, malaise and flatulence are common.

Differential diagnosis
The differential diagnosis of acute watery diarrhoea and of dysentery is shown in Table 10.45 and of chronic diarrhoea in Table 10.12 (p. 664). It is important not to misdiagnose ulcerative colitis as dysentery, because a delayed diagnosis or inappropriate treatment may have serious consequences. The history, examination and basic blood tests do not allow differentiation of these two common causes of bloody diarrhoea. Where there is doubt, particularly in developed countries where the incidence of infective dysenteric illnesses is low, it is reasonable to treat both conditions from the outset (steroids + antibiotics) while awaiting the results of definitive tests such as stool culture and rectal biopsy.

Complications
Most patients recover completely from infective diarrhoea, but occasional complications are:
● Transient lactose intolerance
● Postinfective irritable bowel syndrome
   More unusual complications are:
● Reiter's syndrome, particularly following *Salmonella* or *Yersinia* spp. infection (see pp. 119, 121, 232 and 1119)
● Erythema nodosum (see p. 1158)

Investigation
Investigation depends on the presenting symptoms and is shown in Fig. 10.52. Full supportive treatment may be needed until the diagnosis is made.

10

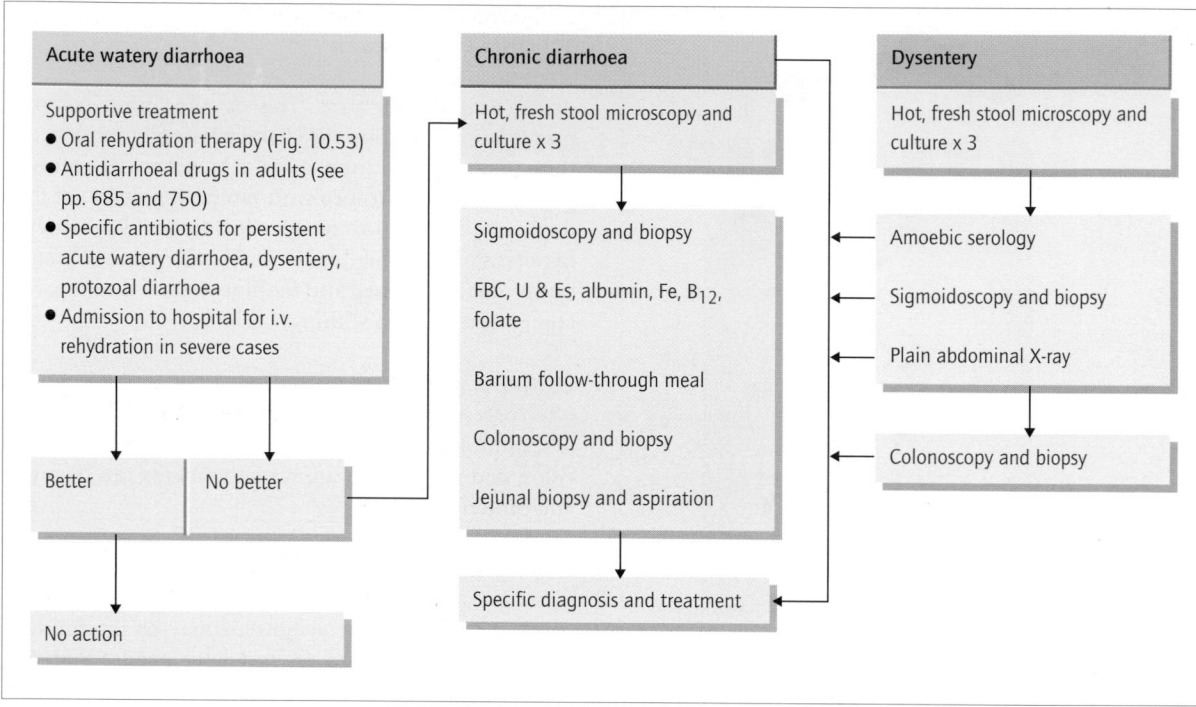

Figure 10.52 Investigation of suspected infective diarrhoea.

Management

Supportive treatment

The cornerstone of treatment is immediate replacement of lost fluid and electrolytes:

- *In patients needing hospital admission:* this is usually achieved by giving intravenous fluids containing Na^+, K^+ and Cl^-
- Elsewhere, *oral rehydration therapy* (ORT), one of the most important medical advances of the 20th century, is used both to prevent and to treat fluid and electrolyte depletion (Fig. 10.53). This has made a major impact on the morbidity and mortality of infective diarrhoea, particularly in developing countries, where its simple composition allows its prompt use, even in very remote areas.

Drugs. Antidiarrhoeal drugs (see p. 685) such as loperamide are not usually indicated and should be avoided in children altogether, and in adults when dysentery is suspected because of the danger of precipitating toxic dilatation of the inflamed colon. They can be used cautiously in adults with persisting watery diarrhoea to reduce stool volume and frequency.

Specific treatment

Antibiotics have a minor role in infective diarrhoea, but may be useful in:

- More prolonged acute watery diarrhoea in travellers (Fig. 10.54)
- Dysentery (e.g. caused by *Salmonella*, *Campylobacter* and *Shigella* spp.) if the patient is seriously ill
- Protozoal chronic diarrhoea caused by *Giardia* spp. or amoebae

Indiscriminate use of antibiotics is not recommended because of the risk of side-effects, prolonging carriage of the organism (e.g. *Salmonella* spp.) and increasing microbial drug resistance.

Certain infections (e.g. cholera, typhoid) must be notified to public health laboratories in Western countries such as the UK so that preventive measures can be rapidly taken.

Preventive treatment

Measures to prevent enteric infection are:

- Personal hygiene, in particular washing hands
- Avoidance of untreated and potentially contaminated water and undercooked, reheated or raw foods
- Vaccination of travellers to areas where they may be exposed to infection (e.g. cholera and typhoid)
- Population measures to improve sanitation, overcrowding and nutrition

Prognosis

In the Western world, most patients make a prompt and

Composition

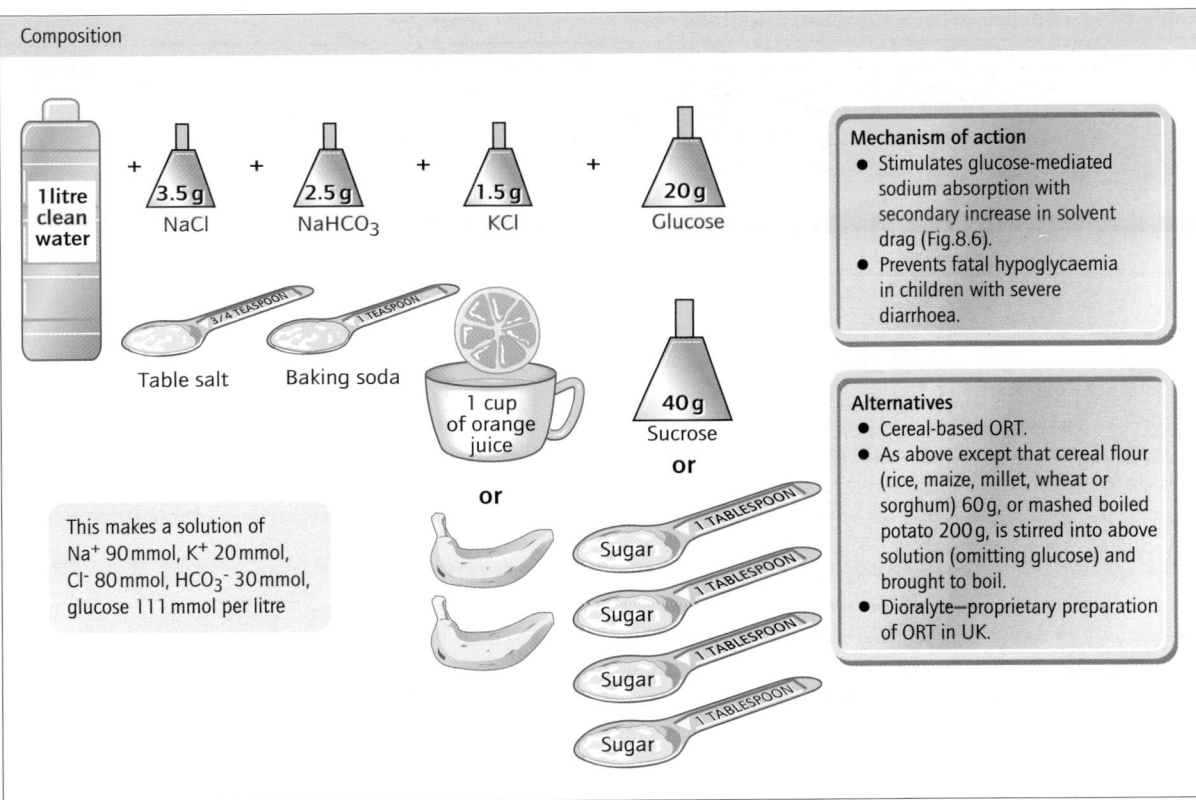

Mechanism of action
- Stimulates glucose-mediated sodium absorption with secondary increase in solvent drag (Fig.8.6).
- Prevents fatal hypoglycaemia in children with severe diarrhoea.

Alternatives
- Cereal-based ORT.
- As above except that cereal flour (rice, maize, millet, wheat or sorghum) 60 g, or mashed boiled potato 200 g, is stirred into above solution (omitting glucose) and brought to boil.
- Dioralyte—proprietary preparation of ORT in UK.

1 litre clean water

+ 3.5 g NaCl

+ 2.5 g NaHCO$_3$

+ 1.5 g KCl

+ 20 g Glucose

Table salt   Baking soda

1 cup of orange juice

40 g Sucrose

or

This makes a solution of Na$^+$ 90 mmol, K$^+$ 20 mmol, Cl$^-$ 80 mmol, HCO$_3^-$ 30 mmol, glucose 111 mmol per litre

or

Sugar   1 TABLESPOON
Sugar   1 TABLESPOON
Sugar   1 TABLESPOON
Sugar   1 TABLESPOON

Figure 10.53 Oral rehydration therapy (ORT).

10

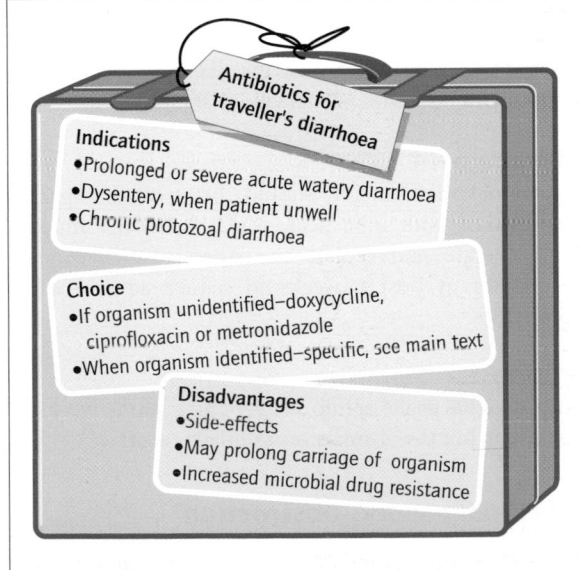

Antibiotics for traveller's diarrhoea

Indications
- Prolonged or severe acute watery diarrhoea
- Dysentery, when patient unwell
- Chronic protozoal diarrhoea

Choice
- If organism unidentified—doxycycline, ciprofloxacin or metronidazole
- When organism identified—specific, see main text

Disadvantages
- Side-effects
- May prolong carriage of organism
- Increased microbial drug resistance

Figure 10.54 Antibiotics for traveller's diarrhoea.

complete recovery from infective diarrhoea with or without specific treatment. In developing countries, morbidity and mortality has fallen markedly since the advent of ORT, but will continue to be high where malnutrition is common, particularly in children.

Specific infections

A full description of the common specific infections is given in Chapter 3.

Bacterial food poisoning

Bacterial food poisoning syndromes are summarized in Table 10.46. All can be diagnosed by identifying the organism in food, vomit and/or stool, are self-limiting, and require no specific drug treatment. Preventive measures include:
- *High standards of public health:* including efficient notification systems to control outbreaks
- *High standards of food preparation by suppliers:* (e.g. animal slaughterhouses, poultry rearers) and *caterers*

Table 10.46 Common bacterial food poisoning syndromes

Organism	Source	Incubation period	Symptoms	Recovery
Staphylococcus aureus	Food contaminated by humans	2–6 h	Vomiting, diarrhoea	A few hours
Bacillus cereus	Spores in food surviving boiling	1–10 h	Vomiting, diarrhoea	A few hours
Salmonella spp.	Eggs, poultry	12–24 h	Diarrhoea, fever, abdominal pain, vomiting	5–14 days
Campylobacter jejuni	Milk, poultry	2–5 days	Bloody diarrhoea, fever, abdominal pain	3–7 days

(adequate refrigeration, good personal and equipment hygiene, avoidance of carriers)
• *Meticulous food preparation at home:* defrost thoroughly, cook adequately, eat immediately and avoid inadequate reheating

Tropical sprue

Tropical sprue is idiopathic persistent malabsorption, particularly of folate and B_{12}, in a patient who is or who has been recently resident in the tropics for more than 4 weeks. It is also known as postinfective tropical malabsorption. It can be endemic or epidemic.

Disease mechanisms

Usually there is an acute diarrhoeal episode such as traveller's diarrhoea or dysentery. This is followed by persisting bacterial overgrowth with various organisms. Later, folate deficiency may worsen mucosal damage. The roles of ingested toxins and other nutritional deficiencies are not clear.

Pathology

The small bowel mucosa shows partial villous atrophy and lymphocyte and eosinophil infiltration in the lamina propria.

Epidemiology

Age. Usually, young adults of 20–40 years of age.

Geography. Indian Subcontinent, South East Asia, Central America.

Clinical features

The main symptoms are diarrhoea, steatorrhoea, abdominal distension, anorexia, lassitude and weight loss after a sudden onset weeks or months earlier with a presumed gastrointestinal infection. Milk may worsen the symptoms because of secondary hypolactasia. Nutritional deficiencies may develop (Table 10.18, p. 680). Often the symptoms improve on leaving the tropics, but recurrences are common.

Differential diagnosis
• Small intestinal infection with parasites (e.g. *Giardia* spp., amoeba, cryptosporidia) or bacteria (e.g. tuberculosis)
• Hypolactasia (primary or secondary)
• Lymphoma
• Non-tropical causes of diarrhoea (Table 10.12, p. 664)

Investigation
Haematology
FBC. There is often a folate- and vitamin B_{12}-deficient megaloblastic anaemia.

Biochemistry
• *Serum calcium, phosphate and alkaline phosphatase:* may reveal biochemical osteomalacia (see p. 280)
• *Serum albumin:* may be low

Microbiology
Small bowel aspiration and stool examination helps exclude specific infections.

Histopathology
Small bowel biopsies suggest the diagnosis by showing inflamed mucosa with partial villous atrophy.

Management
Nutritional deficiencies should be treated. Specific treatment is with folic acid, which helps the mucosa to regenerate and replete the stores. Tetracycline is needed for at least 6 weeks to reduce adverse small bowel flora.

Prognosis
Most patients make a full recovery after some weeks of treatment, but the disorder occasionally recurs.

Intestinal pseudo-obstruction

Intestinal pseudo-obstruction is a rare gut motility disorder in which the clinical features suggest large and/or small intestinal obstruction in the absence of any mechanical cause.

Table 10.47 Causes of intestinal pseudo-obstruction

Primary
Idiopathic

Secondary
Acute
Postoperative
 Ileus
Serious abdominal disorder
 Liver failure
 Acute pancreatitis
 Intestinal ischaemia
 Retroperitoneal haematoma
Metabolic
 Hypokalaemia
 Hypocalcaemia
 Hypomagnesaemia
 Hypothyroidism

Chronic
Neurological
 Diabetes mellitus
 Chagas' disease
 Parkinson's disease
Myopathy
 Dystrophia myotonica
 Polymyositis
Muscle infiltration
 Amyloid
 Systemic sclerosis
Iatrogenic
 Anticholinergics
 Antidepressants
 Phenothiazines
 Opiates

Disease mechanisms

Causes of intestinal pseudo-obstruction are listed in Table 10.47. The idiopathic primary chronic variety is very rare. It is sometimes familial and is associated with oesophageal and urinary tract smooth muscle disorders. Pathological findings depend on the cause. In primary pseudo-obstruction there are abnormalities of the smooth muscle fibres and myenteric plexus.

Clinical features

Acute intestinal pseudo-obstruction. This presents with abdominal discomfort, distension and constipation, which resolves spontaneously with the underlying cause.

Chronic pseudo-obstruction. This presents with continuous or recurrent episodes of pain and distension with constipation, diarrhoea or steatorrhoea (because of small bowel bacterial overgrowth). There may be vomiting, anorexia and weight loss.

Physical signs include abdominal distension, a succussion splash and increased, normal or reduced bowel sounds. Laparotomy scars are common.

The underlying cause of secondary intestinal pseudo-obstruction may be apparent.

Complications

Acute caecal dilatation may progress to perforation. Anorexia and steatorrhoea in chronic disease may lead to death.

Investigation

Secondary causes should be sought (Table 10.47), and the degree of malabsorption and bacterial overgrowth assessed (Tables 10.17 and 10.18, p. 680).

Diagnostic imaging
- *Plain abdominal radiography:* shows gross bowel distension
- *Barium studies* (and sometimes laparotomy): necessary in chronic cases to exclude mechanical obstruction

Management

Acute intestinal pseudo-obstruction. Treatment is of the underlying cause. Nasogastric aspiration and intravenous correction of electrolyte deficiencies may be necessary. Colonoscopy can be used to deflate the dilated large bowel and exclude obstructive lesions. Intravenous neostigmine may be helpful. Caecostomy is performed if perforation seems imminent.

Chronic intestinal pseudo-obstruction. This is difficult to manage if the underlying cause is not reversible. Antibiotics can be given for small bowel overgrowth. Nutritional supplements are often necessary, but long-term parenteral nutrition may be the only option. Surgery is rarely beneficial.

Adverse effects of drugs on the intestine

Laxative abuse

Laxative abuse is defined as surreptitious ingestion of laxatives by patients complaining of diarrhoea.

Disease mechanisms

Prolonged laxative consumption may result in excessive faecal loss of potassium and magnesium leading to ileus and metabolic alkalosis. Anthracene derivatives (e.g. senna) taken for long periods may additionally lead to:
- Melanosis coli (Fig. 10.55)
- Damage to myenteric nerve plexuses, resulting in an atonic dilated large bowel (cathartic colon)

10

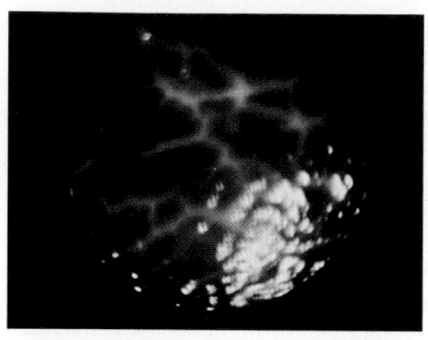

(a)

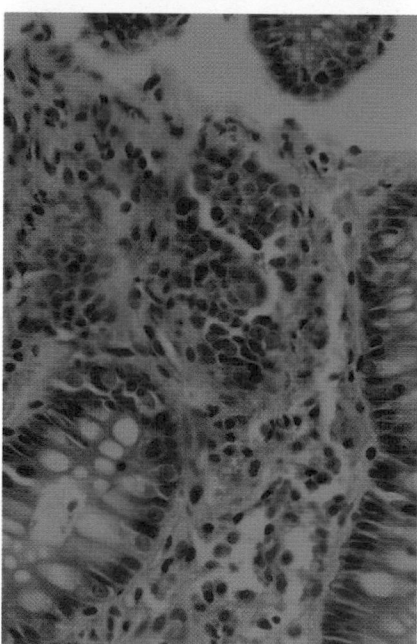

(b)

Figure 10.55 Melanosis coli caused by prolonged laxative ingestion. (a) Colonoscopic appearance. (b) Histological appearance. The brown mucosal pigmentation is caused by excess pigment in macrophages in the lamina propria.

Epidemiology

Prevalence. More common than suspected by doctors.

Age. Adults, 20–60 years of age.

Sex. Most common in women.

Clinical features

The patient usually presents with chronic diarrhoea and/or steatorrhoea, often with weight loss, and a history of extensive investigation and one or more negative laparotomies. Drug ingestion is categorically denied, and there is often a background of anorexia nervosa, bulimia and/or diuretic abuse. On examination there may be cachexia and clubbing.

Investigation

It is essential, if possible, to avoid overinvestigation.

HAEMATOLOGY
No significant findings.

BIOCHEMISTRY
Serum biochemistry may reveal low K^+, low Mg^{2+} and metabolic alkalosis.

DIAGNOSTIC IMAGING
• *Sigmoidoscopy or colonoscopy:* may reveal melanosis coli (Fig. 10.55a)
• *Barium enema:* may show an inert atonic dilated colon

HISTOPATHOLOGY
Rectal biopsy may reveal melanosis coli (Fig. 10.55b).

OTHER
Urine and stool tests for laxatives. The urine and faeces of people taking phenolphthalein-containing laxatives will turn pink on alkalinization with NaOH. The urine and stool can also be tested for senna and magnesium.

Management

Management of people who abuse laxatives is difficult. Some continue to deny purgative abuse even when confronted with the evidence. Most require psychiatric referral. Monitoring of serum electrolyte levels is advisable.

Antibiotic-induced diarrhoea

Many patients given antibiotics develop diarrhoea. Usually it is caused by alterations in colonic bacterial flora. The most commonly identified is overgrowth by *Clostridium difficile* (see below). Other mechanisms may involve allergy or ischaemia.

Pseudomembranous colitis

Pseudomembranous colitis is colitis characterized by the formation of a superficial pseudomembrane. It is associated with infection by *Cl. difficile*.

Disease mechanisms

There is usually a history of recent antibiotic treatment. Occasional outbreaks in wards or old people's homes may be caused by cross-infection in the absence of antibiotic exposure. *Cl. difficile* is present in the stools of about 3% of healthy adults and 40% of neonates. In pseudomembranous colitis, the organism produces enterotoxins and cytotoxins, which, respectively, induce fluid secretion by and have a direct cytotoxic effect on colonic epithelium.

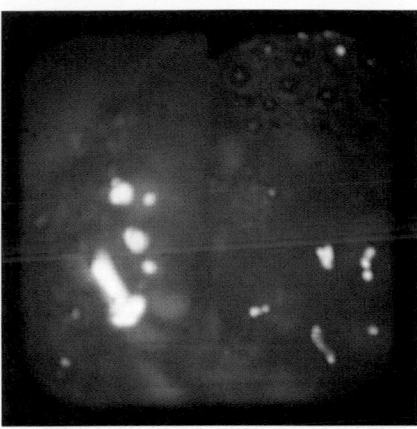

Figure 10.56 Colonoscopic appearance of pseudomembranous colitis. Note the scattered white pseudomembranes.

PATHOLOGY

Macroscopically, the pseudomembranes appear as raised pale plaques with intervening hyperaemic mucosa (Fig. 10.56). Histology shows focal ulceration, with acute inflammation and superficial volcano lesions containing polymorphs, fibrin and necrotic epithelium.

Clinical features

The patient presents with diarrhoea during or after a course of antibiotics. Usually there is no bleeding, but fever, abdominal pain and tenderness are common. The condition may progress to toxic dilatation, perforation and death.

Investigation

• *Sigmoidoscopy and rectal biopsy:* show pseudomembranes in some patients. The rest have more proximal lesions
• *Colonoscopy:* detects the more proximal lesions
• *Stool microscopy:* shows leucocytes
• *Stool cultures:* grow *Cl. difficile*
• *Identification of the toxin:* by demonstrating its cytotoxic effect on cell cultures *in vitro* provides proof of its pathogenicity

Management

Treatment is with oral metronidazole or vancomycin for 10 days, together with fluid, electrolyte and nutritional repletion as necessary. Other antibiotics must be discontinued. A possible role for prevention of antibiotic-induced diarrhoea using probiotics such as *Lactobacillus* remains to be established.

Prognosis

Recovery is usually prompt, but relapses may occur on discontinuing vancomycin.

Intestinal ischaemia

Intestinal ischaemia occurs when there is an acute or chronic reduction in arterial or venous blood flow sufficient to threaten intestinal viability.

Disease mechanisms

Intestinal ischaemia may be caused either by arterial or venous occlusion or by severe hypotension (e.g. in shock).

Causes of arterial occlusion include atheroma and embolus—the latter may be a complication of atrial fibrillation. Venous occlusion is usually by thrombosis, and can be precipitated by infections, malignancy and use of the oral contraceptive pill.

Bowel supplied by the superior mesenteric artery and the splenic flexure of the colon are most commonly involved. Partial ischaemia affects the mucosa more than the serosa and therefore tends to cause malabsorption or ischaemic colitis (diffuse or focal). Complete vascular occlusion causes segmental infarction with necrosis, perforation and/or bleeding. Recovery may leave a fibrous stricture.

Clinical features and management

Presentation can range from the acute form, where there is sudden reduction in blood supply, resulting in gangrene of the affected bowel and death if untreated, through to chronic ischaemia, where symptoms may occur only intermittently at times of high demand for blood flow (e.g. after meals), and no irreversible mucosal damage occurs. The most common clinical pattern is ischaemic colitis in the elderly, which resolves spontaneously in most cases. The features of these different types of intestinal ischaemia are shown in Table 10.48.

Radiation damage to the gut

Radiation damage to the gut is defined as acute or chronic intestinal injury in patients who have had internal or external abdominal or pelvic irradiation.

Disease mechanisms

The gut is particularly radiosensitive because of its rapid epithelial cell turnover. The terminal ileum, distal colon and rectum are most commonly affected because of their relative immobility in the pelvis. Fixity from adhesions after previous surgery places other areas of the bowel at risk.

The acute effects of irradiation range from minor epithelial damage to massive bowel necrosis after overdosage. Chronically, there is progressive ischaemia over some years resulting from an obliterative vasculitis.

10

Table 10.48 Clinical features and management of different types of intestinal ischaemia

Clinical features	Management
Acute intestinal ischaemia Severe abdominal pain, vomiting and rectal bleeding or melaena. Signs are peritonism, absent bowel sounds and shock. Often signs of cardiovascular disease	Urgent resuscitation, laparotomy with excision of non-viable gut, embolectomy and/or revascularization. Intensive postoperative care with antibiotics and heparin. Mortality is high
Chronic intestinal ischaemia Intestinal angina or abdominal claudication: postprandial abdominal pain, weight loss, sometimes malabsorption. Signs are rare. A localized abdominal bruit occasionally	Arterial surgery
Ischaemic colitis Acute pain, usually in the left iliac fossa, fever and dark red rectal bleeding. Signs are localized peritonitis	Usually conservative. Often resolves completely. Sometimes colonic strictures develop

Macroscopically, there may be ulceration, stricturing, infarction and sometimes perforation. Microscopy shows submucosal oedema, telangiectasia, fibrosis and ulceration, as well as vasculitis.

Epidemiology

Prevalence. Incidence varies with the treatment regimen (including dosage), and should decrease as radiotherapy techniques improve.

Age. Usually middle-aged adults.

Sex. Usually, women who have had irradiation for pelvic malignancy; sometimes men who have been treated for prostatic carcinoma and testicular tumours.

Clinical features

Acute radiation damage causes nausea, vomiting, abdominal pain and diarrhoea with blood or mucus, during and immediately after irradiation.

Many years after radiotherapy, chronic radiation damage causes:
● Malabsorption caused by bile-salt malabsorption or stasis-induced small bowel bacterial overgrowth
● Haemorrhage from telangiectasia or ulcerated mucosa
● Chronic proctocolitis
● Obstruction caused by stricture formation
● Perforation
● Fistulation
● Ischaemic infarction

Investigation

Haematology

FBC. Patients with blood loss or malabsorption may be anaemic.

Diagnostic imaging

● *Barium studies:* may show local dilatation, abnormal motility, strictures, ulceration and/or fistulae
● *Sigmoidoscopy and/or colonoscopy:* may show superficial ulceration, friability, telangiectasia and/or bleeding

Histopathology

Mucosal biopsy may be diagnostic.

Other

Tests for malabsorption may be abnormal.

Management

Acute radiation damage

Acute radiation damage is usually treated symptomatically with antidiarrhoeal drugs, bulking agents and/or rectal corticosteroids.

Chronic radiation damage

People with chronic radiation damage may need treatment to correct nutritional deficiencies, and antibiotics and colestyramine for bacterial overgrowth and bile acid malabsorption. Proctocolitis may respond to sulfasalazine or topical corticosteroid, and bleeding to colonoscopic diathermy or laser treatment. Surgery should be avoided if possible because healing of involved bowel is poor and anastomotic leakage is common.

Prognosis

The prognosis is often poor because radiation injury tends to be slowly progressive.

Vascular malformations of the gut

The two most important vascular malformations of the

gut are hereditary haemorrhagic telangiectasia (Osler–Rendu–Weber syndrome) and angiodysplasia. Both may present as difficult to diagnose chronic gastrointestinal blood loss.

Hereditary haemorrhagic telangiectasia (Osler–Rendu–Weber syndrome)

Epidemiology
Prevalence. Rare.

Genetics. Autosomal dominant.

Clinical features
Telangiectasia occur on mucous membranes and skin. Patients present with recurrent nosebleeds, gastrointestinal haemorrhage and/or microcytic anaemia.

Investigation
Mucosal gut lesions can be seen on OGD, colonoscopy or angiography.

Management
Treatment is by endoscopic electrocoagulation or laser, or surgery.

Angiodysplasia
Angiodysplasia is a recently recognized acquired vascular anomaly occurring most commonly in the right colon.

Epidemiology
Prevalence. The true prevalence is unknown because it is usually clinically silent and hard to diagnose.

Age. Associated with ageing.

Disease mechanisms
The cause is unknown, but raised venous pressure may be contributory. There is an association with aortic stenosis and primary biliary cirrhosis. The lesions appear as slightly raised dilated submucosal vessels (Fig. 10.57), which on histology are dilated, distorted and thin-walled.

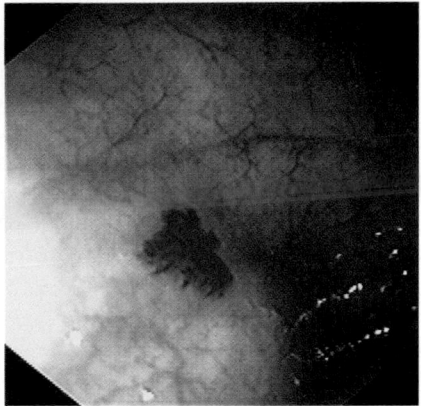

Figure 10.57 Endoscopic appearance of a 3-mm angiodysplasia in the colon. Reproduced from Cotton PB, Williams CB. *Practical Gastrointestinal Endoscopy*, 3rd edn. Oxford: Blackwell Scientific Publications, 1990 with the permission of the authors.

Clinical features
Clinical features are usually chronic bleeding and anaemia. Look for aortic valve disease, which may be associated. Occasionally, haemorrhage is acute and severe.

Investigation
Colonoscopy or high-quality selective arteriography confirms the diagnosis.

Management
The lesions can be treated either colonoscopically with electrocoagulation or laser, or by surgical resection (e.g. right hemicolectomy). Neither approach is necessarily curative as further lesions may develop.

Neuroendocrine disorders

Tumours arising from apud cells (see p. 659) are called apudomas (Table 10.49).

Table 10.49 Clinical features and diagnosis of apudomas (all are rare)

Tumour	Major gastroenterological (and other) features	Diagnostic factor
Gastrinoma (Zollinger–Ellison syndrome)	Peptic ulceration, diarrhoea, steatorrhoea	Gastrin
VIPoma (Verner–Morrison syndrome)	Watery diarrhoea, hypokalaemia, achlorhydria	Vasoactive intestinal polypeptide (VIP)
Carcinoid syndrome	Diarrhoea, flushing, wheezing, endocardial fibrosis, hepatomegaly, pellagra	Urine 5-hydroxyindole acetic acid (5-HIAA)
Medullary carcinoma of the thyroid	Diarrhoea, flushing, local invasion	Calcitonin
Insulinoma	Hypoglycaemia, neuropsychiatric disturbance	(See p. 791)

10

Carcinoid syndrome

Carcinoid tumours arise from apud cells in the intestine. In patients with small bowel tumours and hepatic metastases (or extraintestinal primaries), secretion of a variety of pharmacologically active molecules causes the carcinoid syndrome of diarrhoea, flushing, wheezing and right-sided cardiac signs. Rarely, the tumour occurs as part of multiple endocrine neoplasia (MEN) type I (see p. 864).

Disease mechanisms

An intestinal carcinoid tumour causes carcinoid syndrome only when there are hepatic metastases. This is because pharmacologically active products from the intestinal primary are inactivated on reaching the liver via the portal vein. Functioning carcinoid cells synthesize 5-hydroxyindoles from the essential amino acid, tryptophan. The diversion of tryptophan metabolism away from nicotinamide can cause pellagra. The main secretory products are:

- Tryptophan metabolites: 5-hydroxytryptophan (5-HTP); 5-hydroxytryptamine (5-HT) (serotonin); inactive 5-hydroxyindole acetic acid (5-HIAA)
- Kinins
- Histamines
- Prostaglandins

5-HT, kinins, histamine and prostaglandins cause diarrhoea by their effects on motility and mucosal fluid transport. All except 5-HT cause flushing.

Carcinoid tumours occur most commonly in the appendix (where they are usually benign), and small bowel. Other sites include the rectum, stomach, colon, duodenum and Meckel's diverticulum, as well as the lung, testis and ovary.

Epidemiology

Prevalence. About 2 in 100 000 of the population and only about 10% of these cause carcinoid syndrome.

Age. From middle age onwards.

Clinical features

Carcinoid tumours may present incidentally (e.g. at appendicectomy or postmortem), or with obstruction, perforation or bleeding. Alternatively, there may be (non-functioning) metastatic disease with cachexia and hepatomegaly.

Features of carcinoid syndrome are:
- Flushing, which can cause facial telangiectasia and a violaceous complexion
- Diarrhoea
- Attacks of wheezing

- Endocardial fibrosis causing pulmonary and tricuspid valve dysfunction with right ventricular hypertrophy and failure
- Hepatomegaly caused by metastases
- Rarely, pellagra

Differential diagnosis

Full-blown carcinoid syndrome is easy to diagnose. Rarely, a similar syndrome of flushing and diarrhoea may be produced by medullary carcinoma of the thyroid, phaeochromocytoma or systemic mastocytosis, in which malignant proliferation of mast cells is associated with histamine hypersecretion.

Investigation
Biochemistry
- *24-h Urinary excretion of 5-HIAA* (a breakdown product of 5-HT): usually increased. If it is not, but a neuroendocrine tumour is suspected, a serum gut hormone screen to rule out the other specific neuroendocrine tumours (Table 10.49) is indicated
- *Liver function tests:* performed because of the possibility of hepatic metastases

Diagnostic imaging
- *Chest radiography, ultrasound, CT scan and barium radiology:* used to localize the tumour and to detect metastases
- *Radioisotope scanning:* using radiolabelled octreotide or ^{131}I-meta-iodobenzyl guanidine (^{131}I-MIBG) localizes neuroendocrine tumours in about 50% of patients

Histopathology
Biopsy of liver metastases is diagnostic.

Other
ECG and echocardiography are required to assess right ventricular, pulmonary and tricuspid valve function.

Management
Drugs. Diarrhoea usually responds to anti-5-HT agents (e.g. cyproheptadine) and somatostatin derivatives (e.g. octreotide). Flushing may improve with methyldopa, phenoxybenzamine, corticosteroids, and sometimes chlorpromazine as well as somatostatin. Treatment with cytotoxics is disappointing.

Radioisotopes. Cytotoxic doses of ^{131}I-MIBG can be helpful in patients with metastases that take up this radioisotope.

Surgery. Surgical cure is possible if the tumour is detected before metastasizing. Prolonged palliation can then be achieved by enucleation of hepatic metastases, partial hepatectomy or hepatic arterial ligation, or embolization, with appropriate pharmacological steps to prevent carcinoid crisis.

Prognosis

Carcinoid tumours are slow-growing and, even with multiple metastases, survival may be prolonged: 40% at 5 years and 15% at 10 years.

Other apudomas

The main clinical features of other apudomas are shown in Table 10.49.

Gastrinoma (Zollinger–Ellison syndrome)

Gastrinoma is a rare tumour of gastrin-producing apud cells.

Disease mechanisms

The tumour usually arises in pancreatic islet D cells and, more rarely, in the duodenum or gastric antrum. It is often small (less than 1 cm in diameter). Most are malignant, but slow-growing. There may be multiple tumours.

Excess gastrin secretion causes:
- Acid hypersecretion and therefore peptic ulceration
- Diarrhoea resulting from the inhibitory effect of gastrin on intestinal absorption, the high volume of gastric secretion and intestinal hurry
- Steatorrhoea resulting from inactivation of pancreatic lipase, bile-salt precipitation and small bowel mucosal damage by excess acid

Clinical features

Most people with gastrinoma have dyspepsia because of severe duodenal and even jejunal ulceration, and watery diarrhoea. Some have steatorrhoea, reflux oesophagitis or a complication of peptic ulceration (e.g. haemorrhage, perforation).

About 20% of people with gastrinoma have multiple endocrine adenomatosis (MEA) type I.

Investigation
Biochemistry
- *Serum gastrin:* there is usually a fasting hypergastrinaemia (greater than 1000 pg/ml; normal less than 100 pg/ml)
- *Gastric acid secretion:* can be measured for diagnosis and monitoring of the response to treatment. Most people with gastrinoma have basal acid outputs higher than 15 mmol/h (normal is less than 5 mmol/h) with little rise on maximal stimulation
- *Serum calcium:* should be checked to screen for MEA type I

Diagnostic imaging
- *OGD:* shows florid duodenal bulbar and postbulbar ulceration. There may also be gastric rugal hypertrophy and excess fasting residue
- *Ultrasound, isotope scanning (as for carcinoid), CT scan, selective arteriography, percutaneous transhepatic venous portography with pancreatic venous sampling for gastrin level and/or exploratory laparotomy:* may be used to search for the primary tumour

Management
Drugs. Sustained inhibition of gastric acid secretion can be effectively achieved by PPIs (Table 10.21, p. 686). Cytotoxic doses of ^{131}I-MIBG can help patients in whom the tumour takes up this isotope. 5-Fluorouracil-based chemotherapy sometimes induces remission in metastatic disease.

Surgery. If the tumour can be identified and there are no metastases, the best treatment is excision. If exploratory laparotomy fails to find the primary, highly selective vagotomy will reduce the dosage of antisecretory drugs required.

10

❗ Must know checklist

- Differential diagnosis and investigation of dyspepsia
- Medical treatment of peptic ulceration
- Investigation of dysphagia
- Assessment of nutritional status
- Causes and management of gastrointestinal bleeding

- Investigation of iron-deficiency anaemia
- Investigation and management of diarrhoea
- Positive diagnosis of irritable bowel syndrome
- Medical treatment of inflammatory bowel disease
- Whom to screen for colon cancer

Further reading

Books

Bloom S, ed. *Practical Gastroenterology*. London: Martin Dunitz, 2001.

Farthing MJG, Ballinger AB, eds. *Drug Therapy for Gastrointestinal Disease*. London: Martin Dunitz, 2001.

McDonald J, Burroughs A, Feagan B, eds. *Evidence Based Gastroenterology and Hepatology*. London: BMJ Books, 1999.

Journals

Gastroenterology, Official Journal of the American Gastroenterological Association, Elsevier. http://www2.gastrojournal.org/

Gut, BMJ Publishing Group. http://gut.bmjjournals.com/

Alimentary Pharmacology and Therapeutics, Blackwell Publishing. Print ISSN: 0269–2813 Online ISSN: 1365–2036

Websites

http://www.GastroHep.com
http://www.gastroendonews.com
http://www.medscape.com
http://www.gastroenterology.com

10

Diabetes Mellitus, Lipoprotein Disorders and Other Metabolic Diseases

11

Introduction

This chapter covers a number of conditions of increasing importance in both developed and developing countries. Diabetes mellitus, lipid disorders and obesity all contribute to the pathogenesis of atherosclerotic disease, the major cause of death in developed countries. Social changes, including an energy-rich high-fat diet and lack of physical exercise, have resulted in an increasing prevalence of obesity in both developed and developing countries. It is predicted that this will result in a metabolic time bomb with the prevalence of diabetes increasing rapidly with its associated sequelae.

Structure and function

Intermediary metabolism

The energy substrates of carbohydrates, fats and proteins are inter-related by what is termed intermediary metabolism, under hormonal regulatory control. Metabolic homoeostasis is essential to ensure the supply of substrates to all tissues in the varying conditions of basal state, feeding, exercise and starvation. Insulin has primarily anabolic actions and its effects on metabolism are antagonized by a number of factors including glucagon, corticosteroids, catecholamines and growth hormone.

Control of glucose metabolism (Fig. 11.1)

Glucose production

Approximately 200 g of glucose is produced and used each day, but blood glucose levels are tightly regulated in health within the range of 3.5–8.0 mmol/l. The brain is an obligate consumer of glucose utilizing approximately 100 g/day. After an overnight fast, glucose is being used by peripheral tissues, such as the brain, kidney and intestine. In contrast, skeletal muscle uses little glucose in the fasting state and derives most of its energy from the oxidation of fatty acids.

Total body glucose production mostly occurs in the liver by both glycogenolysis (the breakdown of glycogen) and by *de novo* production of glucose from gluconeogenic precursors. Renal gluconeogenesis makes only a small (5–10%) contribution to total daily glucose production.

Substrate supply when fasting

Liver glycogen is the major body store of carbohydrate for rapid release as glucose. Hepatic glycogenolysis is under hormonal control by insulin, glucagon, catecholamines and cortisol. In the fasted state, insulin levels are low and the effect of glucagon is to increase glycogenolysis. Gluconeogenesis occurs using the gluconeogenic substrates alanine, glutamine, pyruvate, lactate and glycerol (Fig. 11.1). The major source of gluconeogenic substrates is amino acids released from proteins by proteolysis.

If fasting is prolonged, then continued lipolysis releases fatty acids from adipose tissue and they are increasingly used as a fuel supply. In the liver, fatty acids are converted into the ketone bodies acetoacetate and 3-hydroxybutyrate, which can be utilized by peripheral tissues including the brain. Insulin and glucagon have opposing effects on hepatic ketone body synthesis with insulin decreasing and glucagon increasing the formation of ketone bodies.

Postprandial changes

After feeding, blood glucose concentration rises because of absorption of carbohydrate from the intestine. In order to prevent a major rise in blood glucose concentration, hepatic gluconeogenesis must be switched off and glucose disposed to peripheral tissues. Rising blood glucose concentration stimulates the release of insulin and inhibits the release of glucagon, thus altering the ratio of these two antagonistic hormones.

The major effect of insulin is to switch the liver from a

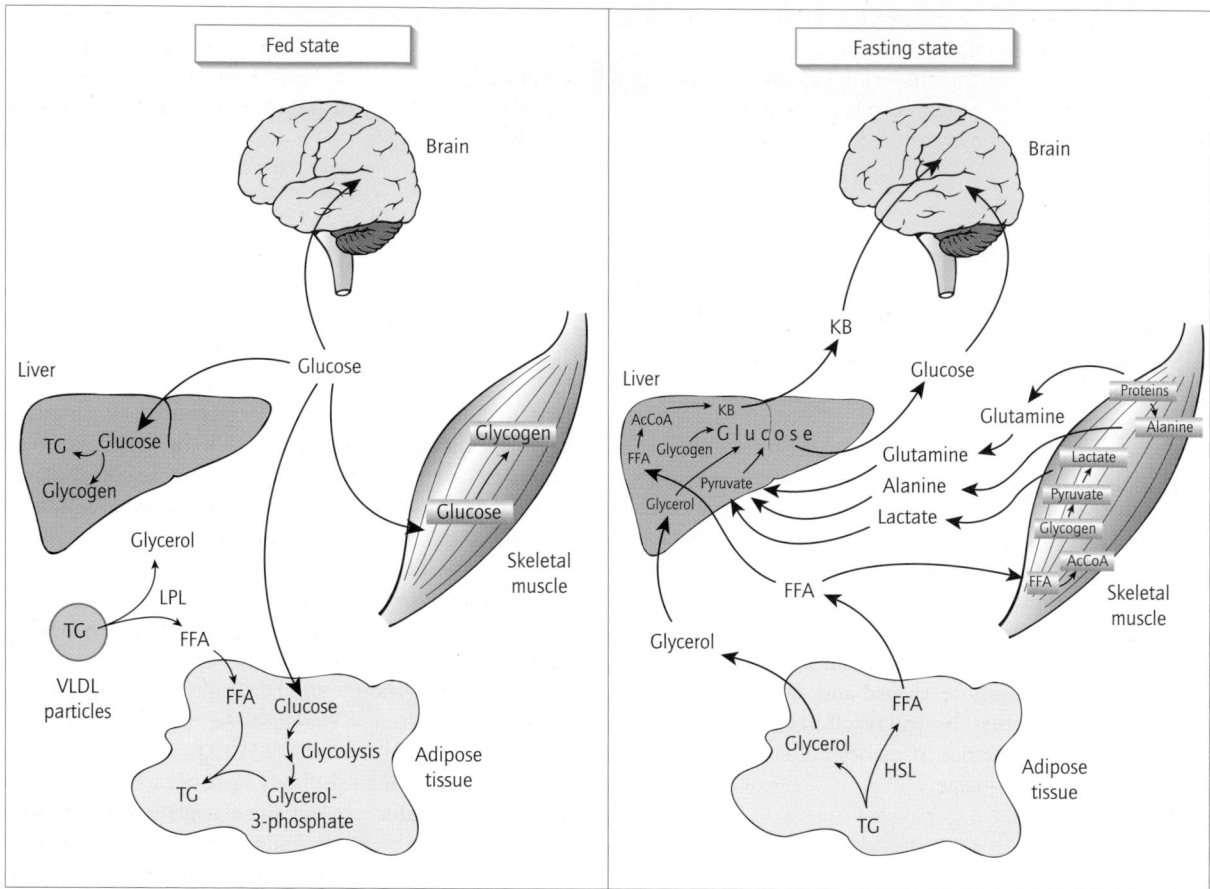

Figure 11.1 Metabolic pathways of fuel substrates in (a) fed and (b) fasted states. Ac CoA, acetyl CoA; FFA, free fatty acids; HSL, hormone-sensitive lipase; LPL, lipoprotein lipase; KB, ketone bodies; TG, triglyceride; VLDL, very low-density lipoprotein.

producer of glucose to a glucose store. Hepatic gluconeogenesis is suppressed by inhibition of glycogen phosphorylase both by the high insulin : glucagon ratio and by direct inhibition of the enzyme by glucose via an allosteric mechanism.

Glucose enters hepatocytes down its concentration gradient, but requires the action of insulin to stimulate entry into skeletal muscle and adipose tissue. In the liver, glucose is converted to glycogen by insulin-induced stimulation of glycogen synthase and is used as a source of glycerol-3-phosphate for use in triglyceride synthesis. During the high insulin concentrations found after a meal, insulin acts on skeletal muscle and adipose tissue to increase glucose uptake, with the larger depot being in skeletal muscle:

● In skeletal muscle, insulin stimulates glucose uptake and increases the activity of glycogen synthase
● In adipose tissue, insulin increases glucose uptake and suppresses lipolysis by inhibiting hormone-sensitive lipase. The action of insulin to suppress lipolysis in adipose

tissue also removes the supply of glycerol as a gluconeogenic precursor in the liver

Catecholamines and cortisol

Catecholamines (norepinephrine, epinephrine) and cortisol both antagonize the action of insulin to lower blood glucose.

Catecholamines have a direct action on the liver to stimulate glycolysis. Catecholamines also have an indirect effect on the liver by stimulating lipolysis in adipose tissue, thus increasing the supply of fatty acids and glycerol to the liver. Oxidation of fatty acids in the liver increases the supply of cytosolic citrate, tending to increase hepatic gluconeogenesis, with glycerol being used as a substrate for gluconeogenesis.

Cortisol increases both proteolysis and lipolysis, thus increasing the supply of gluconeogenic substrates to the liver. Cortisol also reduces the sensitivity of tissues to insulin (insulin resistance), making the same amount of insulin less effective in controlling blood glucose concentrations. An important clinical consequence of these metabolic responses is that under stress situations, such as sepsis or trauma, the increased release of corticosteroids and catecholamines may result in hyperglycaemia.

Metabolic diseases and their management

Diabetes mellitus

Diabetes mellitus (DM) is a cluster of conditions united by chronic hyperglycaemia (raised blood glucose). Diabetes mellitus has been known since ancient times, with descriptions dating back to 1550 BC. Diabetes is named after the Greek root for a siphon, a particularly apt name for a disorder characterized by excessive thirst ('polydipsia') and excessive urination ('polyuria'). The sweet taste of the urine in diabetes mellitus was described in Indian Vedic literature in the 6th century AD, rediscovered in the West in the 17th century AD and shown to be a result of the presence of a sugar in the 18th century AD.

Diabetes mellitus is the most common endocrine disorder and has implications for both the individual and society. Patients with DM often need to make major changes to their lifestyle to manage their condition and they have a reduced life expectancy. Life expectancy is reduced by about 20 years in type 1 DM and by about 10 years in type 2 DM. Morbidity and mortality are both increased in patients with DM because of macrovascular and microvascular complications.

Macrovascular complications
- *Ischaemic heart disease:* angina, myocardial infarction, heart failure, arrhythmia
- *Peripheral vascular disease:* claudication, lower limb gangrene, amputation
- *Cerebrovascular disease:* stroke, transient ischaemic attack

Microvascular complications
- *Retinopathy:* visual loss, blindness
- *Nephropathy:* renal failure, nephrotic syndrome
- *Neuropathy:* sensory, motor and autonomic nerves

DM has significant resource implications for health care systems, mainly because of the cost of treating the associated complications but partly because of the direct cost of managing hyperglycaemia. Hyperglycaemia is important because in the short term it may produce symptoms and in the long term hyperglycaemia is strongly associated with the development of the **microvascular** complications of diabetes.

Classification and terminology

It is recommended that the terms non-insulin-dependent diabetes mellitus (NIDDM) and insulin-dependent diabetes mellitus (IDDM) are no longer used because they may result in people being classified by their treatment modality rather than their disease characteristics. Most people (approximately 85%) with DM have type 2 diabetes, a significant group (10–15%) have type 1 diabetes and the rest a number of secondary causes of DM. It may not be possible to decide which type of DM a person has when they are initially diagnosed.

Type 1 diabetes mellitus
This is characterized by the loss of the insulin-producing pancreatic islet β cells, resulting in absolute insulin deficiency. People with type 1 DM are prone to develop ketoacidosis and require insulin treatment for survival.

Type 2 diabetes mellitus
This is characterized by relative insulin deficiency and insulin resistance, either of which may be predominant at the time of presentation. People with type 2 DM do not require insulin for survival, but may be treated with insulin to improve symptoms of DM or for better metabolic control.

Gestational diabetes mellitus
This is the development of glucose intolerance during pregnancy.

Other types of diabetes mellitus
If the specific cause of DM is known (e.g. postpancreatectomy) then it is classified under **secondary causes or other types of DM** (Table 11.1). The World Health Organization (WHO) revised its classification of DM in 1999, withdrawing the classification of malnutrition-related diabetes mellitus, because there is little evidence to suggest that malnutrition causes DM.

DM is found in many endocrine disorders that should always be considered as possible diagnoses in a patient with newly diagnosed DM. Growth hormone, corticosteroids and catecholamines are all antagonists of the action of insulin and can result in hyperglycaemia if they are produced in excess. Treatment of patients with secondary DM should be directed at the underlying disorder, as this may remove the cause of the hyperglycaemia.

11

Table 11.1 Causes of secondary diabetes mellitus

Iatrogenic
Corticosteroids
Thiazide diuretics

Endocrine
Cushing's syndrome
Acromegaly
Phaeochromocytoma
Thyrotoxicosis

Pancreatic disease
Fibrocalculous pancreatopathy
Chronic pancreatitis
Cystic fibrosis
Haemochromatosis
Pancreatectomy
Pancreatic carcinoma

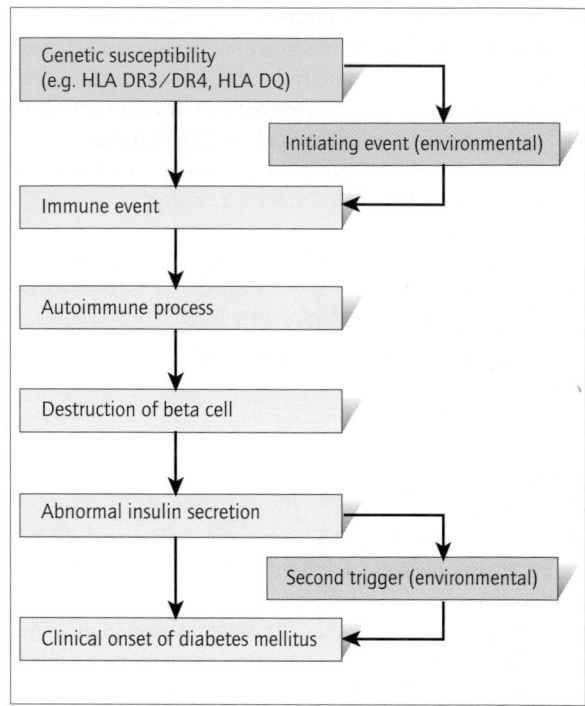

Figure 11.2 A simplified representation of a possible mechanism for the development of type 1 diabetes mellitus (DM).

Disease mechanisms

Type 1 diabetes mellitus

Type 1 DM is almost always an autoimmune disease with selective destruction of the insulin-producing pancreatic β cells, leading to insulin deficiency (Fig. 11.2).

Immunology

Type 1 DM is associated with a variety of other diseases with an autoimmune aetiology such as pernicious anaemia, vitiligo, Graves' disease and Addison's disease. Histological examination of pancreatic tissue from patients with type 1 DM shows evidence of infiltration of the islets of Langerhans by T cells ('insulitis') thought to represent an autoimmune process.

Serum from patients with newly diagnosed type 1 DM has been shown to contain two major groups of autoantibodies: islet cell antibodies (ICAs) and antibodies against glutamic acid decarboxylase (GAD), an enzyme found in pancreatic β cells. These antibodies may be found in serum from patients without clinical diabetes, suggesting that the disease process that results in type 1 DM has an extensive time course and does not necessarily result in clinical disease.

Genes

In white populations, the overall lifetime risk of developing type 1 DM is 0.4%, rising to 5–6% in first-degree relatives of patients with type 1 DM. Concordance rates for monozygotic twins are approximately 50%, while for dizygotic twins about 6%. These two pieces of information suggest a disease with a significant genetic contribu-

tion. Genome-wide searches for susceptibility genes for type 1 DM have revealed at least 10 chromosomal loci linked to type 1 DM. The loci with the strongest effects are the human leucocyte antigen (HLA) region on chromosome 6 and the insulin gene region on chromosome 11. The HLA gene region is complex, containing over 200 genes. HLA haplotypes DR3, DR4 and certain DQ types appear to increase and DR2 to reduce susceptibility to developing the disease. The HLA region contributes approximately 43% and the insulin gene region approximately 10% to the familial inheritance of type 1 DM, with the other loci making smaller contributions.

Environment

The clinical onset of type 1 DM peaks in the spring and autumn months, coinciding with higher incidence of viral infections at these times. It has been hypothesized that viral infections precipitate a final autoimmune insult to the pancreas, leading to clinical symptoms of DM. An alternative explanation is that viral infections decrease insulin sensitivity, which would result in an increased demand for insulin from a pancreas already depleted of insulin-secreting capacity. The pancreas might then decompensate in the face of increased demand.

Type 2 diabetes mellitus

Two metabolic defects are found in people with type 2 DM:

- *Insulin resistance:* or the reduced ability of tissues of the body to respond to physiological insulin concentrations
- *Relative insulin deficiency:* in relation to the increased requirement for insulin produced by the presence of the insulin resistance

Longitudinal studies suggest that insulin resistance occurs many years before the onset of diabetes in many people with a predisposition to type 2 DM. However, the clinical onset of diabetes is associated with declining pancreatic release of insulin. Pancreatic tissue from people with type 2 DM shows infiltration with fibrils of amyloid.

Genes

Twin studies show higher concordance rates for monozygotic than for dizygotic twins suggesting that shared genes, rather than a shared environment, contribute to type 2 DM.

Some populations have a high prevalence of type 2 DM (e.g. Nauruans in the South Pacific). Studies have shown that Nauruans with unsuspected foreign genetic admixture have a lower prevalence of type 2 DM compared to full-blooded Nauru islanders, despite sharing the same environment and cultural practices. This is strong evidence for a genetic effect on type 2 DM aetiology. Some patients with type 2 DM presenting before the age of 25 years have a clear autosomal dominant pattern of inheritance (maturity onset diabetes of young; MODY). Specific genetic defects have been discovered in most families with this pattern of diabetes.

Metabolic factors

Obesity is a major risk factor for the development of type 2 DM. Body fat distribution also seems to be important, with accumulation of abdominal rather than subcutaneous fat being deleterious. Obesity is known to increase the degree of insulin resistance, but the mechanism remains unclear.

Physical activity

Prospective studies have shown that those taking part in regular physical activity are less likely to develop type 2 DM. The effect appears to be independent of any effect the exercise may have on body weight. Exercise probably reduces the risk of type 2 DM by increasing whole body insulin sensitivity.

Fetal nutrition

Epidemiological studies in a number of populations have shown an increased prevalence of type 2 DM in low birth-weight babies compared to higher birth-weight babies. One explanation for this data is that poor fetal nutrition (caused by either poor placental development or lack of access to food by the mother during pregnancy) results in defective pancreatic organogenesis *in utero*. Later in life, with increased demands on the pancreas from the insulin resistance of obesity, the pancreas has a limited reserve; thus, relative insulin deficiency and clinical diabetes ensue.

Epidemiology

Type 1 diabetes mellitus

Type 1 DM most commonly presents in children, although it may occur at any age. The incidence increases from birth, with a peak at age 11–13 years. The sex distribution is equal. There are marked variations in prevalence between countries, with high rates being found in Scandinavia and Malta. There appears to be a seasonal variation in the date of diagnosis, with an increased incidence reported in spring and autumn months. The incidence of type 1 DM appears to be increasing, especially in the under-5 age group.

Type 2 diabetes mellitus

Type 2 DM usually presents in middle-aged or elderly adults, although it is uncommonly diagnosed in children. The sex distribution is roughly equal. The prevalence of type 2 DM increases with age, but varies markedly between different populations. The prevalence is higher in certain ethnic groups: South Asians have a sixfold higher risk and Afro-Caribbeans a threefold higher risk compared to white populations.

Environmental influences are important, with a higher prevalence in urban compared to rural populations of similar ethnic background. In developed countries, type 2 DM is slightly more common in people from lower social classes. Significant temporal trends in prevalence of type 2 DM are occurring (e.g. prevalence of DM in the USA increased by one-third between 1990 and 1998), probably as a result of the increasing prevalence of obesity.

Clinical presentation of diabetes mellitus

Diabetes mellitus should be **suspected** if:

- There are symptoms of diabetes
- Blood tests demonstrate hyperglycaemia
- Glycosuria is found on urinalysis
- A complication associated with diabetes is discovered

Symptoms of diabetes

These include thirst, polydipsia, dry mouth, polyuria, tiredness, blurred vision and unintentional weight loss. In addition, if diabetic ketoacidosis is present, symptoms

11

Diabetes mellitus: Clinical presentations at a glance

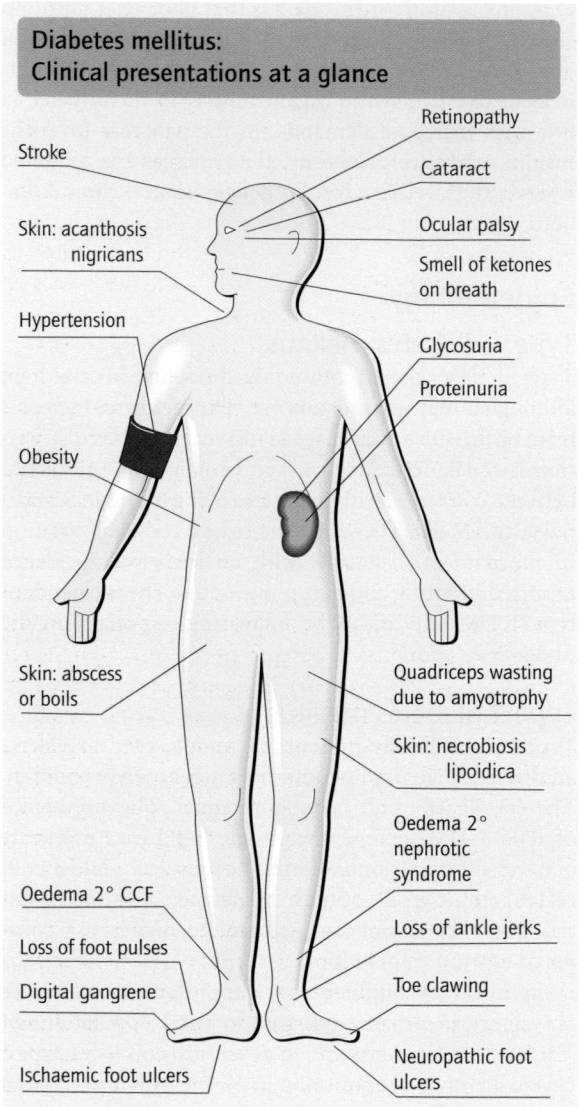

Stroke

Skin: acanthosis nigricans

Hypertension

Obesity

Skin: abscess or boils

Oedema 2° CCF

Loss of foot pulses

Digital gangrene

Ischaemic foot ulcers

Retinopathy

Cataract

Ocular palsy

Smell of ketones on breath

Glycosuria

Proteinuria

Quadriceps wasting due to amyotrophy

Skin: necrobiosis lipoidica

Oedema 2° nephrotic syndrome

Loss of ankle jerks

Toe clawing

Neuropathic foot ulcers

may include nausea, vomiting, shortness of breath, drowsiness and coma (HISTORY & EXAMINATION BOX 11.1).

Hyperglycaemia

In normal individuals, blood glucose concentrations usually fluctuate to a small degree, varying with the amount of time since food was last taken. A **fasting** plasma glucose more than 6 mmol/l or **non-fasting** more than 7.8 mmol/l is potentially abnormal and should be further investigated.

Glycosuria

The presence of an increased glucose concentration in the renal filtrate raises the osmotic pressure of the filtrate. This causes an osmotic diuresis, producing the symptoms of polyuria, dehydration and thirst. Glycosuria does not always indicate the presence of diabetes (and indeed, the absence of glycosuria does not indicate the absence of diabetes). Glucose usually starts to appear in the urine when blood glucose values rise above a threshold between 10 and 13 mmol/l.

Renal glycosuria is a renal tubular disorder in which glycosuria occurs with **normal** blood glucose levels. In this disorder, the glucose in the renal filtrate is unable to be completely reabsorbed because of a reduction in the maximum transport capacity of the glucose-reabsorbing transporters in the renal tubules. It is important to recognize this in order to avoid repeated unnecessary investigations.

Complications

The complications associated with diabetes are discussed in detail below. Opticians may detect the presence of diabetic retinopathy after a visit provoked by blurred vision (HISTORY & EXAMINATION BOX 11.2). Skin infections, including boils and abscesses, are more common in diabetics and such a presentation should prompt a request for a blood glucose test.

11

History & Examination 11.2

General appearance
Does the breath smell of ketones?
Is the patient overweight or obese?
Are there skin changes—necrobiosis lipoidica, acanthosis nigricans?
Are there skin infections—abscesses and boils?
Is there candidiasis?
Is there muscle wasting (amyotrophy)?
Is there evidence of cerebrovascular disease?

Eyes
Is there retinopathy?
Are there cataracts?
Is there an ocular palsy?

Cardiovascular
Is there hypertension?
Are the peripheral pulses present?
Are there bruits?

Feet
Are there foot ulcers?
Is there ischaemia of the feet?
Are there neuropathic changes?
Is there oedema?

Neurological
Is there sensory loss resulting from neuropathy?
Is there loss of reflexes or power resulting from neuropathy?
Are there neuropathic changes in the skin or muscles?

Urine
Is there ketonuria?
Is there glycosuria?
Is there proteinuria?

Investigation

Diagnostic tests

Diabetes mellitus is present if:
- There are symptoms of diabetes and the blood glucose is significantly raised, *or*
- In the absence of symptoms of diabetes, the blood glucose is significantly raised on more than 2 days and there is no acute illness

Diabetes mellitus can usually be diagnosed on the basis of a non-fasting venous plasma glucose of greater than 11 mmol/l if there are symptoms of diabetes. If there are no symptoms of diabetes, it is important to repeat the blood glucose sample on another day because transient hyperglycaemia may occur in stress situations, such as infections. If a non-fasting glucose is borderline it is usual to take a blood glucose after a 10-h fast.

The 1999 WHO agreement on the diagnosis of diabetes mellitus lowered the fasting glucose concentration used for the diagnosis of diabetes to 7.0 mmol/l (venous plasma). It is important to note that the type of blood sample used (venous or capillary, plasma or whole blood) affects the reference values (Table 11.2). Special considerations apply during pregnancy (see p. 777).

A diagnosis of diabetes mellitus is usually lifelong (unless diagnosed during pregnancy or resulting from secondary causes) and has significant implications for driving, employment and life insurance premiums. It is therefore important to ensure the diagnosis is certain before informing a patient. Diagnosis should be based on laboratory blood samples rather than a capillary blood glucose monitor reading, and repeated in asymptomatic people.

If there is still doubt, or a strong clinical suspicion, a 75-g oral glucose tolerance test should be performed and the result interpreted using the criteria in Table 11.2. People with impaired glucose tolerance (IGT) have an increased risk of developing diabetes. Clinical trials in those with IGT have shown that weight loss and increased physical activity reduce the risk of developing diabetes.

Urinalysis to look for the presence of ketonuria should be performed in everyone presenting with symptoms of diabetes and hyperglycaemia. Heavy ketonuria (3+ or more) suggests the possibility of DKA and the need for urgent specialist assessment.

Differentiating type 1 from type 2 diabetes mellitus

Type 1 DM is most likely to present in a child or young

Table 11.2 Diagnosis of diabetes mellitus and impaired glucose tolerance. Revised World Health Organization guidelines (1999)

	Venous plasma (mmol/l)	Venous whole blood (mmol/l)	Capillary whole blood (mmol/l)
Diabetes mellitus			
Fasting	≥7.0	≥6.1	≥6.1
2 h post glucose load	≥11.1	>10.0	≥11.1
Impaired glucose tolerance			
Fasting	<7.0	<6.1	<6.1
and			
2 h post glucose load	≥7.8	≥6.7	≥7.8

adult (under 30 years old) with a short history (weeks) and marked symptoms of weight loss. Ketonuria (2+ or greater) will be found at presentation. A metabolic acidosis may be present (HCO_3^- less than 18 mmol/l or arterial pH less than 7.36). No markers of microvascular complications of DM will be found at diagnosis because hyperglycaemia has not been present for long enough for them to develop. Autoantibodies indicating autoimmune pancreatic damage (ICAs, anti-GAD antibody; see p. 764) should be present, but are not usually measured in routine clinical practice.

Type 2 DM, in contrast, often has an insidious onset. Most people will be asymptomatic, but some may have an acute onset of symptoms. A high index of suspicion for diagnosing DM should be held for people in high-risk groups: family history of type 2 DM, obesity, past history of gestational DM, ethnic groups with increased prevalence of DM (South Asians, Polynesians, Afro-Caribbeans). Ketonuria is absent or minimal (1+). Some may have microvascular complications of DM when first diagnosed, because the asymptomatic prodrome may be as long as 6–10 years.

Long-term complications of diabetes mellitus

Long-term complications of DM are conveniently classified as either macrovascular or microvascular (Fig. 11.3).

Macrovascular complications

In developed countries macrovascular complications are the leading cause of death in people with diabetes—40–50% of people with DM die from these causes. Factors that contribute to the increased risk include:

- Increased prevalence of hypertension in DM
- Unfavourable lipid profile
- Abnormalities in the clotting system
- Effect of hyperglycaemia on progression of atherosclerotic lesions

The relative risk of developing cardiovascular disease with DM is two- to threefold in men and three- to fourfold in women compared to age- and sex-matched controls without DM. Approximately 1 in 5 people having coronary artery bypass grafting have DM. Relative risk of cerebrovascular disease is threefold higher. The relative risk of having a lower limb amputation is up to 15 times higher and approximately half the people having a lower limb amputation have DM.

Microvascular complications

The duration and severity of hyperglycaemia are strongly related to the development of microvascular complica-

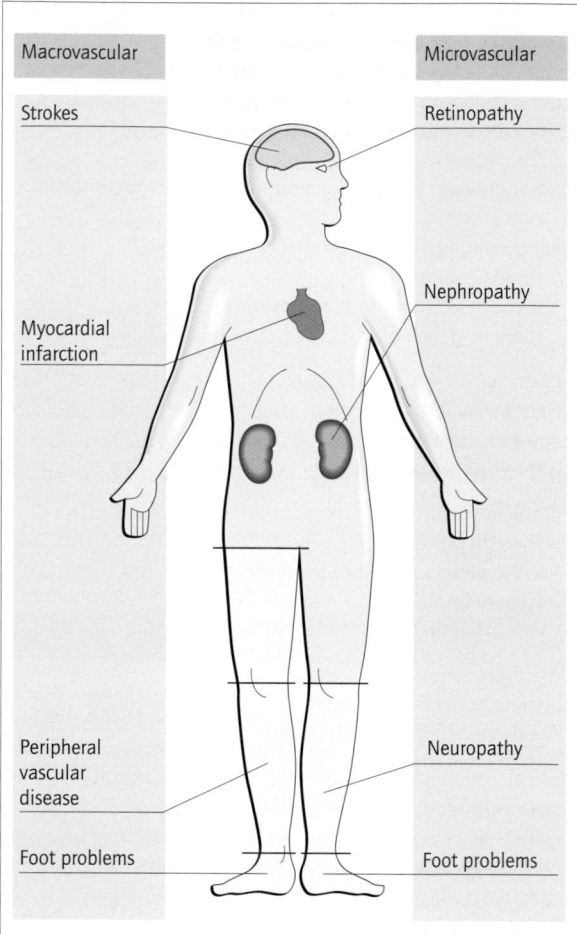

Figure 11.3 Common macrovascular and microvascular complications of DM.

tions. Indeed, the threshold for diagnosing diabetes is based on epidemiological consideration of the risk of developing retinopathy with increasing blood glucose values:

- Diabetic retinopathy is the leading cause of visual loss and blindness in the under-65 age group
- Diabetic nephropathy is the leading cause of end-stage renal failure and the need for renal dialysis in developed countries. Approximately 1 in 6 people starting renal replacement therapy has DM
- Diabetic neuropathy contributes to the pathogenesis of foot ulceration in DM

Management

Management of the patient with diabetes aims to improve the symptoms of hyperglycaemia and to retard the development of complications of DM, but with an acceptable level of side-effects from treatment. A number of clinical trials have established that over the long term the closer to normal that blood glucose is maintained, then the lower the risk of **microvascular** complications of DM. Separate trials have examined this question in both type 1 and type 2 DM. The key trials showing this were the Diabetes Control and Complication Trial (DCCT) for type 1 DM and the UK Prospective Diabetes Study (UKPDS) for type 2 DM. There is little evidence that improving glucose control reduces the **macrovascular** complications of DM. In type 2 DM tight blood pressure control reduces the incidence of stroke and heart failure and the progression of retinopathy. Lipid-lowering therapy has been contentious in DM because early clinical trials had few patients with DM. However, emerging evidence indicates that patients with DM do benefit from lipid-lowering medication.

Education

All patients with diabetes need education about their condition, including the symptoms of hypoglycaemia and how to treat it, the symptoms of hyperglycaemia, and how to manage their diabetes if they are unwell with another illness. Diet plays an important part in the management of DM (Table 11.3). Many learn how to test capillary blood glucose levels so that they can make adjustments to their treatment. Patients with type 1 DM also need education about how to recognize the symptoms of ketoacidosis. All patients with diabetes should be discouraged from smoking because of the high risk of cardiovascular disease that their diabetes already confers on them. People with diabetes are usually required to inform their licensing authority about their condition if they possess a driving licence. Women with diabetes are usually fertile, but need to be aware that metabolic control needs to be optimal before pregnancy to reduce the likelihood of congenital malformation in the fetus. Diabetes is a long-term disorder and health care providers need to inspire and challenge their patients to help them manage their condition.

Monitoring glucose control

Random clinic blood glucose readings

These provide little information apart from indicating asymptomatic hypoglycaemia or marked hyperglycaemia.

Fasting blood glucose readings

In patients with type 2 DM, these are of value because they correlate reasonably well with overall glucose values.

Self-testing of capillary blood glucose

Most people with DM can be taught to use a portable meter, but it does require the discomfort of taking the sample from a finger or ear lobe (Fig. 11.4). The blood

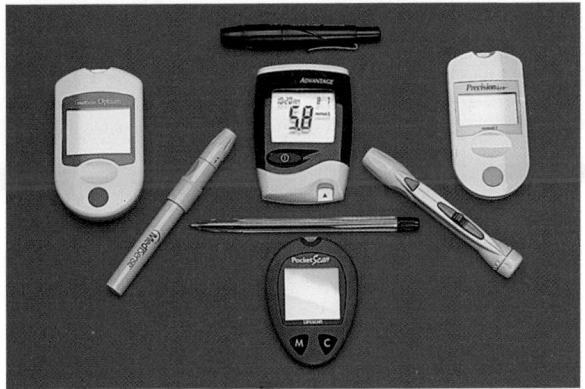

Figure 11.4 A range of capillary blood samplers and capillary blood glucose analysers. A standard ballpoint pen is included as a size comparator.

test strips used with these meters can be costly. Self-monitoring is especially valuable for patients with type 1 DM, who are more likely to have wide variations in their blood glucose concentrations. The information obtained can be used to alter their diet, insulin or exercise regimen. Values obtained from blood glucose meters are often inaccurate at the extremes of their measurement ranges: at glucose concentrations below 3 mmol/l (hypoglycaemia) or above 20 mmol/l.

Glycated haemoglobin assays

Proteins are irreversibly modified in the presence of glucose by a non-enzymatic chemical reaction, which adds a glucose molecule to amino acid side-chains. Haemoglobin protein is glycated at physiological concentrations of glucose producing a number of molecules with altered electrophoretic mobility. The higher glucose concentrations found in DM result in more haemoglobin being glycated and this has been validated as a test to indicate the degree of hyperglycaemia. The glycated haemoglobin isoform most widely used to monitor diabetes control is HbA_{1c}. Because red blood cells have a life-span of 120 days, the glycated haemoglobin assay taken at one point in time gives an indication of the average glucose concentration for the previous 2 months. Glycated haemoglobin assays have been invaluable as a means of assessing glucose control over the medium term and are not significantly affected by manipulating diet or treatment in the week before a clinic appointment. They are not sensitive or specific enough to be used to diagnose DM and should be restricted for use in monitoring people with known diabetes.

Urine testing for glucose

Glycosuria occurs when the renal threshold for glucose is

Diabetes mellitus at a glance

Epidemiology

Prevalence in UK
Type 1 diabetes mellitus (DM) 25 in 10 000
Type 2 DM 200 in 10 000

Age of onset
Type 1 usually under 30 years
Type 2 usually over 30 years

Genetics
Implicated in both type 1 and type 2 DM

Geography
High prevalence of type 1 DM in Scandinavia and Malta; higher prevalence of type 2 DM in South Asians, Afro-Caribbeans, Polynesians

Findings on investigation
Symptoms of DM

plus
Random venous plasma glucose ≥11.1 mmol/l

or
Fasting venous plasma glucose ≥7.0 mmol/l

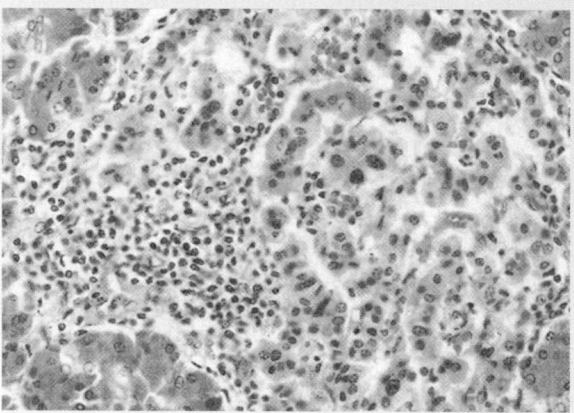

Fig. A Infiltration of islets with chronic inflammatory cells, resulting in insulitis. In recent-onset type 1 DM most islets are insulin deficient, with residual B cells showing 'insulitis' which could be a product of autoimmune destruction. H&E stain, magnification × 300. Both figures reproduced from Williams & Pickup, *Handbook of Diabetes*, 1992 (Blackwell Scientific Publications, Oxford) with the permission of the authors.

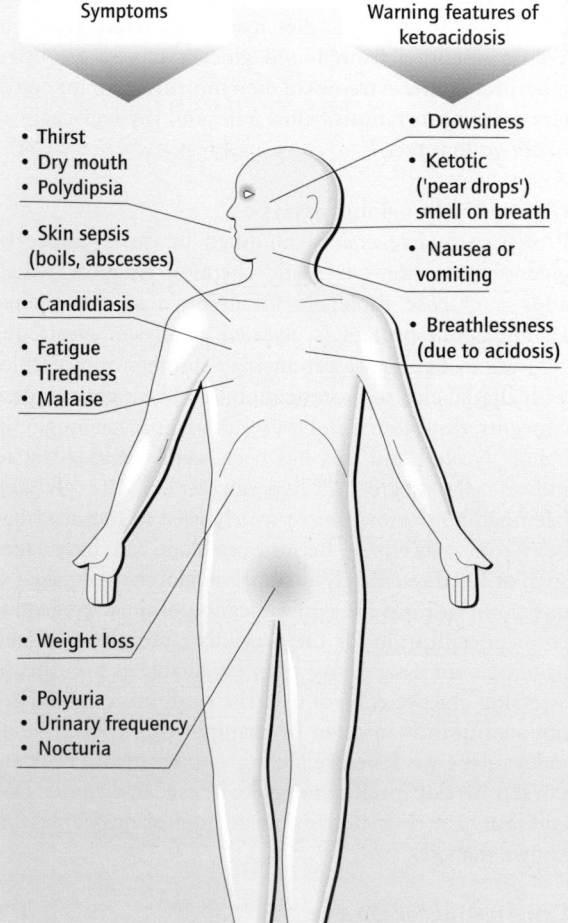

Symptoms

- Thirst
- Dry mouth
- Polydipsia

- Skin sepsis (boils, abscesses)

- Candidiasis

- Fatigue
- Tiredness
- Malaise

- Weight loss

- Polyuria
- Urinary frequency
- Nocturia

Warning features of ketoacidosis

- Drowsiness
- Ketotic ('pear drops') smell on breath
- Nausea or vomiting
- Breathlessness (due to acidosis)

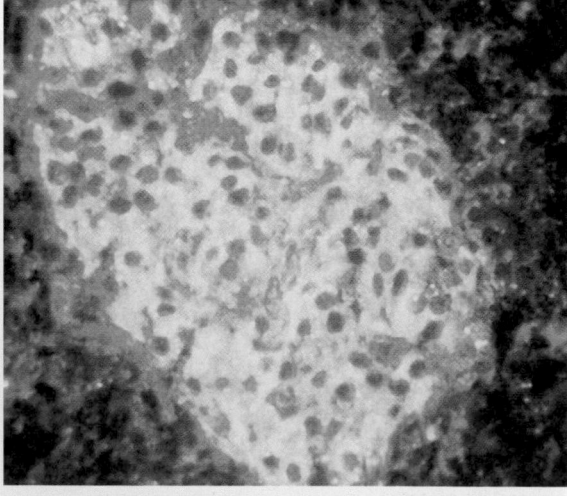

Fig. B Human pancreas stained with anti-human IgG fluoresceinated serum: the cells within the islets are strongly positive.

Urinalysis

Urine should be tested in all people with suspected or newly diagnosed DM. Ketonuria 3 + suggests the possibility of ketoacidosis requiring emergency treatment

Glycated haemoglobin (HbA_{1c} or HbA_1) should not be used for *diagnosis* of DM. It is useful for monitoring glycaemic control

Complications

Long-term complications include:

Microvascular disease
- *Retinopathy*
- *Nephropathy*
- *Neuropathy*

Macrovascular disease
- *Coronary heart disease*
- *Peripheral vascular disease*
- *Cerebrovascular disease*

Table 11.3 Management of diabetes

Supportive care	**Macrovascular complications**
Education of patient, family and/or carers by nurses, dietitians, group education classes, cookery classes, diabetes charities (e.g. Diabetes UK, American Diabetes Association), summer camps for young people with DM	*Prevention* Stop smoking Seek and treat hypertension Seek and treat hyperlipidaemias Optimize weight Take adequate exercise Educate about foot care
Specific treatment *Diet* *Weight:* aim for 5–10% weight loss if obese, or ideal body weight if feasible *Carbohydrates:* restrict intake of refined carbohydrates (e.g. sugar, jams, sweets, chocolate) and some restriction on complex carbohydrates (e.g. rice, pasta, potatoes) *Proteins:* generally little restriction except for calorie control *Fats:* reduce saturated fats and substitute with polyunsaturated or monosaturated vegetable oils *Alcohol:* limit to sensible drinking guidelines of 2–3 units/day; avoid binge drinking	*Screening* Check for evidence of cardiac disease or peripheral vascular disease Check footcare *Specific treatment* Medical and/or surgical treatment of ischaemic heart disease Prophylaxis for transient ischaemic attacks (aspirin) and surgery (endarterectomy) in selected cases Reconstructive surgery or amputation for peripheral vascular disease
Exercise Increase physical activity level if inactive and able to become more active	**Microvascular complications** *Prevention* Good blood glucose control Good blood pressure control Eye examination (acuity, fundoscopy, retinal photography) Look for evidence of nephropathy (microalbuminuria or albuminuria) Examine for evidence of neuropathy (reflexes, sensation, postural hypotension)
Oral hypoglycaemics In type 2 DM if diet and exercise alone are inadequate *Metformin:* if obese *Sulphonylureas:* if slim α-Glucosidase inhibitors *in either group* Combination therapy often required	
Insulin Generally mandatory in type 1 DM May be required for metabolic control in type 2 DM Precise type of insulin and regimen depends on individual patient's lifestyle and requirements	*Specific treatment* Photocoagulation for retinopathy Cataract extraction ACE inhibitors/AT1 antagonists in microalbuminuric nephropathy Plan for renal replacement therapy Symptomatic measures to relieve neuropathic problems
Monitoring glycaemic control Monitor with glycated haemoglobin and/or home blood glucose measurements Feedback results to alter behaviour and/or medical therapy	

11

exceeded; however, this varies between individuals. Some individuals with type 2 DM appear to be able to control their diet with feedback from urinalysis testing. Urinalysis cannot detect hypoglycaemia.

Urine testing for ketones

Mild ketonuria (1+) occurs in all individuals after fasting overnight because of the use of ketone bodies for gluconeogenesis. Heavy ketonuria (3+) is suggestive of the possibility of ketoacidosis. It is useful for patients with type 1 DM to test their urine for ketones if they develop marked and persistent hyperglycaemia because it may indicate incipient ketoacidosis, which may be avoided if early action is taken.

Diet

All patients with DM should receive dietary advice. Dietary change is as effective as medication in reducing hyperglycaemia in type 2 DM. However, maintaining dietary change is difficult and requires regular reinforcement. In the obese, weight loss of 5% of body weight improves metabolic control, both by restricting the intake of carbohydrate and by increasing insulin sensitivity. Patients with DM are advised to follow a healthy eating plan of low fat, increased fibre and restricted carbohydrate intake. This is often achieved by increasing their intake of vegetables, pulses and fruit, and reducing the amount of processed foods. Simple carbohydrates (glucose, fructose, sucrose) from sources such as sugar, confectionery, cake and soft drinks should be restricted, but are not forbidden.

Oral hypoglycaemic agents

Sulphonylureas

This group of drugs acts by binding to receptors on pancreatic β cells, stimulating insulin release (the sulphonylurea receptor is a subunit of a gated K^+ channel). Sulphonylureas rely on the presence of insulin within the pancreas and so eventually become less effective as continuing pancreatic damage reduces the available store of insulin for release. Their main side-effect is hypoglycaemia but they may also cause skin rashes and a metallic taste in the mouth. Examples include glibencamide, gliclazide, tolbutamide, chlorpropamide and glipizide. Glibencamide and chlorpropamide have longer half-lives and are therefore more likely to cause hypoglycaemia. Chlorpropamide taken with alcohol causes a reaction of flushing, vomiting, hypotension and sweating in approximately one-third of people.

Biguanides

The exact mechanism of action of biguanides is uncertain but they reduce hepatic glucose production and increase insulin sensitivity. Metformin is the only available example of this class of drug. Side-effects of metformin include nausea, indigestion, diarrhoea and reduced absorption of vitamin B_{12}. A rare but serious adverse effect of biguanides is lactic acidosis, which has a reported mortality of 50%. Metformin is contraindicated in the presence of renal or hepatic failure because there is reduced metabolism of metformin and an increased risk of lactic acidosis. The biguanide phenformin was withdrawn from use after an unacceptably high incidence of lactic acidosis.

α-Glucosidase inhibitors

These drugs act on the small bowel by inhibiting enzymes involved in the digestion of oligosaccharides to monosaccharides, thus reducing postprandial hyperglycaemia. The undigested oligosaccharides are delivered to the large bowel where they may be fermented by bacteria, resulting in the side-effects of flatulence and diarrhoea.

Thiazolidinediones (glitazones)

Thiazolidinediones reduce blood glucose concentrations by increasing whole body insulin sensitivity, which makes the available endogenous insulin more effective. They bind to a nuclear hormone receptor (PPARγ) and so alter the transcription of insulin-sensitive genes. They have a mild hypoglycaemic action, which is potentiated when they are combined with biguanides or sulphonylureas. Side-effects include skin rashes, fluid retention and gastrointestinal disturbance. Examples include pioglitazone and rosiglitazone. The first available thiazolidinedione, troglitazone, was withdrawn after an excess of deaths from hepatic failure; therefore, it is currently recommended that liver function be monitored in patients taking thiazolidinediones.

Insulin and insulin analogues

Insulin is a polypeptide of 51 amino acids and is absolutely required for the treatment of people with type 1 DM. It may also be used for treating people with gestational DM or type 2 DM. Endogenously produced insulin is synthesized as the prohormone proinsulin. This is then sequentially cleaved by endopeptidases to create mature insulin consisting of an A and a B chain linked by disulphide bonds (Fig. 11.5). In this process, the intervening amino acids are removed as C-peptide.

Insulin was manufactured for many years by purification from animal pancreas glands and this type of insulin is still widely available. However, most insulin now produced is the result of a biotechnological process, whereby genetically engineered bacteria or yeast synthesize human insulin, which is then purified from the culture medium. This technique increases the reliability of production and purity, reduces the risk of prion transfer from animal-derived products and allows for the production of insulins with different amino acid sequences.

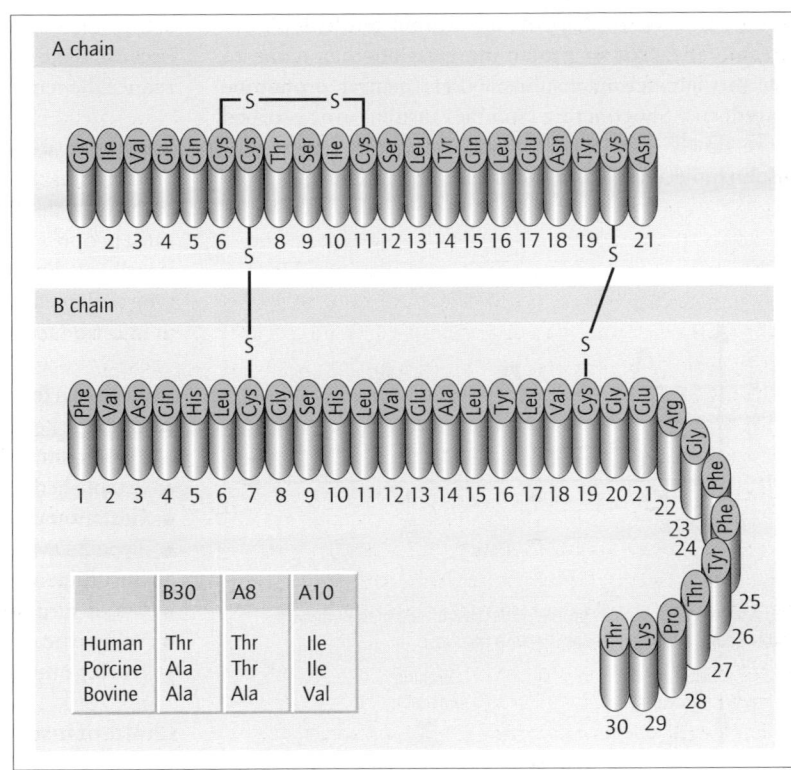

Figure 11.5 Structure of insulin. The amino acids that differ between human, porcine and bovine insulin are shown in blue.

	B30	A8	A10
Human	Thr	Thr	Ile
Porcine	Ala	Thr	Ile
Bovine	Ala	Ala	Val

Table 11.4 Factors affecting insulin absorption rate

Type of insulin	Rapid analogue > soluble > isophane
Site of injection	Abdomen > arm > thigh
Injection technique	Inadvertent intramuscular injection is more rapidly absorbed
Physical activity	Raises skin blood flow increasing absorption
Insulin temperature	Slower absorption if cold from fridge
Volume of insulin	Larger volumes have smaller surface area : volume ratio

Table 11.5 Features of different insulin preparations

Type	Rapid	Short	Intermediate	Long
Synonyms		Soluble Clear	Isophane NPH	
Examples	Aspart Lispro	Actrapid Humulin S Velosulin	Humulin I Insulatard	Glargine
Onset of action (min)	10–20	15–60	60–120	20–40
Peak action (h)	0.4–1.0	2–4	4–8	1–24
Duration of action (h)	3–5	4–8	18–24	24–36

Insulin is a polypeptide so it is inactive given by the oral route and is usually administered by subcutaneous injection. The standard strength for insulin preparations is 100 units/ml. The absorption of insulin from subcutaneous injection sites varies according to the type of insulin, the site of injection, skin temperature, temperature of the insulin, amount of physical activity being taken and the volume of injected fluid (Table 11.4).

Many brands of insulin are available, but are essentially short acting, intermediate acting, insulin analogues or mixtures of these (Table 11.5). Intermediate-acting insulins are cloudy in solution because of the addition of a

11

protein or zinc to delay its absorption into the bloodstream. The protein protamine gives another name to intermediate-acting insulins: NPH (neutral protamine Hagedorn). Short-acting (soluble) insulins are absorbed more slowly than expected because of the tendency of insulin molecules to form relatively stable hexamers. Rapid-acting insulin analogues have a faster onset of action because their amino acid sequences have been altered to reduce the tendency of insulin to form hexamers.

Starting insulin treatment

Starting insulin treatment can be a major milestone because of the fear of self-injecting; however, in practice most people's fears are worse than the reality. If the patient is well, insulin treatment can be started as an outpatient as long as there are support staff available to give instruction in injection technique and blood glucose monitoring.

Indications for insulin therapy

- Diabetic ketoacidosis
- Hyperosmolar non-ketotic diabetic coma
- Established type 1 DM
- Gestational DM where diet is insufficient
- Type 2 DM where diet and oral hypoglycaemic agents are insufficient
- Major surgery in people with DM
- Post myocardial infarction
- During any severe illness where there is a risk of DKA

Choice of insulin

The choice of insulin regimen is often tailored to the individual patient. A common insulin regimen is injection of a biphasic insulin mixture, containing both short-acting and intermediate-acting insulin, before breakfast and before the evening meal (Fig. 11.6). Insulin requirements are often higher in the morning because of higher levels of cortisol, catecholamines and glucagon, which antagonize the action of insulin. Patients with type 1 DM are often treated with a basal-bolus regimen, which uses injection of short-acting insulin before meals and intermediate-acting insulin at bedtime. The aim of a basal-bolus regimen is to try to mimic physiological insulin release; however, it can only be an approximation. Patients with type 2 DM can be treated with a combination of oral hypoglycaemic agents plus a once daily injection of intermediate-acting insulin. The aim is to lower glucose levels overall by suppressing hepatic glucose production with insulin. Choice of an

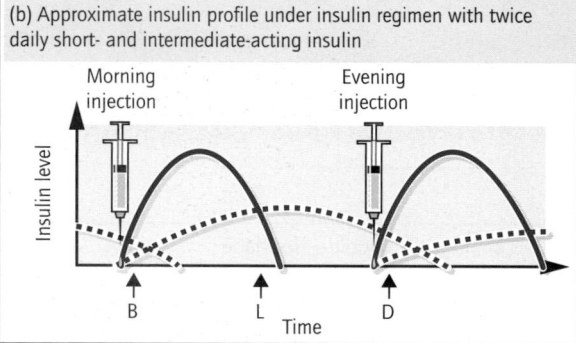

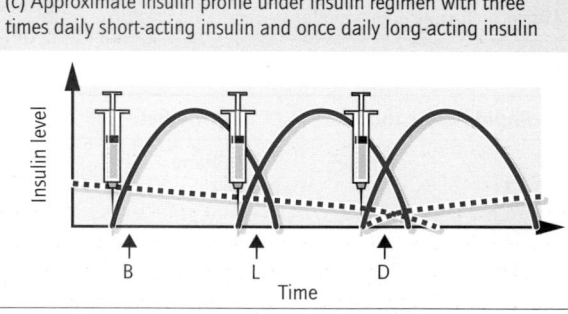

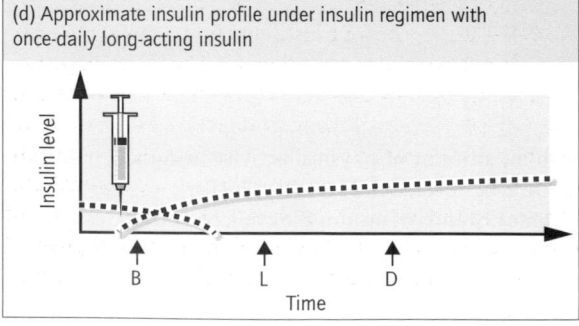

Figure 11.6 (*left*) Schematic representation of insulin profiles during a 24-h period in: (a) a non-diabetic individual, and in three different insulin regimens; (b) twice daily mixture of short- and intermediate-acting insulin; (c) three times daily short-acting insulin with once daily long-acting insulin (particularly useful in allowing flexibility in people with variable daily routines); and (d) once daily long-acting insulin (does not allow good glycaemic control so unsuitable for young people, but may be appropriate occasionally in elderly people where convenience is paramount and good control not essential). B, breakfast; L, lunch; D, dinner.

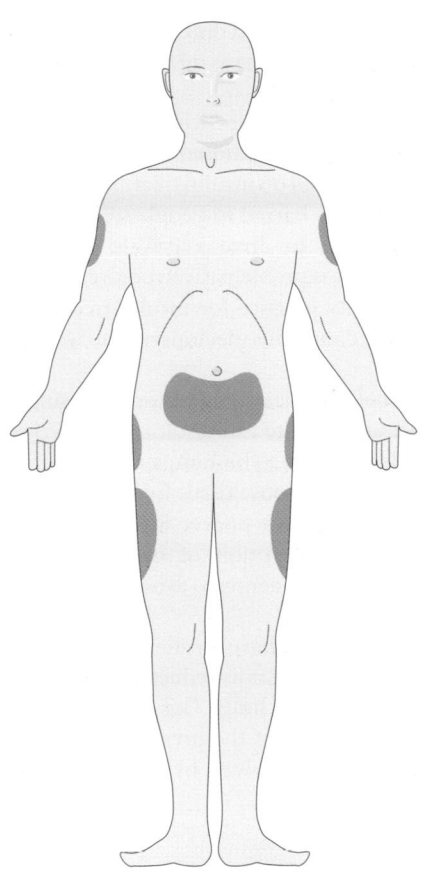

Figure 11.7 Recommended sites for insulin injection.

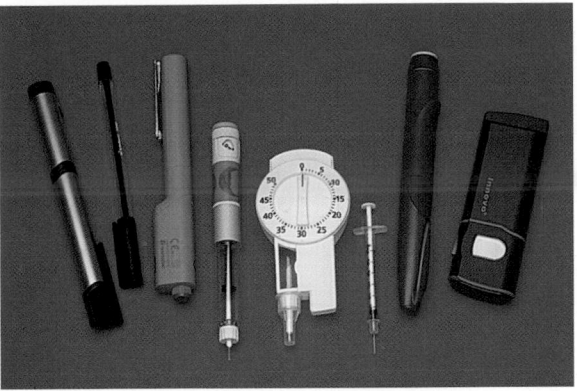

Figure 11.8 A range of insulin injection devices including a traditional insulin syringe, insulin 'pens' and other devices. A standard ballpoint pen is included as a size comparator.

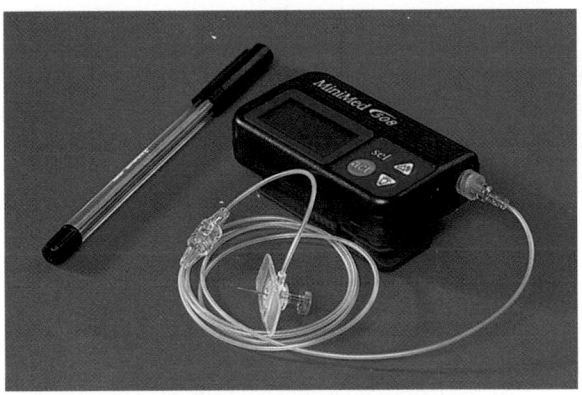

Figure 11.9 An example of an insulin pump device used for continuous subcutaneous insulin infusion. A standard ballpoint pen is included as a size comparator.

insulin regimen and adjusting dosage is a matter of specialist judgement.

Administration of insulin

Insulin is usually injected subcutaneously by the patient (Fig. 11.7). Insulin may be delivered by a traditional insulin syringe, a 'pen' injector or other injector device (Fig. 11.8). Patients with impaired vision or cognitive problems may need to have their insulin administered by carers. An alternative method of insulin administration is an insulin pump that continually infuses insulin subcutaneously at variable rates (Fig. 11.9). This method is unpopular in the UK, but more common in Europe and the USA.

Problems with insulin therapy

Hypoglycaemia. The major adverse effect of insulin treatment is hypoglycaemia. Symptoms of hypoglycaemia derive either from activation of the autonomic nervous system (tremor, sweating, anxiety, pallor, nausea, palpitations) or from dysfunction of CNS (impaired concentration, irritability, confusion, aggression, drowsiness, fitting, coma) or are non-specific symptoms (hunger, weakness, blurred vision). Most episodes of hypoglycaemia are mild, recognized by the subject and self-treated (Table 11.6). Patients with insulin-treated DM are advised to wear an identity bracelet so that they can be easily recognized as having diabetes and being at risk of a hypoglycaemic attack.

Hypoglycaemia occurs because of a mismatch of carbohydrate intake and insulin action—mostly because of the limitations of insulin therapy. Short-acting insulin has a relatively slow onset of action and a slow offset. An injection at 7 a.m. will have peak action between 9 and 11 a.m and may last up to 3 p.m. Therefore, to avoid hypoglycaemia, it is usually necessary to take a carbohydrate-containing snack mid-morning. A major cause of hypoglycaemia is eating late or taking increased physical exercise—a common combination when out on a shopping trip.

11

Table 11.6 Treatment of mild hypoglycaemia

If the patient is fully conscious and able to eat they should take a rapidly absorbed form of carbohydrate:
- 2–4 glucose (dextrose) tablets
- 2 teaspoons of sugar, honey or jam in water or milk
- A small glass of soft drink containing sucrose or glucose

Liquid solutions are more rapidly absorbed than solid forms. If there is no improvement after 5–10 min this should be repeated

A snack containing a source of more slowly absorbed carbohydrate (e.g. fruit, slice of bread, biscuit) should be taken to maintain blood glucose levels if the next meal is not due within 1 h

Table 11.7 Factors increasing hypoglycaemia in people using insulin

Excessive insulin dose
Dose recommended by doctor is too high
Intentional injection of larger or extra dose of insulin
Accidental injection of larger dose

Insufficient carbohydrate
Late meal
Missed meal
Dieting

Increased speed of insulin absorption
Exercise
Altered site of injection
Increased skin temperature from hot bath

Concomitant hypoglycaemic factors
Alcohol
Exercise

Nocturnal hypoglycaemia is a particular problem because the early warning symptoms are not recognized and the degree of hypoglycaemia is usually more severe before sweating, restlessness or even fitting wakes the patient. Patients are usually advised to take a bedtime snack to reduce the chance of nocturnal hypoglycaemia.

Factors that increase the risk of hypoglycaemia are intensive insulin regimens aiming for normoglycemia (e.g. during pregnancy), increased physical activity, alcohol use and duration of diabetes (Table 11.7).

Weight gain. Weight gain is common after starting insulin therapy. Weight gain in patients with type 1 DM is caused by the reversal of the catabolic state of insulin deficiency. Weight gain in patients with type 2 DM is partly caused by gain of the calories previously lost through glycosuria, but

also because of increased hunger from mild hypoglycaemia and continued excess intake of calories.

Social restrictions. People with diabetes are usually required to inform the national driving licence authority that they have started on insulin treatment. Some forms of driving licence are barred to people treated with insulin, although licences to drive a private vehicle are only restricted if there is problematic hypoglycaemia. It is good health and safety practice for insulin-treated employees not to operate dangerous machinery or to work at heights.

Lipohypertrophy. Repeated injection of insulin into the same subcutaneous site can result in the development of lumps under the skin. The lumps are a combination of fibrous tissue and adipose tissue hypertrophy. The blood supply to these regions is poorer, leading to unpredictable (usually worse) absorption of insulin. Injection sites should be rotated frequently to avoid this adverse effect.

Allergy. Some patients have an allergic reaction to insulin injections, which appears as redness around the injection site and generalized itching. This allergy is usually triggered by components of the preservatives in the insulin solution and is often solved by changing the brand of insulin used.

Pregnancy and diabetes mellitus

Diabetes mellitus that is already known about before the pregnancy is discussed below under 'Pregnancy and diabetes'. Hyperglycaemia discovered for the first time during pregnancy is known as **gestational diabetes**.

Pregnancy and diabetes

Most obstetric complications are increased in pregnant women with diabetes. In particular, the risk of congenital malformation, stillbirth and macrosomia (large fetus) are increased. Macrosomia probably arises because maternal hyperglycaemia is transmitted to the fetus, which responds by increasing its release of insulin. The growth factor activity of insulin means that fetal hyperinsulinaemia causes excessive fetal growth and excessive deposition of adipose tissue. In early pregnancy, metabolic changes such as ketonaemia, hyperglycaemia and hypoglycaemia are thought to affect organogenesis and cause congenital malformations. Diabetic complications, such as retinopathy and nephropathy, may worsen during pregnancy. DKA during pregnancy carries a high risk for the fetus with a fetal mortality of up to 50%. After birth, the baby of a mother with diabetes may develop hypoglycaemia and has a higher risk of respiratory distress syndrome.

Before becoming pregnant, women with diabetes are advised to take high-dose folic acid (5 mg/day) because of the increased incidence of fetal neural tube defects. Glucose control should also be improved if necessary before attempting to become pregnant. Oral hypoglycaemic drugs should be stopped because they are suspected to be teratogenic and insulin therapy should be started instead. During pregnancy, frequent visits to a diabetes specialist (e.g. every 2 weeks) are needed because insulin requirements increase by up to threefold. Screening for worsening of diabetic retinopathy should also occur. Macrosomia may prevent vaginal delivery and rates of caesarean section are increased in mothers with diabetes. Immediately following delivery, insulin requirements fall dramatically and insulin dosage needs to be adjusted to prepregnancy values. Diabetes is not a contraindication to breastfeeding, although some oral hypoglycaemic drugs appear in breast milk and should be avoided.

Gestational diabetes

Gestational diabetes is the appearance of glucose intolerance during pregnancy. Hyperglycaemia may occur during pregnancy because of increases in a number of hormones including placental lactogen, progesterone, prolactin and cortisol. Compared to the higher glucose values usually diagnostic of diabetes, the small degree of hyperglycaemia represented by impaired glucose tolerance is significant during pregnancy. Macrosomia and neonatal hypoglycaemia are increased in gestational DM. However, congenital malformations do not appear to be increased, because the hyperglycaemia develops after organogenesis has started.

Risk factors for gestational DM include:
- Obesity
- Family history of type 2 DM
- Previous gestational DM or a large baby (more than 4 kg)

Gestational diabetes is usually asymptomatic and usually develops during the second trimester. Screening for gestational DM should be offered to all pregnant women. The exact method used for diagnosing gestational DM, and at what stage to screen in pregnancy, is still debated. Methods used include the measurement of random or fasting glucose levels or a modified form of the oral glucose tolerance test. Initially, gestational DM is managed by diet, but if glucose values remain above normal, then insulin treatment is started. After delivery, gestational DM usually remits as the hormonal changes reverse. A small proportion of women remain diabetic, so it is usual to arrange a glucose tolerance test 6 weeks after delivery. Type 2 DM develops later in 30–50% of women with previous gestational DM. Weight gain is the most powerful predictor of this metabolic outcome in this group.

Surgery and diabetes

The care of patients with diabetes undergoing an operation is a frequent clinical problem. There are four main concerns:
1 Hypoglycaemia during surgery and/or anaesthesia, impairing recovery from the anaesthetic
2 Hyperglycaemia perioperatively, reducing the normal response to infection and impairing wound healing
3 Increased risk of developing metabolic decompensation (DKA and lactic acidosis)
4 Increased prevalence of cardiovascular disease in people with diabetes

General guidelines for glycaemic control perioperatively

Emergency surgery carries a higher risk of metabolic decompensation because of the release of stress hormones (catecholamines, cortisol, growth hormone) with actions that antagonize the effect of insulin.

Surgery on patients with DKA carries a high mortality. DKA should be considered in the differential diagnosis of patients with diabetes presenting with abdominal pain. Ideally, DKA should be treated before surgery is undertaken if surgery is necessary. For major elective operations, glucose control should be acceptable or improved preoperatively. Aim to maintain blood glucose between 4 and 11 mmol/l in the perioperative period.

It is safer to use glucose and insulin infusion for **all emergency operations**.

Type 2 diabetes mellitus on diet alone

For most procedures, monitor glucose and give insulin temporarily if needed. For emergency operations and operations needing intensive care postoperatively (e.g. coronary artery bypass graft), use insulin and glucose infusion as below.

Type 2 diabetes mellitus on oral hypoglycaemic agents

Metformin should ideally be stopped at least 24 h before surgery because of rare reports of postoperative lactic acidosis in patients taking metformin.

Morning list (nil-by-mouth from midnight)
Omit long-acting sulphonylureas (e.g. glibenclamide, chlorpropamide) the evening before surgery. Other oral hypoglycaemic agents may be taken as normal around the evening meal. Between 6 a.m and 8 a.m. start intravenous infusions of glucose and insulin (Table 11.8).

Afternoon list (nil-by-mouth from 9 a.m.)
Omit all oral hypoglycaemic medication in the morning.

11

Table 11.8 Surgery and diabetes mellitus

Glucose and insulin infusion ('sliding scale')
Start 5% glucose 1 l + 20 mmol KCl over 8 h
Slower infusions of 10% or 20% glucose may be used if fluid
  overload is a problem

Start an intravenous infusion of 50 units of soluble insulin
  made up to 50 ml with 0.9% sodium chloride (1 unit/ml)
  in a syringe pump driver
Deliver the following amounts of insulin according to the
  results of hourly capillary blood glucose measurements

Blood glucose (mmol/l)	Insulin dose (units/h)	Comments
≤4.0	0.5	Increase intravenous infusion of glucose by 30%
4.1–7.0	1.0	
7.1–11.0	2.0	
11.1–14.0	4.0	
14.1–17.0	6.0	
≥17.1	8.0	Check urine for ketones

Special circumstances
If blood glucose is not controlled the dose of insulin used
  should be altered either up or down
These suggested insulin doses are unsuitable for use with
  children
Patients with a history of heart failure or renal disease may
  need fluid restriction
In renal failure with hyperkalaemia, KCl should not be added
  to the infusate

Give 6 units of soluble insulin before breakfast. Between 10 a.m and 12 noon start intravenous infusions of glucose and insulin (Table 11.8).

Type 1 diabetes mellitus and Type 2 diabetes mellitus on insulin

Morning list (nil-by-mouth from midnight)
Patients on twice daily biphasic insulin should take **half** their usual dose of insulin with their evening meal the day before surgery. Patients on a basal-bolus regimen should take their usual dose of soluble insulin with their evening meal, but take **half** their usual dose of long-acting insulin at bedtime. No subcutaneous insulin should be given on the morning of surgery. Between 6 a.m and 8 a.m. start intravenous infusions of glucose and insulin (Table 11.8).

Afternoon list (nil-by-mouth from 9 a.m.)
Patients on twice daily biphasic insulin should take **half** their usual morning dose before a light breakfast. Patients on a basal-bolus regimen should take **half** their usual bed-time dose of long-acting insulin the night before surgery and **half** their usual morning dose of soluble insulin before a light breakfast. Between 10 a.m and 12 noon start intravenous infusions of glucose and insulin (Table 11.8).

Stopping intravenous insulin infusions

Once food and drink can be taken normally it is reasonable to resume the patient's usual treatment regimen. After a major operation, it is sensible to wait until the second attempted meal before deciding that they are eating and drinking normally. Creatinine should be normal before restarting metformin therapy. After complex surgery, it may be best to use insulin temporarily in patients with type 2 DM. Good glucose control is difficult to achieve in patients on 'sliding scales' if they are eating and drinking because the insulin dose always lags behind the rise in blood glucose post meal. If patients are eating and drinking normally, they should be converted to subcutaneous insulin to avoid this problem.

Complications of diabetes mellitus

Retinopathy

Disease mechanisms in diabetic retinopathy
Electron micrography indicates that the earliest change in diabetic retinopathy is thickening of the capillary basement membrane. Ongoing damage leads to the blood vessels becoming leaky, resulting in the loss of blood (blot haemorrhages) or fluid rich in protein and lipid (hard exudates). Some blood vessels become occluded, leading to ischaemia and the release of growth factors that stimulate the formation of new blood vessels. The new vessels lack supporting connective tissue and have a high risk of haemorrhage into the aqueous humour, resulting in sudden loss of vision.

Patterns of diabetic retinopathy
Diabetic retinopathy is classified into different patterns of disease, but these are not necessarily progressive steps from one to the other:
- Background
- Maculopathy
- Preproliferative
- Proliferative
- Advanced

Background diabetic retinopathy. Background diabetic retinopathy is the most common form of diabetic retinopathy. It is not usually seen until after at least 10 years of diabetes in type 1 DM, but may be found at diagnosis in up to 30% of people with type 2 DM. It includes 'dots' (microaneurysms), 'blot' haemorrhages and hard exudates (Fig. 11.10). The earliest visible feature on fund-

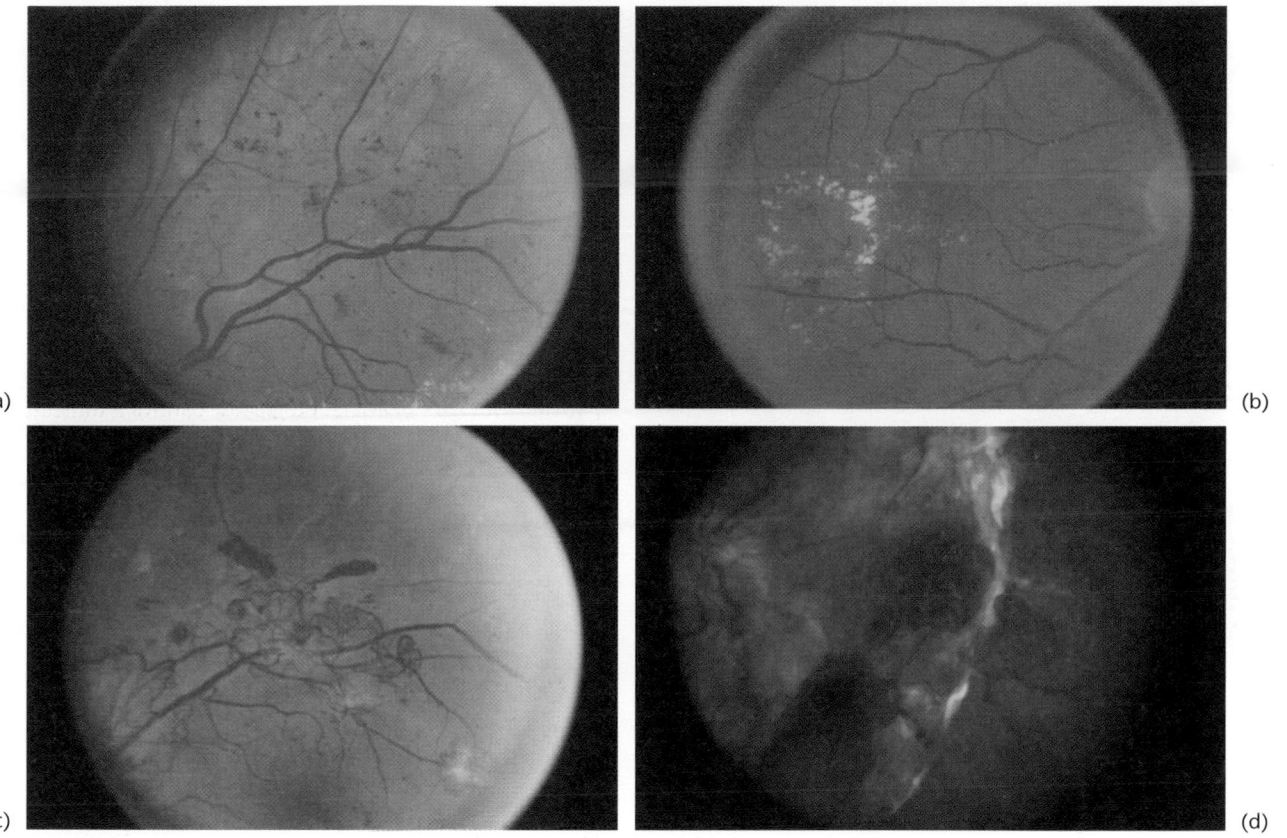

(a)

(b)

(c)

(d)

Figure 11.10 Different forms of diabetic retinopathy. (a) Background retinopathy, showing scattered red 'dots and blots' (microaneurysms and haemorrhages), and exudates. (b) Maculopathy, showing hard exudates encroaching onto the macula. (c) Proliferative retinopathy, showing leashes of new vessels and haemorrhages. (d) Advanced retinopathy, showing retinal detachment. Reproduced from Williams G, Pickup JC. *Textbook of Diabetes*. Oxford: Blackwell Scientific Publications, 1991 with the permission of the authors.

oscopy is the appearance of microaneurysms ('dots') that represent localized dilatation of the retinal capillaries. 'Blot' haemorrhages are small haemorrhages into the deep retinal layer. Hard exudates are white hard-edged areas that represent leakage of plasma containing proteins and lipid. Using fluorescein angiography, the earliest clinical features of diabetic retinopathy are capillary dilatation and capillary occlusion; however, these are not visible on direct fundoscopy.

Maculopathy. This is background diabetic retinopathy affecting the macula and associated with macular oedema. Macular oedema is difficult to detect with direct ophthalmoscopy, but is important because permanent central visual loss may occur if it is left untreated.

Preproliferative retinopathy. This heralds the onset of new vessel formation, which is the characteristic of proliferative retinopathy (see below). Preproliferative changes include cotton wool spots, venous beading and dilated abnormal capillaries. Cotton wool spots represent axonal transport interrupted secondary to ischaemia, but are not unique to diabetic retinopathy and may occur in other conditions.

Proliferative retinopathy. This occurs when new blood vessels are formed, usually from a major vein. These new vessels are liable to bleed and cause visual loss by vitreous or preretinal haemorrhage. New vessels on the optic disc are especially likely to bleed. The blood vessels grow because of the release of growth factors in areas of ischaemic retina.

Advanced diabetic retinopathy. This is the end result of proliferative retinopathy and is usually associated with profound irreversible visual loss. Clinical features are fibrous traction bands, retinal detachment and thrombotic glaucoma.

11

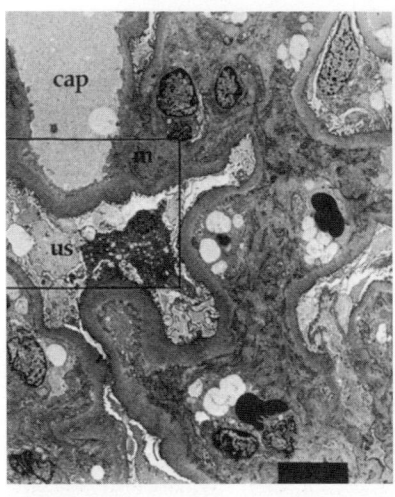
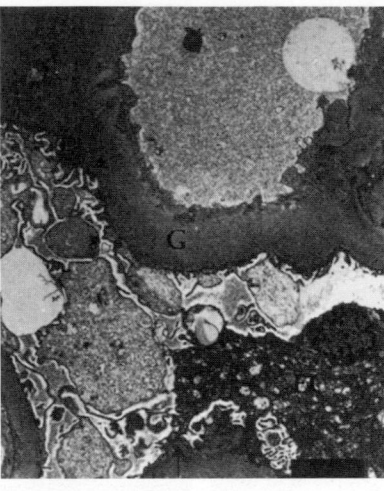

(a)　　　　　　　　(b)

Figure 11.11 Photomicrographs showing glomerular basement membrane thickening, and mesangial expansion in the kidney of a diabetic patient with nephropathy. (a) Magnification × 1700: m, mesangial cell and matrix; us, urinary space; cap, capillary lumen. (b) Magnification × 4300, enlargement of boxed area in (a), foot processes are arrowed: G, glomerular basement membrane; EC, epithelial cell. Reproduced from Williams G, Pickup JC. *Handbook of Diabetes*. Oxford: Blackwell Scientific Publications, 1991 with the permission of the authors.

Nephropathy

Disease mechanisms in diabetic nephropathy

Electron micrography of diabetic nephropathy shows that the glomerular basement membrane is thickened after only 2 years of diabetes (Fig. 11.11). Typically, the kidneys enlarge before the development of diabetic nephropathy because of a combination of enlargement of the glomeruli and of the tubulo-interstitium. The earliest light microscopy change of renal damage is enlargement of the mesangium, which is seen as periodic acid–Schiff (PAS)-positive extracellular material (glomerulosclerosis). If the mesangial enlargement contains nodules, this is known as the **Kimmelstiel–Wilson** lesion and is pathognomic of diabetic nephropathy (Fig. 8.18). The thickened basement membrane is functionally defective: it loses its normal negative charge and becomes more permeable to proteins, resulting in proteinuria. Initially, it is more permeable to small proteins, such as albumin, but the basement membrane eventually allows passage of larger proteins, such as immunoglobulins. Enlargement of the mesangium reduces the available surface area for filtration within the glomerulus and eventually results in the functional loss of nephrons. Renal failure occurs when a significant number of nephrons become non-functional. Glycosylation of proteins within the glomerulus may be one mechanism for the renal damage.

Longitudinal clinical investigation has shown that changes in renal function occur long before persistent proteinuria appears. Early changes include an **increased** renal blood flow, an **increased** glomerular filtration rate, and an **increased** glomerular capillary pressure.

Factors influencing renal function in diabetes

Renal damage may occur in long-standing DM because of:

- Diabetic nephropathy (glomerular damage)
- Renal artery stenosis and ischaemia
- Ascending infection
- Papillary necrosis

Clinical features of diabetic nephropathy

Diabetic nephropathy is characterized by persistent proteinuria, decreasing glomerular filtration rate and increasing blood pressure. In type 1 DM, the incidence of diabetic nephropathy peaks 10–20 years after diagnosis, but is not inevitable, because only about one-third of patients eventually develop overt nephropathy. The first clinical indication of the development of diabetic nephropathy may be the appearance of dipstick-positive proteinuria or worsening hypertension. Once diabetic nephropathy is established, glomerular filtration rate slowly declines, resulting in chronic renal failure and eventually end-stage renal failure.

Neuropathy

Diabetic neuropathies fall into a number of clinical presentations:

- Symmetrical sensory polyneuropathy
- Mononeuropathy and multiple mononeuropathy
- Autonomic neuropathy

Disease mechanisms in diabetic neuropathy

Symmetrical polyneuropathy is related to the duration of DM and to the severity of hyperglycaemia, suggesting a metabolic cause. Na^+/K^+ ATPase activity (required for maintaining the membrane potential of nerve tissue) is reduced in nerves from experimental models of diabetic neuropathy. Entry of glucose into nervous tissue does not depend on insulin so that neural cytoplasmic glucose concentrations closely follow blood concentrations. A number of theories invoking the elaboration of toxic metabolic products of excess cytoplasmic glucose have been proposed. The sudden onset of focal mononeuropathies strongly suggests a vascular cause, although some cases may result from pressure on exposed peripheral nerves (e.g. median nerve).

Symmetrical sensory polyneuropathy

This is the most common form of diabetic neuropathy and there is usually an insidious onset of loss of sensation in feet and occasionally hands ('glove and stocking' distribution). Patients may complain of 'walking on cotton wool'. It may be detected by an inability to feel a 10-g monofilament device, loss of vibration sense and reduced/lost ankle and/or knee jerks. Loss of proprioception in the joints may result in difficulty in walking or loss of balance when visual clues are absent (e.g. walking in dark or bending over to wash the face). Romberg's sign may be positive. Loss of peripheral nerve function also results in wasting of the small muscles of the feet and/or hands (Fig. 11.12).

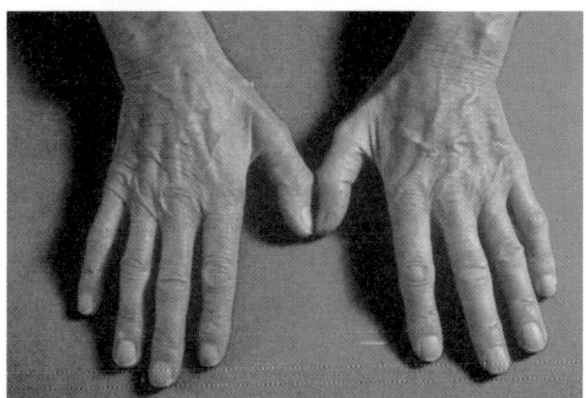

(a)

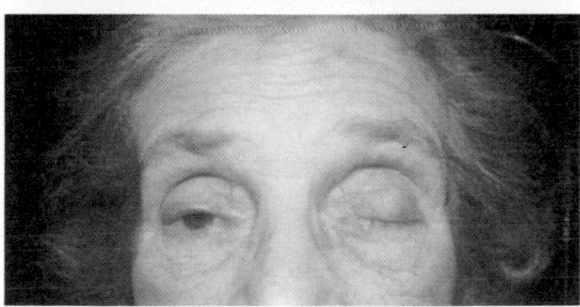

(b)

Figure 11.12 Diabetic neuropathies. (a) Generalized wasting of small muscles of the hands because of diffuse motor neuropathy. (b) Focal cranial nerve palsy causing left ptosis. Reproduced from Williams G, Pickup JC. *Handbook of Diabetes*. Oxford: Blackwell Scientific Publications, 1991 with the permission of the authors.

An acute painful form of sensory neuropathy is relatively rare. It presents with paraesthesiae, burning and electric shock-like pains in the feet and legs. It is often worse at night, disrupting sleep and patients may be unable to tolerate the pressure of bedclothes on their lower limbs. This clinical scenario may be associated with hyperglycaemia and weight loss before the diagnosis of diabetes has been made, but usually gradually improves with reduction of blood glucose. Occasionally—and inexplicably—acute painful sensory neuropathy may be associated with the institution of treatment for hyperglycaemia.

Mononeuropathy and multiple mononeuropathy

Sudden onset focal neuropathies of cranial nerves or peripheral nerves can occur occasionally in patients with DM. Sometimes more than one nerve is affected (mononeuritis multiplex). The cranial nerves most often affected are the oculomotor (IIIrd) and abducens (VIth) nerves and fortunately they often recover spontaneously (Fig. 11.12). Median nerve palsy (carpal tunnel syndrome), ulnar nerve palsy and common peroneal nerve palsy all occur with greater frequency in patients with DM and have a variable clinical outcome.

Proximal motor neuropathy (amyotrophy)

Amyotrophy is characterized by unilateral or bilateral pain and weakness in the quadriceps muscles. Typically, it affects older men with type 2 DM. Marked muscle wasting is often present, accompanied by weakness or difficulty in walking, reduced or absent knee jerks and sometimes extensor plantar reflexes. Poor glucose control is most often present and the condition usually responds to an improvement in glucose control. Many cases have resolved a year after onset. It is important to consider spinal cord compression as a differential diagnosis in the presence of extensor plantar responses.

Autonomic neuropathy

Autonomic nerve damage is a relatively common finding in long-standing DM if specialized autonomic function tests are performed, but it is uncommon as a cause of symptoms. Sympathetic and parasympathetic nervous system dysfunction in different organs results in a variety of clinical syndromes:

- *Cardiovascular:* loss of vagal (parasympathetic) tone produces a resting tachycardia and loss of sinus arrhythmia (the change in heart rate with respiration). Loss of sympathetic activity in arterioles results in peripheral vasodilatation and postural hypotension
- *Gastrointestinal:* delayed gastric emptying may produce symptoms of early satiety or, rarely, recurrent vomiting (gastroparesis). Diarrhoea, typically nocturnal, may be associated with faecal incontinence

11

Table 11.9 Comparisons between purely neuropathic and purely ischaemic diabetic feet

	Neuropathic foot	Ischaemic foot
Symptoms	Painless	Claudication
	Neuropathic pain	Rest pain
Signs	Full, bounding pulses	Weak/absent pulses
	Normal capillary return	Poor capillary return
	Warm skin	Cool skin
	Clawed toes	
	Dry (lack of sweating)	
Ulcer site	Metatarsal heads	Toes
		Heels

● *Atonic bladder:* loss of bladder smooth muscle tone results in incomplete emptying, stasis and an increased risk of urinary tract infection. In severe cases, the bladder is painlessly distended; atonic and overflow incontinence occurs
● *Gustatory sweating:* an unusual symptom whereby eating causes excessive facial sweating
● *Erectile dysfunction:* autonomic dysfunction contributes to erectile dysfunction (impotence)

Foot disease

Foot problems in diabetes can be caused by peripheral vascular disease or peripheral neuropathy, but commonly both are present to some degree. It is essential to assess the severity of each of these factors when presented with a problem diabetic foot (Table 11.9). The most common clinical problem is a non-healing foot ulcer. Ulcers occur because of either increased pressure at points on the foot and/or reduced skin nutrition from poor blood supply. Once an ulcer has formed and the epithelial barrier is breached, then infection may intervene, further compromising the likelihood of healing.

Neuropathic foot ulcer pathophysiology

Small-muscle wasting secondary to peripheral neuropathy results in weakness of the interosseous muscles in the foot. Unopposed action of the long flexors in the foot over time results in clawing of the toes and a high arch. These changes redistribute pressure over the foot, which creates points of high pressure over the metatarsal heads. Callus (hard skin) builds up over the metatarsal heads, but paradoxically this increases shear pressure in the underlying soft tissues, leading to haemorrhage and an inflammatory exudate. Rupture of this region through the overlying skin produces the ulcer (Fig. 11.13).

Ischaemic foot ulcer pathophysiology

In the presence of a limited blood supply, epithelial

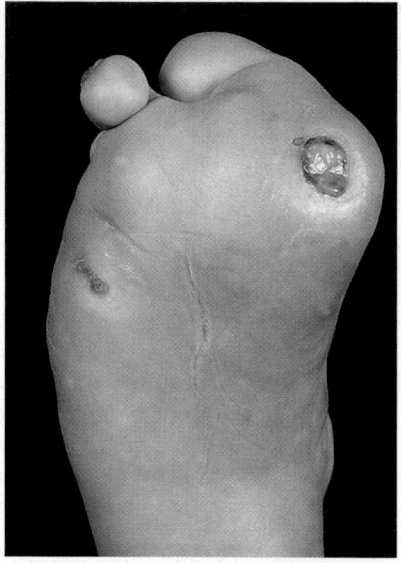

(a)

(b)

Figure 11.13 Neuropathic ulcers. (a) Typical 'punched-out' ulcer under first metatarsal head. Note previous amputations. (Reproduced by kind permssion of Dr Ian Casson, Broadgreen Hospital, Liverpool.) (b) Note particularly thickened callosities caused by high pressure area. (Reproduced from Williams G, Pickup JC. *Handbook of Diabetes*. Oxford: Blackwell Scientific Publications, 1992 with the permission of the authors.)

turnover is reduced (because of lack of oxygen and nutrients), producing skin that is thinner than normal and often flaky (Fig. 11.14). In addition, smoking further reduces the oxygen-carrying capacity of the blood. Skin in this situation is susceptible to damage

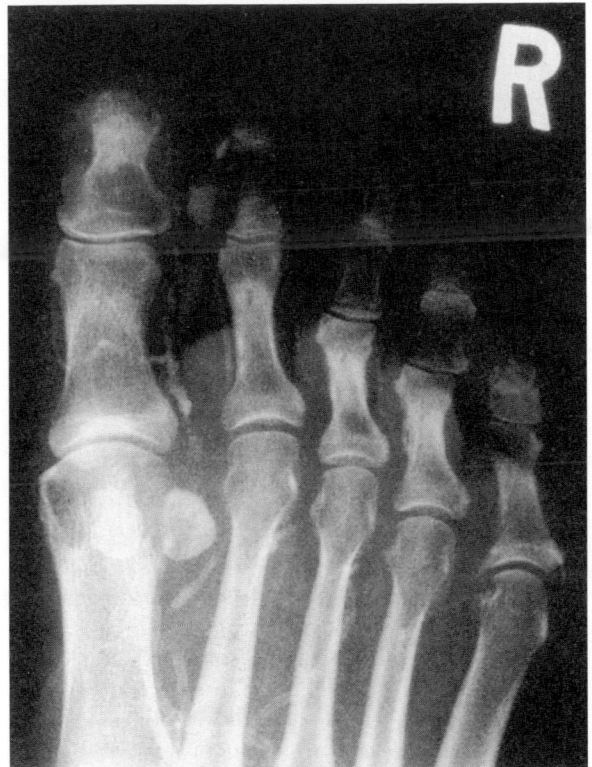

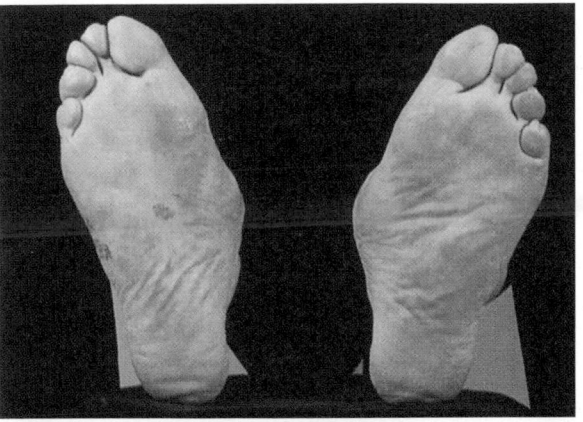

(a)

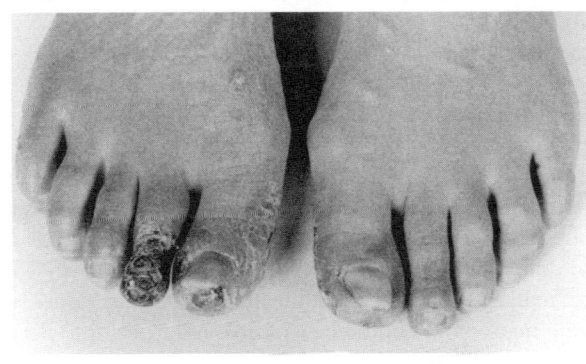

(a)

(b)

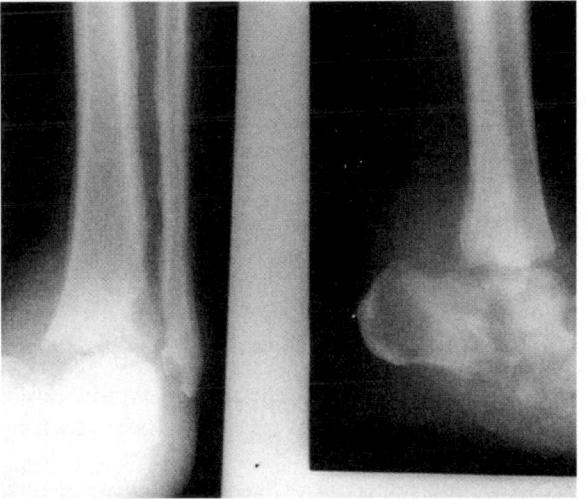

(b)

Figure 11.15 Advanced Charcot's arthropathy. (a) Gross disorganization of small joints in foot. (b) Radiograph of advanced Charcot's arthropathy showing destruction of the ankle and foot joints. Reproduced from Williams G, Pickup JC. *Handbook of Diabetes*. Oxford: Blackwell Scientific Publications, 1991 with the permission of the authors.

Figure 11.14 Ischaemic diabetic feet. (a) Radiograph showing medial artery calcification, a well-recognized feature in diabetics. (b) Digital gangrene typical of diabetic vascular disease. Reproduced from Williams G, Pickup JC. *Handbook of Diabetes*. Oxford: Blackwell Scientific Publications, 1991 with the permission of the authors.

Charcot's arthropathy

This is an unusual complication of neuropathic feet, presenting as a red, hot, swollen foot with or without pain. Infection is often initially suspected because of the cardinal features of inflammation being present. However, the condition can occur in the absence of infection. Radiographs are initially normal, but later show fracture, osteolysis, new bone formation and disorganization of the joint by subluxation (Fig. 11.15). Isotope bone scans show focal increased uptake in the region of bone affected. Subluxation of the joint may further alter pressure over the plantar aspect of the foot, increasing its risk of ulceration.

from external pressure, which results in hypoperfusion and anoxic tissue necrosis. External pressure from new shoes worn for too long is a common precipitant for ischaemic foot ulcers to form around the margins of the foot. The heel is particularly at risk in bed-bound patients (e.g. postoperatively).

11

Surveillance and management of complications

Diabetic eye disease

Patients with diabetes should usually be offered annual eye checks including measurement of visual acuity and retinal examination. Background diabetic retinopathy remains asymptomatic for many years before visual loss occurs. Therefore, screening for retinopathy is valuable because treatment may be instituted before visual loss occurs. Visual loss may occur because of macular oedema (maculopathy) or retinal haemorrhage (proliferative retinopathy). Hyperglycaemia may affect vision by causing swelling of the ocular lens, and cataracts are more common in people with diabetes. Any unexplained visual loss in a patient with diabetes should be assessed by a specialist ophthalmologist, because macular oedema is difficult to detect by direct fundoscopy. Sight-threatening diabetic retinopathy is treated by producing focal laser burns in the retina. This reduces the elaboration of growth factors by the ischaemic retina and causes new vessels to regress and macular oedema to improve. Extensive laser treatment may restrict the peripheral field of vision, but aims to preserve central vision.

Diabetic nephropathy

Surveillance

At an annual review check, patients with DM will usually have urine tested by dipstick for the presence of proteinuria and have their plasma creatinine measured. Proteinuria has other causes, as well as diabetic nephropathy, that should also be considered—the most common being urinary tract infection. If infection is excluded and the patient has long-standing DM, the most likely cause is diabetic nephropathy. The presence of diabetic retinopathy increases the chance that diabetic nephropathy is the underlying diagnosis. In the absence of diabetic retinopathy, and the presence of significant persistent proteinuria, it should not be assumed that DM is the cause—patients with diabetes can also get glomerulonephritis!

Microalbuminuria

In established diabetic nephropathy, the urinary albumin excretion is more than 300 mg/24 h compared to the normal rate of up to 30 mg/24 h. Patients with intermediate albumin excretions of 30–300 mg/24 h (microalbuminuria) have a 20-fold increased risk of developing established diabetic nephropathy. Microalbuminuria probably represents an early stage of glomerular damage, although not all patients with microalbuminuria will progress to established diabetic nephropathy. Increasingly, patients are tested to detect the presence of microalbuminuria, and so to identify those at risk of later developing nephropathy. One useful screening tool is to estimate the urinary albumin excretion by a 24-h urine collection or by measuring the albumin : creatinine ratio in a single urine sample. Patients with microalbuminuria tend to have slightly higher blood pressure and higher rates of cardiovascular disease compared to matched normoalbuminuric diabetics. Both improving glucose control and the use of antihypertensive agents reduces progression of microalbuminuria to diabetic nephropathy. Both angiotensin-converting enzyme (ACE) inhibitors and angiotensin II receptor blockers have been shown to be useful in certain patient groups.

Established diabetic nephropathy

Meticulous control of blood pressure and a low protein diet have been shown to retard the progression of established diabetic nephropathy to end-stage renal failure. However, care must be taken with low protein diets to ensure that the patient does not develop protein malnutrition and for this reason they are not often used. ACE inhibitors are more effective than older antihypertensive drugs that have similar effects on blood pressure. Multidrug treatments are often needed to reduce blood pressure. Patients need to be monitored for problems related to chronic renal failure, such as fluid overload, anaemia and renal bone disease. Regular attendance at a specialist clinic supervised by a renal physician is useful to enable planning for renal replacement therapy.

Diabetic neuropathy

Preventive care

Patients with neuropathy should be offered regular chiropody, because minor trauma, such as incorrect toenail cutting, may lead to the introduction of infection. Areas of callus over points of high pressure should be débrided to reduce shear forces in the tissue beneath. Patients with neuropathy should be educated to inspect their feet daily for evidence of trauma, as they will not necessarily experience pain. It is not unknown for drawing pins to be removed from neuropathic feet at chiropody clinics. Patients should be advised to avoid walking barefoot if they have neuropathy.

Neuropathic foot ulcers

In the presence of cellulitis surrounding a neuropathic ulcer, inpatient treatment with bed rest and antibiotics is indicated. In the absence of cellulitis, redistribution of weight over the foot by surgical shoes, local débridement of callus and antibiotics (if indicated) may allow healing.

Charcot's arthropathy

Immobilization of the foot in a plaster cast is the mainstay of treatment. The affected bones are at high risk of fracture and if this occurs the architecture of the foot is permanently and dramatically damaged, increasing the risk of future foot ulceration.

Painful neuropathy
Symptoms may be improved by a number of agents, including tricyclic antidepressants, gabapentin or carbamazepine; however, the response rate is often below 50%.

Diabetic ischaemic feet
Preventive care
Smokers should be encouraged to stop. Patients should ensure that new shoes are not tight fitting. New shoes should not be worn for more than an hour initially, because trauma from a blister can easily deteriorate into an ulcer.

Ischaemic ulcers
Infection should be treated promptly and any pus drained by chiropody. Footwear should be inspected and changed if inappropriate. Surgical intervention to improve the proximal blood supply should be considered. Peripheral vascular disease in diabetes is often 'distal' in smaller vessels and less amenable to bypass surgery or angioplasty.

Critical ischaemia
Rest pain or gangrene in the foot requires urgent vascular surgical assessment. Foot radiography should be arranged to look for evidence of gas in the soft tissues, because gas gangrene requires urgent surgical débridement to prevent progression.

Blood pressure and lipid-lowering agents
Hypertension is more common in patients with DM. Approximately 50% of people with type 2 diabetes have hypertension and many of the secondary causes of diabetes are associated with hypertension (Table 11.1, p. 764). Because of their increased risk of macrovascular disease, people with DM gain greater benefit from treatment of hypertension than those without DM. Strict control of hypertension, aiming for blood pressure lower than 150/85 mmHg, reduces the chance of stroke, heart failure and the progression of diabetic retinopathy in patients with type 2 DM. Control of hypertension is also an important part of the management of diabetic nephropathy.

Because of the increased prevalence of coronary heart disease in patients with DM, they are more likely to be prescribed lipid-lowering drugs as part of secondary prevention. The use of lipid-lowering drugs in primary prevention of coronary heart disease in people with DM is considered in those calculated to be at high risk (see p. 807)

Erectile dysfunction
Erectile dysfunction is the inability to maintain an erection sufficient for sexual intercourse. Erectile dysfunction is relatively common in men over 60 years, but more prevalent in men over 60 years with diabetes. It may also occur in much younger men with long-standing type 1 DM. A combination of autonomic nerve dysfunction and/or a reduced vascular supply makes erectile dysfunction more prevalent in men with diabetes. Treatment options include sildenafil, intracavernosal injections (of prostaglandins or α-blockers) and vacuum pump devices.

Diabetic ketoacidosis
Diabetic ketoacidosis (EMERGENCY BOX 11.1) is a medical emergency with a reported mortality rate of 5%. DKA is the leading cause of death in patients with type 1 DM under the age of 20 years. Mortality from DKA is high in the elderly as a result of coexisting morbidities.

Disease mechanisms
Risk factors for diabetic ketoacidosis
Diabetic ketoacidosis results from absolute or relative insulin deficiency. DKA may occur because of undiagnosed type 1 DM, omission of insulin or infection. Infections can precipitate DKA because stress hormones (cortisol, catecholamines, growth hormone, glucagon) and cytokines antagonize the action of insulin. Patients with type 1 DM should never omit their insulin, even if they are eating less or vomiting, because DKA will inevitably ensue. If patients with type 1 DM become ill they should follow 'sick day rules': continue taking insulin, monitor blood glucose more closely, monitor urine for ketonuria; if unable to eat take carbohydrate in fluid form (fruit juice, carbonated drinks), increase insulin dose if hyperglycaemia develops. Patients with type 2 DM may also develop DKA under major stress such as postoperatively, after myocardial infarction or if septic

Metabolic changes in diabetic ketoacidosis
Insulin has activity to inhibit lipolysis (breakdown of fats into fatty acids and triglycerides) and to inhibit hepatic glucose production. When insulin deficiency occurs, hepatic glucose production and lipolysis are unrestrained, resulting in hyperglycaemia and increased fatty acid release. Fatty acids released by adipose tissue are taken up by the liver and converted into ketone bodies (Fig. 11.16). Because ketone bodies are strong organic acids, they readily dissociate at physiological pH to produce equimolar quantities of hydrogen ions (H^+) and ketone anions. The resultant metabolic acidosis stimulates the brainstem vomiting and respiratory centres.

11

Emergency 11.1: Diabetic ketoacidosis

Establish the diagnosis
Triad of:
1 *Hyperglycaemia:* glucose usually more than 15 mmol/l
2 *Metabolic acidosis:* pH lower than 7.35, HCO_3^- less than 17 mmol/l
3 *Ketonuria:* ketonuria 3+ or more

Main metabolic features
■ *Hyperglycaemia:* leading to dehydration from osmotic diuresis
■ *Metabolic acidosis:* caused by elevated ketone bodies from insulin deficiency
■ *Hyperkalaemia:* secondary to acidosis, whole-body potassium stores will be low

Mainstays of treatment
Intravenous rehydration
Intravenous insulin
Replacement of low body potassium stores

Initial treatment
1 l 0.9% saline over 30 min
Actrapid insulin 6 units intravenously (Actrapid insulin 20 units intramuscularly if no intravenous access)
Consider treating an underlying cause

Insulin
Start intravenous infusion of soluble insulin at 6 units/h. If blood glucose does not fall, first check patency of intravenous lines and that infusion apparatus working;

if these are satisfactory increase prescribed dose of insulin. Aim to reduce blood glucose by no more than 3–5 mmol/l/h.

Fluid
As a guide, infuse 1 l over first 30 min, then 1 l over 1 h, then 1 l over 2 h, then 1 l over 4 h, then 1 l over 6 h. Consider central venous pressure monitoring in the elderly, those with heart failure or renal failure
Change fluid from 0.9% saline to 5% glucose when blood glucose has fallen below 10 mmol/l, but continue to infuse intravenous insulin

Potassium
Potassium should usually be given from the second bag of fluid, unless the patient is oliguric or K^+ is more than 6 mmol/l. Give 20–40 mmol/l with each litre of fluid (maximum rate of 20 mmol/h). Increase rate of potassium replacement if K^+ falls below 4 mmol/l. Plasma potassium should be measured after 60 min, and then every 2–4 h until stable

Alkali
Consider giving 50 mmol of 1.4% sodium bicarbonate if pH is lower than 7.0, after seeking specialist advice

Precipitating causes
■ Stopping insulin deliberately or running out
■ Infections increasing insulin resistance
■ Myocardial infarction

Dehydration is produced by the hyperglycaemic osmotic diuresis and by this vomiting.

Clinical features

Diabetic ketoacidosis usually develops over a period of a few days. Advice from a telephone helpline increases the use of early preventive action during intercurrent illnesses and may reduce the incidence of DKA. 'Sick day rules' should be part of the education package offered to all patients with diabetes.

Symptoms of DKA include:
● Thirst and polyuria caused by hyperglycaemia
● Vomiting, shortness of breath and abdominal pain caused by acidosis
● General malaise and drowsiness
● Symptoms from an underlying infection (e.g. pneumonia)
Signs of DKA include:
● Smell of acetone on breath (like 'pear drops' or 'nail varnish remover')
● Hyperventilation (Kussmaul's respiration) caused by acidosis

● Dehydration with reduced tissue turgor
● Hypotension and tachycardia caused by hypovolaemia
● Signs of any underlying precipitating illness

Investigations

Investigations should be directed to confirming the diagnosis and looking for an underlying cause. The three most useful **quick** tests are:
● Bedside capillary blood glucose (usually over 17 mmol/l)
● Urinalysis (heavy ketonuria 3+ or greater)
● Acidosis on arterial blood gas (pH usually less than 7.3)
    If DKA looks likely from the results of these quick bedside tests, treatment should be started while waiting for the results of other investigations:
● *Urea and electrolytes:* hyperkalaemia secondary to acidosis is usual and renal failure from dehydration may occur
● *Venous plasma glucose:* usually more than 17 mmol/l, although DKA may occur with smaller glucose values in patients who have not been eating
● *Venous bicarbonate (HCO_3^-):* reduced because of metabolic acidosis

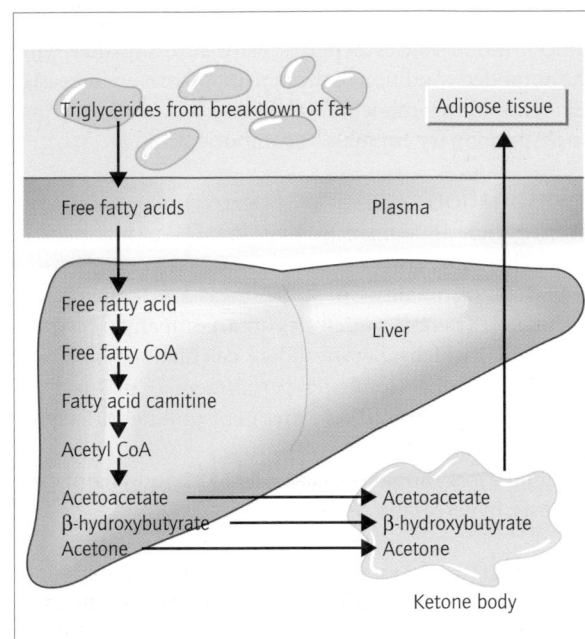

Figure 11.16 Ketogenesis.

- *Full blood count:* acidosis may produce a neutrophilia and does not necessarily indicate an infection
- *ECG and cardiac enzymes:* myocardial infarction may be 'silent' (symptomless) in people with diabetes
- *Urine culture*
- *Chest radiography:* especially if breathless or coughing
- *Blood culture:* in all cases, because hypovolaemia may mask a fever
- *Other tests for sepsis* (e.g. lumbar puncture, throat swab): as indicated by clinical suspicion

Management (EMERGENCY BOX 11.1)
Treatment of DKA has three main features:
1 Replacement of lost fluid
2 Replacement of low body potassium stores
3 Correction of insulin deficiency

Fluid balance
In established DKA, the total body deficit of water is typically 4–5 l. This is accompanied by a total body deficit of sodium ions. The marked dehydration typical of DKA is mainly a result of the osmotic diuresis and vomiting. Intravenous infusion of normal saline replaces the lost fluid and sodium without causing a further rise in blood glucose. Rapid correction of fluid loss should be attempted in young people without cardiac or renal disease, but greater care is needed in the elderly, who may be at risk of pulmonary oedema if fluid overloaded. Care in a high

dependency area with central venous pressure monitoring should be considered.

Potassium replacement
At presentation of DKA, plasma potassium is usually raised as a result of the metabolic acidosis. Hyperkalaemia may be marked, increasing the risk of cardiac arrhythmia and sudden cardiac death. Once insulin therapy has been started, the plasma potassium starts to fall because of a shift of potassium ions from the extracellular to the intracellular space. Total body potassium stores are low and profound hypokalaemia will occur if potassium is not replaced. Intravenous potassium is usually infused once the plasma potassium has fallen into the high-normal range. As a general guide, 20 mmol of potassium chloride are added to each litre of fluid infused, starting with the second bag of fluid. If the plasma potassium concentration falls below 3.5 mmol/l, the rate of potassium replacement should be increased to 40 mmol with each litre of fluid. Frequent plasma potassium measurements are necessary during the first 24 h of treatment of DKA.

Correcting insulin deficiency
Insulin is best given by the intravenous route at low doses by an electrical pump. Administration of insulin by the subcutaneous route should be avoided, because the usual hypovolaemia results in poor absorption into the bloodstream. Small doses of insulin (e.g. 4–6 units/h) are very effective at switching off lipolysis, which is the main source of the metabolic acidosis.

Rapid correction of hyperglycaemia using high doses of insulin may be harmful. High blood glucose in DKA produces an osmotic potential in both brain and plasma. If plasma glucose falls more quickly than brain glucose, an osmotic gradient is produced. Water will flow down this osmotic gradient entering brain tissue and causing it to swell. If this process happens to a significant degree, it causes cerebral oedema and coma. When treating DKA, blood glucose should be lowered by 3–5 mmol/l/h.

Once plasma glucose has fallen to less than 10 mmol/l it is usual to change the infusion fluid to 5% or 10% glucose, but to continue the insulin infusion. This ensures that lipolysis continues to be suppressed so that further ketone bodies are not produced and the acidosis can improve further.

Other measures
Bicarbonate infusion. Conventional treatment of DKA with fluid and insulin replacement will correct the acidosis as it removes the supply of acidic ketone bodies. Excess ketone bodies are excreted by the kidneys. Occasionally, if the acidosis is severe (pH less than 7.0) and not improving, it may be necessary to infuse bicarbonate. Bicarbonate

11

infusion is not given routinely because there is a school of thought that although it improves plasma pH it may worsen intracellular pH and so increase the risk of cardiac arrhythmia.

Nasogastric tube. Aspiration pneumonia contributes to morbidity and mortality in DKA. Patients with reduced consciousness level should be nursed in the prone position if possible. A nasogastric tube should be considered for patients who are vomiting and unable to protect their airway because of their reduced consciousness level.

Urinary catheterization. This is often needed to monitor fluid balance and to ensure continued renal function. Care is needed replacing potassium if there is oliguria and renal impairment.

Cardiac monitoring. Monitoring is useful in the acute stages when there is a risk of arrhythmia resulting from potassium fluxes or acidosis.

Hyperosmolar non-ketotic coma

Hyperosmolar non-ketotic coma (HONK) is characterized by a markedly increased plasma glucose (usually higher than 50 mmol/l) associated with significantly raised plasma osmolality. Ketonuria and acidosis are mild or absent.

Disease mechanisms

In patients with HONK, ketone body levels are not excessively raised as in DKA. It has been suggested that this is a result of marked hyperglycaemia inhibiting excessive lipolysis or the presence of sufficient endogenous insulin to inhibit lipolysis. A common factor in HONK appears to be the consumption of large volumes of glucose-rich drinks in response to thirst. This creates a vicious cycle whereby thirst from hyperglycaemia prompts ingestion of refined carbohydrate, which increases the hyperglycaemia. High glucose concentrations also inhibit pancreatic insulin release (glucose toxicity) and the spiral of worsening hyperglycaemia continues.

Epidemiology

Age. Usually the middle-aged or elderly.

Ethnicity. More common in Afro-Caribbeans.

Clinical features

HONK presents with thirst, polyuria and an impaired level of consciousness. There may also be evidence of a precipitating pathology (e.g. intercurrent infection). Ketonuria is usually mild (1+ to 2+) and acidosis absent or mild (pH usually more than 7.3). The high plasma glucose concentration causes hyperviscosity and, together with the obtunded condition of the patient, there is an increased incidence of thromboembolic disease (deep-vein thrombosis, pulmonary embolus, thrombotic stroke).

Investigation

Investigation is similar to that for DKA, but plasma osmolality must also be checked.

Plasma osmolality must be measured rather than calculated. There is sometimes an accompanying hyperlipidaemia, which may invalidate calculations based on plasma electrolyte levels. Hypernatraemia (plasma Na^+ more than 150 mmol/l) is a frequent finding initially or during treatment.

Blood gases should be measured to exclude significant acidosis, hypercapnia and hypoxia.

Management (EMERGENCY BOX 11.2)

The management of HONK resembles that of DKA, but there are some important differences.

Fluid replacement

Plasma sodium over 160 mmol/l is often associated with impaired conscious level. Initial fluid replacement volumes are similar to those in DKA, but the hypernatraemia may worsen if normal saline (0.9%) is used as the infusate. Half normal saline (0.45%) is often used at some stage in treatment. Monitoring of fluid replacement with a central

---

Emergency 11.2: Hyperosmolar non-ketotic coma

Diagnosis
- *Hyperglycaemia:* blood glucose often more than 50 mmol/l
- *No/minimal acidosis:* pH more than 7.3, HCO_3^- more than 17 mmol/l
- *Minimal ketonuria:* ketonuria 2+ or less
- *Hyperosmolarity:* usually over 350 mOsmol/l

Treatment
Acute management is generally the same as for DKA
Plasma sodium is usually over 150 mmol/l, 0.45% saline is often needed to prevent severe hypernatraemia
Prophylactic anticoagulation with subcutaneous low molecular weight heparin should be given, unless there is a contraindication, because of the high risk of thromboembolism
Patients are more often elderly, with type 2 DM, and can usually be managed long-term with oral hypoglycaemic drugs and diet

venous pressure line is more commonly required than for DKA, because people with HONK are usually older.

Insulin

HONK is more sensitive to insulin than DKA, so less insulin is usually required (e.g. 4 units/h at first, reducing to 1–2 units/h depending on the response).

Plasma potassium

Plasma potassium concentration needs frequent monitoring and correction as appropriate.

Anticoagulation

Heparin should be given in a prophylactic regimen subcutaneously or in a treatment regimen if active thromboembolism (e.g. pulmonary embolus) is suspected.

Prognosis

HONK has a mortality of up to 30% as a result of:

- Associated electrolyte abnormalities (particularly sodium concentration)
- Thrombotic complications caused by hyperviscosity
- General complications of being an unconscious patient
- Infection
- Any underlying condition precipitating HONK

People who survive HONK rarely require continued insulin treatment. They usually have type 2 DM and may be managed by diet, with or without oral hypoglycaemic drugs. A significant number of patients with HONK are known to have type 2 DM, but have defaulted on their diet and/or medication. Testing for cognitive deficit should take place on recovery and an education package started as appropriate.

Hypoglycaemia

Capillary (or arterial) blood glucose concentration less than 3.5 mmol/l is generally taken to indicate hypoglycaemia. Venous blood glucose concentrations less than 3 mmol/l may occur in normal people during an oral glucose tolerance test because of a high arteriovenous difference in blood glucose. Hypoglycaemia most commonly occurs as a result of hypoglycaemic treatment in people with DM, but may also occur spontaneously or through inappropriate use of hypoglycaemic agents in non-diabetic individuals. Causes of hypoglycaemia are listed in Table 11.10.

Hypoglycaemia in diabetes mellitus

Hypoglycaemia is an unwelcome side-effect of treatment in diabetes. It is more common in people treated with insulin than those on oral hypoglycaemic drugs. Hypoglycaemia can significantly affect cognitive and mental

Table 11.10 Causes of hypoglycaemia

Drug related
Diabetes treatment (insulin/sulphonylureas)
Deliberate self-harm using insulin or sulphonylureas
Alcohol intoxication
Intravenous quinine therapy

Liver disease
Liver failure
Primary hepatic carcinoma

Physiological
Reactive hypoglycaemia
Dumping syndrome
Starvation
Prolonged exercise

Endocrine
Hypoadrenalism
Hypothyroidism
Insulinoma

Infection
Septicaemia

Congenital
Neonatal hyperinsulinism (nesidioblastosis)
Hereditary fructose intolerance
Galactosaemia
Glycogen storage disease

function and so influence work performance. Decreased motor coordination during hypoglycaemia can be hazardous if operating machinery or driving. Recurrent or intrusive hypoglycaemia can seriously undermine an individual's confidence. Intensified insulin regimens increase the risk of hypoglycaemia. The benefit of trying to reduce overall glycaemia to prevent long-term complications of diabetes needs to be balanced against the risk of an unacceptable degree or frequency of hypoglycaemia.

- *Insulin therapy:* the most common cause of hypoglycaemia. Factors contributing to its development are shown in Table 11.7 (p. 776).
- *Sulphonylureas:* with longer half-lives are more likely to cause hypoglycaemia (e.g. glibenclamide, chlorpropamide)
- *Metformin therapy:* does not usually cause hypoglycaemia unless combined with excessive alcohol use
- *Diabetic diet:* on its own, does not cause hypoglycaemia

Disease mechanisms

Symptoms of hypoglycaemia are variable and depend on the individual as well as the degree and rapidity of onset of hypoglycaemia (Fig. 11.17). Clinical investigation in people without diabetes has indicated that mild symptoms of hypoglycaemia usually appear when capillary

11

blood glucose falls below 3 mmol/l, but that significant symptoms do not appear until blood glucose has fallen below 2 mmol/l. Hypoglycaemic symptoms have been classified as 'autonomic activation' and 'neuroglycopenia'.

Autonomic activation

When blood glucose concentration falls below approximately 2 mmol/l, hypothalamic autonomic centres become activated and stimulate both sympathetic and parasympathetic pathways; the resultant secretion of catecholamines, cortisol, glucagon and growth hormone act to raise blood glucose concentrations. Autonomic activation produces symptoms of cold sweat, tachycardia, tremor, blurred vision, hunger and altered salivation.

Neuroglycopenia

Mild hypoglycaemia (blood glucose 2–3 mmol/l) causes subtle defects in higher cognitive function such as reasoning ability. At more severe degrees of hypoglycaemia (blood glucose less than 1 mmol/l), neuroglycopenic symptoms include aggression, confusion, slurred speech, double vision and ataxia. This may be wrongly attributed to inebriation by bystanders. If severe hypoglycaemia is sustained, impaired conscious level, fitting and coma ensue. Prolonged severe hypoglycaemia carries a small risk of permanent brain damage or accidental death.

Diagnosis

In a patient with diabetes, clinical features of sweating, confusion and tachycardia should suggest hypoglycaemia: look for cards or a bracelet confirming DM. Hypoglycaemia produces transient neurological signs, such as extensor plantar responses, that resolve when hypoglycaemia is treated. If feasible, test capillary blood glucose with a portable meter at the bedside and send blood for laboratory glucose estimation. Hypoglycaemia should always be considered in the differential diagnosis of an unconscious or confused patient. If there is any doubt, treat immediately for hypoglycaemia without waiting for laboratory results.

Prolonged or severe hypoglycaemia may be followed by a long period of recovery. A headache or 'hung over' feeling may last for many hours afterwards. These symptoms may be the only clue to unsuspected nocturnal hypoglycaemia.

Hypoglycaemia unawareness

Loss of warning symptoms of hypoglycaemia occurs in patients with long-standing diabetes and the reasons for this appear to be multifactorial (Fig. 11.17). This is partly because of the development of autonomic neuropathy reducing the symptoms of autonomic activation. More recently, clinical investigators have shown that repeated

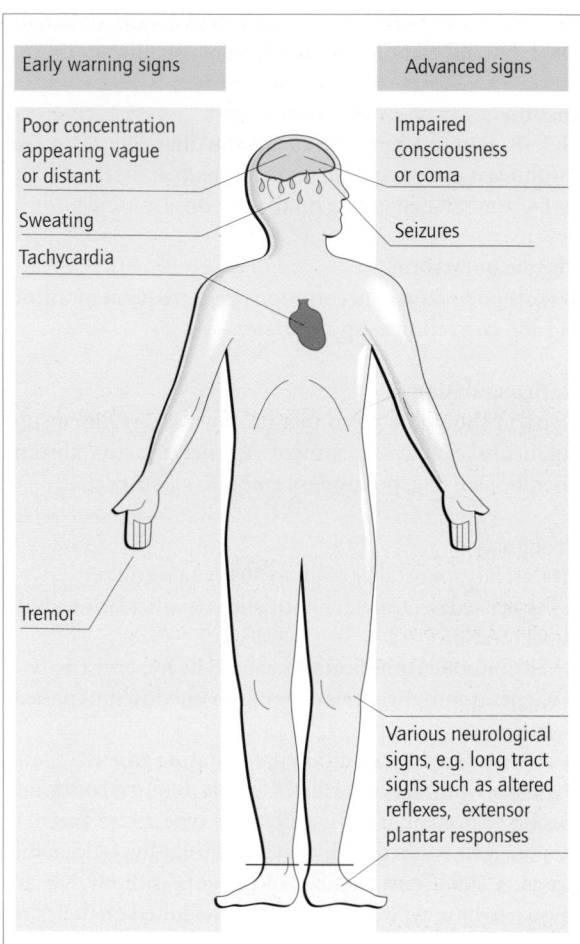

Figure 11.17 Warning signs in hypoglycaemia.

episodes of hypoglycaemia cause adaptation of hypothalamic centres so that the same degree of hypoglycaemia produces a smaller autonomic activation. Loss of autonomic activation symptoms means that action to correct hypoglycaemia is not taken, resulting in more severe hypoglycaemia. Loss of higher mental function and confusion with severe hypoglycaemia will also prevent individuals from treating themselves. Therefore, an individual with hypoglycaemia unawareness may end up in a downward spiral of deepening hypoglycaemia, yet become disabled from acting to treat it and be dependent on other people to recognize and treat the problem.

Management

● *If the patient is conscious, and able to swallow:* give readily absorbed carbohydrate food or drink (Table 11.6, p. 776)
● *If the patient's level of consciousness is reduced so that oral administration is dangerous:* give intramuscular glucagon or intravenous 50% glucose (EMERGENCY BOX 11.3)

Glucagon is a useful treatment as family, work colleagues or friends can be readily taught to give an intramuscular injection. Intravenous glucose needs to be administered by trained personnel—it must be given into a large vein as it may cause phlebitis and if extravasated may cause tissue necrosis.

Coma from hypoglycaemia usually responds within minutes to restoration of blood glucose concentrations. However, severe and/or prolonged hypoglycaemia may take longer to respond.

Emergency 11.3: Severe hypoglycaemia

Diagnosis
Blood glucose less than 3.5 mmol/l
plus
Help from a third party required for treatment

Causes
Patients with diabetes taking insulin or sulphonylureas
Other causes are listed in Table 11.7 (p. 776)

Treatment
If fully conscious:
■ Give oral carbohydrate (Table 11.6, p. 776)
If impaired conscious level:
■ Intravenous glucose
or
■ Intramuscular glucagon

Intravenous glucose
■ 30–50 ml of 50% glucose
or
■ 90–125 ml of 20% glucose
High concentration glucose should be given into a large vein and flushed with saline afterwards to reduce the risk of thrombophlebitis. **Care:** 50% glucose may cause skin necrosis if extravasated. These are recommended doses for adults only. Children should be given smaller doses

Intramuscular glucagon
Glucagon 0.5–1 mg intramuscularly
May be given by paramedical staff or trained family members. No risk of thrombophlebitis. May precipitate vomiting. Ineffective in chronic liver disease as glycogen stores are depleted

Aftercare
After recovery ensure that oral carbohydrate is taken
Consider cause for hypoglycaemic episode
If the conscious level does not improve rapidly with correction of hypoglycaemia, consider the possibility of another cause of coma such as head injury, stroke, deliberate self-harm (e.g. overdose)

Prevention
The risk of hypoglycaemia may be minimized by:
● *Diet:* people using soluble insulin usually need a snack 3–4 h after the injection; nocturnal hypoglycaemia can often be prevented by taking a bedtime snack
● *Education:* late or missed meals, insufficient carbohydrate intake or increased physical exercise increase the risk of hypoglycaemia
● *Therapeutic changes:* changing dose of insulin and/or sulphonylureas, altering type of insulin used or timing of injections

Mild hypoglycaemia is almost inevitable in insulin-treated people and may occur in those taking sulphonylureas. Self-treatment of hypoglycaemia should be part of the education package of all patients with diabetes who are at risk of hypoglycaemia (Table 11.6, p. 776). Everyone treated with insulin should carry readily absorbable carbohydrate with them at all times (e.g. glucose tablets or sweets).

Insulinoma

Insulinomas are rare tumours of the pancreas that cause hypoglycaemia because of unregulated secretion of insulin. Symptoms of hypoglycaemia may be wrongly attributed to anxiety or to neurological disease. Insulinomas classically cause **fasting** hypoglycaemia, although daytime symptoms may also occur. Because anxiety is common and insulinomas are rare, an algorithm (Whipple's triad) should be used to suggest the diagnosis. Whipple's triad states that:
1 Symptoms should be associated with fasting or exercise
2 Hypoglycaemia is demonstrated to be present during the symptoms
3 Glucose relieves the symptoms

Confirmation of the diagnosis requires demonstration of inappropriately high or non-suppressed insulin levels during hypoglycaemia. This is usually done by fasting the patient for a prolonged period (72 h) and monitoring blood glucose concentrations. An important differential diagnosis is factitious hypoglycaemia secondary to insulin injection or use of sulphonylureas. Insulin for injection does not contain C-peptide so elevated C-peptide in the presence of hypoglycaemia suggests an insulinoma as the diagnosis. Sulphonylureas may be detected in blood or urine samples. Investigation and diagnosis of insulinoma is a specialist field.

Most insulinomas are benign tumours and treatment by surgical excision is usually curative. Preoperatively, the tumour may be localized by CT scanning and/or pancreatic angiography. Insulinomas are often small and imaging may fail to locate the tumour, but they may be located at operation by careful palpation of the pancreas

11

by the surgeon. Patients unfit or unwilling to undergo surgery may be treated by diazoxide, which inhibits insulin release by pancreatic β cells.

Obesity and overweight states

Body weight is determined by genetic, environmental, cultural and psychosocial factors. Obesity is a condition in which excess body fat accumulates, such that health may be affected. In healthy adult men of average weight, body fat accounts for 15–20% of total body weight, while for women it is 25–30% of total body weight. It is difficult to measure body fat directly so the body mass index (BMI) is usually used as an indirect measure. BMI is weight (kg) divided by the square of height (m^2). Obesity is usually defined as a BMI of 30 or more (Table 11.11). Epidemiological studies show an increased morbidity and mortality as BMI increases above the desirable range.

Simple obesity

When obesity is not a secondary feature of another disorder, it is classified as simple obesity. Eating in excess of energy requirements is the primary cause, but its origin is contentious. Different schools of thought emphasize either biological or psychological mechanisms driving the overeating.

Secondary obesity

Obesity occurs as an associated feature of a number of conditions, and weight gain may be exacerbated by drug treatments (Table 11.12). These differential diagnoses should be considered in any subject presenting with obesity.

Disease mechanisms

Day-to-day food intake needs to be closely matched to energy expenditure for the maintenance of body weight. When energy intake exceeds expenditure, the excess calories are stored as adipose tissue. Fat is stored subcutaneously, around internal organs, within the omentum and in intramuscular spaces. Fat storage confers a survival value when food is in short supply, allowing a person of normal weight to survive 2 months of total starvation. A plentiful food supply and overconsumption, common in affluent societies, can lead this physiological mechanism to become a health risk.

Hypothalamic control of eating

The physiological urge to eat and the perception of being satiated are controlled centrally by discrete areas of the hypothalamus:

- *Ventrolateral hypothalamus:* 'feeding centre'
- *Ventromedial hypothalamus:* 'satiety centre'

The feeding centre sends signals to the cerebral cortex to stimulate eating and as feeding progresses the satiety centre inhibits the activity of the feeding centre. Both these regions of the hypothalamus receive neural input from another region of the hypothalamus, the arcuate nucleus. The activity of these neural centres is regulated by several peripheral factors, including:

- Rise in plasma glucose and/or insulin that follows a meal
- Leptin released from adipose tissue
- Humoral substances (e.g. cholecystokinin) released from the gut in response to gastric and duodenal distension
- Autonomic nervous system neural input from stretch receptors in the stomach

Damage to the hypothalamic centres by tumour or surgery may result in hyperphagia (overeating) and hence obesity. There is evidence to suggest that the hypothalamic control of feeding is linked to a relatively fixed 'set point' for body adiposity and this may be the reason for the difficulty experienced by previously obese people in maintaining a lower body weight.

Cognitive control of eating

Psychological theories of obesity emphasize the role of learned and cognitive influences on eating behaviour. Hunger is not solely related to metabolic status (time since

Table 11.12 Causes of secondary obesity

Hypothyroidism
Cushing's syndrome
Drug treatments
    Corticosteroids
    Phenothiazines
    Lithium
    Tricyclic antidepressants
    Sodium valproate
    Insulin
Monogenic syndromes associated with hypogonadism
    Prader–Willi syndrome
    Laurence–Moon–Biedl syndrome
Pituitary and hypothalamic disorders

Table 11.11 World Health Organization (WHO) classification of overweight

BMI (kg/m^2)	WHO class	Popular term
<18.5	Underweight	Thin
18.5–24.9	–	Healthy, acceptable
25.0–29.9	Overweight grade 1	Overweight
30.0–39.9	Overweight grade 2	Obese
≥40	Overweight grade 3	Morbidly obese

BMI, body mass index.

last meal), but also to anticipation of nutritional require-ments. For example, many people do not take breakfast, reporting that they do not feel hungry, despite this meal following the longest fast of the day. Most people will feel hungry if offered a special treat, even if they have recently eaten. An early 'psychosomatic theory' of obesity stated that overeating occurs as a response to emotional stimuli. Obesity was thus a result of a learned behaviour (overeat-ing) adopted as a coping response. The 'externality theory' has suggested that obese people are more responsive to external cues to eating such as palatability of food and less responsive to internal satiety and hunger cues (e.g. gastric distension). More recent theories have emphasized the role of voluntary restriction of food intake. A propor-tion of people identified by questionnaire as 'restrained eaters' consciously limit their food intake; however, if given an amount of food thought to exceed their self-imposed limit they abandon restraint and overeat. Such a cognitive loop may underlie the behaviour of people with bulimia nervosa.

Energy intake and expenditure

Most obese people report that they do not overeat; how-ever, even a small increase of energy intake of 5% above weight neutral requirements will lead to weight gain if maintained. Energy intake for weight maintenance is approximately 2500 kcal/day for men and 2000 kcal/day for women. An increase of 5% (100–150 kcal) taken daily would result in an extra 35 000–45 000 kcal over a year, equivalent to the energy contained in 5–7.5 kg of fat tissue.

For adults to maintain a stable weight, their daily energy intake (food) needs to match their daily energy expend-iture. Total daily energy expenditure consists of:
- Energy used to maintain the resting metabolic rate
- Thermic effect of food (see below)
- Energy cost of physical activity

Resting metabolic rate usually accounts for 60–70% of total energy expenditure, the thermic effect of food for 10% and physical activity for a variable proportion. Physical activity accounts for about 20% of total energy expenditure in sedentary people, 30–40% in active people and even higher in professional athletes. Physical activity is the only variable that affects total energy expenditure and is under voluntary control.

Resting metabolic rate. Metabolic studies of obese subjects have excluded a low resting metabolic rate as a cause of common obesity. Resting metabolic rates expressed as units of energy per unit of fat-free mass are the same as for lean people. As obese people are larger, their total daily energy expenditure is higher than that of lean people. A low resting metabolic rate does occur in profound untreated hypothyroidism.

Thermic effect of food. For several hours after ingestion, energy is expended above the resting metabolic rate to power the digestion, absorption and storage of nutrients. Some studies have observed a reduced thermic response to food in obese people, which may be caused by insulin resistance. This effect normalizes with weight loss, sug-gesting that it is a secondary rather than a primary feature of obesity.

Physical activity. Cross-sectional studies show that obese people are less physically active compared to lean people, which contributes to a lower total daily energy expend-iture. Large prospective studies indicate that low physical activity at baseline weight is a risk factor for the sub-sequent development of obesity. Lack of physical activity may make a significant contribution to weight gain in those with poor mobility because of illness or injury.

Epidemiology

Prevalence. In England in 2001 21% of men and 24% of women were obese. In the USA, an estimated 30% of the population are defined as obese. In developed countries, obesity is more common in people from lower socio-economic classes.

Age. Obesity increases with age until 50–60 years.

Sex. Obesity is more prevalent in women.

Geography. The prevalence of obesity is increasing globally. Prevalence rates are much higher in developed countries with high rates in the USA, and southern and eastern Europe.

Genetics. Obesity tends to run in families, but this may be because of shared genetic or environmental factors. Twin studies suggest a genetic contribution to body weight. Studies on adopted children show a significant association between weight status of the adopted child and the natural parents. Genetic research has identified a number of single obesity genes in animal models of obesity, most of which affect feeding behaviour. A number of rare individuals have been identified with similar genetic defects as found in these animal models, usually from consanguineous families and characterized by obesity from infancy. In most people, any genetic influence on obesity is probably polygenic, acting through a number of susceptibility genes.

Clinical features

Clinical examination of obese people should be directed to identifying associated comorbid conditions (Table 11.13) and clinical features of disorders causing secondary obes-ity (Table 11.12). Obesity may present with symptoms of

Table 11.13 Comorbidities associated with obesity

Metabolic
Type 2 diabetes mellitus
Hyperlipidaemia
Insulin resistance

Cardiorespiratory
Hypertension
Coronary heart disease
Sleep apnoea ('Pickwickian syndrome')
Thromboembolic disease
Cerebrovascular disease

Rheumatological
Osteoarthritis
Back pain
Ligament/tendon injury

Gastrointestinal
Gallstones
Reflux oesophagitis
Hepatic steatosis (fatty liver)

Psychological
Depression
Anxiety
Low self-esteem

Cancer risk increased
Endometrium
Breast
Colorectal
Prostate
Ovary

these comorbid conditions. An assessment of the mental state should not be forgotten, especially because morbidly obese people have higher rates of anxiety and depression. Breathlessness is often brought about by the increased work associated with walking with an increased mechanical load and may be compounded by lack of physical fitness, but consider other causes of breathlessness, including obesity hypoventilation syndrome. Body temperature regulation is more difficult in the obese because of the insulating effect of fat and may result in problematic sweating. Ascites may present as 'obesity' and should be considered as a differential diagnosis in people with an increasing waist size.

Quantifiying the obesity
The rate of weight gain should be assessed using historical records and photographs if available. Patients may be unable to recall their previous body weight, but may remember changes in dress size or in the waist size of their trousers. Significant life events such as smoking cessation,

change in physical activity related to change in occupation and retirement or physical illness should be sought.

The degree of obesity should be estimated using the body mass index:

$$\text{BMI} = [\text{weight (kg)}] / [\text{height (m)}]^2.$$

Special scales may be required to accurately weigh the morbidly obese. Fat mass may be estimated by scales incorporating a bioelectrical impedance device and may help individuals using an exercise regimen to differentiate a loss of fat from a gain of lean tissue. Skin-fold thickness, measured over the triceps or subcapsular areas, may be used in specialist centres.

Complications of obesity
Metabolic. Metabolic changes found in obesity include insulin resistance and hyperlipidaemia. The oxidation of free fatty acids is increased and the oxidation of glucose is reduced in obesity and these changes may indirectly cause the insulin resistance of obesity. Tissue insensitivity to insulin in liver, adipose tissue and skeletal muscle contribute to the hypertriglyceridaemia—principally in very low-density lipoprotein (VLDL) particles—found in obesity. Although obesity is a major risk factor for the development of type 2 diabetes, most moderately obese people do not develop diabetes.

Cardiovascular. Cardiovascular disease is the principal cause of death among obese people, as it is among the non-obese. Modifiable risk factors for cardiovascular disease (smoking, hypertension, hyperlipidaemia, physical inactivity) should be addressed at the same time as considering treatment for obesity. There is a link between the degree of obesity and the degree of essential hypertension. Measurement of blood pressure in the overweight should be performed with a correctly sized cuff, because an inappropriately small cuff size will result in spuriously raised blood pressure readings (Fig. 11.18). Weight loss will improve both hypertension and hyperlipidaemia associated with obesity.

Cancer. Obesity increases the risk of a number of cancers (Table 11.13). Epidemiologically, obesity is becoming a major factor in the increasing incidence of certain cancers. It should be remembered that significant **unintentional** weight loss in an obese person may be the first presenting symptom of any cancer. However, unfortunately, obesity makes detection of abnormalities on clinical examination more difficult.

Investigations
Obese people (BMI of 30 kg/m^2 or more) should be assessed by thyroid function tests, fasting or random

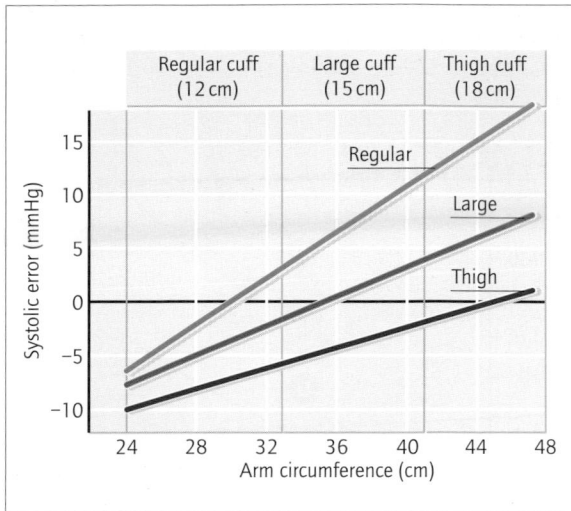

Figure 11.18 Relationship between arm circumference and blood pressure cuff size as related to systolic error of blood pressure measurement. Reproduced from Swales JD, *Textbook of Hypertension*. Oxford: Blackwell Scientific Publications, 1994 with the permission of the author.

glucose, lipid profile and ECG. People with a BMI within the healthy range (18.5–24.9 kg/m^2) should be reassured. These people frequently desire weight loss for cosmetic reasons and should be assessed to exclude an underlying eating disorder (see pp. 980–3). Overweight (BMI 25–29.9 kg/m^2) and obesity (BMI 30 kg/m^2 or more) have a combined prevalence of 40–60% in European countries so specialist investigation should be restricted to those with features to suggest a secondary cause of weight gain, or where the rate of weight gain is excessive. If there are clinical features of a lack of androgenization in men, or menstrual disturbance in women, the gonadal axis should be investigated. Patients suspected to have Cushing's syndrome or hypothalamic or pituitary disease should be assessed by an endocrinologist. Sleep apnoea should be suspected in the morbidly obese.

Management
Treatment choices and goals
The treatment of obesity aims to improve health and to reduce the associated complications of obesity. Patients often request treatment to improve cosmetic appearance and may have unrealistic expectations of treatment programmes. Success should be judged by the reduction in the severity of obesity rather than a return to an 'ideal' body weight. Modest weight loss of 5–10% body weight has been shown to improve blood pressure, dyslipidaemia and hyperglycaemia. Intermediate weight loss goals are useful to encourage adherence to a treatment programme. Long-term changes in lifestyle, both in diet and in physical activity, are required for weight maintenance.

Diet
Dietary treatment of obesity involves a reduction in daily energy intake. Food diaries are useful to make a baseline assessment of diet composition and energy intake. These usually under-report energy intake, but they provide a focus on which to make recommendations for change. An estimate of the patient's energy requirement can be made based on a daily energy consumption of 30–35 kcal/kg of body weight. A reduction in energy intake of 500–1000 kcal/day is usually sufficient to induce weight loss, but a long-term reduction in energy intake of 1000 kcal/day is difficult to maintain. Consider that for many women, whose energy requirements are approximately 2000 kcal/day, this represents a 50% reduction in energy intake. More severe restriction than this will lead to excessive loss of lean tissue, as well as fat tissue and should be discouraged.

The diet should be well balanced and take into account the patient's tastes and lifestyle. Initial weight loss on an energy-restricted diet is more rapid because of loss of glycogen stores in muscle and liver and their associated water content. Continuing weight loss will be slower and it is easy for disillusionment to develop. Weight loss of more than 0.5–1 kg/week should not be expected from a fairly restricted diet of 1000 kcal/day deficit. Despite this, some patients expect to lose much greater quantities of weight than this and will abandon a diet that was working well for 'lack of efficacy'. Support from a slimming club, family members and a professional dietitian can aid motivation.

A number of studies have indicated that people on low-fat diets tend to lose more weight compared to habitual diets, probably because they are less energy dense, although no less palatable. Diets high in fibre are rated as more satiating than low-fibre diets. Current dietetic practice is to recommend a healthy eating plan of reduced fat, increased fibre, increased fruit and vegetable intake along with a reduction in total energy intake.

Cognitive–behavioural treatment
Studies suggest that cognitive–behavioural treatments increase weight loss when used as an adjunct to diet treatment alone. Food diaries may identify situations or emotions that lead to uncontrolled eating. Behavioural treatments aim to reduce exposure to these situations (stimulus control), such as avoiding food shopping when hungry. Cognitive therapy aims to identify false beliefs about body image. For some patients, psychotherapy or drug treatment for depression may be required before a diet treatment plan is adopted.

11

Obesity at a glance

Epidemiology

Prevalence in England
21% of men; 24% of women

Age
Incidence increases with age between 20 and 60 years

Genetics
Twin and adoption studies suggest a genetic contribution

Geography
Higher prevalence in developed countries

Findings on investigation

Anthropometry
Body mass index (BMI) ≥30 kg/m^2

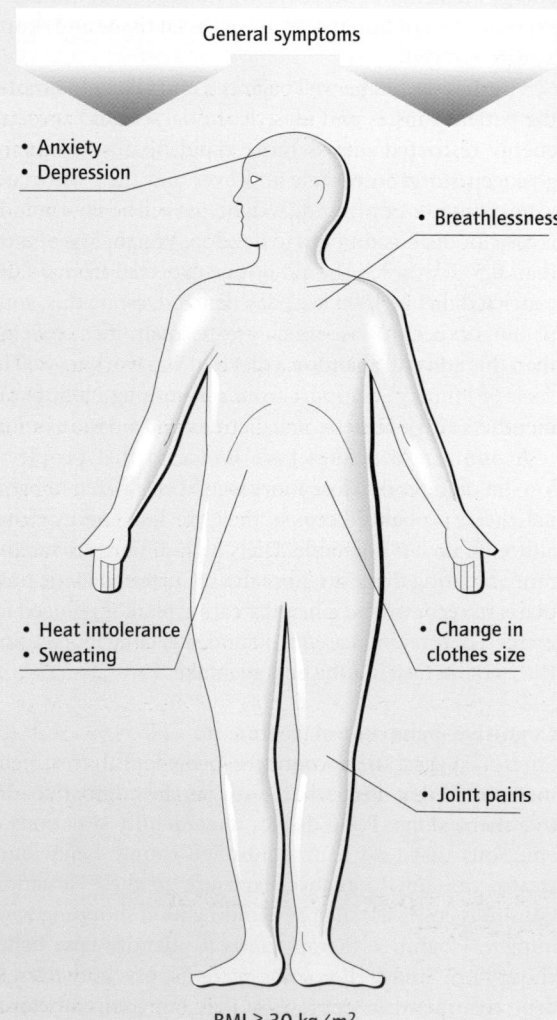

General symptoms

- Anxiety
- Depression

- Breathlessness

- Heat intolerance
- Sweating

- Change in clothes size

- Joint pains

BMI ≥ 30 kg/m^2

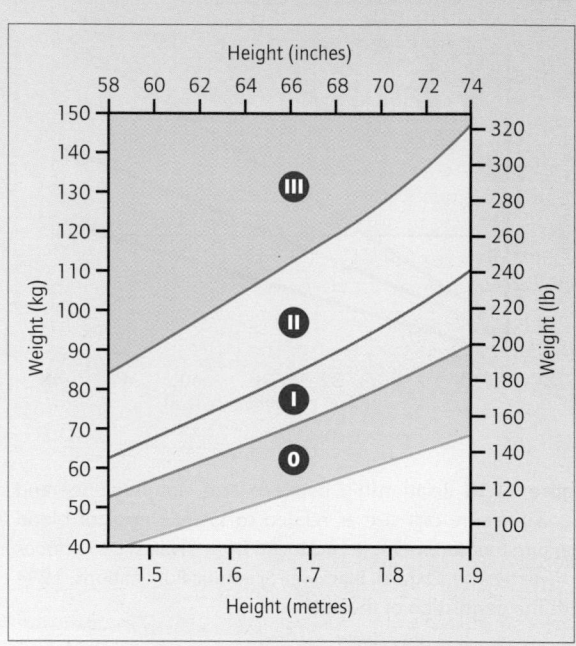

Fig. A Height/weight relationships indicating boundaries of desirable weight (0), mild (I), moderate (II) and severe (III) obesity. Reproduced from Grossman, *Clinical Endocrinology*, 1992 (Blackwell Scientific Publications, Oxford) with the permission of the author.

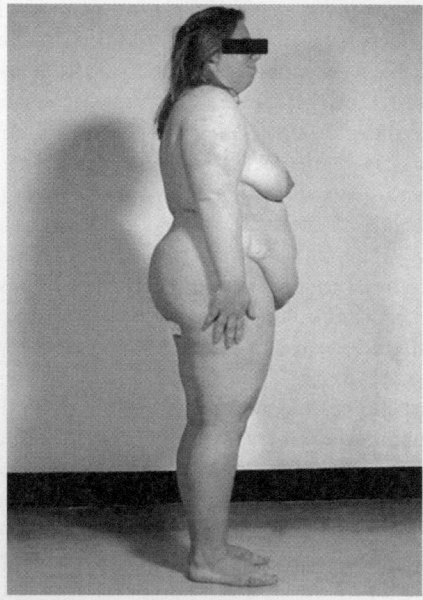

Fig. B Moderately obese female who has a significant risk of heart disease.

Biochemistry	Cardiorespiratory
Role of biochemical investigations to exclude secondary causes of obesity	Hypertension
Impaired glucose tolerance	Coronary heart disease
Hyperlipidaemia	Stroke
	Thromboembolism
	Sleep apnoea
Differential diagnosis	*Gastrointestinal*
Hypothyroidism	Hiatus hernia
Cushing's syndrome	Gallstones
Associated features	*Rheumatological*
Metabolic	Osteoarthritis
Hyperlipidaemia	Back pain
Insulin resistance	
Type 2 DM	

Exercise

Regular aerobic exercise increases daily energy expenditure and will aid weight loss as long as energy intake is not similarly increased. Clinical studies suggest that subjects who increase their physical activity, as well as adhere to a calorie-restricted diet, experience greater weight loss. Importantly, people who continue their increased level of physical activity are more likely to maintain their weight loss after stopping calorie restriction.

Drugs

Drug treatment for obesity should be considered if obesity is accompanied by other risk factors that increase the risks from obesity for that person (e.g. hypertension, sleep apnoea, diabetes). Most drug treatments report median weight losses of 5–10% of initial body weight, but weight is often regained after cessation of therapy. Drug treatments that have been used include:
- *Orlistat:* an inhibitor of intestinal lipases that reduces the digestion of fats in the intestine, thus reducing the energy absorbed from ingested food
- *Sibutramine:* a serotonin and noradrenaline reuptake inhibitor that appears to act both centrally to reduce appetite and peripherally to increase metabolic rate. The noradrenergic actions may increase blood pressure. Interactions with some antidepressants may be a problem for some patients
- *Amphetamines:* fenfluramine and dexamfetamine were once widely used and act by reducing appetite centrally. Amphetamines can cause problems with physical dependency and were withdrawn from licensed use after they were shown to be associated with valvular heart disease

Surgery

Surgical procedures may produce marked weight loss, but surgery is problematic because of the increased operative risk for obese patients and the difficulty in reversing some of the available procedures:
- *Bariatric surgery:* an O-shaped ring is fitted around the gastric body, limiting the stomach capacity. The volume of the ring may be altered by injection or withdrawal of saline so allowing reversal of the procedure
- *Gastroplasty:* the stomach is divided into two compartments by a line of staples, hence reducing its capacity. This method limits food intake by delaying gastric emptying and giving a feeling of fullness after smaller meals, but is a non-reversible procedure
- *Gastric balloon:* a latex (or silicone) balloon is inserted by endoscopy and inflated within the stomach to reduce its capacity. Side-effects include intestinal obstruction, abdominal cramps and vomiting. Reversal is easy by endoscopic deflation and removal of the balloon
- *Jaw wiring:* the jaws are kept shut by attaching pegs to the teeth and wiring the pegs together. The patient is only able to take a liquid diet during this time. This may be an effective technique, but it is still possible to overeat, it is disfiguring and it does not change eating behaviour permanently. Weight may be rapidly regained once the wires are removed

Plasma lipid and lipoprotein disorders

Plasma lipid and lipoprotein disorders—the dyslipidaemias —are associated with increased risks of atherosclerosis-related disease, particularly coronary heart disease

11

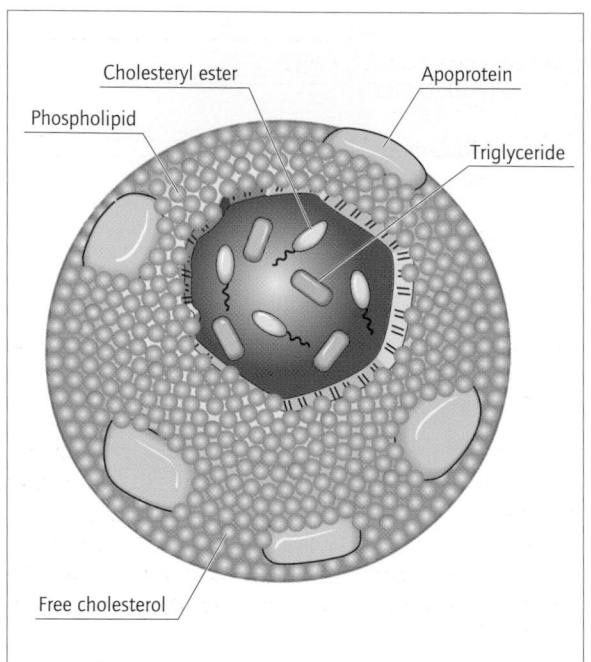

Cholesteryl ester

Apoprotein

Phospholipid

Triglyceride

Free cholesterol

Figure 11.19 Structure of lipoprotein particles.

(CHD). Severe hypertriglyceridaemia is a risk factor for pancreatitis.

Treatment of dyslipidaemia is an important component of the global approach to secondary prevention of CHD and to primary prevention of CHD in those at high risk. Familial lipid disorders, such as familial hypercholesterolaemia and familial combined hyperlipidaemia, are associated with a high relative risk of CHD and merit therapy in their own right. Relatives of individuals presenting with premature CHD and those with known familial lipid disorders should be screened for lipid abnormalities.

Lipid and lipoprotein metabolism

The major plasma lipids, cholesterol and triglyceride, are essential to the overall structure and fuel economy of the body. Cholesterol is a major component of cell membranes and a precursor of steroid hormones and bile acids. Triglycerides (glycerol esterified with three fatty acids) are the body's major energy store, particularly in adipose tissue.

Cholesterol and triglyceride are relatively insoluble in the aqueous environment of the plasma and are transported as lipoproteins, which are multimolecular micelle-like particles (Fig. 11.19). Insoluble cholesterol ester and triglyceride form a lipid droplet at the centre of the lipoprotein with more polar molecules such as free cholesterol, phospholipid and apoproteins on the surface, at the interface with plasma. Apoproteins have not only structural roles, but also important regulatory functions in lipoprotein metabolism (Table 11.14).

The nomenclature of the lipoproteins is based on their separation by density gradient ultracentrifugation (Table 11.15). High-density lipoprotein (HDL) contains the smallest, densest particles and the lowest content of lipid, while chylomicron particles have a high content of lipid, are large and least dense.

Lipoproteins transport absorbed dietary fat and

Table 11.14 Classification and function of apoproteins

Type	Molecular weight (kDa)	Origin	Lipoprotein distribution	Principal function
A-I	29	Liver, intestine	HDL, chylomicrons	LCAT activator
A-II	17	Liver, intestine	HDL, chylomicrons	Structural protein in HDL
A-IV	44	Liver, intestine	HDL, chylomicrons	Non-specific LCAT cofactor
B$_{48}$	241	Intestine	Chylomicrons, chylomicron remnants	Mediates chylomicron formation and secretion by enterocytes
B$_{100}$	513	Liver	VLDL, LDL	Mediates hepatic VLDL formation Ligand for LDL receptor
C-I	6.6	Liver	Chylomicrons, VLDL, HDL	Inhibitor of chylomicron uptake
C-II	9	Liver	Chylomicrons, VLDL, HDL	LPL activator
C-III	9	Liver	Chylomicrons, VLDL, HDL	Inhibitor of LPL
D	19	Liver	HDL	?Involved in cholesterol ester transfer
E	34.1	Liver	Chylomicrons, VLDL, HDL	Ligand for chylomicron receptor and LDL receptor

HDL, high-density lipoprotein; LCAT, lecithin : cholesterol acyltransferase; LDL, low-density lipoprotein; LPL, lipoprotein lipase; VLDL, very low-density lipoprotein.

Table 11.15 Classification of lipoproteins

Class	Diameter (nm)	Density (g/ml)	Electrophoretic mobility	Chemical composition (% of dry mass)				
				Triglycerides	Cholesterol esters	Cholesterol	Phospholipids	Proteins
Chylomicrons	75–1200	0.93	α_2	86	3	2	7	2
VLDL	30–80	0.96–1.006	Pre-β	55	12	7	18	8
IDL	25–35	1.006–1.019	Slow pre-β	23	29	9	19	19
LDL	18–25	1.019–1.063	β	6	42	8	22	22
HDL$_2$	9–12	1.063–1.125	α_1	5	17	5	33	40
HDL$_3$	5–9	1.125–1.210	α_1	3	13	4	25	55

HDL, high-density lipoprotein; IDL, intermediate-density lipoprotein; LDL, low-density lipoprotein; VLDL, very low-density lipoprotein.

endogenously synthesized cholesterol and triglyceride. Lipoprotein metabolism is complex and there are considerable interactions between different lipoproteins with the liver playing a pivotal part (Fig. 11.20). Lipoprotein metabolism may be simplified to three main pathways:

1 *Exogenous pathway:* lipids from food
2 *Endogenous pathway:* lipids synthesized by the liver
3 *Reverse cholesterol transport:* return of cholesterol from tissues to liver

Exogenous pathway

Dietary cholesterol and mono- and diglycerides (from the digestion of triglycerides) are re-esterified in the jejunal enterocyte and packaged with apoprotein B$_{48}$ to form chylomicrons, the largest lipoprotein species (Fig. 11.20). Chylomicrons are transported in intestinal lymphatics and enter the bloodstream via the thoracic duct. Once in the blood they receive additional apoproteins (C and E) by transfer from HDL particles.

Chylomicron triglyceride is hydrolysed by the enzyme lipoprotein lipase (LPL), which acts at the endothelial surface of capillary beds in muscle and adipose tissue. During this process, surface components of chylomicrons (apoproteins, phospholipid and free cholesterol) transfer to the HDL fraction (Fig. 11.20). The free fatty acids and glycerol may be used as metabolic fuel or re-esterified for storage as triglyceride in adipose tissue. Chylomicron remnant particles are relatively rich in cholesterol ester and are removed by the liver through a complex process involving a unique chylomicron remnant receptor, the low-density lipoprotein receptor-related protein (LRP). The major apoprotein ligand interacting with LRP is apoprotein E.

Endogenous pathway

Cholesterol and triglyceride synthesized by the liver are transported by VLDLs (Fig. 11.20). Each VLDL particle contains *one* molecule of apoprotein B$_{100}$ and additional apoproteins (C and E) transfer from HDL particles. VLDL

triglyceride is hydrolysed by LPL and surface components transfer to HDL (in a similar fashion to chylomicron hydrolysis). This process produces intermediate-density lipoproteins (IDLs), which can be removed directly by the liver via LDL receptors (apoB/E receptors). IDL may be further processed by hydrolysis by hepatic lipase to form LDL (Fig. 11.20).

Role of low-density lipoprotein

Low-density lipoprotein is the major carrier of cholesterol in plasma (~70%) and transports cholesterol to peripheral cells for membrane synthesis, to some tissues for hormone production and to the liver for bile acid production. LDL is taken up by cells through the LDL receptor, which is a specific high-affinity receptor that recognizes apoprotein B. Excess LDL is also taken up by the liver through LDL receptors. The activity of LDL receptors in the liver largely controls plasma LDL levels. The LDL receptor pathway, which delivers cholesterol to cells, is important for the maintenance of overall cholesterol homeostasis (Fig. 11.21). A defect in the LDL receptor causes familial hypercholesterolaemia (see p. 801). As cellular cholesterol increases, cellular synthesis of cholesterol is decreased through suppression of the enzyme HMG-CoA reductase and the synthesis of new LDL receptors is inhibited.

Reverse cholesterol transport

Reverse cholesterol transport is the process whereby cholesterol from peripheral tissues is returned to the liver, which is the only major site of cholesterol excretion. HDL, the smallest and most heterogeneous of the lipoproteins, carries approximately 20–30% of plasma cholesterol and is central to reverse cholesterol transport. HDL collects free cholesterol from cell membranes in a regulated process involving transmembrane cholesterol efflux regulatory proteins. Free cholesterol is esterified by the enzyme lecithin : cholesterol acyltransferase (LCAT) which circulates with the HDL particles. Cholesterol esters formed on HDL may return to the liver either by:

11

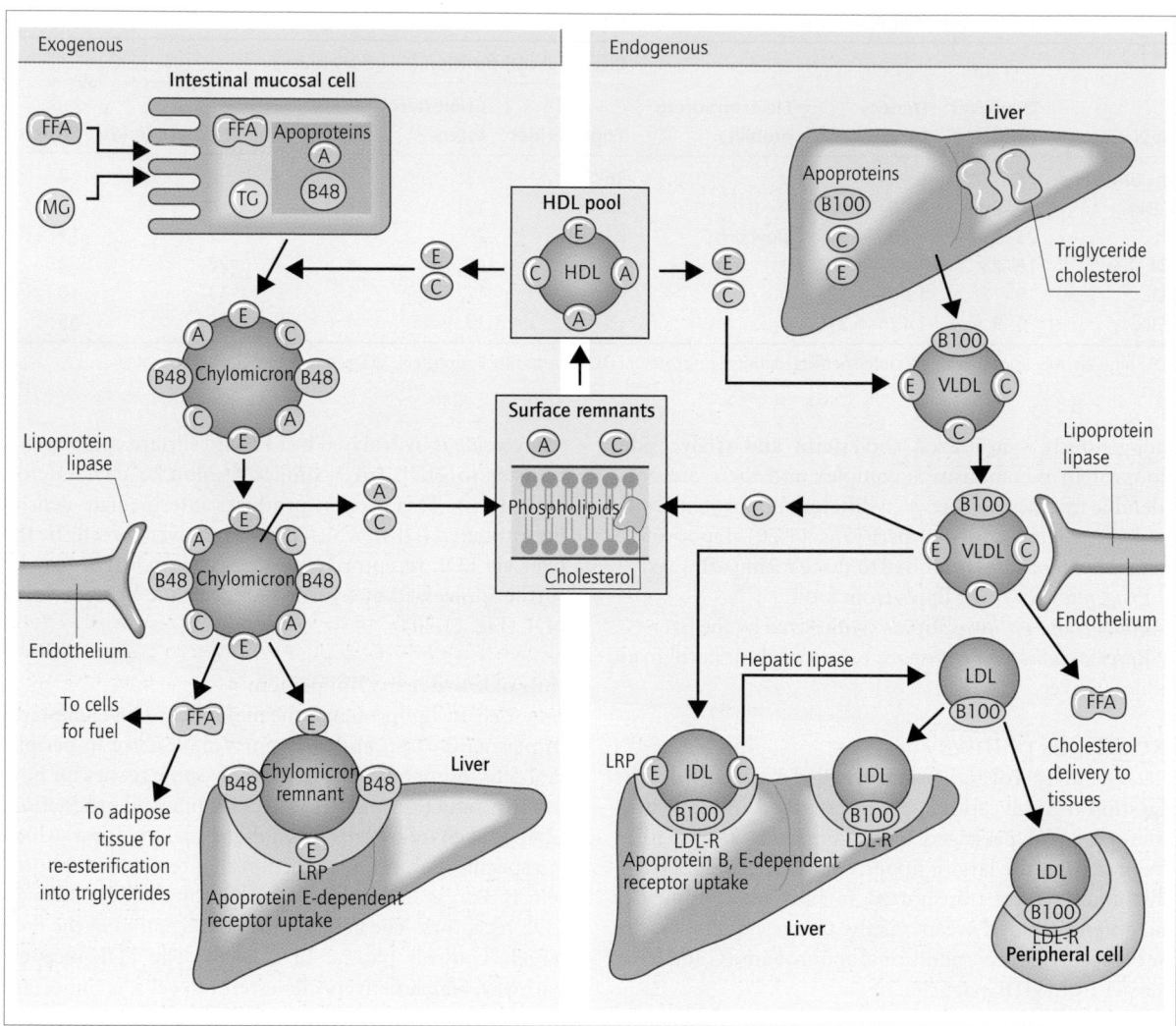

Figure 11.20 Overview of lipoprotein metabolism: exogenous and endogenous pathways. FFA, free fatty acids; LDL-R, LDL receptor; LRP, LDL receptor-related protein; MG, monoglycerides; TG, triglycerides; letters A, B48, B100, C and E refer to apoproteins A, B_{48}, B_{100}, C and E, respectively.

- Transfer to lipoproteins of lower density via cholesterol ester transfer protein (CETP) and then uptake of these lower-density lipoproteins by the liver
- Direct uptake of HDL particles in the liver return by 'scavenger' receptors (SRB1).

Lipids, lipoproteins and atherogenesis

It is clear that increasing plasma cholesterol concentrations are strongly and independently related to risk of atherosclerosis-related disease, particularly CHD. Data from the men screened for the Multiple Risk Factor Intervention Trial (MRFIT) are shown in Fig. 11.22. The relationship between plasma cholesterol and CHD death was continuous, graded and strong across the whole age range and was independent of cigarette smoking and hypertension. A gradient of risk between cholesterol and CHD is seen even in populations where mean plasma cholesterol is low. Essentially, LDL-cholesterol determines the relationship of total plasma cholesterol to CHD risk. The relationship of LDL-cholesterol to the development of the early lesion of atherosclerosis, the fatty streak, is shown in Fig. 11.23.

HDL-cholesterol is strongly and independently related to CHD, but unlike LDL-cholesterol the relationship is inverse. It is not fully understood how increasing HDL-cholesterol appears to protect and low levels increase the risk of CHD. The involvement of HDL in reverse cholesterol transport is likely to be important.

The relationship between plasma triglycerides and

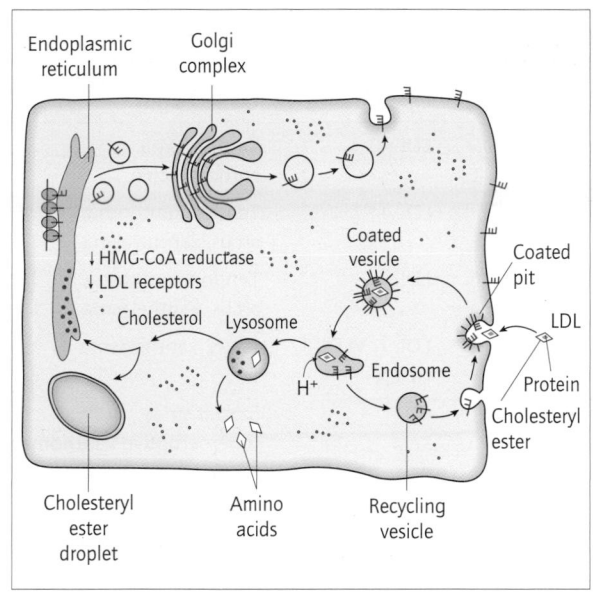

Figure 11.21 The low-density lipoprotein (LDL) receptor pathway.

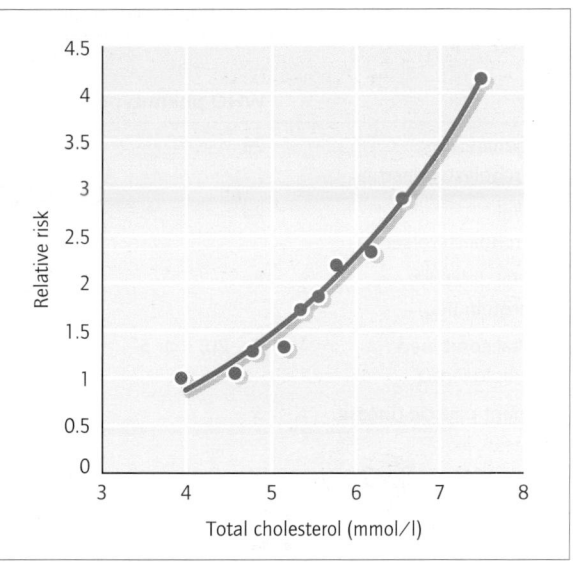

Figure 11.22 Relationship of plasma cholesterol to coronary heart disease (CHD) mortality in the Multiple Risk Factor Intervention Trial (MRFIT) study. Adapted form Stamler J, Wentworth D, Neaton JD. Is relationship between serum cholesterol and risk of premature death from coronary heart disease continuous and graded? *JAMA* 1986; 256: 2823–8.

CHD has remained controversial. Hypertriglyceridaemia can be associated with the accumulation of remnant particles, which are thought to be highly atherogenic. In addition, when triglycerides are raised, LDL subclass distribution is altered towards smaller denser particles, which are thought to be more atherogenic.

Lipoprotein(a) [Lp(a)] is a form of LDL with an additional apoprotein (apoprotein a) attached to it by disulphide bridges. Apoprotein(a) has close structural homology to plasminogen. Lp(a) concentrations are largely genetically determined. Lp(a) is a risk factor for CHD when plasma cholesterol is raised.

Dyslipoproteinaemias

Lipid disorders are classified as either primary or secondary (Tables 11.16 and 11.17). The nomenclature of primary disorders is based, where possible, on the underlying metabolic and/or genetic abnormality. For clarity the WHO phenotype classification is also given.

Lipid and lipoprotein concentrations are normally measured in the fasting state. For most clinical purposes

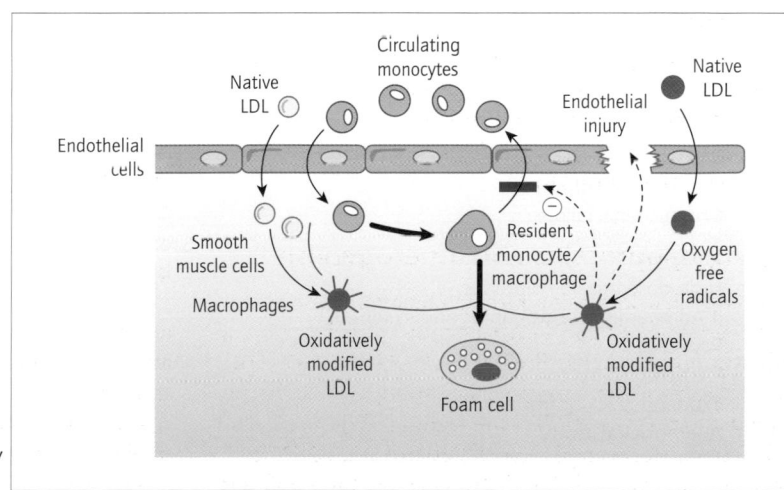

Figure 11.23 LDL-cholesterol and fatty streak formation.

Table 11.16 Classification of primary hyperlipidaemias

Type	WHO phenotype	Typical lipid levels (mmol/l)			Clinical signs
		Cholesterol	Triglycerides	Lipoproteins	
Polygenic hypercholesterolaemia	2a	6.5–9.0	<2.3	LDL ↑	Xanthelasma, corneal arcus
Familial hypercholesterolaemia	2a	7.5–16.0	<2.3	LDL ↑	Tendon xanthoma, arcus, xanthelasma
Familial defective apoprotein B$_{100}$	2a	7.5–16.0	2.3	LDL ↑	Tendon xanthoma, arcus, xanthelasma
Familial combined hyperlipidaemia	2a, 2b, 4 or 5	6.5–10.0	2.3–12.0	LDL ↑, VLDL ↑, HDL ↓	Arcus, xanthelasma
Remnant particle disease	3	9.0–14.0	9.0–14.0	IDL ↑	Palmar striae, tuberoeruptive xanthomas
Familial hypertriglyceridaemia	4, 5	6.5–12.0	10.0–30.0	VLDL ↑	Eruptive xanthomas, lipaemia retinalis, hepatosplenomegaly
Lipoprotein lipase deficiency	1	<6.5	10.0–30.0	Chylomicrons ↑	Eruptive xanthomas, lipaemia retinalis, hepatosplenomegaly
Primary HDL abnormalities					
Hyperalphalipoproteinaemia	–	HDL >2.0	–	HDL ↑	–
Hypoalphalipoproteinaemia	–	HDL <0.9	–	HDL ↓	–

HDL, high-density lipoprotein; IDL, intermediate-density lipoprotein; LDL, low-density lipoprotein; VLDL, very low-density lipoprotein.

Table 11.17 Factors contributing to secondary hyperlipidaemias

Hormonal factors
Pregnancy
Diabetes mellitus
Hypothyroidism

Nutritional factors
Obesity
Anorexia nervosa
Problem drinking

Liver disease
Primary biliary cirrhosis
Extrahepatic biliary obstruction

Renal dysfunction
Nephrotic syndrome
Chronic renal failure

Iatrogenic
High-dose thiazide diuretics
β-Adrenergic receptor antagonists (some)
Retinoids
Corticosteroids
Exogenous sex hormones
Antiretroviral drugs

total cholesterol, total triglyceride and HDL-cholesterol are measured directly. LDL-cholesterol is not measured directly, but calculated by the Friedewald formula (Fig. 11.24).

Familial hypercholesterolaemia

Familial hypercholesterolaemia (FH) is associated with a high risk of premature CHD.

Disease mechanisms
There is a genetic defect in the LDL receptor gene resulting in either absent or defective LDL receptor activity. This reduces the hepatic removal of LDL and prolongs the plasma half-time of LDL, and increases plasma LDL-cholesterol by two- to threefold. Over 400 mutations in the LDL receptor gene have been described.

Epidemiology
Prevalence. Approximately 1 in 500 of the UK population are heterozygotes. The homozygous form is rare and affects approximately 1 in 1 million of the population.

Age and sex. The average age of onset of CHD in untreated heterozygous cases is in the early forties in men and early fifties in women.

$$\text{LDL-cholesterol (mmol/litre)} = \text{total cholesterol} - \text{HDL-cholesterol} - \frac{\text{total triglyceride}}{2.19}$$

Figure 11.24 The Friedewald equation (applicable when total triglyceride less than 4.5 mmol/l).

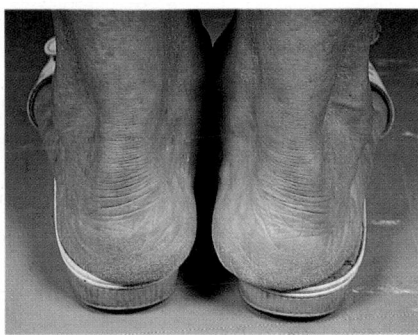

Figure 11.25 Tendon xanthoma in a patient heterozygous for familial hypercholesterolaemia.

Genetics. Autosomal dominant.

Ethnicity. More common (approximately 1 in 100) in some population groups (e.g. South Africans of Dutch descent and Lebanese).

Clinical features

The condition is characterized by a high plasma cholesterol (because of high LDL-cholesterol), premature CHD and tendon xanthomas (Fig. 11.25). Individuals homozygous for FH develop CHD in adolescence.

Tendon xanthomas consist of cholesterol ester-laden foam cells and are typically seen in the extensor tendons on the backs of the hands, over the knuckles and in the Achilles tendons. Sometimes they occur in the patellar tendons and the tendons of the feet. The development of xanthomas is a function of age; approximately 70% of patients have xanthomas by the age of 30 years.

It is important to make the diagnosis, as aggressive lipid-lowering therapy is warranted given the high CHD risk. Family screening is important to identify affected individuals.

Very rarely, the same clinical **phenotype** results from mutations in apoprotein B—familial ligand-defective apoprotein B.

Familial combined hyperlipidaemia

Disease mechanisms

The genetic defect(s) in familial combined hyperlipidaemia (FCH) remains to be determined, although a consistent metabolic finding is overproduction of apoprotein B-containing lipoproteins by the liver. The resulting lipid phenotype depends on the efficiency or otherwise of the lipid catabolic pathways determined by genetic and environmental factors. Obesity and insulin resistance are more common in FCH and contribute to the phenotypic variation. Affected members from the same family may have a raised cholesterol, a raised triglyceride, or both. Apoprotein B concentrations are raised and HDL cholesterol concentrations are low. In addition, remnant particles accumulate and LDL particles are small and dense.

It has been estimated that familial combined hyperlipidaemia accounts for about 10–15% of premature myocardial infarction in Europe and North America. Affected family members have multiple lipoprotein phenotypes.

Epidemiology

Prevalence. Approximately 1 in 200.

Genetics. Uncertain.

Clinical features

FCH is associated with increased CHD risk. There are no specific clinical stigmata; affected individuals may have corneal arcus and xanthelasma, but these signs are not specific. Tendon xanthomas do *not* occur. The diagnosis is often presumptive in a patient with mixed lipaemia, CHD and a family history of CHD. The crux of the clinical diagnosis is the demonstration of multiple lipoprotein phenotypes in the family.

Remnant particle disease

Although rare, this is an interesting disease demonstrating the atherogenicity of lipoprotein remnant particles and the interaction between genetic and other secondary factors (either genetic or acquired).

11

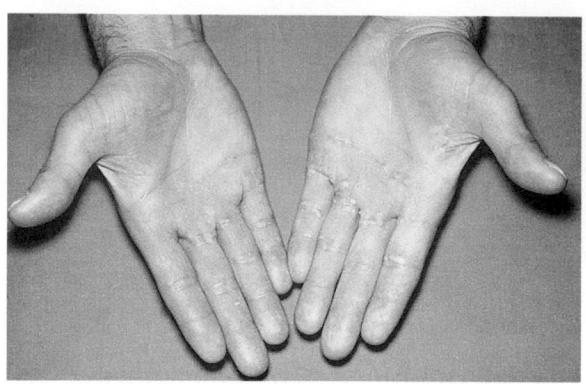

(a)

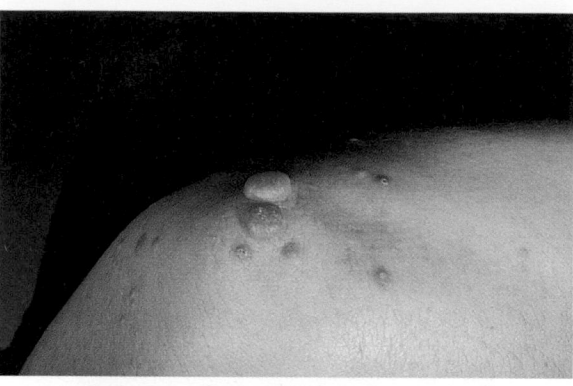

(b)

Figure 11.26 (a) Palmar and (b) tubero-eruptive xanthomas in a patient with remnant particle disease.

Disease mechanisms

There are three common, genetically determined isoforms of apoprotein E. Approximately 70% of all individuals are homozygous for E_3 (the normal allele). Apoprotein E_2 homozygosity occurs in 1% of the population. Apoprotein E_2 is a less efficient ligand for the LDL and LRP receptors. For the remnant particle phenotype to develop, further genetic factors (e.g. FH, FCH) or environmental factors (e.g. obesity, diabetes mellitus, hypothyroidism) are required, which 'stress' the apoprotein E-mediated removal of remnant particles.

Epidemiology

Prevalence. Rare. Affects 1 in 5000–10 000 individuals.

Genetics. The majority (over 90%) of patients with remnant particle disease are homozygous for apoprotein E_2.

Clinical features

The risk of premature CHD and peripheral vascular disease is high in remnant particle disease. The clinical hallmarks are the presence of palmar xanthomas and tubero-eruptive xanthomas (Fig. 11.26).

Plasma cholesterol and triglyceride are both markedly elevated to an approximately equal degree because of the accumulation of remnant particles. Remnants produce a characteristic broad β band on lipoprotein electrophoresis. Apoprotein E_2 homozygosity can be demonstrated by electrophoresis of apoproteins or by sequencing the apoprotein E gene.

Common polygenic hypercholesterolaemia

This diagnosis applies to the *majority* of patients with hypercholesterolaemia.

Epidemiology

Prevalence. Common. Frequency depends on dietary intake of saturated fat and cholesterol.

Genetics. Polygenic. Several common polymorphisms in different gene loci (e.g. apoprotein E, apoprotein B, LDL receptor gene) have been shown to determine differences in plasma cholesterol.

Clinical features

There are no specific clinical features, although corneal arcus and xanthelasma may be present. It is really a diagnosis made after exclusion of secondary causes and the monogenic primary disorders.

Chylomicronaemia syndrome

Chylomicronaemia syndrome is characterized by massive hypertriglyceridaemia (fasting levels more than 11 mmol/l) with the persistence of chylomicrons in the fasting state. Cholesterol levels may be normal (WHO type I) or raised (WHO type V). Usually the syndrome occurs in patients with alcohol excess, diabetes mellitus or on antiretroviral therapy, who often have another genetic hyperlipidaemia such as FCH. Very rarely, it is caused by inborn errors of lipid metabolism such as LPL deficiency.

Clinical features can be dramatic with the development of eruptive xanthomas (Fig. 11.27), hepatosplenomegaly and lipaemia retinalis. In the presence of massive hypertriglyceridaemia, other laboratory measurements (e.g. haemoglobin, bilirubin, liver transaminases) can be affected. Artificially low sodium (approximately 2–4 mmol/l per 10 mmol/l triglyceride) occurs because of the decreased water volume of the plasma. This is termed pseudohyponatraemia (see p. 582).

Chylomicronaemia is associated with an increased risk of pancreatitis. Often, patients complain of inter-

Table 11.18 Classes of lipid-modifying drugs and their mechanisms of action

Drug class	Mechanism of action	Metabolic effects	Plasma lipoproteins		
			LDL	HDL	VLDL
HMG-CoA reductase	Inhibits early stage of cholesterol synthesis	Increased clearance of LDL from plasma by LDL receptors	↓↓↓↓	↑	↓
Fibrates	Increased lipoprotein lipase activity, reduced hepatic VLDL production	Increased VLDL catabolism Increased synthesis of HDL	↓↓	↑↑	↓↓↓
Bile acid sequestrants	Interruption of entrohepatic circulation of bile salts increases hepatic bile acid synthesis from intracellular hepatic cholesterol upregulating hepatic LDL receptors	Increased clearance of LDL from plasma by LDL receptors	↓↓↓	↑	→
Nicotinic acid	Inhibition of lipolysis in fat tissue, reducing free fatty acid flux to liver	Decreased VLDL and LDL synthesis Decreased clearance of HDL	↓↓↓	↑↑↑↑	↓↓↓↓
Fish oils	Inhibit VLDL synthesis		→	→	↓↓↓
Ezetimibe	Inhibits intestinal absorption of dietary and biliary cholesterol	Reduced delivery of cholesterol to liver in chylomicra	↓↓	↑	↓

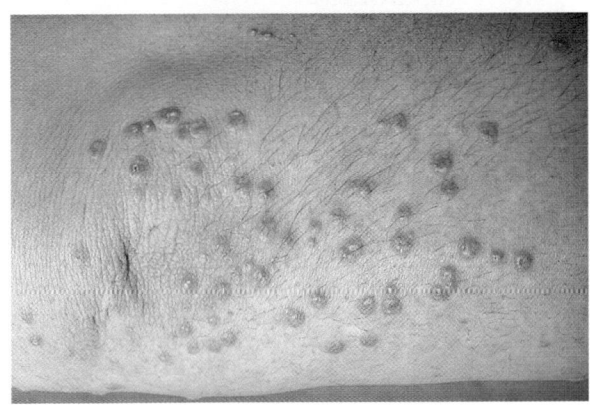

Figure 11.27 Eruptive xanthomas in a patient with chylomi-cronaemia syndrome.

mittent episodes of abdominal pain without full-blown acute pancreatitis. Massive hypertriglyceridaemia may interfere with the assay of amylase producing falsely low levels.

Lipoprotein lipase deficiency

Epidemiology
Prevalence. Rare. Approximately 1 in 1 million.

Genetics. Autosomal recessive.

Clinical features
Lipoprotein lipase deficiency results from genetic defects

in the LPL gene. Over 60 structural defects have been described in the gene. Loss of LPL results in massive hypertriglyceridaemia (50–100 mmol/l). Fasting plasma refrigerated overnight shows a characteristic cream layer. Symptoms and signs are as described for chylomicron-aemia syndrome above. A similar **phenotype** is seen in individuals with an absence of apoprotein C_2, which is necessary for activation of LPL.

Management of dyslipidaemia

The main indications for treatment of dyslipidaemia are the secondary prevention of vascular disease in those with established atherosclerotic disease and the primary pre-vention of vascular disease in those at high risk. Rarely, the major goal of therapy is to reduce the risk of pancreatitis. An additional benefit of therapy in patients with FH is the reduction in size and often the complete disappear-ance of tendon xanthomas. Xanthomas are occasionally symptomatic, probably because of synovitis. Eruptive xanthomas in chylomicronaemia and palmar and tubero-eruptive xanthomas disappear with therapy.

Lipid-lowering therapy is part of the global approach to vascular risk reduction (Table 11.18). Nutritional coun-selling (Table 11.19) and other lifestyle measures such as appropriate physical exercise and smoking cessation are important in all patients (Table 11.20).

Statins
The major therapeutic agents are the HMG-CoA reductase inhibitors known as statins. These drugs (atorvastatin,

11

Table 11.19 Basic principles of lipid-lowering diet

Principle	Amount	Food sources
Decreased total fat; decreased saturated fat	<30% of energy 7–10% of energy	Avoid butter, hard margarine, whole milk, cream, ice cream, high-fat cheese, fatty meats and poultry, sausages, pastries, coffee whitener, products containing hydrogenated oils, palm oil and coconut oil
Increased use of high-protein food (low in saturated fat)		Fish, chicken and turkey; veal, game, spring lamb
Increased complex carbohydrate; increased fruit and vegetable fibre; increased legumes	About 35 g/day of fibre, half derived from fruit and vegetables	All fruit, including dried fruit; all fresh and frozen vegetables; lentils, dried beans, chick peas; unrefined cereal foods, including oats
Decreased dietary cholesterol	<300 mg/day	Allowance of up to 2 egg yolks/week; liver up to twice monthly, other offal avoided
Moderately increased use of mono- and polyunsaturated	Mono: 10–15% of energy Poly: 7–10% of energy	Olive oil, sunflower oil, corn oil and products based on these oils and products

Table 11.20 Management of hyperlipidaemias

Exclude secondary causes of hyperlipidaemia
Glucose tolerance
Thyroid function
Urea and electrolytes
Liver function

Secondary causes of hyperlipidaemia
Treat the primary condition

If lipid abnormality persists
Lipid abnormalities may persist in DM and renal impairment despite the best endeavours and contribute to morbidity from atherosclerosis-related disease
Treatment should then be as for a primary lipid abnormality

Nutritional counselling
Weight loss if overweight
Modify total fat content of the diet, particularly saturated fat
Lipid-lowering modifying diet (Table 11.19)

Chylomicronaemia syndrome
Reduce dietary fat intake to less than 20% of calories; supplementation with medium-chain triglyceride makes the diet more palatable

If dietary and lifestyle measures fail to lead to acceptable lipid levels
For individuals at high risk of premature vascular disease, hypolipidaemic drug therapy (Table 11.18)

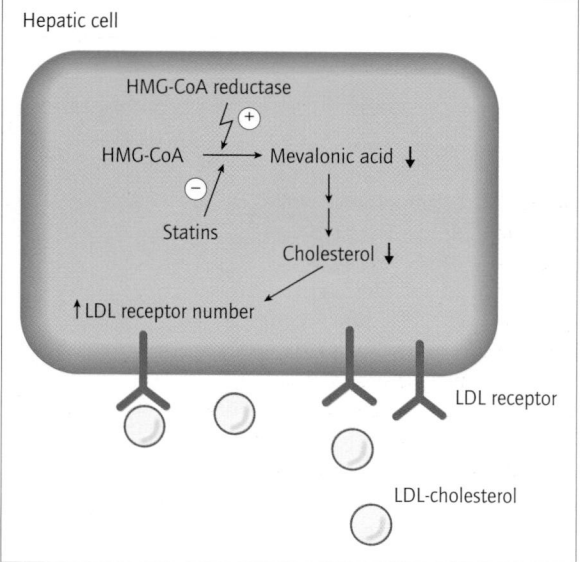

Figure 11.28 Mechanism of action of HMG-CoA reductase inhibitors (statins). Statin drugs reduce the intracellular concentration of cholesterol causing upregulation of hepatic LDL receptors. This increases hepatic uptake of plasma LDL-cholesterol.

fluvastatin, lovastatin, pravastatin and simvastatin) are specific competitive inhibitors of 3-hydroxy-methylglutaryl coenzyme A reductase, the rate-determining enzyme in cholesterol synthesis (Fig. 11.28). Their major site of action is the liver where, as a result of decreased hepatic cholesterol synthesis, the production of LDL receptors is upregulated. This leads to increased LDL uptake by the liver and plasma LDL-cholesterol concentrations decrease by 30–60%. The mechanisms of benefit of statin therapy are not fully understood. However, it is likely that candidate atherosclerotic lesions for myocardial infarction—those which are lipid-rich with a thin fibrous cap—are stabilized and thus less likely to rupture and lead to thrombosis. Arterial endothelial function is also improved by statin therapy.

Table 11.21 Important clinical trials using statin drugs

Trial	Type	Year reported	Drug used	Number of subjects
Scandinavian Simvastatin Survival Study (4S)	Secondary	1994	Simvastatin	4444
Cholesterol and Recurrent Events (CARE)	Secondary	1996	Pravastatin	4159
Long-term intervention with pravastatin in ischaemic disease (LIPID)	Secondary	1998	Pravastatin	9014
West of Scotland Coronary Prevention Study (WOSCOPS)	Primary	1994	Pravastatin	6595
Air Force/Texas Coronary Atherosclerosis Prevention Study (AFCAPS/TexCAPS)	Primary	1998	Lovastatin	6605
Heart Protection Study (HPS)	Primary	2002	Simvastatin	20 536

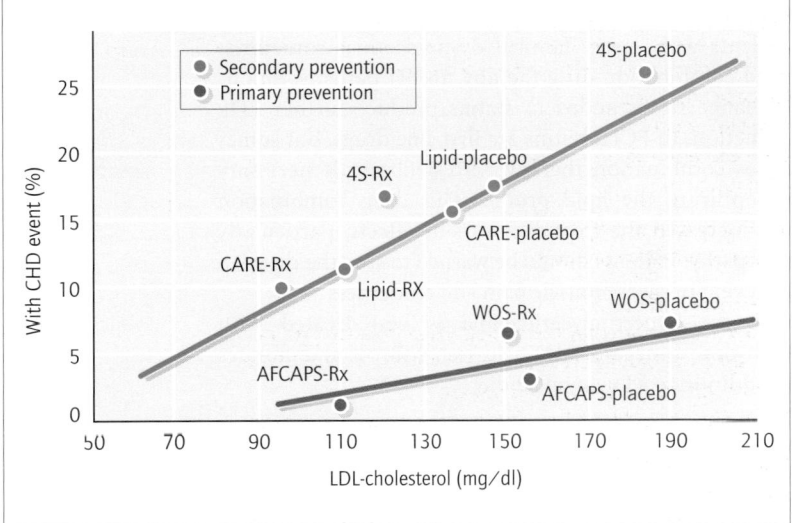

Figure 11.29 Important clinical trials using statin drugs. The graph shows the reduction in coronary heart disease events with some of the different trials. The benefit of each trial is shown in the reduction in events from the placebo group to the treatment (Rx) group. The slope of the lines indicates the magnitude of the benefit and it can be seen that the benefit is greater in secondary prevention than in primary prevention.

Secondary prevention of vascular disease

The introduction of these effective and well-tolerated drugs to clinical practice is based on key clinical trials (Table 11.21; Fig. 11.29), which have made a huge impact on clinical practice. Statins effectively lower the risk of death resulting from CHD, CHD events and stroke in individuals with established CHD across a wide range of plasma cholesterol concentrations. Current UK guidelines give a goal of therapy of total cholesterol less than 5 mmol/l and LDL-cholesterol less than 3 mmol/l in these patients. In the future it is likely that these recommendations will be revised following the Heart Protection Study, which demonstrated similar relative risk reductions across a wide range of LDL-cholesterol concentrations. This suggests that all patients with established vascular disease (including those with carotid and peripheral vas-

cular disease), irrespective of baseline cholesterol, should receive statin therapy.

Primary prevention of vascular disease

Statin therapy has also been shown to reduce the risk of death resulting from CHD, CHD events and stroke in individuals without symptomatic vascular disease (Fig. 11.29). Current guidelines for primary prevention stress the importance of calculation of absolute risk of the individual based on data from the Framingham Prospective Epidemiology Study. Data used to calculate absolute risk include plasma cholesterol or total cholesterol : HDL ratio, age, gender, systolic blood pressure, cigarette smoking and diabetes. Absolute risk may be determined using risk assessment charts (e.g. Joint British Risk Charts, which are now published and updated in the *British*

11

National Formulary) or a computer software package. The absolute risk at which statin therapy is warranted for primary prevention of vascular disease is largely determined by economic considerations. European guidelines suggest that statins should be prescribed for those with a greater than 20% 10-year risk of CHD, while British guidelines use a 30% 10-year risk cut-off point.

When using risk charts it is important to remember that family history is not included. The presence of a family history of premature CHD increases the absolute risk of CHD. Hypertriglyceridaemia also increases the risk category. Risk charts should not be used for familial dyslipidaemias (FH, FCH, remnant particle disease) as these conditions should be treated in their own right given the high CHD risk. Patients with diabetes mellitus without symptomatic vascular disease showed benefit from statin therapy in the Heart Protection Study.

Other drug treatments

Patients with severe familial dyslipidaemias sometimes need combination drug therapy. In FH patients, anion-exchange resins added to statins produce further LDL reduction. In FCH, statins are first-line drugs, but sometimes combination therapy with a fibrate is necessary to optimize the lipid profile. This drug combination has increased the frequency of side-effects, particularly myopathy. Patients should be warned to stop the drugs in the event of severe muscle pain and tenderness.

Severe hypertriglyceridaemia is best treated with high-dose omega-3 fatty acid-rich fish oil and fibrates in addition to a low total fat diet.

The porphyrias

The porphyrias are disorders caused by the overproduction of intermediary compounds, known as porphyrins, as a result of defects in specific enzymes in the haem biosynthetic pathway. In the porphyrias, there is excess production of porphyrins, either in the liver (hepatic porphyrias) or red cells and bone marrow (erythropoietic porphyrias). The result is a spectrum of clinical manifestations, especially neurological symptoms and cutaneous photosensitivity. The acute porphyrias are usually dominantly transmitted and characterized by a tendency to acute attacks of abdominal pain, hypertension and neuropsychiatric distubances including peripheral neuropathies. These attacks can be triggered by alcohol, sex hormones and drugs. Liver disease principally occurs in congenital erythropoietic porphyria and porphyria cutanea tarda.

Pathophysiology

Haem biosynthetic pathways are complex. Briefly, glycine

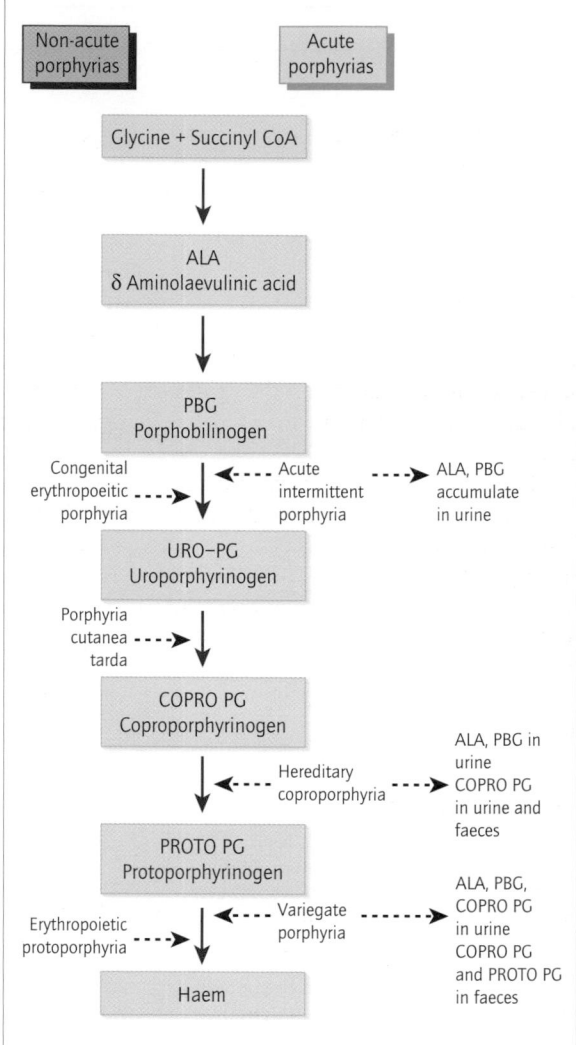

Figure 11.30 The haem biosynthetic pathway and the acute and non-acute porphyrias. If there is a block in the pathway, metabolites above the block tend to accumulate. Both porphobilinogen and uroporphyrinogen can be present in the urine and later metabolites can also accumulate in faeces.

and succinyl–CoA are converted to δ-aminolaevulinic acid (ALA) by δ-ALA synthase. Two molecules of ALA are joined together to form a pyrrole ring and four pyrrole rings are then joined together to create a porphyrin. Porphyrin intermediates are further metabolized to produce haem (Fig. 11.30).

Accumulation of ALA and porphobilinogen (PBG) in acute porphyrias is thought to produce the acute neuropsychiatric and gastrointestinal symptoms. Plasma and urinary ALA and PBG are raised in acute attacks and clinical improvement is associated with falling levels.

Table 11.22 Classification of porphyrias

		Hepatic	Erythropoietic
Acute		Acute intermittent porphyria	
		Hereditary coproporphyria	
		Variegate porphyria	
Non-acute		Porphyria cutanea tarda	Congenital porphyria
			Erythropoetic protoporphyria

Non-acute porphyrias do *not* cause increased ALA or PBG levels (Table 11.22).

All porphyrias (except acute intermittent porphyria) are associated with photosensitivity. Porphyrinogens undergo photo-oxidation in the epidermis to form porphyrins that are deposited and have photosensitizing properties.

The investigation of porphyrias can be confusing, but in all acute forms urinary ALA and PBG are raised. Further distinction is made on detection of abnormal amounts of other porphyrin metabolites in urine and faeces:

- *Acute intermittent porphyria*: no elevation of COPRO PG
- *Hereditary coproporphyria*: COPRO PG in urine and faeces
- *Variegate porphyria*: COPRO PG and PROTO PG in faeces

Hepatic porphyrias

Acute intermittent porphyria

Disease mechanisms
- Enzyme deficiency: hydroxymethylbilane (HMB) synthase, widespread but more common in Scandinavia and the UK
- Autosomal dominant

Clinical features
- Abdominal pain, nausea, vomiting and constipation
- Polyneuropathy: sensory or motor
- Cardiovascular: tachycardia and hypertension
- Psychiatric symptoms: anxiety, depression, disorientation, hallucinations, paranoia
- Other pain symptoms: affecting the limbs, head, neck and chest
- Genitourinary: dysuria and urinary retention
- There is often a family history of porphyria

Heterozygous patients usually remain asymptomatic unless exposed to factors that increase the production of porphyrins. Symptoms rarely occur before puberty.

Common precipitating factors are:
- Alcohol
- Synthetic oestrogens and progestrogens
- Porphyrinogenic drugs (e.g. sulphonamide antibiotics, barbiturates, succinimides)

Investigation
- ALA and PBG are increased in plasma and urine during acute attacks
- Urine turns red-brown on standing during acute attacks
- Faecal porphyrins are usually normal or minimally increased
- HMB synthase measurement in erythrocytes can confirm the diagnosis outside acute attacks and can be used to screen asymptomatic family members

Management
This involves avoiding drugs known to precipitate porphyria, including alcohol and the oral contraceptive pill. Opiates can be given for abdominal pain and phenothiazines for nausea, vomiting, anxiety and restlessness.

A high carbohydrate intake reduces hepatic ALA synthase activity, so intravenous glucose or parenteral nutrition are used. Intravenous haem reduces porphyrin precursor excretion and is thought to lead to more rapid recovery. The rate of recovery depends on the degree of neuronal damage and may take 1–2 days or months to years.

Prevention of further attacks relies on identifying and avoiding precipitating factors.

Variegate porphyria and hereditary coproporphyria

Disease mechanisms
- Autosomal dominant
- Enzyme deficiency:
  Variegate porphyria: protoporphyrinogen oxidase
  Hereditary coproporphria: coproporphyrinogen oxidase

Clinical features
The presentation is like acute intermittent porphyria, but photosensitivity also occurs. Variegate porphyria is common in South Africa (3 in 1000 white South Africans have the disorder). Hereditary coproporphyria is rare.

Investigation
Urinary ALA and PBG are increased in both forms during acute attacks. In variegate porphyria, there is increased faecal protoporphyrin and coproporphyrin, and increased urinary coproporphyrin during attacks. In hereditary coproporphyria, coproporphyrin is increased in urine

11

and faeces and the diagnosis can be confirmed by measuring coproporphyrinogen oxidase activity.

Management

As for acute intermittent porphyria.

Porphyria cutanea tarda

Disease mechanisms

Cases may be acquired or inherited. There is a deficiency of hepatic uroporphyrinogen decarboxylase. Iron and transferrin levels can be raised and mild hepatic iron overload can occur.

Clinical features

The main feature is cutaneous photosensitivity causing bullous eruptions on sun-exposed areas that heal with scarring. Hirsutism, hyperpigmentation and hepatomegaly may occur. Neurological manifestations are not observed.

The most common contributory factor is excessive alcohol intake, although associations with iron, oestrogen and polychlorinated hydrocarbons have been described.

Investigation

Increased urinary uroporphyrin, but normal urinary ALA and PBG.

Management

Contributory factors, especially alcohol use, should be discontinued. Repeated venesection reduces hepatic iron content. Chloroquine or hydroxychloroquine form complexes with the excess porphyrins and promote their excretion.

Erythropoietic porphyrias

Congenital erythropoietic porphyria

Disease mechanisms

- Autosomal recessive (very rare)
- Enzyme deficiency: uroporphyrinogen synthase

Clinical features

Severe cutaneous photosensitivity, beginning in early infancy. There may be secondary infection. Porphyrins are deposited in teeth and bones.

Investigation

Uroporphyrin and coproporphyrin accumulate in bone marrow, erythrocytes, plasma, urine and faeces. The diagnosis is confirmed by deficiency of uroporphyrinogen synthase activity in erythrocytes.

Management

Blood transfusions are often necessary and splenectomy

reduces any haemolysis. Protection from sunlight and prevention of minor skin trauma are important. β-carotene may be useful. Bacterial infections should be treated promptly. Bone marrow transplantation may be curative.

Erythropoietic protoporphyria

Disease mechanisms

- Autosomal dominant
- Enzyme deficiency: partial deficiency of ferrochelatase

Clinical features

Childhood skin photosensitivity occurs and is characterized by redness, swelling, burning and itching on sunlight exposure. Chronic liver disease may be caused by the accumulation of protoporphyrin leading to liver failure and death.

Investigation

Protoporphyrin levels are increased in bone marrow, circulating erythrocytes, plasma, bile and faeces.

Management

Oral β-carotene improves tolerance to sunlight. Colestyramine and other porphyrin absorbents are useful if the liver is involved. Splenectomy is useful if there is haemolysis. Transfusions or intravenous haem therapy may be beneficial. Liver transplantation may be necessary.

Other metabolic diseases

Lysosomal storage diseases

Disease mechanisms

Lysosomes are cytoplasmic organelles containing enzymes involved in hydrolysis. Their major function is the degradation of macromolecules, but they are also involved in the uptake of molecules such as vitamin B_{12}, lipoproteins, peptides, hormones and growth factors. Lysosomal enzymes are glycoproteins synthesized within the endoplasmic reticulum.

Lysosomal storage diseases are rare and are usually autosomal recessive or X-linked recessive disorders. They are characterized by progressive deposition of metabolic substrates in different organs including brain, liver, spleen and bone.

Lysosomal storage diseases have been classified into groups according to the type of macromolecule affected (Table 11.23). These groups include:

- Sphingolipidoses
- Mucopolysaccharidoses
- Mucolipidoses

Table 11.23 Lysosomal storage diseases

	Enzyme deficiency	Stored material	Genetics	Specific manifestations
Sphingolipidoses				
G_{M1} gangliosidosis	β-Galactosidase	Ganglioside G_{M1}	AR	Coarse facies, blindness
G_{M2} gangliosidosis (Tay–Sachs disease)	Hexosaminidase	Ganglioside G_{M2}	AR	Macrocephaly, cherry red spot Increased prevalence in Ashkenazi Jews
Gaucher's disease	β-Glucocerebrosidase	Glucocerebroside	AR	Mental retardation, hepatosplenomegaly Increased prevalence in Ashkenazi Jews
Fabry's disease	α-Galactosidase	Trihexoside	X-linked recessive	Paresthesiae Cutaneous angiokeratoma Renal failure
Niemann–Pick disease	Sphingomyelinase	Sphingomyelin	AR	Hepatosplenomegaly, foam cells in liver and bone marrow
Mucopolysaccharidoses				
Hurler's disease	α-Iduronidase	Dermatan sulphate Heparan sulphate	AR	Coarse facies, corneal clouding, deafness
Hunter's disease	Iduronate sulphatase	Dermatan sulphate Heparan sulphate	X-linked recessive	Coarse facies, deafness
Mucolipidoses				
Mucolipidosis I	*N*-acetyl-neuraminic hydrolase	Sialic acid-rich Glycoproteins	AR	Myoclonus, cherry red spot, foam cells in blood/bone marrow

AR, autosomal recessive.

Clinical features

Frequent clinical features include learning disability, epilepsy, hepatosplenomegaly (causing abdominal distension) and bony abnormalities. In many of the sphingolipidoses, neuronal degeneration is associated with retinal degeneration causing a diagnostic 'cherry red spot' appearance at the macula. Mucopolysaccharidoses are associated with coarse facies, thickened skin, clouded corneas and skeletal abnormalities (dysostosis multiplex). Mucolipidoses are clinically similar to mucopolysaccharidoses.

Investigation

Diagnosis of these rare disorders is an area for paediatricians with an interest in metabolic diseases. Diagnosis depends on demonstrating enzyme deficiency in tissues from the affected individual (e.g. rectal biopsy or skin biopsy). Parental consanguinity is frequently found in the autosomal recessive disorders. Genetic techniques are increasingly used in diagnosis and screening of family members. The high incidence of Tay–Sachs disease in Ashkenazi Jews has resulted in a successful voluntary screening programme to detect carriers of the gene defect. Mucopolysaccharidoses are associated with excess urinary excretion of heparan, dermatan or keratan sulphates. These urinary products are not found in excess in the clinically similar mucolipidoses. Radiography is often necessary to assess skeletal abnormalities.

Disorders of carbohydrate metabolism

Glycogen storage diseases

Disease mechanisms

Glycogen is a high-molecular-weight polymer of glucose residues that functions as a glucose store in many tissues. Liver and skeletal muscle have significant glycogen stores, while neural tissue has very little glycogen content. Glycogen is formed by the enzyme glycogen synthase and is mainly catabolized by glycogen phosphorylase. Glycogen storage diseases are a group of disorders in which glycogen stores increase because of a failure to catabolize glycogen or where the molecular structure of glycogen is abnormal. Most of these conditions are autosomal recessive in inheritance and usually present in childhood. Type 1 (von Gierke's disease) and type 5 (McArdle's disease) are the most common forms (Table 11.24).

Clinical features

Two main presentations are recognized:

1 In infancy with hypoglycaemia and hepatomegaly. Hypoglycaemia occurs because of an inability of the liver to maintain gluconeogenesis in the fasting state and hepatomegaly because of the increased hepatic stores of glycogen.

2 In childhood with muscle weakness, hypotonia and muscle wasting.

11

Table 11.24 Glycogen storage diseases

Type	Disease	Affected tissues	Clinical features	Prognosis
1	von Gierke's	Liver, kidney, intestine	Hepatomegaly, hypoglycaemia, lactic acidosis	High mortality in infant years, good prognosis if survive
2	Pompe's	Liver, skeletal and cardiac muscle	Heart failure, hypotonia	Usually die in first year of life
3	Forbes'	Liver, muscle	Similar to type 1, but milder phenotype	Good
4	Andersen's	Liver	Hepatomegaly, failure to thrive, liver cirrhosis and portal hypertension	Usually die in first 3 years of life
5	McArdle's	Muscle	Muscle cramps, proximal muscle wasting	Normal life expectancy

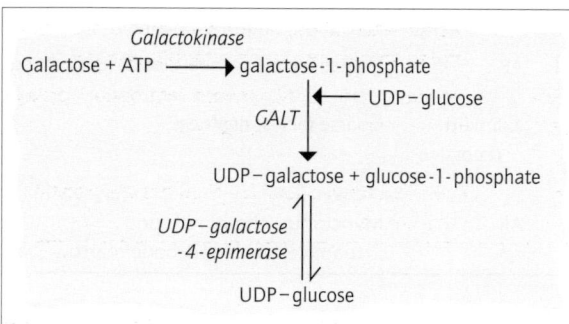

Figure 11.31 Metabolism of galactose. Classic galactosaemia results from galactose-1-phosphate uridyl transferase (GALT) deficiency.

Investigation

Diagnosis frequently requires liver or skeletal muscle biopsy to demonstrate defective enzyme activity. In McArdle's disease, muscle enzymes (creatine phosphokinase, lactate dehydrogenase) are raised after strenuous exercise and myoglobinuria may occur.

Management

Dietary therapy with frequent feeding is a useful therapeutic approach to the hepatic hypoglycaemic disorders. Muscle cramps in McArdle's disease may be prevented by taking glucose before exercise or simply avoiding strenuous exercise. Glucagon is usually an ineffective treatment for the hypoglycaemia because the liver is unable to mobilize the glycogen stores.

Galactosaemia

Disease mechanisms

Lactose, the main carbohydrate in milk, is a disaccharide containing galactose and glucose. After ingestion, lactose is hydrolysed by intestinal lactase and in the liver the absorbed galactose is converted to glucose by a series of enzymatic steps (Fig. 11.31). Deficiency of galactose-1-phosphate uridyl transferase (GALT) produces the clinically most important form of galactosaemia, also known as classic galactosaemia. Its inheritance is autosomal recessive and it occurs in approximately 1 in 50 000 births.

Clinical features

Classic galactosaemia usually presents within days to weeks of birth. Reluctance to ingest breast milk or milk formulas, dehydration, hypoglycaemia and dehydration occur. Jaundice, hepatomegaly and ascites may develop. Cataracts develop over weeks to months. The infant dies within weeks in the absence of treatment.

Galactokinase deficiency results in cataract formation caused by galactitol deposition in the lens, but no other clinical features. Inheritance is autosomal recessive.

Investigation

Raised blood concentrations of galactose and galactose-1-phosphate. Assay of red blood cell GALT activity.

Management

Breastfeeding must be stopped and milk substitutes that do not contain galactose used instead. Survivors require long-term follow-up because they remain at risk of hepatic damage and cataracts.

Hereditary fructose intolerance

Fructose is a normal dietary constituent found in fruits, vegetables and honey. Sucrose (table sugar) is a disaccharide containing fructose and glucose. Fructose is absorbed from the gut by specific fructose transporters and metabolized mainly in the liver. Defects of fructose metabolism lead to raised blood fructose, hypoglycaemia and vomiting soon after fructose ingestion. In children, vomiting, hepatomegaly, jaundice, proteinuria, aminoaciduria and failure to thrive may occur. Avoiding fructose-containing foods removes the symptoms so children learn to avoid sucrose- and fructose-containing food. Consequently, adults with this condition often have little tooth decay.

Hereditary fructose intolerance is caused by deficiency

Table 11.25 Inherited disorders of amino acid metabolism

Amino acid affected	Disorder	Enzyme defect	Clinical manifestations
Phenylalanine	Phenylketonuria	Phenylalanine hydroxylase	Mental retardation, neuropsychiatric dysfunction, hypopigmentation of skin and hair, eczema
Tyrosine	Alkaptonuria	Homogentistic acid oxidase	Dark urine stains nappies, blue-grey cartilage (ochronosis), arthritis
Tyrosine	Albinism	Tyrosinase	White hair, pale skin, pink eyes, easy sunburn
Homocystine	Homocystinuria		
	Type 1	Cystathione-β-synthase	Mental retardation, Marfan-like syndrome, thrombotic tendency
	Type 2	5,10-Methylene tetra-hydrofolate reductase	Mental retardation
Ornithine	Hyperammonaemia	Ornithine transcarbamylase	Mental retardation, neuropsychiatric dysfunction, protein intolerance, ammonia intoxication
Branched chain amino acids (valine, leucine and isoleucine)	Maple syrup disease (branched chain ketoaciduria)	Branched chain keto-acid decarboxylase	Neonatal acidosis, fits, mental retardation, protein intolerance, maple syrup odour
Glycine	Hyperoxaluria (type 1)	Alanine glyoxylate aminotransferase	Recurrent renal calculi (calcium oxalate stones), renal failure

of fructose-1-phosphate aldolase, inherited as an autosomal recessive trait. The condition is sometimes fatal in childhood, but treatment by avoiding fructose results in a good prognosis.

Inherited disorders of amino acid metabolism and storage

Eight of the 20 different amino acids required for polypeptide synthesis are essential; they must be obtained from dietary sources because humans cannot synthesize them. There are more than 70 amino acid disorders, which are typified by catabolic defects (approximately 60) and transport abnormalities (approximately 10).

Disease mechanisms

Disorders of amino acid catabolism result in the accumulation of the intermediary compound in the blood or urine (Table 11.25). This may be the parent amino acid (aminoacidopathy) or products in the catabolic pathway (organic acidaemia). There may be a variety of defective reactions involving some amino acid pathways and there may be an even larger variety of molecular defects (e.g. there are five forms of hyperphenylalaninaemia, seven forms of homocystinuria and seven types of methylmalonic acidaemia).

Epidemiology

Rare, ranging from 1 in 10 000 (cystinuria or phenylketonuria) to 1 in 200 000 (homocystinuria or alkaptonuria).

Collectively, they are found in approximately 1 in 500–1000 live births/year.

Clinical features

Clinical manifestations are varied. Some are asymptomatic (e.g. sarcosinaemia or hyperprolinaemia) and some may be lethal in the untreated neonate (e.g. ornithine carbamoyltransferase deficiency).

Central nervous system dysfunction may occur, resulting in developmental retardation, seizures, alterations in sensation and behavioural disturbances. Protein-induced vomiting, neurological dysfunction and hyperammonaemia occur in disorders of the urea cycle intermediates (e.g. ornithine carbamoyltransferase). Metabolic ketoacidosis is frequent in branched-chain amino acid metabolism disorders (e.g. maple syrup urine disease). There is occasional focal tissue or organ involvement (e.g. liver disease, renal failure, cutaneous abnormalities or eye lesions).

Management

Diagnosis and appropriate treatment can prevent or reduce the effects of these disorders. Treatment often involves reducing the intake of the amino acid that cannot be effectively metabolized. Screening programmes to detect phenylketonuria in newborns have been established in most developed countries. Aminoacidopathies and organic acidaemias can be screened for in the newborn using blood or urine. Genetic defects have been determined for many of these disorders, allowing prenatal diagnosis in affected families.

11

Table 11.26 Genetic disorders of membrane transport

Disorder	Substrate(s)	Tissue manifesting defect	Molecular basis of defect	Major clinical manifestation	Genetics
Amino acid					
Cystinuria	Cystine, lysine, arginine, ornithine	Proximal renal tubule, jejunal mucosa	Mutation of shared di-basic cystine transport protein	Cystine nephrolithiasis	Autosomal recessive
Hartnup's disease	Neutral amino acid	Proximal renal tubule, jejunal mucosa	Neutral amino acid transport protein	Aminoaciduria, pellagra	Autosomal recessive
Sugar					
Renal glycosuria	D-glucose	Proximal renal tubule	Mutation of D-glucose transporter	Glycosuria with normal blood glucose	Autosomal recessive
Anion					
Familial hypo-phosphataemic rickets	Inorganic phosphate	Proximal renal tubule, jejunal mucosa	Mutation of inorganic phosphate transport protein	Rickets/osteomalacia	X-linked dominant
Cystic fibrosis	Chloride	Lung, pancreas, sweat glands	Mutation of ion channel protein	Bronchiectasis, pancreatic failure	Autosomal recessive
Cation					
Renal tubular acidosis	Hydrogen ion	Distal or proximal renal tubule	Mutation of hydrogen ion pump carrier protein	Hyperchloraemic acidosis Type 1: hypokalaemia	Autosomal recessive
				Type 2: bicarbonate wasting	Autosomal recessive
Water					
Nephrogenic diabetes insipidus	Water	Distal renal tubule	Defective vasopressin receptor	Polyuria, polydipsia	X-linked recessive
			Defective aquaporin channel		Autosomal dominant and recessive

Inherited defects of membrane transport

Many molecules require transport systems to cross across cell membranes either because of low permeability of the membrane to the molecule, to increase the rate of transfer or to allow transport against a concentration gradient (Table 11.26). There have been more than 20 inherited disorders of membrane transport reported and most affect the epithelia of the gut and/or the kidney (see p. 527). The molecules affected include amino acids, lipids, sugars, cations, anions and water. These disorders have specific phenotypes and usually have autosomal recessive or X-linked inheritance. The phenotypes vary from benign disorders with no pathological consequences (renal glycosuria) to life-threatening multisystem disorders (cystic fibrosis). The genetic defects associated with these disorders have largely been elucidated.

Amyloidosis

These conditions constitute a heterogeneous group of disorders caused by extracellular protein deposits with a characteristic fibrillar structure. Amyloidosis can be acquired or hereditary and the deposits can be localized or systemic. Focal amyloid deposits may be incidental, particularly in the elderly, but systemic amyloidosis and some local forms are progressive and frequently fatal.

Epidemiology

Clinically significant amyloid deposits occur in a number of common diseases. In Alzheimer's disease, β-protein amyloid deposits are found in the brain and cerebral blood vessels. In type 2 diabetes mellitus, amyloid derived from islet amyloid polypeptide is always present in the islets of Langerhans (Fig. 11.32). β_2-Microglobulin amyloid deposition in the bones and joints ultimately affects

Table 11.27 Classification of the most common types of amyloid and amyloidosis

Type	Fibril protein precursor	Clinical syndrome
AA	Serum amyloid A	Reactive systemic amyloidosis associated with acquired or hereditary chronic inflammatory diseases. Formerly known as secondary amyloidosis
AL	Monoclonal immunoglobulin light chains	Systemic amyloidosis associated with myeloma, monoclonal gammopathy, occult dyscrasia. Formerly known as primary amyloidosis
ATTR	Normal plasma transthyretin Genetically variant transthyretin	Senile systemic amyloidosis with prominent cardiac involvement Familial amyloid polyneuropathy, usually with systemic amyloidosis. Sometimes prominent amyloid cardiomyopathy or nephropathy
$A\beta_2M$	β_2-Microglobulin	Periarticular and, occasionally, systemic amyloidosis associated with renal failure and long-term dialysis
$A\beta$	β-Protein precursors (and rare genetic variants)	Cerebrovascular and intracerebral plaque amyloid in Alzheimer's disease. Occasional familial cases
AIAPP	Islet amyloid polypeptide	Amyloid in islets of Langerhans in type 2 DM and insulinoma

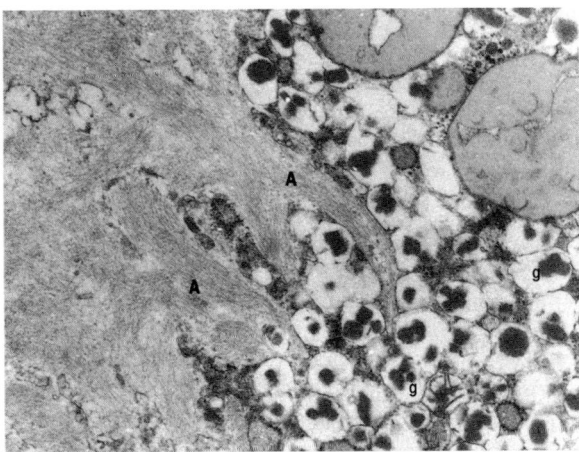

Figure 11.32 Histology of type 2 DM showing amyloid deposition (A) in pancreatic β cells.

most individuals receiving long-term dialysis. Systemic AL amyloidosis, the most frequently diagnosed type, complicates 5–10% of cases of myeloma and other monoclonal B-cell dyscrasias. Systemic AA amyloidosis develops in 1–5% of patients with chronic inflammatory disorders. Hereditary forms of systemic amyloidosis, caused by point mutations in a variety of genes, may account for up to 5% of cases.

Disease mechanisms

Amyloid deposits consist mainly of protein fibrils, the peptide subunits of which differ in the different forms of the disease and constitute the basis for the classification of the clinical amyloidosis syndromes (Table 11.27). All amyloid fibrils share a common, predominantly β-sheet ultrastructure, and stain characteristically with certain histochemical dyes including Congo red. Amyloid fibrils are derived from soluble precursor proteins that tend to be produced either in abnormal **quantity** or in abnormal **forms**.

Many amyloid fibril precursor proteins are plasma proteins, and others are produced locally (e.g. hormone proteins). Amyloid deposits disrupt the structure and function of normal tissues, although accumulation sufficient to cause symptoms may take many years. Macroscopically, amyloidotic organs have a rubbery, waxy consistency, and may be markedly enlarged, especially the liver, spleen, kidneys, heart and tongue. The variety of organs that may be involved, especially in AL amyloidosis, produces a wide spectrum of clinical features.

Clinical features

Amyloidosis is typically identified following a biopsy for organ dysfunction (e.g. of the kidneys, liver, heart or gut). The diagnosis should be specifically considered in certain situations (e.g. proteinuria in a patient with a chronic inflammatory disorder or with a monoclonal gammopathy). In AL amyloidosis, other clinical features may be present, such as carpal tunnel syndrome, peripheral and autonomic neuropathy, and/or restrictive cardiomyopathy. Certain signs are highly characteristic of AL amyloid, including periorbital purpura and macroglossia (large tongue).

AA amyloidosis presents with proteinuria and/or renal impairment in 95% of cases. The spleen and adrenal glands are commonly affected, and the liver in about 25%. Clinically significant cardiac and neuropathic amyloid is very rare, but patients with advanced disease often have gastrointestinal dysfunction. The median prognosis is 5–10 years, but is much improved with successful anti-inflammatory treatment.

11

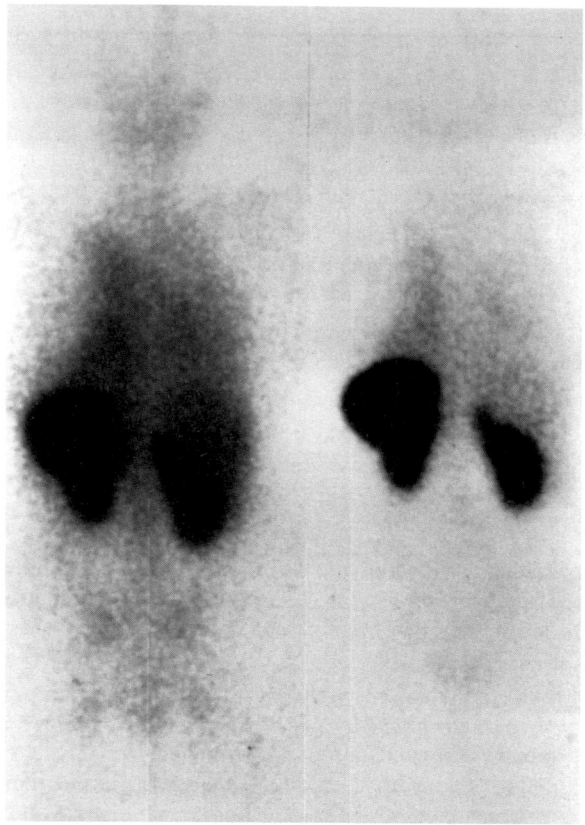

Figure 11.33 Posterior whole-body scintigraphs following intravenous injection of radiolabelled serum amyloid P component (^{123}I-SAP) of a patient with AA amyloidosis complicating rheumatoid arthritis. At presentation with proteinuria (left), the spleen, kidneys and adrenal glands are infiltrated with amyloid. 12 months later, a follow-up scan (right) shows more intense uptake into the same organs indicating that the quantity of amyloid has increased. The remainder of the image is because of tracer in the circulation.

AL amyloidosis often involves the heart, kidneys, skin, gut, liver, muscle (e.g. tongue) and peripheral and/or autonomic nerves. The immunoglobulin light chain amyloid precursor protein differs in every patient, and the deposits may be quite localized or very diffuse. Typical survival is less than 2 years, although chemotherapy to suppress the underlying plasma cell dyscrasia is very effective in some cases.

Typical features of amyloid organ involvement:
- *Kidney:* mild proteinuria to nephrotic syndrome with progressive renal failure
- *Heart:* restrictive cardiomyopathy
- *Skin:* diffuse waxy infiltration with nodules and plaques.

Purpura caused by vascular fragility, characteristically around the eyes in AL
- *Liver:* hepatomegaly, but function is well preserved. Cholestatic picture
- *Gut:* weight loss, dysmotility, bleeding, altered bowel habit and malabsorption. More often resulting from autonomic dysfunction than from severe amyloid infiltration
- *Endocrine:* mild adrenal impairment is common in all systemic types
- *Nervous system:* peripheral neuropathy (sensorimotor) and autonomic neuropathy (postural hypotension, diarrhoea, bladder dysfunction)
- *Joints:* painful arthropathy with swelling, typical in β_2-microglobulin type and occasionally in AL
- *Miscellaneous:* carpal tunnel syndrome, macroglossia, acquired clotting factor IX and X deficiencies are all characteristic of AL amyloidosis

Investigation

Staining biopsy samples with Congo red dye reveals amyloid deposits in affected organs as red-green birefringence under polarized light. The type of amyloid fibril is determined by immunohistochemical staining using antibodies that react with the various fibril proteins.

All amyloid deposits contain a minor non-fibrillar constituent, amyloid P component, derived from a normal plasma protein 'serum amyloid P component' (SAP). SAP binds specifically to all types of amyloid fibril and radiolabelled SAP has been developed as a nuclear medicine tracer for scintigraphic imaging of amyloid deposits *in vivo* (Fig. 11.33).

Radiolabelled SAP scintigraphy provides a macroscopic whole-body survey and permits serial prospective monitoring. SAP scintigraphy is now available routinely at the National Amyloidosis Centre at the Royal Free Hospital, London.

Management and prognosis

The underlying disorder that has led to amyloid deposition must be characterized, monitored and managed as appropriate. No treatment is yet available that specifically causes regression of amyloid deposits. Studies in several different forms of amyloidosis have shown that therapy that succeeds in reducing the supply of the amyloid fibril precursor protein helps to preserve organ function and can prolong survival substantially (Table 11.28). Gradual regression of amyloid has been demonstrated by systematic serial radiolabelled SAP studies under these circumstances. Supportive therapy for failing organ function is vital including dialysis and, in selected cases, renal, cardiac and hepatic transplantation.

Table 11.28 Reducing the supply of fibril precursors in systemic amyloid

Disease	Aim of treatment	Example of treatment
AA amyloid	Suppress acute phase response	Immunosuppression in rheumatoid arthritis, Still's disease (chlorambucil). Colchicine for familial Mediterranean fever, even if clinical episodes not fully suppressed. Surgery for osteomyelitis and rare cytokine-producing tumours
AL amyloid	Suppress production of monoclonal immunoglobulin light chains	Chemotherapy for myeloma and monoclonal gammopathy
Hereditary amyloidosis	Eliminate source of genetically variant protein	Orthotopic liver transplantation for variant transthyrethin-associated familial amyloid polyneuropathy
Haemodialysis amyloidosis	Reduce plasma concentration of β_2M	Renal transplantation

! Must know checklist

- A random venous plasma glucose of greater than 11 mmol/l is abnormal and suggests a diagnosis of diabetes mellitus (DM)

- Obesity is a major risk factor for coronary heart disease, hypertension and type 2 DM

- Intensive treatment aiming to reduce blood glucose concentrations to near normal reduces the appearance of microvascular complications of DM in both type 1 and type 2 DM

- Microvascular complications of DM may be present at diagnosis

- Heavy ketonuria (3+ or greater) strongly suggests the possibility of diabetic ketoacidosis

- In type 2 DM, strict blood pressure control reduces the progression of diabetic retinopathy and the incidence of stroke

- Statins (HMG-CoA reductase inhibitors) reduce total cholesterol by upregulating hepatic low-density lipoprotein receptors

- Polygenic hypercholesterolaemia is the most common form of hypercholesterlaemia, but is a diagnosis of exclusion

- Inherited metabolic diseases are frequently associated with learning disability and epilepsy

- Patients with DM are most likely to die from macrovascular complications

Further reading

Books

Beaudet AL, Scriver CR, Sly WS, Valle D. *Metabolic Molecular Bases of Inherited Disease*, 8th edn. New York: McGraw-Hill, 2002.

Watkins PJ. *ABC of Diabetes*, 5th edn. London: BMJ Publishing Group, 2003.

Williams G, Pickup JC. *Handbook of Diabetes*, 2nd edn. Oxford: Blackwell Science, 1999.

Hoffman GF, Nyham WL, Zschocke J, Kahler SG, Mayatepek E. *Inherited Metabolic Diseases*. Philadelphia: Lippincott Williams & Wilkins, 2002.

Journals

Diabetes Reviews, American Diabetes Association.

International Journal of Obesity, Nature Publishing Group. http://www.nature.com/ijo/

Current Opinion in Lipidology, Lippincott Williams & Wilkins. http://www.colipidology.com/

Websites

http://www.diabetes.org
http://care.diabetesjournals.org
http://www.diabetes.org.uk
http://www.niddk.nih.gov
http://www.idf.org
http://www.diabetes.com.au
http://www.clinicalevidence.org
http://www.ncbi.nlm.nih.gov/omim

11

Endocrine Disease

12

Introduction

Endocrine disorders can present in many different medical specialties or in general practice. Therefore, all doctors need a clear understanding of these disorders. Disorders of the thyroid gland and of the female reproductive system are particularly common, and present routinely to primary care physicians. A skilled general practitioner will spot when the common symptoms of fatigue, weight change or altered mental function signal an endocrine disorder. This is particularly true when such symptoms are brought about by one of the more uncommon pituitary or adrenal disorders.

Worldwide, iodine deficiency has a great impact, causing goitre and hypothyroidism.

The financial cost of treating endocrine diseases ranges from the trivial (e.g. a course of thyroxine, which in the UK costs a few pounds per week) to the alarmingly expensive (e.g. growth hormone and erythropoietin, which in the UK can cost over £200 per week).

Structure and function

Principles of endocrinology

Hormones are chemical messengers released by one cell to act on another, which may be nearby or distant. They may be transported by the bloodstream, by the body fluid or may act locally on adjacent cells. When a blood-borne hormone acts on a distant target tissue, this is termed an 'endocrine' effect. When a hormone acts on cells adjacent to the cells that secrete it, this is termed a 'paracrine' effect. When a hormone acts on the cells that secrete it, then this feedback is termed an 'autocrine' effect.

Hormone functions may be grouped into several categories:
- Reproduction and sexual differentiation
- Growth and development
- Maintenance of the internal environment (homoeostasis)
- Regulation of metabolism and nutrient supply

Secretion of hormones is subject to negative **feedback control**. Feedback loops can involve the hypothalamo-pituitary axis, which detects changes in concentrations of hormones secreted by peripheral endocrine glands, or one gland may sense and respond to changes in a variable that it regulates.

Types of hormones

There are four **chemical classes** of hormones:
- Proteins and polypeptides (the largest group)
- Cholesterol derivatives
- Tyrosine and tryptophan derivatives
- Lipid and phospholipid derivatives

Protein and polypeptide hormones

These are synthesized and packaged within membrane-bound cell structures. During protein synthesis of these hormones, the first few amino acids to be translated from a messenger RNA (mRNA) template form a signal sequence, which interacts with a signal recognition particle on the membrane of the rough endoplasmic reticulum. The entire polypeptide that is translated from the mRNA is called a 'preprohormone'. The signal sequence is cleaved before the end of translation, resulting in a 'prohormone'. This is cleaved by peptidases in the Golgi apparatus into the biologically active hormone. Further

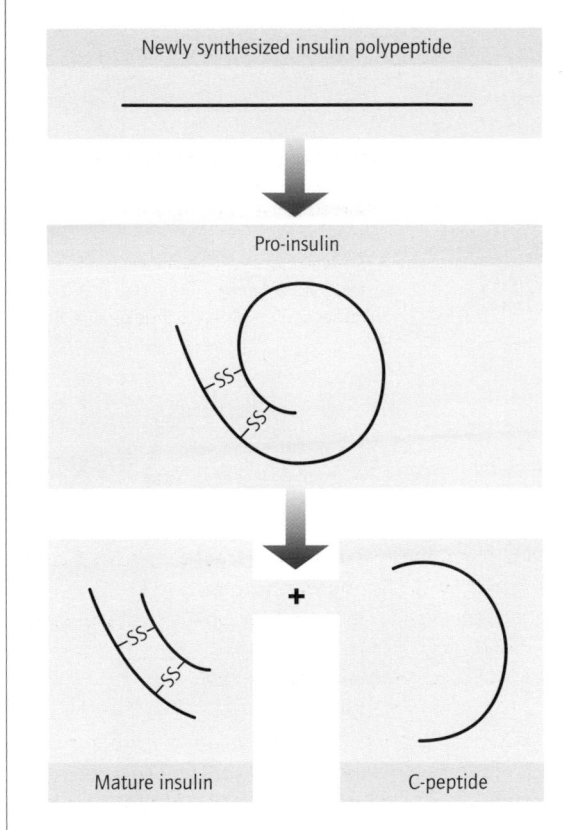

Newly synthesized insulin polypeptide

Pro-insulin

+

Mature insulin   C-peptide

Figure 12.1 Synthesis of insulin. Insulin is produced as a linear polypeptide that then curls on itself allowing disulphide bonds to form. Cleavage then occurs and a C-peptide is removed leaving the mature disulphide-bonded insulin.

post-translational processing can occur including folding and bridging by disulphide bridges, glycosylation (attachment of carbohydrate) and sometimes the assembly of different chains by non-covalent bonding (e.g. α and β chains).

Most peptide hormones are single-chain polypeptides. Insulin is looped into a ring before having part of the joining section of the loop (the C-peptide) cleaved leaving two chains linked by disulphide bridges (Fig. 12.1). The glycoprotein family (luteinizing hormone, LH; follicle-stimulating hormone, FSH; thyroid-stimulating hormone, TSH; and human chorionic gonadotrophin, hCG; see below) have sugar groups attached and two chains (α and β) each. The β subunit is variable, thus allowing the different versions to interact with specific receptors. Peptide hormones are usually released in bursts, which may be regular and pulsatile (e.g. insulin and LH). Growth hormone and prolactin have a tonic level of release with additional superimposed bursts. Peptide hormones can

be released rapidly when required, and can be rapidly metabolized.

Cholesterol derivatives
These include adrenal and gonadal steroids, which share the same basic ring structure, and vitamin D. Steroid hormone synthesis requires specific enzymes that convert cholesterol into the appropriate steroid (see Fig. 12.12).

Tyrosine and tryptophan derivatives
Thyroid hormones are formed by the conjugation of two tyrosine molecules with the help of specific enzymes and iodine (see p. 824).

In the adrenal medulla, tyrosine is made into catecholamines such as norepinephrine (noradrenaline) and epinephrine (adrenaline). The catecholamines are stored in secretory granules in the adrenal medulla and released in response to a neurological or humoral stimulus. Their release is pulsatile and their clearance is rapid. They are not bound to carrier proteins. Catecholamine receptor activation induces a cellular response without the hormones themselves entering the target cell.

Tryptophan is a precursor of serotonin (5-hydroxytryptamine) and melatonin synthesis.

Lipids and phospholipids derivatives
These include the major classes of eicosanoids including prostaglandins, prostacyclins, thromboxanes and leucotrienes.

Hormone transport
More than 90% of steroid and thyroid hormones circulate in the blood as complexes bound to specific plasma globulins or albumin. This is because these hormones are less soluble in aqueous solution than protein and peptide hormones. Unbound (free) hormone is biologically active. Assays of total hormone concentrations do not necessarily reflect changes in free hormone concentration. However, they are often used in clinical practice, because measuring the concentration of free hormone is usually more difficult and more expensive. The half-life of catecholamines is seconds, while that of protein and peptide hormones is minutes, and of steroid and thyroid hormones hours.

Hormone receptors
Most protein and peptide hormone receptors are G-protein coupled receptors. Once a hormone has interacted with its receptor there is dissociation of the intracellular G-protein. This may allow opening of membrane ion channels or activate an enzyme that promotes or inhibits production of a second messenger such as cyclic AMP.

12

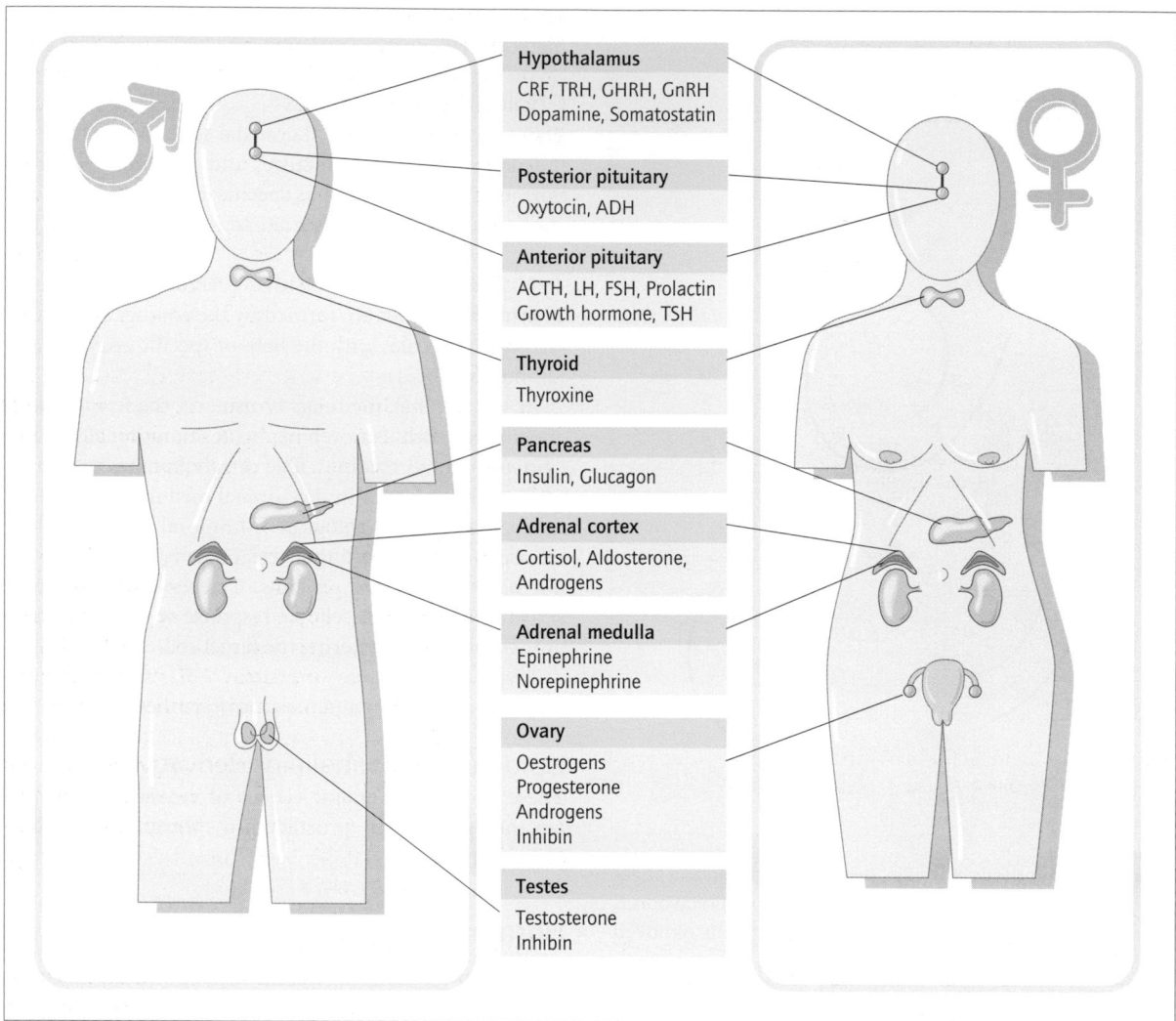

Figure 12.2 Overview of the major endocrine organs and the hormones they produce.

Second messengers can activate serine kinases or phosphatases and trigger other intracellular events.

Growth hormone, insulin and prolactin receptors are either transmembrane proteins with tyrosine kinase activity, or associate with other intracellular molecules with tyrosine kinase activity.

Steroid and thyroid hormones diffuse easily across cell membranes and have intracellular receptors, which are classified by their location. Type 1 receptors are found in the cytoplasm and type 2 receptors in the nucleus.

Hormone receptor regulation

This occurs by up- or downregulation of the number of receptors. Interactions between hormones and their receptors is influenced by the number of receptors, the

hormone concentration and the affinity of the hormone for the receptor.

Endocrine organs and the hormones they produce

Figure 12.2 provides an overview of the major endocrine organs.

Pituitary gland

The hypothalamus and pituitary gland have important roles in the control of the endocrine system. The pituitary gland consists of two main parts, the anterior and the posterior pituitary, which have different embryological origins and different functions.

12

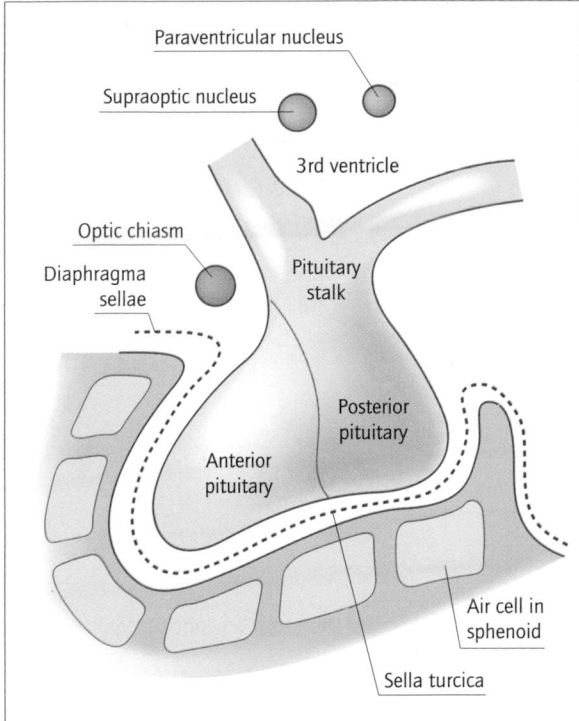

Figure 12.3 Anatomy of the hypothalamus and pituitary gland. This is a cross-sectional sagittal view taken from the left side.

Anatomical relations

The pituitary gland is located in a bony fossa of the sphenoid bone of the skull, the **sella turcica** (Fig. 12.3).

Important anatomical relations may be affected by pituitary enlargement:
- *The optic chiasm:* lies above and in front of the pituitary gland
- *The hypothalamus and third ventricle:* lie above the pituitary gland
- *Cavernous sinuses:* containing nerves to the external ocular muscles of the eye, lie above and lateral to the pituitary gland

Anterior pituitary

The anterior pituitary (adenohypophysis) is derived from an outgrowth of the primitive pharynx (Rathke's pouch). It synthesizes hormones that stimulate other endocrine glands or act on target tissues.

The synthesis of anterior pituitary hormones is controlled by stimulatory or inhibitory factors produced in the hypothalamus that reach the pituitary through the portal blood system linking the two organs. The production of hypothalamic controlling factors is in turn controlled by metabolic, physical, humoral and nervous factors.

Hypothalamic and pituitary hormone production is further controlled by the hormone production of target endocrine glands through feedback inhibitory loops. The anterior pituitary secretes the following hormones.

Adrenocorticotrophic hormone

Adrenocorticotrophic hormone (ACTH) is a polypeptide hormone produced by enzymatic cleavage of a large precursor molecule, the prohormone pro-opiomelanocortin (POMC) (Fig. 12.4). A related peptide, **lipotrophin**, is produced at the same time. ACTH itself may undergo enzymatic breakdown, producing **melanocyte-stimulating hormone** (MSH) and **corticotrophin-like peptide** (CLIP). The metabolic importance of some pro-opiomelanocortin products is not yet clear. ACTH secretion is stimulated by the hypothalamic releasing factor, **corticotrophin-releasing hormone** (CRH), which is inhibited through direct negative feedback by cortisol.

Thyroid-stimulating hormone

Thyroid-stimulating hormone (TSH) is a glycopeptide regulating the production of thyroid hormones by the thyroid gland. Its production is controlled by **thyrotrophin-releasing hormone** (TRH), a tripeptide produced by the hypothalamus. TSH release is controlled through negative feedback by the thyroid hormones.

Growth hormone

Growth hormone is a polypeptide hormone exhibiting pulsatile secretion, particularly during the night. Levels

Figure 12.4 Adenocorticotrophic hormone (ACTH) synthesis is an example of prohormone processing whereby pro-opiomelanocortin is cleaved to ACTH and β-lipotrophin. ACTH can be further processed to α-melanocyte-stimulating hormone (αMSH) and corticotrophin-like intermediate peptide (CLIP). β-lipotrophin is further cleaved to α-lipotrophin and β-endorphin.

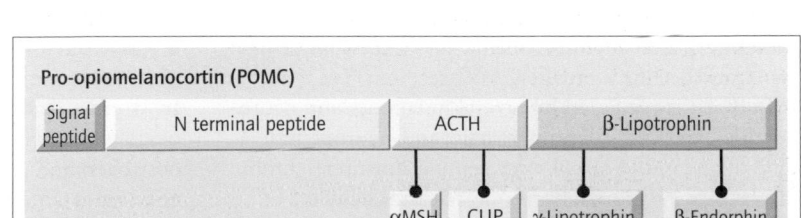

12

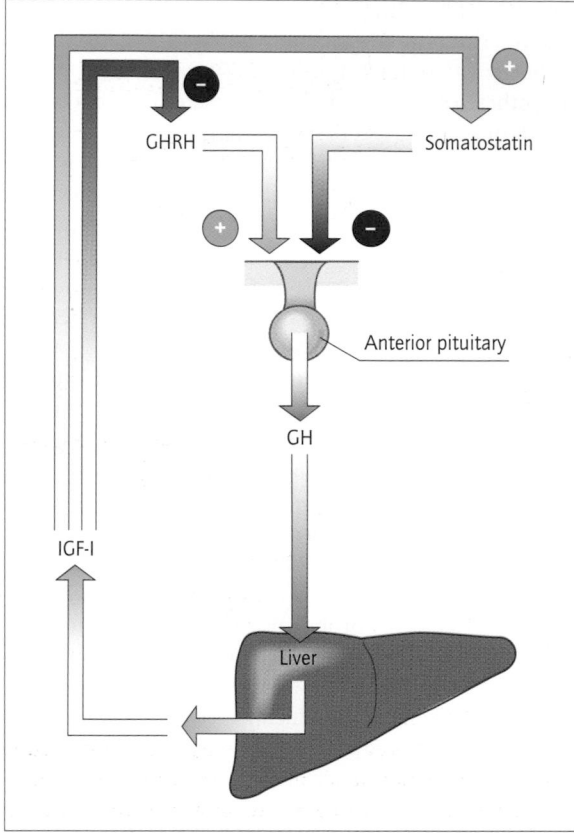

Figure 12.5 Overview of the control of growth hormone.

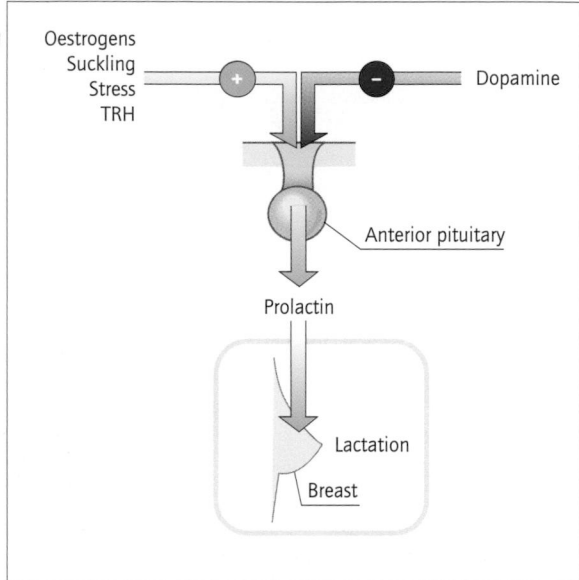

Figure 12.6 Overview of the prolactin control mechanisms.

during the day are low. Its secretion by the anterior pituitary is stimulated by **growth hormone-releasing hormone (GHRH)** and is inhibited by **somatostatin** (Fig. 12.5). Levels of growth hormone increase in response to hypoglycaemia, to the hormones glucagon and vasopressin, and the amino acid, arginine.

The metabolic effects of growth hormone are mainly related to growth. Growth hormone stimulates the hepatic production of insulin-like growth factor-1 (IGF-1), which stimulates growth. Metabolic actions include promoting the retention of substrates for anabolic activity (calcium, phosphorus, nitrogen) and collagen and protein synthesis. Both the frequency and magnitude of growth hormone pulses increase during the adolescent growth spurt, and decline thereafter.

Body fat is regulated by several hormones and neuropeptides, including leptin, ghrelin and neuropeptide Y. One of these, the circulating peptide hormone **ghrelin**, displays strong growth hormone-releasing activity.

Prolactin

Prolactin is a peptide hormone that has considerable structural homology with growth hormone. Its secretion is highest during the night and levels fall after waking and during the morning.

Prolactin secretion is inhibited by **dopamine**, which is synthesized in the hypothalamus and reaches the anterior pituitary via the portal blood system (Fig. 12.6). The principal actions of prolactin are concerned with lactation and development of the mammary duct system. Prolactin secretion increases:

- Slowly during pregnancy
- In response to postpartum stimulation of the breast and nipple
- In response to stress, physical exercise and hypoglycaemia

Gonadotrophins

The gonadotrophins FSH and LH are glycopeptides comprising α and β chains.

Gonadotrophin secretion is:
- Stimulated by the hypothalamic hormone **gonadotrophin-releasing hormone (GnRH)**
- Inhibited in men by **testosterone** and **inhibin**
- Controlled in women by a complex feedback mechanism involving **estradiol** and **progesterone**

In women, FSH stimulates follicle development in the ovary while LH stimulates ovulation and the synthesis of oestrogen and progestogen in the ovary (Fig. 12.7). LH is also important for the maintenance of the corpus luteum.

In men, FSH stimulates development of the testicular seminiferous tubule while LH stimulates testosterone secretion from the testicular Leydig cells (Fig. 12.8).

12

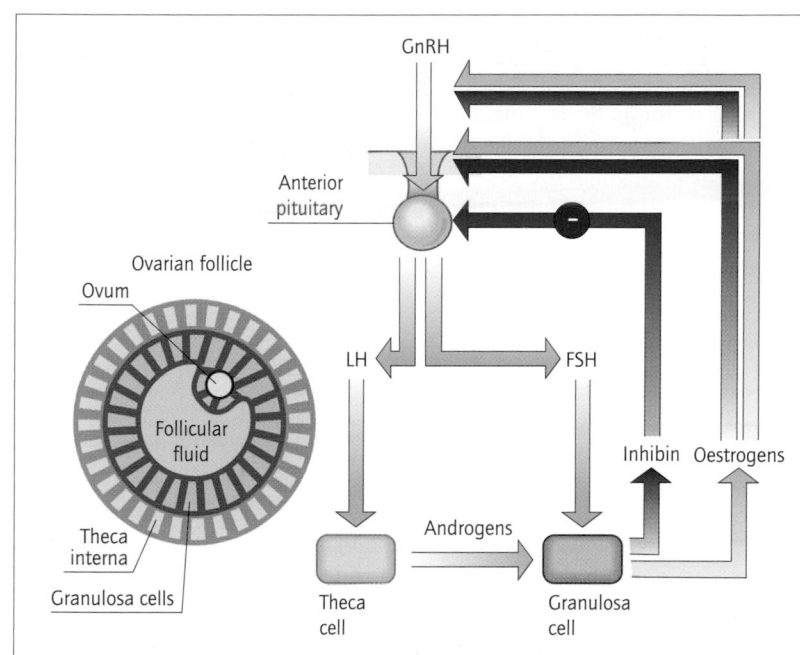

Figure 12.7 Hormonal control of the ovary. Note that theca produces androgens which are converted to oestrogens by the granulosa cell.

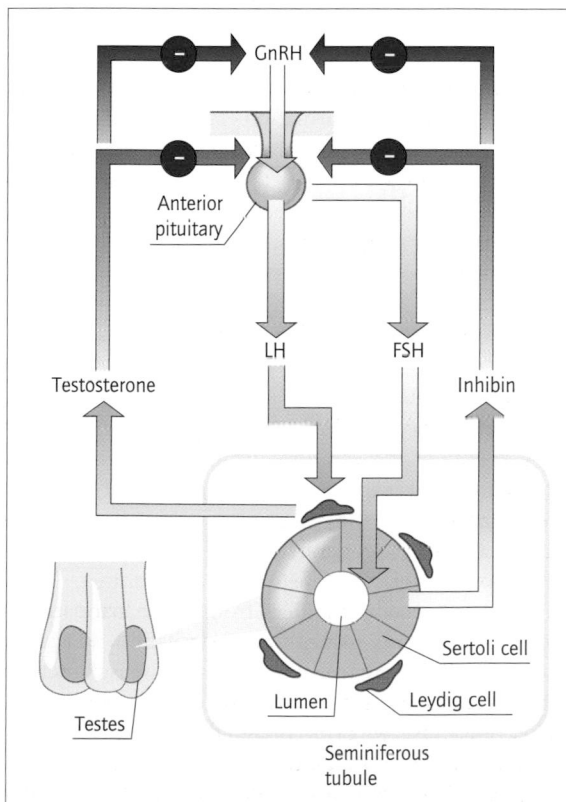

Figure 12.8 Hormonal control of the testis.

Posterior pituitary

The posterior pituitary (neurohypophysis) is of neural origin and contains nerve cells. Nerve axons of the neurohypophysis arise from neurones with their cell bodies in the supraoptic and paraventricular nuclei of the hypothalamus. Vasopressin (antidiuretic hormone, vasopressin) and oxytocin are synthesized in these cell bodies and reach the posterior pituitary via the connecting nerve axons. The hormones are then stored and released from the posterior pituitary.

Vasopressin

Vasopressin is an octapeptide. It acts via the adenylate cyclase system on the renal collecting tubules increasing their permeability to water and therefore reducing urine volume (see p. 507). Because it exists in a free form and does not interact with binding proteins, it has a very short plasma half-life (5 min).

Changes in plasma osmolality detected by osmoreceptors in the hypothalamus are the major determinants of vasopressin secretion. Other important stimulants of vasopressin release include a reduction in plasma volume, stress, exercise, emotional factors, trauma, morphine and nicotine.

Oxytocin

The role of oxytocin in humans is not fully understood. In animals, it has important effects on the breast and uterus during birth and lactation. Synthetic oxytocin is used to induce labour in humans.

12

Thyroid gland

The thyroid gland weighs about 20 g and is located in the front of the neck. It consists of two conical lateral lobes, which extend from the thyroid cartilage to the sixth tracheal ring and are joined by a narrow isthmus between the second and fourth tracheal ring. Posteriorly, the recurrent laryngeal nerves lie between the trachea and the oesophagus.

Thyroid hormones

Thyroxine (T_4) and triiodothyronine (T_3) are stored in association with a glycoprotein called thyroglobulin in the protein-rich colloid of the thyroid follicles. Iodine is an important precursor of thyroid hormones. Iodine ions are avidly taken up by the gland, oxidized and bound covalently to tyrosine residues to form iodotyrosines. This process depends on the enzyme peroxidase, which is inhibited by antithyroid drugs.

T_4 is the major hormone secreted by the thyroid, but T_3 is more active. In peripheral tissues, such as the liver, heart and kidney, and in the anterior pituitary, T_4 is converted to T_3 by deiodination. This process accounts for approximately two-thirds of the T_3 production. In chronic ill health and starvation T_4 is converted to the inactive metabolite reverse T_3.

Less than 1% of the thyroid hormones are free in plasma because they are bound to thyroid binding globulin and, to a lesser extent, to prealbumin and albumin. The level of the free hormones affects metabolism and determines the thyroid status of the individual.

Control of thyroid hormone production

Thyroid hormone production is controlled by **TSH** (Fig. 12.9). TSH secretion is controlled by feedback inhibition by thyroid hormones. TSH secretion is inhibited by high levels and stimulated by low levels of thyroid hormones. It is also controlled by the tripeptide, **TRH**, which is produced in the hypothalamus.

Action of thyroid hormones

Thyroid hormones are essential for normal growth and development and have multiple effects on carbohydrate, protein and fat metabolism. Perhaps their best known action is the stimulation of cellular oxygen consumption, which is evident as an increase in basal metabolic rate.

Free thyroid hormones bind to receptors in cell nuclei and more than 90% of receptor-bound thyroid hormone is T_3. T_3 then induces the formation of mRNA coding for various proteins including enzymes, growth hormone and adrenergic receptors.

Thyroid hormones also have direct effects on mem-

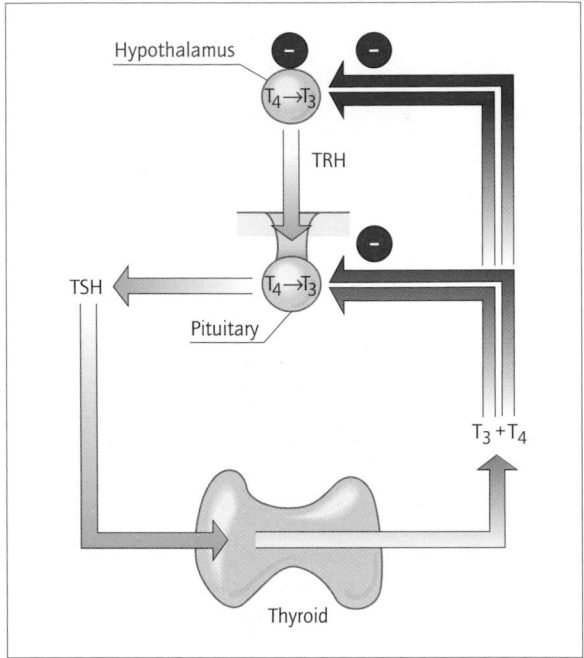

Figure 12.9 Overview of the thyroid feedback mechanism. Hypothalamic and pituitary negative feedback involves the conversion of T_4 to T_3.

brane functions including amino acid transport, calcium uptake and cyclic AMP formation.

Adrenal glands

The left and right adrenal glands lie in the retroperitoneal space attached to the upper poles of the kidneys. Each gland is approximately 2–3 cm wide and 4–6 cm long and is composed of a medulla and cortex.

Adrenal medulla

The adrenal medulla forms part of the sympathetic nervous system and develops from ectodermal neural crest tissue. It receives preganglionic cholinergic nerve fibres from sympathetic nerves. The cells of the medulla can be regarded as postganglionic sympathetic neurones without axons.

The adrenal medulla differs from other sympathetic tissues by producing epinephrine (adrenaline) as well as norepinephrine (noradrenaline). This ability is conferred by the presence of the enzyme phenylethanolamine N-methyltransferase, which is cortisol dependent.

The secretion of catecholamines occurs in response to a variety of stimuli, such as exercise, emotion, surgical trauma, hypoglycaemia and fear. Their actions are mediated through α- and β-adrenergic receptors:

12

The adrenal androgens dehydroepiandrostenedione and its sulphate are weak androgens and have a much lower affinity for the androgen receptor than testosterone. However, they are converted peripherally to the more active testosterone. In males, the amount released from the adrenal glands and converted to testosterone is insignificant compared to the amount secreted by the testis. In females, adrenal-derived testosterone is important in maintaining normal pubic and axillary hair. After the menopause, adrenal androgens may be an important source of oestradiol, because of peripheral conversion.

Mineralocorticoids

Aldosterone is the principal mineralocorticoid produced by the adrenal cortex. Small amounts of deoxycorticosterone and 18-hydroxy-deoxycorticosterone are also produced. Aldosterone acts on the distal renal tubule where it promotes potassium excretion and sodium uptake.

Renin–angiotensin system

The production of aldosterone is controlled mainly by the renin–angiotensin system. The cells of the juxtaglomerular apparatus, which is located close to the afferent arteriole of the glomerulus, secrete renin in response to a depletion of intravascular volume, cardiac failure, hypoalbuminaemia and sodium depletion.

Renin is a proteolytic enzyme that acts on angiotensinogen (which is hepatic in origin) to produce the decapeptide **angiotensin I**. In turn, angiotensin I is converted by angiotensin-converting enzyme (ACE) to the octapeptide angiotensin II; this takes place mainly in lung and vascular endothelium. **Angiotensin II** stimulates aldosterone production. It also has a direct potent vasoconstrictor action.

Glucocorticoids

Cortisol is the principal glucocorticoid, although some corticosterone is also secreted. Cortisol binds to receptors in the cytoplasm of target cells and the ligand–receptor complex is then transported to specific binding sites within the cell nucleus. This leads to production of various mRNA molecules, resulting in protein synthesis and the major actions of the glucocorticoids.

Glucocorticoid and androgen production by the adrenal gland is stimulated by ACTH. Pituitary secretion and release of ACTH is stimulated by CRH. ACTH secretion is also under feedback control by cortisol.

Glucocorticoid secretion varies during the day, the highest levels occurring soon after waking and the lowest levels during the early part of the night. This diurnal rhythm may be interrupted by stressful stimuli, either physical or psychological. Some of the many factors that

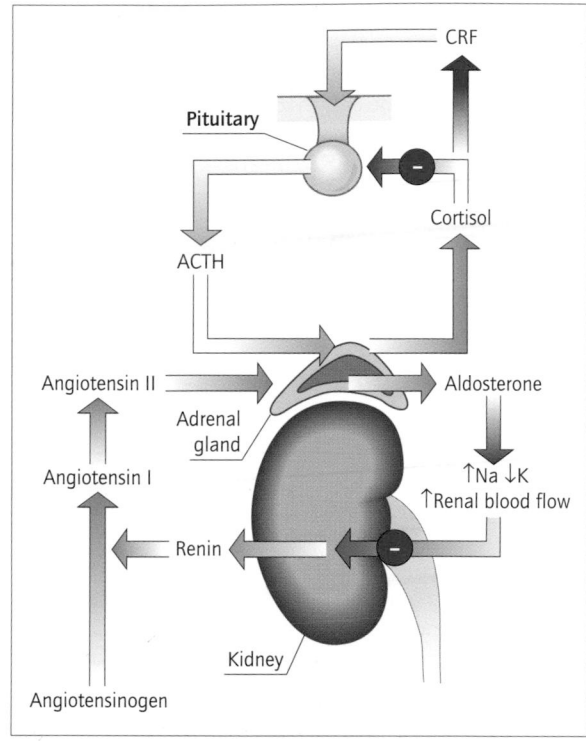

Figure 12.10 Overview of adrenal cortex feedback mechanisms.

- Epinephrine binds to both types of receptors
- Norepinephrine has predominantly α-adrenergic effects

The enzyme catechol-*O*-methyltransferase (COMT), which is found in the liver and kidney, catabolizes circulating catecholamines to normetanephrine and metanephrine. A further enzyme, monoamine oxidase, plays an important part in the conversion of these metabolites to vanillylmandelic acid (VMA), which is the major breakdown product of catecholamines.

Adrenal cortex

The adrenal cortex originates embryologically from mesoderm and comprises approximately 90% of the adrenal gland. It has three distinct anatomical zones. From the outside inwards these are:
- *zona glomerulosa:* produces aldosterone
- *zonas fasciculata and reticularis:* produce glucocorticoids, androgens and oestrogens

The adrenal cortex produces more than 50 known steroids. The principal steroids (Fig. 12.10) are the glucocorticoids (e.g. cortisol) and mineralocorticoids (e.g. aldosterone). In both sexes, the cortex produces small amounts of oestrogen and androgens, but in men adrenal androgens comprise less than 10% of total androgen production.

lead to increased glucocorticoid release are fever, severe illness, trauma, surgery and hypoglycaemia.

Testis

The normal testis weighs 20–45 g and has a volume of 12–25 ml. Its major component is the seminiferous tubules. These join to form the epididymis, which in turn becomes the vas deferens.

The **seminiferous epithelium** lines the seminiferous tubules and is composed of **Sertoli cells**; at the base of tubules are **germ cells**. As the germ cells mature into spermatocytes they pass through the Sertoli cells towards the lumen of the tubule. The Sertoli cell makes a peptide hormone, inhibin, which suppresses FSH release from the pituitary.

Leydig (interstitial) cells are located between the seminiferous tubules and produce testosterone under the influence of LH.

Testosterone has:

- A local (paracrine) action, which is essential for spermatogenesis

- A peripheral action; after conversion to dihydrotestosterone in target organs, it is involved in secondary sexual characteristics (hair follicles, prostate gland, penis, scrotum, larynx, bone epiphyses).

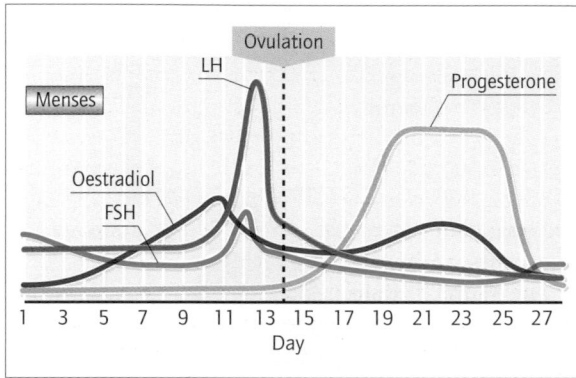

Figure 12.11 Hormonal changes in the menstrual cycle. Note that the luteinizing hormone (LH) surge occurs before ovulation. The rise in progesterone following ovulation is a product of the corpus luteum and can be used as evidence of ovulation.

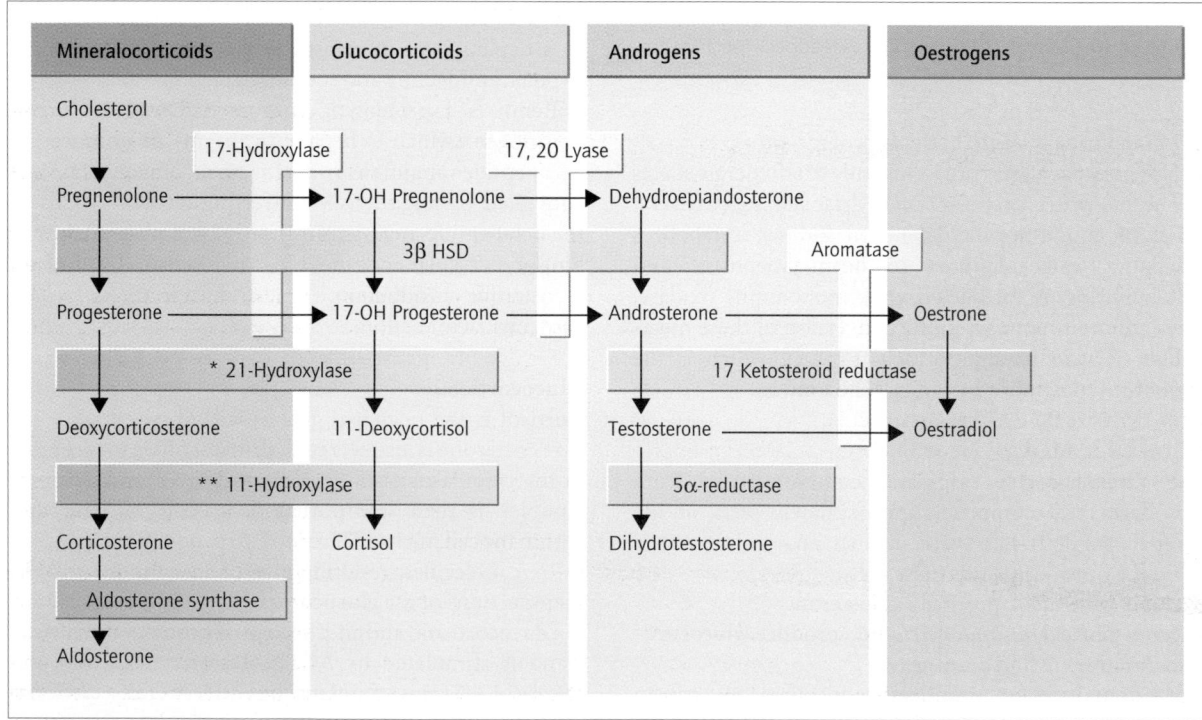

Figure 12.12 Pathways of steroid synthesis. The synthetic pathway of steroids and the enzymes catalysing each step. 17-hydroxylase and 21-hydroxylase activity are mediated by a single microsomal enzyme. The enzymes for sex steroid synthesis occur mainly outside the adrenal gland: aromatase in granulosa cells and fat tissue, 5α-reductase in skin and prostate glands, 17-ketosteroid reductase in gonads. * The most common defect in congenital adrenal hyperplasia is 21-hydroxylase deficiency. ** Site of action of metyrapone (see p. 853) is 11-hydroxylase inhibition.

12

Ovary

The normal ovary weighs 10–20 g and has a volume of 3–7 ml. The ovarian cortex encloses **follicles** of varying maturity; follicle development is dependent on FSH from the pituitary.

Each follicle consists of an **ovum** surrounded by **granulosa cells**, which secrete follicular fluid and convert androgens of thecal origin into oestrogen (aromatization) (see Fig. 12.7). A mature follicle measures at least 16 mm and ruptures under the influence of the mid-cycle LH surge to release the ovum into the pelvic cavity. It later forms a **corpus luteum**, which is the source of progesterone in the luteal phase of the menstrual cycle (Fig. 12.11).

The central medulla of the ovary contains the stroma, which is made up of support tissue and interstitial cells, which synthesize androgens (testosterone and androstenedione) under the influence of LH. These androgens are converted to oestrogens by the granulosa cells, and in peripheral sites. A proportion of the androgens produced will reach the circulation unchanged (Fig. 12.12).

The normal menstrual cycle is 25–34 days. Oligomenorrhoea is defined as a cycle longer than 34 days; amenorrhoea is defined as no menstrual cycle for 6 months.

Table 12.1 Questions to be addressed in suspected endocrine diseases

What endocrine disorder is suggested by the initial symptoms?

Are there any other associated endocrine disorders that should be sought?

Are there other features suggesting an endocrine syndrome?

What was the earliest onset of symptoms?

What is the differential diagnosis?

What biochemical investigations are required?

Should the gland be imaged?

If there is an overactive gland does the patient understand medical and surgical options?

If there is an underactive gland, does the patient understand the timescale of endocrine replacement therapy?

Approach to the patient

History

Endocrine disorders can affect any bodily function so a detailed history must be broad. Symptoms of abnormal endocrine function may be subtle and insidious and be unnoticed by the patient. In order to place the onset of many endocrine disorders, a full history of developmental milestones is required (Table 12.1).

Symptoms

General symptoms of tiredness, lethargy, depression and weight gain are common in the absence of hormone abnormalities, but may be the earliest clue to an endocrine disorder and more specific features relating to each hormone system should be sought.

Weakness, lethargy and depression can be features of hypothyroidism, Cushing's syndrome (excess adrenocortical hormone production), hypothyroidism, sex steroid deficiency or hypopituitarism. Hypothyroidism may be accompanied by dry skin and alopecia, while features of Cushing's syndrome would include thin skin with bruising, purple striae and hirsutism. Weight gain may be generalized in hypothyroidism or truncal in Cushing's syndrome (HISTORY & EXAMINATION BOX 12.1).

Reproductive problems with an endocrine basis

Women

Menstrual disturbance is a common feature of female gonadal disorders. Such disorders can be divided into:
- Low oestrogen states (e.g. primary and secondary hypogonadism)
- Normal oestrogen states (e.g. polycystic ovary syndrome)

Symptoms of oestrogen deficiency include hot flushes, depression and vaginal dryness. Symptoms of hyperandrogenism are hirsutism, acne, alopecia and clitoromegaly. Endocrine disorders cause infertility as a result of anovulation.

Men

Impotence of endocrine origin is suggested by accompanying features of androgen deficiency (e.g. hair loss, gynaecomastia, loss of libido).

Precocious sexual development is usually reported by parents as the early appearance of secondary sex characteristics such as deepening voice and penis enlargement.

Delayed puberty may be associated with hypopituitarism, and growth retardation is usually the first manifestation of pituitary disease in children. If only sex hormones are affected and there are no other endocrine deficiencies, the age of presentation may be higher. A bone age assessment will identify any discrepancy between bone and chronological age and is often the most informative measurement of sex steroid status in children.

12

History & Examination 12.1

General

When were you last completely well?

Have you noticed any change in your energy levels, mood, sleeping pattern, heat tolerance, weight, appetite, skin or hair?

How have your symptoms developed from when you first noticed them until now? (Most endocrine disorders are gradually progressive rather than relapsing)

Cardiovascular

Do you get palpitations? (thyrotoxicosis)

Do you get short of breath? (a sign of heart failure, which is a feature of hypothyroidism)

Gastrointestinal

Do you get constipated? (hypothyroidism)

Do your bowels seem overactive? (thyrotoxicosis)

Neurological

Do your hands shake? (a tremor is a feature of thyrotoxicosis)

Do you get double vision or any problem with your vision? (Graves' disease and pituitary tumour)

Musculoskeletal

Do your muscles feel weak? (thyrotoxicosis, Cushing's syndrome, Conn's syndrome, hypokalaemia)

Female reproductive symptoms

How old were you when you started your periods?

How old were you when you had your menopause?

What is the longest period of time between your periods?

How many periods do you have a year?

Do you have flushes? (a sign of oestrogen deficiency)

Do you find intercourse painful? (a sign of oestrogen deficiency)

Have you noticed any discharge from your nipples? If so is it spontaneous or only on expression?

Male reproductive symptoms

Have you noticed any change in your libido?

Do you have early morning erections?

How often do you shave?

Drug history

What medicines and tonics, either prescribed by a doctor or obtained from elsewhere, do you take?

Do you take an oral contraceptive? If so which one?

Past medical history

Have you had any thyroid surgery? (thyroidectomy)

Family history

Does anyone in your family have any thyroid disorder or diabetes?

Has anyone in your family had a similar illness?

Do any illnesses run in your family?

Drug history

Be aware of factitious hyperthyroidism in those with access to thyroxine or 'diet' treatment. Lithium reduces thyroxine release, causing hypothyroidism. Amiodarone frequently disturbs thyroid function.

Iatrogenic glucocorticoid excess is a common cause of Cushing's syndrome.

Family history

Autoimmune endocrinopathies and multiple endocrine neoplasia may have a positive family history and rare autosomal recessive disorders are more likely with consanguinous parents.

Past medical history

Men and women

Head injury can cause hypopituitarism. Gonadal failure may be related to previous irradiation or cytotoxic therapy.

Women

The timing of onset of hypogonadism is usually relatively precise as there will be a history of primary or secondary amenorrhoea or infertility.

Men

Find out whether there is a history of testicular infection, trauma or maldescent in adult men with hypogonadism.

Examination

General inspection

Note the following:
- Changes in skin, hair quality and fat distribution are features of Cushing's syndrome and hypothyroidism
- Skin pigmentation and postural hypotension are features of Addison's disease
- Bradycardia, signs of heart failure and slow-relaxing reflexes occur in hypothyroidism
- Tachycardia or atrial fibrillation with tremor and possibly pretibial myxoedema are features of hyperthyroidism (HISTORY & EXAMINATION BOX 12.2)

Pituitary signs

Test the visual fields and examine the optic disc for pallor if a pituitary disorder is suspected.

History & Examination 12.2

General inspection

Hands

Are the skin creases pigmented? (a feature of Addison's disease)

Does the patient have a tremor? (a sign of thyrotoxicosis)

Are the hands enlarged? (a feature of acromegly)

Are the nails abnormal? (e.g. Graves' disease)

Skin

Is the skin thin? (a feature of Cushing's disease)

Is there vitiligo? (associated with autoimmunity)

Is the skin dry? (a feature of hypothyroidism)

Is the patient hirsute? (a feature of Cushing's disease and hyperandrogenism)

Is there any bruising? (a feature of Cushing's disease)

Is there evidence of sweating or acne? (hyperandrogenism)

Hair

Is there alopecia? (a feature of hypothyroidism and hyperandrogenism)

Is the hair brittle? (a feature of Graves' disease)

Eyes

Look for lid lag and exophthalmos (features of thyrotoxicosis)

Mouth

Is there any pigmentation? (a feature of Addison's disease)

Is there oral candidiasis? (autoimmune disease, glucocorticoid excess)

Examination of neck

Inspect and palpate for goitre and lymph nodes

Listen for a thyroid bruit

Feel the pulse

Is it slow or fast? What is its character? (bradycardia is a feature of hypothyroidism; tachycardia or atrial fibrillation are features of thyrotoxicosis)

Examination of the thyroid gland

Clinical assessment of the thyroid gland includes:
- Detailed examination of any thyroid swelling
- Examination for signs of hyper- or hypothyroidism and thyroid eye disease

The thyroid gland is first inspected from the front. Thyroid swellings move upwards on swallowing because the gland is enclosed within the pretracheal fascia which blends with the larynx. The thyroid is gently palpated by standing behind the sitting patient holding his or her head slightly flexed. Determine the nature of any swelling. Is the gland uniformly enlarged or nodular, hard or soft, tender or non-tender? Palpation of the thyroid gland during swallowing will help in delineation of the lower border of the gland and indicate whether there is any retrosternal extension.

Benign enlargement of the thyroid (goitre) may displace close anatomical relations. Compression and narrowing of the trachea and oesophagus may cause difficulty in breathing and swallowing.

Carcinoma of the thyroid invades neighbouring structures. Erosion into the trachea or oesophagus may occur and the recurrent laryngeal nerves and the cervical sympathetic chain may be involved, producing hoarseness and Horner's syndrome, respectively. Enlarged cervical lymph nodes caused by secondary deposits may be associated with carcinoma of the thyroid, particularly papillary carcinoma.

Auscultation over an enlarged gland may reveal a bruit caused by increased vascularity. This is a typical feature of Graves' disease.

Examination of reproductive endocrine status

Sexual development is measured by comparing genital development, breast size and pubic hair density with the charts of Tanner (Fig. 12.13).

An assessment of reduced sex steroids is made by observation of body hair distribution and density, although differentiation from normal variation is often difficult. In women, signs of hyperandrogenism include acne, seborrhoea, male pattern baldness and clitoromegaly.

Measurement of testis size is made by comparison with ovoids of known volume (Prader orchidometer). A careful examination of the scrotum for varicocoeles or testicular neoplasms may be most conveniently performed when the patient is standing.

Examination of the ovary is part of the gynaecological assessment and is usually performed by ultrasound.

Progesterone causes a mid-cycle rise in body temperature of about 0.5°C and this can be used to time ovulation.

Investigation

Haematology

A raised white cell count can occur in Cushing's syndrome. A raised mean red cell volume (macrocytosis) is a feature of hypothyroidism.

Biochemistry

Urea and electrolytes

Hyponatraemia reflects the water retention and low

12

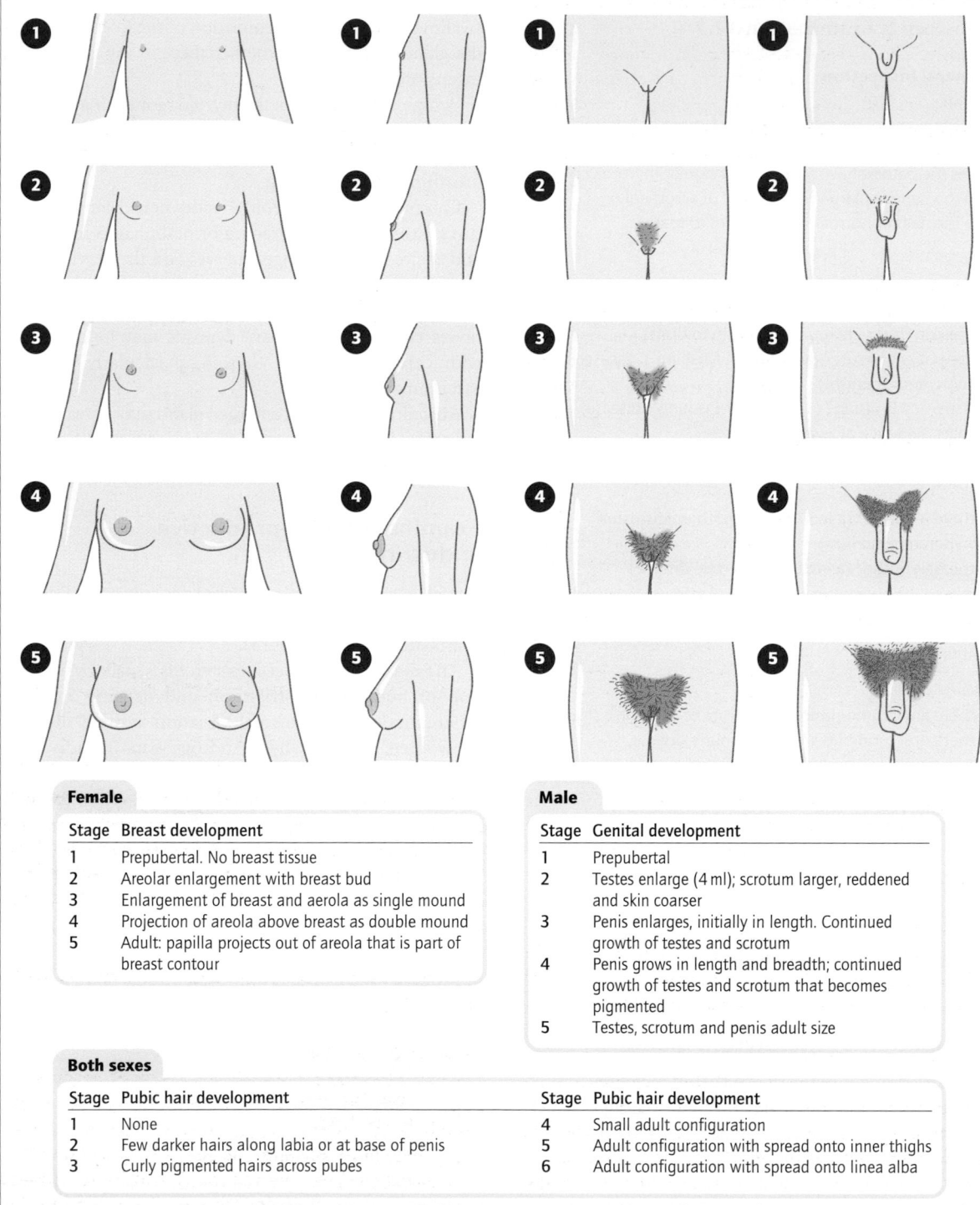

Female

Stage	Breast development
1	Prepubertal. No breast tissue
2	Areolar enlargement with breast bud
3	Enlargement of breast and aerola as single mound
4	Projection of areola above breast as double mound
5	Adult: papilla projects out of areola that is part of breast contour

Male

Stage	Genital development
1	Prepubertal
2	Testes enlarge (4 ml); scrotum larger, reddened and skin coarser
3	Penis enlarges, initially in length. Continued growth of testes and scrotum
4	Penis grows in length and breadth; continued growth of testes and scrotum that becomes pigmented
5	Testes, scrotum and penis adult size

Both sexes

Stage	Pubic hair development	Stage	Pubic hair development
1	None	4	Small adult configuration
2	Few darker hairs along labia or at base of penis	5	Adult configuration with spread onto inner thighs
3	Curly pigmented hairs across pubes	6	Adult configuration with spread onto linea alba

Figure 12.13 Tanner stages of sexual development.

osmolality of inappropriate vasopressin secretion. Conversely, hypernatraemia is consistent with water loss and hyperosmolality in diabetes insipidus. Hyponatraemia with hyperkalaemia are characteristic of mineralocorticoid deficiency in Addison's disease. Conversely, there may be hypernatraemia with hypokalaemia with the mineralocorticoid excess of Conn's syndrome. Hypokalaemia is also a feature of Cushing's syndrome, particularly if resulting from an ectopic source of ACTH.

Pituitary function tests

Plasma prolactin

Clinical suspicion of a prolactinoma is supported by a high plasma prolactin level. Prolactin levels may be moderately raised in association with other pituitary tumours if there is compression of the pituitary stalk. This blocks the normal negative control of prolactin-secreting cells by hypothalamic dopamine.

Serum growth hormone levels

Serum growth hormone levels are used to confirm a diagnosis of acromegaly. Growth hormone levels may exclude acromegaly if undetectable, but a detectable value is non-diagnostic. The glucose tolerance test is diagnostic, as those with acromegaly fail to suppress growth hormone below 2 mU/l and some show a paradoxical rise in response to a 75-g oral glucose load (Fig. 12.14). IGF-1 levels are almost always raised in acromegaly and this can be an appropriate cost-effective initial screening test for acromegaly.

Serum thyroid-stimulating hormone levels

A TSH-secreting pituitary tumour should be suspected when TSH levels are not suppressed in the presence of hyperthyroidism.

Plasma osmolality

Plasma osmolality is higher than 300 mOsmol/kg in moderate to severe diabetes insipidus while the urine is unconcentrated (osmolality less than 280 mOsmol/kg).

Water deprivation test

This is necessary for borderline diabetes insipidus. Oral fluids are withheld for 8 h and urine and plasma osmolality are monitored frequently. In addition, the patient is frequently weighed and the volume of urine is measured. Normally, plasma osmolality is maintained within the normal range and urine osmolality increases to more than 600 mOsmol/kg. In diabetes insipidus, urine osmolality fails to increase and urine output stays high. The test may have to be abandoned if there is excessive urine output and weight reduction. Synthetic vasopressin (desmopressin) can be administered and causes urine concentra-

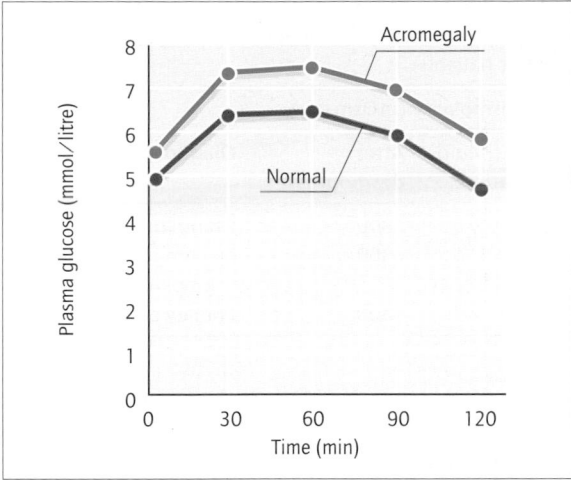

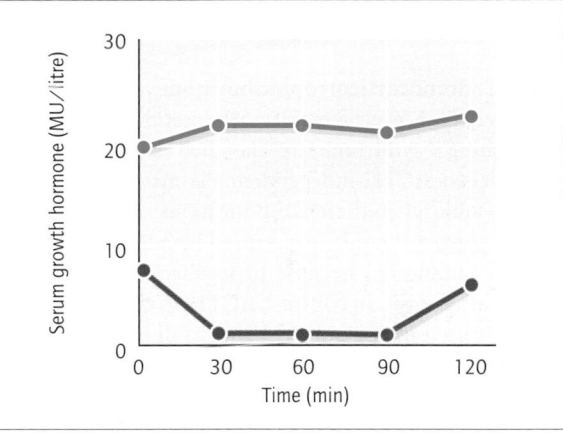

Figure 12.14 Oral glucose tolerance test for the diagnosis of acromegaly. Serum growth hormone concentrations are normally suppressed after an oral glucose load (blue lines) but fail to suppress, or paradoxically rise, in acromegaly (green lines). Glucose tolerance is often impaired in acromegaly but is normal in this case.

tion in cranial but not in nephrogenic diabetes insipidus (Table 12.2).

Insulin tolerance test

The insulin tolerance test (ITT) is used for the diagnosis of hypopituitarism. The stress induced by hypoglycaemia stimulates the release of pituitary hormones—cortisol and growth hormone in particular. Soluble insulin (0.1–0.15 unit/kg) is given intravenously and blood samples are taken at 0, 20, 30, 60, 90 and 120 min to measure glucose, cortisol and growth hormone levels. For the test to be valid, biochemical (blood glucose less than 2.2 mmol/l) and symptomatic (sweating, palpitations) hypoglycaemia must occur. The test must not be performed if the patient has ischaemic heart disease or epilepsy. Because it carries

12

Table 12.2 Water deprivation test for suspected diabetes insipidus. Response to fluid deprivation and desmopressin in polyuric patients

Urine osmolality (mOsm/kg)		
After 8 h fluid deprivation	After desmopressin	Diagnosis
<300	>800	Cranial diabetes insipidus
<300	<300	Nephrogenic diabetes insipidus
>800	>800	Primary polydipsia

risks, it should only be conducted on carefully selected patients by experienced staff in specialized endocrine units. For patients in whom the test is contraindicated, an alternative approach is to use the combined arginine and growth hormone-releasing test.

Plasma adrenocorticotrophic hormone
Plasma ACTH levels are extremely useful and the causes of Cushing's syndrome are classified as either ACTH-dependent or ACTH-independent. Plasma ACTH levels are undetectable when there is autonomous adrenal production of glucocorticoids (e.g. caused by adrenal adenoma, adrenal carcinoma) because of feedback suppression at the hypothalamus. In contrast, ACTH levels are normal or slightly raised in pituitary-dependent disease (Cushing's disease) and may be very high (over 200 ng/l) if there is ectopic ACTH production (Fig. 12.15).

Thyroid function tests
Measurements of free hormone levels (free T_4 and free T_3) are now widely available. In hyperthyroidism, the levels of T_4 and T_3 are elevated and the TSH is abnormally low. Occasionally in hyperthyroidism T_4 is normal but

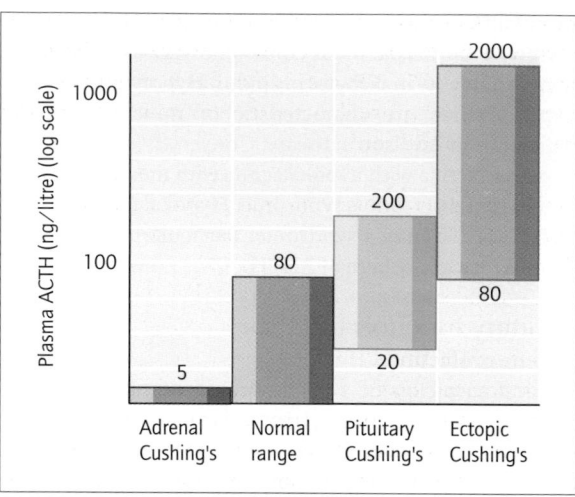

Figure 12.15 ACTH measurements in Cushing's syndrome.

T_3 is raised (so-called T_3 hyperthyroidism). In primary hypothyroidism, the levels of T_4 and T_3 are low and TSH is raised. In secondary hypothyroidism, TSH values are inappropriately low.

The current highly sensitive assay for TSH is very helpful in the assessment of thyroid disease and is the favoured thyroid function test for screening.

Biochemical investigation of Cushing's syndrome
(See p. 852; Table 12.3.)

Does the patient have Cushing's syndrome?
(Screening tests)
Urinary free cortisol concentration. This is measured by radioimmunoassay in a 24-h urine collection and is

---

Screening tests for Cushing's syndrome
1 24-h urinary free cortisol
2 Overnight 1 mg DST
3 Midnight cortisol
4 Low-dose DST

Investigation of ACTH-dependent Cushing's syndrome

Test	Pituitary-dependent disease (%)	Ectopic disease (%)
Serum potassium <3.2 mmol/l	10	100
Suppression of basal cortisol by >50% on high-dose DST	90	10
Exaggerated rise in cortisol on CRF test	95	<1

CRF, corticotrophin-releasing factor; DST, dexamethasone suppression test.

Table 12.3 Investigation of Cushing's syndrome

raised in Cushing's syndrome (more than 250 nmol for men and more than 400 nmol for women). The false-negative rate of 5–10% means that this test should not be used alone. The urinary metabolites of adrenocortical steroids are often normal.

Overnight dexamethasone suppression test. This is a useful outpatient screening test for suspected Cushing's syndrome. Dexamethasone (1 mg) is taken orally at bedtime and a blood sample for plasma cortisol is taken at 9 a.m. the next morning. Normally, plasma cortisol is suppressed (less than 100 nmol/l) in response to this powerful synthetic glucocorticoid; in Cushing's syndrome it is not. False-positives do occur, particularly if the patient is obese or depressed. If the 24-h urinary free cortisol and overnight dexamethasone suppression test are both normal, Cushing's syndrome is unlikely.

Plasma cortisol. Demonstration of loss of the normal diurnal rhythm of cortisol secretion is particularly important. These tests should not be performed immediately after admission as hospital admission itself may lead to a temporary loss of the rhythm. Diurnal rhythm should be checked 1–2 days after admission. Plasma cortisol levels are measured at 9 a.m. and midnight. The patient must not be warned of the midnight test so that he or she is asleep before the venepuncture. In Cushing's syndrome, the circadian rhythm is lost and there is a high concentration of cortisol in the midnight sample. Plasma cortisol level at 9 a.m. may be normal or raised.

Low-dose dexamethasone suppression test. This is a useful test for confirming a diagnosis of Cushing's syndrome. Dexamethasone is given in a regimen of 0.5 mg 6-hourly for 48 h. Normally, this suppresses plasma cortisol levels, but in Cushing's syndrome cortisol levels are not suppressed. Cushing's syndrome, particularly caused by Cushing's disease (a pituitary adenoma producing ACTH; see p. 837), may be intermittent, and this may lead to diagnostic difficulties. If the diagnosis is strongly suspected, the low-dose dexamethasone test may need to be repeated several times.

What is the underlying cause?
Plasma ACTH. This is one of the most important tests to discriminate between the ACTH-dependent and ACTH-independent aetiologies (see above; Fig.12.15; Table 12.3).

Serum potassium. Hypokalaemia below 3.2 mmol/l is found in almost 100% of patients with ectopic secretion of ACTH but fewer than 10% with pituitary-dependent disease.

High-dose dexamethasone suppression test. This test helps in the differentiation of pituitary-dependent Cushing's disease from other causes of Cushing's syndrome. Dexamethasone (8 mg orally) is administered in four divided doses of 2 mg 6-hourly for 48 h. This suppresses plasma cortisol and urinary metabolites by 50% in 90% of patients with Cushing's disease. Rarely, it will cause suppression in the ectopic ACTH syndrome, particularly when the tumour is slow-growing.

Response to corticotrophin-releasing factor. CRF can be used in the differential diagnosis of Cushing's syndrome. The plasma ACTH level following a CRF injection is measured. In Cushing's disease, CRF leads to an exaggerated rise in plasma ACTH. This test may be particularly helpful in equivocal cases of possible Cushing's disease when combined with selective catheterization of veins draining the pituitary gland.

Bilateral inferior petrosal sinus sampling. In Cushing's syndrome, selective venous blood sampling from the inferior petrosal vein with ACTH measurement (in the basal state and in response to intravenous CRF) is often required to locate a pituitary adenoma that is not demonstrable by computerized tomography (CT) or magnetic resonance imaging (MRI) scanning. It may also help in localizing ectopic ACTH production.

Biochemical investigation of adrenal insufficiency
Short Synacthen test
Synacthen (tetracosactrin) is a synthetic form of ACTH. In suspected adrenocortical insufficiency, 250 μg is injected and plasma cortisol levels are measured before, and at 30 and 60 min after the injection. Normally, the plasma cortisol rises to more than 550 nmol/l (Fig. 12.16).

Biochemical investigation of gonadal function
Measurement of luteinizing hormone and follicle-stimulating hormone
These measurements help to differentiate primary from secondary hypogonadism. They are increased in gonadal failure (e.g. because of menopause, premature ovarian failure, testicular damage, Klinefelter's syndrome) and low, although not always undetectable, in hypothalamic or pituitary disease.

Gonadotrophin-releasing hormone test
The GnRH test for pituitary function is now performed less frequently because most central causes of hypogonadism are hypothalamic in origin.

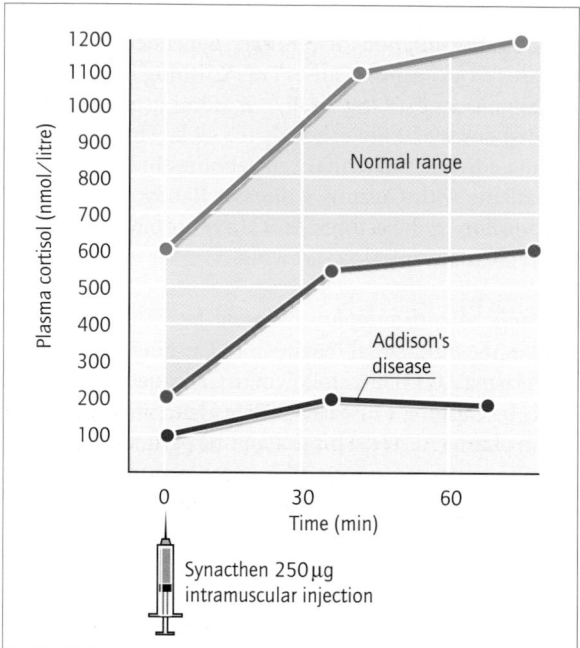

Figure 12.16 Short Synacthen test for Addison's disease showing the normal range for cortisol response to Synacthen.

Sex hormone-binding globulin

Sex hormone-binding globulin (SHBG) binds circulating oestrogen and testosterone and its level is low in obesity and in hyperandrogenic females. Testosterone and androstenedione in the circulation are of combined adrenal and gonadal origin.

Progesterone measurements

Progesterone measurements in the luteal phase can confirm ovulation (see Fig. 12.11).

Immunology

Autoantibodies

Thyroid disease is commonly caused by autoimmune disease. Immune mechanisms are involved in the development of primary myxoedema, Hashimoto's thyroiditis and Graves' disease.

● *Thyroid-stimulating antibodies:* the cause of thyroid overactivity in Graves' disease. They bind to and stimulate TSH receptors on thyroid cells. Measurement of these antibodies is useful in pregnant women with Graves' disease to assess the risk of hyperthyroidism in the newborn.

● *Microsomal antibodies:* present in the blood of most people with autoimmune thyroid disease and high titres

are found in Hashimoto's disease. These IgG antibodies are also found in 10% of otherwise apparently healthy individuals.

● *Adrenal autoantibodies:* can help to define the cause of Addison's disease.

Diagnostic imaging

Pituitary imaging
Lateral skull radiography
This usually shows an expanded pituitary fossa if there is a large pituitary tumour.

Magnetic resonance imaging
This is the best way to assess the extent of a pituitary tumour. In women, a prolactinoma is often small (microadenoma; less than 1 cm) and confined to the sella turcica at presentation, but the abnormality within the pituitary substance can usually be defined using MRI. MRI following gadolinium enhancement localizes ACTH-producing adenomas in up to 80% of cases. At least 10% of the normal population harbour microadenomas and the biochemical investigation of patients is therefore essential.

Adrenal imaging
Computerized tomography
Adrenal size is best assessed by CT. Bilateral adrenal hyperplasia is a feature of ACTH-driven Cushing's syndrome and adenomas of the cortex are found in Cushing's and Conn's syndrome and of the medulla with a phaeochromocytoma. In Addison's disease, the adrenal glands may be atrophic.

Unsuspected masses may be discovered during adrenal imaging. Functional tests should be performed and, if no evidence of secretory activity is evident, surgical removal of masses larger than 4 cm should be considered.

Magnetic resonance imaging
MRI may provide additional information if there is no demonstrable adrenal adenoma on CT scanning.

Thyroid imaging
Radioactive uptake tests
Uptake of a radioactive isotope by the thyroid gland is used to determine the localization, size and function of the gland. A radioisotope of technetium is often used because it has a short radioactive half-life. Uptake studies are useful in the diagnosis of de Quervain's thyroiditis and factitious hyperthyroidism as a result of self-administration of thyroxine (when there is a greatly reduced uptake of tracer). Uptake studies can also determine the distribution of uptake within the thyroid, which is useful in the investigation of a thyroid nodule. A thyroid cyst or a

thyroid carcinoma is apparent as a 'cold' nodule with low isotope uptake. Tracer uptake is diffusely increased in Graves' disease.

Ultrasound

The cystic or solid nature of a thyroid nodule can be confirmed by thyroid ultrasound.

Gonad imaging

Ultrasound

Ultrasound is the most useful gonadal imaging technique. In males, it may define otherwise impalpable testicular tumours or undescended testes in the inguinal canal. In females, pelvic ultrasound is performed either trans-abdominally, through a full bladder, or transvaginally.

Follicular development and ovulation status may be determined by serial ultrasound scans through the menstrual cycle. Measurement of oestrogen-sensitive organs (uterus and endometrium) by ultrasound is often more informative than serum oestrogen concentrations.

Histopathology

Thyroid

Needle aspiration should be performed on thyroid nodules for cytological examination.

Reproductive endocrinology

Karyotype definition using a buccal smear or lymphocytes may reveal Turner's syndrome in the female and Klinefelter's syndrome in the male.

Management

Supportive treatment

Specific instructions must be given to patients receiving replacement glucocorticoids. Intercurrent illness requires at least a doubling of the maintenance dose. Patients should carry a steroid card or medical alert bracelet.

Specific treatment

Endocrine gland hyperactivity

Glandular hyperactivity may be amenable to medical treatment (e.g. prolactinoma, hyperthyroidism). When this is lacking, a surgical option is often necessary (e.g. acromegaly, Cushing's syndrome).

Hormone deficiency

All important hormones are available for administration as therapeutic agents. They are given lifelong or for the life of the gland (e.g. oestrogen replacement therapy).

Diseases and their management

Diseases of the pituitary gland

Pituitary tumours

Disease mechanisms

Excessive autonomous production of growth hormone, ACTH, prolactin, LH, FSH or TSH is usually caused by a benign adenoma of the pituitary gland. Pituitary tumours are almost always benign. They are usually adenomas arising from the anterior pituitary gland.

Epidemiology

Prevalence. Account for approximately 10% of all intracranial neoplasms. Prolactinoma is the most common, followed by non-secreting pituitary tumours. Growth hormone- and ACTH-secreting tumours are moderately rare. TSH- and gonadotrophin-secreting tumours are very rare, accounting for less than 1% of all pituitary tumours.

Sex. Acromegaly affects both sexes equally; Cushing's disease is more common in women.

Clinical features

These vary widely according to the tumour size and whether or not it secretes hormones. Tumours that do not secrete hormones can present with local effects and with signs of hypopituitarism because of damage to hormone-secreting tissue. Symptoms and signs of a pituitary tumour may result from:

- Local expansion of the tumour
- Interference with normal pituitary hormone production (hypopituitarism)
- Excessive hormone production if the tumour is secretory

Local effects
Local effects include:

- Lateral extension of a pituitary tumour may compress nerves to the external ocular muscles.
- Downward extension erodes the pituitary fossa (often asymmetrically) in the sphenoid bone and the tumour may grow through the sphenoid air sinus into the post-nasal space. This may result in cerebrospinal fluid rhinorrhoea (cerebrospinal fluid leaking into the nose).
- Upward extension of the tumour (suprasellar extension) may compress the optic chiasm leading to visual

12

loss. The field loss is bitemporal hemianopia, but the upper temporal quadrants tend to be affected first. Large pituitary tumours may cause headaches, other signs and symptoms of raised intracranial pressure, and epilepsy.

● Hypothalamic pressure may lead to a hypothalamic syndrome with hyperphagia, disordered temperature control and thirst.

Hypopituitarism

A pituitary tumour, especially if it is non-secreting, may present with hypopituitarism, which is characterized by decreased or absent pituitary hormone secretion. Gonadotrophin and growth hormone secretion are characteristically the first to be affected, followed by TSH and ACTH secretion. Prolactin secretion is rarely affected by tumours, but can be reduced in postpartum pituitary necrosis (Sheehan's syndrome) caused by severe obstetric haemorrhage.

The symptoms and signs of hypopituitarism depend on which hormone secretion is affected. In addition, there may be local effects brought about by the enlarged pituitary gland itself. Other conditions associated with hypopituitarism are given in Table 12.4.

Gonadotrophin (LH, FSH) deficiency will lead to the clinical features of hypogonadism (see p. 858). In women, these include decreased libido, amenorrhoea, genital atrophy, reduced body hair and decreased breast size. In men, hypogonadism is characterized by decreased libido and impotence, decreased size and softening of the testes, azoospermia and loss of body hair. In both sexes, the skin develops a fine texture with increased fine creasing, particularly around the eyes and mouth.

ACTH deficiency results in the characteristic pallor of the skin seen in hypopituitarism with secondary adrenal failure. This produces symptoms similar to those described for primary adrenal failure (see p. 856). In primary hypoadrenalism, however, ACTH levels are high, and associated with skin pigmentation.

TSH deficiency results in symptoms of hypothyroidism, which are similar to those of primary thyroid disease (see p. 841). Measurement of TSH differentiates the two types of hypothyroidism.

In **vasopressin deficiency**, large pituitary tumours may cause failure of normal vasopressin production, with resultant cranial diabetes insipidus (see p. 831). When there is extensive pituitary disease with failure of anterior pituitary secretion, its symptoms may be masked because of the associated corticosteroid deficiency. The symptoms may then develop when corticosteroid replacement is started. Polyuria and polydipsia are the major symptoms, and if severe there may be dehydration, exhaustion and coma. Other causes of polyuria are listed in Table 12.5.

Table 12.4 Causes of hypopituitarism

Developmental/congenital
Defects, particularly of midline structures
Kallmann's syndrome (see p. 861)

Infiltrations
Sarcoidosis
Haemochromatosis

Immunological
Autoimmune hypophysitis

Vascular
Sheehan's syndrome
Pituitary apoplexy

Tumours
Pituitary tumours

Injury
Radiation
Surgery
Trauma

Infection
Meningitis
Tuberculosis

Functional
Anorexia, starvation
Stress
Exercise
Depression

Table 12.5 Causes of polyuria

Diabetes mellitus
Diabetes insipidus (cranial or nephrogenic)
Psychogenic polydipsia
Diuretic therapy
Hypokalaemia
Hypercalcaemia

Most cases of diabetes insipidus are cranial, because of decreased production or release of vasopressin.

Diabetes insipidus sometimes results from a resistance of the renal tubules to vasopressin; this is nephrogenic diabetes insipidus (see p. 582), which can be caused by mutations of the vasopressin receptor in the kidney. Diabetes insipidus may result from trauma to the hypothalamus (e.g. after pituitary surgery), and may then be transient and recover spontaneously.

Excessive hormone production

Excessive hormone production is a feature of prolactinoma, acromegaly, Cushing's disease and a TSH-secreting tumour.

12

Table 12.6 Causes of hyperprolactinaemia

Cranial disease
Hypothalamic disease
Pituitary tumour with stalk disconnection
Prolactin-secreting tumour (prolactinoma, acromegaly)

Drugs
Phenothiazines
Metoclopramide
Oestrogens

Endocrine
Hypothyroidism

Stress
Surgical
Illness
Venepuncture

Prolactinoma. Women with prolactinoma present early because hyperprolactinaemia results in amenorrhoea and infertility by reducing gonadotrophin secretion. Galactorrhoea is also common. Men often present late and symptoms include lack of libido, impotence, infertility and galactorrhoea. The hypogonadism associated with hyperprolactinaemia leads to decreased bone mass and osteoporosis. Other causes of hyperprolactinaemia have to be excluded (Table 12.6).

Acromegaly. Excessive growth hormone secretion leads to the clinical condition known as acromegaly. If it occurs before epiphyseal fusion, then it results in gigantism. The clinical progression of acromegaly is shown in Fig. 12.17. As with other pituitary tumours, these result from the local effects of the tumour itself and the effects of excessive hormone production (in this case growth hormone). The clinical appearance suggests the diagnosis, but as the changes, particularly in the face and the hands and feet, are insidious, the diagnosis is often not made until the disease has been present for many years. Previous pictures of the patient often show that the disease has been present for about 10 years.

Cushing's disease. Autonomous ACTH production leads to bilateral adrenal hyperplasia. Cushing's disease as a cause of Cushing's syndrome is discussed elsewhere (see p. 852).

TSH-secreting tumour. This is a very rare cause of hyperthyroidism.

Investigation
(See pp. 831 and 838.)

Management
Prolactinoma
Drugs. Most prolactinomas are amenable to medical treatment and the dopamine agonists bromocriptine and cabergoline are most commonly used, the latter having fewer side-effects. Prolactin levels usually fall, symptoms improve and tumour size decreases.

Dopamine agonists are the first-line treatment, even in patients with large prolactinomas when there are visual symptoms. A clinical response in terms of visual improvement is usually evident within a few weeks. Patients with

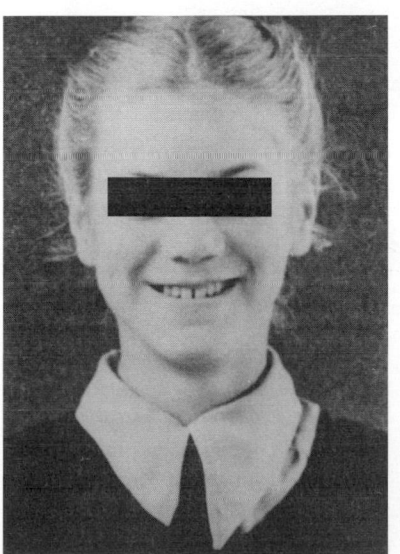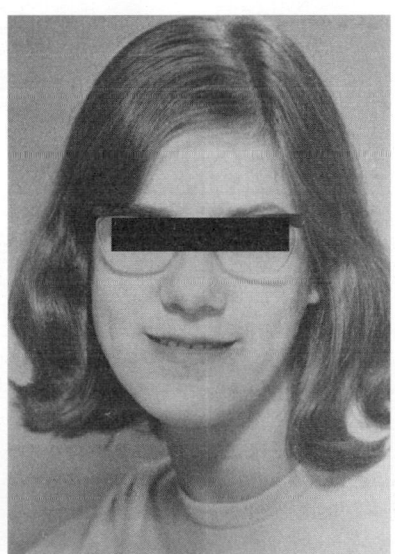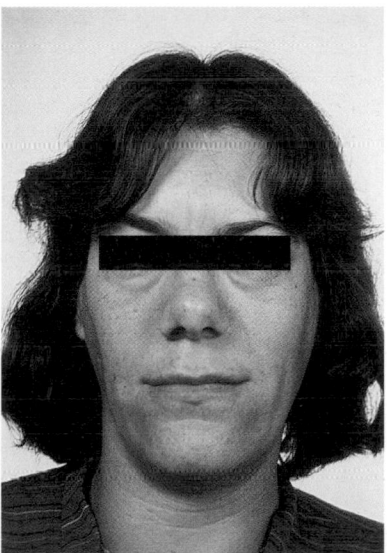

Figure 12.17 Pictorial record of the development of acromegaly.

12

Pituitary tumours at a glance

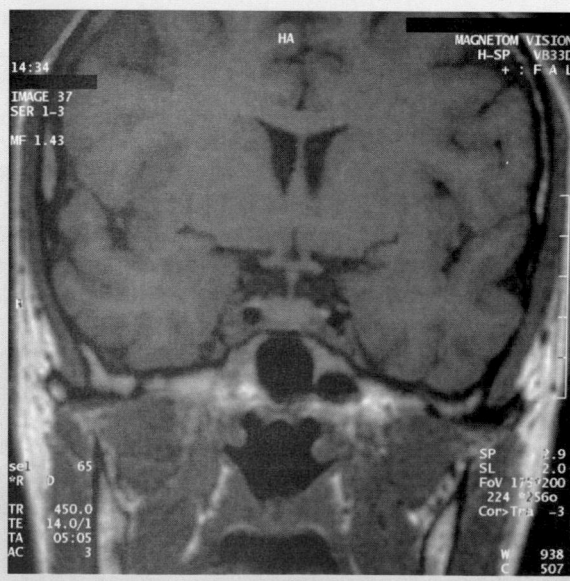

Hypopituitarism

Bitemporal hemianopia

Local mass effect

Syndromes of excess hormone production
- Acromegaly
- Cushing's disease
- Hyperprolactinaemia

Epidemiology
Prevalence
Uncommon

Sex
Prolactinomas are more frequently diagnosed in women

Findings on investigation
Biochemistry
Anterior pituitary hormones and target organ products: LH, FSH, ACTH, prolactin, growth hormone, TSH, thyroxine, cortisol, testosterone, IGF-1

Diagnostic imaging
- *Pituitary CT or MRI*
- *Petrosal sinus venous sampling:* occasionally. Clarifies origin of excess hormone production (e.g. ACTH)

Histopathology
Benign adenomas are the most common

Clinical features
Local mass effect
Hypopituitarism
Hyperprolactinaemia (from stalk disconnection)
Bitemporal hemianopia

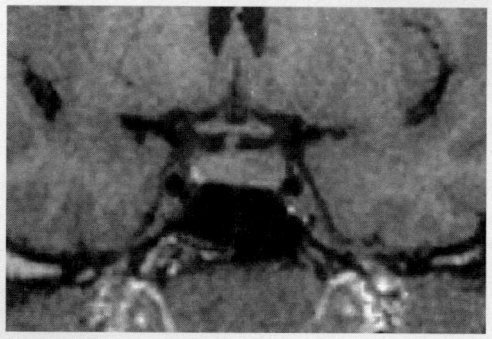

(i)

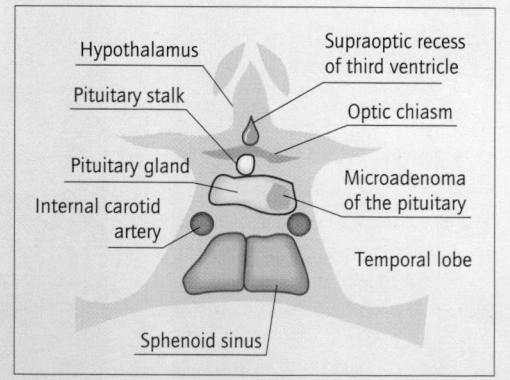

Hypothalamus

Supraoptic recess of third ventricle

Pituitary stalk

Optic chiasm

Pituitary gland

Microadenoma of the pituitary

Internal carotid artery

Temporal lobe

Sphenoid sinus

(ii)

Fig. A Magnetic resonance image showing normal pituitary gland.

Fig. B Magnetic resonance image and line diagram of a microadenoma of the pituitary gland.

12

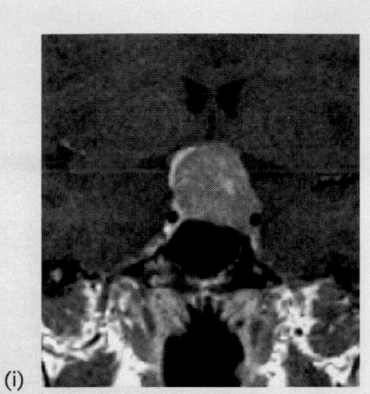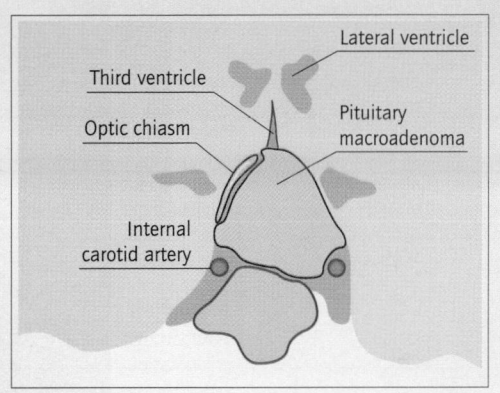

(i) (ii)

Fig. C Magnetic resonance image and line diagram of non-functioning macroadenoma of the pituitary presenting with visual field defect. The 2-cm tumour displaces the optic chiasm to the right with suprasellar extension.

large tumours often need to continue medical treatment indefinitely because the tumour may rapidly expand if medication is stopped. Prolactinomas may also expand during pregnancy. Therefore, women who become pregnant while on treatment need careful monitoring.

Surgery. Patients may require neurosurgical therapy if:
- They are unable to tolerate drug therapy
- There are rapidly progressive visual symptoms
- The tumour continues to grow despite drug therapy

Acromegaly

It is not always easy to manage acromegaly successfully and surgery, radiotherapy and drugs may all be necessary. Treatment is important if there are local effects because of tumour growth. In addition, treatment can in some cases produce regression of the coarse facial features, which patients may find distressing. Treatment is also indicated, particularly in young patients, to reduce the increased risk of cardiovascular disease and mortality associated with acromegaly.

Surgery. The treatment of choice is trans-sphenoidal surgery with preservation of pituitary tissue if possible. Growth hormone levels may return to normal after the surgery, but a surgical 'cure' of a large tumour is often not possible. A realistic expectation of surgery in this situation is optic chiasmal decompression and tumour debulking. Radiotherapy is often given as an adjunct to surgery, especially if growth hormone levels remain high.

Drugs. A minority of patients will respond to treatment with dopamine agonists, such as bromocriptine, with an improvement in well-being and a reduction in plasma

growth hormone levels. Somatostatin analogues such as octreotide have proved a major advance in the therapy of acromegaly. Treatment has resulted in significant reductions of growth hormone and IGF-1, with levels returning to normal in about 40% of patients. Tumour shrinkage occurs during long-term therapy in some patients. Somatostatin analogues have to be given by subcutaneous or intramuscular injection, which is a disadvantage. Gallstone development as a result of inhibition of gall bladder contraction is an important complication of somatostatin therapy. Pegvisomant is a new genetically engineered analogue of human growth hormone that functions as a growth hormone-receptor antagonist. It is given subcutaneously and can normalize IGF-1 in 90% of patients. Data are awaited regarding its effect on tumour size and long-term safety.

Non-secreting pituitary tumour

Surgery. Pituitary surgery is often combined with conventional radiotherapy if complete surgical removal is not achieved.

Cranial diabetes insipidus

Diabetes insipidus is best treated with the long-acting vasopressin analogue DDAVP (desmopressin, 1-desamino-8-D-arginine vasopressin), which is administered intranasally or as an oral preparation. DDAVP is available parenterally for postoperative patients.

Syndrome of inappropriate antidiuretic hormone

Disease mechanisms

A variety of medical disorders cause syndrome of

12

Acromegaly at a glance

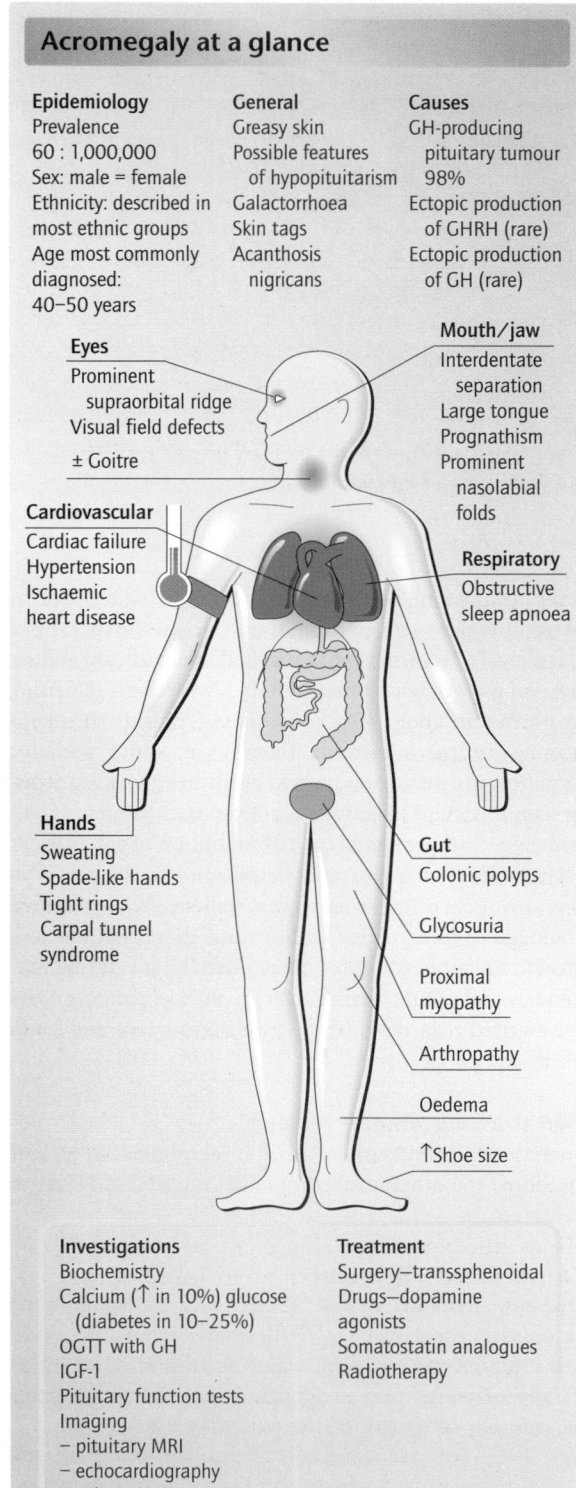

Epidemiology
Prevalence
60 : 1,000,000
Sex: male = female
Ethnicity: described in
most ethnic groups
Age most commonly
diagnosed:
40–50 years

General
Greasy skin
Possible features
of hypopituitarism
Galactorrhoea
Skin tags
Acanthosis
nigricans

Causes
GH-producing
pituitary tumour
98%
Ectopic production
of GHRH (rare)
Ectopic production
of GH (rare)

Eyes
Prominent
supraorbital ridge
Visual field defects
± Goitre

Mouth/jaw
Interdentate
separation
Large tongue
Prognathism
Prominent
nasolabial
folds

Cardiovascular
Cardiac failure
Hypertension
Ischaemic
heart disease

Respiratory
Obstructive
sleep apnoea

Hands
Sweating
Spade-like hands
Tight rings
Carpal tunnel
syndrome

Gut
Colonic polyps

Glycosuria

Proximal
myopathy

Arthropathy

Oedema

↑Shoe size

Investigations
Biochemistry
Calcium (↑ in 10%) glucose
(diabetes in 10–25%)
OGTT with GH
IGF-1
Pituitary function tests
Imaging
– pituitary MRI
– echocardiography
– colonoscopy

Treatment
Surgery–transsphenoidal
Drugs–dopamine
agonists
Somatostatin analogues
Radiotherapy

Table 12.7 Causes of syndrome of inappropriate antidiuretic hormone secretion (SIADH)

Lung disease
Bronchial carcinoma
Tuberculosis
Pneumonia
Abscess

Cranial disease
Especially tumour or haemorrhage

Drugs
Chlorpropamide
Psychotropics

inappropriate antidiuretic hormone secretion (SIADH) (Table 12.7), but the pathogenesis is not clear in many patients. It may be secondary to ectopic vasopressin production or a failure of normal suppression of vasopressin secretion. When associated with drugs, it can be caused either by stimulation of vasopressin secretion (e.g. vincristine, clofibrate) or by increasing renal vasopressin sensitivity (e.g. chlorpropamide, carbamazepine). It is common as a temporary occurrence in postsurgical patients. It can also occur in patients with lung diseases or lung infections. Water retention throughout the body compartments is increased, accompanied by reduced plasma osmolality and inappropriately raised urine osmolality. A similar situation can also arise from excessive vasopressin administration for the treatment of diabetes insipidus.

Epidemiology

Prevalence. A relatively common cause of hyponatraemia.

Age. Increasing prevalence with increasing age.

Clinical features

Patients with SIADH are not hypotensive or hypovolaemic. Most are asymptomatic and the syndrome is identified when urea and electrolytes are measured routinely. If plasma sodium falls below 120 mmol/l, symptoms of confusion, irritability and nausea may develop. As the sodium falls further fits and coma may occur.

Investigation

- Low serum sodium
- Low plasma osmolality
- Urinary osmolality inappropriately higher than plasma osmolality
- Urinary sodium excretion more than 30 mmol/l
- Normal renal, adrenal and thyroid function tests

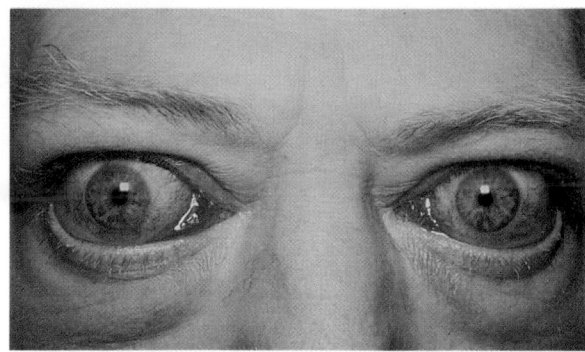

Figure 12.18 Hyperthyroidism (exophthalmos).

inflammatory reaction involving the orbital contents causes forward protrusion of the eyeball. This is revealed by the presence of white sclera between the cornea and the lower eyelid as the patient looks straight forwards (proptosis). Marked proptosis is called exophthalmos (Fig. 12.18); from the side of the patient, its extent from the lateral orbital margin can be measured with a ruler or an exophthalmometer. Occasionally, exophthalmos is asymmetrical. Damage to the cornea (keratitis) may result because of an inability to close the eyelids fully. If severe, conjunctival oedema (chemosis), raised intraocular pressure and papilloedema may develop. Weakness and tethering caused by inflammation of the extraocular muscles leads to ophthalmoplegia. Characteristically, the inferior rectus muscles are affected, leading to a failure of upward and outward gaze and diplopia. If more severe, other muscles may be involved.

Investigation

Haematology
Check the FBC before starting antithyroid therapy, because of the later risk of drug-induced agranulocytosis.

Biochemistry
Thyroid function tests. T_3 is raised, T_4 may also be raised and TSH is suppressed.

Immunology
Thyroid receptor antibodies may be helpful.

Diagnostic imaging
Ultrasound and technetium scanning are used in certain circumstances to help differentiate Graves' disease from adenoma.

Histopathology
In Graves' disease there is scant colloid and follicles are small (Fig. 12.19).

Management
The three main options for the treatment of hyperthyroidism are antithyroid drugs, radioactive iodine therapy and thyroid surgery.

Drug treatment
Antithyroid drugs are the first-line therapy for all patients with hyperthyroidism. Even when the preferred treatment is radioactive iodine or thyroid surgery, it is important to render the patient euthyroid with drugs first, to prevent a thyrotoxic crisis or 'thyroid storm'.

Carbimazole. The most commonly used antithyroid drug in the UK is carbimazole. It inhibits the production and coupling of iodotyrosine, and so inhibits thyroid hormone synthesis. It is given in a high dose (40–60 mg/day) for 4–6 weeks and then reduced to a maintenance regimen of 5–15 mg/day. Some physicians continue carbimazole in a high dose together with a replacement dose of L-thyroxine (the block-and-replace regimen). Most continue carbimazole for 12–24 months and then withdraw it. There may be a relapse when the drug treatment is stopped and this is most common among patients with large vascular goitres, high titres of thyroid-stimulating antibodies and HLA-DR3 haplotype. Patients are advised about the possibility of relapse, and asked to look out for recurrent symptoms of hyperthyroidism. If there is a relapse, then carbimazole can be restarted and the patient is prepared for the more definitive treatment of radioactive

Figure 12.19 (a) Histological appearance of Graves' disease. The follicles are small and lined with hyperplastic columnar epithelium. Colloid within the lumen is sparse or absent. There is also infiltration of the gland with lymphocytes and plasma cells. (b) After treatment with antithyroid drugs the follicles become larger and the lining epithelium flatter.

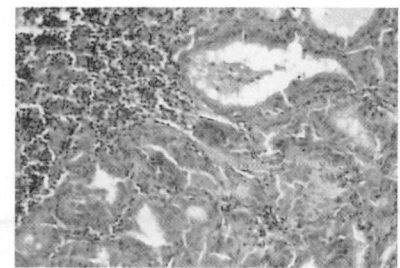

(a)

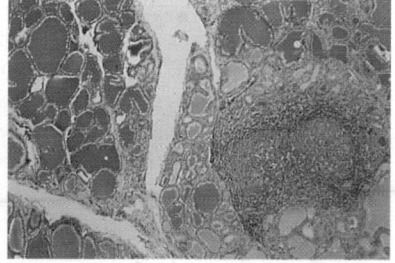

(b)

Hyperthyroidism at a glance

Epidemiology
Age: most common 30–60 years
   of age
Sex: 90% female
Genetics: shows a familial tendency
Geography: more common in
   iodine-replete areas

Causes
Graves' disease*
Toxic multinodular goitre
Toxic adenoma
Iodine induced
TSH-secreting tumour

Eyes
Exophthalmos
Lidlag
Conjunctival
   oedema
Ophthalmoplegia

Neuropsychiatric
Irritability
Psychosis

Nervous system
Hoarse voice
Slow relaxing
   reflexes

Thyroid
Goitre
Bruit*

Cardiovascular
Cardiac failure
Tachycardia
Atrial fibrillation
Systolic
   hypertension

Gut
Increased
   appetite
Increased stool
   frequency
Weight loss

Oligomenorrhoea

Proximal myopathy

Hands
Tremor, sweating
Warm peripheries
Palmar erythema
Onycholysis
Acropachy*

Pretibial
myxoedema*

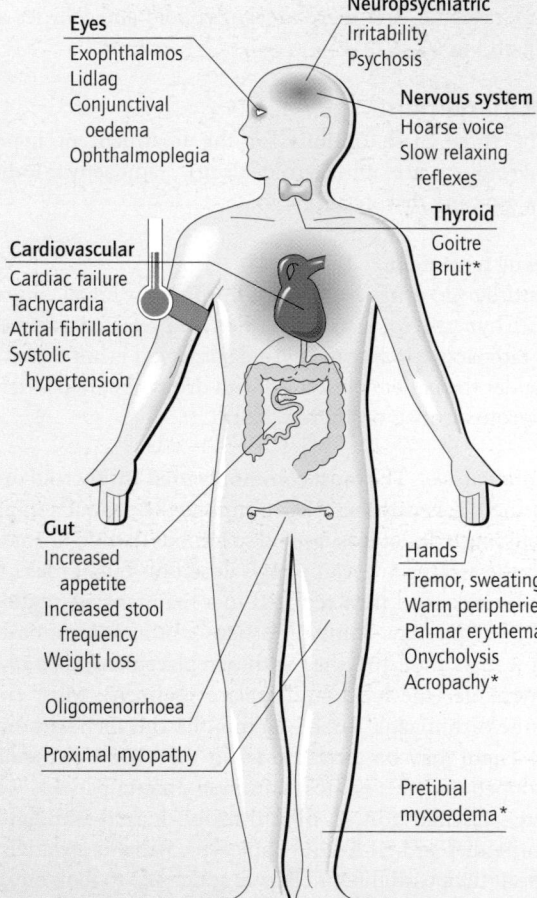

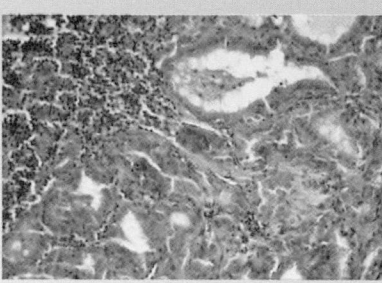

Fig. A Histological appearance of Graves' disease. The follicles are small and lined with hyperplastic columnar epithelium. Colloid within the lumen is sparse or absent. There is also infiltration of the gland with lymphocytes and plasma cells.

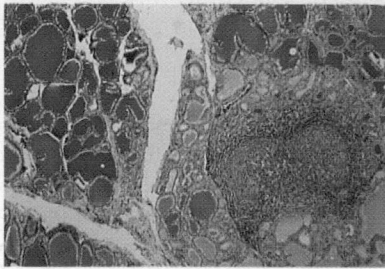

Fig. B After treatment with anti-thyroid drugs the follicles become larger and the lining epithelium flatter.

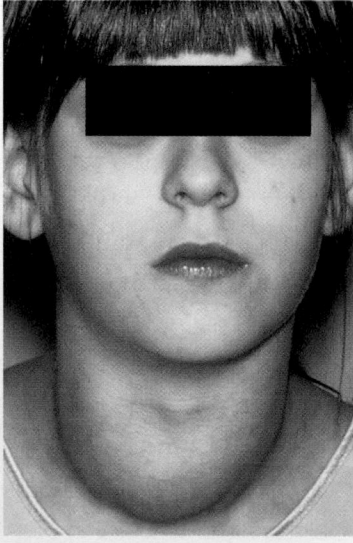

Fig. C Patients with Graves' disease appear thin, nervous, hyperactive and unable to sit still, often with a wide-eyed expression and symmetrical thyroid enlargement that moves on swallowing.

Investigations
Biochemistry—T_4 and T_3
   raised
Immunology—thyroid
   receptor antibodies titre
   raised
Ultrasound + nuclear
   imaging help distinguish
   Graves' and adenoma
Histopathology—small
   follicles and scant colloid
   in Graves'

Treatment options
Education—warn about
   drug side effects
Drugs—carbimazole,
   propylthiouracil,
   propranolol
Surgery—large goitre
   failed medical treatment
I_{131}—indications vary
   depending on cause
   and course of disease;
   patient's age and sex

12

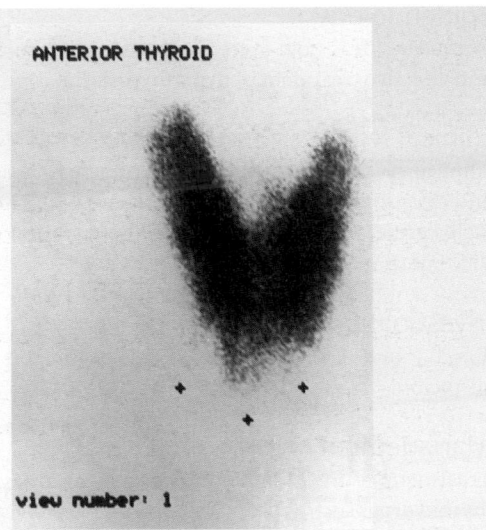

ANTERIOR THYROID

view number: 1

Fig. D Thyroid isotope scan showing typical thyroid enlargement with uniformly increased uptake of ^{99}Te. All photographs reproduced from Grossman (ed.) *Clinical Endocrinology*, 1992 (Blackwell Scientific Publications, Oxford) with the permission of the author.

iodine or surgery, or simply continued on carbimazole. Occasional side-effects of carbimazole include a skin rash and, very rarely, agranulocytosis. Patients are advised to stop carbimazole and seek medical advice if they develop a skin rash or a sore throat (which may be the first sign of agranulocytosis).

Propylthiouracil. This is an alternative antithyroid drug which is used if carbimazole is not tolerated. It is often preferred in pregnancy, because it is probably less teratogenic.

Propranolol. This is useful in the early stages of treatment. It controls distressing palpitations and tremor, and directly reduces the peripheral conversion of T_4 to T_3.

Thyroid surgery
Partial thyroidectomy is considered for:
● Large goitres
● Patients who are unable to tolerate drug therapy
● Patients who relapse repeatedly after drug therapy is discontinued
The patient must be euthyroid before surgery is performed. Some surgeons use oral potassium iodide for 10 days before surgery to reduce the vascularity of the gland.

Complications of partial thyroidectomy include damage to the left recurrent laryngeal nerve and the parathyroid glands. Transient hypocalcaemia is observed in about 10% of patients, but usually recovers spontaneously. This can arise if the parathyroid glands are damaged during surgery or if there is a calcium flux into bones that have experienced calcium loss during the period of hyperthyroidism. Hypothyroidism or recurrent hyperthyroidism may develop later.

Radioactive iodine therapy
Radioactive iodine therapy has conventionally been offered to patients over 40 years of age:
● If the disorder is difficult to control with drugs
● If there is a recurrence after thyroidectomy
Currently, many physicians offer iodine therapy to younger patients. As with surgery, the patient must be made euthyroid before treatment. Once this is performed, the antithyroid drugs are stopped 5–10 days before administration of the radioactive iodine to allow the gland to take up the therapeutic dose.

Sometimes repeated doses of radioactive iodine are needed to control hyperthyroidism, but the main complication is the development of hypothyroidism, which is easily treated. Patients should be made aware of hypothyroid symptoms, particularly weight gain, and should have thyroid function checked soon after receiving radioactive iodine.

Prognosis
Apart from the rare thyrotoxic crisis, hyperthyroidism is completely curable. However, ophthalmic Graves' disease may run a protracted course.

Thyrotoxic crisis
Disease mechanisms
Thyrotoxic crisis is a life-threatening medical emergency. Continued awareness is necessary to prevent thyroid crisis or storm, which is precipitated in severely hyperthyroid patients by a major stress such as an injury, infection or surgery.

12

Epidemiology

Prevalence. It is now exceedingly rare as a result of early and effective treatment of hyperthyroidism.

Clinical features

Clinical features include marked anxiety and agitation, and occasionally frank psychosis. There is a pronounced tachycardia, marked tremor, fever, dehydration and cardiac failure.

Investigation

T_4, T_3, and TSH, but treatment begins on clinical suspicion.

Management

Treatment is urgent and consists of large doses of antithyroid drugs such as propylthiouracil 250 mg every 6 h, or carbimazole 60–80 mg in divided doses, and potassium iodide 15 mg 4–6 hourly (EMERGENCY BOX 12.2). Adrenergic blocking drugs given intravenously (e.g. propranolol 1–5 mg 6-hourly) usefully control cardiac and neuromuscular complications. Other supportive measures include dexamethasone, parenteral fluids, and reducing hyperpyrexia with fans and tepid sponging.

Emergency 12.2: Thyrotoxic crisis

Drug treatment
Propylthiouracil 600–1200 mg orally
or
Carbimazole 60–80 mg orally
Potassium iodide 15 mg 4–6 hourly
Propranolol 1–2 mg intravenously (up to 5 mg) 6 hourly
    or 160–320 mg orally in divided doses

Other treatment
Intravenous fluids
Antipyretics

Prognosis

Poor. A successful outcome depends on prompt recognition and treatment.

Thyroid swellings

Thyroid swellings or goitre are common and may be associated with hyper- or hypothyroidism or normal thyroid function.

Management of the goitre depends on its nature, which is determined by clinical, biochemical and imaging assessments.

Endemic goitre
Disease mechanisms

Endemic goitre is associated with dietary iodine deficiency, but in an endemic area it is likely that other factors contribute to its development. Pregnancy, which is a substantial drain on maternal iodine, and mild disorders of enzymes involved in the production of thyroid hormones probably contribute to the large goitres seen in iodine-deficient areas. People with endemic goitre usually have normal thyroid function, but if iodine deficiency is severe, hypothyroidism may develop. Babies born to mothers with severe iodine deficiency may develop cretinism.

Epidemiology

Prevalence. Iodine deficiency is the major cause of goitre worldwide.

Geography. Mountainous regions and the Far East.

Clinical features

Cretinism is characterized by a severe neurological deficit, hypothyroidism and goitre.

Investigation

TSH. A raised TSH indicates hypothyroidism.

Management

The introduction of dietary iodine supplements (e.g. iodized table salt) has eliminated endemic goitre in developed countries. The introduction of supplements to goitrous areas may unmask Graves' disease and precipitate hyperthyroidism.

Prognosis

Most patients with endemic goitre do not need treatment.

Simple diffuse goitre
Disease mechanisms

Goitre that is not associated with an inflammatory or neoplastic process is common. The pathogenesis of simple goitre is poorly understood. It often develops at puberty, suggesting that oestrogens may be involved.

Epidemiology

Prevalence. Common.

Age. Usually 10–50 years of age.

Sex. Particularly common in women.

Genetics. Shows a familial tendency.

Clinical features

There is a goitre only. Clinically, the patient is euthyroid by definition.

Investigation

T_4, T_3 and TSH are normal.

Management

Often no treatment is necessary, but if the gland is large it can occasionally be reduced in size by treatment with thyroxine. This suggests that the goitre is dependent on TSH stimulation, which is suppressed by the thyroxine.

Prognosis

Occasionally, the goitre gradually enlarges and surgery is required.

Multinodular goitre

Disease mechanisms

The presence of goitrogens in the diet may contribute to the development of multinodular goitre. In parts of Japan, goitre may result from excess dietary iodine related to eating seaweed. Cassava root also contains a goitrogen that may interfere with the incorporation of iodine into thyroid hormones. Individual nodules of a multinodular goitre may become autonomous, and eventually clinical hyperthyroidism may develop.

Epidemiology

Prevalence. Common. Occurs in 5% of women over 50 years of age.

Age. Increasing prevalence with increasing age.

Sex. More common in women.

Geography. High incidence in areas of iodine deficiency.

Clinical features

The goitre may cause symptoms because of its mass effect (Fig. 12.20), and there may be hyperthyroidism. Hypothyroidism is a rare association.

Investigation

Radiographical examination of the thoracic inlet may demonstrate tracheal compression.

Management

Surgery may be required if there are obstructive symptoms (e.g. stridor). Surgery is also offered if there is significant retrosternal extension, because occasionally haemorrhage into a nodule can cause rapidly developing obstructive symptoms. A dominant nodule within a

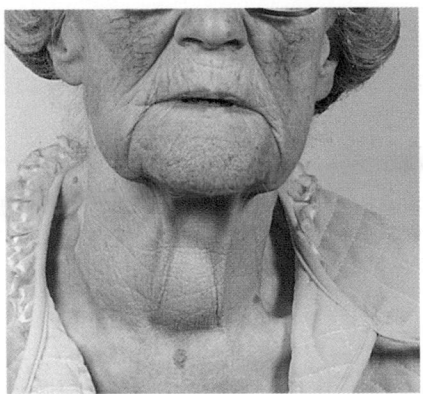

Figure 12.20 Multinodular goitre.

multinodular goitre requires fine needle aspiration to investigate possible malignancy.

Prognosis

The risk of thyroid malignancy is very small.

Thyroid malignancies

Disease mechanisms

Thyroid malignancies are classified as either well-differentiated papillary and follicular carcinomas, or anaplastic carcinomas. Carcinomas generally arise in otherwise normal glands. Approximately 10% of all thyroid malignancies arise from the parafollicular cells of the thyroid. These medullary carcinomas of the thyroid are rare and have distinct endocrine and biochemical properties.

External irradiation to the head and neck predisposes to the development of papillary carcinomas.

In MEN type 2 (see p. 864) medullary carcinoma commonly occurs in association with parathyroid adenomas and phaeochromocytoma; mutations in the *RET* oncogene have been identified.

Epidemiology

Prevalence. Primary malignancies of the thyroid are rare, accounting for less than 1% of all cancer deaths and 1–2% of localized thyroid swellings.

Age. Papillary carcinomas can occur at any age, but the median age is 40 years. Follicular carcinomas usually occur in people over 40 years of age.

Sex. Carcinomas are more common in women.

Genetics. Occasionally, papillary carcinomas are familial. Approximately 15% of medullary carcinomas are familial

12

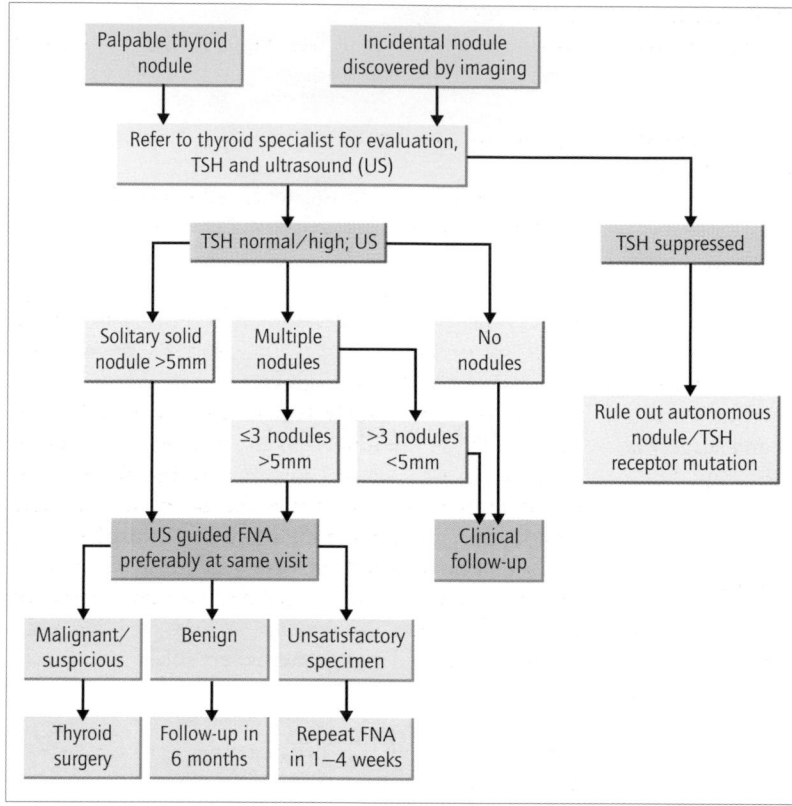

Figure 12.21 Suggested approach to thyroid nodules. FNA, fine needle aspiration.

and inheritance is autosomal dominant as part of Sipple's syndrome or multiple endocrine neoplasia (MEN) type 2 (see p. 864).

Geography. Follicular carcinomas are more common in iodine-deficient areas. Papillary carcinomas are generally seen in areas with a high iodine intake.

Clinical features

The most common presentation of thyroid malignancy is a solitary nodule in one of the thyroid lobes or in the thyroid isthmus. Clinically, it is often difficult to distinguish a nodule resulting from carcinoma from a benign adenoma or a colloid nodule. Often the lump in the neck is first noticed by a relative or the patient becomes aware of the lump when looking in the mirror or washing.

Less frequently, a more aggressive thyroid carcinoma can result in a rapidly enlarging gland, which may be associated with alterations in the voice and difficulty in swallowing and breathing because of extension to adjacent structures. There may be detectable secondary deposits in the cervical lymph nodes.

The presence of a solitary nodule should arouse a high level of clinical suspicion of thyroid malignancy, particularly if there is evidence of spread. However, examination

will often reveal only a solitary nodule with no extra-thyroid spread and no systemic symptoms. A sensible route of investigation is shown in Fig. 12.21.

Investigation
Biochemistry
● *Calcitonin:* produced in large amounts by medullary carcinoma and measurement of plasma calcitonin can be used as a marker for this tumour type
● *Plasma thyroglobulin levels:* can be used as a tumour marker in well-differentiated thyroid carcinomas

Diagnostic imaging
● *Radioactive iodine scan:* a nodule that is 'cold' is more likely to be malignant than a hot nodule.
● *Ultrasound scan:* will determine whether the cold area is solid or cystic. A solid 'cold' nodule is not necessarily a carcinoma.

Histopathology
Fine needle aspiration with cytology should be carried out in a centre with the expertise to confirm the diagnosis.

Management
Surgery is the treatment of choice; the extent of resection

is determined by the physician and thyroid surgeon. A lobectomy and removal of the isthmus may be acceptable if the disease is confined to one lobe.

Radioactive iodine. If the tumour takes up radioactive iodine, it is a useful treatment for residual local and metastatic disease.

Radiotherapy. Radiotherapy may be of benefit for anaplastic tumours.

Prognosis

The progression of malignant thyroid tumours varies and depends on the patient's age at presentation. They tend to grow slowly in younger age groups (under 40 years of age), and more rapidly and invasively in older age groups. Lifelong follow-up is recommended.

Diseases of the adrenal medulla

There is no typical syndrome caused by impaired function of the adrenal medulla because the rest of the sympathetic nervous system can compensate. A tumour of the adrenal medulla (a phaeochromocytoma) may produce large amounts of catecholamines. This tumour is of considerable interest because of its pharmacological effects.

Phaeochromocytoma

The term phaeochromocytoma is derived from the darkening of this tumour when stained with chromium salts.

Disease mechanisms

Phaeochromocytoma can occur as part of multiple endocrine neoplasia (MEN type 2; see p. 864). This syndrome may be familial and inherited as an autosomal dominant trait. In MEN type 2, phaeochromocytoma may coexist with hyperparathyroidism and medullary carcinoma of the thyroid (Fig. 12.26). Some people with MEN have mucosal neuromas on the tongue, buccal mucosa and lips (MEN type 3).

Approximately 5% of patients with phaeochromocytoma have neurofibromatosis (von Recklinghausen's disease). Sturge–Weber disease (hereditary cerebellar ataxia) and von Hippel–Lindau syndrome (cerebello-retinal haemangioblastomatosis) are also associated with a higher than normal prevalence of phaeochromocytoma.

Phaeochromocytomas can arise anywhere in the sympathetic chain but 90% develop in the adrenal medulla; 10% are malignant. Adrenal phaeochromocytomas secrete both epinephrine and norepinephrine, but those arising elsewhere in the sympathetic chain secrete only norepinephrine. Malignant tumours may secrete dopamine.

Epidemiology

Prevalence. Rare. Prevalence is unknown, but estimated to be 0.1–0.3% within the hypertensive population.

Age. Most common in adults 25–55 years of age.

Genetics. Five per cent are inherited either alone or in combination with other traits (MEN type 2).

Clinical features

The typical clinical features of a phaeochromocytoma result from the release of excess amounts of catecholamines into the circulation.

Symptoms are usually paroxysmal and may be precipitated by an emotional disturbance, posture changes or physical exercise. An attack may last from a few minutes to several hours and is characterized by a severe headache, palpitations, tremor and sweating. There may be nausea and vomiting, and pain in the chest or abdomen. If a hypertensive patient has these symptoms suspect a phaeochromocytoma, particularly if he or she has glycosuria.

Investigation

Investigation is aimed at demonstrating catecholamine overproduction.

Haematology

Haematocrit is commonly elevated.

Biochemistry

● *Urine:* 24-h urinary epinephrine and norepinephrine (or the metabolites normetanephrine, metanephrine and VMA) are measured. Various drugs and dietary factors can affect these tests, particularly urinary VMA. The diagnosis is not always straightforward if the tumour is small and if there is paroxysmal release of catecholamines. A 24-h urine collection following a symptomatic episode may be helpful.
● *Plasma:* plasma epinephrine and norepinephrine should be measured after 30 min rest. Epinephrine is raised in adrenal phaeochromocytomas and norepinephrine is raised in ectopic phaeochromocytomas.

Diagnostic imaging

● *CT scanning:* localization of a phaeochromocytoma has become much easier since the advent of CT combined with contrast.
● *Arteriography:* sometimes necessary, and selective venous sampling has been used to locate tumours that cannot be located by CT.
● *Metaiodo-benzylguanidine (MIBG) scanning:* a recent advance. This radionucleotide is taken up by chromaffin

12

tissue and is very useful in the isotopic imaging of phaeochromocytoma.

Histopathology
The tumours are composed of large pleomorphic chromaffin cells.

Management
Drugs
α-**Adrenergic blocking drugs** such as phenoxybenzamine are prescribed as soon as the diagnosis is made and before any invasive imaging, including the administration of contrast during CT scanning. If β-blocking drugs are given before α-blockers, hypertension may be exacerbated as a result of reduced β-receptor-mediated vasodilatation. The combination of α- and β-adrenergic receptor blocking drugs controls hypertension and allows restoration of plasma volume by decreasing vascular tone.

If patients are not treated before invasive procedures, a dangerous hypertensive crisis can occur because of catecholamine release. In addition, pretreatment prevents the profound hypotension that may follow surgical removal of the tumour.

Surgery
Surgery usually cures the patient and normalizes blood pressure. If unsuccessful, hypertension can be controlled with α- and β-adrenergic receptor blocking drugs.

Radiotherapy
Radiotherapy is used for residual malignant tumours, but its effect is generally disappointing.

Metaiodo-benzylguanidine
Therapeutic doses of MIBG have been used recently with some success for metastatic disease.

Prognosis
● Five-year survival is greater than 95% for non-malignant tumours
● Recurrence after surgery is less than 10%
● Surgical cure of hypertension is approximately 75%

Diseases of the adrenal cortex

Cushing's syndrome

Cushing's syndrome is characterized by excess adrenocortical hormone production.

Disease mechanisms
The causes of Cushing's syndrome:
● *Cushing's disease:* caused by an anterior pituitary adenoma producing ACTH

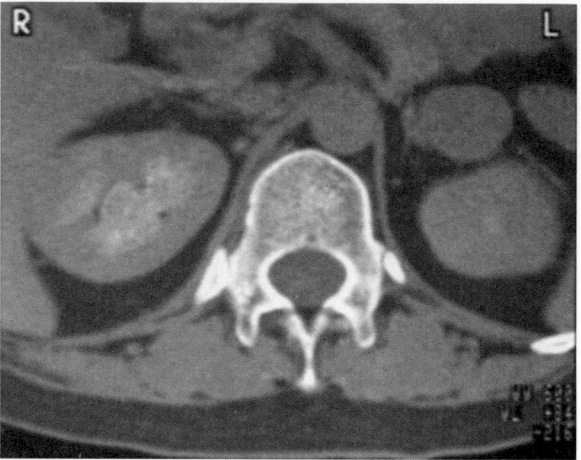

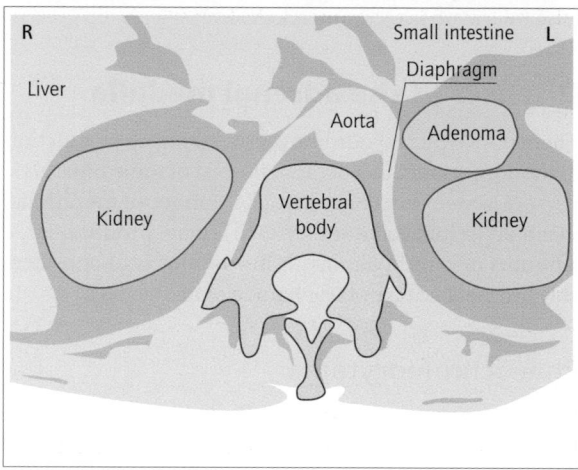

Figure 12.22 Abdominal computerized tomography (CT) scan and line diagram showing adenoma of the left adrenal gland.

● *Ectopic cushing's syndrome:* caused by ectopic ACTH production, is a feature of several carcinomas, most commonly lung carcinomas that produce ACTH
● *Adrenal Cushing's syndrome:* caused by excess steroid production by adrenal adenomas (Fig. 12.22) and carcinomas

Epidemiology
Prevalence. Cushing's syndrome, particularly iatrogenic, is common and often unreported.

Age. Most common in 25–45-year-olds.

Sex. Cushing's disease is more common in females; ectopic Cushing's is more common in males.

Clinical features
Typically, there is a centripetal distribution of body fat, a plethoric 'moon' face, a buffalo hump and a protuberant abdomen. Generalized obesity is not uncommon. Muscle

wasting contributes to the cushingoid appearance. The arms and legs look thin and often the proximal muscles are weak (proximal myopathy). The skin is characteristically thin with purple striae and it bruises easily. Commonly, cushingoid women are hirsute and have acne and a greasy skin. If there is severe virilization with clitoral enlargement, an underlying adrenal carcinoma is highly likely.

Back pain results from osteoporosis and vertebral collapse. Psychiatric features are common and are evident in up to 90% of patients. They range from depression, which is common, to hypomania and frank psychosis. Hypertension and peripheral oedema are common and result from excess mineralocorticoid secretion.

Differential diagnosis
Many of the clinical features of Cushing's syndrome can also be features of chronic alcoholism (alcoholic pseudo-Cushing's syndrome). A careful history of alcohol intake should therefore be obtained and occasionally a blood alcohol level is useful. A drug history must be taken to establish whether or not the patient has received glucocorticoid treatment.

Investigation
Diagnosis of Cushing's syndrome is based on the characteristic clinical features and biochemical investigations. When Cushing's syndrome is suspected and outpatient screening tests are positive, the patient should be admitted to hospital, preferably to a metabolic ward, for more detailed endocrine investigation.

Once a diagnosis of Cushing's syndrome is established, further biochemical and imaging techniques are necessary to identify the underlying cause.

Haematology
There may be polycythaemia, a polymorphonuclear leucocytosis and a low eosinophil count.

Biochemistry
● Glucose intolerance is common and sometimes diabetes mellitus results from the insulin resistance of excess glucocorticoid secretion
● Electrolytes: there may be hypokalaemia as a result of a mineralocorticoid effect
● The full investigation of suspected Cushing's syndrome is discussed above (see p. 832)

Management
Optimum treatment depends on the cause and may involve surgery, radiotherapy and/or pharmacological treatment.

Cushing's disease
Transsphenoidal pituitary surgery. Selective adenectomy is the treatment of choice.

Pituitary radiotherapy. This may be a useful adjunct to pituitary surgery in Cushing's disease if surgery fails to control the hypercortisolaemia. However, it may take some time to be effective if used without surgery.

Bilateral adrenalectomy. Performed if other treatments fail. If all the adrenal tissue is removed, the hypercortisolaemia is cured at the expense of a lifelong need for adrenal replacement therapy.

Adrenal surgery, especially in Cushing's syndrome, carries a significant morbidity and mortality. This can be reduced by treatment with metyrapone to reduce plasma cortisol levels preoperatively to allow partial correction of the metabolic and other features of the syndrome.

If Cushing's disease is treated with bilateral adrenalectomy alone, there is a significant risk of Nelson's syndrome. This is characterized by increasing levels of plasma ACTH (often very high), skin pigmentation and an enlarging pituitary tumour. The syndrome presumably results from an accelerated growth of the pituitary tumour because the partial feedback inhibition of high plasma cortisol levels is removed with adrenalectomy. Pituitary radiation is therefore given after bilateral adrenalectomy for Cushing's disease to prevent Nelson's syndrome.

Metyrapone and ketoconazole. On a long-term basis, these are useful therapeutic options, especially when it is not certain whether Cushing's syndrome results from pituitary-dependent disease or ectopic ACTH production. The dosage of the drug is titrated against plasma and urinary cortisol concentrations.

Ectopic adrenocorticotrophic hormone production
When ectopic ACTH production is caused by a rapidly growing bronchial carcinoma, treatment is often palliative. The adverse effects of hypercortisolaemia can be controlled with metyrapone. Operative removal of benign tumours affects a cure.

Adrenal adenoma and carcinoma
Operative removal following appropriate pretreatment with metyrapone is the treatment of choice. If carcinoma is suspected, pretreatment is restricted to no longer than 2 weeks. Radiotherapy is given postoperatively for malignant tumours. Disseminated adrenal carcinoma is generally unresponsive to conventional cytotoxic therapy.

Iatrogenic Cushing's syndrome
Where possible, steroid dosage should be reduced and steroid-sparing agents substituted.

Prognosis
The prognosis for untreated Cushing's syndrome is poor with early death, often from cardiovascular disease,

12

Cushing's syndrome at a glance

Epidemiology
Prevalence:
10/1 000 000
Age: most common in
25–45 year olds
Sex: pituitary Cushing's:
female predominance
ectopic Cushing's:
male predominance

General
Hirsutism
Thin skin
Easy bruising
Poor wound
healing

Causes
Anterior pituitary
adenoma
Ectopic ACTH
secreting tumour
Adrenal, adenoma/
carcinoma

Neuropsychiatric
Depression
Psychosis

Buffalo
(interscapular)
hump

Face
Moon face
Acne
Plethora

Cardiovascular
Hypertension

Thin limbs

Osteoporosis
± fractures

**Reproductive/
urinary**
Oligo/amenorrhoea
Polyuria
Glycosuria

Proximal myopathy

Abdomen
Violaceous striae
Obesity—
centripetal

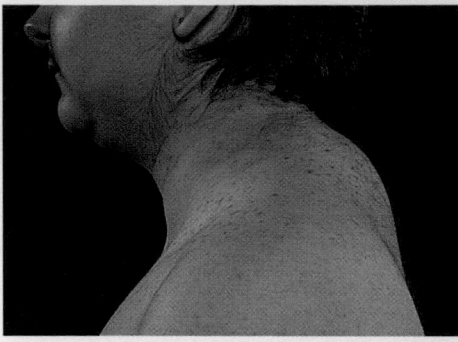

Fig. A Buffalo hump.

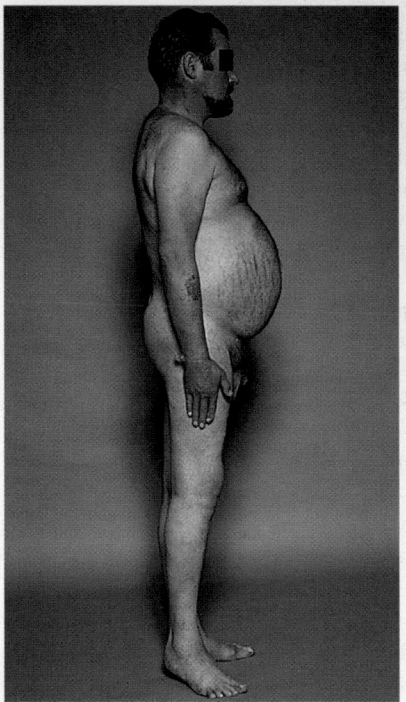

Fig. B Truncal obesity with abdominal striae.

Investigations
Biochemistry
Urinary free cortisol
increased
Diurnal rhythm of cortisol:
absent
Plasma glucose: increased
Plasma potassium:
decreased
Low dose Dex: plasma
cortisol not suppressed
ACTH; high-dose Dex;
CRF test: to establish cause
Haematology: FBC:
polycythaemia, neutrophilia
Imaging: pituitary MRI,
adrenal CT, petrosal sinus
sampling, lung CT

Treatment options
• Drug treatment
metyrapone
• Surgery–pituitary
Cushing's:
Transsphenoidal
resection
Adrenal Cushing's:
adrenalectomy
Ectopic Cushing's:
bilateral adrenalectomy,
removal of ACTH-
secreting tumour
• Radiotherapy–adjunct to
surgery

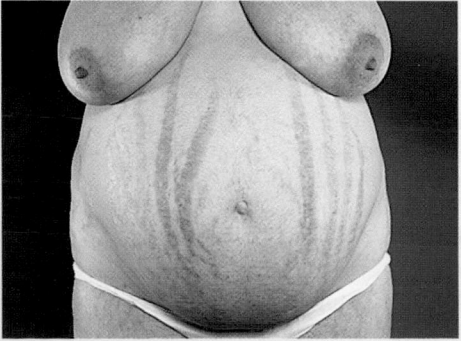

Fig. C Abdominal striae.

thromboembolism or bacterial infection. Untreated Cushing's syndrome carries a 50% mortality at 5 years. Cushing's disease is associated with increased morbidity and mortality and normal pituitary function often has to be sacrificed to obtain a cure.

Primary hyperaldosteronism (Conn's syndrome)

Primary hyperaldosteronism results from overproduction of aldosterone by cells in the zona glomerulosa of the adrenal cortex.

Disease mechanisms
The causes of Conn's syndrome are:
- A solitary adrenal adenoma (85%)
- Bilateral hyperplasia of adrenal glomerulosa cells (15%)

These causes can usually be accurately distinguished (see below). The pathogenesis of adrenal adenoma and hyperplasia is unknown.

Hyperaldosteronism causes hypertension as a result of sodium and water retention.

Epidemiology
Prevalence. Relatively uncommon.

Age. Peak incidence 30–50 years of age.

Sex. More common in females.

Genetics. The rare condition of glucocorticoid-responsive hyperaldosteronism is autosomal dominant.

Clinical features
Conn's syndrome is characterized by hypertension and hypokalaemia (because aldosterone enhances renal potassium excretion). Hypokalaemia causes muscle weakness, a metabolic alkalosis (which in turn causes tetany), polyuria and polydipsia. Malignant hypertension is rare.

Differential diagnosis
Other causes of hypokalaemia need to be excluded (see p. 584). Conn's syndrome should be suspected in anyone with hypertension and hypokalaemia, but the most common cause of hypokalaemia in a hypertensive patient is diuretic therapy.

Investigation
Haematology
Normal.

Biochemistry
Plasma renin and aldosterone. Conn's syndrome is confirmed by demonstrating a high plasma aldosterone concentration not suppressed by saline infusion of 300 mmol over 4 h, and a low plasma renin. This indicates autonomous aldosterone production and feedback suppression of renin (Fig. 12.10). An adenoma and hyperplasia can be distinguished by their different patterns of aldosterone concentrations during the day:
- In the case of an adenoma, aldosterone levels fall throughout the morning
- In contrast, patients with idiopathic bilateral hyperplasia are sensitive to the small increase in renin and angiotensin II that occurs on standing and plasma aldosterone levels rise over the morning

Diagnostic imaging
- *CT scanning:* adenomas of the zona glomerulosa leading to Conn's syndrome may be too small for identification by CT scanning.
- *Radiolabelled cholesterol scanning:* this has been used to distinguish hyperplasia from adenoma. There is bilateral uptake of the tracer in hyperplasia and unilateral uptake with an adenoma.

Venous blood sampling
Selective venous blood sampling for aldosterone under imaging control may help localize an adenoma. The site of each sample can be verified by simultaneous measurement of cortisol and aldosterone.

Management
Treatment of Conn's syndrome depends on the underlying cause.

Surgery
Surgery is generally recommended for an adenoma as it will usually cure the hypertension. Potassium stores should be replaced before surgery and this can be achieved by pretreatment with specific aldosterone antagonists such as spironolactone, and sometimes by potassium supplementation.

Medical treatment
Bilateral adrenal hyperplasia is treated medically. The hypertension and hypokalaemia are controlled using spironolactone. Important side-effects include decreased libido and tender enlargement of the breasts in men. Triamterene and amiloride are alternative drugs. Other antihypertensive agents may also be necessary to control the hypertension.

Prognosis
Long-term cure rates for surgery for a Conn's adenoma vary from 70 to 90%.

12

Secondary hyperaldosteronism

Activation of the renin–angiotensin system results in high aldosterone levels. Causes include renal artery stenosis, decompensated liver disease, accelerated hypertension, cardiac failure and nephrotic syndrome (see p. 515).

Adrenocortical failure (Addison's disease)

Failure of the adrenal cortex to produce normal amounts of glucocorticoid and mineralocorticoid hormones may be primary or secondary.
● Primary adrenocortical failure is caused by disease of the adrenal gland.
● Secondary adrenocortical failure is caused by failure of ACTH production by the pituitary. This may be secondary to pituitary disease, parapituitary disease, hypothalamic disease or withdrawal of chronic corticosteroid therapy. Some rare congenital conditions result from deficiencies of various enzymes in the corticosteroid synthetic pathway (e.g. congenital adrenal hyperplasia).

Primary adrenal failure

Disease mechanisms

Autoimmune destruction of the adrenal cortex is the most common cause of primary adrenocortical failure in Western countries and is responsible for 75% of cases. Tuberculosis accounts for 20% of cases, and rare destructive processes for 5%. The human immunodeficiency virus (HIV) has increased the incidence of hypoadrenalism because of opportunistic infection. In countries with a high incidence of tuberculosis, this is a more important cause than it is in developed countries.

About 70% of patients with idiopathic Addison's disease have antibodies to the adrenal cortex. Destruction of the adrenal cortex may occur in tuberculosis, fungal infections or lymphoma. Waterhouse–Friderichsen syndrome is an acute adrenal crisis caused by destruction of the adrenal cortex by haemorrhage associated with meningococccal infection.

The mineralocorticoid action of adrenal steroids promotes sodium retention and potassium excretion, so deficiency causes sodium loss and hyperkalaemia.

Epidemiology

Prevalence. 1 in 20 000 population.

Sex. Autoimmune Addison's disease is more common in women.

Genetics. May be a family history of Addison's disease or another autoimmune disorder.

Geography. Local prevalence of tuberculosis is important because it suggests the possibility of adrenal gland destruction by the disease.

Clinical features

Early symptoms are vague and include anorexia, lethargy and weakness. Later there is weight loss and hyperpigmentation because of high ACTH levels, which result from the lack of normal negative feedback inhibition by cortisol. Skin melanin is increased and has a characteristic distribution (Fig. 12.23). It is most evident in skin exposed to sunlight and affected by pressure and irritation.

A characteristic feature is pigmentation involving the inside of the cheek or gums, the lips and palmar creases. Dizziness because of postural hypotension, nausea, vomiting and abdominal pain are also late features.

Patient presentation may be precipitated by an intercurrent illness (e.g. infection, trauma or surgery). Such an illness may lead to acute hypoadrenalism (Addisonian crisis) if adrenocortical function is impaired. This is a medical emergency. The clinical features include nausea, vomiting, apathy, confusion and profound weakness. Hypotensive and hypovolaemic shock may develop.

Addison's disease may coexist with other autoimmune disorders, especially thyroid disease, premature ovarian failure and type 1 diabetes mellitus.

Diagnosis is often late because initial symptoms are vague.

Investigation

Haematology

There is often a lymphocytosis and eosinophilia.

Biochemistry

● *Electrolytes:* other features of Addison's disease include hyperkalaemia and hyponatraemia secondary to mineralocorticoid deficiency.
● *Glucose:* occasionally there is hypoglycaemia.
● *Plasma cortisol level:* and its response to an injection of ACTH will confirm a diagnosis of Addison's disease. The cortisol is measured at 9 a.m. In severe Addison's disease, it may be less than the lower limit of the normal range. In less severe disease, it may be normal and the diagnostic procedure is to demonstrate a failure of the plasma cortisol to respond to appropriate stress.
● *Short Synacthen test:* Synacthen (tetracosactrin) is a synthetic form of ACTH. In suspected adrenocortical insufficiency, 250 µg is injected and plasma cortisol levels are measured before, and at 30 and 60 min after the injection. Normally, the plasma cortisol rises to more than 550 nmol/l (Fig. 12.16).
● *Long Synacthen test:* this is performed if there is an impaired response to the injection of Synacthen. In

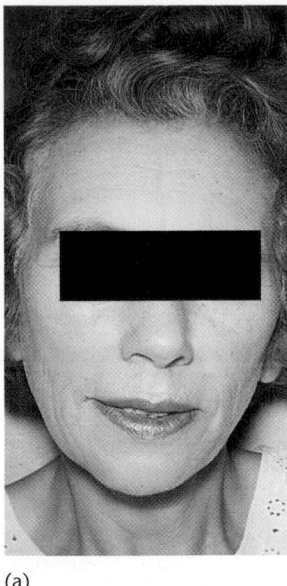
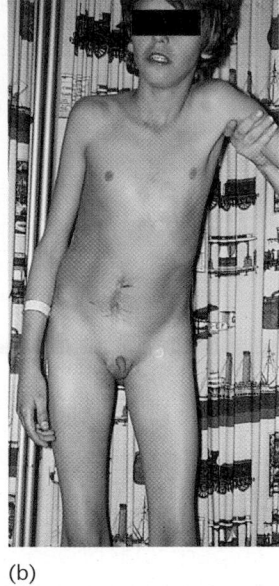
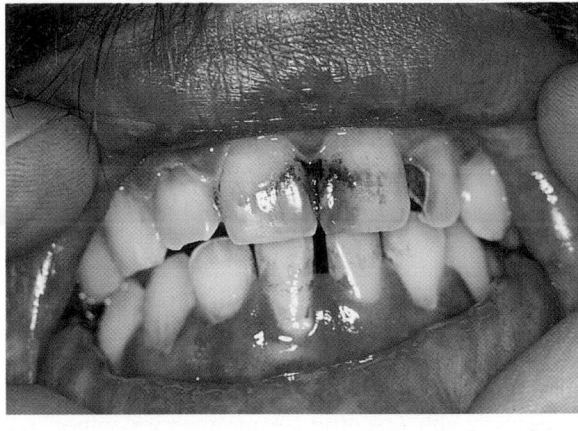

(a)   (b)   (c)

Figure 12.23 (a) Facial appearance in Addison's disease. (b) Acute Addison's disease. Note pigmentation of abdominal scar and general pigmentation. (c) Buccal pigmentation in Addison's disease.

Addison's disease there is no response. If the initial poor response to the short Synacthen test is a result of partial adrenal atrophy secondary to pituitary or hypothalamic disease, cortisol levels progressively rise.

Immunology
Plasma autoantibodies to the adrenal gland can be demonstrated in autoimmune Addison's disease.

Microbiology
Blood culture and occasionally adrenal biopsy can provide evidence of infection such as tuberculosis or fungal infection.

Diagnostic imaging
Adrenal CT may be useful if a non-autoimmune destructive process is considered.

Management
Addisonian crisis
An acutely ill patient with an Addisonian crisis needs immediate treatment; there is no time to wait for the results of the usual investigative procedure (EMERGENCY BOX 12.3). Blood is taken to measure plasma cortisol and urea and electrolytes, and treatment is commenced immediately with intravenous physiological saline and hydrocortisone. In severe Addison's disease 6 l of saline may be required.

Emergency 12.3: Addisonian crisis

Supportive treatment
Patient education
Lifelong replacement therapy is required

Specific treatment
Drug treatment
Hydrocortisone 100 mg intravenously 6-hourly for 24–48 h
Normal (0.9%) saline 2–6 l intravenously in 12–24 h
When stable convert to maintenance hydrocortisone and
   fludrocortisone orally

Other treatment
Monitor for evidence of a precipitating infection and treat
   accordingly

Less severe Addison's disease
Less severe Addison's disease may be treated with oral therapy from the outset. Hydrocortisone is the treatment of choice and it is given to mimic the normal circadian rhythm of plasma cortisol. The usual replacement regimen is 10 mg on waking, 5 mg at midday and 5 mg in the late afternoon. In addition, mineralocorticoid activity is supplied by fludrocortisone 0.05–0.3 mg/day. Adrenal insufficiency following withdrawal of chronic corticosteroid treatment can be avoided by gradually tapering the steroid dosage over weeks.

12

Long-term management

Addison's disease requires lifelong replacement therapy and this must be emphasized to the patient. The replacement therapy must never be stopped. The patient must have an adequate supply of treatment at all times. The patient is also advised to increase the replacement dose during intercurrent stress. This mimics the body's normal response to stress.

A steroid card should always be carried and should give details of the medication and the responsible hospital and physician. Ideally, patients should wear a medical identification bracelet or necklace, such as Medic Alert.

Intercurrent surgery

People on replacement therapy with corticosteroids need particular care during any operative intervention:

● *For minor procedures* (under local anaesthetic): it is best to give an injection of 100 mg of hydrocortisone intramuscularly, although often 100 mg orally will suffice
● *For operative procedures* (involving general anaesthesia): 100 mg of hydrocortisone should be given intramuscularly or intravenously with the premedication and repeated 6-hourly as required until oral medication can be resumed

Prognosis

An acute adrenal crisis is a life-threatening emergency and a treatable cause of death. Before treatment, 80% of patients died within 2 years of diagnosis. Comparable figures for the present are not available.

Disorders of female reproductive endocrinology

The endocrine disorders that involve the ovary (Table 12.9) are:

● Hypogonadism
● Hyperandrogenism
● Disorders of sexual differentiation

Any of these may present with menstrual disturbance or anovulation.

Female hypogonadotrophic hypogonadism

Hypothalamic and pituitary diseases

The gonadotrophs (FH, LSH) fail relatively early in neoplastic, vascular or granulomatous diseases of the pituitary and hypothalamus. Disorders affecting the pituitary are relatively uncommon compared to primary defects of GnRH secretion from the hypothalamus. Pituitary disorders may be distinguished from hypothalamic defects by GnRH stimulation tests, which reveal a diminished LH and FSH response only in pituitary disease.

Table 12.9 Causes of female disorders of reproductive endocrinology

Hypogonadotrophic hypogonadism
Hypothalamic and pituitary diseases
Hyperprolactinaemia
Low body weight
Idiopathic

Hypogonadism with increased gonadotrophins
Gonadal dysgenesis including Turner's syndrome
Premature ovarian failure (autoimmune, idiopathic, iatrogenic)

Hyperandrogenism
Polycystic ovary syndrome
Congenital adrenal hyperplasia
Adrenal and ovarian tumours
Syndromes of extreme insulin resistance

Hyperprolactinaemia

Raised prolactin concentrations suppress hypothalamic secretion of GnRH and therefore induce hypogonadotrophic hypogonadism. In addition, large pituitary tumours may interrupt the portal circulation to gonadotrophs and cause hyperprolactinaemia through stalk compression.

Weight-related amenorrhoea

Weight loss is often accompanied by amenorrhoea of hypothalamic origin. The low body weight is frequently not as severe as in anorexia nervosa, and the menstrual cycle may not restart for several months after regaining the premorbid weight.

Stress- and exercise-related amenorrhoea are frequently mediated through weight loss; swimmers commonly maintain their fat tissue for buoyancy and thus menstruate, whereas runners have low body fat and are more prone to amenorrhoea.

Idiopathic hypogonadotrophic hypogonadism

Many women with amenorrhoea of hypothalamic origin have no obvious cause for hypogonadism.

A single measurement of gonadotrophins may be normal, but inappropriately low for the serum oestrogen concentration. Serial blood sampling demonstrates an absence of gonadotrophin pulsatility. Imaging must be considered to exclude structural lesions.

Treatment of hypogonadism

Treatment of hypogonadism involves:

● Sex steroid replacement
● Treatment for infertility

In women who have not had a hysterectomy, oestrogen must be given in conjunction with cyclical progesterone to avoid endometrial hyperplasia and the risk of uterine carcinoma. Low oestrogen concentrations must not be allowed to persist because of the risk of developing osteoporosis.

Anovulation may respond to oral therapy with the antioestrogen clomifene, or parenteral therapy with gonadotrophins or GnRH administered by a pulsatile syringe pump. All attempts to induce ovulation are best monitored by oestrogen measurements in blood or urine and pelvic ultrasound to reduce the risk of hyperstimulation and multiple pregnancies.

Female hypogonadism with increased gonadotrophins

Gonadal dysgenesis

Disease mechanisms
Mosaicism in Turner's syndrome occurs when a proportion of the cells have a normal 46,XX genotype, leading to a variable expression of the Turner's phenotype. The 46,XO cell lines result from early mitotic non-disjuncture. The gonads are described as streaks and the clinical picture is one of premature ovarian failure. The number of germ cells in the second trimester of gestation is normal, but by birth the ovary has a greatly reduced ovum content, resulting in primary gonadal failure and primary (rarely, secondary) amenorrhoea.

Epidemiology
Prevalence. Turner's syndrome is the most common form of gonadal dysgenesis and occurs in 1 in 2000 live births.

Age. Usually diagnosed in the neonate, but mosaicism may present later with premature ovarian failure and primary amenorrhoea.

Sex. Female.

Clinical features
A 46,XO karyotype is accompanied by a female phenotype characterized by a short stature, sexual infantilism, a webbed neck, a fish-like mouth, epicanthal folds, cubitus valgus, coarctation of the aorta and sometimes neonatal lymphoedema.

Investigation
- *Karyotype*
- *Pelvic ultrasound*
- *Gonadotrophin levels:* LH and FSH levels are high and oestrogen levels are low

Management
Oestrogen replacement therapy is essential and should be started at a low dose (ethinylestradiol 10 µg/day) to minimize side-effects and ensure adequate breast development. Growth hormone treatment for short stature in Turner's syndrome may add 5–10 cm to final height.

Prognosis
Life expectancy is normal.

Premature ovarian failure

Disease mechanisms
Premature ovarian failure describes an early failure of ovarian function as a result of oocyte depletion. Usually the cause is unknown. Some patients have ovarian antibodies, and occasionally other endocrine autoimmunity (e.g. Addison's disease, hypothyroidism, pernicious anaemia). Many people who have been treated for leukaemia and lymphoma develop premature ovarian failure secondary to chemotherapy and radiotherapy.

Epidemiology
Prevalence. 1% of females.

Age. Defined as menopause occurring under 40 years of age.

Genetics. Familial forms are rare.

Clinical features
Premature ovarian failure may present with either primary or, more commonly, secondary amenorrhoea. There are symptoms of oestrogen deficiency (e.g. flushing, dyspareunia).

Investigation
- *Gonadotrophin and oestrogen measurements:* oestrogen levels are low and LH and FSH levels are elevated
- *Pelvic ultrasound*

Management
Treatment of premature ovarian failure with hormone replacement therapy is simple, but patients may require several consultations before understanding the implications of infertility. Ovum donation offers the chance of pregnancy with a donor egg and a partner's sperm.

Prognosis
Only very rare remissions of premature ovarian failure have been reported.

Female hyperandrogenism

Polycystic ovary syndrome

Disease mechanisms
Polycystic ovary syndrome is caused predominantly by

ovarian rather than adrenal hyperandrogenism. Polycystic ovary syndrome is of unknown aetiology, but the heterogeneous clinical and endocrine features probably result from several pathological mechanisms. It is often obesity related.

Epidemiology
Prevalence. Common.

Age. Most common postpubertally and in women 20–30 years of age.

Genetics. Associated with a familial tendency.

Clinical features
Polycystic ovary syndrome most commonly presents with hirsutism, obesity, oligomenorrhoea and infertility because of anovulation.

Investigation
● *Serum LH and/or testosterone concentrations:* characteristically raised in up to 40% of patients.
● *Ultrasound:* greater use of ultrasound has revealed a high prevalence of polycystic ovaries (Fig. 12.24) in women previously thought to have idiopathic hirsutism (hirsutism with no abnormal hormone measurement). Such women are now usually considered to have mild polycystic ovary syndrome.

Polycystic ovary syndrome must be differentiated from less common causes of hyperandrogenism:
● Serum 17-hydroxyprogesterone concentrations are raised in congenital adrenal hyperplasia

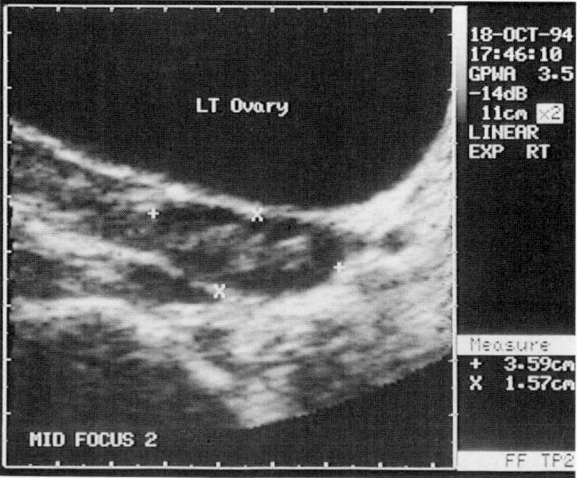

Figure 12.24 The appearance of a polycystic ovary on transabdominal ultrasonography with a 'necklace' of cysts surrounding echodense stroma.

● Serum testosterone concentrations are higher (more than 4 nmol/l) and there is severe hirsutism and a short history if there is an androgen-secreting tumour

Management
Treatment depends on the main symptom:
● *Hirsutism:* usually responds to combined oestrogen and antiandrogen (cyproterone acetate) therapy.
● *Menstrual disturbance:* often responds to the combined oral contraceptive pill.
● *Anovulation:* treated with oral clomifene citrate or parenteral gonadotrophins to induce ovulation.
● *Insulin-sensitizing drugs:* such as metformin and the thiazolidinediones may lead to resumption of normal ovulatory cycles and amelioration of the clinical features. Metformin reduces insulin and testosterone levels and improves prospects for fertility in obese women with polycystic ovary syndrome, but its use should be combined with dietary modification and a regular exercise programme.

Prognosis
Polycystic ovary syndrome may vary in its symptomatology through life, but does not remit. Of those women with polycystic ovary syndrome who present with anovulatory infertility, 80% will respond to ovulation induction.

Congenital adrenal hyperplasia
Disease mechanisms
The most common cause of congenital adrenal hyperplasia is a deficiency of the 21-hydroxylase enzyme, which converts 17-hydroxyprogesterone to deoxycortisol in the cortisol pathway (Fig. 12.12). Low cortisol synthesis increases ACTH stimulation of the adrenal gland, which results in a build-up of 17-hydroxy precursors proximal to the enzyme deficiency. Elevated precursors are diverted to androgen production, which becomes excessive. In about 10% of patients the underlying defect is 11-β-hydroxylase or 3-β-hydroxysteroid dehydrogenase deficiency.

Epidemiology
Prevalence. 1 in 1000 live births.

Age. Commonly presents in the neonate.

Genetics. Congenital adrenal hyperplasia is autosomal recessive and is usually caused by mutations in the gene encoding 21-hydroxylase.

Geography. Various populations (e.g. Eskimos) have an increased prevalence.

Clinical features
Neonatal presentation is with either ambiguous genitalia

12

or a salt-losing crisis. Females have normal internal genitalia and varying degrees of external virilization. The spectrum of virilization depends on the severity of the enzyme block and varies from a penile urethra to, more usually, clitoromegaly. A late-onset variant results in hirsutism alone and may be diagnosed as late as the fifth decade.

Investigation
17-hydroxyprogesterone measurements before and 30 min after 250 μg of intravenous Synacthen. Concentrations of 17-hydroxyprogesterone over 20 nmol/l occur in mild forms and concentrations over 100 nmol/l in severe forms.

Management
Adrenal replacement therapy as in Addison's disease (see p. 857).

Adrenal and ovarian tumours
Disease mechanisms
Adrenal adenomas and carcinomas can produce a variable amount of androgen in combination with other steroids.
   Ovarian tumours can secrete:
- Oestrogen (granulosa-thecal cell tumours)
- Androgens (dysgerminomas, lipoid cell tumours, gonadoblastomas)

Epidemiology
Prevalence. Rare.

Clinical features
The clinical features depend on the relative amounts of androgen, glucocorticoid and mineralocorticoid.

Investigation
- Sex steroid measurements
- CT scan of adrenals
- Pelvic ultrasound

Management
Surgery.

Prognosis
Depends on pathology.

Androgen insensitivity syndrome
Disease mechanisms
Androgen insensitivity syndrome is characterized by the 46,XY karyotype accompanied by an external female phenotype with variable virilization caused by androgen resistance as a result of defects in the androgen receptor.

Epidemiology
Prevalence. 1 in 50 000.

Age. Usually presents in the neonate.

Sex. Male genotype.

Genetics. Inheritance of 46,XY is X-linked recessive.

Clinical features
Complete androgen insensitivity syndrome is the complete form of this disorder. The phenotype is then female and the presentation is often with primary amenorrhoea. Anti-müllerian hormone function is normal, resulting in the formation of testes (usually inguinal), and absent uterus and fallopian tubes.

   In partial forms of the syndrome there is a spectrum of clinical presentations extending from phenotypic females through ambiguous genitalia to normal male phenotypes with oligospermia (Reifenstein's syndrome).

Investigation
- Karyotype
- Testosterone, LH and FSH measurements

Management
The testes are removed because of an increased prevalence of testicular carcinoma. Oestrogen replacement therapy is then required.

Disorders of male reproductive endocrinology

The endocrine disorders that affect the testes (Table 12.10) involve:
- Androgen deficiency (hypogonadism)
- Relative oestrogen excess (gynaecomastia)

Male hypogonadotrophic hypogonadism
Hypothalamic and pituitary disorders
Disease mechanisms
Hypogonadism may be secondary to hypothalamic or pituitary disease, but the relative importance of the different causes of hypogonadotrophic hypogonadism varies between the sexes. Isolated gonadotrophin deficiency is more common in the male, and when associated with anosmia is termed Kallmann's syndrome. Hyperprolactinaemia appears to be more common in women, possibly because the clinical markers (galactorrhoea and amenorrhoea) are more obvious.

   Haemochromatosis, an autosomal recessive disorder of iron accumulation in which hypogonadism results from deposition of iron in the pituitary (not the gonads), affects both sexes equally, but the clinical manifestations occur

12

Table 12.10 Causes of male hypogonadism

Hypogonadotrophic hypogonadism
Hypothalamic and pituitary disease
Isolated gonadotrophin deficiency
Kallmann's syndrome,
Hyperprolactinaemia
Haemochromatosis

Hypogonadism with increased gonadotrophins (testicular failure)
Congenital causes
Testicular agenesis
Cryptorchidism
Klinefelter's syndrome
Androgen resistance
5α reductase deficiency

Acquired causes
Testicular trauma/torsion
Orchitis (mumps, Coxsackie viruses)
Iatrogenic (cytotoxicity, irradiation)

earlier in men because they do not benefit from the protective effect of menstruation on iron stores.

Clinical features

Clinical features of hypogonadism depend on the age of onset of androgen deficiency. Hypospadias, microphallus and cryptorchidism occur *in utero*. In the adult, scant body and facial hair, decreased libido and impaired sexual function are the main presenting features. Prepubertal androgen deficiency results in late closure of the epiphyses, leading to elongated limbs (arm span greater than height and heel-to-pubis length greater than pubis-to-crown).

Investigation

- *Full pituitary function tests:* may be required to test other endocrine axes (see p. 831)
- *Serum testosterone, LH and FSH measurements:* are sufficient to test the pituitary–testicular axis
- *Pituitary MRI*

Management

Androgen replacement therapy is required to prevent osteoporosis and maintain secondary sexual characteristics. Gonadotrophins are required to induce spermatogenesis. Oral testosterone replacement is available, but it is best given parenterally, either by monthly intramuscular injections or by subcutaneous implant every 6 months. Transdermal testosterone is convenient but expensive. Spermatogenesis can be induced only if the testes are free of disease, in which case parenteral gonadotrophins or subcutaneous GnRH administered via a pulsatile syringe pump are required.

Hypogonadism with increased gonadotrophins (testicular failure)

Testicular agenesis

Clinical features

Impaired testicular function produces a spectrum of disorders ranging from a female phenotype with female müllerian structures if the failure occurs before 8 weeks' gestation (46,XY gonadal agenesis) to a male phenotype with absent testes if regression occurs after the critical phase of male differentiation at 13–14 weeks of gestation.

Epidemiology

Prevalence. Rare.

Age. Prepubertal presentation.

Sex. Variable phenotype.

Investigation

- Karyotype
- Pelvic ultrasound

Management

Testosterone replacement therapy.

Cryptorchidism

Disease mechanisms

Cryptorchidism is incomplete descent or maldescent of the testis. The cause is unknown. Testosterone production is reduced and spermatogenesis is defective.

Epidemiology

Prevalence. The incidence is about 3% at birth and less than 1% at 6 months and thereafter.

Age. Usually neonatal or prepubertal.

Clinical features

The patient presents with an undescended testis or androgen deficiency.

Investigation

Testosterone levels are low and LH and FSH levels are elevated.

Management

Androgen replacement therapy and orchidoplasty.

Prognosis

Surgical correction of cryptorchidism does not remove the increased risk of malignancy; 10% of testicular tumours are associated with undescended testes.

Klinefelter's syndrome

Disease mechanisms

The 47,XXY karyotype of Klinefelter's syndrome occurs from aberrant meiosis in either parent. The condition is sporadic and associated with advanced maternal age.

Epidemiology

Prevalence. Uncommon.

Age. Usually presents postpubertally.

Sex. Male.

Clinical features

The prime feature of Klinefelter's syndrome is seminiferous tubule dysgenesis that results in small testes. Testosterone deficiency is responsible for a small phallus, reduced body hair, azoospermia, gynaecomastia and disproportionately long limbs. The past emphasis on a low intelligence is now less obvious as the condition has become more widely recognized with a milder phenotype.

Investigation

- *Karyotype*
- *Testosterone, LH and FSH measurements:* testosterone levels are low and LH and FSH levels are elevated

Management

Androgen replacement.

Acquired testicular diseases

Disease mechanisms

Causes of acquired testicular defects include infections (e.g. mumps, Coxsackie and echoviruses, mycoplasma), radiation, drugs (especially cyclophosphamide) and associated systemic disease, such as renal failure.

Clinical features

These conditions present with androgen deficiency.

Investigation

Testosterone levels are low and LH and FSH levels are elevated.

Management

Androgen replacement.

Gynaecomastia

Disease mechanisms

Enlargement of the male breast tissue can be:
- *Physiological:* in the newborn, at puberty and in the elderly

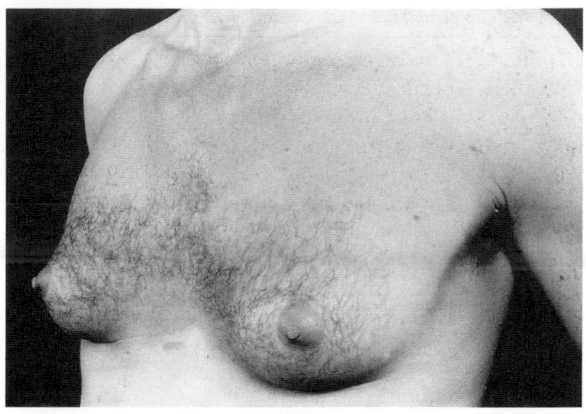

(a)

(b)

Figure 12.25 (a) Gynaecomastia in a 26-year-old man caused by an oestrogen-secreting Leydig cell tumour of the testis. (b) Testicular ultrasound of the same patient, the Leydig cell tumour is arrowed.

- *Pathological:* caused by male breast cancer, where differentiation from adipose deposition is often difficult
- *Gynaecomastia:* with enlargement of breast tissue that can be caused by excess oestrogen (Fig. 12.25a), a deficiency of androgens (Table 12.11) or drugs

Epidemiology

Prevalence. Uncommon.

Age. 15–70 years of age.

Sex. Male.

12

Table 12.11 Causes of gynaecomastia

Oestrogen excess
Testicular (Leydig cell) tumour
Increased peripheral production
   Adrenal tumour
   Congenital adrenal hyperplasia
   Liver disease
   Starvation
   Hyperthyroidism

Testosterone deficiency
Anorchia
Klinefelter's syndrome
Androgen resistance
Acquired testicular failure

Drugs
Oestrogen derivatives
Digoxin
Spironolactone
Cimetidine
Cannabis

Clinical features

Asymmetry is common. Examination of the testes is essential to locate a possible source of oestrogen, such as a tumour and to look for evidence of testicular failure.

Investigation

- *Endocrine screen:* should include gonadotrophins, testosterone, oestradiol and thyroid function
- *Testicular ultrasound:* particularly useful to detect occult testicular tumours (Fig. 12.25b)

Management

A primary cause can be found for about 50% of men with gynaecomastia and specific treatment can be instituted. For idiopathic gynaecomastia, tamoxifen, which is an antioestrogen, has been used, but its effect is variable. Antioestrogen therapy is unlikely to be effective if the breast enlargement has persisted for more than 2 years because the breast tissue will have become organized. Plastic surgery may then be required.

Diseases of multiple endocrine organs

Multiple endocrine neoplasia syndromes

Multiple endocrine neoplasia (MEN) syndromes are autosomal dominant conditions associated with a predisposition to cancers, characteristically in two or more endocrine organs. The affected organs in the two principal forms, MEN types 1 and 2, are shown in Fig. 12.26.

MEN type 1
Disease mechanisms
Carriers of a mutation in the *MEN-1* gene on chromosome 11 will develop characteristic tumours during their lifetime, although manifestations of the disease may differ from one family member to another.

Epidemiology
Prevalence. 2–3 in 100 000.

Age. Variable onset.

Sex. Affects both sexes equally.

Clinical features
Manifestations of disease occur as a result of overproduction of hormones by various tumours, or as a result of tumour growth itself. The tumours are usually benign, but may undergo malignant change at a later age. Clinical features vary and depend on the pattern of organ involvement. They may include hypercalcaemia secondary to hyperparathyroidism, hypoglycaemia resulting from an insulinoma and peptic ulceration because of a gastrinoma.

Investigation
Genetic testing (of family members) allows early detection and reduces morbidity and mortality. Screening tests include serum calcium and parathyroid hormone (± gastrin and prolactin) levels and MRI of the pituitary and pancreas.

Management
This depends on clinical features but may include surgery (e.g. parathyroid, pancreatic) and medical treatment (gastrinoma and prolactinoma).

MEN type 2
Disease mechanisms
This condition is caused by a mutation in the *RET* proto-oncogene.

Epidemiology
Prevalence. 2.5 in 100 000.

Age. Variable onset.

Clinical features
Medullary thyroid carcinoma is the most common tumour in MEN 2 patients and occurs in almost all cases

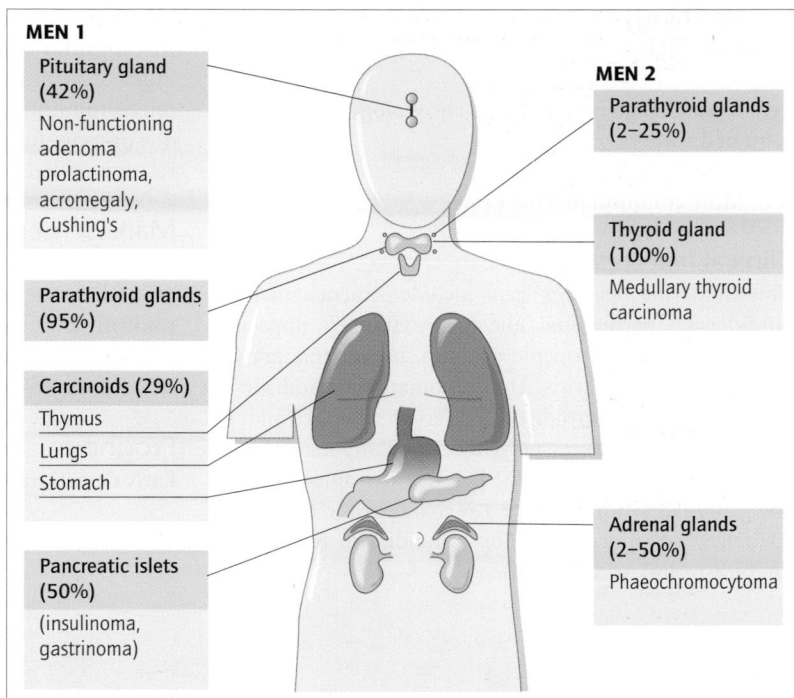

MEN 1

Pituitary gland (42%)
Non-functioning adenoma prolactinoma, acromegaly, Cushing's

Parathyroid glands (95%)

Carcinoids (29%)
Thymus
Lungs
Stomach

Pancreatic islets (50%)
(insulinoma, gastrinoma)

MEN 2

Parathyroid glands (2–25%)

Thyroid gland (100%)
Medullary thyroid carcinoma

Adrenal glands (2–50%)
Phaeochromocytoma

Figure 12.26 Organs affected in patients with multiple endocrine neoplasia (MEN) syndromes.

by 40 years of age. Parafollicular C cells of the thyroid produce calcitonin, but serum calcium levels are normal. MEN 2 may be further subdivided into MEN 2A and MEN 2B. Involvement of the parathyroid glands occurs in MEN 2A, while ganglioneuromas, musculoskeletal abnormalities and eye anomalies are found in MEN 2B. Familial medullary thyroid carcinoma is characterized by medullary thyroid carcinoma as the sole abnormality.

Investigation
Early genetic screening of family members for *RET* gene mutations to detect carriers before the onset of disease symptoms is indicated. Biochemical screening includes serum levels of calcitonin, calcium and parathyroid hormone, and urinary catecholamines.

Management
Prophylactic thyroidectomy in carriers, performed under the age of 6 years, eliminates the risk of medullary thyroid carcinoma. Surgical removal of the adrenal gland(s) is performed for phaeochromocytoma.

Autoimmune polyglandular syndromes
Disease mechanisms
These disorders represent defects in cell- and antibody-mediated immunity. Antibodies against normal cell com-

ponents usually serve as nothing more than markers of the immunological disorder. There is characteristically a lymphocytic infiltrate followed by fibrosis of the organs concerned. Around 20% of cases are familial. There are disease associations with HLA-B8, HLA-DR3 and HLA-DR4. The features of the two key syndromes are listed in Table 12.12.

Table 12.12 Features of autoimmune polyendocrinopathy syndromes (APS)

APS 1	
Hypoparathyroidism	90%
Candidiasis	70%
Addison's disease	60%
Gonadal failure	40%
Hypothyroidism	10%
Other glands: pituitary, pancreatic islets	1%
Other organs: malabsorption, alopecia, B$_{12}$ deficiency, chronic active hepatitis, vitiligo	25%
APS 2	
Addison's disease	95%
Hypothyroidism	70%
Type I diabetes mellitus	50%
Gonadal failure	20%
Other organs: B$_{12}$ deficiency, myasthenia gravis, rheumatoid arthritis, vitiligo	5%

12

Epidemiology

Prevalence. Rare.

Age. Variable age of onset and chronology of development of disorders.

Sex. More common in females.

Clinical features

Non-endocrine features can include mucocutaneous candidiasis, pernicious anaemia, vitiligo, alopecia, immune thrombocytopenic purpura, myasthenia gravis and rheumatoid arthritis. The combination of Addison's disease and hypothyroidism is referred to as Schmidt's syndrome. Autoimmune polyendocrinopathy–candidiasis–ectodermal dystrophy (APECED) or autoimmune polyglandular syndrome type 1 is characterized by a high incidence of mucocutaneous candidiasis, hypoparathyroidism and Addison's disease.

Investigation

Investigation depends on the organs involved. A high index of suspicion is needed with regard to patients with one autoimmune disease, as 5–10% have or will develop one or more further disorders. Autoantibody screening is recommended.

Management

The specific treatment of thyroid disease, Addison's disease, diabetes mellitus, gonadal failure, hypoparathyroidism and hypopituitarism are covered elsewhere. Lifelong follow-up for the detection of new components of the disease is required.

Prognosis

Early detection of new components improves prognosis.

! Must know checklist

- How to manage patients on steroid replacement therapy
- How to diagnose steroid deficiency and interpret short Synacthen tests
- How to interpret thyroid function tests
- How to diagnose and manage an Addisonian crisis
- How to diagnose and manage a hyperthyroid crisis

- How to diagnose and manage myxoedema coma
- Endocrine causes of hypertension
- Endocrine causes of impaired glucose tolerance
- Diagnosis of diabetes insipidus
- Diagnosis of SIADH

Further reading

Books

de Groot L, Jamesson JL, eds. *Endocrinology*. London: Saunders, 2000.

Laycock JF, Wise PH, eds. *Essential Endocrinology*. Oxford: Oxford University Press, 1996.

Levy A, Lightman SL, eds. *Endocrinology*. Oxford: Oxford University Press, 1996.

Nussey SS, Whitehead SA, eds. *Endocrinology: an Integrated Approach*. Oxford: BIOS Scientific, 2001.

Turner H, Wass J, eds. *Oxford Handbook of Endocrinology and Diabetes*. Oxford: Oxford University Press, 2002.

Journals

Clinical Endocrinology, Blackwell Publishing.

Journal of Clinical Endocrinology and Metabolism, Endocrine Society. http://jcem.endojournals.org/

Endocrine Reviews, Endocrine Society. http://edrv.endojournals.org/

Websites

The Society for Endocrinology (UK): http://www.endocrinology.org/

The Endocrine Society (USA): http://www.endo-society.org

Neurological Disease

Introduction

Neurological problems

About 5 million people will have a stroke in the coming year. Other common neurological disorders, such as migraine, epilepsy, dementia, head injury and the neurological complications of acquired immune deficiency syndrome (AIDS), affect many tens of millions of patients throughout the world. About 20% of emergency admissions to medical units are related to acute neurological problems. Some of these disorders are life-threatening, and all of them require informed expert attention. Neurological diseases therefore place substantial demands on health care services.

Changing patterns of disease

The epidemiology of common neurological diseases is changing. The incidence of stroke is declining in the Western world but increasing in other regions such as eastern Europe. Infectious disease of the nervous system such as leprosy and meningitis remains a significant problem worldwide, while other infections, particularly those associated with AIDS, are becoming more common. New conditions such as variant Creutzfeldt–Jakob disease have created new medical challenges and have illuminated society's expectations of doctors.

New developments in treatment

There are now effective agents for the treatment of acute stroke and for its prevention. New therapeutic agents are also available for the treatment of epilepsy, migraine and infections of the nervous system. Therapeutic claims are also made for novel drugs for multiple sclerosis, Alzheimer's disease and motor neurone disease. It remains to be seen whether these will have a role in the standard management of these conditions. However, their advent means that doctors must add a further skill to the mix—the robust critical appraisal of trial data, which may be biased through too close involvement of the pharmaceutical industry in trial design and data analysis.

While there may yet be no disease-modifying treatments for many neurological conditions (e.g. Parkinson's disease, muscular dystrophy, Huntington's disease), symptomatic treatments can make a significant impact. Active focused neurological rehabilitation can achieve a great deal to restore a patient's dignity, independence and quality of life. Furthermore, the identification of gene defects responsible for many neurological conditions will allow prenatal testing in affected families and—if this is what those family members want—prevention of distress and suffering through early termination of affected embryos.

Understanding the causes

Advances in imaging, neurophysiology, molecular biology and pharmacology are rapidly increasing our understanding of the causes and pathophysiology of many neurological problems. This is already leading to faster and more accurate diagnosis and rational drug design, and these benefits are likely to become much more apparent in the coming years.

Social and economic factors and neurological disease

Many neurological conditions, including migraine and epilepsy, affect adults of working age and impact on their economic status; such conditions may have a profound impact on the economic circumstances of individuals. The reverse is also true; social factors such as unemployment and poverty impact not only on the incidence of neurological conditions such as epilepsy and stroke but also on its severity and on the way it is managed by health care systems. The management of patients with neurological diseases therefore requires an awareness of the impact of social factors on disease.

Diagnosis of neurological disorders

The nervous system is the most functionally complex of all the organ systems. Neurological disorders can therefore produce a wide range of symptoms and signs. With some basic knowledge of anatomy and pathology, it is often possible to work out the most complicated clinical problems through careful history-taking and logical thought.

Structure and function

Central nervous system

The central nervous system (CNS) consists of the cerebral hemispheres, the basal ganglia, the thalamus and the hypothalamus, the cerebellum and the brainstem (comprising the midbrain, pons and medulla; Fig. 13.1). The cortical mantle of grey matter deals with conscious thought and cognitive functions. The motor cortex integrates commands from other parts of the cortex, and turns thought into movement by a complex interaction between the pyramidal system, the extrapyramidal system and the cerebellum. In the presence of an intact cortical mantle, the brainstem controls arousal and the level of consciousness. The medulla controls the most primitive functions of respiration and regulation of autonomic functions.

Cranial nerves

The cranial nerves control eye movement (III, IV, VI), the facial, neck and bulbar musculature (V, VII, IX–XII), contain fibres of the autonomic nervous system (III, VII, X) and convey efferent sensory information to the brain (I, II, V, VII–X).

Spinal cord

The spinal cord carries information between the brain

and the periphery and has sophisticated information-processing functions subserving both motor control and integration of incoming sensory information.

Plexuses and roots

Motor (ventral) and sensory (dorsal) roots leave the spinal cord and combine to form spinal nerves; these may then exchange fibres in the brachial (arm) or lumbar (leg) plexus.

Peripheral nervous system

The peripheral motor nerves carry information to the muscles. Depolarization releases acetylcholine, which interacts with the nicotinic acetylcholine receptor to induce muscle contraction. Sensory nerves from skin, muscle and other structures relay information back to the spinal cord.

Autonomic nervous system

The sympathetic (adrenergic) and parasympathetic (muscarinic) systems regulate the action of the heart, lungs and gastrointestinal tract, and control emptying of the bowels and bladder.

Approach to the patient

The nervous system may appear complex, but the principles of diagnosis and management of neurological problems are straightforward (HISTORY & EXAMINATION BOX 13.1).

History & Examination 13.1: Purpose of clinical assessment

To identify the symptoms and what their impact is
To identify the site(s) of the lesion(s)
To establish the likely pathology of the lesion(s)
To plan appropriate investigations
To initiate appropriate treatment(s)
To avoid unnecessary investigations and treatments
To gauge the patient's understanding of his or her symptoms
To understand the patient's expectations

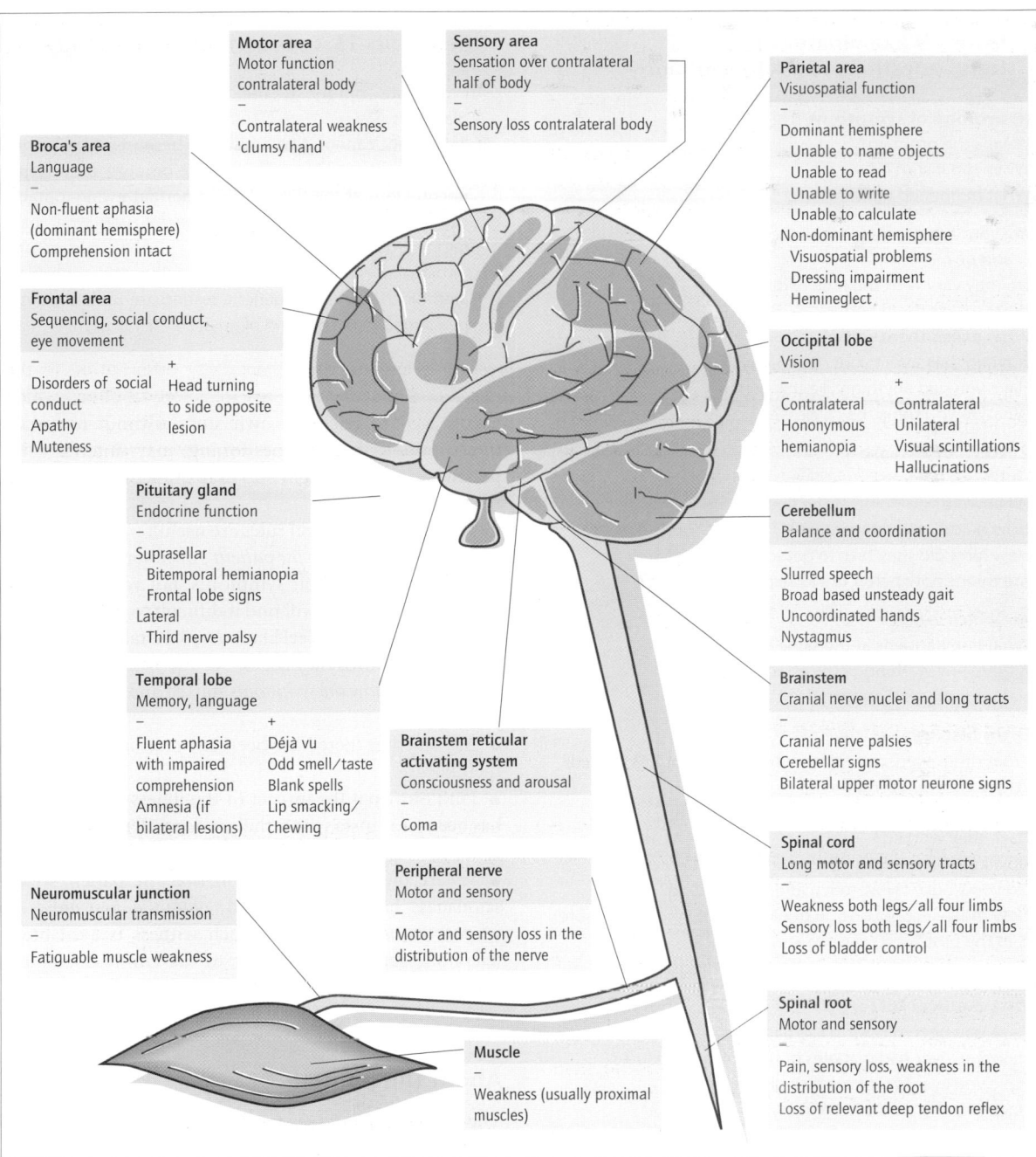

Motor area
Motor function
contralateral body

–

Contralateral weakness
'clumsy hand'

Sensory area
Sensation over contralateral
half of body

–

Sensory loss contralateral body

Parietal area
Visuospatial function

–

Dominant hemisphere
  Unable to name objects
  Unable to read
  Unable to write
  Unable to calculate
Non-dominant hemisphere
  Visuospatial problems
  Dressing impairment
  Hemineglect

Broca's area
Language

–

Non-fluent aphasia
(dominant hemisphere)
Comprehension intact

Frontal area
Sequencing, social conduct,
eye movement

–   +

Disorders of social   Head turning
conduct   to side opposite
Apathy   lesion
Muteness

Occipital lobe
Vision

–   +

Contralateral   Contralateral
Hononymous   Unilateral
hemianopia   Visual scintillations
                   Hallucinations

Pituitary gland
Endocrine function

–

Suprasellar
  Bitemporal hemianopia
  Frontal lobe signs
Lateral
  Third nerve palsy

Cerebellum
Balance and coordination

–

Slurred speech
Broad based unsteady gait
Uncoordinated hands
Nystagmus

Temporal lobe
Memory, language

–   +

Fluent aphasia   Déjà vu
with impaired   Odd smell/taste
comprehension   Blank spells
Amnesia (if   Lip smacking/
bilateral lesions) chewing

**Brainstem reticular
activating system**
Consciousness and arousal

–

Coma

Brainstem
Cranial nerve nuclei and long tracts

–

Cranial nerve palsies
Cerebellar signs
Bilateral upper motor neurone signs

Peripheral nerve
Motor and sensory

–

Motor and sensory loss in the
distribution of the nerve

Spinal cord
Long motor and sensory tracts

–

Weakness both legs/all four limbs
Sensory loss both legs/all four limbs
Loss of bladder control

Neuromuscular junction
Neuromuscular transmission

–

Fatiguable muscle weakness

Muscle

–

Weakness (usually proximal
muscles)

Spinal root
Motor and sensory

Pain, sensory loss, weakness in the
distribution of the root
Loss of relevant deep tendon reflex

Figure 13.1 Structure and function of the nervous system. Symptoms and signs of lesions in different sites in the nervous system. A – sign indicates a loss of function (e.g. weakness), a + sign indicates positive phenomena (e.g. focal seizures).

The four basic questions to answer are:
1 Are the symptoms coming from the nervous system?
2 If so, which part(s) of the nervous system is affected?
3 Is the problem localized to one part of the nervous system or is it generalized?
4 Is there one lesion or are there multiple lesions?

History and examination

The history is the bedrock of diagnosis in neurology. Meaningful examination and effective investigation can only occur on the foundation of a well-executed history. For many common neurological problems (e.g. headaches,

History & Examination 13.2: Useful questions to ask in neurology

Neurological symptoms

What's the problem?
When did it start?
What happened next?

Are your symptoms there all the time, or do they come and go?
Do they vary with the time of day?
What makes them better?
What makes them worse?
How do they affect your day-to-day life?
Have you had anything like this before?
What do you think the cause is?

Pattern of disease

Onset and progression
What were you doing at the time?
How quickly did things start ?
How long did they take to get to their worst?
Are things now better or worse or just the same?

Associated features
What else happens at the same time?
Is there any warning of the attacks?
Has your physical appearance changed?

Drug history

What drugs were you taking when the symptoms started?
Why were you taking them?
What drugs have you taken for the symptoms?
Have they worked?
How long were you on them, and at what dose?
Do you smoke? How much and for how long?
How much alcohol do you drink now? Did you drink more in the past?
Do you take any other non-prescribed drugs?

Past medical history

Have you been unwell in the past?
Have you ever had diabetes or high blood pressure?
Have you ever had fits or convulsions?
Have you ever had a head injury?
Have you ever had meningitis?

Family history

Does anyone else in your family have a similar problem?
Do any other conditions run in the family?

Keypoints 13.1: Diagnosis in neurology

An accurate history is the bedrock of neurological diagnosis
If the patient cannot give a history—because of language problems, cognitive difficulties or because they were unconscious at the time of an important event—obtain a history from someone who can tell you what has happened
Neurological examination, neuroimaging and sophisticated biochemical and genetic testing are useless unless performed in the context of an accurate history

encouraged to tell their own story without too many interruptions. Direct questioning may interrupt the patient's train of thought and may draw them away from the central problem.

The following general rules are useful:

- *Record the history in the patient's own words.* The history is their account of their symptoms, not your interpretation of it. Often, they will find it difficult to put into words what their symptoms feel like, so try to establish what they mean by the words they use.
- Ask about *how the symptoms* started and how they have developed.
- Ask whether there have been any *previous episodes* and their nature.
- Find out what the impact of the illness on the patient has been—for instance on their independence in *activities of daily living* (Table 13.1)
- Where there is any question that the patient's consciousness has been impaired, *obtain a first-hand eye witness account.* Where no such witness is available, a telephone call to a relative or to the family doctor can provide high-quality diagnostic information.

About the patient

The patient's age and sex can help decide which diagnoses are likely:

- *Cerebrovascular disease:* rare in those under 40 years old.
- *Symptoms of multiple sclerosis (MS):* usually start between the ages of 20 and 35 years. MS is extremely rare in childhood, and development of MS in those over 60 is unusual. It is twice as common in women as in men, and is rare in non-white populations.
- *Some genetic diseases* (e.g. Duchenne muscular dystrophy) are sex-linked and may only affect or be much more severe in males.

dizzy spells and blackouts), the examination contributes little to diagnosis, which is based almost completely on the history and investigations (HISTORY & EXAMINATION BOX 13.2; KEYPOINTS BOX 13.1). The patient should be

Table 13.1 Activities of daily living (Barthel Index). Maximum score = 20. The Barthel Index provides a systematic assessment of the impact of neurological disease on performance in activities of daily living, and can also be used to measure progress during rehabilitation

Activity	Score
Feeding (including cutting food)	
Independent	2
Needs help	1
Unable	0
Grooming (face, hair, teeth, shaving)	
Independent	1
Dependent	0
Bowels	
Fully continent	2
Occasional accident	1
Incontinent	0
Bladder	
Fully continent	2
Occasional accident	1
Incontinent (or catheterized)	0
Dressing	
Independent	2
Needs help	1
Dependent	0
Chair/bed transfer	
Independent	3
Minimal help	2
Able to sit, major help to transfer	1
Unable, no sitting balance	0
Toilet	
Independent	2
Needs help	1
Unable	0
Mobility	
Independent walking	3
Minimal help to walk	2
Independent in wheelchair	1
Immobile	0
Stairs	
Independent	2
Needs help	1
Unable	0
Bathing	
Independent	1
Dependent	0

Neurological symptoms

Blackouts: fits or faints or funny turns?

The distinction between epilepsy, which is comparatively rare, and syncope, which is common, can usually be made from the history. Because the patient will have been unconscious for at least some of the attack, corroboration of their history with a first-hand eye witness account is crucial. If the attack was not witnessed, a firm diagnosis may not be possible.

- *Was the patient standing*, *sitting or lying* when the blackout occurred? Simple syncope is unusual in the sitting or lying position.
- *Tongue biting* (especially the side of the tongue) or *urinary incontinence* suggest epilepsy rather than syncope.
- *Speed of recovery:* was the patient fully alert and orientated immediately after the attack (syncope) or were they confused, tired and 'headachy' for several hours (epilepsy)?

Headaches

Headaches are one of the most common reasons for referral to a neurologist. In spite of the fears of many of these patients, brain tumours are only very rarely the cause of such headaches. Headache that has lasted for years is always benign. Headache over weeks or months does sometimes have a serious cause, especially when it is progressive and when there are other symptoms. The character, location and associated symptoms may suggest the diagnosis:

- A 'tight band' around the head suggests tension headache
- Persistent headache with scalp tenderness in a person over 50 years old suggests temporal arteritis
- A unilateral headache with visual disturbance, nausea and photophobia suggests migraine
- A severe sudden onset headache with neck stiffness, photophobia and vomiting suggests subarachnoid haemorrhage
- Generalized headache with neck stiffness, photophobia and vomiting suggests meningitis
- A headache which is worse in the mornings, exacerbated by coughing or sneezing and relieved by being upright suggests raised intracranial pressure

Problems with memory and concentration

Loss of concentration and poor memory is a common complaint. A significant cause is more likely if there is:

- Selective loss of memory for recent events (Alzheimer's disease)
- Memory loss of recent onset with personality change (frontal tumour)
- Disturbed sleep, anhedonia and low mood (pseudo-dementia resulting from depression)

13

Difficulty with language, speech and swallowing

Difficulty in articulating speech that is normal in content (**dysarthria**) must be distinguished from difficulties in language processing (**dysphasia**). Such difficulties may affect the generation of language (**expressive dysphasia**), the understanding of spoken words (**receptive dysphasia**), or both in combination. Weakness of respiratory muscles may lead to inadequate air flow over an otherwise normal larynx (**dysphonia**).

Difficulty in swallowing (**dysphagia**) may be associated with a loss of feeling on the palate and a change in vocal quality when it is a result of disease of the lower cranial nerves. Dysarthria or dysphagia that increase with prolonged effort may be caused by myasthenia gravis. Dysphagia with nasal regurgitation of fluids may be caused by motor neurone disease.

Loss of smell

Loss of smell is a common symptom usually caused by problems such as polyps in the nasal cavity. Neurological causes of anosmia are uncommon and it seldom features in neurological histories, except when it follows head trauma, when it may be caused by shearing of the olfactory nerves as they pass through the cribriform plate into the skull.

Blindness, blurred and double vision

Transient monocular visual loss of sudden onset (**amaurosis fugax**) is usually caused by microemboli, from either the carotid bifurcation or the heart, occluding the retinal blood supply. Patients may describe a grey curtain which descends over their vision for seconds to minutes before rising again. Similar symptoms can be caused by temporal arteritis, where complete and irreversible loss of vision can occur if steroid treatment is not started urgently, and in idiopathic intracranial hypertension. Ocular causes of transient visual loss include acute glaucoma and retinal detachment.

Persisting monocular visual loss of sudden onset is usually vascular in origin, resulting from disease of the central retinal artery or temporal arteritis. When the onset is gradual and no cause is immediately apparent then optic nerve compression (e.g. tumour, ophthalmic artery aneurysm) must be assumed until proven otherwise. Other causes of gradual onset monocular blindness include optic neuritis, vascular disease affecting the optic nerve (e.g. anterior ischaemic optic neuropathy, temporal arteritis) and granulomatous diseases (e.g. sarcoidosis).

Simultaneous complete bilateral visual loss is uncommon; where it does occur it is usually caused by posterior circulation vascular events. With partial bilateral visual loss, the patient may use phrases like 'blind in one eye' to describe being blind to one side because of a homonymous hemianopia.

Blurred vision that is not improved by glasses warrants referral; it may be caused by systemic disorders such as diabetes; ophthalmic disorders such as glaucoma; or neurological disorders such as migraine, optic neuritis or ophthalmoplegia.

Double vision (**diplopia**) is also important and may result from lesions of the IIIrd, IVth or VIth cranial nerves, the midbrain or the pons. Alternatively, local pathology in the orbit may interfere with the function of the extraocular muscles. Diplopia is generally abolished by covering one eye; rarely, diplopia persists when one eye is closed (monocular diplopia) and this may be a result of abnormalities of the cornea, iris, lens or retina. Diplopia may also be caused by myaesthenia gravis, when it is often worse at the end of the day.

Difficulty with hearing/tinnitus

Some loss of hearing is part of normal ageing (**senile presbyacusis**).

Progressive unilateral hearing loss may indicate a lesion of the vestibulocochlear (VIIIth) cranial nerve, and acoustic neuromas often present in this way.

Hearing loss with facial weakness and double vision suggest a space-occupying lesion in the cerebellopontine angle, with involvement of the Vth, VIIth and VIIIth cranial nerves.

Ringing in the ear (**tinnitus**), deafness and paroxysms of disabling vertigo suggests Ménière's disease.

Dizziness and vertigo

Dizziness is one of the most common neurological symptoms. It is essential to differentiate vertigo (a hallucination of movement) from the less specific light-headed 'swimmy' feeling that many patients experience. Patients often find it difficult to make this distinction.

- *Vertigo:* usually caused by disease of the inner ear or brainstem, and may be associated with nausea or vomiting.
- *Light-headedness or giddiness:* a feature of many conditions including postural hypotension, anaemia, anxiety, depression and hyperventilation and commonly has no medical explanation.

Problems with balance

Patients may report 'poor balance' or 'walking as if drunk' or 'dizziness' as a result of disease of the inner ear, the vestibulocochlear (VIIIth) nerve, the brainstem, the cerebellum and its connections and of proprioception. Occasionally, double vision may present as problems with balance.

Difficulties moving the arms or legs

Weakness

Weakness in a limb can be caused by a lesion at any point in the motor pathways from the cerebral cortex to the affected muscle. A weak hand may result from a focal lesion of the contralateral cerebral hemisphere, a nerve root entrapment in the cervical spine, a lesion in the peripheral nerve that supplies the hand or a problem in the muscle itself. A careful history and examination will usually indicate the correct diagnosis.

The same principle applies to weakness in the legs. If just one leg is weak, the problem may be at the level of the peripheral nerve, nerve roots, spinal cord or the contra-lateral cerebral hemisphere. Weakness of both legs may be a result of a lesion in the spinal cord or, less commonly, a symmetrical peripheral neuropathy.

Weakness of proximal muscles is usually caused by muscle disease (e.g. polymyositis or a metabolic myo-pathy as seen in Cushing's syndrome). Patients have difficulty raising their arms (cannot brush their hair) or legs (difficulty with stairs or getting out of low chairs), or problems with truncal muscles (cannot sit up or turn over in bed). People who feel 'tired all the time' are generally suffering from depression, anxiety or stress and probably do not have a neurological disorder. How-ever, patients who develop weakness, diplopia or ptosis that gets worse after exertion or at the end of the day may have a disorder of the neuromuscular junction such as myasthenia gravis.

Clumsiness

The loss of fine control of movements is a non-specific symptom. It may indicate cerebellar disease, loss of sensa-tion in the affected part or a lesion in the cerebral hemi-spheres. Some people with Parkinson's disease report clumsiness in the early stage of their illness.

Difficulty walking

People with dizziness, poor balance, visual disturbance, leg weakness, cerebrovascular disease, muscle disease or extrapyramidal disease may all present with 'difficulty walking'. The pattern of these associated neurological symptoms should help determine the cause of the difficulty. A host of other non-neurological problems (e.g. arthritis) can cause difficulty with walking.

Sensory problems

Sensory loss (numbness)

Loss of sensation in a limb is usually caused by a lesion of a peripheral nerve or nerve root. However, spinal cord disease and lesions in the sensory cerebral cortex can also lead to numbness. The transient neurological dis-turbances that characterize brief episodes of focal cerebral ischaemia (transient ischaemic attacks; TIAs) are usually negative (loss of power and loss of sensation).

Positive sensory symptoms (paraesthesiae, tingling)

Everyone has experienced 'pins and needles' in the legs after prolonged pressure over a peripheral nerve. Positive sensory symptoms can be caused by local damage to peripheral nerves or roots. Paraesthesiae that start in one limb and spread up on to the face over a few minutes are most commonly caused by migraine, although occasion-ally focal seizures can be responsible. The symptom of 'water running over the skin' suggests a lesion in the spinothalamic tract.

Sphincter problems

Patients find sphincter problems particularly distressing. There may be complete loss of bladder and/or bowel control (incontinence), or a sudden inability to pass urine or faeces (retention or constipation). Both may be symp-toms of serious disease in the spinal cord (e.g. extrinsic or intrinsic tumour compressing the cord, central disc prolapse or ischaemia of the cord). Incontinence of urine may occur during a generalized seizure.

Other sphincter problems such as difficulty starting to pass urine (hesitancy), a sudden urge to pass urine (urgency) or socially inappropriate urination (e.g. into flowerpots) may indicate a lesion in the lumbar plexus, spinal cord or frontal lobe, respectively. Bear in mind that there are many non-neurological causes for sphincter dysfunction (e.g. benign prostatic hypertrophy as a cause for urinary retention).

Sexual problems

Many neurological conditions and drugs used in neurology impact on patients' physical and psychological capacity to enjoy sex. Sexual problems may also provide diagnostic clues (e.g. erectile failure in multisystem atrophy).

Pattern of disease

Time course

Because different pathological processes evolve over different timescales, the pace of the illness provides important diagnostic information. The most important questions are 'What happened?' and 'What happened next?' Where symptoms have developed suddenly the patient will be able to relate exactly what they were doing at the time; where the onset has been slower, their answers may be vaguer.

The time course of a patient's symptoms may give significant clues to the underlying disease process:

● *Abrupt onset of symptoms:* suggests a vascular cause (stroke or subarachnoid haemorrhage)

13

● *Relapsing–remitting pattern:* strongly suggests an inflammatory disease such as multiple sclerosis
● *Gradual onset with a relentless progression:* suggests a tumour

Pattern of physical features

There may be a characteristic pattern of physical features:
● A neurological problem affecting different parts of the nervous system at different times is typical of multiple sclerosis
● Episodic headaches with stereotyped visual symptoms and nausea are characteristic of migraine
● Fatiguable limb muscle weakness and difficulty speaking and swallowing that deteriorates as the day goes on is typical of myasthenia gravis
● Slowing down generally with loss of facial expression, slowness of gait, tremor and loss of dexterity is typical of Parkinson's disease

Associated symptoms

Non-neurological symptoms may be relevant in formulating a diagnosis:
● When dealing with dizziness or blackouts ask about cardiovascular symptoms; arrhythmias and reduced cardiac output can cause neurological symptoms
● Recent skin rash, joint pain or gastrointestinal disorders may illuminate the cause of neurological symptoms (e.g. a facial rash in systemic lupus erythematosus; SLE)
● Poor general health and weight loss may be caused by covert malignant disease or by other systemic disorders
● Sleeping patterns may change because of early morning headache or a depressive illness
● Ask whether relatives and friends have commented on any recent change, and whether relatives have noticed the patient's presenting symptoms

Disease impact

Effect on activities of daily living

Neurological diseases are significant because of their impact on the lives of individual patients, and treatment goals should reflect this. It is therefore helpful to chart the progression of a neurological disorder in terms of its effects on the patient's ability to perform activities of daily living using measures such as the Barthel Index (Table 13.1). This 20-point scale may also identify problems not mentioned in the history and can be used to monitor progress.

The clinician should also assess the impact of the disease on the patient in terms of **disability** and **handicap**. **Disability** is what the patient is unable to do. **Handicap** is the impact of that disability on the context of that patient,

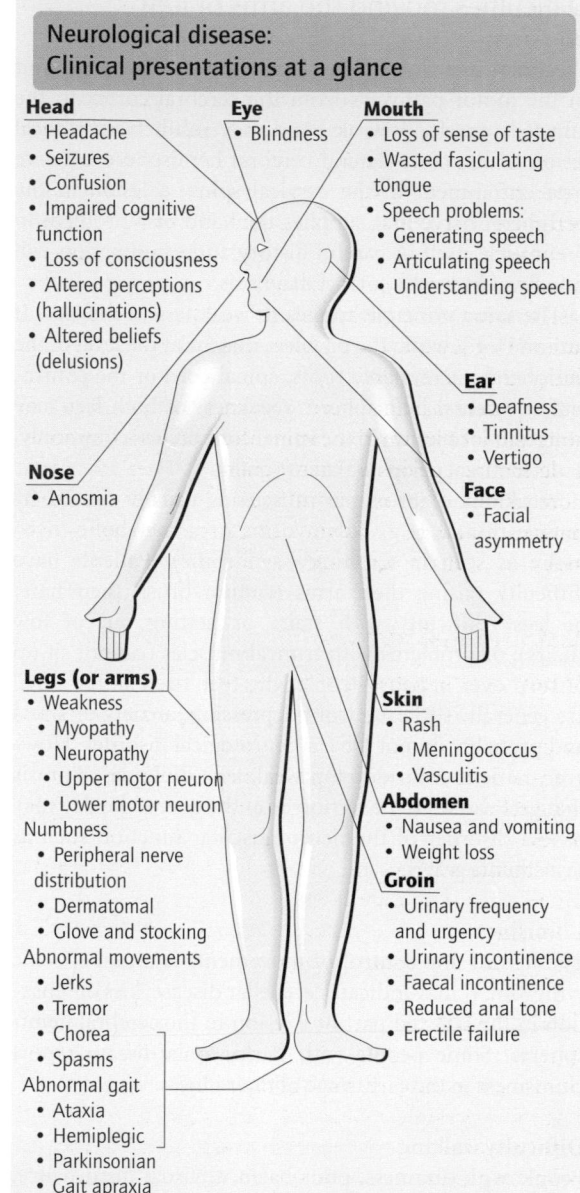

Neurological disease: Clinical presentations at a glance

Head
• Headache
• Seizures
• Confusion
• Impaired cognitive function
• Loss of consciousness
• Altered perceptions (hallucinations)
• Altered beliefs (delusions)

Eye
• Blindness

Mouth
• Loss of sense of taste
• Wasted fasiculating tongue
• Speech problems:
  • Generating speech
  • Articulating speech
  • Understanding speech

Ear
• Deafness
• Tinnitus
• Vertigo

Nose
• Anosmia

Face
• Facial asymmetry

Legs (or arms)
• Weakness
  • Myopathy
  • Neuropathy
  • Upper motor neuron
  • Lower motor neuron
Numbness
  • Peripheral nerve distribution
  • Dermatomal
  • Glove and stocking
Abnormal movements
  • Jerks
  • Tremor
  • Chorea
  • Spasms
Abnormal gait
  • Ataxia
  • Hemiplegic
  • Parkinsonian
  • Gait apraxia

Skin
• Rash
  • Meningococcus
  • Vasculitis

Abdomen
• Nausea and vomiting
• Weight loss

Groin
• Urinary frequency and urgency
• Urinary incontinence
• Faecal incontinence
• Reduced anal tone
• Erectile failure

taking into account its impact on their social role and their occupation. The handicap for a portrait painter rendered blind by optic neuritis is much more than that for a bank teller with the same optic neuritis and the same disability.

Drug history

Many drugs affect the nervous system and so a detailed drug history is essential, especially where there is an altered conscious level. Many neurological problems can be caused by the side-effects of common drugs taken for minor ailments. Movement disorders may be caused by a range of drugs, particularly phenothiazines.

For a patient with a spontaneous intracerebral haemorrhage, a history of oral anticoagulant use not only identifies the cause (iatrogenic bleeding disorder) but also the treatment (reversal of the clotting defect with clotting factor infusion). Stroke in a young patient may be caused by the use of 'recreational' drugs such as cocaine or ecstasy.

For patients with poorly controlled epilepsy, it is vital to know which antiepileptic drugs have been taken in the past, in what dosage with what benefit, and whether the patient has actually been taking their tablets, before any change is contemplated.

If a patient has Parkinson's disease that is difficult to control, it is often worth charting the medication regimen to determine periods of most benefit and periods where more treatment is required. It is also important to check that patients are not inadvertently taking other drugs (e.g. antiemetics) that might make their symptoms worse.

Past medical history

Previous neurological episodes
If a patient has had previous neurological symptoms, attempt to:
- Record the date of onset of each new symptom
- Establish whether the symptoms recover completely or not
- Establish whether the symptoms in the past are the same as the present symptoms
- Find out how the symptoms were interpreted and what investigations were carried out

Other history
Document previous illnesses to determine whether they may have a bearing on this illness:
- Is there previous malignant disease that may have led to metastatic disease or a non-metastatic manifestation of malignancy (paraneoplastic syndrome)?
- Could past symptoms be caused by multisystem disease now involving the nervous system (e.g. SLE, sarcoidosis)?
- Is there previous infective disease, perhaps inadequately treated, now involving the nervous system (e.g. syphilis, tuberculosis, human immunodeficiency virus; HIV)?

Family history

Huntington's disease, Wilson's disease and some forms of muscular dystrophy are single gene disorders showing mendelian inheritance, and a polygenic component is recognized in narcolepsy, multiple sclerosis, stroke and Alzheimer's disease.

Establish the health, age at death and cause of death of all first-degree relatives. Early death of family members may mask a family history. If inherited disease is suspected, a more complete family history is needed with information about grandparents, aunts and uncles. Ask the patient to bring such information on the next visit, or if necessary ask their permission to telephone other family members for full details. Remember that the non-paternity rate in the UK is estimated at approximately 10%.

Neurological examination

The purpose of neurological examination is not to document the status of every facet of neurological function, but rather to test specific hypotheses generated from the history. The correct neurological examination will focus on different parts in different patients, but whichever part is involved the doctor must be able to examine it.

Patients should be examined in a warm well-lit room, in their underwear only. It is not possible to see fasciculation through trousers or test sensation through woolly tights. Every neurological examination should begin with a brief examination of other systems, with particular reference to the state of the vasculature (peripheral and neck pulses and bruits, blood pressure and auscultation of the heart) and of the skin (rashes; ulceration; hair loss).

Conscious level, alertness and cognitive function

The Glasgow Coma Scale (Table 13.2) is used to assess the level of consciousness. The Mini Mental State Exam (HISTORY & EXAMINATION BOX 13.3) tests aspects of 'higher cerebral function' namely orientation, registration, attention, calculation and recall, and language and visuospatial abilities. Isolated problems with specific cortical functions may help localize lesions:
- *Aphasia:* indicates a focal lesion of the dominant hemisphere
- *Visuospatial dysfunction:* indicates a lesion of the non-dominant parietal lobe
- *Amnesia:* usually caused by bilateral temporal lobe lesions

Cranial nerves

A summary of cranial nerve examination is given in HISTORY & EXAMINATION BOX 13.4. The detailed approach to examination of the cranial nerves is given in HISTORY & EXAMINATION BOX 13.5. Causes of cranial neuropathies are discussed in Table 13.35 and on p. 944.

Strength of stimulation	Points
Eye-opening	
Eyes open spontaneously	4
Eyes open to verbal stimulation	3
Eyes open to painful stimulation	2
No eye opening	1
Best verbal response	
Orientated: knows place (hospital) and time (day, month, year)	5
Confused: taking in sentences but disorientated in time and place	4
Inappropriate words: uttering occasional words rather than sentences	3
Incomprehensible sounds: groans or grunts, but no words	2
None	1
Endotracheal tube/tracheostomy	T
Best motor response	
Obeys commands: responds to a simple command such as 'lift your arm'	6
Localizing to pain: responds to painful stimulation of the supraorbital nerve by bringing the hand up beyond the chin	5
Normal flexion to pain: responds to pressure with the shaft of a pen to the fingernail with semipurposeful elbow flexion	4
Abnormal flexion to pain: responds to pressure with the shaft of a pen to the fingernail with movements that do not look like semipurposeful flexion but are not frankly extensor	3
Extending to pain: painful stimulation causes elbow extension and wrist flexion	2
No response to pain	1
Maximum score	*15*

Table 13.2 The Glasgow Coma Scale (GCS). Vague descriptions such as 'stuporose', 'obtunded' and 'comatose' are used differently by different observers and are insensitive to change. The GCS is a not systematic reproducible measure of conscious level comprised of three components: eye opening, best verbal response and best motor response. These components should be reported individually (e.g. GCS 15 (E4V5M6)). In patients with dysphasia, the GCS may be falsely low. Before recording that a patient is unresponsive, ensure that the stimulus is strong enough, that the verbal commands are loud enough and that painful stimuli are strong enough. Record the best response

---

History & Examination 13.3: The Mini Mental State examination of cognitive function

This provides a systematic measure of several cortical functions, weighted towards language function.

1 Orientation
Score 1 point for a correct answer to each of the following questions

Orientation in time

What time is it now?	(1) point
What date is it today?	(1) point
What day is it today?	(1) point
What month is it now?	(1) point
What is the year?	(1) point

Orientation in place

What is the name of this ward?	(1) point
What is the name of this hospital?	(1) point
What is the name of this district?	(1) point
What is the name of this town?	(1) point
What is the name of this country?	(1) point

2 Registration
Name three objects. Score 1 point for each object repeated correctly at the first attempt. Repeat until all three repeated correctly so as to test recall later. (3) points

3 Attention and calculation
Ask the patient to subtract 7 from 100 and then 7 from the result. Repeat this five times, scoring 1 point for each time a correct subtraction is performed in five trials. Alternatively, ask the patient to spell WORLD backwards (5) points

4 Recall
Ask for the three objects repeated in the registration test, scoring 1 point for each correctly recalled. (3) points

5 Language
Show the patient two objects (e.g. a pencil and a watch) and ask him or her to name them. Score 1 point for each correct answer. (2) points

Ask the patient to repeat the sentence 'No ifs, ands or buts'. Score 1 point if the repetition is correct. (1) point

Ask the patient to carry out a complex three-stage command, for example 'Take this piece of paper in your right hand, fold it in half and place it on the floor'. Score 1 point for each correct action. (3) points

On a blank piece of paper write 'Close your eyes' and ask the patient to carry out the written request, scoring 1 point for correct action. (1) point

Ask the patient to write a sentence. Score 1 point if the sentence is sensible and has a verb and a subject. (1) point

Draw a pair of intersecting pentagons, each side 2.5 cm long (see below), and score 1 point if the patient copies the drawing correctly. (1) point

Total score **(30) points**
(Normal ≥24)

History & Examinaton 13.4: Summary of cranial nerve examination

Cranial nerve	Examine
I	Smell
II	Visual acuity, visual fields, fundi, pupil reaction
III, IV, VI	Eye movements, nystagmus, oculocephalic reflex, pupil size, pupil reaction, eyelid position
V	Facial sensation, corneal reflex, muscles of mastication
VII	Muscles of facial expression, taste
VIII	Hearing
IX	Sensation on soft palate
X	Palatal movement, voice quality, cough
XI	Head turning, shoulder shrugging
XII	Tongue movement and appearance

Visual field defects (Fig. 13.3)

• *Homonymous hemianopia or quadrantanopia:* indicate a lesion of the optic tract, the optic radiation or the occipital cortex. Temporal lobe lesions of the optic radiation characteristically cause an upper quadrantanopia while lesions in the parietal lobe cause a lower quadrantanopia. Vascular lesions commonly cause hemianopia of sudden onset; more gradual onset may be caused by tumours, abscesses or by other structural lesions.

• *Bitemporal hemianopia:* indicates a lesion at the optic chiasm, typically a large pituitary tumour.

• *Cortical blindness:* results from bilateral occipital lesions and is commonly caused by hypoxia. Because the optic pathways to the superior colliculi are spared, the pupillary reactions to light are normal.

Pupillary and eye movement disorders

Oculomotor (IIIrd) nerve palsy

Painful IIIrd nerve palsy must be investigated urgently because posterior communicating artery aneurysms and temporal arteritis need immediate treatment. The IIIrd nerve can be compressed as intracranial pressure rises. A drowsy patient with a IIIrd nerve palsy may have critically raised intracranial pressure and be on the point of developing fatal herniation of the medial edge of the temporal lobe through the tentorial hiatus.

Complete ophthalmoplegia

If all eye movements in one eye are lost, consider lesions around the apex of the orbit and cavernous sinus (aneurysm, tumour, cavernous sinus thrombosis, granulomatous

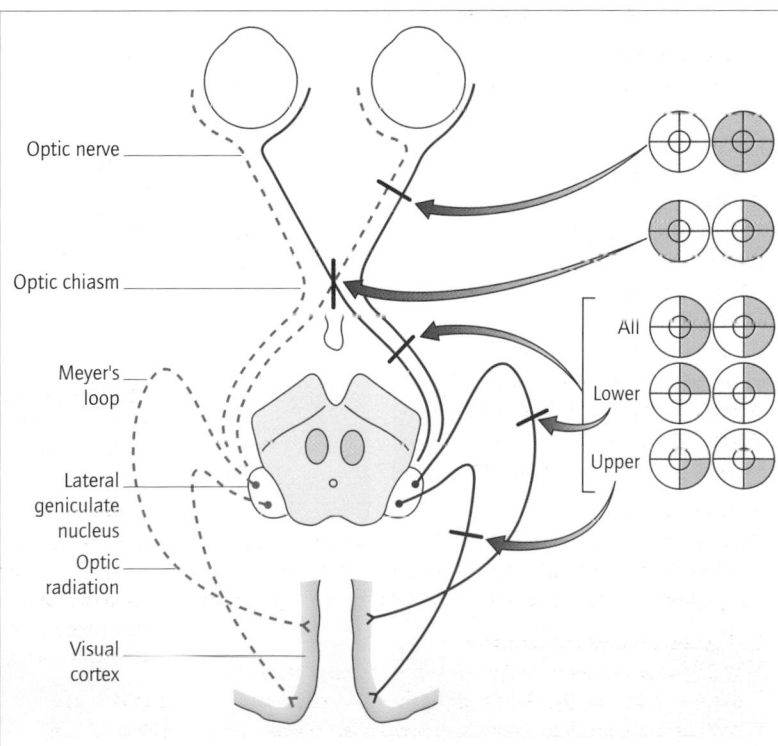

Figure 13.3 Sites of lesions causing different visual field defects.

History & Examinaton 13.5: Cranial nerve examination

Causes of abnormalities of the cranial nerves are given in Table 13.35.

I Olfactory nerve

To test the sense of smell, occlude nostrils in turn and test the ability to smell a non-irritant substance such as coffee or orange zest.

II Optic nerve

Measure corrected **visual acuity** at 6 m using a Snellen reading chart, with any distance glasses on.

- For each eye, record the small number next to the lowest line read as the denominator with the distance to the chart as the numerator.
- If the patient can read the line numbered 24 the acuity is 6/24.
- If no letters can be read, note whether the patient can count fingers, appreciate hand movements or perceive only light and dark.

Examine the **visual fields** by asking the patient to look at the bridge of your nose.

- Place your hands at 10 o'clock and 2 o'clock and ask the patient to indicate the moving finger as each finger is moved in turn and then as they are moved simultaneously.
- Repeat with hands at 8 o'clock and 4 o'clock.
- If the patient only sees movement to one side they have a hemianopia; if they see movements to both sides except when the movements are simultaneous they have visual inattention.
- If the visual loss appears asymmetric, test the eyes separately by confrontation. Each cover one eye and look to the other's uncovered eye; bring a red pin slowly in from the periphery and map the visual field of the patient against your own.

Examine the **optic disc** using an ophthalmoscope; follow the retinal vessels to the optic disc.

- **Papilloedema** (Fig. 13.2) results in a swollen pink optic disc with blurred margins. There may be haemorrhages at the disc margins. It is almost always bilateral. Visual acuity is normal, but the blind spot may be enlarged.

- Unilateral papilloedema is usually caused by vascular or inflammatory disorders of the nerve itself or by a space-occupying lesion in the orbit.
- Papilloedema may be mimicked by:
  (a) hyaline bodies within the optic disc, commonly referred to as 'drusen', which may give the disc a raised appearance
  (b) congenital elevation of the discs in children
- Optic nerve head swelling (**papillitis**) results in a swollen, pink and blurred optic disc. It may be unilateral and is always associated with reduced visual acuity. The pupillary light response is often impaired.
- **Optic atrophy** results in a pale or white optic disc with sharp margins. It is associated with reduced visual acuity.

Eye movements

- To examine eye movements, first inspect eye position and note whether both eyes are straight at rest.
- Ask the patient to report any double vision during testing.
- Test eye movements in all directions of gaze and look for nystagmus.
- Note any drooping of the eyelids (ptosis).
- Using a bright torch, observe the pupil reaction to direct and consensual light and to accommodation.

III Oculomotor nerve

A third nerve palsy results in:

- Partial or complete ptosis because of paralysis of levator palpebrae superioris
- Outwards and downwards deviation of the eye because of the unopposed actions of the lateral rectus and superior oblique muscles
- A dilated pupil that fails to react to light and accommodation because parasympathetic fibres carried in the IIIrd nerve are lost

IV Trochlear nerve

A IVth (trochlear) nerve palsy results in impairment of downward and medial gaze; double vision when reading is a common symptom.

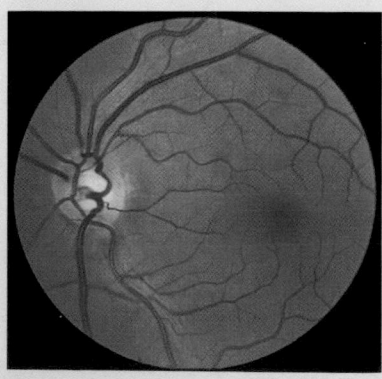

(a)

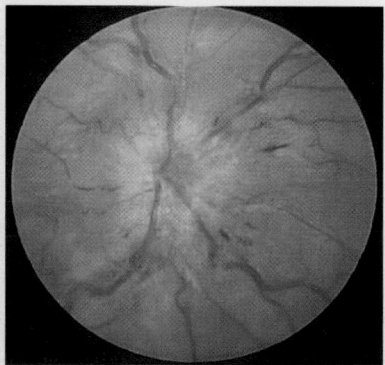

(b)

Figure 13.2 (a) A normal optic disc. The disc should have a clear edge and look like a concave cup. It should be pale yellow in colour. (b) Papilloedema.

V Trigeminal nerve

Test facial sensation using a sterile pin and cotton wool:

- Induce a rapid blink (the corneal reflex) by gently touching the cornea (not the conjunctiva) with a wisp of cotton wool
- Do not let the patient see the approaching stimulus as this itself may induce a blink

Examine the masticatory muscles by:

- Inspecting for wasting of the temporalis and masseter muscles
- Testing jaw opening against resistance

VI Abducens nerve

A VIth (abducens) nerve palsy results in failure of lateral gaze.

VII Facial nerve

Inspect spontaneous movements of the face. Then ask the patient to:

- Raise their eyebrows
- Screw up eyes against resistance
- Smile and to squeeze their lips together

Test taste on the front of the tongue using liquids such as glucose syrup or saline.

VIII Acoustic nerve

Test auditory acuity by whispering numbers in one ear while occluding the other; ask the patient to repeat them out loud.

- For Rinne's test, compare the loudness of a high frequency (>250 Hz) tuning fork when pressed on the mastoid process (bone conduction) and when held in front of the external meatus (air conduction; should be louder unless there is a conductive hearing loss).
- For Weber's test, place the tuning fork on the centre of the forehead and ask the patient in which ear it sounds louder; it should normally be heard in the centre of the head. Localization of the sound to a deaf ear suggests that such hearing loss is conductive rather than sensorineural.

Bulbar examination
IX (glossopharyngeal) and X (vagus) nerves

- Pharyngeal sensation and the gag reflex may be tested by gently touching the back of the pharynx on each side with an orange stick.
- The afferent (sensory) component of the gag reflex is served by the glossopharyngeal nerve.
- The efferent (motor) component of the gag reflex is served by the vagus nerve.
- The vagus maintains the uvula in the midline when the patient says 'ah'.
- The vagus brings the vocal cords together (via the recurrent laryngeal nerves) to produce a nice sharp cough; if the larynx is paralysed, the sharp sound is lost and the cough sounds like a whispered 'HAAAAA'; this is a bovine cough.

XI Accessory nerve

- Examine for wasting of sternomastoid and trapezius.
- Ask the patient to turn their head to the left against resistance to test the right sternomastoid muscle and vice versa.
- Ask the patient to shrug their shoulders against resistance to test trapezius.

XII Hypoglossal nerve

- Inspect the tongue for wasting or fasciculation (best seen with the tongue at rest in the floor of the mouth).
- Then ask the patient to stick out their tongue and record any lateral deviation; it protrudes to the right if there is a right twelfth nerve lesion.

---

disease). Myasthenia gravis and endocrine disease (e.g. dysthyroid eye disease) should be excluded; pupil reactions remain normal in both conditions. Occasionally patients—and senior colleagues—enjoy watching a confused student trying to elicit eye movements in a false ('glass') eye.

Internuclear ophthalmoplegia

Internuclear ophthalmoplegia is demonstrated on lateral gaze; there is a failure of adduction in the adducting eye and nystagmus in the abducting eye (Fig. 13.4). It is caused by a lesion in the median longitudinal fasciculus (MLF), the tract connecting the IIIrd and VIth nerve nuclei. It may be unilateral, in which case the lesion lies in the MLF contralateral to the abducting eye, or bilateral. Causes include multiple sclerosis, Wernicke's encephalopathy and, less commonly, tumours, aneurysms or cerebrovascular disease.

Horner's syndrome (Fig. 13.5)

Interruption of the sympathetic fibres to the pupil causes Horner's syndrome, comprising:

- Ptosis caused by paralysis of Müller's muscle.
- A small pupil (miosis) caused by paralysis of the pupillary dilator muscle. This may be difficult to appreciate when both pupils are small and so is best detected in a darkened room.
- Ipsilateral loss of facial sweating because of loss of sympathetic pseudomotor fibres.
- Apparent retraction of the eye (enophthalmos).

The face

Facial sensation

Unilateral facial sensory disturbance is quite common. If it is confined to one division of the trigeminal nerve, consider demyelination (see p. 920) or a structural lesion.

13

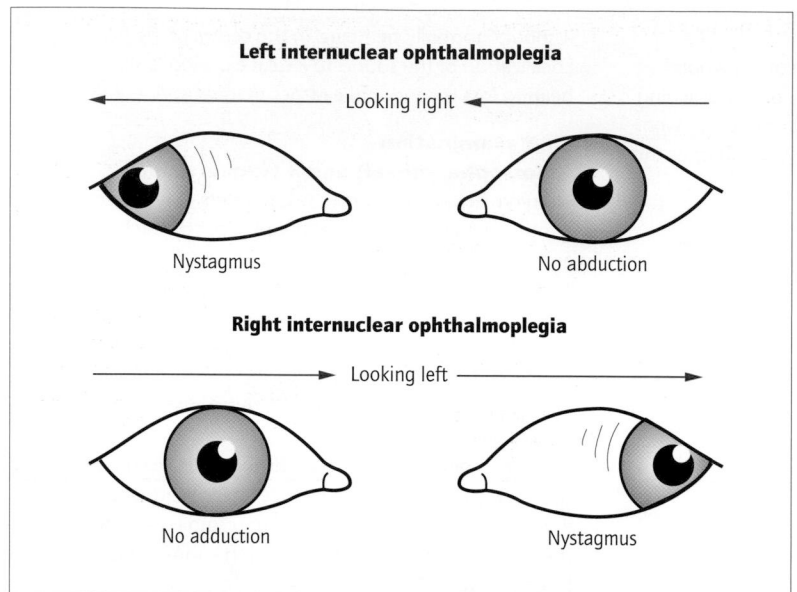

Figure 13.4 Findings in internuclear ophthalmoplegia.

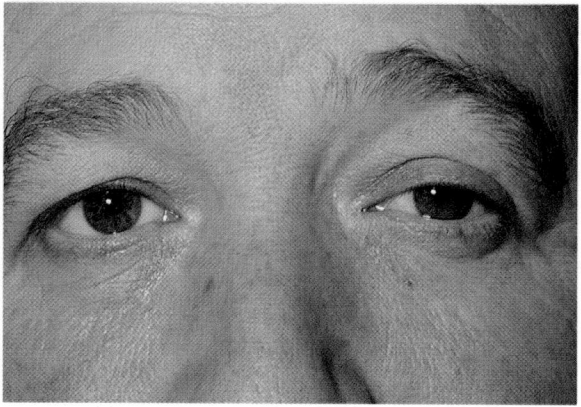

Figure 13.5 Horner's syndrome.

If these have been ruled out, consider an autoimmune inflammatory neuropathy such as Sjögren's syndrome or SLE (see p. 215). Lesions of other cranial nerves (e.g. acoustic neuromas) may expand and involve the Vth nerve, resulting in a combination of deafness, ataxia, ipsilateral facial weakness and loss of the ipsilateral corneal reflex.

Muscles of mastication
Bilateral weakness of jaw opening is not specific to lesions of the motor division of the trigeminal nerve, and can occur in motor neurone disease, myasthenia gravis and myopathies.

Muscles of facial expression
The upper facial musculature receives input from both cerebral hemispheres; the lower musculature from the contralateral hemisphere only. Unlike the lower facial musculature, muscles of the upper part of the face are therefore not completely paralysed by contralateral hemispheric lesions (e.g. tumour, haemorrhage, infarction; Fig. 13.6).

Motor system

The arms and then the legs are examined, with comparison of each part with its opposite (HISTORY & EXAMINATION BOX 13.6).

Spasticity
- A hallmark of upper motor neurone (UMN) lesions
- Caused by interruption of corticospinal inhibitory pathways
- Most marked in flexor muscles in the arms and the extensors of the legs
- Not constant throughout the full range of passive movement
- Elicited by rapid pronation of the arms, flexion of the legs or dorsiflexion at the ankle, when it is felt as a 'catch'

Clonus. This is a series of repeated involuntary contractions of the stretched muscle and is a consequence of spasticity and hyper-reflexia. Ankle clonus is demonstrated by flexing the knee slightly then rapidly dorsiflexing the foot.

Myotonia. This is the inability to relax a muscle after a voluntary contraction. Patients may be unable to release their grip after shaking hands with the examiner. Alternatively, a tap on the thenar eminence using a tendon hammer may

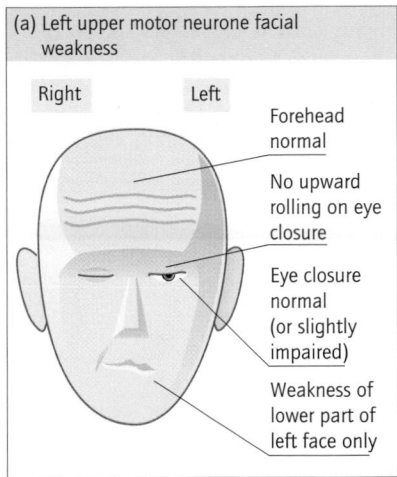

(a) Left upper motor neurone facial weakness

Right · Left

Forehead normal

No upward rolling on eye closure

Eye closure normal (or slightly impaired)

Weakness of lower part of left face only

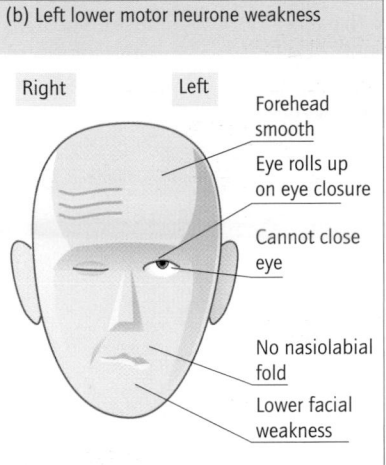

(b) Left lower motor neurone weakness

Right · Left

Forehead smooth

Eye rolls up on eye closure

Cannot close eye

No nasiolabial fold

Lower facial weakness

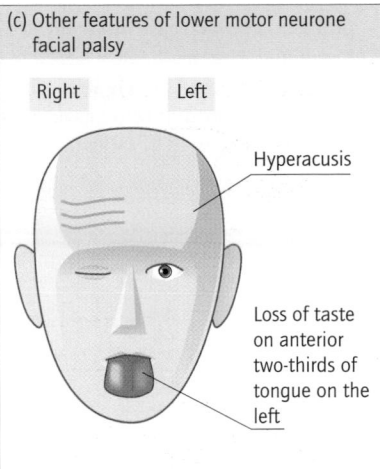

(c) Other features of lower motor neurone facial palsy

Right · Left

Hyperacusis

Loss of taste on anterior two-thirds of tongue on the left

Figure 13.6 Characteristics of facial nerve lesions.

History & Examinaton 13.6: Examination of the motor system

Table A Movements and associated muscles, motor nerves and root levels, in the arms and legs

Joint	Movement	Muscle	Nerve	Root
Shoulder	Abduction	Deltoid	Axillary	C5
Elbow	Flexion	Biceps	Musculocutaneous	C5
	Flexion	Brachioradialis	Radial	C6
	Extension	Triceps	Radial	C7
Wrist	Extension	Forearm extensors	Radial	C6
Finger	Flexion	Forearm flexors	Median (lateral two fingers)	C8
			Ulnar (medial two fingers)	C8
	Extension	Long finger extensors	Radial	C7, C8
	Abduction	Dorsal interossei	Ulnar	T1
Thumb	Abduction	Abductor pollicis brevis	Median	T1
Hip	Flexion	Iliopsoas	Femoral	L1, L2
	Extension	Glutei	Gluteal	L4, L5, S1
Knee	Flexion	Hamstrings	Sciatic	L5, S1
	Extension	Quadriceps	Femoral	L3, L4
Ankle	Dorsiflexion	Tibialis anterior	Deep peroneal	L4, L5
	Plantarflexion	Gastrocnemius	Tibial	S1, S2

Inspection

Arms and legs and axial musculature cannot be inspected adequately if they are covered in clothes, so the patient should be examined in his or her underwear, and the examination room should be warm and well lit. Look for muscle wasting and fasciculation, abnormal limb postures, involuntary movements and tremor.

Passive movement

Feel tone during passive movement.
Examine for:

- *Rigidity:* by passively moving each joint through its full range of movement
- *Spasticity:* best elicited by rapidly moving a joint in one direction
- *Ankle clonus:* may be elicited by flexing the knee slightly and rapidly dorsiflexing the foot

Test muscle power

A systematic brief survey of muscle power (Table A, Figs A–N) will suffice unless there is a specific motor

Continued p. 882

problem, in which case more detailed examination is required. Use the Medical Research Council Scale (Table B) to record muscle strength.

Elicit the deep tendon reflexes and the plantar reflex

Elicit the reflexes listed in Table C. For the plantar reflex stroke a noxious stimulus (such as an orange stick) up the lateral border of the foot and along to the ball of the foot. The normal response is flexion of the great toe. Extension (dorsiflexion) of the great toe and fanning of the little toes suggests an upper motor neurone lesion.

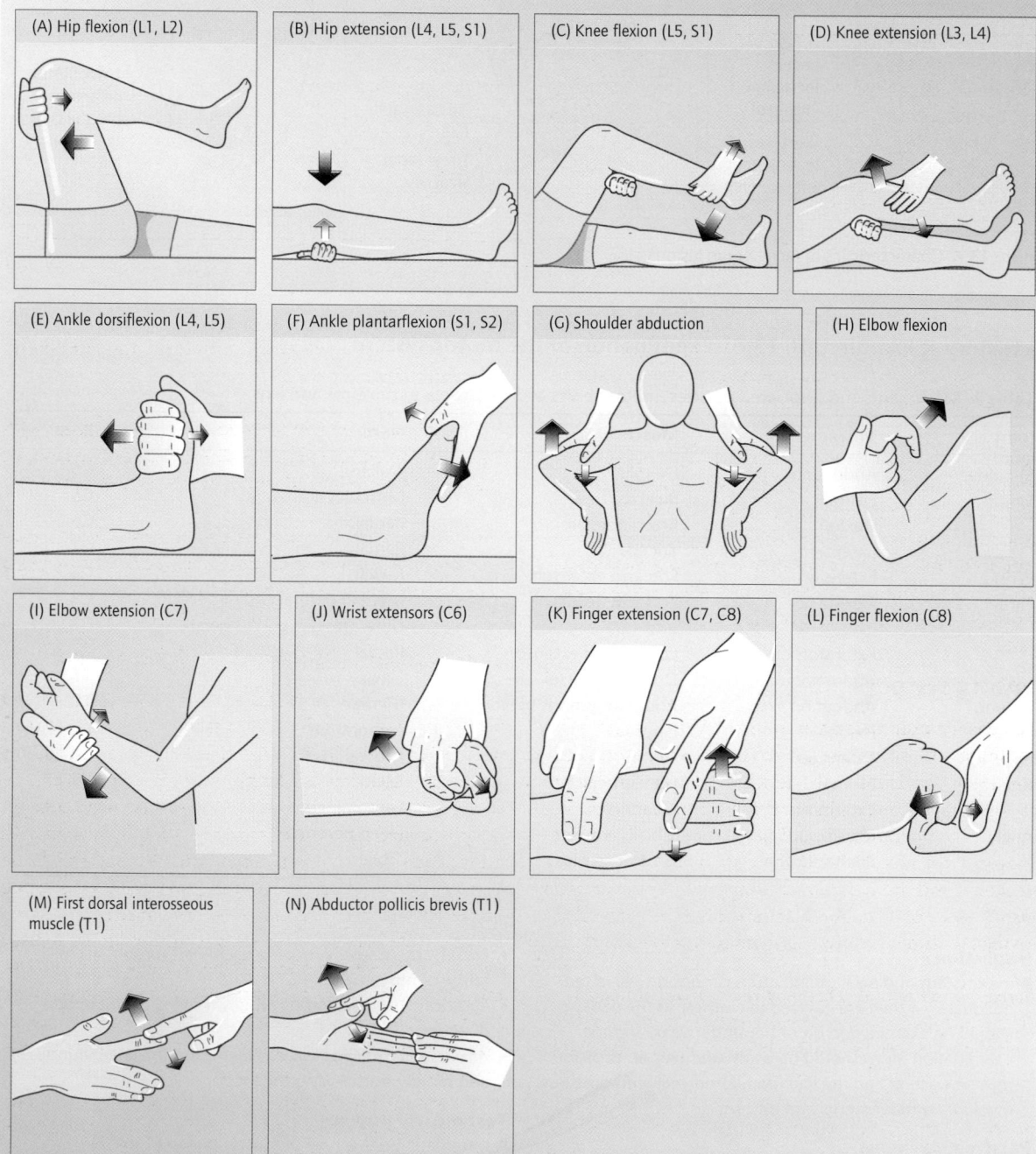

Figs A–N Examination of muscle power.

Table B Medical Research Council (MRC) grading of motor power

No contraction	0
Flicker of contraction	1
Active movement with gravity eliminated	2
Active movement against gravity	3
Active movement against gravity and resistance	4
Normal power	5

Table C Reflexes and their innervations

	Nerve root
Routinely tested	
Biceps	C5, C6
Brachioradialis	C6
Triceps	C7, C8
Abdominal	T7–T12
Knee jerk	L3, L4
Ankle	S1, S2
Occasionally tested	
Jaw jerk	Fifth cranial nerve
Finger flexion	C8
Cremaster	L1
Bulbocavernosus	S3, S4, S5
Anal	S4, S5

lead to a slow and sustained abduction of the thumb (percussion myotonia). It occurs in primary muscle disorders such as myotonic dystrophy.

Rigidity. This is a general increase in muscle tone. Extrapyramidal ('lead pipe') rigidity is present throughout the whole range of passive movement and may be associated with 'cogwheeling' (like moving the joint over a ratchet). This rigidity is not altered by rapid movement, affects both flexors and extensors, and may be exaggerated by simultaneous movements of the contralateral limb.

Sensory system

The sensory examination is more subjective and contributes less to diagnosis. Comparison of sensation side with side or distal limb with trunk may help establish what is normal. Light touch, pin prick, vibration, joint position sense and temperature should be examined (HISTORY & EXAMINATION BOX 13.7). If the patient has no sensory symptoms this need not take long. Where an area of sensory loss exists its boundaries should be mapped by moving the stimulus outwards from numb to normal.

Altered skin sensation. This may result from damage to a peripheral nerve, to the spinal cord or to the cerebral hemispheres. Altered sensation below a level on the trunk may indicate a spinal cord lesion.

Sensory inattention. This may be asymptomatic; it occurs when a patient senses a stimulus when both sides of the body are touched in turn, but reports only one side being touched when the stimuli are simultaneous. A patient with a parietal lobe lesion fails to perceive the stimulus on the contralateral side.

Loss of vibration and/or joint position sense. Occurs with lesions of the dorsal column in the spinal cord, in a dorsal root ganglionopathy and with peripheral neuropathy.

Dissociated sensory loss (loss of pain and temperature sensation with preservation of light touch). Usually caused by a central cord lesion (e.g. syringomyelia; see p. 941).

Coordination, gait and walking speed

Coordination is assessed using the finger–nose and heel–shin tests described in HISTORY & EXAMINATION BOX 13.7. Lesions in the cerebellar hemispheres produce ipsilateral disturbance of arm and leg coordination. In cerebellar disease, tremor is typically worse when a target is approached (intention tremor). Rhythmic repetitive movements (e.g. rapid tapping with the fingers of one hand on the dorsum of the other) and rapid alternating movements (dysdiadochokinesis) are impaired.

Lesions of the midline cerebellum result in loss of balance when sitting and walking. Romberg's sign is an unreliable indication of neurological disease; it tests the ability to stand upright with the feet together and the eyes closed. When positive, balance is restored when the eyes are opened. This is because of loss of postural reflexes or joint position sense in the legs. Patients with cerebellar disease are usually equally unsteady with eyes open or closed.

Gait is assessed at the end of the examination. Observe walking over 10 m and turning, looking for a broad-based gait, loss of arm swing or a series of short steps after

History & Examinaton 13.7: Examination of the sensory system, cerebellar function and gait

Define any area of altered sensation

Ask the patient if they have any patches of lost or altered sensation

If there is, map it out, testing outwards from abnormal to normal

Test light touch sensation

Touch the skin lightly with cotton wool for light touch sensation; avoid stroking, which gives a tickle stimulus

Test pinprick sensation

Use a disposable sterile pin, not venepuncture needles or stylets

Test vibration sense

Use a low frequency (128 Hz) tuning fork placed on a bony prominence (knuckle and lateral malleolus) on each limb. If vibration cannot be felt distally, move the tuning fork more proximally until vibration is perceived.

Test joint position sense

Passively move the distal interphalangeal joint in the fingers and big toe (movement through 2–3° is sufficient). If the movements cannot be felt, test joint position at a more proximal joint such as the metacarpophalangeal joint and ankle.

Test fine finger movement (tests UMN function)

Ask the patient to make 'piano playing' movements of fingers. Inability to move each finger independently or slowness of fine finger movement often indicates either a UMN lesion or an extrapyramidal disorder.

Test coordination and cerebellar function

Finger–nose test

Ask the patient to move an outstretched finger between a target (the examiner's finger) and the patient's nose. Make sure that pain or weakness do not prevent the patient from making the required movement.

Heel–shin test

For the lower limbs, ask the patient to place one heel on the opposite knee and slide the heel down to the ankle and back up.

Rapid alternating movements

Ask the patient to perform rapidly alternating movements (e.g. tapping the fingers of one hand on the back of the other) to detect cerebellar incoordination.

Test balance

Ask the patient to walk a straight line, placing one foot immediately in front of the other ('tandem' or 'heel–toe' walking); truncal ataxia may only be apparent using this test.

Ask the patient to stand without support with their feet in contact with each other both at the heel and the forefoot. Note how steady the patient is. Then ask the patient to close his or her eyes (**Romberg's test**); much worse balance with the eyes closed represents a positive test and indicates a problem with joint position sense.

Observe gait

Ask the patient to walk, and observe posture, arm swing, length of stride and steadiness on turning.

---

turning, these last two being features of Parkinson's disease. Ask the patient to walk with the heel of the next foot placed at the toe of the other (tandem walking) to reveal mild ataxia. Record the time to walk 10 m as a baseline against which to measure future change (normal is less than 10 s).

Investigation

As with examination, the purpose of neurological investigation is not to document every nuance of the human condition but rather to test specific hypotheses regarding the origin of symptoms. Investigations should be used selectively and only after careful consideration.

Blood tests

Full blood count

The full blood count may be altered in infection, arteritis and malignancy:

- Dizziness can be caused by anaemia
- Raised mean cell volume (MCV) occurs with alcohol misuse and with vitamin deficiencies (see p. 1030)
- High haemoglobin may indicate polycythaemia and a thrombotic tendency

In addition, abnormalities of the blood film may indicate specific disorders (e.g. vitamin B_{12} deficiency, malignancy, neuroacanthocytosis).

Erythrocyte sedimentation rate

Marked elevation of the erythrocyte sedimentation rate (ESR) in a patient with a headache strongly suggests temporal arteritis (see p. 908). Other causes include vasculitis (e.g. SLE), granulomatous disease (e.g. sarcoidosis), covert malignancy and lymphoma.

Prothrombin ratio and coagulation screen

Patients with unexplained intracranial haemorrhage should have their prothrombin ratio (PTR) checked. The PTR is also a sensitive test of liver function and is useful in patients with both liver disease and neurological symptoms (e.g. hepatic encephalopathy). Coagulation studies are indicated in young patients with ischaemic stroke to look for thrombophilia (increased clotting).

Vitamin B$_{12}$ and folate

Deficiency of vitamin B$_{12}$ may result in a peripheral neuropathy, optic atrophy, dementia or spinal cord degeneration. The neurological effects of folate deficiency are less clear.

Urea and electrolytes

- Electrolyte disturbance (e.g. hypo- and hypernatraemia) may cause confusion and, if severe, coma
- Hypokalaemia and hypocalcaemia may give rise to muscle weakness
- Hypercalcaemia may cause confusion
- Metabolic disturbance (e.g. uraemia resulting from renal disease) may be a cause of peripheral neuropathy or myoclonus
- Some antiepileptic drugs (e.g. carbamazepine) may give rise to a syndrome of inappropriate antidiuretic hormone (SIADH) production, causing symptomatic hyponatraemia

Glucose

Urgent measurement of blood glucose is mandatory in patients with any disturbance of consciousness. Hypoglycaemia may mimic many neurological conditions, including a hemiplegic stroke. Simple treatment with intravenous glucose or intramuscular glucagon can result in rapid improvement and is often life-saving. Check the glucose of patients with mononeuropathy, polyneuropathy, disorders of consciousness, dementia or cerebrovascular disease.

Cholesterol

Measurement of cholesterol and lipids is relevant in patients with cerebrovascular disease and in certain neuropathies.

Other biochemical changes

Creatine kinase

Creatine kinase is a marker of muscle disease and may be raised in primary muscle conditions such as polymyositis, where it can be used as a marker of the response to treatment.

Thyroid function tests

Depression, confusion and lethargy can be caused by hypothyroidism. Disordered eye movements can be caused by dysthyroid eye disease.

Liver function tests

Hepatic dysfunction can result in confusion, apathy and coma. Some antiepileptic drugs can cause transient disturbance in liver function and this should be monitored. Liver function tests may suggest excess alcohol consumption, which can cause a number of neurological problems. If hepatic encephalopathy is present, the arterial blood ammonia is generally raised.

Serum protein electrophoresis

Abnormalities in the serum proteins in diseases such as myeloma can give rise to severe peripheral neuropathy.

Autoantibodies

The presence of autoantibodies such as antinuclear antibody and antiphospholipid antibody suggests the presence of autoimmune disease.

Syphilis serology

Syphilis can cause a wide variety of neurological syndromes. It should be checked for routinely in many categories of disease, but particularly stroke, dementia, ataxia, ocular disorders, spinal cord lesions and neuropathy.

Human immunodeficiency virus

The range of neurological conditions that may be associated with HIV infection is wide. These syndromes can be the direct result of infection by the virus, or from opportunistic infections (e.g. tuberculosis, toxoplasmosis). Patients and relatives require a careful explanation and counselling about the need for HIV testing and some hospitals provide such a service.

Microbiology

Systemic infections (e.g. urinary tract infections) may worsen function in multiple sclerosis and respiratory compromise (e.g. in muscular dystrophy) may increase susceptibility to infections. Blood, urine and sputum culture are therefore commonly required. Infections of the nervous system usually require cerebrospinal fluid (CSF) for diagnosis; this is collected at lumbar puncture if this is safe (CLINICAL BOX 13.1). Particular culture conditions may be needed for tubercle bacilli, certain other bacteria, viruses or fungi. Other tests (e.g. polymerase chain reaction) may provide a more rapid indication of infection with some agents (e.g. *Meningococcus* spp., herpes simplex), for which urgent treatment is required. Repeated CSF examination may be necessary if tuberculous meningitis is suspected.

Diagnostic imaging

Plain radiography

- *Skull radiography:* detects fractures in patients with head injury.

Clinical box 13.1: Lumbar puncture

Indications

Lumbar puncture is a basic clinical technique important in the investigation and management of:

- Subarachnoid haemorrhage
- Acute meningitis
- Chronic meningeal infiltration or inflammation (e.g. malignant meningitis, sarcoidosis)
- Acute encephalitis
- Transverse myelitis
- Chronic CNS inflammation or infection (e.g. suspected multiple sclerosis, suspected chronic infection such as neurosyphilis, *Borrelia* infection, HIV infection and AIDS)
- Demyelinating peripheral neuropathy (e.g. Guillain–Barré syndrome, chronic inflammatory demyelinating neuropathy)
- Disorders of CSF dynamics (e.g. idiopathic intracranial hypertension, normal-pressure hydrocephalus)

Contraindications

Unless a CT has shown that lumbar puncture is safe (no mass lesions; open basal cisterns), then lumbar puncture should not be performed if there is papilloedema, focal epileptic seizures, dysphasia, hemianopia, hemiparesis, unequal pupils or oculomotor palsy. Lumbar puncture in the presence of a space-occupying intracranial lesion can squeeze the midbrain through the tentorium cerebri and the brainstem through the foramen magnum with devastating consequences.

Technique

Position the patient (Fig. A)

The patient should lie on their side with their knees drawn up to the chest and their neck slightly flexed. The plane of the back should be vertical and parallel to the edge of the bed. Place a pillow between the patient's knees and one under their head to prevent twisting of the trunk.

Identify the space between the spinous processes of L3 and L4 (just below a line joining the iliac crests)

Use either this space or either of the two below (L4/5 or L5/S1)

Take full sterile precautions

Clean the skin around the proposed puncture site three times with antiseptic. Use sterile gloves and a sterile field. Except in experienced hands, the assistance of a nursing colleague is essential.

Local anaesthesia

Any discomfort can be reduced if the local anaesthetic is prewarmed to body temperature. With a 26-gauge needle parallel to the skin, raise a subcutaneous bleb of 2% lidocaine then take a larger bore needle perpendicular to the skin and inject to a total of 2–4 ml with gradual advancement of the needle tip. Aspirate on the syringe every time

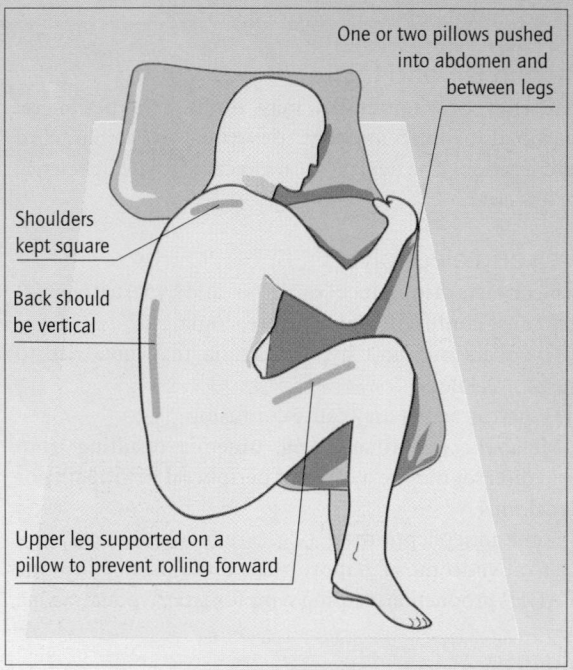

Fig. A Lumbar puncture: patient positioning.

One or two pillows pushed into abdomen and between legs

Shoulders kept square

Back should be vertical

Upper leg supported on a pillow to prevent rolling forward

the needle is advanced to ensure that it has not entered a blood vessel.

Introduce the lumbar puncture needle (Fig. B)

After 1 or 2 min anaesthesia is established; introduce a 9-cm, 18- or 20-gauge lumbar puncture needle held horizontally and pointing slightly cranially (towards the umbilicus). A distinct 'give' may be felt as the needle enters the subdural space. Withdraw the stylet and check for flow of CSF. If not, continue until obstruction or CSF is reached.

Measure CSF pressure

Connect the manometer and measure the pressure of CSF (in centimetres of CSF); this is the 'opening pressure' and is usually less than 25.

Collect CSF samples

Allow 2–3 ml of CSF to drain into each of at least three sterile collection bottles; in some laboratories a further fluoride oxalate tube is required for glucose estimation. Label the tubes in order of collection; in bleeding from subarachnoid haemorrhage the red cell count is constant, but with bleeding induced at the time of the lumbar puncture the red cell count should fall in successive samples.

Withdraw the lumbar puncture needle gently and place a plaster over the puncture. Patients may mobilize immediately after lumbar puncture.

Neurological and neurovascular surgery

Neurosurgery may:
● Provide definitive treatment for lesions including extradural and subdural haematoma; meningioma; cerebral aneurysms; compression of the spinal cord or roots; and hydrocephalus
● Be needed in the management of infectious conditions (e.g. drainage of abscesses in the brain or spinal cord)
● Provide symptomatic relief through a reduction in intracranial pressure in patients with tumours or hydrocephalus; the excision of epileptic foci with improved seizure control in intractable epilepsy; and through carefully placed surgical lesions to control pain in trigeminal neuralgia or to relieve symptoms in Parkinson's disease

Vascular surgery is used, at carotid endarterectomy, in the secondary prevention of stroke, where patients have a severe symptomatic carotid stenosis.

Interventional neuroradiology has an important role in the treatment of cerebral aneurysms and arteriovenous malformations, and in time may replace surgery as the treatment of choice for some of these conditions. However, clinical trials of the long-term efficacy of endovascular treatment of cerebral aneurysms is awaited, and such procedures require an experienced radiologist usually only available at specialist centres.

Diseases and their management

Vascular disease

Stroke and transient ischaemic attack

Stroke and TIA are common and can result from a variety of pathological lesions affecting blood vessels (CLINICAL BOX 13.2). They can be mimicked by a variety of non-vascular problems such as migraine, focal epilepsy and cerebral tumour. Many strokes are potentially preventable.

Epidemiology

Prevalence. Prevalence of stroke-related disability is 800 in 100 000. Annual incidence is 280 in 100 000. Annual incidence of TIA is 35 in 100 000.

Age. Incidence of stroke and TIA rises exponentially with age, and half of all new patients are older than 70 years.

Sex. Slightly more common in females.

Race. No clear association.

Genetics. Some rare causes of stroke [cerebral autosomal dominant arteriopathy with subcortical infarcts and leukoencephalopathy (CADASIL)] are caused by single gene defects (*notch*), but increased risk of stroke is also inherited as a polygenic trait.

Disease mechanisms

The causes of stroke and TIA are listed in Table 13.3. Risk factors for both ischaemic and haemorrhagic stroke include:
● Hypertension, which is by far the most important
● Smoking
● Family history
● Male sex
  Risk factors for ischaemic stroke alone include:
● Diabetes mellitus
● Cardiac lesions giving rise to emboli including atrial fibrillation, valvular heart disease and atheroma of the aortic arch

Most TIAs and ischaemic strokes are caused by emboli:
● Most are clumps of fibrin and platelets, which form on the surface of plaques of atheroma at the origins of the internal carotid and vertebral arteries; these then break off and are carried by the circulation to the brain
● In 10%, the emboli arise from the heart
● About 1 in 5 ischaemic strokes (and perhaps a smaller proportion of TIAs) appear to result from *in situ* formation of atheroma and subsequent occlusion of one of the small deep perforating arteries that supply the internal capsule and the pons; these are lacunar strokes or TIAs

Primary intracerebral haemorrhage is usually caused by rupture of a deep penetrating artery within the brain substance and is related to hypertension. Occasionally, rupture of a cerebral aneurysm or an arteriovenous malformation (AVM) may cause haemorrhagic stroke. Superficial lobar haemorrhages may be a result of other causes such as amyloid angiopathy.

Clinical features

The hallmark of a vascular lesion is the sudden onset of focal symptoms and signs. The speed of onset may need to be confirmed by a witness if the patient is drowsy, confused, amnesic or aphasic. Common manifestations of stroke are discussed on page 895. Ischaemic and haemorrhagic strokes cannot be distinguished on clinical grounds: CT scanning will differentiate between the two. Arterial distributions for some stroke symptoms are given in Table 13.4.

Clinical box 13.2: Classification of stroke

Ischaemic stroke (85% of all strokes)

Large middle cerebral artery territory infarct

Cause. Occlusion of main stem of middle cerebral artery

CT appearance. Infarction of whole territory of middle cerebral artery (Fig. A)

Neurological signs. Hemiplegia, hemianopia, aphasia (if left hemisphere involved), visuospatial disorder (if right hemisphere involved)

Prognosis. 40% die within 30 days of onset; 95% probability of death or disability at 6 months

Cortical infarct (Fig. B)

Cause. Occlusion of small cortical vessel

CT appearance. Infarction of cortex

Neurological signs. Isolated deficit of cortical function (aphasia or hemianopia, or visuospatial disorder or weakness of hand and/or arm alone)

Prognosis. 6% die within 30 days of onset; 45% probability of death or disability at 6 months

Brainstem infarct (Fig. C)

Cause. Small vessel disease or embolus

MRI appearance. Small infarct in the brainstem

Neurological signs. One or more of double vision, unsteadiness, dysphagia, cranial nerve palsies, Horner's syndrome, quadriparesis, hemiparesis, reduced consciousness

Prognosis. 6% die within 30 days; 30% probability of death or disability at 6 months

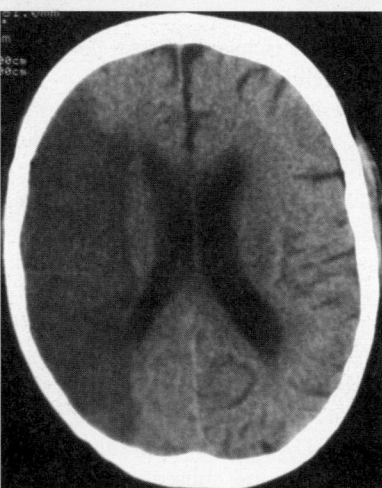

Fig. A Large middle cerebral artery tertiary infarct (CT).

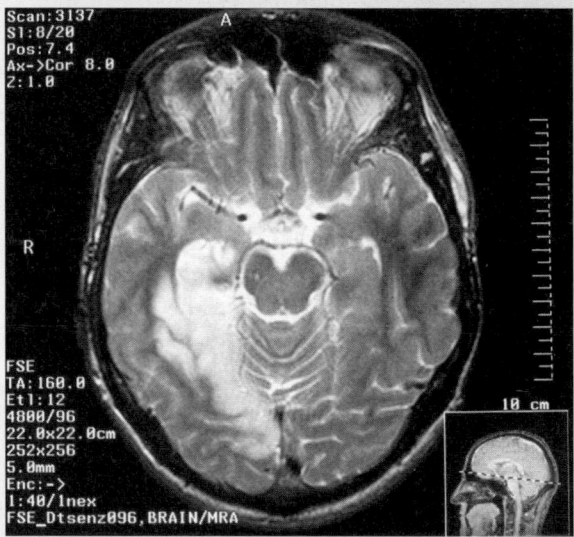

Fig. C Posterior circulation infarct (MRI).

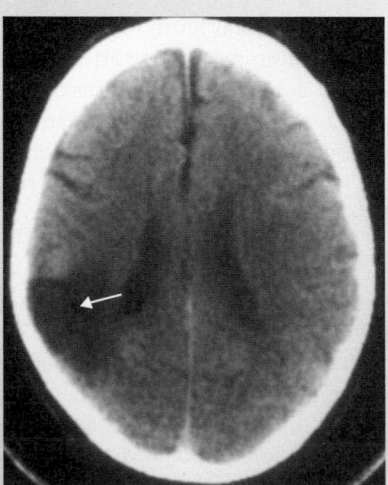

Fig. B Cortical infarct (CT).

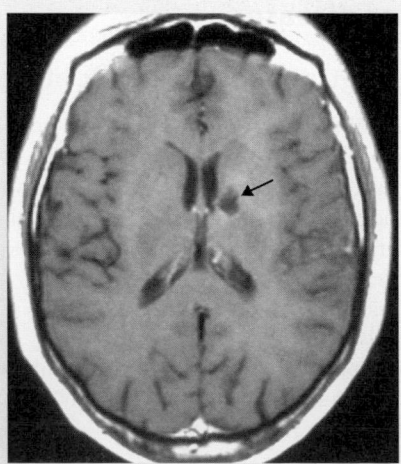

Fig. D Lacunar infarct (MRI).

Lacunar infarct (Fig. D)
Cause. Occlusion of single small deep penetrating artery
CT appearance. Small infarct in basal ganglia and/or internal capsule
Neurological signs. Hemiparesis or hemisensory loss or uni-lateral ataxia without disorder of language, memory or visuospatial function
Prognosis. 3% die within 30 days; 35% probability of death or disability at 6 months

Intracranial haemorrhage (15% of all strokes)
Primary intracerebral haemorrhage (Fig. E)
Cause. Rupture of artery
CT appearance. Haematoma in brain substance

Neurological signs. If severe—coma. If mild—focal neurological deficit, usually indistinguishable from cerebral infarction
Prognosis. 30–50% die within 30 days

Subarachnoid haemorrhage (Fig. F)
Cause. Rupture of cerebral aneurysm or arteriovenous mal-formation
CT appearance. Blood in the subarachnoid space
Neurological signs. Sudden headache, neck stiffness, loss of consciousness, some focal signs if the blood spreads into the brain substance
Prognosis. 50% die within 30 days. High risk of rebleeding within first few weeks

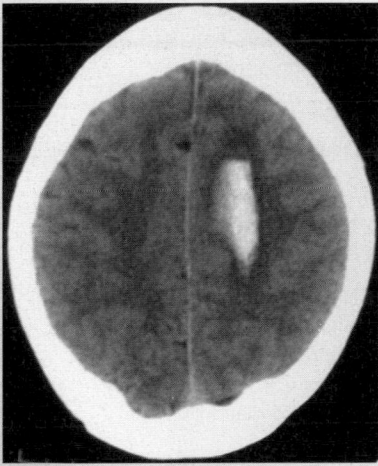

Fig. E Primary intracerebral haemorrhage.

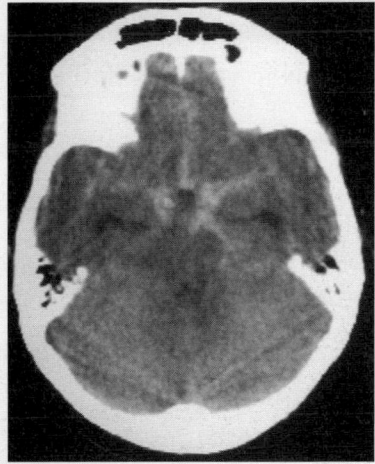

Fig. F Subarachnoid haemorrhage.

Transient ischaemic attack
1 Sudden onset of neurological symptoms that last a few minutes to a few hours (and by definition less than 24 h).
2 Important to exclude other causes of transient focal symptoms:
- Migraine
- Focal epilepsy
- Hypoglycaemia
- Non-ketotic hyperglycaemia
- Arteritis
- Structural brain lesions (e.g. tumour, subdural haematoma, AVM)
3 Non-focal symptoms are not usually caused by TIAs:
- Confusion
- Memory loss
- Loss of consciousness
- Dizziness
- Light-headedness
- Blurred vision
- Generalized weakness

4 Non-focal symptoms may be caused by:
- Cardiovascular disorders (e.g. syncope, arrhythmia)
- Epilepsy
- Metabolic disorders

Keypoints 13.3: Stroke

Stroke is a medical emergency and should be treated as such

Aspirin for acute ischaemic stroke saves as many lives as thrombolysis does in myocardial infarction

Thrombolysis for acute ischaemic stroke may potentially save many more lives

Management in a stroke unit and appropriate secondary prevention saves yet more lives

It is therefore important that stroke patients are looked after properly

Table 13.3 Causes of stroke

ISCHAEMIC STROKE AND TRANSIENT ISCHAEMIC ATTACK

Common causes

Thromboembolic infarcts (about 60%)
Atheroma of carotid and vertebral arteries

Lacunar infarcts (20%)
Disease of small vessels within the substance of the brain

Embolism from the heart (10–20%)
Left atrial thrombus associated with atrial fibrillation
Left atrial myxoma (rare)
Mitral valve endocarditis (bacterial, rheumatic, marantic)
Mitral valve prosthesis
Left ventricular mural thrombus complicating myocardial infarction or left ventricular aneurysm
Cardiomyopathy
Aortic valve endocarditis (bacterial, rheumatic, marantic)
Aortic valve sclerosis
Aortic valve prosthesis
Congenital cardiac disorders
Paradoxical embolism from the venous system through a patent foramen ovale
Atheroma of the aortic arch

Rare causes (1–5% of all ischaemic strokes)

Arteritis
Temporal arteritis
Polyarteritis nodosa
Systemic lupus erythematosus

Rare arterial diseases
Carotid or vertebral dissection
Homocystinuria

Genetically determined causes
CADASIL
Fabry's disease
Mitochondrial disease

Hypercoagulability
Oral contraception

Lupus anticoagulant
Polycythaemia

Infection
HIV, syphilis

Multiple mechanisms
Drug abuse (e.g. cocaine, amphetamine)

PRIMARY INTRACEREBRAL HAEMORRHAGE

Common causes

Ruptured microaneurysm
Hypertension

Small vessel disease
Amyloid angiopathy

Arteriovenous malformation

Haemostatic disorders
Anticoagulant overdose
Thrombocytopenia
Hereditary bleeding disorder

Multiple mechanisms
Drug abuse (e.g. cocaine, ecstasy, amphetamine)

Rare causes
Moya moya disease
Cavernous haemangioma

SUBARACHNOID HAEMORRHAGE

Common causes

Rupture of abnormality
Cerebral aneurysm
Arteriovenous malformation

Rare causes

Rupture of abnormality
Mycotic aneurysm (e.g. subacute bacterial endocarditis)

Haemostatic deficit
Anticoagulant overdose

Symptom	Arterial distribution
Dysphasia	Definitely carotid
Loss of vision in one eye only	Definitely carotid (amaurosis fugax)
Weakness of the face/arm/leg*	Carotid or vertebrobasilar, but more often carotid
Dysarthria or slurred speech	Carotid or vertebrobasilar
Unsteadiness	Carotid or vertebrobasilar
Sensory loss of the face/arm/leg*	Carotid or vertebrobasilar
Visuospatial disorder	Carotid or vertebrobasilar
Quadriparesis	Definitely vertebrobasilar
Hemianopia alone	Definitely vertebrobasilar
Transient bilateral blindness	Definitely vertebrobasilar
Double vision	Definitely vertebrobasilar

Table 13.4 Arterial distributions of focal symptoms occurring with transient ischaemic attack (TIA) or stroke

* Symptoms in the face, arm and leg without aphasia, cortical problems or hemianopia are usually caused by ischaemia in the internal capsule or pons. Symptoms restricted to a limb or to the face are usually caused by cortical lesions.

- Hyperventilation
- Depression

Stroke

A stroke is characterized by a sudden onset, and by symptoms and signs that are definitely focal and that last longer than 24 h (KEYPOINTS BOX 13.3). Other causes of persistent focal deficit should be excluded including cerebral tumour, subdural haematoma and cerebral abscess.

Lateral medullary syndrome of Wallenberg

The lateral medullary syndrome of Wallenberg is a rare neurological syndrome caused by occlusion of the posterior inferior cerebellar artery. This causes infarction of the nuclei of the IXth, Xth and XIth nerves, and of the sympathetic, spinocerebellar and spinothalamic tracts. The signs are:

- Ipsilateral IXth, Xth and XIth nerve palsies, causing dysarthria and dysphagia

---

Ischaemic stroke at a glance

Epidemiology

Prevalence
800 in 100 000

Age
Over 50 years of age

Clinical features

Nervous system
Sudden onset of focal neurological deficit
Preceding transient ischaemic attack (TIA) in 15% of patients

Blood vessels
History of angina; claudication; diabetes mellitus; hypertension
Family history of premature vascular disease

Complications
Dysphagia
Aspiration
Subluxed shoulder
Deep-vein thrombosis
Pneumonia
Depression

Findings on investigation

Blood tests
- *ESR:* usually normal. If abnormal look for treatable cause
- *Cholesterol:* increased
- *Glucose:* increased in 10%

Immunology
Usually normal

Microbiology
Usually normal

Diagnostic imaging
- *CT scan of the brain:* may be normal in 30–40% of patients. Otherwise there is a low-density area of infarction

- *Ultrasound studies of carotid arteries:* may show stenosis or occlusion of the symptomatic artery
- *Chest radiography:* may show cardiomegaly and/or heart failure because of a cardiac source of embolism in 10% of patients

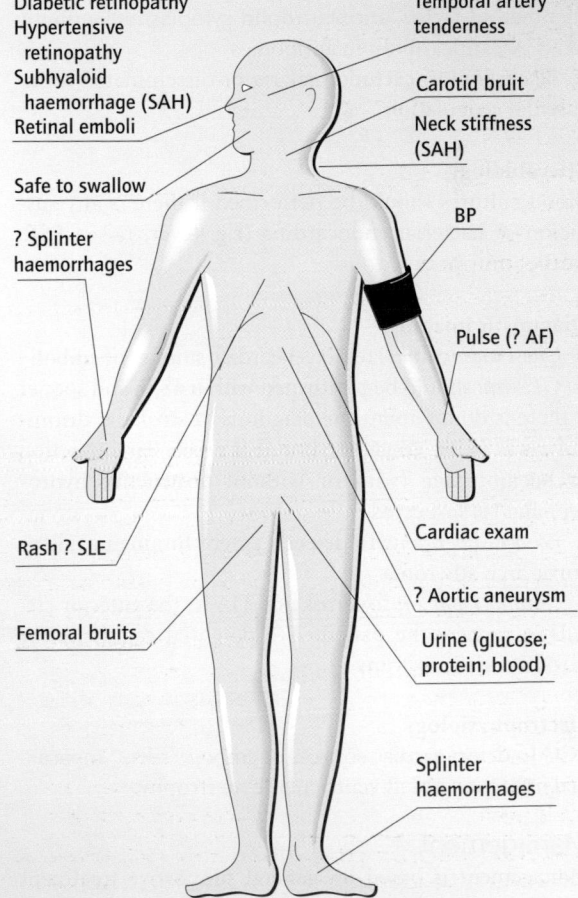

Diabetic retinopathy
Hypertensive retinopathy
Subhyaloid haemorrhage (SAH)
Retinal emboli

Safe to swallow

? Splinter haemorrhages

Rash ? SLE

Femoral bruits

Temporal artery tenderness

Carotid bruit

Neck stiffness (SAH)

BP

Pulse (? AF)

Cardiac exam

? Aortic aneurysm

Urine (glucose; protein; blood)

Splinter haemorrhages

- Ipsilateral Horner's syndrome
- Cerebellar ataxia
- Contralateral loss of pain and temperature (spino-thalamic) sensation below the lesion
- Sometimes, ipsilateral Vth nerve involvement because of damage to the spinal trigeminal nucleus

Investigation
Haematology
- *Full blood count (FBC):* to detect polycythaemia, thrombocytosis or anaemia
- *ESR and C-reactive protein (CRP):* to exclude arteritis or bacterial endocarditis
- *Urea and electrolytes:* to reveal any electrolyte disturbance that might mimic stroke
- *Blood glucose:* as hyper- and hypoglycaemia can mimic stroke, and diabetes mellitus is a risk factor
- *Serum cholesterol:* as this is a risk factor for stroke
- *Syphilis serology:* as syphilis is a rare but treatable cause of stroke
- *Coagulopathy studies:* including proteins C and S and antithrombin III
- *Autoantibodies:* including antinuclear factor (ANF), rheumatoid factor, antineutrophil cytoplasmic antibody (ANCA), anticardiolipin antibodies
- *Blood film:* to exclude malaria or disseminated intravascular coagulation

Microbiology
Blood cultures should be performed if there is any suspicion of bacterial endocarditis (e.g. fever, raised ESR, cardiac murmur).

Diagnostic imaging
- *Chest radiography:* to detect cardiac sources of emboli
- *CT scan:* should be performed within 48 h, and sooner if there is doubt about the diagnosis of stroke; if thrombolysis is being considered; and if cerebellar infarction or haemorrhage (with or without obstructive hydrocephalus) is suspected
- *Echocardiography:* to detect a patent foramen ovale or aortic arch atheroma
- *Carotid Doppler:* for stroke or TIA in the anterior circulation where the patient is a potential candidate for carotid endarterectomy

Electrophysiology
ECG to detect cardiac sources of emboli, 'silent' myocardial infarction or left ventricular hypertrophy.

Management
Management is based on general supportive treatment including management of complications; specific treat-

---

Emergency 13.1: Management of acute stroke

Immediate management
Investigations
FBC, urea and electrolytes, glucose, chest X-ray and ECG
Head CT as soon as possible

Treatment
Aspirin (given rectally if the patient cannot swallow)
Recombinant tissue plasminogen activator (rt-PA) thrombolysis within 3 h of onset for ischaemic stroke
Surgical drainage of hydrocephalus where this complicates cerebellar strokes

Identify and treat any underlying conditions including
- Atrial fibrillation
- Bacterial endocarditis
- Temporal arteritis

Prevent complications arising from immobility
Support a paralysed arm to prevent frozen shoulder
Passive exercises and compression stockings for the paralysed leg to prevent deep-vein thrombosis
Turn the patient regularly to prevent pressure sores
Assess urinary continence, and catheterize if appropriate

Manage any neurological complications
Place in the recovery position if drowsy or unconscious
Arrange early assessment of speech and swallowing by the speech therapist
If there are swallowing difficulties, insert a nasogastric tube or start an intravenous infusion

Rehabilitate
Transfer the patient to a dedicated stroke unit
If there is hemianopia, position the patient with their bedside locker, on the main ward, on their non-hemianopic side

---

ments depending on the type of stroke; and identification and management of reversible risk factors (EMERGENCY BOX 13.1; Table 13.5).

Prognosis
After an **ischaemic stroke** the prognosis depends on the type of infarct (Table 13.3):
- Risk of death within 30 days is 3–50%
- Risk of another stroke within the first year is 5–10%
- Annual risk of stroke thereafter is 5%
- Annual risk of stroke, myocardial infarction or vascular death is 10%

After a **TIA** the prognosis is:
- Risk of death within 30 days is less than 1%
- Risk of a first stroke within the first year is 12%
- Annual risk of first stroke thereafter is 5%

Table 13.5 Secondary prevention following stroke. As well as having a substantial risk of recurrent stroke, patients with transient ischaemic attack (TIA) and stroke have a high risk of myocardial infarction and death from other vascular diseases

All patients (cerebral infarcts and haemorrhages)

Treat hypertension
Unless the blood pressure is markedly elevated (sustained readings greater than 240/120 mmHg) do not lower blood pressure in the first 7 days following stroke
Thereafter, a reduction in diastolic blood pressure of 5–7 mmHg with antihypertensive drugs is associated with a 30–40% reduction in the risk of stroke over the next few years

Stop smoking
Stopping smoking is associated with a substantial reduction in the risk of myocardial infarction and with a probable reduction in the risk of stroke

Reduce saturated fat content of diet
A 10% decrease in plasma cholesterol is likely to reduce the risk of future coronary heart disease events by 20%

Ischaemic stroke and TIA patients only

Antiplatelet drug therapy
Aspirin reduces the risk of further stroke or of myocardial infarction by 25% and of vascular death by 15%. A dosage of 75 mg/day is probably adequate

Anticoagulants
Warfarinization results in a markedly reduced risk of recurrent stroke in those with rheumatic mitral valve disease and atrial fibrillation. It may also be of benefit where the risk of recurrent stroke is somewhat lower (e.g. in non-valvular atrial fibrillation and with bioprosthetic valves)
Avoid anticoagulation in active bacterial endocarditis and in the first 10 days following stroke

Diuretic + ACE inhibitor
The PROGRESS trial demonstrated that combination treatment with a diuretic (indapamide) and an angiotensin-converting enzyme (ACE) inhibitor (perindopril) resulted in reduced vascular events and deaths even in those without high blood pressure

HMG-CoA reductase inhibitor
The MRC/BHF Heart Protection Study demonstrated that treatment with an HMG-CoA reductase inhibitor (simvastatin) following stroke resulted in reduced vascular events even in those without hypercholesterolaemia

Carotid endarterectomy
Where patients have had a carotid distribution event (stroke or TIA) with good recovery and carotid Doppler scans suggest a stenosis of greater than 70% on the relevant side, carotid endarterectomy results in a reduced risk of recurrent stroke *if* it is performed within 6 months. For individual risk assessment see http://www.dcn.ed.ac.uk/model/carotid.asp. In patients who would be candidates for endarterectomy, carotid Doppler scan and surgical referral as appropriate are therefore an important part of the initial stroke work-up

Primary intracerebral haemorrhage

Correct any haemostatic deficit
Rarely, patients with coagulopathies caused by deficiency of clotting factors (e.g. haemophilia) or liver disease may present with intracerebral haemorrhage. These should be treated where possible

Angiography
If the position of the haematoma is not typical of a hypertensive bleed (If it is central rather than peripheral), and if there is no good explanation for the bleed (haemostatic deficit, cocaine use), cerebral angiography should be performed to detect any underlying aneurysm or arteriovenous malformation

● Annual risk of stroke, myocardial infarction or vascular death is 8%

Subarachnoid haemorrhage

Subarachnoid haemorrhage (SAH) accounts for about 5% of all strokes.

Epidemiology

Annual incidence. 10 in 100 000.

Age. Most common in people over 60 years, although can affect any age.

Sex. Slightly more common in females.

13

Disease mechanisms

The causes of SAH are ruptured cerebral aneurysm (90%), ruptured AVM (5%) and, more rarely, mycotic aneurysm associated with subacute bacterial endocarditis and coagulation disorders.

Clinical features

Subarachnoid haemorrhage causes sudden onset severe headache, which reaches a peak within a few minutes; patients may describe it as 'like being hit on the back of the head with a hammer'. It is usually associated with nausea, vomiting and photophobia and the patient may lose consciousness. A focal neurological deficit may be present if there is bleeding into brain parenchyma. Neck stiffness may not be a feature until some hours after the onset, or it may be absent if the bleed is small.

Investigation

CT scanning

This shows blood in the subarachnoid space in 97% of cases if performed early; after a few days CT is less reliable. CT may also give some clue to the site of origin of the haemorrhage, and may identify complications such as hydrocephalus, haematoma and infarction caused by vasospasm.

Lumbar puncture

Where there is evidence of meningeal irritation (headache; nausea; vomiting; neck stiffness) and the CT is normal it is prudent to exclude CT-negative SAH and other causes of meningeal irritation (e.g. meningitis) at lumbar puncture. Uniform blood staining of the CSF and xanthochromia in the supernatant of a centrifuged sample confirms the diagnosis. In the diagnosis of SAH, lumbar puncture is performed at least 8 h after headache onset to allow time for the blood to reach the lumbar subarachnoid space.

Angiography

Once SAH has been confirmed, cerebral angiography is used to determine the presence of cerebral aneurysms to allow identification of neurosurgical ('clipping') or neuroradiological ('coiling') targets.

Management

See EMERGENCY BOX 13.2.

Prognosis

Five to 10% die before they get to hospital and 30–50% of patients die within the first month; 50% of the survivors remain dependent. Early deaths may be because of the effects of the initial bleed; rebleeding from the same aneurysm; cerebral ischaemia caused by vasospasm; and

---

Emergency 13.2: Management of suspected subarachnoid haemorrhage

Immediate management

Investigation
Urgent head CT
Lumbar puncture (at least 8 h after headache onset) if the CT is negative
Neurosurgical referral

Treatment
Nimodipine
Analgesia and antiemetic for pain and nausea, respectively
Ensure adequate fluid intake

Complications
Deteriorating neurological status may be a result of:
- A rebleed
- Vasospasm with cerebral ischaemia
- Hydrocephalus
- Systemic disturbances such as hypoxia or hypotension

Hyponatraemia may occur because of high levels of atrial natriuretic factor
Cardiac arrhythmias or neurogenic pulmonary oedema may develop because of high levels of circulating catecholamines

Patients should therefore be monitored intensively including frequent neurological examination and Glasgow Coma Scale (GCS). Deterioration should lead to a search for systemic causes (hypoxia; hypotension) and if these are not found a repeat CT may demonstrate vasospastic infarction, rebleed or hydrocephalus

---

complications of neurosurgical or neuroradiological interventions.

Cortical venous and dural sinus thrombosis

Epidemiology

Prevalence. Rare.

Sex. More common in females.

Disease mechanisms

The risk factors for cortical venous and dural sinus thrombosis include oral contraception, smoking, pregnancy or labour, dehydration, ecstasy misuse, hypercoagulable states, middle ear infection, sinusitis and Behçet's disease.

Clinical features

The clinical manifestations of cortical venous and dural sinus thrombosis are variable; occlusion of cortical veins

causes focal neurological signs and seizures, whereas occlusion of the dural sinuses causes raised intracranial pressure. The diagnosis should be considered in any patient with:
- Sudden or evolving headache without meningism
- Declining conscious level and seizures, mimicking encephalitis
- A focal neurological deficit mimicking stroke
- Proptosis and ophthalmoplegia (in cavernous sinus thrombosis)
- Headaches, papilloedema and raised intracranial pressure, but normal CT scan, mimicking benign intracranial hypertension

Investigation
- *CT scan:* may show wedge-shaped infarcts that do not correspond with any arterial territory, and there may be small foci of haemorrhage
- *Contrast enhanced CT:* may show the delta sign—dark clot in the lumen of the sagittal sinus where there should be brightly enhancing blood
- *CT venography:* demonstrates the major cerebral venous structures
- *MRI scanning* of brain parenchyma and *MR venography* to examine the cerebral venous system: both sensitive and non-invasive

Management
Treatment aims to reduce intracranial pressure if necessary. If there is significant neurological impairment with reduced conscious level then anticoagulation (intravenous heparin followed by oral warfarin) may be useful. When symptoms are rapidly progressive, thrombolysis may be indicated. Risk factors should be managed as appropriate.

Prognosis
Varies from excellent in mild cases to 60% mortality in those most severely affected.

Episodic disorders

Blackouts and dizzy turns

Epidemiology
Prevalence. Transient neurological symptoms such as 'blackouts' and 'dizzy turns' are very common.

Age. Most common in people over 60 years of age.

Disease mechanisms
A wide variety of mechanisms can cause these disorders (Table 13.6).

Table 13.6 Causes of 'blackouts', vertigo, 'dizzy spells', 'funny turns' and other episodes without loss of consciousness

Blackouts
Neurological
Epilepsy (common)
Convulsive syncope
Non-convulsive seizure
Non-epileptic seizure
Raised intracranial pressure (rare)
Hydrocephalic attacks
Mass lesion

Cardiovascular (syncope)
Reflex syncope (common)
Reflex syncope (postural, micturition, cough, 'emotional')
Reduced cerebral perfusion
Cardiac syncope (arrhythmia, valvular heart disease, cardiomyopathy, shunt)
Hypovolaemia (dehydration, blood loss)
Disordered blood pressure control (autonomic failure)

Altered content of consciousness
Epilepsy
Partial (focal) epilepsies

True rotational vertigo
Labyrinthine and vestibular dysfunction
Ménière's disease
Benign paroxysmal positional vertigo
Vestibular neuronitis
Ototoxic drugs

Brainstem/vestibular nerve lesion
Acoustic neuroma
Demyelination
Brainstem stroke
Space-occupying lesion in or near the brainstem

Focal brainstem ischaemia
Vertebrobasilar TIA

Light-headedness
Global reduction in cerebral perfusion
Presyncope (as in syncope; see above)
Reduced cerebral perfusion (see above)

Other transient symptoms 'funny turns'
Psychogenic
Hyperventilation attacks
Panic attacks
Non-epileptic seizure

Migraine
Basilar migraine

Sleep disorder
Narcolepsy
Obstructive sleep apnoea

Metabolic
Hypoglycaemia

Clinical features

First determine whether the patient loses consciousness during attacks—if so, they are blackouts. When the complaint is of 'dizziness', ask for a more precise description; if it is 'light-headed', 'faint' or 'about to pass out', the attack was probably caused by reduced cerebral perfusion (syncope) and therefore not neurological. If the patient describes vertigo, 'imbalance' or 'altered content of consciousness', the attack was probably neurological.

- *Labyrinthine or vestibular nerve disorder:* causes only vertigo, nausea and nystagmus.
- *Brainstem lesion:* causes diplopia, dysarthria, dysphagia, blurred vision, quadriparesis or cranial nerve palsies in addition to vertigo.
- *Cerebellar lesion:* may cause unsteadiness, imbalance or 'walking as if drunk', but not vertigo.
- *Presyncope:* comprises light-headedness, faintness, sweating and pallor, which are all worse on standing up and aborted by lying flat. Precipitants include heat, crowds, fear and pain.
- *Complex partial seizures:* accompanied by déjà vu, altered smell and/or taste, and vivid memories; stereotyped movements (e.g. lip smacking), automatisms and an open-eyed trance-like state lasting a few minutes may be reported by witnesses (see p. 902).
- *Absence seizures:* most common in children, and characterized by a very brief loss of contact often accompanied by fluttering of the eyelids.

Investigation

The most important investigation is the clinical history. If the diagnosis is clearly vasovagal, cough or micturition syncope and cardiovascular examination is normal, no tests are required. Conversely, if the diagnosis remains obscure after clinical assessment, even an extensive battery of investigations is unlikely to be helpful.

Haematology
- *FBC:* if suspected severe anaemia
- *Urea and electrolytes and glucose:* if suspected hypovolaemia or metabolic disorder

Diagnostic imaging
- *CT scan:* if hydrocephalic attacks or supratentorial mass lesions suspected
- *MRI scanning:* if there is a suspicion of an acoustic neuroma or intrinsic brainstem or cerebellar lesion

Neurophysiology
- *Routine EEG:* rarely helpful
- *Combined EEG, ECG and video monitoring:* can be very helpful if attacks occur with sufficient frequency

Other investigations
Tests of vestibular function. Patients with vestibular or cochlear lesions may require specialist investigations such as caloric testing or electronystagmography.

Management

The management of specific conditions is described elsewhere. For syncopal attacks, patients should be advised to avoid precipitants where possible and to lie down if they feel an attack coming on.

Prognosis

The prognosis depends on the underlying cause. Where no specific diagnosis can be made, the prognosis is good.

Epilepsy

Epilepsy is a tendency to recurrent seizures, so patients with a single seizure do not have epilepsy. There are many seizure types, each with differing clinical features, prognoses and managements (KEYPOINTS BOX 13.4).

Epidemiology

Prevalence. 400–1000 in 100 000 have active epilepsy and 200 in 100 000 have more than one seizure per month. Two to 5% of the population have had at least one seizure. Annual incidence 20–50 in 100 000.

Age. Peak ages of onset are 0–10 years and over 60 years.

Keypoints 13.4: Epilepsy

Even with a good eyewitness account, distinguishing epilepsy from other causes of altered consciousness can be very difficult

If a patient continues to have seizures on medication, they are not getting enough medication—increase the dose

If a patient has disabling side-effects on medication, they are getting too much medication—reduce the dose

If they are continuing to have seizures and have disabling side-effects, they need a change of medication

Drug-resistant epilepsy is unusual in patients whose nervous system is otherwise normal—so remember that non-epileptic seizures (pseudoseizures) are more common than you think

Remember driving and pregnancy

Table 13.7 Causes of seizures

Systemic disturbances	CNS causes
Fever	*Congenital*
	Birth trauma (hypoxia, or intracranial haemorrhage)
Metabolic disorders	Down's syndrome
Hypoxia, hypo- and hyperglycaemia	Lipid storage diseases
Electrolyte imbalance	Tuberous sclerosis
Porphyria	
Pyridoxine deficiency	*Hereditary*
Inborn errors of metabolism	Genetic epilepsy
	Vascular
Organ failure	Cerebral infarction
Hepatic	Primary intracerebral haemorrhage
Renal	Aneurysmal subarachnoid haemorrhage (SAH) and operative
Respiratory	surgery
	Arteriovenous malformation
Toxins	
Alcohol withdrawal or excess	*Trauma*
Drugs (see below)	Diffuse brain injury
Antidepressants (tricyclics, monoamine oxidase	Penetrating injury/depressed fracture
inhibitors)	Haematoma
Antipsychotics (phenothiazines, lithium)	
Analgesics (pethidine, dextropropoxyphene)	*Cerebral tumour*
Anxiolytics (benzodiazepine withdrawal)	Benign or malignant, primary or secondary tumours
Antiarrhythmics (lidocaine)	*Infective*
Antibiotics (penicillins, isoniazid, nalidixic acid)	Bacterial meningitis
Anaesthetic agents (ether, halothane, methohexitane,	Cerebral abscess
althesin)	Viral encephalitis
Recreational drugs (amphetamine, cocaine, opiates,	HIV/AIDS
derivatives of lysergic acid and amphetamines)	*Other*
Radiographical contrast media	Hydrocephalus

Genetics. Some rare forms of epilepsy are inherited as single gene disorders; Baltic myoclonic epilepsy is caused by mutations in the cystatin B gene. Many other epilepsies have a genetic component.

Disease mechanisms

Epilepsy may be secondary to:
- Systemic disturbances
- Drugs
- CNS disorders (Table 13.7)

but in 60% no cause is found.

In those who have a tendency to seizures, attacks may be provoked by:
- Fatigue
- Missed meals
- Hypoglycaemia
- Alcohol
- Stroboscopic light
- Flickering television or computer screens

Seizures can themselves lower the seizure threshold ('kindling'), and this explains the tendency for patients to have 'runs' of seizures interspersed between long seizure-free periods. Tumours are responsible for 1% of cases of epilepsy occurring in those under 30 years, 16% in 50–59-year-olds and 11% in those over 60 years.

Seizure thresholds vary but most people, given a sufficient stimulus, have the capacity to have a seizure. The most common seizure type is partial seizures, which often evolve into secondary generalized seizures.

After a burst of activity, excitatory neurones of the neocortex have a refractory period of reduced excitability. This process is modulated by inhibitory (γ-aminobutyric acid; GABA) and excitatory (glutamate) neurotransmitters. When the reduction in excitability is incomplete, seizures may result from an uncontrolled and recursive recruitment of neighbouring neurones; this process may remain localized (causing a partial seizure) or spread to the entire cortex (causing a generalized seizure).

Clinical features

A first-hand eye witness account is an essential addition to the patient's own description of any attacks. Record the

Table 13.8 Common epilepsy syndromes

GENERALIZED SEIZURES	Intense familiarity *déjà vu* or vivid stereotyped memory
Tonic–clonic epilepsy	Loss of speech
Clinical features	Lip smacking
Falls to ground if standing	Staring into space, uncommunicative for a few minutes
Sudden stiffness and loss of consciousness	Amnesic during attack
Followed by rhythmic jerking of all four limbs	Odd semipurposeful limb movements
May be incontinence and biting of the side of the tongue	May perform complex stereotyped tasks during complex partial seizure
Postictal drowsiness and confusion	
EEG during attack	*EEG during attack*
Generalized spike and wave	Spikes or sharp waves over the temporal lobes, sometimes with rhythmic slowing
Absence seizures	**Partial motor seizures**
Clinical features	*Clinical features*
Brief (5–10 s) loss of contact with surroundings	Turning of head and eyes to one side
Eyes open and staring	Twitching of one hand or arm, or side of face, which may spread from hand to face or from face to hand
Does not fall	Postictal hemiparesis (Todd's paralysis) sometimes occurs
Loses thread of conversation	
Extremely rare in adults	
EEG during attack	*EEG during attack*
Generalized 3-s spike and wave	Focal epileptic activity may be recorded over relevant brain area
PARTIAL SEIZURES	**Partial sensory seizures**
Partial seizures are *simple partial* if consciousness is normal and *complex partial* if consciousness is impaired	*Clinical features*
	Tingling or pins and needles ('positive' sensory phenomena), which may spread over one side of the body (leg to arm, or face to hand to leg) over a few minutes
Temporal lobe seizures	
Clinical features	*EEG during attack*
Onset difficult to describe but may be instantly recognized by the patient, and may have visceral sensory element	Abnormal spike or sharp discharges
Odd unpleasant smell or taste at onset	

evolution of the attack, the circumstances in which the attack occurred, and the speed of onset and recovery.

Diagnosis

Correct diagnosis is essential; once a diagnostic label of epilepsy has been applied it is very difficult to remove. If in doubt make no diagnosis at all instead of falsely labelling someone as 'epileptic'.

A seizure is diagnosed on the basis of:
- A convincing witness account
- The description matching a known seizure type (Table 13.8)
- Exclusion of other causes of funny turns (e.g. syncope, postural hypotension or cardiac arrhythmia; or focal symptoms caused by migraine or TIA)

Epilepsy is diagnosed when more than one seizure has occurred.

Investigation

Haematology

FBC, ESR, urea and electrolytes, liver function tests, calcium and glucose are checked in acutely ill patients with seizures to detect a metabolic cause and before starting anticonvulsant drugs.

Diagnostic imaging

CT will exclude significant space-occupying lesions. MRI will also allow identification of hippocampal atrophy in mesial temporal sclerosis and of areas of grey matter heterotopia (EPILEPSY AT A GLANCE, Fig. B).

Neurophysiology

Ictal (within-attack) EEG is the test of choice for diagnosing epilepsy, but between attacks the EEG may be normal (Table 13.9).

Management

Management aims to identify the cause of the seizures where one exists, to minimize complications and to reduce seizure frequency to the lowest possible level (Table 13.10). Attention to the psychological and social aspects of epilepsy is important, and the involvement of an

Epilepsy at a glance

Epidemiology
Prevalence
Approximately 1 in 100 people have active epilepsy

Age
Peaks in the very young and the elderly

Genetics
Juvenile myoclonic epilepsy is genetically determined
Some epilepsies show autosomal dominant inheritance

Clinical features
Seizures, often partial
Loss or altered awareness
Abnormal sensory symptoms
Tingling and pins and needles of one hand or arm, side of face, spreading from hand to face or vice versa
Abnormal movements, posture

Findings on investigation
Blood tests
• *FBC and ESR:* to detect systemic symptoms of hepatic, renal and respiratory disease
• *Urea and electrolytes, liver function tests, calcium and glucose:* to detect metabolic causes

Diagnostic imaging
• *CT or MRI:* may show structural brain lesions

• *Functional imaging (fMRI, SPECT):* may show increased metabolic activity in brain regions where attacks start

EEG findings
• *Partial motor seizures:* focal epileptic activity over relevant brain area
• *Partial sensory seizures:* abnormal spike or sharp discharges
• *Tonic–clonic epilepsy:* generalized spike and wave
• *Absence seizures:* generalized 3-s spike and wave
• *Juvenile myoclonic epilepsy:* polyspike
• *Temporal lobe seizures:* spikes or sharp waves over temporal lobes

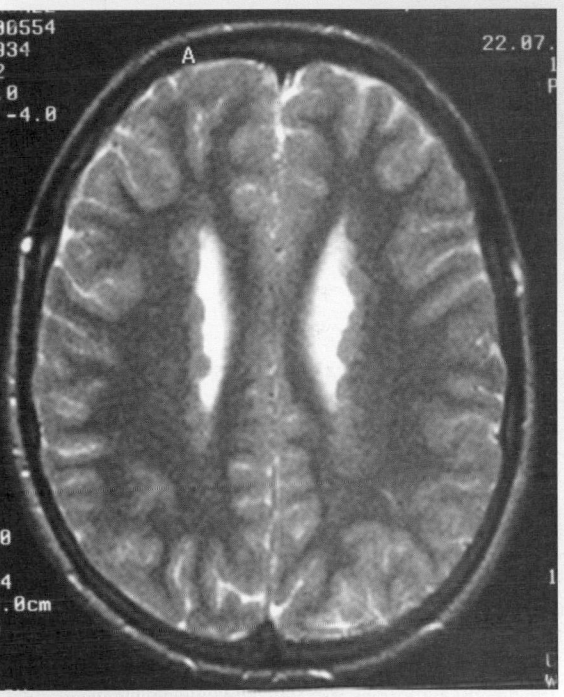

Fig. B MRI showing grey heterotopia on ventricular surface in a patient with treatment-resistant epilepsy.

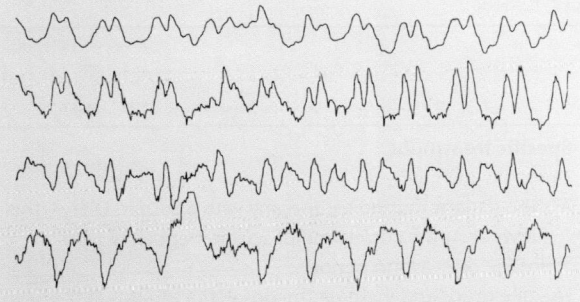

Fig. A Generalized spike-and-wave EEG.

epilepsy nurse practitioner can be invaluable. The management of status epilepticus is discussed in EMERGENCY BOX 13.3.

Who to treat
In adult patients with a single unprovoked seizure or with seizures separated by several years, anticonvulsants may not be necessary. Those with recurrent seizures should be treated unless the attacks are so mild and with such little

impact that the patient prefers their seizures to the side-effects of drugs.

Advice about driving and other activities
• In the UK, responsibility for initiating contact with the DVLA rests with the patient
• For class I licences, patients with daytime seizures will have their licence withdrawn until they have been seizure-free for 1 year

13

Table 13.9 Idiopathic generalized, symptomatic generalized and partial epilepsy syndromes

	Seizure type	Age at onset	EEG	Other features	Approximate remission rate (%)
Idiopathic generalized epilepsy syndromes					
Tonic–clonic epilepsy	Tonic–clonic	3–25 years	Normal or generalized spike and wave	Family history	60
Childhood and juvenile absence seizures	Absence	3–15 years	3-s spike and wave	Family history	70–80
Juvenile myoclonic epilepsy	Tonic–clonic, early morning myoclonus	8–26 years	Polyspike	Family history	Almost 100 with sodium valproate
Symptomatic generalized epilepsy syndromes					
Infantile spasms	Salaam attacks	4 months to 1 year	Hypsarrhythmia	May be associated with severe cerebral underlying abnormality (e.g. damage, tuberous sclerosis)	35–50
Lennox–Gastaut epilepsy	Absence with bilateral myoclonus, tonic seizures, drop attacks	Less than 2 years	Bilateral spike and wave 1–1.25 cycles/s	Mental retardation, unknown cause	35–50
Partial epilepsy syndromes					
Idiopathic partial epilepsy: benign focal motor epilepsy of childhood	Simple motor	8–12 years	Focal spikes	Unknown cause	80
Symptomatic partial epilepsy: complex partial epilepsy	Complex partial with or without tonic–clonic features	Adolescence	Normal or focal abnormality	May be associated with hippocampal sclerosis, tumour	20–40

Table 13.10 Management of seizures and of epilepsy

Supportive treatment

Advice about driving and other activities

Many medical conditions, including epilepsy, impact on driving safety. In the UK, responsibility for informing the driving authorities rests with the patient not the doctor

Following a seizure patients will have their licence revoked for 1 year

However, patients who have only ever had seizures at night may be permitted to drive once this pattern of night-time-only seizures has been established for 3 years

A single seizure leads to a 10-year suspension on class II (heavy goods vehicles and public service vehicle) licences

For other activities (work, swimming, cycling, climbing ladders), patients should be encouraged to make decisions about risk for themselves, based on the likelihood of having a seizure in any given context, and the consequences to their safety if they do have a seizure in that context

Specific treatment

Drugs

Ask the patient to monitor therapy with a Seizure Diary—this allows accurate correlation of seizure frequency with dosage over a long period

Use one drug, and increase the dose until seizures are controlled or side-effects prohibit further dosage increase

If one drug does not work, try another 'first-line' drug as monotherapy

If three first-line drugs have each proved ineffective, move to combination therapy

Consider gradual withdrawal of anticonvulsants after 2 years seizure-free on treatment—but patients who wish to drive generally opt to stay on treatment

Surgery

Where epilepsy is resistant to treatment and disabling, identification of an epileptogenic focus and its surgical resection can in some cases have dramatic benefits

Emergency 13.3: Management of status epilepticus

Definition

- Single seizure lasting more than 30 min, or
- Sequence of seizures lasting more than 30 min without full recovery between

Treatment

- Resuscitate—ensure Airway; Breathing; Circulation
- Exclude hypoglycaemia by checking blood sugar level in capillary (pinprick) blood
- Establish venous access
- Ensure facilities for providing full respiratory support are available
- Give intravenous diazepam

If this does not stop the seizure:

- Start intravenous phenytoin infusion under ECG monitoring
- Failing which seek expert help with view to management in intensive care unit

- Further treatment options while in intensive care unit include propofol and thiopental

Further considerations

What caused the seizures?

- Poor drug compliance
- Drug intoxication or withdrawal
- Central nervous system infection
- Intracranial haemorrhage
- Pseudostatus

In patients already on anticonvulsants, restart their usual drug at the usual dose as soon as possible—usually by nasogastric tube

In patients not already on anticonvulsants, start the drug that will be used for long-term control

Keep the anticonvulsant regimen simple, and do not keep changing things—give the drugs a chance to work

Watch for respiratory depression and metabolic disturbance

Drug	Action	Side-effects	Contraindications
Diazepam	Benzodiazepine—enhances GABA signalling	Hypotension, respiratory depression	Respiratory depression, psychosis, porphyria
Phenytoin	Prevents spread of abnormal activity in neuronal membranes	Cardiac arrhythmias	Sinus bradycardia, heart block, porphyria
Propofol	Barbiturate—enhances GABA signalling	Hypotension, bradycardia, respiratory depression, phlebitis, hyperlipidaemia	
Thiopental	Barbiturate—enhances GABA signalling	Hypotension, respiratory depression, phlebitis	Porphyria

- Patients who have only ever had seizures during sleep may be permitted to drive if such a pattern has been established over 3 years
- For class II licences (HGV, PSV) a single seizure will lead to withdrawal of the licence for at least 10 years
- For other activities (work, swimming, cycling, climbing ladders) advice depends on seizure type and frequency, but should be guided by an assessment of the consequences of having a seizure while engaged in the activity
- Following a simple faint there are no restrictions on driving; following a loss of consciousness likely to be unexplained syncope, with a low risk of recurrence, the patient should be advised not to drive until 4 weeks after the event
- Patients withdrawing from treatment should be advised not to drive until 6 months after withdrawal is complete

Drugs

The dosage of a single drug should be increased until either seizures are controlled or side-effects become intolerable, in which case the patient may be switched to an alternative first-line drug or have a second-line agent added in combination therapy.

Choice of anticonvulsant drug (Table 13.11)

- Sodium valproate, carbamazepine and phenytoin are equally effective for patients with generalized tonic–clonic or partial seizures, but the side-effects of phenytoin restrict its use as a first-line agent
- Valproate and carbamazepine are usually given twice daily and are available in sustained release preparations
- Absence seizures and myoclonic epilepsy respond best to sodium valproate
- Lamotrigine, topiramate, tiagabine, gabapentin and levitiracetam are newer drugs commonly used as add-on therapy for seizures that are resistant to monotherapy
- Clonazepam and clobazam are benzodiazepines that can be used as add-on therapy in patients with generalized seizures (tonic–clonic, absence or myoclonic)

Table 13.11 Drug treatment of epilepsy. *Note*. This information is for guidance only. Full details should be checked in the *British National Formulary* before prescribing

Drug	Action	Indications	Side-effects	Contraindications	Patient monitoring
First-line agents					
Phenytoin	Prevents spread of abnormal activity in neuronal membranes	Generalized seizures	Acute: ataxia, nausea, diplopia, cardiac arrhythmias; chronic: facial hair, acne, gum hypertrophy	Heart block, porphyria	Clinical monitoring essential; drug monitoring *may* be useful if poor compliance is suspected or to confirm toxicity
Carbamazepine	Blockade of voltage-gated sodium channels	All forms of epilepsy Also used in neuralgia	Ataxia, nausea, diplopia; rash; gastrointestinal	Cardiac conduction abnormalities, porphyria and blood disorders, SIADH	
Sodium valproate	Enhances GABAergic transmission	All forms of epilepsy	Gastric irritation, hair loss, disorders of liver function and clotting, jaundice, rashes	Pre-existing liver disease, porphyria	
Second-line agents					
Lamotrigine	Use: dependent blocker of voltage-gated sodium channels	All forms of epilepsy	Rashes, irritability, headache, agranulocytosis	Hepatic or renal impairment	Clinical assessment only
Topiramate	Enhances GABAergic and inhibits glutamatergic transmission through multiple mechanisms	Partial or generalized seizures	Abdominal pain, nausea, anorexia, weight loss	Hepatic or renal impairment	
Gabapentin	Not known	Partial seizures with or without secondary generalization	Somnolence, ataxia, nausea, diplopia; weight gain	Psychotic illness, renal impairment	
Levitiracetam	Unknown	Partial seizures	Drowsiness, dizziness, anorexia, rash	Hepatic or renal impairment	
Tiagabine	Inhibits GABA reuptake	Partial seizures with or without secondary generalization	Diarrhoea, dizziness, fatigue, emotional lability	Hepatic impairment	
Clonazepam	Benzodiazepine	Resistant epilepsy and status epilepticus	Drowsiness, mood changes	Respiratory depression, porphyria	
Phenobarbital/primidone	Enhances GABA transmission	Generalized tonic–clonic, partial, atypical absence, atonic and tonic seizures	Drowsiness, lethargy, ataxia, allergic skin reactions, megaloblastic anaemia	Elderly, frail, children, respiratory, hepatic or renal failure; avoid sudden withdrawal	
Clobazam	Enhances GABA transmission	Adjunct in epilepsy	Drowsiness, confusion, ataxia, dependence	Respiratory insufficiency, sleep apnoea	
Ethosuximide	Inhibits Na and Ca channels	Absence seizures	Gastrointestinal disturbance, weight loss, drowsiness, ataxia, psychosis, agranulocytosis	Hepatic and renal impairment	

- Phenytoin manifests zero-order pharmacokinetics, so dosage should be increased in small increments (25 mg) to avoid toxicity
- Because of differences in bioavailability, anticonvulsants should be prescribed by both their generic and their commercial names

Monitoring therapy

Blood levels have no role in the routine monitoring of anticonvulsant treatment; if the patient is still having seizures the dose is too low, and if they are getting side-effects (impaired concentration, drowsiness, unsteadiness, incoordination and nystagmus) the dose is too high.

If they are still getting seizures and they are getting side-effects then they need a different anticonvulsant, either instead of or as well as their current drug. Watch for chronic anticonvulsant toxicity (Table 13.12), which can affect virtually any body system.

Record seizure frequency. The patient's recollection of the frequency and severity of their seizures can be patchy; a seizure diary allows accurate correlation of seizure frequency with factors such as anticonvulsant dosage.

Changing anticonvulsant. If seizures are not controlled on the first anticonvulsant, change to another first-line agent, withdrawing the first drug after an overlap period of 3–4 weeks. Avoid using more than one anticonvulsant until all first-line treatments have been tried in adequate dosage.

When to stop anticonvulsants. After some years free of seizures, patients may want to find out if their epilepsy has gone away, and if they still need treatment. Actuarial risk of recurrence can be estimated using on-line algorithms (e.g. http://www.dcn.ed.ac.uk/model/epilepsy.asp). Drugs should be withdrawn one at a time, and gradually. Do not stop sodium valproate therapy in patients with juvenile monoclonic epilepsy as relapse is universal. Patients should be advised not to drive for 6 months after a reduction in their anticonvulsant dosage; in practice, most drivers choose to stay on treatment.

Management of epilepsy during pregnancy
(See Table 13.13.)

Table 13.12 Manifestations of chronic anticonvulsant toxicity

Nervous system
Memory and cognitive impairment
Behavioural disturbance
Pseudodementia
Cerebellar atrophy
Peripheral neuropathy

Skin
Erythematous skin rash (carbamazepine, lamotrigine)
Acne (phenytoin)
Hirsutism
Alopecia

Liver
Enzyme induction

Blood/reticuloendothelial system
Megaloblastic anaemia
Thrombocytopenia
Lymphadenopathy

Immune system
IgA deficiency
SLE-like syndrome

Bone
Osteomalacia

Connective tissue disorders
Gum hypertrophy (phenytoin)
Coarsened facial features (phenytoin)

Pregnancy
Obstetric complications
Teratogenicity
Spina bifida (valproate)
Fetal hydantoin syndrome (phenytoin)

IgA, immunoglobulin A; SLE, systemic lupus erythematosus.

Table 13.13 Management of epilepsy during pregnancy

Problems
Anticonvulsants may affect fetus
• Risk of teratogenicity probably doubles
• Phenytoin causes congenital heart disease, cleft lip and palate
• Carbamazepine causes craniofacial problems and spina bifida
• Valproate causes neural tube defects
May be increased seizure frequency and status epilepticus
• Increased plasma and extracellular fluid volume
• Fetal and placental drug metabolism
• Antacids reduce absorption of phenytoin by ~ 50%
Increased obstetric complications
Fertility is reduced by about 30% in women with epilepsy

Preconception
If seizure-free for more than 2 years, consider gradual anticonvulsant withdrawal at least 6 months prior to conception (but note that patients should not drive until 6 months after medication has been withdrawn)
Simplify anticonvulsant regimen to one drug if possible
Discuss teratogenicity
Start oral folic acid supplementation
Check drug levels

During pregnancy
Screen (using α-fetoprotein, ultrasound and amniocentesis) for neural tube defect if on valproate
Monitor drug levels and increase dosage if levels fall
Avoid CBZ and VPA in pregnancy—but after 8 weeks' gestation any teratogenicity will have occurred
Regular (monthly) clinic review

Postpartum
Reduce anticonvulsant dose to prepregnancy levels as appropriate
Reassure the patient that breastfeeding is safe

CBZ, carbamazepine; VPA, valproate.

Surgery

Surgical resection of an identified isolated epileptogenic focus can lead to complete remission of seizures, but the number of patients who are likely to derive benefit from surgery is small.

Prognosis

● Following a first seizure, 50–80% of patients will have a further seizure within 2–3 years
● Two-thirds of patients with epilepsy go into anticonvulsant drug-free remission within 10 years

Transient global amnesia

Disease mechanisms

The cause is unknown.

Epidemiology

Prevalence. Rare.

Age. Usually middle-aged or elderly.

Clinical features

The syndrome is characterized by the sudden onset of an inability to form new memories and lasts for a few hours. During an attack, the patient is fully conscious and alert but is bewildered. They will repeatedly ask questions such as 'Where am I?', and each time they cannot remember the reply. During the attack there may be retrograde amnesia stretching back months or years. Complex actions, including driving a car, can be performed apparently normally. After the attack, amnesia for the attack itself persists, but the period of retrograde amnesia gradually resolves.

Investigation

Detailed investigation is not usually indicated unless the patient has recurrent attacks, associated brainstem symptoms suggesting vertebrobasilar TIA, or frequent stereotyped short-lived attacks with some warning or aura suggesting complex partial seizures.

Management

Reassurance.

Prognosis

Good—most patients have only one or two attacks and there are no long-term sequelae.

Sleep disorders

Sleep disorders can be classified as insomnia, excessive daytime sleepiness and parasomnias.

Epidemiology

Prevalence. Insomnia is very common. Other sleep disorders are fairly rare.

Genetics. Narcolepsy is strongly associated with HLA-DR2.

Disease mechanisms

Insomnia can result from poor sleeping habits (late to bed and late to rise), anxiety, depression, pain and the restless legs syndrome; excessive daytime sleepiness may be primary (e.g. caused by narcolepsy) or secondary (e.g. caused by encephalopathy, intracranial mass lesions, obstructive sleep apnoea, drugs, sedatives). Other sleep disorders (parasomnias) include sleep walking, night terrors and nocturnal enuresis.

Clinical features

Narcolepsy is associated with cataplexy (a sudden loss of muscle tone and collapse in response to emotional stimuli), vivid dreams, hypnapagogic hallucinations and sleep paralysis. There is often a positive family history.

Obstructive sleep apnoea should be suspected in patients with excessive daytime sleepiness who snore loudly, who have morning headaches, who find they are not refreshed by sleep or who are reported to have nocturnal apnoeas.

Investigation

Full blood count, urea, electrolytes, glucose, liver and thyroid function should be checked in patients with excessive daytime sleepiness. Sleep studies (polysomnography), which include EEG, carbon dioxide and oxygen saturation, help confirm the diagnosis of obstructive sleep apnoea.

Management and prognosis

● *Insomnia:* improve sleep hygiene (avoid daytime naps) and use night-time sedatives very sparingly.
● *Obstructive sleep apnoea:* patients should be advised to lose weight and to avoid sleeping on their back; sedative drugs should be avoided and continuous positive airways pressure is often very helpful. The role of uvulopalatopharyngoplasty is not clear.
● *Narcolepsy:* may respond to modafinil.
● *Cataplexy:* may respond to clomipramine.

Headache and facial pain

Recurrent headache is one of the most common neurological problems and is usually caused by tension headache or migraine. Although patients (and sometime doctors) may worry about the possibility of an underlying tumour, the chances are very high that tumour is not the cause.

Epidemiology

Prevalence. Prevalence of severe migraine is 2000 in 100 000. Annual incidence 250 in 100 000. Tension headache is many times more common than migraine, but exact figures are not known. Mild migraine is many times more common than severe migraine.

Age. Any age, but onset of migraine is rare after 50 years of age.

Sex. More common in females.

Genetics. People with migraine often have a first-degree relative with migraine.

Disease mechanisms

The mechanism of tension headache and migraine are not clearly understood. The mechanisms of less common causes of headache include:
- Changes in intracranial pressure
- Meningeal irritation
- Distension, traction or dilatation of the intracranial or extracranial arteries
- Traction, displacement or occlusion of large intracranial veins or their dural envelopes
- Compression, traction or inflammation of the sensory cranial and spinal nerves
- Voluntary or involuntary spasm or inflammation of cranial or cervical muscles

Clinical features

Chronic headache

In most cases clinical examination is normal. Diagnosis is therefore based almost entirely on the history—on the type, character and pattern of the headache (Fig. 13.11). Other possibilities should be considered if the pattern of symptoms and signs does not match one of these common patterns (Table 13.14). Migraine is a unilateral throbbing headache that may be associated with nausea, vomiting, photo- and phonophobia and is often preceded by visual or sensory auras (Fig. 13.12); the pattern of the attacks is often stereotyped (Fig. 13.13).

Sudden severe headache

Sudden severe headache is much less common than chronic headache, and the differential diagnosis lies between SAH (see p. 897), meningitis and cortical venous thrombosis. Neck stiffness may be absent in both SAH and meningitis.

Investigation

Patients with chronic headache and clear clinical features of tension headache or migraine do not require

Table 13.14 Less common causes of acute or chronic headache

Raised intracranial pressure (ICP)
Cerebral space-occupying lesion
- Extradural haematoma
- Subdural haematoma
- Brain tumour
Intermittent raised ICP with Arnold–Chiari malformation, colloid cyst of IIIrd ventricle
Venous sinus thrombosis

Low ICP
Following lumbar puncture

Distension or dilatation of intracranial or extracranial arteries
Unruptured cerebral aneurysm
Arteriovenous malformation
Cough headache
Benign coital headache

Pain syndromes related to specific cranial nerves
Trigeminal neuralgia
Glossopharyngeal neuralgia

Voluntary or involuntary spasm of cranial and cervical muscles
Cervical spondylosis
Spasmodic torticollis

Other causes
Sinusitis
Dental sepsis
Temporomandibular joint dysfunction
Glaucoma
Hypercapnia
High-altitude sickness

investigation. Sudden severe headache warrants referral to hospital for exclusion of SAH by clinical assessment, CT scan and lumbar puncture.

Haematology

In patients over 50 years, the ESR should be checked to rule out temporal arteritis.

Diagnostic imaging

- *CT:* to diagnose SAH. It should be performed urgently in patients with suspected raised intracranial pressure, particularly if the patient has visual obscurations or an impaired conscious level. Normal optic discs do not rule out raised intracranial pressure.
- *Radiography of the sinuses, teeth or temporomandibular joints:* may be necessary if there is a clinical suspicion that the headache has an extracranial cause.
- *Lumbar puncture:* necessary in the investigation of a sudden headache to exclude SAH if the CT scan is normal.

13

Tension headache
Location
Both temples, or diffuse
Character
Dull tight band round head
Pattern
Continuous, 'never free of it', worse in the evening
Other features
Not relieved by analgesia, aggravated by stress

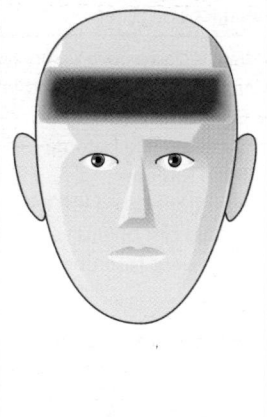

Migraine
Location
One side of head or generalized
Character
Severe, throbbing, banging
Pattern
Episodic, stereotyped, lasts 1–48 h, often at weekends
Other features
Stereotyped pattern. Preceded by visual, sensory, or other aura. Accompanied by photophobia and nausea. Patient may need to lie in a darkened room. Aborted by sleep. Commonly a first-degree relative also has migraine

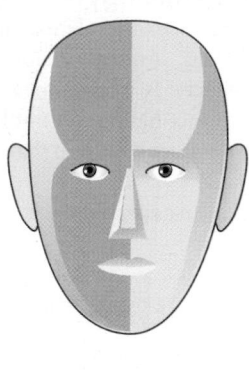

Cluster headache (migranous neuralgia)
Location
Unilateral, centred around one eye
Character
Extremely severe, stabbing, throbbing
Pattern
Episodic, occurs at the same time every day, often in the early hours of the morning, and the attacks are in clusters (i.e. pain once a day for several weeks, and then no pain for months)
Other features
Nausea, photophobia, red eye, nostril feels 'blocked' and eye waters on same side as pain

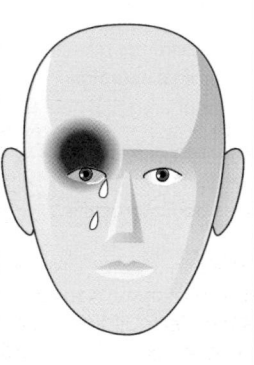

Temporal arteritis
Location
Temples or diffuse
Character
Dull, moderate to severe–sometimes headache is mild or absent, tender scalp, tender temples, 'can't brush hair', 'can't wear hat'
Pattern
Recent onset, continuous
Other features
Over 50 years of age, raised ESR (though a normal ESR does not completely rule out arteritis), aches, pains, and stiffness (polymyalgia rheumatica), episodes of visual loss, pain in jaw on chewing, stroke, weight loss, depression, malaise, pyrexia

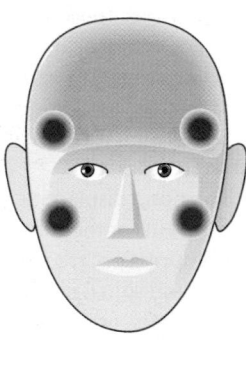

Raised intracranial pressure
Location
Often occipital
Character
Dull
Pattern
Recent onset (within weeks), gradually increasing, present on waking, worse on coughing, bending, straining at stool
Other features
Episodes of blurred/grey vision (visual obscurations), vomiting (a late feature), local neurological symptoms, drowsiness (a late feature), papilloedema (a late feature)

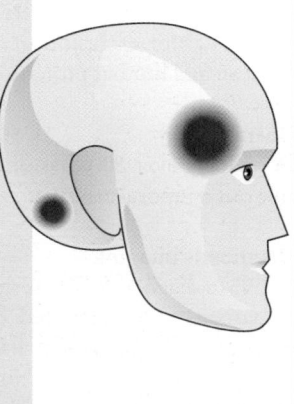

Trigeminal neuralgia
Location
Confined to one division of the fifth cranial nerve
Character
Very severe and very brief (a few seconds) shooting, 'like an electric shock'
Pattern
Precipitated by light, touch, wind, washing, eating
Other features
No abnormal neurological signs, over 40 years of age, relieved by carbamazepine, sometimes occurs in people with multiple sclerosis

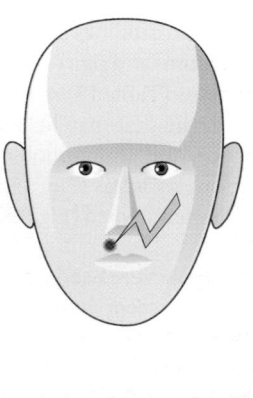

Figure 13.11 Distribution of pain in headache syndromes.

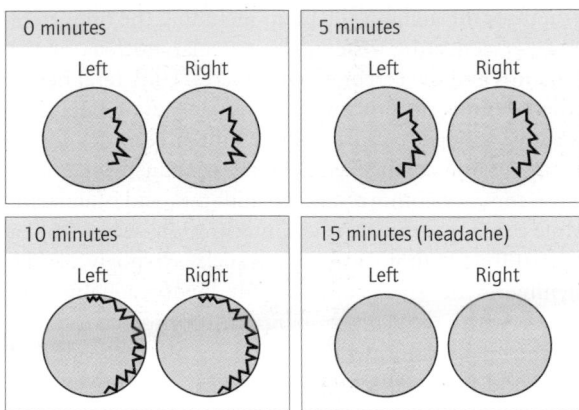

Figure 13.12 Visual aura of migraine. Zigzag lines appear in both eyes in part of the visual field, gradually expand and then disappear, being followed by the headache, which is usually unilateral and associated with nausea and sometimes vomiting.

Duration	Phase	Features
1–30 minutes	Prodrome	'Its going to happen'
30 minutes–72 hours+	Warning	Visual and/or sensory symptoms
	Headache	Nausea and photophobia
	Aftermath	Feels washed out

Figure 13.13 Stereotyped attacks with migraine.

Histopathology

Urgent temporal artery biopsy is mandatory in patients with suspected temporal arteritis. If clinical suspicion is high it should be performed even if the ESR is normal.

Management

The management of different headaches is shown in Tables 13.15 and 13.16. In addition to conventional analgesics and disease-specific treatments, other important interventions include treatment of any underlying depression, patient education and non-pharmacological treatments.

Disorders of consciousness and cognitive function

Coma and brainstem death (HISTORY & EXAMINATION BOX 13.8)

Consciousness depends on the integrity of a number of

Table 13.15 Management of headache

Tension headache
Supportive treatment
Reassure the patient
Advise avoidance of excess caffeine, smoking and alcohol
Advise avoidance of strong analgesics (e.g. dihydrocodeine). Use aspirin or paracetamol instead

Specific treatment
Relaxation therapy
Amitriptyline 10–150 mg at night
Treat any underlying depression

Migraine
Supportive treatment
Reassure the patient that there is no serious underlying cause
Explain good long-term prognosis
Identify and advise avoidance of specific precipitants (e.g. red wine)

Specific treatment
Acute attacks
- Simple analgesics such as aspirin or paracetamol, taken as early in the attack as possible
- Antiemetics if necessary
- Triptans (5-HT$_{1D}$ receptor agonists) are often very effective in severe acute attacks not responding to simple therapy
Prophylaxis
- Where attacks are frequent enough to interfere with work or school, prophylaxis with β-blockers, pizotifen, amitriptyline or sodium valproate may diminish the frequency and severity of attacks

Cluster headache
Supportive treatment
Reassurance of no serious underlying cause

Specific treatment
Acute attacks may respond to a triptan and usually respond to breathing 100% oxygen. Pizotifen prophylaxis may prevent attacks, and attacks may be aborted by verapamil

Temporal arteritis
Specific treatment
Untreated temporal arteritis can cause strokes and blindness; treatment should be started immediately the diagnosis is suspected
Start high-dose oral corticosteroids (60 mg prednisolone) immediately to reduce the risk of irreversible blindness associated with temporal arteritis until the results of a temporal artery biopsy are known
Gradually reduce corticosteroid dosage as symptoms resolve to a target maintenance regimen of 10 mg/day provided the erythrocyte sedimentation rate (ESR) falls with treatment and remains down
Attempt to wean off steroids completely if symptoms controlled and ESR is normal after about 1 year
Sometimes long-term maintenance regimen (e.g. 5–10 mg/day prednisolone) is required

Table 13.16 Migraine treatments

Sumatriptan

5-HT$_1$ agonist

Used for acute treatment of migraine attack

Side-effects. Flushing, dizziness, fatigue

Contraindications. Avoid in patients with a history of ischaemic heart disease or Prinzmetal's angina. Avoid concomitant use with ergotamine-containing agents

Dosage. 50–100 mg orally as soon as possible after onset of attack (maximum dose 300 mg/day) or 6 mg by subcutaneous injector using autoinjector (maximum 12 mg/day)

Pizotifen

Serotonin antagonist with anticholinergic properties

Used in prophylaxis of migraine

Side-effects. Drowsiness, weight gain, dizziness

Contraindications. Caution needed in patients with glaucoma, renal impairment, pregnancy and breastfeeding.

Dosage. 1.5 mg at night. Lower doses may be used if there are troublesome side-effects

structures throughout the brain including the brainstem reticular activating system, the reticular nucleus of the thalamus and the cerebral hemispheres. Unilateral hemisphere lesions do not impair consciousness unless they are large enough to cause midline shift or compression of the upper brainstem (Fig. 13.14). In general, focal lesions cause coma by compressing the midbrain and brainstem, while coma requiring medical intervention results from a more diffuse pathological process such as hypoglycaemia, meningitis or encephalitis. Acute hydrocephalus can present with a rapid onset of impaired consciousness.

Immediate assessment should determine the cause of coma and the need for urgent medical or neurosurgical attention. If neurosurgical attention is required, the patient may require transfer to another hospital and will require appropriate medical support during that transfer.

The level of consciousness is assessed using the Glasgow Coma Scale (HISTORY & EXAMINATION BOX 13.4). Coma may be preceded by the development of focal neurological symptoms (e.g. focal seizures, hemiparesis) and signs and it is crucial to obtain an eye witness account of the

---

History & Examination 13.8: Examination of the comatose patient

Primary survey

Assess and resuscitate

Assess Airway, Breathing, Circulation

Measure blood glucose

Give oxygen

Establish venous access

Monitor ECG, oxygen saturation (SpO$_2$)

Consider naloxone if there is evidence of opiate toxicity (pinpoint pupils, needle 'tracks', reduced respiratory rate)

Consider flumazenil if benzodiazepine overdose is suspected

Take a history

Find out—from ambulance personnel, police or relatives, in person or by telephone—exactly what has happened to the patient. In particular, establish whether there have been focal symptoms, other medical problems and whether the patient is taking any medicines or drugs.

Secondary survey

Detailed clinical examination looking for clues to the cause (cyanosis, rash, neck stiffness, head injury) or for evidence of complications (e.g. fixed dilated pupils)

Priorities in the neurological examination

1 Record the level of consciousness using the Glasgow Coma Scale (Table 13.2).

2 Look for signs of brainstem dysfunction—in particular the pupil size and response to light

3 Look for other signs:
   - Examine the fundi for retinal haemorrhages, subhyaloid haemorrhages and papilloedema
   - Observe eye position for conjugate deviation
   - Test reflexes (corneal, gag, tendon and plantar reflexes)
   - Test for Kernig's sign and neck stiffness

There are clearly limitations to the neurological examination in the unconscious patient, but important information is available: the three most informative signs relate to the pupil response to light, eye movements and the limb response to pain.

Mydriatics should never be used to dilate the pupil of an unconscious patient as this will lead to the loss of one-third of the most useful part of the neurological examination (see above).

Investigation

- *Blood tests.* FBC, urea and electrolytes, liver function tests, calcium, arterial blood gases and pH, also drug screen
- *CT of head.* If there is any doubt as to the cause of the coma
- *EEG.* If there is any possibility that the patient may be unconscious because of an encephalopathy or complex partial status epilepticus
- *Lumbar puncture.* See CLINICAL BOX 13.1

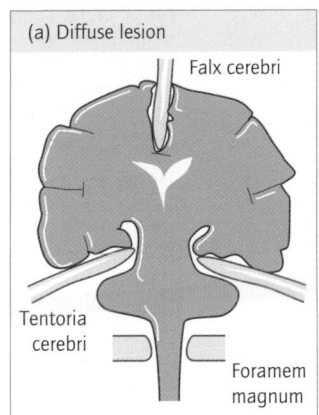
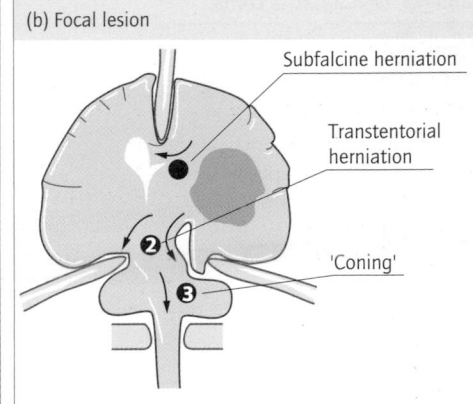

Figure 13.14 Pathophysiology of coma.

evolution of the coma. Such focal disturbance of function usually point to a 'neurosurgical' cause for the coma (e.g. subdural haematoma), but medical conditions such as hypoglycaemia can cause a hemiparesis that resolves on normalization of the blood glucose.

A 'medical' cause of coma is likely if:
● There are no symptoms of focal neurological dysfunction before the coma
● The pupils are equal and reactive to light (see p. 946 for pupil abnormalities)
● The oculocephalic reflex, the caloric responses and the limb response to pain are present and symmetrical

A 'neurosurgical' cause is likely if:
● There are symptoms or signs of focal neurological dysfunction before the coma
● There are asymmetrical pupils or conjugate deviation of the eyes
● There is asymmetry of the oculocephalic reflex, the caloric responses, the limb response to pain or the plantar response

Common medical causes of coma include drugs and alcohol intoxication and diabetic hypoglycaemia. In addition to acute intoxication, coma in alcohol misusers may result from seizures, hypoglycaemia, hepatic encephalopathy, Wernicke's encephalopathy or subdural haematoma complicating head trauma. These alternative diagnoses should be considered before attributing coma in someone said to be 'drunk' to acute alcohol intoxication. SAH may rarely present as coma of sudden onset with no history of antecedent headache, neck stiffness or vomiting. Common causes of coma are summarized in Table 13.17.

Brainstem death
This can only be diagnosed when:
● The patient is unresponsive and requires ventilation

● The coma is brought about by irreversible brain damage **of known cause**
● Sedative or paralytic drugs have worn off and hypothermia or metabolic abnormalities have been corrected
● Brainstem reflexes are absent
● There is no pupillary response to bright light
● There is no corneal reflex
● The oculocephalic response is absent
● There is no response to caloric stimulation
● There is no gag or tracheal reflex
● There are no motor responses in the cranial nerves in response to painful stimulation of limbs
● There is no respiratory effort despite a $P\text{co}_2$ higher than 6.65 kPa off the ventilator

The 'locked-in' syndrome
In some patients, extensive damage to the pons causes quadriplegia and loss of speech while the midbrain and cerebral hemispheres function normally. They are therefore awake, able to hear and think, and have a normal EEG, but are unable to communicate except by vertical movements of their eyes. The cause for this is usually vascular (infarction or haemorrhage), but it may also result from trauma and other destructive lesions of the pons. Some patients recover full functional independence.

Raised intracranial pressure (Table 13.18; EMERGENCY BOX 13.4)

Causes
● Headache that is often present on waking and aggravated by lying flat, coughing, bending or straining
● Brief episodes of loss of vision (visual obscurations), on bending or standing, of sudden onset
● Vomiting
● Neck stiffness, but Kernig's test is negative

Table 13.17 Causes of coma

'Medical' causes (diffuse)

Drug overdose

Alcohol
Intoxication, acute withdrawal
Wernicke's encephalopathy

Organ failure
Cardiac failure/hypotension
Respiratory failure
Hepatic encephalopathy
Renal failure
Anaphylactic shock

Epilepsy
Convulsive status
Non-convulsive (complex partial) status
Postictal state

CNS infection
Encephalitis
Bacterial meningitis
Cerebral malaria

Electrolyte imbalance
Glucose (hypo- and hyperglycaemia)
Sodium (hypo- and hypernatraemia)
Calcium (hypo- and hypercalcaemia)
Oxygen (hypoxia)
Carbon dioxide (hypo- and hypercapnia)
pH (acute acidosis and acute alkalosis)

Endocrine (uncommon cause)
Hypo- and hyperthyroidism
Addison's disease

Vascular
Brainstem stroke

Medically unexplained
Munchausen's syndrome
'Pseudo coma'

'Neurosurgical' causes requiring urgent intervention

Trauma
Penetrating head injury
Head injury with haematoma (subdural, extradural, intracerebral)
Raised intracranial pressure of diffuse brain injury

Vascular
Subarachnoid haemorrhage
Cerebellar haemorrhage or infarction with obstructive hydrocephalus

Raised intracranial pressure
Primary or secondary cerebral tumour
Acute hydrocephalus

Infection
Abscess (intracerebral, extracerebral, extradural)

Table 13.18 Causes of raised intracranial pressure

Focal space-occupying lesion
Tumour
Abscess
Major stroke (e.g. rapidly expanding intracerebral haemorrhage, large infarct with secondary oedema)
Subdural or extradural haematoma

Diffuse brain swelling
Trauma
Encephalitis
CO_2 retention
Acute severe metabolic insult (e.g. severe hypoxia)
Hypertension

Impaired CSF circulation and reabsorption
See Table 13.33

Obstruction to outflow of venous blood
Cerebral venous thrombosis

Unknown
Idiopathic intracranial hypertension

- Papilloedema (not always present)
- False localizing signs with IIIrd or VIth cranial nerve palsy
- Drowsiness and coma (a late sign)

Investigation

The choice of investigation will be determined by the clinical presentation. Such investigation might include:

- *FBC and ESR:* to check for anaemia, infection and vasculitis
- *Urea and electrolytes, glucose, liver function tests, thyroid function tests, calcium and blood levels of alcohol or drugs:* if indicated
- *Urgent blood cultures and antigen tests:* if there is a purpuric rash suggesting meningococcal sepsis
- *Radiography:* for any suspected skull fracture and *CT scan* if there are focal signs, if the coma is unexplained, or if a lumbar puncture is planned
- *EEG:* may suggest hepatic encephalopathy, non-convulsive status epilepticus or unsuspected focal brain lesions
- *Lumbar puncture:* necessary in the diagnosis of meningitis, SAH and encephalitis, but contraindicated in coma until a CT scan has ruled out an intracranial mass lesion

Management and prognosis

The patient should be resuscitated. Use a BM stick to check the blood glucose level and take blood for a laboratory blood glucose level; then examine the patient and get a history. Until the airway is protected, the patient should

Emergency 13.4: Management of raised intracranial pressure

Pathophysiology
Masses cause pressure that pushes brain through bony (foramen magnum) or durally (transtentorial, subfalcine) defined spaces

Raised intracranial pressure reduces blood flow: cerebral perfusion pressure = mean arterial pressure – intracranial pressure.

Clinical features
- Reduced Glasgow Coma Scale score
- IIIrd nerve palsy
- VIth nerve palsy
- Altered breathing pattern or other brainstem functions
- Extensor posturing of the limbs

Treatment
Identify and treat cause

Give (intravenous)
- 200 ml 20% mannitol
- 20 mg frusemide
- 200 ml colloid

Transfer to a high dependency unit or intensive care unit environment

Optimize oxygenation

Treat pyrexia and hyperglycaemia

Elective ventilation

Monitor intracranial pressure with an intraparenchymal intracranial pressure monitor

Nurse with 15° head up tilt

Target end tidal CO_2 to 4–4.5 kPa

Target cerebral perfusion pressure (CPP) to more than 70 mmHg, intracranial pressure to less than 30 mmHg, by:
- increasing mean arterial pressure (MAP) with inotropes
- reducing intracranial pressure with mannitol

Monitor osmolality, plasma sodium

If intracranial pressure continues to rise, consider thiopental

be nursed lying on one side with the topmost leg flexed. Treatment will depend on the cause, but dextrose and thiamine should be given routinely. The prognosis relates to the underlying cause as well as to the depth and duration of coma, but a number of patients with apparently poor prognoses do surprisingly well.

Dementia

Dementia is characterized by a global impairment of intellectual, cognitive and memory function without disturbance of consciousness or alertness. It is a clinical syndrome with many causes, several of which are reversible.

Epidemiology

Prevalence. 250 in 100 000. Annual incidence 50 in 100 000.

Age. Prevalence and incidence rise steeply with age, affecting 5% of those over 65 years and 20% of those over 80 years of age.

Genetics and geography. Some forms of Alzheimer's disease are familial, because of mutations in genes such as presenilin I and II. Dementia is a worldwide problem, most marked in countries where survival beyond the sixth decade is common.

Disease mechanisms

The most common cause of dementia is Alzheimer's disease, a chronic progressive irreversible neurodegenerative condition. One-fifth of cases have a reversible cause (Table 13.19).

Alzheimer's disease is associated with the formation of neurofibrillary plaques and tangles, and 'senile' amyloid plaques in the cerebral cortex and hippocampus. The product of the presenelin gene appears to be involved in the normal processing of amyloid precursor protein.

Clinical features

Dementia causes impairment of language, visuospatial function, memory and social conduct. The earliest features may be an inability to cope at work or gradual self-neglect. Impairment of attention or concentration, or a reduced level of consciousness is not consistent with dementia; rather they describe an acute confusional state (p. 919).

The clinical assessment of disorders of language, visuospatial function and memory are discussed on page 875; more formal assessment by a neuropsychologist is often valuable.

The clinical features of some of the more common types of dementia are as follows:

- *Alzheimer's dementia:* a slowly progressive disease developing over many years, associated with language, visuospatial and memory impairment early in its course.
- *Cerebral arteritis:* patients with arteritis (temporal, granulomatous or that associated with SLE) can present with progressive cerebral impairment indistinguishable from other causes of dementia. It is important to consider the diagnosis because prompt treatment with corticosteroids and/or immunosuppression may reverse symptoms completely.
- *Multi-infarct dementia:* manifests stepwise deterioration and usually accompanied by bilateral UMN signs including a UMN bulbar palsy.

13

Table 13.19 Causes of dementia syndromes

Degenerative disease
Alzheimer's disease
Frontotemporal dementia
Dementia with Levy bodies
Parkinson's disease
Progressive supranuclear palsy
Huntington's disease

Vascular disease
Multi-infarct dementia
Cerebral arteritis
Binswanger's disease

Metabolic disease
Wilson's disease
Hepatic encephalopathy
Hypothyroidism

Toxicity
Alcoholic dementia
Drug intoxication (e.g. benzodiazepines, phenothiazines,
    anticonvulsants)

Deficiency
Thiamine (Wernicke–Korsakoff syndrome)
Vitamin B_{12}
Niacin

Mass lesion
Cerebral tumour
Subdural haematoma

Infection
Tuberculosis, syphilis
Subacute sclerosing panencephalitis
Creutzfeldt–Jakob disease
HIV/AIDS

Inflammation
Advanced multiple sclerosis
Sarcoidosis
SLE

Trauma
Head injury
Boxer's encephalopathy

Pseudodementia
Depression

Hydrocephalus
Obstructive hydrocephalus
Normal-pressure hydrocephalus

● *Depressive pseudodementia:* may be indistinguishable clinically from Alzheimer's disease, although patients often overestimate the extent of their difficulties; it responds to antidepressants.

● *Frontotemporal dementia:* a degenerative dementia characterized by personality change, apathy, blunting of emotions, lack of insight and disinhibition.

● *Dementia with Lewy bodies:* so-called because of the presence at autopsy of Lewy bodies, the neuropathological hallmark of Parkinson's disease. Such patients may have an extrapyramidal movement disorder (with slowness of movement, rigidity and gait disturbance) in association with a dementing illness, fluctuating cognitive function and visual hallucinations.

● *Normal-pressure hydrocephalus* (p. 943)*:* causes memory impairment, urinary incontinence and gait apraxia.

● *Dementia caused by a space-occupying lesion:* usually of recent onset, may be accompanied by papilloedema or focal neurological signs. There is usually no evidence of global cortical impairment.

● *Dementia of neurosyphilis:* may be accompanied by Argyll Robertson pupils, bilateral UMN signs and absent limb reflexes.

● *Dementia of Huntington's disease* (p. 927: begins in early adulthood or middle age and is accompanied by chorea or rigidity.

● *Creutzfeldt–Jakob disease (CJD):* rapidly progressive (over weeks to months), and accompanied by myoclonus, ataxia, muscle wasting and fasciculation, cortical blindness and cerebellar signs. *Variant CJD* is largely restricted to the UK and affects a younger age group. Patients often present with sensory or psychiatric symptomatology. It is more rapidly progressive, and is thought be a transmissible spongiform encephalopathy caused by consumption of beef products from animals with bovine spongiform encephalopathy.

● *Dementia associated with HIV and AIDS seropositivity:* may precede clinical AIDS. It has an insidious onset and may be accompanied by apathy.

Investigation

Investigations should be tailored to the presenting clinical picture, but those outlined below should be considered in all patients.

Haematology

● *White cell count:* may be elevated in infection.
● *Macrocytosis:* may indicate vitamin B_{12} deficiency, alcoholism or hypothyroidism, but vitamin B_{12} should be tested even if the MCV is normal.
● *ESR elevation:* may indicate vasculitis, granulomatous disease, tumour or an infective process.
● *Hypo- or hyperglycaemia:* can mimic dementia.
● *Liver function tests:* disordered in alcoholism, Wilson's disease, hepatic encephalopathy, some infections and granulomatous disease.
● *Serum and urinary copper, and caeruloplasmin (tests*

of copper metabolism): should be carried out in young patients with involuntary movements to exclude Wilson's disease.

- *Thyroid function tests:* necessary to exclude myxoedema and thyrotoxicosis.
- *Autoantibody screen:* may be indicated to exclude SLE and other autoimmune disease.
- *Syphilis serology:* should be checked in all patients, as neurosyphilis is treatable.
- *HIV serology:* dementia is part of AIDS and AIDS-related infections, so any patient with unexplained dementia where there is a plausible risk of HIV should be tested after appropriate counselling.
- *Genetic testing:* it is now possible to test for mutated genes in inherited conditions including Huntington's disease.

Microbiology
CSF analysis for evidence of bacterial, fungal or syphilis infection; markers of CJD; and the presence of oligoclonal bands, which may indicate multiple sclerosis, sarcoidosis or SLE.

Diagnostic imaging
CT or MRI scanning is used to exclude tumours, subdural haematoma or hydrocephalus. Binswanger's disease is a vascular dementia related to small vessel disease affecting the cerebral white matter that shows characteristic white matter changes on CT or MRI.

Histopathology
- *Cytological examination:* of CSF for malignant cells.
- *Temporal artery biopsy:* may be indicated to exclude temporal arteritis if the ESR is elevated.
- *Brain or meningeal biopsy:* may be indicated if granulomatous angiitis is suspected or if there are unusual clinical features suggestive of a treatable cause.

Electrophysiology
EEG is helpful in the diagnosis of CJD and metabolic encephalopathy.

Management (Table 13.20)
To date, the medical treatments available for Alzheimer's disease have been largely disappointing. The progressive intellectual decline and increasing self-neglect and dependence on others that accompanies dementia is commonly a burden not only for the patient, but also for the spouse and the family. The imaginative and appropriate provision of supportive services is essential. Such support may range from sensible advice to salvage a business wrecked by its demented manager, to providing day-hospital or respite care to allow the exhausted family some rest.

Table 13.20 Management of dementia

Supportive treatment
Maintain a stable and safe environment
Treat any underlying infection

Support for the family
Provide information leaflets for the family about the diagnosis and prognosis
Arrange home help to reduce the burden of domestic chores
Arrange domiciliary nursing support to help with bathing/dressing
Arrange social support (e.g. day hospital attendance)
Arrange respite admissions to provide carers with a break
Ensure relevant state social support financial benefits and allowances have been claimed (e.g. Disabled Living Allowance in the UK)
Assess competence to work and to drive a car, and advise on action if not competent to drive
Arrange supervision of financial affairs by lawyer if legally incompetent
Genetic counselling if relevant
Accurate genetic prediction is possible in Huntington's disease, and families at risk should receive genetic counselling before starting a family. Affected fetuses can be diagnosed by amniocentesis and abortion may be offered

Specific treatment
Multi-infarct dementia
Control vascular risk factors, especially hypertension and smoking
Aspirin as antithrombotic therapy

A trial of antidepressants
If there is any suggestion of depression, a trial of antidepressant (SSRI such as sertraline, for at least 8 weeks) therapy should be given

Judicious use of sedatives
In early disease night sedation may worsen symptoms. However, they may be invaluable in the later stages when a reversal of sleep–wake patterns means that the demented person is awake all night and the spouse is unable to sleep

Acetylcholinesterase inhibitors
These drugs are recommended by the National Institute for Clinical Excellence of England and Wales for the management of mild to moderate Alzheimer's disease provided that the MMSE remains above 12 and there is clear evidence of continuing benefit. The magnitude of any benefit is not clear and estimated costs (2001 prices) for England and Wales are £42 million/year

MMSE, mini mental state examination; SSRI, selective serotonin reuptake inhibitor.

Alzheimer's disease at a glance

Epidemiology

Prevalence
1 in 20 over 65 years old, 1 in 5 over 80 years

Age
Most common in older patients

Genetics
Sometimes familial (presenelin mutations)

Clinical features

Social function
Unable to work
Apathetic
Loss of initiative
Withdrawn
Loss of personality

Intellectual ability
Reduced intellect
Reduced reasoning
Concrete thinking
Impaired calculation

Language disorder
Disordered speech
Difficulty reading
Difficulty writing

Visuospatial function
Difficulty with visuospatial tasks

Memory and concentration
Not alert, inattentive
Unable to concentrate
Difficulty retaining new material
Retained memory of past events
May be disorientated in time and place

Findings on investigation

The following screening tests should be normal:
- FBC
- ESR
- Vitamin B$_{12}$
- Thyroid function
- γGT
- Copper studies
- Syphilis serology
- HIV serology
- CSF white cell count, protein, glucose and oligoclonal bands

CT/MRI scan of the brain: normal or shows cerebral atrophy
SPECT scanning: may show hypoperfusion, particularly in anterior temporal lobes
EEG: normal or shows non-specific abnormality

Neuropsychological assessment reveals:
- Acquired impairment of intellect
- Visuospatial disorder
- Language disorder
- Amnesia
- Disorientation

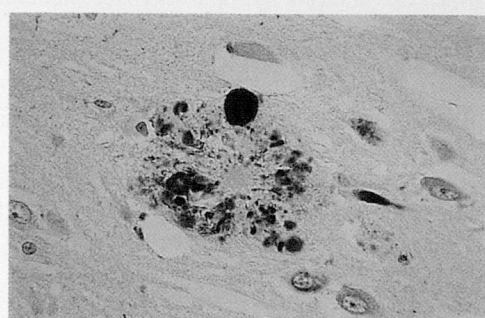

Fig. B Pathology.

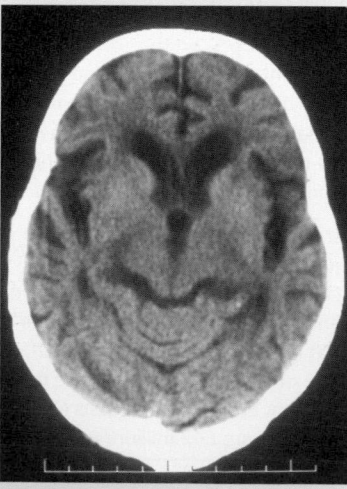

Fig. A CT showing global cerebral atrophy.

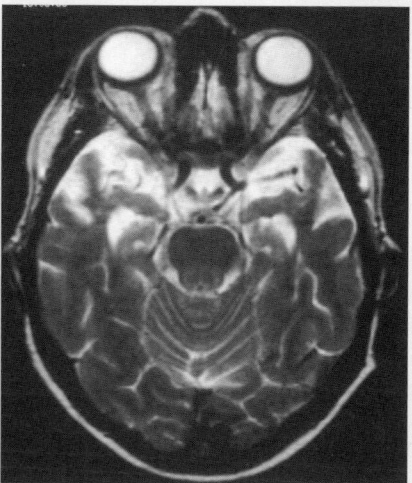

Fig. C MRI showing marked atrophy of temporal lobes in a patient with Alzheimer's disease.

Prognosis

Mean survival after the diagnosis of Alzheimer's disease is 8 years, but survival more than 1 year after a diagnosis of CJD is rare.

Acute confusional states

Acute confusional states are different from dementia and are generally reversible.

Epidemiology

Prevalence. Common.

Age. All ages, but most common in the elderly.

Disease mechanisms

There are many causes of acute confusional state. Many of the conditions leading to coma (Table 13.17) may present with acute confusion in the early stages. The priority is to exclude infection within the CNS.

● *Infection within the CNS:* meningitis (see p. 107), encephalitis (see p. 113) and cerebral abscess (see p. 933) may present with acute confusion. Encephalitis is rare and may be heralded by a seizure.

● *Infection outside the CNS:* a common cause of confusion in the young and the elderly.

● *Acute ischaemic stroke, intracerebral haemorrhage and SAH:* may present with acute confusion of very abrupt onset without focal neurological signs.

● *Alcohol withdrawal syndrome (delirium tremens):* may cause confusion and commonly occurs in patients deprived of their regular intake of alcohol following admission to hospital for other reasons.

● *Drugs:* many prescription drugs cause confusion in the elderly, and confusion in younger patients may result from misuse of street drugs.

● *Metabolic disorders:* leading to abnormalities in glucose, electrolytes, blood gases or acid–base status are common causes of confusion. Wernicke's encephalopathy is caused by thiamine deficiency and can occur in alcoholics, the malnourished (especially the elderly), following prolonged episodes of vomiting (e.g. hyperemesis gravidarum) and as a result of prolonged postoperative intravenous infusions.

● *Non-convulsive status epilepticus:* (usually temporal lobe seizures) can cause a confusional state in the absence of clinically apparent seizure activity. The diagnosis is made at EEG, when intravenous diazepam should cause the EEG to revert to normal as the patient 'wakes up'.

Pathogenesis

Confusion results from impaired attention and registration, and reduced arousal.

Clinical features

Onset is usually rapid (hours to days). Cognitive testing will show disorders of orientation, registration, immediate recall and attention and there may be intermittent drowsiness. There should be no focal signs.

Diagnosis

The disturbed, hallucinating, restless, disorientated and agitated patient usually has an underlying medical rather than psychiatric problem.

● Pyrexia, meningism or raised white cell count in the blood suggests CNS infection or SAH.

● Focal neurological signs or papilloedema suggests an intracranial mass lesion or vascular lesion.

● Wernicke's encephalopathy may present with isolated confusion, but is sometimes accompanied by eye movement disorders (nystagmus, internuclear ophthalmoplegia) and ataxia.

Acute confusion is sometimes wrongly diagnosed in patients who have dysphasia or impaired visuospatial function because of a focal brain lesion.

Investigation

Haematology

● *FBC and ESR:* to look for infection and haematological disorders

● *Urea, electrolytes, glucose, acid–base status, liver function tests and calcium:* to exclude metabolic imbalance as the cause

Microbiology

Culture urine, sputum and blood.

Diagnostic imaging

● *Chest radiography:* often reveals unsuspected pneumonia and occasionally reveals an undiagnosed malignancy

● *CT or MRI scan:* often helpful, and essential if there is any suggestion of CNS infection

Electrophysiology

EEG is often helpful in the detection of encephalopathy and of non-convulsive status epilepticus.

Other investigations

Lumbar puncture. If there is any question of CNS infection a lumbar puncture scan is mandatory, and is safe in the absence of focal symptoms or signs or if the CT scan is normal.

Management

In most patients, a careful clinical assessment and a few well-chosen tests will identify a correctable cause. Where they do not, more detailed investigation is

Emergency 13.5:
Management of acute confusional states

Supportive treatment
Handle the patient calmly
Avoid any drug therapy that may have caused or exacer-
bate the confusion
Nurse in a quiet well-lit single room

Specific treatment
Sedation (only if absolutely necessary)
Use a short-acting benzodiazepine, phenothiazine or
butyrophenone

Suspected Wernicke's encephalopathy
Give high-dose intravenous thiamine. There is a risk of
anaphylaxis, and facilities for treating this should be
available

Suspected alcohol withdrawal
Give oral thiamine
Give prophylaxis against alcohol withdrawal syndrome
with reducing dosage of chlordiazepoxide

required. If there is the slightest suggestion of Wernicke's encephalopathy then intravenous thiamine should be given. As well as specific management of specific causes, attention should also be given to maintaining a safe well-lit environment and providing close supervision of patients to ensure their safety (EMERGENCY BOX 13.5).

Prognosis
Appropriate treatment usually leads to a prompt improvement. Some causes (e.g. Wernicke's encephalo-pathy) are fatal if not treated, and even if treated some amnesia may persist as Korsakoff's psychosis.

Multiple sclerosis

Multiple sclerosis (MS) is an inflammatory condition affecting the myelin sheath of CNS but not peripheral neurones. Axons are probably spared, at least in the early course of the disease. MS may present as benign disease, follow a relapsing and remitting course or show inexor-able progression from the outset.

Epidemiology
Prevalence. 110 in 100 000 in the UK and northern Europe, less in southern Europe and USA and lower still in Africa, Asia and the Far East.

Annual incidence. 5 in 100 000 in the UK.

Age. Usually between 20 and 40 years of age; onset before adolescence or after 60 years is very rare.

Sex. Two-thirds of UK patients are female.

Race and geography. MS mainly affects white people, especially those of Nordic origin. It is very rare in Afro-Caribbeans and Asians. It is more common in tem-perate zones, and rare in the tropics. These geographical variations cannot be completely explained by different racial susceptibilities, as Asians and Afro-Caribbeans who move to temperate zones in early life have an intermediate risk of developing MS.

Genetics. Fifteen per cent of MS patients in the UK have an affected first-degree relative, and people who have a parent with MS have a 1% chance of developing the disease. Concordance rates are 25% for monozygotic compared with 3% for dizygotic twins.

Disease mechanisms
A combination of a genetic predisposition and environ-mental factors, particularly in early life, appear to be important in the aetiology of MS. There is an association with HLA-DR2 in most northern European countries.

There is increased immunological activity in the CNS (CSF lymphocytosis, synthesis of monoclonal antibodies producing oligoclonal IgG bands in the CSF, raised CSF protein and reduced suppressor T cells during a relapse) but the cause of this is not known. The clinical features of MS arise from significant slowing of axonal conduction because of loss of the myelin sheath during relapses; following repair, remyelination may be incomplete, resulting in continuing symptomatology and secondary axonal loss.

Clinical features
Multiple sclerosis can affect:
- *Periventricular deep white matter:* producing euphoria, poor memory and concentration, and occasionally dementia or acute psychiatric disturbance
- *Optic nerve:* producing optic neuritis (a subacute uni-lateral loss of vision with reduced visual acuity, a blind spot or scotoma in the centre of the vision and pain when the eye is moved)
- *Brainstem:* producing double vision, slurred speech, unsteady gait, incoordination of the hands, numbness of the face, unilateral facial weakness, difficulty swallowing and internuclear ophthalmoplegia
- *Spinal cord:* producing weakness, heaviness or stiffness of both legs or all four limbs and sometimes just one limb; sensory loss in the legs that spreads up into the trunk

over a few days; altered sensation; and urinary frequency and urgency

Rarer features of MS include:
- Trigeminal neuralgia
- Paroxysmal motor, sensory and brainstem symptoms
- 'Useless hand' (a hand with normal power but no joint position sense)
- Facial myokymia (continuous rippling movement of the face)

Lhermitte's phenomenon. This is an electric shock-like sensation shooting down the neck and back and into the arms and legs following flexion of the neck. It is caused by a lesion in the cervical spinal cord and may also be caused by spinal cord compression.

Uhthoff's phenomenon. This is loss of function in part of the nervous system associated with a rise in body temperature (e.g. difficulty getting out of a hot bath because of leg weakness). It is strongly suggestive of MS.

Diagnosis

Isolated episodes of inflammation affecting the nervous system have many causes but, by convention, relapsing–remitting MS is only diagnosed where there is **clinical** evidence of at least two attacks separated by at least 8 weeks where other causes have been excluded:
- A patient with loss of vision in his left eye with recovery in 1979 and an UMN weakness of both legs in 1980 has MS because he has had two separate lesions, one of the optic nerve and one of the spinal cord.
- A patient with an episode of slurred speech, double vision and unsteadiness because of a brainstem lesion in 1950 and an episode of weakness in both legs caused by a spinal cord lesion in 1986 also has MS because two different lesions have occurred on two separate occasions.
- A patient with a slowly progressive UMN weakness of both legs because of a spinal cord lesion in 1987 cannot be diagnosed as having MS because she has only one CNS lesion.
- A patient with an episode of blurred vision in her left eye because of a lesion of the optic nerve in 1980 and a further episode of blurred vision in her left eye because of a lesion of the optic nerve in 1986 cannot be diagnosed as having MS because although she had two separate episodes, both affected the same site in the CNS.

Of course, to get two attacks you have to start with one, so there is always a period of uncertainty in making the diagnosis of MS. In such cases, MRI brain imaging can give helpful prognostic information. Furthermore, some forms of MS (e.g. primary progressive MS) do not manifest a relapsing–remitting pattern, and other diagnostic criteria must be used in such cases.

Differential diagnosis

The differential diagnosis of MS includes:
- *Other multifocal diseases that may show a relapsing–remitting pattern:* SLE, polyarteritis nodosa, Behçet's disease, subacute bacterial endocarditis, neurosyphilis, sarcoidosis, AIDS, lymphoma
- *Other progressive multifocal diseases:* Friedreich's ataxia and hereditary ataxias, subacute combined degeneration of the cord caused by vitamin B_{12} deficiency
- *Other lesions affecting a single site in the CNS that may relapse and/or remit:* tumour, arteriovenous malformation of the brain, brainstem or spinal cord, cervical spondylosis

Investigation

Patients who present with gradually progressive neurological symptoms may have a surgically treatable lesion, and it is important to exclude this before confirming the diagnosis of MS.

Haematology
- *FBC and ESR:* to screen for systemic disease
- *Thyroid function tests:* in progressive ataxia, to exclude hypothyroidism; *liver function tests and MCV* to exclude alcoholic cerebellar degeneration
- *Vitamin B_{12}:* for UMN weakness of both legs with or without a sensory loss to exclude subacute combined degeneration of the cord
- *Syphilis serology:* for all patients because neurosyphilis can mimic MS
- *HIV test:* particularly if the patient has risk factors for AIDS or has unexplained progressive symptoms
- *Genetic testing:* for mitochondrial disease, spinocerebellar ataxias or hereditary spastic paraplegias may be appropriate, depending on the clinical presentation

Diagnostic imaging
The primary concern is to exclude a structural lesion as the cause of the symptoms. Therefore, if a patient has symptoms suggesting a spinal cord lesion, the first imaging test should be examination of the relevant part of the spinal cord (by MRI scanning). If a patient has optic neuritis, MRI of the orbits should be performed to exclude a structural lesion of the optic nerve.

Once a structural lesion has been excluded, **cranial MRI** should be performed. Ninety per cent of patients with clinically definite disease will show typical scattered areas of high signal with a periventricular distribution. These changes are not specific for MS and may be seen in vasculitis, sarcoidosis and Behçet's disease. Further confirmatory investigations must therefore be performed (see below).

Electrophysiology

Evoked potentials may show evidence of disseminated asymptomatic lesions and thus make the diagnosis of MS more likely. The visual evoked response (VER), the brainstem auditory evoked response (BAER) and the somatosensory evoked response (SSER) are all sensitive detectors of asymptomatic lesions in the optic nerve, brainstem and spinal cord, respectively. Unfortunately, many lesions besides MS can cause similar abnormalities, so an abnormal VER, BAER or SSER is not diagnostic of MS.

Other investigations

● *CSF examination:* often helpful. The presence of oligoclonal bands restricted to the CSF demonstrates intrathecal antibody production consistent with but not diagnostic of MS, and such bands may be absent in the early stages. MS is unlikely if the CSF protein is more than three times normal, if the white cell count is greater than 100 cells/mm^3 or if the CSF glucose is less than 50% of blood glucose level.
● *Urodynamics, cystoscopy and renal and bladder ultrasound:* patients with urinary symptoms require careful assessment and referral to a specialist urology service where appropriate.

Management (Table 13.21)

Careful investigation should exclude treatable causes of the symptomatology. The diagnosis of MS usually has a profound impact on how patients think of themselves, and often the uncertainty about what the future might hold is as disabling as the direct effects of MS. The diagnosis of MS should not, however, be withheld; where there is reasonable suspicion that it is the cause of a patient's symptoms then this should be discussed openly and frankly in an appropriately unhurried, supportive and informative way.

Attention should be given to any disability and handicap, and symptomatic relief is available for spasticity, dysaesthetic pain and bladder symptoms. Involvement of an MS nurse practitioner can be invaluable. Treatment with oral or intravenous steroids helps speed recovery from acute relapses but has no effect on disease progression. There is currently insufficient evidence to justify the widespread use of immunosuppressive therapies.

Prognosis

Fifty per cent of patients with a single episode of demyelination and an abnormal MRI will develop clinically definite MS within 3 years. American World War II veterans with a diagnosis of MS in 1956 had median survival times of 30 and 40 years for males and females, respectively. For patients with established relapsing–remitting disease, more than half are still able to walk 500 m without assistance 10 years into their illness.

Movement disorders

Parkinson's disease and extrapyramidal disorders

Parkinson's disease (PD) is a neurodegenerative disease affecting dopaminergic neurones of the extrapyramidal system, which causes disturbance of the control of movement and of posture; abnormalities of cognition and mood; and disturbance of the autonomic nervous system. The extrapyramidal system may also be affected in other

---

Multiple sclerosis at a glance

Epidemiology
Prevalence
110 in 100 000 in the UK

Age
Disease of young adults; onset over 60 years of age is rare

Sex
About two-thirds of patients are female

Race
White people

Genetics
15% of cases are familial

Geography
Northern Europe and USA. There is a possible relationship with latitude, being more common in areas further from the Equator

Clinical features
Optic nerve
Optic neuritis (loss of vision in one eye)
Optic atrophy

Brainstem
Diplopia
Internuclear ophthalmoplegia
Sensory loss on the face (cranial nerve V)
Facial weakness (cranial nerve VII)

Slurred speech
Difficulty swallowing

Cerebellum
Slurred speech
Unsteady gait
Nystagmus

Spinal cord
Monoparesis
Paraparesis
Quadriparesis (hemiparesis is rare)
Sensory loss (one arm, one leg, both legs, clearcut sensory level is rare)
Bladder and bowel dysfunction
Sexual dysfunction

Paroxysmal symptoms
Trigeminal neuralgia
Lhermitte's sign
Paroxysmal motor and sensory symptoms

Cerebral hemispheres
Euphoria
Confusion
Dementia

Findings on investigation
Blood tests
Normal

CSF examination
CSF: clear, lymphocyte count may be raised, glucose is normal, protein is normal or slightly raised, and oligoclonal bands (in the CSF but not in the blood) are present in 80–90% of patients but may be absent early in the disease

Cranial MRI scan
Areas of increased signal in the white matter on T$_2$-weighted images, particularly in periventricular regions. However, similar MRI appearances may be seen in late life as part of normal ageing

Evoked potentials (EP)
Visual and brainstem EPs are abnormal in 60–80% of patients

Slurred speech

Optic neuritis
Optic atrophy
Diplopia
Nystagmus
Internuclear ophthalmoplegia

Euphoria

Incoordination
Weakness
Brisk reflexes
Pyramidal weakness

Transverse myelitis

Bladder, bowel, sexual dysfunction

Ataxia
Pyramidal weakness
Brisk reflexes
Upgoing plantars

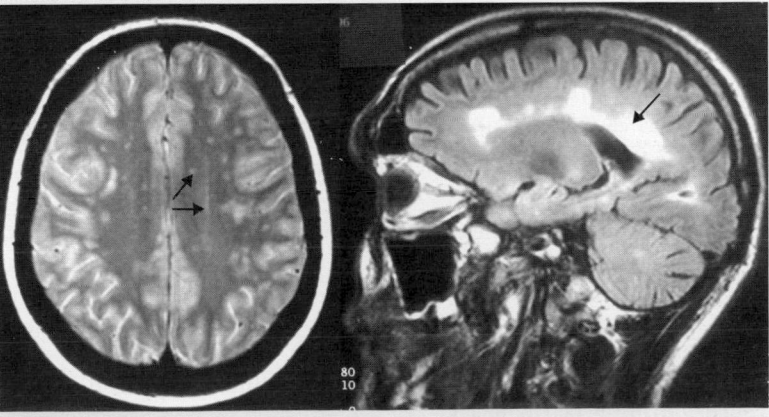

Fig. A MRI showing periventricular white matter lesions in a patient with MS.

Table 13.21 Management of multiple sclerosis (MS)

Principles of treatment

At all times, even as the diagnosis is being made, the patient should have the opportunity to participate fully in the management of their care

Establishing a degree of control over their illness can be invaluable if problems develop over time

Careful explanation of the diagnosis and the relatively benign prognosis (see p. 922) are important

The support of an MS clinical nurse practitioner can be invaluable

Minimization of handicap

Physiotherapy, occupational therapy and adaptations to work and home environments reduce the impact of any impairment on the patient's quality of life and independence

Specific treatment

Suppress inflammation during acute relapse

Intravenous methylprednisolone (1 g/day for 3 days)

Corticosteroids reduce the duration of relapse, but do not influence the long-term outcome

It is not known whether intravenous methylprednisolone is more effective than oral prednisolone

Reduce relapse rates and suppress ongoing disease activity

Interferon-β and glatiramer reduce the appearance of new MRI abnormalities and relapse rate and may have an effect on disease progression in both relapsing–remitting and secondary progressive disease

However, it is not clear that these benefits justify the costs involved

Interferon may also reduce the rate at which patients with a single episode of CNS demyelination progress to clinically definite MS

Azathioprine and intravenous immunoglobulin may reduce relapse rates

Treat symptoms

Carbamazepine or amitriptyline for dysaesthesia or trigeminal neuralgia

Baclofen, tizanidine or dantrolene for spasticity

Anticholinergic drugs (e.g. oxybutinin) for bladder instability

Laxative for constipation

Sildenafil for erectile failure

β-Blockers or rarely functional neurosurgery for tremor

CNS, central nervous system; MRI, magnetic resonance imaging.

Table 13.22 Causes and features of extrapyramidal disorders other than Parkinson's disease

Drugs

Phenothiazines (chlorpromazine, prochlorperazine)

Butyrophenones (haloperidol, droperidol)

Benzamides (metoclopramide)

Tetrabenazine

Reserpine

Toxins

Carbon monoxide exposure

Manganese poisoning

Inherited and metabolic disorders

Wilson's disease

Spinocerebellar ataxia

Neuroacanthocytosis

Hypoparathyroidism

Inherited or degenerative diseases affecting multiple systems as well as the extrapyramidal system

Huntington's disease, often with cognitive and affective abnormalities

Multiple system atrophy involves descending motor pathways, basal ganglia, brainstem, cerebellum and autonomic nerves causing spasticity, parkinsonism, ataxia and postural hypotension

Progressive supranuclear palsy or Steele–Richardson–Olszewski syndrome (involvement of the frontal cortex and its connections to the basal ganglia and brainstem results in dementia, supranuclear gaze palsy, axial rigidity and pseudobulbar palsy)

Encephalitis lethargica

Postencephalitic syndrome

Vascular disease

Diffuse small vessel vascular disease

neurological disorders, but these need to be differentiated from PD because they require different treatment and carry a different prognosis.

Epidemiology

Prevalence. Prevalence of PD is 150 in 100 000. Annual incidence 20 in 100 000 in the UK.

Age. Rarely presents under 50 years of age.

Sex. Probably equal.

Genetics. Rare familial cases may be caused by mutations in the *Parkin* gene family.

Disease mechanisms

While the cause of PD is not known, there appears to be an interaction between genetic and environmental factors; it is one of the few conditions which is less common in cigarette smokers. Other extrapyramidal disorders may have identifiable causes (Table 13.22).

Neurones are lost from the substantia nigra and the locus

ceruleus, and Lewy bodies (intracellular eosinophilic cytoplasmic inclusion bodies containing α-synuclein) are seen in dying neurones.

Clinical features

Extrapyramidal disease is characterized by tremor, rigidity and bradykinesia and postural instability. These features may occur in isolation, as in PD; alongside dysfunction of other CNS systems, as in multiple system atrophy; or as features of more generalized conditions such as multi-infarct dementia or normal-pressure hydrocephalus.

The features of early PD (general slowness, expression-less face, shaking) may be falsely attributed to the effects of age, arthritis, depression, alcohol, stroke or brain tumour, and the correct diagnosis may take some time to establish. PD is often asymmetrical at onset.

Diagnosis

The diagnosis of PD can be made if:
- There is tremor, rigidity and bradykinesia
- Abnormalities are restricted to the extrapyramidal system
- There is no other obvious cause
- There is a good response to L-dopa (levodopa)

If there is tremor, rigidity and bradykinesia in the presence of an obvious underlying cause (such as drugs or toxins), or there are features of disease outside the extrapyramidal system (such as dementia indicating cortical damage, or postural hypotension indicating autonomic failure) then the patient does not have PD. It is better to diagnose an 'extrapyramidal disorder' than 'parkinsonism' in such patients.

Investigation

Those over 50 years who fulfil the diagnostic criteria above do not usually require investigation.

Haematology

Liver function tests, calcium levels, copper, caeruloplasmin and urinary copper to exclude treatable metabolic causes, particularly Wilson's disease.

Diagnostic imaging

CT scan should be performed if only one side is affected, if normal-pressure hydrocephalus is a possibility (p. 943), if the symptoms are progressive or if no definite diagnosis is possible.

Other investigations

Tests of autonomic function and other investigations are required if there is clinical evidence of disease outside the extrapyramidal system (e.g. dementia, UMN signs, symptoms of autonomic dysfunction).

Management

In addition to symptomatic therapies (for constipation, depression or musculoskeletal pain), drug treatment can be highly effective (CLINICAL BOX 13.3). Involvement of a PD nurse practitioner can be invaluable.

Antiparkinsonian therapies

Dopamine signalling can be increased in a number of ways (Table 13.23):
- *L-dopa:* a dopamine precursor that increases synaptic dopamine concentrations by increasing dopamine synthesis. Treatment should begin with a low dose L-dopa combined with a peripheral dopa decarboxylase inhibitor. The dose can be increased if required.
- *Dopamine agonists* (e.g. pergolide, lisuride, bromocriptine, apomorphine, ropinirole, pramipexol): may be used as an alternative to L-dopa as first-line therapy in younger patients. Apomorphine is given by subcutaneous injection and is used for patients with severe troublesome 'on–off' phenomena. All of these agents can cause severe vomiting unless given with a peripheral dopamine antagonist (e.g. domperidone).
- *Amantadine:* may be helpful for dyskinesia.
- *Selegiline* (a monoamine oxidase type B inhibitor) and *entacapone* (catechol-O-methyl transferase; COMT inhibitor): inhibit the breakdown of dopamine and so increase its synaptic concentration.
- *Neuronal transplantation:* seeks to replace the dying dopaminergic cells, and indeed transplanted cells do make meaningful connections with host neurones and are synaptically active; however, it is not yet clear that this therapy will be of general use.

Those who initially respond to L-dopa may find that over time the benefit of each tablet is shorter, with rapid transitions to an unmedicated state; this is the 'on–off' effect. In the first instance, smaller, more frequent dosing may help; in the longer run subcutaneous apomorphine infusion may be required.

Anticholinergic agents (e.g. benzhexol, orphenadrine) may be used if tremor is prominent, but side-effects (confusion, blurred vision, dry mouth) are common in the elderly.

Prognosis

This is a disease of the elderly and, given a median duration from diagnosis to death of 15 years, many patients die with their PD rather than dying of PD.

Chorea, hemiballismus, myoclonus and dystonia

Epidemiology
Prevalence. Taken together, approximately 10 in 100 000.

Parkinson's disease at a glance

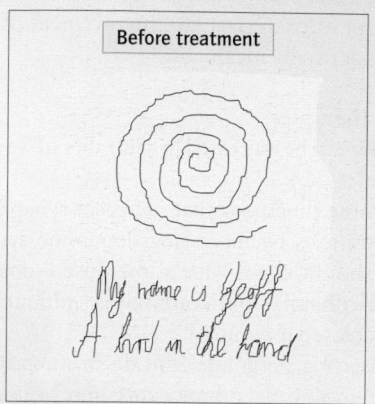

Before treatment

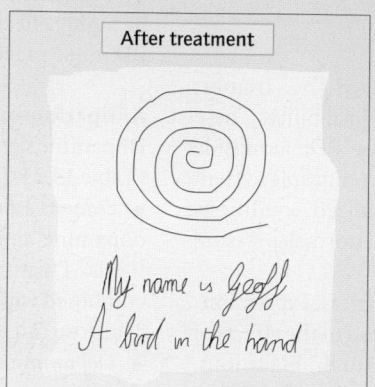

After treatment

Fig. A Writing and spiral by a patient with Parkinson's disease and drawn by the same patient after treatment.

Epidemiology
Prevalence
Approximately 1 in 700

Age
Prevalence increases sharply with age. Usually 50–70 years of age. Very rare in people under 40 years

Clinical features
Nervous system
Resting tremor (5 Hz)
Cogwheel rigidity
Slow movement
Postural instability
Loss of facial expression
Soft monotonous voice

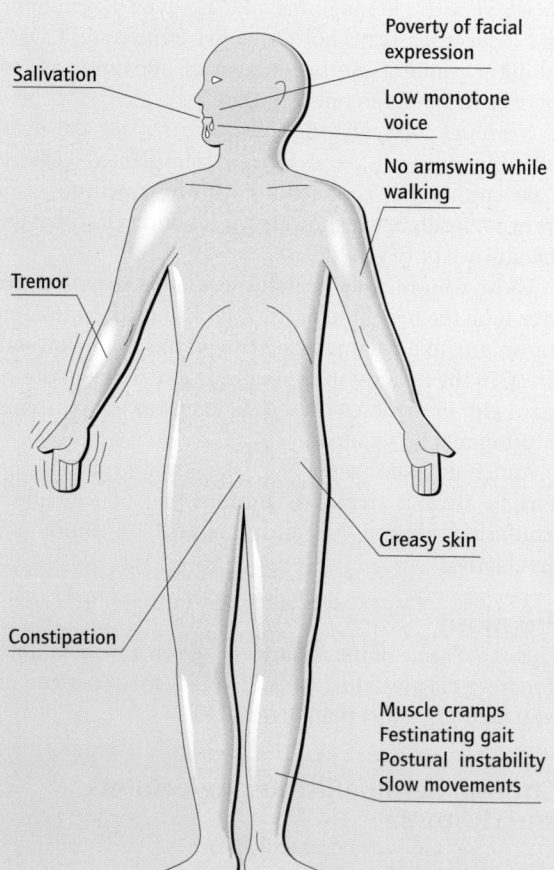

Poverty of facial expression

Salivation

Low monotone voice

No armswing while walking

Tremor

Greasy skin

Constipation

Muscle cramps
Festinating gait
Postural instability
Slow movements

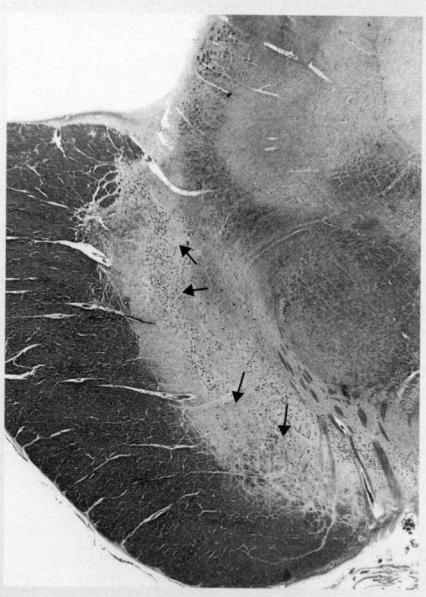

Fig. B Substantia nigra, showing a normal population of large pigmented cells. Klüver–Barrera stain.

Stooped posture
Festinating gait
Loss of arm swing
Cognitive deficits
Mood disturbance
Abnormalities of autonomic function

Skin
Greasy skin

Muscles
Muscle aches
Cramp

Gastrointestinal tract
Excess salivation
Constipation

Findings on investigation
There is no routine diagnostic test
Blood tests and imaging are normal
Positron emission tomography (PET) or single photon emission computerized tomography (SPECT) scanning with various ligands shows altered dopamine metabolism in the basal ganglia

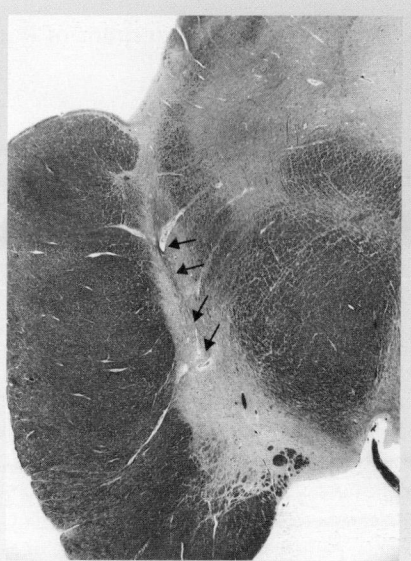

Fig. C Same area as in Fig. B in the case of Parkinson's disease. There is severe depletion of pigmented cells, and the whole area is shrunken. Figures B and C reproduced from Esiri, *Oppenheimer's Diagnostic Neuropathology*, 2nd edn, 1996 (Blackwell Science, Oxford) with the permission of the author.

Age. Age at onset is variable.

Genetics. Huntington's disease (HD) is an autosomal dominant condition resulting from an expanded trinucleotide repeat in the *Huntingtin* gene.

Pathogenesis
In HD it is thought that accumulation of the *Huntingtin* gene product in intracellular inclusions disrupts cellular metabolism and leads to cell death, most marked in the striatum and the cortex.

Clinical features and disease mechanisms
(Table 13.24)
Chorea. Chorea describes continuous irregular random movements that appear semipurposeful and fidgety. All parts of the body appear to be involved at random and the gait has a jerky dance-like quality. There are many causes.

Hemiballismus. This is characterized by sudden and unpredictable throwing movements of one limb, and is usually caused by infarction of the contralateral subthalamic nucleus.

Myoclonic jerks. These are brief jerks of a muscle and are

usually caused by a metabolic disturbance. Unlike chorea, the movements are infrequent and discontinuous. Early morning myoclonus suggests juvenile myoclonic epilepsy, and myoclonus in the context of a rapidly evolving dementia suggests CJD.

Dystonia. This is a slow sustained irregular twisting posture of a limb or the trunk. Some dystonias are focal (affect one limb only), whereas others are generalized:
- Spasmodic torticollis is one form of dystonia in which the head twists to one side.
- Laryngeal dystonia may give rise to isolated dysphonia.
- Recurrent spasms of the mouth and jaw may be caused by oromandibular dystonia.
- Writer's cramp is a dystonia of the hand occurring when the patient tries to write, but not at other times. It is therefore a task-specific dystonia.

Investigation
Haematology
- *Blood film:* to look for acanthocytes
- *Electrolytes:* should be checked in patients with myoclonus
- *Liver function test:* abnormalities may suggest Wilson's disease or another systemic disorder
- *Antinuclear factor:* may indicate that the cause of chorea is SLE

Clinical box 13.3: Management of Parkinson's disease

Supportive treatment

Rehabilitation

Assessments by occupational therapists and physiotherapists are vital to maintain independence in activities of daily living for as long as possible

In the later stages of the disease, family support and day care are very important. The input of a specialist Parkinson's disease nurse practitioner can be invaluable

Specific treatment

Antiparkinsonian drugs (Table 13.23)

- *L-dopa treatment:* start with a low dose of a combination of L-dopa and peripheral dopa decarboxylase inhibitor and increase the dose if the response is inadequate.
- *Dopamine agonists* (e.g. pergolide, lisuride, bromocriptine, ropinirole, cabergoline): may be used as first-line treatments, particularly in younger patients, or as second-line treatments used in combination with L-dopa. Apomorphine is used for severe 'on–off' phenomena but must be given by injection.
- *Selegiline:* a monoamine oxidase inhibitor that may be used as a second-line treatment.
- *Entacapone:* a second-line treatment that inhibits the peripheral breakdown of L-dopa and so increases the amount available to the brain.
- *Anticholinergic agents* (e.g. benzhexol (trihexyphenidyl), orphenadrine): may be useful if there is a prominent tremor, but side-effects are common and these drugs have limited use in the elderly.
- *Amantadine:* may be helpful for dyskinesias.
- *Smaller more frequent doses of L-dopa and decarboxylase inhibitor* (e.g. half a tablet six times a day instead of one tablet three times a day): helpful for troublesome 'on–off' fluctuations.

Drugs for other symptoms

Laxatives for constipation

Antidepressants for depression

Analgesics for muscle aches

β-Blockers for tremor and sweating

Sildafenil for erectile failure

Olanzapine or quetiapine for hallucinations

Domperidone for nausea

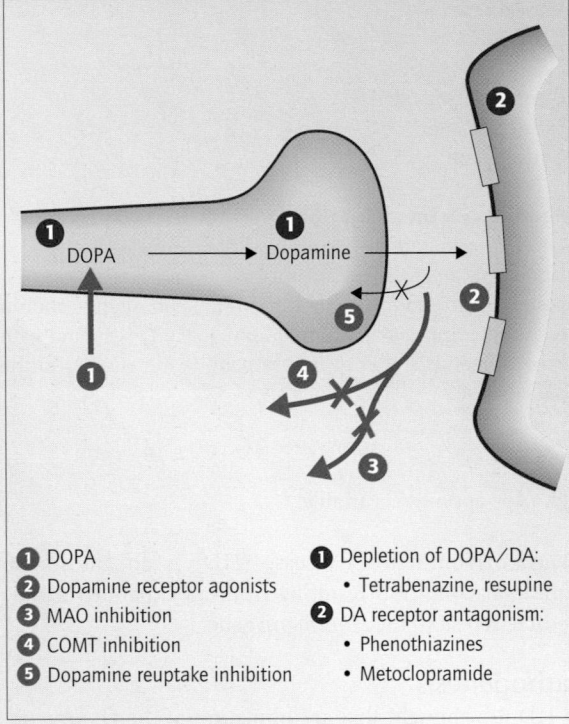

Fig. A Drugs used to treat (blue) or that cause (red) extrapyramidal symptoms.

① DOPA
② Dopamine receptor agonists
③ MAO inhibition
④ COMT inhibition
⑤ Dopamine reuptake inhibition

❶ Depletion of DOPA/DA:
 • Tetrabenazine, resupine
❷ DA receptor antagonism:
 • Phenothiazines
 • Metoclopramide

- *Genetic tests:* for Huntington's disease
- *Anti-streptolysin O (ASO) titres:* for Sydenham's chorea
- *Urinary copper, and blood copper and caeruloplasmin:* to look for Wilson's disease (see below)

Diagnostic imaging

Magnetic resonance imaging brain may confirm infarction in hemiballismus. Atrophy, particularly of the caudate nucleus but often with a degree of global atrophy, is seen in HD.

Management

Summarized in Table 13.25.

Wilson's disease

Epidemiology

Prevalence. 2 in 100 000.

Age. Onset during childhood. Rarely presents in adulthood.

Genetics. Autosomal recessive inheritance resulting from mutations in the gene encoding ATP7B, a copper-transporting-P-type ATPase.

Disease mechanisms

There is failure to excrete copper normally, and it builds

Table 13.23 Antiparkinsonian drugs

Drug	Action	Indication	Side-effects	Contraindications
Co-careldoa (carbidopa and levodopa: Sinemet)	Levodopa is decarboxylated in the brain to form dopamine. Carbidopa and Benserazide are peripheral decarboxylase inhibitors with side-effects caused by systemic dopamine production	Parkinsonism	Involuntary movements, anorexia, postural hypotension	Closed angle glaucoma
Co-beneldopa (benserazide and levodopa: Madopar)		Parkinsonism	Involuntary movements, anorexia, postural hypotension	Closed angle glaucoma
Selegiline	Monoamine oxidase type B inhibitor	Used in conjunction with levodopa to reduce end-of-dose fluctuations	Hypotension, nausea, confusion. May increase side-effects due to levodopa	
Pergolide	Ergot dopamine receptor agonist	Reduces 'off' periods and fluctuations in advanced disease	Hallucinations, confusion, dyskinesia, drowsiness, arrhythmias	Porphyria
Cabergoline	Ergot dopamine receptor agonist	Adjunct to levodopa	Nausea, vomiting, consipation, postural hypotension, Raynaud's phenomenon, hallucinations, dyskinesias	Pregnancy and breastfeeding
Ropinirole	D$_2$ dopamine receptor agonist	Monotherapy, or as an adjunct to levodopa; levodopa dose may be reduced by one-fifth	Nausea, drowsiness, abdominal pain, vomiting and syncope; dyskinesia, hallucinations and confusion; occasionally severe hypotension and bradycardia	Pregnancy and breastfeeding
Pramipexole	Non-ergot dopamine D$_2$ and D$_3$ receptor agonist	Adjunct to levodopa	Hypotension; drowsiness (advise not to drive); nausea, constipation, hallucinations, dyskinesia	Pregnancy and breastfeeding
Apomorphine	Potent stimulator of D$_1$ and D$_2$ receptors	Advanced disease with marked on–off fluctuations. 48 h domperidone pretreatment required	Nausea, vomiting, dyskinesias, postural instability, cognitive impairment, confusion hallucinations, sedation, postural hypotension; local reactions at injection sites	Respiratory or CNS depression, hepatic impairment, neuropsychiatric problems, dementia; pregnancy and breastfeeding
Entacapone	Peripheral COMT inhibitor	Adjunct to levodopa (with dopa-decarboxylase inhibitor); end-of-dose fluctuations; may reduce levodopa dose by one-fifth	Nausea, vomiting, abdominal pain, constipation, diarrhoea, dry mouth, dyskinesias; dizziness	Pregnancy and breastfeeding; hepatic impairment; phaeochromocytoma; history of neuroleptic malignant syndrome or non-traumatic rhabdomyolysis
Amantadine	Non-competitive NMDA receptor antagonist	Adjunct to levodopa; may improve dyskinesia	Anorexia, nervousness, insomnia, convulsions, hallucinations, gastrointestinal disturbance	Epilepsy, peptic ulcer disease, renal impairment, pregnancy, breastfeeding
Trihexyphenidy	Specific muscarinic antagonist	Parkinsonism, drug induced extrapyramidal symptoms	Dry mouth, dizziness, confusion, blurred vision, urinary retention, excitement	Urinary retention, angle closure glaucoma; liable to abuse

Table 13.24 Causes of involuntary movements: chorea, hemiballismus, myoclonic jerks and dystonia

Chorea
Huntington's disease
Drugs
• Oral contraceptive pill
• Treatment of Parkinson's disease
SLE
Sydenham's chorea (in association with rheumatic fever)
Wilson's disease
Polycythaemia
Thyrotoxicosis
Other neurodegenerative disease
• Choreoacanthocytosis
• Spinocerebellar ataxia
• Friedreich's ataxia
• Olivopontocerebellar atrophy
• Dentatorubral pallidoluysian atrophy

Hemiballismus
Vascular lesion (e.g. of the subthalamic nucleus)

Myoclonic jerks
Metabolic upset

• Renal failure
• Hypocalcaemia
• Hepatic failure
• Hypercapnia
Myoclonic epilepsy
Postanoxic brain damage action myoclonus
Alzheimer's disease
Creutzfeldt–Jakob disease
Subacute sclerosing panencephalitis

Dystonia
Idiopathic
Drugs
Wilson's disease
Huntington's disease
Parkinson's disease
'Dopa-responsive' dystonia (young children)
Progressive supranuclear palsy
Mitochondrial cytopathy
Neuroacanthocytosis
Metachromatic leucodystrophy
Ataxia telangiectasia

Table 13.25 Management of other movement disorders: chorea, hemiballismus, myoclonus and dystonia

Supportive treatment
Correct any underlying metabolic disorder
Stop any drugs that may have caused the disorder
Provide patient information about disease-specific
   self-help groups (e.g. in the UK there are separate
   organizations helping patients with chorea, dystonia
   and epilepsy)
Arrange genetic counselling as necessary

Specific treatment
Chorea
Tetrabenazine in small doses (but it can induce depression
   and parkinsonism)
Haloperidol or other neuroleptics such as sulpiride,
   risperidone or olanzapine

Hemiballismus
Chlorpromazine may control the movements

Myoclonic jerks
Myoclonic epilepsy: use sodium valproate or lamotrigine
Other types of myoclonus: sodium valproate, clonazepam

Dystonia
Generalized: use gradually increasing doses of
   anticholinergic agents (e.g. benzhexol). Alternative
   agents include tetrabenazine, benzodiazepines and
   baclofen
Focal (e.g. blepharospasm, torticollis, writer's cramp):
   carefully placed low-dose injections of *Botulinum* toxin into
   the relevant muscles may relieve the symptoms for about

3 months; repeated injections are required, and
   neutralizing antibodies may develop

Drugs
Tetrabenazine
Depletes dopamine from nerve endings
Used in treatment of chorea
Side-effects. Sedation, depression, parkinsonism
Contraindications. Breastfeeding

Botulinum toxin
Clostridium botulinum toxin blocks release of acetylcholine
   from motor neurones, inducing paralysis lasting several
   months
Indications. Essential blepharospasm, hemifacial spasm,
   spasmodic torticollis, spasticity, sialorrhoea, writers' cramp
   and other dystonias
Side-effects. Ptosis, diplopia, facial weakness
Contraindications. Previous adverse reactions to *Botulinum
   toxin*, breastfeeding; safety in pregnancy uncertain
Treatment needs to be repeated at about 4-monthly intervals

Penicillamine
Copper chelating agent
Used in treatment of Wilson's disease
Side-effects. Skin rashes, proteinuria, marrow toxicity
Contraindications. Lupus erythematosus
Patient monitoring. Blood counts, platelets and urine analysis
   should be checked regularly to detect marrow suppression
   and proteinuria

up in the body tissues, first in the liver and then in the brain. The basal ganglia are especially vulnerable.

Clinical features
Patients may present with liver disease in childhood or with the neurological syndrome in adolescence. Neurological symptoms include impaired concentration, declining intellect, behavioural problems, involuntary movements and generalized dystonia, ataxia or an akinetic–rigid syndrome. Patients have a typical smiling facial appearance with drooling, and often have slurred speech. There may be copper deposition in Descemet's membrane of the cornea, giving a greenish brown pigmentary (Kayser–Fleischer) ring, which may only be visible at slit-lamp examination.

Investigation
- *Serum copper and ceruloplasmin:* should be checked in all young patients with a movement disorder and are low in Wilson's disease
- *Urinary copper excretion:* increased
- *Liver biopsy* (using a copper free needle): should be performed to measure the copper content
- *MRI scanning:* may reveal abnormalities in the basal ganglia

Management
Chelating agents are used to increase copper excretion; penicillamine and trientine are potentially toxic and zinc sulphate is safer, if slightly less effective.

Prognosis
If treatment is initiated early, complete recovery is possible. However, if treatment is discontinued disabling relapses can occur.

Essential tremor

Epidemiology
Prevalence. 2000 in 100 000.

Genetics. Sixty per cent have an affected first-degree relative; in many families inheritance is autosomal dominant.

Disease mechanisms
Not known.

Clinical features
Tremor affects the arms (94%), head (titubation, 33%) and voice (16%). The tremor is worse on maintaining a posture and when anxious, and improves following small amounts of alcohol in 70%. Coordination and gait are otherwise normal.

Investigation
- *Thyroid function:* excludes thyrotoxicosis
- *Copper studies:* excludes Wilson's disease (p. 928) if the history is not typical

Management
About 70% of patients improve with propranolol; primidone has similar efficacy.

Prognosis
The condition is only occasionally progressive; however, significant social or physical disability is experienced by one-third of patients.

Cerebellar disorders

Epidemiology
Prevalence. Taken together, approximately 40 in 100 000.

Age. Some disorders affect mainly children, while others affect mainly adolescents or adults.

Genetics. Friedreich's ataxia is autosomal recessive, because of an expanded trinucleotide repeat in the *frataxin* gene.

Disease mechanisms
Many different disease processes can cause cerebellar disorders, including acquired conditions such as paraneoplastic cerebellar degeneration and inherited conditions such as ataxia telangiectasia (Table 13.26). Some ataxias can be caused by spinocerebellar tract degeneration rather than disease of the cerebellum itself.

Clinical features
The main features are:
- Slurred speech (dysarthria)
- Unsteady walking (ataxia)
- Incoordination of hand and arm movements
- Nystagmus

Patients complain of unsteadiness 'as if drunk'. Patients may stumble when trying to change direction and the gait is broad-based. Finger–nose testing may show a tremor that increases in amplitude as the finger nears the target (intention tremor) or misses the target altogether (past-pointing).

Clinical features suggestive of specific disorders:
- *Sudden onset:* suggests stroke (p. 891)
- *Drugs:* may induce cerebellar symptoms even if serum levels are in the 'therapeutic' range
- *Wernicke's encephalopathy:* may be accompanied by confusion, nystagmus, internuclear ophthalmoplegia and absent ankle reflexes

Table 13.26 Causes of cerebellar disorders

Common

Vascular
Cerebellar/brainstem infarct or haemorrhage

Acute toxicity
Acute alcohol intoxication
Anticonvulsants (phenytoin, carbamazepine, valproate)
Sedatives (benzodiazepines, phenothiazines, lithium)

Chronic toxicity
Chronic alcoholic cerebellar degeneration

Multiple sclerosis

Space-occupying lesion
Metastatic tumour
Primary tumour (medulloblastoma or astrocytoma in children, haemangioblastoma in adults)
Cerebellar abscess
Benign tumour (e.g. acoustic neuroma)
Aneurysm of the basilar or other artery

Less common

Degenerative
Creutzfeldt–Jakob disease

Associated with viral infection
HIV
Varicella zoster

Immune mediated
Miller–Fisher syndrome
Paraneoplastic cerebellar degeneration (in association with small cell lung cancer)

Nutritional
Thiamine deficiency causing Wernicke's encephalopathy
Vitamin E deficiency caused by malabsorption (e.g. in coeliac disease)

Endocrine
Hypothyroidism

Genetic
Friedreich's ataxia
Ataxia telangiectasia
Spinocerebellar ataxia
Mitochondrial disease
Episodic ataxia

- *MS (p. 920):* there is usually a history of a relapsing–remitting disorder affecting several sites in the CNS
- *Posterior fossa space-occupying lesions:* cause symptoms and signs of raised intracranial pressure (p. 913)
- *Acoustic neuroma:* causes gradual onset sensorineural deafness
- *Vitamin E deficiency:* may be associated with areflexia,

a history of fat malabsorption or acanthocytosis in a peripheral blood film
- *Friedreich's ataxia:* associated with an onset at less than 25 years of age, UMN signs in legs, absent ankle jerks, absent sensory nerve action potentials and normal motor nerve conduction velocity

Investigation

Patients with impaired consciousness require urgent investigation as cerebellar swelling can obstruct CSF pathways, causing obstructive hydrocephalus, transtentorial herniation and death. With tumours, cerebellar infarcts and cerebellar haemorrhages, this can occur over a few hours, and patients with such lesions who become drowsy require immediate CT scanning.

Haematology
- *Thyroid function tests, antineuronal antibodies and syphilis serology:* indicated if there is no structural lesion on scanning and no clinical evidence of MS or alcoholism
- *Vitamin E levels and antigliadin antibodies:* should be tested in patients with fat malabsorption

Diagnostic imaging
- *Chest radiography or CT:* to look for a bronchial neoplasm
- *MRI of brain:* required to exclude a structural lesion where there is no clear systemic cause such as drugs, alcohol or MS
- *Pelvic ultrasound:* in females, to exclude an ovarian tumour

Other investigations
Once a structural lesion has been ruled out, CSF examination may show oligoclonal bands suggestive of MS, or lymphocytes or malignant cells suggesting an underlying inflammatory or malignant disorder.

Management and prognosis

Depends on the cause (Table 13.27).

Structural lesions of the brain

The presence of a space-occupying lesion has similar consequences regardless of its nature. These fall into the following categories:
- Focal neurological deficits
- Epilepsy (p. 900)
- Raised intracranial pressure (p. 913)
- Hydrocephalus (p. 942)

Cerebral tumours

Epidemiology

Annual incidence. Malignant brain tumour 5–15 in

Table 13.27 Management of cerebellar disorders

Supportive treatment
Rehabilitation
Occupational therapy, physiotherapy and social work
assessment are essential for patients with chronic ataxia

Genetic counselling
Families with hereditary ataxias should be offered genetic
counselling

Specific treatment
Treat any underlying cause
Medical treatment of cerebellar incoordination and ataxia is
usually unrewarding, but propranolol and primidone are
occasionally helpful
Stroke (see p. 891; EMERGENCY BOX 13.1; Table 13.5)
Wernicke's encephalopathy (see p. 931)
Multiple sclerosis (see p. 920; Table 13.21)
Tumours (see Table 13.28)
Replacement of thiamine, vitamin E as appropriate
(Table 13.26)

100 000; metastatic brain tumour 3–15 in 100 000; benign brain tumour 10 in 100 000.

Age. Following a peak in early childhood, when tumours are often located in the posterior fossa, the incidence of all brain tumours increases with age.

Genetics. Bilateral acoustic neuromas and meningiomas occur in type 2 neurofibromatosis, an autosomal dominant condition due to a mutation in *merlin*. Von Hippel–Lindau disease is an autosomal dominant condition causing cerebellar haemangioblastoma and renal carcinoma and is caused by mutation in the *VHL tumour suppressor gene.*

Disease mechanisms

The vast majority of cerebral tumours are of unknown cause.

Cerebral abscess

The annual incidence of cerebral abscess is 1 in 100 000. The clinical manifestations include headache, fever and malaise in a tachycardic, drowsy and confused patient. However, abscesses may occur in the absence of fever or other signs of systemic infection. In addition to the general features of space-occupying lesions described above, there may also be clinical features relevant to the source of the infection or to predisposing factors (e.g. infected sinuses, mastoids or ears; bronchiectasis; congenital heart disease; bacterial endocarditis; tuberculosis; or AIDS).

Extradural and subdural haematoma

Extradural haematoma is usually a consequence of head trauma; tearing of a branch of the middle meningeal artery leads to arterial bleeding into the extradural space. Blood accumulates rapidly, causing mass effect and dysfunction of underlying brain, often with significant midline shift. Without treatment it is often fatal.

While subdural haematoma may also occur acutely, it usually presents 2–5 weeks after head injury. It is caused by tearing of small veins bridging between the brain surface and the dura, and leads to the accumulation of blood in the subdural space. It usually affects patients over 50 years, and while there may initially be a symptom-free period this is followed by the insidious onset of headache, confusion, dementia or evolving focal deficit.

Subdural empyema

Infection in the frontal sinuses or middle ear may extend to the subdural space, causing local pain and tenderness, fever, headache and impaired conscious level. There are often focal signs including hemiplegia, hemisensory disturbance, a unilateral extensor plantar or paralysis of lateral gaze.

Investigation
Haematology
- *FBC:* to check for an elevated white cell count (but in cerebral abscess this may be normal)
- *ESR and CRP*

Microbiology
Blood cultures and culture of abscess material.

Diagnostic imaging
- *CT scanning:* with contrast, will determine whether a space-occupying lesion is present. Patients with subdural empyema may have a 'normal' scan initially, with changes only becoming apparent on repeated scanning 24–48 h later.
- *MRI:* it may be difficult to differentiate tumour from abscess at CT scanning, and in these circumstances MRI may provide better information, particularly for lesions in the posterior fossa.
- *Chest radiography:* helps to identify bronchogenic carcinoma, tuberculosis or chronic lung suppuration.
- *CT scanning of the sinuses and mastoids:* if cerebral abscess or subdural empyema present.

Histopathology
Stereotactic or open biopsy. For tumours and abscesses a histological or microbiological diagnosis should be made on tissue obtained at biopsy.

13

Other investigations
- *Lumbar puncture:* should be avoided because of the risks of tonsilar herniation
- *Screening:* patients with cerebellar haemangioblastomas, and their families, should be screened for renal cell carcinomas (von Hippel–Lindau disease).

Management
Extradural and subdural haematomas are usually drained surgically, and cerebral abscesses should be drained and treated with appropriate antibiotics. The management of a cerebral tumour depends on its type, site and size and on the general condition of the patient (Table 13.28).

Prognosis
The prognosis for promptly treated extradural and subdural haematoma, subdural empyema and cerebral abscess is good, but delays in treatment can be fatal. Epilepsy is a frequent complication of cerebral abscess, subdural empyema and brain tumour. The prognosis for glioblastoma is poor, but patients with a solitary cerebral metastasis may do well following successful excision.

Structural lesions of the spine

Spinal cord lesions

Prompt recognition and treatment of compressive lesions of the spinal cord can prevent the development of severe neurological disability. Rapidly progressive symptoms are a neurological and potentially a neurosurgical emergency, especially if faecal or urinary continence is impaired. Determine when the patient was last able to walk, stand unaided, pass urine and open their bowels (EMERGENCY BOX 13.6).

Epidemiology
Incidence. Uncommon.

Cerebral tumours at a glance

Epidemiology
Incidence
Annual incidence is approximately 1 in 2500

Age
Peaks in fifth decade

Sex
55% occur in men

Genetics
Possible dominant inheritance of neurofibroma and cerebellar heamangioblastoma (von Hippel–Lindau disease)

Clinical features
Epilepsy
Dysphasia
Cognitive defect
Hemiparesis
Personality change
Headache
Papilloedema
Vomiting

Findings on investigation
Blood tests
- *White cell count, ESR and CRP:* may be elevated with cerebral abscess

- *Tumour markers (CEA, CA125, PSA, α-fetoprotein):* may indicate site of primary tumour in metastatic disease

Diagnostic imaging
- *CT:* with or without intravenous contrast to locate site of mass. It is sometimes difficult to differentiate malignant tumours from benign tumours and from cerebral abcesses

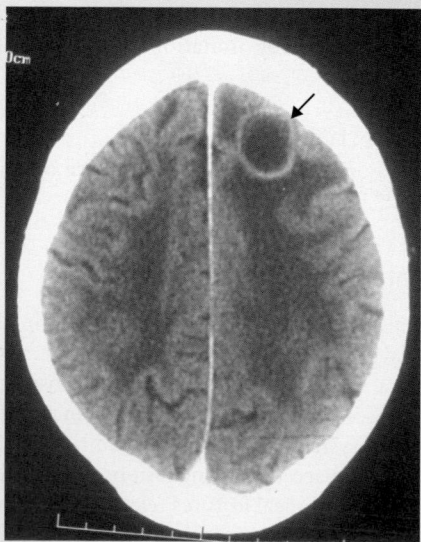

Fig. A CT showing brain abcess.

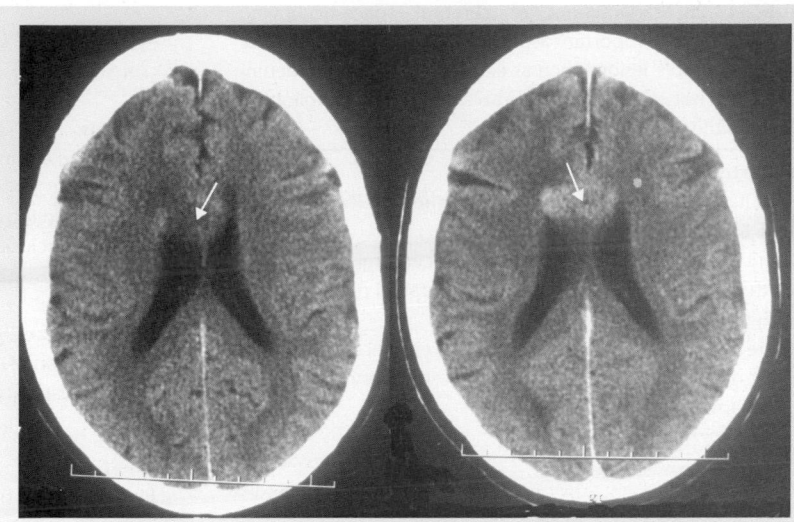

Fig. B CT (pre- and postcontrast) showing glioma.

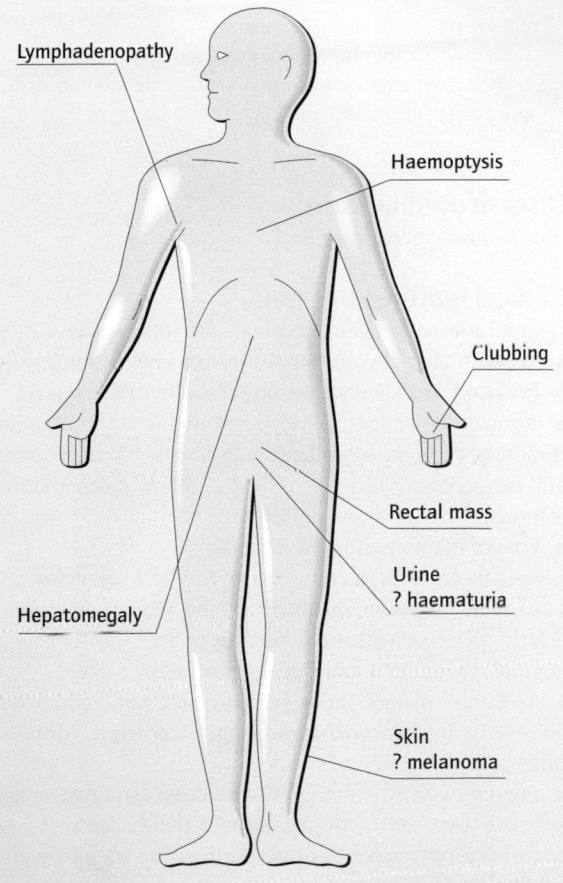

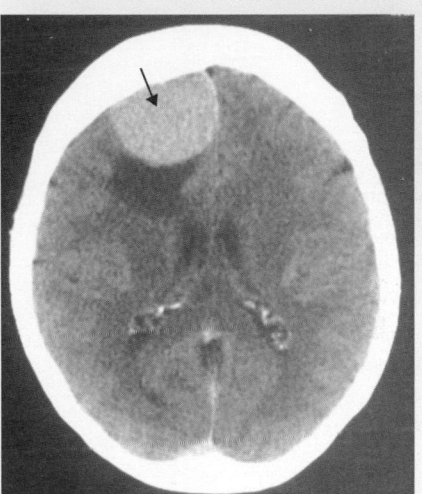

Fig. C CT (postcontrast) showing meningioma.

- *MRI:* provides better resolution than CT, especially in posterior fossa
- *Chest X-ray, liver ultrasound, CT of abdomen and pelvis:* to look for primary tumour in suspected metastatic disease

Tissue diagnosis
Of a peripheral lesion
- Bronchoscopy
- Liver biopsy
- Skin biopsy
- Endoscopy
Brain biopsy
- Open biopsy
- Stereotactic biopsy

13

Table 13.28 Management of cerebral space-occupying lesions. The most important aspect of management is to make sure that curable lesions such as cerebral abscesses or meningiomas are not mistaken for incurable lesions such as glioblastoma multiforme

Supportive treatment
Resuscitation (Airway, Breathing, Circulation)
Correct any electrolyte imbalance
If there is significant brain swelling, treat cerebral oedema with dexamethasone and reduce intracranial pressure (EMERGENCY BOX 13.4, p. 915)
If there is dilatation of the ventricular system because of obstructive hydrocephalus, consider temporary or permanent ventricular drainage

Specific treatment
Glioma
Biopsy
Whole brain radiotherapy
Chemotherapy

Cerebral lymphoma
Biopsy
Chemotherapy

Meningioma
Excision
Consider radiotherapy

Pituitary tumour
Excision
Radiotherapy

Childhood tumours
Medulloblastoma
Biopsy/excision
Radiotherapy

Cerebellar astrocytoma
Biopsy/excision

Cerebral abscess
Stereotactic aspiration
Treat with appropriate antibiotics

Solitary or multiple metastases
Biopsy
Consider excision
Consider radiotherapy

Age and geography. In the developed world, spinal cord compression occurs in older people as a result of cervical spondylosis or metastatic disease. In Africa and South America, tuberculous abscess of the spine is common. Non-compressive spinal cord syndromes include MS in the developed world, human T-cell lymphotropic virus (HTLV-1) infections in the tropics (tropical spastic paraplegia), and AIDS myelopathy where HIV infection is endemic.

Emergency 13.6: Management of suspected spinal cord compression

Diagnosis
Consider the diagnosis in any patient with:
- Spinal pain
- Weakness in legs
Other signs include:
- Sphincter disturbance
- Sensory level
- Loss of reflexes
Look for evidence in the history and examination of malignant disease, which may have metastasized to the cord.

Investigation
- Chest X-ray
- Plain radiography
- Urgent MRI imaging of cord
- Biopsy of extradural compressive lesions

Treatment
- Dexamethasone may reduce cord oedema
- Urgent referral to neurosurgeon and/or radiation oncologist as appropriate

Disease mechanisms
(See Tables 13.29 and 13.30.)

Clinical features (Fig. 13.15)
General clinical features of spinal cord lesions are:
- Weak or absent voluntary movement below the lesion
- Reduced or absent sensation below the affected level
- Abnormal reflex activity: immediately following traumatic cord injury reflexes may be lost (spinal shock), but late excessively brisk reflexes and extensor plantar responses (UMN signs) develop
- Loss of bladder and bowel function
  Specific features of compressive cord lesions include:
- *Chronic degenerative arthritis:* the patient is usually elderly, perhaps with neck pain or stiffness, the onset is gradual and acute deterioration may follow a fall
- *Metastatic disease:* there is usually back pain, tenderness on percussing the spine, or radicular (nerve root compression) pain
- *Pyogenic abscess:* tuberculous infection can cause severe kyphosis because of destruction of the vertebral body; acute bacterial abscesses cause acute severe back pain and tenderness

Specific clinical features of non-compressive cord lesions include:
- *MS* (p. 920): there may be a history of a relapsing–remitting neurological disorder. The onset of symptoms is over days and weeks rather than hours.

Table 13.29 Compressive lesions causing spinal cord syndromes

Common
Chronic degenerative osteoarthritis
Cervical spondylosis

Metastatic malignancy
Metastases to vertebral body from primary tumour in the lung, breast or prostate

Less common
Primary malignant tumour
Myeloma
Lymphoma
Sarcoma

Primary benign tumour
Meningioma
Neurofibroma
Lipoma

Intrinsic cord pathology
Syringomyelia (see p. 941)
Intrinsic tumour

Trauma
Vertebral fracture

Infection
Paraspinal abscess (e.g. acute pyogenic, chronic tuberculosis)

Acute central disc prolapse
Cervical or thoracic disc (rare)

Congenital abnormality
Arnold–Chiari malformation
Spina bifida
Scoliosis

Atlantoaxial subluxation of rheumatoid arthritis

Hypertrophy of dura
Chronic meningitis
Idiopathic hypertrophic pachymeningitis

Table 13.30 Non-compressive lesions causing spinal cord syndromes

Common
Demyelination
MS

Less common
Inflammatory
Acute transverse myelitis

Vascular
Spinal cord infarction

Vitamin deficiency
B_{12} deficiency (subacute combined degeneration of the cord)

Degenerative
Motor neurone disease

Infective
Neurosyphilis
AIDS myelopathy
HTLV-1 myelopathy

Fibrosis
Postradiotherapy to chest, abdomen

Genetic
Friedreich's ataxia
Spinocerebellar degeneration
Hereditary spastic paraplegia

HTVL, human T-cell lymphotropic virus.

- *Acute transverse myelitis:* the onset of symptoms is over minutes or hours. This may occur in the context of recent infection, such as *Mycoplasma pneumoniae*.
- *Vitamin B_{12} deficiency:* causes degeneration of both the pyramidal (corticospinal) and dorsal column (posterior spinothalamic) tracts, causing UMN signs in the legs and loss of vibration sensation and proprioception in the feet. An axonal peripheral neuropathy may also occur, giving absent ankle jerks.
- *Motor neurone disease* (p. 945): shows widespread muscle wasting and fasciculation associated with difficulties with speech and swallowing, and a lack of sensory signs (a mixture of UMN and LMN signs in the arms and legs). The tongue may fasciculate.

- *Acute spinal cord infarction:* usually caused by anterior spinal artery occlusion in elderly patients, there is sudden-onset loss of power and spinothalamic (pain and temperature) sensation below the level of the lesion, usually with preservation of dorsal column sensation (proprioception, vibration and light touch). Loss of spinothalamic sensation in the hands may lead to patients burning themselves without noticing it.
- *Infective:* features of systemic disturbance usually provide evidence of HIV or syphilis infection. HTLV-1 myelopathy may occur in otherwise healthy people.
- *Radiation fibrosis:* there is a history of radiotherapy to near the spinal cord.
- *Genetic:* many genetic disorders including Friedreich's ataxia can affect the spinal cord.

Is the lesion really in the spinal cord?

Patients with brainstem lesions or with bilateral hemisphere lesions may mimic a cord lesion, with UMN and sensory signs in all limbs, but the presence of dysphasia or confusion or cranial nerve palsies places the lesion *above* the spinal cord. UMN signs restricted to one limb are usually caused by intracranial rather than spinal cord pathology.

13

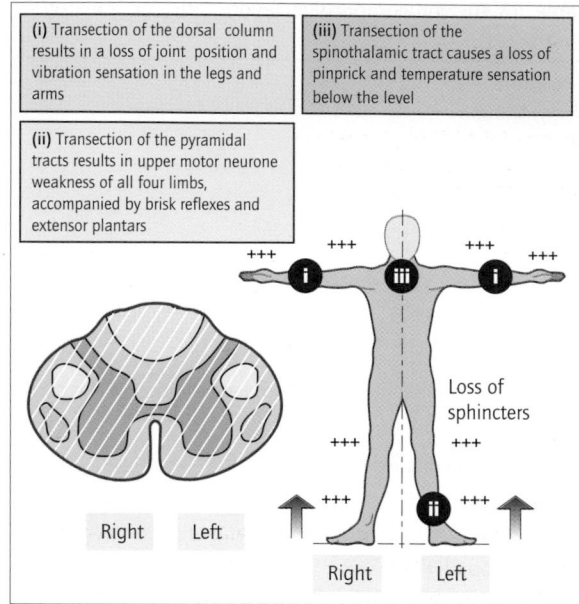

(i) Transection of the dorsal column results in a loss of joint position and vibration sensation in the legs and arms

(ii) Transection of the pyramidal tracts results in upper motor neurone weakness of all four limbs, accompanied by brisk reflexes and extensor plantars

(iii) Transection of the spinothalamic tract causes a loss of pinprick and temperature sensation below the level

Loss of sphincters

Right Left

Right Left

(a)

(i) Pressure on the sensory root at T8 causes pain radiating anteriorly in the root distribution and this may be accompanied by hyperaesthesia

(ii) Transection of the pyramidal tract results in upper motor neurone weakness in the right leg

(iii) Transection of the spinothalamic tract causes a loss of pinprick in the left trunk below the level and in the left leg

Right Left

Right Left

(b)

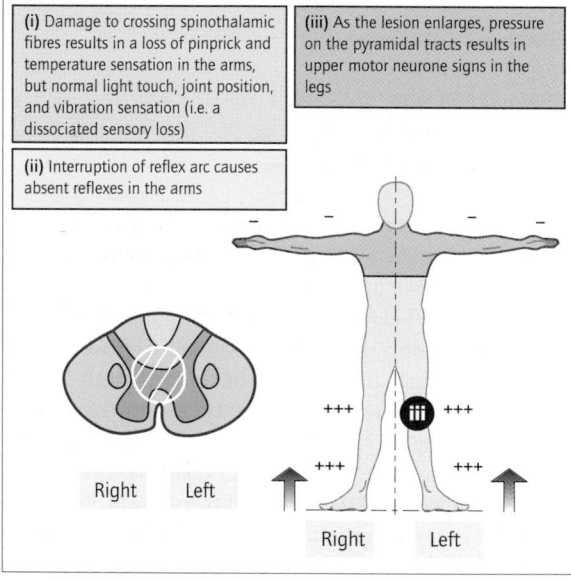

(i) Damage to crossing spinothalamic fibres results in a loss of pinprick and temperature sensation in the arms, but normal light touch, joint position, and vibration sensation (i.e. a dissociated sensory loss)

(ii) Interruption of reflex arc causes absent reflexes in the arms

(iii) As the lesion enlarges, pressure on the pyramidal tracts results in upper motor neurone signs in the legs

Right Left

Right Left

(c)

Figure 13.15 Common patterns of cord lesion. (a) Cord transection. (b) Cord hemisection (Brown-Séquard syndrome) at T8. (c) Cervical central cord syndrome.

Spinal nerve root lesions

Root lesions are rarely associated with serious underlying disease. They are commonly caused by a prolapsed intervertebral disc (PLID) and are a major cause of pain, distress and work absences.

Epidemiology
Prevalence. Prevalence of PLID 300 in 100 000. Annual incidence 150 in 100 000.

Age. Prevalence increases with age.

Risk factors. Trauma, manual occupation.

Disease mechanisms
Root compression may be caused by PLID or facet joint osteoarthritis and hypertrophy causing narrowing of the neural exit foramina (Table 13.31). Herpes zoster is the most common cause of non-compressive root lesions.

Table 13.31 Causes of root lesions

Common compressive lesions
Degenerative osteoarthritis
Cervical spondylosis
Lumbar spondylosis
Lumbar stenosis

Rupture of nucleus pulposus
Acute lumbar disc prolapse

Less common compressive disorders
Primary benign tumour of the nerve root
Neurofibroma

Secondary tumour in the vertebral body
Metastasis from lung, breast, prostate

Compression of roots in the cauda equina
Primary or secondary tumour

Tumour outside the vertebral column
Pelvic, retroperitoneal or thoracic malignancy

Common acute non-compressive root lesions
Infection
Herpes zoster
Lyme disease

Meningitic processes
Chronic infective meningitis
Sarcoidosis

Clinical features

Root lesions cause four cardinal symptoms and signs in the cutaneous distribution (dermatome) and muscles (myotome) supplied by that root:

- Pain
- Weakness
- Sensory loss
- Loss of the tendon reflex

The pain often shoots down the limb and is exacerbated by traction on the root (e.g. bending, neck turning, coughing, straining on the toilet). An aching pain that does not radiate below the knees is often referred pain from diseased facet joints rather than nerve root entrapment pain.

Specific clinical features of spinal nerve root lesions (Fig. 13.16):

- *Cervical spondylosis:* insidious onset, intermittent symptoms, middle-aged or elderly patient
- *Lumbar canal stenosis:* insidious onset, in elderly patients, of numbness and weakness of the legs on prolonged standing or walking; can mimic vascular claudication in that it is relieved by rest
- *Acute disc prolapse:* sudden onset, usually associated with effort
- *Cauda equina syndrome:* sensory loss over the genitalia, perineum and buttocks, with urinary retention and faecal incontinence

Isolated T1 root lesion

An isolated T1 root lesion may result from a cervical rib or an apical chest tumour (Pancoast's syndrome). It causes weakness and wasting of the small muscles of the hand and numbness over the medial aspect of the forearm. There may be an associated ipsilateral Horner's syndrome because of interruption of the sympathetic fibres to the eye.

Investigation of cord and root lesions

Spinal cord and root disorders often coexist and so their investigation and management will be considered together.

Haematology

- *FBC and ESR:* to screen for malignancy and infection
- *Protein electrophoresis:* to detect myeloma
- *Angiotensin-converting enzyme (ACE):* for sarcoidosis
- *B_{12} levels:* for subacute combined degeneration of the cord
- *HTLV and HIV testing:* where this is a likely cause

Diagnostic imaging

- *Plain radiography:* may show destruction of pedicles diagnostic of malignancy. Patients with rheumatoid arthritis who complain of weakness, neck pain, occipital pain or brainstem signs must have flexion–extension views of the neck to look for atlantoaxial subluxation. Radiological evidence of cervical or lumbar spondylosis is so common as to be meaningless.
- *MRI:* the investigation of choice for spinal cord and nerve root lesions, but may be technically difficult in acutely ill patients.
- *CT scanning:* perhaps with contrast myelography, can be useful in the diagnosis of acute central disc prolapse where the patient is unable to tolerate MRI.

Management of spinal cord and root lesions
(Table 13.32)

Acute cord lesions

Seek immediate specialist neurological or neurosurgical advice where there is:

- *Rapidly progressive weakness, especially with sphincter involvement:* emergency discectomy is indicated for acute central disc prolapse, and malignant cord compression may respond to emergency radiotherapy with reversal of the neurological deficit
- *Established paraplegia and loss of sphincter control:* some patients with benign spinal tumours can make an excellent recovery with surgery, despite delayed diagnosis and treatment

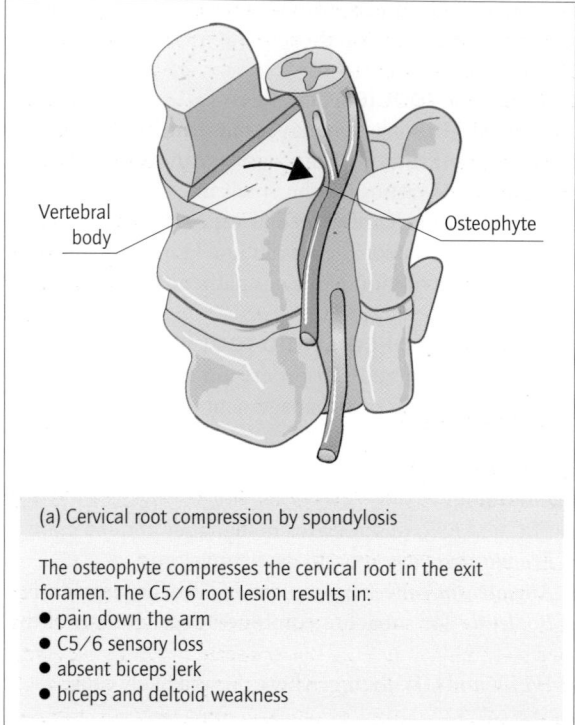

Vertebral body

Osteophyte

(a) Cervical root compression by spondylosis

The osteophyte compresses the cervical root in the exit foramen. The C5/6 root lesion results in:
- pain down the arm
- C5/6 sensory loss
- absent biceps jerk
- biceps and deltoid weakness

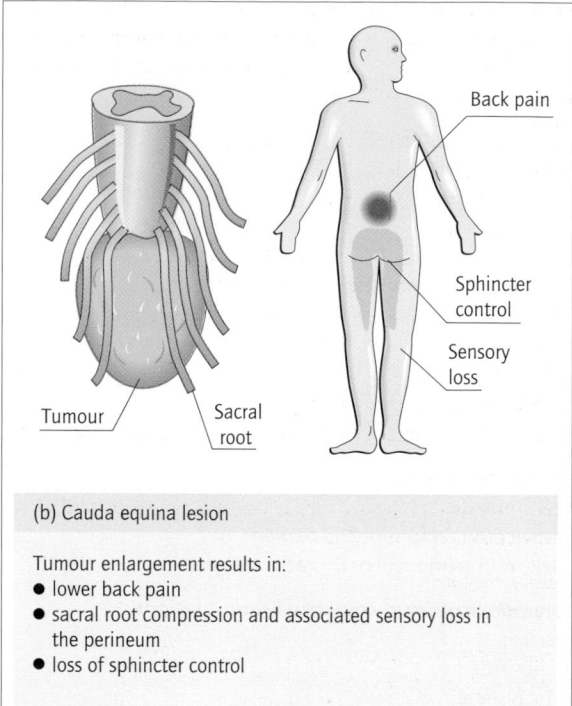

Back pain

Sphincter control

Sensory loss

Tumour

Sacral root

(b) Cauda equina lesion

Tumour enlargement results in:
- lower back pain
- sacral root compression and associated sensory loss in the perineum
- loss of sphincter control

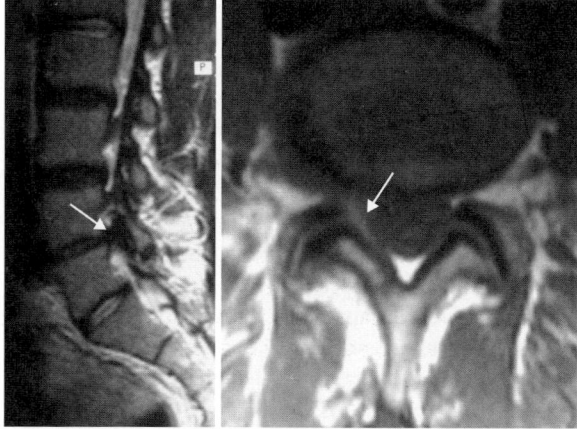

(c) MRI showing lateral disc prolapse.

Figure 13.16 Common patterns of root lesion.

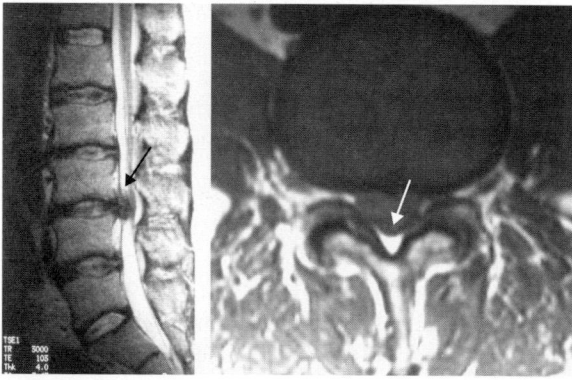

(d) MRI showing central disc prolapse.

Prevent complications:
- Turn regularly to prevent pressure sores
- Use antiembolism stockings and low-dose subcutaneous heparin to prevent deep-vein thrombosis and pulmonary embolism
- Arrange passive exercises by the physiotherapist to prevent contractures
- Pay careful attention to the urinary tract and catheterize if necessary

- If there is quadriplegia, monitor respiratory function and arrange regular chest physiotherapy

Arrange rehabilitation at a specialist spinal rehabilitation unit.

Root lesions without cord involvement
- *Acute PLID:* if there is no evidence of central disc prolapse (bilateral pain or weakness; bladder involvement) treat with analgesia and gradual mobilization. Ninety-five

Table 13.32 Management of cord and root lesions. Immediate specialist referral and urgent imaging is required for all acute cord syndromes and for patients with established cord syndromes who develop involvement of the bladder or faecal incontinence

Supportive treatment
Treat any underlying cause
If there is a malignancy, treat the primary tumour
If there is severe weakness of the legs turn regularly, use antiembolism stockings and low-dose subcutaneous heparin, arrange passive exercises, and pay careful attention to the urinary tract—catheterize if necessary
If there is quadriplegia also monitor respiratory function and arrange regular chest physiotherapy
Arrange rehabilitation at a specialist spinal rehabilitation unit

Specific treatment
Seek immediate specialist neurological or neurosurgical advice and arrange rapid transfer

Dexamethasone
May reduce oedema around the site of compression

Immediate surgical biopsy and/or decompression
May be indicated for confirmed cord compression

Radiotherapy
Provides specific treatment for some tumours and palliative pain-relieving treatment for metastatic tumours

ROOT LESIONS WITHOUT CORD INVOLVEMENT
Supportive treatment
Analgesics for pain
Gradual mobilization as pain allows

Specific treatment
Acute lumbar disc prolapse
Most (~95%) prolapsed lumbar discs will improve spontaneously over 4–6 months. Consider imaging (MRI) and surgical referral at 4 months, or earlier if there are motor symptoms at onset. Central lumbar disc prolapse resulting in bilateral signs or in sphincter disturbance requires immediate neurosurgical referral

Acute cervical disc prolapse
Cervical collar; immediate transfer to a neurological or neurosurgical unit if cord symptoms or signs develop

Benign and malignant tumours affecting the roots
Establish histological diagnosis and then consider definitive or palliative therapy

Herpes zoster
Use specific antiviral agents (e.g. aciclovir) early in the attack

per cent of root compression will resolve as the prolapsed disc dessicates, but for those who remain symptomatic after 4 months specialist referral is indicated.

- *Acute cervical disc prolapse:* give analgesia and apply a rigid cervical collar to reduce pain and muscle spasm. Seek urgent advice if pain is severe or if features of cord compression develop.
- *Benign or malignant tumour affecting the roots:* establish the histological diagnosis by biopsy and treat as appropriate.
- *Herpes zoster:* antiviral agents such as aciclovir may speed healing and reduce the risk of postherpetic neuralgia if started early in an attack.

Syringomyelia

Epidemiology
Prevalence. 7 in 100 000. Annual incidence 0.4 in 100 000.

Disease mechanisms
A central fluid-filled cavity develops in the spinal cord (syringomyelia) and it may extend to the brainstem (syringobulbia). It may be associated with congenital abnormalities at the foramen magnum (e.g. Arnold–Chiari malformation) or occur secondary to a tumour of the cord or to trauma. The expanding cavity compresses sensory fibres crossing the midline on their way to join the lateral spinothalamic tract; later, it may also compress the corticospinal tracts.

Clinical features
There is loss of pain and temperature, but not light touch, proprioception or vibration sensation (dissociated sensory loss) at the segmental levels of the syrinx, often described as being like a cape over the patient's shoulders. There is also reflex loss at the same levels of the lesion. Often the early symptoms and signs are asymmetrical. Patients may complain of stiffness and weakness in the legs and of neck pain. As symptoms progress UMN signs may develop in the legs.

Investigation
MRI scanning of the cord will reveal the syrinx and any associated pathologies (Fig. 13.17).

Management
Surgical treatment of associated structural abnormalities or drainage of the syrinx with a syringoperitoneal shunt may relieve pain and arrest progression of the neurological deficit.

Prognosis
The rate of progression varies considerably, and the condition may arrest spontaneously.

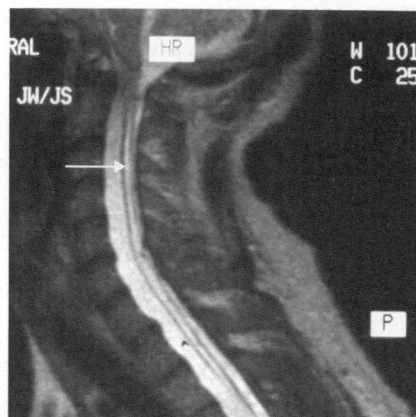

Figure 13.17 MRI showing syringomyelia.

Disorders of cerebrospinal fluid dynamics

Hydrocephalus

Epidemiology
Prevalence. Rare.

Age. Children are particularly affected. Normal-pressure hydrocephalus commonly affects the elderly.

Disease mechanisms
Hydrocephalus is defined as increased ventricular volume, usually associated with increased CSF pressure. There are numerous causes (Table 13.33).

The normal volume of CSF is approximately 200 ml; the choroid plexuses of the ventricular system produce 500 ml of CSF each day, which circulates through the foraminae of Luschka and Magendie to the subarachnoid space where it is reabsorbed by the arachnoid granulations in the walls of major venous sinuses (Fig. 13.18).

While lesions at different sites in the CSF circulation pathways will have different effects, obstruction at any level from the lateral ventricles (e.g. colloid cyst of third ventricle obstructing the foramen of Monro) to the arachnoid granulations (e.g. by clotted blood following subarachnoid haemorrhage) causes ventricular enlargement and hydrocephalus.

Clinical features
If hydrocephalus develops before closure of the skull sutures (about 2 years of age), the skull will be enlarged. While long-standing hydrocephalus can be asymptomatic,

Table 13.33 Causes of hydrocephalus

Obstruction to flow of CSF (obstructive hydrocephalus)
Third ventricle block
Colloid cyst (which may cause intermittent block)
Hemisphere tumour

Aqueduct block
Congenital aqueduct stenosis
Blood clot from intraventricular haemorrhage or SAH
Midbrain tumour

Posterior fossa block
Tumour
Cerebellar haematoma or infarction
Arnold–Chiari malformation
Dandy–Walker malformation

Non-obstructive causes (communicating hydrocephalus)
Impaired CSF reabsorption
SAH
Meningitis
• Acute bacterial
• Chronic infective (e.g. tuberculous meningitis)
• Chronic inflammatory (e.g. sarcoidosis)
• Malignant

Excessive CSF production
Choroid plexus papilloma (rare)

Secondary to cerebral atrophy
Cerebral atrophy of any cause

Unknown
Normal-pressure hydrocephalus

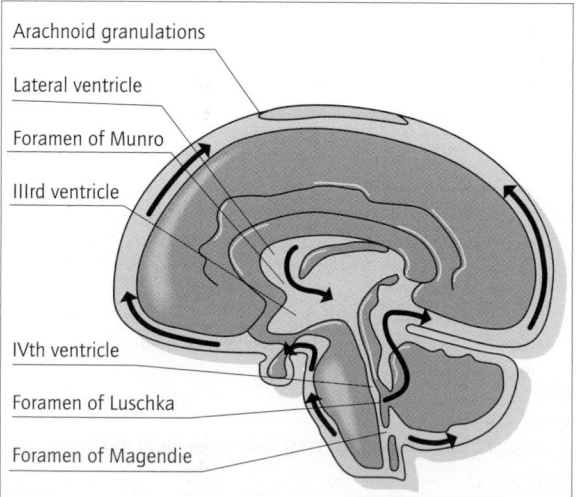

Figure 13.18 Intracranial cerebrospinal fluid dynamics.

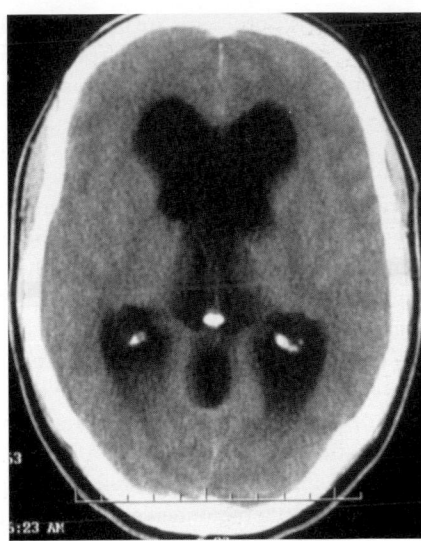

Figure 13.19 CT showing acute hydrocephalus.

acute dilatation of the ventricular system or rises in CSF pressure are almost always symptomatic.

Obstructive hydrocephalus

Obstructive hydrocephalus presents with the symptoms and signs of raised intracranial pressure (p. 913). There may be impaired consciousness, gait abnormalities, seizures, pituitary dysfunction (third ventricle pressure effects on the hypothalamus) and bilateral UMN signs.

Normal-pressure hydrocephalus

Normal-pressure hydrocephalus is characterized by ventricular enlargement without a sustained increase in CSF pressure. The following clinical features are required to make the diagnosis:

- Dementia
- Gait apraxia (the patient has normal power and sensation, is unable to walk but can 'cycle' their legs in the air on the bed)
- Urinary incontinence

Many elderly patients have some of these problems and have a dilated ventricular system resulting from cerebral atrophy. It is therefore essential to provide objective evidence that reducing CSF volume (by repeated lumbar puncture) has a reproducible effect on robust measures of impairment, such as the timed 10 m walk.

Investigation
Diagnostic imaging
CT scanning confirms the presence of hydrocephalus (Fig. 13.19) and, from the pattern of ventricular enlargement, will help determine the site of the obstruction to CSF flow.

Table 13.34 Management of disorders of cerebrospinal fluid dynamics

Obstructive hydrocephalus
Temporary (ventricular access device with external ventricular drainage) or permanent (ventriculoperitoneal or ventriculoatrial shunting) may be required

Idiopathic intracranial hypertension
Immediate control of symptoms usually obtained by serial lumbar puncture
Exclude cerebral sinus thrombosis with CTV or MRV
Identify and discontinue drugs associated with IIH (OCP, vitamin A, tetracyclines)
Measure and monitor visual fields

In longer term, usually responds to weight loss and diuretics (e.g. acetazolamide)
Continuing headache or progressive visual loss indicates need for permanent CSF drainage procedure such as lumboperitoneal shunting or optic nerve sheath fenestration

CTV, CT venogram; IIH, idiopathic intracranial hypertension; MRV, MR venogram; OCP, oral contraceptive pill.

Other investigations
CSF examination. Where there is no obvious cause, CSF should be taken for culture (including testing for tuberculous and fungal infection), biochemistry (for evidence of inflammation) and neuropathology (for evidence of malignant meningitis).

Management (Table 13.34)
Long-standing compensated hydrocephalus is often best managed conservatively. Patients with symptomatic hydrocephalus may require surgical drainage (with a ventriculoperitoneal shunt). True normal-pressure hydrocephalus may also respond to surgical drainage. However, complications including the development of subdural haematoma, ventriculitis, bacterial colonization of shunt plasticware and shunt malfunction dictate that such procedures should only be used in patients who are likely to derive significant benefit.

Prognosis
CSF shunting can be life saving in hydrocephalus, and some patients may go on to lead a normal life. While normal-pressure hydrocephalus may also improve with CSF shunting, the complications of the procedure can offset the benefits.

Idiopathic intracranial hypertension

The previous term 'benign intracranial hypertension' has been discarded because it implied a rather tame, non-threatening disease; however, if untreated the condition can lead to complete blindness.

Epidemiology

Prevalence. Rare.

Age. Young and middle-aged women.

Sex. Seventy-five per cent of patients are female.

Disease mechanisms

This condition of unknown aetiology usually occurs in obese females; it may be drug-related (e.g. tetracyclines, oral contraceptives, vitamin A overdosage) or related to endocrine dysfunction (e.g. Addison's disease), and in some patients it may be associated with cortical venous thrombosis.

Clinical features

Patients present with headaches typical of raised intracranial pressure with papilloedema, but without focal neurological signs. There may be episodes of visual loss caused by waves of increased intracranial pressure reducing retinal perfusion. Visual fields should be charted at each clinic visit to ensure there is no progressive field defect.

Investigation

● *Urgent CT scan:* required to exclude a mass lesion or obstructive hydrocephalus.
● *Lumbar puncture:* CSF should be obtained by lumbar puncture if the CT scan is normal. The diagnosis is confirmed if the pressure is elevated, the CSF is acellular and its protein level is normal.
● *CT* or *MR venography:* required to exclude thrombosis of the cerebral sinuses.

Management (Table 13.34)

Where present, venous thrombosis should be treated (see p. 899). Most patients respond to weight loss and carbonic anhydrase inhibitors such as acetazolamide. Those whose symptoms progress may require neurosurgical treatment in the form of optic nerve fenestration or thecoperitoneal shunting.

Prognosis

With appropriate treatment only a few patients develop persistent visual loss.

Diseases of cranial nerves

The examination of the cranial nerves is described in HISTORY & EXAMINATION BOXES 13.6 and 13.7 and common patterns of deficit are discussed on pp. 875–880. Common causes of cranial nerve problems are given in Table 13.35. Cranial nerve dysfunction may result from compression, impaired vascular supply or from inflammation.

Compression

Brain swelling may lead to herniation of the uncus downwards through the tentorium cerebri and compression of the oculomotor (IIIrd) nerve as it passes over the free edge of the tentorium. This is the cause of a fixed dilated pupil and indicates severe brain swelling requiring immediate treatment (see EMERGENCY BOX 13.4). The abducens (VIth) nerve has a long intracranial course and may be compressed or stretched by raised intracranial pressure. Conversely, patients may experience a transient VIth nerve palsy following lumbar puncture.

More distally, the oculomotor nerve runs in close proximity to the posterior communicating artery and expanding aneurysms of the posterior cerebral artery (PCA) may cause a IIIrd nerve palsy (ptosis; fixed eye; dilated unreactive pupil) with pain around the eye on that side. Similarly, the optic nerve may be compressed by aneurysms of the carotid, anterior communicating or ophthalmic arteries causing a visual field defect or a monocular visual loss.

Neuromas of the auditory (VIIIth) nerve may spread out from the internal auditory meatus and grow in the space between the anterolateral aspect of the cerebellum and the posterolateral aspect of the pons (the cerebellopontine angle). As well as causing deafness because of involvement of the auditory nerve, there may also be compression and dysfunction of the facial (VIIth) and the trigeminal (Vth) nerve.

Intermittent or pulsatile compression from aberrant loops of blood vessel is thought to be the cause of some cases of trigeminal neuralgia (trigeminal [Vth] nerve) and hemifacial spasm (facial [VIIth] nerve); surgical decompression may give dramatic relief of symptoms in those patients unresponsive to medical treatment (gabapentin; carbamazepine; amitriptyline).

Impaired vascular supply

Each nerve carries with it its own blood vessels or vasa nervorum, and occlusion of the arterial supply to a nerve causes it to cease to function. In the majority of cases function returns, usually over 4–8 weeks. The oculomotor (IIIrd) and abducens (VIth) nerve are most often affected, and causes include diabetes, hypertension, arteriosclerosis and, less commonly, vasculitides including temporal arteritis. Such 'medical' causes of IIIrd nerve palsies may be painful, but the pupillary response to light is almost always normal. However, this clinical distinction is often difficult to make with certainty, and so it is reasonable to exclude a posterior communicating artery aneurysm in all patients presenting with a IIIrd nerve palsy.

Inflammation

An inflammatory demyelinating neuropathy can affect cranial nerves, either in isolation or as part of a more generalized neuropathy.

Bell's palsy is a benign, self-limiting, lower motor neurone facial weakness of unknown cause and is the most common lesion of a single cranial nerve. All facial muscles on that side are affected. It needs to be differentiated from more serious causes of a peripheral lesion, and from facial weakness resulting from a central lesion (e.g. hemisphere or brainstem), by the absence of other symptoms or signs.

Bilateral lower motor neurone facial weakness can be difficult to spot and sometimes the only clue is that the patient is unable to smile. Other causes of VIIth cranial nerve lesions:

- Guillain–Barré syndrome
- HIV infection
- Lyme disease
- Nerve infiltration resulting from lymphoma
- Sarcoidosis

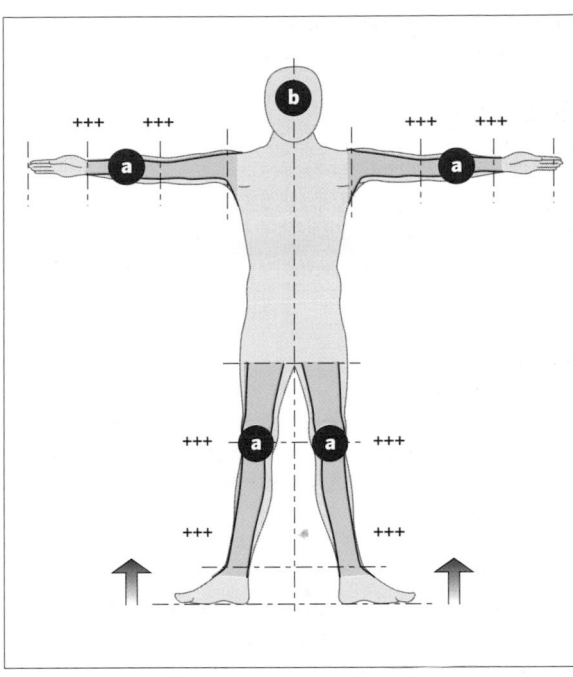

Figure 13.20 Symptoms and signs of neuromuscular disease.

Upper and lower motor neurone problems affecting the lower cranial nerves

Bulbar palsy is caused by the lower motor neurone involvement of the lower cranial nerves and results in slurred speech, difficulty swallowing, choking and hoarseness. It can be a feature of motor neurone disease or of a tumour in the medulla and it is characterized by a wasted fasciculating tongue. Bulbar palsy may also occur with myasthenia gravis, syringobulbia and with inflammation of the basal meninges (e.g. tuberculous meningitis, sarcoidosis).

Pseudobulbar palsy is caused by bilateral upper motor neurone lesions (strokes in both cerebral hemispheres, motor neurone disease and multiple sclerosis) and is characterized by:

- Stiff slow tongue movement, without tongue wasting
- A nasal voice
- A very brisk jaw jerk
- Emotional lability with abrupt onset of inappropriate weeping or occasionally inappropriate laughing

Psudobulbar palsy is often associated with upper motor neurone signs in the arms and legs (spasticity, brisk reflexes and extensor plantar responses).

Diseases of peripheral nerves and the neuromuscular junction

The recognition of these disorders is important because

they may be rapidly progressive, they may herald underlying malignancy or they may have profound genetic implications for relatives.

Motor neurone disease

Epidemiology
Prevalence. 6 in 100 000. Annual incidence 2 in 100 000.

Age. Motor neurone disease (MND) is rare under 50 years, and the incidence rises with age.

Genetics. Ten per cent of cases have an affected first-degree relative, and some of these kindreds have mutations in the gene encoding superoxide dismutase.

Disease mechanisms
There is degeneration of upper and lower motor neurones. While the cause for this is not known, it may involve excitotoxicity and impaired free radical scavenging.

Clinical features
Limb weakness (Fig. 13.20a)
MND commonly starts with progressive weakness, wasting and fasciculation of initially one but soon all four limbs. Reflexes are often very brisk, even when the limb is severely wasted, and there may be increased tone, clonus

Table 13.35 Cranial nerve lesions

I   Causes of loss of smell

Local damage to the nasal mucosa (common)
Smoking, nasal obstruction (infection, polyps)

Olfactory nerve damage (rare)
Head injury (bilateral loss)
Subfrontal meningioma (unilateral loss)

IIa   Causes of papilloedema

Causes	Probable mechanism
Common	
Space-occupying lesion, obstructive hydrocephalus, cerebral venous thrombosis/cavernous sinus thrombosis, hypertension	Increased intracranial pressure causes stagnation of venous return from nerve head and/or interrupted axonal transport
Rare	
Benign intracranial hypertension	Decreased CSF absorption
Papilloma of choroid plexus	Increased CSF production
Guillain–Barré syndrome	High CSF protein content obstructing CSF absorption
Granulomatous disease (e.g. sarcoidosis)	Uncertain
Carbon dioxide retention	?Vasodilatation

IIb   Causes of optic nerve head swelling (papillitis, usually unilateral)

Cause	Probable mechanism
Anterior ischaemic optic neuropathy	Ischaemia of nerve head reducing normal axoplasmic flow
Optic neuritis	Inflammatory processes near nerve head

IIc   Causes of optic atrophy

Optic nerve compression (e.g. by tumour)
Demyelinating disease (e.g. multiple sclerosis)
Central retinal artery occlusion
Secondary optic atrophy following papillitis or papilloedema
Associated with retinal disease (e.g. retinitis pigmentosa)
Syphilis
SLE
Sarcoidosis
Leber's hereditary optic atrophy
Traumatic transection of the optic nerve

IIIa   Third nerve

Posterior communicating artery aneurysm
Temporal arteritis
Critically raised intracranial pressure (patient on the point of developing fatal tentorial herniation)
Diabetes mellitus

IIIb   Causes of pupil abnormalities

Normal reaction to light	Impaired reaction to light
Small pupil	
Old age; Horner's syndrome; pontine lesion	Opiates; pilocarpine eyedrops (for glaucoma); Argyll Robertson pupils of neurosyphilis and diabetes mellitus (react to accommodation but not to light)
Large pupil	
Normal finding in children	Atropine eyedrops; second cranial (optic) nerve lesion; IIIrd cranial (oculomotor) nerve lesion; Holmes–Adie pupil (myotonic pupil that constricts slowly to light and dilates slowly in the dark); post anoxia (e.g. after cardiac arrest)

IIIc   Causes of Horner's syndrome

Brainstem
Demyelination
Tumour
Infarct
Haemorrhage
Outflow at T1
Brachial plexus tumour
Apical lung tumour (Pancoast's)
Carotid artery
Carotid artery dissection

IV   Fourth nerve

Head trauma
Microinfarction of blood supply to nerve (vasa nervorum)
Diabetes mellitus
Metastatic tumour

V   Structural lesions affecting the branches of the fifth cranial nerve

Division	Lesion site
Lower two divisions	Tumour in the nasopharynx
Ophthalmic division	Lesion in cavernous sinus or orbit
All three divisions	Pontine lesions (e.g. tumour, haemorrhage, infarction)

VI   Sixth nerve

Microinfarction of blood supply to nerve (vasa nervorum)
Diabetes mellitus
Raised intracranial pressure
Multiple sclerosis

Table 13.35 (*Cont'd*)

VII Causes of seventh cranial nerve lesions	Motor neurone disease
Unilateral lower motor neurone (LMN) facial weakness	Demyelination
Idiopathic (Bell's palsy)	Lesions at jugular foramen
Herpes zoster	Lesions in retropharyngeal or retroparotid space (e.g.
Diabetes mellitus	nasopharyngeal carcinoma)

VII Causes of seventh cranial nerve lesions

Unilateral lower motor neurone (LMN) facial weakness

Idiopathic (Bell's palsy)
Herpes zoster
Diabetes mellitus
Sarcoidosis
Lyme disease
Fracture of petrous temporal bone
Acoustic neuroma
Middle ear infection
Large parotid gland
Tumour
Malignant tumours

Bilateral LMN facial weakness

Guillain–Barré syndrome
Sarcoidosis
Myasthenia gravis
Myopathy (especially myotonic dystrophy)
Lyme disease

Upper motor neurone (UMN) facial weakness

Contralateral hemisphere stroke or tumour
Multiple sclerosis

VIII Causes of eighth cranial nerve lesions

Mode of onset	Cause
Unilateral, sudden	Vascular lesion to the cochlea
Unilateral, gradual	Acoustic neuroma or other lesion at the cerebellopontine angle (e.g. aneurysm, meningioma, metastatic tumour, dermoid cyst)
Bilateral, subacute	Ototoxicity caused by drugs, especially aminoglycosides

IX Ninth nerve lesion

Tumour or vascular lesion in the medulla
Acoustic neuroma
Syringobulbia

Motor neurone disease
Demyelination
Lesions at jugular foramen
Lesions in retropharyngeal or retroparotid space (e.g.
nasopharyngeal carcinoma)

X Tenth nerve lesion

Tumour or vascular lesion in the medulla
Syringobulbia
Motor neurone disease
Demyelination
Lesions at jugular foramen
Basal meningitis
Tumour in or surgery to the chest damaging the recurrent
laryngeal nerve

XI Eleventh nerve lesion

Tumours high in the spinal cord
Motor neurone disease
Syringomyelia
External compression in the posterior triangle of the neck
Operative damage

**Jugular foramen syndrome with unilateral involvement of
ninth, tenth and eleventh cranial nerves on the same side**

Metastatic tumour in bones of skull base
Neurofibromas
Glomus tumours in region of jugular foramen

**Bilateral weakness and wasting of sternomastoids,
mimicking eleventh nerve lesions**

Myotonic dystrophy

XIIa Twelfth nerve lesion

Brainstem tumours
Vascular damage
Basal meningitis
Tumours of skull base
Carotid dissection
Following carotid endarterectomy

**XIIb Bilateral twelfth nerve lesions (LMN) with weakness,
wasting and fasciculation of the tongue**

Motor neurone disease

and extensor plantars. This combination of upper and lower motor neurone features is strongly suggestive of MND.

Bulbar involvement (Fig. 13.20b)

MND can cause slurred speech, difficulty swallowing, choking, nasal regurgitation of food and fluid, a hoarse voice and a bovine cough. UMN bulbar palsy (pseudobulbar palsy) causes increased jaw jerk, a slow stiff tongue and weakness of the pharyngeal muscles. Lower motor neurone bulbar palsy causes a wasted fasciculating tongue (Fig. 13.21), a bovine cough, and weak pharyngeal and laryngeal muscles.

Respiratory involvement

Involvement of the intercostal muscles and the diaphragm may lead to type II respiratory failure. There may be wasting and fasciculation of the intercostal muscles.

13

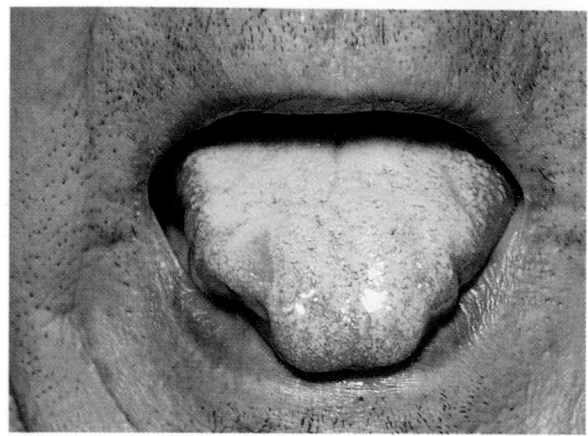

Figure 13.21 Wasted tongue in motor neurone disease.

Other features
MND is accompanied by normal eye movements and normal sensation, and sphincter control is preserved. Muscle cramps may occur. While intellect and higher cerebral function are usually preserved, a subset of patients may have a degree of frontal dementia that may preceed the onset of MND.

Investigation
Haematology
- *FBC and ESR:* to screen for underlying malignancy
- *Thyroid function:* to exclude dysthyroid myopathy
- *Glucose:* to rule out diabetic amyotrophy
- *Syphilis serology:* to exclude tabes dorsalis
- *Creatine kinase:* to rule out inflammatory myopathy, but may be up to twice the upper limit of normal in MND

Diagnostic imaging
- *MRI of brain:* in patients presenting with isolated bulbar features, this will exclude posterior fossa mass lesions
- *MRI of the cervical and lumbar spine:* may be needed to rule out cervical spondylosis

Neurophysiology
Nerve conduction studies and EMG. Nerve conduction studies are usually normal in early disease; later there may be reduced amplitude of the compound motor action potential. EMG shows widespread denervation and reinnervation. It is important to exclude a motor neuropathy.

Other investigations
CSF, which is normal in MND, should be examined to exclude inflammatory and infective disorders.

Management (Table 13.36)
There is no disease modifying treatment, but riluzole may

Table 13.36 Management of motor neurone disease

Supportive treatment
Sensitive discussions about diagnosis and prognosis
Involvement of a specialist motor neurone disease nurse practitioner
Psychological support by a neurologist throughout the illness
Careful attention to and documentation of the patient's wishes
Provision of aids and appliances to maintain independence

Specific treatment
Inability to swallow saliva
Anticholinergic drugs (e.g. hyoscine patch)
Portable suction

Inability to cough
Physiotherapy

Inability to swallow
Liquidize food
Nasogastric tube feeding or gastrostomy

Inability to breathe/respiratory failure
Avoid intubation
Non-invasive positive-pressure ventilation systems may improve sleep quality and improve daytime functioning

Inability to communicate
Speech therapy assessment
Communication aids

Inability to drive a car
Modifications to car

Problems with activities of daily living
Occupational therapy and physiotherapy assessment
Wheelchair, ramps, stairlift, bath aids

Pains (often ill-defined)
Identify cause and treat
Tricyclic antidepressant

Disease modifying treatment
Riluzole is a glutamate inhibitor that appears to slow disease progression. Side-effects include nausea, vomiting, somnolence, headache, dizziness, vertigo, abdominal pain, circumoral paraesthesia, alterations in liver function tests and neutropenia

slow the progression of the disease. Patients who develop cognitive difficulties, headache or daytime somnolence because of sleep apnoea and respiratory failure may benefit from non-invasive nocturnal ventilation.

A sympathetic, caring and team approach including, where available, dedicated MND nurse practitioners may help to soften the impact of this inexorably progressive disease.

Table 13.37 Causes of generalized peripheral neuropathy

Metabolic
Diabetes mellitus
Chronic renal failure
Porphyria
Amyloid

Toxins
Alcohol
Lead
Drugs (e.g. vincristine, isoniazid, nitrofurantoin)

Deficiency states
Vitamin B_1 (beri-beri, alcoholism)
Vitamin B_6 (patients on isoniazid)
Vitamin B_{12}, vitamin E (fat malabsorption)

Inflammatory
Guillain–Barré syndrome (acute)
Chronic inflammatory demyelinating neuropathy (chronic)
Sarcoidosis

Autoimmune
SLE
Polyarteritis nodosa (mononeuritis multiplex)
Rheumatoid arthritis
Sjögren's syndrome
Cryoglobulinaemia

Non-metastatic complication of malignancy
Carcinoma of the bronchus and other malignancies
Monoclonal gammopathies (associated with IgG, IgM, and
  IgA paraproteinaemias) and isolated plasmacytomas

Infective
Leprosy
Diphtheria
AIDS
Borrelia (Lyme disease)

Hereditary
Hereditary sensory motor neuropathy
Mitochondrial disease
Neuroacanthocytosis
Adrenoleucodystrophy
Other hereditary neuropathy

Prognosis

Median survival is 3 years from symptom onset, and shorter if bulbar signs are present.

Peripheral neuropathy

Peripheral neuropathy describes dysfunction of lower motor neurones and sensory neurones, either alone or in combination. While disorders of peripheral nerves are commonly seen in neurology clinics, their causes are poorly understood and often no cause can be found.

Epidemiology

Prevalence. Common.

Genetics. Hereditary motor and sensory neuropathies can be caused by mutations in the genes for peripheral myelin protein, myelin protein zero or connexin 32.

Geography. The most common cause worldwide is leprosy.

Disease mechanisms

Many infections, deficiency states, toxins and metabolic disturbances can cause a neuropathy of peripheral or autonomic nerves (Table 13.37). Inherited neuropathies may be caused by defects in proteins of the myelin sheath.

Pathophysiology

The three main mechanisms underlying generalized neuropathies are:
1 *Demyelinating:* loss of the myelin sheath, often the result of immune-mediated damage
2 *Axonal:* loss of nerve cells, often related to metabolic or toxic processes (e.g. alcohol)
3 *Vasculitis*

Clinical features

The features of a motor neuropathy are distal weakness and wasting in the hands and feet (Fig. 13.22). The feature of a sensory neuropathy is sensory loss in the hands and feet ('glove and stocking'). Some forms of peripheral neuropathy show features of autonomic failure including postural hypotension, loss of sinus arrhythmia, reduced sweating, diarrhoea, impotence and, if severe, retention of urine or constipation.

Investigation

Investigation aims to demonstrate pathology in the peripheral nerves, and then to attempt to identify the cause. Extensive tests are required to screen for infective and metabolic causes and to rule out other illnesses that may give rise to neuropathy as a secondary phenomenon (Table 13.38).

Neurophysiology

Nerve conduction studies confirm that a neuropathy is present and may help to distinguish between demyelinating and axonal neuropathies.

Histopathology

Nerve biopsy may be helpful, especially if infection (e.g. leprosy), vasculitis or demyelinating neuropathy is suspected.

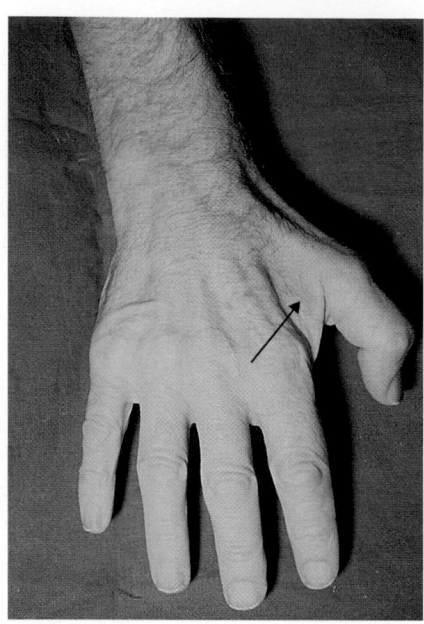

Figure 13.22 Wasting of first dorsal interosseous in ulnar neuropathy.

Table 13.38 Investigation of peripheral neuropathy

Blood tests
Full blood count and ESR
Urea and electrolytes
Blood glucose
Vitamin B_{12}
Liver function tests
Thyroid function tests
Protein electrophoresis
Autoantibodies
HIV and syphilis serology
Diagnostic genetic testing
• Hereditary motor and sensory neuropathies
• Spinocerebellar ataxias

Urine
Bence Jones protein
Porphyrins

Radiology
Chest X-ray
Skeletal survey
Abdominal ultrasound (if paraneoplastic neuropathy suspected)
Mammography (if paraneoplastic neuropathy suspected)
CT chest, abdomen and pelvis (if paraneoplastic neuropathy suspected)

Neurophysiology
Nerve conduction studies

Pathology
Sural nerve biopsy

Table 13.39 Management of peripheral neuropathy

Supportive treatment
Splint weak muscles and joints

Specific treatment
Treat the underlying cause
Rigorous control of blood glucose in patients with diabetic neuropathy
Vasculitic neuropathies may respond to corticosteroids and immunosuppressive therapy (e.g. azathioprine, cyclophosphamide)
Demyelinating neuropathies may respond to treatment with intravenous immunoglobulin and/or plasma exchange
Toxins and metabolic causes may respond to correction of the underlying problem
Genetic counselling may be indicated for the genetic neuropathies

Management

Physiotherapy and occupational therapy have important roles including the provision of splints to support weak joints (e.g. the use of ankle/foot orthoses). Treatment of the underlying cause is summarized in Table 13.39.

Guillain–Barré syndrome

Guillain–Barré syndrome (GBS) is the most common acute neuropathy (annual incidence 1.5 in 100 000); early recognition and appropriate management are essential because death can result from respiratory failure or autonomic dysregulation.

Pathophysiology

Antibodies raised in response to infection cross-react with particular sugars (gangliosides) found on Schwann cell membranes, resulting in inflammation and an autoimmune inflammatory demyelinating polyradiculopathy.

Clinical features

GBS begins a few days after an acute infection, with distal tingling and then weakness; there may be back pain. The weakness is accompanied by areflexia and may progress rapidly to a complete flaccid quadriparesis with respiratory paralysis, and 25% of patients require ventilation. Autonomic involvement can lead to cardiac arrhythmias and labile blood pressure.

Investigation and monitoring

• *Blood tests (FBC, electrolytes,* Campylobacter *and viral serology):* generally normal, although there may be evidence of recent infection. Antiganglioside antibodies may be detected in serum.
• *Vital capacity and blood gases:* respiratory function

should be monitored by measuring vital capacity (not peak expiratory flow) and arterial blood gases; respiratory support may be required if vital capacity falls below 1 l or if there is CO_2 retention.

● *Lumbar puncture:* shows elevated CSF protein but the white cell count is normal; if the white cell count is elevated, consider alternative diagnoses.
● *Neurophysiological tests:* often show marked slowing of nerve conduction velocities, but sometimes distal velocities are normal and it is only proximal velocities that are reduced (increased 'F-wave' latency).

Management
Respiratory function, ECG, fluid balance and blood pressure must be monitored. Vital capacity should be measured hourly in the first instance, with ventilation if required. Treatment with either plasma exchange or intravenous immunoglobulin speeds recovery. Patients may have a prolonged period of paralysis requiring ventilation; they will require considerable psychological support and should receive daily physiotherapy to prevent flexion contractures, heparin as deep vein thrombosis prophylaxis, and analgesia if required.

Prognosis
Two-thirds of patients will eventually recover completely, but there is significant mortality (8%), principally from respiratory failure or pulmonary embolism.

Chronic inflammatory demyelinating polyneuropathy
Epidemiology
Prevalence. 1 in 100 000.

Disease mechanisms
Like GBS, chronic inflammatory demyelinating polyneuropathy (CIDP) is caused by immune-mediated demyelination; however, it is distinguished from GBS in that, by definition, it continues to worsen for at least 2 months from onset; preceding infection is less commonly identified, and the natural history is of a chronic progressive course.

Clinical features
Clinical features are similar to those of GBS, but respiratory muscle, cranial nerve and autonomic involvement is less common in CIDP.

Investigation
● *CSF:* shows elevation of CSF protein, and there may also be a CSF pleocytosis, unlike GBS
● *Nerve conduction studies:* show slowed conduction
● *Nerve biopsy:* may help define the precise aetiology

Management
Supportive measures include respiratory support if necessary, prevention of infection and pressure area care in the immobile patient. Specific measures include plasma exchange or high-dose immunoglobulin, and CIDP may also respond to oral corticosteroids. Long-term low-dose corticosteroids may prevent relapse.

Prognosis
Recovery from the acute episodes is normal. Some patients accumulate mild persistent disability with recurrent episodes.

Mononeuropathies
Epidemiology
Prevalence. 40 in 100 000. Annual incidence 40 in 100 000.

Disease mechanisms
Mononeuropathy (dysfunction of a single peripheral nerve) is usually caused by local compression or trauma. However, the nerve concerned may have increased vulnerability to such lesions because of an otherwise subclinical generalized neuropathy.

Clinical features
Commonly involved nerves include:
● *Median nerve compression at the wrist* (carpal tunnel syndrome): causes pain in the hand, especially at night, which may be relieved by rubbing or shaking the hand. There can be sensory loss in the lateral side of the hand and weakness and wasting of the thenar eminence muscles (abductor pollicis brevis, opponens pollicis, flexor pollicis brevis). Carpal tunnel syndrome is more common in pregnancy, hypothyroidism, rheumatoid arthritis and acromegaly.
● *Ulnar nerve compression at the elbow:* results in sensory loss in the medial side of the hand and wasting of the small hand muscles.
● *Common peroneal nerve compression:* at the head of the fibula causes foot-drop and sensory loss on the dorsum of the foot.
● *Lateral cutaneous nerve of thigh compression* (meralgia paraesthetica): at the inguinal ligament causes tingling and pain in the outer aspect of the thigh.

Investigation
Nerve conduction studies can confirm the site of the nerve lesion.

Management
Most patients improve spontaneously. Carpal tunnel syndrome may respond to surgical decompression and weight loss may cure meralgia paraesthetica.

13

Prognosis
Most compression neuropathies resolve spontaneously.

Mononeuritis multiplex
Epidemiology
Prevalence. 40 in 100 000.

Disease mechanisms
Causes include diabetes mellitus, polyarteritis nodosa, SLE and rheumatoid arthritis. Rarer causes include sarcoidosis, paraproteinaemia, carcinomas, leprosy, AIDS and intravenous drug abuse.

Clinical features
More than one peripheral nerve is affected at the same time. Enough nerves may be affected for the features to be indistinguishable from those of a peripheral neuropathy.

Investigation
- *Nerve conduction studies:* confirm that several peripheral nerves are involved
- *Nerve biopsy:* may be necessary to confirm the diagnosis

Management
Treat the underlying cause where possible. Whatever the cause, there may be a response to immunosuppressive therapy.

Prognosis
This depends on the underlying cause.

Brachial plexus lesions
Disease mechanisms
Lesions of the brachial plexus can be caused by trauma, malignant infiltration, radiation fibrosis or inflammation.

Clinical features
Complete lesions give rise to a wasted, weak, numb and areflexic arm; partial lesions may also cause pain in the arm. **Brachial neuritis** (neuralgic amyotrophy) is characterized by severe pain in the shoulder for 1–3 days followed by the development of weakness and wasting of the shoulder and upper arm muscles as the pain resolves; reflexes may be absent. While the cause is unknown, it is thought to be caused by inflammation of the plexus, and may follow some infective episode.

Investigation
- *Nerve conduction studies:* assist in localizing the lesion
- *Chest radiography* (p. 315)*:* may identify any apical lung lesion (e.g. Pancoast's tumour)

- *MRI of the brachial plexus:* differentiates fibrosis from malignancy

Management and prognosis
There may be slow recovery following trauma, but for infiltrative and fibrotic conditions progressive disease is likely. While oral corticosteroids may shorten the duration of brachial amyotrophy, this usually resolves spontaneously in 3–12 months.

Hereditary neuropathies
Epidemiology
Prevalence. 40 in 100 000.

Disease mechanisms
Hereditary motor and sensory neuropathy (HMSN) has at least 15 different recognized forms:
- Inheritance may be autosomal dominant or recessive, or X-linked
- May be caused by damage to the myelin sheath (demyelinating, HMSN I, III) or to axons (axonal, HMSN II)
- Identified causes include mutations in the genes for peripheral myelin protein 22, myelin protein zero and connexin 32
- Other inherited neuropathies are secondary to metabolic disturbance; for instance, Refsum's disease (autosomal recessive) is caused by a mutation in the gene for phytanoyl-CoA hydroxylase, and leads to accumulation of phytanic acid accumulates in the central and peripheral nervous system.

Clinical features
In HMSN I (autosomal dominant) there is pes cavus, and slowly progressive distal leg weakness, atrophy and sensory loss starting in the late teens. In HMSN II (autosomal dominant) the findings are similar, but onset is in late middle age. HMSN III (Déjérine–Sottas disease, autosomal recessive) is a severe demyelinating neuropathy of infancy and childhood and is associated with marked hypertrophy of peripheral nerves. Other HMSNs may be associated with tremor, ataxia or other neurological features.

Investigation
- *Nerve conduction studies:* indicate whether axonal or demyelinating
- *Biochemical tests:* may identify a relevant metabolic disturbance
- *DNA testing:* may establish a molecular diagnosis
- *Nerve biopsy:* may be indicated if molecular diagnosis is not possible

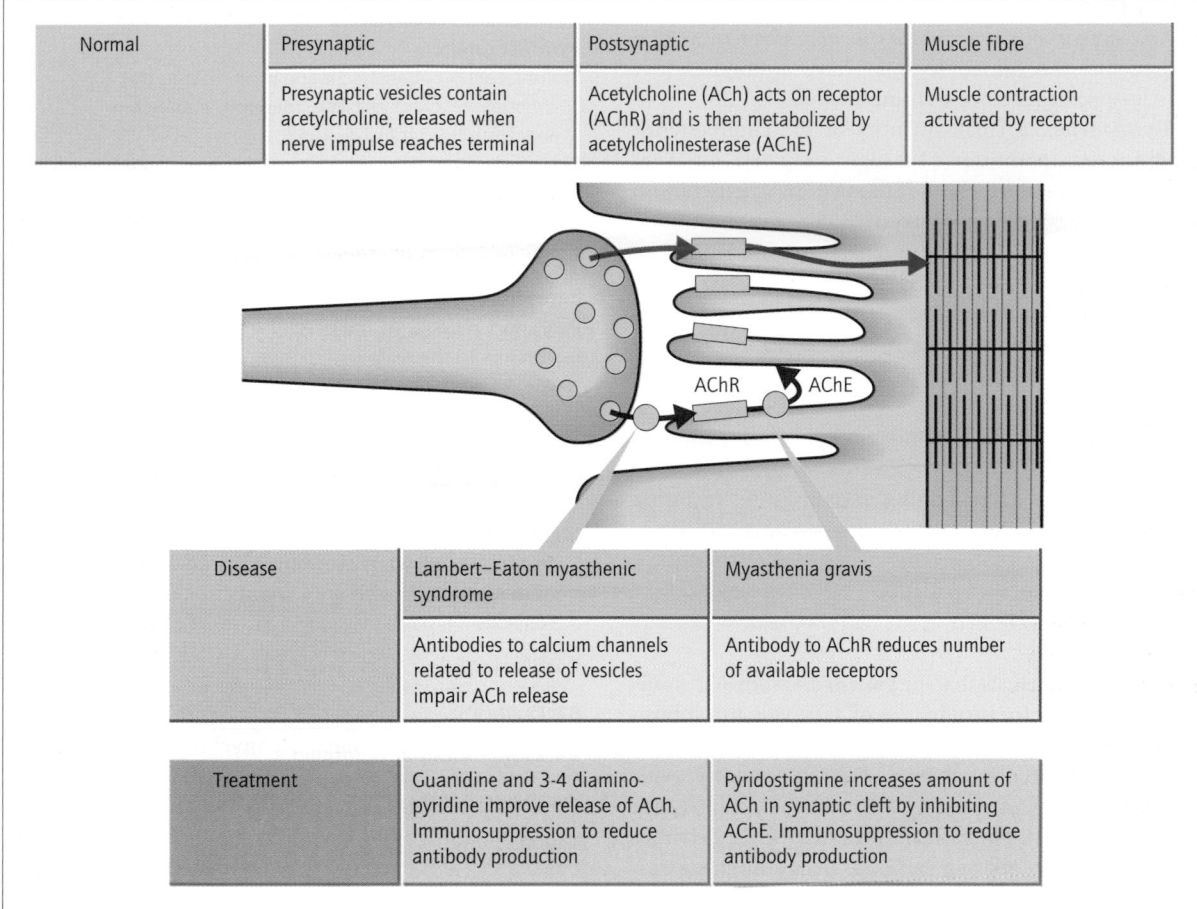

Normal	Presynaptic	Postsynaptic	Muscle fibre
	Presynaptic vesicles contain acetylcholine, released when nerve impulse reaches terminal	Acetylcholine (ACh) acts on receptor (AChR) and is then metabolized by acetylcholinesterase (AChE)	Muscle contraction activated by receptor

Disease	Lambert–Eaton myasthenic syndrome	Myasthenia gravis
	Antibodies to calcium channels related to release of vesicles impair ACh release	Antibody to AChR reduces number of available receptors
Treatment	Guanidine and 3-4 diamino-pyridine improve release of ACh. Immunosuppression to reduce antibody production	Pyridostigmine increases amount of ACh in synaptic cleft by inhibiting AChE. Immunosuppression to reduce antibody production

Figure 13.23 Pathophysiology of myasthenia gravis and Lambert–Eaton myasthenic syndrome.

Management and prognosis

Physiotherapy and provision of support splints are helpful. The disorder is usually only slowly progressive, and patients commonly cope well with minor disability. Genetic counselling may be helpful where this is available.

Myasthenia gravis

Epidemiology

Prevalence. 10 in 100 000. Annual incidence 0.5 in 100 000.

Age. Bimodal, with peaks in young adulthood (women) and late middle age (men).

Genetics. There is an association with the HLA-A1,B8,DR3 (8.1) haplotype.

Disease mechanisms

Circulating autoimmune antibodies bind to and block nicotinic acetylcholine receptors at the neuromuscular junction (Fig. 13.23). Some drugs, including penicillamine, may cause myasthenia gravis and others, including gentamicin and tetracycline, may worsen pre-existing disease. There may be an associated thymoma, particularly in patients over 40 years of age; conversely, younger patients may have thymic hyperplasia.

Clinical features (Fig. 13.20)

Patients complain of weakness, double vision, drooping eyelids, impaired voice and difficulty swallowing that worsen as the day progresses. At examination there may be fatiguable weakness of ocular, bulbar, respiratory or limb muscles. The pupils remain normal, reflexes are preserved and there is no sensory loss. In ocular myasthenia the only affected muscles are the ocular muscles.

13

Investigation

- *Anti-acetylcholine receptor antibodies:* positive in 85% of patients; the remainder may have antibodies to a muscle-specific receptor tyrosine kinase.
- *Tensilon test:* a small quantity of the cholinesterase inhibitor edrophonium (Tensilon) is given intravenously; this prevents the breakdown of acetylcholine, thereby increasing synaptic acetylcholine concentrations, restoring normal neuromuscular transmission and abolishing weakness, diplopia and ptosis. However, acetylcholine concentrations are also increased at muscarinic synapses and atropine must be available to reverse any symptomatic bradycardia. In addition, false-positive results are common.
- *CT or MRI of mediastinum:* required to exclude a thymoma.
- *EMG:* shows decrementing responses to repetitive stimulation.
- *Vital capacity and arterial blood gases:* should be monitored in acutely ill patients.

Management

In acute disease, check that the patient's swallowing is safe, and give heparin for prophylaxis of deep-vein thrombosis if mobility is lost. Respiratory support may be required for respiratory failure. Anticholinesterase drugs may provide immediate relief of symptoms; where it does not then immunomodulatory treatment with steroids, intravenous immunoglobulin, plasma exchange or azathioprine may be required (Table 13.40). Thymectomy is indicated for patients under 40 years whose symptoms are not controlled by anticholinesterase drugs or where CT has suggested the presence of a thymoma.

Prognosis

With appropriate treatment the prognosis is good.

Lambert–Eaton myasthenic syndrome

Disease mechanisms

Lambert–Eaton myasthenic syndrome is caused by circulating antibodies to presynaptic voltage-gated calcium channels, leading to impaired recruitment of synaptic vesicles following depolarization (Fig. 13.23). About half of cases occur as a paraneoplastic phenomenon, usually in association with small cell carcinoma of the bronchus; the remainder occur as a pure autoimmune condition.

Clinical features

The main feature is fatiguable limb weakness, but this may improve with repetitive use of a muscle and towards the end of the day. Other features include absent reflexes and autonomic features such as dry mouth or impotence.

Table 13.40 Treatment of myasthenia gravis

Pyridostigmine

Prolongs action of acetylcholine by inhibiting the anticholinesterase enzyme, therefore enhancing neuromuscular transmission

Side-effects. Bradycardia, increased sweating and salivary secretion, depolarizing block (cholinergic crisis) in excessive dosage

Contraindications. Intestinal or urinary obstruction

Edrophonium bromide (Tensilon)

Very short action anticholinesterase inhibitor

Indications. In the diagnosis of myasthenia gravis and to assess whether a patient with established disease is receiving adequate treatment

Side-effects. As for pyridostigmine. Side-effects may be relieved by injection of atropine, and this should always be available when an edrophonium test is performed

Contraindications. Patients with respiratory impairment may deteriorate following injection of edrophonium. Full intubation and respiratory support facilities should be available

Corticosteroids

Azathioprine

Intravenous immunoglobulin

Plasma exchange

Thymectomy

Absent reflexes may return if the relevant muscle groups are exercised (post-tetanic accentuation). Bulbar and ocular features are rare.

Investigation

- *EMG:* shows increased response to repeated stimulation
- *Chest CT:* to look for underlying malignancy

Management and prognosis

The neurological syndrome may improve if an underlying tumour is removed. 3,4-Diaminopyridine may reduce the symptoms, and immunomodulation with prednisolone, azathioprine, intravenous immunoglobulin or plasma exchange may be helpful.

Muscle disease (Table 13.41)

Primary muscle disorders

Most muscle disorders have greatest impact on proximal limb and truncal musculature. The characteristic symptoms are of difficulty raising the arms above the head, getting up from low chairs, climbing stairs and sitting up in bed.

Table 13.41 Other causes of muscle disorders

Anterior horn cell disease (spinal muscular atrophy)	Dystrophia myotonica
Infantile (Werdnig–Hoffman type)	Glycogen storage diseases
Juvenile (Kugelberg–Welander type)	
Adult spinal muscular atrophy	*Periodic paralysis*
	Hypokalaemic periodic paralysis
Mitochondrial disease	Hyperkalaemic periodic paralysis
Mitochondrial myopathy with ophthalmoplegia	
Mitochondrial encephalopathy with lactic acidosis and	*Non-metastatic effect of malignancy*
stroke-like episodes	Paraneoplastic myopathy
Mitochondrial myopathy with myoclonus,	
epilepsy and typical 'ragged-red fibres' on	*Electrolyte imbalance*
muscle biopsy	Hypokalaemia
	Hypocalcaemia
Inflammatory muscle disease	
Polymyositis	*Endocrine disease*
Dermatomyositis	Hypo- or hyperthyroidism
Inclusion body myositis	Hypo- or hyperparathyroidism
	Addison's disease
Genetically determined muscle disease	Cushing's syndrome
Duchenne and Becker muscular dystrophies	Acromegaly
Emery–Dreifuss muscular dystrophy	
Limb girdle muscular dystrophy	*Drugs and toxins*
Carnitine palmitoyl-transferase deficiency	Alcohol
Myophosphorylase deficiency	Corticosteroids
Phosphofructokinase deficiency	Clofibrate
Acid maltase deficiency	Zidovudine
	HMG-CoA reductase inhibitors (e.g. simvastatin)

Polymyositis and dermatomyositis

(See p. 222.)

Duchenne and Becker's muscular dystrophy

Epidemiology

Prevalence. Rare.

Age. Childhood (Duchenne) or adult (Becker).

Sex. Males only.

Genetics. X-linked recessive because of mutations in *Dystrophin*.

Disease mechanisms

Dystrophin is subject to many mutations; those in one region are associated with the more common and more aggressive Duchenne muscular dystrophy, while those of another are associated with the less severe Becker's dystrophy.

Clinical features (Fig. 13.20)

Symptoms typically begin after the affected boy has learned to walk; they may develop strategies to overcome their proximal weakness, such as 'climbing' their arms up their legs to rise from the floor (Gower's manoeuvre).

Management

There is no treatment. Genetic counselling in affected families gives parents the option of prenatal testing with abortion of affected fetuses.

Prognosis

In Duchenne muscular dystrophy, most patients use wheelchairs by their teens and die in their twenties. Becker's muscular dystrophy is much less severe, and most patients die with their disease rather than because of it.

Dystrophia myotonica (myotonic dystrophy)

Epidemiology

Prevalence. 10 in 100 000.

Genetics. Autosomal dominant trinucleotide repeat

Table 13.42 Neurological manifestations of systemic disease

Non-metastatic neurological effects of malignancy	*Nerve*
Cortex, hemispheres	Painful sensory neuropathy
Metabolic encephalopathy	
Limbic encephalitis	*Muscle*
Opsoclonus myoclonus	Acute painful myopathy after a binge
Electrolyte disorder from ectopic ACTH/ADH/parahormone secretion	Chronic painless myopathy
Vascular (hypercoagulability)	**Neurological manifestations of AIDS**
Stroke	*Cortex, hemispheres*
Venous sinus thrombosis	Dementia
Opportunistic infection	Encephalopathy
Fungi, toxoplasma	Seizures
Retinal degeneration	Aseptic meningitis at seroconversion
	Opportunistic infection
Cerebellum	• Cytomegalovirus
Autoimmune cerebellar degeneration	• Herpes simplex
	• Fungi
Spinal cord	• Tuberculosis
Necrotizing myelopathy	• Progressive multifocal leucoencephalopathy
	Mass lesions
Peripheral nerve	• Toxoplasmosis
Neuropathy	• Lymphoma
	Stroke
Neuromuscular junction	• Infarct
Lambert–Eaton myasthenic syndrome	• Haemorrhage
Myasthenia gravis (thymoma)	
	Eye
Muscle	CMV retinopathy
Dermatomyositis	
Non-inflammatory myopathy	*Spinal cord*
	Vacuolar myelopathy
Neurological manifestations of alcohol	Infection
Cortex/hemispheres	
Dementia	*Peripheral nerve*
Wernicke–Korsakoff syndrome	Acute Guillain–Barré syndrome
Seizures	Chronic inflammatory demyelinating neuropathy
Hallucinosis (withdrawal)	Mononeuritis multiplex
Coma	Painful sensory neuropathy
• Postictal	Cauda equina syndrome
• Hepatic encephalopathy	
• Wernicke's encephalopathy	*Muscle*
	Polymyositis
Eye, optic nerve	Pyomyositis (multiple abscesses)
Tobacco/alcohol amblyopia	Myositis resulting from zidovudine therapy
Methanol blindness	
	Neurological effects of acquired hypothyroidism
Brainstem	*Cortex*
Ophthalmoplegia in Wernicke's encephalopathy	Depression
	Confusion
Cerebellum	Coma
Acute intoxication	
Chronic cerebellar atrophy	
Ataxia as part of Wernicke's encephalopathy	

CMV, cytomegalovirus.

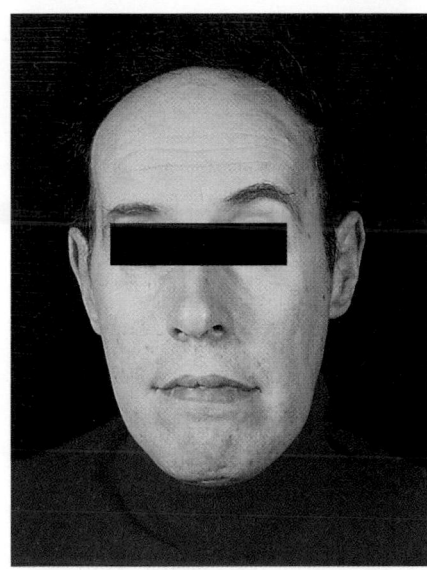

Figure 13.24 Typical facies of myotonic dystrophy.

disorder affecting the *Myotonic dystrophy protein kinase* gene of variable penetrance.

Clinical features (Fig. 13.20)
These include distal muscle weakness and wasting, frontal balding, cataracts, ptosis, type 1 diabetes and a typical facial appearance (Fig. 13.24). Patients have difficulty relaxing muscles after use; this may reveal itself as an inability to let go after shaking hands.

Investigation
- *EMG:* findings are typical
- *DNA testing:* shows the expanded trinucleotide repeat

Management
Procainamide or phenytoin may be used for the weakness, and some patients require a cardiac pacemaker. Genetic counselling in affected families gives parents the option of prenatal testing with abortion of affected fetuses.

Prognosis
Slowly progressive.

Systemic disorders and the nervous system

Changes in the periphery such as pregnancy, systemic diseases, drugs and toxins can all impact on the functioning of the nervous system; the more common of these effects are summarized in Table 13.42.

! Must know checklist

- What is the most important source of information in reaching a diagnosis in neurology?

- Describe the characteristic lesions causing the immediate, slow and very slow development of neurological symptoms

- Describe the difference between upper and lower motor neurone weakness

- What is the role of drug monitoring in treatment for epilepsy?

- From whom does one obtain a history of cognitive impairment or altered consciousness?

- Describe the modes of action available for the treatment of Parkinson's disease

- Differentiate between clinical and biological significance in the interpretation of drug treatment trials

- Is CT scanning sufficient to make the diagnosis of brain tumour?

- Describe treatment options in patients with stroke

- What sources of information, help and advice are there for patients newly diagnosed with a neurological condition?

Further reading

Books

Bradley WG, Daroff RB, Fenichel RB *et al.* eds. *Neurology in Clinical Practice.* Oxford: Butterworth Heinemann, 2003.

Brazis PW, Nasden JC, Biller J *et al. Localization in Clinical Neurology.* London: Lippincott Williams & Wilkins, 2001.

Patten JP. *Neurological Differential Diagnosis.* Berlin: Springer-Verlag, 1995.

Poolos NP. *Handbook of Neurologic Differential Diagnosis.* Oxford: Butterworth Heinemann, 2001.

Rosenberg RN. *The Molecular and Genetic Basis of Neurological Disease.* Oxford: Butterworth Heinemann, 2003.

Journals

Journal of Neurology, Neurosurgery and Psychiatry, BMJ Publishing Group. http://jnnp.bmjjournals.com/

Brain, Oxford University Press. http://brain.oupjournals.org/

Stroke, American Heart Association. http://www.strokeaha.org/

Web sites

The Neurological Alliance: http://www.neurologicalalliance.org.uk/

British Epilepsy Association: http://www.epilepsy.org.uk/

Brain and Spine Foundation: http://www.bbsf.org.uk/

DVLA Driving regulation: http://www.dvla.gov.uk/drivers/dmed1.htm

Epilepsy recurrence risk calculator: http://www.dcn.ed.ac.uk/model/epilepsy.asp

Carotid surgery risk calculator: http://www.dcn.ed.ac.uk/model/carotid.asp

The Cochrane Collaboration: http://www.cochrane.org/

Journal of Neurology, Neurosurgery and Psychiatry: http://jnnp.bmjjournals.com/

Association of British Neurologists: http://www.theabn.org

Stroke information: http://www.strokecentre.org/

Evidence-based neurology

There are data from meta-analyses or from large well-designed randomized controlled trials to suggest a clinically significant benefit for the following interventions. Up-to-date information is available from the Cochrane Collaboration's website.

Condition	Intervention	Endpoint	Odds ratio/outcome*
Stroke	Stroke unit care	Death or dependency at final review	0.75 (0.65–0.87)
Ischaemic stroke	Aspirin 160–300 mg	6 months death or dependency	0.94 (0.91–0.98)
	Alteplase within 3 h	6 months death or dependency	0.58 (0.46–0.74)
Secondary prevention of stroke	Aspirin	Further fatal or non-fatal vascular events	0.78 (0.74–0.82)
	Perindopril 4 mg ± indapamide	Recurrent stroke	0.78 (0.62–0.83)
	Carotid endarterectomy for severe symptomatic stenosis	Disabling stroke or death	0.48 (0.27–0.73)
Relapsing–remitting multiple sclerosis	Interferons	Frequency of relapses	0.80 (0.73–0.88)
		Progression of disability	0.69 (0.55–0.87)
Motor neurone disease	Riluzole	Death or tracheostomy	0.88 (0.75–1.02)
Alzheimer's disease	Galantamine 32 mg	Cognitive function at 6 months	ADAS-Cog improvement of –4.0 (–3.0 to –5.0)
	Rivastigmine 6–12 mg		ADAS-Cog –2.1 (–1.5 to –2.6)
	Donepezil 10 mg		ADAS-Cog –2.9 (–2.2 to –3.6)

* An odds ratio less than 1.00 indicates that the intervention is superior to control.

Psychological Medicine

Introduction

Psychiatric disorders are more common amongst medical and surgical patients than in the general population. However, psychiatric services are often separate from general hospital services. This separation reflects the artificial division between the mind and the body in our thinking. All illnesses have biological, psychological and social components. For example, following a myocardial infarction, a patient may have to make significant life changes. In addition, the risk of a depressive illness is increased, and this in turn is associated with a poorer cardiac prognosis.

Recent advances in understanding the causes, course and management of a number of physical disorders highlight the relevance of psychological and social factors, and demonstrate the need for an integrated approach to patient care. Such an approach should be routine practice in the assessment and management of all patients. Specialist mental health care for general hospital patients is provided by liaison psychiatry services.

described as occurring in the 'mind'. However, the mind is not separate from the brain. For example, memory and behaviour can be altered by physical brain damage. Also, emotions are accompanied by physical changes, such as the activation of the sympathetic nervous system which is associated with anxiety.

The brain has anatomical, physiological and psychological levels of organization. Anatomical and physiological processes can be studied objectively. However, mental processes can only be inferred from an individual's behaviour, what he or she reports and from the measurement of associated physiological processes. When the mental state of a patient is assessed, the observer attempts, as far as possible, to know what the patient's experiences feel like. This involves detailed questioning and empathy—feeling oneself into the situation of the other person. For example, a patient may describe visual hallucinations. These cannot be seen or measured, but the interviewer can attempt to create in his or her own mind what the experience is like.

Structure and function

The brain is a unique bodily organ. Unlike other organs, such as the heart, liver and kidneys, it cannot be transplanted into another person. Apart from physical appearance, the brain contains all the things that mark someone out as an individual. Hence, a brain transplant would be the transplant of another body around the brain.

The functions of the brain include sensory, motor and autonomic control, as well as the 'higher functions' of thinking and feeling. These mental processes may be

Approach to the patient

The aims of a psychiatric assessment are to:
- Obtain a detailed history and mental state examination
- Make a provisional diagnosis
- Decide upon a comprehensive plan of management

Establishing a good working relationship with the patient at the outset of the consultation, not just in psychiatry but in all branches of medicine, is essential for obtaining a full and accurate history. It should take precedence over eliciting 'factual' information, particularly if such information concerns a sensitive issue (e.g. sexual abuse).

This information can be obtained at a later date if the patient feels that he or she is being dealt with empathically and non-judgementally. Questions about such sensitive issues mean that a psychiatric assessment is best carried out in a private interview room.

History and examination

History taking

Important questions to ask when taking a psychiatric history from a medical patient are listed in HISTORY & EXAMINATION BOX 14.1.

About the patient

Document the patient's age, sex, marital status, racial and cultural background, and present occupation. The mode of presentation should also be recorded. Was the patient referred by his or her GP, social services or the police?

Current symptoms

The type of symptoms, their duration and the extent to which they disrupt the patient's daily routine all need to be recorded in detail.

Emotional reactions to physical illness, such as anxiety, fear or depression, are common. Hospital attendance, whether as an inpatient or as an outpatient, is a new and often frightening experience for many people.

Ask about any recent marital, family, financial or occupational stresses.

Past medical and psychiatric history

The patient's symptoms are placed in the context of their previous history. Record details of:
- Previous illnesses
- Hospital admissions
- Treatments prescribed

Family history

Family history is important for both genetic and

History & Examination 14.1: Important questions to ask when taking a history from a medical patient

Symptoms
How long have they been present?
Do they affect your mood?
Are there other factors that affect how you feel?

Pattern of disease
Is there any pattern?
Does your mood worsen with your physical symptoms?
Does your mood vary with the time of day or show any other pattern?

Disease impact
How do you cope with your illness?
What are the main areas of your life that have been affected?
What support do you get?

Past medical and psychiatric history
What illnesses have you had?
Have you been a hospital inpatient at any time? If so, why and when?

Family history
What physical or psychiatric illnesses do you or members of your family have?
Has any member of your family ever misused or had any problems with drugs or alcohol?
Has any member of your family committed suicide?
How have you in the past and how do you now get on with your parents and brothers and sisters?

Personal history
Have you had or do you have any problems with your marriage or your family, or at work?
Have you had or do you have any financial problems?

Forensic history
Have you been convicted of any criminal offence?
Have you spent any time in prison or on probation?

Drug history
What medicines (prescribed or not prescribed) do you take?
Do you use any recreational (illicit) drugs? If so, what and how often?
Do you drink alcohol? If so, what and how often?

Premorbid personality
What are your hobbies and interests?
How would your friends describe you?
What sort of person are you?
How do you cope with pressure?
How do you get on with other people such as your family, friends and work colleagues?

Collateral history
Do you have a relative or close friend I could speak to who knows how things have been recently?

environmental reasons. Ask the patient whether any of his or her family have physical or psychiatric disorders, or have misused drugs or alcohol, or have committed suicide.

Past and present relationships with family members can influence the outcome of a physical illness and need to be discussed.

Personal history

The personal history is a biographical account, beginning with birth and early development, and continuing through childhood and adolescence to adulthood. It should cover:

- Birth and developmental milestones
- Early family life
- Educational attainments
- Occupational history
- Psychosexual development (sexual abuse, sexual orientation, number of partners)
- Interpersonal relationships

An account of marital and other family relationships may identify chronic interpersonal difficulties, which may have a major influence on physical symptoms, especially as perpetuating or maintaining factors.

Social history

The personal history leads into an up-to-date account of the current social situation, including home, family and work. This is an opportunity to ask about the impact of illness on a patient's life. Ask about finances and debt, which can be a major source of stress.

Forensic history

Past criminal offences and periods in prison or on probation may be relevant.

Current medication

Many drugs prescribed for physical illnesses can affect mood. Drugs prescribed for psychological illnesses can have physical side-effects.

Tobacco, alcohol and substance misuse

The CAGE questionnaire is a useful screening instrument for excessive alcohol use (see p. 977). The identification of potentially harmful use of alcohol or recreational (illicit) drugs should lead to a more detailed assessment of these problems.

Premorbid personality

Attempting to make an assessment of a person's personality before the onset of his or her illness is often the most difficult but revealing aspect of the history. It commonly explains important behaviour such as non-compliance with treatment.

A personality assessment is based on:
- The nature and quality of interpersonal relationships: marital, family, friends and work colleagues
- Hobbies and interests
- Beliefs, attitudes and general outlook (e.g. pessimistic or cheerful)
- Emotional response coping strategies (e.g. anger, denial, dependence)
- Gender identity, body image, self-esteem

Physical examination

A physical examination is essential for all patients regardless of whether the presenting symptoms are physical or psychological. A number of physical diseases may first present with psychological features (e.g. hypothyroidism, diabetes mellitus and temporal lobe epilepsy).

Drugs used for the treatment of psychiatric disorders can have important physical adverse effects that may be detected on physical examination, such as the movement disorders associated with neuroleptic medication (see p. 983).

Mental state examination

The mental state examination is described in detail in HISTORY & EXAMINATION BOX 14.2. It comprises an assessment of:
- Appearance and general behaviour
- Emotional state and suicidal ideation
- Thought and speech
- Abnormal perceptions and experiences
- Cognitive state
- Insight
- The interviewer's reaction to the patient

Emotional state

A patient's emotional state (also called mood or affect), both observed and reported, should be recorded in detail as the most common psychiatric disorders seen (and missed!) in physically ill patients are anxiety-related disorders and depressive disorders. Note how a patient's mood varies during the course of an interview and any inconsistencies between the observed and reported emotional state.

Physical effects

Explore the physical effects of the emotional state. Feelings of anxiety are associated with activation of the sympathetic nervous system and the release of adrenaline. Depressed mood is associated with a number of bodily or 'somatic' symptoms; ask about sleep disruption, appetite and weight, energy, concentration, interest and enjoyment.

14

History & Examination 14.2: Mental state examination

Appearance and general behaviour

Look for signs of self-neglect

Note any abnormalities of movement or posture

Look for signs of over- or underactivity

Note degree of cooperation with assessment

Note defence mechanisms (e.g. hostility, denial)

Affect and mood

Record the patient's emotional state, both observed and
   reported, in detail and note inconsistencies between
   the two

Note:
- The prevailing mood
- Reactivity during the interview
- Incongruity of mood

Ask:
- Do you get depressed or feel sad or low?
- Do you feel elated?
- Do you get anxious or fearful?

Ask about:
- Somatic symptoms of depression
- Suicidal ideation

Flow of thought and speech

Comment on the rate, volume and tone of speech. Listen for:
- Pressure of speech (fast and difficult to interrupt)
- Retardation of speech (slow and often inaudible)

Content of thought and speech

Ask:
- Do you have any worries? If so, what are they?
- Are your thoughts preoccupied by anything? If so, by
  what?
- Do you have any irrational fears of specific situations or in
  relation to any external objects (e.g. lifts, queues, spiders)?

Form of thought and speech

Listen to how ideas are linked together. Record examples.
   Listen for:
- Flight of ideas (a rapid shift from one idea to the next)
- Loosening of associations (logical connections between
  ideas break down)
- Neologisms (new words, e.g. 'blattered')

Abnormal perceptions and experiences

Ask about derealization and depersonalization. 'Do you
   ever feel that you are unreal or that everything around
   you is unreal?'

Observe for and ask about hallucinations or illusions

Note any abnormal behaviour during the interview that
   suggests that the patient is experiencing hallucinations or
   illusions. These are most commonly auditory or visual but
   can occur in any sensory modality

Ask: 'Have you ever heard voices or noises when no one is
   there?'

Observe for and ask about passivity experiences

Do you ever feel that your body or mind is being controlled
   by someone or something else?

Do you attribute your thoughts or actions to an external
   source?

Cognitive state

Assess:
- Conscious level
- Orientation in time, place and person (ask: 'What time is
  it? Where are we? Who are you?')
- Attention and concentration (comment on the patient's
  concentration; ask the patient to perform a task that does
  not involve learning new information, e.g. subtracting
  serial 7s from 100, or spelling 'WORLD' backwards)
- Registration, or immediate recall (ask for the immediate
  recall of a series of digits; a normal digit span is 5–9)
- Short-term memory: learning of new material (first
  ensure that the patient has registered the information
  for memorizing (usually a name and address) by repeating
  it, then ask him or her to recall the information 5 minutes
  later)
- Long-term memory, both general and autobiographical
  (ask the patient to tell you what has happened to him or
  her recently; ask for recall of items of general knowledge)

Insight

Ask patients to explain their understanding of their symptoms, and whether they see themselves as ill and in need
   of treatment

Suicidal ideation

All patients should be asked about suicidal ideation. There
is no evidence that asking patients about suicidal ideation
increases the risk that they will harm themselves. Not asking increases the risk that you will miss suicidal ideation
that they might act upon. Patients are often embarrassed
to discuss the subject:

- It can help to normalize the experience with questions
such as: 'It is common when people feel as bad as you that
they have thoughts about ending their own life. Has this
happened to you?'
- Also, lead into the subject: 'Do things get so bad that
you sometimes wish you could go to sleep and not wake
up again?'

Thought and speech

Much of what we infer about someone's thinking comes from what they say. We can separate the examination of thought and speech into *how* someone speaks, or flow (e.g. speed, volume and tone), *what* they say (content) and how ideas are linked together (form).

Thought content

The definitions of a phobia, an obsession and a delusion are as follows:

- A **phobia** is an irrational fear of a specific situation or external object that would not normally be regarded thus
- An **obsession** is a thought, idea, image or impulse that repeatedly intrudes upon consciousness. Although regarded as absurd, it is recognized by the patient as a product of his or her own mind. Attempts are made to suppress it
- A **delusion** is a firmly held false belief that is inconsistent with one's social, cultural and religious background

Abnormal beliefs, especially delusions, are best elicited by asking open-ended questions, although specific probing is often required. Note whether a delusion is consistent with a patient's emotional state. Delusions in depressive disorders often have a negative content, with ideas of guilt and unworthiness. Patients with elated mood (mania) will often have inflated self-esteem and grandiose ideas. Delusions in schizophrenia and organic mental disorders are often persecutory in nature.

Abnormal perceptions and experiences

Hallucinations, illusions, passivity experiences, and derealization and depersonalization are abnormal perceptions and experiences that are defined as follows:

- A **hallucination** is an abnormal perception occurring in the absence of an external stimulus (Fig. 14.1)
- An **illusion** is a misinterpretation of an external stimulus (Fig. 14.1)
- **Passivity** is the experience that one's body actions, thoughts, feelings and impulses are being controlled by someone or something (e.g. a computer)
- **Depersonalization** and **derealization** are the feelings that one is unreal or that everything around one is unreal

Note any abnormal behaviour during the interview that might suggest that a patient is experiencing hallucinations or illusions. These are most commonly auditory or visual, but can occur in any sensory modality. Visual hallucinations or illusions indicate that an organic cause for symptoms is likely.

Cognitive state

An assessment of cognitive state (HISTORY & EXAMINATION BOX 14.2) is an important part of the mental state examination. This is because an organic cause for

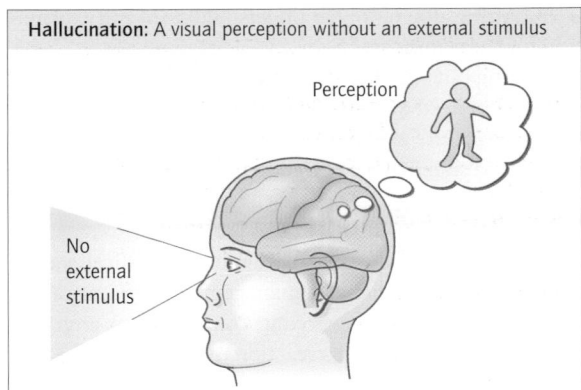

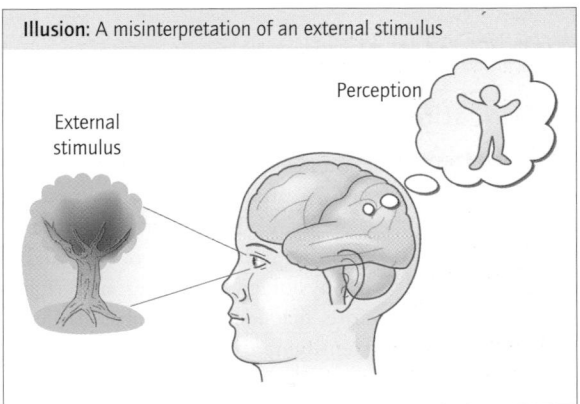

Figure 14.1 Abnormal perceptions.

psychiatric symptomatology must be considered for every patient. The bedside examination of cognitive state is a screening test. A positive finding indicates that a more rigorous examination and appropriate physical investigations are required. When interpreting bedside tests of attention and memory, remember to consider the patient's likely premorbid abilities. It is necessary to assess:

- Conscious level
- Orientation in time, place and person
- Attention and concentration
- Memory—including immediate recall (registration), and short- and long-term memory

Concentration may be impaired in a variety of non functional (non-organic) disorders (e.g. affective disorders and schizophrenia). This makes any subsequent assessment of memory difficult to interpret.

Cognitive impairment, especially in an elderly person with a probable diagnosis of dementia, may significantly impair the whole of history taking. This emphasizes the importance of taking a collateral history.

Insight

A person's insight into his or her illness can be assessed by:

● Enquiring after his or her understanding of and explanation for the symptoms
● Finding out whether the patient sees himself or herself as ill and in need of treatment
● Finding out whether the patient understands the nature and significance of treatments

Interviewer's reaction to a patient

The relationship between a patient and medical staff is an essential component of management. It occasionally breaks down, leaving everyone confused and angry. A critical evaluation of one's reaction to a patient during the first interview may be of use in averting such situations.

Differential diagnosis

Classification of mental disorders

In physical medicine we have greater knowledge of the pathological changes that underlie clinical symptoms than in psychological medicine. This is partly because of the complexity of the brain and our lack of knowledge of the structural and physiological changes underlying mental illness. Therefore, diagnosis in physical medicine usually depends on identifying the cause of a condition, whereas diagnosis in psychological medicine often depends on the identification of symptoms. Conditions with similar symptoms are then classified together (e.g. mood disorders or psychotic disorders).

Diagnostic hierarchy

When considering the differential diagnosis of mental illness it is helpful to use a diagnostic hierarchy, where a diagnosis in one group of conditions takes precedence over those in the groups below (Table 14.1). Organic disorders, including conditions secondary to alcohol and substance misuse, take precedence over all other groups. Next are the psychotic disorders such as schizophrenia, followed by the mood disorders, and finally the neurotic disorders such as anxiety-related conditions.

Table 14.1 Diagnostic hierarchy of psychiatric disorders. A diagnosis in one group takes precedence over those in the groups below

---

1 Organic mental disorders and conditions secondary to alcohol and substance misuse
2 Psychotic disorders, including schizophrenia
3 Mood disorders, including depressive disorder and bipolar affective disorder
4 Neurotic disorders, including anxiety-related disorders

If a patient has psychotic symptoms, such as auditory hallucinations, that can be explained by substance misuse, the mental disorder is classified as one of the group of organic disorders rather than as a condition such as schizophrenia. It is important to consider a possible organic mental disorder in all cases, as such a condition may require emergency medical treatment of the underlying cause.

When considering a differential diagnosis of mental illness it should be remembered that a patient may have more than one condition, such as depressive disorder in combination with alcohol misuse.

Investigation

A list of general investigations that might be considered in a case of mental disorder in a medical patient is given in Table 14.2. Investigations should not be carried out routinely, but should be carried out according to the clinical presentation.

Table 14.2 General investigations

Corroborative information
Observations of medical staff
Collateral history from relatives, friends and other health professionals
Previous medical, psychiatric or primary care records

Laboratory investigations
Haematology
● *FBC:* to detect anaemia, infection, and a raised MCV in alcohol misuse
● *ESR:* to reveal evidence of infection

Biochemistry
● *Urea and electrolytes:* to reveal electrolyte disturbances and dehydration
● *Calcium:* hyper- and hypocalcaemia are possible causes of psychiatric disorders
● *Thyroid function tests:* hyper- and hypothyroidism are possible causes of psychiatric disorders
● *Liver function tests:* to detect liver dysfunction in alcohol misuse
● *Urinary drug screen:* to detect illicit drug use

Microbiology
MSU, blood cultures, virology, lumbar puncture: to detect infection

Diagnostic imaging
● *Chest radiography:* to reveal chest infection and malignancy
● *CT or MRI head scan:* to detect intracranial pathology
● *EEG:* to investigate possible epileptic seizures

CT, computerized tomography; EEG, electroencephalography; ESR, erythrocyte sedimentation rate; FBC, full blood count; MCV, mean cell volume; MRI, magnetic resonance imaging; MSU, mid-stream urine.

Information gathering

Assessment of psychiatric disorders usually relies more heavily on a period of observation (history and mental state assessment as well as nursing observation) and obtaining a collateral history than on physical investigations. Information gathering is therefore an important aspect of investigation.

Physical investigations

Physical investigations are often an essential part of the diagnostic process. This is particularly true in the elderly in whom anxiety, depression or psychotic symptoms (e.g. auditory or visual hallucinations, or persecutory ideas) may be the presenting symptoms of an underlying physical illness:

- Stroke
- Chest, urinary tract and other infections
- Urea and electrolyte disturbance
- Dehydration

In younger patients, a number of physical disorders may present with psychological symptoms:

- Thyroid disease, which may present with depression
- Neurological diseases (e.g. multiple sclerosis, Parkinson's disease)
- Drug-induced disorders caused by prescribed medication (e.g. corticosteroids, oral contraceptive), alcohol or illicit drugs (e.g. amphetamines can cause a syndrome that is often difficult to distinguish from an acute episode of schizophrenia)

Principles of management

The management of any psychiatric disorder must be comprehensive and requires a team approach to physical, psychological and social treatments (Table 14.3). Consideration of the possible causative factors often helps in devising a management plan and ensures that psychological and social as well as physical factors are considered. These can be divided chronologically into those factors that predispose to an illness, precipitate its manifestation and perpetuate the symptoms.

Predisposing factors

Predisposing factors may determine an individual's vulnerability to psychiatric disorder and physical illness.

Personality can be defined as those enduring characteristics of behaviour, thinking and emotion that determine how an individual relates to his or her environment. It is affected by a variety of factors:

- Genetic make-up

Table 14.3 General management of psychiatric disorders in medical patients

Physical
Management of underlying physical illness in organic mental disorders
Psychotropic medication (e.g. antidepressants, neuroleptics)
Electroconvulsive therapy (ECT) for severe depression

Psychological
Counselling to allow ventilation of feelings and to enhance patient's own coping skills
Psychotherapy to tackle underlying emotional and behavioural problems

Social
Ensure appropriate environment for care
Family education and support
Staff education and support
Assistance with accommodation, finances, employment, etc.

- Development *in utero*
- Birth and early childhood experiences

Individual personality traits are significant determinants of a person's ability to cope with the stresses associated with being physically ill and to cooperate with what are often protracted and distressing treatments. Other factors that predispose an individual to both physical illness and psychiatric disorder include:

- Chronic physical illness
- Long-standing marital disharmony and other relationship problems
- Childhood sexual abuse
- Loss of parents (death or separation) during childhood
- Social stresses such as financial difficulties and unemployment

Precipitating factors

Precipitating factors may be physical, psychological or social and occur shortly before the onset of an illness. The relationship between stressful life events and the onset of psychiatric disorder, especially schizophrenia and mood disorders, is well established. Similarly, life events are often associated with a relapse or exacerbation of physical illness. Conversely, the sudden onset of physical illness, with the uncertainty of outcome it often brings, commonly results in an anxiety-related disorder or depressive disorder.

Perpetuating factors

Factors that maintain psychiatric disorder in those with physical disorders include the severity of the illness suffered, the nature of the treatments, the prognosis and the disruption caused to everyday life, especially in terms of work and relationships. Psychological factors may be severe enough to influence the course and prognosis of the physical illness itself.

Diseases and their management

There are a number of ways in which physical and psychiatric disorders can interact (Table 14.3). Medical patients may have coincidental physical and psychiatric disorders; hence a working knowledge of the range of common psychiatric disorders is required.

Psychiatric complications of physical illness

Psychiatric complications of physical illness include disease- or treatment-induced organic mental disorders, and psychological reactions to physical illnesses and their treatments (Table 14.4).

Organic mental disorders

Organic mental disorders are those where the symptoms are attributable to an independently diagnosable cerebral or systemic disease. The possibility that a patient's psy-

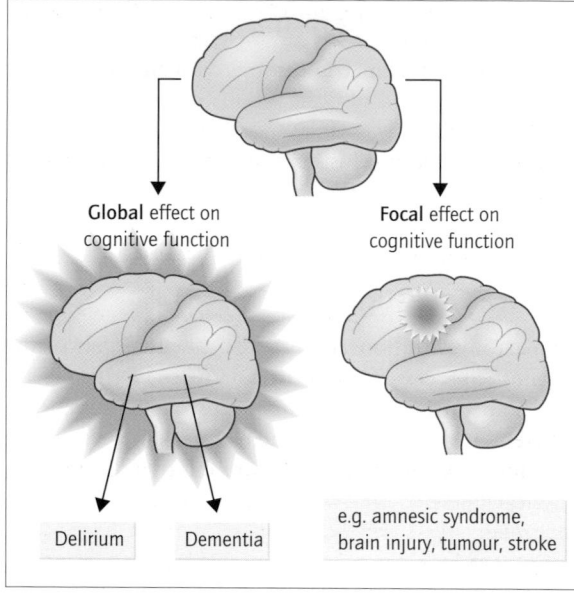

Figure 14.2 Organic mental disorders.

chiatric symptoms may be organic (physical) in origin should always be considered. The organic disorders can be divided into those that have a global effect on cerebral functions (delirium and dementia), and those that have focal effects while leaving other functions relatively intact (e.g. following trauma or stroke; Fig. 14.2).

Delirium

Delirium (also known as acute confusional state or acute organic reaction) is a state of impaired consciousness

Table 14.4 Psychiatric disorders in the physically ill

Classification	Disorder
Psychiatric complications of physical illness	Global organic mental disorders (delirium, dementia)
	Focal organic mental disorders (e.g. amnesic syndrome, consequences of trauma)
	Psychological reactions to physical illness
Somatic presentations of a psychiatric disorder	Medically unexplained symptoms
	Simulated disorders
Physical complications of psychiatric disorder	Deliberate self-harm
	Alcohol misuse and dependence
	Substance misuse and dependence
	Eating disorders
	Adverse effects of psychotropic medication
Psychiatric disorder and physical illness coexisting independently	Psychotic disorders (including schizophrenia)
	Mood disorders (including depressive disorder and bipolar affective disorder)
	Anxiety-related disorders
	Personality disorders

associated with disturbances of behaviour, affect, thought and perception. It should be considered in any medical patient with a sudden deterioration in mental state.

Epidemiology
Prevalence. Delirium occurs in 10–15% of medical inpatients.

Age. It can occur at any age but is more common in the very young (immature brain) and the elderly (ageing brain). On admission to hospital 10–15% of elderly patients have delirium, and an additional 10–40% develop it during their hospital stay.

Causes
Delirium has many possible causes, both intra- and extracerebral. It is important to consider the effects of drugs, either prescribed or misused, as a possible cause.

In the elderly, the most common causes are infections (particularly chest and urinary tract infections) and cerebral hypoxia (which is usually atherosclerotic in origin).

Disease mechanisms
The causative factors in delirium have a global adverse effect on the central nervous system. To exert this effect, extracerebral factors must breach the blood–brain barrier.

Clinical features
Delirium usually develops suddenly and rarely lasts more than a few days. It follows a fluctuating course. Symptoms occur in all areas of cognitive functioning. The level of consciousness (and therefore confusion) varies, often being worse at night. Hallucinations and illusions are common and are usually visual; although transient, they are often frightening and can lead to the rapid development of persecutory ideas. A thorough physical and mental state examination at regular intervals is an essential part of both assessment and management. Certain clinical features help to distinguish delirium from dementia (see DELIRIUM AT A GLANCE).

Investigation
Investigations should be carried out, as appropriate, to identify the underlying cause of the delirium (Table 14.2). In elderly patients, an underlying infection is a common cause of delirium. Appropriate investigations and possible findings in such a case might include:
- *FBC:* to identify infection, blood dyscrasias and vitamin deficiencies
- *ESR:* to indicate an inflammatory process
- *Mid-stream urine:* to identify a urinary tract infection
- *Chest radiography:* to identify a chest infection or neoplasia

Management
Management of a patient with delirium includes identifying and treating the underlying cause. Current medication should be reviewed and stopped where possible. Symptomatic relief may also be necessary, especially if the patient is restless, paranoid, frightened and unable to sleep or in pain. The patient should be nursed in quiet and well-lit surroundings.

It is essential to keep a fluid balance chart to avoid dehydration, and to prescribe adequate pain relief and appropriate sedation. Haloperidol in small doses (see p. 983) is a safe and effective sedative and is less likely to cause confusion in the elderly than benzodiazepines.

Prognosis
Prognosis is variable, depending on identification and treatment of the underlying cause.

Dementia
Dementia is a syndrome of acquired global impairment of higher mental functions (personality, intellect and memory), but without impairment of consciousness. Certain clinical features help to differentiate dementia from delirium (see DELIRIUM AT A GLANCE). Patients with dementia are more vulnerable to delirium than those with normal brains, and hence the two conditions often occur simultaneously in medical patients.

Epidemiology
Prevalence. Approximately 10% of those aged 65 years and over, and 20% of those aged 80 years and over, are affected.

Age. Any age, but primarily the elderly. Mean age of onset is the mid-seventies.

Sex. Two-thirds of patients with Alzheimer's disease are female.

Genetics. Unknown, but a pattern of polygenic or autosomal dominance is evident in some families with Alzheimer's disease.

Disease mechanisms
The two most common types of dementia in the elderly are Alzheimer's disease and vascular dementia. The cause of Alzheimer's disease is unknown, but genetic factors appear to be involved. Vascular dementia results from cerebral ischaemic changes caused by hypertension, generalized atherosclerosis or stroke. Other less common causes of dementia include infection (e.g. HIV, prion disorders), repeated trauma, alcohol and normal-pressure hydrocephalus.

14

14

Delirium at a glance

Signs and symptoms
Impaired and fluctuating conscious level
Impaired attention and concentration
Global disturbance of cognition
Psychomotor disturbances
Altered sleep–wake cycle
Emotional disturbance
Course: transient, sudden onset, fluctuating course

Causes

Cause	Example
Primary cerebral	Tumours (primary and secondary)
	Infections (especially meningitis)
	Abscesses (especially caused by *Listeria*)
	Extra- and subdural haematoma
	Subarachnoid haemorrhage
	Trauma
Systemic	Infections (especially chest and urinary tract)
	Vitamin deficiencies (especially B_1, B_6, B_{12})
	Metabolic (hypo- or hypernatraemia, uraemia, hypoxia, hypercalcaemia, hepatic and/or renal dysfunction)
	Endocrine (hypo- or hyperglycaemia)
Drug-induced (therapeutic)	Antidepressants
	Hypnotics (e.g. benzodiazepines/barbiturates)
	Opiate analgesics (e.g. heroin, codeine, methadone)
	Dopaminergics (e.g. chlorpromazine)
	Anticholinergics
	β-Blockers
	Cardiac glycosides
	H_2 receptor antagonists (e.g. cimetidine)
	Isoniazid
	Non-steroidal anti-inflammatory drugs
	Corticosteroids
Drug-induced (misuse)	Alcohol
	Opiate analgesics
	Stimulants (e.g. cocaine, amphetamines)
	Hallucinogens (e.g. cannabis, solvents, LSD)
	Hypnotics (e.g. benzodiazepines/barbiturates)
Drug withdrawal	Alcohol (delirium tremens)
	Opiates
	Stimulants (e.g. cocaine)
	Hypnotics (e.g. benzodiazepines/barbiturates)
	LSD

Investigations
FBC
ESR
Urea and electrolytes
Calcium and phosphate
Liver function tests
Thyroid function tests
Urinalysis, including drug screen and microscopy, culture and antibiotic sensitivity (MC & S)
Blood cultures
Chest X-ray
CT head

Management
Identify and treat underlying cause
Stop non-essential medication
Fluid balance chart
Analgesia
Low-dose sedation if necessary
Repeated physical and mental state examination
Nurse in quiet and well-lit environment

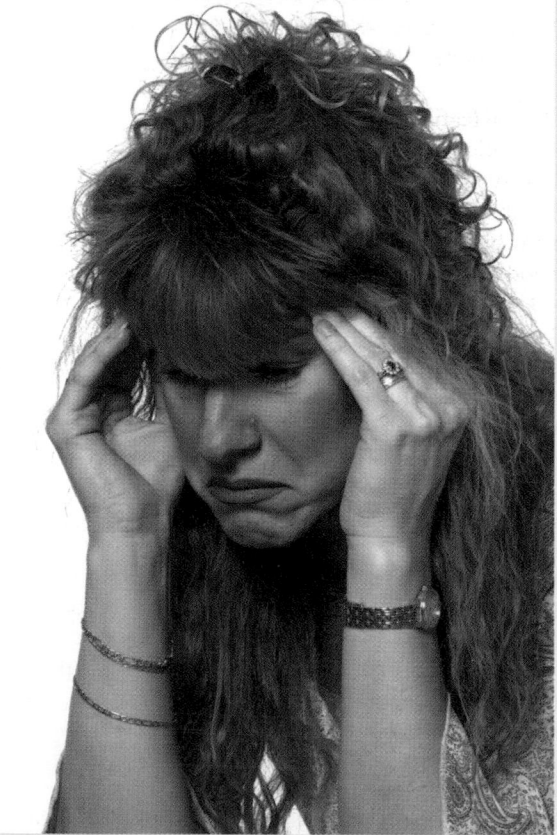

Fig. A Patients with delirium suffer from low mood and perplexity.

Differential diagnosis of delirium and dementia

	Delirium	Dementia
Onset	Acute	Usually insidious
Duration	Transient	Persistent
Course	Fluctuating over hours	Stable over days, worse at night, lucid intervals
Conscious level	Reduced	Normal
Sleep–wake cycle	Disrupted	Often normal
Perception	Impaired (illusions, hallucinations)	Normal early, misidentifications and hallucinations later
Autonomic changes	Common	Uncommon
Psychomotor changes	Common	Uncommon

14

In Alzheimer's disease there is global atrophy of the brain. Neuropathological features include neuronal loss, granulovacuolar degeneration, neurofibrillary tangles and neuritic plaques (senile plaques). Neuritic plaques contain an amyloid core. The gene coding for amyloid is closely related to a chromosome 21 locus for a familial form of Alzheimer's disease. There are biochemical changes in a number of neurotransmitters, including a reduction in acetylcholine. This is associated with decreased choline acetyltransferase, the enzyme needed to synthesize acetylcholine.

Clinical features

Dementia usually develops gradually and the most common symptom is poor memory. However, presentation is highly variable and often characterized by changes in many higher functions, including personality, behaviour, mood, thinking and intellect.

Alzheimer's disease and vascular dementia can often be distinguished clinically. However, the two may coexist in the same patient. A definitive diagnosis may not be made until postmortem.

- *Alzheimer's disease:* characterized by a slow and progressive course in which there is an early loss of memory and a global deterioration of higher functions.
- *Vascular dementia:* causes a stepwise deterioration of mental and physical function, associated with successive vascular events. There may be a relative preservation of personality. Physical examination may identify hypertension and neurological signs.

Many patients with dementia come to medical attention when they present with a superimposed medical problem (e.g. a chest infection or hip fracture).

Investigation

Treatable causes of dementia are rare, but appropriate investigations at initial referral are discussed below.

Haematology. FBC, ESR, vitamin B_{12} and folate levels: vitamin deficiencies and anaemias are treatable causes of dementia.

Biochemistry. Thyroid function tests: patients with hypothyroidism may present with dementia.

Diagnostic imaging
- *Chest radiography:* to identify malignancy
- *CT scan of the head:* to identify vascular disease, space-occupying lesions and the extent of cortical atrophy

Management

Psychological and social support. Treatment is usually symptomatic and supportive; the main aims are to optimize a patient's level of functioning and to support him or her at home for as long as possible. Most patients with dementia are cared for at home rather than in institutions.

An evaluation of daily living skills by an occupational therapist and of appropriate community-based supports by a social worker is essential. Such assessment should take place in the patient's own home environment, where he or she probably functions best.

Drug treatment

- Neuroleptic medication (e.g. haloperidol) or hypnotics (chloral hydrate or short-acting benzodiazepines such as temazepam) in small doses are particularly helpful for agitated and disturbed behaviour or poor sleep—but care is needed as medication can actually increase confusion.
- Drugs are available for the treatment of mild to moderate Alzheimer's disease (e.g. donepezil, rivastigmine, galantamine). These drugs inhibit acetylcholinesterase, the enzyme that breaks down acetylcholine, and in some patients help to slow cognitive decline. Such drugs should only be initiated by specialists.

Prognosis

The prognosis is poor, but helped by adequate provision of the treatment strategies discussed above.

Focal organic disorders

Focal organic disorders occur as the result of discrete brain injuries. Causes include trauma, tumours and strokes. How such disorders are managed often depends on the nature of the symptoms. For example, dysphasic disorders are predominantly managed by neurological services, but severe behavioural problems may require psychiatric services. Amnesic syndrome may come to the attention of psychiatric services, particularly when it occurs as a result of alcohol misuse.

Organic amnesic syndrome

The amnesic syndrome describes a prominent memory impairment, while other cognitive functions are relatively intact.

Causes

The most common cause is alcohol-related thiamine deficiency, which is also known as Korsakoff's psychosis. A variety of other causes, both thiamine- and non-thiamine-related, have also been described:
● *Thiamine-related:* alcohol misuse and/or dependence, malabsorption syndromes, gastric carcinoma, hyperemesis gravidarum
● *Non-thiamine-related:* infections (especially tuberculosis and syphilis), subarachnoid haemorrhage, tumours, trauma, carbon monoxide poisoning

Disease mechanisms

The amnesic syndrome results from degenerative changes in areas of the brain that are involved in the laying down and retrieval of memories. Specifically, these include structures around the third ventricle: the mammillary bodies, the hippocampus and the medial aspect of the thalami.

Clinical features

Memory impairment occurs in clear consciousness and is not part of a dementia. There is a defect of short-term memory (learning new material), but immediate recall (registration) is intact. There will be anterograde and retrograde amnesia around the time of the original insult to the brain and a reduced ability to recall past experiences in reverse order to their occurrence. The memory deficit is often compensated for by confabulation (filling in gaps in the memory with false information). The onset may occur acutely, following an episode of delirium (Wernicke's encephalopathy).

Investigation

Appropriate investigations are required to confirm or exclude a suspected treatable cause.

Management

Profound memory deficit makes independent living virtually impossible. Neurorehabilitation may maximize a patient's abilities. Treatment with thiamine (vitamin B_1) occasionally results in improvement.

Prognosis

Prognosis depends on the cause of the underlying lesion; however, with degenerative changes improvement is unlikely. Patients with alcohol-related amnesic syndrome may show some gradual improvement if they remain abstinent.

Acute behavioural disturbance

Organic mental disorders can be associated with acute disturbed or violent behaviour by a patient. The management of such behaviour is discussed in EMERGENCY BOX 14.1. A key element of management is risk assessment, taking into account risk to the disturbed patient, staff, other patients and yourself. Remember that the patient may be frightened by experiences such as illusions, hallucinations and persecutory delusions. General measures, such as a calm and reassuring approach, are important. Sedation may be required in some situations, but only after general measures have been tried.

Psychological reactions to physical illness

The onset of a physical illness, or deterioration in an ongoing condition, results in a number of psychological tasks that a patient must overcome. Tackling these tasks produces some of the most common psychological symptoms experienced by general hospital patients. If these tasks are not tackled successfully then they may lead to persistent distress and precipitate a psychiatric disorder, such as anxiety-related or depressive disorders.

In the context of physical illness some degree of worry is normal. Other common reactions include uncertainty about the future, a feeling of loss of control, a sense of isolation and thoughts of 'Why me?'. More pronounced reactions include:
● Anxiety-related disorders (see p. 990)
● Depressive disorder (see p. 987)
● Adjustment disorders and the grief reaction
● Abnormal illness behaviour

Adjustment disorder and the grief reaction

Adjustment disorder is a state of distress and emotional

Emergency 14.1: Acute behavioural disturbance

Risk assessment
Assess degree of risk to patient, staff and other patients
Do not place yourself at risk of harm
Collect sufficient staff to manage the situation safely
Call security staff if necessary

General measures
Approach the patient in a calm and reassuring manner
Try talking the patient down
Move the patient to a private and quiet environment, such as a side room on the ward
Treat the underlying cause of the disturbance
Consider constant nursing supervision
If restraint is required, ensure that there are sufficiently trained staff to minimize harm to the patient and staff

Sedation
Offer oral medication
If this is unsuccessful, or the patient refuses, consider intramuscular (i.m.) medication
If the patient has not previously been on neuroleptic medication, use a benzodiazepine drug (e.g. lorazepam 1–2 mg i.m.)
If the patient is on regular benzodiazepines, try a neuroleptic (e.g. haloperidol 2.5–5 mg i.m.)
If sedation is still required after 30 minutes then give repeat medication
Have flumazenil available to reverse the effects of a benzodiazepine if necessary
Have procyclidine available to treat the motor adverse effects of neuroleptics

disturbance arising in the period of adaptation to a significant life change or to the consequences of a stressful event. Adjustment disorder is common in a general hospital and affects one-quarter of medical patients.

The grief reaction, or mourning, is a specific form of adjustment that occurs following a loss, such as bereavement. Other losses that medical patients may experience include the loss of health with the onset of a disorder or the actual or functional loss of a bodily organ. The grief reaction follows a number of stages (Fig. 14.3):
- *Shock and disbelief:* a state of emotional numbness and a sense of disbelief.
- *Yearning and longing:* the individual may experience a lost person in dreams, illusions and hallucinations.
- *Despair:* depressed mood and anger are common at this stage.
- *Acceptance:* the individual adapts intellectually and emotionally to the loss. Feelings of depression may persist. The grief reaction usually takes place over 6 months to 1 year after a death, but feelings of sadness may persist for many years, particularly around the time of anniversaries.

General management of adjustment disorder is supportive, with the aim of facilitating adjustment to a new situation. Patients should be given a clear explanation of their illness, the treatment and prognosis. They should be allowed to express their feelings and encouraged to explore coping resources. Adjustment disorder should be distinguished from anxiety-related or depressive disorders, where the symptoms are more pronounced and prolonged, and specialist assessment may be required (for further discussion of common emotional reactions to life-threatening illness, see Chapter 16).

Abnormal illness behaviour

Abnormal illness behaviour describes a range of behaviours that occur in response to a physical illness. These include excessive concern about physical health, a search for different medical opinions and a cure, and disability out of proportion to the physical disease. A careful assessment of the patient, and consideration of psychological and social causes, will help to suggest a management plan. Specialist psychiatric advice may be helpful.

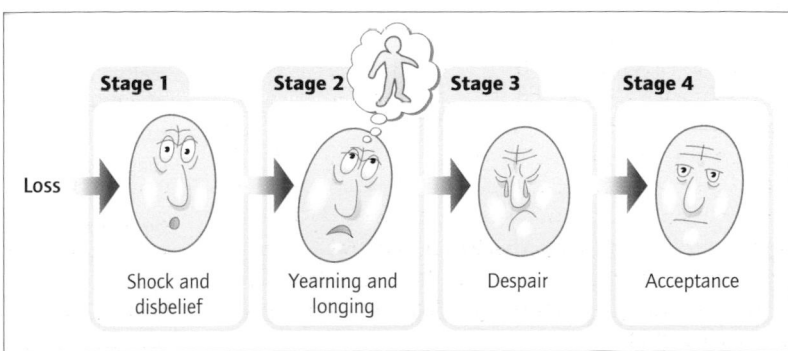

Figure 14.3 Stages of the grief reaction.

14

Somatic presentation of a psychiatric disorder

Medically unexplained symptoms

A large number of patients throughout health services have physical symptoms that cannot be accounted for by organic disease. Various terms, which are often unsatisfactory and confusing, have been used to describe these symptoms. Physicians and psychiatrists tend to use different terms when diagnosing medically unexplained symptoms:

- Physicians tend to describe syndromes reflecting their area of specialist interest, such as 'irritable bowel syndrome' in gastroenterology, and 'fibromyalgia' in neurology
- Psychiatrists describe syndromes that are often based on causative hypotheses, such as 'somatization disorder' (p. 972) or 'dissociative disorder' (see p. 973)

There is no entirely satisfactory classification system, but 'medically unexplained symptoms' can be used as an umbrella term.

Epidemiology

Prevalence. Between one-quarter and one-half of new medical outpatients experience bodily symptoms that cannot be explained by organic disease. Such patients constitute a smaller proportion of inpatients (1–2%), but this group often has more persistent symptoms and a greater use of medical services.

Age, sex and race. No known associations.

Disease mechanisms

Many medically unexplained symptoms are the somatic (bodily) symptoms of anxiety or depression (see pp. 987 and 990); however, the precise cause of many symptoms is unknown and biological, psychological and social factors probably all play a part. We all experience bodily sensations, but only a small proportion of these are interpreted as symptoms of disease. We may then respond in a number of ways, such as ignoring the symptoms or seeking medical help. Causative factors can act at any point in this process:
- *Predisposing:* personality factors, such as excessive health concern; childhood and family experiences of illness; knowledge and beliefs about illness; previous major physical illness
- *Precipitating:* benign or minor pathology; autonomic arousal; side-effects of medication; physiological consequences of alcohol or caffeine; stressful life events; chronic difficulties
- *Perpetuating:* reaction of others, including health professionals; psychiatric disorder; problems in coping; iatrogenic factors

Clinical features

A number of psychiatric syndromes that include medically unexplained symptoms are described below. However, many patients do not fit easily into diagnostic categories, or may fulfil the criteria for more than one diagnosis.

Somatization disorder

Chronic multiple and variable physical symptoms for which no adequate physical explanation can be found. Patients refuse to accept medical reassurance and have impaired social functioning as a result of their problems.

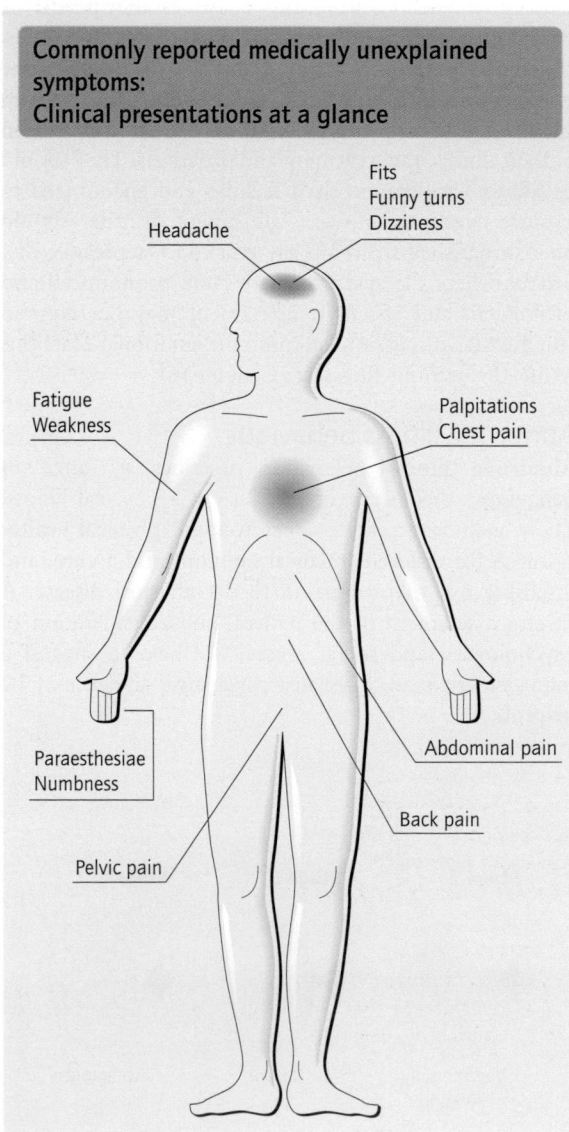

Commonly reported medically unexplained symptoms:
Clinical presentations at a glance

Fits
Funny turns
Dizziness

Headache

Fatigue
Weakness

Palpitations
Chest pain

Paraesthesiae
Numbness

Abdominal pain

Back pain

Pelvic pain

Hypochondriacal disorder
A persistent preoccupation with the possibility of a serious disease, with a refusal to accept medical reassurance.

Dissociative (conversion) disorder
Previously called 'hysteria'. Patients have the signs and symptoms of a disorder (e.g. amnesia, paralysis, convulsions), but no evidence for a physical disorder to explain the symptoms. There is often evidence for an associated psychological problem—'dissociation' implies a loss of the normal integration of psychological functions, and 'conversion' implies the transformation of psychological distress into physical symptoms.

Investigation
Appropriate investigations for the patient's presenting problem should be carried out (Table 14.2). A balance needs to be struck between missing disease and the potential harm of excessive investigations. While physical investigations are often a necessary part of patient reassurance, overinvestigation can reinforce a person's belief that there must be a physical explanation for his or her symptoms. Misdiagnosis is relatively uncommon. A review of previous medical notes is often helpful, particularly where patients have been referred to various specialities with medically unexplained symptoms.

Management
Recent stresses and chronic worries should be identified and simple practical advice should be given where possible. Where there is an underlying psychiatric disorder, this should be treated appropriately. Patients with more severe and persistent problems should be referred to specialist psychiatric services. Antidepressant drugs are most useful when the patient is depressed; however, they may also be helpful when there is no mood disorder. A number of brief psychological interventions have been shown to be of benefit. Generally, it is best to start with the simplest measures and review progress. For those with chronic problems, the aims of treatment may be less

14

Medically unexplained symptoms at a glance

Signs and symptoms
Commonly reported medically unexplained symptoms

Psychiatric syndromes with medically unexplained symptoms
Somatization disorder
Hypochondriacal disorder
Dissociative (conversion) disorder

Medical conditions with medically unexplained symptoms
Irritable bowel syndrome
Fibromyalgia
Atypical chest pain
Chronic fatigue syndrome

Causes
Predisposing: personality factors, previous experience of illness, beliefs about illness
Precipitating: normal bodily sensations, minor pathology, adverse effects of drugs, stress and autonomic arousal
Perpetuating: psychiatric illness, reactions of others, iatrogenic

Investigation
Exclude disease, but avoid unnecessary investigations
Identify treatable psychiatric disorder

Management
General
Acknowledge reality of the problem
Give reassurance

Correct misconceptions about disease
Give a positive explanation for symptoms (e.g. in terms of autonomic arousal)
Encourage return to normal functioning
Treat any psychiatric disorder
Do not suggest:
• There is nothing wrong
• Symptoms are 'all in the mind'

Specialist referral
Appropriate where there is:
• Severe disability
• Persistent problem
• Psychiatric disorder requiring specialist treatment
• Suicidal ideation

Specific treatments
Behavioural and lifestyle changes
Graded increase in activity
Relaxation techniques
Reduction in alcohol and caffeine

Psychotherapy
Cognitive–behavioural therapy
Brief psychodynamic therapy
Problem-solving therapy

Antidepressants

ambitious; infrequent but planned long-term follow-up may lead to a slow improvement and limit the use of medical resources.

Prognosis

For most patients, the symptoms are transient and usually respond to simple reassurance and explanation. Those with chronic symptoms have a worse prognosis.

Simulated disorders

Simulated disorders involve the intentional production or feigning of either physical or psychological symptoms or disabilities. The prevalence of feigned symptoms is difficult to determine as patients may present themselves at several different hospitals and commonly discharge themselves when challenged or when asked to see a psychiatrist. The two main groups of simulated disorders are factitious disorders and malingering. The causes of these disorders are often unclear, but they are distinguished partly by the presumed motivation for the behaviour.

Clinical features
Factitious disorders

Factitious disorders (also known as Munchausen's syndrome or hospital addiction syndrome) are characterized by the conscious, deliberate and surreptitious feigning of physical or psychological symptoms to simulate disease. The intentional production of physical symptoms may include the self-infliction of wounds. The imitation of pain and the insistence of the presence of bleeding may be so convincing and consistent that repeated investigations and operations are performed despite repeated negative findings, often at different hospitals. The motivation for this behaviour is usually obscure and presumably internal, with patients having an unexplained psychological need to assume the sick role. Individuals with this behaviour usually have other abnormalities of personality and relationships.

Malingering

This is characterized by intentional production of physical or psychological symptoms, motivated by identifiable external incentives (e.g. evading the police or criminal proceedings, financial compensation or obtaining drugs).

Management

Patients should be confronted about their behaviour, but also offered support. A joint medical and psychiatric approach is ideal, with the aim of shifting the focus from physical symptoms to psychological help.

Physical complications of psychiatric disorder

Physical complications of psychiatric disorder include deliberate self-harm, alcohol misuse and dependence, other drug misuse and dependence, eating disorders and the effects of psychotropic medication.

Deliberate self-harm

Under 65 years of age, deliberate self-harm (DSH) is the most common reason for hospital admission for women and the second most common for men (after ischaemic heart disease). The most common method of DSH is self-poisoning with over-the-counter analgesic medication, often consumed with alcohol. Other methods include cutting, attempted hanging and asphyxiation by car exhaust.

A major concern is the poor prognosis of patients following DSH (see p. 976); 10% will commit suicide over the next 10 years. Hospital attendance or admission is an important opportunity for intervention as one-quarter of all suicides attend a general hospital after a non-fatal act of self-harm in the 12 months before they die.

These patients often arouse difficult feelings in medical and nursing staff, such as anger at what may be perceived as an unnecessary use of medical resources. There may also be considerable anxiety related to the refusal by patients of essential medical and nursing procedures.

Epidemiology

Prevalence. The incidence of self-harm has risen over the past 50 years, with a current estimate of 400 in 100 000 population per annum. In the UK there are 150 000 hospital attendances following self-poisoning each year.

Age. The mean age of the self-harm population is in the early thirties for both sexes. The peak age of presentation is 15–24 years for women and 25–34 years for men.

Sex. Although there were once 2–3 times as many episodes in females, the self-harm rates are now only slightly more common in women than men.

Geography. Associated with urban deprivation and lower socioeconomic status.

Contributing factors. In many cases, DSH is an impulsive act, precipitated by a recent life stress against a background of chronic social and interpersonal difficulties. In a minority of cases, DSH is carried out with high suicidal intent, particularly by people with chronic physical or psychiatric disorders.

Clinical features

Individual characteristics associated with non-fatal DSH and suicide can guide risk assessment. These factors should be judged in the context of a wider clinical assessment of the act, the patient's social circumstances and mental state. Current suicidal intent should be explored.

Management

Assessment of suicide risk

The aims of the initial management of a patient following DSH include the assessment of suicidal intent at the time of the act and the assessment of ongoing suicidal risk.

Patients often express ambivalence about their intentions. However, some features of the history are more likely to be associated with high suicidal intent.

Associated mental disorders

Of patients who deliberately harm themselves, one-third will have had previous contact with psychiatric services and one-third will receive a psychiatric diagnosis following DSH, although the rate of disorders may be higher. Common mental health problems in people attending with DSH include adjustment disorder, depressive disorder, anxiety-related disorders, alcohol and substance

14

Deliberate self-harm at a glance

Signs and symptoms

Characteristics associated with non-fatal deliberate self-harm
Female
Younger
Marital status: single, divorced, young wife
Unemployed
Urban environment
Lower socioeconomic class

Characteristics associated with suicide
Male
Older—especially over 45 years
Unemployed or retired
Socially isolated
Poor physical health—especially chronic or painful illnesses
Poor mental health—especially schizophrenia, bipolar affective disorder, depressive disorder, alcohol or substance misuse

Features indicating high suicidal intent
Evidence of planning
Preparation for a final event (e.g. leaving a note, making a will)
Act performed alone
Act unlikely to be discovered
Precautions taken to avoid discovery
No effort to get help
All available drugs taken
Expectation of a fatal outcome

Questions to explore ongoing suicidal risk
Has anything changed as a result of what you did?
Do you still feel the same?
Do you regret what you did?
Do you still feel hopeless?
What would make you try again?
What would you do if you went home now?
Can you guarantee me your safety?

Causes

Psychiatric disorders
Physical disorders
Acute and chronic life stresses:
• Relationships
• Financial
• Housing
• Employment or studies
• Social isolation
• Legal

Management

Minimize physical harm from the act
Assess the degree of suicide risk
Detect any underlying psychiatric disorder
Explore recent stresses and coping resources
Follow local protocol
Establish aftercare plan on discharge

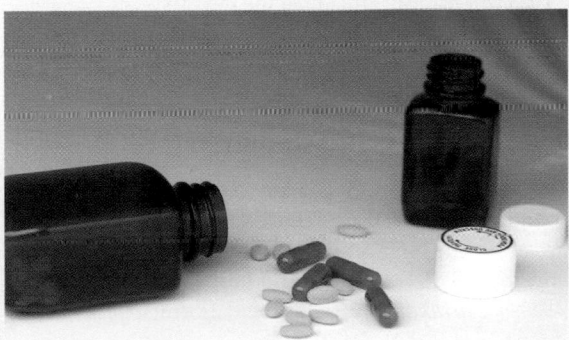

Fig. A Overdose is the commonest method of deliberate self-harm.

misuse, and personality disorder. An important minority have schizophrenia or bipolar affective disorder.

Stresses and coping
Attention should be paid to the circumstances surrounding the overdose. Current stresses and available coping resources help guide the risk assessment and subsequent management.

Policies
It is essential that all hospitals have a locally agreed policy for the assessment and management of DSH. All hospital attendances following DSH should lead to a specialist psychosocial assessment. Direct discharge from an accident and emergency department should only be considered if a psychosocial assessment and aftercare plan can be arranged prior to discharge.

Medical admission
Many DSH patients will have a brief admission to either an accident and emergency ward or a general medical ward. This gives the patient 'time out' from the circumstances that may have precipitated the DSH and the chance to discuss the incident and make plans for the future. The value of one-off interviews should not be underestimated as many DSH patients do not attend follow-up appointments.

Psychotherapy
There is insufficient evidence to recommend specific clinical interventions following DSH, although brief psychotherapeutic interventions appear promising.

Prognosis
Following DSH:
- 15% will repeat over the next year
- 1% will commit suicide in the following year
- 10% will commit suicide in the next 10 years

A history of psychiatric disorder is associated with a particularly poor prognosis.

Alcohol misuse and dependence

Alcohol misuse causes a wide range of physical, psychological and social problems, and places a significant burden on the NHS. Inpatient costs account for 2–12% of the total NHS expenditure on hospitals.
- *Sensible drinking limits:* for men, 21 units/week or less; for women, 14 units/week or less.
- *Hazardous drinking:* where an individual's drinking pattern poses a health risk.
- *Harmful (or problem) drinking:* where alcohol contributes to physical, psychological or social harm.

- *Alcohol dependence syndrome:* this represents a severe form of harmful drinking. It consists of a combination of physical and psychological factors.

In view of the burden alcohol places on the NHS, hospitals must have strategies for the early identification and management of hazardous and harmful drinking.

Epidemiology
Prevalence. 1 in 5 women and 1 in 3 men in the UK regularly drink more alcohol than the sensible limits. Twenty per cent of patients admitted to hospital for illnesses unrelated to alcohol are hazardous drinkers.

Age. Heaviest drinking occurs in the late teens and early twenties.

Sex. About 75% of patients are male.

Race. Prevalence is lower in certain racial groups (e.g. Jews and Japanese people).

Genetics. Studies of adopted children who have an alcoholic natural parent confirm that as adults they have a fourfold higher incidence of alcohol dependence syndrome than the general population.

Geography. There has been an increase in consumption in the UK and most of the rest of Europe over recent decades.

Contributing factors. The cause of alcohol misuse and dependence is a complex interaction of biological, psychological and social factors.
- *Physical:* approximately 20% of people with chronic alcohol dependence may inherit some genetic predisposition; the evidence is stronger for men than women.
- *Psychological:* the pleasurable effects of intoxication can reinforce drinking behaviour. It may also have a role in anaesthetizing painful feelings.
- *Sociological:* there may be reinforcement from the social situation where drinking takes place; people who lack other sources of pleasure or social contact may be especially susceptible to this. The amount of alcohol consumed per head of population is directly related to the availability and cost.

Clinical features
Screening. A simple screening questionnaire is the CAGE (HISTORY & EXAMINATION BOX 14.3). If a patient answers two or more questions positively, this should trigger a more detailed assessment. For all patients, an estimate of the weekly consumption of units of alcohol should be made. One unit contains 8 g of alcohol and is equivalent to a glass of wine, a measure of spirits or one half pint of

> ### History & Examination 14.3: History taking in alcohol and substance misuse
>
> **The CAGE screening questionnaire for alcohol dependence**
> Have you ever felt you ought to cut down on your drinking?
> Have people *annoyed* you by criticizing your drinking?
> Have you ever felt bad or *guilty* about your drinking?
> Have you ever had a drink first thing in the morning (an '*eye*-opener') to get rid of a hangover?
>
> **History taking**
> *Reasons for referral or help seeking*
> Current use:
> • Drugs used
> • Amount and pattern of use, including a typical day
> • Features of tolerance, withdrawal and dependency
> Chronological history of use:
> • Age first used
> • Subsequent use—amounts, frequency, maximum use
> • Abstinence and relapse
> Complications of use:
> • Physical
> • Psychological
> • Social—including relationships, family, occupational, legal
> Previous treatment history:
> • GP
> • Specialist services—inpatient and outpatient
> • Voluntary agencies
> • Self-help groups

normal strength lager. However, careful questioning is needed to establish the volume and strength of alcoholic drinks. One can of high strength lager may contain 4–5 units of alcohol.

Complications of alcohol misuse. The many complications of alcohol misuse can be divided into neurological, psychiatric and social. History taking therefore needs to be comprehensive.

Withdrawal symptoms. Features range from mild discomfort to life-threatening.

Wernicke's encephalopathy. This has a classic triad of symptoms, confusion, ataxia and eye signs (nystagmus and ophthalmoplegia), and may be associated with peripheral neuropathy. However, it does not always present with a 'pure' clinical picture. Wernicke's encephalopathy carries a high risk of irreversible brain damage and may lead on to Korsakoff's psychosis (see p. 970). A presumptive diagnosis should be made and treatment instigated in any patient undergoing alcohol detoxification who experiences ataxia, confusion, memory disturbance, hypothermia, hypotension, ophthalmoplegia, nystagmus, coma or unconsciousness. Patients with malnutrition secondary to alcohol misuse should also be considered for prophylactic treatment.

Investigation
The most common abnormal serological investigations in harmful or hazardous drinking are as follows.

Haematology
FBC. Raised mean cell volume (MCV) without anaemia.

Biochemistry
Liver function tests. Raised gamma-glutamyl transferase.

Management
Patients who experience withdrawal symptoms need to be detoxified. This can be carried out on an outpatient basis if the patient is responsible, has adequate social support and has no past history of withdrawal fits, epilepsy or other medical problems of special concern.

Subsequent management is best coordinated by a specialist alcohol team. People who misuse alcohol can then be offered the most appropriate treatment—whether it be individual counselling, or group, couple or family therapy. Many find voluntary organizations such as Alcoholics Anonymous a useful additional support. Residential treatment programmes are appropriate for a minority.

In younger patients with no physical complications and good family and social supports, it may be possible to achieve controlled drinking, but this needs close monitoring.

Prognosis
At follow-up, 30–40% of problem drinkers have either successfully abstained from alcohol or practise controlled drinking.

The mortality rate for people who misuse alcohol is 2–3 times that of the normal population. The mortality rate for untreated delirium tremens is 10–15%.

Substance misuse and dependence

Substance misuse occurs when a drug is used in a way that is socially unacceptable, illegal or harmful. Misused drugs include the following:
● *Stimulants:* amphetamines, cocaine
● *Hallucinogens:* cannabis, LSD, solvents
● *Opiates:* heroin, morphine, pethidine, codeine, methadone
● *Hypnotics:* benzodiazepines, barbiturates

Alcohol dependence at a glance

Signs and symptoms
Features of the dependence syndrome
Although originally described for alcohol, the dependence syndrome can also be applied to other drugs of misuse
1 Subjective awareness of a compulsion to use a drug
2 Tolerance to the effect of the drug
3 Withdrawal symptoms
4 Use of the drug to avoid withdrawal symptoms
5 Stereotyped pattern of drug use
6 Prominence of drug use over other behaviours
7 Rapid reinstatement after abstinence

Symptoms of alcohol withdrawal
Early withdrawal:
- Occur up to 12 h after the last drink
- Symptoms include: nausea, sweating, insomnia, anxiety

Moderate withdrawal:
- Signs more marked
- Transient auditory hallucinations can occur in clear consciousness

Withdrawal fits:
- Can occur from 12 to 48 h after the last drink
- More likely with a previous history of withdrawal fits or epilepsy

Delirium tremens (DTs):
- Usually 72 h after the last drink
- Clinical features include: tremor, confusion, agitation, restlessness, fearfulness, illusions, hallucinations, autonomic disturbance, sweating, pyrexia, dehydration
- More likely with higher alcohol consumption, severe withdrawal symptoms on presentation, long history of dependency, past history of DTs, older age, concomitant physical illness

Neuropsychiatric and social complications of alcohol misuse and dependence
Neurological
Wernicke's encephalopathy
Korsakoff's psychosis
Alcoholic dementia
Epilepsy
Peripheral neuropathy
Cerebellar degeneration
Central pontine myelinolysis
Machiafava–Bignami syndrome

Psychiatric
Depressive disorders
Anxiety-related disorders
Deliberate self-harm and suicide
Sexual problems, especially impotence
Morbid jealousy syndrome (delusions of infidelity directed towards one's spouse)

Alcoholic hallucinosis (auditory hallucinations occurring in clear consciousness)

Social
Deteriorating relationships—marital, family, friends, work colleagues
Problems with work and finances—absenteeism, poor performance, loss of job and income
Increased risk of accidents at home and work, and on the road
Associated with crime—delinquency, violence, burglary, drink driving

Causes
Physical: genetic, tolerance to effects leading to higher intake
Psychological: pleasurable effects of intoxication, reduction of painful feelings, learned behaviour
Social: social reinforcement, availability

Investigation
Full blood count, including mean cell volume
Liver function tests, including gamma-glutamyl transferase

Management
Withdrawal symptoms
Reducing schedule of chlordiazepoxide to reduce intensity of unpleasant withdrawal symptoms, and to prevent seizures and DTs
A typical regimen would be 20 mg four times daily on day 1, reducing over 9 days and discontinuing on day 10
Increased initial doses may be required in severe withdrawal, and less in mild withdrawal (e.g. 60 mg/day)

Withdrawal seizures
Usually self-limiting
Lorazepam 2 mg intravenously for recurrent or prolonged seizures

Psychotic symptoms
Consider haloperidol (1.5–5 mg 2–3 times daily), in combination with chlordiazepoxide

Vitamin prophylaxis
Incipient Wernicke's encephalopathy: intravenous vitamin B + C (Pabrinex)
Low-risk group: thiamine 200 mg 4 times daily and vitamin B complex strong 30 mg/day

Long-term management
Specialist referral
Voluntary organizations
Psychotherapy
Rehabilitation

Substance misusers, especially those who inject, have high rates of associated physical illness. In addition, many medical patients have coincident substance misuse. Substance misuse, particularly opiate misuse, should be considered when a person behaves in a bizarre or aggressive manner or where unexplained patient–staff conflict occurs. Substance misusers may present with the direct pharmacological action of the drug itself (e.g. overdose), physical complications related to administration (e.g. injection abscesses) and with drug-seeking behaviour. It should be remembered that many patients use a combination of drugs.

Epidemiology

Prevalence. Approximately one-third of adults in England and Wales have used illicit drugs at some point in their lives. There are trends in the use of different drugs. Cannabis is the most frequently reported lifetime drug of use. The other most commonly reported drugs used are hallucinogens (e.g. LSD), amphetamines, cocaine and ecstasy. The reported lifetime prevalence of opiate use is about 1%. The point prevalence of opiate use is higher in urban areas, with estimates of problem drug use of 3–4% in central London.

Age. The prevalence of substance misuse is more common in younger age groups.

Sex. Substance misuse is more common amongst men. About 67–75% of opiate misusers are male.

Contributing factors. As for alcohol misuse, the cause of substance misuse in an individual is a complex interaction of biological, psychological and social factors.
● *Physical:* there is less evidence for a genetic basis to substance misuse and dependence than with alcohol dependence. Relatives of those with opiate dependence have higher rates of alcohol and substance misuse, and psychiatric disorder. Tolerance of drug effects may lead to increased use in order to achieve the same desired effect.
● *Psychological:* the capacity of the drug to produce a pleasant sensation, and hence reinforce its use, depends upon individual and drug factors. The expectation of effect may be important. There may also be learned cues that precipitate use (e.g. when socializing with friends).
● *Sociological:* an individual is influenced by the views of family, friends and wider society. Use also depends on availability.

Clinical features

Opiate use is a recognized cause of both psychological and physical morbidity and mortality. Opiate misusers

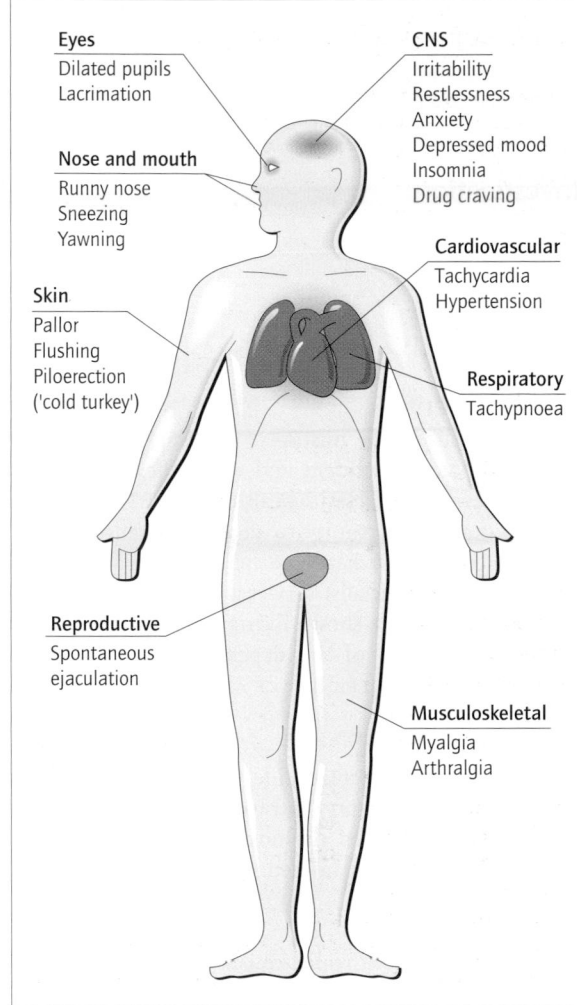

Figure 14.4 Symptoms of opiate withdrawal.

often present first to general medical services, either with a disease for which they have an increased susceptibility (e.g. infective endocarditis, tuberculosis, hepatitis and HIV infection) or with complications of repeated intravenous injection (e.g. abscess or venous thrombosis). Long-term dependence commonly leads to malaise and physical weakness. The symptoms of opiate withdrawal are unpleasant, but not life-threatening in an otherwise healthy person (Fig. 14.4).

Acute intoxication with stimulant drugs, such as amphetamines or cocaine, is characterized by a state of agitation and excitement associated with dizziness, dilated pupils, a tremor, hyperpyrexia and cardiac arrhythmias. A transient psychosis similar to schizophrenia can occur with prolonged usage. Cocaine induces increased energy associated with an increase in blood pressure and heart rate. There have been reports of abnormalities of cardiac conduction and paranoid reactions. Cocaine withdrawal is characterized by a dysphoric mood, irritability and agitation.

Investigation
Biochemistry
Urinary drug screen.

Microbiology
Hepatitis and HIV serology.

Management
For many substance misusers, medical admission or attendance at the accident and emergency department may be the only contact with health services. This provides an important opportunity to detect substance misuse, assess and treat immediate medical problems, and to facilitate referral to specialist services. Questions to explore substance misuse are shown in HISTORY & EXAMINATION BOX 14.3. Features of the dependence syndrome are shown in ALCOHOL DEPENDENCE AT A GLANCE.

Opiate overdose
Opiate overdose is potentially life-threatening and prompt intervention is necessary. Intravenous naloxone can be life-saving and is often diagnostic as the level of consciousness will improve immediately.

Medical inpatients
Medical inpatients with opiate misuse should be discussed with specialist services for advice on the management of drug dependency. Prescribing a substitute opiate such as methadone may be considered after careful assessment and where there is evidence of distressing opiate withdrawal. Non-opiate alternatives can be given for the symptomatic relief of mild withdrawal symptoms.

Withdrawal symptoms
Patients may report withdrawal symptoms and request prescriptions for drugs. However, it is neither necessary nor ideal to prescribe controlled drugs in the majority of cases. The risks of doing so include accidental overdose and similar requests by other patients.

Psychiatric complications
Many substances of misuse, both in intoxication and withdrawal, can give rise to acute psychiatric complications. Management is aimed at treating specific symptoms rather than being drug-specific. The optimal treatment is to allow the effects to wear off, although additional medication may be required. The patient should be approached in a calm and reassuring manner. Vital signs and the state of hydration should be monitored.

Prognosis
The prognosis depends primarily on the individual's motivation. One study found that only 50% of opiate misusers were abstinent after 6 months.

Eating disorders
There is no obvious discontinuity between normal and disordered eating. Ninety per cent of women have been on slimming diets and 10% have used vomiting or laxatives in an attempt to lose weight. Hence, as well as the recognized disorders of anorexia and bulimia nervosa, there are also subthreshold disorders, and disorders with a mixture of anorectic and bulimic symptoms. Eating disorders occur in both sexes, but are much more common in women than men.

Anorexia nervosa
Epidemiology
Prevalence. 0.5–1% of females between 14 and 25 years suffer from anorexia nervosa. The prevalence is greater among the higher social classes and in developed countries.

Age. The peak age of onset is the mid to late teens.

Sex. Ninety-five per cent of patients are female.

Contributing factors. The causes of anorexia nervosa are multifactorial involving physical, psychological and social factors.

Physical. Family and twin studies indicate a genetic susceptibility to anorexia nervosa. There is also an increased incidence of affective disorder in families of patients with anorexia nervosa.

Psychological. There are no definite personality types associated with the eating disorders; however, certain traits, such as low self-esteem and perfectionism, are more common and play a significant part in perpetuating the disorders. It has been suggested that, for individuals with anorexia nervosa, an inability to cope with the problems of adolescence, particularly sexuality and family conflict, is dealt with by a regression to childhood (a prepubertal state brought about by weight loss).

Social. Social and cultural pressures on women influence attitudes to weight and shape. The prevalence is higher in Western societies where thinness is perceived as attractive and desirable. This attitude is reinforced among certain occupational groups (e.g. actors, dancers). Family dysfunction has been suggested as being important in the development of eating disorders. However, when the disorder is established in a family, it is often difficult to conclude whether family problems preceded or followed the onset.

Clinical features

There are three components to the diagnosis of anorexia nervosa:

1 *Core psychopathology:* patients experience a tremendous drive to lose weight and find being at normal weight abhorrent. Weight is below a minimally normal weight for age and height. Patients' sense of identity is closely tied to their weight. Psychological symptoms secondary to starvation include depressed mood, social withdrawal, preoccupation with food, restlessness and poor sleep.

2 *Abnormal eating behaviour resulting in weight loss:* patients severely restrict their intake of food beyond normal dieting. Other weight-reducing behaviours may include self-induced vomiting, excessive exercise and abuse of laxatives, diuretics and amphetamines.

3 *Endocrine disturbance and physical features:* amenorrhoea occurs in the majority of women. The physical consequences of anorexia nervosa are shown in ANOREXIA NERVOSA AT A GLANCE.

Presentation to general medical or gynaecological outpatient departments with weight-related amenorrhoea is common. The psychological component to the weight loss is often recognized, but appropriate intervention is often neglected. It is important therefore to focus history taking at initial presentation on eating habits and beliefs, the meaning of thinness and the family's attitude to food.

Investigation

The investigations carried out depend on the situation and severity of the illness. Other causes of weight loss, both physical and psychiatric (e.g. schizophrenia, depressive disorder and obsessive–compulsive disorder), must be excluded. However, extensive investigations over a long period of time can collude with the patient's avoidance of the real psychological issues.

Haematology
FBC, ESR.

Biochemistry
● Urea and electrolytes, liver function tests, calcium and phosphate, thyroid function tests
● Reproductive hormone assay
● Trace elements including zinc, copper and magnesium

Diagnostic imaging
● ECG
● Bone densitometry
● Pelvic ultrasound: maturity of reproductive organs

Management

Medical outpatients. Staff should be alert to the possibility of anorexia nervosa in women presenting with unexplained weight loss, abdominal and gynaecological symptoms, fatigue and wanting to lose weight when underweight. Patients with an identified eating disorder should be referred to psychiatric services.

Medical inpatients. Inpatient treatment is necessary for patients at an extremely low weight (less than 70% of expected weight for height) and severe physical complications. In such cases there should be joint management between medical and psychiatric teams, with specialist dietetic advice. Refeeding and gradual weight gain are the main focus of treatment. Nasogastric feeding may be required initially to ensure an adequate intake of energy and nutrients. The content of nutrition should be informed by regular serum biochemical investigations (see p. 982). Life-threatening cardiac failure can be caused by a sudden fall in serum phosphate early in refeeding. When a patient is at a medically safe weight, he or she should be transferred to a specialist eating disorders unit. Treatment may be carried out under mental health legislation.

Specialist treatment. Treatment must address both the behavioural and psychological aspects of the disorder. The goals are weight gain to a normal healthy weight, resumption of normal eating behaviour, and dealing with individual and family conflicts.

Prognosis

Approximately 35% of patients make a complete recovery, 35% make a partial recovery and 25% run a chronic course. With effective treatment, the long-term mortality can be reduced to approximately 5% at 20-year follow-up. Without treatment, the mortality at this stage is 15–20%. Thirty per cent of patients with anorexia nervosa subsequently develop bulimia nervosa.

Bulimia nervosa
Epidemiology

Prevalence. 1–2% of adolescent girls and young women. Up to 20% of normal women binge-eat once a month.

Age. Usually 20–35 years (an older age group than for anorexia nervosa).

Sex. Predominantly female.

14

14

Anorexia nervosa at a glance

Signs and symptoms
Psychopathology—drive to lose weight, symptoms of starvation
Abnormal eating behaviours—dietary restriction, exercise, self-induced vomiting, laxatives, diuretics
Endocrine disturbance and physical complications

Causes
Physical: genetic susceptibility
Psychological: personality factors such as low self-esteem, perfectionism; maladaptive coping strategy for emotional problems (e.g. family, sexual maturity); developmental regression to prepubertal state
Social: cultural pressures; more common in certain social and occupational groups

Investigations
FBC
ESR
Urea and electrolytes
Calcium and phosphate
Thyroid function tests
Liver function tests
Reproductive hormones
Trace elements: zinc, copper, magnesium
ECG
Bone densitometry
Pelvic ultrasound

Management
Outpatient
Consider in cases of otherwise unexplained weight loss, fatigue and abdominal symptoms

Inpatient
Admission required in cases of extreme low weight and dangerous physical complications
Cautious refeeding
Repeated examination and investigations

Specialist
Regain and maintain normal weight
Resume normal eating
Psychotherapy to address underlying emotional issues

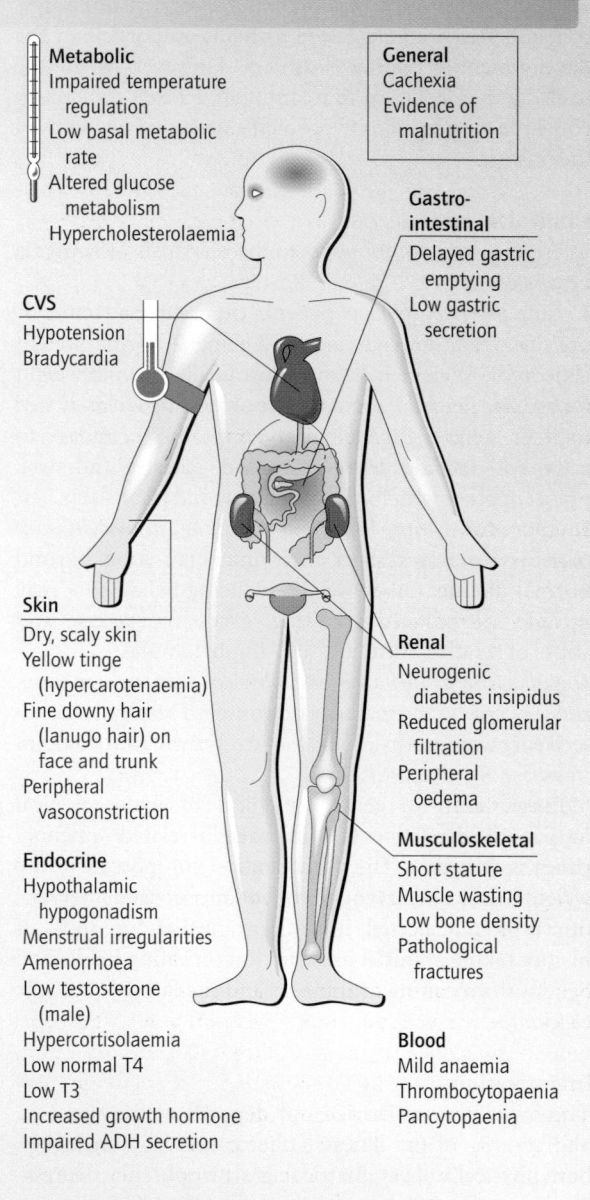

Metabolic
Impaired temperature regulation
Low basal metabolic rate
Altered glucose metabolism
Hypercholesterolaemia

General
Cachexia
Evidence of malnutrition

Gastro-intestinal
Delayed gastric emptying
Low gastric secretion

CVS
Hypotension
Bradycardia

Skin
Dry, scaly skin
Yellow tinge (hypercarotenaemia)
Fine downy hair (lanugo hair) on face and trunk
Peripheral vasoconstriction

Renal
Neurogenic diabetes insipidus
Reduced glomerular filtration
Peripheral oedema

Musculoskeletal
Short stature
Muscle wasting
Low bone density
Pathological fractures

Endocrine
Hypothalamic hypogonadism
Menstrual irregularities
Amenorrhoea
Low testosterone (male)
Hypercortisolaemia
Low normal T4
Low T3
Increased growth hormone
Impaired ADH secretion

Blood
Mild anaemia
Thrombocytopaenia
Pancytopaenia

Contributing factors. Factors are similar to anorexia nervosa. Overall, heritability of bulimia nervosa appears to be less than for anorexia nervosa. Higher rates of alcohol abuse are found among first-degree relatives of those with bulimia nervosa. Bulimic women often report a poor relationship with their parents. Depression is common and may precede the onset of the illness. Binge-eating and vomiting can be seen as a metaphor for the underlying emotional confusion and an inappropriate attempt to deal with unpleasant emotions.

Clinical features

● *Core psychopathology:* individuals judge themselves in terms of their weight and shape, rather than feeling they have any intrinsic value.

● *Abnormal eating behaviour:* the primary feature is binge-eating, where an individual consumes a larger than normal quantity of food in a discrete period of time. This is associated with a feeling of being out of control. Patients compensate for binge-eating by engaging in behaviours to prevent weight gain, such as self-induced vomiting, laxative abuse, exercise and dietary restriction.

● *Physical symptoms:* weight is often normal or only slightly under- or overweight. Bulimia nervosa is associated with menstrual irregularities and infertility. Generally, physical signs are few. Signs of repeated self-induced vomiting include enlarged salivary glands, dental erosion and calluses on the dorsum of the hands.

Investigation

Biochemistry
● Urea and electrolytes
● Calcium and phosphate

Diagnostic imaging
● ECG
● Pelvic ultrasound

Management

Medical. Bulimia nervosa should be considered in patients with unexplained abdominal and gynaecological symptoms. Repeated vomiting or laxative use is a cause of hypokalaemia.

Specialist. In contrast to anorexia nervosa, most patients can be treated as outpatients. Psychotherapy is the treatment of choice. The principles of treatment are education, behavioural methods to regain normal eating habits and addressing the underlying emotional causative factors. Selective serotonin reuptake inhibitor antidepressants have been shown to reduce the frequency of binge-eating.

Prognosis

Prognosis is good if uncomplicated by personality difficulties and drug and alcohol misuse.

Side-effects of psychotropic medication

The physical side-effects of psychotropic medication should be considered in patients presenting with unexplained physical symptoms. The main categories of psychotropic medication are neuroleptics, mood stabilizers, antidepressants, and anxiolytics and hypnotics. They and their side-effects are discussed in detail in Tables 14.5–

Table 14.5 Neuroleptics

Action
Postsynaptic dopamine receptor blockade in the basal ganglia

Indications
Neuroleptics have both antipsychotic properties and a calming and sedating effect on behaviour
Indicated for organic brain syndromes, schizophrenia, mania and depression, accompanied by psychomotor disturbance or psychotic symptoms

Contraindications
Coma or severe central nervous system depression
Past history of neuroleptic malignant syndrome
Bone marrow suppression
Closed-angle glaucoma (chlorpromazine)

Side-effects
Anticholinergic: blurred vision, dry mouth, tremor, urinary retention, constipation
Antiadrenergic: postural hypotension, cardiac arrhythmias, ejaculatory failure
Extrapyramidal: acute dystonia, akathisia, parkinsonism, tardive dyskinesia
Metabolic: weight gain, amenorrhoea, galactorrhoea

14.8, which present brief information relating to some of the commonly used drugs in psychological medicine. However, the information, especially that relating to side-effects and contraindications, is not complete. Fuller information and regimens should be checked in a formulary such as the *British National Formulary*.

Neuroleptics (Table 14.5)

Neuroleptics (also known as antipsychotics, or major tranquillizers) are mainly used in the treatment of psychotic disorders (see p. 985). Neuroleptics are derived from a number of chemically distinct groups and differ in their ability to block different neuroreceptors. This blockade is also the cause of their adverse effects. Their primary therapeutic mode of action is thought to be mediated by the postsynaptic blockade of dopamine receptors in the basal ganglia. Chlorpromazine was the first widely used neuroleptic. More recently introduced 'atypical' neuroleptics have less propensity to cause extrapyramidal side-effects.

Neuroleptic malignant syndrome

The neuroleptic malignant syndrome is usually of sudden onset and is characterized by autonomic instability, hyperpyrexia and muscle rigidity. Untreated, it has a mortality of 20%. Admission to a general medical ward is essential. Initial treatment involves discontinuation of the neuroleptic medication, prescription of a dopamine

14

Table 14.6 Mood stabilizers

Lithium

Action

Lithium affects a number of intracellular processes, in particular regulation of calcium and sensitivity of a number of neurotransmitter receptors, but its precise mechanism of action is unknown

Indications

Lithium is used in the treatment and prophylaxis of bipolar affective disorder and recurrent depressive disorder

Contraindications

Pre-existing renal impairment, sick sinus syndrome

Side-effects

Therapeutic range: nausea, metallic taste, fine tremor, nephrogenic diabetes insipidus, hypothyroidism, weight gain

Toxic range: vomiting, diarrhoea, coarse tremor, ataxia, seizures, coma, death, distal tubular degeneration

Lithium toxicity carries a high morbidity and mortality and is associated with irreversible neurological and renal damage

Monitoring of patients

Lithium serum levels must be monitored regularly every 3–4 months, once stabilized on the appropriate dose

The serum level should be 0.5–1.2 mmol/l

Thyroid function should be checked every 4–6 months

Carbamazepine

Action

Carbamazepine has multiple effects on the CNS, particularly on neuronal excitability; its role in the treatment of affective disorder is, however, obscure

Indications

Carbamazepine is used in the treatment and prophylaxis of manic depressive disorder and recurrent depressive disorder

Contraindications

Pre-existing liver disease, blood dyscrasias

Drug-specific side-effects

Therapeutic range: fine tremor, blood dyscrasias, acute renal failure

Toxic range: coarse tremor, ataxia, confusion

Monitoring of patients

Carbamazepine serum levels must be monitored regularly every 3–4 months, once stabilized on the appropriate dose

The serum level should be 20–50 mmol/l

FBC should also be monitored at similar intervals

Table 14.7 Antidepressants

Action

Tricyclics and SSRIs block presynaptic reuptake of noradrenaline and/or serotonin. MAOIs and RIMAs block catabolism of noradrenaline, serotonin, tyramine and dopamine

Indications

A widely used and highly effective treatment for depressive disorders

Contraindications

Tricyclics: recent myocardial infarction, heart block, mania, porphyria

MAOIs: hepatic impairment, cerebrovascular disease, phaeochromocytoma, porphyria

Side-effects

Anticholinergic: blurred vision, dry mouth, tremor, urinary retention, constipation

Antiadrenergic: postural hypotension, cardiac arrhythmias, ejaculatory failure

Other effects: low seizure threshold, weight gain, sedation

Drug-specific side-effects

Tricyclics: cardiac arrhythmias, overdose often fatal

MAOIs: liver toxicity, dependence, hypertensive crisis

SSRIs: nausea, sexual dysfunction

RIMAs: transient sedation, nausea, headaches

MAOI, monoamine oxidase inhibitor; RIMA, reversible inhibitor of monoamine type A; SSRI, selective serotonin reuptake inhibitor.

agonist (e.g. bromocriptine or dantrolene) and general supportive measures.

Mood stabilizers (Table 14.6)

The mood stabilizers are used for treatment and prophylaxis in bipolar affective disorder. They fall into two main groups: lithium and the anticonvulsants. Anticonvulsants (e.g. carbamazepine) have mood-stabilizing properties, and an increasing number are being used for the treatment of bipolar affective disorder.

Regular monitoring of lithium blood levels is essential to avoid toxicity. If lithium toxicity is suspected, take blood to ascertain the serum lithium level, stop lithium immediately and ensure a high fluid intake with extra sodium to stimulate an osmotic diuresis. Dialysis may be necessary if toxicity is severe. Lithium toxicity carries a high morbidity and mortality and is associated with irreversible neurological and renal damage.

Antidepressants (Table 14.7)

Antidepressants fall into a number of broad categories of chemical compound.

Tricyclic cardiotoxicity

The tricyclics (e.g. dothiepin (dosulepin), amitriptyline and imipramine) are dangerous in overdose, particularly because of their cardiotoxicity. Gastric lavage should be performed if the patient presents early. The mainstay of treatment is supportive, although cardiac monitoring is essential at first, usually in the intensive care unit.

Monoamine oxidase inhibitor-induced hypertension

Monoamine oxidase inhibitors (MAOIs) can cause hypertensive reactions if a tyramine-free diet is not strictly adhered to. Hypertensive crises should be treated by parenteral administration of an α-adrenoreceptor blocker (e.g. phentolamine 5 mg intravenously).

Selective serotonin reuptake inhibitors

The selective serotonin reuptake inhibitors (SSRIs), such as fluoxetine, paroxetine and sertraline, have overcome many of the problematic side-effects associated with both tricyclic antidepressants and MAOIs, but can give rise to troublesome gastrointestinal side-effects, particularly nausea, vomiting and sexual dysfunction. If the symptoms are severe or persistent, the drug should be stopped and alternatives considered.

Anxiolytics and hypnotics (Table 14.8)

Barbiturate and benzodiazepine dependence

Problems of chronic dependence on barbiturates and benzodiazepines are widespread and present a major challenge to medicine, especially in general practice.

If a patient taking an anxiolytic (usually a benzodiazepine) is admitted to hospital, the drug must not suddenly be discontinued as this can result in a severe withdrawal syndrome characterized by confusion, agitation and visual hallucinations.

Table 14.8 Anxiolytics and hypnotics

Action
Activation of benzodiazepine receptors potentiates the action of γ-aminobutyric acid (GABA), the major inhibitory neurotransmitter

Indications
Extensively used in most branches of hospital medicine and general practice. Benzodiazepines are highly effective for treating anxiety disorders and insomnia, particularly when used in short courses for well-defined reasons (e.g. following a bereavement)

Side-effects
Dependence with rebound anxiety, withdrawal syndrome, memory impairment

Psychiatric disorder and physical illness coexisting independently

Psychiatric disorder and physical illness are both common and so considerable independent overlap is inevitable. However, psychiatric disorder is still stigmatizing, even among the medical profession, with the result that the physical symptoms of a person with a psychiatric disorder are often ignored or trivialized. Conversely, although psychiatric disorders are common, they often go undetected in medical patients.

Physical illness, particularly if it requires hospitalization, can be particularly stressful for those with a psychiatric disorder. It is therefore essential that all past and present psychiatric disorders and treatments are adequately documented on admission and that any current psychotropic medication is continued.

In addition to those described above, the main groups of psychiatric disorders encountered in medical patients are:

- *Psychotic disorders:* particularly schizophrenia
- *Mood disorders:* depressive disorder, bipolar affective disorder
- *Anxiety-related disorders:* generalized anxiety disorder, panic disorder, phobic anxiety disorder, obsessive–compulsive disorder and reactions to stress, including adjustment disorder (see p. 970) and post-traumatic stress disorder
- *Personality disorders*

Psychotic disorders

Schizophrenia

Schizophrenia is the most common of the psychotic disorders. It is a major cause of distress, both to individual sufferers and to their families, and carries a high mortality.

Epidemiology

Prevalence. The lifetime prevalence is 0.5–1%.

Age. The mean age of onset is 28 years in men and 32 years in women.

Sex. Equal distribution.

Genetics. Adoption studies consistently demonstrate a 10–20% incidence if one parent has schizophrenia and a 49% incidence if both parents have the disorder.

Disease mechanisms

The syndrome of schizophrenia may represent the end-point of a number of different causal pathways. Evidence for physical causative factors comes from genetic studies as well as such findings as:

- An excess of winter births suggests a role for viral infections
- Excess obstetric complications
- Enlarged cerebral ventricles
- Abnormal cells in the frontal and temporal regions
- Increased rates of 'soft' neurological signs
- Neurochemical abnormalities

Those with a lower inherited predisposition to schizophrenia may require additional environmental triggers for the onset of the disorder, whereas those with a higher genetic load may develop the illness with minimal additional environmental factors.

The onset of the disorder in adolescence or adult life may be because of the requirement of cerebral maturation before schizophrenia can manifest itself. There are increased rates of premorbid behavioural and cognitive problems in children who later develop schizophrenia.

Social factors, in particular stressful life events and family life in which the atmosphere is one of hostility or overinvolvement (high expressed emotion), are important precipitants for relapse.

Clinical features

Schizophrenia is a syndrome characterized by fundamental and characteristic disturbances of thinking, perception and mood, occurring in clear consciousness. The disturbance involves the most basic functions that mark a person out as a unique individual. Schizophrenic symptoms fall into two groups:

- *Positive symptoms:* occur in acute schizophrenia and can be considered as occurring in addition to normal psychological function. They include delusions, hallucinations and thought disorder.
- *Negative symptoms:* occur in chronic schizophrenia and can be considered as diminished psychological functioning. Individuals may have a flattening and lack of reactivity in their mood, problems with attention, appear apathetic and have a reduced output and content of speech.

The pattern of illness varies between individuals, but is most commonly one of acute relapses against a background of persistent chronic symptoms.

The history should include a collateral account from a family member or reliable informant. Information should include any recent changes in behaviour or level of functioning, either socially or occupationally.

A physical examination is essential to exclude an organic cause.

Investigation

Physical investigations should be considered to rule out drug-induced or organic psychotic conditions, especially in patients presenting with their first episode of illness.

Haematology
- FBC
- ESR

Biochemistry
- Urea and electrolytes
- Liver function tests
- Thyroid function tests
- Urinary drug screen to detect drug misuse, especially use of amphetamine, which can cause a syndrome that mimics schizophrenia

Diagnostic imaging
CT scan of the head to exclude intracranial pathology.

Neurophysiology
EEG to exclude temporal lobe epilepsy.

Management

Management of schizophrenia incorporates medical, psychological and social approaches, which are usually coordinated by a community mental health team. Neuroleptic medication (oral or depot) is particularly useful for treating 'positive' symptomatology, but is of little benefit for 'negative' symptoms (Table 14.5). Noncompliance with medication is a well-recognized cause of relapse.

Psychological and social support, of both the patient and the family, are essential given the chronic course of the illness and the associated social deterioration.

Prognosis

Factors associated with a poor prognosis are:

- Early onset
- Insidious onset
- Lack of a precipitant
- Lack of an affective component
- Positive family history
- Low IQ
- Lower social class
- Abnormal premorbid personality
- Predominance of 'negative' symptoms
- Poor response to neuroleptics

Schizo-affective disorder

Schizo-affective disorder is a confusing term usually reserved to describe the illness of a small group of patients in whom the clinical picture is equally dominated by symptoms of both schizophrenia and a mood disorder (mania or depressive disorder).

Schizo-affective disorder often presents as an acute episode which responds well to neuroleptic medication.

Delusional disorder

Delusional disorder is characterized by a well-organized set of delusions in an individual whose occupational and social functioning is otherwise normal.

This disorder often presents later in life than schizophrenia. Response to neuroleptic medication is limited.

Mood (affective) disorders

The fundamental disturbance in these disorders is a change in mood to either depression (with or without anxiety) or elation. The disorders tend to be recurrent and the onset of individual episodes is often related to stressful events. Unlike schizophrenia, individuals usually return to a normal level of psychological and social function between episodes of acute illness.

Depressive disorder

The term depression can be used in a number of ways, including a synonym for sadness, as a pathological symptom or as an illness in its own right. The distinction between normal sadness and depressive disorder depends upon the severity and chronicity of symptoms, and the effect on an individual's level of psychological and social functioning. Depressive episodes may be single or recurrent. A depressive episode can be graded as mild, moderate or severe.

Epidemiology
Prevalence. Depressive disorder is common; however, the estimated prevalence depends on the diagnostic criteria used. Lifetime prevalence is approximately 15%. Depressive disorders are twice as common in medical patients than in the general population.

Age. The mean age of onset is 27 years.

Sex. Twice as common in women.

Genetics. 20% of first-degree relatives of a person with depressive disorder have a mood disorder.

Social class. No relationship between depressive disorder and social class has been identified.

Disease mechanisms
Depressive disorder covers a heterogeneous range of disorders with different causes. For some, there is an inherited vulnerability. Depressed mood is accompanied by neurochemical changes, including serotonin, nora-

Table 14.9 Physical illness and depressive disorder

Depressive disorders are particularly common in the following groups:
- Illnesses affecting the brain (e.g. stroke, head injury)
- Acute, painful or life-threatening illnesses (e.g. myocardial infarction)
- Chronic, painful, disabling and disfiguring illnesses (e.g. rheumatoid arthritis)
- Major and unpleasant treatments (e.g. surgery, chemotherapy)
- Elderly people

Physical disease
Certain illnesses have been specifically linked to depression, with the assumption that there is a physical effect related to the disease or treatment. These include:
- Tumours (primary and secondary)
- Infections and postinfection states
- Hypothyroidism
- Hyperparathyroidism
- Cushing's syndrome
- Vitamin deficiencies (especially B_1, B_6, B_{12})
- Neurological disorders (especially multiple sclerosis and Parkinson's disease)
- Autoimmune rheumatic diseases

Drug-related
Drug-induced depressive disorder is common and may relate to direct or indirect CNS toxicity. Iatrogenic causes include:
- Endocrine agents (e.g. corticosteroids, oral contraceptive pill)
- Antihypertensives (e.g. propranolol, nifedipine)
- Antiarrhythmics (e.g. lidocaine, procainamide)
- Antibiotics (e.g. penicillins, tetracycline)
- Antiparkinsonian drugs (e.g. levodopa, amantadine)
- Anticonvulsants (e.g. carbamazepine, vigabatrin)
- Antineoplastic drugs (e.g. interferon, vincristine)
- Antihistamines (e.g. cimetidine)

drenaline and, possibly, dopamine. Predisposing factors include separations from caregivers in childhood and parental violence. In at least 70% of cases there is an identifiable stressful trigger to an episode of depressive disorder. Perpetuating factors that prevent recovery include chronic stresses, such as physical illness, social isolation, unemployment and housing problems.

The relationships between depressive disorder and physical illness are described in Table 14.9.

Clinical features
Symptoms of a depressive episode include:
- Depressed mood
- Loss of interest and enjoyment
- Reduced energy and fatigue

- Poor concentration and attention
- Reduced self-esteem and self-confidence
- Ideas of guilt
- A pessimistic view of the future
- Disturbed sleep
- Reduced appetite and weight loss

In cases of physical illness, some of the symptoms that might otherwise be indicative of depressive disorder might be directly caused by the physical illness or treatment (e.g. weight loss or difficulty sleeping). In such cases, more emphasis is placed on the cognitive symptoms of depressive disorder in making a diagnosis. An enquiry about mood should always include an assessment of suicidal ideation.

The degree of interference with normal social and occupational activities is a guide to the severity of an episode of depressive disorder. A severe depressive episode may be accompanied by psychotic symptoms (delusions and hallucinations) that are congruent with low mood. Delusions often involve ideas of sin, poverty or disaster, for which the patient may assume responsibility. Auditory hallucinations are usually of defamatory or accusatory voices.

Investigation

For many cases of depressive disorder, physical investigations are not required unless physical disease is suspected. It is important to exclude thyroid dysfunction as a cause in women.

Haematology
- FBC
- Differential cell count
- ESR

Biochemistry
- Urea and electrolytes, including calcium
- Thyroid function tests
- Liver function tests

Diagnostic imaging
CT scan to exclude intracerebral pathology.

Neurophysiology
EEG to exclude temporal lobe epilepsy.

Management

Mild to moderate episodes of depression may respond to either antidepressant medication (Table 14.7), or psychotherapeutic approaches (Table 14.10), or a combination of the two. Severe depression requires antidepressant medication, and neuroleptic medication if psychotic symptoms are present.

When a patient is prescribed an antidepressant, he or

Table 14.10 Psychotherapy

Definition

The treatment of emotional, behavioural or personality problems by psychological means

Characteristics of psychotherapies

A confiding relationship with a helping person

A rationale that includes an explanation of the patient's distress and the methods of relieving it

New information about the nature of the problem

Hope that therapy will provide help

An increased sense of mastery

Facilitation of emotional arousal

Classification

Different forms of psychotherapy can be classified according to their rationale. Commonly used psychotherapies with medical patients are described below

Counselling

Supportive and non-judgemental listening, to help the patient find solutions to personal difficulties

Less stressful than other kinds of psychotherapy

Used to help patients to adjust to a life crisis, such as bereavement, or to cope with physical illness

Behavioural psychotherapy

Based on learning theory

Focus is on changing behaviour, rather than feelings or thoughts

Often used in obsessive–compulsive disorder, phobias and some sexual disorders

Cognitive psychotherapy

Concerned with the way in which behaviours or feelings are dependent on thoughts. For example, a negative interpretation of events may contribute to depressive disorder

Used in the treatment of anxiety, depressive disorders and medically unexplained symptoms

Psychodynamic psychotherapy

Concerned with the way in which a person's mental representation of himself or herself and the world may lead to problems in current personal relationships

Used in depressive disorder, eating disorders and personality disorders

Systemic therapy (family therapy)

Considers problems in the social context in which they arise

May be used where an individual's illness impacts significantly on the family

she should be told that it is usually 2–3 weeks before the antidepressant effect becomes apparent. A course of antidepressants should be continued for at least 6 months to 1 year after recovery to minimize the risk of relapse on

Table 14.11 Electroconvulsive therapy (ECT)

Action
Induces changes in neurotransmitter enzymes similar to antidepressant/mood stabilizer medication

Indications
Serious depressive illness (actively suicidal, psychomotor agitatory retardation/stupor, psychotic features, not responsive to drug treatment)
Mania not responding to drug treatment
Schizophrenia (acute episode not responding to drugs)

Side-effects
Short-term memory disturbance

Contraindications
Intracranial space-occupying lesion
Recent cerebrovascular accident
Anaesthetic contraindications (e.g. recent myocardial infarction)

Course
Often 4–8 treatments, given 2–3 times/week

discontinuation. For patients with recurrent depressive disorder, a severe depressive episode or ongoing stresses, it may be appropriate to continue the antidepressant for longer.

For severe episodes of depressive disorder, particularly where the patient is unresponsive to antidepressants or where a faster response is required, a course of electroconvulsive therapy (ECT) may be appropriate (Table 14.11).

Prognosis
Individual episodes of depressive disorder typically last between 3 and 12 months. Recovery is usually complete between episodes. Fifty per cent of depression is recurrent.

Bipolar affective disorder

Bipolar affective disorder (manic–depressive disorder) is characterized by repeated episodes of mood disorder, with at least one episode of elation (mania).

Epidemiology
Prevalence. The lifetime prevalence is 1.2%.

Age. The mean age of onset is 21 years.

Sex. Sex ratio of 1 : 1.

Genetics. 20–25% of first-degree relatives of a person with bipolar disorder have a mood disorder.

Social class. No relationship between bipolar affective depressive disorder and social class has been identified.

Contributing factors. Bipolar affective disorder has a relatively high genetic contribution, with a heritability of 0.8. Episodes of illness are often precipitated by stressful life events.

Clinical features
In this disorder, patients have repeated episodes of mood disturbance, although individual patients have different patterns of illness. Characteristically, recovery is complete between episodes. Symptoms of a depressive episode are described above (see p. 987). Symptoms of a manic episode include:
- Persistent elevation of mood, out of keeping with circumstances
- Mood may vary from joviality to uncontrolled excitement
- Occasional irritability and suspiciousness
- Increased energy and overactivity
- Speech is fast and difficult to interrupt (pressure of speech)
- Decreased need for sleep
- Loss of normal social inhibitions
- Poor attention and concentration, with marked distractability
- Inflated self-esteem
- Grandiose or overoptimistic ideas

Investigation
Investigations should be carried out where indicated to exclude a potential physical cause for the first presentation of the disorder, particularly thyroid disease in female patients (see p. 987). Additional investigations are required for the monitoring of lithium therapy (Table 14.6).

Management
The main physical treatment for bipolar affective disorder is a mood stabilizing drug (Table 14.6). Neuroleptic drugs may also be used, either in the treatment of an acute relapse of the illness where there are psychotic symptoms, or as a prophylactic medication in patients who are intolerant of mood-stabilizing drugs. Antidepressant drugs should be used with caution as there is a risk that they might precipitate a manic episode. ECT may be used in the treatment of manic or depressive episodes, particularly when the patient is suicidal, psychotic, stuporose or not responding to medication (Table 14.11).

Prognosis
There is wide variation in the long-term outcome of the disorder, with a trend towards shorter remissions and longer depressive episodes after middle age. Patients with four or more episodes per year ('rapid cycling') have a particularly poor prognosis. Bipolar affective disorder carries a 15% risk of suicide.

Anxiety-related disorders

Anxiety-related disorders are common. All of the disorders described below have anxiety as either the primary symptom (generalized anxiety disorder and panic disorder), or a major component of the illness (phobic anxiety disorder, obsessive–compulsive disorder, post-traumatic stress disorder). In addition, anxiety symptoms commonly occur in many other psychiatric conditions, particularly depressive disorder.

Anxiety can be a normal healthy response to a situation where there is a perception of threat, the 'fight or flight' response. It also acts as an important motivational drive that improves performance. However, anxiety becomes pathological when the optimal level of anxiety is exceeded, when it becomes pervasive or when it occurs in inappropriate situations.

Epidemiology

Prevalence. Generalized anxiety disorder and panic disorder have a lifetime prevalence of 5% and 3%, respectively. Anxiety-related disorders are twice as common in medical patients than in the general population.

Age. The mean age of onset is early adulthood.

Sex. Two-thirds of patients with generalized anxiety disorder, panic disorder or phobic anxiety disorder are female; there is an equal sex distribution for obsessive–compulsive disorder and post-traumatic stress disorder.

Genetics. Genetic factors are thought to be important in the anxiety-related disorders, with panic disorder and obsessive–compulsive disorder having a higher heritability than the other disorders.

Disease mechanisms

Individuals may have a constitutional predisposition to excess anxious arousal. This may be because of inherited factors, or the effect of environmental factors on the developing brain. Physical factors implicated in the cause of anxiety-related disorders include abnormal regulation of the central adrenergic system in panic disorder, and structural and functional brain abnormalities in obsessive–compulsive disorder. Vulnerability may be acquired in later life as the result of traumatic experiences of overwhelming anxiety and helplessness.

Whether a certain event will precipitate an anxious response depends on an individual's interpretation of the situation. This, in turn, will depend on their past experiences and their perceived ability to cope. Although the immediate cause of the anxiety is psychological, the response is biologically mediated.

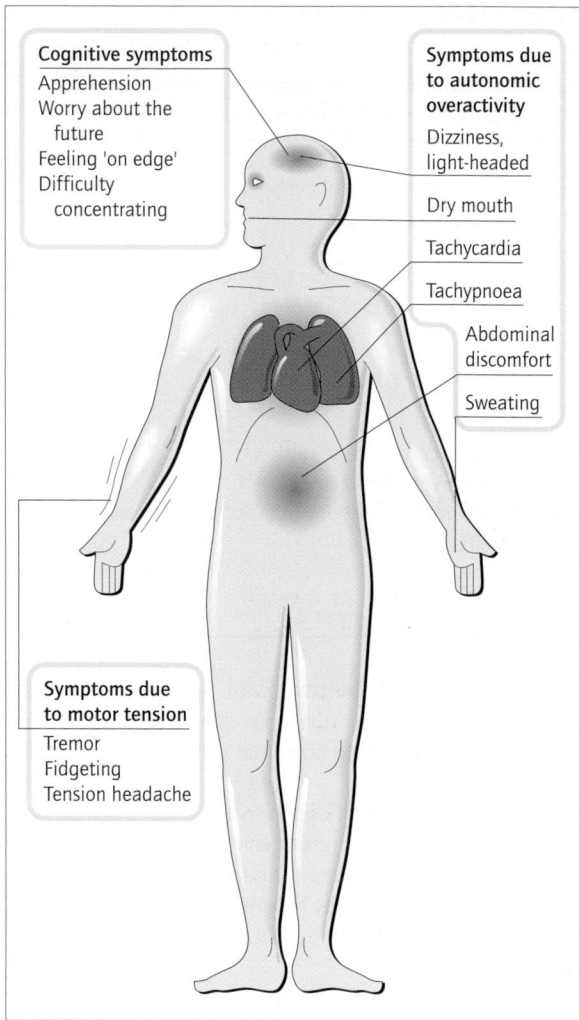

Figure 14.5 Symptoms of anxiety.

Anxiety is associated with a number of physical disorders, including hypoglycaemia, hyperthyroidism, phaeochromocytoma, carcinoid tumours, cardiac disease and caffeinism. It also occurs as part of withdrawal from drugs that suppress the CNS, including alcohol and benzodiazepines.

Clinical features (Fig. 14.5)

Patients may present to medical clinics with the symptoms of anxiety (e.g. complaints of palpitations in cardiology, or abdominal symptoms in gastroenterology).

Generalized anxiety disorder

Patients describe primary symptoms of anxiety for most days for several weeks at a time.

Panic disorder

Anxiety occurs in discrete episodes, or 'panic attacks'. These are unpredictable and not restricted to any particular situation (unlike phobic anxiety disorder). Panic attacks are often accompanied by a fear of dying or losing control.

Phobic anxiety disorder

Anxiety is provoked in certain well-defined situations that are not objectively dangerous. The fear experienced is recognized as irrational by the individual, but it cannot be reasoned away and leads to an avoidance of situations where the feared object or event may be encountered.

● *Simple phobias:* circumscribed fears of specific objects, situations or activities. Common fears include particular animals such as spiders or dogs. In general medical patients, phobias that may be encountered include a fear of blood or injury (including needlesticks), dentistry and of exposure to specific diseases such as AIDS.

● *Social phobia:* a fear of humiliation or embarrassment in front of others, which results in avoidance of social situations.

● *Agoraphobia:* a fear of situations from which there is no easy escape (usually to home). Extreme avoidance leads to some patients becoming housebound.

Obsessive–compulsive disorder

Characterized by obsessions and/or compulsions or rituals (a repetitive and purposeless behaviour performed in response to an obsession) that are not secondary to another disorder and are of sufficient severity to interfere with normal social and occupational functioning. They cause marked distress to the individual, who sees them as absurd, although recognizes them as products of his or her own mind. Attempts to suppress them result in increasing anxiety, which can only be relieved by performance of the compulsive act. The most commonly encountered obsessions and compulsions concern dirt and contamination, pathological counting and compulsive checking and hoarding.

Post-traumatic stress disorder

This arises as a response to an exceptionally catastrophic or threatening event. The traumatic event is re-experienced in recurrent and intrusive distressing recollections, dreams and flashbacks. This often occurs against a background of emotional blunting and a sense of numbness. Commonly there is fear and avoidance of situations that would remind the individual of the event. There is usually a state of autonomic hyperarousal and hypervigilance. Post-traumatic stress disorder may follow medical illness (such as a myocardial infarction) and interventions perceived as traumatic.

Investigation

Investigations may be required when an underlying physical disorder is suspected as a cause for anxiety-related symptoms.

Haematology

● FBC
● ESR

Biochemistry

● *Urea and electrolytes*
● *Thyroid function tests:* to exclude hyperthyroidism
● *Vanillylmandelic acid:* to exclude phaeochromocytoma
● *Blood sugar:* to exclude hypoglycaemic episodes

Management

Behavioural and cognitive psychotherapies are the mainstay of treatment for anxiety disorders (Table 14.10). Reassurance together with relaxation training is an important basis for most treatment strategies.

Benzodiazepines (p. 985) are a useful adjunct to psychological treatment but, because of the rapid development of dependence, these should be used only for short periods. β-Blockers often help those with prominent somatic symptoms in the early stages of treatment. Antidepressants (p. 984) also have an anxiolytic action and are prescribed for the treatment of anxiety-related disorders.

Prognosis

Overall response to treatment is good but very variable, depending on the severity of the illness and the presence of complicating factors (e.g. personality, alcohol and substance misuse).

Personality disorders

Personality disorders and factors that influence their development are described above (see p. 965). Personality disorder occurs when the habitual behaviour of individuals causes long-standing difficulties for themselves or those around them. Individuals with personality disorders often have difficulties in personal relationships, either at home or at work or both. Personality disorder can be seen as the extreme end of a spectrum of personality. Hence, the definition of a 'disorder' is arbitrary and based upon the cultural norms of society. Classification systems describe a number of personality disorders, two of which are more likely to be encountered in medical practice: dependent personality disorder and emotionally unstable personality disorder.

Epidemiology

Prevalence. In general, personality disorders are more

common in medical patients than in the general population. Estimates of general population rates depend on the definitions used, with up to 1% having a severe personality disorder, and 10% having a mild disorder or problematic personality traits. This rate increases to 20% of general practice attenders, with a similar rate likely in medical patients.

Age. An individual's personality develops in adolescence and persists into adult life.

Sex. Emotionally unstable personality disorder is more common in women.

Contributing factors. A common problem in personality disorder is the appropriate control of emotional responses, which may be related to adverse childhood experiences.

Clinical features

Dependent personality disorder

This is characterized by an undue dependence on others, feelings of helplessness when left alone and preoccupation with a fear of being abandoned. In medical practice, such patients may paradoxically appear to be very demanding, because of their inability to make decisions and their need to keep in contact with the people they depend upon, such as health professionals. Demands for help and reassurance may interfere with appropriate medical treatment.

Emotionally unstable personality disorder

This is characterized by a difficulty in controlling emotions, which may become overwhelming. Individuals may have outbursts of anger, or use self-destructive behaviours to reduce tension.

Management

The treatment of choice for most people with a personality disorder is long-term psychotherapy (Table 14.10). Drug treatments, such as low-dose neuroleptic medication or a mood stabilizer, may be useful if the clinical picture is characterized by impulsive behaviour and aggressive outbursts.

Patients with personality disorder often arouse strong feelings in medical staff, including anger, helplessness and confusion. It is important to recognize these feelings and not to let them interfere with appropriate medical care. Successful management depends on firm and consistent handling by medical and nursing staff. Presenting patients with the options and helping them to accept responsibility for treatment decisions is often a successful method of reducing patient–staff and staff–staff conflicts.

Prognosis

Personality disorder tends to persist through adult life. Benefiting from treatment depends on the patient's ability to sustain a therapeutic relationship and continue with long-term treatment.

! Must know checklist

With reference to medical patients, at the end of a psychiatry rotation a student must be able to:

■ Carry out a psychiatric assessment in a patient with physical illness, including history, mental state examination and appropriate physical examination

■ Suggest and justify a differential diagnosis, supported by a discussion of possible causative factors

■ Suggest a management plan, including physical, psychological and social investigations and treatments

■ Describe the presentation and possible causes of delirium

■ Describe the range of psychological reactions to physical illness

■ Discuss the presentation and management of medically unexplained symptoms

■ Describe the assessment and management of a patient following deliberate self-harm

■ Describe the presentation and management of alcohol and substance misuse in medical patients

■ Describe the physical complications of eating disorders

■ Briefly describe the common psychiatric disorders that may coexist with physical illness

Further reading

Books

Guthrie E, Creed F, eds. *Seminars in Liaison Psychiatry*. London: Gaskell, 1996. [Another helpful textbook on general hospital psychiatry, which discusses clinical issues as well as research and service provision.]

Johnstone EC, Freeman CPL, Zeally AK, eds. *Companion to Psychiatric Studies*. Edinburgh: Churchill Livingstone, 1998. [A good reference book for general psychiatry. However, it contains much more than is required for undergraduate psychiatry.]

Lloyd GG. *Textbook of General Hospital Psychiatry*. Edinburgh: Churchill Livingstone, 1991. [A readable text for those who want to know more about psychiatry in general hospital patients.]

Mayou R, Bass C, Sharpe M. eds. *Treatment of Functional Somatic Symptoms*. Oxford: Oxford University Press, 1995. [An excellent reference book for finding out more about medically unexplained symptoms.]

Peveler R, Feldman E, Friedman T. *Liaison Psychiatry: Planning Services for Specialist Settings*. London: Gaskell, 2000. [Of interest to those who want to find out more about the psychiatric problems in particular hospital settings, e.g. the accident and emergency department.]

Journals

British Journal of Psychiatry, HighWire Press. http://bjp.rcpsych.org/

General Hospital Psychiatry, Elsevier. http://www.sciencedirect.com/science/journal/01638343

Journal of Psychosomatic Research, Elsevier. http://www.sciencedirect.com/science/journal/00223999

Websites

Royal College of Psychiatrists: www.rcpsych.ac.uk [Professional body for psychiatrists from the UK and Ireland, and around the world. Includes patient information leaflets on common psychiatric disorders.]

American Psychiatric Association: www.psych.org [Professional body for psychiatrists from the US and around the world.]

Centre for Evidence-Based Mental Health: www.cebmh.com [Organization that promotes the teaching and practise of evidence-based mental health care. Site includes useful tools and resources.]

Mentality: www.mentality.org.uk [Organization that promotes mental health, linked to the Sainsbury Centre for Mental Health.]

Mental Health Foundation: www.mentalhealth.org.uk [UK charity that aims to improve the support available for people with mental health problems.]

Depression Alliance: www.depressionalliance.org [UK charity offering help to people with depression, run by sufferers themselves.]

Eating Disorders Association: www.edauk.com [UK charity with information on eating disorders and their treatment.]

14

Haematological Disease

15

Introduction

Haematology, the science of blood and its diseases, is concerned with:

- The number and function of the **blood cells**: red cells (erythrocytes), white cells (leucocytes) and platelets
- Molecules crucial to the function of blood, whether intracellular (e.g. **haemoglobin**) or extracellular in plasma (e.g. **coagulation factors, red cell antibodies**)
- The process of **haematopoiesis**, which regulates production and replacement of blood cells throughout life, via **haematopoietic stem cells** and their progeny, the erythrocyte, leucocyte and platelet **lineages**
- The process of **haemostasis**, which prevents fatal loss of blood from severed blood vessels
- The **transfusion** (transplantation) of blood cells and their precursors from one individual (the donor) to another (the recipient)
- All the **diseases** that affect the above functions
- All types of **therapy** directed at these diseases

Structure and function of the blood

Haematopoiesis (blood formation)

Origin and sites of haematopoiesis

In human embryos, blood cells first appear in the extra-embryonic yolk sac and embryonic aorta–gonad–mesonephros (AGM) area 15 days postconception. This **primitive or embryonic** phase of haematopoiesis, composed of nucleated red cells filled with embryonic haemoglobins, never reappears in later life. **Definitive haematopoiesis** occupies fetal liver and spleen between 2 and 7 months, and finally the bone marrow between 5 and 9 months postconception. In normal adult life, active haematopoiesis retreats to the skull, vertebrae, ribs, sternum and pelvis (the axial skeleton). During extra-uterine life, haematopoiesis reoccupies all potential marrow spaces if there is increased demand for replacement blood cells (e.g. in haemolytic anaemia). If this demand is great enough —or the haematopoietic stem cells are abnormal— **extramedullary haematopoiesis** recolonizes liver and spleen.

Huge numbers of blood cells (250×10^9 red cells plus 63×10^9 white cells in an adult male) must be replaced every day. These numbers escalate during infection, bleeding or other stresses. Even when demand is extreme, tight control of cell production must be maintained. The productive capacity and control of haematopoiesis depend on a hierarchy of **haematopoietic stem cells (HSCs)** divisible into three 'compartments': at the top sit 'pluripotent' HSCs (Fig. 15.1). Pluripotent HSCs generate all blood cell lineages and can **self-renew** (replicate as new pluripotent self-renewing cells). A small number of pluripotent HSCs (perhaps even a single cell) can fully repopulate a bone marrow damaged by disease or therapy. This regeneration may occur spontaneously, by expansion of dormant HSCs, or therapeutically, after infusion of a person's own HSCs (HSC autograft) or those of a compatible donor (HSC allograft, or bone marrow transplant). After infusion into a vein, HSCs 'home' to environments rich in bone marrow stromal cells

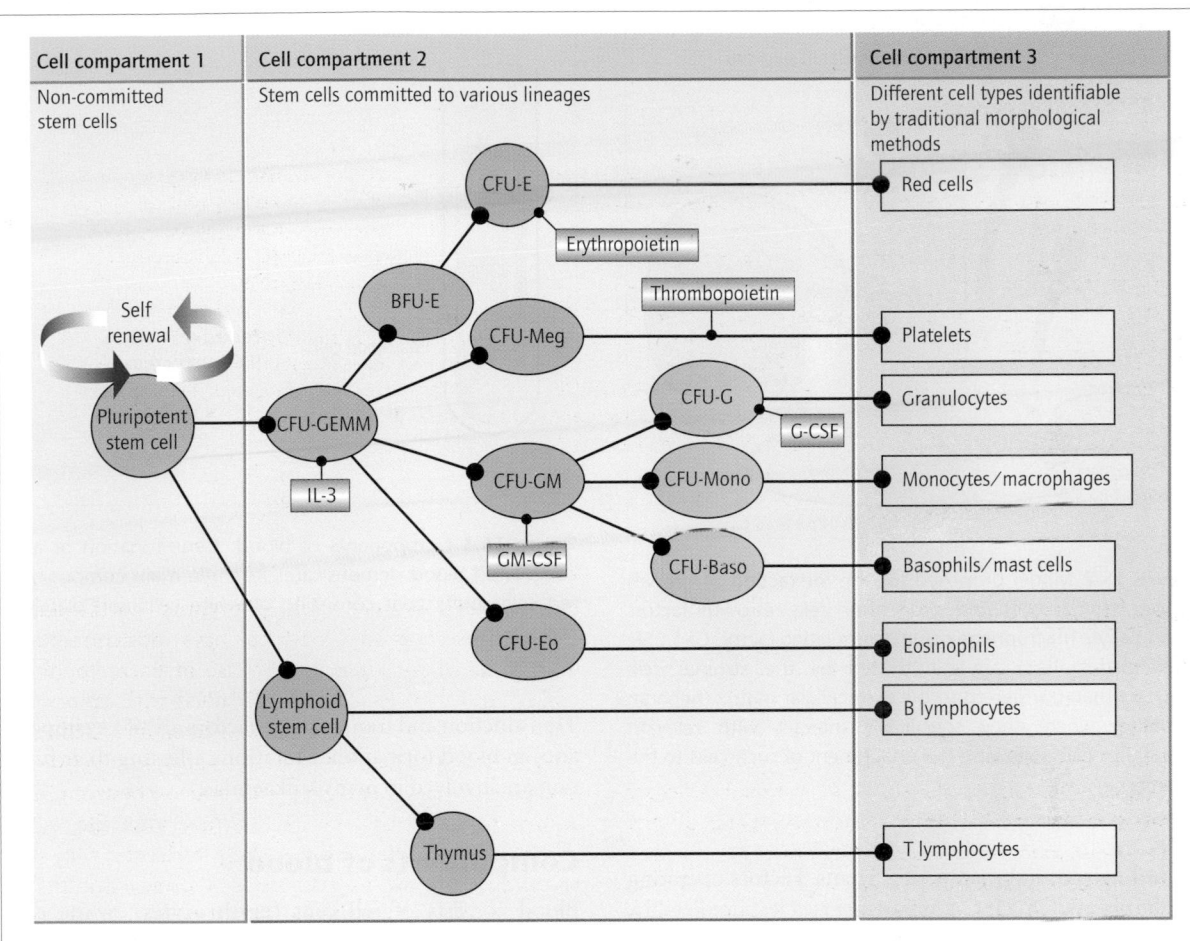

Cell compartment 1	Cell compartment 2	Cell compartment 3
Non-committed stem cells	Stem cells committed to various lineages	Different cell types identifiable by traditional morphological methods

Figure 15.1 Bone marrow pluripotent stem cell development. Diagram to show how non-committed stem cells develop into stem cells committed to the various lineages and lead to the formation of different cell types identifiable by traditional morphological methods. Baso, basophil; BFU-E, burst forming unit-erythroid; CFU, colony forming unit; CFU-E, colony forming unit-erythroid; Eos, eosinophil; G, granulocyte; GEMM, granulocyte, erythroid, monocyte, megakaryocyte; Meg, megakaryocyte; Mono, monocyte.

(Fig. 15.2) where they regenerate haematopoiesis. Recent research appears to show that multipotent HSCs retain **plasticity**—an ability to differentiate, not only into blood cells but other tissue cells such as hepatocytes or neurones under different growth conditions. Because HSCs can be harvested from bone marrow or peripheral blood, this suggests interesting future therapies.

Haematopoietic growth factors

Haematopoiesis depends upon: (a) sufficient normal HSCs; (b) their close association with normal bone marrow stromal cells; and (c) survival, proliferation and differentiation signals given by **haematopoietic growth factors** binding to specific surface receptors on pluripotent and lineage-committed HSCs (Fig. 15.2). They include:

- *Interleukin-3 (IL-3) and stem cell factor (SCF, also called kit-ligand):* promote proliferation of the pluripotential HSC compartment
- *Granulocyte colony-stimulating factor (G-CSF):* promotes granulocyte production and also translocates HSCs from the bone marrow to the peripheral blood, enabling their collection (harvesting) for cryopreservation and subsequent allo- or autografting
- *Erythropoietin (Epo):* drives proliferation and maturation of red cell precursors
- *Thrombopoietin (Tpo):* drives megakaryocyte and platelet production

The actions of haematopoietic growth factors on later, committed HSCs are predictable: Epo deficiency causes lack of red cells (anaemia) and increased Epo causes red cell excess (polycythaemia). Epo and G-CSF are,

15

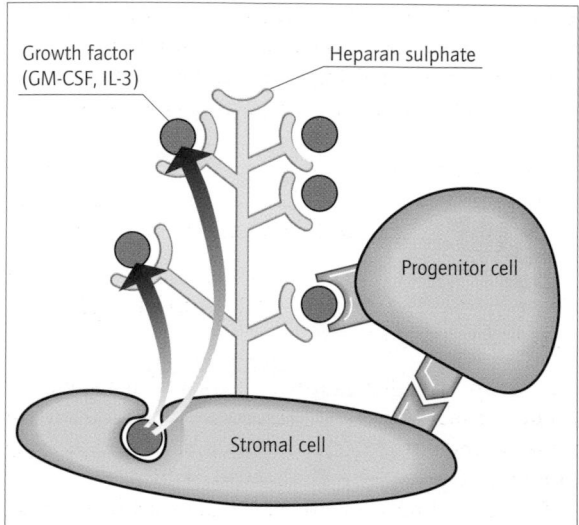

Figure 15.2 Model proposed for the interaction of growth factor, stromal cells and progenitor cells. Growth factors (granulocyte macrophage colony-stimulating factor, GM-CSF; interleukin-3, IL-3) are synthesized by the stromal cell. They are then transferred to the extracellular matrix (heparan sulphate) where they specifically interact with relevant progenitor cells following the attachment of such cells to the stromal cell.

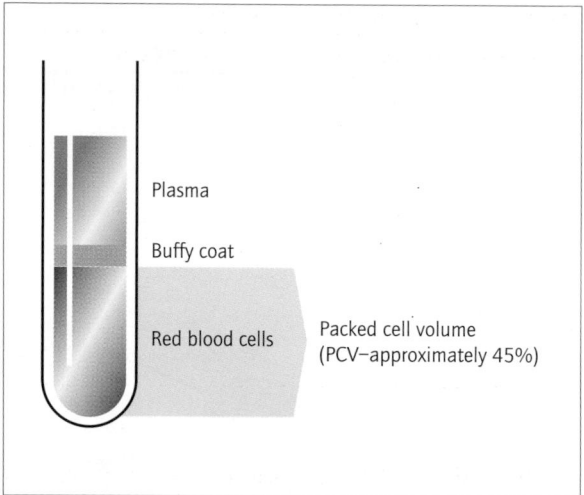

Figure 15.3 Components of blood. Centrifugation of anti-coagulated blood demonstrates its three main components: red cells, buffy coat consisting of white cells and platelets, and plasma.

accordingly, useful therapeutic agents. Factors operating on the pluripotent HSC compartment act less predictably, in concert with many other signals: hence IL-3 and SCF have not yet proved useful as therapy.

Haematopoietic transcription factors

The binding of growth factors to specific receptors leads to coordinated expression of combinations of genes—genetic blueprints—that result in mature functioning red cells, white cells or platelets. First, the specific membrane signal ('make cells of type X') is **transduced** by a cascade of chemical messengers that carries it to the cell nucleus, where it causes activation of specific **transcription factors** that bind to DNA promoters and activate all the genes needed to produce cells of that type. Some transcription factors vital to haematopoiesis are:
- *SCL/Tal-1:* when this gene is lost ('knocked out') in a mutant mouse, haematopoiesis never even starts in the embryo
- *GATA-2:* loss causes failure of definitive haemato-poiesis in the embryo
- *GATA-1:* loss causes total arrest of red cell and platelet production in the embryo
- *EKLF:* loss causes a severe thalassaemia-like failure of erythropoiesis

Transduction and transcription factors are of key importance in blood formation. Mutations affecting their function are involved in many leukaemias.

Components of blood

Blood consists of **red cells** (**erythrocytes**), **white cells** (**leucocytes**) and **platelets** (**thrombocytes**) suspended in blood **plasma**.

If blood clotting is prevented by adding a calcium chelator (ethylenediaminetetra-acetic acid [EDTA] or citrate), the cells can be sedimented by centrifugation. Plasma normally constitutes 55% of the blood volume, cells accounting for 45% (Fig. 15.3).

When blood clots in a tube, a fibrin mesh traps the cells and retracts. The resulting supernatant is called **serum** and differs from plasma, having lost its content of fibrinogen. This eases the study of other plasma proteins, particularly antibodies—hence the study of antibody reactions in human blood is called **serology**.

Red cells (erythrocytes)

The **function of red blood cells** (RBCs) is to transport oxygen from the lungs to the tissues.

Red cell proliferation and maturation

Cells of the pluripotent HSCs and early erythroid progenitor compartments (BFU-E, CFU-E) cannot be recognized by microscopy. Which combination of signals

Table 15.1 Normal haematological values

Haematological parameter		Value
Haemoglobin	Men	13–17 g/dl
	Women	12–16 g/dl
Red blood cell count (RBC)	Men	$4.5–6.0 \times 10^{12}$/l
	Women	$3.8–5.2 \times 10^{12}$/l
Mean cell volume (MCV)		78–95 fl
Packed cell volume (PCV)	Men	40–52%
	Women	37–47%
Reticulocyte count		0.2–2.0%
White blood cell count (WBC)		$4–11 \times 10^9$/l
Platelets		$150–400 \times 10^9$/l

and transcription factors causes a pluripotent HSC to 'commit' to erythrocyte differentiation (**erythropoiesis**) is not yet known, although a shift from [SCL/Tal-1 + GATA-2] effects to [GATA-1 + EKLF] effects, accompanied by increasing sensitivity to Epo (see below), plays an important part.

The earliest recognizable erythroid cells in bone marrow aspirates are large **proerythroblasts**, which have intensely basophilic (blue-staining) cytoplasm, and are therefore close to terminal differentiation into mature erythrocytes. Their trademark basophilia is caused by very high cytoplasmic globin messenger RNA (mRNA) concentration: they are haemoglobin factories.

Proerythroblasts divide into smaller normoblasts as **haemoglobin** accumulates. The cytoplasm stains pink (eosinophilic) as haemoglobin replaces mRNA, and the nucleus becomes pyknotic (densely stained) before being extruded. The erythrocyte then passes the **marrow–blood barrier** and enters the circulation as a **reticulocyte**—which for about 24 h retains some stainable RNA and is hence countable. Therefore the **reticulocyte count** (normally approximately 1% of the red cell total, or approximately 50×10^9/l) represents marrow production of new red cells per 24 h and is a useful measure of erythropoiesis (for the normal range see Table 15.1).

Erythropoietin

Tissue oxygen concentration governs the rate of erythropoiesis via Epo, which drives proliferation of the erythroid precursor cell compartment (Fig. 15.1).

Epo is mainly secreted in the **kidney** by tubular and interstitial cells that sense tissue **hypoxia** (low oxygen tension). In chronic renal failure, severe anaemia, resulting from suppressed erythropoiesis, occurs because of failure of this mechanism.

Tissue hypoxia is commonly caused by:
- Decreased circulating haemoglobin (**anaemia**), the carrier of oxygen to the tissues

- Reduced haemoglobin **oxygenation** because of poor cardiopulmonary function or life at high altitude

In each case, renal hypoxia increases erythropoietin production to **increase** erythropoiesis. This occurs whatever the starting haemoglobin concentration, so people with cardiopulmonary disease or who live at high altitude may develop abnormally high haemoglobin concentrations of more than **18 g/dl** (**polycythaemia**).

Circulating red blood cell (erythrocyte, red blood cell)

The mature red cell is a biconcave disc with a diameter of 7.5 μm. It picks up oxygen in the alveolar capillaries of the lungs and transports it to the tissues, where it picks up carbon dioxide for transport back to the lungs.

The red cell must be extremely **deformable** to transit small capillaries of less than 7 μm in diameter, where its membrane 'moulds' to the capillary wall, minimizing the distance that O_2 (alveolar) has to travel to meet haemoglobin. To survive circulation, the RBC must pass even narrower channels in the spleen, an endurance test that weeds out ageing or abnormal red cells.

RBC deformability depends not only on a normal RBC membrane and cytoskeleton, but also on the availability of sufficient cellular energy reserves to maintain the intracellular ionic environment (cation pump). Because it does not contain a nucleus, the red cell relies entirely on preformed proteins and the adenosine triphosphate (ATP) produced by glycolysis for its metabolic needs. The splenic endurance test stresses red cell metabolism to the limit. Eventually, after about **100 days** in the circulation, the red cell's metabolic pool runs out, it can no longer pass the splenic test, is culled and its contents recycled by splenic macrophages.

The inheritance of malfunctioning membrane components, or enzymes critical to ATP production, can therefore reduce red cell survival (typically to approximately 10 days). Premature destruction of red cells is called **haemolysis**.

Erythrocyte membrane and cytoskeleton

The red cell membrane is a typical lipid bilayer composed of phospholipids, molecules resembling tuning forks with hydrophobic 'prongs' pointing inwards and hydrophilic 'handles' pointing outwards (Fig. 15.4). Cholesterol is inserted between the phospholipids.

A protein cytoskeleton forms a network of fibrils on the inner surface of the red cell membrane. This network consists of tetramers of the contractile protein **spectrin**, linked by **actin** fibrils. Together these proteins confer the red cell's unique shape, flexibility and deformability. Spectrin is anchored to the membrane bilayer by attachment to a transmembrane protein, **band 3 protein** (an ion channel), via the protein **ankyrin**.

15

15

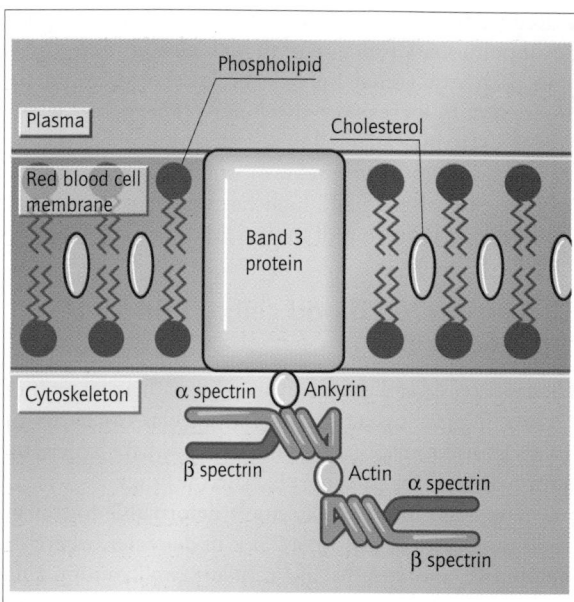

Figure 15.4 Human red cell membrane. A simplified diagram showing the relationship between the red cell membrane and the cytoskeleton of the red cell. Abnormal cytoskeletal proteins (e.g. in hereditary elliptocytosis and hereditary spherocytosis) and various plasma factors (e.g. in uraemia and liver disease) affect red cell shape.

Red cell antigens

The red cell membrane carries many molecules capable of inducing immune responses and therefore known as **blood group antigens**. These antigens are expressed on carbohydrates or proteins. Most, including the most important, have no known function apart from immune recognition. These antigens are grouped into **23 blood group systems**, each of which is inherited independently as maternal and paternal alleles, or 'haplotypes' of linked alleles.

Blood groups are important because an individual who lacks a RBC antigen (antigen-negative) can produce antibodies to it, if transfused with antigen-positive red cells. RBC antibodies can lead to a **haemolytic transfusion reaction**: if **antigen-positive RBCs** are transfused again, the **blood group-specific antibodies** present in the plasma of the immunized recipient bind and destroy them (via complement activation or phagocytosis). The consequent rapid destruction of large numbers of red cells in the circulation can cause severe systemic symptoms including hypotensive shock, acute renal failure and disseminated intravascular coagulation (DIC) (EMERGENCY BOX 15.1). This can be fatal.

Another way that RBC immunization occurs is across the placental interface between mother and fetus. If the

---

Emergency 15.1: Incompatible blood transfusion (wrong blood)

To prevent it:
- Identify the patient (blood recipient) correctly—name, date of birth, hospital or accident and emergency department number
- Fill out the request form fully and accurately
- Label the sample tube fully and accurately **in writing** with the recipient's details **after** adding their blood to the tube
- Blood for transfusion collected from the blood bank only by trained staff
- Two trained staff members should check that the details on the blood label match those of the recipient **at the bedside**
- Observe the patient throughout the transfusion

Symptoms of incompatible blood transfusion (blood transfusion reaction)
- Hypotension (shock)
- Chest, back or abdominal pain
- Agitation and fear
- Fever
- Dark urine (intravascular haemolysis)
- Bleeding (disseminated intravascular coagulation; DIC)
- Rigors
- Rash

If there are symptoms of a blood transfusion reaction:
- **Stop the transfusion immediately**, detach the giving set from the patient
- Attach a new giving set, keeping the line open to infuse saline
- Check the identity of the patient against the details on the blood bag label
- Monitor the patient closely to support vital functions, airway, etc.
- Take new blood samples (FBC, coagulation screen, urea and electrolytes, direct antiglobulin test, re-cross-match) and send to laboratory with the blood unit and giving set associated with the reaction

---

fetus inherits a paternal red cell antigen that the mother lacks, the small numbers of fetal red cells that pass into the maternal circulation may immunize her against it. Transfer of maternal IgG back across the placenta results in destruction of the antigen-positive fetal RBCs, causing **haemolytic disease of the newborn**.

ABO (or ABH) blood group system

This is coded by three allelic genes: A, B and O (Table 15.2). The A and B genes code for specific enzymes that convert a precursor (H antigen) into A and B antigens. The O gene

Table 15.2 ABO blood group system

Blood group (phenotype)	Genotype	Red cell antigen	Antibodies	Frequency in UK (%)	Blood suitable for transfusion
O	OO	H	Anti-A, anti-B	46	O
A	AA or AO	A	Anti-B	42	A or O
B	BB or BO	B	Anti-A	9	B or O
AB	AB	A and B	None	3	AB or O

has no effect, so that in group O individuals the H antigen persists unchanged. ABO antigens are oligosaccharides widely expressed on bacteria. Universal exposure (in early postnatal life) to gut bacteria causes the key property of ABO antigens: **no red cell exposure is needed** to immunize us against them. From early infancy we all possess cytotoxic plasma IgM antibodies against ABO antigens that we lack, called **naturally occurring ABO antibodies** (Table 15.2). **ABO-mismatched** transfusions cause the most dangerous (complement-mediated intravascular) reactions, accordingly named **major haemolytic transfusion reactions**.

Rhesus (Rh) blood group system

This complex system of protein antigens is encoded by allelic genes (Cc, Dd, Ee) at three closely linked loci inherited as haplotypes (e.g. *CDe/cde*). Individuals are termed Rh-positive (85% of the UK population) if their red cells carry the *D* antigen, or Rh-negative (15% of the UK population) if they carry **only** the *d* antigen. Rhesus (D) positive individuals may therefore inherit a single (Dd) or double (DD) dose of the D antigen.

Rh antibodies are immune IgG antibodies (they do not occur without immunization) and result from antigen exposure during transfusion or pregnancy. It is therefore important to avoid transfusing a Rh-negative recipient (*d*) with the strongly immunogenic *D* antigen (with Rh-positive blood). Because Rh antibodies are IgG, they do not cause the violent intravascular haemolysis seen in ABO-mismatched transfusions; red cells they opsonize are phagocytosed by extravascular macrophages in liver and spleen.

Red cell metabolism

Red cell metabolism (Fig. 15.5) is focused on production of:
- **ATP** to provide energy for maintenance of red cell

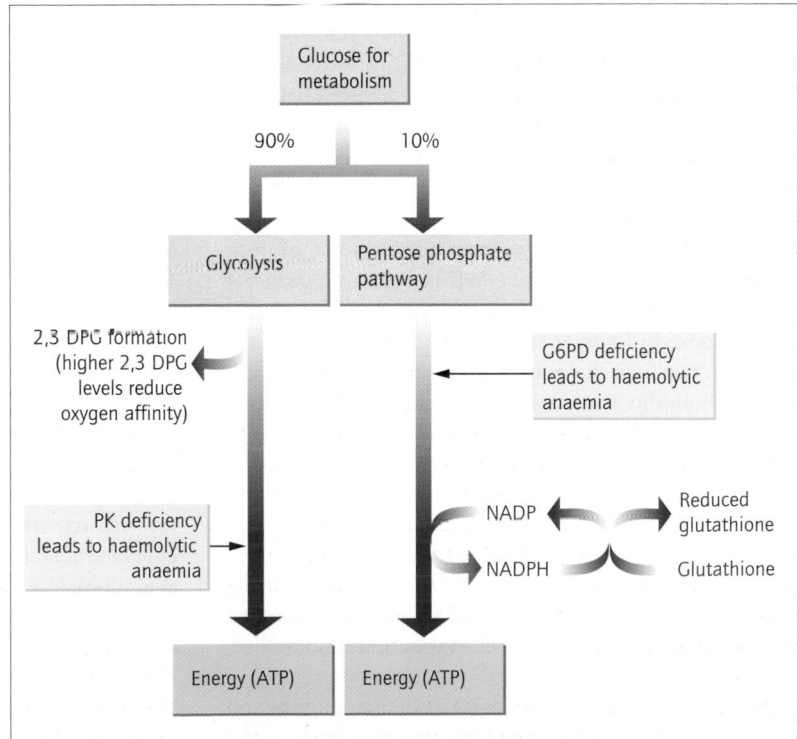

Figure 15.5 Red cell metabolism. Glycolysis and the pentose phosphate pathway are complex biochemical pathways with many intermediary products. These are acted upon by a series of enzymes. Deficiency of any one of these enzymes may affect red cell metabolism, but in practice only two are important: glucose-6-phosphate dehydrogenase (G6PD) deficiency and pyruvate kinase (PK) deficiency.

shape, deformability and function, particularly the cation pump that governs cell size via Na^+ and K^+ gradients
● The reducing agent nicotinamide adenine dinucleotide phosphate (**NADPH**) to block oxidative damage to the vulnerable ferrous ion of haemoglobin and other intracellular components
ATP is produced by anaerobic glycolysis (via the **glycolytic pathway**), while NADPH is the result of aerobic glycolysis (via **the pentose phosphate pathway**).

Glycolytic pathway. Approximately 90% of glucose metabolism occurs by anaerobic glycolysis, which results in the production of two molecules of ATP per molecule of glucose. In addition, reducing power in the form of NADH is produced.

Pentose phosphate pathway. Maintaining membrane components and haemoglobin in a reduced or functional state requires reductive potential. The most important source of this is red cell **reduced glutathione**.

Reduced glutathione (Glu-Cys-Gly) is responsible for the reduction of a variety of substances including haemoglobin, hydrogen peroxide and disulphides, and in the process is constantly consumed. The resulting oxidized glutathione requires continual recycling by glutathione reductase and NADPH (Fig. 15.5), the key product of the pentose phosphate pathway.

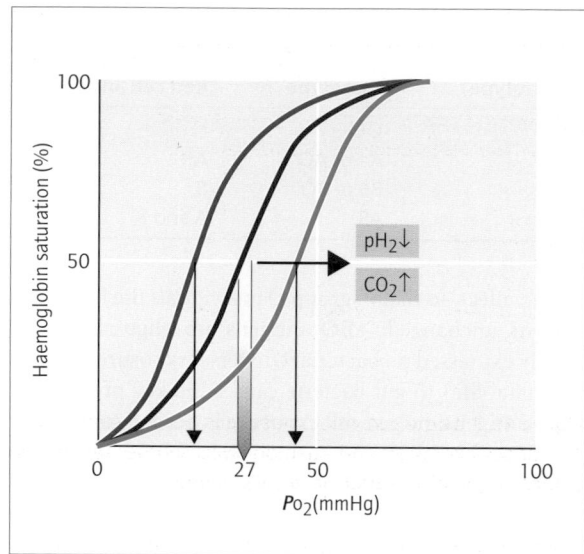

Figure 15.6 Haemoglobin oxygen dissociation curve. The P_{50} is the partial pressure of oxygen at which haemoglobin is 50% saturated, and is normally 27 mmHg (red curve). P_{50} values increase (reflecting decreased oxygen affinity) as the pH decreases (the Bohr effect) and as carbon dioxide concentration increases (green curve). P_{50} values decrease when oxygen affinity increases (e.g. high affinity haemoglobins).

Haemoglobin—the 'molecular lung'

The erythrocyte is red because of the absorption spectrum of **haemoglobin (Hb)**. The intra-erythrocytic concentration of Hb is supersaturated by molecular packing, enabling very efficient carriage of oxygen from the lungs to the tissues, and carbon dioxide from the tissues to the lungs. These key respiratory molecules bind reversibly to Hb.

All human haemoglobin molecules consist of four globin chains: **two α-like** and **two β-like** chains. The major haemoglobins produced during definitive haematopoiesis are composed of two α chains plus two γ chains in the fetus ($\alpha_2\gamma_2$ = **fetal haemoglobin, HbF**), and two α plus two β chains in the adult ($\alpha_2\beta_2$ = **adult haemoglobin, HbA**). Each globin chain is bound covalently to the pigment haem, an iron-containing porphyrin composed of four pyrrole rings joined by methene bridges.

Haemoglobin's vital property of combining loosely and reversibly with oxygen depends on the ferrous (Fe^{2+}) atom of the haem molecule. Each Fe^{2+} atom combines with one molecule of oxygen. Oxidation of Fe^{2+} to Fe^{3+} (forming methaemoglobin) eliminates this reversibility and renders the molecule useless.

During oxygen uptake (forming **oxyhaemoglobin**) and release (forming **deoxyhaemoglobin**) haemoglobin under-

goes conformational change. On combining with oxygen the β chains rotate together by about 0.7 nm—like the expansion–contraction of a 'molecular lung', accounting for many of haemoglobin's properties (e.g. only the deoxy conformation of sickle haemoglobin will polymerize; see pp. 1040–3). In the reduced state **2,3-diphosphoglycerate (2,3-DPG)** binds to the globin tetramer and stabilizes it, reducing its oxygen affinity. Because reduced O_2 affinity equals increased O_2 delivery to the tissues, an increase in red cell 2,3-DPG is a major adaptive response to anaemia.

The binding of oxygen to any haem group depends on oxygenation of the other three haem groups. The binding of the first oxygen molecule to haem is weak, but that of the three successive molecules is increasingly strong. The effect of this **haem–haem interaction** is that the affinity for the last oxygen molecule is 20 times stronger than for the first.

These complex cooperative interactions are essential for efficient oxygen transport and give rise to the vital characteristic of the oxygen dissociation curve of Hb (Fig. 15.6): its sigmoidal shape which maximizes O_2 uptake in the lungs and O_2 delivery to the tissues.

Bohr effect

The effect of pH on the oxygen dissociation curve of haemoglobin is known as the Bohr effect.

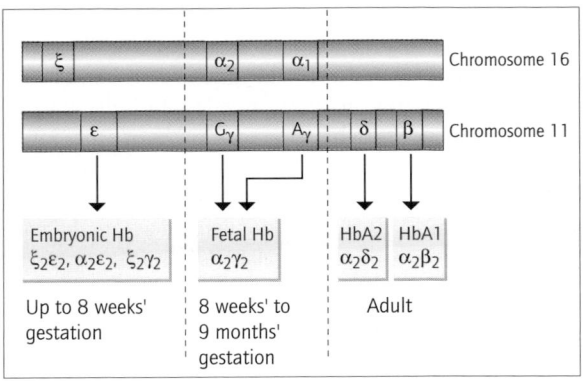

Figure 15.7 Organization of the human globin gene cluster. The genes expressed and haemoglobins synthesized during embryonic, fetal and adult life are illustrated.

An increase in the hydrogen ion concentration (a decrease in the pH) shifts the oxygen dissociation curve to the right because it decreases the oxygen affinity of haemoglobin. Oxygen is therefore released preferentially at sites of lowered pH (in hypoxic tissues).

Why fetal haemoglobin?
Fetal haemoglobin (HbF) binds poorly to 2,3-DPG and fetal blood pH is low, so the amount of oxygen carried at any partial pressure is greater than in adult blood. This **increased oxygen affinity** ensures that HbF can 'steal' O_2 from maternal HbA across the placental interface, thus maintaining an adequate oxygen supply to fetal tissues.

Haemoglobin synthesis
Haemoglobin production in humans is characterized by three major switches in haemoglobin composition (Fig. 15.7):

1 Until the end of the second month postconception, fetal red cells contain the embryonic haemoglobins Hb Gower 1 ($\xi_2 \epsilon_2$), Gower 2 ($\alpha_2 \epsilon_2$) and Hb Portland ($\xi_2 \gamma_2$). These haemoglobins, composed of the α-like globin ξ and the β-like globin ϵ, characterize the primitive or embryonic phase of haematopoiesis, and disappear at the end of this period. From the third to the ninth month postconception, the dominant haemoglobin is HbF ($\alpha_2 \gamma_2$), whatever the timing of birth—so premature infants born at 30 weeks of gestation will maintain synthesis of HbF for another 10 weeks.

2 From 9 months postconception, γ-chain synthesis reduces to a trace and HbF is progressively replaced by adult haemoglobin.

3 By the time an infant is 1 year old, the life-long adult haemoglobin pattern is fully established. HbA ($\alpha_2 \beta_2$) comprises more than 95%, while the minor haemoglobin HbA$_2$ ($\alpha_2 \delta_2$) accounts for approximately 2.5%, and a trace of HbF (approximately 1%) remains, confined to a minority population of red cells called F cells.

This complex switching process involves the turning off and on of genes located in the α-like gene cluster on **chromosome 16** and the β-like gene cluster on **chromosome 11** (Fig. 15.7). The mechanism of the switch, not fully understood, involves transcription factors EKLF and GATA-1 interacting with **locus control regions** (LCRs) upstream of the α- and β-gene clusters.

Haemoglobin metabolism
Ageing or damaged red cells are removed from the circulation by the macrophages of the spleen, liver and bone marrow (the reticuloendothelial system). Globin is separated from the haem and recycled, while the haem ring is split and its iron is retained for use in further haemoglobin synthesis. Haem is then converted to bilirubin, which is bound to glucuronic acid in the liver by the enzyme glucuronyl transferase. Conjugated bilirubin is then excreted in bile and enters the small intestine where it is converted to stercobilin. Some is reabsorbed into the plasma and is later excreted by the kidney as urobilinogen. If there is increased red cell turnover (e.g. because of haemolytic anaemia), bilirubin and urobilinogen excretion increase, with a rise in plasma unconjugated (indirect-acting) bilirubin.

Haemoglobin concentration of the blood
Anaemia
The haemoglobin concentration of blood [Hb] is expressed as **grams per litre** (g/l) or **grams per decilitre** (g/dl).

The range of haemoglobin concentrations found in a **population** depends on:
● Living altitude (oxygen tension: therefore, high altitude = higher haemoglobin levels)
● Average dietary content of nutrients required for haemoglobin and red cell manufacture (haematinics)
● Prevalence of common endemic parasitic diseases that reduce haemoglobin (e.g. hookworm, malaria)
For the range of [Hb] found in the UK (Western Europe, Sea Level) see Table 15.1.

The haemoglobin concentration in an **individual** depends on:
● Age
● Sex
● Pregnancy
● Haematinic content of diet
● Presence of diseases that **steal** (e.g. malaria), **lose** (by bleeding, e.g. colonic carcinoma) or **suppress** (e.g. infection) haemoglobin

Anaemia is an abnormally low haemoglobin concentration—but how do we define abnormality?

15

- By comparison with the 'parent' population; called *'Gaussian'* normality because of the typical distribution curve of values in a population. By this definition, an abnormally low haemoglobin is more than two standard deviations below the mean. In many resource-poor populations, low haemoglobin levels are so prevalent, resulting from poor diet and parasites, that this definition would make them 'normal'.
- By comparison with a 'normal' range consistent with good health: this can be called *'diagnostic'* normality because a lower value can be universally diagnosed as anaemia. By this definition, an abnormally low haemoglobin is one below the lower limit of the accepted normal range. This definition of anaemia is used in this chapter.
- By comparison with previous haemoglobin levels in the same individual. A haemoglobin concentration of 13.5 g/dl in a male may be normal by the above definitions, but if 6 months ago it was 17 g/dl, it still needs investigation (see p. 1027). This definition depends on serial measurements in an individual over time.

Consensus 'diagnostic' **normal ranges** for haemoglobin concentration [Hb] at sea level:
- *Males:* 13–18 g/dl (130–180 g/l). Therefore, anaemia = Hb < 13 g/dl
- *Non-pregnant females:* 12–17 g/dl (120–170 g/l). Therefore, anaemia = Hb < 12 g/dl
- *Pregnant females:* 11–16 g/dl (110–160 g/l). Therefore, anaemia = Hb < 11 g/dl

Ranges for other red cell indices are given in Table 15.1.

White cells (leucocytes)

The **function of white cells** is defence against microbiological attack.

White cell proliferation, differentiation and maturation

This begins with commitment of pluripotent HSC to the myeloid–lymphoid lineage (Fig. 15.1), a 'decision' driven by growth factor signals and transcription factor expression, as described for erythroid cells, but involving different growth factors (G-CSF, granulocyte macrophage colony-stimulating factor; GM-CSF) and transcription factors (PU.1, C/EBPs). Further development to mature lymphocytes of the T, B and natural killer (NK) subtypes is governed by lymphoid-specific factors and cell–cell interactions after cells leave the bone marrow and move to the thymus (T cells) and lymph node follicles (B cells).

The early progenitors in which these key differentiation steps occur are not identifiable in bone marrow smears. Late precursors—myeloblasts and monoblasts—are the earliest identifiable cells in the myeloid (phagocyte) series. Differentiation then diverges into the **granulocyte series** (promyelocytes → myelocytes → band forms → mature polymorphonuclear neutrophils, eosinophils or basophils) and the **monocyte–macrophage** series. Many band forms and mature polymorphs are retained in the bone marrow as reserve defenders to be released at times of acute infection, when band forms and metamyelocytes may appear in the peripheral blood. Because the granulocyte series (in words or pictures) is conventionally read across the page (as above) this is confusingly called 'left shift'.

Granulocyte colony-stimulating factor

Understanding of this cytokine has followed its use in therapy. Not only does G-CSF recruit HSCs to proliferate and differentiate into granulocytes, but it enhances the transcription of many genes that encode molecules concerned with cell motility, phagocytosis and intracellular killing of micro-organisms, 'arming' the granulocyte with extra weaponry. In addition, G-CSF stimulates early pluripotent HSCs, capable of complete haematopoietic regeneration, to leave the bone marrow and wander into the peripheral blood, where they can be harvested by cell separators. This source of marrow-repopulating cells (**autologous stem cells**) can be used to protect the patient against the toxic effects of high-dose cytotoxic chemotherapy.

White blood cell types

Five types of white cell (**polymorphonuclear neutrophils, eosinophils, basophils, monocytes** and **lymphocytes;** Table 15.3) circulate in the blood and can be seen in a stained normal blood film.
- *Neutrophils, eosinophils and basophils* are named according to the specific staining characteristics of the cytoplasmic granules they contain. Because of their granules they are collectively referred to as granulocytes.
- *Monocytes* have indented nuclei, and faintly granulated pale blue cytoplasm.
- Most *lymphocytes* are smaller than granulocytes, with a high ratio of nucleus : cytoplasm (which often forms only a thin rim around the nucleus). They lack specific cytoplasmic granules.

Polymorphonuclear neutrophils [shorter names in common use: polymorphs, neutrophils or granulocytes (US)]

The function of polymorphonuclear neutrophils (PMNs) is to phagocytose and kill micro-organisms.
- *Normal PMN count:* $2–10 \times 10^9$/l, increasing rapidly during infection
- *Increased PMN count:* $>10 \times 10^9$/l = **polymorph leucocytosis** (US; **granulocytosis**)
- *Reduced PMN count:* $<2 \times 10^9$/l = **neutropenia** (US; **granulocytopenia**)

Table 15.3 White cell types (ranked in usual order of frequency in peripheral blood). For images see websites listed on p. 1077

Neutrophil (polymorphonuclear leucocyte, granulocyte [US])
On microscopy of a stained blood film, neutrophils have translucent (neutral-staining) cytoplasmic granules, and multilobed (polymorph) nuclei resembling strings of beads. During acute infections, fewer nuclear lobes may be seen (left shift)

Lymphocyte
On microscopy, lymphocytes have a high nuclear : cytoplasmic ratio (often resembling 'bare' rounded nuclei). During infections (e.g. viral illnesses) they may show more cytoplasm, which may be blue (basophilic): these are termed 'reactive' lymphocytes

Monocyte
Monocytes are larger than neutrophils and lymphocytes, with a lobulated nucleus and greyish 'ground-glass' cytoplasm on stained blood films

Eosinophil
Eosinophils typically show orange cytoplasmic granules large enough to distinguish individually, and a bilobed 'aviator-glasses' nucleus

Basophil
Basophils are rare cells (a typical blood film may not show any). Their blue–black cytoplasmic granules tend to obscure the nucleus

Despite their confusing names, PMNs are easy to identify on stained blood smears: their unique 'polymorphic' nucleus, 2–5 lobes like a string of beads, allows the cell to exit capillaries and reach the tissues through endothelial pores—a process termed **diapedesis**. Their cytoplasm is packed with translucent granules that stain weakly (hence 'neutrophilic').

The circulating pool of PMNs is in transit; other PMNs form a **marginating pool** rolling along vessel walls, waiting for a signal to diapedese. A further **reserve pool** is stored in the bone marrow for rapid release in emergencies.

Chemotaxis
Exposure to micro-organisms, tissue damage or foreign bodies provokes local cells to release **chemokines**, cell–cell signalling molecules that attract motile cells to move in the direction of the signal. The key chemokine for PMNs is **IL-8**. The PMN responds by rapid amoeboid movement (**chemotaxis**) toward the signal. Large numbers of PMNs form the first wave of defenders to reach the danger area.

Micro-organism recognition and binding
PMNs work best when their targets are coated by **opsonins**. Potent opsonins are specific antimicrobial antibodies that bind the target with their **Fab** ends and to PMN surface Fc receptors via their **Fc** ends, forming a bridge between PMN and target. The antibody Fc terminal may recruit **complement** molecules, also potent PMN opsonins, to the microbe surface.

Phagocytosis and killing
Bound micro-organisms are engulfed by the PMN membrane (**phagocytosis**) and internalized in the resulting **phagosome**. The PMN starts to rapidly consume oxygen (the **oxygen burst**) as it turns on the **NADPH–oxidase** membrane complex, a molecular machine that generates the **reactive oxygen** species $[O^-]$, $[OH^-]$ and $[H_2O_2]$. These enter the phagosome, which also fuses with lysosomes. The combination of toxic oxygen and lysosomal enzymes kills the microbe.

Eosinophils

The **function of eosinophils** is defence against multicellular parasites (e.g. helminths) and participation in IgE-mediated immune responses.
- *Normal eosinophil count:* **0.05–0.35 × 10⁹/l**
- *Increased eosinophil count:* **>0.35 × 10⁹/l = eosinophilia**
- *Reduced eosinophil count:* **<0.05 × 10⁹/l = eosinopenia**

Eosinophils are easily recognizable on blood films by their bilobed nuclei and large orange-stained cytoplasmic granules, but how they carry out their function remains obscure. Eosinophils have a separate system of growth factors (**IL-5**), chemokines (**eotaxin**) and opsonins (**IgE**) and, although capable of phagocytosis, attack their targets by external secretion of cytotoxic molecules (e.g. **arylsulphatase**). In almost all types of microbial infection, they disappear rapidly from the blood (presumably into the tissues) resulting in eosinopenia. Eosinophilia is seen in allergic reactions (to drugs or environmental factors) and endo- or ectoparasitic infections.

Basophils

The **function of basophils** is still unknown a century after their discovery.
- *Normal basophil count:* **0.00–0.09 × 10⁹/l**
- *Increased basophil count:* **>0.1 × 10⁹/l = basophilia**

Basophils contain high levels of histamine and heparin and are involved in allergic (IgE-mediated) responses: sustained basophilia is usually a sign of chronic myeloid leukaemia.

Monocytes (mononuclear phagocytes = monocytes in the blood, macrophages in the tissues)

The **function of monocytes** is to phagocytose invading microbes and other foreign material, process resulting peptides, and present them bound to surface MHC-2 complexes for recognition and response by T and B lymphocytes. They are hence **antigen-presenting cells**, which also secrete a wide range of cytokines (**IL-1 and IL-6, tumour necrosis factor**) to stimulate inflammatory and immune responses.

- *Normal monocyte count:* 0.4–1.1 × 10⁹/l
- *Increased monocyte count:* >1.1 × 10⁹/l = **monocytosis**
- *Decreased monocyte count:* <0.4 × 10⁹/l = **monocytopenia**

Blood monocytes are in brief transit *en route* to the tissues where they are destined to become site-specific tissue macrophages: about 50% become liver macrophages (Kupffer cells); 15% lung (alveolar) macrophages; and 35% other types (e.g. brain microglia). Monocyte and macrophage proliferation and terminal differentiation proceeds under the influence of specific growth factors (**GM-CSF** and **M-CSF**).

Lymphocytes

The **function of lymphocytes** is to recognize non-self antigens, and to generate the adaptive **cellular** (**T lymphocyte**) and **humoral** (**B lymphocyte**) immune responses to them.

- *Normal lymphocyte count:* 1.0–4.0 × 10⁹/l
- *Increased lymphocyte count:* >4.0 × 10⁹/l = **lymphocytosis**
- *Decreased lymphocyte count:* <1.0 × 10⁹/l = **lymphopenia**

Lymphocytes originate from the pluripotent HSCs in the bone marrow via committed lymphoid progenitor cells under complex growth factor, cytokine and transcription factor control. They then migrate to the secondary lymphoid organs (thymus for T cells, lymph node follicles for B cells) where they further differentiate into mature antigen-specific T and B cells. Blood lymphocytes are 80% T cells and 20% B cells. There are no morphological differences between the two types, which can be distinguished by marking with diagnostic antibodies against their surface antigens (cell surface phenotype). As immune-recognition cells, they carry surface molecules of the MHC-1 and -2 classes (tissue-type antigens). These, the origin and multiple functions of lymphocytes are discussed in Chapter 1.

Platelets

The **function of blood platelets** is to prevent haemorrhage by forming platelet plugs at sites of blood vessel damage.

- *Normal platelet count:* 150–400 × 10⁹/l
- *Increased platelet count:* >400 × 10⁹/l = **thrombocytosis**
- *Decreased platelet count:* <150 × 10⁹/l = **thrombocytopenia**

Platelets are produced in the bone marrow by cytoplasmic budding from **megakaryocytes**, in turn derived from the pluripotent HSCs via committed megakaryocyte precursors (**CFU-Meg**). Proliferation, maturation and platelet budding are all governed by the platelet growth factor **Tpo**. Platelets function in cooperation with cells of the

Table 15.4 Normal adult differential white cell count

White cell	Absolute number (×10⁹/l)	Relative number (%)
Neutrophils	2.0–7.5	40–75
Lymphocytes	1.5–4.0	20–45
Monocytes	0.1–0.8	2–10
Eosinophils	0.04–0.45	1–6
Basophils	<0.1	1

vessel wall and coagulation factors in **haemostasis**, the defence system against bleeding (see below).

Thrombocytopenia is termed mild (100–150 × 10⁹/l), moderate (50–100 × 10⁹/l) or severe (<50 × 10⁹/l): spontaneous bleeding (e.g. typical skin purpura of thrombocytopenia) is unlikely unless the platelet count is <50 × 10⁹/l.

For a list of normal white cell ranges see Table 15.4. For causes of abnormal white cell counts see Table 15.5.

Haemostasis

Haemostasis is a complex defence mechanism that prevents death from bleeding when blood vessels are breached. If it happens in the wrong place, at the wrong time, then it is expressed as potentially lethal thrombosis. This imposes a critical need for tight control of the process —the reason why haemostasis is so complex. Haemostasis operates in a series of phases.

Primary haemostasis—the initial platelet plug

Platelet adhesion

Vessel wall trauma results in damaged **vascular endothelial cells** and exposes the underlying **subendothelium**. Platelets adhere to the site, as a result of interaction between platelet membrane receptor **glycoprotein Ib**, the giant polymer **von Willebrand factor** (**vWF**), and subendothelial **collagen** (Fig. 15.8).

Platelet aggregation

Adherent platelets expose fibrinogen receptors (**glycoprotein IIb–IIIa**) that bind plasma **fibrinogen**, cross-linking more platelets. The resulting platelet aggregate blocks the defect in the vessel wall and provides an expanse of platelet membrane on which coagulation reactions can proceed.

Secondary haemostasis—generation of fibrin clot by the coagulation pathway

The primary platelet plug disintegrates unless strengthened

Table 15.5 Causes of quantitative white cell abnormalities

Cause	Example
Neutrophilia	
Abnormal distribution because of acute inflammation	Acute infection, myocardial infarction, diabetic ketoacidosis, exercise, stress, drugs (e.g. corticosteroids, adrenaline)
Increased production	Chronic myeloid leukaemia, myeloproliferative disorders, non-haematological malignancies
Decreased destruction	Splenectomy
Neutropenia	
Decreased production	Deficiency states (e.g. vitamin B_{12}, folate deficiency), drugs (especially cytotoxic agents), bone marrow infiltrations
Abnormal distribution	Acute infection, viraemia, endotoxaemia, anaphylactic shock
Increased destruction	Immune causes (e.g. systemic lupus erythematosus, lymphoproliferative disorders), hypersplenism
Eosinophilia	
Allergy	Asthma, allergic rhinitis, drug reactions
Parasitic infection	Tropical pulmonary eosinophilia, schistosomiasis, trichinosis, strongyloidiasis
Haematological malignancy	Chronic myeloid leukaemia, Hodgkin's disease
Unknown aetiology	Certain skin diseases (e.g. pemphigus, dermatitis herpetiformis), hypereosinophilic syndrome
Basophilia	
Haematological malignancy	Chronic myeloid leukaemia, polycythaemia rubra vera
Allergy	Urticaria
Monocytosis	
Haematological malignancy	Acute/chronic monocytic leukaemias, chronic myeloid leukaemia, Hodgkin's disease
Infection	Protozoal and rickettsial infection
Lymphocytosis	
Infections	Infectious mononucleosis, pertussis
Lymphoid malignancy	Chronic lymphatic leukaemia, non-Hodgkin's lymphoma
Lymphopenia	
Glucocorticoid excess	Corticosteroid therapy or acute stress
Malignancy	Hodgkin's disease, disseminated visceral neoplasia

by a fibrin net. The **coagulation pathway** (Fig. 15.9a,b) that generates fibrin can be divided into three substages.

Clot initiation

The receptor molecule **tissue factor** (TF), exposed on damaged endothelial and extravascular cells in the damage zone, binds and activates **factor VII**.

TF–factor VIIa complexes bind and activate **factor X**. Acting like a starter motor, this cleaves a small amount of thrombin (from prothrombin), which activates the

Figure 15.8 (*right*) Platelet adhesion to damaged endothelium. The adhesion of platelets to damaged vascular endothelium is mediated by multimeric von Willebrand factor (vWF: Ag). It binds to glycoprotein Ib on the platelet membrane as well as to subendothelial collagen. Deficiencies of glycoprotein Ib (Bernard–Soulier syndrome), IIb/IIIa (Glanzmann's thrombaesthenia), and vWF: Ag (von Willebrand's disease) all result in haemorrhagic disorders.

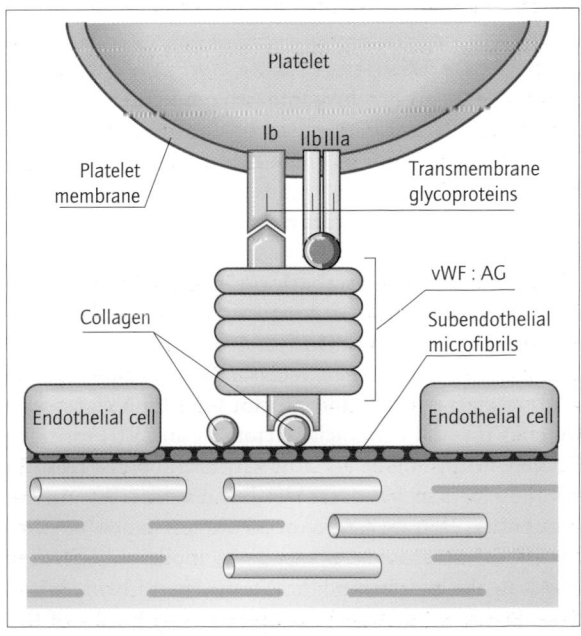

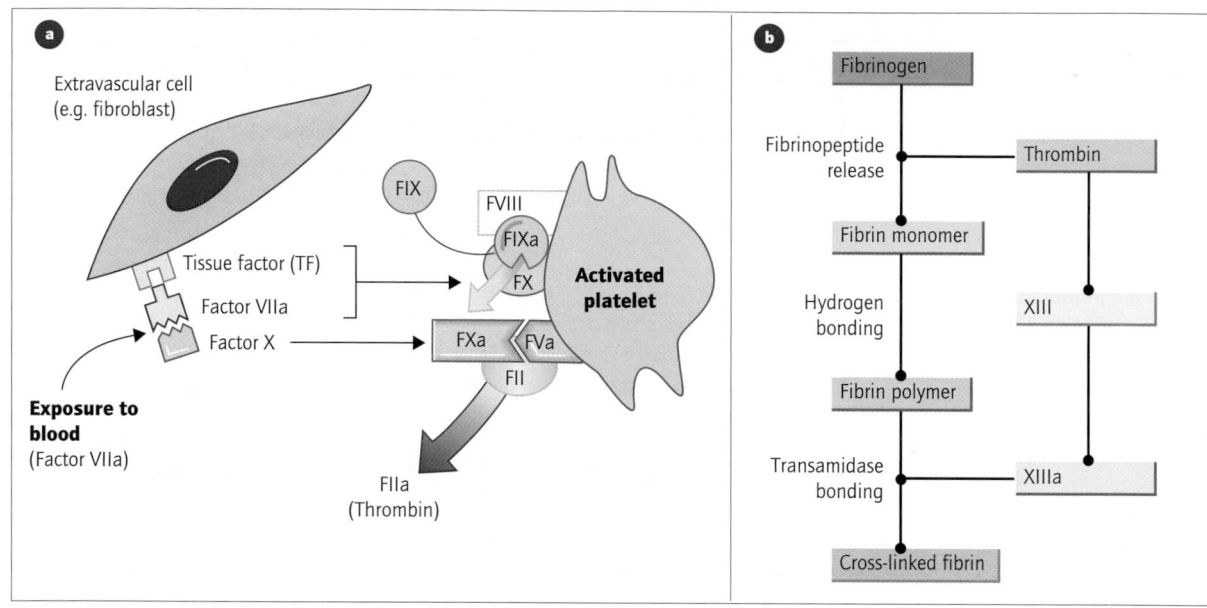

Figure 15.9 (a) The cell-based pathways for the formation of thrombin. (b) Conversion of soluble fibrinogen into a cross-linked fibrin clot. Thrombin specifically cleaves small peptides from α and β chains of fibrinogen. The resultant fibrin is stabilized by activated factor XIII (XIIIa).

cofactors **factors VIII** and **V**, and the enzyme **factor IX**. If this activation is sufficient, coagulation proceeds to the next stage (the 'engine' is started).

Clot amplification

If the 'engine' starts up, **factors VIIIa** and **IXa** form a membrane complex that increases **factor Xa** generation 10-fold. The location of this factor Xa on the platelet surface enables it to hop over to the next phase.

Clot propagation

Factor Xa forms **prothrombinase** complexes with **factor Va** on platelet surfaces, speeding **thrombin** generation from **prothrombin**. Thrombin cleaves fibrinogen to form a durable fibrin clot, and binds to it, promoting further clot growth. This is a secure barrier against bleeding.

Where has the 'intrinsic pathway' gone?

It has been known for at least 20 years that there are no separate intrinsic and extrinsic clotting pathways to clot formation acting in the circulating blood. They were *in vitro* artefacts. In real life, **all clot formation starts with factor VIIa**, and the crucial **factors IX and VIII** form the 'main clotting engine'—that is why haemophilia (A or B; see p. 1070) is such a severe bleeding disorder. Because the laboratory 'clotting screen' occurs in test-tubes (*in vitro*) the otherwise obsolete two-pathway model still serves to illustrate the logic behind these tests (Fig. 15.10).

Clot regulation and removal

Two further systems regulate and eventually remove the clot.

Clot regulation: the protein C system and antithrombin (Fig. 15.11)

Thrombin formed around healthy vascular endothelial cells puts a brake on coagulation by binding to a receptor, **thrombomodulin**, which retargets it to **protein C**. Thrombin and thrombomodulin activated **aPC** knocks out factors Va and VIIIa, slowing thrombin formation. To get at factors Va and VIIIa in their membrane complexes, aPC needs a cofactor, **protein S**.

Thrombin is restricted to the clot by a direct thrombin inhibitor, **antithrombin (AT)**. To work efficiently, AT must bind to heparin-like **proteoglycans** on healthy endothelial cells.

Fibrinolysis (Fig. 15.12)

Clots contain the seeds of their own destruction, **plasminogen**. This is cleaved by **tissue plasminogen activator (tPA)** secreted by healthy vascular endothelial cells (VECs), or **urokinase** on the surface of macrophages, to the fibrinolytic enzyme **plasmin**. Plasmin cleaves fibrin into the D-**dimer** fragment specific to cleavage of cross-linked fibrin. This removes the clot, and plasmin also activates repair of the original vessel damage (angiogenesis).

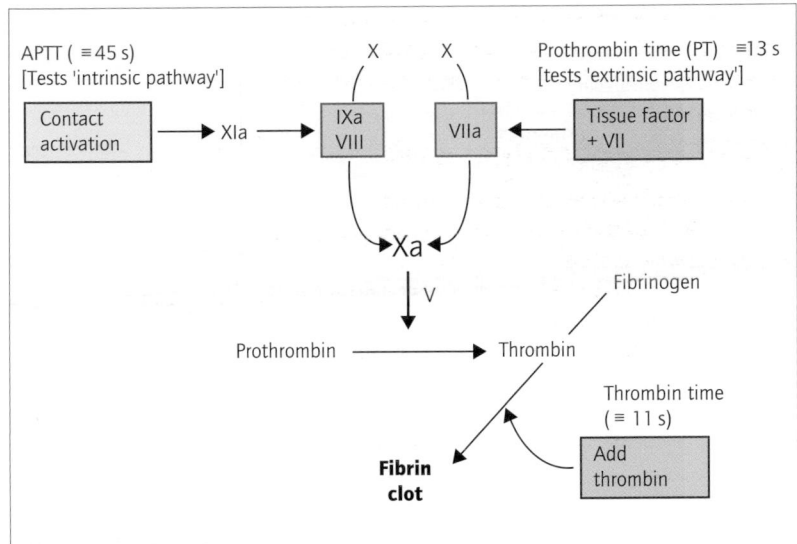

Figure 15.10 How clotting tests 'screen' haemostasis.

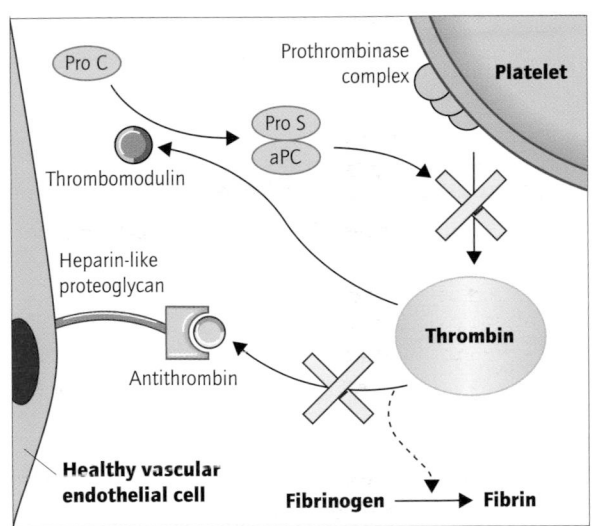

Figure 15.11 Natural anticoagulant mechanisms.

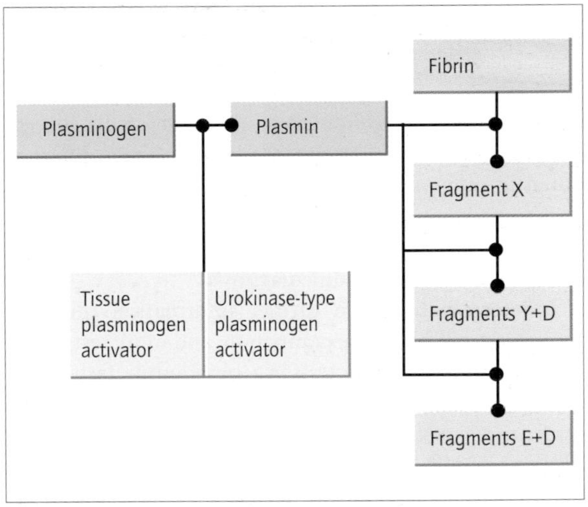

Figure 15.12 Fibrin digestion. Plasmin cleaves fibrin into a number of soluble fragments called fibrin degradation products (FDPs).

Approach to the patient

The diagnostic pathway

The task is to make a **diagnosis** that fits the patient's symptoms and leads to accurate assessment of: (a) the best therapy (if any); and (b) the likely course of the disorder —its **prognosis**. The patient's initial (presenting) complaint suggests possible diagnoses, haematological or otherwise —the **differential diagnosis**. It is best to consider several diagnoses, not to jump too early to a conclusion. The intent of the history taking and examination detailed below is to rank these possible diagnoses in order of probability.

Next, the patient is investigated with a variety of tests. The initial probability (from the history and examination) of each possible diagnosis on the list is its **pretest probability**. Simple division into *high*, *moderate* and *low* probability is useful. Selected tests should be capable of clearly increasing or decreasing this probability. Test

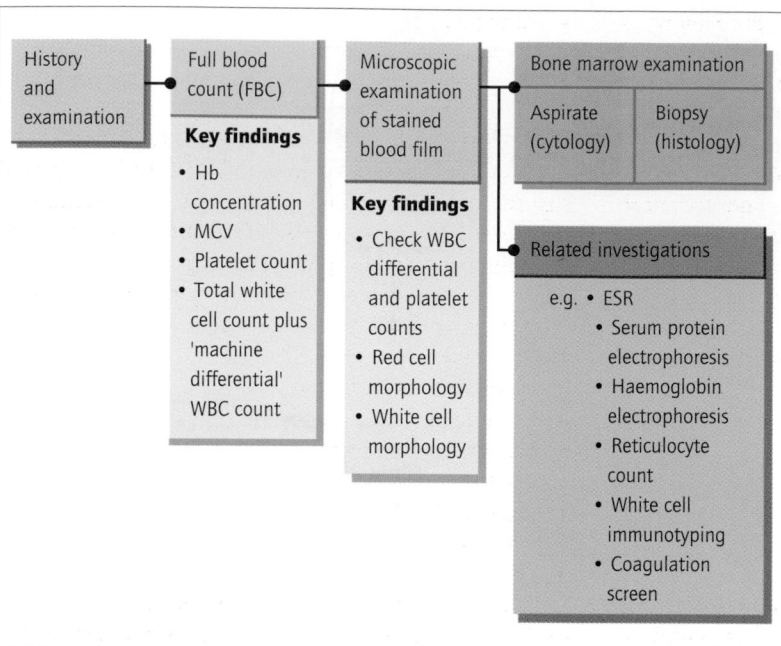

Figure 15.13 Sequence of steps in haematological investigation.

results should be computed in the light of the pretest probability (many tests give results that mean different things in different clinical situations). We end up with a **post-test probability**, which may be:

● High enough to **confirm** a diagnosis
● Low enough to **exclude** a diagnosis
● **Indeterminate**, when further information must be extracted from history, examination, and more tests

Many clinicians order tests in a 'blunderbus' fashion, as if one of them *must* produce the diagnosis. This might sometimes work, but humans and their diseases are usually too complex for this approach. It is more reliable (and economical) to follow the principles suggested above.

History

The patient's history is the most important 'investigation' in making a diagnosis, and the results of all tests must be considered in the light of it (Fig. 15.13). The key part of the history is the **presenting complaint**, the dominant problem that brings the patient to the clinician. Patients can be helped to define the presenting complaint as clearly as possible, but should not be strongly prompted or 'led' towards what the clinician thinks is wrong. Once the presenting complaint has been carefully noted, a **systematic enquiry**, consisting of specific questions put by the clinician, is made to detect related symptoms that the patient has not volunteered but may recall on questioning (HISTORY & EXAMINATION BOXES 15.1 AND 15.2).

**History & Examination 15.1:
General questions addressed by
the initial clinical history**

Who is the patient?
What are their presenting complaints (symptoms) and how do they affect their life and functioning?
Is the patient (or their family/carer) aware of any pre-existing illness or disorder?
What is the patient's ethnic and genetic heritage, and occupation?
Has the patient travelled abroad recently? Where?
What is the patient's understanding of his or her symptoms?
What are the patient's expectations of treatment?
What medications are they taking/have they taken?

About the patient

The patient's **age**, **sex** and **ethnicity** increase or decrease the probability of certain disorders. A few examples (among many):

● Being female reduces the likelihood of having haemophilia, and therefore increases the probability that lifelong bleeding symptoms are caused by von Willebrand's disease

- African ethnic heritage increases the probability of having sickle cell disease
- Clonal myeloid disorders (myelodysplasia) are most common in people over 60 years of age, so being 15 years old reduces the probability of having this disorder
- Being a member of a Hindu Indian ethnic community entails a high likelihood of veganism, and therefore increases the probability of vitamin B_{12} deficiency

This does *not* mean that it is *impossible* for a female to have haemophilia, a fair-haired northern European sickle cell disease, a 15-year-old myelodysplasia or a vegan folate deficiency, but that laboratory tests must give strongly positive results to elevate their **low pretest probability** to diagnostic **post-test probability** levels, before we could make such a diagnosis.

Presenting symptoms of haematological disease

Haematological disease causes **failure of function** of one or more components of the blood. The symptoms of blood diseases are directly caused by this loss of function.

Anaemia (reduced red blood cell function)

Loss of red cell function *can* occur without anaemia (e.g. carbon monoxide poisoning) but in the vast majority of disorders, **reduced RBC function = anaemia**. Because of the 100-day lifespan of red cells in the circulation, many forms of anaemia progress gradually, with a steadily falling haemoglobin concentration, so that the patient may find it difficult to date the onset of symptoms.

The function of the red cell is oxygen transport, so anaemia leads to symptoms of reduced tissue oxygen delivery. The heart and lungs (if healthy) can increase oxygen delivery independently of the haemoglobin level, so they efficiently compensate for milder degrees of anaemia (Hb more than 8 g/dl) in patients for whom high levels of energy expenditure are rare.

Early symptoms of anaemia (more than 8 g/dl)
- Reduced exercise tolerance and performance
- Loss of interest in leisure pursuits
- Sleepiness
- Mild depression

Below 8 g/dl (at higher values in patients with compromised cardiorespiratory function), more severe symptoms develop at rest.

Later symptoms of anaemia (less than 8 g/dl)
- Breathlessness on minimal effort or at rest
- Swollen ankles
- Headache
- Palpitations

- Chest pain
- Leg pain (claudication)
- Others notice pallor

Infection (reduced white blood cell function)

Because the function of white blood cells is to defend against microbiological attack, loss of function is expressed as an **increased risk of infection**. Because of the short lifespan of neutrophils in the circulation, **neutropenia** can develop very acutely, so the symptoms may be of short duration and have had a sudden onset.

Symptoms of neutropenia
- Skin infections: boils or cellulitis
- Painful mouth or throat
- Swollen gums
- Fevers and chills
- Diarrhoea

Symptoms of hypoimmunoglobulinaemia
In lymphomas and chronic lymphocytic leukaemia, reduced immune function resulting from hypoimmunoglobulinaemia and reduced cell-mediated immunity develops despite an increased white cell count (composed of abnormal lymphocytes).
- Recurrent bacterial pneumonia
- Herpes zoster infection (shingles)

Symptoms of asplenia
A variety of blood disorders cause loss of spleen function (asplenia), either as part of the disease process (e.g. sickle cell diseases) or after therapeutic surgical splenectomy. Asplenia results in vulnerability to acute overwhelming septicaemia with encapsulated bacteria (e.g. *Pneumococcus*).
- Rapid onset of fever and chills (rigors)
- Collapse

Bleeding (reduced platelet or coagulation function)

At platelet counts between 100 and 150×10^9/l, bleeding is unlikely. At platelet counts between 50 and 100×10^9/l, easy bruising is likely. Platelet counts in the $10-50 \times 10^9$/l range are usually associated with bruising and skin purpura, and in severe thrombocytopenia (platelets less than 10×10^9/l), skin bruising, purpura and mucosal blood blisters ('wet purpura') often coexist.

Symptoms of thrombocytopenia
- Skin rash (purpura)
- Bruises
- Nosebleeds (epistaxis)
- Oral bleeding or 'blood blisters'
- Heavy periods (menorrhagia)

History & Examination 15.2: Important specific questions (and their implications)

About the patient

What is your ethnic origin, or ethnic heritage?
(? haemoglobinopathies)

What is (or has been) your occupation? (? exposure to leukaemogens)

Do you smoke cigarettes, if so how many per day?
(? secondary polycythaemia)

How many units of alcohol do you tend to drink per week?
(? macrocytosis)

Do you follow a special diet—for example, a vegetarian or vegan diet? (? iron deficiency, megaloblastic anaemia)

Have you travelled abroad? If yes, where and when?
(? malaria)

About the symptoms

The answer 'yes', to any of the below, raises the probability of a blood disorder

Questions relating to anaemia (red blood cell deficiency or dysfunction)

Do activities you used to enjoy, or do with ease, now tire you out?

Do you find you're doing less and less as a result?

Do you get breathless going up stairs? Do you have to stop before reaching the top?

When did you first notice these changes? Was it months ago, weeks ago or very recently?

Do you ever get attacks of yellow jaundice?

See also questions on menstruation (below)

Questions relating to haemoglobinopathies

Do you get aches and pains in your bones and joints? What tends to provoke these?

Have you ever had pain in the bones so bad you had to go to hospital?

Have you always tired easily compared to your classmates/friends/siblings?

Do people tell you that your eyes look yellow?

Have you ever had to have blood transfusions?

Have you ever had ankle ulcers?

Questions relating to infection (white blood cell deficiency or dysfunction)

Has your doctor had to give you antibiotics for an infection recently? If so, what were the symptoms?

Have you had a sore throat, mouth or gum? Mouth ulcers? Toothache?

Have you been troubled by septic skin spots or boils?

Have you had any trouble with pain around the back passage, or piles?

Any recent skin rashes, shingles, thrush?

Any fevers, chills, or night sweats that forced you to wake up and change?

When did you first notice these things? Was it months ago, weeks ago or very recently?

Any high-risk sexual or drug-using behaviours (asked sensitively, in a confidential setting, after gaining the patient's trust)?

Questions relating to bleeding (platelet or coagulation deficiency or dysfunction)

• *Bruises*

Do you always have at least one bruise?

Do you get bruises bigger than a 50p piece (UK) [or quarter (US)]?

Do you get bruises that you can feel as swellings?

When did you first notice these bruises?

• *Bleeds*

Do you get nosebleeds that run like a tap, so you have to get a bowl, not just a tissue? How often?

Have you ever had to go to hospital for a nosebleed?

Have you ever bled from anywhere else: coughed up blood, vomited blood, passed dark stools, bled from the back passage, passed blood in your urine?

When did these bleeds first happen?

• *Menstruation.* These questions also apply to anaemia in a woman (asked sensitively, in a confidential setting, after gaining the patient's trust)

Do you bleed for more than 7 days every month?

Do you have to wear double protection?

Do you have to protect your bed with a towel during your period?

Do you have to cancel social engagements during your period because the bleeding is so heavy?

• *Bleeding on surgical or obstetric challenge*

Have you ever bled into the next day, or had to go back to the dentist with bleeding, after any dental treatment or tooth extraction?

Have you ever had your tonsils or adenoids out? If so, did you have to go back to theatre, or have a blood transfusion, because of bleeding?

Has this happened after any other kind of surgery?

Did you bleed a lot after the delivery of any of your babies? Did they have to take you back to theatre/perform a D & C/give a blood transfusion?

• *Bleeding in the family*

Have any family members had similar problems with bleeding?

Are any family members registered as having haemophilia or other bleeding disorders?

Questions relating to invasive (malignant) blood disorders (e.g. acute and chronic leukaemia, lymphoma, myeloma)

Have you noticed any swellings, lumps or bumps anywhere on your body? Can you show me where?

Have you noticed any enlarged glands in your neck, under your arms or in your groin?

Have you noticed that your abdomen (stomach, belly) is swollen (full, lumpy)? Do you feel full up as soon as you start to eat?

Have you noticed any swelling of your legs?

Have you been getting pain in your bones/back/ribs/anywhere?

About medications

Are you taking any drugs prescribed by a doctor either regularly or as required, and for how long?

Are you taking any drugs you have bought over the counter?

A variety of drugs can cause haematological problems:

- *Agranulocytosis (severe neutropenia):* antithyroid drugs, antibiotics, antirheumatic drugs, anticonvulsants
- *Thrombocytopenia:* gold, thiazide diuretics, quinine, heparin
- *Aplastic anaemia:* chloramphenicol, gold, phenylbutazone
- *Autoimmune haemolytic anaemia:* methyldopa
- *Oxidative haemolytic anaemia:* a number of drugs cause haemolysis in glucose-6-phosphate dehydrogenase (G6PD) deficient patients: antimalarials (e.g. primaquine), sulphonamides (e.g. sulfasalazine), antibacterials (e.g. isoniazid) and quinine

- Prolonged bleeding after surgery
- Vomiting, coughing or passing blood
- Headache and collapse (resulting from intracranial bleeding in severe thrombocytopenia)

Failure of haemostasis may also occur because of inherited or acquired coagulation factor deficiencies.

Symptoms of coagulation factor deficiency
- Bruises
- Painful muscle swellings
- Painful joint swelling and loss of mobility
- Poor wound healing
- Prolonged bleeding after minor trauma or surgery

Symptoms of pancytopenia (bone marrow failure)

When the whole range of bone marrow function fails (e.g. in leukaemia), all the cells of the blood decrease and the symptoms consist of a combination of anaemia, infection and bleeding as above. Because white cells and platelets have a shorter lifespan in the circulation than red cells, symptoms of bleeding and infection usually develop before those of anaemia.

Lumps and swellings

Enlarged glands may be caused by lymphoma or leukaemia, but may signal infection or other malignancies. **Abdominal swelling** and/or **fullness** may be caused by **splenomegaly** in lymphoma and related diseases (e.g. non-Hodgkin's lymphoma, chronic lymphocytic leukaemia) or myeloproliferative disorders (e.g. chronic myeloid leukaemia, myelofibrosis). **Abdominal pain** may be caused by **splenic infarction** in splenomegaly.

Pain

Back pain, particularly if continuous, worse in bed at night, and provoked by minimal movement (such as turning over in bed) may signify myeloma bone disease. Acute episodes of excruciating pain involving back, limbs, chest or the whole body are typical of sickle cell disease. Bone pain preventing a child from walking, when combined with symptoms of pancytopenia, suggest acute leukaemia. Pain in the calf or thigh may be caused by deep-vein thrombosis (DVT), and if accompanied by pleuritic chest pain may signify pulmonary embolism.

Weight loss and fever

Significant weight loss (more than 10% body weight) may occur in lymphoma and chronic leukaemia. Cachexia can be a late effect of malignant blood diseases, or because of disseminated carcinoma or tuberculosis, which can infiltrate bone marrow failure causing pancytopenia. **Fever** may be caused by the blood disease itself, but it is safer to assume it is a result of infection until proven otherwise. When weight loss, fever and drenching night sweats are present (without infection) in Hodgkin's disease, they are termed '**B**' **symptoms** and worsen prognosis.

Systematic enquiry in haematological disease

The systematic enquiry should start by asking about symptoms of blood disorders (described above) that the patient has *not* volunteered. Further questioning should focus on the following.

Drug history

The patient should be questioned about all medication, whether prescribed or bought over the counter. Herbal, traditional or alternative therapies taken should also be detailed. In appropriate situations the patient should be sensitively asked about recreational drug use, or drug sharing. Patients may not regard unprescribed agents as 'real' drugs. Particular agents with impacts on blood function include the following.

Aspirin

Associated with bleeding, particularly in pre-existing mild

bleeding disorders. Large numbers of over-the-counter remedies still contain aspirin.

Antiepileptic agents

May be associated with folate deficiency and macrocytic anaemia.

Combined (oestrogen-containing) oral contraceptives

A risk factor for venous thromboembolic disease.

Antidepressive, antipsychotic, antithyroid and antirheumatic drugs

These widely prescribed classes of drugs have been associated with severe neutropenia (termed **agranulocytosis** when provoked by drugs). The drug information sheet may recommend blood count monitoring.

Past medical history

Previous medical disorders may provide clues to the aetiology of the current haematological disorder:
- A history of peptic ulceration in a patient with microcytic anaemia caused by iron deficiency
- A history of gastrectomy in a patient with macrocytic anaemia caused by vitamin B_{12} deficiency

Family history

A positive family history suggests an inherited disorder, and justifies drawing a family tree highlighting affected members. Screening for the disorder in question can be offered to living first-degree relatives. In **bleeding disorders**, a sex-linked inheritance pattern may be evident, increasing the pretest probability of **haemophilia**.

A family history of immune disorders (e.g. of thyroid or adrenal, or vitiligo) is associated with pernicious anaemia.

Examination

Physical examination should always be performed 'wearing wide-angle lenses', not restricting attention to a single system, and always including measurement of temperature, pulse and blood pressure. However, it is rational to focus on the typical **clinical signs** of blood disorders if the history raises the possibility of one. The clinical examination consists of a series of tests that serve to raise or lower the likelihood of one or other of the differential diagnoses. These characteristic signs are listed in HISTORY & EXAMINATION BOX 15.3.

First impressions

- *How ill does this patient look?* Blood diseases can cause

life-threatening bleeding, infection or other acute crises. If the patient is dangerously ill, the tempo of investigation and diagnosis must be fast. Pallor, sweating, a 'drawn' face, restlessness and anxiety, and reduced conscious level are all danger signs.
- *Stature and body habitus?* Inherited blood disorders often cause short stature and/or delayed puberty: Sickle cell anaemia causes shortening of the vertebral column and lengthy limbs, so the sitting height is normal but the standing height tall; haemophilia may cause valgus knee deformity with limping.
- *Are they in pain?* A patient in pain often finds history taking and clinical examination taxing. It may be necessary to defer some aspects until pain is relieved.
- *Ethnic origin?* The first impression may suggest this, but it is always more reliable to **ask the patient**.

Signs of anaemia

- *Pallor.* Skin colour depends on skin pigmentation and capillary tone, so can mislead: but failure of palmar creases to 'stand out' with a russet colour when the fingers are gently extended is a helpful sign. Mucous membranes of the lips and tongue, and conjunctiva (visible when the lower eyelid is gently eased down by the examiner's thumb), are the most reliable sites to look.
- *Jaundice (icterus).* Using the same manoeuvre, assess the sclera for yellow tint: the combination of pallor with jaundice strongly increases the likelihood of a **haemolytic anaemia**.
- *Signs of cardiovascular compensation.* Increasingly severe anaemia may be associated with signs of a hyperdynamic circulation (e.g. tachycardia, systolic flow murmur) or cardiac failure (e.g. gallop rhythm, basal crepitations, ankle oedema).

Signs of infection

- *Fever.* Thermometer reading over 37.5°C: may be associated with rigors (shaking) or muscular pains. A danger sign.
- *Oropharyngeal ulceration and mucositis.* The mucosae of the oral cavity, gums, tongue and pharynx should be examined *with a bright torch*. Painful **ulcers** suggest neutropenic infection. **Gingivitis** and gum swelling typify acute leukaemia. White **plaques** of 'thrush' signify candidal mucositis in immunosuppressed patients.
- *Skin sepsis.* Localized boils or spreading subcutaneous infection with spreading redness (cellulitis).
- *Sepsis syndrome.* Hypotension, restlessness, dyspnoea and changes in mental function, with or without fever, are danger signals of overwhelming sepsis in neutropenic or asplenic patients.

Signs of bleeding

● *Bruising.* In health, these are common on the outer surfaces of arms and thighs: but bruising elsewhere on the body, or bruises larger than 3 cm across, particularly if palpable as bumps, increase the likelihood of a bleeding disorder.

● *Purpura.* Small red skin spots, often seen in crops mixed with bruises. They **do not blanch on pressure** (the famous 'glass test' successfully used by children on younger siblings), which distinguishes purpura from erythema. They signify **thrombocytopenia** and always need investigation: the 'glass test' is designed to recognize purpura in meningococcal sepsis (DIC; see p. 1074). In the elderly patient, senile purpura are flat bloodstains in thin atrophic skin over the dorsae of hands and forearms, and rarely indicate a blood disorder—but perform a blood count if they are extensive or of recent onset.

● *Mucosal bleeding.* Blood may be seen trickling from peridontal fissures of the gums, or the nares. Purpura may be present over the soft palate. 'Blood blisters' in the mouth signify a marked bleeding tendency. Bleeding from a postextraction dental socket in haemophilia can resemble a flabby bunch of grapes.

● *Intramuscular and joint bleeding.* Severe pain and swelling in muscles and joints (particularly the knee) may indicate bleeding: significantly increases the likelihood of haemophilia.

● *Retroperitoneal bleeding.* The patient may complain of back pain, pain mimicking appendicitis or referred pain along the femoral nerve because of nerve compression in the ileopsoas muscle, and may hold the leg on the affected side in flexion, with an absent knee jerk reflex. Seen in haemophilia and anticoagulant-induced bleeding.

● *CNS bleeding.* Lateralizing signs suggesting a space-occupying lesion may indicate an intracranial bleed. The retina (our only way of directly visualizing the CNS) should be examined for haemorrhages, which are a sign that low-volume CNS bleeding is already occurring, and major intracranial haemorrhage is threatened.

Lymphadenopathy and splenomegaly

Examining lymph node zones

Lymph node enlargement (lymphadenopathy) is best detected by examining each node bearing area in sequence, beginning with the head and neck and working down. Enlarged lymph nodes (more than 1×1 cm) should be measured with a tape. Note if the node has lost: (a) its normal bean-shaped outline; (b) its normal mobility (becoming fixed to underlying tissues or matted with other nodes)—these are signs of pathological enlargement.

● *Head and neck.* The preauricular, occipital, posterior and anterior cervical, submandibular, supra- and infra-clavicular, and scalene node areas are best examined with the patient sitting up and the examiner standing behind them. Palpation should be gentle.

● *Axillae.* The patient is asked to lie flat, and the five spaces of the axilla (apex, medial [chest] wall, lateral [arm] wall, anterior and posterior folds) palpated in turn, with the patient's elbow supported.

● *Abdominal and para-aortic nodes.* Using a gentle bimanual technique, palpate the central abdomen either side of the midline. Enlarged abdominal nodes can be felt as poorly defined masses. This is quite difficult.

● *Pelvic, inguinal and femoral nodes.* The same gentle technique is used in both pelvic fossae. Palpation along the inguinal ligament and the femoral triangle may reveal enlarged nodes, although these are common in normal sexually active individuals.

Lymphadenopathy—local or generalized?

A single node (or contiguous nodes in a single zone) may be enlarged; or there may be generalized lymphadenopathy (enlarged lymph nodes in all areas).

Finding local lymphadenopathy should lead to a search for lesions in the anatomical field drained by the affected nodal group (e.g. in cervical lymphadenopathy, examine the oropharynx for evidence of infection or tumour: in axillary lymphadenopathy, examine the breasts for masses). Early lymphoma, particularly Hodgkin's disease, may involve a single lymph node zone. However, the younger the patient, the more likely that infection is the cause of lymphadenopathy. Tuberculous adenitis can also be localized.

Generalized lymphadenopathy is found in lymphoproliferative disease (e.g. chronic lymphocytic leukaemia) but also in systemic infections (e.g. infectious mononucleosis, HIV infection) and autoimmune disease (e.g. sarcoidosis, systemic lupus erythematosus).

Splenomegaly

Enlargement of the spleen (splenomegaly) is an important finding in a wide range of haematological, inflammatory and infective disorders.

● *Examining the spleen.* The key word is *gently*. Any 'digging' or 'thumping' entails a (low) risk of rupturing the spleen, and the more likely problems of: (a) abdominal 'guarding', obscuring splenomegaly; (b) failing the clinical exam. A massively enlarged spleen extends, banana-like, across the midline into the **right iliac fossa**, so begin fingertip palpation for the splenic tip there. The dipping fingertips move upwards into the **left hypochondrium** and, if the spleen is enlarged, will encounter the tip

History & Examination 15.3: General findings in the clinical examination

Does the patient look: (a) well; (b) unwell; or (c) acutely sick and distressed?

Does the effort of undressing and getting on the couch cause breathlessness?

Is the patient in pain (or other distress), or do certain movements cause pain?

These findings indicate the likely severity of disease and the urgency of finding the diagnosis: they also indicate the need for *gentleness and consideration* during the examination

Clinical examination

Specific findings suggesting anaemia (red cell disorders)
• *Skin*
Pale palmar creases that stay pale when the fingers are gently dorsiflexed*
Spider naevi (liver disease/portal hypertension)
Jaundice (haemolysis)
• *Mucous membranes*
Pale lips, gums and conjunctivae*
Sore red tongue (glossitis—folate or B_{12} deficiency)
• *Musculoskeletal system*
Evidence of rheumatoid arthritis (anaemia of chronic disease)
• *Cardiorespiratory system*
Evidence of compensatory adaptation to anaemia: tachypnoea, tachycardia, forceful apex beat, cardiac flow murmur (aortic, mid-systolic)
• *Abdomen*
Hepatosplenomegaly (haemolysis)
Splenomegaly (haemolysis/portal hypertension)
Masses (stomach, colon, uterus)
Rectal tumour (only perform rectal examination if white cell disorders are excluded: otherwise it may result in local sepsis)
• *Neurological system*
Evidence of peripheral neuropathy or long-tract spinal cord disease (megaloblastic anaemia)
Optic atrophy, dementia, psychosis (megaloblastic anaemia)

Specific findings suggesting haemoglobinopathy (sickle cell disease or thalassaemia)
• *Skin*
Painful ankle ulcers (or scars of healed ulcers) around the medial or lateral malleoli. May be small and punched-out or large and disfiguring
• *Mucous membranes*
Pallor
Jaundice
• *Musculoskeletal system*
Evidence of skeletal distortion by bone marrow hypertrophy (e.g. maxillary overgrowth, frontal skull bossing) or delayed epiphyseal fusion (e.g. sitting height low in proportion to standing height)

Arthritis with or without arthrodesis of hip and shoulder joints resulting from aseptic necrosis
Tender painful bone areas
• *Cardiorespiratory system*
Hyperdynamic circulation with cardiac flow murmur
Evidence of cardiomyopathy with cardiac failure (e.g. iron overload in thalassaemia)
• *Abdomen*
Massive hepatosplenomegaly (thalassaemia)
• *Neurological system*
Evidence of ischaemic stroke (sickle cell disease)

Findings indicating opportunistic infection (white cell disorders)
• *Skin*
Septic spots
Boils
Ulcers
Abscesses
Shingles (herpes zoster)
• *Mucous membranes*
Cold sores (herpes simplex)
Gingivitis and periodontitis
Mouth ulcers
Pharyngitis/tonsillitis
Herpetic lesions of lips and nostrils
• *Cardiorespiratory system*
Pneumonia
Lung abscess
• *Abdomen*
Perianal sepsis
Painful piles
• *Neurological system*
Fever (over 37.5°C)
Meningeal irritation

Findings indicating abnormal bleeding (platelet or coagulation disorders)
• *Skin*
Petechiae (tiny pinpoint red–purple spots)
Purpura (larger confluent purple spots)
Bruises
Haematomas (palpable bruises)
Skin haemorrhages do not blanch on pressure
• *Mucous membranes*
Petechiae and purpura
Blood blisters
Gingival and tooth-socket bleeding
• *Musculoskeletal system*
Acutely swollen, very painful joint, consider haemarthrosis (haemophilia)
Chronically swollen malaligned dysfunctional joint, consider chronic haemophiliac arthropathy

Acute tender muscle swelling, consider intramuscular haematoma (haemophilia)
- *Abdomen*

Evidence of gastrointestinal bleeding (melaena)

Evidence of retroperitoneal haemorrhage (abdominal pain mimicking appendicitis)
- *Neurological system*

Evidence of intracerebral or subarachnoid bleeding

Retinal haemorrhages

Findings indicating invasive (malignant) blood disorders (leukaemias, lymphomas, myeloma)
- *Skin*

Maculopapular skin infiltrates

Skin tumours

Any of the signs indicated above (bone marrow failure)
- *Mucous membranes*

Gum infiltrates

Tonsillar enlargement

Any of the signs indicated above (bone marrow failure)
- *Soft tissues*

Enlarged lymph nodes (lymphadenopathy)

Examination for lymphadenopathy should follow a routine:

With the patient sitting on the edge of the couch, examine the cervical, submandibular and supraclavicular lymph node groups from behind, gently using both hands

Now ask the patient to resume the reclining position and examine both axillae, gently supporting the patient's arm to explore the medial and lateral compartments of the axilla, together with the anterior and posterior axillary folds

Gently examine the inguinal and femoral node compartments

Examination for abdominal and pelvic nodes is performed as part of the abdominal examination (see below)

Normal lymph nodes may be felt in slim individuals: they are small, mobile and bean-shaped

Abnormal lymph nodes are typically more than 1 cm in diameter, lose their normal shape, and are often fixed to the soft tissues and other nodes ('matted')

- *Musculoskeletal system*

Bone tenderness, particularly of sternum, ribs or vertebrae (elicit gently by tapping or light pressure)
- *Abdomen*

Hepatic enlargement or splenomegaly. Detecting splenomegaly requires careful technique:

Always palpate gently, because muscle guarding will hide the spleen

Start from the midline in the suprapubic area and work slowly upward (to the left of the umbilicus) toward the left costal margin, trying to feel the spleen tip

As you do so, ask the patient to take moderately deep breaths in order to feel the tip moving with respiration

If you do not find it, try again starting on the right side of the umbilicus (some spleens grow across the midline)

If you still cannot find it, ask the patient to turn on to their right side and palpate gently under the left costal margin with your right fingertips while gently pulling the patient's left lower ribs toward you with your left hand (preferably get a clinical tutor to demonstrate this technique)

Finally, percuss gently (by light tapping) in the costal margin and over the ribs in the left mid-axillary line, seeking dullness

If you still cannot find it, state confidently 'I cannot detect an enlarged spleen'—but consider confirming this with abdominal ultrasonography

Abdominal lymphadenopathy. Mesenteric lymphadenopathy is sometimes detectable, resembling a 'sack of potatoes' in the middle of the abdomen

Pelvic lymphadenopathy can be detected by gentle palpation in the pelvic fossae

Para-aortic lymphadenopathy can sometimes be felt as a deep midline fullness on very gentle bimanual palpation

These techniques are usually only informative if the nodes are massively enlarged
- *Neurological system*

Cranial nerve lesions

Space-occupying intracranial lesions

Symmetrical peripheral neuropathies (amyloid and other paraproteinaemias)

* For these signs, *compare* with yourself or a colleague

---

moving with respiration. Measure the distance between the spleen tip and the left costal margin with a tape.

- *If the spleen is not found.* Ask the patient to turn on their right side. Then either: (a) cup your left hand around the lower ribs on the left and gently pull them towards you, while using your right fingertips to search for the spleen beneath them; or (b) move around behind the patient and place your right palm on the left costal margin, 'hanging' the fingers over it so their tips are in the left hypochondrium. Ask the patient to breath deeply, and you may feel the spleen tip by these methods.

- *Spleen or kidney?* An enlarged left kidney may mimic splenomegaly. The two can be distinguished by gentle percussion over the mass, the left hypochondrium and the lower ribs in the mid-axillary line: the percussion note will remain dull in splenomegaly ('you can't get above it') but becomes resonant with a renal mass. A gastric air bubble may interfere with this sign.

Enlargement of the spleen and/or liver may be a feature of lymphoproliferative disorders (e.g. Hodgkin's disease and non-Hodgkin's lymphoma) and myeloproliferative disorders (e.g. polycythaemia, chronic myeloid leukaemia

Table 15.6 Causes of splenomegaly

Aetiology	Example
Infection	
Acute bacterial	Septicaemia
	Infective endocarditis
	Typhoid
Acute viral	Infectious mononucleosis, viral hepatitis
Chronic bacterial	Brucellosis, TB
Parasitic	Malaria, schistosomiasis, kala-azar
Inflammation	Rheumatoid arthritis, SLE, sarcoidosis
Haematological	Leukaemia, lymphoma, myeloproliferative disorders, haemoglobinopathies, chronic haemolytic anaemia
Venous congestion	Portal hypertension (liver disease), hepatic and portal vein thrombosis
Other mechanisms	Metabolic storage diseases, amyloidosis

Causes of massive splenomegaly include: chronic malaria and kala-azar (endemic areas). In the UK, chronic myeloid leukaemia and myelofibrosis are more common. Rarely, Gaucher's disease.

[CML] and myelofibrosis [MF]). CML and MF can cause **massive splenomegaly** (defined as a spleen extending across the midline; Table 15.6). A common cause of massive enlargement in malaria-hyperendemic areas is hypertrophic malarial splenomegaly (tropical splenomegaly).

Moderate splenomegaly (10–20 cm) occurs at an earlier stage of the above disorders, and also in:
• A variety of other haematological disorders (e.g. haemolytic anaemia, thalassaemia)
• Association with infections (bacterial, viral or parasitic)

The presence of splenomegaly or hepatomegaly may need to be confirmed by ultrasonography or computerized tomography (CT) scanning, which may also provide further helpful diagnostic information (e.g. liver texture suggestive of hepatitis, cirrhosis or carcinoma) or may reveal the presence of previously unsuspected lymph nodes. For causes of hepatomegaly see Table 9.3, p. 604.

Completing the examination

Patients with severe neutropenia are at risk of invasive bacterial infection in the **perianal tissues** and the ischiorectal spaces (ischiorectal abscess). This area should be inspected for redness and swelling if a patient complains of local pain or pain on defecation, but an internal rectal examination must **not** be performed: it causes severe pain and spread of the organisms into the bloodstream.

The patient's **calves, ankles and feet** should always be examined. Because venous pressure is highest at the ankle, it is often the first place that purpura develop in thrombocytopenia, and the site of swelling, oedema and pain in

DVT. Malleolar skin ulcers, or their residual scars, can be seen in sickle cell anaemia. Local skin infection also seems common in this area, and ischaemic or platelet-induced peripheral cyanosis may affect the toes.

Further examination of the nervous system, heart and lungs, and other organ systems should now be carried out and the findings added to those above.

Investigation

The investigation includes all tests, whether imaging, blood test analyses, biopsy of blood-related tissues such as bone marrow and lymph nodes, intended to lead to a diagnosis. Specific tests for specific diseases will be discussed in the relevant sections below, but a basic set of **initial 'screening' tests** provide useful starting information and are universally applicable (HISTORY & EXAMINATION BOX 15.4).

Haematology
Full blood count
When an automated analyser processes an EDTA-anticoagulated full blood count (**FBC**) sample, it measures, calculates and reports many variables, but the **important** ones are:
• Haemoglobin concentration (**Hb conc, g/dl**)
• Mean cell volume (**MCV, femtolitres/fl**)
• Total white blood cell count (**WBC**)
• Absolute neutrophil count
• Absolute lymphocyte count
• Platelet count

Less informative are the other red cell indices: haematocrit (PCV) is an alternative way of measuring [Hb]: mean cell haemoglobin (MCH) and mean cellular haemoglobin concentration (MCHC), when low indicates a low MCV. A differential WBC expressed as percentage is less useful than absolute neutrophil and lymphocyte counts.

Simple diagnosis using the full blood count
1 *Is the patient anaemic?* Compare the [Hb conc] with the normal ranges given on p. 997 (Table 15.1).
2 *If the patient is anaemic, what is the MCV?*
• If the MCV is < 78 fl the anaemia is microcytic (iron deficiency or thalassaemia trait)
• If the MCV is > 100 fl the anaemia is macrocytic (megaloblastic anaemias, thyroid disease)
• If the MCV is normal (80–100 fl) the anaemia is normocytic (anaemia of inflammation, bone marrow failure)
Microcytic anaemias are always **hypochromic** (low red cell Hb content). This is the reason that a low MCV is always matched by a low MCH and MCHC.

Haematological disease: Clinical presentations at a glance

Family history
- Bleeding tendency
- Thrombotic tendency
- Anaemia
- Sickle cell

Past medical history
- Symptoms since childhood
- Work exposure to carcinogens

Retinopathy
- Sickle cell disease
- Retinal haemorrhage (thrombocytopenia)

Sclera/conjunctivae
- Jaundice (haemolysis)
- Pallor (anaemia)

CNS
- Haemorrhage
- Stroke
- Dementia

Oral cavity
- Pale mucosa
- Sore red tongue
- Gum infiltration (leukaemia)
- Bleeding/ blood blisters (thrombo- cytopenia)

Peripheral lymphadenopathy

Hepatomegaly
- Lymphoma
- Haemolytic anaemia
- Sickle cell disease
- Thalass- aemia

Gallstones
- Pigment + stones (haemolytic anaemias)

Arthritis
- Haemophilia
- Sickle cell disease

Splenomegaly
- Infection
- Malaria
- Lymphoma
- Leukaemia
- Myeloproliferative disease

Bruises
- Any haemostatic disorder

Purpura
- Thrombocytopenia
- Haemophilia

Ankle ulcers
- Sickle cell disease

Urine abnormalities
- Red urine
  Red cells = haematuria
  Haemoglobin only = IV haemolysis
- Bence Jones protein (myeloma)
- Haemosiderinuria = IV haemolysis

Drug use
- Aspirin
- Antithyroid
- NSAIDs
- Oxidants (haemolysis)
- Chemotherapy

History & Examination 15.4: Next steps—how to investigate

Differential diagnosis

As a result of the detailed verbal answers and clinical findings elicited by the history and examination, the clinician constructs a list of possible diagnoses

This list, ranked in order of likelihood (of 'best fit' with the clinical findings) is the differential diagnosis

Always try to construct such a list: try to avoid jumping to a single conclusion too soon

Pretest likelihood

The rank of each possible diagnosis on the differential list represents the 'pretest likelihood' that that particular diagnosis is the correct one

Even a rough ranking (e.g. into high, intermediate or low likelihood) is helpful

When ranking the differential list, the 'goodness of fit' of symptoms and signs with a particular diagnosis should be combined with the incidence of that diagnosis in people who share the age, gender and ethnic origin of the patient

Purpose of initial investigations

To raise or lower the pretest likelihood of each diagnosis on the list, so that:

Some possibilities are 'excluded' by attaining very low post-test likelihoods

One possibility attains a sufficiently high post-test likeli- hood that it becomes the 'working diagnosis'

Initial investigations that carry out this purpose are:

If the history and examination suggests a red cell or white cell disorder, or a haematological malignancy, perform a **full blood count**

If they suggest a bleeding tendency, perform a **full blood count** plus **coagulation screen**

Confirmatory ('definitive') testing

In haematology, the next stage is often to confirm a diag- nosis by detailed study of blood cells, their chromo- somes or DNA, or by specific assay of plasma proteins

These definitive tests often consume resources: they require the time of skilled laboratory scientists and/or are expensive

Therefore, they should only be performed at the 'working diagnosis' stage, not at the 'differential diagnosis' stage

Macrocytic and **normocytic** anaemias are nearly always **normochromic** (normal red cell Hb content).

Answering questions 1 and 2 therefore gets us halfway towards the cause of anaemia—by reading two numbers!

3 *Is the WBC increased or decreased?* Compare the WBC with the normal range (Table 15.1).

4 *If the WBC is increased, which cell type is responsible?* Compare the absolute neutrophil, lymphocyte, monocyte and eosinophil counts with the normal ranges (Table 15.4).

15

5 *If the WBC is decreased, which cell type is lacking?* As for question 4.

Answering questions 3–5 allows an initial classification into neutrophilia/neutropenia, lymphocytosis/lymphopenia, etc. Because each of these categories has a short list of common causes, this now becomes the differential diagnosis, and further tests should focus on increasing or decreasing the likelihood of each item on the list.

6 *Is the platelet count low (thrombocytopenia) or high (thrombocytosis)?* Compare the platelet count with the normal range (Table 15.1). Thrombocytopenia correlates with bleeding symptoms, while thrombocytosis (particularly more than $1000 \times 10^9/l$) can lead to both bleeding and thrombosis. Both have a short differential diagnostic list.

Reticulocyte count

Reticulocytes normally comprise approximately 1% ($25–100 \times 10^9/l$) of circulating red cells. They increase in number if there is increased red cell production (e.g. following haemorrhage or in response to haemolysis). Any reticulocyte count over 7% (more than $300 \times 10^9/l$) is proof of a haemolytic anaemia. In anaemia, an increased reticulocyte count shows that the bone marrow is functioning, but percentage reticulocyte counts may be misleading in severe anaemia (2% of little is not very much), so an absolute reticulocyte count is preferred (see p. 997).

Blood film microscopy

Microscopy of a stained peripheral blood film is necessary if any part of the FBC is abnormal, or if the clinical findings suggest a blood disorder or malaria. Key observations are:
- Confirming the automated FBC findings
- Checking the correctness of automated identification of white cell types
- Identification of **abnormal white cells** (e.g. leukaemic blasts)
- Recognition of **red cell abnormalities** (e.g. sickled cells, oval macrocytes)
- Recognition of a **leukoerythroblastic** film (granulocyte and red cell precursors in the peripheral blood)
- Detection of intracellular **parasites** (malaria)

Bone marrow aspirate and trephine biopsy

Bone marrow aspiration, in which fluid is drawn by syringe through a hollow needle inserted into the medullary cavity of the posterior iliac crest, obtains a marrow sample that is stained and microscopically examined in the same way as a peripheral blood smear. The detailed cytology of normal and abnormal marrow cells can be assessed in this way. The marrow cells obtained by aspiration are still viable, so can also be subjected to cytogenetic, cell culture and molecular studies.

Microscopy of stained films obtained by bone marrow aspirate is a key diagnostic test in the presence of:
- Macrocytic anaemia (? megaloblastic anaemia)
- Unexplained anaemia (? myelodysplasia or infection)
- Persisting neutropenia
- Thrombocytopenia (? immune thrombocytopenic purpura or leukaemia)
- Significant (high or rising) paraproteinaemia (? myeloma)

Bone marrow trephine biopsy, in which a small core of bone marrow (about the size of a matchstick minus the head) is removed from the posterior iliac crest using a trephine (cutting) needle, is often performed immediately following aspiration. Because the biopsy is then fixed and decalcified before sectioning and histological examination, the cells are no longer viable and individual cell detail is lost; however, the complete architecture and structure of the marrow is preserved for analysis. The trephine gives a more accurate measure of total marrow cellularity than the aspirate, and is therefore vital in assessing bone marrow failure with pancytopenia. A trephine biopsy for marrow histology, in addition to the aspirate, is vital in the following settings:
- Abnormal white cells in the blood (? acute/chronic leukaemia, myelodysplasia, lymphomas)
- Pancytopenia (? aplastic anaemia)
- Leukoerythroblastic blood film (? bone marrow infiltration by cancer or myelofibrosis)
- Any situation where the marrow aspirate is 'dry'

Because both marrow aspirate and trephine take a very small sample from a very large organ, both are subject to *sampling artefact* and may misrepresent or miss disease altogether, particularly if a disorder involves the marrow in a focal ('patchy') way.

Sickle solubility test (sickle screening test)

This rapid test for the presence of haemoglobin S (HbS; which forms a precipitate when exposed to a reducing agent) is the most *misunderstood* test in haematology. It does **not** mean that the patient has sickle cell disease, only that their blood contains *some* HbS. It cannot distinguish between the harmless heterozygous state (HbAS, sickle cell trait) and the sickle diseases HbSS, HbSC or $HbS\beta^0$ thal. To do that requires the following test.

Haemoglobin electrophoresis

Separates all the haemoglobin species present in a blood sample by their differing mobility in an electric field. Common haemoglobin variants can be recognized by their position on celluloid or agar gels (which takes about 24 h), or preferably—because of its speed—by their elution profile on high-pressure liquid chromatography (HPLC).

Direct antiglobulin test

The direct antiglobulin test (DAT) recognizes anti-red cell antibodies bound to the surface of circulating red cells by bridging them with an antibody against human antibodies, causing the red cells to agglutinate if the test is positive. It is used: (a) if there is evidence of a haemolytic anaemia (when a positive DAT indicates autoimmune haemolytic anaemia); or (b) if there is suspicion of an antibody-mediated blood transfusion reaction (when a positive DAT confirms the diagnosis).

Coagulation screening tests

These tests should be performed **if there is any evidence of a bleeding disorder** in the patient or a first-degree relative. They effectively increase or decrease the likelihood of a bleeding disorder and guide investigation towards a specific cause. Using them to 'screen' whole populations (e.g. everyone attending hospital) is, by contrast, a misleading waste of time.

Prothrombin time

Prothrombin time (PT) tests the **tissue factor** (TF) driven 'extrinsic' clotting pathway. Usually expressed as a ratio, the international normalized ratio (**INR: normal = less than 1.2**). An INR of more than 1.2 indicates a deficiency of *any* or *all* of coagulation **factors VII, X, V, II and fibrinogen**. The higher the INR, the more severe the deficiency.

Activated partial thromboplastin time

Activated partial thromboplastin time (APTT) tests the contact activated 'intrinsic' clotting pathway. Usually expressed as a ratio, the **APTTr**. An APTTr of more than 1.2 indicates a deficiency of *any* or *all* of coagulation factors (XII), XI, IX, VIII, X, V, II and fibrinogen. The higher the APTTr, the more severe the deficiency. Factor (XII) is in brackets because its deficiency does **not** cause bleeding.

Thrombin clotting time

This tests fibrinogen. Expressed as a time (seconds). TCT more than 14 s indicates **fibrinogen** deficiency (hypofibrinogenaemia), or interference with fibrin polymerization by an abnormal fibrinogen molecule (dysfibrinogen) or a paraprotein.

Simple diagnosis using the coagulation screen (Fig. 15.10) The three tests make diagnostic sense when their results are viewed together. **Five** main patterns occur:
1 *INR ↑, others normal.* Factor VII deficiency. This is a rare inherited disorder, but because factor VII is very sensitive to oral anticoagulant therapy this pattern can be seen during the first few days of treatment with coumarin drugs such as warfarin.

2 *APTTr ↑, others normal.* Factor (XII), XI, IX or VIII deficiency. This pattern is seen in haemophilia A (factor VIII deficiency) and haemophilia B (factor IX deficiency), severe inherited bleeding disorders.
3 *INR ↑ and APTTr ↑, TCT normal.* Vitamin K deficiency or established oral anticoagulant therapy (deficiency of factors II, VII, IX and X).
4 *TCT ↑, others normal.* Indicates hypofibrinogenaemia, or interference with fibrin formation (e.g. by paraprotein). The TCT is more sensitive to fibrinogen abnormalities than the INR or APTTr.
5 *All abnormal (usually with ↓ platelet count).* Hepatic failure or disseminated intravascular coagulation (DIC).

Fibrin D-dimer assay

This detects a plasmin-mediated breakdown product of fully formed fibrin (clot). An increased level indicates the formation of clot in the circulation in DIC (D-dimers ↑↑) and DVT/pulmonary embolism (D-dimers ↑).

'Routine investigations' and thinking

Thought applied (as above) to the results of simple initial tests, which are usually available within 24 h of sampling, can lead rapidly and logically to diagnosis (which usually requires confirmatory tests, described below for specific disorders). The basic tests are often performed as a 'routine', but the thinking sadly is not.

Biochemistry

Haematinic assays

Iron, folate and cobalamin (vitamin B_{12}) assays. Serum haematinic levels in health are given in Table 15.7 and in different haematological disorders in Table 15.8.

Other biochemical changes

- Hypercalcaemia is common in **myeloma**
- Renal failure (↑ creatinine ↑ urea ↑ K^+) is a major risk in **myeloma** with heavy renal Bence Jones (light chain) excretion

Table 15.7 Normal serum haematinic levels

Haematinic	Level
Serum iron	18–48 µmol/l (men)
	120–30 µmol/l (women)
Serum total iron-binding capacity (TIBC)	45–72 µmol/l
Serum ferritin	20–250 µg/l (men)
	15–150 µg/l (women)
Serum folate	3–15 ng/ml
Red cell folate	150–500 mg/ml
Serum vitamin B_{12}	160–1000 pg/ml

Disease	Serum iron	TIBC	Percentage transferrin saturation	Ferritin
Iron deficiency	↓	↑	↓↓	↓
Chronic disease	↓	→ or ↓	↓	→ or ↑
Sideroblastic anaemia	↑	→	↑	↑↑
Haemochromatosis	↑	→	↑	↑↑
Ineffective erythropoiesis	↑	→	↑	↑↑
Hypoproteinaemia	↓	↓	→	→

Table 15.8 Serum iron, total iron-binding capacity (TIBC) and ferritin in different diseases

↓, Decreased; ↑, increased; →, normal.

- Hyperuricaemia (with **gout** or renal impairment) occurs in myeloproliferative disorders and (with hyperphosphataemia) in **tumour lysis syndrome** after chemotherapy of acute leukaemia

Immunology

Paraprotein (monoclonal gammopathy) detection and quantification

A **paraprotein** is an abnormal monoclonal immunoglobulin produced by a malignant clone of antibody-producing B cells (usually plasma cells). It appears as a single dense band (sometimes termed a 'spike' or 'M-band') on serum electrophoresis. Paraproteins are usually composed of entire immunoglobulin molecules, their clonal nature indicated by the possession of a single light-chain type (κ or λ). Often, the malignant clone produces excess free light chains (**Bence Jones protein**). Some produce light chains only (light-chain myeloma) or nothing at all (non-secretory myeloma).

Paraproteins are often found on screening fit elderly individuals: their incidence increases with each passing decade over 60 years. Many of these are of low concentration (less than 10 g/l) and will never develop into an overt plasma cell tumour (myeloma), but this cannot be predicted with certainty, so clinical follow-up with serial paraprotein quantification is needed. Because the eventual outcome of this situation is unknown, it is termed monoclonal gammopathy of undetermined significance (**MGUS**).

The immunoglobulin class of the paraprotein is associated with specific disorders:
- MGUS (IgG, IgA, IgM)
- Myeloma (IgG, IgA, IgD)
- Waldenström's macroglobulinaemia (IgM)
- Chronic lymphoproliferative disorders (IgM)
- IgG/IgA paraproteins over 80 g/l or IgM over 40 g/l are associated with **hyperviscosity syndrome**

Bence Jones protein detection and quantification
Urine should always be tested for the presence of free light chains when a serum paraprotein is detected. If found, they should be quantified in a 24-h urine collection. High levels of more than 2 g/24 h (especially of λ light chains, which are more nephrotoxic) are a risk factor for **renal failure** and **amyloidosis**.

Microbiology

Isolation of bacteria, fungi, viruses and other pathogens

Many patients with blood diseases are vulnerable to infection with opportunistic organisms because of: (a) neutropenia caused by the disease or chemotherapy; (b) asplenism; or (c) poor cell-mediated immunity because of lymphoma or immunosuppressive therapy. Culture and isolation of organisms from blood, secretions, venous access sites and devices, or from skin, lung or other tissue biopsies is often needed to guide antibiotic, antifungal or antiviral therapy.

Immunocompromised patients with fever need urgent microbiological investigation including blood cultures from peripheral and central lines, and sputum, urine and stool cultures. However, because of the high degree of risk, **empirical** antibiotic or antifungal therapy must start before the microbiological results are available, later being modified in the light of culture results.

Occasionally, culture of a **bone marrow** aspirate is indicated to detect infection with **mycobacteria** when miliary or cryptic tuberculosis is suspected.

Serological and nucleic-acid-based diagnosis and monitoring of transfusion-associated infection. In patients who require life-long therapy with blood or blood products, past or (rarely) present infection with transfusion-associated viruses (HIV, hepatitis B and C) are a risk. Serological surveillance, and viral serotype and load estimations are vital to patient safety and management.

Diagnostic imaging

Haematologists are heavy users of imaging because of the need to define the level of dissemination of malignant diseases of the blood (which tend to involve many sites and can invade all body compartments) and detect lesions caused by opportunistic infection, bleeding and thrombosis.

Radiology

Chest radiography

- Lung infiltrates in opportunistic pneumonia, sickle cell acute chest syndrome, tumour invasion
- Abscess formation in fungal infection
- Wedge shadows in pulmonary embolism
- Hilar and mediastinal lymphadenopathy or thymic enlargement in leukaemia or lymphoma (particularly Hodgkin's disease)
- Lytic bone disease (myeloma) in ribs, clavicles

Skeletal radiography

- Lytic bone disease (holes in the bones) and associated pathological fractures in myeloma—particularly the axial skeleton (skull, ribs, vertebrae, pelvis)
- Aseptic necrosis of the hip in sickle cell disease
- Joint damage and cartilage loss in haemophilia

Ultrasound

- Confirmation of spleen and liver size
- Gallbladder stones in haemolytic anaemias
- DVT (Doppler compression technique)
- Detection of lymphadenopathy/tumour masses in inaccessible sites (abdominal, pelvic, retroperitoneal)
- Ultrasound-guided biopsy

Nuclear medicine

- Lung (V/Q) scans for pulmonary emboli
- Scans using labelled blood cells (e.g. blood volume studies in polycythaemia)

Computerized tomography and magnetic resonance imaging

- Detection of lymphadenopathy/tumour masses in inaccessible sites (abdominal, pelvic, retroperitoneal, CNS)
- Cord compression in myeloma
- Cerebral infarction (thrombosis or sickle cell anaemia)
- Cerebral infection (abscess, meningitis)
- Joints in sickle cell disease and haemophilia (magnetic resonance imaging; MRI)
- CT-guided biopsy

Histopathology

Bone marrow trephine biopsy (see p. 1018)

Indicated in any potential clonal or infiltrative marrow disease (leukaemia, lymphoma, myeloproliferative disease, leukoerythroblastic film) because: (a) it reveals cells that may not be aspirated (hence invisible on aspirate smears, e.g. carcinoma cells); and (b) it gives a more accurate estimate of the percentage infiltration with abnormal cells and general cellularity.

Lymph node aspiration and biopsy

If enlarged lymph nodes cannot be explained by proven local or systemic infection (reactive lymphadenopathy), diagnosis requires pathological examination of a node biopsy. **Fine needle aspiration** biopsy with cytological examination of the aspirate is the first step. If the findings indicate lymphoma, **excision biopsy** of a complete node may be necessary for accurate classification of the tumour, while in other diseases (e.g. head and neck carcinoma) excision is unnecessary and potentially harmful.

General principles of management

Supportive treatment

Communication and consent

Leukaemia and related malignant disorders provoke anxiety, depression and potential despair in patients and their families, and therapy is dangerous and arduous. **Breaking bad news** about the diagnosis in a way that meets the individual patient's concerns requires formal training in this skill. Life-long inherited diseases (sickle cell anaemia, thalassaemia, haemophilia) demand a comprehensive approach to care, supporting the patient and affected family throughout life, including reproductive advice and carrier diagnosis. For these reasons, the multidisciplinary team should include members with counselling skills. Both spoken and written information should be employed to address the needs of patients and their families. Patient support groups provide additional help. **Valid consent** by the patient to all invasive diagnostic procedures and therapies, particularly blood or blood product transfusion and chemotherapy, must be secured: this too will often involve written information, counselling skills and as many interviews with patients and their families as it takes. The resulting consent must be clearly documented.

Transfusion: blood component support

In blood disease there is failure of production or function of one or more key cells or molecules that normally protect the individual from anaemia, infection or bleeding. Deficiency can often be corrected by simple treatment of the underlying cause (e.g. iron or vitamin therapy), when waiting for the replenished bone marrow to respond is all that is required and transfusions would be wrong. In acute leukaemia, therapy at first worsens bone marrow failure, and the patient must be supported with red cell and platelet transfusion through inevitable periods (lasting about 28 days) of severe pancytopenia. In aplastic anaemia, in which therapy may only be partly successful, the pancytopenia may require support for months to years. In thalassaemia major, regular red cell transfusions must be life-long; and in severe haemophilia, regular infusions of clotting factors will also be required in the long term.

In view of these differing needs, the basic resource of donated whole blood is processed to create different blood components, each with specific purposes.

Red cells

The purpose of red cell transfusion is to increase the haemoglobin concentration [Hb] from a level causing symptoms to one that does not. In anaemia (unless correctable, e.g. iron deficiency, and **not** in sickle cell anaemia) transfusion is justifiable when [Hb] falls below **7 g/dl** (if there is cardiovascular disease, less than 9 g/dl). Each unit of red cells (**approximately 300 ml**) raises [Hb] by **0.7–1.0 g/dl**. Except in special situations, transfusion aims at [Hb] no higher than **9–10 g/dl**. The reason for red cell transfusion must always be written in the casenotes.

Platelets

The purpose of platelet transfusion is to increase the platelet count from a level causing bleeding to one that does not. There is a less clear-cut relationship between the platelet count and the bleeding risk: some patients with immune thrombocytopenia and platelet count less than 10×10^9/l will not bleed at all; a sick patient with platelets of 40×10^9/l may bleed; and surgery requires a platelet count of 100×10^9/l. Platelet transfusion depends on the clinical assessment of bleeding and related risk.

Frozen plasma

The purpose of infusing (thawed) plasma is to correct deficiencies of several clotting factors in acute situations (e.g. hepatic failure, massive blood transfusion, anticoagulant overdose).

Clotting factors

The purpose of clotting factor concentrates is to correct a deficiency of a single factor (e.g. factor VIII in haemophilia A) in order to arrest bleeding. Plasma-derived concentrates are being replaced by synthetic recombinant clotting factors as the treatment of choice.

Risks of transfusion

Acute haemolytic (ABO) transfusion reaction. Incompatible transfused red cells are destroyed by the recipient's anti-A or anti-B antibodies (see p. 998 and EMERGENCY BOX 15.1).
- *Usual cause:* transfusing red cells intended for a different person (**wrong blood**), when the risk of ABO mismatch

is **1 in 3**. Only a few millilitres of ABO-incompatible cells are needed to cause this reaction. This potentially lethal catastrophe is *avoidable* by good procedures in: (a) sample labelling; (b) blood bank practice; and (c) bedside pre-transfusion checks.
- *Symptoms:* acute fear; flushing; pain at drip site; back and/or abdominal pain.
- *Signs:* fever; hypotension; bleeding; red urine (resulting from haemoglobin—microscopy shows no red cells).
- *Management:* **stop the blood**; keep the drip open; resuscitate and support the circulation (EMERGENCY BOX 15.1).

Fluid overload. A good reason to avoid transfusing an anaemic patient, when iron or vitamin B_{12} would do, is that anaemic people usually have an expanded blood volume. Transfusing too much, or too fast, leads to acute cardiac decompensation.
- *Symptoms:* breathlessness; cough
- *Signs:* basal crepitations; ↑ jugular venous pressure (JVP); tachycardia
- *Management:* oxygen, diuretic therapy

Rhesus-type (IgG-mediated) transfusion reaction. Immune IgG anti-red cell antibodies react with incompatible transfused cells to cause phagocytosis in the reticuloendothelial system and antibody-dependent cellular cytotoxicity. The result is rapid extravascular destruction of the cells (over 24–48 h), without the explosive intravascular events of ABO incompatibility. It is unpleasant for the patient, renders the transfusion useless and is a reportable untoward event.
- *Symptoms:* fever, chills, malaise.
- *Signs:* jaundice, [Hb] rapidly falls to pretransfusion level.
- *Management:* symptomatic. Get the selection of blood for transfusion right next time.

Transfusion-transmitted infection. In order of magnitude, current UK risk estimates of acquiring infection from a single blood component unit are:
- **Hepatitis B:** 1 in 100 000
- **Hepatitis C:** 1 in 400 000
- **HIV:** 1 in 4 million;
- **New variant Creutzfeldt–Jakob disease (vCJD) prion** (hypothetical): unknown

These figures, achieved by rigorous donor selection and testing, suggest that the widespread fear of transfusion-transmitted infection is misplaced. However, in this area of medical practice *tolerance* of risk is even lower than the *incidence*. Recently, all blood components in the UK have been leucodepleted, and plasma products sourced outside the UK, in an attempt to evade the hypothetical risk of vCJD transmission.

Iron overload (transfusion haemosiderosis). Each unit of red cells contains 250 mg iron: this intravenous iron load cannot be excreted. Patients on chronic long-term transfusion regimens (e.g. thalassaemia major) will develop endocrine failure and die of cardiac iron toxicity in their mid-teens unless constant chelation therapy is administered.

Haemopoietic stem cell transplantation

HSCs are capable of repopulating, and thereby replacing, a damaged or abnormal bone marrow (see p. 994). They exist in low numbers in the marrow itself, and enter the circulating blood when induced to do so by administration of the cytokine G-CSF, or during the period of marrow regeneration that follows myelosuppressive chemotherapy. HSCs can therefore be **harvested** from patients or normal donors by:
- Marrow aspiration from multiple sites (general anaesthetic required)
- Leukapheresis (separation of nucleated cells) from blood by automated cell separators after G-CSF or chemotherapy. The cells obtained this way are termed **peripheral blood stem cells** (**PBSCs**).

When required, the HSCs are infused via a vein in the same way as a blood transfusion and spontaneously 'home' to the bone marrow niche environment, where they engraft and proliferate. Harvested HSCs can be used immediately, or cryopreserved to be stored or transported. They are used in two ways:

1 *Autologous HSC infusion (autograft).* Performed in patients with haematological malignancies (and some solid tumours) as part of a course of treatment, if their disease is considered to be sensitive to **high-dose chemotherapy**. The patient's own HSCs are harvested and stored. The patient can then be treated with a dose of chemotherapy that would otherwise cause dangerous marrow suppression. The stored HSCs are infused as soon as the chemotherapeutic agent has left the circulation, and normal blood counts return in 11–14 days.

2 *Allogeneic HSC transplantation.* This is a true transplant in which HSCs harvested from a **normal donor**, who may be **related** or **unrelated** to the patient, are infused and repopulate the marrow of a **recipient** with a bone marrow disease. Because the bone marrow is an immune effector organ, there is a risk that the recipient will reject the transplant. There is also a risk that the transplanted marrow will attack its new host causing **graft-vs.-host disease** (**GVHD**), which may be mutilating or fatal. In order to minimize the risk of these severe complications, the donor and recipient must be closely matched at the molecular level for their **human leucocyte antigen** (**HLA**) types. In addition, the pre-existing stem cells must be eliminated by an appropriate **conditioning regimen** (involving high-dose chemotherapy, radiotherapy or anti-HSC antibodies, depending on the underlying disease). Finally, continued **immunosuppression** with ciclosporin A must be given to prevent GVHD. Allogeneic HSC transplantation is a challenging therapy that must only be carried out in specialist centres. It is used in carefully selected and counselled patients with the following disorders:
- Haematological malignancies, particularly acute myeloid leukaemia (AML)
- Aplastic anaemia
- Thalassaemia major
- Sickle cell anaemia
- Severe immunodeficiency diseases

Antimicrobial agents

Administration of combined broad-spectrum antibiotics —at the **first sign of fever, without waiting for culture results**—is a life-saving therapeutic rule in neutropenic and immunosuppressed haematology patients. In the 1970s it transformed the survival of patients undergoing leukaemia therapy, and has made the era of bone marrow transplantation possible.

Palliative care

Not all malignant blood disorders respond to therapy, and even fewer are reliably cured. The development of expertise in palliative (symptom-relieving) care, first in the hospice movement and then by acute hospital-based palliative care teams, has greatly improved symptom control and quality of life for these patients (see Chapter 16).

Specific treatment

Treatment aims

Treatment should only be embarked upon if both doctor and patient have a shared and clearly stated concept of the aim of the therapy: what is it intended (and likely) to achieve?

Haemato-oncology

Curative intent. Some malignant blood diseases are potentially curable. They share the feature of a high 'growth fraction' (the proportion of malignant cells dividing rapidly, and therefore sensitive to cytotoxic chemotherapy). About 70% of younger patients with acute lymphoblastic leukaemia and Hodgkin's disease will enter long-term remission with a high chance of eventual cure. There is also a reasonable chance of long-term survival in younger patients with acute myeloid leukaemia and high-grade non-Hodgkin's lymphoma (approximately 50%). In these diseases, intensive therapy with curative intent is given.

15

Palliative intent. Many malignant blood diseases are not yet curable. They tend to be chronic disorders with a sluggish tumour growth rate (low growth fraction) and therefore limited sensitivity to cytotoxic chemotherapy. Myeloma, chronic lymphocytic leukaemia, and low-grade non-Hodgkin's lymphomas fall into this group. In these diseases, therapy is given with palliative intent—to control symptoms and preserve the quality of life for as long as possible. Cytotoxic and other disease-modifying treatment is usually low dose, but sometimes high dose and intensive if it provides longer and/or better symptom control.

Haemoglobinopathies

Supportive therapy and its complications. Careful use of red cell transfusions are the basis of therapy, but lead to iron overload. Iron chelation therapy is crucial to fend off the toxic effects of iron. Until recently the only effective chelator (desferrioxamine) had to be given by prolonged subcutaneous infusion, a therapy at the limits of patient bearability. New oral iron chelators (e.g. deferiprone) have been a useful new development.

Disease modification. Hydroxyurea (hydroxycarbamide) is a myelosuppressive agent (reduces bone marrow proliferation) that partly derepresses haemoglobin F synthesis in adult red cell precursors. Increased intra-erythrocytic HbF is a potent antisickling agent. About half of patients with sickle cell anaemia who are able to tolerate chronic hydroxyurea therapy will have fewer crises, higher haemoglobin and consequent improvement in quality of life. The search is on for more effective agents.

Autoimmune disorders

Immunosuppressive therapy. Careful use of corticosteroid therapy is the central approach to autoimmune thrombocytopenia and haemolytic anaemia—the key is to select only patients who need treatment, because many patients whose bone marrow output is able to keep pace with the autoimmune platelet or red cell consumption do not have severe cytopenias or symptoms. However, if treatment is indicated, a full dose of 1 mg/kg prednisone is needed for reliable response. Once response is achieved, the steroid dose is tapered and ideally withdrawn after 6–8 weeks, avoiding long-term steroid side-effects: in about 50% of steroid-responsive cases, the disease remains in remission. Intravenous high-dose immunoglobulin (IVIG) is used if a rapid response is needed, but its effect lasts only 3–4 weeks.

Splenectomy. If autoimmune thrombocytopenia or haemolytic anaemia do not respond well to corticosteroid therapy or a good response is followed by relapse, splenectomy is the standard therapy, with a 60% long-term remission rate. However, the life-long vulnerability of splenectomized patients to overwhelming septicaemia with encapsulated bacteria mandates long-term penicillin prophylaxis.

Bleeding disorders

Replacement therapy. In the inherited single-gene (single clotting factor) deficiencies haemophilia A and B, treatment of severely affected individuals should begin in infancy as prophylaxis—regular infusions of the missing factor in a recombinant form (genetically engineered) if national financial health resources permit. Most adult patients in richer economies, and all patients with access to therapy in others, rely on (currently safe, highly screened and antivirally treated) plasma-derived concentrates. These agents are so effective in eliminating the acute and chronic complications of haemophilia that therapeutic improvement focuses on the *delivery* of care, which should be as closely tailored to the patient's life as possible.

Thrombotic disorders

Antithrombotic therapy. Haematologists are mainly concerned with the therapy of venous thromboembolic disease (VTED), particularly in its recurrent form, using anticoagulants.

Acute therapy: heparin. Heparin is the drug of choice in the initial treatment, but the original standard therapy (intravenous unfractionated heparin in a hospital bed, with frequent monitoring tests) is being replaced by low-molecular-weight heparin (LMWH) therapy administered subcutaneously at home without tests.

Continued therapy: coumarin. Oral coumarin drugs such as warfarin remain the standard for continued therapy of VTED, aiming to prevent recurrence. Six months' therapy is usual after a first VTED and long-term therapy for recurrence. Regular monitoring with the INR test ensures safe and protective intensity of anticoagulation. It is likely that oral drugs requiring less monitoring (e.g. ximelagatran) will start to begin to replace coumarins in some patients over the next few years.

Drugs

Cytotoxic chemotherapy

The purpose of cytotoxic therapy (also known as anti-leukaemic, antitumour or myelosuppressive therapy) is to kill abnormal cells, thereby reducing the size of the malignant clone. If this reduction is enough, the patient enters remission. Remission (defined as a complete lack of detectable malignant cells) is a vital endpoint in therapy because cure is not possible without it. Unfortunately, many patients relapse after a period of remission because reduction of the malignant clone was insufficient. For this reason, ways of increasing the dosage of chemotherapy (including haemopoietic stem cell infusions—known as bone marrow transplants) have been introduced. Cytotoxic drug classes useful in haematological malignancies are as follow.

Alkylating agents
- *Typical drugs:* chlorambucil and cyclophosphamide
- *Mechanism of action:* DNA damage
- *Side-effects:* (a) early: pancytopenia, mucositis, hair loss, cystitis; (b) late: infertility, secondary leukaemia
- *High-dose option?* Yes

Antimetabolites
- *Typical drugs:* methotrexate, cytosine arabinoside
- *Mechanism of action:* mimic nucleic acid precursors
- *Side-effects:* (a) early: pancytopenia, hair loss, mucositis; (b) late: few
- *High-dose option?* Yes

Anthracyclines
- *Typical drugs:* daunorubicin, doxorubicin
- *Mechanism of action:* cross-link DNA
- *Side-effects:* (a) early: mucositis, pancytopenia, hair loss, nausea; (b) late: cardiotoxicity
- *High-dose option?* No

Vinca alkaloids
- *Typical drug:* vincristine
- *Mechanism:* spindle poison
- *Side-effects:* (a) early: abdominal pain, neuropathy; (b) late: neuropathy
- *High-dose option?* No

Combination chemotherapy

As can be seen above, the therapeutic effects of cytotoxic agents are summative (all suppress HSCs, which is the key to remission) while the toxicities, although similar, show just enough difference to be able to combine agents *without* lethal summation of toxicity. Lasting remissions were first obtained (in Hodgkin's disease) by exploiting this fact with a drug combination. Since then, combination therapy has been the central approach to treatment. Typically, *cycles* of combination chemotherapy are given with gaps for recovery, the whole course of therapy (6–8 cycles) being termed a chemotherapeutic *regimen*. High-dose therapy, however, usually consists of a single agent.

Biological (disease-modifying) agents

Interferon-α has been used in chronic myeloid leukaemia (CML) and myeloma. In a proportion of patients it limits the progression of the disorder, at the cost of side-effects of general malaise and depression. In about 30% of patients with CML, a slow decrease—even disappearance—of the malignant clone occurs. Recently, the introduction of a 'designer' drug (imatinib), an **inhibitor** of the mutant transduction factor found in CML, has led to impressive early responses. In myeloma, the **antiangiogenic** drug thalidomide has produced good disease responses in about 50% of treated patients. These new classes of therapy will undoubtedly expand in the future.

Immunosuppressive agents

Corticosteroids are discussed above. In aplastic anaemia, where cell-mediated immunity seems to play a part in stem cell suppression, **antilymphocyte globulin** (ALG, a horse antibody against human lymphocytes) is used. The oral immunosuppressive agent **ciclosporin** can be tried in steroid-resistant autoimmune disorders and has a central role in post bone marrow transplantation in preventing GVHD.

Haematinics

Ferrous sulphate. This is the basic iron replacement agent for iron-deficiency anaemia. Full-dose therapy (200 mg three times daily) can be poorly complied with: 200 mg once or twice daily works if taken consistently for 3–6 months, taking a full course is more important than the daily dose. No other forms of iron are recommended, although parenteral iron is available for special situations (e.g. exacerbation of Crohn's disease by oral iron).

Hydroxocobalamin. This is the parenteral form of vitamin B_{12}. In pernicious anaemia, 1 mg (1 ml) is administered as 3-monthly maintenance therapy by intramuscular injection.

Folic acid. 5 mg daily by mouth is given in folate deficiency, and to prevent exhaustion of folate supplies in chronic haemolytic anaemias (e.g. sickle cell disease).

Diseases and their management

Anaemia

The causes of anaemia (Table 15.9) are:
- Defective red cell production
- Increased red cell destruction
- Red cell loss through haemorrhage

Mechanism	Examples
Defective red cell production	
Defective haem production	Lead toxicity
Defective globin production	Thalassaemia
Marrow hypoplasia	Idiopathic or drug-induced aplastic anaemia
Marrow invasion	Lymphoma, metastatic cancer
Impaired DNA synthesis	Vitamin B_{12} deficiency, folate deficiency
Increased red cell loss	
Haemolysis	Red cell membrane defect, autoimmune haemolytic anaemia
Acute haemorrhage	
Chronic haemorrhage	Iron-deficiency anaemia

Table 15.9 Pathophysiological classification of anaemia

A simple diagnostic approach to anaemia is given on p. 1016.

Microcytic anaemias

Microcytic anaemia is defined as anaemia associated with a low MCV (less than 78 fl). It is always hypochromic (MCH less than 27 pg) as well. In microcytic anaemia, each red cell contains less haemoglobin than it should. This occurs because of shortage of one of the building blocks of haemoglobin: iron deficiency (acquired, very common); globin chain deficiency (thalassaemia, inherited, common); or haem deficiency (lead poisoning, acquired, rare).

Iron-deficiency anaemia

Epidemiology

Incidence. 10–15% of all women of reproductive age.

Prevalence. 500–600 million people worldwide.

Age. All ages.

Sex. More common in women.

Ethnicity. All ethnic groups, but most common in the developing world.

Genetics. N/A.

Geography. A worldwide marker of poverty.

Disease mechanisms

The diagnosis of iron deficiency anaemia is never enough in itself; the underlying cause must be found. In a **woman of reproductive age**, iron deficiency is nearly always caused by imbalance between her dietary intake of iron and her iron losses (monthly menstrual loss plus one or more pregnancies), so that detailed investigation is not indicated unless there are symptoms (e.g. abdominal pain, rectal blood loss) suggesting another cause. However, in **all males and postmenopausal women**, the development of iron deficiency must be *assumed to be caused by an early curable gastrointestinal malignancy* (particularly colorectal carcinoma) until proven otherwise by full gastrointestinal investigation, including endoscopy.

After crossing the intestinal mucosal cell and entering the portal circulation, iron is transported in serum bound to transferrin.

Transferrin-bound iron is taken up by cells expressing transferrin receptors (particularly erythroblasts and hepatocytes). It is then either incorporated into haemoglobin, myoglobin or iron-containing enzymes, or taken up by the two storage proteins, ferritin and haemosiderin, which together constitute the storage compartment (Fig. 15.14).

Ferritin is a water-soluble complex of ferric hydroxide and a protein, apoferritin. It is present in minute amounts in the serum, where its concentration correlates with total body iron.

Haemosiderin is found mainly in macrophages, is water insoluble, and is formed from aggregates of altered ferritin. It can be seen as brown granules in unstained tissue and stains strongly with Prussian blue in bone marrow smears.

Control of iron absorption and turnover
- *The nature of dietary iron:* haem iron—blood in the diet—is best absorbed
- *Gastric juice and vitamin C:* acids favour absorption by converting ferric ions to ferrous ions
- *Iron deficiency and increased erythropoiesis:* regardless of the cause, they enhance the rate of intestinal mucosal iron uptake and transfer to the plasma

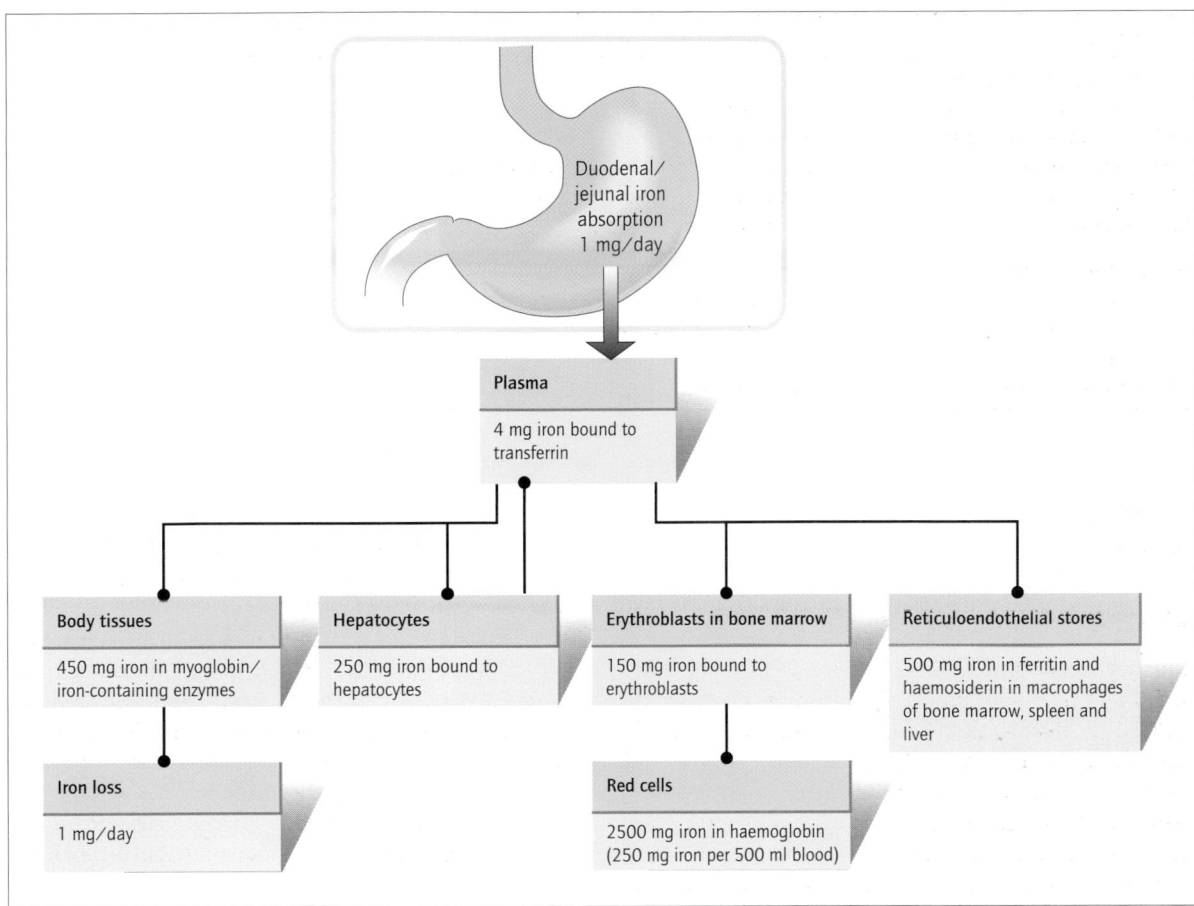

Figure 15.14 Adult distribution of total body iron (4 g).

Clinical features

Symptoms. For symptoms of anaemia see p. 1009.

Diagnosis. This is based on the presence of a microcytic anaemia accompanied by a low serum ferritin, and confirmed by a response to iron therapy.

Investigation

Haematology

- *FBC:* anaemia with MCV less than 78 fl. Increased platelet count (thrombocytosis) is often seen, particularly in the case of chronic blood loss.
- *Blood film:* pale hypochromic red cells and 'pencil' cells (see IRON-DEFICIENCY ANAEMIA AT A GLANCE, Fig. A).

Biochemistry

Serum iron measurements. Iron ↓: total iron-binding capacity (TIBC) ↑: transferrin saturation ↓: ferritin ↓.

Management

Give iron by oral therapy to: (a) correct the haemoglobin (usually increases by 1 g/dl/week if iron is taken); and (b) replace iron stores (this takes an additional 3 months' therapy after the [Hb] is corrected). The underlying cause is sought and treated.

Prognosis

Despite the apparently straightforward solution, many women have persisting or recurring iron deficiency throughout their life. Indeed, many women (in Western societies as well as in the developing world) spend their whole life iron-deficient, having had deficiency in childhood (magnified by iron-consuming growth spurts), adolescence (magnified by puberty) and adulthood (menstrual loss plus childbearing). It is not so easy to treat this chronic deficiency, and if a full 6-month course is not taken to replace stores, the iron deficiency will recur. It is reasonable to advise continuing iron supplements even after the full course is taken.

Iron-deficiency anaemia at a glance

Epidemiology
Prevalence
500–600 million people worldwide

Age, sex and ethnicity
Common in children, women of reproductive age and cultural vegans

Genetics
N/A

Geography
Poor countries with malnutrition and hookworm infestation
Incidence
Most common in women of reproductive age (menstruation plus multiple pregnancies)

Findings on investigation
Haematology
• *Full blood count:* Hb less than 13 g/dl (males), less than 12 g/dl (females): mean cell volume (MCV) less than 78 fl
• *Blood film:* hypochromic red blood cells (RBCs): 'pencil cells' (Fig. A)

Biochemistry
Ferritin ↑, serum iron ↓, total iron-binding capacity (TIBC) ↑, transferrin saturation ↓

Diagnostic imaging
Iron deficiency should be investigated by endoscopy for gastrointestinal cancer in:
All men
All postmenopausal women
Anyone with gastrointestinal symptoms

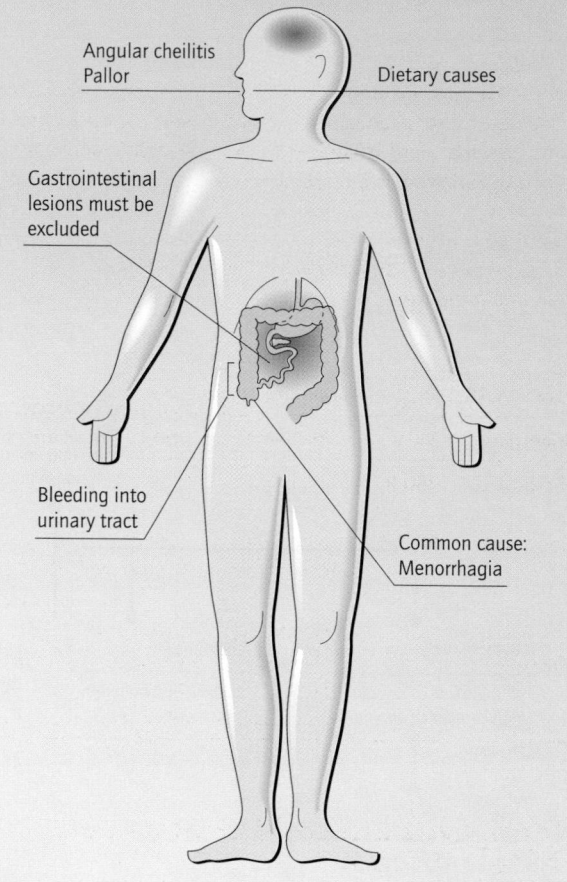

Angular cheilitis
Pallor

Dietary causes

Gastrointestinal lesions must be excluded

Bleeding into urinary tract

Common cause: Menorrhagia

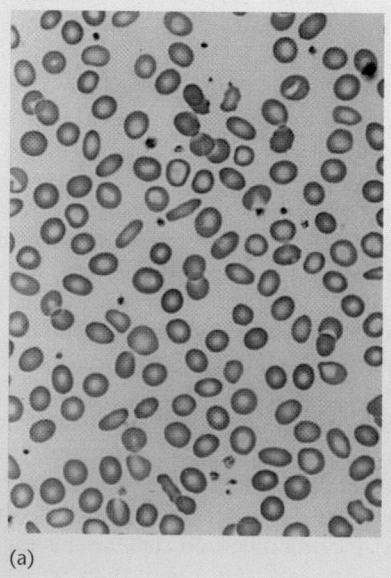

(a)

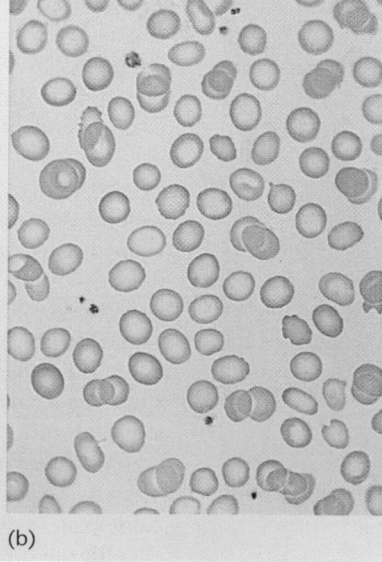

(b)

Fig. A Iron-deficiency anaemia. Peripheral blood films showing hypochromic, cells with poikilocytosis. (a) Pencil cells. (b) Hypochromasia.

Histopathology
Bone marrow cytology is needed in people with other potential causes of anaemia: in iron deficiency, there is absent iron staining (Perls' stain), erythroid hyperplasia and poorly haemoglobinized RBC precursors

Clinical features
Symptoms associated with reduced oxygen transport
Tiredness and sleepiness

Loss of interest in usual pursuits
Breathlessness on effort
Palpitations

Mucocutaneous
Mucosal pallor
Angular stomatitis
Koilonychia (very rare)
Brittle hair and nails

Table 15.10 Diagnostic approach to anaemia

Anaemia	MCV	Platelets	White cell count	Diagnosis
Microcytic	<80 fl			Iron deficiency
				Thalassaemia
Normocytic	80–96 fl	Normal	Normal	Anaemia of chronic disorder, rheumatoid arthritis
		Low/normal	Abnormal	Marrow invasion by cancer (leucoerythroblastic anaemia)
				Haematological malignancy
		Normal	Increased	Chronic haematological malignancy
Macrocytic	>96 fl	Normal	Normal	Vitamin B_{12} or folate deficiency, liver disease, haemolysis
		Low	Normal/low	Vitamin B_{12} or folate deficiency, acute haematological malignancy
		Normal/low	Abnormal	Myelodysplastic syndromes

15

Normocytic anaemia: anaemia of chronic disease

This normocytic normochromic anaemia is as common as iron-deficiency anaemia in **hospitalized** patients. It lacks a name valid in all circumstances, because it can also develop rapidly in acute infections and inflammatory states.

Epidemiology
Incidence. About 10–15% of all hospitalized patients.

Age. More common in those over 65 years. Many people under 80 years have normocytic anaemia, but it is not 'normal for age'.

Sex. Equal.

Ethnicity. All ethnic groups.

Genetics. N/A.

Geography. Worldwide.

Disease mechanisms
Anaemia of chronic disease is normocytic or mildly microcytic. It is associated with impaired iron mobilization from iron stores (iron block), probably a cytokine (IL-1) mediated defence mechanism aimed at depriving micro-organisms of iron, which is a key growth factor for many pathogenic organisms. The defensive iron block is also provoked by any activation of the cytokine inflammatory response. Chronic infections (e.g. tuberculosis), carcinoma and connective tissue disorders (e.g. rheumatoid arthritis) are typical causes (Table 15.10).

Clinical features
The clinical picture is non-specific and largely that of the underlying chronic disorder.

Diagnosis
Anaemia (usually in the range 8.0–10.0 g/dl) in the presence of any chronic or subacute inflammatory or malignant disorder. The anaemia is usually normocytic normochromic (MCV 78–100 fl) but may be mildly hypochromic (MCV less than 78 fl). The anaemia is **refractory** (will not respond to haematinic therapy).

Investigation
Haematology
- *FBC:* normochromic or mildly hypochromic anaemia. White cell and platelet counts are usually normal, but may both be elevated in acute infection or inflammation.
- *Bone marrow examination:* confirms the iron block by demonstrating increased iron in reticuloendothelial cells (bone marrow macrophages) and absent iron granules in erythroid precursors. Marrow examination is only

performed in cases where the clinical and blood findings are unclear.

Biochemistry

Iron status. Iron stores, as reflected in serum ferritin, are normal or increased, but serum iron is low. TIBC is normal, or mildly reduced, so that the percentage iron saturation is not as markedly reduced as in iron deficiency (Table 15.8).

Management

Management may involve doing nothing (accepting that iron block is a form of defence reaction that is difficult to subvert), but if symptoms of anaemia are compromising the patient's quality of life, blood transfusion is the only reliable way of correcting the anaemia apart from successful treatment of the underlying chronic disorder. Trials with erythropoietin have had limited success.

Prognosis

Depends on the underlying pathology. In some patients, the normochromic anaemia will respond rapidly (e.g. to antibiotic therapy of chronic urinary tract infection). In others (e.g. in rheumatoid arthritis), the chronic normochromic anaemia may last for many years or never abate.

Macrocytic anaemias

Megaloblastic anaemia

Megaloblastic anaemia is characterized by distinctive morphological features in red and white cell precursors in the marrow ('megaloblasts').

Megaloblastic anaemia usually results from vitamin B_{12} and/or folate deficiency, but occasionally occurs in the absence of such deficiencies. The investigation of megaloblastic anaemia is outlined in Fig. 15.15.

The physiological features of vitamin B_{12} and folic acid are outlined in Table 15.11, and the causes of vitamin B_{12} and folate deficiency are listed in Table 15.12.

Dietary B_{12} deficiency
Epidemiology
Incidence. Relatively common in UK vegans. Apparently rare in the Indian Subcontinent.

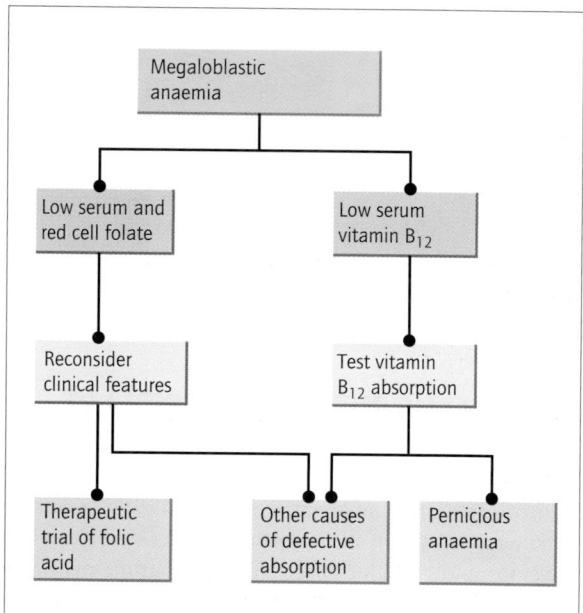

Figure 15.15 Investigation of megaloblastic anaemia.

Table 15.11 Physiological features of vitamin B_{12} and folic acid

Feature	Vitamin B_{12}	Folic acid
Structure	Molecule with red absorption containing cobalt	Molecule with yellow absorption spectrum with three parts spectrum (pteridine, glutamic acid and para-aminobenzoate)
Molecular weight	1400	450
Dietary source	Animal products (e.g. meat, dairy produce)	Widely distributed; abundant in green vegetables
Heat stability	Heat stable	Readily destroyed by heat
Site of absorption	Terminal ileum (bound to intrinsic factor)	Upper gastrointestinal tract
Transport	Bound to transcobalamins (TC), mainly TCI. Increased TCI (e.g. in myeloproliferative disorders) cause increased B_{12} levels	Present in plasma as tetrahydrofolate; active intracellular forms require presence of vitamin B_{12}
Daily requirement	1–3 mg/day	100 mg/day
Body stores	2–3 mg (sufficient for 3–4 years)	10 mg (sufficient for 4 months)
Function	Cofactor for folate metabolism	Involved in pyrimidine and purine synthesis and in amino acid interconversion (e.g. homocysteine to methione)

Table 15.12 Causes of vitamin B$_{12}$ and folate deficiency

Cause	Example
Vitamin B$_{12}$ deficiency	
Nutritional deficiency	Vegan diet
Gastric malabsorption	Pernicious anaemia, gastrectomy
Intestinal malabsorption	Ileal resection, Crohn's disease, stagnant loop syndrome caused by an anatomical blind loop, intestinal stricture, or jejunal diverticulosis, tropical sprue
Folate deficiency	
Nutritional deficiency	Alcoholism, old age, psychiatric disturbance
Malabsorption	Coeliac disease, Crohn's disease
Excessive use	Haemolytic anaemia
Increased requirements	Myeloproliferative disorders, pregnancy
Folate-antagonist drugs	Methotrexate, trimethoprim, anticonvulsants (mechanism unclear)

Age. Usually over 20 years.

Sex. Predominantly women.

Ethnicity. Punjabi, Gujarati or other culturally vegan groups.

Genetics. N/A

Geography. Indian Subcontinent, East Africa, UK.

Clinical features
A strict vegan diet that eliminates all foods of animal origin is potentially lacking vitamin B$_{12}$, particularly in countries where industrial washing of vegetables is widespread. Elective vegans may supplement their diet with non-animal sources of B$_{12}$ (e.g. Marmite) but cultural vegans may require dietary supplementation with oral hydroxycobalamin tablets. A full dietary history will always reveal the aetiology but remember that vegans can also develop pernicious anaemia like anyone else (see below).

Diagnosis
Macrocytic anaemia with a serum B$_{12}$ level less than 200 ng/l in a vegan.

Investigation
Haematology
- FBC shows anaemia and macrocytosis (more than 100 fl)
- Blood film reveals oval macrocytes
- Bone marrow examination may not be required if dietary veganism is clear

Biochemistry
Serum B$_{12}$ assay less than 200 ng/l. Look for associated iron deficiency (see above), folate deficiency (see below) and osteomalacia (see below), which may all be features of similar diets (although the vegan diet contains vegetables rich in folate, this may be inactivated by overcooking). Consider offering testing to other family members (who share the same diet).

Management
Daily oral B$_{12}$ supplement in the form of cyanocobalamin 50 μg tablets, or Marmite.

Pernicious anaemia

Epidemiology
Incidence. 25 cases/100 000 people over 40 years of age per year.

Age. Average 60 years.

Sex. More common in women.

Ethnicity. All ethnic groups, but more common in people of African heritage.

Genetics. Positive family history for 30% of patients.

Geography. Worldwide.

Pathogenesis
Classic ('Addisonian') pernicious anaemia (PA) results from a local 'autoimmune' gastritis leading to atrophy of parietal cells. Autoantibodies against intrinsic factor are found in 55% of patients and their presence is diagnostic. Gastric parietal cell antibodies are much less specific, being found in many conditions. Rare patients have poor B$_{12}$ absorption because of **past gastrectomy** or damage to the **terminal ileum**, for example by Crohn's disease.

Clinical features

PA may present at a late and dangerous stage: its insidious onset and slow progress means that cardiovascular compensation may delay overt symptoms until the anaemia becomes critical (less than 5 g/dl). Such a patient will have pallor (sometimes lemon-tinted because of hyperbilirubinaemia), exhaustion, congestive cardiac failure with incipient pulmonary oedema, with glossitis (a beefy red tongue). Hyperbilirubinaemia signifies the haemolytic element in megaloblastic anaemia.

Awareness of the disease and the sensitivity of automated MCV measurement in the FBC has led to earlier diagnosis, often at the asymptomatic (macrocytic but not yet anaemic) stage of the disorder, so that the 'classic' presentation described above is now a rarity.

Gastrointestinal features of weight loss, diarrhoea and constipation because of impaired growth of the proliferative cells of the gut are common. There is a small increased risk of carcinoma of the stomach in males, but it is not sufficient to justify regular routine endoscopy.

An important subgroup of patients present with neurological effects of B_{12} deficiency, **without any macrocytosis or megaloblastic change**. Neurological manifestations include peripheral neuropathy, optic atrophy, subacute combined degeneration of the cord (posterior column and pyramidal tract involvement) and mental abnormalities such as irritability, somnolence and dementia.

Diagnosis

A plasma B_{12} level less than 200 ng/l (see below) plus poor absorption (less than 25%) of a dose of oral B_{12} that is fully corrected by addition of intrinsic factor to the oral B_{12} dose (the Schilling test) confirms the diagnosis of PA. Technical difficulties with the Schilling test have led to many clinicians relying on the combination of low plasma B_{12} plus positive intrinsic factor antibodies to confirm the diagnosis in practice.

Investigation

Haematology

- *FBC:* reveals a macrocytic anaemia (red cell MCV more than 100 fl). If severe there is an accompanying leucopenia and thrombocytopenia.
- *Blood film:* shows **oval** macrocytes, marked variation in red cell size (anisocytosis, with RBC fragments) shape (poikilocytosis), and hypersegmented (more than 4 lobes per cell nucleus) polymorphs. In alcoholic macrocytosis the macrocytes are round, and the other features are not seen.
- *Bone marrow aspirate:* hypercellular, with erythroid hyperplasia and increased early erythroid precursors

(so-called left shift in the erythroid series). Individual erythroid precursors are large and dysplastic, with fine open chromatin: these are the megaloblasts. Granulocyte development is also affected and giant dysplastic metamyelocytes are characteristic. Strictly, the diagnosis of megaloblastic anaemia cannot be made without seeing these characteristic cells on a bone marrow smear.

Biochemistry

Serum vitamin B_{12} assay and vitamin B_{12} absorption measurements (Schilling test) are necessary to confirm the diagnosis. Serum vitamin B_{12} is assayed radioisotopically: a low level (less than 200 ng/l) suggests deficiency.

Immunology

Parietal cell and intrinsic factor antibodies are useful confirmatory findings in PA. Parietal cell antibodies are positive in 90% of patients with PA, and in about 15% of the normal ageing population. Intrinsic factor antibodies are more specific for PA, but are absent in up to 50% of patients.

Histopathology

All proliferating cells show megaloblastosis, including the cells lining the gastrointestinal tract (buccal mucosa, tongue, small intestine), cervix, vagina and uterus.

Management

Malabsorption of vitamin B_{12}, irrespective of aetiology, is treated with **1 mg hydroxocobalamin** administered by intramuscular injection every 3 months for life. Initially 5–6 doses are given over 3 weeks.

Prognosis

The haematological response of vitamin B_{12} deficiency to treatment is rapid with immediate reticulocytosis and haemoglobin levels rising by approximately 1 g/week. Clinical symptoms improve almost immediately, while megaloblastic changes and any accompanying leucopenia and thrombocytopenia revert to normal within a few days. The only consequence of B_{12} deficiency that may show poor improvement, if recognition and treatment are delayed, is the neuropathy.

Megaloblastic anaemia resulting from folate deficiency

Epidemiology

Incidence. Unknown.

Age. All age groups.

Sex. Equal incidence.

Ethnicity. All ethnic groups.

Genetics. N/A.

Geography. Worldwide.

Pathogenesis

Folate deficiency occurs in six main settings:

1 Decreased dietary intake (often associated with iron deficiency)
2 Malabsorption (e.g. coeliac disease)
3 Acute starvation (which may even occur in hospitalized patients)
4 Increased folate requirement of pregnancy
5 Increased folate requirement because of rapid red cell turnover in haemolytic anaemias (e.g. sickle cell anaemia)
6 Chronic therapy with antiepileptic agents (e.g. phenytoin)

Clinical features

The onset of macrocytic anaemia may be more rapid than in the case of B_{12} deficiency because the body stores of folate are short-lasting. The classic instance is **megaloblastic anaemia of pregnancy**, when acute severe anaemia with life-threatening pulmonary oedema may occur late in the third trimester. Severe ethanol toxicity may also cause acute folate deficient anaemia. In **malabsorption** syndromes, chronic folate deficiency is associated with gastrointestinal symptoms, general growth retardation and a variety of other vitamin deficiencies. In dietary deficiency, the common association with iron deficiency means that macrocytosis is suppressed by iron deficiency and the anaemia becomes normocytic normochromic: in this case **neutrophil hypersegmentation** may be the only sign in the peripheral blood film.

Diagnosis

- Macrocytic anaemia with oval macrocytes and/or hypersegmented neutrophils
- Megaloblastic erythropoiesis on bone marrow examination
- Low serum folate (less than 2.5 µg/l)

Investigation

Haematology
As for PA, with particular attention to microscopy of the blood film. Look for evidence of haemolytic anaemia (direct antiglobulin test, Hb electrophoresis).

Biochemistry
Folate assay on serum (normal range 2.5–10 µg/l). The red cell folate assay rarely seems to provide additional useful information and is no longer often performed.

Look for other biochemical evidence of malabsorption (e.g. low serum albumin; ↓ corrected calcium, ↑ alkaline phosphatase [osteomalacia]; increased faecal fat excretion [steatorrhoea]).

Histopathology
Jejunal biopsy may be required to demonstrate coeliac disease.

Diagnostic imaging
Contrast studies of the gastrointestinal tract may be useful in malabsorption.

Management

Oral folic acid tablets (5 mg) are given once daily in established folate deficiency anaemia. In malabsorption, daily doses of up to 15 mg may be required. Before prescribing folate doses of 5 mg or above, vitamin B_{12} deficiency must be excluded (or treated) because folate can provoke neuropathy if it is present. Combined vitamin B_{12} and folate treatment is safe during the investigation of a presumed megaloblastic anaemia if blood and bone marrow samples have been obtained.

For prophylaxis during pregnancy, a daily dose of 400 µg is given, unless there is a high risk of neural tube defects, when at least 800 µg/day is indicated.

Non-megaloblastic macrocytic anaemia

The most frequent cause of a macrocytic anaemia that does not show features of megaloblastic haematopoiesis on inspection of peripheral blood or bone marrow smears is **chronic excess ethanol ingestion**. Ethanol alone rarely elevates the MCV above the range 100–108 fl, and an additional factor such as folate deficiency (e.g. resulting from poor diet in an ethanol abuser) should be sought if the MCV is above this range. **Non-alcoholic liver disease** and **hypothyroidism** can also cause macrocytic anaemia without megaloblastic change: check for B_{12} deficiency in hypothyroidism because autoimmune PA can be associated with autoimmune thyroiditis.

Haemolytic anaemias

Disease mechanisms

Haemolysis means premature red cell destruction, shortening the circulating lifespan of RBCs to less than 100 days. The main causes of haemolysis are listed in Table 15.13. Haemolysis may exist without anaemia, because the bone marrow can increase its output of red cells fivefold and thereby compensate for a moderately increased rate of red cell loss from the circulation (e.g. red cell lifespan 20–50 days). However, many cofactors (e.g.

15

Table 15.13 Main causes of haemolysis

Cause	Example
Extrinsic trauma to the red cell membrane	
Autoimmune	Warm autoimmune haemolytic anaemia
	Cold autoimmune haemolytic anaemia
Alloimmune	Haemolytic disease of the newborn and transfusion reactions
Mechanical	Cardiac abnormalities (such as prostheses and perivalvular leaks)
Microangiopathic	Toxins or chemicals
	Malignancy
Intrinsic defects of the red cell	Hereditary spherocytosis
membrane or cytoskeleton	Hereditary elliptocytosis
	Paroxysmal nocturnal haemoglobinuria
Defective red cell enzymes	Glucose-6-phosphate dehydrogenase deficiency
	Pyruvate kinase deficiency
Haemoglobinopathies	
Structural variant	Sickle-cell disease
Quantitative abnormality	Thalassaemia

Pernicious anaemia at a glance

Epidemiology

Incidence
250/million/year (over 40 years)

Age
Average age at diagnosis: 60 years

Sex
More common in women

Ethnicity
All, but often occurs at an earlier age in women of Afro-Caribbean descent

Genetics
Affected family member in 30% of patients. Also associated with thyroid disease

Geography
Worldwide

Findings on investigation

Haematology
- *FBC:* macrocytic anaemia (MCV > 100 fl). Leucopenia and thrombocytopenia if severe
- *Blood film:* oval macrocytes, anisocytosis, poikilocytosis and hypersegmented polymorphs
- *Bone marrow aspirate:* hypercellular, with erythroid hyperplasia. Megaloblasts (large early erythroid precursors with abnormal nuclear chromatin) or giant metamyelocytes (enlarged neutrophil precursors with horseshoe nuclei) must be seen to confirm the diagnosis

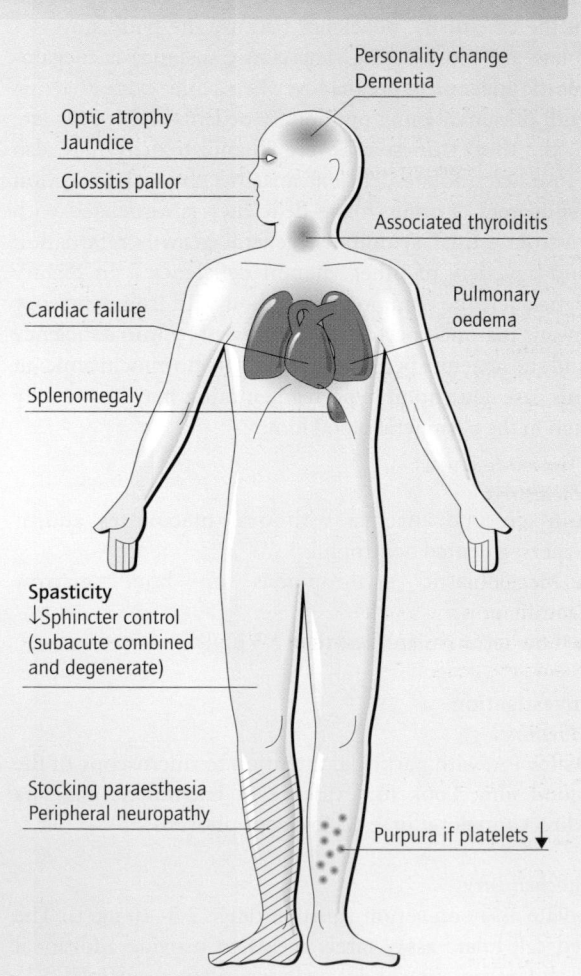

Personality change
Dementia

Optic atrophy
Jaundice

Glossitis pallor

Associated thyroiditis

Cardiac failure

Pulmonary oedema

Splenomegaly

Spasticity
↓Sphincter control
(subacute combined and degenerate)

Stocking paraesthesia
Peripheral neuropathy

Purpura if platelets ↓

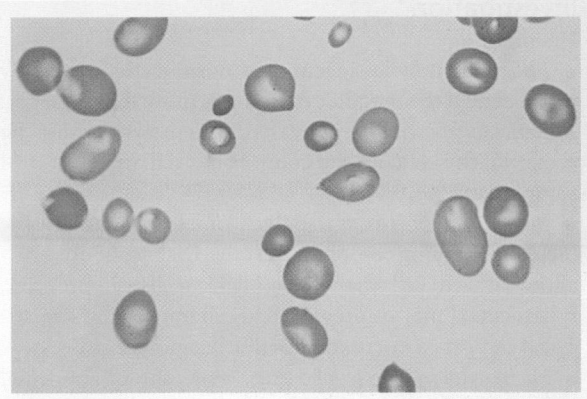

Fig. A Peripheral blood film showing oval macrocytosis, poikilocytosis and anisocytosis. A proportion of the red cells are very large (macrocytes) but a number of smaller irregular cells are also present. Note also the lack of platelets.

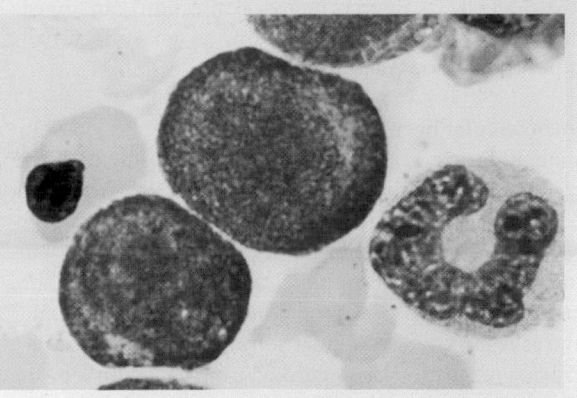

Fig. B Bone marrow showing megaloblastic proerythrocytes and a giant metamyelocyte with a 'horseshoe' nucleus.

Biochemistry
- *Serum vitamin B$_{12}$:* low (less than 200 ng/l)
- *Lactic dehydrogenase:* raised because of intramedullary haemolysis resulting from ineffective erythropoiesis
- *Serum bilirubin:* raised (haemolysis)

Immunology
- *Parietal cell antibodies:* positive in 90% of patients with pernicious anaemia (PA), and in about 15% of the normal ageing population
- *Intrinsic factor antibodies:* more specific for PA, but are absent in up to 50% of patients

Clinical features
Haematology
Anaemia

Mucocutaneous
Glossitis (sore red tongue)
Lemon tint to the skin (anaemia and jaundice, typical of any haemolytic anaemia)

Cardiac
Angina
Congestive cardiac failure

Gastrointestinal
Anorexia
Weight loss
Diarrhoea
Constipation

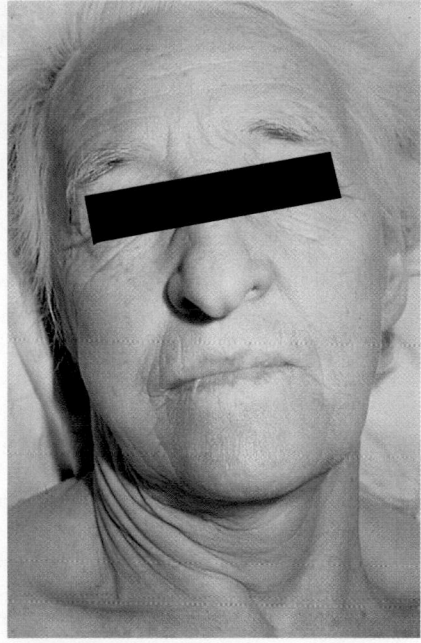

Fig. C Facial appearance in pernicious anaemia. Note lemon tint, pallor and angular cheilosis. Reproduced from Hoffbrand & Pettit, *Essential Haematology*, 3rd edn, 1993 (Blackwell Scientific Publications, Oxford) with the permission of the authors.

Neurology
Peripheral neuropathy
Optic atrophy
Subacute combined degeneration of the spinal cord
Dementia
Mental abnormalities

15

folate deficiency, intercurrent viral infection) can impede this bone marrow compensation, so anaemia usually supervenes at some stage.

Intravascular haemolysis

Violent forms of red cell destruction result in intravascular haemolysis: the red cell bursts in the circulation, releasing haemoglobin into the blood plasma. This overwhelms the haemoglobin-binding plasma proteins (**haptoglobins**), which are rapidly cleared from the circulation. Free Hb now appears in the blood (**haemoglobinaemia**) and is lost in the glomerular filtrate (**haemoglobinuria**), causing red urine—distinguished from haematuria by the absence of intact red cells in the urinary sediment. The renal tubular cells attempt to reabsorb Hb and thereby fill with stainable iron (**haemosiderinuria**). If the intravascular haemolysis is part of an explosive (IgM-mediated) immune reaction, as in ABO-incompatible red cell transfusion ('wrong blood'), it provokes a life-threatening systemic reaction with acute renal failure and disseminated intravascular coagulation.

Extravascular haemolysis

A subtler form of red cell destruction is mediated by IgG red cell antibodies. Binding of IgG to the red cell membrane leads to recognition and clearance by macrophages of the reticuloendothelial system in the spleen, liver and bone marrow. Red cell contents are not released into the circulation but are recycled by the phagocytic system. The responsible IgG antibodies may be alloantibodies (e.g. Rhesus disease of the newborn) or autoantibodies (e.g. autoimmune haemolytic anaemia; AIHA—sometimes termed warm-antibody AIHA because IgG antibodies react best with red cells at 37°C). The IgG can be detected on the red cell surface by the direct antiglobulin test (DAT).

In haemolytic anaemias caused by **red cell membrane defects** (including sickle cell disease), the red cell destruction occurs mainly by the extravascular route. This is also the case in most **red cell enzymopathies**, excepting G6PD deficiency, in which acute intravascular haemolysis can be provoked by exposure to an oxidizing drug (e.g. sulphonamides).

Increased red cell breakdown products

In all forms of haemolytic anaemia, the turnover of haem increases, reflected in the levels of unconjugated and conjugated bilirubin processed by the liver and excreted in the bile. As a result, in long-term chronic haemolytic states, oversaturation of bile results in **pigment gallstones** and consequent gall bladder disease.

Investigation

Haematology

- *FBC:* haemolytic anaemia is normocytic or mildly macrocytic if the reticulocyte count is more than 5%.
- *Reticulocyte count:* increased. Haemolysis must be present if the reticulocyte count is more than $250 \times 10^9/l$ (more than 7%).
- *Blood film microscopy:* polychromasia caused by the presence of young basophilic red cells. Diagnostic abnormalities of red cell shape (e.g. sickle cells, elliptocytes, spherocytes) may be present. Red cell fragments (schistocytes) indicate a **microangiopathic** haemolytic process.
- *Haemoglobin electrophoresis:* may show abnormal haemoglobin (e.g. HbS).
- *Red cell enzyme assay:* may reveal G6PD deficiency.
- *Bone marrow examination:* shows compensatory erythroid hyperplasia. If AIHA is secondary to a lymphoma or chronic leukaemia, abnormal cells may be seen.
- *Haemoglobinuria:* in intravascular haemolysis.

Biochemistry

- Hyperbilirubinaemia (more than 20 µmol/l, mostly unconjugated)
- Reduced or absent serum haptoglobin
- Increased urinary urobilinogen
- Increased serum lactic dehydrogenase (LDH)
- Positive urinary haemosiderin in intravascular haemolysis

Immunology

A positive DAT (sometimes still referred to as the direct Coombs' test) detects anti-RBC antibody bound to circulating red cells, indicating the presence of immune haemolysis.

Diagnostic imaging

Ultrasound of the gallbladder will detect pigment stones and any consequent cholecystitis.

Autoimmune haemolytic anaemia

Epidemiology

Prevalence. 1 in 100 000.

Age. Any age, including childhood, but most frequent over 50 years.

Sex. More common in females.

Ethnicity. All.

Geography. Worldwide.

Table 15.14 Causes of warm-reacting antibody (often IgG) and cold-reacting antibody (often IgM)

Cause	Example
Warm-reacting antibody	
IgG (± complement fixation) directed against very 'public' antigen	Idiopathic
	Lymphoproliferative disorders (or common) erythrocyte (e.g. chronic lymphocytic leukaemia, non-Hodgkin's lymphoma)
	Autoimmune rheumatic diseases (e.g. systemic lupus erythematosus)
Haptens	Drugs (e.g. quinine) sulphonamides, chlorpromazine, penicillin
Immune complexes	
Autoantibodies	
Cold-reacting antibody	
Immunoproliferative disease producing monoclonal IgM that reacts with the red cells at low temperatures	Cold haemagglutinin disease
Autoantibody with anti-I and anti-I specificity	*Mycoplasma* infection, infectious mononucleosis
IgG directed against P blood group system	Paroxysmal cold haemoglobinuria

Disease mechanisms

Autoimmune haemolytic anaemia is caused by an auto-antibody to the patient's own red cells. The antibodies are active either at body temperature (37°C—'warm antibody' = IgG) or at room temperature (15°C—'cold antibody' = IgM; Table 15.14). Cold antibody AIHA often causes red cell autoagglutination on blood films and is therefore sometimes called cold agglutinin disease. Haemolysis is usually extravascular, resulting from phagocytosis of antibody- and/or complement-coated red cells by the spleen and liver.

Clinical features

Depending on its cause and severity, the clinical picture ranges from chronic anaemia to fulminating haemolysis leading to cardiovascular collapse and death. Mild jaundice and moderate splenomegaly are typical of chronic warm AIHA. Worsening of haemolysis on exposure to cold (or even normal ambient) temperatures is typical of cold antibody (IgM) AIHA.
- *Primary AIHA:* occurs without evidence of an underlying disease
- *Secondary AIHA:* occurs in the context of an existing autoimmune disorder (rheumatoid arthritis, SLE) or lymphoma or chronic leukaemia (non-Hodgkin's lymphoma or CLL)
- *Mycoplasma-associated (acute) cold agglutinin AIHA:* associated with atypical pneumonia and cold agglutinins (anti-I antibodies)
- *Drug-induced AIHA:* e.g. methyldopa, cephalosporin antibiotics

Diagnosis

Anaemia with reticulocytosis and positive DAT.

Investigation
- *FBC:* shows anaemia, mild macrocytosis; WBC and platelets usually normal.
- *Reticulocyte count:* increased (more than $100 \times 10^9/l$).
- *Blood film:* shows polychromasia. Microspherocytes (small dense spherical red cells) may be seen in the peripheral blood film. They are formed by partial phagocytosis in the spleen, which removes part of the red cell membrane. Red cell agglutination may be seen in cold antibody AIHA.
- *DAT:* a positive test detects immunoglobulin and/or complement on the red cell membrane.
- *Cold agglutinins* (IgM antibodies directed against the red cell I antigen): detected in warm separated serum in cold AIHA.

Management

Warm (IgG-mediated) AIHA usually responds to corticosteroids (e.g. prednisone 1 mg/kg body weight) by reducing the rate of red cell destruction and increasing the haemoglobin level. Splenectomy may work if there is no response. In possible drug-induced AIHA, the suspected drug is stopped.

Cold haemagglutinin disease is relatively unresponsive

to corticosteroid therapy and splenectomy. Treatment includes control of the underlying disorder (e.g. with anti-*Mycoplasma* antibiotics) and warming the patient.

Haemoglobinopathies

Haemoglobinopathies are genetic disorders of haemoglobin caused by abnormalities of globin genes. Whether the person with a haemoglobinopathy has a disease depends entirely on the **gene dose** they inherit. A single abnormal allele, inherited from one parent, rarely causes disease but results in an asymptomatic **heterozygote** carrier state (a trait). If a person inherits abnormal alleles from both parents, they are affected **homozygotes** who usually suffer from severe anaemia, together with other features arising from abnormal red cell structure and function.

Haemoglobinopathies can be divided into two broad groups:
1 *Reduced synthesis of globin chains (the thalassaemias):* these disorders are caused by a wide range of gene lesions affecting both α-globin and β-globin genes, which share the property of reducing or eliminating effective globin chain synthesis.
2 *Structural haemoglobin variants:* caused by single nucleotide/amino acid substitutions (haemoglobin S, haemoglobin C, haemoglobin E and more than 200 other variants, many of which have no clinical effect). Clinically important structural variants **all affect β-globin chains**, because these are encoded by a single gene on each parental chromosome. Because α-globin chains are encoded by four genes (two per parent), single nucleotide substitutions in α-globin genes rarely cause disease.

Thalassaemias

Thalassaemia is caused by inherited globin gene abnormalities that result in underproduction or absence of either the β-globin or the α-globin chain. The resulting reduction in haemoglobin level causes variable degrees of anaemia (the most severe forms being incompatible with life) together with an imbalance in globin chain synthesis that may be mild or severe enough to lead to haemolysis, cell death in the bone marrow and consequent massive bone marrow hypertrophy and iron overload.

α-Thalassaemia
Epidemiology
Prevalence. Carried by many millions worldwide, depending on ethnicity.

Age. Congenital.

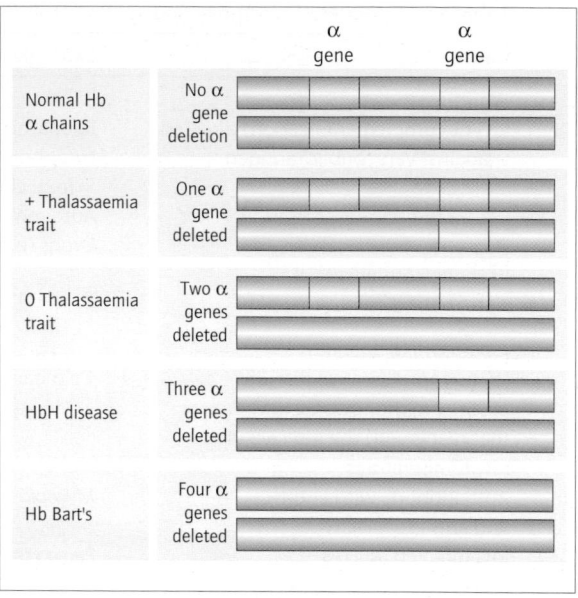

Figure 15.16 Genetic basis of α-thalassaemia. The clinical subtypes of α-thalassaemia are determined by the number of α genes expressed.

Sex. Equal.

Ethnicity. Frequency varies, but may be found in any.

Geography. Worldwide: highest in Africa (mostly α⁺) and South East Asia (China, Thailand, Vietnam: mostly α⁰). Also found in Middle Eastern and Mediterranean populations, and wherever individuals from any of these zones have migrated.

Genetics and pathogenesis
The synthesis of the haemoglobin α chain is controlled by four α-globin genes, two on each chromosome 16. α-Thalassaemia usually results from gene deletions (Fig. 15.16).

Clinical syndromes
The clinical subtypes are determined by the number of expressed α genes:
● *Deletion of all four α genes:* results in α^0 chain production so that neither HbF nor HbA are synthesized (see Fig. 15.16). Hb Bart's (γ_4) self-assembles, but cannot transport oxygen. The fetus develops severe congestive heart failure (Bart's hydrops fetalis) and dies *in utero* or at term. This causes severe maternal morbidity and distress: it was the first haemoglobinopathy to be prevented by antenatal diagnosis (see below).
● *Deletion of three α-globin genes:* results in HbH disease,

in which excess α chains are synthesized and precipitate within the red cell as β_4 molecules or as HbH. Clinically, HbH disease is a thalassaemia intermedia.

● *Deletion of two α genes:* results in α-thalassaemia trait, which is asymptomatic.
● *Deletion of a single α gene:* a 'silent carrier' state indistinguishable from normal.

Investigation
● *HbH disease:* clinically a thalassaemia intermedia: moderate anaemia (haemoglobin 8–10 g/dl), marked microcytosis, anisocytosis and poikilocytosis
● *Deletion of two α genes:* typical findings are a normal haemoglobin level, a low red cell MCH (less than 25 pg) and MCV, and a high red cell count.

Management and prognosis
Hb Bart's is incompatible with life, but is readily preventable by antenatal diagnosis. HbH disease requires little medical intervention apart from prophylactic folic acid. Regular red cell transfusion is not needed, but transfusion may be required in pregnancy or to support surgery. Iron overload rarely requires chelation therapy. α-Thalassaemia trait does not require any treatment, but genetic counselling of carriers of reproductive age is important.

β-Thalassaemia
Epidemiology
Prevalence. Carried by many millions worldwide.

Age. Congenital.

Sex. Equal.

Ethnicity. Frequency varies, but may be found in any.

Geography. Worldwide, but highest heterozygote rates (5–15%) occur in the Mediterranean littoral (Cyprus, southern Italy and Greece). However, effective antenatal diagnostic programmes have much reduced the incidence of **homozygous thalassaemia major** in these areas. β^0 is also found in African, Middle Eastern and South East Asian ethnic groups. The β^+ gene (not associated with thalassaemia major) is widely carried by individuals of African heritage.

Genetics and pathogenesis
In β-thalassaemia, β-globin chain synthesis is reduced (β^+-thalassaemia) or absent (β^0-thalassaemia).

Many different DNA lesions have been reported in and around the β gene. These defects include mutations in regulatory boxes, nonsense mutations causing chain termination, frameshift mutations, defective RNA splicing and deletions. Inheritance of various pairs of defects causes variation in clinical severity (see below).

α-Globin chain synthesis is normal in β-thalassaemia, leading to excess unpaired α chains: these combine with δ and γ chains to form increased HbA2 and HbF (helpful in diagnosis), and with each other to form toxic tetramers (α_4) that result in premature destruction of red cell precursors in the marrow (ineffective erythropoiesis).

β-Thalassaemia syndromes
The many potential pairings of β-thalassaemia genes, both with normal and other thalassaemic variants, result in three clinical syndromes: **thalassaemia major** (severe, transfusion-dependent anaemia); **thalassaemia intermedia** (life-long anaemia but infrequent transfusion needs); and **thalassaemia minor** (the asymptomatic carrier 'trait').

β-Thalassaemia major (Cooley's anaemia) occurs in individuals homozygous for the β^0 gene.

Clinical features
Affected individuals present in the first year of life with failure to thrive and grow because of severe anaemia. If not enlisted in an effective transfusion and iron chelation regimen, they will develop:
● Hepatosplenomegaly
● Bone marrow expansion with disfiguring bone deformity (e.g. facial bones)
● Pigment gallstones resulting from high rate of bilirubin production
● Cardiac damage and endocrinopathies resulting from iron overload

Investigation
● *FBC:* anaemia (Hb may be as low as 2–3 g/dl). Mild reticulocytosis (4–10%) indicates ineffective erythropoiesis
● *Blood film:* target cells, hypochromia, microcytosis, red cell fragments, nucleated red cells
● *Haemoglobin electrophoresis:* HbA1 is absent, HbF is greatly increased (from less than 1% to 80–100% of Hb)
● *Iron status:* ferritin and serum iron levels are increased because of increased iron absorption, and multiple blood transfusions result in gross iron overload
● *Radiography:* bone X-rays show medullary expansion because of marrow hypertrophy (e.g. 'hair-on-end' appearance of skull X-ray)

Management
Regular (4–6-weekly) red cell transfusion aiming to keep Hb more than 10 g/dl to suppress marrow hypertrophy

15

and iron absorption from the gut (hypertransfusion regimen). Continuous iron chelation using subcutaneous desferrioxamine infusions. Allogeneic bone marrow transplantation in young patients with matched allogeneic donors. Counselling and antenatal diagnosis should be made available.

Prognosis

Untreated, about 80% of patients die in infancy as a result of severe anaemia. If iron chelation is suboptimal, death from cardiac failure occurs in late teens or early twenties. With best treatment patients survive to adulthood.

β-Thalassaemia intermedia

Clinical features

Similar to β-thalassaemia major, but less severe. Bone deformity and hepatosplenomegaly may occur. Patients usually maintain their haemoglobin at 6–9 g/dl without transfusion. The blood film appearances are similar to those of thalassaemia major. Iron overload may occur because of increased iron absorption.

Management and prognosis

Intermittent transfusion or splenectomy may be indicated in some patients. Most patients survive to adulthood and have a full lifespan.

β-Thalassaemia minor (β-thalassaemia trait)

Describes the heterozygous state (one normal β-globin gene plus either a $β^0$ or $β^+$ gene).

Clinical features

Affected individuals are asymptomatic and are often diagnosed incidentally. They are carriers with respect to thalassaemia major and therefore should always be provided with reproductive advice and access to antenatal diagnosis and fetal selection if their partner is also a carrier of any β-globin haemoglobinopathy.

Investigation

- *FBC:* haemoglobin levels are 11–12 g/dl (sometimes lower in pregnancy). MCV less than 78 fl. Mimics iron deficiency.
- *Haemoglobin electrophoresis:* shows increased HbA_2 (3–7% of total haemoglobin).
- *Iron status:* usually normal.

Management and prognosis

Patients remain well and do not require any specific therapy apart from genetic counselling. Folic acid supplements should be given during periods of increased bone marrow stress (e.g. during pregnancy).

Sickle cell haemoglobinopathies

Sickle cell anaemia (SCA) refers to the homozygous (disease) state HbSS. **Sickle cell disease (SCD)** refers to all patients with double-gene diseases involving HbS (HbSS, HbSC, HbS/$β^0$ Thal, HbSO^{Arab}, etc.). **Sickle cell trait** refers to the asymptomatic healthy HbAS heterozygote.

Epidemiology

Prevalence. In tropical Africa up to 25% are heterozygous HbAS. In the UK, 20% of West African and 10% of Afro-Caribbean ethnicity carry a single copy of the sickle cell gene. The incidence of newborns with SCD in tropical Africa is at least 200 000/year, but the majority die before 5 years from infection. There are at least 5000 patients in the UK.

Sex. Equal sex distribution.

Genetics. Homozygous inheritance of the HbS gene (HbSS) results in SCA. Double heterozygous states involving one HbS gene results in SCD (see above). Heterozygous inheritance (HbAS) results in sickle cell trait.

Geography. The sickle cell gene occurs everywhere, but highest frequencies are in tropical Africa, Caribbean, USA, South America and Europe—anywhere along the routes of the enforced African diaspora. It also occurs in the Middle East, parts of India and Mediterranean countries.

Sickle cell anaemia

The disorder results from a point mutation in the sixth codon of the β-globin gene leading to substitution of valine for glutamic acid. Homozygotes have SCA: more than 75% of their haemoglobin is HbS. Deoxygenated HbS forms self-organizing polymers, leading to red cell distortion, shortened red cell survival (haemolytic anaemia) and blockage of the microcirculation causing infarction and tissue death. SCA is therefore characterized by anaemia, asplenism and acute and chronic organ damage resulting from vaso-occlusion (vascular obstruction by sickle cells) and consequent infarction.

Clinical features

There is extraordinary clinical variability in SCA, with many affected individuals remaining well without major organ damage; some living lives punctuated with recurrent agonizing pain crises and consequent hospital admissions; and some developing remorseless progressive damage to lungs, heart or kidneys. The usual course is of periods of mild or no symptoms (despite the anaemia)

—this is called 'the steady state'—punctuated by crises of one type or another. Types of crisis:

- *Pain crisis:* the most common event. Agonizing pain commences in the back or limbs but rapidly becomes generalized. The pain will last 10 days. Opiate analgesia is usually required.
- *Splenic sequestration:* extremely rapid fall in Hb (often to 2–3 g/dl) with rapid spleen enlargement. Early recognition and red cell transfusion is vital in this life-threatening situation.
- *Asplenic septicaemia:* with asplenic malaria, this is responsible for the extreme death rate in children with SCA in Africa (? more than 90% before age 15—the true rate is unknown). Life-long oral penicillin prophylaxis (125 mg twice daily in children, 250 mg twice daily in adults) gives protection from pneumococcal sepsis, and is mandatory after diagnosis in infancy.
- *Acute chest syndrome:* the most commonly fatal form of sickle crisis in Western societies. Usually provoked by infection, sickle vaso-occlusion in the lung circulation causes rapidly spreading infarction and consolidation with a vicious cycle of hypoxia and further sickling. Treated with oxygen, positive airways pressure and blood transfusion (often exchange transfusion) to acutely reduce circulating HbS.
- *Cerebral infarction:* stroke is a major complication of SCA in childhood. It tends to recur unless affected children receive long-term transfusion to suppress the HbS content of their blood.
- *Priapism:* painful persisting penile erection. Severe cases can result in permanent loss of erectile function. Treatment of severe cases (only partially effective) is surgical drainage, heparin and red cell exchange transfusion.

Investigation

Haematology

- *FBC:* there is usually an anaemia with a haemoglobin level of 6–8 g/dl and an elevated reticulocyte count of 10–20%. Symptoms of anaemia may be less than expected because HbS is a low-affinity Hb that releases oxygen readily in the tissues.
- *Blood film:* shows sickle cells and target cells.
- *Haemoglobin electrophoresis*: is always required to confirm SCA, which is characterized by the migration of a single band between HbA2 and HbA.

Management

Sickle cell anaemia is managed by preventing infections that may precipitate haemolytic and aplastic crises. This includes life-long penicillin 250 mg twice daily because of the risk of infection from hyposplenism. Life-long folic acid is also necessary. Long-term oral hydroxyurea (HU) therapy has been shown to increase haemoglobin levels

---

Emergency 15.2: Sickle cell crisis

Pain crisis

Give adequate analgesia (e.g. parenteral morphine) as soon as the patient confirms they have sickle cell disease and are in pain

Clinical examination of the chest, cardiovascular system, abdomen and nervous system

Measure temperature, blood pressure, pulse and respiratory rate

Use pulse oximetry to measure oxygen saturation

Blood samples for FBC, urea and electrolytes, blood culture and blood grouping

Chest X-ray if pain is in the chest. Otherwise, do not X-ray painful bones at the outset of the crisis

Ensure airway and give 24% oxygen at 4 l/min by mask

Give 1 l fluid 6-hourly, by mouth if possible, intravenously if not (vascular access may be difficult)

Give broad-spectrum antibiotics if there is fever (more than 37.5°C)

Overwhelming infection caused by hyposplenism

Pneumococcal, meningococcal or haemophilus septicaemia

Peak risk in childhood

May present with shock, seizures, meningeal irritation, coma or severe diarrhoea

Key is to recognize it and start immediate intravenous broad-spectrum antibiotic

Acute splenic sequestration

Peak risk in childhood

Presents with signs of rapidly developing anaemia (change in mental state, sleepiness, breathlessness)

Key finding is a rapidly enlarging spleen

Volume support with crystalloid and red cell transfusion

Surgery and blood transfusion in sickle cell disease

Never plan or carry out surgery, or give a blood transfusion, in a sickle cell patient without haematological advice

---

and reduce the number of crises in severely affected HbSS individuals who respond (not all do) by increasing intra-erythrocytic HbF levels. Candidates for HU need careful selection and explanation of risks and benefits. Many will decline HU therapy because of the need for regular blood tests, concerns about long-term toxicity and effects on fertility.

Sickle cell crisis is treated with rest, rehydration, analgesia and broad-spectrum antibiotics (EMERGENCY BOX 15.2). Exchange transfusion may be required in the event of a severe crisis (e.g. respiratory distress syndrome, stroke) or recurrent painful crises.

Surgery is hazardous if carried out without appropriate

Sickle cell anaemia at a glance

Epidemiology

Prevalence

In the UK, 25% of African descent and 10% of Afro-Caribbean descent have sickle cell trait (heterozygous AS). In tropical Africa, about 1 in 100 births results in a child with sickle cell disease. There are at least 5000 people with sickle cell anaemia in the UK

Sex

Equal sex distribution

Genetics

Homozygous for haemoglobin S gene (HbSS)

Geography

Gene originated in malarious zones (tropical Africa, Mediterranean, India) and followed diaspora to Caribbean, Europe, USA, Brazil

Findings on investigation

Haematology

- *FBC:* haemoglobin level usually 6–8 g/dl
- *Reticulocyte count:* increased
- *Blood film:* sickle cells and target cells
- *Haemoglobin electrophoresis:* shows migration of a single band (HbS) between HbA2 and HbA. HbS more than 70%
- *Screening test* (e.g. Sickledex): detects insolubility of deoxygenated HbS. Used to detect the presence of HbS (does not distinguish between sickle trait [AS] and sickle cell anaemia [SS])

Clinical features

Acute pain crisis

Sudden unpredictable onset of severe pain lasting 7–14 days
Bones: dactylitis (hand–foot syndrome) in children, dorsolumbar spine and limbs in adolescents and adults (but can affect any bone)
Chest (rib) pain (see chest syndrome)
Abdomen (girdle syndrome)
Needs strong analgesia

Acute sickle chest syndrome

Most common fatal event. Often starts with chest pain
Progressive bilateral shadowing on chest X-ray
Hypoxia and respiratory failure
Can be treated with respiratory support and red cell transfusion

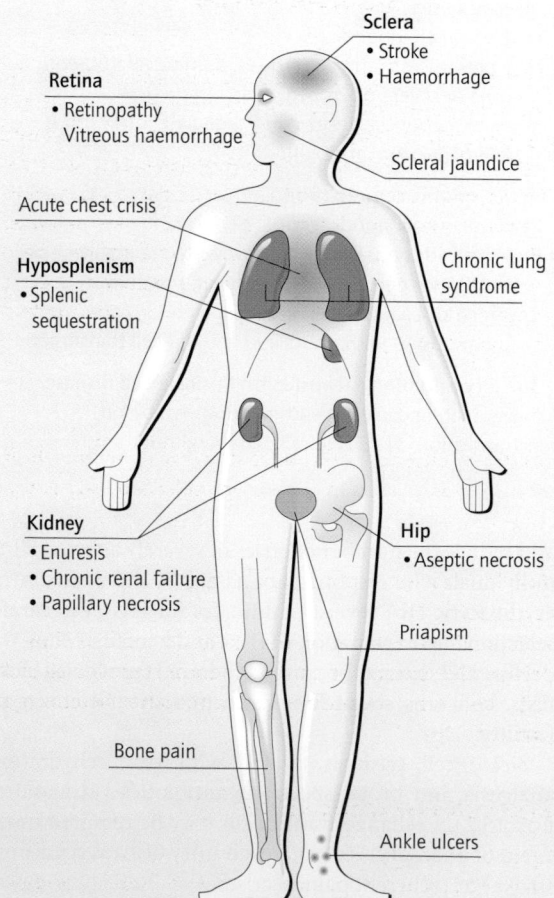

Sclera
- Stroke
- Haemorrhage

Retina
- Retinopathy
  Vitreous haemorrhage

Scleral jaundice

Acute chest crisis

Hyposplenism
- Splenic sequestration

Chronic lung syndrome

Kidney
- Enuresis
- Chronic renal failure
- Papillary necrosis

Hip
- Aseptic necrosis

Priapism

Bone pain

Ankle ulcers

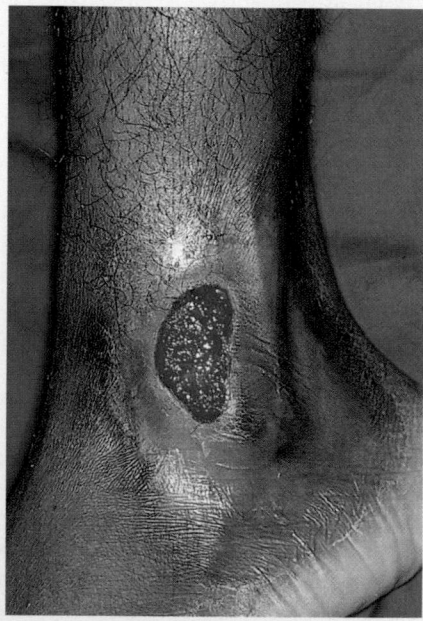

Fig. A Typical sickle ulcer, lateral malleolous.

Infection (hyposplenism)
Acute septicaemia
Osteomyelitis

Splenic sequestration
Rapid worsening of anaemia (→ less than 5 g/dl) with enlarging spleen
Treatment: urgent red cell transfusion

Stroke
Most common in children (occlusive vasculopathy)

Chronic complications
Renal: failure of concentrating ability, progressive renal failure (5%)

Lung: progressive fibrosis with respiratory failure (5%)
Joints: aseptic necrosis of hip and/or shoulder (25%)
Erectile failure: caused by priapism (10% of males)
Chronic bone pain syndrome (10%)

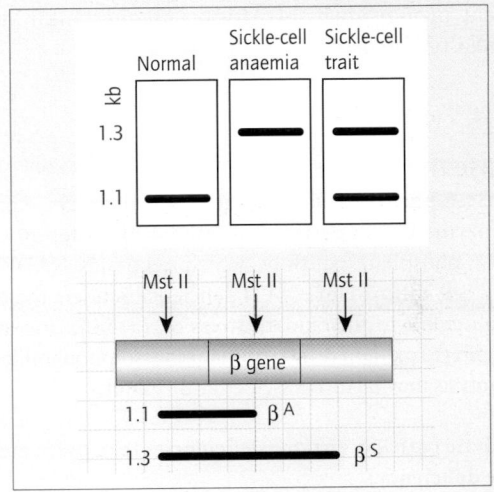

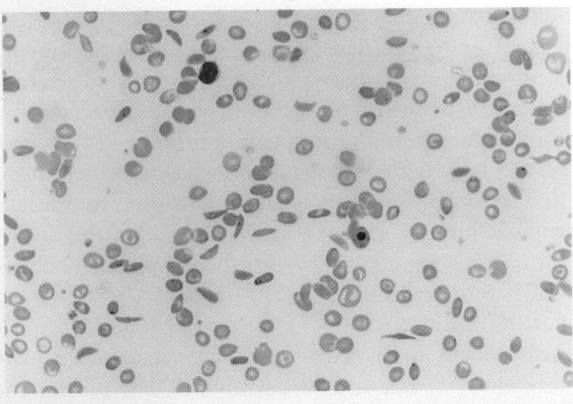

Fig. B Peripheral blood film showing sickle-shaped cells, polychromasia and target cells. Many of the red cells appear irregular and elongated—sickle cells. Target cells are present, together with a nucleated red cell: these indicate functional hyposplenism present in sickle-cell disease.

Fig. C Prenatal diagnosis. Trophoblast DNA, obtained by sampling at 6–9 weeks of gestation is used to detect the base substitution. Different fragment lengths are produced depending on the presence of a normal (HbA) or sickle (HbS) gene. Restriction enzyme analysis of fetal DNA reveals a single 1.3 kb band in homozygotes, a 1.3 kb band in heterozygotes, and a single 1.1 kb band corresponding to the normal β gene in normal individuals. Using the polymerase chain reaction this test can be performed in less than 6 hours, with as little as 0.25 µg of DNA.

precautions in patients with SCA. Strict attention to adequate hydration and oxygenation before and during anaesthesia is essential. Preoperative exchange transfusion is widely recommended before major surgical procedures.

Other sickle cell disorders

HbSC disease results from inheritance of a HbS gene from one parent and a HbC gene from the other. The clinical features are similar (although usually milder), to those of homozygous SCA (HbSS), but because the haemoglobin level is often close to normal, blood viscosity is higher than in SCA: the consequences are: (a) SCD patients may not be regarded as at risk—many are told they have 'sickle trait'; (b) crises, when they do occur, can be explosive; and (c) there is a greater tendency to thrombosis such as pulmonary embolism and a higher incidence of retinopathy.

HbS/β⁰ thalassaemia presents with a similar clinical picture to that of SCA. Persistent splenomegaly is more common.

Antenatal screening with specialist counselling

Antenatal screening with specialist counselling of prospective parents is extremely important for all sickle cell disorders, including asymptomatic heterozygous carriers (HbAS).

Red cell enzymopathies

Epidemiology
Prevalence. G6PD deficiency: many millions worldwide. Others: rare.

Age. Congenital, life-long.

Sex. G6PD deficiency more common in males (X-linked).

Genetics. G6PD deficiency X-linked: glycolytic pathway deficiencies autosomal recessive.

Ethnicity. May be seen in any, but G6PD deficiency most frequent in individuals of African, Mediterranean and South East Asian descent.

Geography. Worldwide.

Disease mechanisms

Glucose-6-phosphate dehydrogenase deficiency

The enzyme G6PD performs a rate-limiting step in the pentose phosphate pathway, which generates NADPH, the red cell antioxidant. G6PD deficiency renders the red cell vulnerable to the oxidant stress of: (a) infection and fever; and (b) oxidant drugs (primaquine, sulphonamides). Haemolysis may be intravascular and violent.

Glycolytic pathway enzyme deficiencies (e.g. pyruvate kinase deficiency)

These deficiencies reduce the ATP energy supply to the red cell and thereby limit its survival in the circulation, causing chronic extravascular haemolytic anaemia.

Clinical features

General features of haemolytic anaemia, with an evident provoking cause in G6PD deficiency.

Investigation

Haematology
- *FBC:* anaemia (usually normocytic).
- *Blood film:* polychromasia. Red cells may show 'bitemarks' (G6PD deficiency) or 'sputnik' projections (pyruvate kinase deficiency). Reticulocytosis.
- *RBC enzyme assay:* in the most common type of G6PD deficiency, the enzyme decays over the lifespan of the red cell, so in the immediate aftermath of a haemolytic crisis (when a high proportion of residual red cells are new), the G6PD assay may be normal: it should be performed later. Other red cell enzyme assays are performed in a specialist laboratory.

Management

- Withdraw provoking drug and treat underlying infection
- Give folate supplementation
- Red cell transfusion only if anaemia severe (less than 5 g/dl)
- Splenectomy may benefit some glycolytic pathway deficiencies: an expert decision

Microangiopathic haemolytic anaemia

Epidemiology

Incidence. 5 in 1 000 000/year

Age. Any age, including childhood.

Sex. Equal.

Ethnicity. All.

Geography. Worldwide.

Disease mechanisms

Red cells are smashed as they pass through abnormal blood vessels, causing intravascular haemolysis. The most common site of damage is the microcirculation, where inflammatory change in the vascular endothelium provokes the red cell damage. In **haemolytic–uraemic syndrome** (HUS) platelet and endothelial damage is related to toxigenic *Escherichia coli* infection, while in **thrombotic thrombocytopenic purpura** (TTP) it is related to inherited or acquired deficiency of a protease that normally controls platelet adhesion to vascular endothelium by cleaving very large (and very sticky) forms of vWF produced by disturbed endothelial cells.

Clinical features

Acute severe intravascular haemolytic anaemia: (a) with thrombocytopenia and CNS symptoms (encephalitis and coma) in **TTP**; (b) with diarrhoea and renal failure in **HUS**; (c) in the context of pregnancy in **eclampsia** and haemolysis, elevated liver enzymes and low platelet count (**HELPP**) syndrome; and (d) with uncontrolled **severe (malignant) hypertension**.

Investigation

Haematology
- *FBC:* anaemia, thrombocytopenia
- *Blood film:* red cell fragments (schistocytes)

Biochemistry
- *LDH elevation:* often a sensitive marker of response to therapy
- *Urea and creatinine:* markers of renal failure

Microbiology

Stool culture for verotoxin-secreting *E. coli*, *E. coli* 0.157 (these organisms may be few and only detectable by DNA methods).

Diagnostic imaging

Brain CT may be negative in TTP, even in the presence of coma.

Management

- Plasma exchange (PEX) is effective in most cases of TTP. A sequence of many exchanges may be required.
- Renal replacement therapy is indicated in many cases of HUS.
- Delivery of the infant is indicated in eclampsia and HELPP.
- Control of hypertension in hypertensive states.

Prognosis

- *TTP:* 80% respond to PEX and 60% do not recur, but non-responders often have a fatal outcome
- *HUS:* 60% fully recover with supportive therapy, with chronic renal impairment or death in the remainder (mainly older patients)
- *Eclampsia, HELPP, malignant hypertension:* good outcome with rapid recognition and treatment

White blood cell disorders

Leucocytosis (WBC ↑)

Disease mechanisms

An increased WBC results from three broad causes:
1 Microbial infection (e.g. bacteria, viruses, fungi)
2 Inflammation of non-infective origin (e.g. trauma, surgery, cancer, connective tissue disorders)
3 An abnormal leucocyte population (e.g. leukaemia)

Clinical features

These are determined by the underlying disorder: the features of leukaemias and lymphomas can be found in the relevant sections below.

Investigation

The first question addressed by investigation is: 'What type of white cell is responsible for this increased WBC count?' The second, 'What is the underlying disease', may require extensive tests outside the remit of this chapter.

Haematology
- *FBC:* infection or inflammation usually cause WBC of $10-30 \times 10^9$/l. Counts more than 30×10^9/l usually indicate leukaemia. Rarely, an infective or inflammatory state causes a WBC of more than 30×10^9/l, sometimes confusingly termed a 'leukaemoid reaction'. Modern cell counters also give a differential count identifying the type of cell accounting for the increase, but this must always be checked by microscopy.
- *Blood film:* the morphology of the dominant white cell type (neutrophil, lymphocyte or abnormal cell) is decided by microscopy. Cytology of the cells may give additional clues:

(a) intense neutrophil granulation and 'left shift' typical of infective or inflammatory neutrophilia
(b) large basophilic 'atypical' lymphocytes in infectious mononucleosis
- *Bone marrow aspirate and trephine:* indicated if abnormal cells are present on the blood film. Immune phenotyping, chromosomal analysis and other tests may also be performed.

Management

Depends on the underlying cause.

Leucopenia (WBC ↓)

Disease mechanisms

There are two broad causes of a low WBC:
1 Reduced ('central') production of normal leucocytes by the bone marrow (e.g. drug-induced agranulocytosis, aplastic anaemia; see p. 1047)
2 Increased ('peripheral') destruction (or removal from the circulating blood; e.g. the early stage of severe infection, hypersplenism)

Clinical features

When production of leucocytes is stopped, the patient becomes vulnerable to **opportunistic** infection, particularly pneumonia and skin or subcutaneous infection. The most dramatic example is drug-induced agranulocytosis, in which exposure to a drug (sulphonamides, antithyroid agents, antipsychotic drugs) results in acute immune-mediated destruction of all cells of the neutrophil series in marrow and blood. When there is increased peripheral destruction of leucocytes alone, this vulnerability is usually not so marked, although a **primary** infection may be responsible for the problem. A striking case is HIV infection, which causes lymphopenia by a direct cytotoxic effect; the lymphopenia then predisposes the patient to further opportunistic infection.

Investigation

Haematology
- *FBC:* reduced WBC. The differential count indicates the cell type that is lacking.
- *Blood film:* morphology confirms the specific cytopenia (e.g. absolute lack of neutrophils in agranulocytosis).
- *Leucocyte immunophenotyping:* may demonstrate CD4 cell cytopenia in HIV infection.
- *Bone marrow aspirate/trephine:* demonstrates bone marrow infiltration or aplasia if this is the cause.

Management

- **Stop all drug treatment** that coincided with the fall in WBC

- **Antibiotic therapy** if active primary or secondary infection indicated by fever (see EMERGENCY BOX 5.3)
- **Growth factor therapy** with G-CSF is indicated in drug-induced agranulocytosis
- **Specific therapy** for disease processes infiltrating or suppressing the bone marrow

Platelet disorders

Thrombocytopenia (platelets ↓)

A reduced platelet count is a common finding in many disorders, because the lifespan of circulating platelets is reduced in:

- All types of infection
- Any disorder causing widespread activation of the haemostatic system (e.g. major trauma)
- Complications of pregnancy (e.g. pre-eclampsia)

In addition, the platelet count may be reduced by the 'pooling' of platelets in the spleen in splenomegaly (e.g. **portal hypertension** caused by liver disease). Reduction of platelet lifespan is also seen in autoimmune disorders, because of specific antiplatelet antibodies (see below).

Beware of two common laboratory artefacts that can mimic thrombocytopenia:

1 *A small clot in the blood sample:* the laboratory will usually check for one
2 *Platelet clumping caused by a reaction with the anticoagulant EDTA:* this will only be apparent if a blood film is examined

Autoimmune thrombocytopenic purpura
Epidemiology
Incidence. 1 in 1000/year (estimate).

Age. Any age, including childhood.

Sex. More common in females.

Ethnicity. All.

Genetics. None: an acquired disorder.

Geography. Worldwide.

Disease mechanisms
There are acute (self-limiting) and chronic forms of immune thrombocytopenic purpura (ITP). Acute ITP is the usual form in children and often follows viral infection, remitting spontaneously as the infection is cleared. Chronic ITP mostly affects adults.

Clinical features
The typical symptom is **purpura** (see p. 1009 for symptoms and signs of thrombocytopenia). There may be other bleeding symptoms (e.g. epistaxis, gum bleeding or menorrhagia). Severe bleeding (e.g. intracranial, retinal or abdominal haemorrhage) is relatively uncommon.

Diagnosis
Depends on finding thrombocytopenia without red or white cell abnormalities, combined with a normal or increased number of megakaryocytes in the bone marrow (this combination shows that the low platelet count is caused by **peripheral destruction**). Primary autoimmune thrombocytopenic purpura (AITP) should be distinguished from secondary AITP occurring with connective tissue disorders, lymphoma or CLL by further tests, because treatment will differ.

Investigation
Haematology
- *FBC:* normal Hb (unless major bleeding). Normal WBC. Low platelet count.
- *Blood film:* red and white cells normal. Platelets reduced, may be bigger than normal.
- *Bone marrow:* normal or increased megakaryocytes. No evidence of abnormal cell infiltration.

Immunology
- *Antiplatelet antibodies:* rarely a useful test because platelets bind immunoglobulin in many disorders (e.g. infection)
- *Antinuclear factor/DNA antibodies:* may show associated connective tissue disease

Management
Treatment is rarely needed for acute self-limited AITP in children: bleeding (see below) is rare, and the condition usually spontaneously remits in 1–4 weeks.

Chronic AITP should be treated if:
- There is evidence of active bleeding, particularly mucosal bleeding, at any platelet count
- Platelet count is persistently less than 5×10^9/l
- Platelet count is less than 100×10^9/l and surgery is needed

There are three effective therapies, which may be combined:
- *Corticosteroids* (e.g. prednisolone 1 mg/kg/day): this rapidly inhibits platelet removal by the spleen (platelets rise in approximately 48 h) and more slowly reduces autoantibody production. If a response is achieved, the dose is maintained for 4 weeks, then reduced (tailed) and stopped.
- *Intravenous immunoglobulin (IVIG) infusion* (total dose 2 g/kg, given over 2–5 days): this expensive therapy usually raises the platelet count in 12–24 h and is therefore preferred if there is serious bleeding (e.g. into the CNS).

- *Splenectomy:* necessary if thrombocytopenia is resistant to corticosteroids, or if withdrawal of corticosteroids is followed by relapse. Eighty per cent of patients respond to splenectomy.

Prognosis

Acute ITP commonly has a self-limited course with spontaneous remission occurring within days to weeks. In chronic ITP symptoms usually stabilize, and the platelet count slowly improves with time. Even in this group, death from haemorrhage is rare.

Thrombocytosis (platelets ↑)

An increased platelet count (more than $400 \times 10^9/l$) is also a common finding. Platelets increase as part of the inflammatory response to:

- Cancer
- Ischaemia
- Blood loss and anaemia
- Trauma (e.g. surgery)

Thrombocytosis (often more than $1000 \times 10^9/l$) may also occur as part of a myeloproliferative disorder, particularly **essential thrombocythaemia (ET)**. These are described on p. 1057.

Platelet function disorders

These disorders are described on p. 1068.

Bone marrow failure

In bone marrow failure states, haematopoiesis fails as a result of stem cell damage. This damage may be caused by destruction or suppression by cytotoxic drugs used in cancer therapy, by γ-irradiation or by autoimmune responses triggered by viral infection or other, unknown, mechanisms. The result is a predictable fall in the circulating numbers of red cells, white cells and platelets in the peripheral blood to levels that threaten oxygen transport, microbiological defence and bleeding.

Aplastic anaemia

Epidemiology
Incidence. 1–2 in 1 000 000/year.

Age. All ages.

Sex. More common in males.

Ethnicity. All.

Geography. More common in the Middle East, Indian Subcontinent and South East Asia: this may be a result of viral (hepatitic) exposure.

Genetics. Some cases are associated with recessive disorders affecting HSCs (e.g. Fanconi's anaemia).

Disease mechanisms
Bone marrow suppression may result from T-cell- or antibody-mediated destruction of stem cells ('seed') or bone marrow stroma ('soil'). This would explain the approximate 50% response rate to immunosuppressive therapy (ALG).

Hypoplastic and aplastic anaemia result when bone marrow erythroid precursors are depressed (hypoplasia) or virtually absent (aplasia). Pure red cell aplasia affects erythropoiesis only, while aplastic anaemia affects all lineages and causes pancytopenia.

Clinical features
The clinical features are those of anaemia, neutropenia or thrombocytopenia. They depend on the severity of marrow hypoplasia. Severe aplastic anaemia with marked neutropenia and thrombocytopenia resembles acute leukaemia clinically, and life-threatening infections (see EMERGENCY BOX 15.3) and bleeding episodes are common.

Emergency 15.3: Fever in a neutropenic patient

Problem

Fever (more than 37°C for 2 h or longer) may be the only sign of life-threatening infection in a patient with neutropenia (polymorph count less than $1.0 \times 10^9/l$)

The most common causative organisms are Gram-positive bacteria

The most dangerous causative organisms are Gram-negative bacteria

Action

Take blood and urine cultures

Immediately start therapy with a combination of intravenous broad-spectrum antibiotics that cover both Gram-negative and Gram-positive pathogens (e.g. gentamicin plus tazocin): do not wait for culture results

If the patient is already on antibiotics, a new second-line combination is commenced

If the patient has been neutropenic and febrile for many days, consider antifungal therapy

G-CSF therapy may improve neutrophil counts in this situation

Diagnosis

Aplastic or hypoplastic anaemia is diagnosed on the basis of a pancytopenia in the absence of other abnormalities with an 'empty marrow' seen on bone marrow trephine biopsy sections.

Differential diagnosis of pancytopenia includes aplastic anaemia, acute leukaemia, bone marrow infiltration by lymphoma, carcinoma, myeloma or myelofibrosis, hypersplenism, megaloblastic anaemia, systemic lupus erythematosus and paroxysmal nocturnal haemoglobinuria.

Investigation

Haematology

- *FBC:* reveals a pancytopenia, and most red cells are normocytic, although some macrocytosis may be present. There is a reduced or nil reticulocyte count.
- *Bone marrow aspiration:* reveals hypocellular particles, in which stromal elements (macrophages and fibroblasts) may be prominent. A trephine reveals hypoplasia or aplasia showing reduced cellularity and increased fat spaces.

Management

Mild or moderate hypoplastic anaemia requires supportive treatment, which includes blood and platelet transfusions, and management of infection.

Severe aplastic anaemia is treated with rabbit or horse antithymocyte globulin (ATG) and ciclosporin. Bone marrow transplantation is best reserved for young patients (less than 30 years of age) who have an HLA-identical sibling.

Prognosis

The course of aplastic anaemia varies from spontaneous recovery to rapid deterioration and death. Poor prognostic features are:

- Platelet count less than $l0 \times 10^9/l$
- Neutrophil count less than $0.5 \times 10^9/l$
- Reticulocyte count less than $10 \times 10^9/l$
- Hypocellular marrow less than 20% haemopoietic cells
  More than 50% of patients in whom all these features persist for longer than 3 weeks will die within 3 months unless effective therapy (ALG, ciclosporin or allogeneic bone marrow transplantation) is given.

Bone marrow failure because of infiltration

Haemopoietic stem cell failure can occur secondary to invasion of the bone marrow (intramedullary) space by malignant cells of haematological (e.g. leukaemia, lymphoma, myeloma) or non-haematological (e.g. prostate, breast) cancers. In these situations, a particular combination of findings on microscopy of the peripheral blood smear (the presence of nucleated red cell precursors and early members of the myeloid series) is often found and suggests the diagnosis. This is called a **leukoerythroblastic** blood film (also seen when the marrow is infiltrated by abnormal fibrotic tissue in myelofibrosis; discussed below).

Bone marrow failure because of infection

Certain disseminated infections tend to involve the bone marrow, when they may result in bone marrow failure.

Mycobacteria (particularly atypical mycobacteria, but also *M. tuberculosis*) and HIV virus are the most often seen.

Haematological malignancies

Acute leukaemia

Disease mechanisms

The causative aetiology of acute leukaemia is not yet known, but agents that damage DNA (e.g. radiation, carcinogenic drugs) are risk factors. The mechanism involves mutations or translocations involving oncogenes, or transcription factors, that affect cell replication and apoptosis. A multistep chain of several such events culminates in the development of a clone of cells with a growth advantage over their normal counterparts. This advantage consists of uncontrolled replication, escape from normal cell death mechanisms (apoptosis) or both. The resulting leukaemia cells are 'blocked' in early differentiation (blast cells) and multiply. They replace normal haemopoiesis causing bone marrow failure with pancytopenia. They also act as tumour cells, invading tissues and sites outside their normal distribution and causing mass lesions and organ failure.

Classification of acute leukaemia

There are two types of acute leukaemia, defined by the lineage to which the blast cells belong:

- Acute lymphoblastic leukaemia (ALL)
- Acute myeloblastic leukaemia (AML)

Clinical features

Both types of acute leukaemia present as bone marrow failure, with symptoms and signs of anaemia, infection and bleeding. General malaise and bone pain (ribs and sternum in adults: limb pains making walking painful in childhood) are frequent. Organomegaly (e.g. a thymic mass in T-cell ALL), lymph node enlargement and splenomegaly may occur because of the accumulation of blast cells. Occasionally, symptoms of central nervous system invasion (cranial nerve lesions, paraparesis) may be present.

Diagnosis

Depends on the presence of a hypercellular ('packed') marrow with more than 30% blast cells, or the finding of proven myeloid or lymphoid blast cell infiltrates in a site outside the bone marrow (extramedullary leukaemia).

Distinguishing AML and ALL is vital, because therapy is different. This is done by:

- *Blast cell morphology:* blood and bone marrow smears
- *Blast cell cytochemical staining:* (e.g. Sudan black positivity = AML)
- *Blast cell immunophenotyping:* using a panel of lineage-specific monoclonal antibody 'markers'
- *Cytogenetic study of blast cells in marrow/blood* (by karyotyping): demonstrates leukaemia-specific chromosome abnormalities
- *Molecular diagnosis:* by fluorescence *in situ* hybridization (FISH), PCR or other DNA technique demonstrates leukaemia-specific DNA sequences

Investigation

Haematology

- *FBC:* may show a pronounced leukocytosis (total WBC $30–200 \times 10^9$/l) but the WBC may be in the normal range or even low. There is reduction of normal cell types (pancytopenia) with anaemia, neutropenia and thrombocytopenia.
- *Blood film:* leukaemic **blast** cells are usually seen, and may attain counts of 50×10^9/l or more.
- *Bone marrow examination:* must be performed to make the diagnosis. Must show massive hypercellularity. Blast cells must amount to more than 30% of the nucleated cells.
- *Coagulation screen:* may show ↑ INR, ↑ TT (see Fig. 15.10) and ↓ fibrinogen resulting from disseminated intravascular coagulation—this is very dangerous and needs urgent platelet and plasma support.

Biochemistry

- *Hypercalcaemia and hyperuricaemia:* may be present
- *Increased hepatic transaminases;* may indicate liver infiltration
- *Urea and creatinine:* may be high, indicating renal impairment

Microbiology

The finding of fever (over 37.5°C) compels blood cultures, and immediate broad-spectrum antibiotic therapy while waiting for the results (see EMERGENCY BOX 15.13).

Cytology

Cerebrospinal fluid examination for the presence of leukaemic blasts is a vital part of the work-up for ALL, but the timing of this test must be carefully determined by an expert clinician.

Diagnostic imaging

- *Chest X-ray:* essential in febrile patients: the most common site of opportunistic infection is the lungs
- *Ultrasound or CT study:* may be required to define extramedullary mass lesions
- *MRI:* of the CNS if symptoms suggest leukaemic infiltration

Acute myeloid leukaemia

Epidemiology

Incidence. 0.5 in 10 000/year.

Age. Incidence increases sharply with age. Maximal incidence over 70 years.

Sex. Equal.

Ethnicity. All.

Geography. Worldwide.

Genetics. Most cases show acquired chromosome abnormalities affecting the leukaemic clone.

Management

Aims of therapy:

1 Prevention of death from bone marrow failure by **supportive therapy**.

2 Induction of **complete remission**, defined as non-detectability of leukaemic blasts (5% or less in the bone marrow) plus return of normal cell counts. Remission induction is not the same as cure, because even after blasts apparently disappear, part of the leukaemic clone survives below the limit of detection. However, achieving remission is a vital step, without which cure is impossible.

3 **Continuation** of cytotoxic therapy, which may include high-dose phases with stem cell support from the patient themselves (autograft) or from a histocompatible donor (allograft) to eliminate residual cells of the leukaemic clone, resulting in a high chance of cure.

Remission induction therapy consists of a combination of profoundly myelosuppressive drug agents, typically including the antimetabolite **cytosine arabinoside** and an antileukaemic antibiotic of the **anthracycline** class. One subgroup of AML (acute promyelocytic leukaemia) is sensitive to the vitamin A derivative all-*trans*-retinoic acid (ATRA), so this may be added. This first cycle of AML therapy usually suppresses all bone marrow activity for 4 weeks, during which the patient is utterly dependent for survival on supportive care. At the end of this period, the bone marrow regenerates, either normally (remission—approximately 90%) or with persistent leukaemia (approximately 10%).

Acute leukaemia at a glance

Epidemiology
Incidence
Age-specific: ALL peak (approximately 4 years old) 80/million/year; over 10 years of age, 10/million/year. AML: under 50 years, 10/million/yr; over 50 years, 60/million/year

Age
ALL peak age = 4 years; AML peak age = 70 years

Sex
Slightly more males in every age group

Ethnicity
No significant differences

Findings on investigation
Haematology
• *FBC:* usually (not always). ↑↑ WBC composed of leukaemic blast cells. Normal cells reduced, with anaemia, neutropenia and thrombocytopenia
• *Blood film:* leukaemic blasts, recognized by high nuclear : cytoplasmic ratio and undifferentiated morphology
• *Bone marrow aspirate:* must be hypercellular, and blast cells exceeding 20% of total nucleated cells to confirm the diagnosis. The type of leukaemia is assigned according to morphology of the blasts (plus cell markers)
• *Cell markers:* cytochemical and immunological markers confirm whether the diagnosis is ALL or AML
• *Chromosome studies:* often give important prognostic information

Cytology
Cerebrospinal fluid examined for blasts in ALL

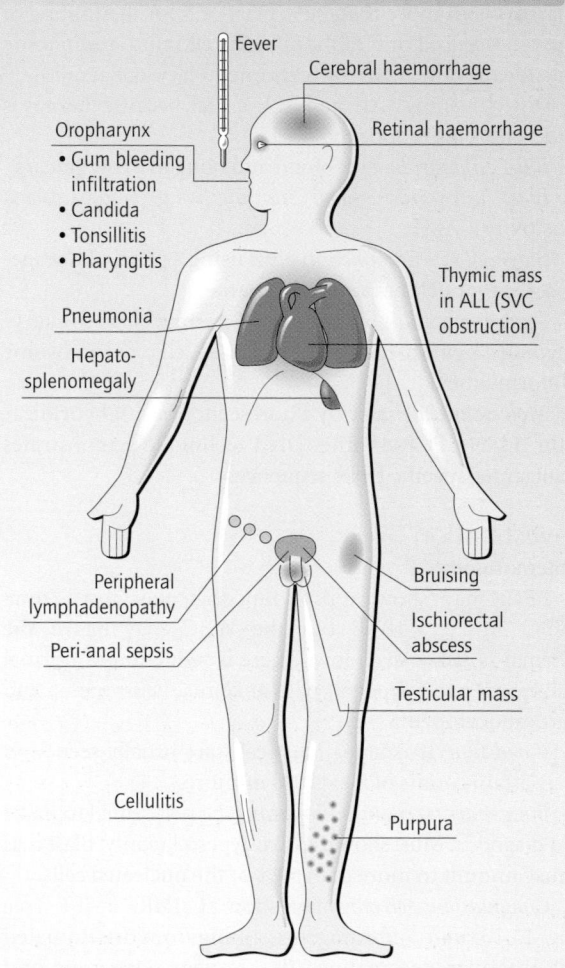

Fever
Cerebral haemorrhage
Retinal haemorrhage
Oropharynx
• Gum bleeding infiltration
• Candida
• Tonsillitis
• Pharyngitis
Pneumonia
Hepato-splenomegaly
Thymic mass in ALL (SVC obstruction)
Peripheral lymphadenopathy
Peri-anal sepsis
Bruising
Ischiorectal abscess
Testicular mass
Cellulitis
Purpura

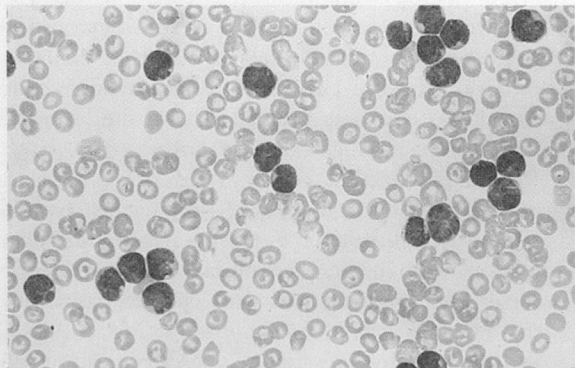

Fig. A ALL (L1 subtype) peripheral blood film showing rather small blasts with a high nuclear/cytoplasmic ratio.

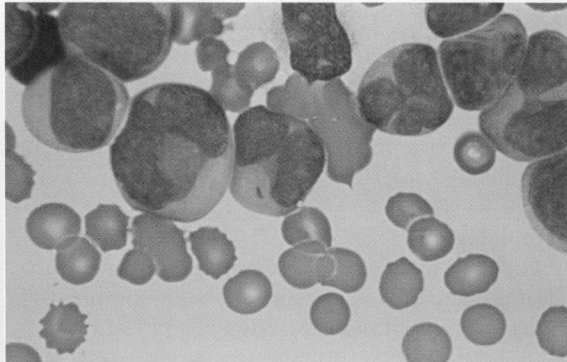

Fig. B AML (M5—acute monoblastic leukaemia). A bone marrow aspirate showing blasts with irregular nuclei and prominent nucleoli. Note the central blast contains a single small Auer rod—a diagnostic feature of AML.

Imaging
Chest X-ray examined for thymic mass in ALL
Clinical features

Haematology
Anaemia
Bruising and purpura
Mucosal bleeding (e.g. gums)
Bone pain (e.g. child refusing to walk)

Dermatology
Purpura
Skin sepsis
Leukaemic skin infiltration

Tumour masses
Thymic mass in T-ALL
Lymph node enlargement
Hepato- and/or splenomegaly
Orbital mass
Gum hypertrophy

Immunology
Septicaemia and other infections, particularly in neutropenic patients

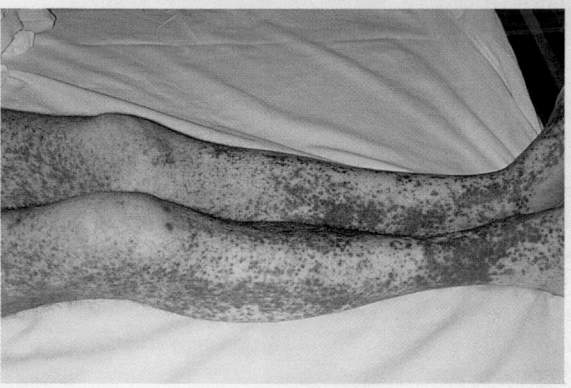

Fig. C Purpura of the lower limbs due to severe thrombocytopenia associated with AML.

15

Continuation therapy consists of a further three or four cycles of similar drug combinations. The individual drugs are usually varied to prevent the leukaemic clone developing drug resistance. Continuation therapy may be completed with high-dose cytotoxic drug and/or total body irradiation therapy supported by auto- or allo-stem cell infusion.

Prognosis
In younger AML patients (under 65 years) treated according to standard protocols, stages 1 and 2 are currently achieved in approximately 90%, and 3 in approximately 50% of cases.

In patients over 65 years, results are much worse, and the nature and intensity of therapy must be carefully judged and discussed.

Acute lymphoblastic leukaemia
Epidemiology
Incidence. 0.5 in 10 000/year.

Age. Peak incidence 1–5 years. Then occurs infrequently in all age groups until the rate rises again over 60 years.

Sex. Equal.

Ethnicity. All.

Geography. Worldwide.

Genetics. Most cases show acquired chromosome abnormalities affecting the leukaemic clone, including an important subgroup with the Philadelphia (Ph[1]) chromosome.

Management
Aims of therapy:
1 and 2 identical to AML therapy (above).
3 *CNS therapy:* because ALL often infiltrates the meninges of the brain and spinal cord, ALL therapy includes an extra sequence of intrathecal chemotherapy (must only be given by specially trained and accredited staff) and in some cases (or if CNS leukaemia has been diagnosed on lumbar puncture) cranial irradiation.
4 *Intensification therapy:* with 2–3 spaced 'blocks' of myelosuppressive combination therapy similar to those used in AML.
5 *Maintenance therapy:* with oral drugs, which lasts for 2 years (maintenance therapy is not used in AML).

Remission induction therapy in ALL usually consists of continuous high-dose corticosteroid therapy plus weekly injections of the vinca alkaloid vincristine. An anthracycline may be added. Remission usually occurs in about 4 weeks.

Maintenance therapy consists of daily 6-mercaptopurine and weekly methotrexate.

Prognosis
More than 90% of patients with ALL achieve complete remission. Children between 2 and 10 years of age have a

70–80% cure rate after maintenance therapy, but that for adult ALL is only about 25%.

Myelodysplastic syndromes

Epidemiology
Identical to AML (see above).

Disease mechanisms
Myelodysplastic syndromes (MDS) refers to a group of blood disorders that share the following features:
- Reduced numbers of red cells, white cells or platelets (cytopenias) in marrow and peripheral blood
- Morphological and functional abnormalities (dysplasia) of white cells and platelets: infection and bleeding may be worse than expected from the counts
- Clonal haematopoiesis (all blood cells are progeny of a single abnormal stem cell)

In addition, some types of MDS have increased blast cells in the marrow and/or blood, with a high risk of progression to AML.

Diagnosis
There are four types of MDS.

Good prognosis:

1 *Refractory anaemia (RA):* refractory refers to lack of response to haematinic therapy (the anaemia is transfusion-dependent)

2 *Refractory anaemia with ringed sideroblasts (RARS):* primary sideroblastic anaemia

Bad prognosis:

3 *Refractory anaemia with excess blasts (RAEB):* 50% transform to AML within a few years

4 *Chronic myelomonocytic leukaemia (CMML)*

Clinical features
Clinical features are characteristically anaemia, neutropenia, monocytosis and thrombocytopenia, either singly or in combination. There is no underlying illness to account for the findings. Patients usually present with anaemia, infection or bleeding secondary to pancytopenia.

Investigation
Haematology
- *FBC:* anaemia (normocytic or macrocytic). WBC may be low, normal or high. Platelets low or normal.
- *Blood film:* characteristic appearance of neutrophils, with hypogranulation (empty appearance) of cytoplasm. In CMML, there is a marked monocytosis.
- *Bone marrow aspirate and trephine:* hypercellularity with: (a) more than 5% myeloblasts in RAEB; (b) monocytosis in CMML; and (c) erythroid cells with complete rings

of iron-laden mitochondria surrounding the nucleus on iron-staining.

Management
Usually supportive, with palliative intent:
- Regular red cell transfusion is arranged for refractory anaemia
- Platelet transfusions and antibiotics may be required for cytopenia or poor function
- Oral low-dose chemotherapy may control counts in CMML
- Intensive anti-AML chemotherapy for fitter patients transforming to AML, but outcome is much worse when AML follows MDS
- Allo-BMT from HLA-compatible siblings offers the possibility of cure to a minority of younger patients

Prognosis
The natural history of MDS is variable, but there is high morbidity and mortality resulting from bone marrow failure and transfusion-related iron overload. Approximately 30% transform into AML.

Chronic myeloid leukaemia

Epidemiology
Incidence. 1 in 100 000/year.

Age. 35–50 years.

Sex. Slightly more common in males.

Ethnicity. All.

Genetics. Acquired chromosomal defect (Philadelphia chromosome).

Geography. Worldwide.

Disease mechanisms
Exposure to ionizing radiation and benzene are factors in rare cases ($\uparrow$ incidence in atom bomb survivors).

Most cases are apparently spontaneous.

In CML, normal haematopoiesis is replaced by a clone of cells containing an abnormal chromosome 22, the Philadelphia (Ph[1]) chromosome. This acquired abnormality affects the pluripotential stem cell, because the Ph[1] chromosome is present in red cells, granulocytes, megakaryocytes and some lymphocytes in CML.

The Ph[1] chromosome is produced by the translocation of material between chromosome 9 and chromosome 22. Translocation of the *c-abl* oncogene from chromosome

9 results in the creation of a fusion gene (*bcr-abl*) on chromosome 22. Transcription and translation of this hybrid gene results in a hybrid abnormal signalling kinase, which seems to drive the overproduction of myeloid cells.

Clinical features

Uncontrolled proliferation and accumulation of myeloid cells causes most of the clinical features. Hypermetabolic manifestations include weight loss, anorexia, lassitude and sweating. Splenomegaly is prominent, often larger than 10 cm at diagnosis, and may cause discomfort. Other features include hepatomegaly, anaemia because of bone marrow suppression, hyperuricaemia and gout.

The clinical course follows a sequence of phases:
1 Stable **chronic phase** lasting 3–5 years.
2 **Accelerated phase** with increasing white cell counts and splenomegaly. Myelofibrosis may develop.
3 Terminal **blast crisis** (median duration 2–4 months) with rapidly progressive and poorly treatable acute myeloid or lymphoid leukaemia.

Investigation

Haematology
- *FBC:* anaemia. The WBC is increased, often massively (e.g. 250×10^9/l). Thrombocytosis is common.
- *Blood film:* the dominant feature is neutrophilia, with numerous myelocytes and basophils.
- *Neutrophil alkaline phosphatase:* low or absent in contrast to raised levels in leukaemoid reactions.

Management

- The initial aim of therapy in the chronic phase is to control hypercellularity and keep the patient symptom-free. The best myelosuppressive drugs for this purpose are **hydroxyurea** and **cytosine arabinoside**, with allopurinol to prevent hyperuricaemia.
- A further aim is to suppress the CML clone. This allows normal haematopoiesis to repopulate the marrow, and reduces the risk of transformation to accelerated or blastic phases, hence prolonging life. **Interferon-α** therapy does this in about 20% of patients. Promising is the new agent **imatinib**, a 'designer drug' that inhibits the abnormal signalling kinase produced by the CML translocation. Suppression of the CML clone by this agent backs up the theory that the abnormal kinase 'drives' CML. However, the effect is lost if interferon or imatinib therapy is stopped, so neither provides a cure.
- **Allogeneic bone marrow transplant** from a histocompatible donor is the treatment of choice, the only treatment that offers a chance of cure. Only a minority of patients can access such a donor, and allo-BMT is a dangerous therapy for patients over 50 years old.

Prognosis

Death from CML usually results from terminal acute transformation with associated infection or haemorrhage at a mean of 5–7 years from diagnosis: imatinib may improve this outlook. Unlike the chronic phase, the terminal phase is rarely responsive to therapy.

Chronic lymphocytic leukaemia

A chronic leukaemia caused by excess production of a clone of abnormal lymphocytes, involving the blood, bone marrow and lymphoid tissues. Sometimes classified as a lymphoproliferative disorder, and sometimes (if it predominantly involves lymph nodes) as a low-grade lymphoma. Haematologists prefer to call it a chronic leukaemia.

Epidemiology

Prevalence and age. The most common leukaemia in the West. Age-dependent. 1 in 10 000/year over 60 years, rising to 2 in 1000/year over 75 years.

Sex. Two-thirds are male.

Genetics. Acquired clonal chromosome defects (e.g. trisomy 12) may be present.

Geography. In the West, CLL > non-Hodgkin's lymphoma (NHL): elsewhere, NHL > CLL.

Disease mechanisms

Chronic lymphatic leukaemia is a clonal proliferation of normal-looking but functionally useless B lymphocytes. The clone originates in a poorly understood minor subset of B cells that weakly express surface immunoglobulin. In progressive CLL they slowly accumulate in the blood, marrow and lymphoid tissues, compromising normal marrow and immune function (via hypoimmunoglobulinaemia).

Clinical features

The natural history of CLL is bimodal: many asymptomatic patients are diagnosed coincidently on routine FBCs and the disorder progresses slowly or not at all. Others present with a high lymphocyte count, lymphadenopathy and heavy bone marrow invasion, with symptoms of general malaise, bone marrow failure and immunodeficiency. In these patients, splenomegaly and hepatomegaly may be found.

15

Chronic lymphocytic leukaemia at a glance

Epidemiology
Incidence
200/million people over 60 years

Age
Rarely seen in people under 40 years old

Sex
Male : female 2 : 1

Ethnicity and geography
In Europe and North American populations, CLL > NHL: in others, NHL > CLL

Genetics
Acquired clonal chromosome defects (e.g. trisomy 12)

Findings on investigation
Haematology
- *Full blood count:* normochromic or haemolytic anaemia

common. ↑ WBC because of lymphocytosis (more than 10×10^9/l). ↓ Platelet count because of bone marrow infiltration or autoimmune thrombocytopenic purpura (AITP)
- *Blood film:* excess small lymphocytes and 'smear' cells

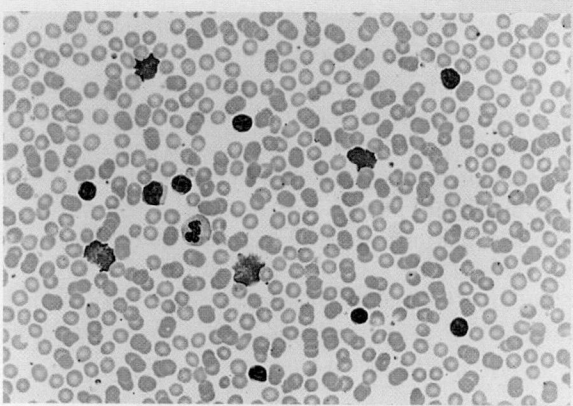

Fig. A Chronic lymphatic leukaemia (CLL). Blood film showing immature B lymphocytes and smear cells. In this low-power field most of the cells are typical CLL lymphocytes. These are small cells with a high nuclear cytoplasmic ratio in which the nuclei contain very heavily clumped chromatin. One rather larger lymphocyte is present and some lymphoid heterogeneity is often present in CLL. At least four damaged lymphocytes are present—smear cells.

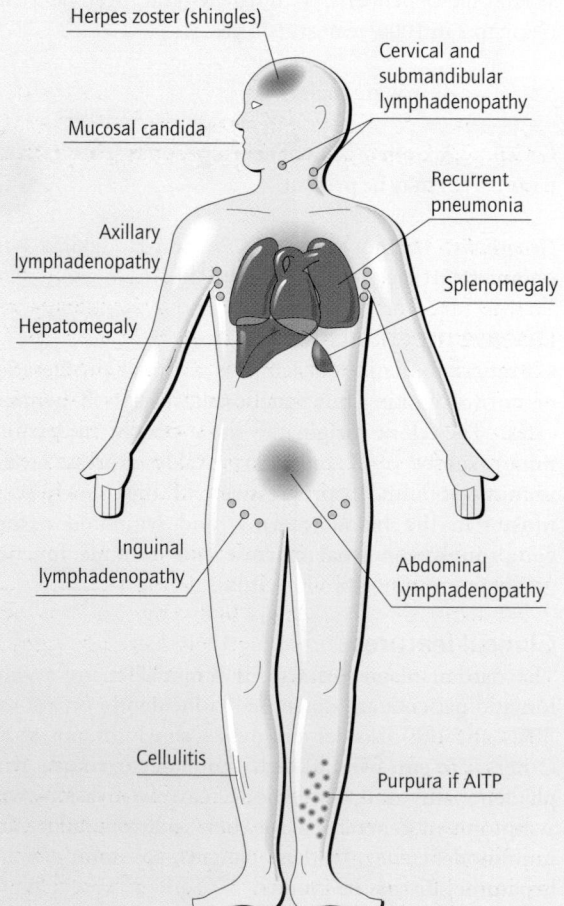

Herpes zoster (shingles)
Cervical and submandibular lymphadenopathy
Mucosal candida
Recurrent pneumonia
Axillary lymphadenopathy
Splenomegaly
Hepatomegaly
Inguinal lymphadenopathy
Abdominal lymphadenopathy
Cellulitis
Purpura if AITP

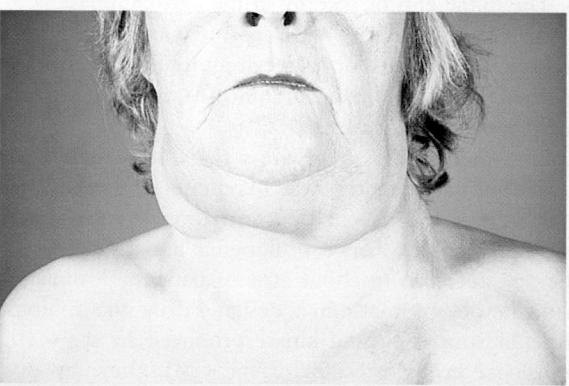

Fig. B Chronic lymphatic leukaemia: bilateral cervical lymphadenopathy in a 67-year-old woman. Haemoglobin 12.5/dl; white blood count 150×19^9/l (lymphocytes 146×10^9/l); platelets 120×19^9/l. Reproduced from Hoffbrand & Pettit, *Essential Haematology*, 3rd edn, 1993 (Blackwell Scientific Publications, Oxford) with the permission of the authors.

• *Bone marrow aspirate and trephine:* varying degrees of marrow infiltration with small lymphocytes
• *Cell markers:* essential test to show clonality and typical CD5⁺ B-cell phenotype

Immunology
Immunoglobulin quantitation reveals hypoimmunoglobulinaemia in 60%

Diagnostic imaging
• *Chest X-ray:* to detect opportunistic pneumonia secondary to hypoimmunoglobulinaemia
• *CT:* of chest and abdomen to detect the extent of lymphadenopathy and splenomegaly

Clinical features
Lymphadenopathy may be absent, localized or massive
Splenomegaly often found, may be massive
Systemic symptoms: anorexia, weight loss (more than 10% body weight), fever and night sweats. In late stages cachexia may develop
Bone marrow involvement: anaemia, neutropenia (susceptible to infections), thrombocytopenia (easy bruising)

Immune suppression with opportunistic infection (e.g. shingles)
CLL is often diagnosed coincidentally on routine FBC in an asymptomatic elderly patient

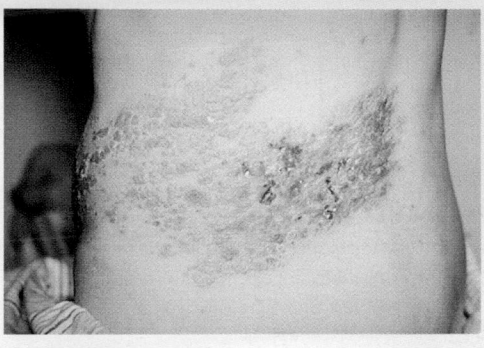

Fig. C Chronic lymphatic leukaemia: herpes zoster infection in a 68-year-old female. Reproduced from Hoffbrand & Pettit, *Essential Haematology*, 3rd edn, 1993 (Blackwell Scientific Publications, Oxford) with the permission of the authors.

Recurrent opportunistic infections are common, especially pneumonia. Aggressive herpes zoster (shingles), often with severe scarring and pain, is also common.

Secondary autoimmune haemolytic anaemia (in 5–10% of patients) or autoimmune thrombocytopenia (in 1–2%) sometimes develops, and may be the presenting feature.

Diagnosis
Depends on the demonstration of a peripheral blood lymphocytosis (more than 7×10^9/l) composed of B cells with a unique phenotype (weak expression of surface immunoglobulin, and coexpression of the [usually T cell] marker CD5).

Investigation
Haematology
● *FBC:* lymphocytosis (more than 7×10^9/l up to 500 $\times 10^9$/l). Anaemia or thrombocytopenia may be present.
● *Blood film:* typical small lymphocytes. Many are smashed while making the film: 'smear' or 'basket' cells.
● *Marrow and trephine:* the CLL infiltrate varies from patchy to diffuse and massive. The bigger the infiltrate, the worse the prognosis.

Immunology
Immunoglobulin assays. Sixty per cent of patients have

hypogammaglobulinaemia, usually with deficiency of IgG and IgA (the IgA deficiency is linked to the risk of pneumonia).

Management
Many patients are asymptomatic when diagnosed on routine blood counts, and require no active therapy: premature treatment at this stage shortens healthy life. The patient and their primary care team are advised to rapidly treat bacterial and herpetic infections, and the patient kept under clinical review—so-called 'watchful waiting'. If the CLL progresses, with severe hypoimmunoglobulinaemia, monthly intravenous immunoglobulin reduces infective episodes.

If troublesome mass effects develop from lymphadenopathy, chemotherapy with the alkylating agent chlorambucil or the purine analogue fludarabine, is given with palliative intent to reduce symptoms. Corticosteroids are also used to treat associated AIHA or AITP.

Prognosis
The prognosis of CLL depends on its progression. Many patients with non-progressive CLL will die of other age-related diseases. In the progressive form, careful therapy may help the patient to a good quality of life for 5 years or so, but CLL is incurable and the patient eventually dies from opportunistic infection or organ failure.

15

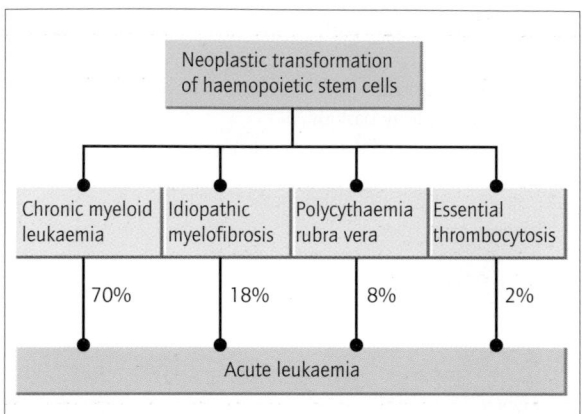

Figure 15.17 Interrelationships between myeloproliferative disorders. Intermediate myeloproliferative disorders having features of more than one type of myeloproliferative disease may occur.

Myeloproliferative disorders

This group of chronic diseases are classed together because they share the basic feature of overproduction of blood cells, and may 'transform' into each other (Fig. 15.17). They are clonal disorders: the progeny of a single haematopoietic stem cell replaces the normal polyclonal population of blood cells. CML is sometimes classified as a member of this group (see p. 1052), but its specific genetic basis gives it independent status. MPD are divided into three main types depending on the most prominent finding:

1 *Overproduction of red cells:* polycythaemia rubra vera (PRV)
2 *Overproduction of platelets:* essential thrombocythaemia (ET)
3 *Overproduction of bone marrow matrix (stromal) elements:* with disturbed function, in idiopathic myelofibrosis.

The most common transitions are from PRV or ET into myelofibrosis. As myelofibrosis develops, the cell counts fall and severe anaemia and thrombocytopenia may develop.

Polycythaemia rubra vera

A chronically increased haemoglobin concentration above the normal range (more than 18.0 g/dl in males, more than 16.0 g/dl in females) because of primary bone marrow overproduction of red blood cells. PRV is a clonal myeloproliferative disease, so the platelet count and leucocyte count may also be abnormally high.

Epidemiology

Incidence. 1 in 100 000/year.

Age. Older age groups: average age at diagnosis is 60 years.

Sex. Equal.

Ethnicity. All.

Geography. Symptoms may be suppressed where iron deficiency is endemic.

Genetics. Abnormal chromosomes may be found in myeloid cells: acquired.

Disease mechanisms

Polycythaemia is caused by an increased total volume of red cells in the body (sometimes mistermed the red cell 'mass'). The clonal change affecting the bone marrow stem cell enables unregulated proliferation of red cell precursors.

Diagnosis

● Proof of increased total red cell volume by radio-isotopic dilution tests
● Lack of any detectable cause of **secondary** polycythaemia (Table 15.15)
● Evidence of multilineage bone marrow hypertrophy on blood or bone marrow examination

Additional features that can help distinguish PRV from secondary polycythaemia:
● Splenomegaly
● Evidence of autonomous (erythropoietin-independent) erythroid precursor proliferation
● Low or normal plasma erythropoietin level

Clinical features

Nearly 50% of patients present with arterial or venous thrombosis including stroke, coronary thrombosis, digital ischaemia, superficial thrombophlebitis and DVT, including thrombosis in the splenic, hepatic and portal veins.

Neurological features include loss of concentration, memory impairment, headaches and dizziness.

Excessive bruising or bleeding may follow trauma and results from abnormal platelet function. Haemorrhage from peptic ulceration may lead to iron-deficiency anaemia.

Approximately 10% of patients experience an attack of gout during the illness. Splenomegaly largely excludes secondary polycythaemia; massive splenomegaly suggests the development of myelofibrosis. Pruritus affects 15% of patients at presentation and is especially noticeable after a bath.

Table 15.15 Causes of polycythaemia

Pathogenesis	Disorder
True polycythaemia	
Primary	Polycythaemia rubra vera
Secondary	
Appropriate erythropoietin increase	High altitude, congenital cyanotic heart disease, pulmonary disease, hypoventilation (including obesity), high-affinity haemoglobins, heavy smoking
Inappropriate erythropoietin increase	Renal disease (hypernephroma, cysts), hepatoma, cerebellar haemangiomas, uterine fibromas (large)
Relative polycythaemia	
Unknown	Stress or pseudopolycythaemia
Dehydration	Vomiting, diarrhoea, diuretics

Investigation

Haematology
- *FBC:* high [Hb] conc, increased white cell and platelet counts
- *Bone marrow examination:* erythroid hyperplasia with increased megakaryocytes
- *Red cell volume:* over 25% greater than predicted by sex and weight (more than 40 ml/kg in men, or more than 35 ml/kg in women = polycythaemia)

Biochemistry
- *Serum uric acid and vitamin B_{12}:* usually elevated
- *Blood gases:* an arterial oxygen saturation of less than 92% is against PRV: it indicates secondary (epo-driven) polycythaemia

Diagnostic imaging
Abdominal ultrasound, intravenous pyelogram and CT scan. To exclude underlying renal pathology (? secondary polycythaemia) and to find splenomegaly.

Management
- *Venesection* (removal of 400 ml venous blood every 1–2 weeks): initially used to reduce the haemoglobin concentration to normal, but may aggravate thrombocytosis. Chronic venesection (2–4 weekly) causes iron deficiency, which may help to control the red cell volume, but has unwanted effects reversed by low-dose iron replacement.
- *Aspirin antiplatelet therapy:* often added if the platelet count is more than 500×10^9/l, to prevent vascular occlusion and transient ischaemic attacks.
- *Myelosuppressive therapy with hydroxyurea:* often required to achieve long-term normalization of blood counts.
- *Regular follow-up:* vital to monitor hydroxyurea therapy and to observe for evidence of transformation (see below).

Prognosis
The median survival is 13–16 years. PRV may transform to myelofibrosis and AML, with a poor prognosis.

Essential thrombocythaemia

Chronic elevation of the platelet count above 500×10^9/l, associated with megakaryocytic hypertrophy in the bone marrow.

Epidemiology
Incidence. 1 in 100 000/year.

Age and sex. Bimodal distribution: seen in young, mainly female patients and in older patients of both sexes.

Ethnicity. All.

Geography. Probably worldwide.

Genetics. Abnormal (clonal) chromosome pattern may be found in myeloid cells: acquired.

Disease mechanisms
In this variant of MPD it is the total platelet volume in the marrow and blood that escapes normal regulation and progressively increases. A clonal change at the level of the myeloid stem cell is thought to be responsible. The consequent high platelet count ($500–1000 \times 10^9$/l or above) leads to increased risk of both bleeding and thrombosis. If the platelet count is controlled, the disorder has a good prognosis and transformation to myelofibrosis or leukaemia is unusual.

Diagnosis
See above.

15

Clinical features

Patients may present with transient cerebral ischaemic attacks (TCIAs) or with stroke. Two specific features of ET are:

1 *Digital ischaemia and cyanosis with normal peripheral pulses:* caused by platelet aggregation in small vessels

2 *Erythromelalgia:* red hyperaemic fingers and toes affected by an unpleasant burning or itching sensation (probably caused by platelet granule release in microcirculation)

Investigation

Haematology

- *FBC:* normal Hb. Normal WBC. Platelet count persistently above 500×10^9/l.
- *Blood film:* clearly increased platelets.
- *Bone marrow and trephine:* aspirate shows increased megakaryocytes and large masses of aggregated platelets. Trephine biopsy shows some increase in general (multilineage) cellularity. Fibrosis not increased.

Management

The aim of management is to control the thrombosis risk by limiting the platelet count (usually to 500×10^9/l or below) and/or using antiplatelet therapy. The intensity of such therapy is tailored to the patient's risk factor profile for arterial thrombosis; for example, an elderly patient with hypertension and diabetes needs active therapy for ET, while a young fit person with a platelet count of less than 1000×10^9/l may be offered low-dose aspirin alone.

- Aspirin 150 mg to prevent platelet thrombi
- If platelet count rises to over 1000×10^9/l (or at any elevation in the presence of symptoms), suppression of the platelet count by **hydroxyurea** is effective in the older age group.
- In younger patients, the non-myelosuppressive drug **anagrelide**, which prevents platelet budding from megakaryocytes, may be preferred because of the theoretical risk of carcinogenesis by hydroxyurea in long-term use
- Both hydroxyurea and anagrelide are potentially teratogenic so **interferon-α** is substituted preconception

Idiopathic myelofibrosis

Chronic progressive haemopoietic failure caused by infiltration of the marrow space by fibrosis (and eventually new bone). Starts as hyperproliferation of the megakaryocytic cell lineage, often with increased WBC and platelet counts in the blood: pancytopenia resulting from marrow failure develops over several years as the marrow is replaced by fibrosis. Extramedullary spread of myelofibrotic haematopoiesis to spleen and elsewhere is typical.

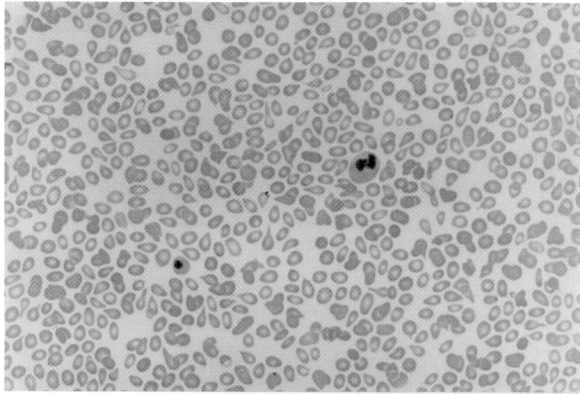
(a)

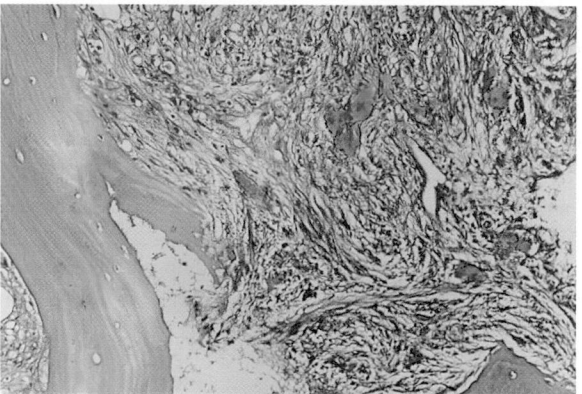
(b)

Figure 15.18 Idiopathic myelofibrosis. (a) Typical peripheral blood appearances in myelofibrosis. Many of the red cells have the elongated teardrop appearance (teardrop poikilocytes). A nucleated red cell is present and is part of the leukoerythroblastic picture typical of myelofibrosis. (b) Bone marrow trephine stained with reticulin showing complete replacement of the intertrabecular space by dense connective tissue. The dense fibres represent reticulin and are grossly increased. Megakaryocytes are abundant and are responsible for stimulating the fibrosis.

Epidemiology

Incidence. 1 in 1 000 000/year.

Age. Older age groups: average age at diagnosis is 60 years.

Sex. Equal.

Ethnicity. All.

Geography. Probably worldwide.

Genetics. Abnormal chromosomes rarely found because of difficulty getting viable cells from fibrotic marrow.

Disease mechanisms

Marrow fibrosis results from uncontrolled release of growth factors (e.g. platelet-derived growth factor) from abnormal (clonal) megakaryocytes. Simultaneously, production of platelets becomes ineffective with thrombocytopenia, and any platelets produced are functionally useless. Abnormal myelofibrotic marrow tissue migrates to extramedullary sites, particularly to the spleen which may become massively enlarged. Myelofibrosis can supervene in the late stages of PRV, ET and CML.

Clinical features

The most common presentation is with severe anaemia, weight loss, symptoms resulting from splenomegaly, pruritus and haemorrhage secondary to acquired platelet dysfunction. Complete marrow failure with severe pancytopenia may supervene. Transformation to AML (often the otherwise rare megakaryoblastic type) is more common than with other MPD, occurring in 15% of cases.

Investigation
Haematology
- *FBC:* anaemia, usually normocytic or mildly macrocytic. WBC and platelet counts may be high (early stages) or low (late stage).
- *Peripheral blood film:* a leucoerythroblastic film, with typical 'tear-drop' poikilocytes.
- *Bone marrow and trephine:* aspiration is frequently unsuccessful—a 'dry tap'—because of the fibrosis. Trephine biopsy is vital and reveals the hypercellularity and infiltration with fibrosis (Fig. 15.18) and—in late stages—with new bone (osteomyelosclerosis).
- *Neutrophil alkaline phosphatase:* unlike CML, idiopathic myelofibrosis is associated with normal–high neutrophil alkaline phosphatase.

Chromosomes
Ph¹ chromosome is absent.

Management
Palliative supportive care includes:
- Regular red cell transfusion, with iron chelation therapy in younger patients, is the keystone of care
- Platelet transfusion for bleeding
- Myelosuppression with hydroxyurea may control counts and/or splenomegaly during hypertrophic phase
- Analgesia for bone pain
- Occasionally, splenectomy for high transfusion requirement or splenic pain—this is a very difficult expert decision, because the operation is dangerous in myelofibrosis

Prognosis
The course of idiopathic myelofibrosis is of slow but remorseless deterioration, with a median survival of 1–5 years. The most common causes of death are bone marrow failure, cardiac iron overload, infection and leukaemic transformation.

Lymphoma

Hodgkin's disease

Hodgkin's disease (HD), despite being the first lymphoma described, is still incompletely understood. It probably consists of a clonal B-cell tumour ('Hodgkin's cells') mixed with a large population of non-malignant cells (eosinophils, T cells, macrophages) that seem to be 'reacting' to the abnormal clone; often these outnumber the tumour cells, and their morphology suggests response to a viral infection. HD spreads differently from other lymphomas: stepwise from one anatomical group of lymph nodes to the next ('contiguous') group via lymphatics. Marrow and blood involvement are very uncommon, another striking difference from non-Hodgkin's lymphomas.

Epidemiology
Incidence. 2 in 100 000/year.

Age. Peak incidence 18–28 years, mainly resulting from the nodular sclerosing (NS) subtype. A second small peak after 60 years involves the diffuse subtype.

Sex. Equal overall, but in NS female more common than male.

Ethnicity. All.

Geography. Probably worldwide.

Genetics. Clonal chromosome abnormalities rarely found.

Disease mechanisms
An atypical response to Epstein–Barr virus (EBV) may play a part. Positive serology to this herpesvirus, and evidence of persisting or dormant EBV infection in tumour cells strongly suggests that EBV is part of a multistep process of lymphomagenesis, particularly in younger patients. HD occurrence as an opportunistic lymphoma in transplant recipients and HIV-infected persons also suggests a viral aetiology.

Histologically, HD forms several different patterns. The most common in younger patients is NS HD, in which the 'reaction' to the tumour cells forms dense bands of fibrosis in affected nodes: it has the best prognosis. In patients over 60 years, Hodgkin's cells dominate and the reactive cell population is absent or weak: it has a poor prognosis. Generally, the bigger the reactive population, the better the prognosis.

Diagnosis

Requires the detection of Hodgkin's cells (multinucleate Reed–Sternberg cells or mononuclear types) in the typical background of reactive types. Expert histopathology is needed.

Clinical features

Typically there is painless, sometimes massive, rubbery lymphadenopathy, commonly affecting cervical and supraclavicular lymph nodes, less often axillary or inguinal nodes. One-third of patients present with systemic symptoms (loss of more than 10% body weight, drenching night sweats or fever). These are termed 'B' symptoms: they worsen the prognosis and may indicate more systemic therapy. Opportunistic infections (herpes zoster/shingles, cryptococcosis) may occur in late or heavily treated HD.

Investigation

Investigation in HD (and in other lymphomas) has two purposes: first, to confirm the **diagnosis** ('What is it?'); secondly, to **stage** the disease ('Where is it?'). The main purpose of staging is to distinguish local HD involving a single node area (Stage I) from HD extending to nearby lymph node groups (Stage II), to distant lymph nodes and spleen (Stage III) or to extralymphoid tissues such as bone marrow or liver (Stage IV). If systemic symptoms are absent, the suffix A is added (e.g. Stage IA); if present, the suffix B (e.g. Stage IIIB).

Haematology
- *FBC:* normocytic anaemia, sometimes neutrophil leucocytosis and eosinophilia
- *ESR:* raised
- *Bone marrow trephine biopsy:* if HD infiltration is present, it indicates Stage IV disease

Biochemistry
- *Liver function:* alkaline phosphatase may be increased. This finding suggests liver invasion by HD
- *LDH:* may be increased. Suggests disseminated (Stage IV) disease

Immunology
T-lymphocyte subsets. T-helper cell deficiency may occur in disseminated disease, with consequent immunodeficiency.

Diagnostic imaging
- *Chest X-ray:* essential. Shows enlargement of paratra-cheal nodes (particularly important when disease presents as cervical node mass), mediastinal or hilar nodes, or lung parenchyma.
- *Abdominal ultrasound:* to show hepatosplenomegaly.
- *CT of thorax, abdomen and pelvis:* staging test: shows HD extension into para-aortic and pelvic node groups.

Histopathology
Lymph node biopsy. Fine needle aspiration is unhelpful in HD because of the mixed cell infiltrate. Excision biopsy of a whole node is needed. Expert interpretation confirms the diagnosis and allows classification of the HD type according to the Rye classification (NS type, good prognosis; mixed cellularity type, intermediate prognosis; lymphocyte-depleted type, bad prognosis).

Management

The treatment selected for HD depends on the stage of the disease, and is **individualized** for each patient by an expert lymphoma team. As in acute leukaemia, therapy aims to remove all detectable disease (complete remission)
- *Localized HD* (Stages IA and IIA): can be cured by **extended field radiotherapy** (irradiation of the involved nodes plus contiguous node-bearing areas). Lasting remission is achieved in approximately 80%, and relapsing patients can still be cured ('salvaged') by chemotherapy.
- *Disseminated HD* (Stages III, IV and any stage with proven B symptoms): can be treated and sometimes cured with **combination chemotherapy** regimens. Lasting remission is obtained in approximately 50%, and some relapsing patients can be salvaged by high-dose therapy with HSC support.

Prognosis

Patients with HD who achieve complete and lasting remissions are effectively cured, with a normal lifespan. Some relapsing patients can also be cured with additional therapy. Patients who do not achieve remission, or who relapse with unresponsive disease, will die of HD or its associated immunosuppression. Unfortunately, patients who receive chemotherapy plus radiotherapy have a 5–10% chance of developing a secondary malignancy (e.g. therapy-related AML) a few years after treatment, because this therapy is carcinogenic. Patients who receive chemotherapy have reduced fertility.

Non-Hodgkin's lymphomas

These are malignant tumours of T or B lymphocytes affecting lymph nodes. The tumour cells resemble lymphocyte types seen in normal lymph nodes, and the histological pattern in the malignant node is often a caricature of the normal appearance. The complicated classification systems that pathologists use (and frequently change) are based on these resemblances. A simple version will be used here.

Epidemiology
Incidence. All types of NHL combined are a common form of cancer (1 in 1000/year).

Age. Strongly age-related: increasing incidence over 60 years.

Sex. Probably equal.

Ethnicity. Some types increased in people of African heritage.

Geography. Different zonal incidence (e.g. Burkitt's lymphoma in malaria hyperendemic areas).

Genetics. Acquired subtype-specific clonal translocations, often involving oncogenes, probably part of a multistep lymphomagenic process.

Disease mechanisms
Non-Hodgkin's lymphoma is a tumour of lymph nodes, but may arise anywhere in the body (including the gut and brain) because lymphoid tissue is so widely distributed. NHL is a clonal proliferation of B cells (B-NHL, common) or T cells (T-NHL, rare). Its precise aetiology is unknown, but a multistep oncogenic process has been mapped in some types (e.g. Burkitt's lymphoma, a rare high-grade tumour). The first step in Burkitt's lymphoma seems to be 'immortalization' of normally short-lived B-cell precursors by EBV infection; the second, massive expansion of the immortalized cells by chronic malaria reinfection; the third, a chromosome translocation (t8/14) that activates the oncogene c-*myc* in a clone within this now-vulnerable cell population, initiating explosive malignant expansion. It is thought that many NHL may arise via analogous multistep processes.

Clinical features
The key presenting feature of all NHL is **lymphadenopathy**, which may be **localized** to a single node-bearing area of the body or **generalized** to many. There is often enlargement of other lymphoid organs such as the spleen and liver.

Lymphomas follow one of two clinical patterns: they grow rapidly (high-grade lymphomas) or slowly (low-grade lymphomas).

High-grade non-Hodgkin's lymphoma (rare)
This usually begins with the rapid enlargement of lymph nodes at a single site. It invades local non-lymphoid tissues (including the CNS), causing space-occupying effects. T-cell high-grade lymphomas often involve the skin. If not treated early, it soon disseminates. It includes some of the fastest growing human malignancies (e.g. Burkitt's lymphoma), which behave like acute leukaemia. This rapid growth rate makes high-grade NHL sensitive to chemotherapy and therefore curable.

Low-grade non-Hodgkin's lymphoma (common)
Insidious lymph node enlargement, often at several anatomical sites, often involving the spleen, bone marrow and blood by the time the diagnosis is made. Although not rapidly fatal, it progresses remorselessly and eventually causes death by immune failure or invasion of vital organs. Slow growth rate makes it generally incurable by therapy, which is given with palliative intent.

Diagnosis
Requires demonstration of invasion of enlarged lymph nodes and/or other tissues by clonal B or T cells.

Investigation
Haematology
- *FBC:* normochromic anaemia is common. Increased WBC if lymphoma cells in blood.
- *Blood film:* abnormal lymphoma cells may be seen or detected by marker studies.
- *Bone marrow and trephine:* infiltration by lymphoma cells may be evident morphologically.
- *Cell marker studies:* abnormal B and T cells can be detected in low numbers, and their clonal nature demonstrated. Clonal B cells carry a single immunoglobulin light chain type (κ or λ); clonal T cells are either CD4$^+$ or CD8$^+$.
- *Molecular studies:* in difficult cases, to show clonal rearrangement of B- or T-cell receptor genes.

Biochemistry
- *Liver function tests:* elevated alkaline phosphatase and/or alanine aminotransferase suggest liver infiltration
- *Urea and electrolytes:* may show renal impairment because of retroperitoneal nodes compressing the renal tract

Immunology
Immunoglobulin assays. May show hypoimmunoglobulinaemia or a paraprotein (usually IgM).

Diagnostic imaging
Radiography, ultrasound, CT and MRI. May all be useful in staging NHL, in a similar way to HD (see above).

Histopathology/cytology
- *Fine needle aspiration:* of an enlarged lymph node is

15

a useful first step. Clear-cut demonstration of a clonal lymphoid population by marker or molecular studies can sometimes confirm the diagnosis.

● *Excision biopsy:* of a complete involved lymph node is required for full pathological classification. Expert advice, particularly in the case of head and neck lymphadenopathy, must be obtained prior to excision biopsy.

Management
High-grade non-Hodgkin's lymphoma
Rapid growth rate makes high-grade NHL sensitive to chemotherapy and therefore curable. Intensive combination therapy (e.g. cyclophosphamide, doxorubicin, vincristine and prednisolone; CHOP) is given as a series of cycles, aiming at complete remission as in acute leukaemias. The remission rate is approximately 50%. Relapsed cases may sometimes be salvaged by high-dose therapy with stem cell support.

Low-grade non-Hodgkin's lymphoma
Slow growth rate entails resistance to therapy, which is given as low doses of single (usually oral) drugs with palliative intent. Some localized (Stage I) low-grade NHL may be curable by surgery plus radio- or chemotherapy. As with CLL (see above), a **watchful waiting** technique saves the patient from unnecessary therapy and toxicity.

Individualized therapy
In real life, not all NHL fall neatly into one of the above clinical categories (they are of intermediate grade). The pros and cons of therapy are considered carefully for every individual with the disease.

Prognosis
Prognosis for individual patients is variable and depends on precise histology, stage and tumour sensitivity.

High-grade non-Hodgkin's lymphoma
Complete remission can be obtained in 60–80% of patients. However, 20–40% of patients will relapse and their outlook is poor. Those who do not obtain remission usually die within 3–7 months.

Lymphoma at a glance

Epidemiology
Incidence
All types combined, approximately 40/million/year

Age
More common in those over 50 years

Sex
No known sex differences

Ethnicity and geography
Complex relationship with type of lymphoma (e.g. Burkitt's lymphoma in Africa)

Genetics
Many types of lymphoma are associated with specific acquired clonal chromosome translocations

Findings on investigation
Haematology
● *Full blood count:* normochromic anaemia common. ↑ WBC may be caused by lymphoma cells in blood (particularly in low-grade lymphoma). ↓ Platelet count if bone marrow infiltration
● *Blood film:* circulating lymphoma cells may be seen
● *Bone marrow aspirate and trephine:* essential staging tests show lymphoma infiltrate in 80% low-grade and 20% high-grade lymphomas

● *Cell markers:* essential test to show clonality and B- or T-cell origin
● *Molecular diagnostics:* may be needed to prove clonal nature of tumour or confirm specific translocations

Biochemistry
● *Liver function tests:* alkaline phosphatase ↑ suggests liver infiltration by lymphoma
● *Urea and creatinine:* if elevated, suggest urinary tract obstruction by enlarged lymph nodes

Diagnostic imaging
● *Chest X-ray:* to detect mediastinal lymphadenopathy and lung infiltration
● *CT:* chest and abdomen to detect the extent of lymphadenopathy

Histopathology
● *Cytology:* fine-needle aspiration of an enlarged lymph node often indicates lymphoma
● *Histology:* excision biopsy of a complete enlarged node, or other tissue infiltrate, is often essential for complete diagnosis and staging. This may include biopsy of lymph nodes, bone marrow or liver

Clinical features
Lymphadenopathy is the key feature, with painless enlargement of single or multiple lymph nodes

Symptoms and signs of a space-occupying tumour in any body compartment (e.g. brain, abdomen), because lymphoma can involve any organ

Systemic symptoms: anorexia, weight loss (more than 10% body weight), fever and night sweats

Bone marrow involvement: anaemia, neutropenia (susceptible to infections), thrombocytopenia (easy bruising)

Immune suppression with opportunistic infection (e.g. shingles)

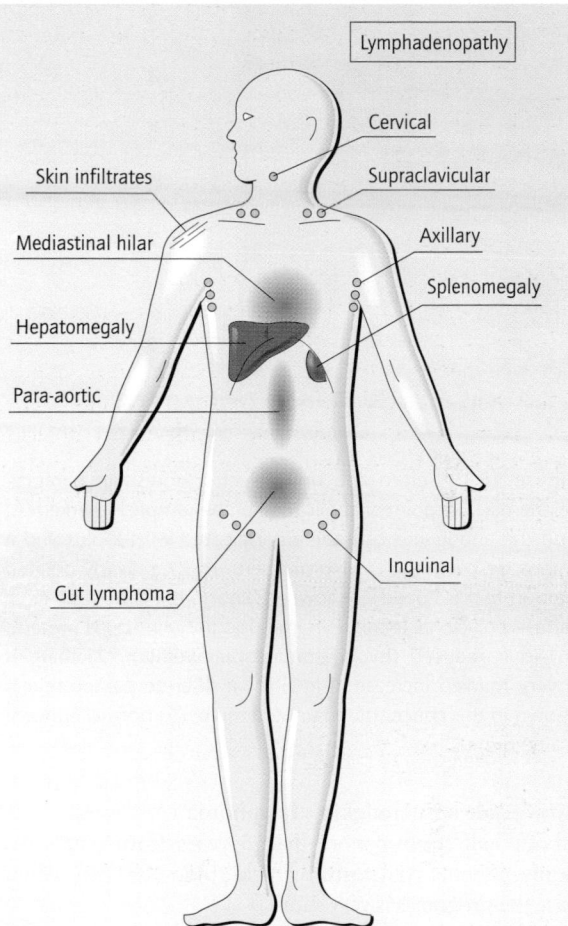

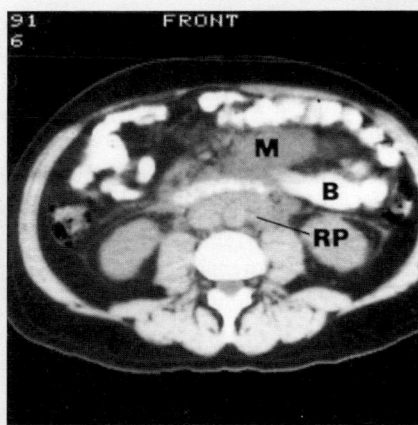

Fig. A CT scan of the abdomen showing enlarged mesenteric (M) and retroperitoneal (RP; para-aortic) lymph nodes. B, bowel.

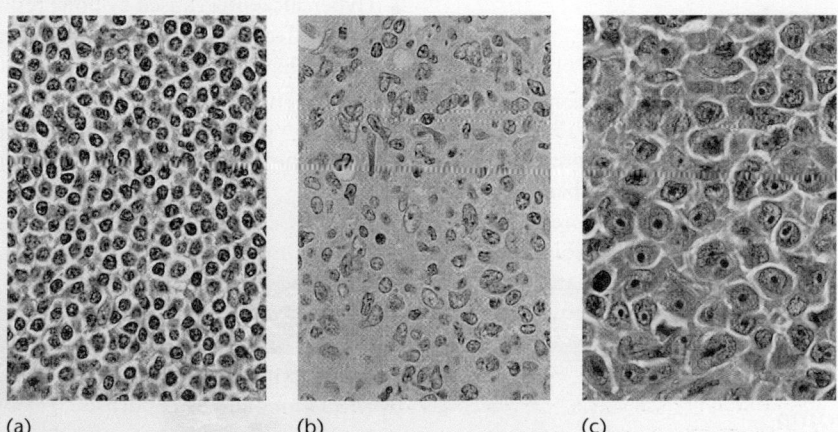

(a)   (b)   (c)

Fig. B Non-Hodgkin's lymphoma: high-pose view of lymph node biopsies showing: (i) lymphocytic lymphoma showing predominantly small lymphocytes with round nuclei containing densely clumped heterochromatin; (ii) centrocytic lymphoma showing medium-sized cells with nuclear pleomorphism but characteristically having a cleaved nucleus and pale indistinct cytoplasm. The nuclei have a light chromatin pattern and may contain nucleoli; (iii) immunoblastic lymphoma showing large neoplastic cells with a single prominent nucleolus and abundant darkly staining cytoplasm. All figures reproduced from Hoffbrand & Pettit, *Essential Haematology*, 3rd edn, 1993 (Blackwell Scientific Publications, Oxford) with the permission of the authors.

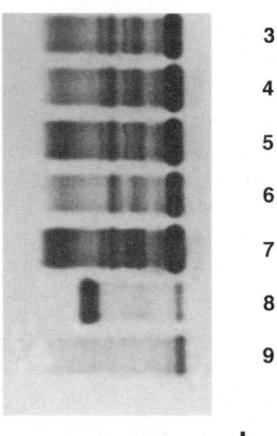

− +

Figure 15.19 Serum and urine electrophoresis in paraproteinaemia. The point of application of the sample is marked (A) and the anode and cathode are indicated with a plus and a minus, respectively. (1) Normal serum; (2) a clearly defined paraprotein (M band) is shown; (3) normal; (4) normal; (5) a diffuse polyclonal increase in immunoglobulin (Ig) is present; (6) Ig is reduced (hypogammaglobulinaemia); (7) there is a very marked increase in IgG; (8) a discrete paraprotein is shown in this concentrated urine sample; (9) normal concentrated urine.

Low-grade non-Hodgkin's lymphoma
About half survive more than 5 years from diagnosis. Some patients transform to high-grade NHL, in which case the prognosis is very short.

Multiple myeloma and other paraproteinaemias

Multiple myeloma is a malignant tumour of plasma cells. Plasma cells, terminal cells of the B-cell lineage, secrete immunoglobulins (antibodies), so myeloma is typically associated with the presence of a **paraprotein** (clonal immunoglobulin molecules that form a **band** in the gamma region on serum protein electrophoresis) in the blood. Other clonal disorders of B cells, which do not behave like myeloma, can also be associated with a paraprotein: these are also classified (with myeloma) as **paraproteinaemias** (Fig. 15.19).

Multiple myeloma

Epidemiology
Incidence. 3 in 100 000/year. Appears to be increasing.

Age. Peak incidence is during the seventh decade (only 2% of patients are under 40 years old).

Sex. Males account for two-thirds of cases.

Ethnicity. Increased incidence in people of African heritage.

Geography. Worldwide.

Genetics. A variety of acquired abnormalities affecting the immunoglobulin heavy chain genes.

Disease mechanisms
Multiple myeloma (also known as **plasma cell myeloma** or **myelomatosis**) is a malignant disease caused by expansion of a single clone of bone marrow plasma cells. Its aetiology is unknown; rare cases occur in individuals exposed to atomic radiation.

Diagnosis
Requires **two** of the following:
1 Lytic lesions (holes seen on X-ray) in the bones
2 Plasma cell infiltration of the bone marrow (more than 20% of nucleated cells)
3 Presence of a paraprotein in the blood and/or paraprotein light chains (Bence Jones protein) in blood or urine

Clinical features
These are caused by:
● Invasion of the marrow of the axial skeleton (skull, ribs, sternum, vertebrae, pelvis) by myeloma cells, causing **lytic bone disease** (holes in the bones) and eventual bone marrow failure
● Bone resorption at these sites, driven by cytokines secreted by the myeloma cells, causing additional bone destruction and generalized **osteoporosis**
● **Hypercalcaemia** caused by bone resorption
● Toxic effects of glomerular filtration of free paraprotein light chains (Bence Jones protein) on renal function (**myeloma kidney**)
● Tendency of paraprotein light chains to self-organize to form **amyloid** (in approximately 5% of patients)

Bone pain
This is the most common presenting symptom, usually affecting the spine or ribs. The pain is constant and occurs at rest but is worsened by movement, particularly bending or torsion of the spine (e.g. turning in bed). The pain steadily gets worse and does not remit. Bone pain is caused by lytic lesions and osteoporosis.

Pathological bone fractures
Osteoporosis causes vertebral collapse with spinal kyphosis and loss of height. Spread of myeloma tissue from vertebrae into the spinal canal causes **spinal cord compression** (an emergency needing rapid diagnosis, decompression and myeloma therapy). Fractures of long bones (e.g. femur) also occur.

Hypercalcaemia

Occurs because of rapid bone resorption; causes nausea and vomiting, altered level of consciousness, renal impairment. Constitutes an emergency.

Anaemia and pancytopenia

Caused by marrow invasion by malignant plasma cells.

Infection

Hypoimmunoglobulinaemia (caused by suppression of normal B-lymphocyte function by the malignant clone) leads to pneumonia and other infections, as in CLL (see above).

Renal failure

The renal glomeruli filter free immunoglobulin light chains, which form obstructive casts in the renal tubules, causing rapid nephron loss. Hypercalcaemia, dehydration, infection and amyloid may all contribute to the damage. About 20% of myeloma patients, mainly those excreting λ light chains, present this way.

Amyloidosis

Free immunoglobulin light chains (usually of the λ type) sometimes self-organize into the abnormal proteinaceous (β-pleated sheet) tissue called amyloid, which then infiltrates skin (causing bruising and purpura), tongue (risking asphyxiation), kidney (adding to renal problems) or heart (with cardiac failure and death).

'Smouldering' myeloma

Sometimes a patient is found to have a paraprotein and an excess of plasma cells in the blood, but **no** evidence of bone disease, marrow failure, renal impairment or other damaging effect. It is reasonable to deal with this situation with 'watchful waiting' as in asymptomatic CLL or static low-grade NHL. Treatment of myeloma is purely palliative—there is no point palliating symptoms that do not exist.

Investigation

Haematology

- *FBC:* anaemia and/or thrombocytopenia occur in approximately 60%.
- *Blood film:* blue background staining and rouleaux formation (paraprotein effects). There may be a leucoerythroblastic blood picture (marrow infiltration). Myeloma cells are sometimes seen.
- *Bone marrow and trephine:* there is plasma cell infiltration (more than 20% nucleated cells).

Biochemistry

- *Corrected plasma calcium:* may show hypercalcaemia
- *Urea and electrolytes:* may show renal failure

Immunology

- *Protein electrophoresis:* usually shows a single narrow heavily stained band in the gamma region of the strip. This is the paraprotein. About 10% of myelomas do not secrete a full paraprotein: some secrete light chains only (which do not show up on an ordinary protein strip, but can be detected by other methods) and some nothing at all (non-secretory myeloma).
- *Urinalysis:* will detect free clonal light chains (Bence Jones proteinuria) in nearly all cases.
- *Immunofixation:* a sensitive method of detecting and typing paraprotein: The relative frequencies of different types of paraprotein in myeloma are IgG (55%), IgA (25%), Bence Jones protein (18%), IgD or IgE (1%) and biclonal (1%).
- *Immunoglobulin quantification:* detects deficiency of normal (polyclonal) immunoglobulin.
- *β_2-Microglobulin:* a useful marker of the activity of the disease (high = active = bad)

Histopathology

Demonstration of amyloid tissue infiltration by Congo red staining or birefringence in polarized light.

Diagnostic imaging

- *Radiography of the axial skeleton (skeletal survey):* required to detect lytic lesions in the bones and generalized osteoporosis
- *MRI of the spine and spinal cord:* sensitive detection of vertebral myeloma and spinal cord compression

Management

Urgent initial supportive treatment may include:

- Immediate rehydration for renal failure
- Bisphosphonate drugs for hypercalcaemia
- Red cell transfusion for anaemia
- Antibiotics for infection
- Analgesia for pain
- Surgical decompression of the spinal cord

Specific antimyeloma treatment should follow initial stabilization. It is carefully individualized for:

- The age and physical health of the patient
- The myeloma tumour 'load' estimated from the amount of paraprotein, the severity of bone and organ damage, and the likely speed of growth indicated by the Hb and platelet count and β_2-microglobulin level

In a frail patient with a low myeloma load, single-agent oral therapy with the alkylating agent **melphalan**, plus oral bisphosphonate to limit bone disease, is a valid plan. In a fit patient with a high load of myeloma and evidence of severe bone or renal disease, intravenous combination chemotherapy to control rapidly the tumour load would be appropriate, perhaps followed by high-dose therapy and stem cell infusion. Many patients fall

15

Myeloma at a glance

Epidemiology

Incidence
50/million/year (men), 30/million/year (women)

Age
Peak incidence over 60 years: only 2% of patients are under 40 years old

Sex
Two-thirds of patients are male

Ethnicity
Twice as common in people of Afro-Caribbean descent

Geography
Worldwide

Findings on investigation

Haematology
- *FBC:* normocytic anaemia. Thrombocytopenia in 30% of patients (bad prognostic sign)
- *Blood film:* rouleaux formation and blue background staining (both caused by paraprotein) are common. Leukoerythroblastic blood picture in 10%
- *Bone marrow examination:* plasma cell infiltration of the bone marrow (more than 20% of nucleated cells)

Biochemistry
Serum calcium, urea and creatinine are commonly raised

Immunology
- *Protein electrophoresis and urine analysis:* reveals the presence of a paraprotein and/or Bence Jones proteinuria
- *Paraprotein quantitation:* measures the paraprotein level and its rate of increase
- *Immunoglobulin assays:* demonstrates associated hypo-immunoglobulinaemia (reduction of normal Ig)

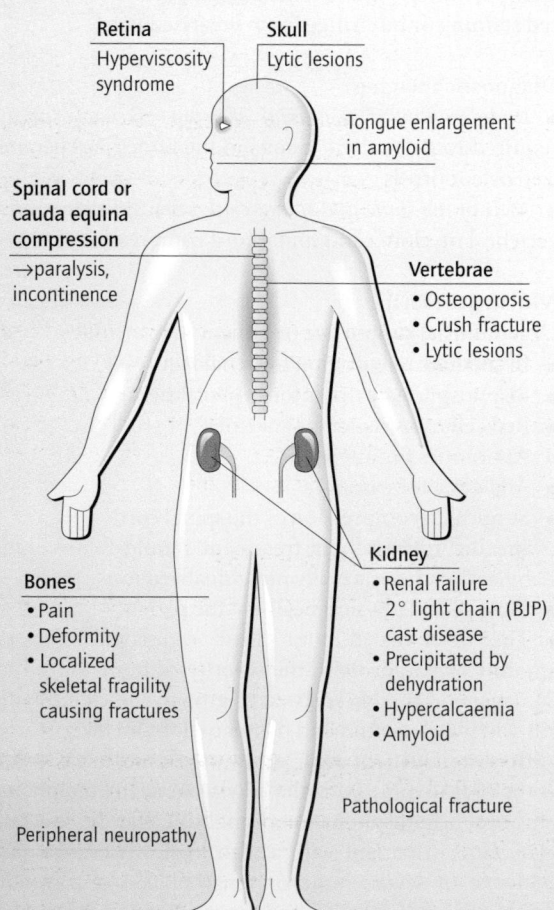

Retina
Hyperviscosity syndrome

Skull
Lytic lesions

Tongue enlargement in amyloid

Spinal cord or cauda equina compression
→paralysis, incontinence

Vertebrae
- Osteoporosis
- Crush fracture
- Lytic lesions

Bones
- Pain
- Deformity
- Localized skeletal fragility causing fractures

Kidney
- Renal failure 2° light chain (BJP) cast disease
- Precipitated by dehydration
- Hypercalcaemia
- Amyloid

Pathological fracture

Peripheral neuropathy

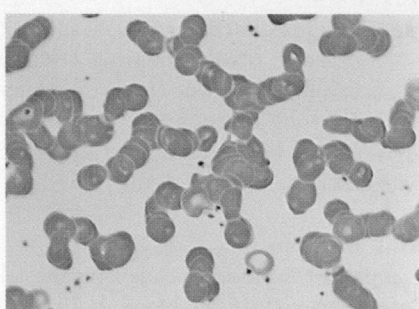

Fig. A Blood film showing rouleaux formation, which is a common finding in multiple myeloma.

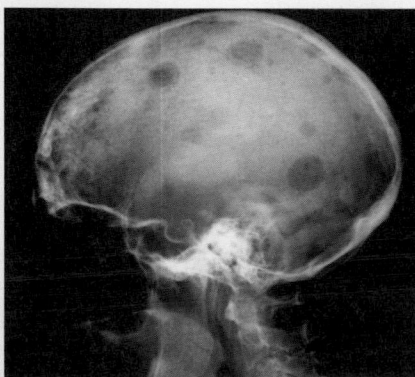

Fig. B Radiograph showing multiple small 'punched out' osteolytic lesions (rounded lucent areas) of multiple myeloma in the skull.

- *β₂-Microglobulin assay:* related to number of myeloma cells; high β₂-microglobulin is a bad prognostic sign

Diagnostic imaging
- *Radiography:* a skeletal survey is vital to detect lytic lesions in the bones. Most relevant bones are skull, ribs, vertebrae and pelvis (the axial skeleton)
- *MRI of the spinal canal:* confirms clinical evidence of spinal cord compression

Histopathology
Bone marrow trephine. Replacement by plasma cells. Reticulin may be increased

Clinical features
Musculoskeletal
Bone pain
Pathological fractures
Vertebral collapse
Kyphosis and loss of height

Neurology
Spinal cord compression

Haematology
Anaemia
Thrombocytopenia

Immunology
Infections of the respiratory tract as a result of hypoimmunoglobulinaemia

Renal
Protein (light chain) cast disease (myeloma kidney)
Renal tubular atrophy and degeneration
Pyelonephritis

Metabolic
Hypercalcaemia
Amyloid
Cryoglobulinaemia

Vascular
Hyperviscosity syndrome

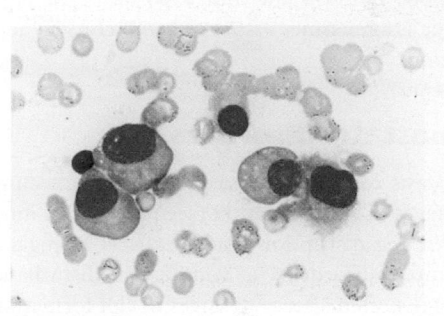

Fig. C Bone marrow aspirate in myeloma. This high-power field shows five plasma cells, together with a small lymphocyte. Note the very basophilic cytoplasm with a paler area corresponding to the Golgi apparatus. The nucleus has a typically eccentric location.

between these extremes and require carefully individualized therapy.

Recently, myeloma has been shown to respond to the antiangiogenic agent **thalidomide** in about 50% of cases. In addition to bone protective action, bisphosphonates also seem (via anticytokine activity) to inhibit myeloma cells. Further development of these and related drugs may provide more treatment options in the future.

Prognosis
About 60% of patients respond to chemotherapy. They rarely attain complete remission (which would require complete disappearance of the paraprotein); the typical response is stabilization of the paraprotein level and slowing of signs of progression—the **plateau** phase. Chemotherapy is stopped once plateau is achieved. All patients on plateau are likely to eventually relapse and require more treatment. Eventually, the myeloma will become resistant to all therapy. This sequence may take 2–10 years or even longer, so given further advances in therapy there is time for the outlook to improve.

This poor outlook has led to the exploration of high-dose therapy with stem cell infusion. This increases the speed of response and may prolong plateau phase, but does not appear capable of curing the disease. In young fit patients (a small minority) allogeneic stem cell transplantation introduces a chance of cure.

Other paraproteinaemias
Monoclonal gammopathy of undetermined significance
This elegant term is applied to the finding of a low-level paraprotein **alone** (e.g. IgG band less than 20 g/l), without increased plasma cells in the marrow or any symptom, sign or investigational finding suggesting myeloma activity. It is a very common finding in patients over 65 years, and might be found in up to 1% of individuals over 80 years. Approximately 1 in 10 monoclonal gammopathy of undetermined significance (MGUS) will progress to smouldering or overt myeloma on follow-up.

Waldenström's macroglobulinaemia

This chronic lymphoproliferative disease is defined by the presence of an IgM paraprotein in the serum. IgM paraproteins (macroglobulins) are not associated with myeloma-type bone disease. Instead, the abnormal cells (lymphocytoplasmoid cells) infiltrating the marrow and lymph nodes resemble those of a low-grade non-Hodgkin's lymphoma, and the disease is treated similarly. If the IgM paraprotein attains plasma levels of 40 g/l or more, its molecular bulk causes **hyperviscosity syndrome** with circulatory disturbances of brain and visual function, and bleeding. Urgent removal of the IgM paraprotein by plasmapheresis is indicated. IgM paraproteins may also sludge on cooling (cryoproteins) causing digital, nasal and earlobe cyanosis on cold exposure. IgM paraproteinaemia is sometimes associated with chronic hepatitis C infection.

Haemostatic disorders

Haemostasis can fail because of problems affecting any of the stages of clot formation (see p. 1004). In inherited disorders, the disruption usually affects a single stage. In acquired disorders, a widespread disturbance of haemostasis often affects all stages of clot formation and removal. Symptoms and signs of haemostatic disorders are described in detail on pp. 1011, 1013 and in HISTORY & EXAMINATION BOX 15.3.

Disorders of primary haemostasis (platelet plug formation)

If formation of the platelet plug is delayed, abnormal bleeding tends to be immediately obvious from cuts, surgical incisions or mucous membranes (e.g. epistaxis).

Platelet disorders

Thrombocytopenia
The most common platelet disorder is lack of them, described on p. 1046.

Abnormal platelet function
Primary haemostasis may fail if the platelet count is normal but platelet function reduced.

Inherited platelet function disorders. These are rare. Affected individuals have a life-long mild to moderately severe bleeding tendency, which tends to improve in adult life, but will always pose difficulties with surgery and childbirth.
- *Glanzmann's thrombocythaemia:* recessively inherited deficiency of platelet fibrinogen receptors
- *Bernard–Soulier disease:* recessively inherited deficiency of platelet von Willebrand factor receptors
- *Platelet storage pool deficiency and transduction disorders:* a larger group of dominantly inherited mild bleeding disorders in which platelet activation mechanisms are disturbed

Acquired platelet function disorders. These are common. Evidence of a newly developed bleeding tendency is seen in the setting of systemic disease or drug therapy. The bleeding disorder may prevent or complicate management of the underlying disease.
- *Aspirin therapy:* blocks platelet metabolism. Effect lasts for 7 days after aspirin is withdrawn.
- *Ethanol toxicity:* high blood alcohol levels reduce platelet function.
- *Renal failure (uraemia):* retained metabolites impair platelet function, corrected by dialysis.
- *Myelodysplasia or myeloproliferative disease:* see pp. 1052 and 1056.
- *Disseminated intravascular coagulation:* breakdown products of fibrin block platelet function.

Clinical features
See HISTORY & EXAMINATION BOX 15.3. Easy bruising and mucosal haemorrhage (epistaxis, menorrhagia) are typical.

Investigation
Haematology
- *FBC:* platelet count may be normal or moderately reduced
- *Blood film:* May show abnormal platelet granulation or size
- *Skin template bleeding time:* performed by an experienced operator, will be more than 9 min
- *Whole blood platelet function analysis:* if available, is more sensitive than bleeding time in showing low platelet function
- *Platelet aggregometry:* pattern of aggregation to different platelet activators gives definitive diagnosis (e.g. in Glanzmann's thrombocythaemia, platelet fibrinogen receptor deficiency)

Management and prognosis (EMERGENCY BOX 15.4)
- *Patients with hereditary platelet defects:* require registration with a haemophilia centre for advice and therapy in case of bleeding or surgery. Minor bleeds can be arrested by firm pressure. Major bleeds or surgical challenges require platelet transfusion. The prognosis is good if access to expert treatment is assured.
- *Patients with acquired platelet defects:* require effective treatment of the underlying cause, with platelet transfusion in case of dangerous bleeding or surgical challenges.

Von Willebrand's disease

An inherited bleeding disorder caused by deficiency

> ## Emergency 15.4: Severe unexpected haemorrhage
>
> **Definition**
> Sudden, unexpected and ongoing loss of 2 l of blood or more
>
> **Problems**
> If not resolved, mortality 50%
> Loss of circulating volume (hypovolaemia) is immediate threat and also leads to further bleeding via disseminated intravascular coagulation
> If losses replaced with crystalloid or bank blood, dilutional thrombocytopenia and coagulopathy develop
>
> **Actions**
> Ensure good vascular access: maintain blood volume with saline or plasma expanders
> Notify blood bank of situation (many hospitals operate a 'code red' for this event)
> Send two cross-matched samples to blood bank
> If red cells must be given prior to compatible blood issue by the blood bank, give ABO group-compatible uncross-matched blood. Outside hospital (e.g. trauma/obstetrics) 'flying squad' group O rhesus negative blood may be given
> To counter dilutional thrombocytopenia and/or coagulopathy, give 1 l of fresh plasma and two adult doses of platelet concentrate for every 6 units of blood transfused

(Type 1 von Willebrand's disease; vWD) or abnormality (Type 2 vWD) of the large adhesive plasma protein von Willebrand factor (vWF).

Epidemiology
Prevalence. Not accurately known. In northern Europe, up to 1 in 1000. The most common inherited bleeding disorder.

Age. Congenital: symptoms slowly improve with age.

Sex. Equal.

Ethnicity. Rare in individuals with African heritage.

Genetics. Dominant inheritance in Type 2. Dominant with variable penetrance in Type 1, with complex relation to ABO blood group. Abnormalities of the vWF gene are usually found in Type 2, but only in a few Type 1.

Disease mechanisms
Von Willebrand factor links platelets to the damaged vessel wall during initial platelet adhesion, by binding to a specific platelet receptor. Reduced vWF participation delays platelet plug formation.

Diagnosis
Can be difficult: many tested for excess bleeding have vWF levels around the lower end of the normal range, particularly blood group O individuals, who have a lower range of vWF levels.

Requires the combination of:
- A history of excessive mucosal bleeding, or bleeding on surgical challenge
- A family history of similar bleeding in a first-degree relative
- A reduced level of vWF antigen and/or vWF functional activity in the blood

Clinical features
- Easy bruising
- Epistaxes (nosebleeds that run like a tap)
- Menorrhagia
- Early excess bleeding during dentistry or surgery
- Peripartum bleeding (Type 2)
- Joint, muscle and CNS bleeds are very rare

Investigation
Haematology
- *Coagulation screen:* may show ↑ APTTr, but often normal
- *Skin bleeding time:* may be more than 9 min, but often normal
- *Whole blood platelet function analysis:* abnormal
- *Platelet aggregometry:* abnormal response to Ristocetin
- *VWF assay:* antigen (vWF: Ag) less than 50%; function (vWF: Rcof) less than 50%

Management
Type 1 vWD. The vWF content of plasma is increased (often to normal) by injection of the synthetic vasopressin analogue desmopressin (DDAVP; 0.4 µg/kg), which is the treatment of choice because it poses no risk of blood-transmitted infection. Infusion of blood-derived vWF is only required for major surgery, when the vWF level needs to be sustained at 100% for several days, and DDAVP cannot be repeated more than twice in any 4-day period (risk of hyponatraemia).

Type 2 vWD. The vWF molecule is abnormal, so boosting it with DDAVP is no help. Blood-derived vWF concentrate is given to treat bleeds and cover surgery and childbirth.

Prognosis
The vast majority live normal lives. The term 'disease' is **clinically** misleading.

Disorders of secondary haemostasis (clot formation)

The establishment of a durable clot at the site of vascular damage effectively seals it. A durable clot depends on the concerted action of the plasma coagulation factors in thrombin generation (see p. 1006). Deficiency of any or all of the key coagulation factors will retard clot formation and render the clot vulnerable to premature breakdown. Abnormal bleeding is not as immediate as that seen in disorders of primary haemostasis and may be delayed for several hours after surgery or trauma, but once it starts it persists until corrective treatment is given.

Inherited disease: haemophilia

Haemophilia is the most severe inherited bleeding disorder. An identical clinical disorder occurs because of deficiency of either factor VIII (haemophilia A) or factor IX (haemophilia B or Christmas disease). The reason that deficiencies of two different proteins result in an identical clinical picture is that the frail abnormal clot that forms in haemophilia results from low activity of the key complex formed by factors VIII and IX (see Fig. 15.9a).

Haemophilia A (factor VIII deficiency)

Epidemiology
Incidence. 1 in 10 000 male births.

Age. Congenital bleeding (infant may bleed during delivery).

Sex. Males. Not impossible, but very rare in females.

Ethnicity. All, equally.

Genetics. X-linked recessive.

Geography. Worldwide.

Disease mechanisms
Haemophilia A results from deficiency of factor VIIIC, arising from a number of different factor VIII gene lesions (Fig. 15.20). Nearly half of all cases are caused by a major chromosomal inversion (the intron 22 inversion) that renders the gene untranslatable. Nearly half occur sporadically, in families with no history of haemophilia.

The generation of sufficient thrombin to form an effective durable clot depends on a functioning complex of factors VIIIa and IXa. If deficiency of factors VIII or IX prevents this, the clot does not seal the vessel wall. The severity of the disorder depends on the plasma level of

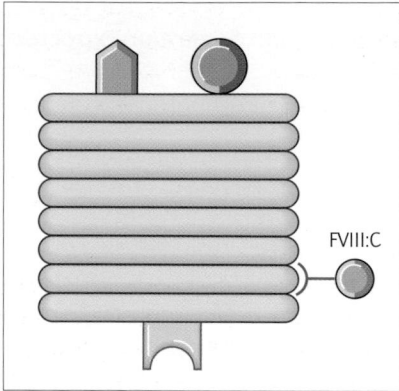

Figure 15.20 Diagram of the factor VIII complex. vWF: Ag is a multimer of up to 80 units, each of molecular weight 270 000. Factor VIIIC is bound to vWF: Ag via specific receptors.

factor VIII. Most patients have severe haemophilia (factor VIII less than 2% normal); others have moderate (factor VIII 2–5%) or mild (factor VIII more than 5%) variants.

Clinical features
Recurrent haemorrhage into joints (haemarthrosis) and muscles (intramuscular haematoma), beginning when the child starts to walk, occurs in severe haemophilia. Typically, a sequence of bleeds affects a single joint (target joint). Resulting permanent damage affecting knees, elbows, ankles and wrists leads to severe arthritis (chronic haemophiliac arthritis) and disability by mid-teens in the untreated or inadequately treated patient. Spontaneous dangerous haemorrhage may occur into the gastrointestinal and urinary tracts, tongue and retroperitoneal space. Intracerebral bleeding, occurring spontaneously or following trauma, is the most common cause of death.

Until the development of recombinant factors VIII and IX, factor VIII concentrate was manufactured from multiple donations of human plasma, exposing the recipient to blood-borne viruses. Successive epidemics of hepatitis B, C and HIV therefore occurred in haemophilia, and the clinical features of these disorders may dominate in individual patients. The risks of blood-borne infection are now minimized (see below).

Investigation
Haematology
Coagulation screen: ↑ APTTr with normal INR and TCT
Factor VIII assay: less than 2% (severe), 2–5% (moderate), 5–35% (mild)

Biochemistry
Liver function tests. ↑ ALT may indicate chronic hepatitis B or C.

Management

Mild haemophilia. Desmopressin (DDAVP) injection (see vWD above) also boosts factor VIII level in mild haemophilia because vWF is the carrier protein for factor VIII.

Severe and moderate haemophilia. The impact of severe haemophilia on individuals and their families requires a model of treatment called comprehensive care, in which every aspect (bleeding, joint and muscle rehabilitation, surgery, genetics, treatment of associated infections, dentistry, surgery, social care, etc.) is delivered by a specialized clinical team.

Central to care is prompt treatment of bleeds with effective doses of factor VIII concentrate, often self-injected or by a family member. Prophylactic factor VIII therapy, aiming to prevent bleeds, is best practice in severe haemophilia. It is sometimes begun in infancy after inserting a permanent vascular access device. The concentrate used should be recombinant (non-plasma-derived) factor VIII if available. High doses of factor VIII are used to enable surgery.

Haemophilia B (factor IX deficiency, Christmas disease)

Epidemiology
Incidence. 2 in 100 000 male births.

Age. Congenital bleeding (infant may bleed during delivery).

Sex. Males. Not impossible, but very rare in females.

Ethnicity. All, equally.

Genetics. X-linked recessive.

Geography. Worldwide.

Disease mechanisms
Haemophilia B results from deficiency of factor IX, arising from a number of factor IX gene lesions. Most cases occur in families with a history of haemophilia.

Identical to haemophilia A (see above) except that the factor VIII level is normal: a **factor IX** assay demonstrates the causative deficiency.

Management
Comprehensive care as for haemophilia A, but therapy is intravenous **factor IX concentrate**. Desmopressin does not work in haemophilia B.

Prognosis of haemophilia A and B
Before effective factor replacement began in the early 1960s, the median age of death for boys with severe haemophilia was approximately 16 years. Life expectancy for both types normalized by the early 1980s, but then fell back again because of the HIV epidemic of the later 1980s. At present it is approaching normal again because of improved blood safety. These figures apply to wealthy societies; in the developing world access to treatment is patchy at best, and prognosis is worse.

Acquired disease

Acquired deficiencies tend to affect more than one coagulation factor.

Vitamin K deficiency
Epidemiology
Incidence. Haemorrhagic disease of the newborn (HDN) 1 in 10 000 births if vitamin K prophylaxis not given.

Age. HDN in newborn. Older patients are vulnerable to vitamin K starvation.

Sex. Equal.

Ethnicity. All.

Genetics. N/A.

Geography. Worldwide.

Disease mechanisms
Vitamin K is:
- Required as a cofactor for the synthesis of the functional forms of coagulation factors II (prothrombin), VII, IX and X (these are termed the vitamin-K-dependent coagulation factors; Fig. 15.21)
- Fat-soluble: its absorption depends on normal biliary function and intestinal absorption of fat
- Present at very low levels in human breast milk
- Stored in the liver, but this reserve is only sufficient for 1 week or so
- Antagonized by the commonly used coumarin anticoagulant drugs (e.g. warfarin)

Vitamin K deficiency can therefore develop rapidly in:
- Biliary obstruction (gallstones, pancreatic cancer)
- Malabsorption syndromes
- Pancreatic failure
- Starvation (even in hospital)
- Early or late neonatal period in exclusively breastfed babies (HDN)
- Overanticoagulation with coumarin drugs (e.g. warfarin)

Haemophilia at a glance

Epidemiology

Incidence
1 in 10 000 males (haemophilia A), 1 in 50 000 males (haemophilia B)

Age
From birth

Sex
Males

Ethnicity
All

Genetics
X-linked recessive inheritance

Geography
Worldwide

Findings on investigation

Haematology
Full blood count: normal
Clotting studies
• Prolonged activated partial thromboplastin time (APTT), normal prothrombin time (INR) and thrombin time (TCT)
• Low factor VIII:C (or factor IX:C in haemophilia B
• Severe: less than 2 iu/dl
• Moderate: 2–5 iu/dl
• Mild: 5–40 iu/dl
• vWF: Ag normal
Bleeding time and platelet function normal

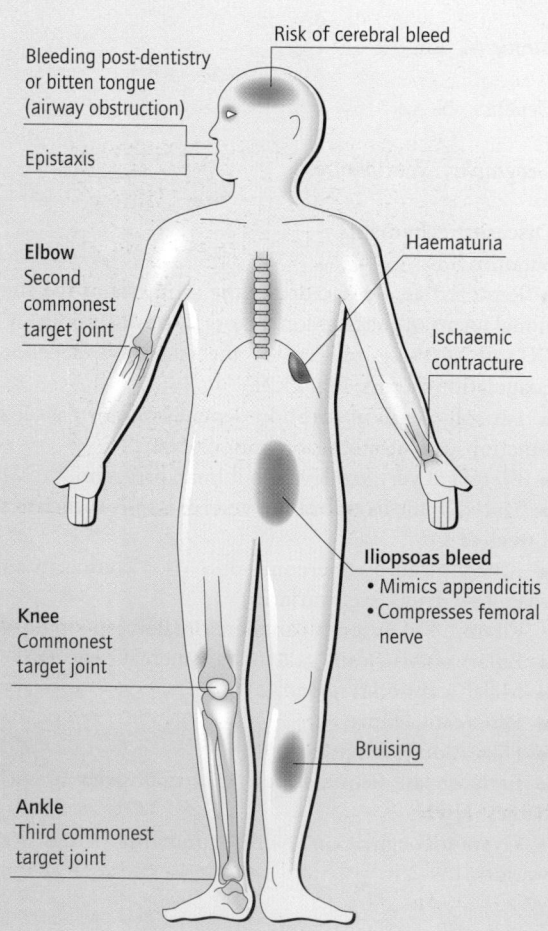

Bleeding post-dentistry or bitten tongue (airway obstruction)

Epistaxis

Risk of cerebral bleed

Elbow
Second commonest target joint

Haematuria

Ischaemic contracture

Iliopsoas bleed
• Mimics appendicitis
• Compresses femoral nerve

Knee
Commonest target joint

Bruising

Ankle
Third commonest target joint

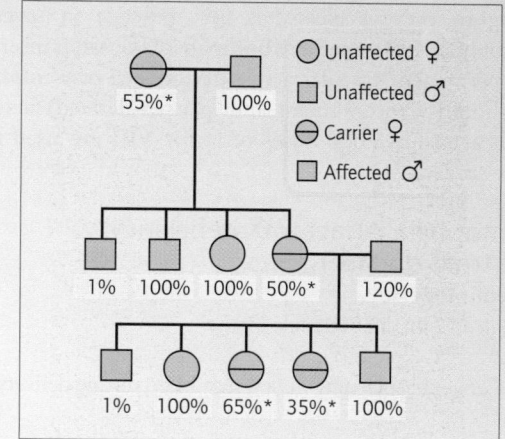

Fig. A A typical family tree in a family with haemophilia. Note the variable levels of factor VIII activity in carriers (*) due to random inactivation of X chromosome (lyonization). The percentages show the degree of factor VIII activity as a percentage of normal. Reproduced from Hoffbrand & Pettit, *Essential Haematology*, 3rd edn, 1993 (Blackwell Scientific Publications, Oxford) with the permission of the authors.

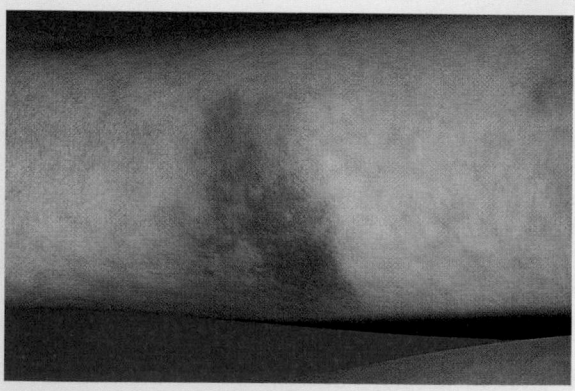

Fig. B Abnormal bruising in severe haemophilia A.

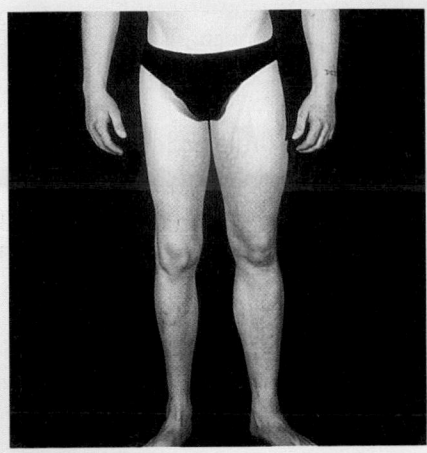

(i)

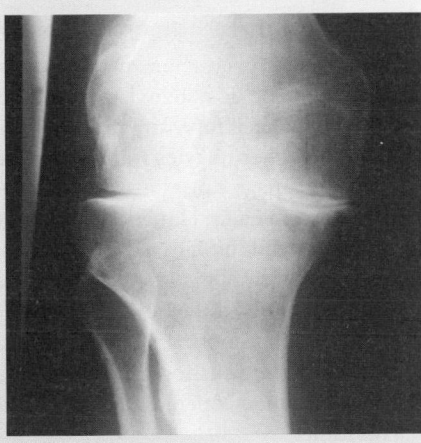

(ii)

Fig. C (i) Haemophilia: target joint in otherwise fit patient. In this patient the right knee is a target joint damaged by repeated haemarthroses. As a result the muscles of the thigh are wasted. The patient has been promptly treated with on-demand factor VIII over the years. (ii) Chronic haemophilia arthropathy. Radiograph of the right knee joint showing marked narrowing of joint space, subchondral cyst formation and osteoarthritic changes. Progressive damage despite on-demand therapy is the rationale for prophylaxis.

Inhibitor studies: detect alloantibodies against factor VIII in approximately 15% of severely affected individuals. Makes therapy complex

Molecular and genetic diagnosis: gene lesions responsible for haemophilia can be determined in affected individuals and their female relatives, enabling antenatal diagnosis and reproductive choice for carriers

Diagnostic imaging

Radiography of knees, ankles, elbows show erosive arthropathy (haemophilic arthropathy) if patients sustained recurrent joint bleeds with suboptimal therapy

Ultrasound or CT scan to demonstrate cerebral or retroperitoneal bleeds

Clinical features

Risk of fatal haemorrhage

Affecting airway: tongue or palatal bleeds

Intracranial

Post surgery or dentistry in unprepared patients

Musculoskeletal

Acute haemarthrosis: severe joint pain and swelling

Acute intramuscular haematoma

Nerve entrapment syndromes

Chronic haemophilic arthropathy

Resulting joint deformities and disability

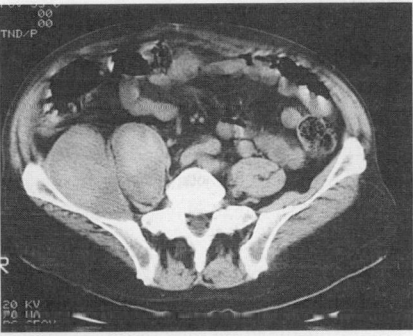

Fig. D CT scan of the pelvis showing iliopsoas (retroperitoneal) haematoma.

Diagnosis

Awareness of the possibility of vitamin K deficiency is crucial. A high INR (more than 1.5), corrected to normal within 24 h by parenteral vitamin K, is diagnostic. The INR is very sensitive to the factor VII level—and to vitamin K deficiency.

Clinical features

Skin bruising, often on a jaundiced background. Gastrointestinal haemorrhage may complicate vitamin K deficiency resulting from cholestasis. Babies with HDN also have heavy bruising, and sometimes present with gastrointestinal, pleural, pericardial or CNS bleeding. Other features of biliary and/or pancreatic disease (abdominal pain, masses) or malabsorption (steatorrhoea, small stature) may be present.

Investigation

Haematology

Coagulation screen: ↑ INR (more than 1.5); usually ↑ APTTr; normal TCT

Factor assays: not usually required

15

15

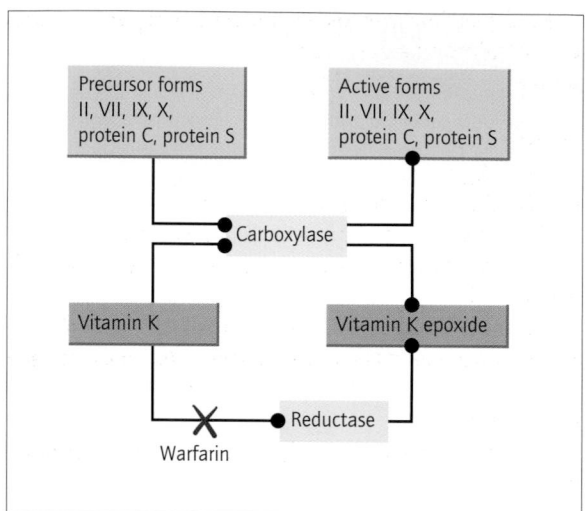

Figure 15.21 Role of vitamin K in the activation of coagulation factors. Vitamin K is required for γ carboxylation of glutamic acid residues in factors II, VII, IX and X, and in proteins C and S. Carboxylation is essential for functional activity of these various factors. Oral anticoagulants prevent the conversion of vitamin K epoxide to its active form.

Biochemistry
Liver function tests: ↑ bilirubin indicates cholestasis
Tests for malabsorption

Management
Haemorrhagic disease of the newborn. Prevented by:
- Intramuscular injection of 1 mg vitamin K (phytomenadione) at birth
- Two doses of oral vitamin K in the first postnatal week, plus a third at 1 month in exclusively breastfed babies

Cholestasis and malabsorption. Coagulation must be corrected before any surgery for cholestasis—otherwise severe perioperative bleeding may result.
    If immediate correction is required:
- In coumarin anticoagulation with dangerous (e.g. intracerebral) bleeding, prothrombin complex concentrate (contains factors II, VII, IX and X) is infused after discussion with an expert
- In cholestasis or emergency surgery, fresh-frozen plasma (FFP; 15 ml/kg) is infused
    If a short delay is acceptable:
Vitamin K (phytomenadione) 1–5 mg depending on size of patient, by **slow** intravenous injection, will correct clotting within 24 h.

Prognosis
Excellent if the deficiency is prevented, or recognized and treated. Not good if intracerebral bleeding has already begun. In cholestasis, prognosis clearly depends on the underlying cause.

'Global' acquired disorders of haemostasis

Some acquired disorders cause multiple effects on all the components of the haemostatic system (the vessel wall, platelets, coagulation and fibrinolysis). This causes worse bleeding than deficiency of any single factor.

Hepatocellular disease and portal hypertension
Epidemiology
See Chapter 9, p. 628.

Disease mechanisms
Every protein of the coagulation, natural anticoagulant (see below) and fibrinolytic systems is synthesized by hepatocytes in the liver. Therefore, any disorder that kills or functionally impairs hepatocytes will disrupt blood clotting. Hepatocyte damage causes intrahepatic cholestasis, adding vitamin K deficiency. Until the late stage of hepatic failure, synthesis of inhibitors of fibrinolysis is affected more than that of fibrinolytic activators, with a marked increase in circulatory fibrinolytic (clot-busting) activity. Finally, portal hypertension traps platelets in the spleen, and thrombopoietin production by the liver is reduced, with resulting thrombocytopenia. All these effects favour abnormal bleeding.

Clinical features
Bruising, epistaxis, gastrointestinal haemorrhage (e.g. from gastro-oesophageal varices), cerebral haemorrhage, in the context of cirrhosis and hepatic failure.

Investigation
Haematology
- *FBC:* anaemia, thrombocytopenia
- *Coagulation screen:* ↑ INR (more than 1.5); usually ↑ APTTr, ↑ TCT
- *Fibrinogen assay:* usually ↓ (less than 1.5 g/l)
- *Factor assays:* factor V (hepatic synthesis but not vitamin K-dependent) less than 50%; distinguishes hepatocytic failure from simple vitamin K deficiency

Biochemistry
Liver function tests are deranged.

Management and prognosis
Vitamin K and FFP are used to treat serious or threatened bleeding as in vitamin K deficiency (see above). In addi-

tion, platelet transfusion may be required. Treatment with prothrombin complex concentrate and/or antifibrinolytic drugs may sometimes help, but could also provoke DIC (see below), so should only be given by an expert. Treatment (or transplantation) of the diseased liver may be the only effective solution to the bleeding problem. The prognosis of liver disease of this severity is poor.

Disseminated intravascular coagulation

Systemic activation of haemostasis, triggered by a severe clinical insult, that overwhelms regulatory mechanisms and causes haemostatic failure, with both thrombosis and bleeding.

Disease mechanisms

Haemostasis works best on localized damage to blood vessels. Diffuse vascular damage, caused by trauma, blood loss or invasion of the circulation by foreign cells or microbes, can 'overdrive' the haemostatic system into chaotic activation and failure—DIC. DIC always has some **underlying cause**. The initial phase of DIC consists of formation of microvascular thromboses in kidneys and lungs, causing varying degrees of acute renal failure and adult respiratory distress syndrome (ARDS). In the second phase, which may supervene rapidly, widespread activation of fibrinolysis lyses microthrombi but destroys coagulation factors and platelets, all of which are rapidly consumed and depleted. This severe **consumption coagulopathy** leads to uncontrolled bleeding from wounds and spontaneous haemorrhage into tissues, gut and brain.

Diagnosis

Depends on clinical recognition of thrombotic and bleeding events in an appropriate clinical context (see below), accompanied by a typical set of findings on investigation.

Clinical features

Clinical features of the underlying cause:
- Trauma
- Pregnancy, labour, postpartum
- Sepsis—fever, hypothermia, shock
- Metastatic carcinoma
  Clinical features of thrombi in the microvasculature:
- Acute renal failure
- ARDS
- Delirium, altered conscious level, coma
- Digital gangrene, progressing to limb ischaemia and gangrene
- Haemorrhagic infarction of the adrenals (Waterhouse—Friderichsen syndrome)
  Clinical features of consumption coagulopathy:
- Widespread bruising and purpura

- Fresh bleeding from old wounds and skin puncture sites
- Gastrointestinal bleeding
- Retroperitoneal bleeding

Investigation
Haematology
- *FBC:* thrombocytopenia
- *Blood film:* red cell fragments may be present
- *Coagulation screen:* usually (but not always) ↑ INR, ↑ APTTr, ↑ TCT
- *Fibrinogen assay:* usually reduced (less than 1.5 g/l)
- *Fibrin degradation products (FDP or D-dimers):* increased

Biochemistry
Urea, creatinine and electrolytes show evidence of renal failure.

Microbiology
Blood cultures for DIC-causing organisms (e.g. meningococcus).

Management
Treatment of the underlying cause is paramount. Without reducing or removing the DIC trigger, supportive therapy cannot keep pace with worsening haemostatic failure. This may mean:
- *In DIC complicating pregnancy* (most common cause, placental abruption): delivery of the infant and placenta
- *In DIC with sepsis:* immediate broad-spectrum parenteral antibiotics (as soon as blood cultures drawn)
- *In hypovolaemic shock:* rapid correction with plasma expanders
  Supportive transfusion to reduce bleeding while treating the underlying cause:
- Fresh frozen plasma
- Platelet transfusion
- Fibrinogen infusion (sometimes, with expert guidance)

Prognosis
This is very variable and clearly depends on successful treatment of the underlying cause.

Thrombosis and thrombophilia

Virchow's triad theory proposed that thrombosis (haemostasis in the wrong place) required any two of:
1 Blood flow stasis
2 An abnormal vessel wall
3 A change in blood 'clottability' (now termed hypercoagulability)
Haematology is concerned with the third member of the triad, which is particularly important in **venous thromboembolic disease** (VTED).

Thrombophilia refers to an inherited or acquired state leading to an increased risk of VTED.

Epidemiology

Incidence. Some inherited thrombophilias are common: factor V Leiden is found in 5% of people in the UK. Others are rarer (e.g. antithrombin deficiency approximately 1 in 1000). In general, thrombophilia is much more common than haemophilia.

Age. Increasing age is a risk factor for VTED. Rare homozygous protein C deficiency presents in the neonate, but in all other inherited thrombophilia the median age of first thrombosis is 45 years.

Sex. Equal.

Ethnicity. Factor V Leiden predominantly affects northern European individuals.

Genetics. Inherited thrombophilia acts as an autosomal dominant trait.

Geography. Both VTED and thrombophilia are more common in Europe and the USA.

Disease mechanisms

Clot regulation (see Fig. 15.11) depends on controlling thrombin via two mechanisms: direct inhibition by antithrombin, and negative feedback regulation by the protein C pathway. Inherited thrombophilias change proteins with roles in thrombin control, in directions that increase thrombin activity.

Inherited thrombophilia

- Factor V Leiden
- Prothrombin gene mutation
- Protein C deficiency
- Protein S deficiency
- Antithrombin deficiency

Acquired thrombophilia

Acquired thrombophilia usually involves interference with thrombin control arising from underlying disease processes or autoantibodies. The most important is antiphospholipid syndrome, in which an autoantibody reacting with cell membranes is associated with enhanced thrombin generation.

- Antiphospholipid syndrome
- Antithrombin deficiency secondary to nephrotic syndrome
- Hyperhomocysteinaemia (e.g. smoking, folate or B_{12} deficiency)

Inherited and acquired thrombophilias interact with life events that increase the risk of VTED. These are:

- Pregnancy and puerperium
- Surgery, particularly lower limb orthopaedic procedures
- Trauma and immobility, particularly spinal injury
- Circulatory diseases (cardiac failure, stroke, myocardial infarction)
- Oestrogen therapy

The likelihood that an individual will sustain a thrombotic event is therefore a **multifactorial** risk. When deciding how (or whether) to protect someone against VTED, or in performing diagnostic imaging for DVT, all the factors listed above are computed in a clinical risk score.

Diagnosis

The diagnosis of thrombophilia depends on finding a known inherited or acquired risk factor in an individual with a **personal or familial history** of recurrent venous thrombosis. Finding a known risk factor in someone without such a history is much less significant or helpful.

Clinical features

VTED usually presents as:

- DVT of the leg, either distal (calf veins only) or proximal (popliteal vein or above)
- Pulmonary embolism (PE) caused by embolization of clot from proximal DVT

In addition, thrombophilia may present as:

- Atypical venous thrombosis in axillary, mesenteric or cerebral veins
- Recurrent mid-trimester fetal loss (secondary to placental thrombosis)
- Recurrent DVT

Investigation

The key investigation is objective confirmation of the presence of a DVT. This is because **clinical** diagnosis (by symptoms and signs) is incorrect in approximately 70% of cases. If a personal or family history is being taken, only proven DVTs count.

Haematology

In an individual with proven recurrent DVT, or DVT in the context of other family members with proven DVT:

- *Coagulation screen:* may show ↑ APTTr that does not correct on addition of normal plasma; evidence of an antiphospholipid antibody (lupus inhibitor)
- *D-dimer assay:* used (along with clinical risk score and imaging) to diagnose DVT
- *Assays:* protein C, protein S, antithrombin

- *Molecular analysis:* factor V Leiden, prothrombin gene mutation

Biochemistry
Homocysteine assay. High levels of this thrombosis-associated amino acid are a risk factor.

Immunology
Anticardiolipin assay. Detects antiphospholipid antibody.

Diagnostic imaging
Venography, ultrasound, spiral CT or MRI. May be needed to confirm the presence of a DVT.

Management
For treatment of proven acute DVT or PE (see Chapter 6).

Prevention of deep-vein thrombosis and pulmonary embolism
This is a very effective approach to individuals with proven thrombophilia. Patients who have already sustained more than one proven DVT or PE should be on continuous coumarin anticoagulant therapy. Individuals who have sustained a single proven DVT may require thromboprophylactic therapy (e.g. subcutaneous low-dose heparin in one of its forms) to safely undergo one of the life-events associated with increased risk.

❗ Must know checklist

- How bone marrow stem cells provide new mature blood cells

- The normal human haemoglobins, and abnormal haemoglobin variants causing disease

- The normal limits of haemoglobin concentration, neutrophil, lymphocyte and platelet counts

- The consequences of abnormally low haemoglobin concentration, neutrophil and platelet counts

- How to classify a case of anaemia using the mean cell volume

- The human ABO and Rhesus blood group systems and what they mean in blood transfusion

- The hazards of blood transfusion

- The different clinical impacts of: (a) acute versus chronic leukaemia; (b) low-grade versus high-grade lymphoma

- How to examine a patient for: (a) lymphadenopathy; (b) hepatomegaly and splenomegaly; (c) signs of anaemia; and (d) signs of abnormal bleeding

- How to use the coagulation screen to locate the underlying cause of abnormal bleeding

---

Further reading

Books
Hoffbrand AV, Pettit JE, Moss P. *Essential Haematology*, 4th edn. Oxford: Blackwell Publishing, 2001.
McClelland DBL. *Handbook of Transfusion Medicine*, 3rd edn. Norwich: The Stationery Office, 2001.
Provan D, Chisholm M, Duncombe, A, Singer C, Smith A. *Oxford Handbook of Clinical Haematology*. Oxford: Oxford University Press, 1998.
Sackett DL, Straus S, Richardson S, Rosenberg W, Haynes RB. *Evidence-based Medicine: How to Practice and Teach EBM*, 2nd edn. London: Churchill Livingstone, 2000 (chapter on Diagnostic Testing and Screening).
Stamatoyannopoulos G, Majerus P, Perlmutter RM, Varmus H. *The Molecular Basis of Blood Diseases*, 3rd edn. Philadelphia: WB Saunders, 2001.

Journals
Current Opinion in Hematology, Lippincott Williams & Wilkins. http://www.cohematology.com/
Blood Reviews, Elsevier Science. www.harcourt-international.com/journals/blre
Hematology, American Society of Hematology. www.asheducationbook.org
British Journal of Haematology, Blackwell Science.

Websites
Directory. Hardin MD: *Blood Diseases and Hematology*: www.lib.uiowa.edu/hardin/md/hem.html
On-line journal. Bloodline: www.bloodline.net
Basic atlas. How to do morphology: Digital image study sets: http://medocs.ucdavis.edu/420A/course.htm
Comprehensive atlas. Atlas of Hematology: http://pathy.med.nagoya-u.ac.jp/atlas/doc/atlas.html
Web lectures. http://www.med-ed.virginia.edu/courses/path/innes

15

Palliative Medicine **16**

Introduction

The aims of medical care form a continuum, ranging from complete cure at one end to symptom control at the other. Palliative medicine is the branch of medicine that specializes in symptom control. It addresses the needs of the patient with advanced incurable illness. For such patients, the primary aim of treatment is no longer to prolong life but to make life as comfortable and meaningful as possible. Relief of symptoms is the priority. These patients often have far advanced cancer; however, a large proportion have non-malignant disease, such as end-stage renal failure, chronic obstructive pulmonary disease, end-stage cardiac failure, motor neurone disease or acquired immune deficiency syndrome (AIDS).

This chapter applies to all terminally ill patients, but it must be appreciated that most experience has been gained from the management of patients with advanced cancer. An estimated 1 in 3 people will develop cancer during their lifetime. Survival from cancer varies enormously, depending on the type and stage of the cancer. Metastatic spread is common. Typical sites are the lymph nodes, bone, liver, lung and brain. Approximately 65% of patients with cancer will die from their disease. Cancer accounts for 25% of all deaths in the UK and cancer deaths form a substantial proportion of early deaths (33% of those dying between the ages of 5 and 65 years). In the UK most cancer deaths still occur in hospital.

Aims of palliative medicine

People with advanced incurable illness have complex problems. The practice of palliative medicine therefore focuses on the whole patient rather than taking a disease-orientated approach. It does this by:
- Addressing psychological, social, spiritual and financial needs as well as physical symptoms
- Providing effective symptom control

- Offering control, independence and choice, to allow participation in decisions about the management of problems—including negotiating the most appropriate place to die (home, hospice or hospital)
- Supporting 'the family' (all those who are important to the patient) as well as the patient
- Providing bereavement counselling for the family
- Providing support and expert advice to the professionals and other carers involved in management

No one individual can command all the skills necessary to achieve these goals; a team approach is therefore essential. The aim is to provide an integrated seamless service to the patient and his or her 'family'. Close liaison between the hospital, community and hospice is essential.

The multidisciplinary palliative care team might include a palliative medicine physician, clinical nurse specialists (Macmillan nurses), social workers and counsellors. This specialist team should be seen as part of a broader team, which includes the patient and his or her family as well as the other professionals involved in ongoing care (e.g. the hospital consultant/ward sister and GP/district nurse). In the home, the GP and district nurse are the key workers; in the hospital, the consultant and the ward staff. The palliative care team does not generally take over the care of the patient, but rather facilitates the best use of all the disciplines and local resources to maximize the quality of care. It has expertise in symptom control and is familiar with all local facilities, thus putting it in a position to advise and act as a resource for the patient's professional and lay carers. The multidisciplinary specialist team within the hospice is larger and more complex, and includes senior and junior doctors, nurses, specialist social workers, counsellors, physiotherapists, clergy, bereavement workers and complementary therapists.

In addition to clinical work, formal and informal teaching of students, doctors, nurses and other carers is an essential part of any team's work.

Communication

A substantial number of medical students graduate without ever having had any active participation in the management of dying patients. It is not surprising therefore that many doctors have difficulty in communicating with terminally ill patients and their families. Terminal illness can be seen as a failure and can generate feelings of inadequacy, fear and despair in doctors. These fears lead to the use of certain tactics in order to keep patients at a safe emotional distance. These include the following:

• *Premature reassurance:* for example, when a patient complains of pain, the doctor quickly reassures him or her that it can be relieved, but does not explore what the patient feels about the pain
• *Selective attention:* for example, when a patient complains of losing weight and constipation, and says 'I am worried', the doctor ignores the worry and discusses bowel habit
• *Changing topics:* for example, when a patient says that he or she feels his or her condition is deteriorating, the doctor ignores the statement and proceeds to ask about pain control
• *Closed questions:* for example, the doctor says to the patient: 'You're feeling much better today, aren't you?'

The principles of good communication are to deal with the patient's concerns before professional concerns, to ensure full coverage of one topic before proceeding to the next, to obtain a list of all the problems before giving advice or attempting any solution, to watch for non-verbal as well as verbal clues, and to clarify and summarize what the patient reports.

It is not a question of 'What should the patient know?', but an assessment of 'What does the patient want to know?'.

Common emotional reactions to life-threatening illness

Anxiety

Anxiety is a normal reaction to serious illness. The most common emotional reaction to a life-threatening illness is fear, and many anxieties are based on fears that can be resolved. Common fears are concerned with:

• Unrelieved symptoms, especially pain
• Death and the process of dying
• Dying alone
• Uncompleted tasks (e.g. a will has not been made)
• Loss of and separation from family, job, income
• Loss of dignity because of confusion, incontinence and loss of control
• Altered body image

• Retribution in the afterlife
Find out what the fears are so that they can be addressed.

Clinical features

Recognize and accept normal levels of anxiety, but look for features of clinical anxiety:

• Presence of an anxious mood most of the time
• Difficulty distracting a patient from his or her worries
• Awareness on the patient's part that the mood is different from normal worrying
• Feelings of tenseness and restlessness
• Insomnia
• Autonomic hyperactivity (e.g. palpitations, sensation of choking)
• Panic attacks
In such patients anxiolytics may be helpful.

Denial

Assess whether or not the denial is causing harm (e.g. refusal of necessary medication, psychological turmoil). For many patients, denial is a successful coping strategy. Removing it may cause unnecessary distress.

Anger

Anger can be displaced onto staff and/or relatives. It is important not to react to anger but to try to accept and understand. It needs to be explained to the relatives that the patient is not really angry with them, but is displacing the anger he or she feels towards the disease onto them.

Despair and depression

Despair is a normal reaction to a life-threatening illness and should be recognized and acknowledged. However, it is important not to miss clinical depression.

Clinical features

Features of clinical depression include:

• Common somatic symptoms of depression (e.g. weight loss, anorexia, lethargy), but they carry less weight because they are often a manifestation of the terminal illness itself
• Presence of the depressed mood most of the time
• Difficulty in distracting the patient
• Awareness on the patient's part that the mood is different from normal sadness
• Lowering of interest and enjoyment of social activities
• Crying, irritability, poor concentration, poor sleep
• Feelings of guilt
• Suicidal ideas
Such patients should be treated with antidepressants.

16

Principles of symptom control

Adopt a positive, but realistic, attitude and assure the patient that a considerable amount can be achieved. A problem-orientated individualized approach is essential. For each symptom, diagnose its cause, explain it to the patient, discuss the possible treatments, set realistic objectives, treat appropriately, anticipate changes, keep relatives informed and supported, and never say 'There is nothing more I can do.' This statement is negative, unhelpful and untrue.

Diagnose the cause of the symptom

Both physical and psychological aspects should be taken into account. An accurate diagnosis is important in palliative medicine, but the emphasis lies on careful history and examination, as investigations can be impractical and distressing in the very ill (HISTORY & EXAMINATION BOX 16.1). Investigations should only be carried out if they will significantly alter the management of the patient.

Treatment of the same symptom varies considerably depending on the underlying pathology. For example, vomiting in a patient with cancer may result from many causes, including raised intracranial pressure, drugs, hepatomegaly or intestinal obstruction. Each of these causes requires specific management.

Many symptoms are multifactorial in origin. Recognize the contributory factors and address each as far as possible.

History & Examination 16.1: History and examination of a patient referred for palliative care

Acquire a detailed past history
Full information is needed from both the patient and from specialist teams that are or have been involved in the patient's care. It is very helpful to know *precisely* what has been said to the patient regarding diagnosis, extent of disease and prognosis and to have reports of recent investigations, blood tests, etc. This helps to give the clinician an in-depth picture of the patient's illness, previous problems and treatments. It is important to be open minded and if necessary question previous assumptions made about the cause(s) of the patient's symptoms. The clinician should be aware that previous assessments may be incorrect

Take a full history as in any medical consultation
In particular try to:
- Understand the impact the illness has made on the patient—allow the patient to tell 'his or her own story'
- Prioritize, from the patient's perspective, the symptom control issues that need to be addressed
- Elicit any fears or misconceptions the patient has about his or her disease and/or past treatments
- Find out if, and what, the patient knows about his or her diagnosis, the extent of disease and the prognosis

Offer the patient the chance to discuss broader emotional and psychosocial concerns about his or her illness
The patient can then be referred to suitable professionals for further support
- *Emotional problems:* sadness, depression, despair, anxiety and fear. Common fears include a fear of an uncertain future, a distressing death, losing control and independence
- *Social problems:* isolation, unsuitable accommodation, financial concerns

- *Sexual problems:* relationships, the patient's role in a family and his or her sexuality
- *Spiritual and religious problems:* people often search for meaning in their lives when faced with an advanced illness. Some patients have specific needs based on their religious beliefs

Examine the patient
The patient should be fully examined as in any medical consultation, taking into account any clues given in the history to likely pathology. In patients referred for palliative care, additional consideration should be given to the following areas

General
Assess general state of the patient—how unwell is he or she?
Is the patient in pain?
Is the patient dying?

Mood and cognition
Is the patient sad, depressed, anxious or frightened?
Is the patient confused, agitated or distressed?

Mouth
Does the patient have *Candida*?

Respiratory
If the patient is dying, does he or she have retained secretions and noisy breathing?
If the patient is dying, has the pattern of breathing changed (tachypnoea or Cheyne–Stokes respiration)?

Abdominal and/or rectal examination
Is there constipation?
Is there diarrhoea (could it be overflow)?

Skin
Is there any evidence of bed sores?

Symptomatic relief must be given, even if the diagnosis is tentative and it is not appropriate to investigate further. Very often a therapeutic trial will indicate the cause. For example, a trial of corticosteroids can be given to a confused patient with suspected brain metastases who is too unwell to undergo a computed tomography (CT) scan. A response suggests metastatic disease.

Explain the symptom to the patient
Fear is an important factor in the patient's interpretation of any symptom. Explanation will reassure the patient, giving him or her confidence in the doctor's ability to control it.

Discuss the treatment options
Patients should be given adequate and accurate information about the treatment options so that they can make informed choices.

Set objectives that are realistic
Both patients and staff get frustrated if unachievable objectives are set.

Treat appropriately
Ensure that prescriptions of drugs are:
- *Rational* (e.g. use laxatives and not analgesics for the pain of constipation)
- *Regular* (e.g. laxatives, antiemetics and analgesics must be given regularly for persistent symptoms)
- *The right dose* (e.g. there is no maximum dose of morphine)
- *Given at the right interval* (e.g. sustained-release morphine preparations should be prescribed 12- or 24-hourly; immediate-release morphine sulphate should be prescribed 4-hourly)
- *Given by the correct route* (e.g. rectally, transdermally, subcutaneously or intramuscularly if the patient is vomiting). Keep the regimen simple, and explain it to the patient, in writing if appropriate. Supervise it carefully.

Anticipate
Symptoms can change rapidly in the context of advanced illness, and distress may be avoided if such changes are anticipated. A deterioration that makes it impossible to continue with oral medication should be anticipated to ensure that injectable preparations are available. This is particularly important in the home care setting and can avert an unnecessary crisis.

Common symptoms in patients with advanced disease

The common symptoms in our unit are shown in Table 16.1.

Table 16.1 Prevalence of common symptoms in patients with advanced cancer at Edenhall Marie Curie Centre

Symptom	Prevalence (%)
Pain	70
Fatigue	80
Dyspnoea	50
Anorexia	70
Dysphagia	10
Nausea and vomiting	40
Constipation	50
Depression	30
Anxiety	30

Pain

Pain is especially feared by cancer patients and is also a significant problem in about 40% of patients with progressive neurological diseases such as multiple sclerosis and motor neurone disease. It can be modified or alleviated in all patients. Proper pain assessment leads to effective management.

Diagnose the cause of the pain
Most patients with advanced disease have pain at more than one site. Each pain should be evaluated individually.

To establish the cause of any pain, it is essential to take a careful history, particularly noting:
- Site of pain and any radiation
- Type and severity of pain
- When the pain started and any subsequent changes
- Exacerbating and alleviating factors
- Previous history of analgesic use

Physical examination often confirms the diagnosis. It may be appropriate to X-ray or scan a patient, or perform some other form of investigation, if management will be altered by the results.

Always assess how significant the pain is for patients (how it affects them; how it alters their lifestyle).

Pain may result from a malignant or non-malignant cause. In about one-third of patients with advanced cancer who complain of pain, the underlying pathology is non-malignant.

Common causes of pain
Bone pain
Bone pain is common in patients with cancer and can be caused by metastatic disease or by local infiltration by adjacent tumour. It is characteristically a deep gnawing pain made worse by movement. The bone is often tender on percussion.

16

Visceral pain

Visceral pain is most commonly caused by tumour in the lung or internal organs of the abdomen and pelvis. It may:
- Be a deep-seated pain arising from complex pathology associated with soft-tissue infiltration
- Result from stretching of a capsule (e.g. stretching of the liver capsule is a common source, causing right hypochondrial pain, which can be severe and may be worsened by a local bleed into a deposit, and is accompanied by tender hepatomegaly)
- Result from distension of a hollow organ (e.g. small and large intestines, bladder, ureters) causing severe spasmodic pain that may be colicky in nature

Nerve pain

Nerves may be infiltrated or compressed. Pain resulting from nerve destruction may be burning and lancinating, and associated with abnormal sensations (e.g. hyperaesthesia); that caused by nerve compression is more often a deep ache.

Destruction of nerve plexuses, nerve roots or peripheral nerves may result in deafferentation pain (pain associated with sensory changes in the painful area).

Pain that arises centrally (from the brain or spinal cord) often manifests as unilateral spontaneous pain and hypersensitivity, associated with disagreeable dysaesthesiae.

Nerve compression and nerve destruction may coexist.

Myofascial pain

Musculoskeletal pains are common in patients with cancer, and can be particularly troublesome in patients with progressive neurological disease (e.g. multiple sclerosis and motor neurone disease). Musculoskeletal pain radiates in a non-dermatomal pattern. Typically, there are localized hypersensitive areas of muscle known as trigger points, which are tender to pressure.

Superficial pain

Bed sores may be unavoidable in weak, debilitated patients and cause distressing superficial pain.

Realistic objectives

Realistic objectives should be set. For nearly all patients, pain can be significantly modified, and complete pain relief can be achieved in many. For a few, pain can prove intractable and unresponsive to most treatments. These patients provide the greatest challenge and all avenues of achieving pain relief must be explored.

Realistic goals are:
- *Freedom from pain at night:* should always be achievable
- *Freedom from pain at rest:* usually achievable
- *Freedom from pain on mobility:* may not be achievable

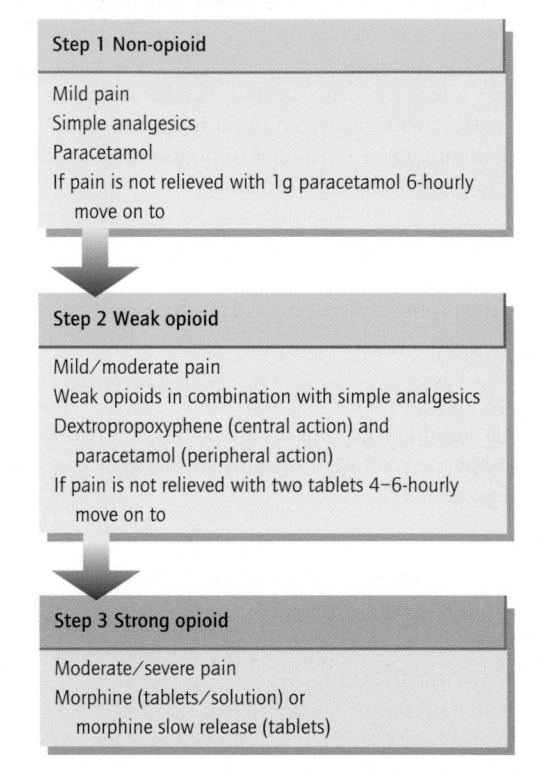

Figure 16.1 Three-step regimen for treating pain.

Treat appropriately

This clearly depends on its cause. Not all pain requires analgesia; for example, the pain of urinary retention is best treated by catheterization. When analgesics are indicated, however, they must be prescribed correctly.

Analgesic treatment of pain

The variety of analgesics available for treating pain can be daunting, but the authors advocate the following simple three-step regimen (based on the WHO analgesic ladder) shown in Fig. 16.1. It is better to use a few drugs effectively than many ineffectively.

Principles of prescribing opioids

Opioids are used to suppress pain and, if possible, to prevent any breakthrough pain. This requires regular prescribing. The pain is caused by advanced disease and is unlikely to remit. The dosage should be adequate and titrated upwards until the pain is controlled. Medication should be prescribed as required for any breakthrough pain.

Strong opioids of choice

The gold standard has always been morphine. It is

Table 16.2 Strong opioids: prescribing oral morphine

Immediate-release morphine preparations

These are quick-acting preparations, available as tablets or solution

Prescribed 4-hourly, although a double dose often given at bedtime (omitting 4 a.m. dose) to avoid patient being woken

Prescribed less frequently if renal impairment present

Flexible drug, dose can easily be adjusted and patient's response assessed

Used when patient first starts on strong opioids

Sustained-release morphine preparations

These are long-acting preparations, available as tablets or soluble granules

Both 12- or 24-hourly preparations are available

Used when patient's pain is stable on the immediate-release preparation

Breakthrough or episodic pain

Extra doses of immediate-release morphine are used for 'breakthrough or episodic' pain which occurs before next regular dose is due

Slow-release preparations must not be used for breakthrough pain

Getting the dose right

Doses of immediate-release morphine are reviewed and the regular prescription adjusted every 24 h (or sooner if pain severe)

Regular dose is titrated up in line with the total 'breakthrough' doses given in the preceding 24 h

This process is repeated until the patient remains pain free between doses or until the 'breakthrough' doses have no further effect

If residual pain remains, a co-analgesic will need to be considered

Maintenance regimen

If patient stabilizes on immediate-release morphine, convert to slow-release preparation

Conversion from immediate- to slow-release morphine preparations is performed on a mg for mg basis

The total immediate-release morphine given per 24 h is given as either a single dose (24-hourly preparation) or divided by two (12-hourly preparation)

Table 16.3 Strong opioids: alternative opioids

Transdermal fentanyl

Transdermal preparation applied every 3 days

Useful in patients unable to swallow or absorb oral opioids or in whom compliance is a problem

Inactive metabolites and not as dependent as morphine on the kidney for its excretion

Long-acting opioid of choice in renal failure

Hydromorphone

Inactive metabolites, therefore suitable alternative opioid for the morphine intolerant

Useful in patients with renal impairment

Methadone

Long-acting opioid acting on broad range of opioid receptors, *N*-methyl-D-aspartate (NMDA) receptors and serotoninergic receptors

Role in neuropathic pain that is relatively insensitive to morphine

Long action because of its lipophilicity results in accumulation, which makes it a difficult drug to use

Table 16.4 Indications for parenteral opioids

Indications for parenteral opioids

The last few hours/days of life when the patient is unable to swallow

Dysphagia

Nausea and vomiting

Gut obstruction

Inability to tolerate taste or the number of tablets

If regular injections are required, consider a continuous subcutaneous infusion.

available in both immediate-release and sustained-release preparations (Table 16.2). Typically in our unit, two-thirds of patients are on the equivalent of 30 mg morphine or less 4-hourly and over 80% are on 60 mg or less 4-hourly.

Alternative opioids can have advantages over morphine. They are used in specific circumstances that exploit their relative lack of active metabolites or their route of administration (Table 16.3).

Remember:
- If a patient has significant pain, adequate effective analgesics should be started early
- Valuable time wasted using ineffective moderate analgesics can mean that patients with a short prognosis may spend a substantial portion of their remaining life with uncontrolled pain
- Opioids are the most effective strong analgesics

Routes of administration

The oral route is always preferable if the patient is able to swallow, but at times it may be necessary to give opioids rectally, parenterally or transdermally (Table 16.4).

Small-volume injections are preferred and diamorphine hydrochloride is therefore the drug of choice for parenteral use because it is highly soluble. Subcutaneous injections are effective and this is the route of choice.

16

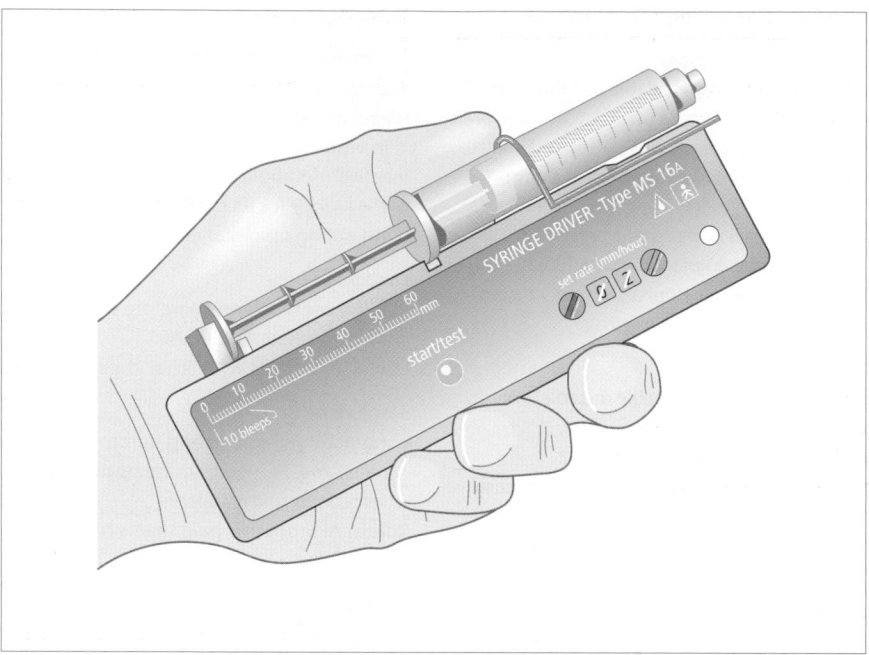

Figure 16.2 Subcutaneous infusion pump. A subcutaneous infusion pump is a small battery-driven device that will inject the contents of a syringe over a 24-h period. It can be used in the home and in the inpatient setting.

Dose conversion

Diamorphine undergoes first-pass metabolism in the liver and the subcutaneous dose should therefore be approximately half to one-third of the oral dose. If the patient is going to require more than 2–3 injections, a subcutaneous infusion pump should be considered (Fig. 16.2).

Fears of prescribing opioids

Opioids are safe and effective and should not be withheld from patients in pain. There are many fears about prescribing opioids, which can compromise effective pain management (Table 16.5).

Side-effects of opioids

Opioids do have some predictable side-effects (Table 16.6).

Opioid-resistant pain

Some pains are either partially sensitive or insensitive to opioids. These pains need to be managed with an additional or alternative drug or some other technique.

Bone pain

Although partially sensitive to opioids, bone pain frequently needs additional treatment with a non-steroidal anti-inflammatory drug (NSAID). In patients at risk of NSAID-associated gastric and duodenal ulceration, prostaglandin analogues (e.g. misoprostol) or proton pump inhibitors may be used prophylactically or COX-2 inhibitors should be considered. If the pain is localized radiotherapy may be suitable. Surgical fixation may be indicated if there is a pathological fracture or a high risk of this occurring.

Nerve pain

Nerve pain is very often insensitive to opioids. Corticosteroids are useful in nerve compression. Nerve infiltration, irritation and destruction may respond to drugs that alter neurotransmission (e.g. low-dose tricyclic antidepressants, anticonvulsants). Consider radiotherapy and nerve blocks.

Liver capsule pain

Liver capsule pain is partially opioid sensitive. Corticosteroids should be considered because they may reduce the liver swelling and relieve capsular stretching.

Colic

Treat colic caused by constipation with laxatives. If colic is caused by tumour obstruction, antispasmodics will be required.

Meningeal pain and raised intracranial pressure

Corticosteroids are the drug of choice. Radiotherapy should be considered.

Table 16.5 Fears of prescribing opioids

Addiction

'Patients will become dependent on opioids'

Many studies have shown that 'psychological' addiction does not occur. Commonly patients can reduce and/or stop their opioid if their pain is controlled by another method such as by a nerve block or surgical fixation. Chemical dependence does occur (as with many drugs) and this must be considered when morphine is reduced. In these instances, morphine should be gradually reduced. It must never be stopped abruptly

Tolerance

'I must not start morphine too early in case the patient becomes used to it and the dose will need increasing'

Tolerance has been shown to occur, but only to a minor degree when opioids are taken over a long period. For practical purposes it is not relevant. If the dosage of opioid needs to be increased, it is because of an increase in pain secondary to advancing tumour

Respiratory depression

'I cannot use morphine in frail patients or those with respiratory problems because it precipitates respiratory depression'

This does not occur with careful attention to dosage. Opioids are used in the palliative care setting for dyspnoea because they reduce ventilatory demand and therefore the sensation of breathlessness

Hastening death

'I can't prescribe morphine until the patient is very close to death. I like to reserve morphine until the very end'

Opioids do not hasten death. Indeed, relieving pain may allow the patient to start to eat again and enjoy life

Indicating death is imminent

'Morphine signals imminent death'

A prescription of morphine is often perceived by the patient as an unspoken sign that death is imminent. The physician should always be aware of this, explaining that when an opioid is prescribed the intention is to treat pain and that opioids are not reserved only for the terminal phase of illness

Lymphoedema

Physical treatment (e.g. massage and compression hosiery) has an important role. NSAIDs and corticosteroids can be helpful.

Muscle spasm

Muscle spasm can be treated with benzodiazepines or baclofen.

Infection

The most appropriate treatment for pleuritic chest pain secondary to infection or the cellulitic pain of an infected ulcer is antibiotics.

Joint and myofascial pain

NSAIDs should be used in conjunction with opioids. Local injections of corticosteroid into joints and trigger points may be of value.

Superficial pain

Patients with bed sores need to be kept off the pressure areas with regular turning. An effective patient support system (e.g. pressure-relieving mattress) is crucial.

Psychological factors

Pain may be aggravated by psychological factors. Management directed only at physical factors may fail to control pain adequately in some patients. Coexistent depression or anxiety must be treated and, if appropriate, counselling and diversionary activities should be offered.

Complementary therapies

Although scientifically unproven, certain complementary therapies seem to benefit some groups of patients. If patients perceive these therapies as adding to their overall well-being, carers should support them, provided the treatment does not harm patients or interfere with their conventional management. The authors find hypnosis,

Table 16.6 Predictable side-effects of morphine and diamorphine

Side-effect	Approximate frequency (%)	Suitable action
Constipation	>95	*Regular laxative* is essential and should be prescribed prophylactically
Nausea and vomiting	30	*Prescribe antiemetic.* The first choice is haloperidol. If the patient is primed to vomit (e.g. because of gastrointestinal tumour, already nauseated) prescribe prophylactic antiemetic when starting opioids. Usually self-limiting if caused by opioid alone and so antiemetic can be withdrawn after 10–14 days
Drowsiness	20	*Wears off* in about 5 days on a stable dose. Not a reason to withhold opioids
Other side-effects		A dry mouth is very common and should be treated with simple local measures. Confusion and hallucinations are rare (<1% of patients) and other causes should be excluded

acupuncture, aromatherapy, art therapy and relaxation therapy useful in many patients.

Injection techniques for cancer pain

Nerve blocks have a place in palliative care, but should only be offered if there is a reasonable chance of success and not as a 'last resort'. They are highly effective when used judiciously in a selected group of patients; approximately 4% of patients with pain will benefit.

Various 'injection techniques' can be used. Some of these techniques need expertise and specialized equipment, but simple techniques can be performed at the bedside. Side-effects can occur, especially with the major neurolytic procedures (e.g. intraspinal neurolysis for nerve root pain can produce urinary and faecal incontinence).

If pain is resistant to analgesic treatment or if the side-effects of analgesics are distressing, nerve blocks should be considered. They may prove helpful for:

- Unilateral pain
- Localized pain
- Pain resulting from involvement of one or two nerve roots
- Abdominal pain arising from the 'upper' gut
- Rib pain

Weakness

Weakness is a common and distressing symptom in patients with advanced illness. When caused by general debility it is very difficult to treat. Reversible causes, such as cord compression and cerebral metastases, in patients with cancer must be excluded (ONCOLOGICAL EMERGENCIES IN PALLIATIVE MEDICINE AT A GLANCE).

Management

It is important to acknowledge the problem and explain to the patient that the weakness results from the illness. This allows realistic goals to be set, which in itself can reduce the patient's distress. Simple practical measures such as providing a wheelchair can allow the patient who has difficulty walking to get to the dayroom and to venture further afield.

Corticosteroids can be useful for some patients, but their effect (increase in energy and sense of well-being) is temporary, lasting only a few weeks. They should not therefore be introduced too early, and their short-term benefit must be weighed against possible side-effects such as proximal myopathy and peptic ulceration.

Dyspnoea

Dyspnoea is a subjective difficulty in breathing. It is experienced by:

Table 16.7 Causes of dyspnoea in terminal disease

Cancer
Primary tumour
Parenchymal or lymph node metastases
Lymphangitis carcinomatosis
Malignant effusion
Massive ascites splinting the diaphragm

Other causes
Infection
Anaemia
Postradiotherapy or postchemotherapy fibrosis
Congestive cardiac failure
Chronic obstructive airways disease
Dysfunction of respiratory muscles because of progressive neurological disease
Anxiety

- 50% of patients with advanced cancer
- 60% of patients with motor neurone disease
- 70% of patients with lung cancer

When assessing the patient, consider the causes given in Table 16.7.

Management

Coexistent medical problems such as infection and congestive cardiac failure are treated conventionally. Management of dyspnoea caused by tumour is outlined below. Explanation should always precede prescription, and can itself lead to improvement. Severe dyspnoea resulting from large airway compression causes stridor, is extremely distressing and requires prompt action (ONCOLOGICAL EMERGENCIES IN PALLIATIVE MEDICINE AT A GLANCE).

Drugs

Drug treatment of dyspnoea in terminal illness includes:
- Corticosteroids for lymphangitis, bronchospasm, large bulk tumour and superior vena cava obstruction
- Bronchodilators for bronchospasm
- Low-dose morphine to reduce the sensation of dyspnoea
- Anticholinergics to dry up secretions
- Anxiolytics for anxiety and increased muscle tone

Other treatment

Other treatment includes:
- Attention to the environment (e.g. upright position, cool fan, calm surroundings, advice against tight clothes)
- Radiotherapy
- Transfusion
- Aspiration of fluid from the chest or abdomen

Oncological emergencies in palliative medicine at a glance

Reversible problems which are commonly underdiagnosed include:

Superior vena cava obstruction

Symptoms
Dyspnoea, oedema of face, neck and arms, headache

Cause
Tumour mass compressing superior vena cava

Management
Immediate steroids
Urgent radio- or chemotherapy ± venous stent and anticoagulation

Stridor

Symptoms
Severe dyspnoea

Cause
Tumour mass compressing upper airways

Management
Steroids, radiotherapy/chemotherapy ± stent

Cord/cauda equina compression

Symptoms
Back pain, progressive or acute
Weakness in legs, sensory loss and/or urinary retention/incontinence

Cause
Extradural compression by tumour mass arising in vertebral body, or direct spread of paraspinal tumour mass

Management
Time is of the essence: if left untreated cord compression becomes irreversible.
Immediate steroids and urgent investigation with MRI of spine
Then radiotherapy usually follows, but sometimes neurosurgical intervention may be necessary

Hypercalcaemia

Symptoms
Malaise, anorexia, nausea, vomiting, constipation, thirst, polyuria, drowsiness, confusion

Cause
Tumour-related humoral factors
Often but not necessarily associated with bone metastases

Management
Fluids and bisphosphonates, together with treatment of underlying malignancy if possible (e.g. chemotherapy, hormones)

Acute renal failure

Symptoms
Oliguria, anuria, or symptoms of uraemia, e.g. confusion, twitching

Cause
Ureteric obstruction due to pelvic/para-aortic tumour mass
Drugs, especially NSAIDs

Management
Obstruction: ultrasound scan of the kidneys
Steroids, radiotherapy/chemotherapy and/or ureteric stents
Drugs: stop offending drug

Fractured bone

Symptoms
Severe pain, immobility
Usually pathological fracture

Cause
Bone metastasis or local invasion

Management
If prognosis >1 month consider surgical fixation

Urinary retention

Quite common and often missed

Symptoms
Difficulty passing urine, abdominal pain, but sometimes, in patients who are unable to communicate, only manifestation is agitation

Cause
Drugs, cord compression, local obstruction, general debility

Management
Catheterization

16

Table 16.8 Causes and management of dysphagia

Type of dysphagia	Implication	Cause	Management
Solids then liquids	Obstruction	Tumour mass, external compression	Corticosteroids, radiotherapy, laser dilatation, stent
Solid and liquids simultaneously	Neuromuscular	Terminal neuromuscular dysfunction in very weak patients	
		Progressive neurological disease	Dry secretions, anticholinergics ± PEG feeding
		Perineural tumour infiltration with head and neck tumours that damage cranial nerves (V, IX, X)	Corticosteroids ± PEG feeding
Painful	Mucosal causes	*Candida* (only 50% of patients with oesophageal *Candida* have clinically apparent oral *Candida*)	Antifungals
		Postradiotherapy	Analgesia
Psychogenic			Counselling, anxiolytics

- Counselling
- Alternative methods (e.g. hypnotherapy, relaxation tapes)

Anorexia

Approximately 70% of all patients with advanced cancer have anorexia. Its incidence in patients with non-malignant disease is unknown. It is important to decide whose problem it is—the patient's or his or her carers'.

Causes of anorexia are:
- Disease load
- Fear of vomiting
- Presentation of food (too much, unappetizing)
- Constipation
- Oral problems (thrush may present atypically as sores, ulcers or a dry mouth, or as classical white patches)
- Oral tumour
- Offensive smell from tumour
- Biochemical abnormality (hypercalcaemia, uraemia, hyponatraemia)
- Drugs, radiotherapy
- Depression or anxiety

If the above factors have been attended to and it is still felt to be a problem for the patient, try corticosteroids as an appetite stimulant.

Dysphagia

Dysphagia occurs in only approximately 10% of cancer patients. It is a common problem in patients with progressive neurological disease, occurring in approximately 60% of patients. It is vital to explain the cause of the dysphagia, and advise the patient about diet (soft or liquid diet) (Table 16.8). Any concurrent pain should be treated. If the patient is not in the terminal phase (commonly patients with progressive non-malignant neurological disease) and all other avenues have been exhausted, consideration should be given to percutaneous endoscopic gastrostomy (PEG) feeding. It is better to discuss this option sooner rather than later to allow the patient to make an informed decision.

Nausea and vomiting

Approximately 40% of patients with advanced cancer experience nausea and vomiting. Rational treatment is based on the assessment of the most likely underlying cause. Antiemetics are often indicated and in the majority of patients with advanced illness they should provide satisfactory symptom control. Most antiemetics act at one of the three sites shown in COMMON CAUSES OF NAUSEA AND VOMITING IN PATIENTS WITH ADVANCED DISEASE AT A GLANCE.

Sometimes more than one antiemetic will be necessary to control the symptoms. If so, it is common sense to combine drugs that act at different sites (a neuroleptic with an antihistamine). The choice of drug clearly depends on the cause of vomiting.

Hypercalcaemia

The normal range of serum calcium is 2.1–2.6 mmol/l if the serum albumin level is normal, but many people with cancer have low albumin levels. The calcium result should be adjusted according to the level of albumin (low albumin artificially lowers serum calcium).

Hypercalcaemia is not unusual in people with advanced malignancy, in particular in those with squamous cell carcinoma, breast cancer, prostate cancer, myeloma or lymphoma. It may develop insidiously or acutely, the most common symptoms being associated with the

Common causes of nausea and vomiting in patients with advanced disease at a glance

Drugs (e.g. opioids)
Management
Stop offending drug if possible

Cerebral primary/metastases, meningeal metastases ± cerebral oedema
Management
Steroids ± radiotherapy
Antiemetic acting on vomiting centre (NB neuroleptics lower the threshold for fitting and therefore should be avoided)

Biochemical uraemia, hypercalcaemia, hyponatraemia, abnormal liver function
Management
Treat cause if reversible
Use centrally acting antiemetic

Gastric irritation due to drugs or blood
Management
Stop offending drug if possible, give proton pump inhibitor or H2 receptor antagonist

Gastric stasis secondary to drugs or gastric stasis due to squashed stomach caused by massive hepatomegaly or ascites
Management
Prokinetic antiemetic ± antacid
Consider ascitic drainage

Constipation
Management
Laxatives

Bowel obstruction proximal or distal
Management
See Table 16.9

Pharyngeal irritation due to tumour or *Candida*
Management
Tumour: steroids
Candida: antifungals

Anticancer treatments such as chemotherapy or radiotherapy especially if involve upper gut
Management
HT3 antagonists

Psychosocial, anxiety, fear
Management
Counselling, anxiolytics

Vestibular causes (associated vertigo)
Management
Labyrinthine sedatives, e.g. antihistamines

Sites of action of antiemetic drugs

Site of action	Class of drug	Example
Centrally acting		
Chemoreceptor trigger zone	Neuroleptic	Haloperidol
Vomiting centre	Antihistamine	Cyclizine
Peripherally acting	Prokinetic	Domperidone
Broad spectrum	Phenothiazine	Levomepromazine

gastrointestinal tract and central nervous system (see ONCOLOGICAL EMERGENCIES IN PALLIATIVE MEDICINE AT A GLANCE).

Hypercalcaemia is associated with a very poor prognosis in patients with chemotherapy- or hormone-resistant tumours. However, its treatment plays an important part in the palliation of the distressing symptoms. The serum calcium level can be satisfactorily reduced in the majority of patients with oral rehydration and an intravenous infusion of bisphosphonate (usually over a few hours). Occasionally, intravenous hydration may be needed. Bisphosphonates can be repeated if necessary at a future date. As always, the patient's overall condition must be taken into account when making decisions about treatment.

Bowel obstruction—medical management in terminally ill patients

Obstruction may be proximal (obstruction of the stomach or small bowel), in which case the predominant symptom is vomiting, or distal (small bowel or colon), when the predominant symptoms are colicky pain and abdominal distension. Surgery should be considered but is rarely

Table 16.9 Medical management of bowel obstruction in terminally ill patients

Diet
Small meals; no restrictions

Nausea and vomiting
Centrally acting antiemetic (e.g. cyclizine and/or haloperidol) via syringe pump
If high obstruction with large-volume vomiting or severe abdominal distension, consider whether octreotide is warranted

Reverse obstruction
Clear constipation if present using faecal softeners. Consider high-dose corticosteroids. Chemotherapy can be helpful in selected cases. Consider stents

Pain
Diamorphine in appropriate dose in syringe pump according to previous analgesic requirement and level of pain. Halve the oral dose to get equivalent subcutaneous dose

Colic
If persists despite the above measures, add anticholinergic to the syringe pump

Table 16.10 Drugs suitable for use in the syringe driver in the terminal phase

Indication	Drug
Analgesic	Diamorphine (dosage according to need)
Antiemetic	Haloperidol
	Cyclizine
	Levomepromazine at low doses
Terminal secretions	Hyoscine hydrobromide
	Hyoscine butylbromide
	Glycopyrronium
Terminal agitation	Midazolam
	Levomepromazine at higher doses

indicated in obstruction caused by advanced malignancy with high-bulk disease. Intravenous fluids and nasogastric tubes are rarely necessary; the aim is symptom control with drugs (Table 16.9).

Nausea is often more distressing than vomiting. The aim is to eliminate nausea and reduce vomiting to a maximum of once or twice a day. Avoid gastrokinetic antiemetics such as metoclopramide or domperidone as they will exacerbate symptoms. Cyclizine and levomepromazine are usually effective.

Constipation

Constipation is common in debilitated patients and can be exacerbated by the use of opioids. The need to treat constipation is often a consequence of failing to use prophylactic laxatives. Virtually all patients on opioids should have a regular laxative. A rectal examination is essential if any patient complains of constipation to assess for impaction.

Care of the dying patient

When a patient who has advanced illness enters into the terminal phase (normally a day or so before death), all medication should be reviewed; *all* drugs should be stopped apart from those aimed at symptom control.

Communication is vital; anticipate problems and changes in the patient's condition and explain them to the patient and his or her carers. Reassure them that symptoms will remain controlled and that the patient will be kept comfortable. Often it is appropriate to use a syringe pump to administer medications (Fig. 16.2; Table 16.10).

Analgesia

Analgesia should be continued even if a patient becomes unconscious. The patient may still perceive pain. In addition, abrupt withdrawal of opioids can result in an unpleasant withdrawal reaction. If a patient is on regular opioids, he or she needs to be continued at an equivalent dosage subcutaneously. If the patient will require more than a few injections, a syringe driver should be started.

Agitation

Agitation can be a problem and causes must be looked for and treated appropriately; for example, retention of urine requires catheterization.

It is not uncommon for patients to become agitated and confused shortly before death. If a tranquillizer is indicated, use subcutaneous midazolam or levomepromazine, either as single doses or as a subcutaneous infusion using a syringe driver. Both can be combined with diamorphine in a syringe driver if necessary.

Terminal secretions ('death rattle')

Terminal secretions can be controlled using subcutaneous hyoscine or glycopyrronium as required. Either can be added into the syringe driver together with diamorphine and sedative.

Crises

Occasionally it may be appropriate to prescribe drugs

for a crisis. For example, if it is likely that the patient may have a major bleed (e.g. haemoptysis or haematemesis), prescribe midazolam as a 'crisis injection' to be given to rapidly sedate the patient in the event of such an emergency. Such crises can greatly distress the patient and his or her family and need to be handled with speed and sensitivity.

The rules of symptom control should always be followed, even at this stage of the illness. Symptoms should be evaluated and appropriate treatment instituted. It is important to anticipate problems and to communicate well with all concerned. A 'peaceful' death leads to far fewer bereavement problems for the family.

Religious considerations

People with different faiths have different needs at the time of death. The professionals involved at this time need an understanding of the different religions and beliefs and associated rituals so that they can provide maximum support. Staff should not hesitate to consult with the patient and his or her carers about specific needs.

Bereavement

Support offered to the family both during a patient's illness and at the time of his or her death not only helps the family to cope better, but reduces the likelihood of future complications.

Evidence suggests that there is a higher physical and psychiatric morbidity, and possibly an increased mortality, in those recently bereaved.

People avoid grieving individuals because:
- They feel helpless, awkward or embarrassed
- They do not wish to feel sad themselves
- They fear releasing strong emotions

Important risk factors for abnormal bereavement reactions

Factors associated with an increased risk of difficult bereavement include:
- A close, dependent or ambivalent relationship
- Concurrent stress at the time of bereavement
- Memories of a 'bad' death (e.g. uncontrolled symptoms)
- Perception of a low level of support (perception is more important than the actual support in determining outcome)
- Strong feelings of guilt and reproach
- Lack of opportunity to say goodbye and things left unsaid (e.g. as a result of a sudden or traumatic death or absence at the time of death)

Conclusions

The assessment and treatment of patients with palliative care needs are particularly challenging. There is a clear imperative to accurately assess patients and speedily attend to their physical symptoms. This requires significant skill in patients with a complex illness. The picture is made even more difficult when one takes into account the considerable emotional and social problems patients and families face when trying to cope with a life-threatening illness. All physicians will treat patients who have palliative care needs and so they should be familiar with the palliative approach to patient care and be able to respond to the diverse needs of such patients.

16

! **Must know checklist**

- Understand the principles of palliative medicine and be aware that they are applicable to people with a wide variety of life-threatening illness

- Have an understanding of palliative care delivery including the concept of the multidisciplinary approach

- Be able to assess patients' physical, emotional, social and spiritual needs and be aware of the wider dimension of the family

- Understand the importance of hope and that this may have other goals than cure

- Understand the importance of diagnosing and treating the cause of each symptom

- Be aware of the common symptoms in patients with advanced progressive illness and their management

- Have a working knowledge of analgesics and their use and side-effects

- Be able to weigh up the benefits and burdens of treatment

- Be familiar with the major problems encountered by patients and families during the dying process

- Be aware of the risk factors for abnormal bereavement reactions

Further reading

Books

Doyle D, Hanks G, MacDonald N, eds. *Oxford Textbook of Palliative Medicine*, 3rd edn. Oxford: Oxford University Press, 2003.

Fallon M, O'Neill B, eds. *ABC of Palliative Care*. London: BMJ Books, 1998.

Kaye P. *A to Z of Hospice and Palliative Medicine*. UK: EPL Publications, 1992.

Twycross R, Wilcock A. *Symptom Management in Advanced Cancer*, 3rd edn. Oxford: Radcliffe Medical Press, 2001.

Journals

Palliative Medicine, Arnold.
http://www.arnoldpublishers.com/journals/pages/pal_med/02692163.htm

Journal of Pain and Symptom Management, Elsevier.
http://www.elsevier.nl/inca/publications/store/5/0/5/7/7/5/index.htt

European Journal of Palliative Care, Hayward Medical Communications.
http://www.ejpc.co.uk/ejpchome.asp?FR = 1

Websites

www.palliativedrugs.com
www.hospice-spc-council.org.uk

16

Poisoning

17

Introduction

Poisoning is very common. In some hospitals up to 10% of acute medical admissions are related to poisoning.

Occasionally, poisoning occurs accidentally at work when patients are exposed to toxic substances such as cyanide or organophosphate insecticides. However, in the majority of cases patients have poisoned themselves. The agents used most frequently are those readily available in the home. Over-the-counter drugs (paracetamol, aspirin) and commonly prescribed drugs (sedatives, hypnotics and psychotropic drugs) are the most common poisons ingested (with or without alcohol). Poisoning resulting from illicit drugs is increasingly common, and opiate poisoning is responsible for the great majority of deaths in such cases. Ingestion of household products, such as bleach, descaling agents, solvents, weedkiller and the like, is much less common but still occurs, particularly in children.

The motivating factors in acts of self-poisoning are varied; however, the majority do not constitute genuine suicide attempts. Nevertheless, all patients with self-poisoning should be assessed to ascertain whether they represent a true suicide risk. The most common drugs involved in fatal poisoning episodes are analgesics, anti-depressants and tranquillizers.

Approach to the patient

Over 80% of patients are awake and alert on arrival at hospital and are capable of giving a full history (HISTORY & EXAMINATION BOX 17.1). The following points in the history should be noted:

- What poison is involved, and in what quantity? Note many patients take more than one drug and/or alcohol

- When and how were they exposed to it (e.g. was it ingested, inhaled or injected)?
- What symptoms have been experienced since exposure?
- Significant past medical history including psychiatric history, allergies and regular medications
- Was poisoning self-inflicted, and if so what was the degree of suicidal intent?
- In children, how the poison was obtained, with particular attention to quantity taken and spillage, and consideration of child protection issues

---

History & Examination 17.1: History of the poisoned patient

What poison(s)?
How much?
When and how exposed to the poison?
Symptoms
Past medical history
Past psychiatric history
Drug and allergy history
Suicide risk

If the patient is unsure of the nature of the poison, every attempt should be made to establish its identity. Relatives or work colleagues (and sometimes the police) should be dispatched to the scene of the poisoning to collect evidence of any possible poison that the patient may have been in contact with. Empty and unlabelled drug bottles can provide valuable information.

Approximately 20% of patients will have an altered consciousness level, which varies from mild drowsiness to unconsciousness. Poisoning should enter into the differential diagnosis of any patient brought to hospital with altered consciousness or coma.

When no history is available and poisoning is suspected,

History & Examination 17.2: Examination of the poisoned patient

General
Quickly assess Airway, Breathing and Circulation

Appearance
Is the patient alert, semiconscious or unconscious?
How is the patient clothed?
Are there any clues as to the poison: smells, liquids or bottles?
Is there a suicide note?
Is alcohol or another organic solvent obvious?

Look at the skin
Are injection marks present?
Are burns or blisters present?
Is the patient sweaty?

Look at the eyes
What are the pupil sizes?

Look in the mouth
Are corrosive burns present?

Look at the cardiovascular system
What is the heart rate? Is it regular?
What is the blood pressure?

Look at the respiratory system
Is brady- or tachypnoea present?
Are there crackles or wheeze?

Look at the abdomen
Is there tenderness, especially in the epigastrium or over the liver?

Look at the nervous system
What is the Glasgow Coma Score?
Is nystagmus present?
Are there cerebellar signs?

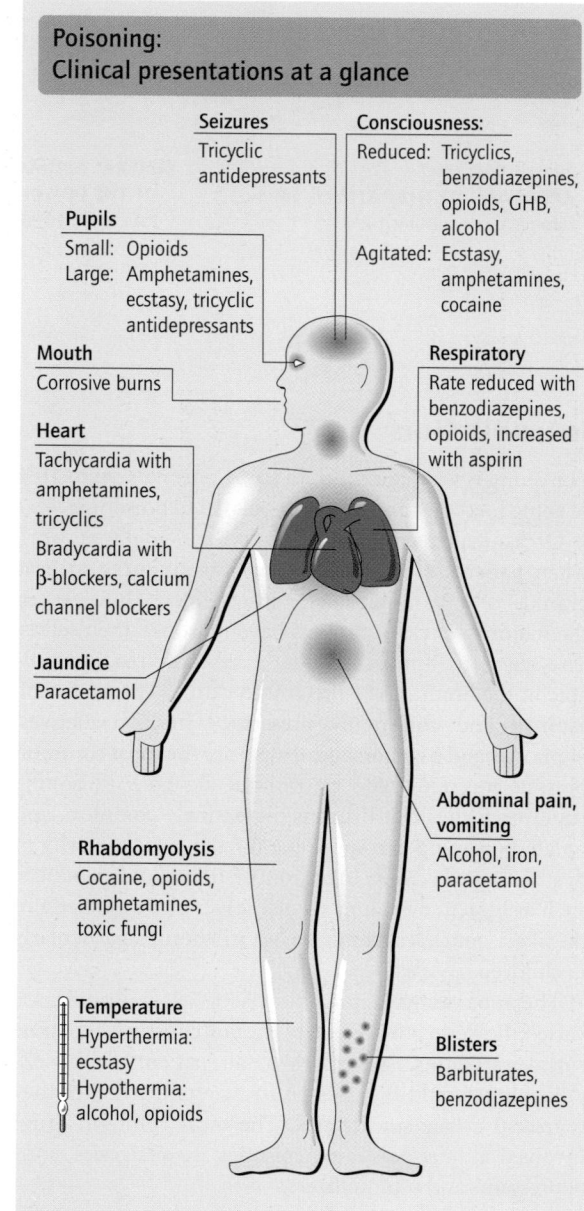

Poisoning: Clinical presentations at a glance

Seizures
Tricyclic antidepressants

Consciousness:
Reduced: Tricyclics, benzodiazepines, opioids, GHB, alcohol
Agitated: Ecstasy, amphetamines, cocaine

Pupils
Small: Opioids
Large: Amphetamines, ecstasy, tricyclic antidepressants

Mouth
Corrosive burns

Respiratory
Rate reduced with benzodiazepines, opioids, increased with aspirin

Heart
Tachycardia with amphetamines, tricyclics
Bradycardia with β-blockers, calcium channel blockers

Jaundice
Paracetamol

Abdominal pain, vomiting
Alcohol, iron, paracetamol

Rhabdomyolysis
Cocaine, opioids, amphetamines, toxic fungi

Temperature
Hyperthermia: ecstasy
Hypothermia: alcohol, opioids

Blisters
Barbiturates, benzodiazepines

clinical signs may give an indication of the nature of the poison (HISTORY & EXAMINATION BOX 17.2).

Elimination of poisons

It is now no longer recommended that patients be subjected routinely to gastric lavage or induced vomiting. It has been shown that poisons are not successfully eliminated by these manoeuvres. Gastric lavage in particular has potentially serious complications and is no longer recommended unless a life-threatening overdose has been taken (see p. 980) and the procedure can be performed within 1 h of ingestion.

Charcoal

Activated charcoal is the only general purpose adsorbent recommended and is usually only given once. Ten parts charcoal to one part poison has to be used for maximum efficiency and it has most benefit when given as early as possible after ingestion of the poison. In fact, poisons information centres now recommend activated charcoal is reserved for those poisoned patients who present within 1 hour of ingestion, and that even in these charcoal is not mandatory.

Table 17.1 Effects of other poisons

Poison	Mechanism of toxicity	Clinical effects	Management	Specific antidote (if applicable)
Lithium	Direct CNS effects	Acute: tremors, rigidity, nystagmus and convulsions Chronic: diarrhoea, nausea, vomiting	Supportive. Haemodialysis may be required	
β-Blockers	Direct myocardial depressant	Bradycardia, hypotension	Careful fluid management Pacing	Glucagon
Verapamil and diltiazem	Direct myocardial depressant, AV blockade	Bradycardia, hypotension, heart block	Supportive. Pacing	Glucagon
Organophosphates	Inhibit cholinesterase	Initial restlessness, vomiting, colic and sweating. Later muscle weakness and flaccid paralysis. Coma	Remove ongoing exposure, supportive Ventilation and removal of bronchial secretions may be needed	Atropine (large doses may be needed) Pralidoxime
Iron	Locally very irritant to upper gastrointestinal tract	Nausea, vomiting and abdominal pain, followed by acute gastrointestinal haemorrhage, encephalopathy, renal and liver failure	Supportive. Removal of iron tablets by purgation or endoscopy	Desferrioxamine
Cyanide	Disables cytochrome P450 system	Dizziness, syncope, coma, convulsions and cardiorespiratory arrest	Supportive	Dicobalt edetate, sodium thiosulphate, sodium nitrite
Paraquat	Nephrotoxic and creates O_2 free radicals to give pulmonary toxicity	Nausea and vomiting, burning in the mouth, acute renal failure, pneumonitis and pulmonary fibrosis	Supportive. Avoid high O_2 concentrations	
Digoxin	Increases AV block and promotes cardiac irritability	Acute: arrhythmias and as chronic Chronic: nausea, vomiting, diarrhoea and confusion	Keep $[K^+]$ 4.5–5 mmol/l Pacing Antiarrhythmics DC shock	Fab digoxin antibodies (Digibind)
Corrosives	Local burns	Painful local tissue damage to the mouth, larynx, oesophagus and stomach	Supportive. Gastric lavage is dangerous	
Monoamine oxidase inhibitors	CNS effects. Also increase circulating catecholamines	Increased sympathetic activity, blood pressure is labile. Progressive muscle twitching and spasm, convulsions	Supportive. Sometimes general anaesthesia needed	
Selective serotonin reuptake inhibitors	Increase CNS effects of serotonin	Serotonin syndrome: alteration in mental state, hyperactivity, autonomic instability, rhabdomyolysis, hyperthermia	Supportive	
Ethanol	Sedative by central action, inhibits gluconeogenesis	Coma, metabolic acidosis	Supportive. Watch for hypoglycaemia	
Ethylene glycol	Accumulation of toxic metabolites inhibits cellular respiration	Coma, metabolic lactic acidosis	Supportive. Haemofiltration	Ethanol, fomepizole

AV, arteriovenous; CNS, central nervous system.

17

Forced alkaline diuresis

This procedure is potentially lethal and is rarely undertaken. It should only be considered in a carefully monitored environment such as an intensive care unit. The indications for its use are few: severe aspirin and phenobarbital poisoning being the main ones. Serum levels should be obtained and serious poisoning confirmed before forced alkaline diuresis is contemplated.

Haemoperfusion and haemodialysis

These are occasionally necessary for some forms of poisoning when taken in potentially lethal quantities (e.g. lithium).

General management of the poisoned patient

The management of a poisoned patient is supportive, to ensure as near physiological normality as possible, and to give specific antidotes when indicated.

Airway and breathing

Control of the airway and ventilation is of paramount importance in the unconscious patient. Problems are most frequently encountered in patients poisoned with opiates or sedatives. Arterial blood gases should be performed early to aid management decisions.

Circulation

Intravenous access is recommended for all except the mildest cases of poisoning. Patients are often normovolaemic, and hypotension, if present, is caused by drug-induced vasodilatation or via a negative inotropic effect:
● If systolic BP is over 90 mmHg—observe
● If systolic BP is under 90 mmHg—judicious fluid administration may help, although close monitoring of the central venous pressure is important

Normovolaemic patients with persistent hypotension may need inotropic support. Rhythm disturbances giving rise to cardiac compromise should be treated using standard guidelines. For all arrhythmias, including life-threatening, underlying hypoxia, metabolic, electrolyte and acid–base disturbance should be corrected as soon as possible.

Disability and convulsions

Intravenous diazepam or lorazepam is the treatment of choice for convulsions. Underlying hypoxia and hypoglycaemia should be corrected.

Hypothermia

Temperatures below 35°C are common in the poisoned patient. The two most common mechanisms are ingestion of drugs that alter temperature control (e.g. tricyclic antidepressants or alcohol) and prolonged exposure to a cold environment in a patient incapacitated by poison. Rewarming is usually successfully and gently achieved with a hot air-blown blanket. Careful attention to oxygenation and fluid and electrolyte balance is particularly important in these patients.

Management for some common specific poisons

Details of the management of specific poisons are available 24 h a day from the National Poisons Information Service and Toxbase (Table 17.2).

Table 17.2 Poisons information centres

Toxbase: www.spib.axl.co.uk/	
UK National Poisons	0870 600 6266
Information Service	
Belfast	028 9024 0503
Birmingham	0121 507 5588/9
Cardiff	029 2070 9901
Dublin	Dublin 837 9964/837 9966
Edinburgh	0131 536 2300
London	020 7635 9191
Newcastle	0191 282 0300

Paracetamol

There are approximately 200 deaths annually in the UK from paracetamol poisoning. Doses of 15 g or more can be lethal.

Mechanism of toxicity

Normally paracetamol is inactivated in the liver by conjugation. In therapeutic doses, 85% is conjugated with glucuronide and sulphate and approximately 10% is oxidized to an intermediate metabolite that then undergoes conjugation with glutathione. In overdose, glutathione stores are depleted allowing build-up of the toxic intermediate metabolite. This hydroxylamine metabolite can directly affect both liver and renal cells, producing acute

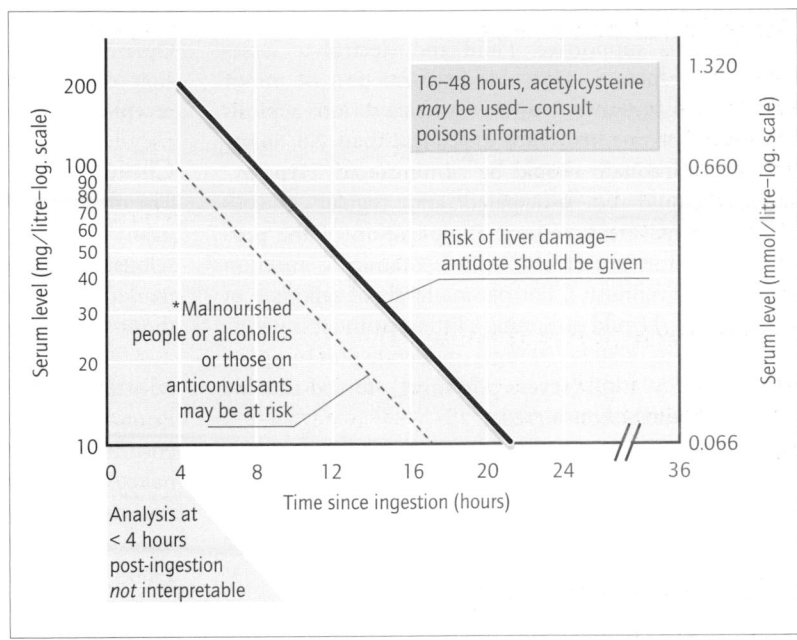

Figure 17.1 Paracetamol overdose treatment graph.

hepatic and renal tubular necrosis. The aim of treatment is to raise intracellular glutathione levels; the most useful agent available to promote this is *N*-acetylcysteine.

Clinical features

These are usually delayed for 18–24 h when vomiting and upper abdominal pain are common. Signs of acute liver damage are usually not present until 36–48 h after ingestion. Coma is an unusual early feature and other drugs should be suspected (e.g. co-proxamol). Uncommonly, an early metabolic acidosis can occur, which needs to be vigorously treated.

Management

Gastric lavage should be performed in all patients who have taken a significant overdose (more than 7.5–10 g) within 1 h, but most present after this. Patients who have alcohol problems or who are taking anticonvulsants are at greater risk of hepatotoxicity, and treatment should be started as soon as possible. Serum levels should be estimated 4 h after ingestion.

Using a chart similar to the one shown in Fig. 17.1, the serum level is plotted. For levels above or near the line, treatment should be started. For those patients at higher risk, the lower treatment line should be used. *N*-Acetylcysteine is infused at varying rates over 20 h.

Oral methionine is an alternative to acetylcysteine; however, treatment is less effective especially when there is vomiting. For patients presenting after 4 h with a significant overdose, *N*-acetylcysteine should be started immediately while serum paracetamol levels are awaited. This can always be stopped if treatment is not necessary. The earliest sign of liver damage is a prolonged prothrombin time and this, together with arterial blood gases, urea and electrolytes and liver function tests, should be monitored regularly. Patients with progressive liver damage should be discussed with the local liver unit.

Aspirin

The incidence of aspirin poisoning is decreasing, in parallel to its decline in over-the-counter sales. The lethal adult dose is 20–25 g. The way in which it poisons the body is complex, affecting acid–base status, oxidative phosphorylation and glucose metabolism.

Clinical features

Initial common symptoms include nausea, vomiting, epigastric pain, tinnitus, irritability, agitation and sweating. Hyperventilation gives rise to a respiratory alkalosis in the early hours following exposure but a metabolic acidosis that develops more slowly becomes the major acid–base disturbance. Most patients are awake on admission and altered consciousness and coma indicate very severe poisoning or the involvement of another poison. The vomiting, sweating and hyperventilation lead to dehydration, and electrolyte disturbances are common. Hypoglycaemia and hypoprothrombinaemia can also occur. Early detection of these complications and correction are needed.

17

Management

Treatment is supportive. Fluid and electrolyte losses should be replaced. This aids in correction of minor acid–base disturbance. However, when a serious acidosis has been documented, with a pH less than 7.0, intravenous bicarbonate should be administered. Hypoglycaemia should be anticipated and regular glucose measurements are necessary. Prolongation of the prothrombin time is corrected with a vitamin K injection (10 mg intravenously). For plasma levels of salicylate of 250–500 mg/l (mild poisoning), little treatment is necessary. For levels of 500–750 mg/l (moderate poisoning) or more than 750 mg/l (severe poisoning), forced alkaline diuresis should be considered.

Tricyclic antidepressants

Self-poisoning with tricyclic antidepressants accounts for over 300 deaths/year in adults in the UK.

Mechanism of toxicity

The action of tricyclic antidepressants on the heart and central nervous system produces potentially fatal complications of overdose. The anticholinergic actions of these drugs produce dilated pupils, sinus tachycardia, hallucinations, urine retention and ileus. Their action on the central nervous system causes coma and convulsions, whereas the cardiotoxic action produces hypotension and arrhythmias that can be resistant to treatment. Metabolic acidosis is common and it is exacerbated by hypotension and hypoxia.

Management

Charcoal and gastric lavage are recommended if the patient presents within 1 h of ingestion. Supportive therapy with constant monitoring of ventilation, acid–base status, fluid balance and cardiac function is necessary. Metabolic acidosis should be corrected with sodium bicarbonate and hypokalaemia with potassium supplements.

Cardiac arrhythmias not causing haemodynamic compromise should be treated by correcting underlying hypoxia, acidosis or electrolyte imbalance. Administration of bicarbonate until the arterial pH is at or above the upper limit of normal may allow arrhythmias to resolve. Direct current cardioversion is the treatment of choice for tachyarrhythmias causing haemodynamic impairment.

Bradyarrhythmias may need cardiac pacing.

Opiates

Opiates such as heroin, methadone and morphine are commonly taken in overdose, often accidentally, and account for 600 deaths/year in the UK.

Mechanism of toxicity

Opiates in overdose cause coma and respiratory depression to the point of apnoea via central actions on opioid receptors.

Clinical features

The diagnosis of opiate poisoning should be considered in any patient who presents with unexplained altered consciousness. The presence of pinpoint pupils, needle-track marks and a reduced respiratory rate should further raise the possibility.

Management

Priority must be given to maintaining the airway and ensuring adequate ventilation. The opiate antagonist naloxone should be given in all cases as soon as the diagnosis is confirmed or suspected. An initial dose of 400 µg intravenously should be followed by further doses at 2-min intervals up to a maximum of 2.0 mg. Improvement usually occurs within minutes. Naloxone has a short elimination half-life and a naloxone infusion may be required. Intramuscular naloxone lasts longer and may be appropriate for agitated patients who leave the department after intravenous naloxone has reversed their overdose.

Ecstasy and amphetamines
Mechanism of toxicity

Amphetamines are sympathomimetic and thus have cardiovascular stimulant effects. Ecstasy also acts centrally, binding to dopamine receptors, and releases serotonin to produce mood alteration and release antidiuretic hormone.

Clinical features

The most common features are of restlessness, agitation and confusion, accompanied by sinus tachycardia. Ecstasy toxicity may also present in two other ways: first with hyperthermia, dehydration, cardiac arrhythmias or cardiac arrest. Disseminated intravascular coagulation and rhabdomyolysis may follow. The second presentation includes confusion or coma caused by cerebral oedema, convulsions and hypervolaemic hyponatraemia.

Management

In mild cases, supportive treatment and observation are usually all that is needed. Fluid resuscitation, anticonvulsant treatment and cooling may be needed. Dantrolene, a calcium-channel blocker, may help reduce muscle spasms and assist cooling. If cerebral oedema and hypervolaemic hypernatraemia are present, ventilation and fluid restriction in the intensive care unit may be needed.

Carbon monoxide

Carbon monoxide is one of the most common poisons to cause death in this country—either intentionally or accidentally.

Mechanism of toxicity

Carbon monoxide causes cell death by disrupting the cytochrome P450 enzyme system. Exposure to a large dose causes critical interruption of the metabolism of all cells and is rapidly fatal. Chronic lower dose exposure produces a progressive acidosis.

Clinical features

The diagnosis is often not suspected unless there is a clear history of exposure. Sources of carbon monoxide are fires, heating systems, car exhausts and, rarely, paintstripper (via the liver). Risk of poisoning is highest when exposure occurs in a poorly ventilated environment. Initially, symptoms are very non-specific and include headache, dyspnoea, weakness and nausea and vomiting. In severe poisoning, drowsiness, coma, convulsions and cardio-vascular collapse can occur. The cherry-red skin colour is a late sign and is most commonly seen in fatalities.

Management

All patients need maximal oxygen therapy, either with a tight-fitting face mask, or if semiconscious or comatose via an endotracheal tube. Carboxyhaemoglobin levels should be measured along with blood gases, as acidosis is a key prognostic indicator. Normal levels are less than 6%, and levels of 15% or more at any time after exposure indicate significant poisoning. Levels over 40% are associated with coma, and those of 60% or more with cardiovascular collapse.

The use of hyperbaric oxygen therapy is controversial. Indications for its consideration (to reverse carbon monoxide binding to haemoglobin, and increase elimination) are:

- Conscious patient with levels of 20% or more
- Neurological symptoms other than headache at any time since exposure
- Pregnancy
- Cardiac arrhythmias

A list of available hyperbaric facilities can be obtained from the Hyperbaric Medical Centre (DDRC, Plymouth: 01752 261910 (24 h)).

General considerations

Table 17.3 shows preventative measures to minimize the risks of poisoning. It is important to remember that we do not necessarily have the right to treat a poisoned patient if he or she refuses. In such circumstances, assessment of mental competence is essential, and would involve senior help, psychiatrists and relatives.

Table 17.3 Preventative measures

Children
Keep medicines out of reach
Keep chemicals and cleaning fluids in a locked cupboard
Education about toxic plants, berries and mushrooms

Adults
Low-risk prescribing (e.g. avoiding tricyclic antidepressant medicines in those likely to self-poison)
Blister packs
Reducing amount of medicine in repeat prescriptions (e.g. 1 week as opposed to 4 weeks' worth)
Access to self-help: Samaritans, mental health services
Ensuring all patients have an adequate suicide risk assessment after an episode of poisoning
Health and safety measures when toxic chemicals are transported or used in the workplace

Keypoints 17.1: Poisoning

Poisoning is common
All patients should have assessment of suicide risk
Patients need a thorough assessment for the varied clinical effects of poisons
Usually careful observation and supportive treatment are all that is required
Gastric emptying procedures are of limited or no value
Specific antidotes may be useful
Definitive advice is available from the National Poisons Information Service and Toxbase

17

! Must know checklist

- Poisoning is a very common reason for attendance at, and admission to, hospital

- All patients should be assessed for suicide risk

- Initial assessment and management should follow Airway, Breathing and Circulation

- Gastric lavage is not useful unless a potentially life-threatening overdose and can be undertaken within 1 h of ingestion

- Activated charcoal can adsorb some poisons successfully if given within 1 h of ingestion

- Induced vomiting does not successfully eliminate poison

- *N*-Acetylcysteine is effective in reducing the toxic effects of a paracetamol overdose

- Toxbase provides up-to-date and easily accessible information about management and antidotes

Further reading

Books

Lester M, Haddad LM, Shannon MW, Winchester JF, eds. *Clinical Management of Poisoning and Drug Overdose*. London: Harcourt, 1997.

Journals

Position statement and practice guidelines on the use of gut decontamination in the treatment of acute poisoning. American Academy of Clinical Toxicology, European Association of Poisons Centres and Clinical Toxicologists. *J Toxicol Clin Toxicol* 1999; 37(6): 731–51.

Position statement and practice guidelines on the use of multidose activated charcoal in the treatment of acute poisoning. American Academy of Clinical Toxicology, European Association of Poisons Centres and Clinical Toxicologists. *J Toxicol Clin Toxicol* 1997; 35(7): 695–762.

European Resuscitation Council. Part 8. Advanced challenges in resuscitation. Section 2: toxicology in ECC. European Resuscitation Council. *Resuscitation* 2000; 46: 261–6.

Websites

Toxbase: www.spib.axl.co.uk

17

Skin Disease

18

Introduction

The global prevalence of skin disease is high, but the problems of developed and developing countries differ. Worldwide, the morbidity and mortality of cutaneous illness is caused by the infectious diseases leprosy, tuberculosis, onchocerciasis, leishmaniasis, trypanosomiasis and filariasis, which affect many millions of people. Travel and immigration mean that some of these diseases are seen in dermatological practice in developed countries.

Acquired immune deficiency syndrome (AIDS) is a new infectious disease and has cutaneous manifestations in almost all patients. It is as much a problem in developing countries as in the developed world.

The main inflammatory skin diseases in developed countries are eczema, psoriasis and acne. They are not lethal, but can cause severe morbidity, particularly in an image-orientated society. Body image-related pressures lead to cosmetic dermatological concerns, and also lie behind the recreational exposure to ultraviolet light, which is associated with melanoma, non-melanoma skin cancer and premature actinic (solar) ageing of the skin. In an ageing society, the cumulative effect of skin exposure to ultraviolet light is increasing the demand for dermatological expertise.

Structure and function

The skin is a large and complex organ (Fig. 18.1). It has several different structures and many cell types with multiple functions (Table 18.1). Regional variations relate to the different functions of the skin at different sites and contribute to the focality of some dermatoses (e.g. acne is found on the face and upper trunk where sebaceous glands are prominent). Sexual and racial variations are appreciable. The skin is not a static organ, but constantly regenerates and changes throughout life.

The epidermis derives from the surface of the early embryonic gastrula. It is separated from the underlying mesoderm-derived dermis by the basement membrane. The dermis is essential for inducing epidermal structures and maintaining the epidermis. The neural crest contributes pigment-producing melanocytes. Structural cells contribute physically to the complex organization of the skin. Trafficking cells are derived from bone marrow and interact with the structural elements in the orchestration of the diverse functions of the skin.

The hair cycle

Human hair growth is cyclical (Fig. 18.2) and not synchronous. Each scalp hair may last over 3 years growing at a rate of 1 cm/month (**anagen**). An individual hair may abruptly enter **catagen** at any time; the end of the hair forms a club over about 6 weeks and then enters telogen, which may last 6 months and during which the hair may be shed.

About 1% of hairs are in catagen at any time, but an illness or physiological change such as pregnancy can cause many more to enter this phase, resulting in a partial moult of longer hairs (**telogen effluvium**). Patients should be reassured that they have not lost viable hair follicles and that the hair will return to normal within a few months.

The normal fingernail grows 1 mm/week and the normal big toenail 1–2 mm/month (Fig. 18.3).

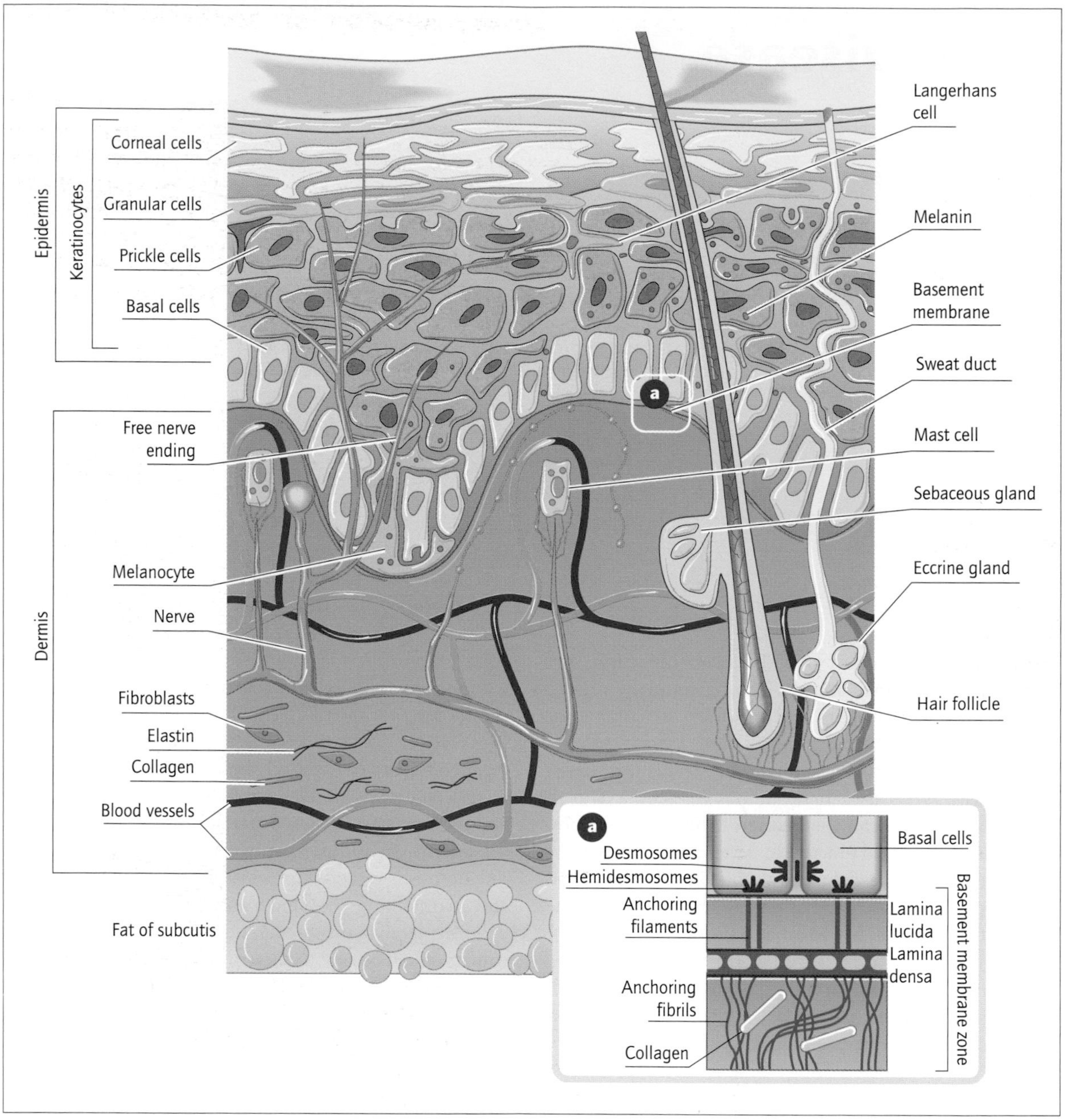

Figure 18.1 Normal adult skin.

Table 18.1 Functions of the skin

Function	Examples
Physicomechanical protection	Ultraviolet and ionizing radiation; trauma
Immunological protection	Antigen recognition and presentation; immunological effector organ
Inflammatory and reparative	Triple response of Lewis
Sensation	Touch, pain
Control of homoeostasis	Core temperature; water loss
Chemical synthesis, metabolism and excretion	Vitamin D, bile salts, cytokines, hormones
Psychosexual	Individual recognition, sexual attraction

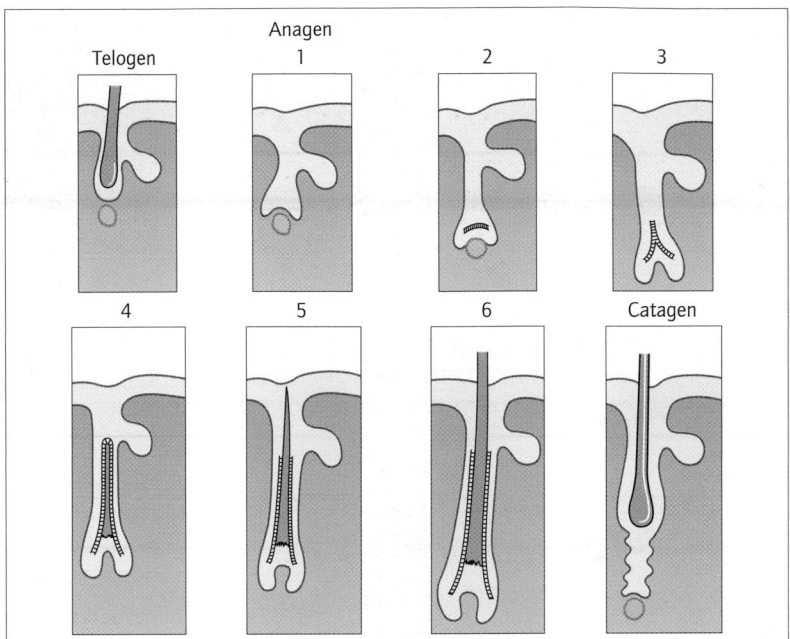

Figure 18.2 Phases in the hair cycle. Courtesy of Dr A. Messenger, Sheffield. Reproduced from Champion *et al.* (eds) *Textbook of Dermatology*, 5th edn. Oxford: Blackwell Scientific Publications, 1992 with the permission of the authors.

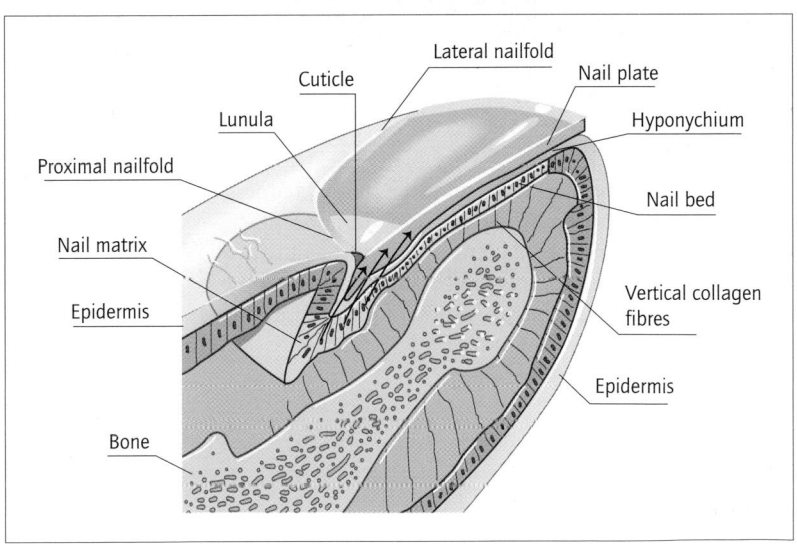

Figure 18.3 Structure and relationships of the nail.

Approach to the patient

History

Dermatology is a visual subject, but an accurate history is essential (HISTORY & EXAMINATION BOX 18.1) because:

1 It is possible to recognize patterns of disease from the history alone

2 It is vital to assess the impact of the disease on the patient

Details of occupation, personal and family medical history are frequently of diagnostic importance. Sexual practices and drug use should be carefully and tactfully asked about because they contribute increasingly to the prevalence of skin diseases. It is also important to find out how an individual's skin reacts to the sun (Table 18.2) and how much lifetime sun exposure has accumulated.

18

Table 18.2 Classification of skin sensitivity to the sun

Type I	Always burns
Type II	Usually burns, sometimes tans
Type III	Sometimes burns, usually tans
Type IV	Always tans
Type V	Asian
Type VI	Afro-Caribbean

History & Examination 18.1: Issues to be addressed by the history and examination in dermatology

What are the symptoms and what is their effect on the patient?

Which part of the skin is involved?

What is the diagnosis?

What are the correct investigations?

What is the suitable treatment?

Are unnecessary investigations and treatments being avoided?

What is the patient's understanding and expectations of his or her symptoms and treatment?

Skin symptoms

Skin symptoms are itch, rash, lump or bump, redness, scaling, flushing, soreness, pain, cosmetic appearance, hair loss and nail changes. Patients usually present with a rash or a lump or bump. It is important to ask about the temporal and spatial characteristics of the presenting symptoms (HISTORY & EXAMINATION BOX 18.2):

- When did the rash/bump appear?
- Where did it spread?
- When did it ulcerate and bleed?

Disease impact

Skin diseases can affect people's lives profoundly. If hands and feet are involved, an individual's capacity to work (at a job or at home) or to walk can be impaired. Social and sexual functioning can be gravely disrupted by real or perceived cosmetic disfiguration. Severe itch and dryness interfere with sleeping and washing. Skin cancer kills young people.

Drug history

It is essential to know what other remedies have been used (e.g. for eczema, acne, psoriasis or a wart) and how effective they have been. Cutaneous reactions to drugs are

History & Examination 18.2: Important questions to ask a patient with a skin disorder

About the patient

How old are you?

What is your ethnic/racial background?

What is your occupation?

Are you heterosexual, homosexual or bisexual?

How much time have you spent/do you spend in the sun?
  Do you tan or burn (Table 18.2)?

Symptoms

What are your symptoms?

Which part of your skin is involved?

Pattern of disease

Onset and progression

When did the symptoms start?

How have they changed with time?

Associated features

Are your symptoms associated with your lifestyle, work, home?

Have you noticed any changes affecting your hair, eyes, mouth, nails, genitals, joints?

Have you noticed any general symptoms?

Disease impact

How do your symptoms affect you at work and at home (mobility, your social life, your sexual life, your personal hygiene or your sleep)?

Drug history

What prescribed treatments and over-the-counter and bathroom cabinet preparations do you take?

What treatments have you been using for your skin and what effect have they had?

Family history

Does anyone in your family have atopy (e.g. asthma, eczema or hay fever), psoriasis, skin cancer, especially melanoma?

Does anyone in your family have a serious illness?

Past medical history

Have you had any skin disorder in the past (e.g. eczema, psoriasis, moles, skin cancer)?

Have you had any other disorder such as asthma, hay fever, diabetes, rheumatic disease, sexually transmitted disease?

common and all other medications should therefore be listed, with special attention to over-the-counter or bathroom cabinet agents, which are not always acknowledged by patients as 'drugs'.

Family history

The genes that determine susceptibility to common skin disorders are widely distributed in the general population. It is useful to know whether there is a history of such conditions in first-degree relatives.

Examination

It is mandatory to examine the whole of the skin in a good light with the patient lying supine on an examination couch. This also allows a general medical examination when relevant. A description of the presenting features should include the distribution pattern, site and individual characteristics of any lesions using the appropriate terminology (CLINICAL EXAMINATION AT A GLANCE). A differential diagnosis can then be established. Skin signs must be interpreted, bearing in mind the state (Table 18.3) and age of the patient.

Erythema (redness) signifies increased blood flow and vascular dilatation. **Purpura** occurs when red blood cells leak into skin because the vessel wall is weakened (e.g. scurvy) or damaged (e.g. vasculitis), or because blood is under pressure (e.g. heart failure, suction, love bites).

Clinical examination at a glance

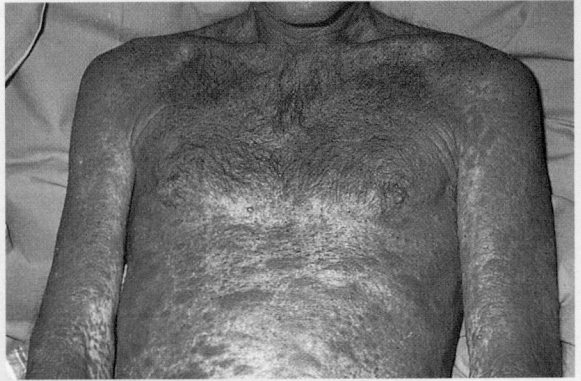

Fig. A Confluent erythema and erythematous nodules (drug eruption and histoplasmosis—AIDS).

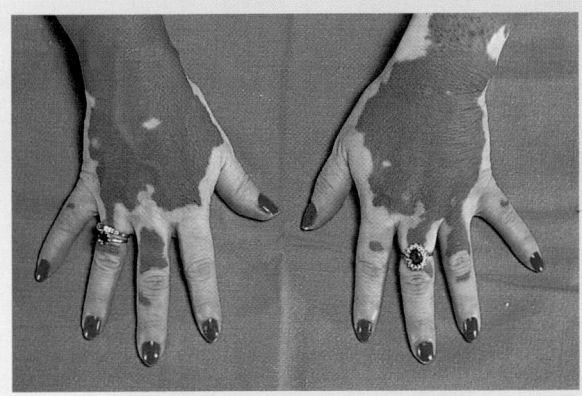

Fig. B Macules and patches of hypopigmentation (vitiligo).

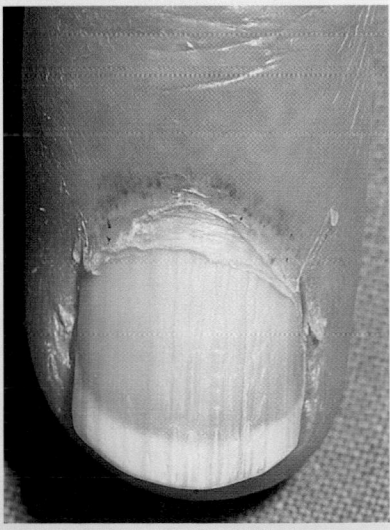

Fig. C Nailfold telangiectasia (systemic sclerosis).

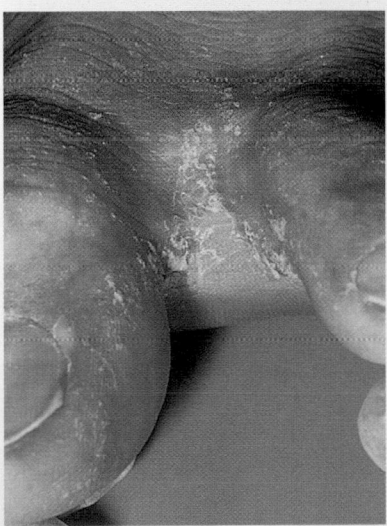

Fig. D Interdigital scale (Norwegian scabies).

18

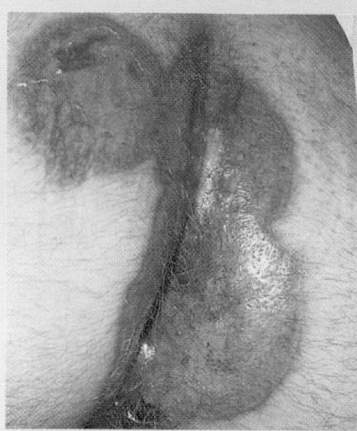

Fig. E Perianal erosion (herpes simplex—AIDS).

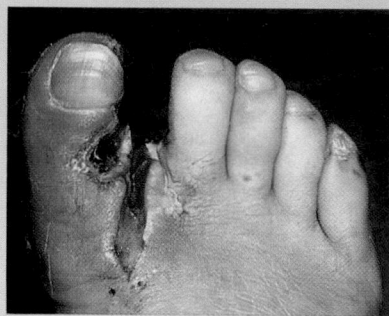

Fig. F Interdigital ulcer (diabetes mellitus).

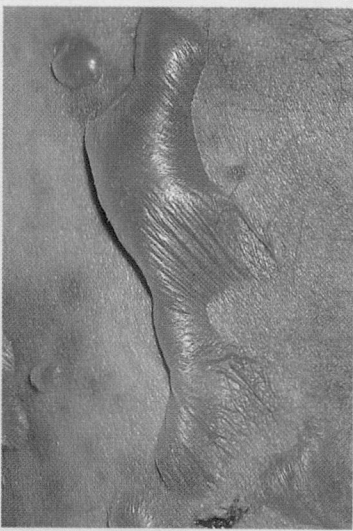

Fig. G Vesicles and bulla (bullous pemphigoid).

Fig. H Café au lait patch (polyostotic fibrous dysplasia).

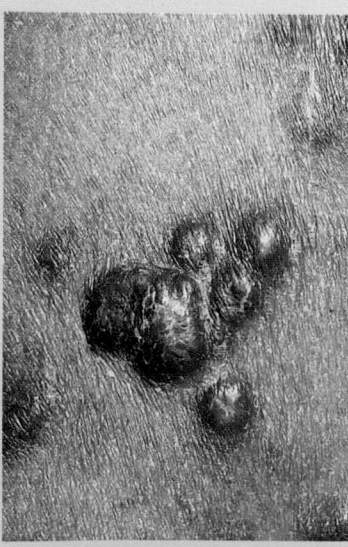

Fig. I Papules and nodules (Kaposi's sarcoma—AIDS).

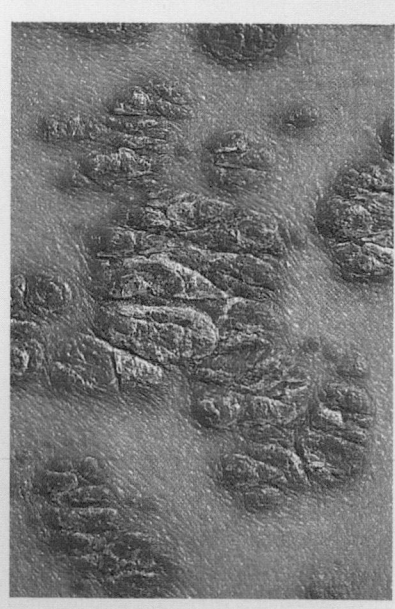

Fig. J Hyperkeratotic (scaly), erythematous plaques (psoriasis).

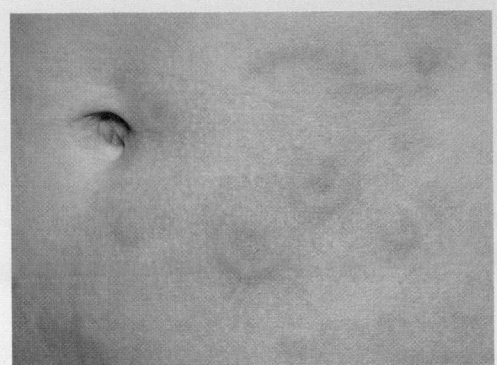

Fig. K Urticarial wheals (acute urticaria).

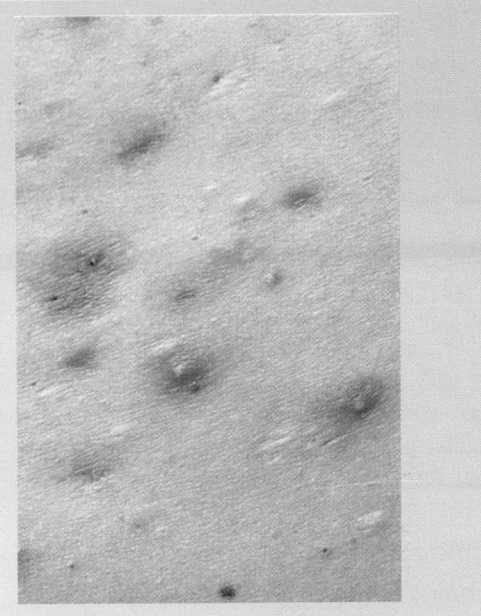

Fig. L Comedones, pustules and scars (acne vulgaris).

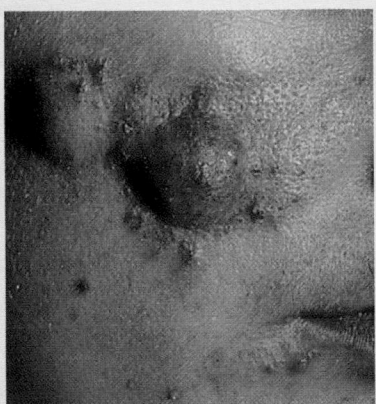

Fig. M Cysts (pyoderma faciale).

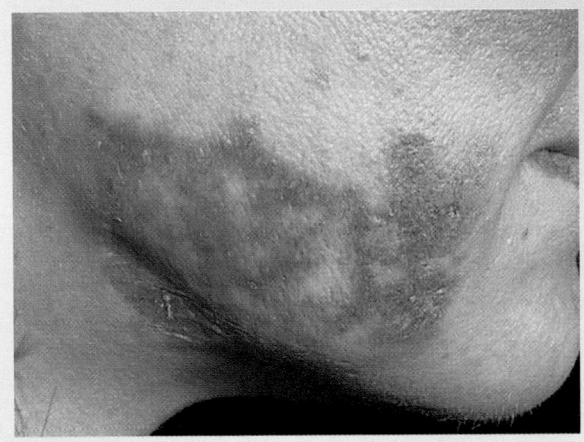

Fig. N Erythema, atrophy, scarring (discoid lupus erythematosus).

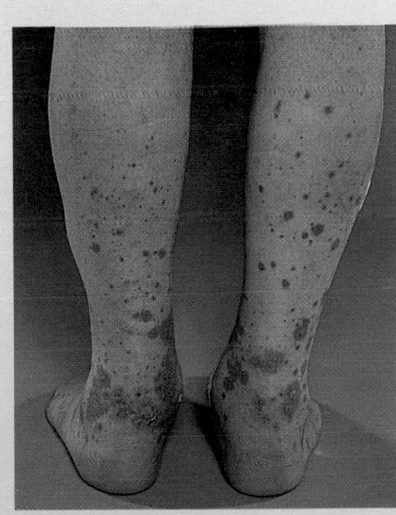

Fig. O Palpable purpuric papules (allergic vasculitis of the leg).

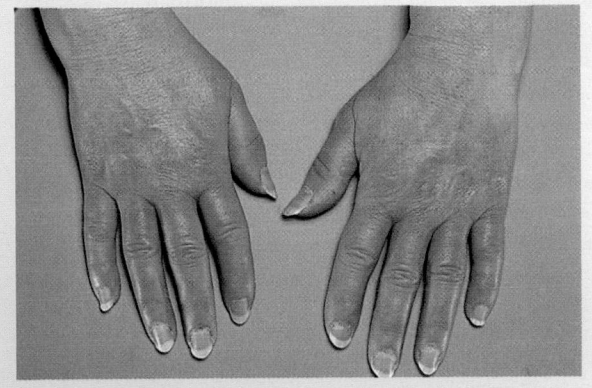

Fig. P Sclerosis (sclerodactyly—systemic sclerosis).

Table 18.3 Skin changes in and around pregnancy

Change	Comment
Increased pigmentation	Affects areolae, genitalia, linea alba, chloasma
Melanocytic naevi	Increased number, increased pigmentation
Increased hair loss	Dramatic shedding of hair postpartum (telogen effluvium), subtler thinning 3 months postpartum; both regrow
Spider naevi	Increased number in first and second trimesters; regress postpartum

The haematological causes of purpura are discussed in Chapter 15. Palpable purpura is differentiated from macular purpura and results from inflammation in the lesion caused by vasculitis.

Ageing and sun-induced changes in the skin

As in other organs, disease processes in the skin and its appendages occur against a background of age-related and degenerative changes. The skin is additionally influenced by the cumulative effect of environmental factors, especially solar radiation.

It is difficult to separate the consequences of inherently degenerative ageing processes from the effects of chronic actinic damage. However, with advancing years, both the epidermis and dermis thin. Thinning of the dermis is caused partly by a reduction in both the quality and quantity of collagen. Endocrinological factors produce changes in skin collagen after the menopause in women and postmenopausal hormone replacement stems the collagen loss.

The clinical sequelae include:
- *Senile purpura:* less mechanical support for blood vessels, so minor trauma causes dermal bleeding, manifest as senile purpura, and age-related attenuation of phagocytosis explains their relative persistence
- *Dry skin, xerosis and pruritus:* as sweat and sebaceous gland activity decline with age
- *Sebaceous gland hyperplasia:* without increased sebum production this may result in small shiny white papules on the forehead and cheeks, often mistaken for basal cell carcinoma
- *Hair thinning:* occurs on the body and the scalp in both sexes, but hair also loses its strength and lustre
- *Greying:* caused by diminished melanogenesis and fewer melanocytes in the hair follicle papilla
- *Longitudinal ridging:* common as nails become opaque, discolored and brittle

Solar damage

The most pernicious environmental influence on the skin is the sun. Chronic solar damage to the cellular elements

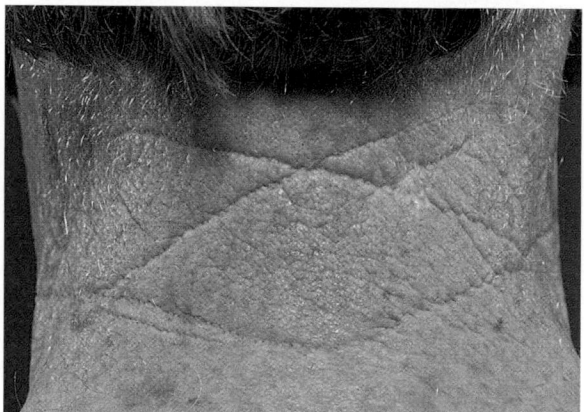

Figure 18.4 Actinic damage. Rhomboidal creases (solar elastosis).

of the epidermis is manifest as **dysplastic** or even frank **malignant** change (see p. 1142). The effect of ultraviolet radiation on immunocompetent (e.g. Langerhans') cells may be as important as the direct carcinogenic effect of damage to DNA: overall dampening of the cutaneous immune system favours the development of neoplasia.

Solar elastotic degeneration describes a loss of collagen with proliferation of abnormal elastin in the dermis. It causes the yellow wrinkled appearance of skin that has lost its turgor, elasticity and mechanical support. **Crow's feet** around the eyes, **rhomboidal creases** (Fig. 18.4) on the nape of the neck and **triradiate scars** on the forearm are the clinical corollaries. **Senile comedones** are also characteristic of solar elastosis. They are most numerous around the eyes and on the cheeks.

Investigation

Appropriate special investigations are necessary if there is diagnostic doubt or if it is important to confirm an apparently obvious diagnosis (e.g. malignancy, contagious infection, medicolegal controversy).

Histopathology

Histology of the skin is central to dermatological practice

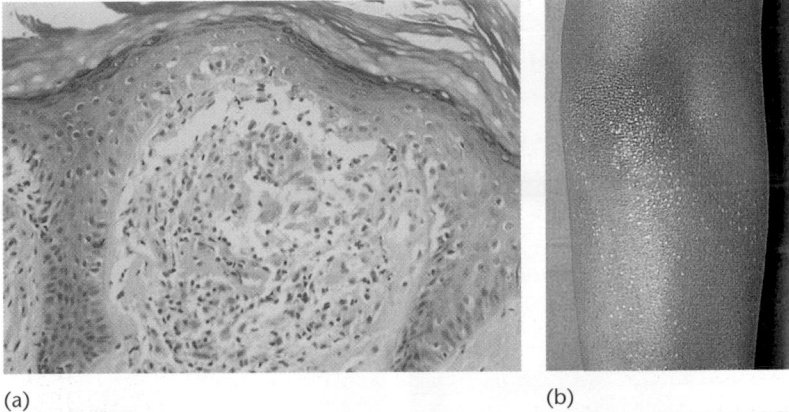

(a)

(b)

Figure 18.5 (a) Photomicrograph of skin showing: histology (haematoxylin and eosin) papillary dermal inflammatory cell infiltrate of lichen nitidus; (b) clinical photograph of lichen nitidus (micropapular variant of lichen planus).

and depends on providing the pathologist with an appropriate specimen. A biopsy may be:

- *Excisional:* if a cure is attempted (e.g. for basal cell carcinoma)
- *Incisional:* if a diagnosis is sought (e.g. bullous pemphigoid)

A generous ellipse of skin is taken through a representative lesion to include normal neighbouring skin and all components of the lesion from the epidermis down to the subcutis. A disposable skin punch is often used instead of a scalpel.

The specimen is fixed, usually in formalin, and a request form is completed. This must include relevant clinical information including a differential diagnosis and the site from which the skin has been removed.

The standard histopathological orientation of skin is vertical and the standard stain is haematoxylin and eosin (Fig. 18.5), but alternatives may be suggested by the clinician or pathologist.

Immunopathology

Immunofluorescence and immunocytochemistry are an important part of diagnosis in inflammatory and bullous disorders:

1 *Direct immunofluorescence* (Fig. 18.6): refers to incubation of skin with fluorescently tagged antibodies (e.g. against other immunoglobulins)

2 *Indirect immunofluorescence:* involves reacting patient's sera with normal human skin or other epithelial substrate such as monkey oesophagus. Fluorescent antihuman globulin antibodies are then used to establish the pattern of immunofluorescence and the titre of antibodies in the sera

3 *Immunocytochemistry:* uses antibodies against specific cell products or receptors that identify a particular cell type and its state of activation

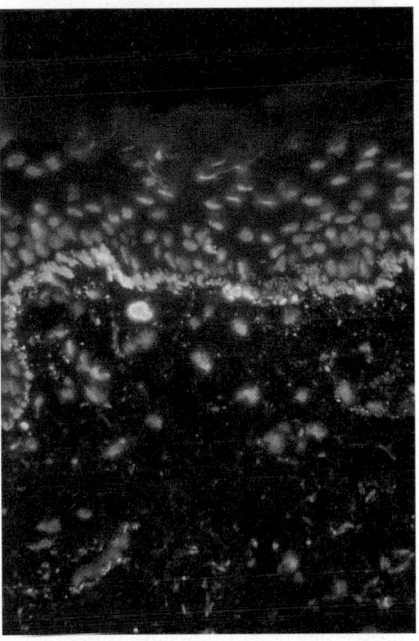

Figure 18.6 Direct immunofluorescence of lupus erythematosus showing speckled basement membrane zone deposition of IgM. Courtesy of B.S. Bhogal, Institute of Dermatology. Reproduced from Champion *et al.* (eds) *Textbook of Dermatology*, 5th edn. Oxford: Blackwell Scientific Publications, 1992 with the permission of the authors.

Wood's light

Wood's light (ultraviolet, wavelength 360 nm) enhances contrast and produces specific patterns of fluorescence in certain dermatoses (Fig. 18.7). It is standard apparatus in the outpatient department (Table 18.4).

18

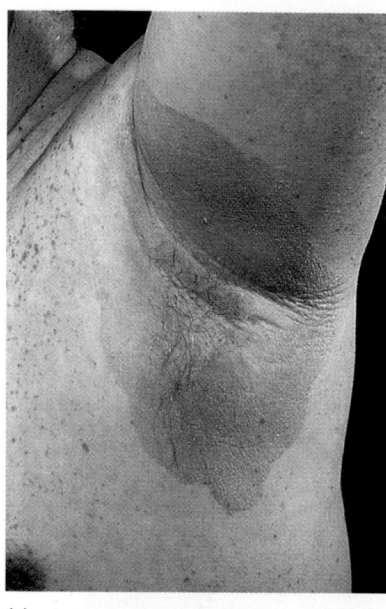

(a)

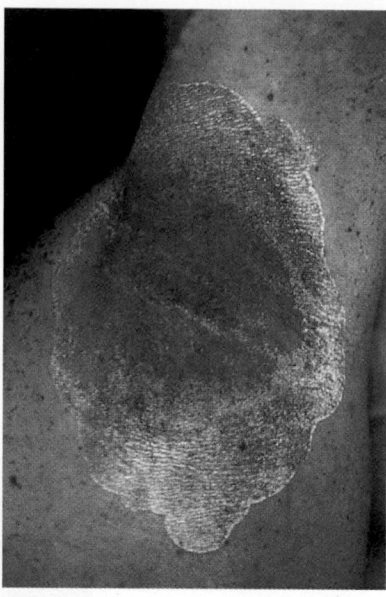

(b)

Figure 18.7 Erythrasma: (a) normal light; (b) coral pink axillary fluorescence, resulting from proporphyria III elaborated by *Corynebacterium minutissimum* in erythrasma, under Wood's light.

Table 18.4 Patterns of fluorescence with Wood's light

Fluorescence	Coral pink	Erythrasma
		Porphyrins in teeth/urine
	Green	Tinea capitis
Contrast	Hypopigmentation	Vitiligo
		Ash leaf macules of tuberous sclerosis

Microbiology

It is often useful to take a swab for microscopy, culture and sensitivity to antibiotics. Skin scrapings, nail clippings or hair samples may be examined for fungi (after clearing of keratin with potassium hydroxide) and sent for culture on special media.

General principles of management

In the skin, a range of pathological processes (infection, inflammation, fibrosis, dysplasia and neoplasia) result in thousands of named diseases, but some general principles of management can be expounded.

Supportive treatment

In general, supportive treatment includes:
- Moisturizing the skin and avoiding soap
- Avoiding the sun and wearing a sunscreen
- Providing reassurance and psychological support

Specific treatment

Specific treatments may be dietary, or involve the use of drugs, phototherapy or surgery.

Diet

Essential fatty acids (e.g. in oily fish and evening primrose oil) may be useful in inflammatory dermatoses.

Drugs

Brief information relating to some of the commonly used drugs in skin diseases is given in Tables 18.5 and 18.6. However, the information, especially that relating to side-effects and contraindications, is not complete. Fuller information is given in a formulary (e.g. *British National Formulary; BNF*). Drug regimens should also be checked in the *BNF*.

Phototherapy

Ultraviolet B (UVB) phototherapy may be useful in psoriasis, eczema and some other dermatoses (e.g. pityriasis lichenoides). PUVA is psoralens plus ultraviolet A (UVA) photochemotherapy (Table 18.7). The patient takes the plant-derived 8-methoxypsoralens or soaks in a bath containing another psoralens derivative before prescribed exposure to UVA. The mechanism is a controlled phototoxic reaction. Its main use is for psoriasis, eczema, mycosis fungoides and vitiligo.

Surgery

Surgical procedures are used for diagnosis and as a curative treatment for skin tumours.

18

Table 18.5 Topical treatments

	Action	Indications	Side-effects
Emollients and soap substitutes			
Paraffin, emulsifying ointment, aqueous cream and other proprietary preparations	Hydrate skin	Dry scaly dermatoses, pruritus	May contain preservatives and other ingredients that irritate or sensitize (e.g. lanolin)
Shampoos			
Alphosyl, Polytar	Contain detergents and tar	Dermatitis, psoriasis	Irritant
Betadine	Contains detergents and antibacterials	Folliculitis	Irritant
Selsun (selenium sulphide), Nizoral (ketoconazole)	Contain antifungals	Seborrhoeic dermatitis, pityriasis versicolor	Irritant
Sunscreens			
PABA, cinammate, oxybenzone, titanium dioxide	Sun protection	Photodermatoses, prevention of actinic damage	Irritant, allergic contact sensitivity
Topical steroids (corticosteroids)			
>0.5%, 1% and 2.5% hydrocortisone (mild), Eumovate (moderate), Betnovate (potent), Dermovate (very potent)	Anti-inflammatory	Inflammatory dermatoses. Use as a lotion, cream or ointment, or with an antibacterial (e.g. Betnovate, clioquinol) or antifungal (e.g. hydrocortisone, clotrimazole), or with tar or dithranol	Striae, infection, atrophy, tinea incognito, systemic absorption, allergic contact sensitivity
Topical antibiotics			
Fucidic acid, mupirocin, neomycin, clindamycin, erythromycin, metronidazole		Infections, acne, rosacea	Irritant
Topical antifungals			
Clotrimazole, ketoconazole, nystatin		Tinea, seborrheic dermatitis	Irritant
Topical keratolytics			
Benzoyl peroxide, salicylic acid		Acne, warts, hyperkeratosis	Irritant
Topical retinoids			
Retinoic acid, isotretinoin	Downregulate collagenase and elastase. Affect regeneration and repair; isotretinoin is sebostatic	Photodamage, acne	Irritant, photosensitivity
Topical cytotoxics			
5-fluorouracil	Cytotoxic	Actinic keratoses, Bowen's disease	Irritant

18

Table 18.6 Systemic treatments

	Action	Indications	Side-effects	Contraindications
Systemic antibiotics				
Oxytetracycline, doxycycline, lymecycline, minocycline, erythromycin, flucloxacillin		Infections, acne, rosacea	GI upset, candidosis	Stained teeth (tetracyclines)
Metronidazole				
Systemic antifungals				
Griseofulvin, itraconazole, terbinafine		Tinea	Hepatitis	
Antihistamines				
Hydroxyzine (sedating), chlorpheniramine (sedating), terfenadine (non-sedating), cetirizine (non-sedating)	Anti-H_1 histamine receptor blockade	Pruritus, eczema, urticaria, sedation	Drowsiness	Driving, alcohol
Anti-inflammatory drugs				
Dapsone	Unknown	Leprosy, dermatitis herpetiformis, vasculitis, pyoderma gangrenosum, bullous dermatoses	Haemolysis, hepatitis, bone marrow suppression, angina in the elderly	G6PD deficiency
Hydroxychloroquine	Unknown	Lupus erythematosus, polymorphic light eruption	Retinopathy, lichenoid rash	Lichen planus
Systemic retinoids				
Isotretinoin, acitretin	Affect regeneration and repair; isotretinoin is sebostatic	Acne, psoriasis	See p. 1123	Pregnancy

Table 18.7 Phototherapy with UVB and PUVA

	UVB	PUVA
Action	Immunosuppressive	Immunosuppressive, antihyperproliferative
Indications	Psoriasis, occasionally eczema	Psoriasis, vitiligo, mycosis fungoides, atopic dermatitis
Contraindications	Photosensitivity	Photosensitivity
Side-effects	Burning	Burning, skin cancer, cataract
Monitoring of patients	Total cumulative dose	Total cumulative dose. Regular examination of the skin. Protect eyes with sunglasses. Protect genitals
Recommended adult dose	Sufficient to cause minimal erythema	The dose of psoralen is 0.6 mg/kg given 2 h before UVA and is repeated 2–3 times/week for 6–8 weeks

Diseases and their management

Acute inflammatory dermatoses

Urticaria

Epidemiology, aetiology and pathogenesis
Urticaria (hives) is very common; there are several types (Table 18.8). The mechanism is mast cell degranulation with the release of histamine and other vasoactive mediators causing erythema and oedema.

Usually, the trigger mechanisms are unknown, but type I immunological mechanisms are thought to be involved. Urticarial vasculitis (5% of all urticarias) is conceived as a type III (serum sickness) immune complex condition. It is associated with systemic lupus erythematosus (SLE) and hepatitis B. Causes of common urticaria are given in Table 18.9.

Clinical features
Itchy erythematous wheals constitute urticaria; deeper swelling causes angio-oedema. The lesions of urticarial

Table 18.8 Types of urticaria

Type	Features
Common urticaria	Lesions last for several hours
Acute	
Chronic	
Angio-oedema	Deeper dermal and subdermal involvement
Contact urticaria	Immediate response to allergens (e.g. foods)
Physical urticaria	Lesions last several minutes, but less than 1 h
Dermographism	In response to a scratch or trauma
Cholinergic	In response to heat or exercise
Cold	
Aquagenic	
Heat	
Solar	
Urticarial vasculitis	Lesions last several days or longer. Purpura
Hereditary angio (neurotic)-oedema	C1 esterase inhibitor deficiency

vasculitis last longer than 24 h and may be tender and purpuric.

Hereditary angioedema caused by congenital (autosomal dominant) deficiency of C1 esterase inhibitor is suspected when there is a family history of whealing and angio-oedema in response to trauma. Often patients have abdominal pain. Angio-oedema can affect the face, lips and neck, and threaten laryngeal patency.

Diagnosis of the type of urticaria can be difficult and is largely based on careful history taking. Approximately 70% of patients with urticaria have common urticaria. The differential diagnosis of urticaria includes insect bites, the prodrome of pemphigoid, toxic erythema and erythema multiforme.

Investigation
If urticaria other than common urticaria is suspected, other investigations may be indicated.

Haematology
Full blood count (FBC), eosinophil count and erythrocyte sedimentation rate (ESR).

Biochemistry
Thyroid function tests.

Immunology
Antinuclear antibody (ANA), complement levels and hepatitis serology if indicated clinically.

Histopathology
Biopsy of urticarial vasculitis shows a leucocytoclastic vasculitis.

Microbiology
Stool sample for ova, cysts and parasites.

Table 18.9 Causes of common urticaria (most are idiopathic)

Cause	Example
Drugs	Aspirin, codeine, morphine, non-steroidal anti-inflammatory drugs
Foods	Fish and shellfish, eggs, nuts, tomatoes
Additives	Tartrazine, benzoates
Inhalants	Pollen, spores, house dust
Infections	Focal sepsis (e.g. urinary tract infection, upper respiratory tract infection, hepatitis, *Candida* spp., protozoa, helminths)
Systemic disease	Systemic lupus erythematosus, reticuloses, carcinoma

Management
Withdraw the offending agent (Table 18.9). Non-sedating antihistamines by day are supplemented by sedating antihistamines at night. The patient should be warned about drowsiness, alcohol and driving (Table 18.6). Systemic steroids are usually avoided.

Hereditary angio-oedema
Methyltestosterone, danazol and tranexamic acid have been used as prophylaxis in hereditary angio-oedema. Fresh plasma is used before and during surgery and in an attack. Respiratory obstruction is managed by intubation or tracheostomy and adrenaline 500 µg, 1/1000, 1 mg/ml i.e. 0.5 ml (adult dose) intramuscularly and hydrocortisone 200 mg or more intravenously.

Urticarial vasculitis
The treatment of urticarial vasculitis depends on the cause, but sometimes oral corticosteroids or other non-specific immunosuppressants are needed (Table 18.10).

Table 18.10 Immunosuppressants

Azathioprine, prednisolone, methotrexate, ciclosporin,
  mycophenolate
Indications. Connective tissue disease; bullous disease;
  eczema; psoriasis

Recommended adult doses
Azathioprine: 50–150 mg daily
Prednisolone: 10–60 mg daily
Methotrexate: 2.5–30 mg/week
Ciclosporin: 1–5 mg/kg/day

Insect bites (papular urticaria)

Disease mechanisms and clinical features

Allergic hypersensitivity to the bites of blood-sucking
insects is a common cause of an itchy eruption. Grouped
papular, sometimes vesicular lesions with a punctum
at the apex of each papule suggest the diagnosis. There
may be secondary infection and severe postinflammatory
hyperpigmentation.

Differential diagnosis

Consider lice or scabies (see p. 1141), but the source may
be furniture (e.g. bed bugs, *Cimex lectularius*), the house
and pets (e.g. fleas, *Ctenocephalides felis*) or pets alone (e.g.
sarcoptic mange, *Cheyletiella* spp.).

Management

Oral antihistamines and topical steroids are prescribed,
but the priority is to establish the source of the bites.
Examine the pet or the house, but leave their treatment to
the vet or the environmental health officer.

Lichen planus

Disease mechanisms

The cause is unknown, but a viral or autoimmune pathogenesis has been proposed. There is an association with
liver disease.

Clinical features

Lichen planus is a pruritic eruption of violaceous polygonal papules topped by characteristic white lines called
Wickham's striae (Fig. 18.8). Often there is oral involvement and sometimes nail dystrophy with scarring of the
nail bed (pterygium) and of the scalp causing alopecia. A
micropapular form (lichen nitidus) is recognized (Fig. 18.5).

Investigation

Skin biopsy histology shows epidermal basal cell attack by
a lymphoid infiltrate to give a saw-tooth appearance of the
dermo-epidermal junction.

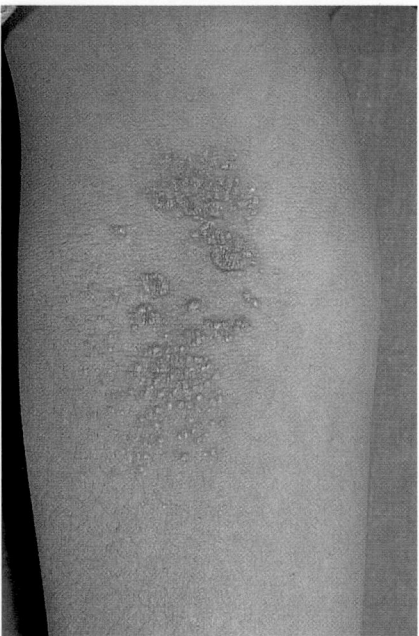

Figure 18.8 Lichen planus. Polygonal papules with superficial
shiny scale (Wickham's striae).

Management and prognosis

Topical steroids hasten resolution and decrease itch.
Sometimes prednisolone has to be given to save the hair
or nails. The eruption is usually self-limiting. Orogenital
lichen planus, particularly when erosive or atrophic,
should be followed up long term because of the risk of
malignant change.

Pityriasis rosea

Epidemiology and disease mechanisms

Pityriasis rosea is common in young adults, and a viral
aetiology is suspected.

Clinical features

There is an eruption of itchy oval erythematous patches
with a collarette of scale (Fig. 18.9). Typically, a larger
lesion appears (the herald patch) before the florid rash.

Investigation

Serology to exclude secondary syphilis.

Management and prognosis

Oral antihistamines and topical steroids until it resolves
within 4–8 weeks.

Chronic inflammatory dermatoses

Psoriasis is characterized by a variable course but may be

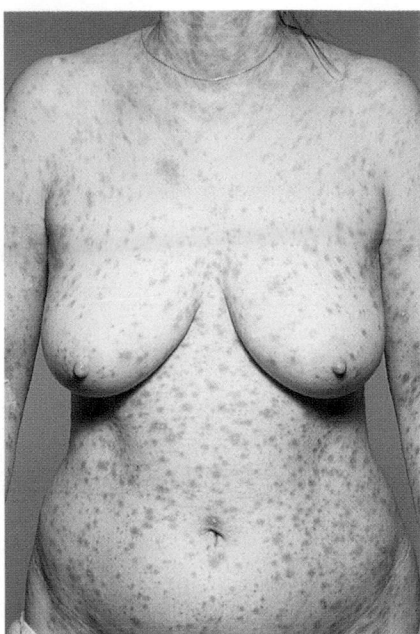

Figure 18.9 Pityriasis rosea. Oval scaly patches. Herald patch centre right chest.

Table 18.11 Classification of eczema

Endogenous eczema	Exogenous eczema
Atopic eczema	Irritant contact dermatitis
Pityriasis alba	Allergic contact dermatitis
Seborrhoeic eczema	Photodermatitis
Stasis eczema	Photoallergic dermatitis
Asteatotic eczema	(phytophotodermatitis)
Pompholyx	
Discoid eczema	
Lichen simplex	
Neurodermatitis	
Nodular prurigo	
Eczematous drug reactions	
Perianal dermatitis	
Autosensitization	
Eczema-like eruptions with systemic disease (children)	
Wiskott–Aldrich syndrome	
X-linked agammaglobinaemia	
Hyper IgE syndrome	
Chronic granulomatous disease	
Phenylketonuria	
Histiocytosis X (Letterer–Siwe disease)	
Acrodermatitis enteropathica (zinc deficiency)	

acute (e.g. more lesions, pustulation, erythroderma, worsening arthritis). Acute guttate psoriasis (a subtype characterized by the appearance of small scaly patches) may be precipitated by a streptococcal sore throat and other infections. It is often self-limiting. Eczema and psoriasis are discussed in this section, but some episodes of eczema, particularly contact dermatitis and photodermatitis, may be acute and self-limiting. Other eczematous dermatoses such as seborrhoeic dermatitis and atopic eczema are characterized by a fluctuating course and acute-on-chronic episodes. In atopic eczema, deterioration may be precipitated by cutaneous superinfection.

Eczema and dermatitis

These terms are synonymous. Eczema is subdivided aetiologically or clinically (Table 18.11). The hallmark is intercellular epidermal oedema (spongiosis on histology). Pruritus is invariable. Lesions are ill-defined at their edges with normal skin, and infection is common. The physical signs are listed in Table 18.12.

Atopic eczema

Epidemiology

Prevalence. About 3% of children under 5 years of age have atopic eczema in the UK.

Table 18.12 Physical signs of acute and chronic eczema

Acute	Chronic
Erythema	Lichenification
Oedema	Scaling
Vesicles	
Serum exudation/crusts	

Disease mechanisms

Atopic eczema is a relapsing condition usually beginning in infancy and sometimes continuing into later life (ECZEMA AT A GLANCE). Atopy means an inherited tendency to develop an altered state of immune reactivity—type I hypersensitivity. A personal or first-degree family history of asthma, hay fever, conjunctivitis or eczema and an elevated IgE defines the atopic and is very common (25%). Although type I hypersensitivity mechanisms explain some of the pathology in asthma, rhinitis and conjunctivitis, they do not suffice in atopic eczema where the pathogenesis is still largely unknown (Table 18.13).

Clinical features

Ill-defined erythematous scaly patches occur on the face and in flexural sites. Scratching and rubbing lead to infection, skin thickening and lichenification.

18

Table 18.13 Possible pathogenesis of atopic eczema

Mechanism	Evidence
Type I hypersensitivity	Increased IgE, foods (egg and milk), pollen, house dust mite
Intrinsic pruritus	Clinical
Ichthyotic tendency	Clinical and familial
Vascular pharmacological reactivity	Histamine/prostaglandins/neuropeptides
Altered cell-mediated immunity	Susceptibility to cutaneous infections (e.g. warts, molluscum, HSV, vaccinia), decreased cytotoxic T-cell function, decreased T-suppressor cell function

Investigation

Atopic dermatitis is a clinical diagnosis.

Microbiology

Swabs to investigate for staphylococcal or herpetic superinfection.

Immunology

IgE is usually elevated.

Management

Atopic eczema may be difficult to manage. A miserable baby with tired and anxious parents can lead to an explosive situation. Topical emollients and bath additives are the mainstay together with oral antihistamines (Table 18.14). Coal tar paste and mild topical steroids can be applied under light bandages. Infection is treated topically or systemically. In the older child or adult it is reasonable to use stronger topical steroids. Topical

Eczema at a glance

Epidemiology

Prevalence

Very common: 3% of children under 5 years have atopic dermatitis/atopic eczema (dermatitis and eczema are synonymous) and 25% of the population have an atopic diathesis. One million elderly people have leg ulcers associated with stasis dermatitis.

Findings on investigation

Diagnosis of the type of eczema is a clinical process and does not usually require special investigation, with the exception of suspected contact dermatitis (see Fig. F).

Clinical features

Acute
Erythema
Oedema
Vesicles
Serum exudation/crusts

Chronic
Lichenification
Scaling

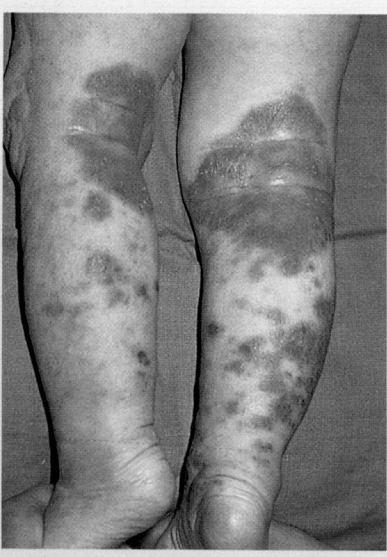

Fig. A Atopic-like dermatitis (Wiskott–Aldrich syndrome).

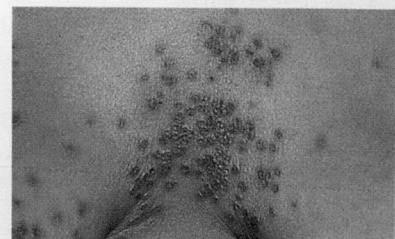

Fig. B Eczema herpeticum. Erosions and crusts.

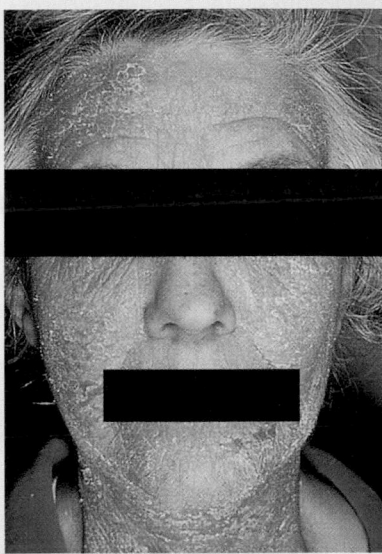

Fig. C Severe seborrhoeic dermatitis. Reproduced from Champion *et al.* (eds), *Textbook of Dermatology*, 5th edn, 1992. Oxford: Blackwell Scientific Publications with the permission of the authors.

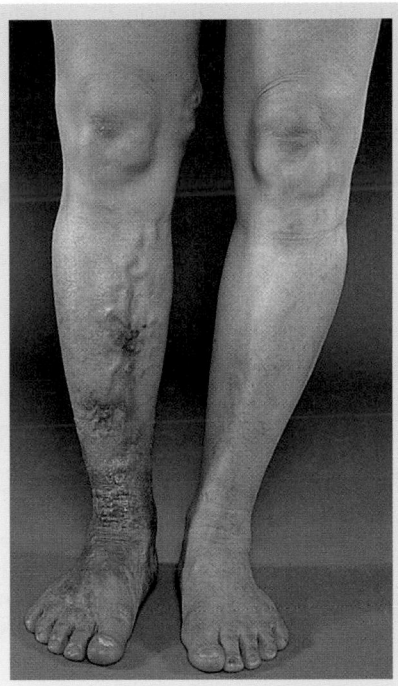

Fig. D Varicose eczema (stasis dermatitis).

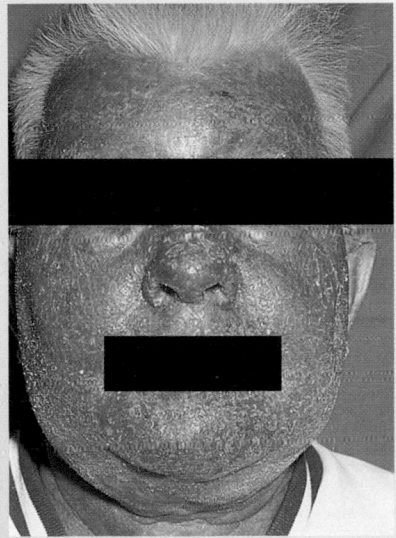

Fig. E Acute contact dermatitis.

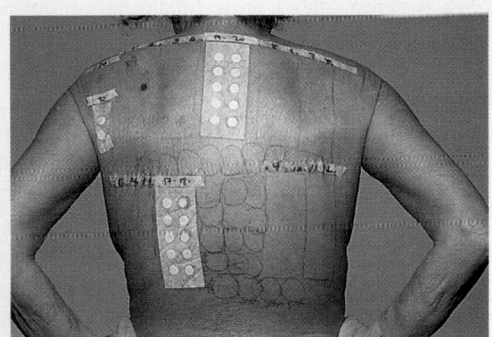

Fig. F Contact dermatitis under evaluation by patch testing.

Table 18.14 Atopic eczema treatment

| Supportive | Specific | |
	Topical	Systemic
Emollients	Tar (refined coal and wood tars)	Antibiotics
Antihistamines	Steroids	Antiviral agents
Diet (oily fish, evening primrose oil)	Antibiotics	PUVA
Chinese herbs (under evaluation)	UVB	Azathioprine, ciclosporin A, prednisolone

18

tacrolimus is a promising innovation. UVB phototherapy or PUVA have a place. Some severe atopics may require azathioprine, prednisolone or ciclosporin.

Eczema herpeticum results when herpes simplex virus has supervened and is an emergency that may require hospitalization and treatment with systemic aciclovir.

Prognosis

The condition resolves in 40% after the age of 5 years and in up to 90% by 15–20.

Other types of endogenous eczema

Nodular prurigo, lichen simplex and neurodermatitis

Lichen simplex is a patch of eczema in response to repeated trauma or scratching. **Neurodermatitis** implies that increased itch is the pathogenetic trigger.

Nodular prurigo is more severe and more widespread than neurodermatitis with greater pruritus; it is related to the atopic diathesis. Topical steroids and bandaging are indicated.

Stasis eczema

Stasis eczema (varicose eczema, lipodermatosclerosis) usually results from failure of the calf muscle pump and consequent venous hypertension. Diminished tissue perfusion and pericapillary deposition of fibrin and haemosiderin result in itchy or painful indurated scaly purpuric areas, particularly over the inner shin and medial malleolus. As episodes of acute inflammation subside, hyperpigmentation remains. There may be oedema.

Stasis eczema is often complicated by contact dermatitis, autosensitization, cellulitis and ulceration:
- *Contact dermatitis:* either allergic resulting from antibiotics and anaesthetics, or irritant resulting from keratolytics and antiseptics, it may be caused by the constituents of topical medications. Patch testing is necessary
- *Autosensitization:* secondary generalization of chronic stasis eczema perhaps caused by 'sensitization' to epidermal antigens. This tends to localize on the face, neck and extensor regions of the arms and thighs. Often there is a history of trauma approximately 1 week before generalization. There may be recurrent exacerbations of the secondary lesions

Asteatotic eczema

Asteatotic eczema occurs on the legs of elderly patients with a dry skin. There is a glazed crazy-paving effect. It responds to emollients.

Discoid eczema

Discoid eczema is characterized by itchy, symmetrical, coin-shaped lesions on the extensor surfaces of the limbs and feet. The lesions are differentiated from those of ringworm, which have an active border, and from those of mycosis fungoides, which are asymmetrical and persistent. Discoid eczema responds to emollients, topical steroids and systemic antihistamines.

Pompholyx

Pompholyx is acute vesicular eczema on the palms and soles. The vesicles look like sago seeds. It responds to potassium permanganate soaks and topical steroids, but may recur.

Seborrhoeic dermatitis

Seborrhoeic dermatitis is a common itchy, scaly, erythematous dermatosis with a particular predilection for the scalp, face, chest, back, axillae and groins. It is very common in human immunodeficiency virus (HIV) infection. It is thought to be an abnormal cutaneous reaction to *Pityrosporum* yeasts and usually responds to topical steroids plus an antiyeast agent such as nystatin or clioquinol. When the scalp is affected (dandruff), ketoconazole shampoo is helpful.

Contact dermatitis

Epidemiology and disease mechanisms

Contact dermatitis is a major industrial and occupational category of diseases. It may be allergic or irritant. Almost anything in the environment can be an irritant and many substances are sensitizers including medicaments (Table 18.15). Allergic contact dermatitis is the archetypal type IV cell-mediated immunological reaction (see p. 50).

Investigation

Patch testing. A battery of common allergens is applied to a quiet (non-inflamed) back. The patches are removed at 48 h and the reactions read. The patient is seen again at 72 h and late responses recorded. Interpretation (false-negatives, false-positives and significance of positives) and management can be difficult.

Management and prognosis

Withdrawal of the offending agent is vital but allergic contact dermatitis may persist despite this.

Prevention

Often atopic, irritant and allergic factors coexist (e.g. with hand eczema). The use of cotton gloves inside rubber gloves for all wet and dirty work is recommended. Barrier creams are important in industrial and domestic prophylaxis.

Table 18.15 Causes of irritant and allergic dermatitis

Irritant dermatitis	Allergic dermatitis
Soaps and detergents	Nickel (jewellery, clasps)
Hairdressing chemicals	Chromate (cement, leather)
Soluble cutting oils	Cosmetics
Coolants	Acrylates (dentists, printers)
Rubber chemicals	
Formaldehyde (household goods)	
Plants (primula)	
Lanolin	
Topical medicaments and dressings	
(e.g. preservatives, antibiotics, local anaesthetics)	

Psoriasis

Epidemiology

Prevalence. Occurs in 2% of the population, but only approximately 1% of the total will have severe psoriasis with arthritis.

Genetics. A polygenic susceptibility is thought to exist. Human leucocyte antigen (HLA) Cw06 is associated with skin disease and B27 with arthritis.

Disease mechanisms

Attacks of psoriasis may be precipitated by infections (e.g. with *Streptococcus* spp.), stress and drugs.

Epidermal keratinocyte and T-cell cytokine-mediated interactions contribute to the dual pathological features of epidermal hyperproliferation and cutaneous inflammation (PSORIASIS AT A GLANCE).

Clinical features

Psoriasis is characterized by red, silver-scaled lesions, which may be guttate, nummular or plaques. The scalp is frequently involved, as are the nails with pitting, onycholysis, dystrophy, subungual hyperkeratosis and even complete shedding. Pustulosis may occur, particularly on the palms and soles. Occasionally psoriasis presents as erythroderma.

Reiter's syndrome

Reiter's syndrome (arthritis, urethritis and conjunctivitis; see p. 265) is part of the same continuum as psoriasis in genetically predisposed individuals. Skin lesions are similar to those of psoriasis. Patients have cobblestoned thickened yellow palms and soles, pustular lesions (keratoderma blenorrhagica) and psoriatic penile lesions (circinate balanitis).

Investigation

Histopathology

Skin biopsy. Irregular epidermal hyperplasia, suprapapil-

Table 18.16 Psoriasis treatment

	Specific	
Supportive	Topical	Systemic
Emollients	Tar (refined coal	PUVA
Oily fish diet	and wood tars)	Methotrexate
	Dithranol	Acitretin
	Topical steroids	Re-PUVA
	Calcipotriol	Ciclosporin
	UVB	Hydroxyurea
	Bath PUVA	Sulfasalazine

lary thinning, leucocyte infiltration and epidermal pustulosis typify psoriasis.

Management and prognosis

A hierarchical approach to management is presented in Table 18.16.

Acne vulgaris

Epidemiology

Prevalence. Common.

Age. Common from adolescence onwards with 1% (male) to 5% (female) of adults still requiring treatment until 40 years of age.

Disease mechanisms

Acne vulgaris is a chronic disorder of the pilosebaceous apparatus with increased androgen-dependent sebum production: the fundamental abnormality. Ductal hypercornification, a deranged symbiotic relationship with normally commensal micro-organisms (*Propionibacterium acnes*) and cutaneous inflammation also occur. The rate of sebum excretion is related to the severity of the acne. Approximately 80% of women with acne have polycystic

18

Psoriasis at a glance

Epidemiology

Prevalence
2% of the population

Genetics
Probably a polygenic susceptibility

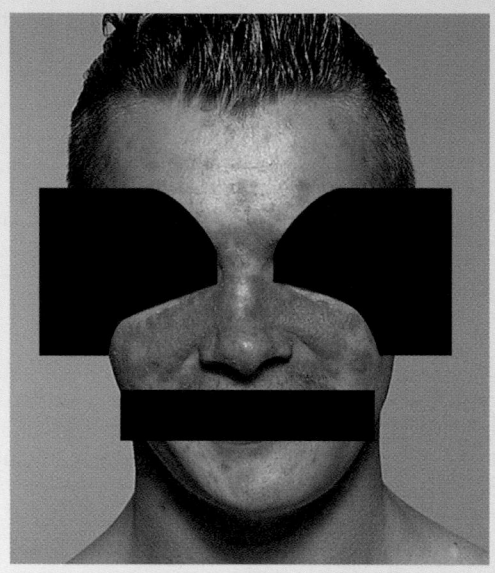

Fig. C Sebopsoriasis (clinical overlap with seborrhoeic dermatitis; compare with ECZEMA AT A GLANCE, Fig. C, p. 1117).

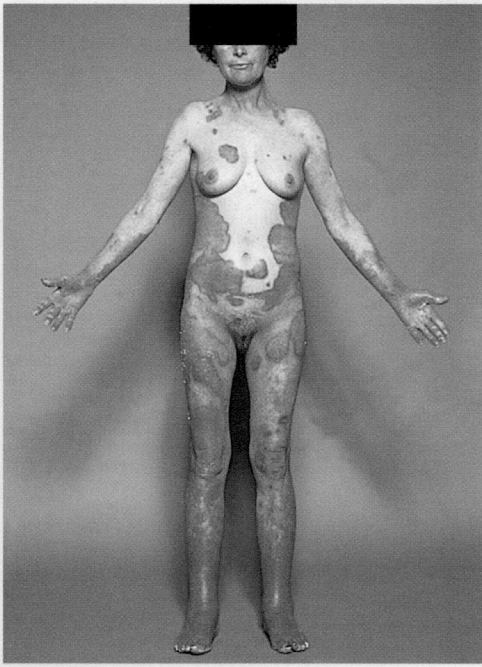

Fig. A Near erythrodermic psoriasis.

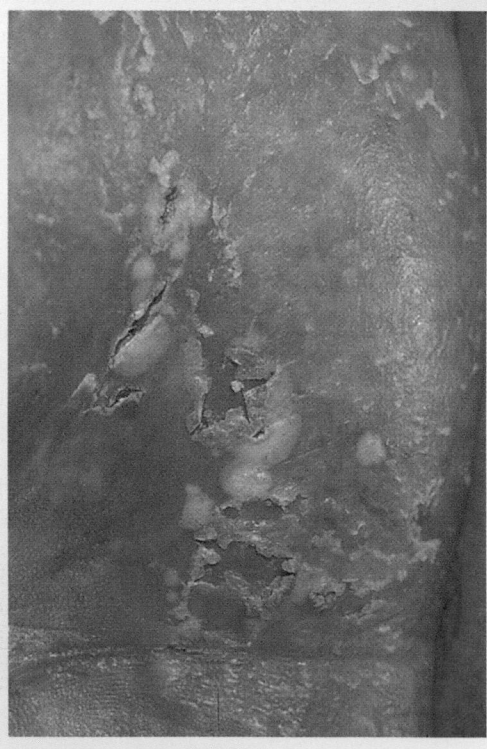

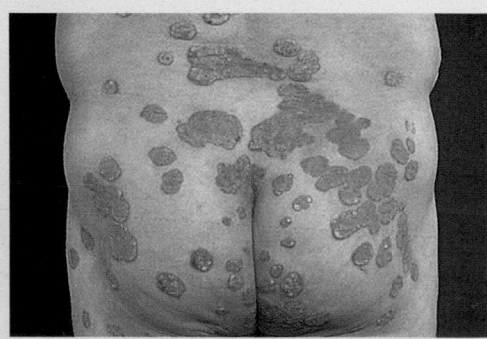

Fig. B Chronic plaque psoriasis.

Fig. D Palmoplantar psoriasis (pustular hypothenar eminence).

18

Findings on investigation
Diagnosis of psoriasis and its variants is a clinical process and does not usually require investigation, although occasionally a biopsy may be performed

Histology
Irregular epidermal hyperplasia, suprapapillary thinning, leucocyte infiltration and epidermal pustulosis

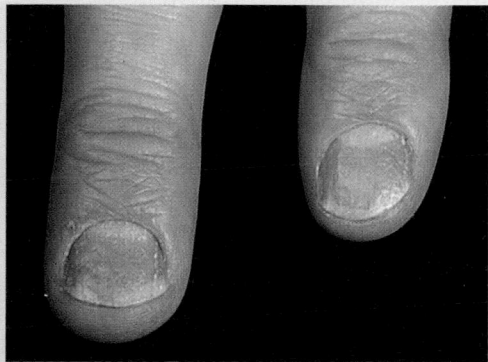

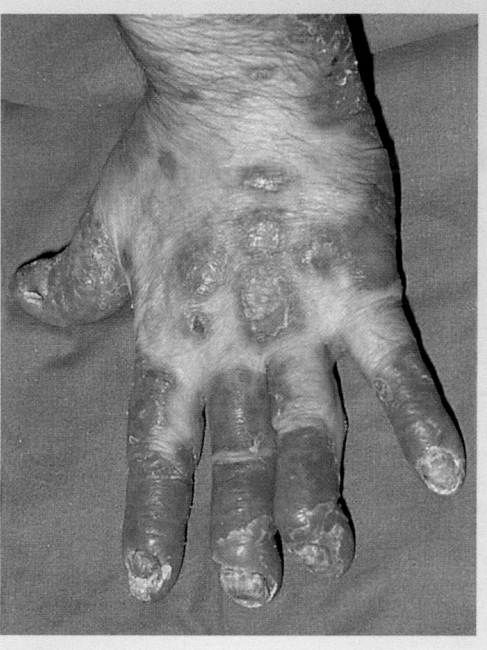

Fig. E Nail involvement in psoriasis. Note dystrophy, pits and irregular yellowing onycholysis.

Fig. F Psoriatic arthropathy (arthritis mutilans); severe nail dystrophy.

ovaries on ultrasound scanning, but most do not have the other features of the polycystic ovary syndrome. There is no evidence for systemic endocrine abnormalities in males. Both men and women with acne may have an amplified target organ response. The endocrine factors are summarized in Table 18.17.

Clinical features
The clinical features of acne are seborrhoea, comedones, papules, pustules, nodules, cysts and scars (Fig. 18.10). The lesions are distributed on the face, neck, back and

Table 18.17 Endocrine factors in the pathogenesis of acne vulgaris

Menstruation
Pregnancy
Neonatal
Adolescence
Polycystic ovary syndrome
Cushing's syndrome
Virilizing neoplasms
Congenital adrenal hyperplasia
Iatrogenic (corticosteroids, androgens)

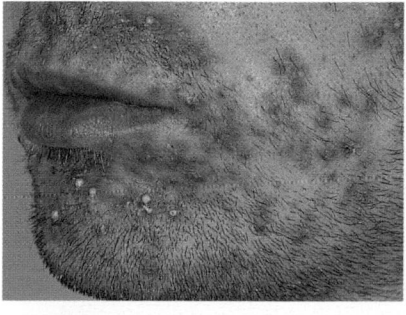

(a)

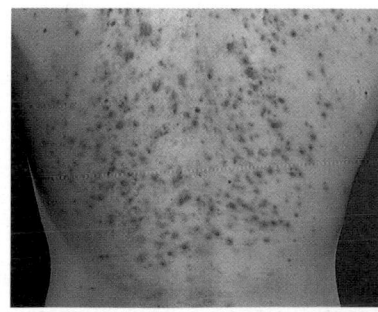

(b)

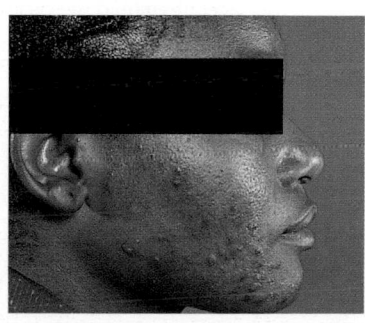

(c)

Figure 18.10 (a–c) Acne vulgaris (seborrhoea, comedones, papules, pustules, nodules, scars and postinflammatory hyperpigmentation).

Table 18.18 Acne vulgaris

Physical treatments
Comedo removal
UV light
Intralesional steroids
Scar excision
Dermabrasion
Collagen injections

Topical treatments
Disinfectants
Betadine
Chlorhexidine

Topical keratolytics
Benzoyl peroxide
Retinoids
Salicylic acid

Topical antibiotics
Erythromycin
Clindamycin

Other topical treatments
Zinc sulphate
Azelaic acid
Nicotinamide
Adapalene
Isotretinoin

Oral antibiotics
Tetracyclines (oxytetracycline 500 mg twice daily,
    minocycline 100 mg once daily, lymecycline 300 mg
    daily or doxycycline 100 mg once daily)
Erythromycin 500 mg twice daily
Treat for 6 months minimum
Not with meals (except erythromycin)
Concomitant topical treatments not contraindicated
Side-effects: gastrointestinal, photosensitivity, benign
    intracranial hypertension and renal impairment

Hormonal treatments
Contraceptive pill (appropriate choice, see Table 18.19)
Cyproterone acetate (high dose, cyclical)
Prednisolone

chest. Pyoderma faciale is acute severe facial acne (CLIN-ICAL EXAMINATION AT A GLANCE, Fig. M, p. 1107). Acne fulminans is acute severe acne with fever and arthralgia.

Investigation
Investigations are only very rarely indicated if Cushing's syndrome or virilization are suspected. Pelvic ultrasound will demonstrate polycystic ovaries.

Management and prognosis
Treatment depends on the severity of the condition and an objective record of severity helps follow-up (Table 18.18). Up to 5% of all women and 1% of all men 25–40 years of age may need treatment.
● *Mild acne:* topical therapy only
● *Moderate–severe acne:* both topical and systemic therapy, with antibiotics and/or, for women, hormonal manipulation with a suitable combined oral contraceptive pill (Table 18.19)
● *Severe nodulocystic (conglobate) acne:* failure to respond to other treatments is an indication for isotretinoin (13-*cis*-retinoic acid)

Acne is usually self-limiting. With the exception of isotretinoin, treatment does not alter the natural history. Therefore treatment should continue throughout the course of the disorder. Topical therapies are needed long term and antibiotics should be given for at least 6 months and repeated courses or long-term treatment may be necessary. Maintenance topical treatment is needed after oral therapy is stopped. Combined therapy is *not* irrational because there are several pathogenic factors.

Isotretinoin and acne
Very small amounts of vitamin A are essential; larger amounts are very toxic. Isotretinoin is a synthetic retinoid that is profoundly sebostatic (Table 18.20).

Hidradenitis suppurativa

Hidradenitis suppurativa is the apocrine equivalent of acne vulgaris. In mild forms, patients have recurrent boils in apocrine areas (axillae, groins, breasts, behind the ears).

Type	Theoretical effect on acne	Examples
Androgenic	Worsen acne	Norgestrol
		Norethindrone
		Norethisterone
Anti-androgenic	Improve acne	Ethynodiol diacetate
		Megestrol acetate
		Cyproterone acetate
		Desogestrol
		Levonorgestrol

Table 18.19 Synthetic androgenic and antiandrogenic progestagens

Table 18.20 Isotretinoin

Action. Affects all four aetiological factors operating in acne. Sebum production is strikingly reduced by 75–90%

Indications. Severe, usually cystic or conglobate, acne not responsive to conventional treatment (systemic antibiotics at the right dose for 6 months plus topical treatment) or hormonal treatment in women

Side-effects. Correspond to the hypervitaminosis A syndrome (eating polar bear liver). The most important side-effect is teratogenesis. Major embryopathic changes if conception occurs on isotretinoin

Contraindications. Women must agree to avoid pregnancy during and for some months after a course of isotretinoin: the half-life is about 22 days. Pregnancy during therapy is an indication for termination because of the risk of devastating teratogenesis

Dosages

1.0 mg/kg/day for 4–6 months (120–150 mg/kg, total)

Side-effects are common, but it is important that the target dose is achieved

Some patients require longer treatment, others need a higher dose

Most patients need no further treatment

Side-effects

Eczema, cheilitis, conjunctivitis

Arthralgia, myalgia, diffuse interstitial skeletal hyperostosis (DISH)

Benign intracranial hypertension

Elevated liver function tests and blood lipids

Teratogenesis

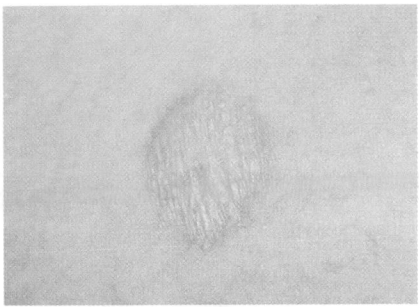

Figure 18.11 Lichen sclerosus.

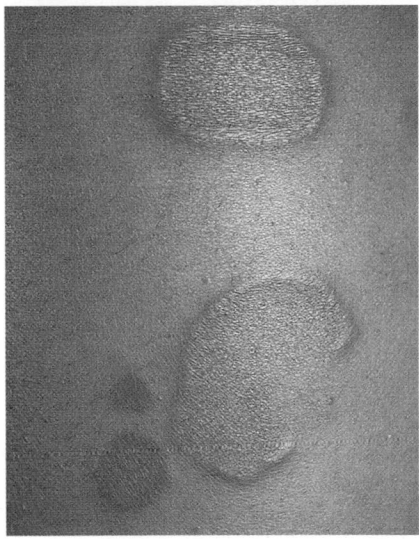

Figure 18.12 Granuloma annulare.

Chronic nodulocystic involvement of the groins with suppuration and fistula formation can occur.

Hidradenitis can respond indifferently to antibiotics, hormonal manipulation and isotretinoin. Surgery may be necessary.

Lichen sclerosus

Lichen sclerosus is an uncommon inflammatory dermatosis that may affect all areas of skin, but has a particular predilection for the genitalia. Characteristic lesions are wrinkled plaques of pink papules leading to whiter, more atrophic, ivory patches (Fig. 18.11; Fig. 18.70, p. 1166).

Granuloma annulare

Granuloma annulare (Fig. 18.12) is an idiopathic degenerative condition characterized by erythematous ring-shaped lesions with an elevated edge. When focal and acral it is sometimes related to trauma (e.g. on the foot), but when diffuse and generalized it may be a hallmark of underlying diabetes mellitus. Potent topical steroids are sometimes an effective treatment, but granuloma annulare can be self-limiting.

Immunobullous disorders

Bullous pemphigoid

Epidemiology

Prevalence. Common.

Age. Most common in the elderly.

Disease mechanisms

It is thought to be brought about by autoimmunity against the hemidesmosome of the basement membrane (Fig. 18.1), but the trigger is unknown. There may be an association between seronegative disease and malignancy, in which mucosal lesions are more common.

Clinical features

The primary lesions are often not blisters, the patient

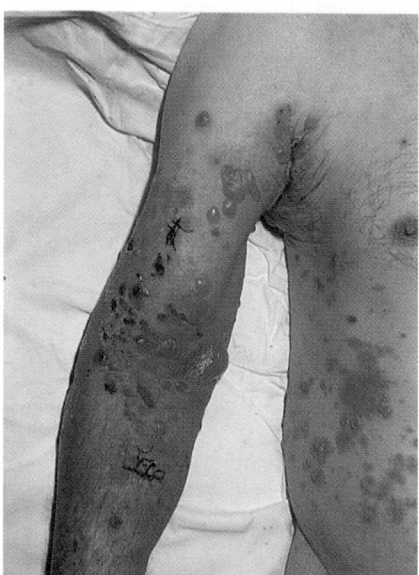

Figure 18.13 Bullous pemphigoid. Tense blisters (bullae) on an erythematosus and urticated base.

first developing erythematous, urticated and eczematous areas on the trunk and limbs (Fig. 18.13; CLINICAL EXAMINATION AT A GLANCE, Fig. G, p. 1106). Tense blisters then appear in these sites.

Investigation

The diagnosis is confirmed by histological evidence of a subepidermal blister with positive direct immunofluorescence of perilesional skin, where IgG and C3 are demonstrated at the basement membrane zone (BMZ). Circulating antibodies to the BMZ are often found in the serum.

Management and prognosis

Most patients respond well to prednisolone 40–60 mg/day, which is given until the blisters begin to heal and no new blisters are appearing. The dosage is reduced over a few weeks and many patients remain free of lesions after treatment is stopped. Azathioprine is often introduced (50–150 mg/day) as a corticosteroid-sparing agent.

Mucous membrane cicatricial pemphigoid

This is a rare variant of bullous pemphigoid. Blisters affect the skin and the mucous membranes, predominantly the palate and gingivae, sometimes the oesophagus with dysphagia. Healing with scarring occurs; conjunctival blistering with the formation of symblepharon can cause blindness.

Direct immunofluorescence is usually positive (Fig. 18.14), but circulating antibodies to the BMZ are rarely found.

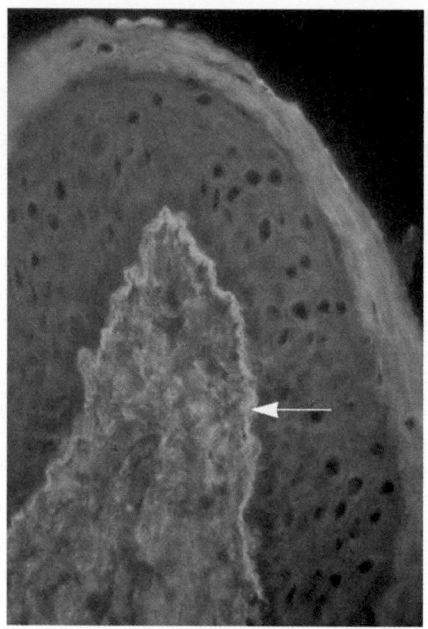

Figure 18.14 Bright green immunofluorescence of IgG at the basement membrane zone (BMZ) (indicated by arrow) in a patient with pemphigoid. Reproduced from Champion *et al.* (eds) *Textbook of Dermatology*, 5th edn, Oxford: Blackwell Scientific Publications, 1992 with the permission of the authors.

The response to corticosteroids is disappointing, but dapsone or another sulpha drug may be helpful. Regular FBCs are mandatory with dapsone because haemolytic anaemia and agranulocytosis can occur.

Pemphigus vulgaris

Epidemiology

Prevalence. Rare.

Age. Most common in the 45–50-year age group.

Disease mechanisms

Pemphigus is a direct result of antibody-mediated attack on the interepidermal cell desmosomal structure (Fig. 18.1).

Clinical features and investigation

Involvement may be confined to the oral mucosa. The blisters are intraepithelial and therefore rupture readily, leaving raw erosions (Fig. 18.15). Skin lesions may not appear for some months.
- *Histology:* shows an intraepidermal blister with acantholysis (separation of prickle cells)
- *Direct immunofluorescence:* demonstrates intercellular IgG and C3 (Fig. 18.16)
- *Circulating antibodies:* found in the serum and the titre correlates with disease severity

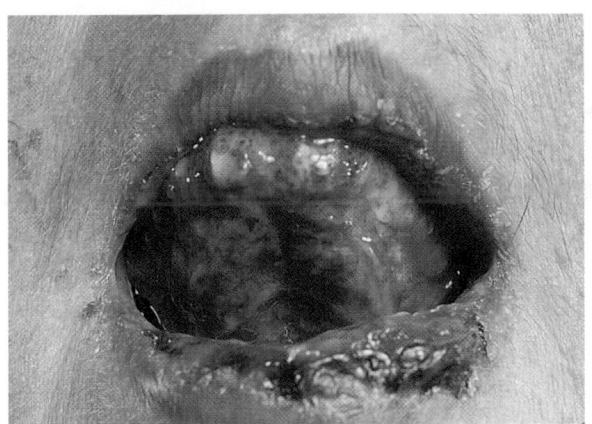

Figure 18.15 Pemphigus vulgaris. Severe mucocutaneous erosions.

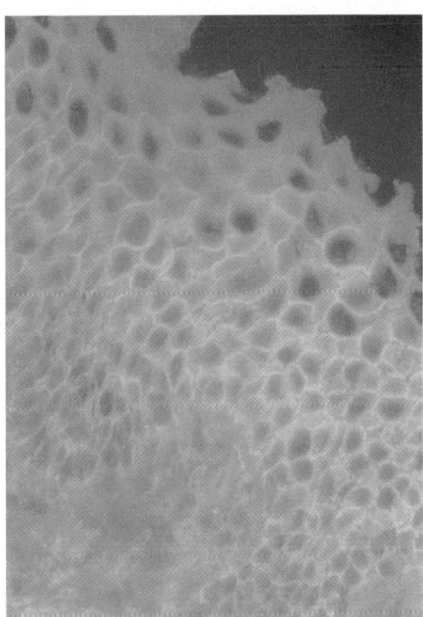

Figure 18.16 Bright green immunofluorescence of IgG in the intercellular space in a patient with pemphigus vulgaris. Reproduced from Champion *et al.* (eds) *Textbook of Dermatology*, 5th edn. Oxford: Blackwell Scientific Publications, 1992 with the permission of the authors.

Management and prognosis

Before the use of systemic corticosteroids, pemphigus vulgaris was invariably fatal. High doses are usually employed, starting with 80–120 mg prednisolone. Iatrogenic side-effects are common and contribute to the mortality. Other drugs used include azathioprine, dapsone and gold. Potent topical steroids are used for the mucocutaneous lesions.

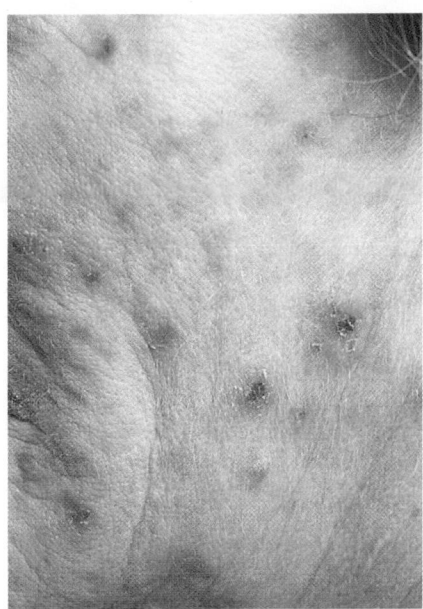

Figure 18.17 Dermatitis herpetiformis. Excoriations and erosions.

Dermatitis herpetiformis

Epidemiology

Prevalence. Very rare.

Age. Occurs in young adults with a second peak of incidence in old age.

Disease mechanisms

An association with the HLA B8, DR3 and DQw2 haplotype suggests an autoimmune basis but circulating antibodies are not found.

Clinical features and investigation

Intensely itchy groups of small blisters on an urticarial base occur over the elbows, knees, buttocks or face; often only excoriations may be seen (Fig. 18.17).
- *Histology:* reveals subepidermal blisters and microabscesses in the dermal papillae
- *Positive direct immunofluorescence:* shows IgA in the papillary tips
- *Intestinal biopsy:* may be necessary because patients often have a gluten-sensitive enteropathy, which may be clinically silent and inapparent on simple screening (e.g. FBC, serum iron, and folate and red cell folate)

Management and prognosis

The itch and rash respond to dapsone within a few days. A strictly controlled gluten-free diet means most patients can be off dapsone in 2 years.

Table 18.21 Causes of erythroderma

Eczema
Psoriasis
Drugs
Mycosis fungoides (Sézary syndrome)
Reactions to sunlight
Toxic erythema
Toxic shock syndrome
Staphylococcal scalded skin syndrome
Toxic epidermal necrolysis
Infestations (scabies and lice)
Congenital disorders

Table 18.22 Causes of hyperpigmentation

Melasma/chloasma
Addison's disease
Acromegaly
Nelson's syndrome
Pregnancy/menstruation
Oral contraceptives
Lymphoma
Renal failure
Haemochromatosis
Amyloid
Pellagra
Drugs

Table 18.23 Disorders associated with vitiligo

Alopecia areata
Halo naevus
Malignant melanoma
Thyroid disease
Pernicious anaemia
Addison's disease
Diabetes mellitus
Myasthenia gravis

Erythroderma

Erythroderma is a state of complete confluent cutaneous inflammation that may develop acutely or insidiously. Causes are listed in Table 18.21. A clinical diagnosis is not always apparent and a biopsy is often needed.

Patients may require hospital management of the haemodynamic and metabolic effects caused by the failing homoeostatic function of the skin. Toxic epidermal necrolysis is discussed on p. 1167.

Disorders of pigmentation

Hypo- and hyperpigmentation are common complications of all inflammatory dermatoses. Both are more readily apparent in racially pigmented skin. Hyperpigmentation particularly complicates some photosensitive reactions to drugs, chemicals and plants.

Hyperpigmentation

Some congenital and acquired lesions of the melanocyte are described elsewhere (see p. 1145). Fanconi's syndrome (pancytopenia with congenital defects) and Albright's syndrome (ostotic fibrous dysplasia with precocious puberty) may be associated with hyperpigmented areas of skin, which sometimes appear as *café au lait* patches (CLINICAL EXAMINATION AT A GLANCE, Fig. H, p. 1106).

Hyperpigmentation can occur in some endocrine conditions. The patchy pattern on the cheeks seen in women during pregnancy or on the contraceptive pill is called melasma or chloasma. Other causes are listed in Table 18.22. Among the drugs that cause hyperpigmentation are phenothiazines (blue–grey), antimalarials (blue–grey), amiodarone (grey) and cytotoxics. Minocycline can cause a blue–black discoloration.

Hypopigmentation

Hypopigmentation may be genetic:

- In albinism, melanization cannot occur as a result of tyrosinase deficiency
- Hypopigmented ash leaf patches may be found in tuberous sclerosis
- Congenital circular, whorled or streaked hypopigmentation (naevus depigmentosus of Ito) may be associated with mental retardation

Vitiligo

Epidemiology

Prevalence. May be as high as 1%.

Race. Affects all racial skin types.

Disease mechanisms

Although vitiligo is associated with organ-specific autoimmune disease (Table 18.23) and antimelanocytic antibodies can be found in the blood, the aetiology remains obscure.

Clinical features

Hypopigmented macules appear on sun-exposed areas (CLINICAL EXAMINATION AT A GLANCE, Fig. B, p. 1105), areas that were previously hyperpigmented (e.g. face, axillae, groins) and areas exposed to trauma or friction (Koebner phenomenon). Hairs within a lesion are amelanotic. Wood's light shows stark white lesions.

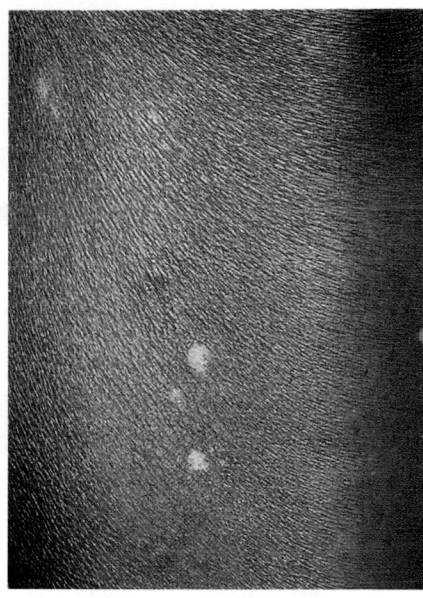

Figure 18.18 Idiopathic guttate hypomelanosis. Macular hyperpigmented lesions.

Management and prognosis

Treatment is unsatisfactory, but the priorities are protection from the sun and cosmetic camouflage advice. Up to 20% of younger patients may spontaneously repigment, but it is usually an unsatisfactory patchy perifollicular repigmentation. Some patients respond to PUVA.

Idiopathic guttate hypomelanosis

Idiopathic guttate hypomelanosis can be mistaken for vitiligo. It is common in coloured skins and may be a postinflammatory phenomenon. In white skin it may be a sign of actinic damage (Fig. 18.18).

Photodermatology

Figure 18.19 shows the electromagnetic spectrum. All ultraviolet C (UVC) is absorbed by the atmosphere. UVA and B reach the skin and penetrate it, depending on several factors (Table 18.24). Some of the effects of sun on the skin are beneficial (e.g. stimulation of vitamin D

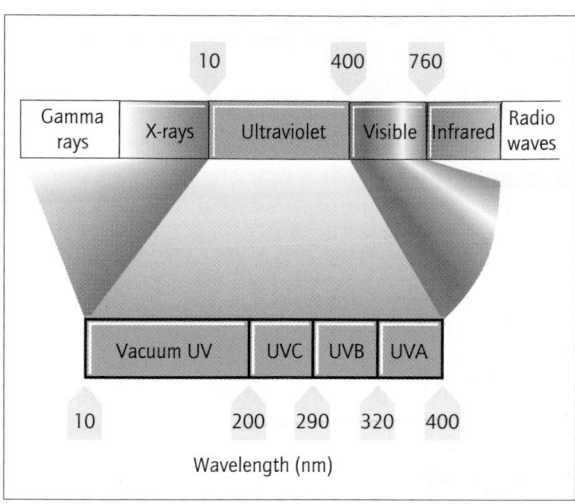

Figure 18.19 The electromagnetic spectrum, with emphasis on the wavelengths of ultraviolet light.

Table 18.24 Factors affecting how much UVA and UVB reach the skin and its penetration

Non-cutaneous	Cutaneous
Altitude	Melanin
Season	Epidermal thickness
Time of day	Hair (scalp)
Reflection (snow, water, sand)	

synthesis). Other effects are harmful and are listed in Table 18.25.

Photodermatoses

Clinical features

Several photodermatoses are recognized. Sites affected are the forehead, cheeks, ears, nose, chin, anterior chest 'V' and hands. Sites spared are periorbital, retroauricular and submental sites.

Polymorphic light eruption

This is very common in young women. Erythema, papules, urticarial wheals and plaques develop usually a

Table 18.25 Harmful effects of UV light

Relation to time	Effect
Immediate	Erythema, pigmentation (oxidation of melanin)
Days	Erythematous sunburn, delayed pigmentation (melanogenesis)
	Epidermal hyperplasia, Langerhans' cell dysfunction
	Melanocyte carcinogenesis
Years	Photoageing, keratinocyte carcinogenesis

18

day or more after sun exposure. Sun avoidance and sunscreens are essential. Prophylactic PUVA (before holidays) can be offered.

Solar urticaria

Solar urticaria is rare, but is characterized by an immediate urticarial response to sun exposure. It fades in the shade.

Actinic prurigo

Actinic prurigo is a problem of childhood and adolescence. It is a very itchy persistent papulonodular response to sunlight and may scar. Sun avoidance and protection are therefore essential.

Hydroa vacciniforme

Hydroa vacciniforme is a rare childhood photodermatosis characterized by blisters that crust and heal with scarring. Sun avoidance and sunscreens are mandatory.

Actinic reticuloid

Actinic reticuloid is a chronic actinic dermatitis in middle-aged men. There is erythema and lichenification. Often there is superimposed contact sensitivity.

Light-aggravated dermatoses

Light-aggravated dermatoses include:
- Atopic eczema
- Psoriasis (10%; most improve)
- Lupus eythematosus
- Lichen planus
- Acne (most improve)
- Pellagra
- Porphyrias

Porphyrias

Porphyrias are metabolic disorders and are described on p. 808. They result from enzyme deficiencies in the synthesis of haem. Skin disease results from precursor deposition in the cutis.

Porphyria cutanea tarda (Fig. 18.20) may be familial or sporadically affect young women (associated with alcohol and the contraceptive pill) or middle-aged men (associated with alcoholism). There is an association with viral hepatitis (B and C) and HIV. Skin fragility and photosensitive blistering with scarring occur on exposed sites, especially the hands. Hypertrichosis occurs on the face. There is a deficiency of uroporphyrinogen decarboxylase activity. Uroporphyrin III is found in urine and faeces. Treatment is by the avoidance of alcohol, oestrogen and sunlight, venesection and low-dose hydroxychloroquine.

Other porphyrias that affect the skin are erythropoietic

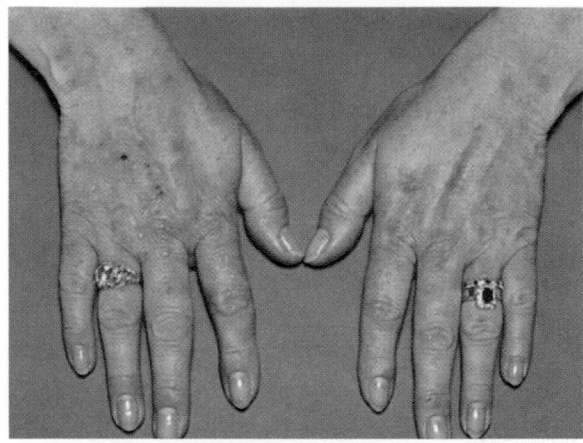

Figure 18.20 Porphyria cutanea tarda. Blisters, erosions and scars on dorsal aspect of hands.

protoporphyria (burning pain on sunlight exposure, scarring but no blistering); congenital erythropoietic porphyria (werewolf syndrome—severe photosensitivity, scarring, hypertrichosis and red fluorescence of urine and teeth); variegate porphyria (South African, drug-provoked, photosensitive blistering, neuropsychiatric attacks).

Disorders of hair and nails

Diffuse non-scarring alopecia

The differential diagnosis of diffuse non-scarring alopecia is given in Table 18.26.

Androgenetic alopecia in men is physiological and consists of focal frontal and vertical loss with eventual confluence of baldness and occipital sparing. In women, the picture is more diffuse thinning. Women should be screened for endocrine and thyroid disturbance and iron deficiency.

Minoxidil 2–5% lotion is of variable efficacy. In women, the antiandrogen cyproterone acetate given with ethinyl oestradiol to regulate the menstrual cycle has some effect.

Alopecia areata refers to focal areas of complete but non-scarring alopecia (Fig. 18.21). It sometimes occurs in association with organ-specific autoimmune disease. Topical or intralesional corticosteroid may help. The prognosis cannot be predicted. Patients with nail pits may do worse, as do those with more widespread hair loss (alopecia totalis, universalis).

Scarring alopecia

The differential diagnosis of scarring alopecia is important. Skin biopsy is essential. Diagnosis must be prompt

Table 18.26 Causes of diffuse non-scarring alopecia

Endocrine disorders
Androgenetic alopecia
Telogen effluvium
Hypothyroidism
Hypopituitarism
Virilizing syndromes (e.g. adrenal or ovarian tumours,
     congenital adrenal hyperplasia, polycystic ovary syndrome)

Skin diseases
Erythroderma
Psoriasis
Seborrhoeic dermatitis
Alopecia areata

Nutritional
Iron deficiency

Chronic illness
HIV infection
Renal disease
Liver disease
Malignant disease

Drugs
Lithium
Anticoagulants
Cytotoxics
Immunosuppressants

Table 18.27 Causes of scarring alopecia

Infection/infestation
Tinea capitis (Fig. 18.22) and kerion
Staphylococcal folliculitis/folliculitis decalvans
Syphilis
Herpes simplex and zoster

Skin disease
Lupus vulgaris
Lichen planus (Fig. 18.23)
Sarcoid
Lupus erythematosus (especially DLE; Fig. 18.24)
Scleroderma
Basal cell carcinoma
Metastatic carcinoma

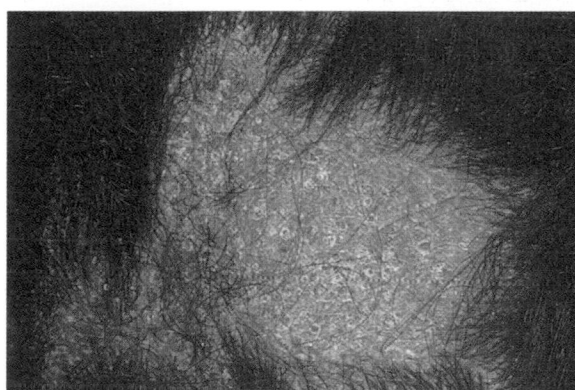

Figure 18.22 Tinea capitis. Erythema, scale, hair loss and scarring. An inflammatory mass is called a kerion.

if a treatable infection or another cause is to be found (Table 18.27; Figs 18.22–18.24). Topical or systemic corticosteroids are used in lichen planus or discoid lupus erythematosus (DLE). Hydroxychloroquine is used in DLE.

Hirsutes

Hirsutes is the appearance of coarse terminal hair in women in areas where it is normal in postpubertal men (Fig. 18.25). A virilizing tumour is rare but examine for deepening of the voice and clitoromegaly. Idiopathic hirsutes is very common and is diagnosed when there is no endocrine abnormality. Often it occurs with other features of cutaneous virilism, acne and androgenic alopecia.

Treatment includes depilation and antiandrogens (cyproterone acetate and spironolactone).

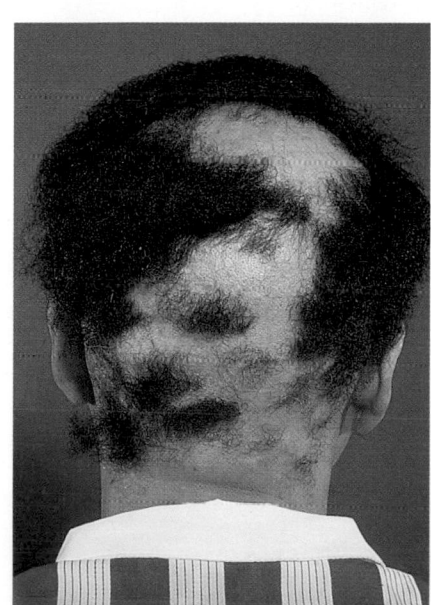

Figure 18.21 Alopecia areata.

18

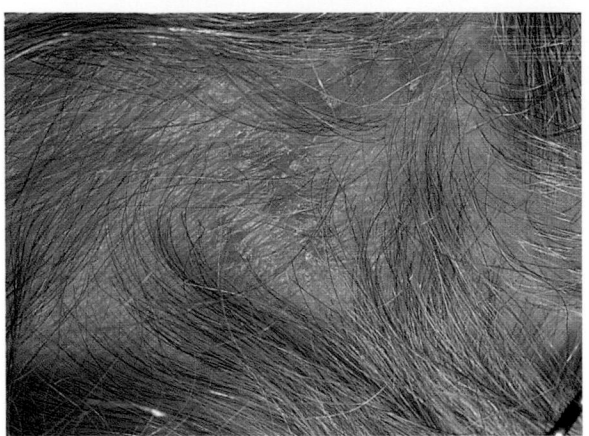

Figure 18.23 Cicatricial (scarring). Lichen planus.

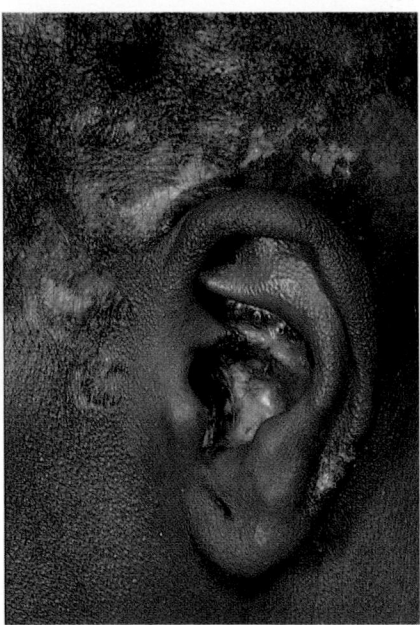

Figure 18.24 Discoid lupus erythematosus. Erythema, atrophy, scarring and hair loss.

Hypertrichosis

Hypertrichosis is the appearance of excess (usually finer vellus) hair in non-androgen-dependent areas. Causes are listed in Table 18.28.

Nail disorders

Causes of different types of nail changes are given in Table 18.29. Nail changes may indicate underlying illness (Figs 18.26 and 18.27).

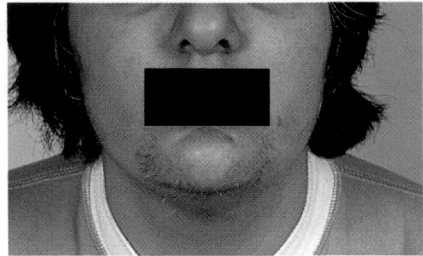

Figure 18.25 Hirsutes of the chin and cheeks.

Table 18.28 Causes of hypertrichosis

Localized
Becker's naevus (trunk)
Spina bifida occulta (base of spine)
Postinflammatory (trauma, porphyria cutanea tarda, arthritis)
Occlusion
Hypertrichosis lanugosa (lymphoma)

Generalized
Hypothyroidism
Malnutrition
Anorexia nervosa
Drugs (ciclosporin, corticosteroids, phenytoin, PUVA)

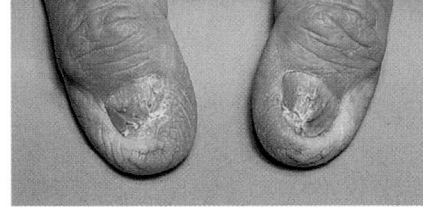

Figure 18.26 Scarring nail dystrophy. Lichen planus.

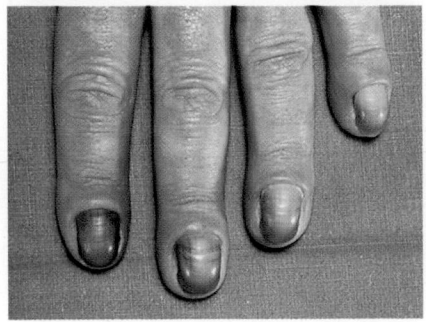

Figure 18.27 Yellow nail syndrome.

Table 18.29 Causes of nail changes

Nail change	Cause
Pits	Psoriasis (PSORIASIS AT A GLANCE, Fig. E, p. 1121)
	Eczema
	Alopecia areata
Ridges	Psoriasis (PSORIASIS AT A GLANCE)
Nicks	Darier's disease (see p. 1155)
Dystrophy	Psoriasis (PSORIASIS AT A GLANCE, Figs E and F, p. 1121)
	Raynaud's phenomenon
	Arterial disease
	Lichen planus (Fig. 18.26)
	Onychomycosis (Fig. 18.48)
White spots	Trauma
Red, white and blue bands	Darier's disease (see p. 1155)
Longitudinal black bands	Race: Afro-Caribbeans
	Lichen planus
	Melanoma
Black spots	Trauma (haemorrhage)
	Naevi
	Melanoma
Red spot	Glomus tumour
Onycholysis	Psoriasis (PSORIASIS AT A GLANCE, Figs E and F, p. 1121)
	Drugs
Paronychia	Proximal or lateral nailfold infection (often *Candida* spp. and bacteria)
Grooves	Acute illness (Beau's lines: recurrent (e.g. febrile) illnesses, myocardial infarction, pulmonary embolus)
	Psoriasis (PSORIASIS AT A GLANCE, Fig. E, p. 1121)
White bands	Arsenic poisoning
	Hypoalbuminaemia
Leuconychia	Cirrhosis
	Diabetes mellitus
	Cardiac failure
	Anaemia
Yellow nail syndrome (curved nail, reduced growth, peripheral lymphoedema; Fig. 18.27)	Bronchiectasis
	Bronchogenic carcinoma
Blue nails	Wilson's disease
Longitudinal melanonychia	Malnutrition
	Addison's disease
Koilonychia (spoon-shaped nails)	Iron deficiency
Splinter haemorrhages	Trauma
	Autoimmune rheumatic disease
	Endocarditis
Ragged cuticles	Autoimmune rheumatic disease (CLINICAL EXAMINATION AT A GLANCE, Fig. C, p. 1105)
Nailfold telangiectasia	Autoimmune rheumatic disease (CLINICAL EXAMINATION AT A GLANCE, Fig. C, p. 1105)

Finger clubbing

In clubbing the distal phalanx is broadened (Fig. 18.28), there is increased transverse and longitudinal curvature and increased vascularity and soft tissue, and the base angle between the nail and fold is more than 180°. Causes of clubbing are listed in Table 18.30.

Vascular disorders

Peripheral vascular disease resulting from **atherosclerosis** and **Buerger's disease** may lead to digital ulceration and nail dystrophy. The pulses may be diminished or absent and the distal skin is cold and hairless.

18

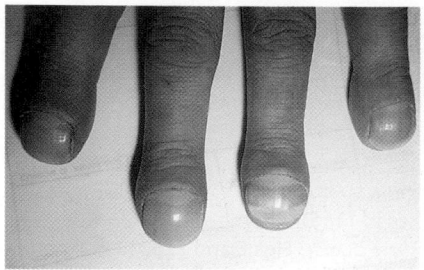

Figure 18.28 Clubbing associated with bronchial carcinoma. Causes: lung disease, cardiac disease, gut disease, idiopathic familial, vascular disorders, thyroid acropachy (see Table 18.30). Reproduced from Champion *et al.* (eds) *Textbook of Dermatology*, 5th edn. Oxford: Blackwell Scientific Publications, 1992 with the permission of the authors.

Table 18.30 Causes of clubbing

Lung diseases
Bronchiectasis
Cystic fibrosis
Pulmonary tuberculosis
Carcinoma of the bronchus
Mesothelioma
Fibrosing alveolitis
Asbestosis

Cardiac diseases
Congenital heart disease (cyanotic)
Bacterial endocarditis
Atrial myxoma

Gut diseases
Crohn's disease
Tropical sprue
Cirrhosis

Idiopathic/familial

Vascular disorders
Axillary artery aneurysm

Hyperthyroidism
Acropachy

Venous insufficiency

Venous insufficiency causes lipodermatosclerosis, stasis eczema and venous ulceration of the lower legs. Other causes of leg ulcers are given in Table 18.44 on p. 1157 and in LEG ULCERATION AT A GLANCE. The management of venous ulceration is addressd by Table 18.31 and requires collaboration with vascular surgeons to define and rectify potentially operable defects.

Table 18.31 Venous ulceration. Other causes of leg ulceration are given in Table 18.44

Management
Hinges on correcting the aetiological factors and avoiding complications
Good trials of interventions in leg ulceration are difficult to design and are few
The most significant therapeutic measures are exercise, leg elevation and dressings

Main measures
Weight loss
Treat constipation
Exercise the limb
Elevate the limb when at rest
Compressive bandaging

Other measures
Mild to moderate potency steroids may be applied to non-ulcerated skin
Trauma must be avoided
Possible sensitization to topical applications must always be borne in mind: contact dermatitis becomes much more likely when ulceration has supervened because the range of preparations available for leg ulcers is extensive
The patient may have an elemental or vitamin deficiency, which should be corrected. Elderly people living alone often have deficiencies such as protein, vitamin C or zinc
Cellulitis, often caused by *Staphylococcus aureus* or *Streptococcus* spp., should be treated with a systemic antibiotic, which may need to be continued long term. Otherwise bacterial colonization does not necessarily impair wound healing. This is probably not true of *Pseudomonas aeruginosa*, but this is most appropriately treated topically

Dressings
A clean exudate is desirable
Many of the occlusive dressings retain exudate on the ulcer bed (e.g. Gellperm, Granuflex). Slough delays healing
There are numerous topical cleansing and debriding agents that encourage clean granulation upon which healthy re-epithelialization can occur (e.g. Debrisan, Hioxyl, Varidase). The more traditional ones, such as non-adherent (N/A) dressings and paraffin gauze, should remain the mainstay of treatment

Skin grafting
If a clean granulating ulcer base can be achieved, there is a place for skin grafting. Multiple pinch grafts from the thigh are popular and successful in many units

Raynaud's phenomenon

Disease mechanisms

Causes of Raynaud's phenomenon are listed in Table 18.32.

Clinical features

Raynaud's phenomenon is episodic painful digital ischaemia in response to cold or emotional stimuli. It is characterized by classical sequential colour changes of white, blue and red (Fig. 18.29). Idiopathic Raynaud's phenomenon is diagnosed in young women who have no features of an underlying disorder on clinical evaluation or investigation. Raynaud's phenomenon is more likely to be secondary to an underlying disease, usually as a harbinger of systemic sclerosis, if it is especially severe and persistent or if it begins for the first time in early adulthood.

Management

Treatment is avoidance of cold, using heated gloves and systemic vasodilators, of which the mainstay is nifedipine.

Table 18.32 Causes of Raynaud's phenomenon

Idiopathic
Cervical rib
Vibrating tools
Autoimmune rheumatic disease
Arteritis (e.g. giant cell arteritis)
Drugs (e.g. β-blockers and ergot alkaloids)
Hyperviscosity syndromes

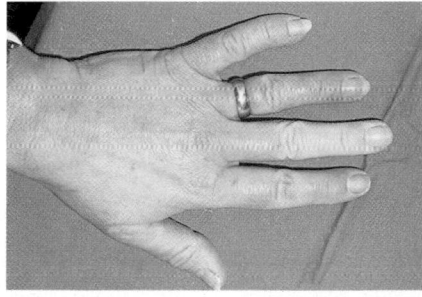

Figure 18.29 Raynaud's phenomenon. Digital pallor of left middle finger. Causes: idiopathic, cervical rib, vibrating tools, autoimmune rheumatic disease, arteritis, drugs (β-blockers, ergot alkaloids), hyperviscosity syndromes.

Perniosis (chilblains)

Perniosis or chilblains are common, sore, itchy, inflammatory lesions of the skin resulting from an abnormal reaction to a moderate degree of cold. There is evidence that suggests the lesions have a vasospastic basis. If the problem is severe, the treatment of choice is probably nifedipine.

Rosacea

Rosacea is a disorder of unknown aetiology, but associated with instability of the facial vasculature, which leads to flushing and the secondary development of inflamed papules and pustules (Fig. 18.30). It is exacerbated by alcohol.

Avoidance of precipitants is helpful. For unknown reasons it responds to tetracycline antibiotics.

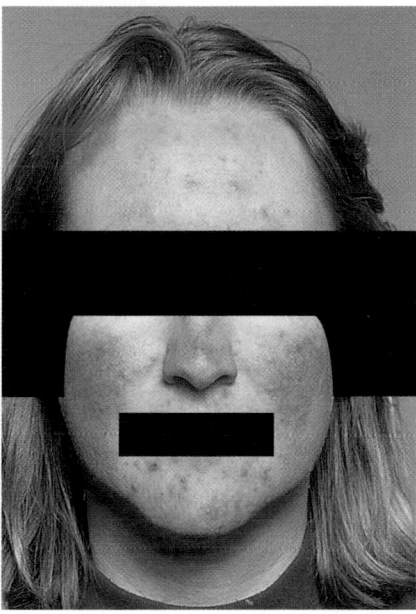

Figure 18.30 Rosacea. Facial erythema, papules, pustules and telangiectasia.

Livedo reticularis

Livedo reticularis is a network of cutaneous cyanosis (Fig. 18.31). Some causes are listed in Table 18.33.

Erythema ab igne is reticulate livedo occurring as a response to chronic heat exposure (e.g. from a hot water bottle or electric fire in the elderly).

Vasculitis

Vasculitis has many causes and some of these have been discussed elsewhere (see p. 220). The characteristic clinical features in the skin range from erythema, livedo reticularis and urticaria, to palpable purpuric papules and nodules, and necrosis and infarction. The signs reflect the calibre of vessel involved, the nature of the inflammatory response, and the severity of the vasculitic insult.

18

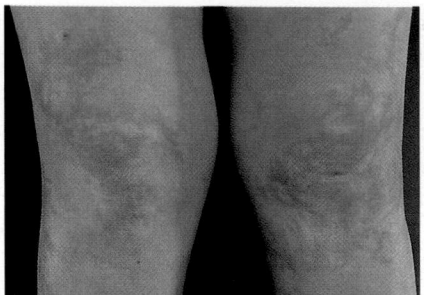

Figure 18.31 Livedo reticularis. Network of cyanotic vascularity in the knees. Causes: lupus erythematosus, polyarteritis nodosa, drugs.

Table 18.33 Causes of livedo reticularis

Physiological (cutis marmorata in young girls)
Vasculitis (as in autoimmune rheumatic disease)
Cholesterol emboli
Thrombocythaemia
Cryoglobulinaemia
Paralysis
Heart failure
Hyperviscosity
Drugs (e.g. amantadine)
Idiopathic

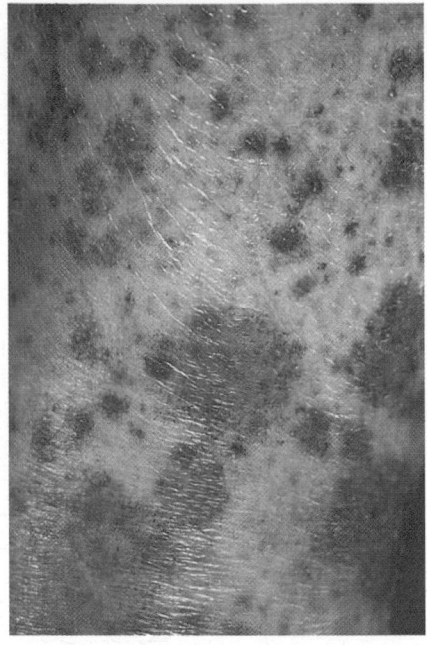

Figure 18.32 Purpura (cryoglobulinaemia).

Allergic vasculitis

Allergic vasculitis usually affects the limbs in the context of fever, malaise, arthralgia and gastrointestinal symptoms (CLINICAL EXAMINATION AT A GLANCE, Fig. O, p. 1107). The most common clinical pattern is acute self-limiting palpable purpura (Fig. 18.32), but it may be chronic or recurrent and other types of vasculitic lesion may be present. The cause is often not discovered, but infections (e.g. streptococcal, tuberculosis, subacute bacterial endocarditis and meningococcal septicaemia), connective tissue disease, neoplasia and drugs should be excluded.

The term **Henoch–Schönlein purpura** (anaphylactoid purpura) should be reserved for the syndrome in children that probably represents a response to a viral infection and in which nephritis may be predominant (see p. 221).

Lymphoedema

Lymphoedema is oedema brought about by inadequate lymphatic drainage (Fig. 18.33). Causes include congenital lymphatic abnormalities, cancer and its treatment, erysipelas and filariasis.

Lymphoedema is managed by:

- Eliminating the underlying cause (e.g. treat chronic infection with long-term antibiotics)
- Using exercise, massage, compression hosiery, pneumatic compression, skin toilet and surgery to increase lymphatic drainage

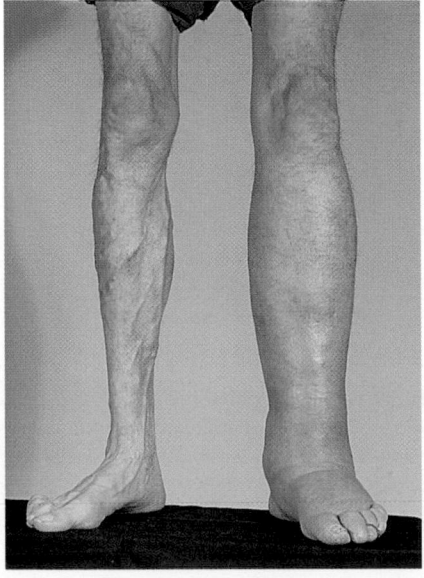

Figure 18.33 Lymphoedema of the leg and foot. Swelling and deep crevices. Reproduced from Champion *et al.* (eds) *Textbook of Dermatology*, 5th edn. Oxford: Blackwell Scientific Publications, 1992 with the permission of the authors.

Table 18.34 Gram-positive cocci and the skin infections they cause

Examples of staphylococcal skin infections	Examples of streptococcal skin infections
Folliculitis	Ecthyma
Sycosis barbae	Erysipelas
Furunculosis	Cellulitis
Ecthyma	Impetigo
Impetigo	Scarlet fever
Cellulitis	Necrotizing fasciitis
Staphylococcal scalded skin syndrome (SSSS)	Erythema nodosum
Vasculitis	? Kawasaki disease
? Kawasaki disease	Superinfects other dermatoses (e.g. leg ulcers)
Toxic shock syndrome (TSS)	
Superinfects other dermatoses (e.g. atopic eczema, HSV, leg ulcers)	

Skin infections

The paediatric exanthems and the cutaneous manifestations of HIV infection are discussed on pp. 143 and 1164 and in Table 18.53. Most skin infections are caused by Gram-positive cocci and are listed in Table 18.34.

Staphylococcal infections (*Staphylococcus aureus*)

Folliculitis

Folliculitis is an infection of hair follicles resulting in a pustular eruption. It is more common in warm moist climates and when occlusive clothes are worn.

Management is with topical antiseptics often diluted in the bath water and an appropriate antibiotic, usually flucloxacillin or erythromycin. Scarring is rare, but post-inflammatory pigment changes may occur (Table 18.35).

Sycosis barbae

Sycosis barbae is a more severe folliculitis. Infected follicles in the beard area coalesce to form a plaque dotted with pustules. Topical or systemic antibiotics are required.

Table 18.35 Treatment of staphylococcal skin infections

Specific treatment	If recurrent, exclude:
Topical	Nasal carriage
Fucidic acid	Iron deficiency
Mupirocin	Diabetes mellitus
Neomycin	Immunodeficiency
Systemic	
Flucloxacillin	
Erythromycin	
Teicoplanin	
Vancomycin	

Furunculosis

Furuncles are boils. The infection is deeper seated than folliculitis and may require incision and drainage. Scarring occasionally occurs if it is not treated early with an appropriate antibiotic (Table 18.35). Recurrent furunculosis should lead to the suspicion of nasal carriage of staphylococci. A carbuncle is a more extensive subcutaneous infection.

Impetigo

Impetigo is caused by staphylococci able to elaborate a toxin that cleaves the upper layers of the epidermis (Fig. 18.34). The eruption is therefore vesicobullous, and

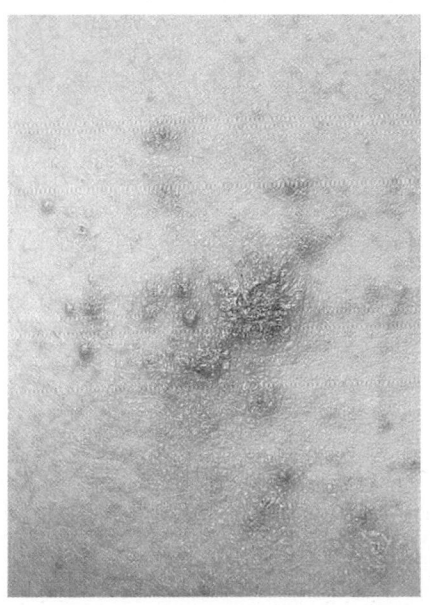

Figure 18.34 Impetigo. Vesicopustules with golden crust.

18

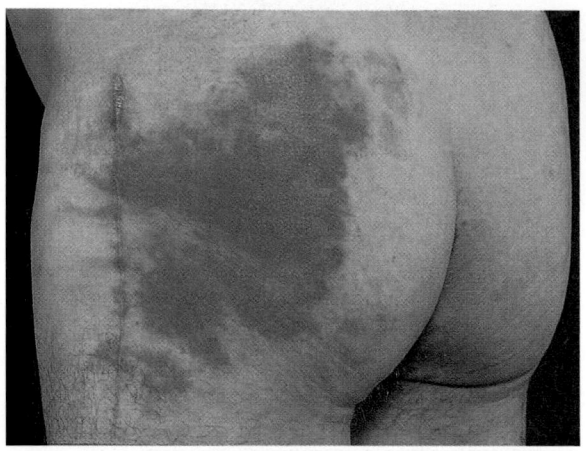

Figure 18.35 Cellulitis complicating hip replacement operation site.

often on the face (perioral, ears, nares) and in the armpits. Vesicles rupture to form a crust. The crusts should be soaked off and topical fucidic acid or mupirocin applied several times a day. Systemic antibiotics are sometimes given. Impetigo does not scar.

Non-bullous impetigo may be caused by streptococci.

Cellulitis

Cellulitis is infection of subcutaneous connective tissue and may be acute or chronic. Oedema and lymphoedema are predisposing factors and recurrent attacks may be caused by successive destruction of local lymphatic architecture. Tender swelling with ill-defined erythema around a wound or ulcer or oedema are the physical signs (Fig. 18.35). Oral antibiotics should be prescribed, often in long courses, and prophylactically (Table 18.36).

Staphylococcal scalded skin syndrome

In staphylococcal scalded skin syndrome (SSSS) there is a generalized skin reaction to a toxin-producing staphylococcus. It is characterized by generalized erythema and exfoliation in an unwell child. The organism cannot be cultured from the denuded skin. Sometimes SSSS occurs in immunocompromised adults (e.g. those being treated for leukaemia or lymphoma). The important differential diagnosis is **toxic epidermal necrolysis** (TEN; p. 1167), which is usually a result of an adverse reaction to a drug. The level of the skin split is deeper in the epidermis in TEN than SSSS and this can be established by biopsy.

Management

The patient should be admitted to hospital so that systemic antistaphylococcal treatment can be given and fluid, electrolyte and nutritional balances can be monitored.

Toxic shock syndrome

Toxic shock syndrome (TSS) is described on p. 125. Staphylococcal toxins are implicated in TSS.

Streptococcal infections

Ecthyma

Ecthyma is pyogenic ulceration of the skin with adherent crusts. It is associated with poor hygiene and nutrition and may complicate insect bites or scabies infestation. Its microbiology is similar to impetigo (see above) with streptococci and staphylococci implicated and often both may be present. Systemic antibiotics are usually needed (Table 18.36).

Erysipelas

Erysipelas is infection of the deep dermis and subcutis (Fig. 18.36). Pain draws attention to sharply defined bright erythema, often on the face or limb; there may be desquamation. There may be a red streak of lymphangitis and enlarged local lymph nodes if it involves the arm or leg. The patient is usually unwell. Hospitalization and intravenous antibiotics (penicillin) are usually indicated. Subsequently, prophylactic penicillin may be offered. A portal of entry should be sought (e.g. tinea pedis).

Scarlet fever

Scarlet fever is caused by upper respiratory tract infection

Specific treatment	Investigations
Topical (often not sufficient)	Swab
Fucidic acid	ASOT
Mupirocin	DNAase
Neomycin	Do not fail to consider the possibility of:
	(a) complications of *Strep.* infection
Systemic (often intravenous)	(b) necrotizing fasciitis
Penicillin	
Ampicillin	
Erythromycin	

Table 18.36 Treatment of streptococcal skin infections

18

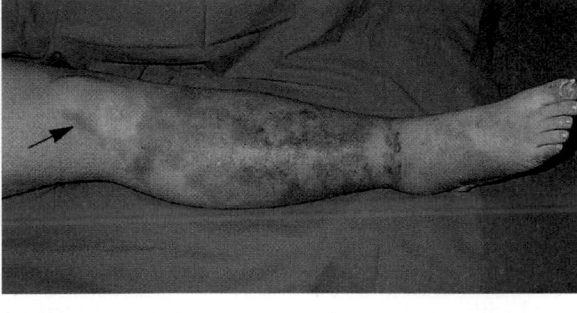

Figure 18.36 Erysipelas. Note superior linear track of lymphangitis indicated by arrow.

with erythrogenic toxin-producing streptococci. The toxin causes the cutaneous vasodilatation.

Necrotizing fasciitis

Necrotizing fasciitis is a serious synergistic infection involving streptococci, staphylococci, Enterobacteriaceae and obligate anaerobes. Alternatively, the syndrome may be caused by *Streptococcus pyogenes* alone. The infection may begin in a wound in an unwell patient, but often there is no obvious portal of entry in a healthy individual. The first sign is usually a dusky induration with rapid progressive painful necrosis of skin, connective tissue and even muscle.

Prompt diagnosis is essential, but antibiotics are rarely completely successful and surgical debridement is necessary. There is an appreciable mortality. The infection usually occurs on a limb, but can affect the scrotum (Fournier's gangrene) where other Gram-negative organisms may be involved.

Progressive (Meleney's) synergistic gangrene

Progressive synergistic gangrene complicates wound healing, trauma, instrumentation diabetes, cancer and HIV. It is usually a mixed streptococcal–staphylococcal infection. Debridement and intravenous antibiotics are indicated.

Complications of streptococcal infections

Nephritis, but not rheumatic fever, may follow streptococcal skin infections. Although the overall incidence has declined, it is still advisable to treat all the streptococcal skin infections mentioned above with systemic penicillin or erythromycin.

Hypersensitivity to *Streptococcus* has been implicated in erythema nodosum (Fig. 18.37), some vasculitides and guttate psoriasis. Diagnosis of streptococcal disease is not always possible by culture of the organism. The antistreptolysin (ASO) and anti-DNAase titres may be helpful.

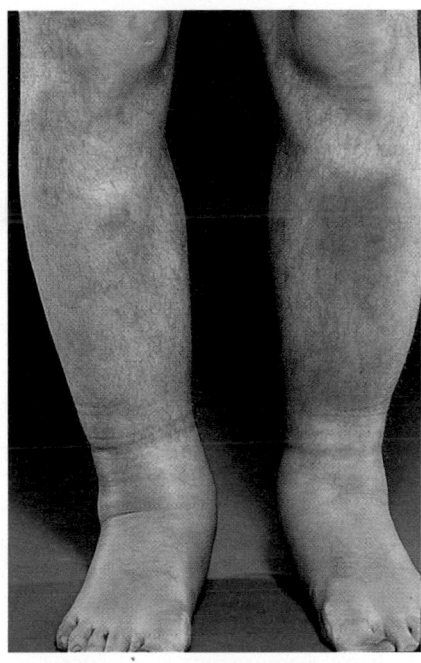

Figure 18.37 Erythema nodosum. Causes: streptococcal infection, sarcoid, tuberculosis.

Mycobacterial infection

Cutaneous tuberculosis

Cutaneous tuberculosis is now relatively rare in the UK. Occasionally, **lupus vulgaris** (Fig. 18.38) may be seen in immigrants. Tuberculosis must be excluded in patients

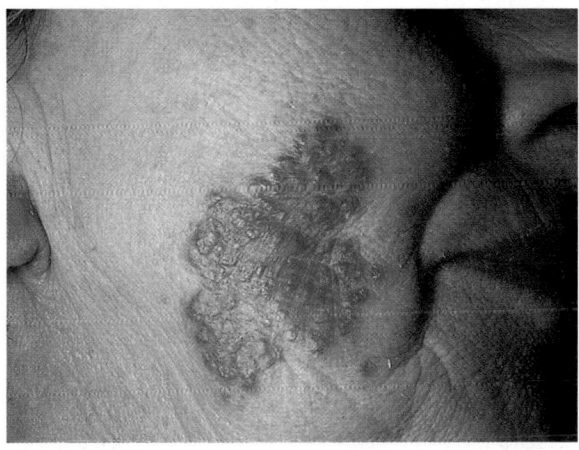

Figure 18.38 Lupus vulgaris of the cheek. Erythematous indurated granulomatous plaque. Courtesy of Professor J.A.A. Hunter, Edinburgh Royal Infirmary. Reproduced from Champion *et al.* (eds) *Textbook of Dermatology*, 5th edn. Oxford: Blackwell Scientific Publications, 1992 with the permission of the authors.

18

presenting with erythema nodosum (Fig. 18.37). A full general examination, chest radiography, tuberculin testing and skin biopsy are needed.

Atypical mycobacterial infection

Atypical mycobacterial infection can cause skin lesions in AIDS and other immunosuppressed states. *Mycobacterium marinum* can result in an indolent granulomatous ulcer (swimming pool or fish-tank granuloma) in otherwise well people. *M. ulcerans* is an important cause of limb ulceration in Africa (Buruli ulcer) or Australia (Searle's ulcer).

Other bacterial infections

Borreliosis (Lyme disease)

Lyme disease is a zoonosis caused by the spirochaete *Borrelia burgdorferi* after the bite of the *Ixodes ricinus* (UK) or *I. dammini* (USA) tick. This causes a spreading indurated annular erythema (erythema chronicum migrans), which may become very large. Arthritis, cardiac disease or neurological disease may occur many weeks later. Diagnosis is by serology for the spirochaete, and treatment is with oral amoxicillin or doxycycline or intravencus cephalosporin or penicillin.

Erythrasma

Erythrasma is suggested by a well-defined wrinkled patch with a reddy brown discoloration seen in intertriginous areas (groins, axillae and breasts). It may cause maceration between the toes. The organism is *Corynebacterium minutissimum*, which fluoresces coral pink under Wood's light (Fig. 18.7), and responds to topical imidazoles or systemic erythromycin.

Pitted keratolysis

Pitted keratolysis occurs on dirty macerated feet shod with unsuitable occlusive trainers. It is caused by *Micrococcus sedentarius*, which produces pitted erosions and brown discoloration of the soles and heels.

Pitted keratolysis is improved by better hygiene and footwear, potassium permanganate soaks and topical clindamycin or topical fusidic acid.

Erysipeloid

Erysipeloid is an infection of the hand caused by *Erysipelothrix rhusiopathiae* after handling contaminated raw fish or meat. A slowly evolving, red, oedematous process affects the hand and fingers over several weeks.

The organism is sensitive to penicillin.

Anthrax

Cutaneous *Bacillus anthracis* infection is very rare. It causes a painless necrotic ulcer with surrounding oedema and regional lymphadenopathy at the site of contact with infected hides, bone meal or wool. It is painful and causes systemic upset with regional lymphadenopathy.

Treatment is with doxycycline or ciprofloxacin.

Pseudomonas infection

Pseudomonas aeruginosa can cause otitis externa, toe web infections, necrotic ulcers, paronychia (the nails may appear green or black) and a specific folliculitis (associated with systemic symptoms) after recent immersion in hot tubs or whirlpool baths.

Viral infections

Herpes simplex virus (HSV) infection

Any skin or mucosal site may be infected with and show recurrence of herpes simplex virus (HSV Type 1) infection. The lesions are painful vesicles and crusts on an erythematous base that heal and resolve over 2 weeks (Fig. 18.39). Genital infections are more often caused by HSV Type 2 (see p. 163).

Diagnosis is clinical, but may be supported by viral culture, electron microscopy and serology.

Management includes:

- Aciclovir cream to treat the primary infection
- Oral aciclovir if the infection is severe and in the immunosuppressed
- Treatment of secondary infection with topical and sometimes systemic antibiotics
- Prophylaxis with oral aciclovir if indicated

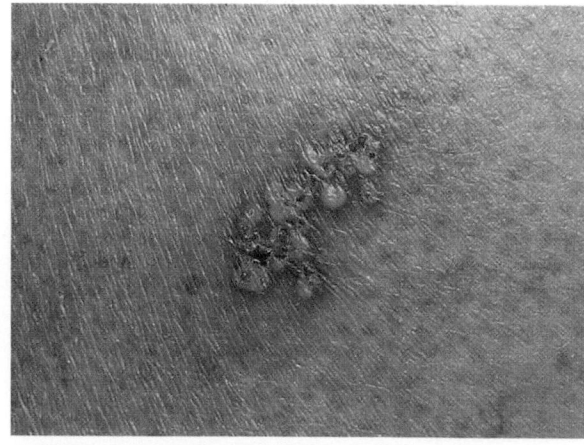

Figure 18.39 Herpes simplex. Erythema and vesicles.

Herpes zoster virus (HZV)
Chickenpox

Chickenpox is usually a disorder of childhood, when

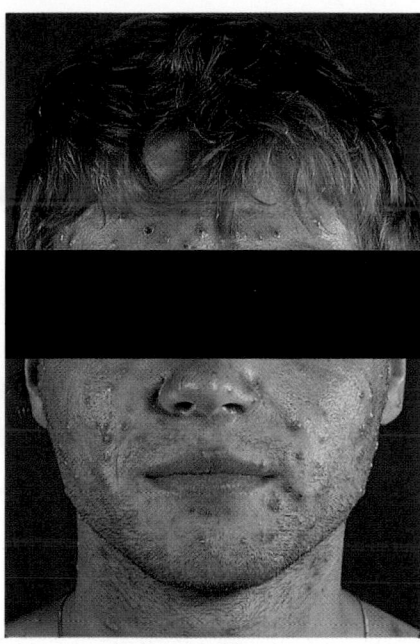

Figure 18.40 Chickenpox. Crops of vesicles and pustules.

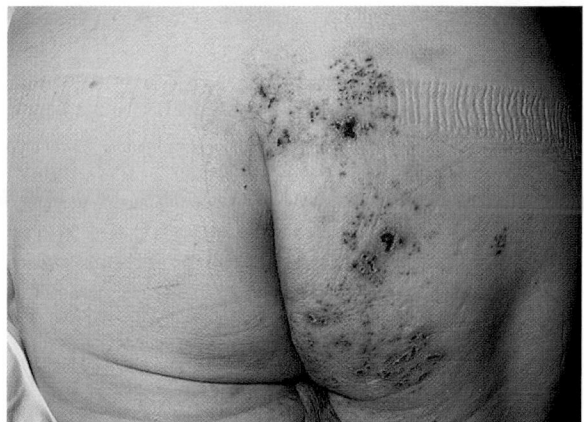

Figure 18.41 Shingles. Healing with pain, crusts and scars.

there is little or no prodrome, but may occur in adults when the prodrome can be severe. The rash is centripetal and also affects the oral mucosa with crops of lesions at different stages of development (macules, papules, vesicles and crusts) over 10 days (Fig. 18.40). Treatment is conservative, but topical and even systemic antibiotics may be needed to counter bacterial superinfection. Topical steroids may prevent scarring.

Shingles

Disease mechanisms. Shingles results from reactivation of HZV. In lymphoproliferative disorders, zoster may be severe and recurrent. Underlying malignancy is found no more frequently than in the normal population. Physical trauma to the involved dermatome may be the most common trigger.

Clinical features. Paraesthesiae and pain precede the eruption. Sometimes there is no sensory prodrome and very rarely there is pain and no eruption (*zoster sine herpete*). Post-herpetic neuralgia may persist for years. The rash is variable, but usually asymmetrical. Erythematous oedematous papules and vesicles arise in one crop, become haemorrhagic and necrotic, and then scab and heal with superficial scarring (Fig. 18.41). Outlying lesions are found in most patients if looked for. Severe generalization can occur in people with immune deficiency. Recurrent zoster is rare and rarely at the same site.

Investigation. Diagnosis is clinical, but shingles can be confused with HSV so viral culture, electron microscopy and serology are useful.

Management. Potent analgesics may need to be given to control the pain. Topical steroids and antibiotics are used to control cutaneous inflammation and secondary bacterial infection, respectively. Post-herpetic neuralgia is a consequence of the main insult of zoster, to the nerves and not the skin; it can be intractable. A short course of oral prednisolone from the onset may reduce the risk. Ophthalmic zoster may cause conjunctivitis or rarely optic neuritis. Zoster of S2 and below may present with acute retention of urine and constipation, and haemorrhagic cystitis. In these instances, as for motor zoster, zoster encephalomyelitis, purpura fulminans and zoster in the immunologically compromised, systemic therapy with aciclovir is indicated and may save sight, sphincter function, facial expression and even life. Oral aciclovir probably reduces the time course of the cutaneous eruption, but whether it affects the development of post-herpetic neuralgia is doubtful.

Hand, foot and mouth disease

Hand, foot and mouth disease is an acute epidemic self-limiting infection with a coxsackievirus with vesicular lesions in the mouth and on the palms and soles.

Orf

Orf is caused by a poxvirus that causes an ulcerative stomatitis in sheep. Farmers and vets may develop a large tender nodule on the hands or face. Secondary erythema multiforme is almost universal.

Treatment with antibiotics is usually required for secondary infection.

18

Warts

Warts are caused by human papillomavirus (HPV) of which there are many types: HPV1, 2, 4 cause common warts and verrucas; HPV 16 and 18 are associated with cervical cancer.

HPV has a fastidious requirement for human epidermal cells in a particular stage of differentiation. It causes a proliferation of keratinocytes, which partially keratinize and therefore sequester the virus from immunological elimination. Lesions may be sporadic, recurrent or persistent (Fig. 18.42).

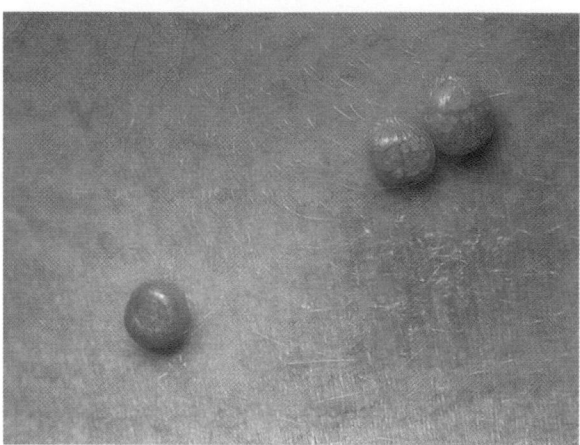

Figure 18.43 Molluscum contagiosum. Dome-shaped papules with central umbilication.

Fungal infections

Candidosis

Candidosis is usually an intertriginous infection (affecting the axillae, submammary folds [Fig. 18.44], crurae and digital clefts). It is a common cause of vulvovaginitis in women. In the immunocompetent, it may also affect the mucosa and genitalia. It is treated with topical nystatin, imidazole or clioquinol.

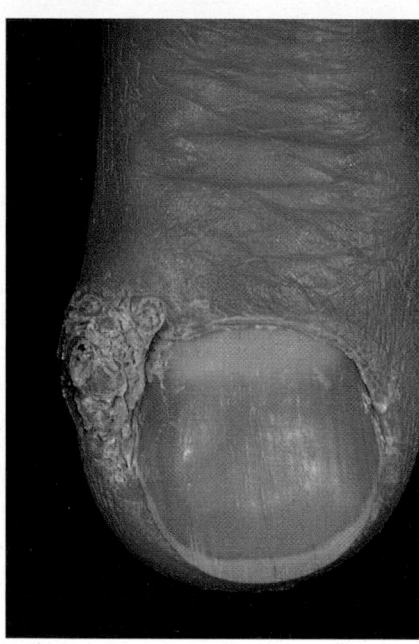

Figure 18.42 Periungual viral wart. Papillomatosis, hyperkeratosis and loss of dermatoglyphics.

Management

Treatment is with keratolytics (such as salicylic acid or retinoic acid) or cryotherapy. Cautery and surgical excision may result in lower treatment success rates and scarring. Persistent warts can be treated by laser or intralesional bleomycin.

Molluscum contagiosum

Molluscum contagiosum is caused by a poxvirus. The typical lesion is an umbilicated dome-shaped papule or nodule (Fig. 18.43). Lesions are common on the trunk in children and usually resolve spontaneously. Cryotherapy is the treatment of choice in adults and is occasionally tolerated by a child.

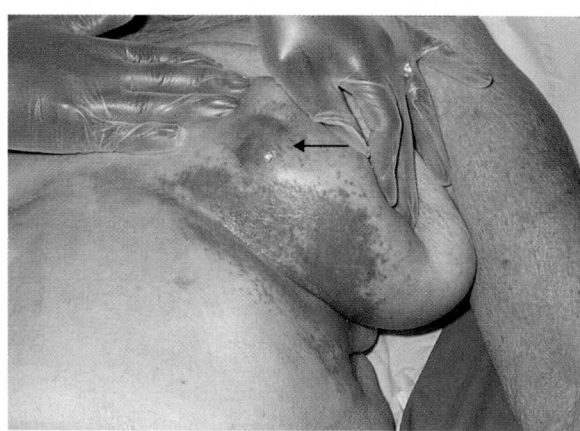

Figure 18.44 Candidosis. Erythematous, almost eroded intertrigo. Note satellite lesions and nodular breast carcinoma (arrow).

Pityriasis versicolor

Pityriasis versicolor is a superficial infection of the horny layer by the *Malassezia* yeasts. It is characterized by small confluent scaly depigmented patches, which are often apparent for the first time after tanning (Fig. 18.45).

18

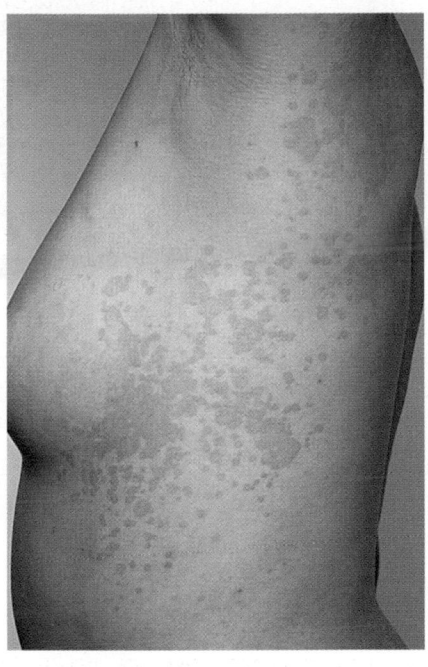

Figure 18.45 Pityriasis versicolor. Petaloid, scaly macules.

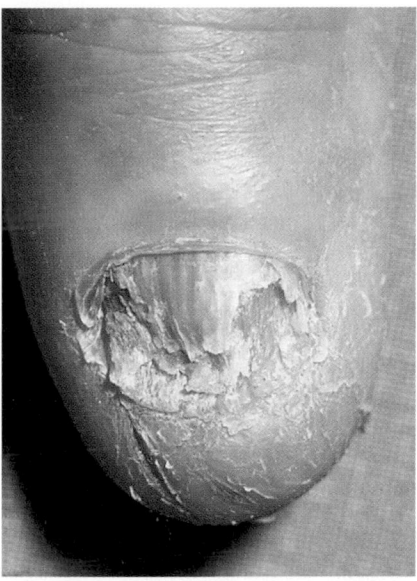

Figure 18.47 Onychomyosis. Tinea unguium/gross nail dystrophy. Linear burrows in web space.

Treatment is with a topical imidazole or with selenium sulphide shampoo. Occasionally, an oral antifungal such as itraconazole is used.

Dermatophytosis

Dermatophytosis is the term for ringworm infection. Lesions are red, scaly and itchy. The groins and feet are common sites (Fig. 18.46); the lesions are then not necessarily circular and scaly, but are macerated and moist with a scaly edge. The nails may be involved (onychomycosis; Fig. 18.47).

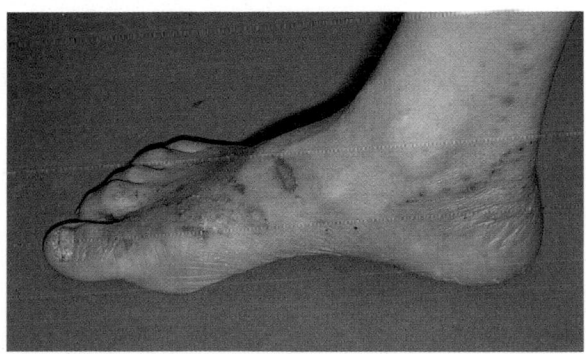

Figure 18.46 Tinea pedis. Well-marginated erythematous scaly eruption (moccasin pattern).

Scarring may occur on the scalp because of an infected inflammatory plaque called a kerion. *Microsporum* spp. form spores around hair (ectothrix) and fluoresce green under Wood's lamp, whereas *Trichophyton* spp. invade the hair shaft (endothrix) and do not fluoresce.

Conventional treatment is with a topical imidazole or griseofulvin or terbinafine orally. Systemic therapy is necessary for scalp or nail infections. Oral ketoconazole is not widely prescribed because of liver toxicity. Newer imidazoles are safer (Tables 18.5 and 18.6).

Skin infestations

Scabies

Scabies must always enter the differential diagnosis of pruritus. Typically, the rash is symmetrical, involving the fingers (Fig. 18.48), backs of hands, axillae, breasts and buttocks. Most of the lesions may be excoriated papules and nodules, but with care, burrows may usually be identified. Sites to examine carefully are digital clefts, around the nipples and the genitalia. By taking a skin scraping, burrow contents may be examined under a microscope. The presence of the female mite (*Sarcoptes scabiei*) or her eggs confirms the diagnosis (Fig. 18.49). Apposition of skin surfaces for several minutes is needed to transmit the infestation, so sexual contact is the usual means of spread.

18

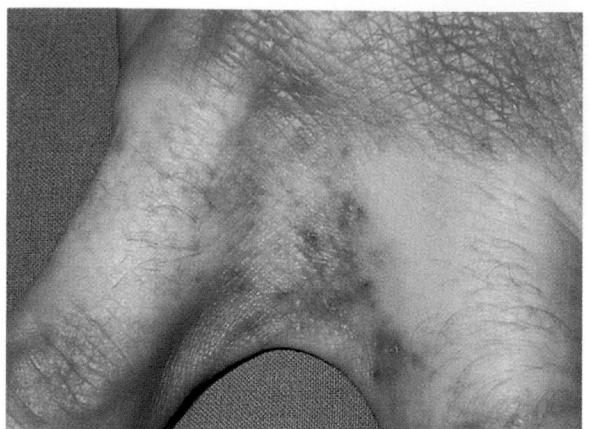

Figure 18.48 Scabies.

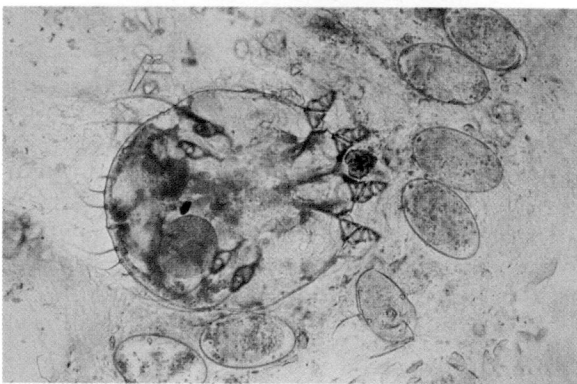

Figure 18.49 *Sarcoptes scabiei*, the scabies mite. Female with eggs. Reproduced from Champion *et al.* (eds) *Textbook of Dermatology*, 5th edn. Oxford: Blackwell Scientific Publications, 1992 with the permission of the authors.

Pediculosis (lice)

Pediculosis pubis is caused by *Phthirus pubis*, the crab louse, so named because of its appearance.

Pediculosis capitis is caused by the head louse, which sucks blood from the scalp and lays eggs that are cemented to the hair shaft (nits). Bites become itchy excoriations.

Pediculosis corporis is caused by a very similar louse, the clothing or body louse, which lives in the seams of clothing and lays its eggs there. It is sometimes responsible for a widespread itchy excoriated dermatosis (vagabond's disease).

Management

Infestations are managed by topical insecticides (malathion, permethrin, γ-benzene hexachloride). Secondary eczema and infection should also be treated. The insecticide is applied to cool dry skin all over the body.

In scabies in adults and people without HIV, the head can be omitted. Usually, patients sleep with the treatment on their skin and wash it off in the morning. It is usual to repeat the treatment the following night. It is mandatory to advise patients to suggest that their partners and cohabitants are treated at the same time and that they should attend for full sexually transmitted disease and genitourinary clinic screening.

Skin tumours

There are many cell types in skin that contribute to the large number of recognized benign and malignant skin tumours. In practice, only a few types of skin tumour are common, but skin cancer is the most common of all cancers in the UK, reflecting the proliferative nature of the epithelium and environmental exposure. Causes of skin tumours are listed in Table 18.37.

Table 18.37 Causes of skin tumours

UV light
Thermal injury
X-radiation
Hydrocarbons
Arsenic
Immunosuppression (e.g. renal transplantation)
Human papillomaviruses (HPV)
Human T-cell lymphotropic virus I (HTLV-I)
Bartonella henselae—bacillary angiomatosis
Human herpes virus 8 (HHV8)–Kaposi's sarcoma
Genetic predisposition

Epithelial tumours

Epidermoid cysts

Epidermoid cysts (misnomer, sebaceous cyst; they are filled with keratin not sebum) are smooth papules or nodules with a central punctum. They are common on the head, neck, ears or back and may become secondarily infected if traumatized. Treatment is by excision.

Gardner's syndrome is an autosomal dominant disorder in which epidermoid cysts are associated with premalignant gastrointestinal polyposis.

Pilar cyst

Pilar cysts (wens) are usually familial, multiple and occur on the scalp. There is no punctum, but the cysts contain keratin. Occasionally, the lesions may grow to a large size and ulcerate, simulating squamous carcinoma (Cock's peculiar tumour). Treatment is by excision.

Basal cell papilloma

Basal cell papillomas (seborrhoeic warts, senile warts) are

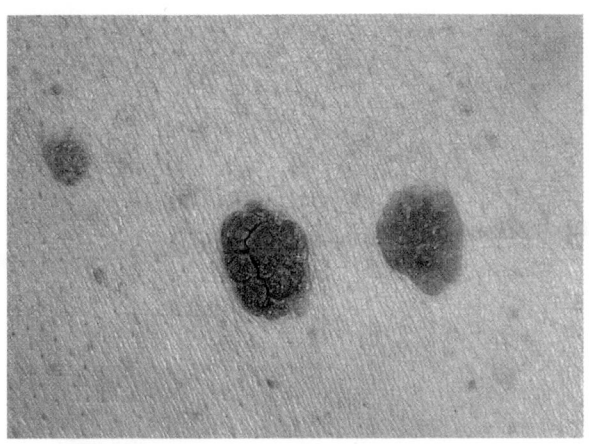

Figure 18.50 Basal cell papillomas. Tan to black, warty, flat papules and nodules.

flesh-coloured, tan, brown or black, round, broad-based, flat-topped greasy lesions (Fig. 18.50). They are common on the trunk and face with increasing age. If necessary, treatment is by cryotherapy or curettage and cautery.

Very rarely, eruptive symptomatic basal cell papilloma may signify internal malignancy (Leser–Trélat sign).

Other epithelial tumours
- *Viral warts:* discussed on p. 1140.
- *Dermatosis papulosa nigra:* describes a very common profusion of tiny pigmented filiform epidermal proliferations on the face and neck of people with dark skin.
- *Epidermal naevus:* a congenital lesion, which usually occurs as a thickened plaque that histologically may contain any hamartomatous elements of skin. Occasionally, it may be part of a systemic syndrome in association with other defects.
- *Sebaceous naevus:* the elements are predominantly derived from sebaceous glands and may be complicated by transformation to basal cell carcinoma in later life. Plastic excision is usually recommended in early adulthood. Benign appendageal tumours are common.
- *Syringomas:* small flesh-coloured ovoid lesions on the cheeks and around the eyes.
- *Trichoepitheliomas:* small, rounded and translucent, they occur around the nose and mouth.
- *Sebaceous hyperplasia:* small pearly microcysts on the face and forehead, which may be confused with basal cell carcinoma.

Keratoacanthoma
Keratoacanthoma is a rapidly growing nodular lesion on the light-exposed skin of the hand or face. It reaches its maximum size in 1–2 months when it appears as a smooth dome-shaped lesion with a central crater filled with keratinaceous material. It can spontaneously involute to leave scarring but should be treated as a suspected squamous carcinoma.

Multiple keratoacanthomas, sebaceous neoplasia and gastrointestinal malignancy constitute the **Muir–Torré syndrome**.

Solar (actinic) keratosis
A keratosis is a palpable, scaly, often erythematous lesion (see SQUAMOUS CELL CARCINOMA AT A GLANCE, Figs A and C) that shows epidermal dysplasia on histology and has a recognizable, albeit low, risk of developing into Bowen's disease or squamous carcinoma. It may be associated with actinic damage, X-ray exposure, thermal damage (in blast-furnace workers), arsenic ingestion, immuno-suppression after organ transplantation and topical hydrocarbon exposure.

Cryotherapy or topical 5-fluorouracil or diclofenac cream are used for treatment.

Bowen's disease
Intra-epidermal carcinoma (Bowen's disease) presents as a single red scaly patch (SQUAMOUS CELL CARCINOMA AT A GLANCE, Fig. B), which may be mistaken for eczema or psoriasis, but it does not itch and does not respond to topical steroids. Sometimes there are multiple lesions. It is associated with exposure to one or more of the agents associated with keratosis (see above) and can be treated in the same way, but surgical curettage or excision is often favoured for the single lesion.

Histology shows a disorganized epidermis with abnormal keratinocytes and atypical mitotic figures. The condition can progress to squamous cell carcinoma.

Basal cell carcinoma/epithelioma
Disease mechanisms
Basal cell carcinoma/epithelioma (BCE) is an extremely common neoplasm on the face, head and neck of elderly people (BASAL CELL EPITHELIOMA AT A GLANCE). Although it is extremely rare for it to metastasize, its indolent growth may lead to delayed presentation and deep invasion, particularly into embryological fusion borders. This can lead to high rates of recurrence after conventional treatments. Actinic damage is the greatest risk factor for BCE, but sometimes multiple BCEs are associated with previous X-ray treatment of ankylosing spondylitis (spine) and tinea capitis (scalp). Rarely, multiple BCEs are caused by **Gorlin's syndrome**, which is characterized by the presence of multiple BCEs in a young adult, palmar pits, bifid ribs and dental anomalies with jaw cysts.

Management
Excisional biopsy, curettage and cautery and radiotherapy are conventional approaches, but recurrence rates may be

Basal cell epithelioma at a glance

Epidemiology
Prevalence
100 000 cases in the UK, 2001; 90% of non-melanoma skin cancers

Age
More common in the elderly

Race
Races with fair complexion

Other
Associated with chronic exposure to UVB and, more rarely, exposure to non-ionizing radiation and inorganic arsenic

Clinical features
Lesions commonly at sides of the nose and around the orbit
Slow-growing, pearly, flesh-coloured translucent smooth papules or nodules with rolled edges or plaques
Surface telangiectasia
Frequent central necrosis with crusting or ulceration
More rarely, cystic or pigmented lesions

Management
Cryosurgery
Curettage/cautery
Excisional surgery (± grafting)
Mohs' micrographic surgery (± grafting)
Chemosurgery (intralesional 5-fluorouracil)
Radiotherapy

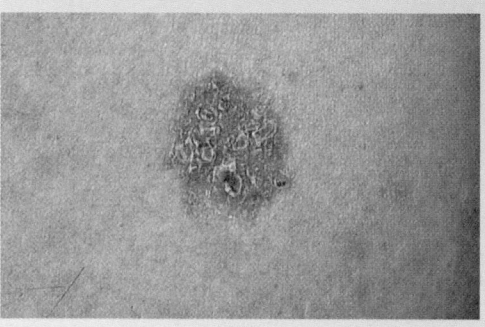

Fig. C Superficial basal cell carcinoma on back of shin. Red scaly patch.

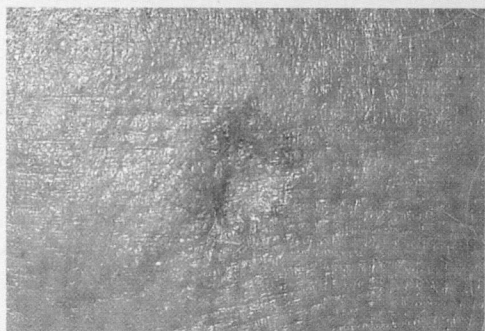

Fig. D Morphoeic basal cell carcinoma on the face. Irregular plaque.

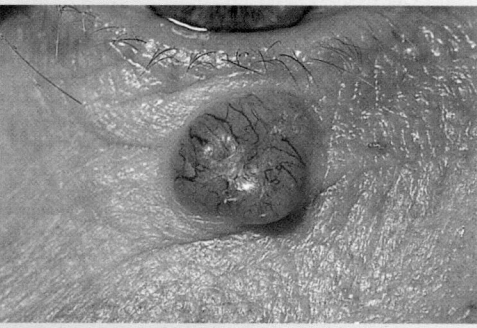

Fig. A Basal cell carcinoma below the right eye. Nodule.

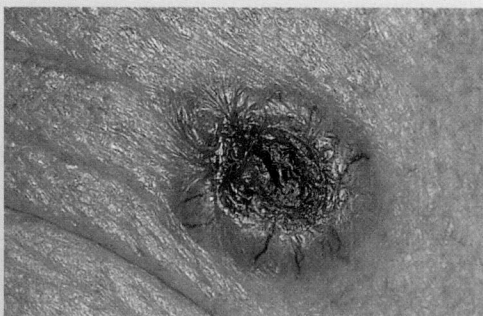

Fig. B Classical crateriform basal cell carcinoma. Ulcerating nodule.

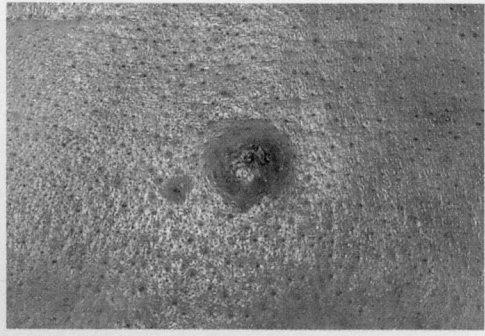

Fig. E Pigmented basal cell carcinoma. Courtesy of Dr R.C.D. Staughton.

5–20%, depending on the chronicity and site of the lesion. Tumours around the eye and furrows of the nose invade embryological fusion planes early. The best results (99.5% cure) are those achieved by Mohs' micrographic surgery with subsequent plastic repair, but this painstaking technique is reserved for specially selected cases. Late presentation or failed treatment is complicated by fungation, involvement of other structures (such as the eye and lacrimal apparatus), deep invasion with destruction of cartilage, bone and periosteum, and effectively incurable disease.

Squamous cell carcinoma

Squamous cell carcinoma occurs in sun-exposed areas in elderly people (SQUAMOUS CELL CARCINOMA AT A GLANCE). Risk factors are those discussed in Table 18.37, but also include pipe smoking (for lip tumours) and chronic inflammation. Venous ulceration, lupus vulgaris, lichen planus, lichen sclerosus and epidermolysis bullosa may be complicated by squamous cell carcinoma (e.g. Marjolin's ulcer of the leg). The best-known occupational cancer in the past was cancer of the scrotum in chimney sweeps, which was related to exposure to the hydrocarbons in soot. Features of the congenital condition xeroderma pigmentosum (photosensitivity leading to atrophy, pigmentary changes and skin malignancy caused by a DNA repair defect) are given in Table 18.43.

Squamous cell carcinoma most commonly presents as a spreading invasive ulcer, but it may present as a rapidly growing nodule.

The differential diagnosis of mouth and leg ulcers is given in Tables 18.44 and 18.55, respectively. Ulcers on the lip may also be caused by herpes simplex and syphilis. The nodular form on the face and hand may be difficult to differentiate from keratoacanthoma.

Squamous cell carcinoma may be very destructive locally, but can also metastasize to the lymph nodes and other organs. Treatment must therefore be ablative and long-term follow-up is necessary.

Melanocytic tumours

The assessment of a patient with a solitary or multiple pigmented lesions is a common, but not always straightforward, exercise (Table 18.38). There should be a high index of suspicion and a low threshold for excision and biopsy if the lesion cannot be confidently diagnosed clinically.

Freckles

Freckles (ephelides) are light-induced pigmented macules in which the number of melanocytes is unchanged, but the number of melanosomes per melanocyte is increased.

Table 18.38 Assessment of pigmented lesions

History
Congenital or acquired
Change in size, shape, colour, bulk
Itch or bleed
Family history
Sun exposure
Skin type

Examination
Irregular size, shape, pigmentation, surface
Ulceration

Phenotype
Numerous other naevi
Atpical naevi
Atypically distributed naevi
Actinic damage

Lentigines

Lentigines look similar to freckles, but also occur on non-sun-exposed areas and do not vary in colour with sun exposure. They are caused by a focal increase in the number of melanocytes. Congenital disorders associated with lentigines include **Peutz–Jeghers** and **LEOPARD** syndromes (Table 18.43).

Senile lentigo

Senile lentigo (liver spot) is a large tan-coloured lesion on sun-exposed areas of elderly people.

Melanocytic naevus

Melanocytic naevi (moles) are localized collections of melanocytes. Most people have up to 10. The clinical and histological features are shown in Fig. 18.51. They begin to appear in childhood and may later progress from junctional to compound and intradermal. At puberty and during pregnancy 'junctional activity' is evident from changes in colour, size and shape.

Halo naevus

Halo naevus is a mole with an area of vitiligo around it and is associated with the same conditions as vitiligo (Table 18.23).

Congenital melanocytic naevus

Congenital melanocytic naevi are large pigmented lesions (Fig. 18.52) that are present from birth. They are common anywhere, but a bathing trunk distribution is recognized. There is a risk of malignant melanoma developing in large lesions (and, it is now thought, in small lesions). Problems in quantifying this risk include defining how big is big

18

(5 cm is usually taken as the cut-off point) and ascertaining that small lesions are congenital.

Spitz naevus

This is a rapidly growing but benign pigmented smooth dome-shaped nodule, which may remit spontaneously in a 4–10-year-old child. Spindle cell naevus (of Reid) is a similar lesion in adults. It is often dense black and occurs on the thighs of women.

Dysplastic naevus

The features of dysplastic naevi that may be associated with an increased risk of melanoma are given in Table 18.39. Often what a histopathologist describes as dysplastic may not equate with a clinically characterized dysplastic naevus (Fig. 18.53). The dysplastic/atypical naevus syndrome is the presence of multiple dysplastic naevi (often larger than 2 cm) in the context of a personal or first-degree family history of melanoma.

Table 18.39 Features of atypical/dysplastic naevi that may be associated with an increased risk of melanoma

Criteria	Feature
Clinical	Larger than 5 mm, single or multiple, irregular shape, size, surface, colour, familial, sporadic
Histological	Atypical basal melanocytes, collagen changes, lymphocytic infiltrate

Lentigo maligna (melanoma)

Lentigo maligna (Hutchinson's freckle) is a slow-growing pigmented macule on the face in older people. Histologically it is an intra-epidermal melanoma, but can become invasive at any stage (lentigo maligna melanoma). Treatment is by excision (with plastic repair if necessary).

Malignant melanoma

Epidemiology

Prevalence. 5000 new cases (doubling every decade) and 1500 deaths in the UK in 2000. UK lifetime risk is 1 in 200.

Sex. Most common on the legs in women and on the back in men.

Race. Rare in Afro-Caribbeans and Asians, common in Scots and Australians.

Disease mechanisms

A genetically determined susceptibility to excessive ultraviolet light exposure is proposed (MALIGNANT MELANOMA AT A GLANCE).

Risk factors for melanoma are:
- Family history (melanoma, atypical naevus syndrome)
- Skin type (I–II), freckling tendency
- Sun exposure (severe sunburn, short sharp exposures in childhood)
- Total numbers of all naevi (more than 50)
- Numbers of atypical naevi
- Distribution of naevi (e.g. scalp, buttocks feet, iris lentigines)
- Congenital naevi
- Depletion of the ozone layer

Clinical features

The clinical subtypes of melanoma are summarized in MALIGNANT MELANOMA AT A GLANCE. Many melanomas do not arise from an existing mole. The earliest growth of superficial spreading melanoma is in the horizontal plane so presentation is usually as a new or abnormal freckle. Melanoma invades locally and metastasizes early.

On examination, assess the phenotype for sun damage and other risk factors (freckles, and numbers and types

---

Squamous cell carcinoma at a glance

Epidemiology

Prevalence
1 in 2000 population/year in the USA; 10% of non-melanoma skin cancers

Age
More common in the elderly

Race
Races with fair complexion

Risk factors
Type I–II skin; sun exposure; actinic keratoses; non-ionizing radiation; arsenic; immunosuppression (HIV, renal transplant); human papillomavirus; xeroderma pigmentosum; chronic inflammation (venous ulceration, leprosy, lupus vulgaris)

Clinical features
Hyperkeratotic and crusting lesions
Ulcerated nodule or superficial erosion
Verrucous papule or plaque

Management of pre-cancer
Careful evaluation of patients with numerous keratoses especially scalp and ears
Cryotherapy

Topical 5-fluorouracil
Topical retinoids
Systemic retinoids
Sunscreens

Management of established cancer
Surgical excision (± grafting)
Mohs' micrographic surgery (± grafting)
Radiotherapy
Prophylaxis (as above)

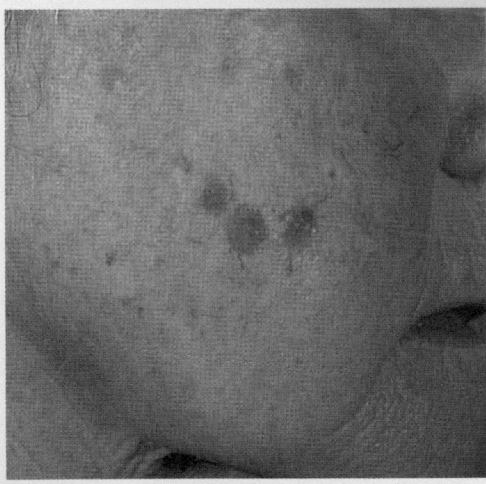

Fig. A Actinic keratoses on cheek. Red scaly patches.

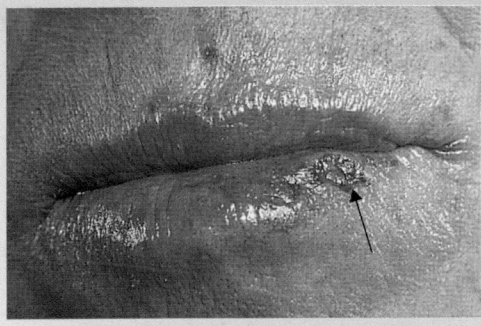

Fig. D Squamous cell carcinoma of the lip (early ulcer).

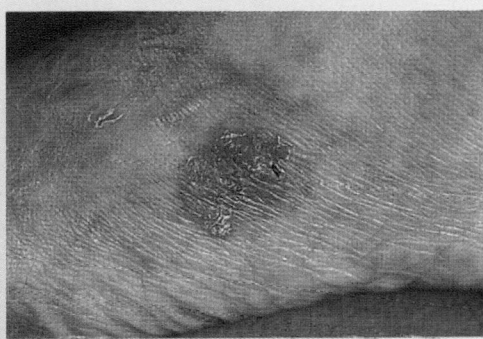

Fig. B Bowen's disease. A red scaly patch of intra-epidermal carcinoma *in situ* on histology.

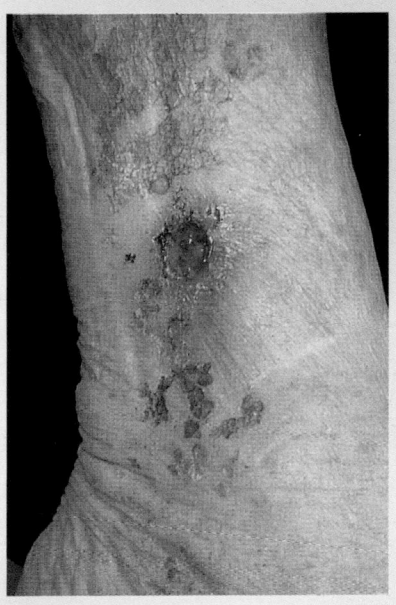

Fig. E Squamous cell carcinoma of the leg (Marjolin's ulcer) complicating long-standing venous disease.

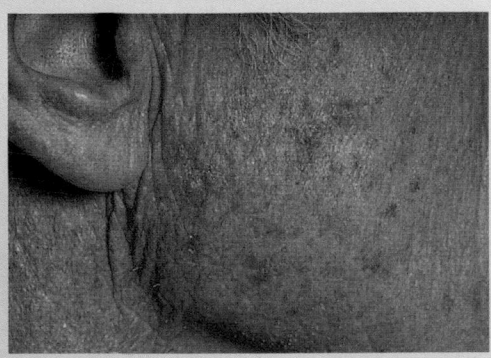

Fig. C Actinic keratoses. Biopsy showed that the central lesion was a squamous cell carcinoma.

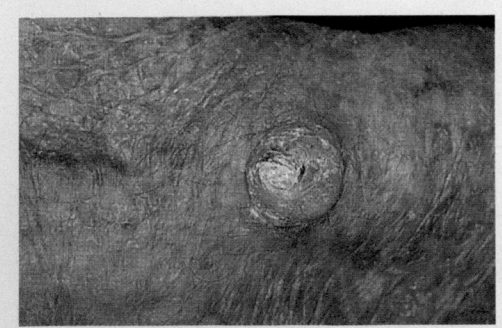

Fig. F Nodule of squamous cell carcinoma.

18

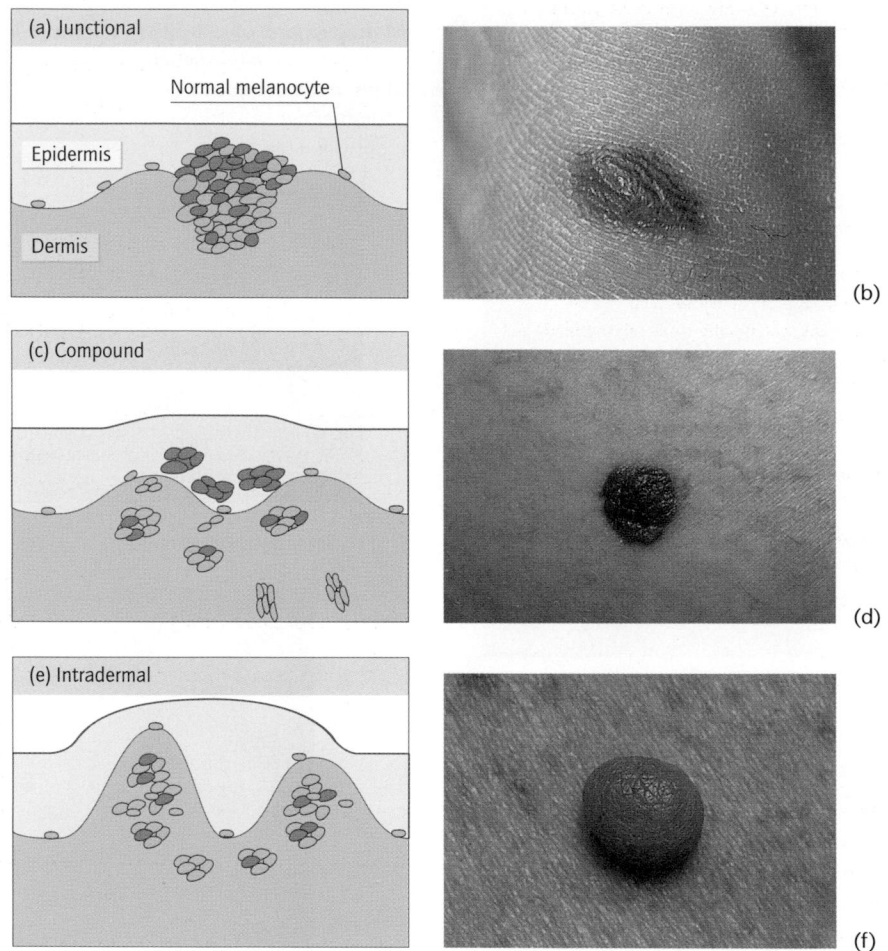

Figure 18.51 Cartoons and clinical pictures of melanocytic naevi. (a,b) Junctional melanocytic naevus. (c,d) Compound melanocytic naevus. (e,f) Intradermal melanocytic naevus.

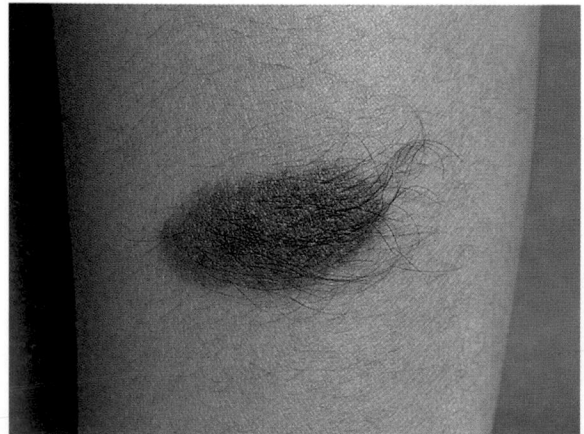

Figure 18.52 Congenital melanocytic naevus.

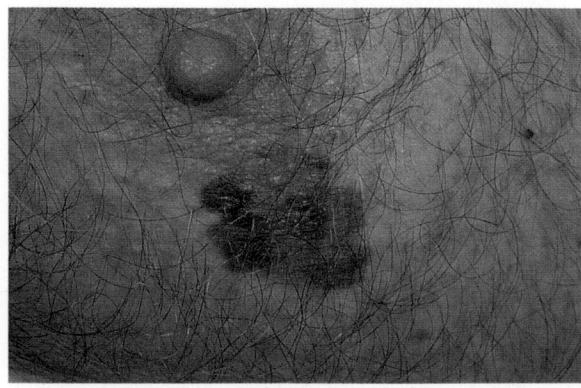

Figure 18.53 Dysplastic naevus. Large, irregular edge, irregular pigmentation.

Table 18.40 Management of malignant melanoma

Prevention

Individual advice (sunbeds, sunburn, sunscreen, hats, shirts, trousers)

Vigilance (new or changed freckles or moles)

Publicity ('mole patrol')

GP awareness

Pigmented lesion clinics

Specific treatment

Excise with primary closure and regular follow-up

Best managed by specialists (usually general or plastic surgeons working with an oncologist and dermatologist)

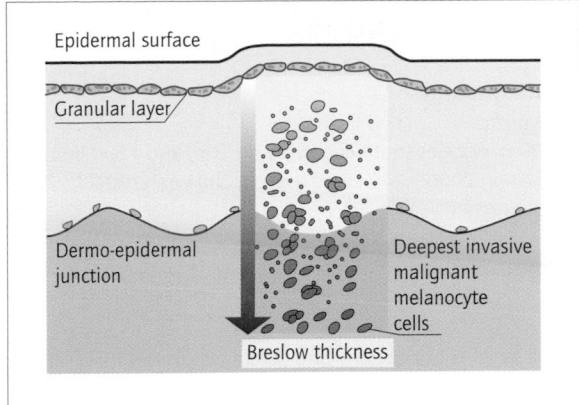

Figure 18.54 Breslow thickness is measured from the granular layer in the epidermis down to the deepest tumour cell in the dermis.

Table 18.41 Correlation of Breslow thickness with prognosis

Depth of invasion (mm) (Breslow)	Approximate 5-year survival (%)
0.0–0.5	100
0.6–1.0	98
1.1–1.5	90
1.6–2.0	80
2.1–3.0	60
>3.0	50

Table 18.42 Clarke's levels

Level	Histopathological characteristics of tumour
I	Intra-epidermal only (*in situ*)
II	Invasion into the upper layers of papillary dermis
III	Filling and distorting of the papillary dermis with tumour cells
IV	Invasion of the reticular dermis
V	Invasion into subcutaneous tissue

and distribution of naevi). Examine the lymph nodes and liver.

Most benign pigmented lesions can be diagnosed with confidence and the patient reassured. Any suspicion or doubt should lead to biopsy and/or appropriate referral.

Investigation

Histopathology. Skin histopathology is the crucial investigation.

Management

Thick melanoma, melanoma with secondary spread and recurrent melanoma are best managed by specialists with an interest and expertise in its treatment. This usually means general or plastic surgeons working with an oncologist and dermatologist (Table 18.40).

Melanoma should be excised with primary closure. The mandatory wide (5 cm) excision and grafting policy is now obsolete and surgery for malignant melanoma is as follows:

- *Less than 0.5 mm Breslow* (Fig. 18.54): adequate excision is now common practice
- *Less than 2 mm Breslow:* 1 cm margin
- *More than 2 mm Breslow:* 1 cm versus 3 cm margin (trial in progress)

Some patients with thicker tumours may benefit from sentinel node biopsy and regional lymph node dissection, but this is controversial. Other treatments are surgical or laser debulking, amputation, isolated limb perfusion with chemotherapy, systemic chemotherapy including with cytokines, and radiotherapy.

Prognosis

The pathology should be staged (Breslow thickness, Fig. 18.54, Table 18.41; and Clarke's level, Table 18.42) and the prognosis decided. Treatment of established melanoma is often not curative and the prognosis is grim. The prognosis is related to the depth of the lesion on first presenta-

tion. Considerable effort should therefore be directed to prevention and early diagnosis.

Vascular and lymphatic tumours

Capillary naevi

Capillary naevi (salmon patch) are classically seen on the nape of the neck from birth in many babies, but may occur on the face. They usually disappear by 1 year of age.

Port-wine stain

Port-wine stain (naevus flammeus) is a capillary naevus seen from birth on the face and neck. It does not change

18

Malignant melanoma at a glance

Epidemiology

Prevalence
5000 new cases (doubling every decade) and 1500 deaths in the UK in 2000. UK lifetime risk 1 in 200

Sex
More common on legs in women and on back in men

Race
Rare in Afro-Caribbeans and Asians, common in Scots and Australians

Genetics
Dysplastic naevus syndrome

Risk factors

Family history of melanoma and dysplastic naevus syndrome
Skin type (I–II) and freckling tendency
Sun exposure (severe sunburn and short sharp exposures)
Total numbers of all naevi (>50)
Numbers of atypical naevi
Distribution of naevi (scalp, buttocks, feet, iris lentigines)
Congenital naevi
Depletion of the ozone layer

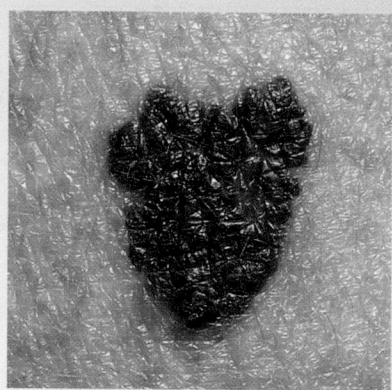

Fig. C Superficial spreading melanoma (back).

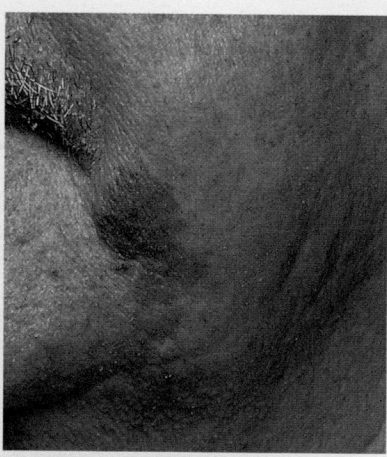

Fig. A Lentigo maligna (Hutchinson's freckle).

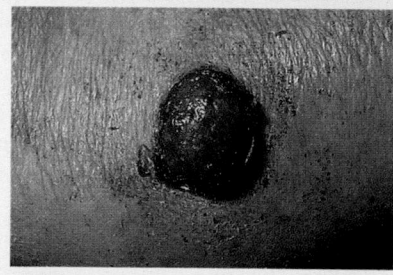

Fig. D Nodular melanoma (arm).

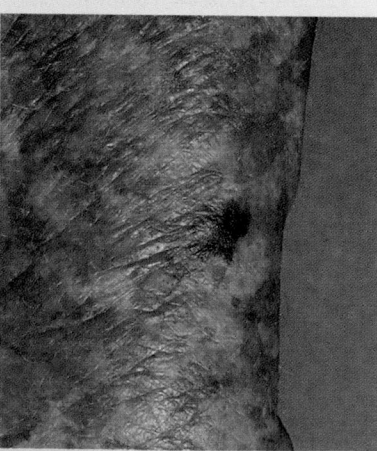

Fig. B Area of actinic damage (arm) containing superficial spreading melanoma.

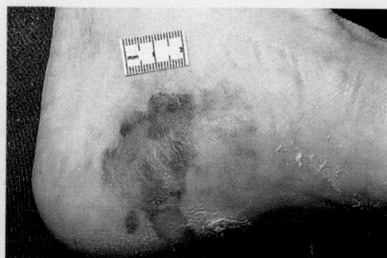

Fig. E Acral lentiginous melanoma (foot). Reproduced from Champion *et al.* (eds), *Textbook of Dermatology*, 5th edn, 1992. Oxford: Blackwell Scientific Publications with the permission of the authors.

18

Findings on investigation
Melanoma is a clinicopathological diagnosis. Other investigations are only indicated if symptoms and signs suggest disseminated disease at presentation

Histopathology
Excisional biopsy and Breslow thickness staging are an essential part of determining management and prognosis

Surgical treatment
<0.5 mm Breslow: complete excision
<2 mm Breslow: 1 cm margin
2 mm Breslow: 1 cm versus 3 cm margin (under investigation)

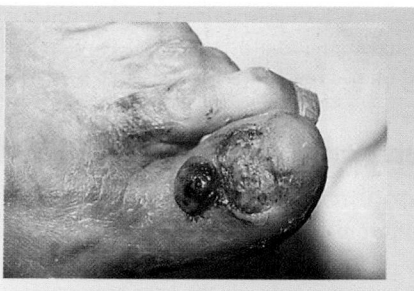

Fig. F Subungual melanoma causing destruction of the nail. Note the pigmentation of the nailfold. Reproduced from Champion *et al.* (eds), *Textbook of Dermatology*, 5th edn, 1992. Oxford: Blackwell Scientific Publications with the permission of the authors.

during life and can be cosmetically distressing. If the naevus is in the distribution of the ophthalmic division of the trigeminal nerve, there may rarely be an associated intracranial vascular anomaly with a neurological deficit such as epilepsy (Sturge–Weber syndrome).

Cosmetic treatment is now possible with the tunable dye laser.

Cavernous haemangioma
Cavernous haemangioma (strawberrry naevus) is a round bulbous tumour on the face, neck or trunk. It appears in the first month, but involutes by 6 years of age.

Campbell de Morgan's angioma
Campbell de Morgan's spots (cherry angiomas) are small (1–2 mm) tortuous vascular dilatations, which are common on the trunk in later life.

Venous lakes
Venous lakes occur in elderly people on the face, lips and ears, and are caused in part by loss of vascular support from connective tissue.

Telangiectasia
Telangiectasia refers to dilated capillaries. It may be essential and related to weathering on the face, or a physical sign of other dermatoses (CLINICAL EXAMINATION AT A GLANCE, Fig. C, p. 1105). If it is arborizing and in dependent regions it may reflect horizontal capillary dilatation caused by chronic venous hypertension.

Spider naevus
Spider naevi are arteriolar dilatations that blanch on pressure. They are classically found in the area drained by the superior vena cava and may increase in number during pregnancy and with oral contraception, but then involute.

They may be a sign of chronic liver disease, thyrotoxicosis or autoimmune rheumatic disease.

Angiokeratoma
Angiokeratomas occurring on the scrotum (Fordyce's angiokeratoma) are common and benign and are 2–4 mm, bright red papular lesions. The possibility of angiokeratoma corporis diffusum (Anderson–Fabry disease; Table 18.43) should be considered where similar, but smaller and more obviously hyperkeratotic lesions occur in a bathing trunk distribution. It is diagnosed by demonstrating glycolipid deposition in skin blood vessels on histology or by measuring a reduced level of the enzyme α galactosidase A in plasma.

Glomus tumour
Glomus tumour (glomangioma) is a pink or purple tender nodule and may be multiple.

Pyogenic granuloma
Pyogenic granuloma is an aberrant healing vascular response to trauma. It often occurs on the hands, fingers and face, and may be complicated by bleeding after recurrent trauma. It is not always pyogenic and is not truly granulomatous.

Lymphangioma circumscriptum
Lymphangioma circumscriptum is a localized hamartomatous lymphatic dilatation with deep vesicles looking like frog's spawn. It may be apparent from birth or appear at any age, and tends to persist.

Kaposi's sarcoma
Classical Kaposi's sarcoma occurs in elderly male central Europeans, Italians or Jews, and is solitary and acral, consisting of purple nodules, which may ulcerate.

18

AIDS-related Kaposi's sarcoma and epithelioid angiomatosis (haemangiomatosis), which may be similar, are described on p. 1164.

Dermal connective tissue tumours

Dermatofibroma

Dermatofibroma (histiocytoma) probably represents an aberrant healing response to mild trauma such as an insect bite. It is very common on the legs, appearing as a small

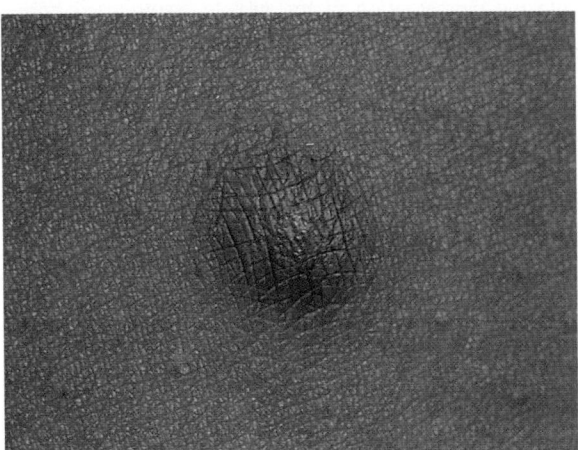

Figure 18.55 Dermatofibroma/histiocytoma. Firm pigmented papule.

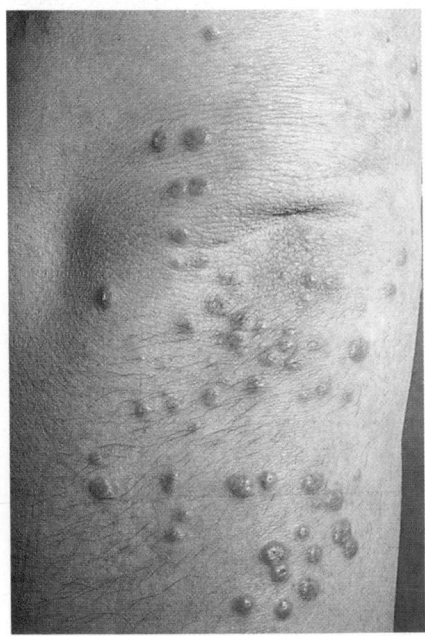

Figure 18.56 Extensive eruptive xanthomas in a patient with chylomicronaemia syndrome. Yellow infiltrated papules.

round brown papule or nodule (Fig. 18.55), and may be falsely suspected of being a melanoma.

Xanthoma

Xanthomas can be classified clinically as in Table 11.16, which includes the possible correlations with primary hyperlipidaemia, hyperlipidaemia secondary to other disease, and pancreatitis. They consist of yellow tumours representing massive abnormal lipid deposition within dermal cells (Figs 18.56–18.58).

Lipoma

Lipomas are fluctuant, but well-defined subcutaneous tumours and are common. Multiple painful lipomas (**Dercum's disease**) are rarer.

Metastases

Metastases from solid tumours are not uncommon in the skin and their appearance tends to reflect the prevalence of the responsible cancer: lung, gut and breast cancer are the usual causes.

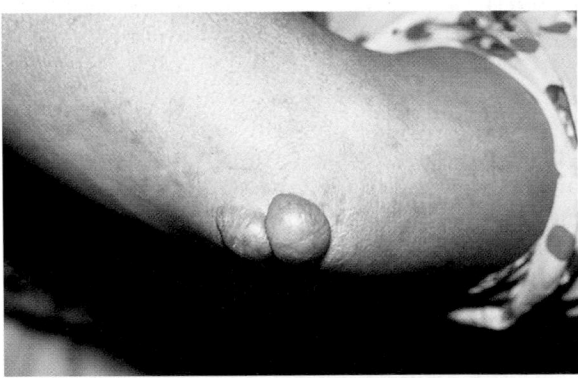

Figure 18.57 Tuberous xanthoma in a patient with hypercholesterolaemia.

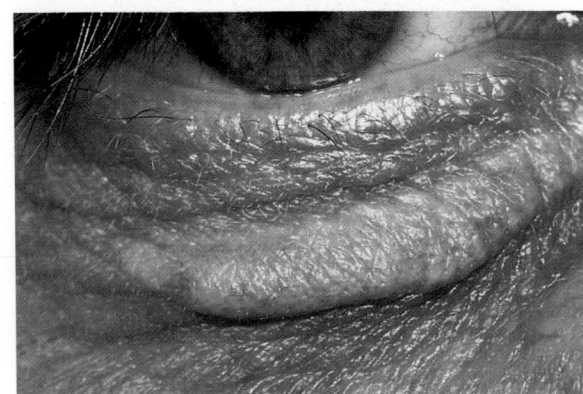

Figure 18.58 Xanthelasma. Most patients do not have a hyperlipidaemia.

Lymphoma
Mycosis fungoides
Mycosis fungoides is a cutaneous T-cell lymphoma where there is slowly evolving infiltration of the skin with T-helper cells (Fig. 18.59). The cause is not known.

Clinical features
The following stages are recognized:
- Fixed itchy scaly patches (like eczema or psoriasis)
- Fixed geographical plaques
- Nodules, tumours and ulcers
- Lymph node or systemic organ involvement

A variant is the **Sézary syndrome** in which the patient is erythrodermic and there is lymphadenopathy and abnormal cells (Sézary cells) with cerebriform nuclei in the blood. The differential diagnosis of erythroderma is given in Table 18.21.

Management and prognosis
The prognosis is good. Treatments include topical steroids, PUVA, topical nitrogen mustard and electron beam therapy. With more advanced disease, therapy is more radical (radiotherapy, chemotherapy, extracorporeal photochemotherapy) and the outlook is bleak.

Adult T-cell lymphoma/leukaemia
A cutaneous prodrome of granulomatous papules and nodules (from which proviral DNA can be recovered) precedes and accompanies adult T-cell lymphoma/leukaemia (ATLL) resulting from human T cell lymphotropic virus-1 (HTLV-I).

Hodgkin's disease
Hodgkin's disease and non-Hodgkin's lymphoma may involve the skin and, it is argued, may originate in the skin.

Other lymphomas
Cutaneous B-cell lymphomas and those derived from cutaneous macrophages usually present as nodules and tumours with variable systemic involvement and variable response to treatment (radiotherapy and chemotherapy).

Hereditary and congenital disorders

There are many inherited diseases of skin or inherited disorders characterized by skin manifestations (Table 18.43). Although rare, they are important because they may be associated with significant morbidity or handicap and may be amenable to antenatal screening and genetic counselling. The molecular basis of increasingly more of these diseases is understood (X-linked ichthyosis–steroid sulphatase defect: epidermolysis bullosa simplex keratins 5 and 15 mutations), but it is to be hoped that the new molecular genetics will allow the description of the basic defect in many more of them.

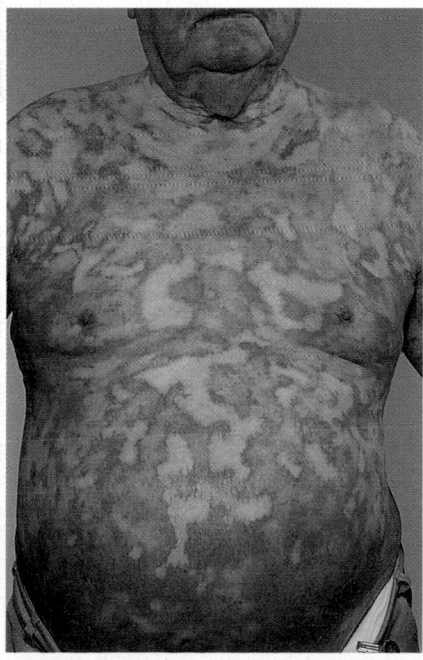

Figure 18.59 Mycosis fungoides. Advanced plaque stage.

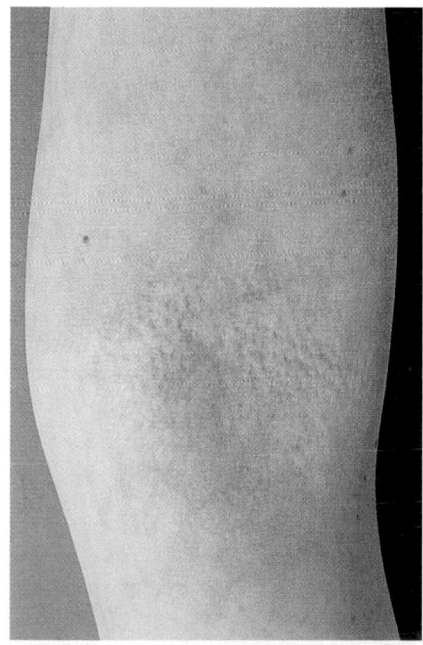

Figure 18.60 Pseudoxanthoma elasticum. Chicken skin appearance of antecubital fossa. Patient presented with gastrointestinal haemorrhage and had angioid streaks on fundoscopy.

18

Table 18.43 Some congenital diseases with cutaneous manifestations

Syndrome	Inheritance and cause	Skin features	Other manifestations
Xeroderma pigmentosum	Autosomal recessive defect of DNA repair	Photosensitivity, pigment changes, keratoses, skin cancers	
Peutz–Jeghers syndrome	Autosomal dominant	Perioral pigmented macules	Gastrointestinal polyps with malignant potential
Tuberous sclerosis	Autosomal dominant	Angiofibromas, periungual fibromas, shagreen patches, ash leaf patches	Epilepsy, mental retardation
LEOPARD syndrome		**L**entigines	**E**CG abnormalities, **O**cular hyperteleorism, **P**ulmonary stenosis, **A**bnormal genitals, **R**etarded growth, **D**eafness
Anderson–Fabry disease	Sex-linked Sphingolipid metabolism decreased with reduced α-galactosidase	Angiokeratoses, skin pain, dysaesthesia, cyanosis, flushing	Neuropathy, cardiac and renal disease
Von Recklinghausen's syndrome	Autosomal dominant	*Café au lait* spots, axillary freckling, neurofibromas	Acoustic neuroma, sarcoma, retinal Lisch nodules, epilepsy
Hereditary haemorrhagic telangiectasia (Osler–Weber–Rendu disease)	Autosomal dominant	Facial and mucosal telangiectasia	Epistaxis, gastrointestinal bleeding
Pseudoxanthoma elasticum	Autosomal dominant and recessive. Classification of elastin	'Chicken skin' affecting neck, antecubital fossae (Fig. 18.60)	Angioid retinal streaks, mitral valve prolapse, angina, claudication, myocardial infarction, cerebral haemorrhage, gastrointestinal bleeding
Ehlers–Danlos syndrome	Autosomal dominant and recessive. Disorders of collagen biosynthesis	Skin fragility with tissue paper scars, hyperelasticity	Hyperextensible joints, easy bleeding
Klippel–Trenaunay syndrome		Port-wine stain of limb	Bone hypertrophy, arteriovenous fistulae
Cutis laxa		Lax pendulous skin, premature ageing	
Incontinentia pigmenti	Sex-linked dominant	Vesicular, verrucous skin lesions, pigmented patches	Eye, skeletal and CNS defects

Epidermolysis bullosa

Epidermolysis bullosa (Fig. 18.61) describes a group of diseases in which blisters arise either spontaneously or as a consequence of mild trauma to the skin or in the mouth and oesophagus. Sometimes they are called the mechanobullous disorders to distinguish them from the immunobullous diseases described on p. 1123. The inset in Fig. 18.1 correlates the level of the split and therefore the BMZ defect (as identified to date) with the main types.

In general, blistering over traumatized sites (hands and feet) and in the mouth leaves erosions, which may heal to form milia. Nails and hair may be lost. Because of the level of the split the dystrophic types heal with scarring and sometimes mutilating contractures and fusion of fingers (syndactyly). Squamous cell carcinoma may develop.

Management of a severely affected child may be difficult and is largely symptomatic. Antenatal diagnosis with monoclonal antibodies to BMZ components is becoming possible.

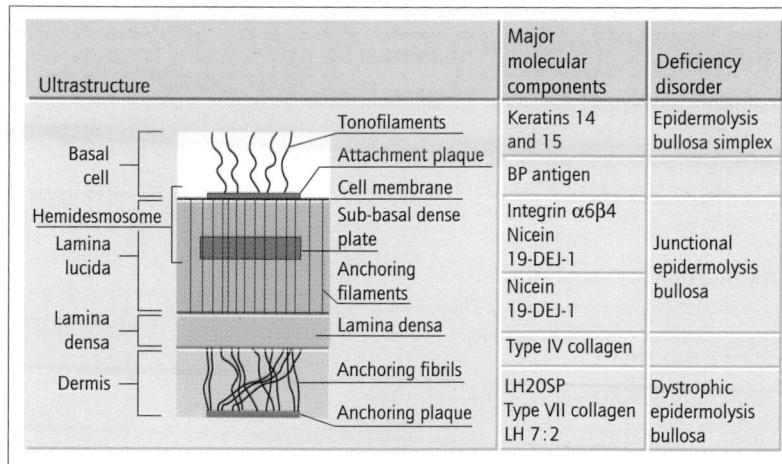

Figure 18.61 Summary of epidermolysis bullosa. Reproduced from Moss & Savin, *Dermatology and the New Genetics*. Oxford: Blackwell Science, 1995 with the permission of the authors.

Disorders of keratinization

The disorders of keratinization are a broad group of conditions characterized by abnormal epidermal proliferation and maturation. Psoriasis is an example in which the abnormality is probably polygenic (see p. 1119).

Ichthyoses

The ichthyoses are characterized by a generalized persistent non-inflamed scaling (like fish scales):
- *Autosomal dominant ichthyosis vulgaris:* very common and responds to emollients
- *Acquired ichthyosis:* may signify Hodgkin's disease or another internal malignancy

Keratosis pilaris

Keratosis pilaris is a common hyperkeratotic condition of hair follicles. It results in small spiky follicular lesions, often on the upper arms and legs.

Keratosis follicularis (Darier's disease)

Keratosis follicularis is an autosomal dominant condition in which greasy crusted papules occur and coalesce on the face, neck, upper trunk and in the groin. They may become secondarily infected. On the palms and soles there are small pits and the nails show red, white and blue banding, with V-shaped nicks in the free ends.

Conventional treatment is with topical steroid, antibiotic and antifungal combinations. The cause is unknown, but there is evidence for an abnormality in the handling of vitamin A, which is an important modulator of epidermal growth and differentiation. The synthetic retinoid acitretin is useful in this condition.

Hereditary palmoplantar keratoderma

There are a large number of hereditary palmoplantar keratodermas (thickening—tylosis—of the skin of the palms and soles). One very rare autosomal dominant type is associated with carcinoma of the oesophagus.

The skin and systemic disease

Non-specific skin manifestations

Hair and **nail** manifestations are discussed on pp. 1128 and 1130, **Raynaud's phenomenon**, **vasculitis** and **livedo reticularis** on p. 1133. The causes of facial flushing are listed in Table 18.48.

Toxic erythema

Toxic erythema is a non-specific diagnosis of a generalized erythema in response to illness, infection or a drug. It may be maculopapular (as in the classical example of a patient with infectious mononucleosis who is given ampicillin) or confluent. There are more specific characteristic erythemas or exanthems of childhood disorders (see p. 143). Rarely, TEN may supervene (see p. 1167).

Erythema marginatum is a very rare reticulate erythema in rheumatic fever. A diurnal angulated macular erythema is seen in Still's disease.

Leg ulcers

The most common causes of leg ulcers are venous insufficiency, arterial disease and diabetes mellitus, but other important causes are listed in Table 18.44 (see also LEG ULCERATION AT A GLANCE and Table 18.31). **Pyoderma gangrenosum** is a painful ulcerated lesion that usually occurs on a limb (Fig. 18.63). Causes are ulcerative colitis, Crohn's disease, seronegative rheumatoid arthritis and myelomatosis. It may be very difficult to treat and

Leg ulceration at a glance

Epidemiology

Prevalence

Up to 1 million people in the UK have chronic leg ulceration. Worldwide, the idiopathic tropical ulcer is even more common

Findings on investigation

Investigation may be necessary to confirm the cause
Doppler studies (arterial pressures)

Skin biopsy
Systemic investigations

Complications

Contact dermatitis
Infection

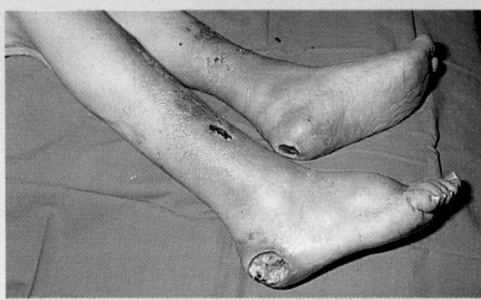

Fig. C Calcific vasculopathy causing leg ulceration (chronic renal failure and replacement therapy).

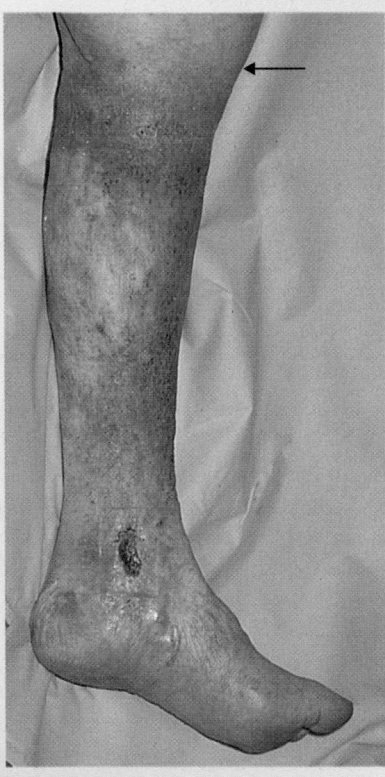

Fig. A Venous ulceration. Note the margin of allergic contact dermatitis due to rubber in the compression bandaging (arrow).

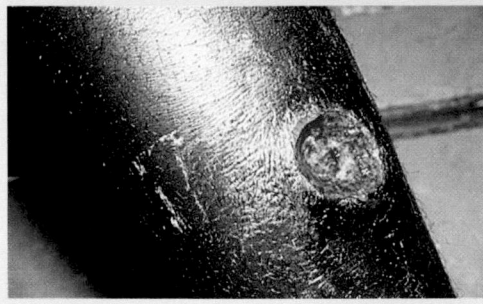

Fig. D Tropical ulcer. Aetiology uncertain: malnutrition and infection incriminated. Courtesy of Institute of Dermatology, London. Reproduced from Champion *et al.* (eds), *Textbook of Dermatology*, 5th edn, 1992. Oxford: Blackwell Scientific Publications with the permission of the authors.

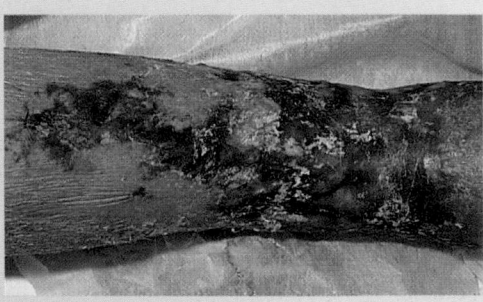

Fig. B Cholesterol emboli. Necrotic ulcers.

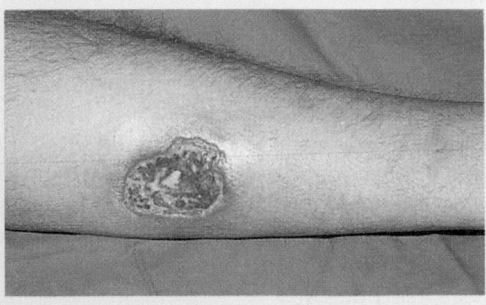

Fig. E Pyoderma gangrenosum (rheumatoid arthritis). Ulcer with indurated edge.

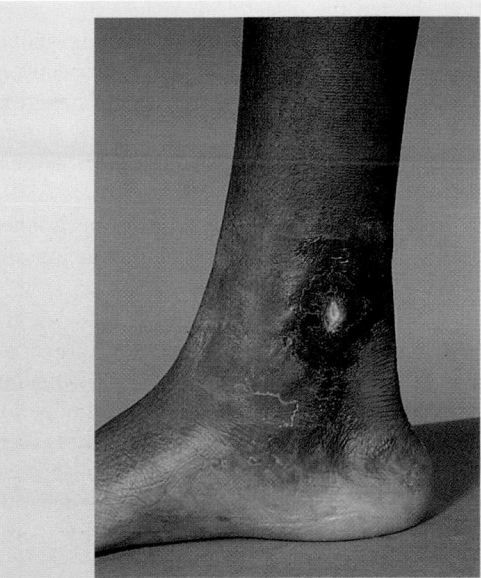

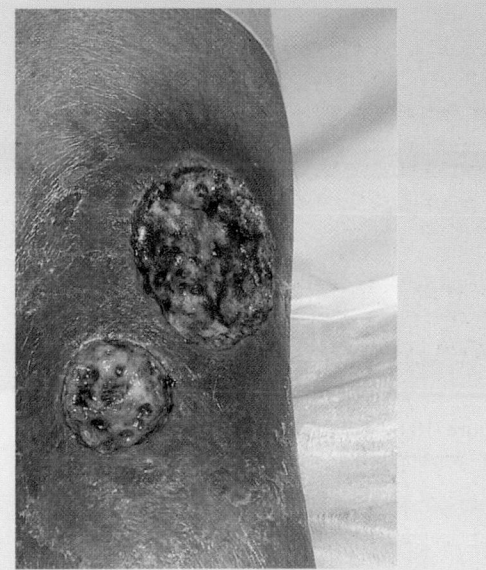

Fig: F Haemolysis (sickle cell anaemia). Chronic ulcer.

Fig. G Vasculitis (cytomegalovirus—AIDS).

Table 18.44 Causes of leg ulcers

Trauma
Venous insufficiency
Arterial disease
Hypertension (Martorell's ulcer)
Cholesterol emboli
Diabetes mellitus
Pyoderma gangrenosum
Haemoglobinopathy and haemolysis
Tropical ulcer
Tuberculosis
Leishmaniasis
Vasculitis
Gout
Renal failure
Hyperparathyroidism
Protein C or protein S deficiency
Immunobullous diseases
Skin cancer (SQUAMOUS CELL CARCINOMA AT A GLANCE, Fig. E, p. 1147)
Necrobiosis lipoidica
Neuropathy

Table 18.45 Causes of erythema multiforme

Infection
Herpes simplex, mycoplasma pneumonia, psittacosis, hepatitis B, orf, infectious mononucleosis, histoplasmosis

Autoimmune rheumatic diseases
Lupus erythematosus or SLE (Rowell's syndrome), PAN

Drugs

Tumours
Carcinoma, leukaemia

Endocrine
Pregnancy and premenstrual

Sarcoid

heals with scarring. Prednisolone is the most commonly used treatment.

Erythema multiforme

Disease mechanisms

The triggers of erythema multiforme include herpes simplex infection, mycoplasma, orf and drugs, such as non-steroidal anti-inflammatory agents (Table 18.45); often it is idiopathic.

Clinical features

Erythema multiforme (Fig. 18.62) is an acute erythema characterized by a symmetrical eruption of raised annular (target) lesions, particularly on the hands and feet. With increasing severity it becomes more centripetal. Fever and lassitude herald the appearance of the rash, which may vary from a few red raised patches, usually on the hands, to a widespread mucocutaneous picture of 'target' lesions, blisters and erosions. There may be a systemic upset and

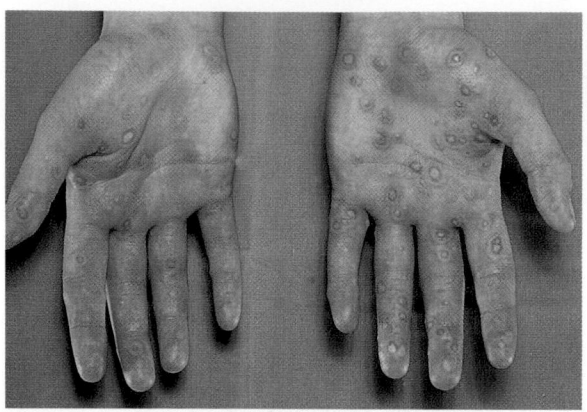

Figure 18.62 Erythema multiforme. Target lesions. Causes: HSV, mycoplasma, orf, SLE (see p. 1157).

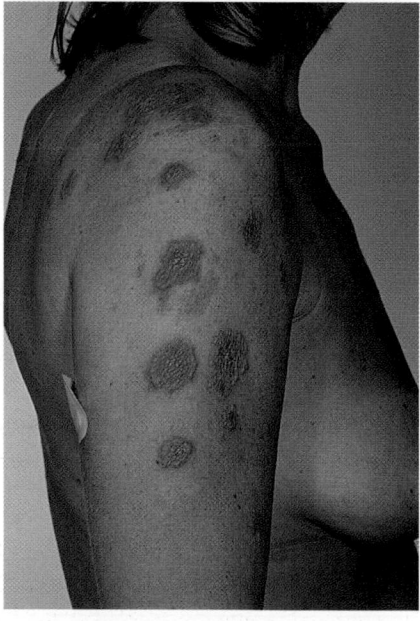

Figure 18.63 Pyoderma gangrenosum. Vesicobulbous and nodular lesions. Causes: rheumatoid arthritis, inflammatory bowel disease, myeloma.

oculo-orogenital involvement. If there is fever, tachycardia and a severe rash with blistering and mucocutaneous involvement (**Stevens–Johnson syndrome**), there is an appreciable mortality. Drugs are often the cause. Erythema multiforme may blister, especially in Stevens–Johnson syndrome.

Management

Intensive support may be necessary, with attention to fluid and electrolyte balance. Oral corticosteroids prob-ably neither shorten the disease nor reduce its severity. Herpes simplex and mycoplasma pneumonia should be treated with aciclovir and penicillin, respectively. Often a cause cannot be found so treatment has to be symptomatic with a moderately potent topical steroid. Systemic corticosteroids are usually given in Stevens–Johnson syndrome.

Recurrent or chronic erythema multiforme is often thought to be caused by herpes simplex infection and long-term prophylactic aciclovir may be useful.

Erythema nodosum

Erythema nodosum (Fig. 18.38) is a tender erythematous nodular eruption that evolves and resolves over a period of 6 weeks with the colour changes of a bruise. It often occurs on the shins, and does not scar. A full history, examination and investigation should be carried out, bearing in mind the large number of causes (Table 18.46). Many cases will be idiopathic.

Table 18.46 Causes of erythema nodosum

Infection
Streptococcal infections, tuberculosis, cat-scratch disease, psittacosis, *Yersinia*, kerion, histoplasmosis, blastomycosis, coccidioidomycosis, erythema nodosum leprosum

Sarcoid

Inflammatory bowel disease
Crohn's disease, ulcerative colitis

Drugs

Neoplasia
Leukaemia, Hodgkin's disease

Acanthosis nigricans

Acanthosis nigricans describes velvety hyperkeratotic papillomatous lesions in the flexures and intertriginous areas. Causes are:
● Endocrine disorders (acromegaly, Cushing's disease, Addison's disease, hypothyroidism, insulin-resistant diabetes mellitus, polycystic ovary disease)
● Drugs (corticosteroid treatment)
● Obesity
● Familial
● Internal malignancy

Generalized pruritus

Generalized pruritus is a common presenting symptom in dermatology and there is a broad non-dermatological differential diagnosis. Causes and suitable investigations are given in Table 18.47.

Table 18.47 Causes of generalized pruritus (without diagnostic skin lesions) and recommended investigations

Pathology	Disorder	Investigation
Metabolic and endocrine	Hypothyroidism	Thyroid function
	Hyperthyroidism	Thyroid function
	Diabetes mellitus	Blood glucose
	Diabetes insipidus	Sodium osmolality
Haematological	Iron deficiency	Full blood count, iron, total iron-binding capacity, ferritin, faecal occult blood, gynaecological assessment (fibroids)
	Polycythaemia rubra vera	Full blood count
	Lymphoma	Full blood count, CXR
	Leukaemia	Full blood count
	Myeloma	Urea, Ca, serum, electrophoresis
Neoplasia	Lung	CXR
	Abdomen	Ultrasound
	Central nervous system	CT scan
Infestation	Pediculosis, scabies	Eosinophils, stool
	Intestinal parasites	
Renal	Chronic renal failure	Full blood count, urea, creatinine
Hepatic	Obstructive biliary disease	Liver function
Drugs	Opiates, alcohol, gold	
Miscellaneous	Senile pruritus	
	Psychogenic	

Table 18.48 Causes of facial flushing

Endocrine
Carcinoid syndrome
Phaeochromocytoma
Medullary carcinoma of the thyroid
Zollinger–Ellison syndrome
Angioneurotic oedema
Menopause and postmenopause

Foods
Alcohol
Glutamate, nitrite, capsicum

Drugs
Bromocriptine, nifedipine, tamoxifen

Skin disease
Rosacea, urticaria, erythromelalgia

Specific skin manifestations

Gastrointestinal disease

Crohn's disease

Crohn's disease can affect any part of the gastrointestinal tract from the mouth to the anus, including the lips and perianal skin. There may be a granulomatous cheilitis, ulcers in the mouth and perianal abscess and fistula formation. Clubbing, erythema nodosum and pyoderma gangrenosum may occur.

Ulcerative colitis

Ulcerative colitis may be associated with clubbing, erythema nodosum, pyoderma gangrenosum and leg ulcers.

Dermatitis herpetiformis

Dermatitis herpetiformis is associated with partial villous atrophy and often with frank coeliac disease. It is an immunobullous disease and is described on p. 1125.

Gastrointestinal malignancy

- Palmoplantar keratoderma
- Gardner's syndrome
- Peutz–Jeghers syndrome
- Muir–Torré syndrome

Liver disease

Skin signs of liver disease are jaundice, spider naevi, leuconychia, pruritus, xanthomas, lichen planus and striae.

Pancreatic disease

Skin signs of pancreatic disease are:

- Grey Turner's sign (bruising on the flank in acute pancreatitis)

18

Table 18.49 Skin manifestations of nutritional disease

Skin sign	Features	Nutrient deficiency
Scurvy	Purpura, perifollicular cork screw hairs	Vitamin C
Pellagra	Photosensitive dermatitis (Casal's necklace)	Nicotinic acid
Acrodermatitis enteropathica	Neonatal perioral, perianal and acral dermatitis	Zinc
Glossitis and angular cheilitis	Sore tongue and lips	B complex
Hyperkeratosis	Itch and dryness	Essential fatty acids
Kwashiorkor/marasmus	Exfoliation	Protein/calorie

Table 18.50 Skin manifestations of endocrine disorders

Disorder	Skin signs
Diabetes mellitus	Neuropathic foot ulceration, candidiasis, staphylococcal skin infections, diabetic dermopathy, necrobiosis lipoidica diabeticorum (Fig. 18.64), generalized granuloma annulare, xanthomas, injection site lipoatrophy and hypertrophy
Hypothyroidism	Cold, dry skin (peaches and cream), fine thin hair, eyebrow loss
Hyperthyroidism	Hot, moist skin, diffuse hair loss, thyroid acropachy (clubbing)
Autoimmune thyroid disease	Vitiligo, pretibial myxoedema
Cushing's syndrome	Striae, moon face, buffalo hump, acne, hirsutes, truncal obesity
Addison's disease and Nelson's syndrome	Vitiligo, hyperpigmented scars, palmar creases, pigmented oral macules

- Cullen's sign (periumbilical bruising in acute pancreatitis). Differential diagnosis: rupture of the common bile duct, ectopic pregnancy, perforated duodenal ulcer, hepatoma, bleeding diathesis
- Reticular livedo
- Panniculitis resulting from fat necrosis in acute pancreatitis
- Necrolytic migratory erythema in glucagonoma syndrome

Nutritional diseases
Skin signs of nutritional disease are listed in Table 18.49.

Endocrine diseases
The skin signs of endocrine diseases are listed in Table 18.50 (Fig. 18.64).

Metabolic disease
Tophaceous gout may present with painful dactylitis or a nodule on the ear. The porphyrias are considered on p. 808. Xanthomas (Figs 18.56–18.58) and their differential diagnosis are discussed on p. 1152 and in Table 11.16.

Haematological disease
The skin signs of haematological disorders are listed in Table 18.51.

Sarcoidosis
Sarcoidosis is a multisystem granulomatous disease of unknown aetiology. The most common of its numerous cutaneous manifestations are:

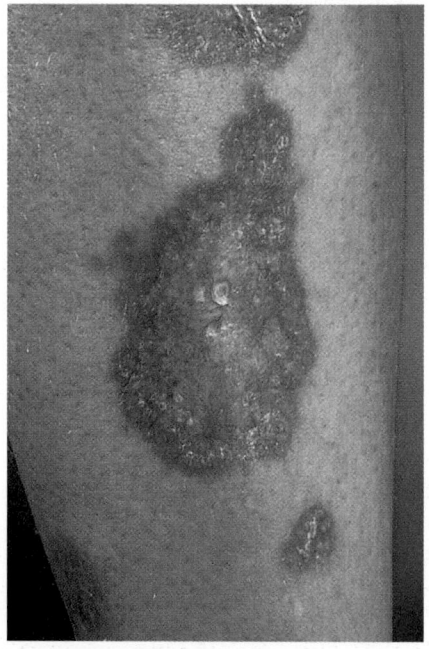

Figure 18.64 Necrobiosis lipoidica diabeticorum. Atrophic plaques. Causes: diabetes mellitus.

- Erythema nodosum (Fig. 18.38)
- Lupus pernio (Fig. 18.65)
- Dactylitis
- Papules, nodules and plaques
- Scarring alopecia

Table **18.51** Skin manifestations of haematological disorders

Skin sign	Haematological disorder
Purpura	Thrombocytopenia
Leuconychia	Anaemia
Jaundice (lemon-yellow tinge)	Haemolytic anaemia
Leg ulcers	Haemolysis (e.g. thalassaemia and fibrinolytic disorders—proteins C and S)
Pyoderma gangrenosum	Monoclonal gammopathy
Vasculitis	Monoclonal gammopathy and myeloma
Leukaemic infiltration (especially myelomonocytic types)	Leukaemia
Granulomatous	Human T-cell lymphotropic virus type I (HTLV-I/ATLL) adult T-cell lymphoma leukaemia papules
Urticaria pigmentosa	Mast cell leukaemia
Non-melanoma skin cancer	Chronic lymphatic leukaemia

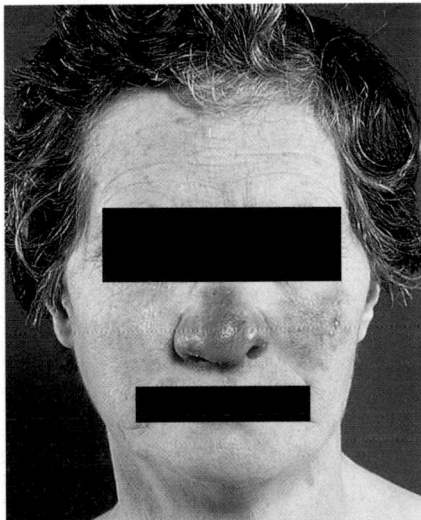

Figure 18.65 Sarcoidosis (lupus pernio of the nose and cheek). Infiltrated plaques and nodules.

Wegener's granulomatosis

Wegener's granulomatosis is a rare necrotizing arteritis that results in granulomatous destruction of the respiratory tract and glomerulonephritis (see p. 221). It may present with crusting of the external nares, and there may be erythema, urticaria, vasculitis, and granulomatous nodules and plaques in the skin.

Lichen myxoedematosus (scleromyxoedema)

Lichen myxoedematosus is a rare infiltrative condition characterized by an eruption of small papules on a background of erythematous thickened skin. It is associated with paraproteinaemia and, unless treated with cyclophosphamide or melphalan, may be fatal.

Amyloidosis

About 40% of patients with primary and myeloma-associated systemic amyloidosis have cutaneous lesions. They result from deposition of immunoglobulin light chain material derived from a circulating paraprotein.

Mucocutaneous features of amyloidosis include:
- Macroglossia
- Carpal tunnel syndrome
- Waxy purpuric mucocutaneous lesions

Systemic (reactive) amyloidosis is rarely associated with skin lesions.

Primary cutaneous amyloidosis is usually localized and is either nodular (caused by plasma cell infiltration and the deposition of light chain material) or macular/papular (lichen amyloidosis in which keratin filaments constitute the amyloid material).

Autoimmune rheumatic disease

Systemic lupus erythematosus

Malar butterfly rash, discoid rash, photosensitivity and oral ulcers are four cardinal American College of Rheumatology criteria for the diagnosis of SLE (see p. 212).

A particular site to examine for skin signs in SLE is the hand. Patients may have red scaly patches over the digits and nail, and nailfold changes (CLINICAL EXAMINATION AT A GLANCE, Fig. C, p. 1105; Table 18.29). Raynaud's phenomenon (Fig. 18.29) and cutaneous vasculitic lesions may also occur.

Discoid lupus erythematosus

Clinical features. Discoid lupus erythematosus (DLE) usually involves the face and other sun-exposed areas. The lesions are red scaly patches, which heal with scarring (CLINICAL EXAMINATION AT A GLANCE, Fig. N, p. 1107). There may be scarring alopecia (Fig. 18.24).

18

Patients may have arthralgia (25%), Raynaud's phenomenon (15%) (Fig. 18.29) and haematological and serological abnormalities (approximately 50%). About 5% of patients are eventually diagnosed as having SLE. Lupus erythematosus is a spectrum of disease.

Investigation. Diagnosis is clinical, but confirmed by skin biopsy:
- *Skin biopsy:* shows degeneration of the basal layer of the epidermis, degenerative changes in dermal connective tissue and a lymphocytic infiltrate
- *Immunofluorescence:* shows IgG, IgA, IgM and complement at the dermo-epidermal junction of lesional but not uninvolved skin

Management. This comprises sun avoidance, sunscreens and potent topical steroids. Antimalarials (hydroxychloroquine and mepacrine) may be effective, but ocular toxicity can occur with hydroxychloroquine.

Systemic sclerosis

Disease mechanisms. Systemic sclerosis (see p. 225) is a disease of unknown aetiology, but agents implicated in its development include vinyl chloride, silica (including from silicone implants), epoxy resin, bleomycin, rapeseed oil and aniline.

Clinical features. Raynaud's phenomenon (Fig. 18.29) heralds scleroderma and vasculitic involvement of other organs. It is much more common in women than in men, and patients have sclerodactyly and characteristic facies. Features of sclerodactyly are tight shiny skin or waxy swollen sausage fingers (CLINICAL EXAMINATION AT A GLANCE, Fig. P, p. 1107), dorsal erythematous patches, digital ulceration, calcinosis, loss of pulp space, flexion deformity, muscle wasting, nail dystrophy, periungual erythema and telangiectasia, and ragged cuticles (CLINICAL EXAMINATION AT A GLANCE, Fig. C, p. 1105). Sclerodermatous facies are characterized by perioral radial furrowing, microstomia and telangiectasia. Other symptoms indicating organ and systemic involvement are dysphagia (oesophageal hypoperistalsis), abdominal pain and diarrhoea (small bowel involvement and bacterial overgrowth), shortness of breath with a restrictive pattern (pulmonary fibrosis), arthralgia (erosive arthritis and osteoporosis), dry eyes (Sjögren's syndrome), muscle weakness, ECG abnormalities, proteinuria and renal failure. Other causes of scleroderma are porphyria cutanea tarda, phenylketonuria, leprosy and carcinoid syndrome.

Investigation. Antinuclear antibodies are detected in nearly all patients. Anticentromere antibody is found in up to 70% of patients with the **CREST syndrome** (calcinosis, Raynaud's phenomenon, oesophagitis, sclerodactyly and telangiectasia).

Management. Management of the patient with systemic sclerosis involves:
- Arresting the progression of the disease
- Providing symptomatic relief

No single agent or combination of drugs has proven efficacy, but prednisolone, penicillamine, colchicine and cyclophosphamide have been used.

The predominant symptoms arise from digital vascular insufficiency and the upper gastrointestinal tract. Cold avoidance and vasodilators (e.g. nifedipine) prevent and cure digital ulceration. Antibiotics may be prescribed prophylactically. Sometimes it is necessary to infuse prostacyclin or calcitonin gene-related peptide. Some patients may still lose a digit to amputation.

Anti-H_2 blockers, proton pump inhibitors and antacids are helpful for dysphagia.

Most patients do well, even with some degree of organ involvement. Patients may die from renal or pulmonary disease. There is a suspicion that systemic sclerosis is associated with internal malignancy (e.g. breast), but this has not been proven.

Localized scleroderma

Localized scleroderma (**morphoea**; Fig. 18.66) may be circumscribed, linear or facial (en coup de sabre). Patients rarely have systemic involvement even if the disorder is generalized. Colchicine may be useful.

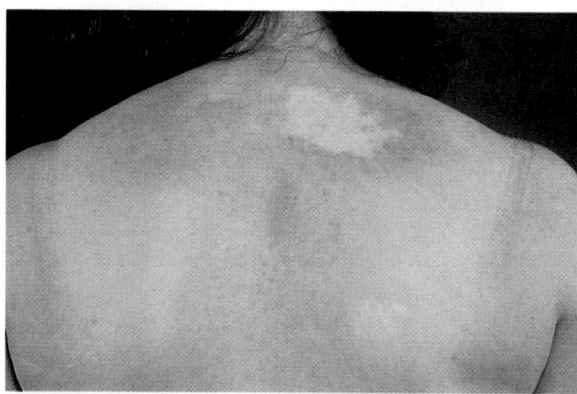

Figure 18.66 Localized scleroderma (morphoea). Plaques on back.

Vasculitis
See p. 1133.

Dermatomyositis
Clinical features. In dermatomyositis (see p. 222)

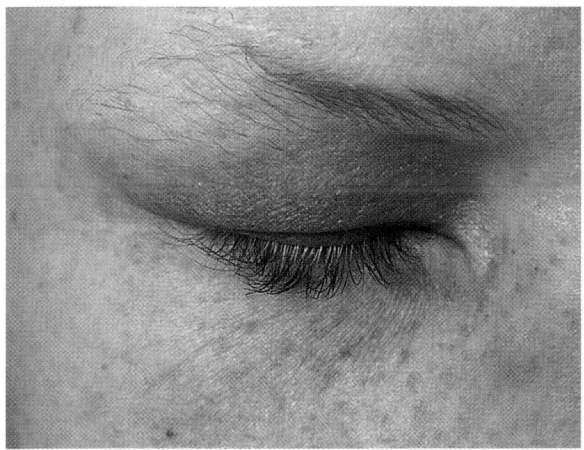

Figure 18.67 Dermatomyositis. Lilac heliotropic rash on eyelids.

oedematous maculopapular erythematous plaques are seen over the knuckles, finger joints, elbows and knees. The eyelids may be swollen and show a characteristic violet discoloration (Fig. 18.67). Muscle weakness is proximal and symmetrical. It may affect speech, swallowing and ventilation. Involved muscles are often oedematous, and may calcify.

Investigation
- *Serum creatine phosphokinase and aldolase:* elevated
- *Electromyography:* abnormal
- *Anti-Jo1 antibodies:* may be present

Management and prognosis. Treatment is with oral corticosteroids, endeavouring to avoid a confounding myopathy, and cytotoxics (e.g. methotrexate). Dermatomyositis is more strongly associated with internal malignancy with increasing age. Approximately 20–40% of patients over 50 years of age have an underlying cancer. The prognosis is poor even when there is no associated malignancy.

Malignant disease and the skin

Solid tumours, metastases, leukaemia and lymphoma have been discussed above. Table 18.52 lists the recognized skin manifestations of malignant disease.

Paget's disease of the nipple
Paget's disease of the nipple is an eczematous eruption of the areola associated with spread from an intraductal breast carcinoma.

Extramammary Paget's disease
Extramammary Paget's disease is a similar manifestation

Table 18.52 Cutaneous associations of malignant disease

Feature	Cause
Invasion of skin by neoplastic cells	Metastases and infiltration by reticuloses and leukaemic cells
	Paget's disease
Non-specific skin markers	Infections (e.g. varicella-zoster in lymphoproliferative disease)
	Purpura, petechiae and ecchymoses (e.g. leukaemia and dysproteinaemias)
	Viscosity syndromes (Raynaud's, acral infarction, erythromelalgia, polycythaemia rubra vera and dysproteinaemias)
Accepted skin markers	Acanthosis nigricans
	Dermatomyositis
	Hypertrichosis lanuginosa
	Endocrine (e.g. ectopic ACTH, Nelson's syndrome, acromegaly)
	Necrolytic migratory erythema (glucagonoma)
	Episodic facial flushing
	Pyoderma gangrenosum
	Erythema multiforme and nodosum
	Erythema elevatum diutinum
	Nicotine stains
	Radiodermatitis
	Acquired ichthyosis
	Generalized pruritus
	Urticaria pigmentosa
Genetic syndromes	Palmoplantar keratoderma/tylosis
	Gardner's syndrome
	Peutz–Jeghers syndrome
	Muir–Torré syndrome

18

of carcinoma of perineal glandular tissue around the anus or on the genitalia.

Leukaemia

Leukaemia can present in the skin with purpura resulting from thrombocytopenia. Ulcers may result from infiltration. Monocytic leukaemia causes specific infiltrated lesions (Table 18.51).

HIV infection and AIDS

Skin disease is an important corollary of AIDS and HIV infection. The incidence of several cutaneous diseases is increased in people who are HIV positive or who have AIDS. The percentage of people with HIV who have skin manifestations and the number of manifestations increase as HIV infection progresses. The incidence and severity sometimes correlate with the absolute numbers of T-helper cells and the prognostic significance of some disorders is well recognized. HIV infection can affect the behaviour of other dermatological conditions such as psoriasis. Skin diseases associated with HIV are listed in Table 18.53. The majority of the cutaneous complications of AIDS are reversed by successful treatment.

Hairy leucoplakia

This is probably caused by Epstein–Barr virus. It is usually asymptomatic, but patients have often noticed the development of a roughened patch along the lateral margin of their tongue (Fig. 18.68). Other intraoral sites have been reported. The differential diagnosis includes trauma, *Candida*, leucoplakia, lichen planus and white sponge naevus. Biopsy may be necessary.

Hairy leucoplakia also occurs in other immuno-compromised people and has been reported in healthy individuals.

Seborrhoeic dermatitis

Seborrhoeic dermatitis is a common itchy scaly erythematous dermatosis with a predilection for the scalp, face, chest, back, axillae and groin. It is common in the later stages of HIV infection, when it can be very severe and generalized, even amounting to erythroderma.

Psoriasis

Psoriasis may worsen or appear for the first time in a person with HIV, and may be severe.

Classical or incomplete **Reiter's syndrome** has been reported in AIDS and in association with AIDS-related complex.

AIDS-related Kaposi's sarcoma

AIDS-related Kaposi's sarcoma (KS) is multicentric and

Table 18.53 Cutaneous manifestations of HIV infection and AIDS

Inflammatory dermatoses
Seroconversion toxic erythema
Psoriasis
Seborrhoeic dermatitis
Eosinophilic pustular folliculitis
Generalized granuloma annulare
Papular eruption of HIV
Severe drug reactions

Infections
Tinea and onychomycosis
Candidosis
Hairy leucoplakia
Papulonodular demodiciosis
Atypical primary, secondary and late syphilis
Bacterial folliculitis
Bacillary haemangiomatosis
Condyloma acuminata (viral warts)
Molluscum contagiosum
Cutaneous atypical mycobacterial infection
Herpes simplex
Herpes zoster

Other skin manifestations
Cutaneous and nail hyperpigmentation
Porphyria cutanea tarda
Atypical pityriasis rosea
Atypical atopic type dermatitis and xerosis
Acquired ichthyosis and keratoderma
Yellow nail syndrome
Severe aphthous stomatitis

Neoplasia
Kaposi's sarcoma
Cutaneous lymphoma
Melanoma and non-melanoma skin cancer

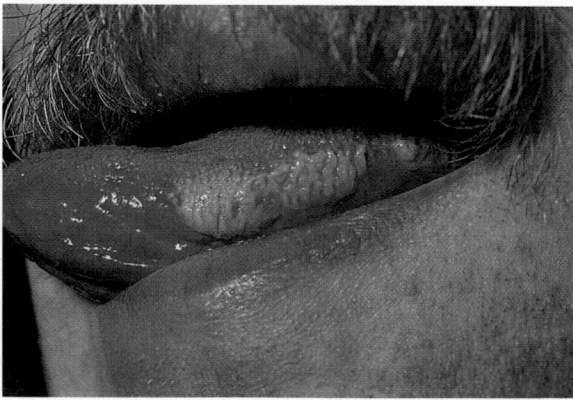

Figure 18.68 Hairy leucoplakia.

often involves the face, oral mucosa, palate and genitalia. The characteristic lesion is a purple nodule, which may ulcerate (CLINICAL EXAMINATION AT A GLANCE, Fig. I, p. 1106). The common differential diagnosis includes naevi, histiocytoma and pyogenic granuloma. KS is caused by infection with HHV8.

Bacillary angiomatosis

Bacillary angiomatosis has some clinical similarity to KS and is also associated with HIV infection (Fig. 18.69). It is caused by infection with the cat-scratch organism *Bartonella henselae*.

Immunodeficiency syndromes that may be associated with cutaneous changes similar to those seen with HIV are listed in Table 18.54.

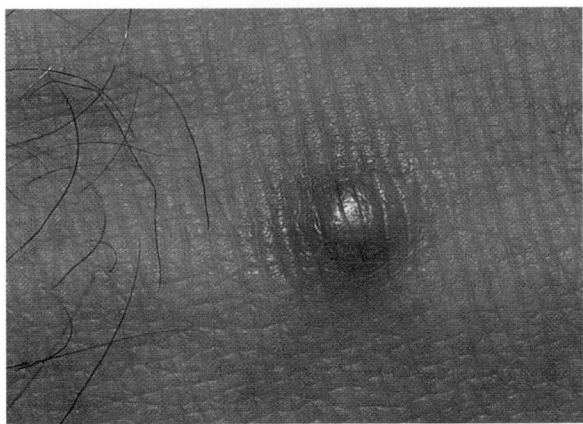

Figure 18.69 Bacillary angiomatosis. Purple nodule on cheek, mimicking Kaposi's sarcoma.

Table 18.54 Immunodeficiency syndromes with cutaneous manifestations

Congenital
Di George's syndrome
Ataxia telangiectasia
Wiskott–Aldrich syndrome
Agammaglobulinaemias
T- and B-cell immunodeficiencies

Acquired
Malnutrition
Alcohol
Malignancies
Congenital infections
Iatrogenic immunosuppression
Graft-vs.-host disease

Orogenital disorders

Mouth

Traumatic changes occur along the line of occlusion.

Candida

Candida is an extremely common intraoral pathogen complicating immunosuppression resulting from infection (e.g. HIV), disease (e.g. diabetes mellitus) or drugs (e.g. oral antibiotics or cytotoxics). White detachable deposits and plaques are the usual physical signs.

Mouthwashes or nystatin lozenges or a systemic imidazole are effective treatments, but *Candida* may recur, depending on the context.

Leucoplakia

Leucoplakia is a common non-specific disturbance of oral mucosal keratinization. Smoking and poor dental hygiene are associated factors. It may result from syphilitic atrophic glossitis, but small white mucous patches may occur anywhere in the oral cavity during secondary syphilis.

Erythroplakia

Erythroplakia describes red patches in the mouth. It may be more indicative of premalignancy or malignancy than leucoplakia and should therefore be biopsied.

Lichen planus

Lichen planus is characterized by Wickham's striae and is more common on the buccal mucosa than the tongue, although all intraoral sites may be involved. Approximately 30% of patients have extraoral lichen planus, and approximately 10–50% of all patients with lichen planus have oral lesions. Erosive or atrophic lichen planus may progress to malignancy.

Oral ulceration

Oral ulceration is common and the differential diagnosis of mouth ulcers is given in Table 18.55.

Behçet's syndrome

Behçet's syndrome is characterized by painful orogenital ulceration and variable involvement of other systems as follows:
● Oral ulcers (90–100%)
● Genital ulcers (60–90%)
● Ocular manifestations (keratitis, uveitis, optic neuritis) (50–90%)
● Pustules, pyoderma gangrenosum, erythema nodosum, arthritis (20–50%)
● Central nervous system involvement (e.g. vasculitis, thrombophlebitis) (10–20%)

18

Table 18.55 Differential diagnosis of oral ulceration

Lichen planus
Behçet's syndrome
Herpes simplex and other viruses
Stevens–Johnson syndrome
Aphthous stomatitis
Reiter's disease
Pemphigus
Mucous membrane pemphigoid
Lupus erythematosus
Syphilis
Oral cancer

- Pulmonary infarction (10–40%)
- Renal involvement (10%)
- Budd–Chiari syndrome (10%)

Vulva

Vulval dermatoses can be severely symptomatic with itch, dyspareunia and somatopsychic symptoms. Seborrhoeic dermatitis, psoriasis and lichen planus can affect the vulva and are discussed on pp. 1118, 1119 and 1114, respectively.

Viral warts

Vulval warts are usually caused by HPV types 6 and 11, which are probably not associated with malignancy. They are common and all patients presenting with them should be screened for sexually transmitted diseases and have colposcopy and a cervical smear examination. Their partners should be examined for genital warts and managed accordingly. Treatment is usually with liquid nitrogen therapy.

Bowenoid papulosis

Bowenoid papulosis (warty lesions with the histological appearance of Bowen's disease) may affect the vulva and is associated with HPV 16 and 18.

Lichen simplex

Lichen simplex refers to a chronic eczematous process exaggerated and propagated by scratching in response to itch. Treatment is topical steroid.

Lichen sclerosus

Lichen sclerosus (see p. 1123) is an idiopathic chronic inflammatory dermatosis with subsequent atrophy (Figs 18.11 and 18.70). It can cause intense itching. Characteristically the lesions are shiny white and red-rimmed

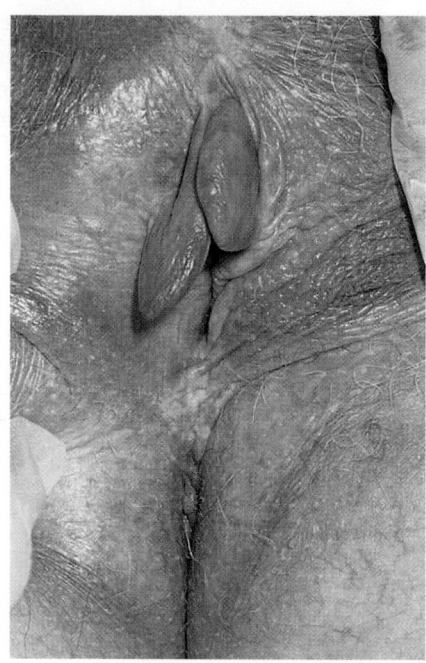

Figure 18.70 Vulval lichen sclerosus. Note loss of vulval architecture. Courtesy of Dr R.C.D. Staughton.

with central telangiectasia, purpura and erosions. There may be atrophy of the labia and clitoris. Lichen simplex and lichen sclerosus may be difficult to distinguish by the non-expert and may coexist in the same individual.

Potent topical steroids may relieve the symptoms of lichen sclerosus. Punch biopsy is an important part of management because it may develop into intraepithelial neoplasia and, very rarely, frank invasive carcinoma. However, many women may have had unnecessary mutilating vulval surgery for this condition.

Vulval intra-epithelial neoplasia

Vulval intra-epithelial neoplasia (VIN) is suspected clinically when there are hard white plaques or erosions. Some posterior lesions of VIN may extend into the anal canal. The invasive potential of VIN is probably small. HPV types 16 and 18 are associated with VIN and cervical intra-epithelial neoplasia (CIN) and invasive squamous cell carcinoma. Cryotherapy is the treatment of choice, but liaison with a gynaecologist is desirable.

Other causes of vulval itching

Additional causes of vulval itching include urinary incontinence and vaginal discharge often resulting from *Candida*. All women with pruritus vulvae should be screened for diabetes mellitus.

Penis

The penis is a common site for seborrhoeic dermatitis, psoriasis and viral warts.

Balanitis resulting from *Candida* or other microbials may be a presenting feature of diabetes mellitus.

Lichen sclerosus

Lichen sclerosus of the penis may result in phimosis and even retention of urine. It is a common medical reason for a circumcision. The severest form of damage is balanitis xerotica obliterans. The clinical features are described on p. 1123.

Zoon's balanitis

Zoon's balanitis is an idiopathic lymphocytic inflammatory condition of the penis. It will respond to topical corticosteroids, but circumcision is the most effective treatment.

Penile intra-epithelial neoplasia

Bowen's disease (squamous cell carcinoma *in situ*; see p. 1143) can affect the penile shaft. Erythroplasia of Queyrat is the eponym for Bowen's disease of the glans penis or mucosal prepuce. Fixed red scaly (shaft) or shiny (glans) lesions of the penis should be regarded with suspicion and biopsied. Bowenoid papulosis (see p. 1166) may also affect the penis.

Anus

Common anorectal diseases such as haemorrhoids and fissure *in ano* as well as poor hygiene and faecal incontinence predispose to localized perianal itching (pruritus ani). Physical irritation by harsh toilet paper, contact dermatitis from local anaesthetic preparations, threadworms, lice, *Candida*, tinea and erythrasma should be considered. Psoriasis, lichen planus, lichen sclerosus and seborrhoeic dermatitis can all affect the perineum. All patients should have a rectal examination to exclude carcinoma.

Psychogenic dermatoses

Skin disease is responsible for much psychosomatic morbidity. In some instances, however, the skin may be the presenting site of psychological or psychiatric disturbance.

Dermatitis artefacta

Dermatitis artefacta refers to peculiar self-inflicted lesions in accessible sites. The patient is usually a young woman and is unable to give a believable account about how the lesions developed, and often has other artefactual ill-nesses. The skin heals with topical treatment under occlusion if the patient can be kept from interfering with the wounds. Confrontation rarely works, but a sympathetic rapport and reassurance are essential.

Acne excoriée

Acne excoriée describes picked acne spots: the picking is usually denied. It can be difficult to manage. A small dose of trifluoperazine may help if it is severe.

Trichotillomania

Trichotillomania is a type of traction alopecia. The hair is pulled deliberately by the patient, usually an infant or young woman.

Delusions of parasitosis

Delusions of parasitosis occur when the patient presents with the unshakeable belief that he or she is infested with a parasite, and there are no physical signs of infestation, although there may be some excoriations. Often patients bring a bag or matchbox containing dust, debris and hair to the clinic. Sometimes collusion in the delusion has been achieved, usually with a spouse. Suicide is a real possibility.

Psychotherapeutic support is essential with avoidance of confrontation. Pimozide can be very useful, but treatment has to be long term.

Dys(cogno)morphophobia

This is a disorder of perception of body image. It may not be frankly delusional, but is more often obsessional. It is common for girls to imagine their acne is very much worse than it is. Excessive concern over unwanted facial hair and anxiety over scalp hair fall are also common.

Pruritus ani, vulvodynia penodynia and scrotodynia

In men, severe discomfort on sitting down, pruritus ani and itchy burning scrotum in the absence of overt dermatological disease are not uncommon. Women too may have severe symptomatology from the perineum with no obvious disease. Such vulvodynia requires careful evaluation.

Iatrogenic skin disease

Drugs cause many skin disorders. The types of drug rash and some of their causes are listed in Table 18.56.

Toxic epidermal necrolysis (Lyell's syndrome)

This is a serious life-threatening idiosyncratic reaction caused either by a drug or an intercurrent illness. Widespread skin loss compromises cutaneous homoeostasis, and shock, cardiovascular collapse, infection and failure

Table 18.56 Drug causes of skin disease

Skin disease	Drug causes
Toxic erythema	Penicillins, cephalosporins, thiazides
Toxic epidermal necrolysis	Penicillins, phenytoin
Erythema multiforme	Sulphonamides, penicillins, phenytoin, non-steroidal anti-inflammatory drugs (NSAIDs)
Eczema	Thiazides, β-blockers, aminophylline, sulphonamides
Photosensitivity	Tetracyclines, phenothiazides, amiodarone, thiazides, hypoglycaemics
Urticaria	Aspirin, codeine, morphine, contrast media, penicillins
Pigmentation	Tetracyclines (especially minocycline), oral contraceptives, antimalarials, amiodarone, phenytoin
Fixed drug eruptions	Phenolphthalein, NSAIDs, paracetamol, codeine, barbiturates

of thermoregulation contribute to a high mortality. Mucocutaneous involvement is common.

Patients are managed in the intensive care unit or in a burns unit. Scarring may occur if the patient survives. The use of systemic corticosteroids is controversial. Ciclosporin and intravenous gamma globulins may be useful.

Contact sensitivity

Contact sensitivity is a common problem, especially in the management of stasis eczema and ulceration (see pp. 1118, 1132 and 1155), but complicates the use of topical medicaments at any site (e.g. the external auditory meatus and the genitalia). Often the possibility of contact sensitivity is overlooked by the physician when a presenting problem is followed up and found to have worsened. Sensitivity may be to an active ingredient (e.g. neomycin) or a preservative (e.g. parabens). Potential common sensitizers are listed in Table 18.15.

Immunosuppression

The management of people with malignant disease, particularly lymphoma and leukaemia, and the increase in organ transplantation, has produced a population of patients who are acutely or chronically immunosuppressed. This is reflected in an increased incidence of cutaneous disease in these patients, especially infections and tumours. The cutaneous complications of renal transplantation include:

- Viral warts
- Actinic keratoses
- Basal cell carcinoma
- Squamous cell carcinoma

Radiotherapy

- Radiodermatitis (acute/chronic)
- Basal cell carcinoma

! Must know checklist

- Basic skin biology including wound healing and carcinogenesis

- Take and present a suitable and accurate history

- Examine the skin systematically and be able to describe the physical signs

- Diagnosis and management of dermatological emergencies and 'skin failure' (e.g. toxic epidermal necrolysis, erythema multiforme, acute urticaria, angio-oedema)

- Diagnosis and management of common and important inflammatory diseases of the skin (atopic eczema, contact dermatitis, psoriasis, acne, urticaria, blistering eruptions, drug eruptions, leg ulcers)

- Diagnosis and management of skin cancer (melanoma, basal cell carcinoma, squamous cell carcinoma)

- Diagnosis and management of common and important cutaneous infections (bacterial, viral and fungal) and infestations (scabies and lice)

- Diagnosis and management of cutaneous complications of acquired (HIV) and iatrogenic (transplantation, immunosuppressive and cytotoxic medication) skin disease

- Diagnosis of cutaneous manifestations and presentations of systemic disease, including internal malignancy

- The side-effects of topical and systemic drugs used in dermatological medicine

Further reading

Books

Champion RH, Burton JL, Burns DA, Breathnach SM, eds. *Textbook of Dermatology*, 6th edn. Oxford: Blackwell Scientific Publications, 1998.

Du Vivier A. *Atlas of Clinical Dermatology*. London: Churchill Livingstone, 2002.

Harper J, Oranje A, Prose N. *Textbook of Paediatric Dermatology*. Oxford: Blackwell Science, 2000.

Litt JZ. *Drug Eruption Reference Manual*. New York and London: Parthenon, 2001.

McKee P. *Pathology of the Skin*. London: Mosby, 1999.

Journals

British Journal of Dermatology, Blackwell Publishing.

Journal of Investigative Dermatology, Society for Investigative Dermatology. http://www.jidonline.org/

Journal of the American Academy of Dermatology, American Academy of Dermatology. http://www2.us.elsevierhealth.com/

Websites

www.aad.org/medical_reference.html

www.lib.uiowa.edu/hardin/md/derm.html

http://telemedicine.org/ids.html

Index